Anesthetic Pharmacology: Physiologic Principles and Clinical Practice

A Companion to Miller's Anesthesia

Anesthetic Pharmacology: Physiologic Principles and Clinical Practice

A Companion to Miller's Anesthesia

Alex S. Evers, MD
Henry E. Mallinkrodt Professor and Chairman
Department of Anesthesiology
Professor of Internal Medicine and Molecular Biology and Pharmacology
Washington University School of Medicine
St. Louis, Missouri

Mervyn Maze, MB, ChB
Sir Ivan Magill Professor of Anaesthetics
Department of Anaesthetics and Intensive Care
Faculty of Medicine, Imperial College London
London, United Kingdom

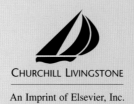

CHURCHILL LIVINGSTONE

An Imprint of Elsevier, Inc.

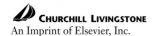 CHURCHILL LIVINGSTONE
An Imprint of Elsevier, Inc.

The Curtis Center
Independence Square West
Philadelphia, Pennsylvania 19106

Notice

Anesthesia is an ever-changing field. Standard safety precautions must be followed, but as new research and
clinical experience broaden our knowledge, changes in treatment and drug therapy may become necessary
or appropriate. Readers are advised to check the most current product information provided by the
manufacturer of each drug to be administered to verify the recommended dose, the method and duration of
administration, and contraindications. It is the responsibility of the licensed prescriber, relying on experience and knowledge of the patient, to determine dosages and the best treatment for each individual patient.
Neither the publisher nor the author assumes any liability for any injury and/or damage to persons or property arising from this publication.

Library of Congress Cataloging-in-Publication Data

Anesthetic pharmacology : physiologic principles and clinical practice : a companion to
  Miller's Anesthesia / [edited by] Alex S. Evers, Mervyn Maze.
    p. ; cm.
  ISBN 0-443-06579-9
    1. Anesthetics—Physiological effect.   2. Pharmacology.   I. Evers, Alex S.   II. Maze, Mervyn
III. Anesthesia.
  [DNLM: 1. anesthetics—pharmacology.   2. Analgesics—pharmacology. QV 81 A5787 2004]
RD82.A687 2004
617.9'6–dc21   2003055211

Acquisitions Editor: Natasha Andjelkovic
Developmental Editor: Agnes Hunt Byrne
Publishing Services Manager: Joan Sinclair
Project Manager: Mary Stermel
Book Designer: Gene Harris

Printed in HongKong
Last digit is the print number: 9   8   7   6   5   4   3   2   1

Contributors

Takashi Akata, M.D., Ph.D.,
Assistant Professor
Department of Anesthesiology and Critical Care
  Medicine
Faculty of Medicine
Kyushu University, Japan
Vascular Reactivity

Michael Avidan, M.B.B.Ch.
Assistant Professor
Department of Anesthesiology
Washington University School of Medicine
St. Louis, Missouri
Agents Affecting Coagulation and Platelet Function

Lindsey R. Baden, M.D.
Instructor of Medicine
Harvard Medical School
Clinical Research Director
Division of Infectious Diseases
Brigham and Women's Hospital
Boston, Massachusetts
Antimicrobial Therapy

Jeffrey R. Balser, M.D., Ph.D.
Chairman
Department of Anesthesiology
The James Tayloe Gwathmey Professor of Anesthesiology
  and Pharmacology
Vanderbilt University School of Medicine
Nashville, Tennessee
Cardiac Rhythm

Juliana Barr, M.D.
Assistant Professor
Department of Anesthesia
Stanford University School of Medicine
Staff Anesthesiologist and Intensivist
Department of Anesthesiology Service
Veterans Administration Palo Alto Health System
Palo Alto, California
Sedatives, Anxiolytics, and Amnestics

Manfred Blobner, M.D.
Associate Professor and Attending Anethesiologist
Klinik für Anaesthesiologie der Techischen Universität
  München
Klinikum rechts der Isar
Munich, Germany
Neuromuscular Blocking Agents and Reversal Drugs

Frances Bonnet, M.D.
Professor
Paris VI
Department of Anesthesiology
UFR Saint-Antoine
Tenon
Department of Anesthesiology
Assistance Publique—Hôpitaux de Paris
Paris, France
Analgesics: Receptor Ligands—α_2 Adrenergic Receptor
  Agonists

Walter A. Boyle, III, M.D.
Associate Professor of Anesthesiology and Surgery
Division Chief, Adult Critical Care
Department of Anesthesiology
Washington University School of Medicine
Medical Director, Surgical Intensive Care Unit
Barnes-Jewish Hospital
St. Louis, Missouri
Vascular Reactivity

Julia C. Buckingham, B.Sc., Ph.D., D.Sc.
Professor of Pharmacology and Division Head
Department of Neuroendocrinology
Division of Neuroscience and Psychological Medicine
Faculty of Medicine
Imperial College School of Medicine
London, United Kingdom
Hypothalamic-Pituitary-Adrenal Axis

M. Catherine Bushnell, Ph.D.
Professor
Department of Anesthesia
McGill University Faculty of Medicine
Montreal, Quebec
Canada
Neural Substrates for Behavior: Pain

Eugene Campbell, M.B., Ch.B.
Specialist Registrar
Department of Gastroenterology
Birmingham Heartlands Hospital
Birmingham, United Kingdom
Antimotility and Antisecretory Agents

Jerry G. Collins, M.D.
Professor of Anesthesiology
Lecturer in Pharmacology
Yale University School of Medicine
New Haven, Connecticut
Sensory Processing: Spinal Cord

Dean A. Cowie, M.B., FANZCA
Staff Specialist in Anaesthesia
Department of Anesthesia
Austin Health, Heidelburg
Melbourne, Australia
Anticonvulsant Drugs

Florence Crestani, Ph.D.
Research Scientist
Institute of Pharmacology and Toxicology
University of Lurich
Sedatives, Anxiolytics, and Amnestics

Albert Dahan, M.D., Ph.D.
Associate Professor
Staff Anesthesiologist
Department of Anesthesiology and Physiology
Leiden University Medical Center
Leiden, The Netherlands
Lung Function

M. Frances Davies, Ph.D.
Directory of Faculty Development
Research Associate
Department of Anesthesia
Stanford University School of Medicine
Palo Alto, California
Sedatives, Anxiolytics, and Amnestics

Timothy M. DeLorey, Ph.D.
Senior Scientist
Department of Pharmacology
Molecular Research Institute
Mountain View, California
Sedatives, Anxiolytics, and Amnestics

Charl de Wet, M.B., Ch.B.
Assistant Professor
Department of Anesthesiology
Washington University School of Medicine
St. Louis, Missouri
Myocardial Protection

George Despotis, M.D.
Associate Professor
Departments of Anesthesiology, Pathology and
    Immunology
Washington University School of Medicine
St. Louis, Missouri
Agents Affecting Coagulation and Platelet Function

Hugh Dorman, M.D., Ph.D.
Professor
Department of Anesthesiology
Medical University of South Carolina College of Medicine
Charleston, South Carolina
Agents Used to Treat Myocardial Ischemia

Talmage D. Egan, M.D.
Associate Professor
Department of Anesthesiology
University of Utah School of Medicine
Salt Lake City, Utah
Common Pharmacodynamic Drug Interactions in
    Anesthetic Practice

Helge Eilers, M.D.
Assistant Professor
Attending Physician
Department of Anesthesia and Perioperative Care
University of California, San Francisco, School of
    Medicine
Attending Physician
Department of Anesthesia and Perioperative Care
San Francisco, California
Sensory Processing: Peripheral Nociceptors

Charles W. Emala, M.D.
Associate Professor San Francisco General Hospital
Department of Anesthesiology
College of Physicians and Surgeons of Columbia
    University
New York, New York
Bronchodilators, Corticosteroids, and Anti-Inflammatory
    Agents

N.J. Emptage, Ph.D.
Lecturer in Pharmacology
Department of Pharmacology
University of Oxford
Oxford, United Kingdom
Synamptic Transmission

Alex S. Evers, M.D. (editor)
Henry E. Mallinckrodt Professor and Chairman
Department of Anesthesiology
Professor
Departments of Internal
Medicine and Molecular Biology and Pharmacology
Washington University School of Medicine
Anesthesiologist-in-Chief
Barnes-Jewish Hospital
St. Louis, Missouri
Inhalational Anesthetics

David Feldman, M.D., Ph.D.
Director of Heart Failure and Cardiac Transplantation
Division of Cardiology Department of Medicine
Ohio State University College of Medicine
Columbus, Ohio
Agents Used to Treat Myocardial Ischemia

Heidrun Fink, M.D.
Resident
Klinik für Anaesthesiologie der Technischen Universität
    München
Klinikum rechts der Isar
Munich, Germany
Research Fellow, Department of Anesthesia and Critical
    Care
Massachusetts General Hospital and Harvard Medical
    School
Boston, Massachusetts
Neuromuscular Blocking Agents and Reversal Drugs

Pierre Fiset, M.D.
Associate Professor
Department of Anesthesia
Associate Member
Department of Pharmacology and Therapeutics
McGill University Faculty of Medicine
Staff Anesthesiologist
Department of Anesthesia
Royal Victoria Hospital
Montreal, Quebec Canada
Neural Substrates for Behavior: Pain

Pierre Foëx, D.M., M.A., D.phil, FRCA, FANZCA
Emeritus Nuffield Professor of Anaesthetics
Nuffield Department of Anaesthetics
University of Oxford
Honorary Consultant
Nuffield Department of Anaesthetics
Oxford Radcliffe Hospitals
Oxford, United Kingdom
Myocardial Performance

Susan Garwood, M.B., Ch.B., B.Sc., FRCA
Associate Professor
Department of Anesthesiology
Yale University School of Medicine
New Haven, Connecticut
Diuretics

Adrian W. Gelb, M.B., Ch.B., D.A., FRCPC
Professor and Chair
Department of Anesthesia
Professor
Departments of Clinical Neurological Sciences, and
    Pharmacology and Toxicology
The University of Western Ontario Faculty of Medicine
Chief
Department of Anesthesia
London Health Sciences Centre and St. Joseph's Health
    Care London
London, Ontario, Canada
Anticonvulsant Drugs

Jean-Antoine Girault, M.D.
Research Director
INSERM U536 and "Pierre et Marie Curie" University
Paris, France
Signal Transduction Mechanisms: Receptor-Effector
    Coupling

Marye J. Gleva, M.D.
Assistant Professor
Cardiovascular Division
Department of Internal Medicine
Washington University School of Medicine
St. Louis, Missouri
Antiarrhythmic Agents

David P. Glick, M.D.
Assistant Professor
Department of Anesthesia & Critical Care
The University of Chicago
Pritzker School of Medicine
Chicago, Illinois
Autonomic Function

Anne Carol Goldberg, M.D., FACP
Associate Professor
Department of Internal Medicine
Division of Endocrinology, Metabolism, and Lipid
    Research
Washington University School of Medicine
St. Louis, Missouri
Drugs Affecting Lipid Metabolism

Neil L. Harrison, Ph.D.
Professor and Director
C.V. Starr Laboratory for Molecular Neuropharmacology
Department of Anesthesiology
Weill Medical College of Cornell University
New York, New York
Intravenous Anesthetics: Barbiturates, Etomidate, Propofol,
    Ketamine, and Steroids Clinical Pharmacology

Hugh C. Hemmings, Jr., M.D., Ph.D.
Professor of Anesthesiology, Vice-Chair for Research
Department of Anesthesiology
Associate Professor
Department of Pharmacology
Weill Medical College of Cornell University
Attending Anesthesiologist
Department of Anesthesiology
New York Presbyterian Hospital—New York Weill Cornell
    Center
New York, New York
Signal Transduction Mechanisms: Receptor-Effector
    Coupling

Helen E. Higham, M.B., Ch.B., FRCA
Research Fellow and Honorary Consultant Anaesthetist
Nuffield Department of Anaesthetics
Oxford University
Oxford, United Kingdom
Myocardial Performance

Laureen L. Hill, M.D.
Assistant Professor
Department of Anesthesiology
Washington University School of Medicine
St. Louis, Missouri
Vasodilators

Kirk Hogan, M.D., J.D.
Associate Professor
Department of Anesthesiology
University of Wisconsin Medical School
Madison, Wisconsin
Pharmacogenetics and Pharmacogenomics of Drug Action

Charles W. Hogue, Jr., M.D.
Associate Professor
Chief, Division of Cardiothoracic Anesthesiology
Department of Anesthesiology
Washington University School of Medicine
St. Louis, Missouri
Antiarrhythmic Agents

Richard C. Hubbard, M.D.
Executive Director Clinical Development
Pfizer Research and Development
Ann Arbor, Michigan
Analgesics: Nonsteriodal Anti-Inflammatory Drugs

Peter C. Isakson, Ph.D.
Vice President
R&D Strategy & Senior Science Fellow
Pharmacia Corporation
Peapack, New Jersey
Analgesics: Nonsteriodal Anti-Inflammatory Drugs

Eric Jacobsohn, M.B., Ch.B., MPHE, FRCPC
Associate Professor
Departments of Anesthesiology and Division of
    Cardiothoracic Surgery
Director, Cardiothoracic Critical Care
Washington University School of Medicine
St. Louis, Missouri
Myocardial Protection

Vesna Jevtovic-Todorovic, M.D., Ph.D.
Associate Professor of Anesthesiology
Department of Anesthesiology
University of Virginia Health System
Charlottesville, Virginia
Neuroprotective Agents

Christopher D. John, B.Sc., Ph.D.
Lecturer
Department of Neuroendocrinology
Division of Neuroscience and Psychological Medicines
Imperial College School of Medicine
London, United Kingdom
Hypothalamic-Pituitary-Adrenal Axis

Judy R. Kersten, M.D.
Professor
Departments of Anesthesiology and Pharmacology and
    Toxicology
Medical College of Wisconsin
Froedtert Memorial Lutheran Hospital
Zablocki Veterans Affairs Medical Center
Milwaukee, Wisconsin
Cardiovascular Pharmacology of Positive Inotropic Drugs

Evan D. Kharasch, M.D., Ph.D.
Assistant Dean for Clinical Research
Professor and Director of Research
Department of Anesthesiology
Adjunct Professor in Medicinal Chemistry
University of Washington School of Medicine
Seattle, Washington
Principles of Drug Biotransformation

Donald D. Koblin, Ph.D., M.D.
Professor
Department of Anesthesia and Perioperative Care
University of California, San Francisco School of Medicine
Attending Anesthesiologist
Department of Veteran Affairs Medical Center
San Francisco, California
Inhalational Anesthetics

Jelveh Lameh, Ph.D.
Assistant Adjunct Professor
Department of Biopharmaceutical Sciences
University of California, San Francisco
Senior Scientist
Department of Pharmacology
Molecular Research Institute
Mountain View, California
Sedatives, Anxiolytics, and Amnestics

Spencer S. Liu, M.D.
Clinical Professor
Department of Anesthesiology
University of Washington School of Medicine
Staff Anesthesiologist
Virginia Mason Medical Center
Seattle, Washington
Analgesics: Ion Channel Ligands/Sodium Channel
    Blockers/Local Anesthetics

Andrew B. Lumb, M.B., B.S., FRCA
Senior Clinical Lecturer in Anaesthesia
University of Leeds
Consultant Anaesthesiologist
St. James's University Hospital
Leeds, United Kingdom
Lung Function

Alex Macario, M.D., M.B.A.
Assistant Professor
Department of Anesthesiology and Health Research and
    Policy
Stanford University School of Medicine
Palo Alto, California
Pharmacoeconomics

Ken Mackie, M.D.
Professor
Department of Anesthesiology
Adjunct Professor
Department of Physiology and Biophysics
University of Washington School of Medicine
Seattle, Washington
Analgesics: Cannabinoids

Nándor Marczin, M.D., Ph.D.
Assistant Professor
Department of Anaesthetics and Intensive Care
Pecs University
Pecs, Hungary
MCR Clinician Scientist Fellow
Department of Cardiothoracic Surgery
National Heart and Lung Institute
Imperial College at Harefield Hospital
Clinical Research Fellow
Department of Anaesthetics
Royal Brompton and Harefield NHS Trust
Heart Science Center
Harefield Hospital
Harefield, United Kingdom
Immunosuppressants

J. A. Jeevendra Martyn, M.D., Ph.D.
Professor of Anaesthesiology, Harvard Medical School
Director, Clinical and Biochemical Pharmacology
    Laboratory
Anesthetist, Department of Anesthesia and Critical Care
Massachusetts General Hospital
Anesthetist-in-Chief
Shriners Hospital for Children
Boston, Massachusetts
Neuromuscular Blocking Agents and Reversal Drugs

Mervyn Maze, M.B., Ch.B., FRCP, FRCA, FMedSci
    (editor)
Sir Ivan Magill Professor of Anaesthetics, Chair
Department of Anaesthetics and Intensive Care
Faculty of Medicine, Imperial College London
Professor of Biological Sciences
Faculty Life Sciences, Imperial College London
Director of Research and Development and Campus Dean
Chelsea & Westminster NHS Healthcare Trust
London, United Kingdom
Neural Substrates for Behavior: Consciousness
Analgesics: Receptor Ligands—α_2 Adrenergic Receptor
    Agonists

Susan McDonald, M.D.
Fellow, Cardiothoracic Anesthesiology
Department of Anesthesiology
Washington University School of Medicine
St. Louis, Missouri
Agents Affecting Coagulation and Platelet Function

Howard L. McLeod, Pharm.D.
Director, Pharmacology Core
Siteman Comprehensive Cancer Center
Associate Professor
Departments of Internal Medicine, Genetics, and
    Pharmacology
Washington University School of Medicine
St. Louis, Missouri
Chemotherapeutic Agents

Berend Mets, M.D., M.B., Ch.B., Ph.D., FRCA, FFASA
Professor and Chair
Department of Anesthesiology
Milton S. Hershey Medical Center
Pennsylvania State University
Hershey, Pennsylvania
Sympathomimetic, Sympatholytic Drugs,
    Parasympathomimetic, and Parasympatholytic Drugs

Charles F. Minto, M.B., Ch.B.
Senior Lecturer
Department of Anaesthesia
University of Sydney
Sydney
Staff Specialist Anaesthetist
Department of Anaesthesia and Pain Management
Royal North Shore Hospital
St. Leonards, NSW, Australia
Pharmacokinetic and Pharmacodynamic Principles of Drug
    Action
Common Pharmacodynamic Drug Interactions in
    Anesthetic Practice

Hanns Möhler, Ph.D.
Professor and Director
Institute of Pharmacology and Toxicology
University of Zürich'
Swiss Federal Institute of Technology (ETH) Zürich
Chair of Pharmacology
Department of Chemistry and Applied Biosciences
Zürich, Switzerland
Sedatives, Anxiolytics, and Amnestics

Terri G. Monk, M.D.
Professor
Department of Anesthesiology
University of Florida College of Medicine
Gainesville, Florida
Diuretics

Jonathan Moss, M.D., Ph.D.
Professor and Vice Chairman for Research
Department of Anesthesia & Critical Care
The University of Chicago
Pritzker School of Medicine
Chicago, Illinois
Autonomic Function

Istvan Nagy, M.D., Ph.D.
Lecturer
Department of Anaesthetics and Intensive Care
Faculty of Medicine, Imperial College London
London, United Kingdom
Sensory Processing: Primary Afferent Neuron/Dorsal Root
    Ganglia

Rupert P. M. Negus, M.A., M.B., B.S., MRCP, Ph.D.
Department of Gastroenterology
St. Mary's Hospital
London, United Kingdom
Liver Physiology

Laura E. Nelson, Ph.D.
Reserarch Fellow
Department of Anaesthetics and Intensive Care and
    Biological Sciences
Imperial College London
London, United Kingdom
Neural Substrates for Behavior; Consciousness

John W. Olney, M.D.
Professor of Psychiatry and Neuropathology
Department of Psychiatry
Washington University School of Medicine
St. Louis, Missouri
Neuroprotective Agents

Paul S. Pagel, M.D., Ph.D., FACC
Professor and Director of Cardiac Anesthesia
Department of Anesthesiology
Medical College of Wisconsin
Milwaukee, Wisconsin
Cardiovascular Pharmacology of Positive Inotropic Drugs

Chris Papageorgio, M.D.
Hematology/Oncology Fellow
Department of Internal Medicine
Washington University School of Medicine
St. Louis, Missouri
Chemotherapeutic Agents

Robert A. Pearce, M.D., Ph.D.
Professor and Associate Chair for Academic Affairs
Department of Anesthesiology
Betty J. Bamforth Research Professor of Anesthesiology
Affiliate Professor of Anatomy
Affiliate Professor of Physiology
University of Wisconsin Medical School
Madison, Wisconsin
Signal Transduction Mechanisms: Ion Channels

Ronald G. Pearl, M.D., Ph.D.
Professor and Chairman
Department of Anesthesia
Stanford University School of Medicine
Palo Alto, California
Pulmonary Vasodilators

Misha Perouansky, M.D.
Associate Professor of Anesthesiology
University of Wisconsin, Madison
Madison, Wisconsin
Signal Transduction Mechanisms: Ion Channels

Imre Rédai, M.D., FRCA
Assistant Professor of Anesthesiology
Department of Anesthesiology
College of Physicians & Surgeons Columbia University
Assistant Attending Anesthesiologist
New York Presbyterian Hospital
New York, New York
Sympathomimetic, Sympatholytic Drugs,
    Parasympathomimetic, and Parasympatholytic Drugs

Joseph G. Reves, M.D.
VP for Medical Affairs
Dean, College of Medicine
Professor
Department of Anesthesiology
Medical University of South Carolina
Charleston, South Carolina
Agents Used to Treat Myocardial Ischemia

Andrew S. C. Rice, M.B., B.S., M.D., FRCA
Senior Lecturer in Pain Research
Department of Anaesthetics and Intensive Care
Faculty of Medicine, Imperial College London
Honorary Consultant Anaesthetist
Chelsea & Westminster NHS Healthcare Trust
London, United Kingdom
Analgesics: Cannabinoids

C. D. Richards, B.Sc., Ph.D.
Professor of Experimental Physiology
Department of Physiology
University College London
London, United Kingdom
Synaptic Transmission

D.A. Richards, B.Sc., Ph.D.
Research Associate
Department of Physiology
University of Wisconsin
Madison, Wisconsin
Synaptic Transmission

Stephen Robinson, M.D., FRCP
Consultant Physician
Department of Metabolic Medicine
St. Mary's Hospital
London, United Kingdom
Insulin

Carl Rosow, M.D., Ph.D.
Associate Professor of Anaesthesia
Harvard Medical School
Anesthetist
Department of Anesthesia and Critical Care
Massachusetts General Hospital
Boston, Massachusetts
Analgesics: Receptor Ligands and Opiate Narcotics

Robert H. Rubin, M.D., F.A.C.P. F.C.C.P.
Gordon and Marjorie Osborne Professor of Health Sciences
    and Technology
Harvard Medical School
Associate Director, Division of Infectious Disease
Brigham and Women's Hospital
Director, Center for Experimental Pharmacology and
    Therapeutics
Harvard Univeristy-Massachusetts Institute of Technology
    Division of Health Sciences and Technology
Boston, Massachusetts
Antimicrobial Therapy

Uwe Rudolph, M.D.
Assistant Professor of Molecular Neuropharmacology
Institute of Pharmacology and Toxicology
University of Zürich
Zürich, Switzerland
Sedatives, Anxiolytics, and Amnestics

Francis V. Salinas, M.D.
Clinical Assistant Professor
Department of Anesthesiology
Virginia Mason Medical Center
Clinical Assistant Professor of Anesthesiology
University of Washington School of Medicine
Seattle, Washington
Analgesics: Ion Channel Ligands/Sodium Channel
    Blockers/Local Anesthetics

Sunita Sastry, M.B., B.S., M.S., M.D.
Assistant Professor
Department of Anesthesia
Stanford University School of Medicine
Stanford, California
Pulmonary Vasodilators

Michael M. Schachter, BSc, MB, BS, MRCP
Senior Lecturer
Department of Clinical Pharmacology
Faculty of Medicine, Imperial College London
Honorary Consultant, St. Mary's NHS Healthcare Trust
London, United Kingdom
Hypothalamic-Pituitary-Adrenal Axis

Thomas W. Schnider, P.D., Dr. med.
Chairman, Institute of Anesthesiology
Kantonsspital
St. Gallen, Switzerland
Pharmacokinetic and Pharmacodynamic Principles of Drug
    Action

Andreas Scholz, P.D., Dr. med.
Electrophysiological Laboratory
Physiological Institute
Justus-Liebig-University
Giessen, Germany
Analgesics: Ion Channel Ligands/Sodium Channel
    Blockers/Local Anesthetics

Jens Scholz, M.D., Ph.D.
Professor and Chair
Department of Anesthesiology and Intensive Care Medicine
University Hospital Kiel
Kiel, Germany
Antiemetics

Mark Schumacher, Ph.D., M.D.
Assistant Professor
Department of Anesthesia and Perioperative Care; and Oral
    and Maxillofacial Surgery
University of California San Francisco
Attending Physician
Department of Anesthesia and Perioperative Care
Moffitt-Long Hospitals
San Francisco, California
Sensory Processing: Peripheral Nociceptors

John W. Sear, M.A., Ph.D., FFARCS, FANZCA
Professor in Anesthetics
Nuffield Department of Anaesthetics
University of Oxford
Honorary Consultant Anaesthetist
Nuffield Department of Anaesthetics
John Radcliffe Hospital
Fellow of Green College
University of Oxford
Oxford, United Kingdom
Intravenous Anesthetics: Barbiturates, Etomidate, Propofol,
    Ketamine, and Steroids\
Clinical Pharmacology

Robert N. Sladen, M.B., Ch.B., MRCP (UK), FRCP (C)
Medical Director
Cardiothoracic and Surgical Intensive Care Units
Columbia Presbyterian Medical Center
Professor and Vice-Chair
Department of Anesthesiology
College of Physicians & Surgeons of Columbia University
New York, New York
Renal Physiology

Martin R. Smith, B.Sc., MRCP
Specialist Registrar in Diabetes & Endocrinology
Department of Metabolic Medicine
St. Mary's Hospital
London, United Kingdom
Insulin

Neil Soni, M.B., Ch.B, M.D., FFARCS
Consultant in Anaesthetics and Intensive Care Unit
Magill Department of Anaesthesia
Chelsea & Westminster NHS Healthcare Trust
London, United Kingom
Honorary Senior Lecturer
Department of Anaesthetics and Intensive Care
Faculty of Medicine, Imperial College London
London, United Kingdom
Electrolytes Solutions and Colloids

Christoph Stein, M.D.
Professor and Chairman
Department of Anesthesiology and Intensive Care Medicine
Freie Universität Berlin
Campus Benjamin Franklin, Charité-Universitätsmedizin
  Berlin
Berlin, Germany
Analgesics: Receptor Ligands and Opiate Narcotics:
  Mechanisms of Drug Action

Joseph Henry Steinbach, Ph.D
Russell and Mary Sheldon Professor of Anesthesiology
Professor of Anatomy and Neurobiology
Department of Anesthesiology
Washington University School of Medicine
St. Louis, Missouri
Neuromuscular Function

Markus Steinfath, M.D., Ph.D.
Klinik für Anästhesiologie und Operative Intensivmedizin
Universitätsklinikum Schleswig-Holstein, Campus Kiel
Kiel, Germany
Antiemetics

Gary R. Strichartz, Ph.D.
Professor of Anaesthesia (Pharmacology)
Department of Biological Chemistry and Molecular
  Pharmacology
Harvard Medical School
Vice Chairman for Research
Department of Anesthesiology, Perioperative and Pain
  Medicine
Brigham and Women's Hospital
Pain Research Center/BWH
Boston, Massachusetts
The Generation and Propagation of Action Potentials

John A. Summerfield, M.D., FRCP
Professor of Medicine
Division of Medicine
Faculty of Medicine, Imperial College School London
London, United Kingdom
Liver Physiology

Richard S. Teplick, M.D.
Associate Professor of Anesthesia
Harvard Medical School
Vice-Chairman
Department of Anesthesia, Perioperative and Pain Medicine
Director, Division of Critical Care
Brigham and Women's Hospital
Boston, Massachusetts
Antimicrobial Therapy

Elizabeth Theogaraj, B.Sc.
Postgraduate Student
Department of Neuroendocrinology
Division of Neuroscience and Psychological Medicine
Imperial College School of Medicine
London, United Kingdom
Hypothalamic-Pituitary-Adrenal Axis

Isao Tsuneyoshi, M.D., Ph.D.
Consultant
Department of Anesthesiology and Critical Care Medicine
Kagoshima University School of Medicine
Sakuragaoka, Kagoshima, Japan
Vascular Reactivity

Peter H. Tonner, M.D., Ph.D.
Klinik für Anästhesiologie und Operative Intensivmedizin
Universitätsklinikum Schleswig-Holstein, Campus Kiel
Kiel, Germany
Antiemetics

Kevin K. Tremper, M.D., Ph.D.
Professor and Chair
Department of Anesthesiology
University of Michigan Medical School
Chair
Department of Anesthesiology
University of Michigan Health System
Ann Arbor, Michigan
Red Blood Cell Substitutes

Robert P. Walt, M.D., FRCP
Senior Clinical Lecturer
Department of Medicine
Birmingham University
Director of Gastroenterology
Department of Gastroenterology
Birmingham Heartlands and Solihull NHS Trust (Teaching)
Birmingham Heartlands Hospital
Birmingham, United Kingdom
Antimotility and Antisecretory Agents

Denham S. Ward, M.D., Ph.D.
Senior Director
Department of Surgical Support Services
Strong Memorial Hospital
Professor
Department of Electrical Engineering
University of Rochester
Professor and Chairman
Department of Anesthesiology
University of Rochester School of Medicine and Dentistry
Rochester, New York
Lung Function

David C. Warltier, M.D., Ph.D.
Professor of Anesthesiology, Pharmacology, Toxiocology,
  and Medicine
Division of Cardiovascular Diseases
Vice Chairman for Research
Departments of Anesthesiology, Pharmacology, and
  Toxicology, and Medicine (Division of Cardiovascular
  Disease),
Medical College of Wisconsin
Milwaukee, Wisconsin
Cardiovascular Pharmacology of Positive Inotropic Drugs

Charles Weissman, M.D.
Professor and Chairman
Department of Anesthesiology and Critical Care
  Medicine
Hebrew-University-Hadassah School of Medicine
Jerusalem, Israel
Nutritional Supplements

Brian J. Woodcock, M.B. Ch.B., M.R.C.P., F.R.C.A
Assistant Professor
Department of Anesthesiology
University of Michigan Medical School
Ann Arbor, Michigan
Red Blood Cell Substitutes

Ling-Gang Wu, Ph.D.
Assistant Professor
Departments of Anesthesiology and Anatomy and
  Neurobiology
Washington University School of Medicine
St. Louis, Missouri
Neuromuscular Function

Paul B. Zanaboni, M.D., Ph.D.
Associate Professor of Anesthesiology and Cardiothoracic
  Surgery
Department of Anesthesiology
Washington University School of Medicine
St. Louis, Missouri
Vasodilators

Acknowledgments

The success of any multiauthored text is dependent on the expertise and commitment of the contributors. We are fortunate to have assembled authors who are truly experts in their various fields, and we express our gratitude at their willingness to participate in this project and for the scholarly chapters that they have produced. We also thank our assistants, Patti Wanko and Elizabeth Ogden, for their organizational and secretarial contributions, and Allan Ross, Acquisition Editor, and Agnes Byrne, Developmental Editor, for their perseverance and support. Above all, we deeply thank our wives, Dr. Carol Evers and Dr. Janet Wyner, for their patience and support through the many nights and weekends that went into editing this book.

Alex S. Evers, M.D.
St. Louis, Missouri

Mervyn Maze, M.B., Ch.B.
London, United Kingdom

Preface

Recent years have seen the beginning of a revolution in our understanding of how anesthesia is produced and how the drugs used by anesthesiologists work at a molecular level. Concomitantly, the clinical practice of anesthesia has become increasingly more complex and demanding. The result of these developments has been a growing chasm between clinically sophisticated anesthesiologists, who may be inadequately versed in basic and molecular pharmacology, and anesthetic researchers, who are well versed in the mechanistic details of anesthetic drug action, but are inadequately informed about the clinical context in which these drugs are used. We have assembled this textbook with the aim of bridging this chasm. With this goal in mind, we designed this book to provide:

■ Anesthesia trainees with a broad integrated introduction to the basic science and clinical use of drugs used in anesthesia.
■ Anesthesia clinicians with enhanced understanding of the mechanisms of drug action and with a conceptual framework to approach new agents.
■ Basic scientists with a clinical context to understand the relevance of their work and to direct investigations to clinically important problems.

We hope that this book also will foster clinical studies to resolve therapeutic deficiencies and discrepancies.

This book is organized into three sections. The initial section, "Principles of Drug Action," provides detailed theoretical and practical information about pharmacokinetics, pharmacodynamics, and cell signaling pathways. It also provides an introduction to several topics including pharmacoeconomics and pharmacogenetics. The second section, "Physiologic Substrates of Drug Action," focuses on the physiology of processes central to the actions of agents used in anesthesia and provides a detailed review of molecular, cellular, and integrated physiology. The goal of this section is to facilitate understanding of the targets and mechanisms of drug action. The third and final section, "Pharmacologic Basis of Clinical Practice," covers the various classes of drugs organized according to their primary purpose. The emphasis of this section is on drugs primarily used in anes-

thesia, but it also deals with such drugs as antibiotics and chemotherapeutic agents, which are frequently encountered by the anesthesiologist and may have significant implications for anesthetic practice and interactions with anesthetic agents. Each chapter has the same structure and includes the following sections: Mechanisms of Action, Clinical Pharmacology, Adverse Effects, Practical Aspects of Drug Use, and Dosage and Administration.

For trainees, the book can be read as a whole and will provide an in-depth background in anesthetic pharmacology, including all the information needed for specialist training examinations. For readers interested in specific organ systems or classes of drugs, individual chapters are designed to stand on their own. Finally, the "Practical Aspects of Drug Use" section at the end of each chapter can serve as a quick reference for practical questions of immediate importance.

We expect that the scientific revolution in understanding the molecular details of anesthetic drug action will continue, bringing with it better versions of existing drugs, as well as new drugs working via novel mechanisms. We hope that this book provides the conceptual framework for incorporating new agents into your thinking and practice. Toward this aim, we have tried throughout to highlight existing deficiencies in the therapeutic armamentarium and potential opportunities for new therapeutic modalities.

This book arose from a suggestion by Dr. Ronald Miller that his textbook, *Anesthesiology*, could no longer provide the depth of pharmacologic detail that anesthesia practitioners and students required. We have designed this book to complement the information contained in Dr. Miller's general text. The similar size and binding of *Anesthetic Pharmacology: Physiologic Principles and Clinical Practice* emphasize that this text can be viewed as a companion to *Anesthesia*.

Alex S. Evers, M.D.
St. Louis, Missouri

Mervyn Maze, M.B., Ch.B.
London, United Kingdom

Foreword

In the last 20 years, both the scope and complexity of peri-operative medicine and specifically anesthetic practice have dramatically increased. Coping with the challenge of caring for patients with greater acuity and intricacy of disease requires a keen knowledge and intellectual flexibility to improve our approaches to clinical disease processes and pharmacology. Both the number of drugs and their specificity have markedly increased. For example, in the first edition of *Anesthesia,* published in 1981, only seven drugs were listed (Table 46–1) for all eventualities in providing advanced cardiac life support. In contrast, there are ten drugs listed for the tachycardia algorithm alone (Table 75–13) in the fifth edition of *Anesthesia*, published in 2000. This example is indicative of the explosion in the development and registration of new target-specific drugs based on a more complete understanding of the complex mechanisms governing drug action.

Despite the completeness of *Anesthesia,* it was decided that a separate text was needed to provide the depth of pharmacologic information to satisfy the needs of the sophisticated clinician. Of prime importance would be the inclusion of creative full color illustrations to facilitate coordination between mechanisms of action and clinical pharmacology. To have two internationally renowned anesthesiologist-pharmacologists, Drs. Alex Evers and Mervyn Maze, assured the excellence of *Anesthetic Pharmacology: Physiologic Principles and Clinical Practice.*

Ronald D. Miller, M.D.
Professor and Chair, Department of Anesthesia
and Perioperative Care
Professor of Cellular and Molecular Pharmacology
University of California San Francisco

Table of Contents

Principles of
Drug Action

Pharmacokinetic and Pharmacodynamic Principles of Drug Action

Thomas W. Schnider PD, MD • Charles F. Minto, MBChB

Basic Pharmacokinetic Parameters
Compartment Models
Special Compartment Models
Drug Input
Effect Compartment Concept
   Pharmacodynamic Models
Tolerance

Indirect Models
Predictors of Onset
Predictors of Offset
Drug Accumulation
Dose Equivalence: Principles of Calculation
Interpatient Variability
Principle of Target Controlled Infusion

Achieving the appropriate drug effects at any time during surgery, at the end of surgery, and after surgery is an important objective of anesthesia. The main drugs used to induce general anesthesia are the hypnotics, analgesics, and muscle relaxants, which are given to ensure unconsciousness, to provide analgesia and suppress the hemodynamic response, and to suppress reflex movements, respectively. The dose of each drug is titrated against the individual patient's response to achieve the intraoperative therapeutic goals. The patient should lose consciousness rapidly after induction, the level of analgesia should follow closely the level of surgical stimulation, and at the end of the operation the drug effect should dissipate so that the patient wakes up, has no residual muscle relaxation, and is pain free. Unfortunately, at the end of an operation the desired intraoperative drug effects are viewed as "side effects," e.g., excessive sedation and respiratory depression.

From a pharmacologic perspective, anesthesia is concerned with controlling the time course of drug effect. This is dependent on the site and rate of input of the drug, the distribution of the drug within the body, the elimination of the drug from the body, and the sensitivity of the patient to the drug. Innumerable anatomic, physiologic, and chemical factors influence these processes. If we knew quantitatively all of the factors affecting the distribution, elimination, and sensitivity to a drug in an individual patient, we could predict the time course of drug effect exactly. However, we

only know a minority of all the aspects of the dose-response relationship and, unfortunately, an understanding of one important factor generally does not explain the bigger picture. For example, the higher lipid solubility of fentanyl is sometimes used to explain its faster onset of effect compared with morphine. Although it is not possible to quantify the speed of onset with this knowledge, it might be tempting to categorize opioids based this property. However, we know that there must be other important factors because alfentanil has a faster onset of effect than fentanyl, despite its lower lipid solubility.

Mathematic models are commonly used to relate the administered drug dose to the measured drug concentration (a *pharmacokinetic* model) and to relate the measured drug concentrations to the measured drug effects (a *pharmacodynamic* model). After a model that describes the time course of effect in an individual patient has been developed, factors that are responsible for an individual's deviation from the average response are included into the model, that is if they are statistically justifiable. With such models the time course of the drug effect for other dosing regimens and other patients can be predicted. Inversely, the dose, dose interval, or infusion rate that is required to achieve a desired concentration and desired effect level can also be calculated.

This chapter focuses on the pharmacokinetic and pharmacodynamic (PK/PD) principles necessary for understanding the time course of drug effect.

Basic Pharmacokinetic Parameters

The first basic PK parameter considered here is volume of distribution (V_d). In the simplest case, the amount of drug administered intravenously is related to the concentration measured in the plasma. Thus the apparent V_d can be calculated with the formula: $V_d = \dfrac{Amount}{Concentration}$, which assumes that the drug is administered into a single well-mixed compartment. If a drug remains unbound in the plasma and does not distribute into other tissues, the V_d would be the same as the plasma volume. However, most drugs leave the plasma and distribute into and bind to other tissues. If the binding capacity of the tissue is very high, the relative amount of drug circulating in the plasma will be low. It is possible for the calculated V_d to be much larger than the whole body volume. For instance, the V_d of furosemide is 7.7 L/70 kg, but chloroquine is 13,000 L/70 kg. Therefore it is better to refer to this volume as an *apparent* V_d because it does not correspond with a real anatomic volume. Usually the apparent *initial* volume of distribution is reported, which, for an intravenous bolus dose, is calculated according to the above formula using the concentration "back-extrapolated" to time zero.

The second basic pharmacokinetic parameter is clearance (Cl). Clearance is often defined as the volume of plasma that must be completely cleared of the drug per unit time; that is, clearance has the same units as flow. Figure 1–1 shows the elimination rate and concentrations for 30 minutes after an intravenous bolus dose. More drug is cleared from the plasma per unit of time at the beginning when the concentration is high, i.e., *the elimination rate is proportional to the concentration* ($ER \propto C$). From this relationship, we obtain another helpful definition: clearance is the proportionality constant, which relates the rate of elimination to the measured concentration ($ER = Cl \cdot C$). The amount of drug (A) eliminated during any time interval Δt is given by the equation: $A_{\Delta t} = ER \cdot \Delta t = Cl \cdot C \cdot \Delta t$. Note that $C \cdot \Delta t$ is the area under the concentration curve in the Δt interval. By summing all the $C \cdot \Delta t$ elements, the complete area under the concentration time curve (AUC) will be the result. Mathematically, this is expressed by the integral: $AUC = \int\limits_{0}^{\infty} C(t) \cdot dt$. The total amount of drug eliminated between time zero and infinity must be the same as the dose. Therefore we can rewrite the above equation as follows:

$$Dose = Cl \cdot AUC \qquad (1)$$

which gives us an estimate of clearance obtained using noncompartment methods:

$$Cl = \frac{Dose}{AUC} \qquad (2)$$

We can also calculate the V_d by noncompartment methods, using so-called "moment analysis." The first moment is given by $t \cdot C(t)$, which is the product of the

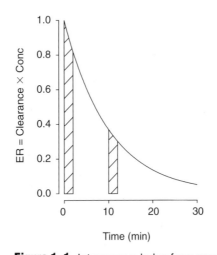
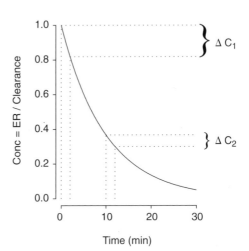

Figure 1–1. Intravenous bolus for a one-compartment model; volume of distribution = 10 L, clearance (Cl) = 1 L/min, elimination rate constant, $k = Cl/V = 0.1\,min^{-1}$, dose = 10 mg. The elimination rate (ER) decreases over time (*left*). $ER = k \times$ amount remaining in the central compartment at any time. The amount in the central compartment equals the concentration multiplied by the volume of the central compartment. The area under the curve shaded between 0 and 2 minutes (*left*) equals the amount of drug eliminated in this interval. The area under the curve shaded between 10 and 12 minutes (*left*) equals the amount of drug eliminated in this interval. The total area under the elimination rate (mg/min) against time (min) curve equals the dose administered (mg). The right graph shows the concentration changing over time. The total area under the concentration (mg/mL) against time (min) curve equals the dose divided by clearance (*right*). At any time, the rate of decrease of concentration (the slope of the concentration vs. time curve) divided by the concentration is a constant, i.e., it is an exponential process. Note that the change in the concentration in the interval from 0 to 2 minutes (ΔC_1) is greater than 10 to 12 minutes (ΔC_2).

elapsed time, t, and the concentration at time t. Analogous to the calculation of AUC, the area under the moment curve is $AUMC = \int_0^\infty t \cdot C(t) \cdot dt$ from which we can calculate V_d as:

$$V_d = Cl \cdot \frac{AUMC}{AUC} = Cl \cdot MRT \qquad (3)$$

This term, $AUMC/AUC$ provides the mean residence time (MRT), defined as the arithmetic average of the times that each drug molecule remains in the body. Practically, moment analysis makes only minimal assumptions about how the drug is distributed and eliminated, because the parameters are estimated based on the measured concentrations. However, the analysis theoretically requires concentration measurements until "infinite time." Because a limited number of concentration measurements are available, the area under the curve from the last measurement until infinity must be extrapolated, which introduces some assumptions. If the extrapolated area under the curve forms a significant percentage of the total area under the curve (area under data + area under extrapolated curve), then we have less confidence in the estimated parameters. To analyze data after different types of drug input, e.g., oral dosing or intravenous infusions, modifications to the above formulae are necessary.

The determination of the basic pharmacokinetic parameters clearance, volume of distribution, and mean residence time by noncompartment methods represents the gold standard by which the estimates of other approaches should be compared. Unfortunately, these parameters alone are insufficient. To facilitate rational drug selection and the development of rational dosing guidelines, a thorough understanding of several other important concepts is required.

Compartment Models

It is helpful to think of compartment models in terms of a hydraulic model.[1] The cross-sectional area of the bucket represents the volume of distribution, the height of water in the bucket represents the drug concentration, and the amount of water added to the bucket represents the amount of drug added to the body. Thus for a given amount of water added to the bucket (dose), the water level (concentration) will be higher when the cross-sectional area (volume of distribution) is smaller, and the water level (concentration) will be lower when the cross-sectional area (volume of distribution) is larger. If a single hole is made in the bucket (representing drug elimination), the water level will decrease in an exponential manner, i.e., the rate of change in the height of water will be proportional to the height of water at any time.

The pharmacokinetics of many drugs are poorly described by a single bucket, because many drugs used in anesthesia distribute extensively into different body compartments. We can make a better model by connecting other buckets to the central bucket by means of small connecting hoses of different diameters. When water is now added to the central bucket, the water level decreases because of two

processes: water runs out the bottom of the central bucket (drug elimination) and water runs between the central bucket and the peripheral buckets (drug distribution).

It is customary to differentiate between different phases of the decrease in concentration following an intravenous bolus dose. The "distribution phase" usually refers to the initial rapid decrease in concentrations, and the "elimination phase" usually refers to the later slower decline in concentrations. However, as is apparent from the hydraulic model, these two processes actually occur simultaneously, rather than sequentially. As described above, the rate of elimination is proportional to the concentration. Thus it is during the initial high concentrations of the "distribution phase" (when the drug is moving from the central to the peripheral compartments) that the *elimination rate* is greatest. Also, it is during the "elimination phase" that the rate of decline of concentrations is slowed by the *distribution* of drug from the peripheral compartments back into the central compartment.

To derive the parameters of a compartment model, assumptions must be made about the structure of the model. The compartment models that are normally used are called mammillary models. This means that the drug is administered into the central compartment; the peripheral compartments are connected to the central compartment; drug is eliminated from the central compartment; and no drug is eliminated from the peripheral compartments. Other types of models exist (e.g., catenary models) in which the compartments are connected in a chainlike manner. Because the shape of the curve changes with the number of compartments, the model that best fits the data must be selected based on objective statistical criterion. Nonlinear regression is used to estimate the model parameters, so that the model predictions accurately describe the measured concentrations.

Compartment models can be parameterized in several different ways. A common method involves ordinary differential equations. The underlying idea is that drug elimination and drug distribution between the compartments is described by rate constants (k), which are commonly assigned subscripts to indicate the direction of drug movement. The central volume of distribution (V_1) and five rate constants ($k_{10}, k_{12}, k_{13}, k_{21}, k_{31}$) describe a three-compartment model. Another common method is to use a polyexponential equation, e.g., $C(t) = Dose \cdot (A_1 \cdot e^{-\lambda_1} + A_2 \cdot e^{-\lambda_2} + A_3 \cdot e^{-\lambda_3})$. In this case, a plot of the natural logarithm of the concentrations that are observed after an intravenous bolus versus time reveals three distinct slopes, which are equal to λ_1, λ_2 and λ_3. Although a different equation is required to describe the concentrations after an intravenous infusion, the same coefficients (A_1, A_2, A_3) and hybrid-rate constants (λ_1, λ_2 and λ_3) are used. Another common method is to use three volumes (V_1, V_2, V_3) and three clearances (Cl_1, Cl_2, and Cl_3). Other combinations of parameters are possible. However, for a one-, two- or three-compartment model, the number of parameters required is always twice the number of compartments. With one full set of parameters, all of the other parameters can be calculated.

Figure 1–2 illustrates two drugs, which both have a steady-state volume of distribution (V_{dss}) of 100 L. However, the drug on the left is described by a one-compartment model and the drug on the right is described by a two-

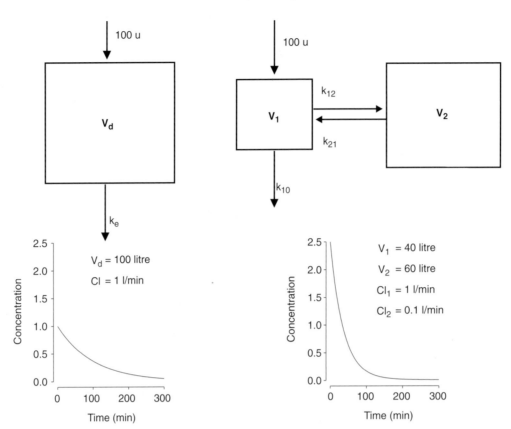

Figure 1–2. Intravenous bolus for one- and two-compartment models. The concentrations decline exponentially, shown over the first 5 hours. Both drugs have a steady-state volume of distribution (V_{dss}) of 100 L. The rate of movement of drug (mg/min) in the directions of the arrows are governed by the product of the amount of drug in the compartment (units = mg) and the rate constants (units = min^{-1}). The direction of movement is indicated by the subscripts, e.g., k_e and k_{10} are the elimination rate constants from the central compartment one (the central compartment) to the outside (compartment zero), k_{12} is the rate constant governing the rate of drug movement from compartment one to compartment two (the peripheral compartment), and k_{21} is the rate constant governing the rate of drug movement from compartment two to compartment one. After administration of 100 units (u) bolus to the one-compartment model, the initial concentration is given by 100 u/100 L = 1 u/L. After administration of 100 units bolus to the two-compartment model, the initial concentration is given by 100 u/40 L = 2.5 u/L (see bottom graphs). The drug is assumed to mix instantaneously in the central compartment. Both drugs have the same clearance. Thus the total area under the curve over all time will be identical. The predicted concentrations for the one-compartment model (*bottom left*) can be completely described by two parameters, V_d (which for the one-compartment model is the same as V_{dss}) and Cl, both of which can be estimated by noncompartment techniques. However, the predicted concentrations for the two-compartment model (*bottom right*) cannot be described by V_{dss} and Cl_1 alone, two more parameters are required.

compartment model. Both drugs also have the same clearance ($Cl = Cl_1$). The two-compartment model has a volume of distribution at steady-state, V_{dss}, which is divided between two compartments and is given by $V_{dss} = V_1 + V_2$, whereas the one-compartment model has a V_{dss} equal to its initial volume of distribution (in this case, labeled V_d). As illustrated in Figure 1–2 (*bottom*), the measured drug concentrations for the two-compartment model (drug elimination and distribution) are different from the one-compartment model (drug elimination only).

It should now be obvious that, although very important, the basic pharmacokinetic parameters (V_{dss}, Cl, and MRT) obtained by noncompartment methods do not adequately describe the pharmacokinetic behavior of drugs that are best described by multicompartment models. It is possible for two drugs with identical steady-state volume of distribution

and clearance to have completely different concentrations following the same dosing history. For multicompartment models, all model parameters must be known to calculate the predicted concentrations. Even when all of the parameters are available, it is nearly impossible to make correct inferences about the pharmacokinetic behavior of a drug without the aid of computer simulations.[2]

So far we have not mentioned a very popular pharmacokinetic parameter: the half-time or half-life. For a one-compartment model, the meaning of the half-time is unambiguous and it can be calculated easily. Plotting the natural logarithm of the drug concentrations following an intravenous bolus on the *y*-axis against time on the *x*-axis will obtain a straight line with slope −*k*. In any time interval equal to $t_{1/2}$, the concentration, *C*, will decrease by one half from *C* to *C*/2). Thus

$$k = \frac{\Delta y}{\Delta x}$$

$$k = \frac{\log_e(C) - \log_e(C/2)}{t_{1/2}}$$

$$t_{1/2} = \frac{\log_e(2)}{k}$$

$$t_{1/2} = \frac{0.693}{k} \tag{4}$$

For a one-compartment model, $t_{1/2}$ describes the time required for the concentrations to decrease by one half, which is unchanged for any combination of boluses or infusions, and is unchanged by the duration of drug administration. We can also call it the "elimination half-life," and quite correctly imply that it is also the time to eliminate half of the drug from the body. Thus, for a one-compartment model, the "context sensitive half-time" (see later) equals the elimination half-life, and does not change with the duration of the infusion.

However, for drugs that are described by multicompartment pharmacokinetics, the concept of half-time is more complicated. Instead of a single exponential process with one half-time, the pharmacokinetics are described by two or more exponential processes. Thus for each of the exponential terms (λ_1, λ_2, and λ_3), a half-time can be calculated as:

$t_{1/2,i} = \dfrac{0.693}{\lambda_i}$. Often these are referred to as the α, β, and γ

half-lives. Importantly, the time for the concentration to decrease by 50% is dependent on the preceding dosing history and can vary with the duration of drug administration. For multicompartment models, the time for the concentration to decrease by half does not equal the time to eliminate half of the drug from the body, and the time required to eliminate half of the drug from the body is not the same as the "elimination half-life." For this reason, the expression "terminal half-life" is preferred to "elimination half-life." Other concepts are required, because a single parameter, such as one half-time, cannot represent the entire time course of the concentration of a drug described by multicompartment pharmacokinetics. Concepts such as "context-sensitive half-time" and "relative decrement time" are better suited and will be discussed later in this chapter.

Several factors influence the estimated parameters, including obvious problems, such as errors in the dose, errors in the timing of the samples, and errors in measuring the drug concentrations. However, design issues are also important. Factors such as the site of sampling (e.g., arterial vs. venous), the method of administration (e.g., bolus vs. infusion), and the number and timing of samples, in particular the duration of sampling, also have an important influence on the parameter estimates. In general, the longer the sampling time the more "compartments" can be detected. Based on many hours of sampling, a three-compartment model is commonly reported for many drugs to describe their pharmacokinetics. Sometimes the three compartments are assigned physiologic significance, i.e., the central compartment is thought to correspond with the vascular space; the second compartment with the rapidly equilibrat-

ing, high-perfusion tissues, such as muscle; and the large third compartment with the slowly equilibrating, low-perfusion tissues, such as fat. Based on measurements obtained for 6 to 7 days after 30 minutes of isoflurane and sevoflurane, five-compartment models were reported.[3] The five compartments were referred to as: (1) the central compartment, (2) the vessel-rich group, (3) the muscle group, (4) the fourth compartment, and (5) the fat group. It is important to remember that these models were developed to describe the time course of measured concentrations at a single site (e.g., plasma, or end-tidal) and that no drug concentrations were actually measured in the "vessel rich group," "the fourth compartment," "muscle," or "fat." Conversely, in physiologic models, mathematic models for each organ are based on careful studies of measured concentrations relevant to each organ.

Special Compartment Models

The assumption that the rate of elimination (and drug movement between the compartments) is proportional to the concentration in the relevant compartments implies that the concentration at any time is linearly related to the dose or infusion rate, respectively. Or simply, the models imply that doubling a bolus dose or doubling an infusion rate will double the concentrations. But this might be an invalid assumption for some drugs. A prerequisite for linearity is that the elimination and transport processes are not saturated. However, when the enzyme system responsible for elimination becomes saturated, the rate of drug elimination reaches a maximum and becomes concentration independent. The pharmacokinetics of alcohol is a well-known example for nonlinear kinetics within the "therapeutic" range.

The elimination rate (ER) for a one-compartment model with nonlinear kinetics is described as

$$ER = \frac{V_m \cdot C_u(t)}{K_m + C_u(t)} \tag{5}$$

where $C_u(t)$ is the concentration of unbound of drug at time t and K_m is the Michaelis-Menton constant, which is the concentration at which the rate is half maximum, V_m. Two extremes can be distinguished. Firstly, when the C_u is much smaller than K_m, the process not saturated and the elimination is proportional to the concentration (linear kinetics). Secondly, when C_u is much greater than K_m, the elimination rate approaches V_m and is concentration independent. These extremes are expressed in Equation 1.6.

$$\text{if} \quad : C_u << K_m$$
$$\text{then} \quad : ER = \frac{V_m}{K_m} \cdot C_u(t) = Cl \cdot C_u(t)$$
$$\text{if} \quad : C_u >> K_m$$
$$\text{then} \quad : ER = V_m \tag{6}$$

If the amount of drug excreted by specific routes (e.g., into the bile and urine) is also known, more complex compartment models can be developed with more than a single site of elimination. Sometimes the pharmacokinetics of a metabolite can be of interest, particularly if the metabolite is active clinically. To develop a compartment model for both the parent compound and the metabolite, it is necessary to measure the concentrations of both substances. The underlying principle is that a fraction of the parent compound is converted into the metabolite, which is then described by its own pharmacokinetic model.[4] The accuracy of the model will be improved if the kinetics of the metabolite can be investigated (by administering pure metabolite without parent compound) in the same subjects in a crossover study design).

Drug Input

In theory, an intravenous bolus dose is an infusion with an infinite rate, i.e., the total amount of drug is instantaneously injected at $t = 0$. The bolus dose concept is appealing because it makes the mathematics of the pharmacokinetic model somewhat easier. Another requirement is that the injected drug is instantaneously mixed (or "well-stirred") within the central compartment, so that the drug concentration is maximal at $t = 0$. However, neither of these two assumptions is true. In practice, a bolus dose is a rapid infusion with a finite rate. For example, a 100 mg bolus of propofol administered over 15 seconds is really an infusion rate equal to 400 mg/min. The use of "infusion rate" equations rather than "bolus dose" equations has the advantage of avoiding maximum predicted concentrations at $t = 0$. However, in reality, mixing is still not instantaneous. The drug must return to the heart, pass through the pulmonary circulation and then through the systemic circulation before it is detected at an arterial sampling site. Even during an infusion at "steady-state," the drug concentrations in different parts of the circulation may not be the same, particularly if the drug is rapidly metabolized. Traditional compartment models only poorly describe arterial concentrations during the first minute or so. More complex recirculatory models[5] or hybrid physiologic models[6] are required to more accurately describe the concentrations in different parts of the circulation.

With a constant infusion rate, IR, the concentration rises gradually towards a steady-state. This is the result of two processes, as defined in the following equation for a one-compartment model.

$$\frac{dA}{dt} = IR - ER \tag{7}$$

This differential equation states that rate of change in the amount (A) of drug in the compartment is equal to the rate of drug entering the compartment (the infusion rate) minus the rate of drug leaving the compartment (the elimination rate). This equation indicates how differential equations are used to describe complex models. The concentration in the compartment is then obtained by dividing the amount in the compartment by the volume of the compartment. During the infusion, the elimination rate increases in proportion to

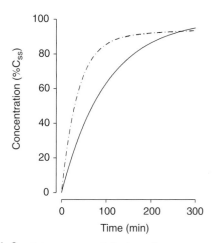

Figure 1–3. Intravenous infusion for one- and two-compartment model. Parameters for both drugs are identical to Figure 1–2. The half-time for the one-compartment model is 69 minutes and the two half-times for the two-compartment model are 25 minutes and 460 minutes. Both drugs in this simulation have the same clearance, and the infusion rate is the same. The steady-state concentration (100 u/L) is given by the product of rate (100 u/min) and clearance (1 L/min). For the one-compartment model (*solid line*), the following relationship is observed: after 1, 2, 3, 4, and 5 half-lives, 50%, 75%, 87.5%, 93.75%, and 97% of steady-state concentration is achieved. For the two-compartment model (*dashed line*), this relationship is no longer true; despite the longer terminal half-time (460 minutes), the initial approach toward the steady-state level is more rapid. Without knowing the respective coefficients (see text), it is not possible to predict the relative contribution of each exponential process. In this example, A_1/λ_1 accounts for 90% of the area under the curve and A_2/λ_2 accounts for only 10% of the area under the curve. Thus the shorter half-time is of greater significance initially.

the increasing concentration, whereas the input rate is constant. Therefore, the concentration will increase until the elimination rate equals the infusion rate (Fig. 1–3) at which time a steady-state concentration is achieved (theoretically only after an infinite time). The concentration at any time, t, during the infusion is described by the following equations.

$$C(t) = \frac{R}{k_{10} \cdot V_1}\left(1 - e^{-k_{10} \cdot t}\right)$$

$$C(t = \infty) = \frac{R}{k_{10} \cdot V_1} = \frac{R}{Cl_1} \tag{8}$$

The first line only applies to a one-compartment model, but the second line is also true for two- and three-compartment models.

Another important category of drug administration is absorption from an extravascular site, such as the buccal area, gastrointestinal tract, the muscles, the skin and the respiratory tract. For the intravenous route, the rate of input is precisely known. In contrast, for the extravascular routes the rate of input of the drug into the circulation is influenced by a variety of different physical and chemical processes. Factors such as the formulation of the drug, its molecular weight, its lipid solubility, its pKa, the pH value of the tissue, and the blood supply to the site will all affect the rate of absorption. Importantly, there may be a significant delay between drug administration and the commencement of absorption from the site (referred to as the lag time or t_{lag}), and only some fraction of the total dose may be absorbed. The bioavailability, F, can be calculated when data are available for both intravenous (iv) and extravascular (ev) administration of the same drug. The calculation assumes that clearance remains constant when the two routes are compared:

$$Dose_{iv} = Cl \cdot AUC_{iv}$$

$$F \cdot Dose_{ev} = Cl \cdot AUC_{ev}$$

$$F = \left(\frac{AUC_{ev}}{AUC_{iv}} \right) \cdot \left(\frac{Dose_{iv}}{Dose_{ev}} \right) \quad (9)$$

Thus by definition the bioavailability of a drug given intravenously is 100%, whereas only a fraction (F) of this might reach the systemic circulation when given by an extravascular route. For example, if some of an orally administered drug passes the gastrointestinal tract without being absorbed, and some undergoes first-pass metabolism,

the area under the curve for the oral route will be smaller than the intravenous route (given the same dose) and the bioavailability will be less than 100%.

Figure 1–4 shows a compartment model that describes the time course of the concentration after extravascular administration of a drug. It shows the impact of changing the bioavailability (F) or absorption rate on the concentration in the central compartment. The mathematic expression for such a model must include two separate pharmacokinetic processes: the absorption rate and the elimination rate. The rate of decrease in the amount of drug in the extravascular site equals the rate of absorption from the site. The rate of change in the amount of drug in the central compartment equals the rate of absorption from the extravascular site minus the rate of elimination from the central compartment. This can be expressed in the following two differential equations:

$$\frac{dA_{ev}}{dt} = -k_a \cdot A_{ev}(t)$$

$$\frac{dA_1}{dt} = k_a \cdot A_{ev}(t) - k_{10} \cdot A_1(t) \quad (10)$$

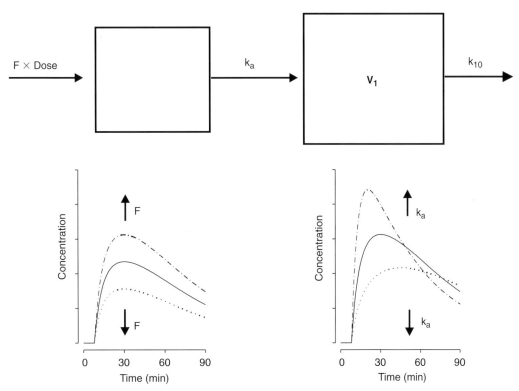

Figure 1–4. Extravascular dose and one-compartment model. The fraction of the absorbed dose is described by the bioavailability, F. Increasing the F by one-third (*dashed line*) or decreasing F by one-third (*dotted line*) will increase or decrease the concentrations proportionally (*left*). The rate of increase and decrease of the concentration in the central compartment (V_1) is determined by the absorption rate constant (k_a) and the elimination rate constant (k_{10}). Usually k_a is greater than k_{10}. (If k_a is very small compared with k_{10}, then "flip-flop" kinetics exist and the slow terminal half-time is due to the slow absorption process, rather than a slow elimination process.) Increasing the k_a (*dashed line*) will increase the maximum concentration (C_{max}), which will occur earlier (t_{max}), and decreasing k_a (*dotted line*) will decrease the maximum concentration (C_{max}), which will occur later (t_{max}) (*right*). If the dose, bioavailability, and clearance are unchanged, the area under the three curves will be the same. In both graphs, the absorption begins after a lag time (t_{lag}) of several minutes.

Figure 1–5. Effect site model. Concentrations are measured in the central compartment, which is not the site of drug effect. An additional effect-site compartment (a one-compartment model) is added to the model (*top*). This model describes the delay between concentration in the central compartment and the effect without changing the pharmacokinetic model developed to describe the concentrations in the central compartment. The volume of the effect-site is a tiny fraction of the volume of the central compartment and k_{1e} is a tiny fraction of k_{e0}. If the rate constant, k_{e0}, is large (a short $t_{1/2}\,k_{e0}$), then the effect-site equilibrates rapidly with the central compartment. At steady-state, the concentration in the effect-site equals the concentration in the central compartment. A 10-minute remifentanil infusion (*middle*) shows the increase and decrease of remifentanil concentrations (*solid line*) and the decrease and increase in the spectral edge frequency (*dashed line*). The counterclockwise loop is seen when the effect is plotted against the concentration in the central compartment (*bottom*). For the same level of effect, the concentration is higher during onset than during offset, because central compartment concentrations are the driving force for the movement of drug to and from the effect-site. It is important to plot the effect on the *y*-axis with the baseline effect at the origin, otherwise the direction of the loop is reversed. The *dashed line* shows the nonlinear static relationship between the concentration and effect in the effect site compartment, which is usually described by an E_{max} pharmacodynamic model.

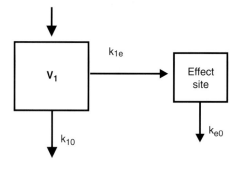

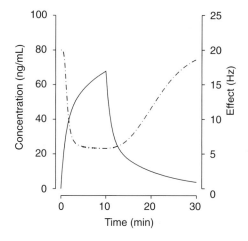

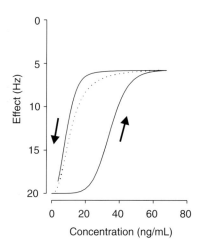

where A_{ev} denotes amount of drug in the extravascular site, k_a represents the absorption rate constant, k_{10} represents the elimination rate constant from the central compartment, and the amount of drug in the extravascular site at $t = 0$ is $F \times Dose$. Again, the concentration in the central compartment is then obtained by dividing the amount in the compartment by the volume of the central compartment. Data from oral dose studies are often summarized with two parameters, the time (t_{max}) of the maximum concentration (C_{max}), which are compound descriptors of the absorption and distribution/elimination processes. In some circumstances it is possible to estimate the absorption half-life based on t_{max}. Often the absorption process is more complex and adequate description requires a model with more than a single absorption rate constant.[7] To detect the appropriate form of the absorption process, "deconvolution" methods are used to analyze data obtained after both intravenous and extravascular routes of administration in the same individuals.

Effect Compartment Concept

After an intravenous bolus dose, it takes time to establish an effect. This is most obvious when substances whose effect can be measured objectively and continuously are used, such as muscle relaxants. The drug must be transported close to the site of effect, penetrate into the tissue, bind to a receptor, and elicit some intracellular process, which eventually will be called the *effect*. All of these steps are time consuming and introduce a delay between the time course of the plasma concentration and the time course of the effect.

Figure 1–5 shows the effect of a brief remifentanil infusion on the electroencephalogram. The concentration versus effect curve forms a counterclockwise hysteresis loop. If the concentration in the central compartment produced the effect without delay, the concentration versus effect curve would be a simple curve, i.e., there would be no loop. Thus the loop is present because the concentration was measured at the wrong site, i.e., in the case of remifentanil, the blood is not the site of drug effect.

Hull and colleagues[8] and Sheiner and co-workers[9] introduced the effect compartment concept based on data from studies with muscle relaxants. Unfortunately, the effect-site concentration cannot be measured directly. It is not a real "measurable" concentration, but rather a virtual concentration in a virtual compartment. For any concentration in this virtual compartment, there is a corresponding effect. This relationship between concentration and effect in this compartment is usually nonlinear (see section on pharmacodynamic models later in this chapter) and static (does not explicitly depend on time). If the concentration in the central compartment is maintained at a constant level, the model assumes that at equilibrium the concentration in the effect-site equals the concentration in the central compartment. If the blood concentration is measured, it is assumed that the effect-site is in equilibrium with the blood concentrations at steady-state. If the unbound plasma concentrations (likely to be different to the blood concentration) are measured, it is assumed the effect-site is in equilibrium with the unbound plasma concentrations at steady-state.

An important property of this virtual compartment is that it is has negligible volume and contains only a negligible amount of drug. The delay is mathematically described by a single parameter, k_{e0}, the effect-site equilibration rate constant, which is a first order process. When k_{e0} is large, the rate of equilibration is rapid and the effect-site concentrations will rapidly approach the central compartment concentrations. Conversely, when k_{e0} is small, the rate of equilibration is slow and the effect-site concentrations will only slowly approach the central compartment concentrations. This can be expressed as an equilibration half-life, where $t_{1/2}k_{e0} = \dfrac{Log_e(2)}{k_{e0}} = \dfrac{0.693}{k_{e0}}$, so that a rapid rate of equilibration (a large k_{e0}) gives a short equilibration half-life and vice versa.

The concept has been depicted differently by various authors. Sometimes the rate constant k_{e0} is directed out of the effect compartment, sometimes k_{e0} is directed back to the central compartment, sometimes a rate constant k_{1e}, which is negligibly small, is used to describe the rate at which drug moves from the central compartment to the effect-site compartment. Independent of the graphical representation of the effect compartment, the key principles are the same: (1) the effect-site is a hypothetical compartment where there is no delay between concentration and effect; (2) the time course of the concentration in the central compartment is not effected by the addition of the effect-site to the pharmacokinetic model; and (3) at equilibrium the concentration in the effect-site is equal to the concentration in the central compartment.

Pharmacodynamic Models

Traditionally, pharmacodynamics describes the relationship between the drug dose and the drug effect. Thus the traditional view includes factors that influence both the dose versus concentration relationship and the concentration versus effect relationship. However, in this chapter, pharmacodynamics focuses on the relationship between the effect-site concentration and drug effect.

It is often observed that very low concentrations of drugs have almost no measurable effect. When the concentration is increased further, the effect also increases further until a maximal effect is reached. Even an excessive increase of the concentration does not result in more effect. This relationship is mathematically shown by a nonlinear function, such as:

$$E = E_0 + (E_{max} - E_0) \cdot \left(\frac{C^\gamma}{C_{50}^\gamma + C^\gamma} \right) \qquad (11)$$

where E denotes effect, E_{max} the maximal effect, E_0 the baseline effect, C the drug concentration, and C_{50} the concentration needed for 50% of maximal effect. The parameter γ affects the gradient and shape of the curve. This hyperbolic or sigmoid (depending on γ) curve suggests a receptor-mediated effect. It is a saturable effect, similar to the oxygen binding to hemoglobin that was described by Hill.[10]

The measured drug effect must be quantifiable to be described with a pharmacodynamic model. It is important to specify the drug effect exactly. For example, we can use depression of the twitch height to measure the drug effect of muscle relaxants; we can use changes in blood pressure as a measure of side effect; sometimes we have to use a surrogate measure of drug effect, because the clinical effect is difficult to measure directly (e.g., the electroencephalographic effects of opioids and hypnotics). If a drug effect is assessed as a yes/no response, a model that describes the probability of a positive response can be used. The minimum alveolar concentration (MAC) concept relates the alveolar concentration to the probability that patients move after skin incision. The MAC value is the concentration (C_{50}) that will result in a positive response in 50% of patients. With this well-established concept, volatile agents can be compared with respect to response to intubation ($MAC_{intubation}$), skin incision ($MAC_{skin\ incision}$), and waking up (MAC_{awake}). The mathematic formula for the probability, P, looks similar to the above E_{max} model:

$$P = \frac{C^\gamma}{C_{50}^\gamma + C^\gamma} = \frac{C^\gamma}{MAC^\gamma + C^\gamma} \qquad (12)$$

Some drugs exhibit a linear concentration effect relationship. This can happen because the drug effect is not saturable or because the high dose range could not be investigated due to unacceptable side effects. In this event, a linear model, such as $E = E_0 + \gamma \cdot C$, will describe the pharmacodynamics more appropriately. Log-linear models ($E = E_0 + S \cdot Log(C)$) have also been used to describe the concentration effect relationship, but this type of model is not popular because of several shortcomings.[11]

Pharmacodynamic parameters

Efficacy

The efficacy is the maximal effect, which can be achieved with a drug. To assess a drug's efficacy the concentration must be increased until no further increase in the effect is observed, i.e., E_{max} is achieved. For instance, the efficacy of paracetamol in treating a severe pain (e.g., from a major surgical incision) is less than that of morphine. Even at toxic

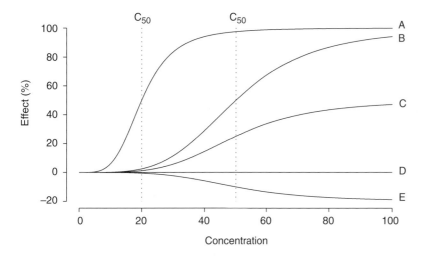

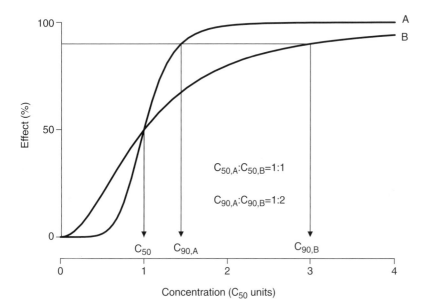

Figure 1–6. Pharmacodynamics: the concentration response relationship. The curves are all calculated with Equation 1.11. Five drugs (A, B, C, D, E), which differ in maximum effect and potency, are shown (*top*). All drugs have the same gradient parameter, $\gamma = 4$. A linear concentration scale (not logarithmic) is shown. Drugs A and B are full agonists. Drug C is a partial agonist. Drug D has no effect, and might be a competitive antagonist. Drug E is an inverse agonist. The C_{50} for drug A is 20 units. The C_{50} for drugs B, C, and E is 50 units. Drugs B and A have the same efficacy, but drug A is more potent than drug B. A relative potency of two drugs is not constant at different levels of effect if the gradient of the pharmacodynamics is different (*bottom*). Drugs A and B have the same potency, i.e., the same C_{50}. However, in this example, if an effect of 90% of the maximal effect is desired, the concentration of drug B will be twice that of drug A.

doses of paracetamol, the analgesia would be inadequate. Based on their efficacy, drugs can be described as full agonists, partial agonists, antagonists, or inverse agonists (Fig. 1–6, *top*). Classically, drugs are assigned to one of these categories. Opiates studies have shown that whether a drug behaves as full or a partial agonist can depend on the intensity of the stimulus. In rodents, Dirig and Yaksh[12] have shown that at low-intensity stimuli morphine and sufentanil are full agonists, whereas at a high-intensity stimuli sufentanil still acts as a full agonist, but morphine acts like a partial agonist.

Potency

The potency is determined by the position of concentration effect curve relative to the concentration-axis (see Fig. 1–6). Potency is often reported in terms of mass of drug (mg or μg), although it is probably better to compare the concentrations in terms of number of drug molecules present at the site of effect (molar potency). Based on an E_{max} model, the C_{50} can be considered a measure of the potency relative to another drug, one with a higher C_{50} has a lower potency and vice versa. A similarly established model-parameter is not available when the concentration is linearly related to the effect.

Notably, with the classical E_{max} model, the relative potencies of two drugs for different levels of effect are not the same when the γ, efficacy, or both, of the two drugs are different (see Fig. 1–6, *bottom*). For some drugs, potency is still reported based on intravenous bolus doses. This has many potential problems, because the dose-effect relationship is heavily effected by the pharmacokinetics of the drugs being compared. Separate description of the pharmacokinetic and the pharmacodynamic properties is preferred.

If the potency is reported as a concentration-based parameter (rather than a dose-based parameter), it can be used together with the pharmacokinetic parameters for simulation of the dose-effect relationship. Potency is clinically irrelevant if the total amount of drug can be administered conveniently. From the perspective of a standard PK (effect-site) model and standard PD (E_{max}) model, changing the potency of a drug has no effect on the rate of onset or offset of drug effect, provided the dose is scaled accordingly.

Gradient γ

If the gradient of the concentration versus effect curve is very steep, a small change of the concentration causes a major change in the effect.

Tolerance

A graph of the observed drug effect versus measured plasma concentration during an intravenous infusion often shows a counterclockwise hysteresis loop, which indicates a time delay between the time course of the concentration and the effect. However, it is possible that the concentration-effect plot shows a *clockwise* loop when the effect is measured at increasing and decreasing concentration steps over a significant period of time. This indicates that the drug becomes less effective with time, i.e., tolerance is developing. The time required to develop tolerance depends on the drug. For most opioids used in anesthesia acute tolerance has been described either in animals or human.[13–17] Investigation of tolerance must carefully differentiate between real tolerance effects and time effects. This is achieved by the investigation of a placebo group, where drug independent time effects can be observed. Because tolerance development and effect-site equilibration occurs simultaneously, the pharmacokinetic model must account for both factors.[18] Thus tolerance can be modeled with an effect compartment, which models the agonist effects of the drug, and a tolerance compartment, which models the effects of a *virtual* antagonistic metabolite. Similar to the k_{e0} for the effect compartment, the temporal aspect of this antagonistic action is characterized by an equilibration rate constant.

Indirect Models

Although the hypothetical effect compartment model is often used to account for the time lag between concentration and effect, computer simulations have shown that in some cases the effect compartment model lacks parsimony, biologic plausibility, and extrapolation capability.[19] Many drug responses may be considered indirect in nature, because the drug acts to stimulate or inhibit the production or loss of endogenous substances that mediate the drug effect. In these cases, indirect response models may be more appropriate. This type of model was first applied to account for the anticoagulant effects of warfarin.[20,21] Renewed interest in the indirect nature of this relationship has been stimulated by Jusko and colleagues' presentation of four basic models of indirect pharmacodynamic responses.[19,22–25] This general scheme is shown in Figure 1–7. Indirect response models are popular because they provide a reasonable description of the mechanism of action for many drugs.

Predictors of Onset

The time to the peak effect-site concentration (t_{peak}) is a dose independent pharmacokinetic parameter (Fig. 1–8). It is, however, dependent on both the plasma pharmacokinetic parameters and the rate of equilibration between the plasma and the effect site. Thus t_{peak} is an important descriptor of onset of drug effect, which is particularly useful when comparing drugs of the same group. We note, however, that t_{peak} only coincides with the time of peak effect when a submaximal dose is given. With "supramaximal" doses, the maximum effect will occur prior to t_{peak}. However, even if a drug is administered by infusion, and supramaximal doses have been administered, it is still possible to determine t_{peak} by simulations based on the PK/PD model.[26–28]

Figure 1–7. Indirect response models. The concentration in the site of drug effect either stimulates or inhibits the rate of production (k_{in}^0, a zero order rate constant) or rate of elimination (k_{out}) of the response (R) variable. For example, consider the effect of warfarin on the prothrombin time (R). A step increase in the effect-site concentration of warfarin would cause a step decrease in the synthesis rate (k_{in}^0) of prothrombin (the relationship may be nonlinear). However, there will still be a delay in the effect. This response variable has its own kinetic model, and a step decrease in k_{in}^0 is analogous to a step decrease in an infusion rate for a one-compartment model; time is required before a new steady-state level of R is achieved.

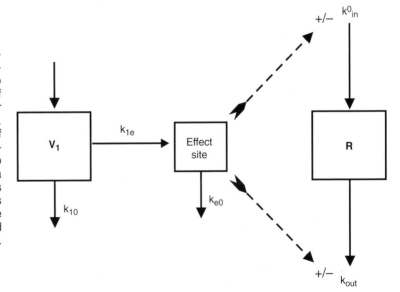

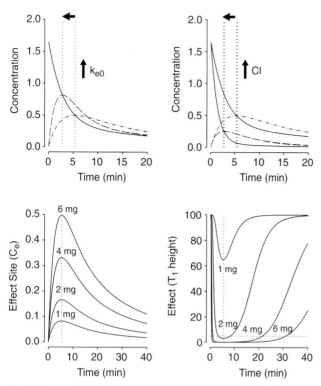

Figure 1–8. Onset of drug effect after intravenous bolus dose. A pharmacokinetic and pharmacodynamic model for vecuronium is used to illustrate the principles. An increase in k_{e0} (shorter $t_{1/2}\ k_{e0}$) results in a more rapid equilibration between the central compartment and the effect site (*top left*). This results in an earlier t_{peak}, the time of peak effect-site concentration (*arrow*). A more rapid decrease in concentrations in the central compartment (e.g., increase in clearance) also results in an earlier t_{peak} (*top right*, the k_{e0} is not changed in this simulation). Increasing the dose increases the effect-site C_{peak}, but does not change the effect-site t_{peak} (*bottom left*). Increasing the dose does not change the time of the maximum effect for submaximal doses (*bottom right*). However, the time to 95% depression of twitch height is shorter, and the duration of effect is longer, for doses greater than the D_{95} (the dose causing 95% suppression of the twitch height).

Neither the central volume (V_1) nor volume of distribution at steady-state (V_{dss}) is a useful parameter for calculating the bolus dose required to achieve a desired effect. The use of V_1 or V_{dss} result in calculated loading doses that are either too small or too large, respectively. In contrast, the t_{peak} concept has been used to calculate optimal initial bolus doses.[29] The volume of distribution at the time of the peak effect-site concentration (Vd_{pe}) following an intravenous bolus dose is calculated as:

$$Vd_{pe} = \frac{V_1}{C_{peak}/C_0}, \tag{13}$$

where V_1 is the central volume of distribution, C_0 is the concentration at the $t = 0$ (as predicted by the pharmacokinetic model), and C_{peak} is the predicted effect-site concentration at the time of the peak effect-site concentration. Using Vd_{pe} we can calculate the loading dose to achieve the effect-site concentration (C_{peak}) associated with a desired effect at t_{peak} as:

$$\text{Loading dose} = C_{peak} \cdot Vd_{pe} \tag{14}$$

In this way, drugs can be compared by calculating the time to a specified effect using the full PK/PD model.

Predictors of Offset

Using computer simulations, Youngs and Shafer[30] found that no single parameter of the pharmacokinetic model predicted fast recovery. They showed that the implications of a change in a single parameter on the time course of onset and offset of drug effect could only be predicted if all the other parameters of the pharmacokinetic model remain unchanged. For example, if all the other parameters of the model were fixed a small V_1, or big Cl_1, or both, predicted rapid recovery. However, a large Cl_1 can be completely offset by other parameters of the pharmacokinetic model. Because no two drugs differ only by one parameter, comparison is not possible on a parameter by parameter basis. Nevertheless, the most commonly quoted and traditional descriptor of drug offset is the drug's "terminal" half-life,[31] which using the above notation for a three-compartment model can be calculated as $\log_e(2)/\lambda_3$. Unfortunately, if we know only one (or even all three) of the half-times, we cannot calculate the rate of decline of the drug concentrations; a computer and all six parameters are necessary to complete this calculation. However, some insight into the relative contribution of each half-time can be obtained relatively easily by calculating A_1/λ_1, A_2/λ_2, and A_3/λ_3 as a percentage of the total area under the curve $(A_1/\lambda_1 + A_2/\lambda_2 + A_3/\lambda_3)$.[2]

Shafer and Varvel[32] introduced the concept of recovery curves based on simulations for the purpose of rational opioid selection. Hughes and colleagues[33] subsequently coined the expression "context sensitive half-time." This concept provides a graphical insight into the pharmacokinetic behavior of many drugs. For many drugs the time required for the concentration to decrease by 50% increases with the duration of the infusion (Fig. 1–9). Although providing an insight into the pharmacokinetics of a drug in a way that simply is not possible by inspection of the model parameters, the context sensitive half-time may not be clinically relevant, because the percentage decrease in concentration required for recovery from drug effect is not necessarily 50%. Bailey generalized this concept to "relative decrement times," which incorporates the pharmacodynamic model into the simulations.[34,35]

Bailey extended these concepts further by evaluating the duration of drug effect when drug effect is assessed in a binary, response/no response fashion.[34,36] The mean effect time (MET) is the area under the probability of drug effect curve as a function of time after drug administration is discontinued, assuming that the probability of responsiveness to surgical stimulation was reduced to 10% (C_{90}) during the infusion. As noted by Bailey, the pharmacodynamic analysis of binary data is mostly assessed by logistic regression of data pooled from multiple patients. With this methodology, the gradient of the pharmacodynamic model is often relatively low, reflecting high interindividual variability. If the slope of the individual concentration-response relationship is steep, and if the anesthesiologist has titrated

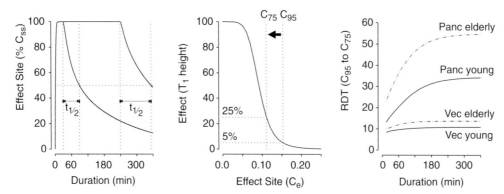

Figure 1–9. Offset of drug effect. The rate of decline of concentrations for a one-compartment model is always the same whatever the dosing history or duration of infusion. This is generally not true for drugs described by multicompartment pharmacokinetic models. Steady-state effect site concentrations (C_{ss}) are maintained for pancuronium (panc) in the elderly for 30 minutes and 240 minutes (*left*). The time taken for the concentration to decrease by half depends on the duration of the infusion. In the context of a 30-minute target-controlled infusion of pancuronium, the effect-site concentration takes about 70 minutes to decrease by half. In the context of a 240-minute target-controlled infusion of pancuronium, the effect-site concentration takes about 114 minutes to decrease by half. A series of such simulations can be performed to construct a curve showing the time taken for the concentration to decrease by half for a large range of infusion rates. The simulations can be performed for both the central compartment concentrations and the effect-site concentrations. However, the time taken for the concentrations to decrease by half (from whatever starting value) may have absolutely no clinical relevance. For example, if the relaxant concentration is extremely high, when the concentrations decrease by half the patient may still have no recovery of neuromuscular block. The concentration response curve for vecuronium (vec) in the young is shown (*middle*). If we infuse vecuronium to maintain the single twitch at 5% of control (TOFC = 1) and we give anticholinesterase when single twitch is 25% of control (TOFC = 4), then we can use these two endpoints to calculate the clinically relevant percentage decrement for vecuronium (~27%). Relevant decrement time curves for pancuronium and vecuronium in the young and elderly are shown (*right*).

the dose to effect, the time to offset of drug effect may be much shorter than that predicted by the MET.

Drug Accumulation

When a drug is administered at regular intervals, there is always some drug remaining in the body before the next dose is given. Theoretically, some drug remains in the body forever, because the amount of drug in the body after a single intravenous bolus dose is given by $(Dose/V_1) \times e^{-(Cl/V_1) \cdot l}$ (for a one-compartment model), which only equals zero at infinite time. When a fixed dose of a drug is given at frequent intervals, the concentration will gradually increase toward a steady-state concentration, and the total amount of drug in the body will accumulate. This is true for all drugs and, with regard to this behavior, claims that some drugs are "non-cumulative" are misleading.

The "cumulation ratio" (CR) is defined as the ratio of the peak amount of drug in the body at the "cumulation plateau" (peak at steady-state) to the peak amount of drug in the body after a single dose.[37] The following equation for CR is based on intravenous bolus dosing, and only applies to a one-compartment model:

$$CR = \frac{1}{1 - 2^{-(\tau/t_{1/2})}} \qquad (15)$$

Thus the CR depends entirely on the ratio of dosing interval (τ) to half-life ($t_{1/2}$). When the dosing interval equals the half-life, CR equals 2, i.e., the peak levels at steady-state or plateau are twice those after a single intravenous dose. When the dosing interval is less than the $t_{1/2}$, CR is greater than 2, and when the dosing interval is more than the $t_{1/2}$, CR approaches unity. This ratio is sometimes referred to as the accumulation factor and accumulation index.

Once neuromuscular blockade recovers spontaneously, small doses of relaxant are usually administered to keep relaxation at a certain level of effect. Generally, the duration of effect of the first additional dose is shorter than that of identical doses administered later. This phenomenon has been called "cumulation" in the neuromuscular literature.[38] This is a different phenomenon to the accumulation described above. Indeed, this longer duration of effect after later doses does not occur with a one-compartment model. Rather, it is a property of drugs that are described by multicompartment pharmacokinetic models, and occurs for the same reasons that the "context-sensitive half-time" changes with duration of infusion.

Dose Equivalence: Principles of Calculation

Switching from one drug to another of the same class can be desirable for different reasons. In pain therapy, changing the route of administration between the intravenous, oral, transcutaneous, epidural, and intrathecal routes is not uncommon. Sometimes, the change of route also necessitates changing the drug. Possibly a department decides that a new drug has a better risk/benefit ratio, or is just significantly cheaper with no obvious change in risk/benefit ratio, and changes to the new drug. In a whole variety of situations, it becomes necessary to calculate equipotent doses of a new drug, which unfortunately is more difficult than believed by most clinicians. Most often recommendations regarding equivalent dosing are empirical,[39,40] mostly because of lack of detailed PK/PD models. Often a "potency ratio" ratio (between different routes or between different drugs) or observed total drug consumption are used to develop the new dosing regimen. Although both factors contain some information regarding appropriate dosing neither alone is sufficient. The "one ampoule = equipotent dose" philosophy has caused more than one clinician to claim that the drug simply is ineffective. Obviously, the amount of drug in one ampoule is not necessarily equipotent to others in its class. However, even if one ampoule is equipotent for an intravenous bolus dose, it might not be equipotent when given by infusion. The time course of effect of two different drugs may be entirely different, even if an "equipotent bolus dose" or "equipotent infusion rate" is used.

To understand the principles involved, we will use PK/PD modeling to calculate the equipotent doses of two opioids with which anesthesiologists are familiar: fentanyl and alfentanil. For both of these drugs, an effect-site model has been developed using the electroencephalogram (EEG) as a sensitive and continuous measure of drug effect.[41] This research also provides us with the C_{50} value for each drug (the steady-state concentration required to produce 50% depression in the spectral edge of the processed EEG). We assume that this also provides us with a guide to the relative C_{50} for other clinically relevant measures of drug effect, such as the concentration associated with spontaneous respiration during anesthesia and the concentration required to obtund the response to intubation.[42] The C_{50} is 6.9 ng/mL for fentanyl and 520 ng/mL for alfentanil, which is approximately 75 times greater. If we want to give an intravenous bolus dose of alfentanil that is similar to 50 µg fentanyl, does this mean that we should give 75 times (3.75 mg) as much? Those familiar with both drugs will know from their clinical experience that a single bolus of 50 µg of fentanyl is an appropriate dose, which generally permits spontaneous breathing during general anesthesia. In contrast, 3.75 mg alfentanil will render the patient apneic and, in conjunction with a modest dose of hypnotic, is probably enough to render most patients unresponsive to intubation. These two doses are certainly not equipotent!

Based on our understanding of the effect-site concept, we can use Equation 1.14 to determine the intravenous bolus dose required to give a concentration equal to the C_{50} for both drugs at the time of peak effect-site concentration (t_{peak}). First we must calculate the Vd_{pe}. The ratio of the peak effect-site concentration to the initial concentration in the central compartment at $t = 0$ (C_{peak}/C_0) is 0.16 and 0.33 for fentanyl and alfentanil, respectively. Dividing the central volume of distribution by this ratio gives Vd_{pe} for each drug: fentanyl, 12.7/0.16 = 76.9 L; alfentanil, 2.18/0.33 = 6.6 L. The dose to

achieve the respective C_{50} at t_{peak} is calculated as $C_{50} \times Vd_{pe}$, which gives a dose of 530 µg for fentanyl and 3.43 mg for alfentanil. Thus based on the effect-site model and the steady-state C_{50}, we have calculated that only 6.5 times as much alfentanil as fentanyl (not 75 times!) is required for an equipotent intravenous bolus dose at the time of the peak effect-site concentration. Returning to the original example (50 µg fentanyl), we conclude that this is equipotent to an intravenous bolus dose of approximately 325 µg (6.5 × 50 µg) alfentanil at t_{peak}. Thus from the perspective of a single intravenous bolus dose, there is almost "twice as much opioid" in a 1,000 µg ampoule of alfentanil compared with a 100 µg ampoule of fentanyl. However, the time course of effect is certainly different. The t_{peak} for alfentanil is much earlier at approximately 1.5 minutes compared with 3.7 minutes for fentanyl, necessitating a change in the timing of events if one wishes to compare the clinical effectiveness of these two doses at their peak. Although these two doses are equipotent at their peak effect, they are certainly not equipotent for the entire duration of a short anesthetic.

Is this equipotent bolus dose ratio (~6.5:1) also applicable for intravenous infusions or should the steady-state C_{50} ratio of 75:1 be used? Based on our understanding of infusion pharmacokinetics, we can use Equation 1.8 to determine the infusion rate that will result in a concentration equal to the C_{50} for both drugs at steady-state. First we must know the clearance for each drug, which is 0.71 L/min and 0.19 L/min for fentanyl and alfentanil, respectively. Then we calculate the dose to achieve the respective C_{50} at steady-state as $C_{50} \times Cl$, which gives an infusion rate of approximately 300 µg/h for fentanyl and approximately 6 mg/h alfentanil. Thus based on the steady-state C_{50} and clearance, approximately 20 times more alfentanil than fentanyl (not 75 times!) is required for an equipotent intravenous infusion at steady-state conditions. However, these infusion rates may not be particularly useful in clinical practice, because it takes about 24 hours for fentanyl, and about 5 hours for alfentanil, to attain 90% of their steady-state concentrations (Fig. 1–10, *left*).

To maintain equi-effective steady-state concentrations of fentanyl and alfentanil, the relative infusion rates required vary over time, gradually approaching the steady-state ratio of ~20:1 the longer the targeted concentrations are maintained (see Fig. 1–10, *right*). If we use a alfentanil:fentanyl infusion rate ratio of 10:1 to 20:1, based on 100 µg/h for fentanyl, we obtain an infusion rate of 1 to 2 mg/h for alfentanil, which agrees with clinical experience.

In this example, for which we have well-defined PK/PD models, we find that there is no simple "equipotent ratio" on which we can base "equipotent dosing" when switching between fentanyl and alfentanil. We have assumed that the relative potency based on the steady-state EEG concentration-response relationship is true for other clinical measures of drug effect. We have also assumed that the relative gradients for other measures of effect are similar for the two drugs. We have found that although the steady-state potency differs by a ratio of 75:1, the intravenous bolus dose potency at t_{peak} differs by 6.5:1, and the infusion rate required to maintain equipotent concentrations varies over time between approximately 10:1 and 20:1. We can also compare the cumulative dose, which after 6 hours of equipo-

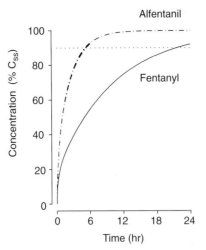

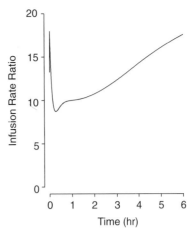

Figure 1–10. Equipotent infusion rates. Simulation showing approach to steady-state concentration (C_{ss}) for constant rate infusions of fentanyl and alfentanil (*left*). A constant rate infusion is calculated that will achieve an equipotent effect at steady state, which is only achieved after many hours (90% of C_{ss} shown by dotted line). The relative magnitude of effect will change over time, because the drugs have different PK and approach steady state at different rates. A target controlled infusion uses the three-compartment model parameters for each drug to calculate the infusion rates to rapidly attain and maintain the desired equipotent concentration. The relative rates (alfentanil rate/fentanyl rate) required for an equipotent effect change significantly over time (*right*).

tent infusion rates varies by a factor of 12 : 1. Thus we cannot simply compare two C_{50} and use the ratio to guide the doses required for one drug based on the doses for the other drug.

If the PK/PD of two drugs are very different, and if the administration mode (oral vs. intravenous) is also different, recommended equipotent doses are likely to be inaccurate. For example, switching from morphine to methadone is clinically difficult[45–47] and equi-analgesic dose ratios are difficult to define.[40] As discussed earlier, from a PK/PD point of view it is questionable whether the notion of a single "equi-analgesic" dose ratio is appropriate. With simulation based on good PK/PD models, an "equi-effective dosing strategy" can be determined, which will provide optimal initial dosing guidelines. However, for many drugs, these well-defined PK/PD models are simply not available. Thus sometimes our best effort is to make decisions based on clinical experience using "equipotent ratios," which are often based on hourly or daily cumulative dose requirements, and then carefully titrate to the desired drug effect.

Interpatient Variability

Accurate dosing is challenging because there is considerable interpatient variability in both pharmacokinetics and pharmacodynamics. It is not uncommon to find at least a two-fold variation on the concentrations resulting from the same dosing scheme in different individuals (this is as true for volatile agents as it is for intravenously administered drugs). There is at least a fivefold range in the concentration required to cause the same effect in different individuals;

this range can be significantly greater if tolerance has developed in some individuals. In addition, this PK/PD variability is usually reported in carefully controlled experimental studies in volunteers, who are generally very healthy. It is likely that the variability encountered in routine clinical practice is significantly greater.

Interestingly, in clinical practice it is sometimes possible to completely ignore this interindividual variability. For some drugs, we routinely "dose high," particularly when there the risk for adverse hemodynamic consequences is minimal. For example, we routinely give 2 to 3 times the ED_{95} for muscle relaxants, and if we wait a sufficient time, all patients are paralyzed. Thus the one dose works for everyone. However, if we monitor the level of block, the interpatient variability is easily observed in the duration of effect and in the infusion rate required to maintain the desired effect.

If there are significant adverse hemodynamic consequences from a relative overdose, we usually try harder to titrate to the desired endpoint. Our ability to titrate during the onset of drug effect is more or less effective depending on the delay between administering the drug and observing the effect of the drug (acting at its "effect-site"). If the delay is relatively short, by monitoring the effect of the drug we can attempt to give a dose titrated to the patient's individual requirements. If the delay is relatively long, or if we only have one opportunity to give the correct dose (e.g., a "single shot spinal"), based on our experience, we guess the right dose, give it, and treat the adverse effects accordingly.

If we are trying to titrate the dose to a clinical endpoint (e.g., loss of lash reflex), the rate of administration is extremely important. If the rate of administration is too rapid, by the time we observe the clinical endpoint, we will already have given an excessive dose and the effect will be much greater than desired. If the rate is too slow, a large total dose will still be given, but there will be minimal "overshoot" and the time to achieve the desired endpoint will be unnecessarily prolonged. Recent work by Gentry and colleagues[48] explores these concepts based on a PK/PD model for thiopentone. Their simulations suggest that the optimum rate for induction with thiopentone is approximately 100 mg/min.

In anesthesia, dosing proportional to body weight is customary, although in many instances it is not based on good PK/PD evidence. Conversely, when weight is not a significant covariate on clearance, it is possible that scaling the clearance does not deteriorate the PK/PD description[50] and therefore scaling the infusion rate by weight at least does not harm the patient. Often clearance is not simply scaled by weight, but also changes according to other patient covariates.[27,51–53] Despite these more complex models, most recommendations for bolus doses and infusion rates are still given as amount per kilogram (e.g., mg/kg or µg/kg) and amount per kilogram per time (e.g., mg/kg/h or µg/kg/min), respectively. These weight-proportional dosing schemes assume that all of the volumes and clearances of the compartment model are scaled linearly by weight, i.e., tripling the weight will triple the volume of distribution and triple the clearance. Although it seems reasonable to assume that a 40 kg adult needs a smaller drug dose than a 120 kg adult, and that the liver, kidneys, blood volume, muscle, and fat mass are different, it is less certain that all these factors are scaled linearly by weight. This seems even less likely when we compare a 10 kg infant with a 40 kg adult. However, weight-proportional dosing is an easy way to remember approximate drug doses, one which seems to be firmly entrenched in the practice of anesthesia. In other areas, e.g., oncology, dosing is typically based on body surface area. Although this is more complicated, the same shortcomings apply.[50] Dose recommendations can also be derived empirically by giving different doses to patients and measuring the effect.[55]

One of the goals of PK/PD analyses is to try to explain as much of the interindividual variability in the dose-response relationship as possible. However, even with a sophisticated analysis, only the information that is in the study data can enter the PK/PD model.[56] If only young healthy volunteers aged between 20 and 25 years are investigated in a study, detection of a significant influence of age on the dose-response relationship cannot be expected and extrapolation to 80-year-old patients would be unwise! Even when a large range of patients is studied, less than half of the interindividual variability can be explained by careful analysis of covariates such as age, weight, height, sex, body surface, and lean body mass.[27,52,53,57] With these models, dosing guidelines can be derived rationally[32,58] and comparison between drugs and extrapolation to other drugs is possible.[59]

Table 1–1 shows the PK/PD parameters for remifentanil.[27] Based on this complex mathematic model, the dose or infusion rate based on individual covariates can be calculated. The impact of changing patient age and lean body mass on the equi-effective intravenous bolus dose, the time of the peak effect-site concentration after a bolus, and the equi-effective infusion rates are not obvious without the aid of computer simulations.[58]

Principle of Target Controlled Infusion

In 1983, Schüttler and colleagues[60] used a computerized infusion system to administer constant concentrations of etomidate and alfentanil. Since that time other systems have been developed at other centers and their performances have been evaluated for a variety of drugs, including alfentanil,[61] fentanyl[62] and propofol.[63] The desired concentration is referred to as the *target concentration* (which can refer to either the plasma or the effect-site), and the pumps have been more recently called target controlled infusion (TCI) systems. In addition to the commercially available system for propofol (Diprifusor; AstraZeneca, Waltham, Mass), different computer programs for setting up TCI systems for research purposes are freely available from the respective authors. A syringe pump, a computer with a serial communication port, and the computer program to controls the pump are all that is required. Many of the noncommercial TCI systems have built in drug libraries, which allow the user to select from a variety of different drugs and different pharmacokinetic models.

TABLE 1–1.

Remifentanil Pharmacokinetic and Pharmacodynamic Parameters

Parameter	Equation
V_1 (L)	$5.1 - 0.0201 \times (\text{Age} - 40) + 0.072 \times (\text{Lean body mass} - 55)$
V_2 (L)	$9.82 - 0.0811 \times (\text{Age} - 40) + 0.108 \times (\text{Lean body mass} - 55)$
V_3 (L)	5.42
Cl_1 (L/min)	$2.6 - 0.0162 \times (\text{Age} - 40) + 0.0191 \times (\text{Lean body mass} - 55)$
Cl_2 (L/min)	$2.05 - 0.0301 \times (\text{Age} - 40)$
Cl_3 (L/min)	$0.076 - 0.00113 \times (\text{Age} - 40)$
k_{e0} (min^{-1})	$0.595 - 0.007 \times (\text{Age} - 40)$
E_0 (Hz)	20.0
E_{max} (Hz)	5.5
C_{50} (ng/mL)	$13.1 - 0.148 \times (\text{Age} - 40)$
γ	2.44

To attain and maintain a target concentration, a high initial infusion rate is required, which then decreases continually over time. This has nothing to do with decreasing anesthetic requirements over time. Rather, this decrease in infusion rate is necessary to maintain a constant concentration, and is a feature of multicompartment pharmacokinetic models. The reason for this can be understood by once again referring to the three-bucket hydraulic model. In the beginning, the tap filling the central bucket must be opened widely to rapidly fill the central bucket to the desired water level. To keep the water at this desired level, the tap must be adjusted so that the rate in equals the rate out, which initially is by three routes—by elimination from the hole in the central bucket, and by distribution to the other two buckets). As the two peripheral buckets fill (one faster than the other), the rate of loss by distribution to the other buckets gradually reduces to zero, until the rate in equals the rate of loss from the hole in the central bucket alone (when the water level in all three buckets is at the same level). Compared with the "10, 8, 6" scheme proposed by Roberts and co-workers,[64] which decreases the infusion rate in steps at 10-minute intervals during the first 30 minutes (as the second bucket fills), TCI systems change the infusion rate much more frequently, e.g., every 10 seconds.

A variety of different algorithms has been used in these programs to calculate the required infusion rate.[65–67] However, most modern systems use a simple analytic solution for this calculation.[68] Calculation of the infusion rate for effect-site control is more complex, but solutions have been presented and are already implemented in research systems.[28,69] Neither the computer nor the actual TCI software is critical, but rather the selection of the pharmacokinetic model with the best performance. Ideally, the pharmacokinetic model should explain some of the interindividual variability by individualizing the pharmacokinetic parameters according to the patient's covariates. Actually this is one of the main advantages of TCI systems: that these systems have no difficulty handling any complexity of the pharmacokinetic model, such as the model shown in Table 1–1. However, complexity is no guarantee of excellence, and the *prospective* evaluation of any pharmacokinetic model is absolutely necessary.[69,71]

There will always be some difference between the concentrations predicted by the TCI system and the real (measured) drug concentrations, because of the unexplained pharmacokinetic variability between patients. However, even if we had an on-line measure of the arterial concentration, we would not be that much wiser. We never know in advance what concentration any given patient will require because of the large pharmacodynamic variability. Thus the main purpose of the TCI system is to attain and maintain a steady-state concentration, which can be increased or decreased depending on the desired effect in an individual patient. Provided the model performs with minimal bias, good precision, does not diverge from the target, and does not wobble about the target,[72] the TCI system facilitates the anesthesiologists ability to titrate to and maintain the desired level of effect. Targeting the effect-site is the logical extension of current TCI technology.[73]

A thorough understanding of the PK/PD principles discussed in this chapter will facilitate both the rational selection of individual drugs from a group of drugs with similar effects, but different pharmacokinetic properties, and the development of rational dosing strategies.

References

1. Mapleson WW: Pharmacokinetics of inhaled anaesthetics. In Prys-Roberts C, Hug CC Jr, (eds): Pharmacokinetics of Anaesthesia. Malden, Mass, Blackwell Scientific, 1984.
2. Shafer SL, Stanski DR: Improving the clinical utility of anesthetic drug pharmacokinetics. Anesthesiology 76:327–330, 1992.
3. Yasuda N, Lockhart SH, Eger EI, et al: Comparison of kinetics of sevoflurane and isoflurane in humans. Anesth Analg 72:316–324, 1991.
4. Szenohradszky J, Caldwell JE, Wright PM, et al: Influence of renal failure on the pharmacokinetics and neuromuscular effects of a single dose of rapacuronium bromide. Anesthesiology 90:24–35, 1999.
5. Henthorn TK, Avram MJ, Krejcie TC, et al: Minimal compartmental model of circulatory mixing of indocyanine green. Am J Physiol 262:903–910, 1992.
6. Upton RN, Ludbrook GL: A physiological model of the induction of anaesthesia with propofol in sheep. 1. Structure and estimation of parameters. Br J Anaesth 79:497–504, 1997.
7. Mandema JW, Kaiko RF, Oshlack B, et al: Characterization and validation of a pharmacokinetic model for controlled-release oxycodone. Br J Clin Pharmacol 42:747–756, 1996.
8. Hull CJ, Van Beem HB, McLeod K, et al: A pharmacodynamic model for pancuronium. Br J Anaesth 50:1113–1123, 1978.
9. Sheiner LB, Stanski DR, Vozeh S, et al: Simultaneous modeling of pharmacokinetics and pharmacodynamics: application to d-tubocurarine. Clin Pharmacol Ther 25:358–371, 1979.
10. Hill AV: The possible effects of the aggregation of the molecules of haemoglobin on its dissociation curves. J Physiol (Lond) Proc Physiol Soc 40:iv–vii, 1910.
11. Holford NH, Sheiner LB: Understanding the dose-effect relationship: clinical application of pharmacokinetic-pharmacodynamic models. Clin Pharmacokinet 6:429–453, 1981.
12. Dirig DM, Yaksh TL: Differential right shifts in the dose-response curve for intrathecal morphine and sufentanil as a function of stimulus intensity. Pain 62:321–328, 1995.
13. Mandema JW, Wada DR: Pharmacodynamic model for acute tolerance development to the electroencephalographic effects of alfentanil in the rat. J Pharm Exp Ther 275:1185–1194, 1995.
14. Kissin I, Brown PT, Robinson CA, Bradley ELJ: Acute tolerance to the hypnotic effect of morphine in rats. Anesth Analg 73:619–621, 1991.
15. Askitopoulou H, Whitwam JG, Al-Khudhairi D, et al: Acute tolerance to fentanyl during anesthesia in dogs. Anesthesiology 63:255–261, 1985.
16. Vinik HR, Kissin I: Rapid development of tolerance to analgesia during remifentanil infusion in humans. Anesth Analg 86:1307–1311, 1998.
17. Guignard B, Bossard AE, Coste C, et al: Acute opioid tolerance: intraoperative remifentanil increases postoperative pain and morphine requirement. Anesthesiology 93:409–417, 2000.
18. Shi J, Benowitz NL, Denaro CP, Sheiner LB: Pharmacokinetic-pharmacological modeling of caffeine: tolerance to pressor effects. Clin Pharmacol Ther 53:6–14, 1993.
19. Dayneka NL, Garg V, Jusko WJ: Comparison of four basic models of indirect pharmacodynamic responses. J Pharmacokin Biopharm 21:457–478, 1993.
20. Sheiner LB: Computer-aided long-term anticoagulation therapy. Comput Biomed Res 2:507–518, 1969.
21. Nagashima R, O'Reilly RA, Levy G: Kinetics of pharmacologic effects in man: the anticoagulant action of warfarin. Clin Pharmacol Ther 10:22–35, 1969.
22. Jusko WJ, Ko HC: Physiologic indirect response models characterize diverse types of pharmacodynamic effects. Clin Pharmacol Ther 56:406–419, 1994.
23. Verotta D, Sheiner LB: A general conceptual model for non-steady state pharmacokinetic/pharmacodynamic data. J Pharmacokin Biopharm 23:1–4, 1995.
24. Sheiner LB, Verotta D: Further notes on physiologic indirect response models. Clin Pharmacol Ther 58:238–240, 1995.

25. Jusko WJ, Ko HC, Ebling WF: Convergence of direct and indirect pharmacodynamic response models. J Pharmacokin Biopharm 23:5–8, 1995.

26. Shafer SL, Varvel JR, Gronert GA: A comparison of parametric with semiparametric analysis of the concentration versus effect relationship of metocurine in dogs and pigs. J Pharm Biopharm 17:291–304, 1989.

27. Minto CF, Schnider TW, Egan TD, et al: Influence of age and gender on the pharmacokinetics and pharmacodynamics of remifentanil. I. Model development. Anesthesiology 86:10–23, 1997.

28. Gentilini A, Frei CW, Glattfelder AH, et al: Identification and targeting policies for computer-controlled infusion pumps. Crit Rev Biomed Eng 28:179–185, 2000.

29. Wada DR, Drover DR, Lemmens HJ: Determination of the distribution volume that can be used to calculate the intravenous loading dose. Clin Pharmacokinetics 35:1–7, 1998.

30. Youngs EJ, Shafer SL: Pharmacokinetic parameters relevant to recovery from opioids. Anesthesiology 81:833–842, 1994.

31. Sear JW: Recovery from anaesthesia: which is the best kinetic descriptor of a drug's recovery profile? Anaesthesia 51:997–999, 1996.

32. Shafer SL, Varvel JR: Pharmacokinetics, pharmacodynamics, and rational opioid selection. Anesthesiology 74:53–63, 1991.

33. Hughes MA, Glass PS, Jacobs JR: Context-sensitive half-time in multicompartment pharmacokinetic models for intravenous anesthetic drugs. Anesthesiology 76:334–341, 1992.

34. Bailey JM: Technique for quantifying the duration of intravenous anesthetic effect. Anesthesiology 83:1095–1103, 1995.

35. Bailey JM: Context-sensitive half-times and other decrement times of inhaled anesthetics. Anesth Analg 85:681–686, 1997.

36. Schnider TW, Shafer SL: Evolving clinically useful predictors of recovery from intravenous anesthetics [editorial; comment]. Anesthesiology 83:902–905, 1995.

37. Hull CJ: Pharmacokinetics for Anaesthesia. Woburn, Mass, Butterworth-Heinemann, 1991.

38. Bevan DR, Bevan JC, Donati F: Muscle Relaxants in Clinical Anesthesia. St. Louis, Mosby Year-Book Medical, 1998.

39. Lawlor PG, Turner KS, Hanson J, et al: Dose ratio between morphine and methadone in patients with cancer pain: a retrospective study. Cancer 82:1167–1173, 1998.

40. Ripamonti C, Groff L, Brunelli C, et al: Switching from morphine to oral methadone in treating cancer pain: what is the equianalgesic dose ratio? J Clin Oncol 16:3216–3221, 1998.

41. Scott JC, Stanski DR: Decreased fentanyl and alfentanil dose requirements with age: A simultaneous pharmacokinetic and pharmacodynamic evaluation. J Pharmacol Exp Ther 240:159–166, 1987.

42. Egan TD, Muir KT, Stanski DR, Shafer SL: The EEG versus clinical measures of opioid potency: Defining the EEG-clinical potency fingerprint with application to remifentanil. Anesthesiology 85:A349, 1995.

43. Garzone PD, Kroboth PD: Pharmacokinetics of the newer benzodiazepines. Clin Pharmacokinet 16:337–364, 1989.

44. Walker MC, Tong X, Brown S, et al: Comparison of single- and repeated-dose pharmacokinetics of diazepam. Epilepsia 39:283–289, 1988.

45. Fainsinger R, Schoeller T, Bruera E: Methadone in the management of cancer pain: a review. Pain 52:137–147, 1993.

46. Mercadate S: Methadone in cancer pain. Eur J Pain 1:77–85, 1997.

47. Ripamonti C, Zecca E, Bruera E: An update on the clinical use of methadone for cancer pain. Pain 70:109–115, 1997.

48. Gentry WB, Krejcie TC, Henthorn TK, et al: Effect of infusion rate on thiopental dose-response relationships: Assessment of a pharmacokinetic-pharmacodynamic model. Anesthesiology 81:316–324, 1994.

49. Dundee JW, Hassard TH, McGowan WA, et al: The "induction" dose of thiopentone: A method of study and preliminary illustrative results. Anaesthesia 37:1176–1184, 1982.

50. Gepts E, Shafer SL, Camu F, et al: Linearity of pharmacokinetics and model estimation of sufentanil. Anesthesiology 83:1194–1204, 1995.

51. Maitre PO, Vozeh S, Heykants J, et al: Population pharmacokinetics of alfentanil: The average dose-plasma concentration relationship and interindividual variability in patients. Anesthesiology 66:3–12, 1987.

52. Schuttler J, Ihmsen H: Population pharmacokinetics of propofol: a multicenter study. Anesthesiology 92:727–738, 2000.

53. Schnider TW, Minto CF, Gambus PL, et al: The influence of method of administration and covariates on the pharmacokinetics of propofol in adult volunteers. Anesthesiology 88:1170–1182, 1998.

54. Ratain MJ: Body-surface area as a basis for dosing of anticancer agents: science, myth, or habit? J Clin Oncology 16:2297–2298, 1998.

55. Kopman AF: The onset/offset profiles of rapacuronium and succinylcholine are not identical. Anesthesiology 91:1554; discussion 1555–1556, 1999.

56. Wright PM: Population based pharmacokinetic analysis: Why do we need it; what is it; and what has it told us about anaesthetics? Br J Anaesth 80:488–501.

57. Schnider TW, Minto CF, Shafer SL, et al: The influence of age on propofol pharmacodynamics. Anesthesiology 90:1502–1516, 1999.

58. Minto CF, Schnider TW, Shafer SL: Pharmacokinetics and pharmacodynamics of remifentanil. II. Model application. Anesthesiology 86:24–33, 1997.

59. Lemmens HJ, Dyck JB, Shafer SL, Stanski DR: Pharmacokinetic-pharmacodynamic modeling in drug development: application to the investigational opioid trefentanil. Clin Pharmacol Ther 56:261–271, 1994.

60. Schüttler J, Schwilden H, Stoekel H: Pharmacokinetics as applied to total intravenous anaesthesia: Practical implications. Anaesthesia 38(Suppl):53–56, 1983.

61. Ausems ME, Stanski DR, Hug CC: An evaluation of the accuracy of pharmacokinetic data for the computer assisted infusion of alfentanil. Br J Anaesth 57:1217–1225, 1985.

62. Alvis JM, Reves JG, Govier AV, et al: Computer-assisted continuous infusions of fentanyl during cardiac anesthesia: comparison with a manual method. Anesthesiology 63:41–49, 1985.

63. White M, Kenny GN: Intravenous propofol anaesthesia using a computerized infusion system. Anaesthesia 45:204–209, 1990.

64. Roberts FL, Dixon J, Lewis GT, et al: Induction and maintenance of propofol anaesthesia: A manual infusion scheme. Anaesthesia 43(Suppl):14–17, 1988.

65. Shafer SL, Siegel LC, Cooke JE, Scott JC: Testing computer-controlled infusion pumps by simulation. Anesthesiology 68:261–266, 1998.

66. Jacobs JR: Algorithm for optimal linear model-based control with application to pharmacokinetic model-driven drug delivery. IEEE Trans Biomed Eng 37:107–109, 1990.

67. Jacobs JR: Analytical solution to the three-compartment pharmacokinetic model. IEEE Trans Biomed Eng 35:763–765, 1998.

68. Bailey JM, Shafer SL: A simple analytical solution to the three-compartment pharmacokinetic model suitable for computer-controlled infusion pumps. IEEE Trans Biomed Eng 38:522–525, 1991.

69. Shafer SL, Gregg KM: Algorithms to rapidly achieve and maintain stable drug concentrations at the site of drug effect with a computer-controlled infusion pump. J Pharmacokinet Biopharm 20:147–169, 1992.

70. Coetzee JF, Glen JB, Wium CA, Boshoff L: Pharmacokinetic model selection for target controlled infusions of propofol: Assessment of three parameter sets. Anesthesiology 82:1328–1345, 1995.

71. Vuyk J, Engbers FH, Burm AG, et al: Performance of computer-controlled infusion of propofol: an evaluation of five pharmacokinetic parameter sets. Anesth Analg 81:1275–1282, 1995.

72. Varvel JR, Donoho DL, Shafer SL: Measuring the predictive performance of computer-controlled infusion pumps. J Pharm Biopharm 20:63–94, 1992.

73. Wakeling HG, Zimmerman JB, Howell S, Glass PS: Targeting effect compartment or central compartment concentration of propofol: what predicts loss of consciousness? Anesthesiology 90:92–97, 1999.

2

Signal Transduction Mechanisms

Hugh C. Hemmings, Jr., MD, PhD • Jean-Antoine Girault, MD

RECEPTOR-EFFECTOR COUPLING

General Principles
  Extracellular Signals
  Receptors
  Receptor Regulation
Cell Surface Receptors: Structure and Function
  G Protein–Coupled Receptors
  Ligand-Gated Ion Channels
  Enzyme-Linked Cell Surface Receptors

Second Messengers and Protein Phosphorylation
  Cyclic Adenosine 3′:5′-Monophosphate
  Cyclic Guanosine 3′:5′-Monophosphate/
   Nitric Oxide
  Calcium Ion and Inositol Triphosphate
  Protein Phosphatases

General Principles

Signal transduction or cell signaling concerns the mechanisms by which biologic information is transferred between cells. Functional coordination in multicellular organisms requires intercellular communication among individual cells in various tissues and organs. Adjacent cells can communicate directly by specialized plasma membrane junctions (gap junctions). Long range cell-to-cell communication is possible through the involvement of extracellular signaling molecules (such as hormones and neurotransmitters) that are synthesized and released by specific cells, diffuse or circulate to target cells, and elicit specific responses in target cells that express receptors for the particular extracellular signal. The responses to the extracellular signal are generated by diverse signal transduction mechanisms that frequently involve intracellular signals (second messengers) that transmit signals from activated receptors to the cell interior, resulting in changes in the expression of genes and the activity of enzymes. These intercellular and intracellular signaling pathways are essential to the growth, development, metabolism, and behavior of the organism.[1,2]

At the level of individual cells, signaling is crucial in division, differentiation, metabolic control, and death. Cell signaling pathways are involved in the pathophysiology of many diseases. Cancer is a disease of signaling malfunction due to inactivation of a growth-inhibiting (tumor suppres-

sor) pathway, or to activation of a growth-promoting (oncogene) pathway by genetic mutation. Diabetes results from defects in insulin signaling involved in blood glucose homeostasis. Cell signaling pathways are also involved in the mechanisms of action of many drugs, including local and general anesthetics. For example, the drug STI 571, an inhibitor of the tyrosine kinase Abl, is effective in treating specific leukemias in which Abl is activated by mutation. Knowledge of basic cell signaling mechanisms is therefore essential for understanding many pathophysiologic and pharmacologic mechanisms. Progress in this area has been enhanced by completion of a draft sequence of the human genome, which includes at least 3,775 genes (or 14.3% of genes) involved in signal transduction.[3]

Extracellular Signals

Communication by extracellular signaling is usually classified based on the distance over which the signal acts. In *autocrine* signaling, the signaling cell is its own target. This situation occurs with many growth factors that are released by cells to stimulate their own growth. *Paracrine* signaling involves the release of extracellular signals that affect target cells in close proximity to the signaling cell, as occurs through neurotransmitters in neuromuscular transmission and synaptic transmission. *Endocrine* signaling involves

TABLE 2–1.

Receptor Classification

Cell-surface receptors

G protein coupled: receptors for hormones, neurotransmitters (biogenic amines, amino acids) and neuropeptides
Activate/inhibit adenylyl cyclase
Activate phospholipase C
Modulate ion channels

Ligand-gated ion channels: receptors for neurotransmitters (biogenic amines, amino acids, peptides)
Mediate fast synaptic transmission

Enzyme-linked cell surface receptors

Receptor guanylyl cyclases: receptors for atrial natriuretic peptide, Escherichia coli heat-stable enterotoxin

Receptor serine/threonine kinases: receptors for activin, inhibin, transforming growth factor (TGF)-β

Receptor tyrosine kinases: receptors for peptide growth factors

Tyrosine kinase-associated: receptors for cytokines, growth hormone, prolactin

Receptor tyrosine phosphatases: ligands unknown in most cases

Intracellular receptors

Steroid receptor superfamily: receptors for steroids, sterols, thyroxine (T3), retinoic acid, and vitamin D

the release of hormones, which are extracellular signals that usually act on distant target cells after being transported by the circulatory system from their sites of release. This classification is not strict in that many signals function in more than one manner; for example, epinephrine functions as both a neurotransmitter and a hormone.

The cellular response to an extracellular signal requires its binding to a specific receptor (Table 2–1), which is coupled to changes in the functional properties of the target cell. The particular receptors expressed by the target cell determine its sensitivity to various signals and are responsible for the specificity involved in cellular responses to

various signals. Receptors can be classified by their cellular localization (Fig. 2–1). Most signaling molecules are hydrophilic and interact with *cell surface receptors* that are directly or indirectly coupled to various effector molecules. The majority of hormones and neurotransmitters are water-soluble (hydrophilic) signaling molecules that interact with cell-surface receptors, including peptides, catecholamines, amino acids, and their derivatives. Prostaglandins are the major class of lipid-soluble signaling molecules that interact with cell surface receptors. A number of lipid-soluble (hydrophobic) signaling molecules diffuse across the plasma membrane and interact with *intracellular receptors*. Steroid hormones, retinoids, vitamin D, and thyroxine are transported in the blood bound to specific transporter proteins, from which they dissociate and diffuse across cell membranes to bind to specific receptors in the nucleus or cytosol. The hormone-receptor complex then acts as a ligand-regulated transcription factor to modulate gene expression by binding to *cis*-acting regulatory DNA sequences in target genes that alter their transcription and thereby regulates target cell function. However, recent evidence suggests that receptors for the steroid estrogen also act at the plasma membrane by coupling to G protein to modulate intracellular Ca^{2+} and cyclic adenosine $3':5'$-monophosphate (cAMP) levels. Nitric oxide (NO), and possibly carbon monoxide (CO), are members of a new class of gaseous signaling molecules that readily diffuse across cell membranes to affect neighboring cells. NO, which is unstable and has a short half-life (5–10 seconds), acts as a paracrine signal because it is able to diffuse only a short distance before breaking down. Cell surface receptors can also bind to insoluble ligands, such as the extracellular matrix of cell adhesion molecules, and these interactions are crucial to cell development and migration.

Signal transduction pathways have a number of common properties with important functional implications.[4] *Signal amplification* occurs as a result of sequential activation of catalytic signaling molecules. This enables sensitive physiologic responses to small physical (several photons) or chemical (a few molecules of an odorant) stimuli, as well as graded responses to increasingly larger stimuli. *Specificity* is imparted by specific receptor proteins and their association with cell type–specific signaling pathways and effector mechanisms. *Pleiotropy* results from the ability of a single extracellular signal to generate multiple responses in a target cell, for example, the opening of some ion channels, the closing of others, activation or inhibition of many enzymes, modification of the cytoskeleton, or changes in gene expression. Signal *integration* occurs as the cascades of reactions triggered by different signals interact at multiple levels (crosstalk), both positively and negatively, to produce a unique cellular response distinct from that of any single signal. *Feedback* loops can occur in signaling pathways in which a component can negatively (or positively) influence the activity of an earlier (upstream) component. Activation of signaling pathways can lead to *long-lasting effects* on cellular function as a result of changes in gene expression, which provides a molecular basis for learning and memory.

A *modular* organization of signaling proteins is an emerging theme in signal transduction. Modules are domains of proteins that are usually involved in protein interactions.

They direct protein interactions through their ability to specifically recognize other modules. Examples include PDZ, SH2, and SH3 domains (see later). Larger proteins can contain multiple modules that appear to impart higher selectivity for a given protein–protein interaction and to provide a scaffold to help bring multiple partners together in a signaling complex. These interactions are important in a number of pathways that involve the *translocation* of signaling proteins to a different cellular location. For example, activation of phosphatidylinositol-3 kinase by receptor tyrosine kinases generates phosphatidylinositol-3,4,5-trisphosphate at the plasma membrane, which binds in pleckstrin homology (PH) domains in proteins like Akt, a

serine kinase, causing Akt to translocate to the plasma membrane, where it is phosphorylated and activated by another protein kinase.

Receptors

Signal transduction begins with receptor proteins in the plasma membrane, which sense changes in the extracellular environment. As a result of the interactions between receptors and their ligands, signals are transduced across the plasma membrane (see Fig. 2–1). Ligand binding to a recep-

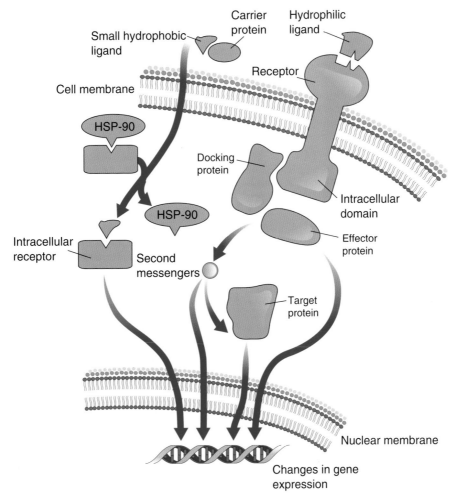

Figure 2–1. *Extracellular signaling.* Ligands bind to either cell surface receptors or intracellular receptors. Most signaling molecules are hydrophilic and therefore unable to cross the plasma membrane. They bind to cell surface receptors, which in turn generate one or more intracellular signals (second messengers) inside the target cell or change the activity of effector proteins (e.g., G proteins, protein kinases, ion channels) through their intracellular effector domains. Receptor activation can result in direct changes in the activity of intrinsic enzymatic activities of the receptor intracellular domain, or indirectly through association of the receptor with intracellular mediators, which in turn regulate the activity of effector proteins. Some effectors translocate to the nucleus to control gene expression (e.g., transcription factors) or to other subcellular compartments. Some small signaling molecules, by contrast, diffuse across the plasma membrane and bind to receptors inside the target cell, either in the cytosol (as shown) or in the nucleus. Many of these small signaling molecules are hydrophobic and nearly insoluble in aqueous solutions; therefore, they are transported in the bloodstream and other extracellular fluids bound to carrier proteins, from which they dissociate before entering the target cell. HSP-90, heat shock protein-90.

tor protein causes a change in the shape (conformation) of the protein, which is transmitted to the cell interior. This can result in the stimulation of an enzyme activity or function that is intrinsic to the receptor (e.g., protein kinase activation, ion channel opening). Other receptors interact with downstream signaling proteins that couple the change in receptor conformation to a change in the activity of an interacting protein, as illustrated by the G protein–coupled receptors (GPCR).

Diverse cellular functions are independently regulated in part by the existence of distinct extracellular signals. Receptors bind the signaling molecule with high affinity and specificity. Additional specificity is imparted by the existence of distinct receptors coupled to different intracellular signaling pathways that respond to the same extracellular signal. Thus a single extracellular signal can elicit different effects on different target cells depending on the receptor subtype and the signaling mechanisms present. A good example is the neurotransmitter acetylcholine, which stimulates contraction of skeletal muscle, but relaxation of smooth muscle. Differences in the intracellular signaling mechanisms also allow the same receptor to produce different responses in different target cells.

The intracellular receptors are all structurally related and act by directly regulating the transcription of specific genes. In contrast, there are three known classes of cell surface receptors, defined by their signal transduction mechanisms: GPCRs, ligand-gated ion channels, and receptor-linked enzymes (see Table 2–1). These cell surface receptor proteins act as signal transducers by binding the extracellular signal molecule and converting this information into an intracellular signal that alters target cell function. *GPCRs* interact with specific G proteins in the plasma membrane, which in turn activate or inhibit an enzyme or ion channel. GPCRs constitute the largest family of cell-surface receptors, and they mediate the cellular responses to diverse extracellular signals including hormones, neurotransmitters, and local mediators. There is also remarkable diversity in the number of GPCRs for the same ligand. Examples include the multiple receptors for epinephrine, dopamine, and the opioids. *Ligand-gated ion channels* (ionotropic receptors) are involved primarily in fast synaptic transmission between excitable cells. Specific neurotransmitters bind to these receptors and transiently open or close the associated ion channel to alter the ion permeability of the plasma membrane and thereby the membrane potential. The nicotinic acetylcholine receptor at the neuromuscular junction is the classic example of a ligand-gated ion channel. The *enzyme-linked cell surface receptors* are a heterogeneous group of receptors that contain intracellular catalytic domains or are closely associated with intracellular enzymes. This receptor class includes the receptor tyrosine kinases, receptor guanylyl cyclases, receptor tyrosine phosphatases, and receptor serine/threonine kinases, in which ligand binding to the receptor activates intrinsic catalytic activity.

The activation of many receptors leads to changes in the concentration of intracellular signaling molecules, termed *second messengers*. These changes are usually transient, which is a result of the tight regulation of the synthesis and degradation (or release and reuptake) of these intracellular signals. Important second messengers include cAMP, guanosine 3′:5′-monophosphate (cGMP), 1,2-diacylglycerol, inositol 1,4,5-trisphosphate (IP_3), and Ca^{2+}. Changes in the concentrations of these molecules following receptor activation are coupled to the modulation of the activities of important regulatory enzymes and effector proteins. The most important second messenger-regulated enzymes are protein kinases and phosphatases, which catalyze the phosphorylation and dephosphorylation, respectively, of key enzymes and proteins in target cells. Reversible phosphorylation alters the function or localization of specific proteins. It is the predominant effector mechanism involved in mediating cellular responses to almost all extracellular signals.

Receptor Regulation

The number and function of cell surface receptors are subject to regulation by several mechanisms. Many receptors undergo *receptor desensitization* in response to prolonged exposure to a high concentration of ligand, a process by which the number or function of receptors is reduced, such that the physiologic response to the ligand is attenuated (tachyphylaxis). Receptor desensitization can occur by several mechanisms, including receptor internalization, down-regulation, or modulation. Receptor internalization by endocytosis is a common mechanism for desensitization of hormone receptors (e.g., insulin, glucagon, epidermal growth factor). The hormone–receptor complex is sequestered by receptor-mediated endocytosis, which results in translocation of the receptor to intracellular compartments (endosomes) that are inaccessible to ligand. This is a relatively slow process that usually terminates the hormone signal. Cessation of agonist stimulation allows the receptor to recycle to the cell surface by exocytosis. In other cases the internalized receptors are degraded and are no longer available for recycling, a process known as receptor down-regulation. Receptors must then be replenished by protein synthesis. Receptor down-regulation in response to prolonged agonist stimulation can also occur at the level of receptor protein synthesis or of receptor mRNA regulation caused by changes in gene transcription, mRNA stability, or both. Regulated endocytosis and delivery of α-amino-3-hydroxy-5-methylisoxazole-4-propionic acid (AMPA)-type glutamate receptors may be involved in the activity-dependent regulation of synaptic strength.[5]

A more rapid and transient form of receptor desensitization involves receptor modulation by phosphorylation (see later), which can rapidly change receptor affinity, signaling efficiency, or both. For example, the β-adrenergic receptor is desensitized as a result of phosphorylation of a number of sites in its intracellular carboxy-terminal domain by cAMP-dependent protein kinase, protein kinase C (PKC), and β-adrenergic receptor kinase (βARK), a G protein–coupled receptor kinase (GRK). The former kinase is activated as a result of β-receptor stimulation of adenylyl cyclase and results in homologous or heterologous desensitization, whereas the latter kinase is active only on β-receptor occupied by ligand and therefore results in only homologous desensitization. Phosphorylation by βARK leads to the binding of β-arrestin to the receptor. These processes both serve to uncouple the active ligand-receptor complex from interacting with G_s, creating a negative feedback loop for modulation of β-receptor activity. In other instances, receptor phosphorylation can affect ligand affinity or associated ion channel kinetics rather than G protein coupling.

Cell Surface Receptors: Structure and Function

G Protein–Coupled Receptors

A variety of signals, which include hormones, neurotransmitters, cytokines, pheromones, odorants, and photons, produce their intracellular actions by a pathway that involves interaction with receptors that activate heterotrimeric guanine nucleotide (GTP)-binding proteins (G proteins).[6,7] G proteins act as molecular switches to relay information from activated receptors to the appropriate effectors.[8,9] An agonist-stimulated receptor can activate several hundred G proteins, which in turn activate a variety of downstream effectors, including ion channels and enzymes, to alter the levels of cytosolic second messengers such as Ca^{2+}, cAMP, and inositol triphosphate. GPCRs form a large and functionally diverse membrane-spanning receptor superfamily; 616 (2.3% of total genes) members have been identified. Heterotrimeric G proteins belong to several gene families, but all in the human genome consist of a large α subunit and a smaller β/γ subunit dimer. GPCR crosses the membrane seven times (hence the alternate terms seven-transmembrane domain, heptahelical, or serpentine receptors; Fig. 2–2*B*). They transduce a wide variety of extracellular signals, such as light, odorant molecules, biogenic amines, and peptides. GPCRs have an important role in pharmacology—more than two thirds of all nonantibiotic drugs target GPCRs—and are thus critical to anesthesiology.[10]

The binding of extracellular signals to their specific receptors on the cell surface initiates a cycle of reactions to promote guanine nucleotide exchange on the G proteins that involves three major steps: (1) the signal (ligand) activates the receptor and induces a conformational change in the receptor; (2) the activated receptor turns on a heterotrimeric G protein in the cell membrane by forming a high affinity ligand–receptor–G protein complex, which promotes guanine nucleotide exchange of GTP for GDP bound to the α subunit of the G protein, followed by dissociation of the α subunit and the βγ subunit dimer from the receptor and each other; and (3) the appropriate effector protein(s) is then regulated by the dissociated G protein α or βγ (or both) subunits, which thereby transduces the signal. The dissociation of the G protein from the receptor reduces the affinity of the receptor for the agonist, and the system returns to its basal state as the GTP bound to the α submit is hydrolyzed to GDP and the trimeric G protein complex reassociates and turns off the signal. A number of different isoforms of G protein α, β, and γ subunits have been identified that mediate the

stimulation or inhibition of functionally diverse effector enzymes and ion channels (Table 2–2). Among the effector molecules regulated by G proteins are adenylyl cyclase, phospholipase C, phospholipase A_2, cyclic GMP (cGMP) phosphodiesterase, and Ca^{2+} and K^+ channels. These effectors then produce changes in the concentrations of a variety of second messenger molecules or in the membrane potential of the target cell.

Despite the diversity in the extracellular signals that stimulate the various effector pathways activated by G protein–coupled receptors, these receptors are structurally homologous, which is consistent with their common mechanism of action. Molecular cloning and sequencing have shown that these receptors are characterized by seven hydrophobic transmembrane α helical segments of 20 to 25 amino acids connected by alternating intracellular and extracellular loops. The structural domains of G protein–coupled receptors involved in ligand binding and in interactions with G proteins have been analyzed by deletion analysis, in which segments of the receptor are sequentially deleted, by site-directed mutagenesis, in which specific single amino acid residues are deleted or mutated, and by constructing chimeric receptor molecules, in which recombinant chimeras are formed by splicing together complementary segments of two related receptors. For example, the agonist isoproterenol binds among the seven transmembrane α helices of the $β_2$ adrenergic receptor near the extracellular surface of the membrane. The intracellular loop between α helices 5 and 6 and the C-terminal segments is important for specific G protein interactions.

Heterogeneity within the GPCR signaling pathway exists at both the level of the receptors and at the level of the G proteins. A single extracellular signal may have several closely related receptor subtypes. For example, six genes for α-adrenergic receptors, three genes for β-adrenergic receptors, and five genes for muscarinic cholinergic receptors have been identified. Likewise, G proteins consist of multiple subtypes. The 16 homologous α subunit genes are classified as subtypes (G_s, G_i, G_k, G_q, and so on) based on structural similarities. The different α subunits have distinct functions, coupling with different effector pathways. The different β and γ subunit isoforms may also couple with distinct signaling pathways. Heterogeneity in effector pathways makes divergence possible within GPCR-activated pathways. This effector pleiotropy can arise from two distinct mechanisms: (1) a single receptor can activate multiple G protein types, or (2) a single G protein type can activate more than one second messenger pathway. Thus a single type of GPCR can activate several different effector pathways within a given cell, whereas the predominant pathway may vary between cell types.

The structure and function of the adrenergic receptors for epinephrine and norepinephrine and their associated G proteins can be used to illustrate important principles of GPCRs (see Fig. 2–2). β-Adrenergic receptors are coupled to the stimulation of adenylyl cyclase, a plasma membrane-associated enzyme that catalyzes the synthesis of cAMP. cAMP was the first second messenger identified and has been found to exist in all prokaryotes and animals. The G protein that couples β-adrenergic receptor stimulation to adenylyl cyclase activation is known as G_s, for stimulatory

Part I Principles of Drug Action

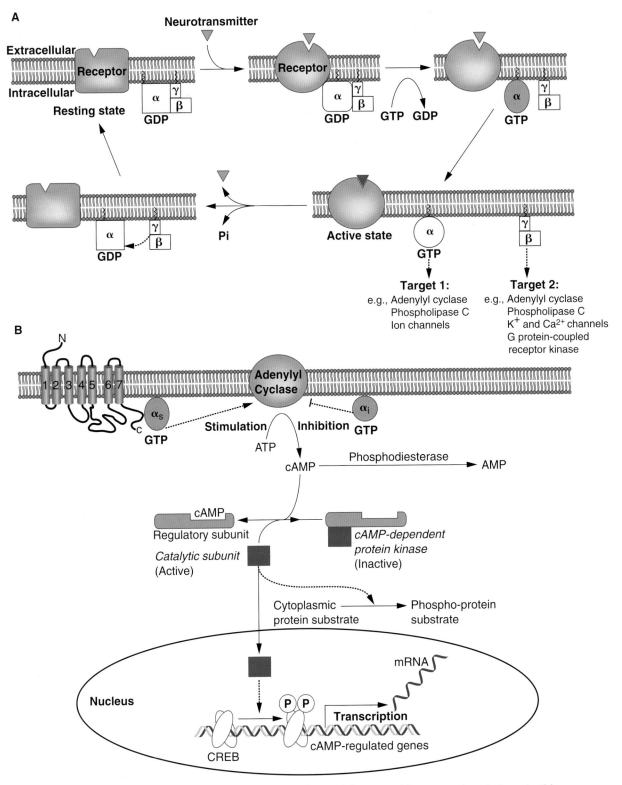

A

Neurotransmitter

Extracellular

Receptor

Intracellular

Resting state

GDP

GDP

GTP GDP

GTP

Pi

GDP

Active state

GTP

GTP

Target 1:
e.g., Adenylyl cyclase
Phospholipase C
Ion channels

Target 2:
e.g., Adenylyl cyclase
Phospholipase C
K$^+$ and Ca^{2+} channels
G protein-coupled
receptor kinase

B

N

1 2 3 4 5 6 7

C

α_s

GTP

Adenylyl Cyclase

Stimulation

Inhibition α_i

GTP

ATP

cAMP

Phosphodiesterase

AMP

cAMP

Regulatory subunit

Catalytic subunit
(Active)

*cAMP-dependent
protein kinase*
(Inactive)

Cytoplasmic
protein substrate

Phospho-protein
substrate

mRNA

Nucleus

P P

Transcription

CREB

cAMP-regulated genes

Figure 2–2. *G protein–coupled receptors. A,* General features. Many receptors belong to this class, including those for neurotransmitters, hormones, odorants, light, and Ca^{2+}. These receptors associate with heterotrimeric G proteins composed of three subunits: α, β, and γ. They are not transmembrane proteins but are associated with the membrane by covalently bound fatty acid molecules. In the resting state, GDP is bound to the α subunit, which is closely attached to the βγ complex. When the neurotransmitter binds to the receptor, the conformation of the receptor changes, inducing a change in the conformation of the α subunit, which expels GDP and replaces it by GTP. The GTP-bound α subunit is no longer capable of interacting with the receptor or βγ. GTP-bound α and βγ interact with specific targets that differ for each isoform α or βγ subunits. After a short time GTP is hydrolyzed to GDP and α-GDP reassociates with βγ. At about the same time, the neurotransmitter leaves its receptor, which returns to its resting state. G

Figure 2–2, cont'd. protein, guanine nucleotide-binding protein; Pi, inorganic phosphate. *B,* The adenylyl cyclase/protein kinase A (PKA) pathway. cAMP is formed from ATP by a class of transmembrane enzymes, adenylyl cyclases. A cytosolic form of adenylyl cyclase has also been described recently. Transmembrane adenylyl cyclases are activated by two related subtypes of G protein α subunits, α_s (stimulatory, which is ubiquitous) and α_{Olf} (olfactory, which is found in olfactory epithelium and a subset of neurons). Adenylyl cyclases are inhibited by α_i (inhibitory). In addition, some adenylyl cyclases can be stimulated or inhibited by $\beta\gamma$, or Ca^{2+} combined with calmodulin. Cyclic adenosine 3':5'-monophosphate (cAMP) is inactivated by hydrolysis into AMP by phosphodiesterases, a family of enzymes that is inhibited by theophylline and related methylxanthines. cAMP has only two known targets in vertebrates: one is a cAMP-gated ion channel that is most prominently found in olfactory neurons, and the other is cAMP-dependent protein kinase that is present in all cells. cAMP-dependent protein kinase is a tetramer composed of two catalytic subunits and two regulatory subunits (only one of each is shown). When cAMP binds to the regulatory subunits (two molecules of cAMP bind to each regulatory subunit), they dissociate from the catalytic subunits. The free active catalytic subunit phosphorylates numerous specific substrates including ion channels, receptors, and enzymes. In addition, the catalytic subunit can enter the nucleus, where it phosphorylates transcription factors. One well-characterized transcription factor phosphorylated in response to cAMP is cAMP-responsive element binding protein (CREB). In the basal state, CREB forms a dimer that binds to a specific DNA sequence in the promoter region of cAMP-responsive genes, called CRE (cAMP-responsive element). CREB is unable to promote transcription when it is not phosphorylated, whereas phospho-CREB strongly stimulates transcription. Genes regulated by CREB include immediate-early genes *c-Fos* and *c-Jun*. CREB is also activated by Ca^{2+} calmodulin-dependent protein kinase.

G protein. Epinephrine-stimulated cAMP synthesis can be reconstituted in phospholipid vesicles using purified β-adrenergic receptors, G_s and adenylyl cyclase, which demonstrates that no other molecules are required for the initial steps of this signal transduction mechanism. In the resting state, G_s exists as a heterotrimer consisting of α_s, β, and γ subunits with GDP bound to α_s. Agonist binding to the β-adrenergic receptor alters the conformation of the receptor and exposes a binding site for G_s. The agonist-activated receptor binds the GDP-G_s complex, thereby reducing the affinity of α_s for GDP, which dissociates, allowing GTP to bind. The α_s subunit bound to GTP then dissociates from the G protein complex, which exposes a binding site for adenylyl cyclase, to which it binds and activates. The affinity of the receptor for agonist is reduced following dissociation of the complex, leading to agonist dissociation and a return of the receptor to its inactive state. Activation of adenylyl cyclase is rapidly reversed following agonist dissociation from the receptor because the lifetime of active α_s is limited by the intrinsic GTPase activity of α_s that is stimulated by binding to adenylyl cyclase. The bound GTP is hydrolyzed to GDP, which returns the α subunit to its inactive conformation. The α_s subunit then dissociates from adenylyl cyclase, which renders it inactive, and reassociates with $\beta\gamma$

to reform G_s. Nonhydrolyzable analogues of GTP, such as GTPγS or GMPPNP, prolong agonist-induced adenylyl cyclase activation by preventing inactivation of active α_s. The mechanism of action of cholera toxin and pertussis toxin, which are adenosine diphosphate (ADP)-ribosyltransferases, involves selective ADP ribosylation of α_s or α_i, respectively, which inhibits its GTPase activity and results in prolonged $G_{s\alpha}$ activation or $G_{i\alpha}$ inactivation.

The activity of adenylyl cyclase can also be negatively regulated by specific receptors coupled to the inhibitory G protein, G_i. An example is the α_2-adrenergic receptor, which is coupled to inhibition of adenylyl cyclase through G_i. Thus the same extracellular signal, epinephrine in this example, can either stimulate or inhibit the formation of the second messenger cAMP depending on the particular G protein that couples the receptor to the cyclase. G_i, like G_s, is a heterotrimeric protein consisting of an α_i subunit and β and γ subunits, which can be the same as those in G_s. Activated α_2 receptors bind to G_i and lead to GDP dissociation, GTP binding, and complex dissociation, as occurs with G_s. Both the released α_i and the $\beta\gamma$ complex are thought to contribute to adenylyl cyclase inhibition, α_i by direct inhibition, and $\beta\gamma$ by direct inhibition and indirectly, by binding to and inactivating any free α_s subunits. Activated G_i can also open K^+ channels, an example of how a single G protein can regulate multiple effector molecules. A similar G protein regulatory cycle applies to other G protein subtypes as well.

One of the hallmarks of signal transduction by GPCRs, as well as other receptor/second messenger systems, is their ability to amplify the extracellular signal. Amplification is possible because the receptor and G protein are able to diffuse in the plasma membrane, which allows each agonist-bound receptor complex to interact with many inactive G_s molecules and convert them to their active state. Further amplification occurs when each active $G_{s\alpha}$/GTP complex activates a single adenylyl cyclase molecule, which then catalyzes the formation of many cAMP molecules in the period before the GTP is hydrolyzed, the complex dissociates, and the adenylyl cyclase is inactivated.

Ligand-Gated Ion Channels

Signals that use G protein-linked receptors are involved in functions that operate with time courses of seconds to minutes, as occurs with slow synaptic transmission or neuromodulation, in which receptor activation is coupled indirectly through a series of steps to a specific change in effector function. In contrast, signals that require rapid transduction, such as fast synaptic transmission, use ligand-gated ion channels, in which binding of the signal to the receptor directly causes an immediate conformational change in the receptor-ion channel complex that opens the associated ion channel (see Chapter 3) and selectively changes its ion permeability independent of a second messenger. The ligand binding site and the ion channel are part of the same molecule or macromolecular complex. Current models support a common structural pattern for the ligand-gated ion channel superfamily consisting of a pentamer of subunits surrounding a central ion pore.[11] Ion channel activation is dependent on the continued occupation of receptor by the ligand and is

TABLE 2–2.

Diversity of G Protein–Coupled Receptor Signal Transduction Pathways: G Proteins and Their Associated Receptors and Effectors

G Protein	Representative Receptors	Effectors	Effect
G_s	β_1, β_2, β_3-adrenergic, D_1, D_5-dopamine	Adenylyl cyclase Ca^{2+} channels	Increased cAMP Increased Ca^{2+} influx
G_i	α_2-adrenergic; D_2; m_2, m_4 Muscarinic; μ, δ, κ opioid	Adenylyl cyclase Phospholipase A_2 K^+ channels	Decreased cAMP Eicosanoid release Hyperpolarization
G_k	Atrial muscarinic	K^+ channel	Hyperpolarization
G_q	m_1, m_3 muscarinic; α_1-adrenergic	Phospholipase C β	Increased IP_3, DG, Ca^{2+}
G_{olf}	Odorants	Adenylyl cyclase	Increased cAMP (olfactory)
G_t	Photons	cGMP phosphodiesterase	Decreased cGMP (vision)
G_o	?	Phospholipase C Ca^{2+} channels	Increased IP_3, DG, Ca^{2+} Decreased Ca^{2+} influx

cAMP, adenosine $3',5'$-monophosphate; cGMP, guanosine $3',5'$-monophosphate; DG, 1,2,-diacylglycerol; G_s, stimulation; G_i, inhibition; G_k, potassium regulation; G_q, phospholipase C regulation; G_{olf}, olfactory; G_t, transducin; G_o, other; IP_3, inositol triphosphate.

rapidly reversible on ligand dissociation. This allows ligand-gated ion channels to mediate rapid onset and rapidly reversible cell signaling.[12]

Ligand-gated ion channels allow the conversion of extracellular chemical signals directly into electrical signals in excitable cells such as neurons and muscle. The ionic selectivity of the ion channel and the membrane potential of the target cell determine whether the ligand-gated ion channel has an excitatory or an inhibitory effect on neuronal excitability or synaptic transmission (see Chapter 3). Excitatory neurotransmitters, which include acetylcholine and glutamate, open cation selective channels that allow Na^+ influx, which depolarizes the membrane. Inhibitory neurotransmitters, which include γ-aminobutyric acid (GABA) and glycine, open Cl^- selective channels that hyperpolarize the membrane or prevent depolarization. A subclass of ligand-gated ion channels includes receptors for intracellular messengers that control Ca^{2+} channels on organelle membranes involved in the regulation of intracellular Ca^{2+} concentration (e.g., the ryanodine receptor and IP_3 receptors; see later).

Although their ligand binding specificities and ion channel selectivities differ, the ligand-gated ion channels that respond to acetylcholine, serotonin, GABA, and glycine consist of structurally homologous subunits and constitute a receptor superfamily. They are heteropentameric membrane-spanning proteins that consist of homologous subunits that interact to form a central transmembrane ion channel. Multiple isoforms of each subunit exist that interact in different combinations to form receptor-ion channel complexes with distinct ligand affinities, sensitivities to drugs and channel conductance, and kinetic properties. Glutamate-gated ion channels (AMPA, kainate, *N*-methyl-D-aspartate [NMDA] subtypes) constitute a distinct family of receptors that also consist of multiple subunit isoforms.

Extensive structural and functional information is available for the nicotinic acetylcholine (ACh) receptor,[13] which can be isolated in large quantities from fish electric organs. This receptor contains four subunit types, which exist in the stoichiometry $\alpha_2\beta\gamma\delta$ (Fig. 2–3A). Each subunit of the nicotinic ACh receptor, GABA receptor, and glycine receptor contains four hydrophobic transmembrane domains in its carboxy-terminal region in similar positions within the subunit, with similar deduced membrane topology (see Fig. 2–3B). A long intracellular loop is located between the third and fourth transmembrane segments and may mediate interactions with the cytoskeleton. The second transmembrane segment is the most hydrophilic of the four, and lines the aqueous ion channel. A large extracellular domain extends over the entire amino-terminal half of the subunit.

Molecular cloning techniques have identified a large number of isoforms of the five different subunit types that constitute the $GABA_A$ receptor (α_1–α_6; β_1–β_4; γ_1–γ_3; ε; δ;

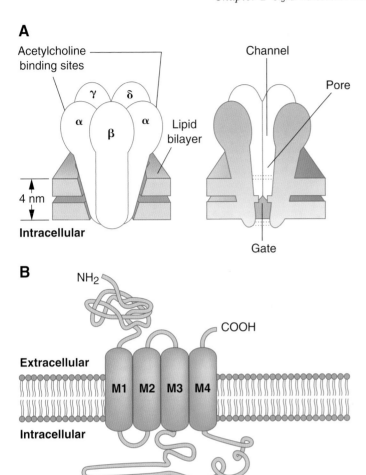

Figure 2–3. *Ligand-gated ion channel superfamily. A,* The nicotinic acetylcholine receptor, a representative ligand-gated ion channel. Five homologous subunits (α, α, β, γ, δ) combine to form a transmembrane aqueous pore. The pore is lined by a ring of five transmembrane α helices, one contributed by each subunit. The ring of α helices is probably surrounded by a continuous rim of transmembrane β sheet, made up of the other transmembrane segments of the five subunits. In its closed conformation the pore is thought to be occluded by the hydrophobic side chains of five leucine residues, one from each α helix, which form a gate near the middle of the lipid bilayer. The negatively charged side chains at either end of the pore (dotted lines) insure that only positively charged ions pass through the channel. Both of the α subunits contain an acetylcholine binding site; when acetylcholine binds to both sites, the channel undergoes a conformational change that opens the gate, possibly by causing the leucine residues to move outward. *B,* Transmembrane topography of each of the four subunit types of the nicotinic acetylcholine receptor. M1–M4 represent the four transmembrane domains of the receptor subunit. A region of the intracellular loop of each subunit is phosphorylated by cyclic adenosine 3′:5′-monophosphate–dependent protein kinase, protein kinase *C,* and a protein-tyrosine kinase. Phosphorylation of the receptor in this region increases its rate of rapid desensitization. (Modified from Hemmings HC Jr: Cell signaling. In Hemmings HC Jr, Hopkins PM (eds): Foundations of Anesthesia: Basic and Clinical Sciences. London, Mosby, 2000, pp 21–36.)

and ρ subunits), an important target for general anesthetics, benzodiazepines, and anticonvulsants.[11,14] Each isoform is homologous and has the general structure shown in Figure 2–3*B.* Experimental expression of specific subunit isoforms in cultured cells has identified pharmacologic differences produced by various subunit combinations. For example, benzodiazepine sensitivity can be altered depending on the specific α or γ subunit isoform present. Alternative splicing of subunit mRNA precursors has also been shown to generate a second isoform of each γ subunit, which may contain an additional phosphorylation site. The many alternative combinations of GABA$_A$ receptors have been shown to have a complex anatomic distribution within the central nervous system, which may have important functional and pharmacologic implications.

The ligand-gated glutamate receptors are functionally divided into NMDA (activated by NMDA) and non-NMDA receptors; the latter can be distinguished by their sensitivities to AMPA and kainate.[15] Expression cloning was used to identify the first non-NMDA receptor subunit structure, from which a family of homologous non-NMDA receptor subunits has been identified (GluR1–GluR7 and KA1–KA2). These subunits have four deduced hydrophobic transmembrane domains, similar to GABA$_A$ receptor subunits, but the amino-terminal domains are significantly longer. More than one type of subunit is required to express glutamate-gated cation channel function, which suggests that the functional form of the receptor exists as an oligomer. Alternative splicing results in additional subunit heterogeneity, as seen with the GABA$_A$ receptor. NMDA receptors possess many unique properties among ligand-gated ion channels, which include voltage sensitivity (in addition to glutamate sensitivity), the requirement of glycine as a co-agonist, slow kinetics, and blockade by Mg^{2+}. Identification of the structure of an NMDA receptor subunit by expression cloning (NR1) again revealed a topology consisting of four similar transmembrane domains. Additional subunits have since been identified (NR2A–NR2C). Although NR1 can produce the above physiologic properties in homomeric form, NR2A–NR2C are only functional in a heteromeric form with NR1. The NR2 subunits differ considerably from NR1 in amino acid sequence and subunit lengths due to variable carboxy-terminal extensions. Although the multiple glutamate receptors overall show considerable sequence diversity, the similarities in their four transmembrane sequences justifies their inclusion as a distinct subgroup in one superfamily with the nicotinic ACh receptors.

Ligand-gated ion channels are important targets for drugs, and of anesthetics in particular,[16] in part because of their specialized functions dictated by distinct combinations of receptor subtypes, their differing electrophysiologic properties and pharmacologic sensitivities, and their specialized anatomic localizations. Thus the structural diversity of these receptors is reflected in a rich pharmacologic diversity. Important examples include the actions of neuromuscular blocking drugs on nicotinic ACh receptors at the neuromuscular junction (see Chapter 32), of barbiturates (see Chapter 23) and benzodiazepines (see Chapter 24) on GABA$_A$ receptors, and of phencyclidine derivatives (e.g., ketamine) on NMDA receptors (see Chapter 23).

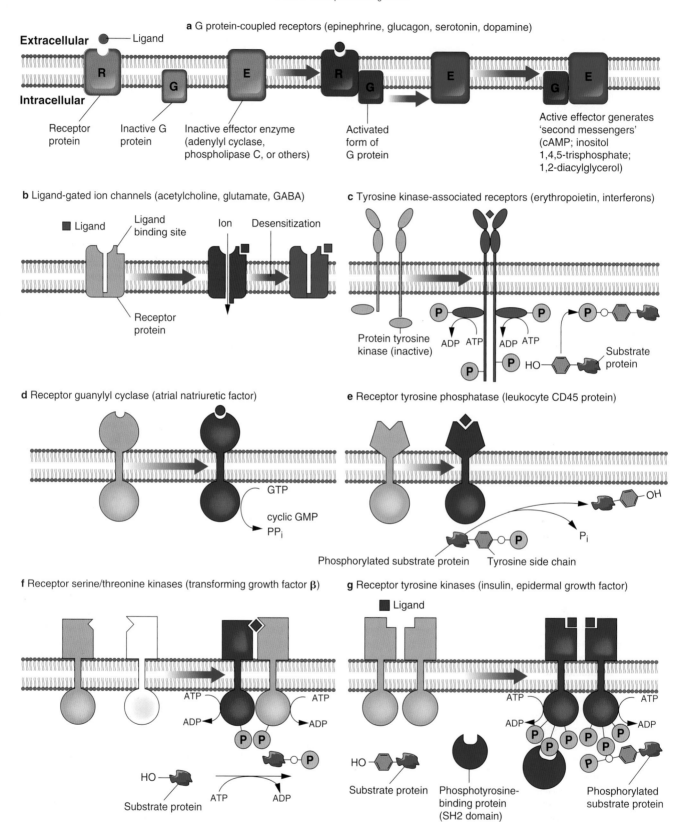

Figure 2–4. *Cell surface receptor types.* Common ligands for each receptor type are shown in parentheses. *A,* G protein-coupled receptors. Ligand binding triggers activation of a het-erotrimeric G protein, which then binds to and activates an enzyme that catalyzes synthesis of a specific second messenger or regulates an ion channel. cAMP, cyclic adenosine 3':5'-monophosphate. *B,* Ligand-gated ion channels. A conformational change triggered by ligand binding opens the channel for ion flow. Continuous occupation of the receptor can result in desen-sitization of the receptor because of closure of the ion channel. GABA, γ-aminobutyric acid. *C–G,* Enzyme-linked cell surface receptors. *C,* Tyrosine kinase-associated receptors. Ligand binding

Figure 2–4. cont'd. causes formation of a homodimer or heterodimer, triggering the binding and activation of a cytosolic protein tyrosine kinase. The activated kinase phosphorylates tyrosines in the receptor; substrate proteins then bind to these phosphotyrosine residues and are phosphorylated. ADP, adenosine diphosphate; ATP, adenosine triphosphate. *D,* Activated receptors are monomers with guanylyl cyclase activity that generate the second messenger cyclic guanosine 3':5'-monophosphate (cyclic GMP). *E,* Ligand binding to other receptors activates intrinsic tyrosine phosphatase activity; these receptors can remove phosphate groups from phosphotyrosine residues in substrate proteins, thereby modifying their activity. *F,G,* The receptors for many growth factors have intrinsic protein kinase activity. Ligand binding to these receptors causes either identical or nonidentical receptor monomers to dimerize and activates their enzymatic activity. Activated receptors with serine/threonine kinase activity are heterodimers *(F),* whereas those with tyrosine kinase activity are heterodimers or homodimers *(G).* In both cases, the activated dimeric receptor phosphorylates several residues in its own intracellular domain. Receptor tyrosine kinases also can phosphorylate certain substrate proteins, thereby altering the activity of these proteins; it is not known whether receptor serine/threonine kinases phosphorylate specific substrate proteins. Specific phosphotyrosine residues in receptor tyrosine kinases function as recognition sites for binding proteins containing SH2 domains. (Modified from Hemmings HC Jr: Cell signaling. In Hemmings HC Jr, Hopkins PM (eds): Foundations of Anesthesia: Basic and Clinical Sciences. London, Mosby, 2000, pp 21–36.)

Enzyme-Linked Cell Surface Receptors

Enzyme-linked receptors are transmembrane proteins that couple an extracellular ligand binding domain with an intracellular catalytic domain through a single transmembrane domain. The enzyme activity is either contained within the intracellular domain of the receptor (intrinsic activity) or is associated with the intracellular domain of the receptor (associated activity). Although this is a heterogeneous group of receptors, most possess a single transmembrane domain and are associated with the activation of protein kinase activity (Fig. 2–4). The known enzyme-linked receptors can be divided into five classes: receptor tyrosine kinases, tyrosine kinase-associated receptors, receptor tyrosine phosphatases, receptor serine/threonine kinases, and receptor guanylyl cyclases.

The best-known receptors in this family are the *receptor tyrosine kinases*, which include the receptors for many peptide/protein growth factors,[17] including epidermal growth factor (EGF), platelet-derived growth factor (PDGF), nerve growth factor (NGF) and related neurotrophins, fibroblast growth factors (FGFs), insulin, and insulin-like growth factor-1 (IGF-1). Signaling through receptor tyrosine kinases is central to many of the cell–cell interactions that regulate embryonic development, tissue maintenance, and repair.[18,19] Their activity is tightly regulated; pertubation caused by mutations results in deregulated kinase activity and malignant transformation.[20] Ligand

binding to the extracellular domain of most receptor tyrosine kinases induces dimerization and activation of the tyrosine kinase intrinsic to the intracellular domain, which catalyzes the phosphorylation of the receptor itself (autophosphorylation) and of specific intracellular proteins, which leads to specific physiologic effects and changes in gene expression. Receptor dimerization is thought to play an important role in the activation of the intracellular tyrosine kinase activity because it allows cross-phosphorylation of the two intracellular domains.[19] The autophosphorylated tyrosines on the receptors create high affinity binding sites for specific intracellular signaling proteins in the target cell, resulting in changes in their localization or activity. These interacting proteins usually contain Src homology-2 domains (SH2 domains), which recognize phosphorylated tyrosine residues in the receptor. Binding of these proteins frequently results in their phosphorylation on tyrosine and subsequent activation, or in their interaction with other signaling molecules. Receptor tyrosine autophosphorylation thereby triggers the assembly of a transient intracellular signaling complex that is involved in the signal transduction process (Fig. 2–5). Some proteins in these complexes appear to function only as scaffolding (or adaptor) proteins that bring together other signaling molecules.[21] Some of the proteins that interact with tyrosine phosphorylated receptors through their SH2 domains are phospholipase Cγ, GTPase activating proteins (GAPs), c-Src-like nonreceptor tyrosine kinases, and phosphatidylinositide 3OH-kinase. Activation of phosphatidylinositide 3-OH kinase activates another pleiotropic signaling pathway by phosphorylation of membrane lipids to form phosphatidylinositol-3,4-bisphosphate and phosphatdylinositol-3,4,5-trisphosphate, which recruits the serine/threonine kinase Akt to the membrane by binding to its PH domain. This allows Akt activation by PDK-1, an Akt kinase, and leads to the phosphorylation of Akt substrates involved in regulating programmed cell death (apoptosis) and cell growth.

Ras proteins are small G proteins involved in transducing mitogenic signals from activated receptor tyrosine kinases to the nucleus to stimulate cell growth and differentiation (see Fig. 2–5). In contrast to the larger heterotrimeric G proteins, the small G proteins are monomeric and consist primarily of the GDP/GTP binding domain. They are involved in many functions, such as regulation of the cell cycle and cytoskeleton.[22,23] Ras activation by growth factor receptor tyrosine kinases requires the adapter proteins Grb2, Shc, and Sos, which couple receptor activation to Ras activation. Binding of growth factor to its cell surface receptor leads to its autophosphorylation. An SH2 domain in Grb2 specifically interacts with a phosphotyrosine residue on the intracellular portion of the activated receptor tyrosine kinase (e.g., EGF receptor) or on the adapter protein Shc. Grb2 then binds and activates Sos through two SH3 domains on Sos, thereby linking the receptor with Sos, a guanine nucleotide exchange factor (GEF) that activates Ras by stimulating release of GDP and subsequent GTP binding. The active GTP-bound form of Ras then recruits the Raf-1 protein kinase to the membrane, which results in its activation. Activated Raf-1 protein kinase then initiates a protein kinase cascade that involves phosphorylation and activation of mitogen-activated protein kinase (MAPK, also called ERK kinase), which then phosphorylates and activates MAPK by

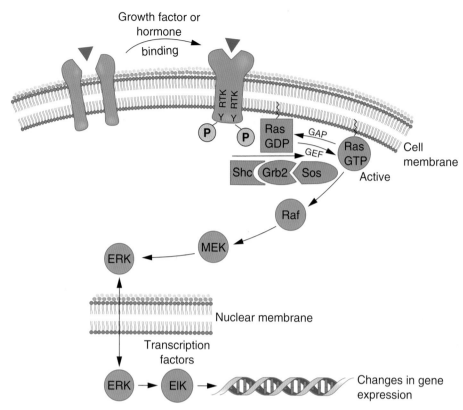

Figure 2–5. *Cell-signaling pathways mediated by the mitogen-activated protein (MAP) kinase pathway.* Binding of a hormone such as insulin leads to dimerization, autophosphorylation, and activation of a receptor tyrosine kinase (RTK). On receptor stimulation, the adaptor protein Shc binds to activated, tyrosine-phosphorylated receptors and becomes phosphorylated. Tyrosine-phosphorylated Shc subsequently interacts with the SH2 domain of Grb2, which binds by its SH3 domains to the guanine nucleotide exchange factor (GEF) Sos, which activates Ras. Sos enhances GDP dissociation from Ras promoting its activation by rebinding GTP; Ras then slowly hydrolyzes GTP to GDP and becomes inactive. Ras in turn activates Raf-1, a serine-threonine protein kinase. Raf-1 phosphorylates and activates MEK (also called) MAP kinase kinase, a bifunctional protein tyrosine and protein serine/threonine kinase. MEK (extracellular signal-regulated kinase [ERK] kinase) activates ERK (MAP kinase) by phosphorylation on both tyrosine and threonine. MAP kinase itself phosphorylates and activates cytoplasmic proteins such as S6 kinase, which stimulates protein synthesis and insulin-stimulated protein kinase p90^{rsk}, which activates protein phosphatase-1, and nuclear transcription factors such as Elk-1 and c-Jun. Ras functions as a GDP/GTP-regulated binary switch at the inner surface of the plasma membrane to relay extracellular signals to the cytoplasmic signaling cascades. A linear pathway exists between the activation of receptor tyrosine kinases, Ras, a serine/threonine kinase cascade (Raf→MEK→ERK) and transcription factors to provide a link between the cell membrane and the nucleus.

phosphorylation of both thoerine and tyrosine residues (an unusual dual-specificity kinase). Activated MAPK signals downstream by phosphorylating various effector molecules such as phospholipase A$_2$ and transcription factors involved in gene regulation.[24] The MAPK pathway is a highly conserved eukaryotic signaling pathway involving a kinase cascade that couples various receptor signals to cell proliferation, differentiation, and metabolic regulation. Activated GTP-Ras is slowly converted to the inactive, GDP-bound form by its intrinsic GTPase activity, which can be accelerated by a GAP.

Tyrosine kinase-associated receptors are comparable to the receptor tyrosine kinases, but instead of activating an integral tyrosine kinase activity, they work through associated nonreceptor tyrosine kinases. This diverse group of receptors includes those for some hormones (prolactin,

growth hormone, for leptin), lymphocyte antigen receptors, many cytokines, interferons, and growth factors (e.g., erythropoietin). The associated tyrosine kinases belong to the c-Src family (e.g., Src, Fyn, Yes, and Lck) or the Janus family (e.g., JAK1 and JAK2) of nonreceptor tyrosine kinases. Similarly, integrins, which are receptors for extracellular matrix proteins, associate with the tyrosine kinase FAK (focal adhesion kinase). These receptors are thought to function like the receptor tyrosine kinases, except that the tyrosine kinase domain is a separate entity that interacts with the receptor noncovalently. As with the receptor tyrosine kinases, ligand binding usually induces receptor dimerization, tyrosine kinase activation, and phosphorylation of distinct sets of substrate proteins.

Receptor tyrosine phosphatases are a large and diverse group of membrane-bound enzymes that reverse the action of tyrosine kinases by catalyzing the dephosphorylation of specific phosphotyrosine residues. Receptor tyrosine phosphatases include an extracellular domain of variable length and composition, a single membrane-spanning domain, and one or two intracellular catalytic domains. CD45, the prototype of this family, has a single transmembrane domain and is activated by cross-linking with antibodies to the extracellular domain. The natural ligand for CD45, or for most other members of this family, are unknown.

Receptor serine/threonine kinases constitute a family of receptors for the transforming growth factor-β (TGF-β) family of signaling proteins, including activin and inhibin. These receptors consist of a single transmembrane domain with an integral serine/threonine protein kinase domain within the intracellular portion of the receptor.

Another class of receptors are linked to the activation of proteolytic enzyme cascades. Receptors for Fas ligand and tumor necrosis factor (TNF), which are able to trigger apoptosis, associate with various intracellular proteins that activate, *inter alia*, aspartate-specific proteases (caspases).

The *receptor guanylyl cyclases* are discussed later.

Second Messengers and Protein Phosphorylation

Work by Sutherland and his colleagues in the late 1950s on the hormonal control of glycogen metabolism in the mammalian liver revealed that epinephrine and glucagon stimulated glycogenolysis by increasing the synthesis of the intracellular second messenger cAMP. Subsequently, Krebs and his colleagues discovered a protein kinase in skeletal muscle that was activated by physiologic increases in the levels of cAMP, and demonstrated that epinephrine stimulated glycogenolysis through activation of this protein kinase. Since this groundbreaking work, the mechanisms of action of a number of additional extracellular signals have been found to involve second messengers, regulation of protein phosphorylation, or both. This process can involve either direct activation of a receptor-associated protein kinase or an alteration in the level of a second messenger, which then in turn regulates a specific protein kinase or protein phosphatase (Fig. 2–6). Thus the regulation of the state of phosphorylation of specific substrates by a variety of protein kinases represents a final common pathway in the molecular mechanisms through which most hormones, neurotransmitters, and other extracellular signals produce their biologic effects.[25]

Protein phosphorylation involves the covalent modification of key substrate proteins by phosphoryl transfer, which in turn regulates their functional properties. All protein phosphorylation systems have three components in common: (1) a substrate protein (phosphoprotein) that can exist in either the dephosphoform or phosphoform, (2) a protein kinase that catalyzes phosphoryl transfer from the terminal (γ) phosphate of adenosine triphosphate (ATP) to a specific hydroxylated amino acid of the substrate protein (serine, threonine, or tyrosine), and (3) a protein phosphatase that catalyzes dephosphorylation of the phosphory-lated substrate protein (see Fig. 2–6). Several

second messengers are involved in the control of protein phosphorylation by extracellular signals. These second messengers include cAMP, cGMP, Ca^{2+} (together with calmodulin), and 1,2-diacylglycerol, each of which is capable of activating one or more distinct protein kinases.

Protein kinases can be divided into two major classes, protein-serine/threonine kinases and protein-tyrosine kinases, and a minor class of dual specificity kinases. The protein-serine/threonine kinases can be further divided into those that are regulated by known second messengers (e.g., cAMP, cGMP, and Ca^{2+}) and those that are not (the Ca^{2+} independent and cyclic nucleotide independent protein kinases and the receptor serine/threonine protein kinases). Almost 2% of human genes encode for protein kinases (501 genes), most of which are protein-serine/threonine kinases (395 genes), whereas there are 15 serine/threonine and 56 tyrosine phosphatase genes.[1]

Cyclic Adenosine 3′:5′-Monophosphate

cAMP, the first intracellular messenger identified, operates as a signaling molecule in all eukaryotic and prokaryotic cells. A variety of hormones and neurotransmitters have been found to regulate the levels of cAMP. Adenylyl cyclases form a class of membrane-bound enzymes that catalyze the formation of cAMP, usually under the control of receptor-mediated G protein–coupled stimulation (by α_s and α_{Olf}) and inhibition (by α_i). The rapid degradation of cAMP to adenosine 5′-monophosphate by one of several isoforms of cAMP phosphodiesterase provides the potential for rapid reversibility and responsiveness of this signaling mechanisms. Most of the actions of cAMP are mediated through the activation of cAMP-dependent protein kinase and the concomitant phosphorylation of substrate protein effectors on specific serine or threonine residues.

The widespread distribution of cAMP-dependent protein kinase throughout the animal kingdom and in all cells led to the hypothesis that the diverse effects of cAMP on cell function are mediated through the activation of this enzyme, which has been shown to be the principal intracellular receptor for cAMP. Other known receptors for cAMP are the hyperpolarization-activated cyclic nucleotide-gated (HCN) channels. cAMP-dependent protein kinase exists as a tetramer composed of two types of dissimilar subunits, the regulatory (R) subunit and the catalytic (C) subunit. In the absence of cAMP, the inactive holoenzyme tetramer consists of two R subunits joined by disulfide bonds, bound to two C subunits (R_2C_2). The binding of cAMP to the R subunits of the inactive holoenzyme decreases their affinity for the C subunits and leads to the dissociation from the holoenzyme of the two free C subunits expressing phosphotransferase activity. Each R subunit contains two binding sites for cAMP, which activate the kinase synergistically and exhibit positively cooperative cAMP binding.

The phosphorylation of specific substrates brought about by cAMP-dependent protein kinase represents the next step in the molecular pathway by which cAMP produces its biologic responses. Substrates for cAMP-dependent protein kinase are characterized by two or more basic amino acid residues on the amino-terminal side of the phosphorylated residue. The identification and characterization of the

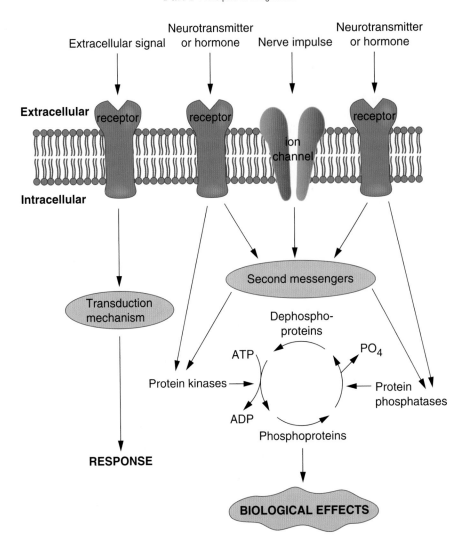

Figure 2–6. *Schematic diagram of cellular regulation by extracellular signals acting through protein phosphorylation.* A generalized scheme for cell surface receptor-mediated signal transduction is shown on the left. Extracellular signals (first messengers), which include various neurotransmitters, hormones, growth factors, and cytokines, produce specific biologic effects in target cells through a series of intracellular signals. Cell membrane receptors for many extracellular signals are coupled to the activation of protein kinases, either directly by activating a protein kinase intimately associated with the receptor, or indirectly through changes in the intracellular levels of second messengers. Protein kinases are enzymes that transfer a phosphoryl group from adenosine triphosphate (ATP) to serine, threonine, or tyrosine residues. Prominent second messengers involved in the regulation of protein kinases include cyclic adenosine 3':5'-monophosphate (cAMP), cyclic guanosine 3':5'-monophosphate (cGMP), Ca^{2+}, and 1,2-diacylglycerol. Other protein kinases are themselves regulated by phosphorylation and participate in kinase cascades (see Fig. 2–5). The activation of individual protein kinases causes the phosphorylation of specific substrate proteins (phosphoproteins) in target cells. Specificity of the sites phosphorylated is conferred by the surrounding amino acid sequence. In some cases these substrate proteins, or third messengers, are the immediate effectors for the biologic response, and in other cases they produce the biologic response indirectly, through additional intracellular messengers (e.g., the mitogen-activated kinase [MAP] kinase cascade). Protein phosphatases are also subject to regulation by extracellular signals acting directly, or through second messengers (e.g., Ca^{2+} acting on Ca^{2+}/CaM-dependent protein phosphatase-2B), or by the phosphorylation of specific protein phosphatase modulator proteins. Many, if not all, membrane receptors and ion channels are themselves regulated by phosphorylation/dephosphorylation. (Modified from Hemmings HC Jr: Cell signaling. In Hemmings HC Jr, Hopkins PM (eds): Foundations of Anesthesia: Basic and Clinical Sciences. London, Mosby, 2000, pp 21–36.)

specific substrate(s) phosphorylated in response to cAMP are important goals in the study of agents whose actions are mediated by cAMP. The various substrates for cAMP-dependent protein kinase present in different cell types explain the diverse tissue-specific effects of cAMP. They include ion channels, receptors, enzymes, cytoskeletal proteins, and transcription factors (e.g., cAMP-responsive element binding protein [CREB]).

Cyclic Guanosine 3':5'-Monophosphate/Nitric Oxide

cGMP is a key intracellular signaling molecule in virtually all animal cells that is involved in signal transduction pathways activated by NO and the natriuretic peptides.[26,27] Various tissues contain multiple forms of guanylyl cyclase and cGMP phosphodiesterase, the two enzymes that regulate the intracellular concentration of cGMP. Guanylyl cyclases exist in both soluble and particulate (cell surface) forms. Soluble forms of the enzyme are activated by NO formed from L-arginine by activation of NO synthase or donated by exogenous nitroglycerin or nitroprusside. Nitric oxide signaling is important in the control of vascular tone, neurotransmission, and macrophage function. Soluble guanylyl cyclase contains a heme moiety, which binds NO and other oxidants to stimulate enzyme activity. The family of NO synthases includes constitutive neuronal and endothelial forms and an inducible macrophage form. The endothelial and neuronal isoforms of NO synthase are dependent on Ca^{2+}/calmodulin for activation, whereas the inducible form is constitutive and Ca^{2+}-independent. Nitric oxide is thought to be the endogenous regulator of guanylyl cyclase activity that mediates the action of several vasodilators, including acetylcholine, bradykinin, and substance P (Fig. 2–7). These transmitters stimulate the production of a diffusible mediator known as endothelium-derived relaxing factor (EDRF), which has been identified as NO or a closely related molecule.

The NO/guanylyl cyclase signaling pathway has received considerable attention as the first example of a signaling system that involves a gaseous signaling molecule. Recent evidence suggests that CO can also act as a signaling molecule to stimulate guanylyl cyclase. Because it readily diffuses within a restricted volume across cell membranes, NO formed in one cell is able to activate guanylyl cyclase in the same cell as a second messenger (autocrine effect), as well as in neighboring cells as a transmitter (paracrine effect), but its diffusion is limited by its high chemical reactivity and short half-life. NO donors, inhibitors of NO synthase and NO itself, are providing new approaches to the management of a number of diseases, including sepsis, adult respiratory distress syndrome, pulmonary hypertension, ischemia, and degenerative diseases.

Particulate forms of guanylyl cyclase serve as cell surface receptors for a variety of different peptide ligands, including the natriuretic peptides (e.g., atrial natriuretic peptide [ANP]). These receptors contain a single transmembrane domain flanked by an extracellular peptide binding domain and intracellular guanylyl cyclase and protein kinase-like catalytic domains. Some forms of particulate guanylyl cyclase also appear to be sensitive to intracellular Ca^{2+}.

The cellular responses to cGMP are mediated in specific tissues by regulation of cGMP-regulated phosphodiesterase, cGMP-gated ion channels, and cGMP-dependent protein kinase. cGMP-dependent protein kinase is a protein-serine/threonine kinase that is either a soluble dimer of identical subunits (type I) or a membrane-bound monomer (type II). cGMP-dependent protein kinase is activated by increases in intracellular cGMP, the formation of which is catalyzed by guanylyl cyclase. The primary mechanism of inactivation of cGMP-dependent protein kinase results from hydrolysis of cGMP by cyclic nucleotide phosphodiesterase, of which there is a form specific for cGMP. Each subunit of type I cGMP-dependent protein kinase contains a cGMP-binding domain and a catalytic domain, which is homologous to cAMP-dependent protein kinase catalytic subunit. On binding of cGMP, a conformational change occurs in the enzyme that exposes the active catalytic domain; the mechanism of activation of the type II kinase has not been determined. In contrast to cAMP-dependent protein kinase, which is present in similar concentrations in most mammalian tissues, cGMP-dependent protein kinase has an uneven tissue distribution. Relatively high concentrations of the type I enzyme are found in lung, heart, smooth muscle, platelets, cerebellum, and intestine; the type II enzyme is widely distributed in the brain and intestine. In vitro, cGMP-dependent and cAMP-dependent protein kinases show similar substrate specificities. Although many physiologic substrates for cAMP-dependent protein kinase have been identified, only a few specific physiologic substrates for cGMP-dependent protein kinase have been found.

Calcium Ion and Inositol Triphosphate

Along with cAMP, Ca^{2+} controls a wide variety of intracellular processes.[28] Ca^{2+} entry through Ca^{2+} channels or its release from intracellular stores triggers hormone and neurotransmitter secretion, initiates muscle contraction, and activates many protein kinases and other enzymes. The concentration of free Ca^{2+} is normally maintained at a very low level in the cytosol of most cells ($<10^{-6}$M) compared with the extracellular fluid ($\sim10^{-3}$M) by a number of homeostatic mechanisms. A Ca^{2+}-ATPase in the plasma membrane pumps Ca^{2+} from the cytosol to the cell exterior at the expense of ATP hydrolysis, a Ca^{2+}-ATPase in the endoplasmic and sarcoplasmic reticulum concentrates Ca^{2+} from the cytosol into intracellular storage organelles and a Na^+/Ca^{2+} exchanger, which is particularly active in excitable plasma membranes, couples the electrochemical potential of Na^+ influx to the efflux of Ca^{2+} (Na^+ driven Ca^{2+} antiport). Although mitochondria have the ability to take up and release Ca^{2+}, they are not widely believed to play a major role in cytosolic Ca^{2+} homeostasis during normal conditions.

Changes in intracellular free Ca^{2+} concentration can be induced directly by depolarization-evoked Ca^{2+} entry down its electrochemical gradient through voltage-dependent Ca^{2+} channels (as in neurons and muscle) and by extracellular signals that activate Ca^{2+}-permeable ligand-gated ion channels (e.g., the NMDA receptor), or directly by extracellular signals coupled to the formation of IP_3 (Fig. 2–8). IP_3 is formed in response to a number of extracellular signals that

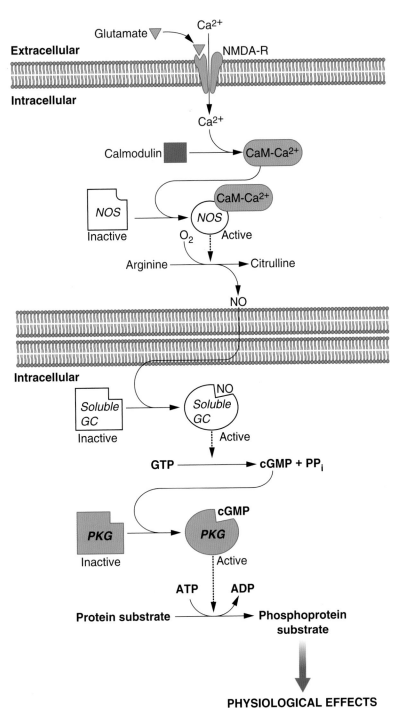

Figure 2–7. *Nitric oxide as a signaling molecule.* Nitric oxide (NO) is a gas that is highly diffusible and chemically reactive. In the nervous system it is used as a locally active intracellular or inter-cellular messenger. The enzyme responsible for the formation of NO is NO synthase (NOS). It is activated by Ca^{2+} complexed to calmodulin. In neurons, opening of glutamate receptors of the *N*-methyl-D-aspartate (NMDA) subtype is a major source of Ca^{2+} influx that can lead to the activation of NOS; NOS is a complex enzyme that uses molecular oxygen, O_2, to generate NO by transforming arginine into citrulline. Nitric oxide can cross membranes readily and diffuse to neighboring cells. Thus the rest of the cascade depicted in the figure can take place in a cell different from that in which NO was gen-erated, as symbolized by the *broken line*. A major target of NO is soluble guanylyl cyclase. This enzyme is activated by NO and uses GTP to form cyclic guanosine 3′:5′-monophosphate (cGMP), a second messenger that remains within the cell in which it is produced. cGMP exerts its effects by activating several enzymes, one of which is cGMP-dependent protein kinase. Phosphorylation of specific proteins by cGMP-dependent protein kinase accounts for some of the physiologic effects of NO. ADP, adeno-sine diphosphate; ATP, adenosine triphosphate; GC, guanylyl cyclase; NMDA-R, *N*-methyl-D-aspartate subtype of glutamate receptor; PKG, cGMP-dependent protein kinase.

interact with G protein–coupled cell surface receptors (G_q, G_{11}) coupled to the activation of phospholipase C.[29]

Phospholipase C hydrolyzes phosphatidylinositol-4,5-bisphosphate to IP_3 and diacylglycerol; further degradation of diacylglycerol by phospholipase A_2 can result in the release of arachidonic acid. All three of these receptor regulated metabolites are important second messengers. IP_3 increases intracellular Ca^{2+} by binding to specific IP_3 recep-tors on the endoplasmic reticulum, which are coupled to a Ca^{2+} channel that allows Ca^{2+} efflux into the cytosol. IP_3 receptors are similar to the Ca^{2+} release channels (ryanodine receptors) of muscle sarcoplasmic reticulum that release Ca^{2+} in response to excitation. Diacylglycerol remains in the plasma membrane where it activates PKC, whereas arachi-donic acid, in addition to its metabolism to biologically active prostaglandins and leukotrienes, can also activate PKC. The Ca^{2+} signal is terminated by hydrolysis of IP_3 and by the rapid reuptake and extrusion of Ca^{2+}.

Ca^{2+} carries out it second messenger functions primarily after binding to intracellular Ca^{2+} binding proteins, of which *calmodulin* is the most important. Calmodulin is a ubiqui-tous multifunctional Ca^{2+} binding protein, highly conserved between species, which binds four atoms of Ca^{2+} with high affinity. Ca^{2+} can also bind to C2 domains found in several

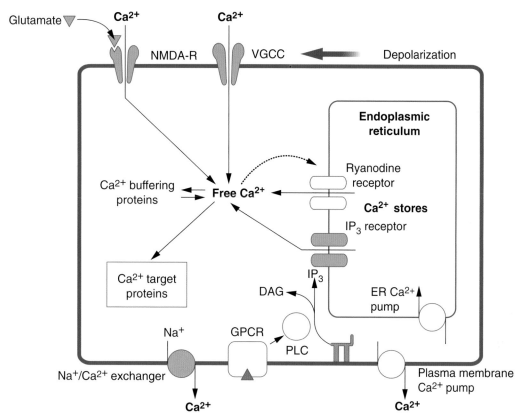

Figure 2–8. *Pathways by which Ca^{2+} can enter the cytosol as a second messenger in response to extracellular signals. A,* Ca^{2+} enters a nerve terminal from the extracellular fluid through voltage-gated Ca^{2+} channels when the nerve terminal membrane is depolarized by an action potential. *B,* Binding of an extracellular signaling molecule to a cell-surface receptor generates inositol trisphosphate, which stimulates the release of Ca^{2+} from the endoplasmic reticulum. Ca^{2+} is a divalent cation whose concentrations are relatively high in the extracellular space (approximately 1.2 mM) and more than 10,000 times lower within the cytosol (approximately 100 nM). In resting conditions, the plasma membrane is impermeable to Ca^{2+}. In neurons, it can penetrate through specific channels that include voltage-gated Ca^{2+} channels (VGCC) and glutamate receptors of the *N*-methyl-D-aspartate (NMDA) subtype. When these channels are open, in response to depolarization in the case of VGCC or in the presence of glutamate in the case of NMDA receptor, Ca^{2+} flows readily into the cytosol following both its concentration gradient and the electrical potential. Ca^{2+} can also be released into the cytosol from internal stores (the endoplasmic reticulum). Two types of Ca^{2+} channels are responsible for the release of Ca^{2+} from internal stores: one is the IP$_3$ receptor the opening of which is triggered by inositol-1,4,5-trisphosphate (IP$_3$), a second messenger generated by phospholipase C from phosphatidylinositol 4,5-bisphosphate; and the other is the ryanodine receptor, named after ryanodine, a drug that triggers its opening. Opening of ryanodine receptors is triggered by Ca^{2+} itself by a mechanism called Ca^{2+}-*induced Ca^{2+} release,* which can give rise to propagation of waves of Ca^{2+} release along the endoplasmic reticulum. In the cytosol, Ca^{2+} is mostly bound to specific binding proteins. Some of them function as buffering proteins, preventing excessive increases in cytosolic free Ca^{2+}. Others are the actual targets of Ca^{2+}, which account for the potent biologic effects of this cation. Among the best-characterized targets are calmodulin and calmodulin-related proteins, which undergo a conformational change enabling them to interact with, and activate, a number of enzymes. Ca^{2+} can also bind to another type of protein domain called C2. Free Ca^{2+} in the cytosol is maintained at very low levels by several highly active processes that include Ca^{2+} pumps and Ca^{2+} exchangers. The Ca^{2+} pumps have a high affinity but a low capacity for Ca^{2+} and are used for fine tuning of Ca^{2+} levels. They are located on the plasma membrane and the membrane of the endoplasmic reticulum, and their energy is provided by adenosine triphosphate (ATP) hydrolysis. Na$^+$/Ca^{2+} exchangers, whose driving force is provided by the Na$^+$ gradient, have a large capacity, but a low affinity for Ca^{2+}. DAG, diacylglycerol; ER, endoplasmic reticulum; GPCR, G protein–coupled receptor; NMDA-R, *N*-methyl-D-aspartate subtype of glutamate receptor; PLC, phospholipase /C/.

proteins (PKC, phospholipase A$_2$, synaptotagmin). Most calmodulin-regulated enzymes appear to be activated by a similar mechanism. Calmodulin does not bind to the enzyme in the absence of Ca^{2+}; however, in the presence of micromolar concentrations of Ca^{2+}, calmodulin undergoes a marked conformational change exposing hydrophobic binding sites. The exposed hydrophobic domain of the Ca^{2+}/calmodulin complex interacts with a calmodulin-binding domain present in a variety of effector proteins, including the Ca^{2+}/calmodulin-dependent protein kinases, which along with PKC mediate most of the effects of Ca^{2+} in cells. Ca^{2+}/calmodulin-dependent activation of protein kinases was originally observed for phosphorylase kinase and myosin light chain kinase (see Chapter 22, Section A). Subsequently, Ca^{2+}/calmodulin-dependent protein phosphorylation was found to be widespread in various tissues. Ca^{2+}/calmodulin kinases I and II, myosin light chain kinase, and phosphorylase kinase appear to be responsible for most Ca^{2+}/calmodulin-dependent protein kinase activity.

Ca^{2+}/calmodulin kinase I has a widespread species and tissue distribution, and like phosphorylase kinase or myosin light chain kinase exhibits a limited substrate specificity. In contrast to other Ca^{2+}/calmodulin kinases, the isozymes of Ca^{2+}/calmodulin kinase II exhibit a relatively broad substrate specificity. This kinase is therefore referred to as the multifunctional Ca^{2+}/calmodulin-dependent protein kinase.

PKC is a family of serine/threonine protein kinases that consists of 12 structurally homologous phospholipid-dependent isoforms with conserved catalytic domains, which are distinguished by their variable N-terminal regulatory domains and cofactor dependence.[30] PKC was first purified from brain as a cyclic nucleotide-independent protein kinase that could be activated by a Ca^{2+}-dependent protease. The holoenzyme was subsequently found to be activated by the addition of Ca^{2+}, diacylglycerol, and membrane phospholipid. PKC has been shown to be the intracellular receptor for, and to be activated by, the tumor-promoting phorbol esters. The Ca^{2+}-dependent or conventional isoforms of PKC (cPKC) are components of the phospholipase C/diacylglycerol signaling pathway. They are regulated by the lipid second messenger 1,2-diacylglycerol, by phospholipids such as phosphatidylserine, and by Ca^{2+} through specific interactions with the regulatory region. Binding of diacylglycerol to the C1 domain of cPKC isoforms (α, β1, β2, γ) increases their affinity for Ca^{2+} and phosphatidylserine, facilitates PKC translocation and binding to cell membranes, and increases catalytic activity. The novel PKC isoforms (nPKC; δ, ε, η, θ, μ) are similar to cPKCs, but lack the C2 domain and do not require Ca^{2+}. The atypical isoforms (αPKC; ζ, λ) differ considerably in the regulatory region, and do not require Ca^{2+} or diacylglycerol for activity. The cPKC holoenzyme contains a hydrophobic regulatory domain that interacts with Ca^{2+}, phospholipids (C2), and diacylglycerol and phorbol esters (C1). A hydrophilic C-terminal catalytic domain can be cleaved from the holoenzyme by proteolysis to yield a fragment that is catalytically active in the absence of Ca^{2+}, diacylglycerol, and phospholipid, illustrating the negative modulatory role of the regulatory domain. PKC has a broad substrate specificity, which differs from those of both cyclic nucleotide-dependent and Ca^{2+}/calmodulin-dependent

protein kinases. Additional specificity may be provided by specific targeting subunits that may localize PKC near its important substrates.

PKC is activated by micromolar concentrations of Ca^{2+} and membrane phospholipids of which phosphatidylserine is the most active. Addition of low concentrations of diacylglycerol increases the affinity of cPKC for Ca^{2+}. cPKC and nPKC isoforms are activated by an increase in the concentration of diacylglycerol produced by receptor-stimulated phosphatidylinositol turnover. The activation of the kinase by diacylglycerol, although dependent on micromolar concentrations of Ca^{2+}, does not appear to be dependent on increases in intracellular Ca^{2+}. Tumor-promoting phorbol esters appear to substitute for diacylglycerol in the activation of PKC. The hydrolysis of phosphatidylinositol-4,5-bisphosphate produces diacylglycerol and IP$_3$, and the latter compound mobilizes Ca^{2+} in cells. Activation of PKC results from the synergistic actions of increases in the intracellular concentrations of both Ca^{2+} and diacylglycerol. The contributions of each second messenger may vary, however, depending on the cell type or receptor-mediated event. Activation of PKC, which is predominantly a cytosolic enzyme, leads to its translocation to the plasma membrane, where it undergoes protease-mediated down-regulation in the presence of continuous stimulation. Translocation of PKC may be important in targeting the enzyme to specific substrates and cellular compartments.

Protein Phosphatases

The phosphorylation of specific sites on proteins is transient and regulated by protein phosphatases in addition to protein kinases (see Fig. 2–6). Rather than simply reversing the phosphorylation catalyzed by protein kinases, protein phosphatases exhibit distinct substrate specificities and are tightly regulated; regulation of both protein phosphorylation and dephosphorylation increases the complexity and flexibility of this regulatory mechanism.[31] The protein phosphatases involved in the dephosphorylation of most of the known proteins phosphorylated on serine or threonine residues are accounted for by four enzymes: type 1 protein phosphatase (protein phosphatases-1) and type 2 protein phosphatases (protein phosphatase-2A, -2B, and -2C). Protein phosphatase-1, -2A, and -2B share homologous catalytic subunits, and are complexed with one or more regulatory subunits. Protein phosphatase-2C is distinct and relatively minor in most tissues. Protein phosphatase-1, -2A, and -2C all exhibit relatively broad substrate specificities, whereas protein phosphatase-2B appears to be more restricted. Multiple forms of both cytosolic and membrane-bound (receptor) phosphotyrosine-protein phosphatases have been demonstrated, which are distinct from the phosphoserine/phosphothreonine-protein phosphatases.

Protein phosphatases, like protein kinases, experience tight physiologic regulation. Protein phosphatase-2B (also known as calcineurin), which is a prominent calmodulin-binding protein in the brain, is activated by Ca^{2+} plus calmodulin. Protein phosphatase-1 is regulated indirectly by cAMP, which stimulates phosphorylation and activation of two potent and specific inhibitor proteins (DARPP-32 and phosphatase inhibitor-1). This provides a positive feedback mechanism for amplifying the effects of cAMP, and a mechanism for cAMP to modulate the phosphorylation state of substrate proteins for protein kinases other than cAMP-dependent protein kinases. Protein phosphatase-1 is also regulated by its interaction with phosphatase inhibitor-2. A complex of protein phosphatase-1 with phosphatase inhibitor-2 (together known as the Mg^{2+}-ATP-dependent protein phosphatase) is inactive, but is activated by incubation with glycogen synthase kinase-3 plus Mg^{2+}-ATP. Tissue-specific targeting subunits also serve to localize protein phosphatase-1 to important subcellular sites of action in many tissues.

Acknowledgments

The thoughtful contributions of Steven Robicsek, MD, PhD, are gratefully acknowledged.

References

1. Cell-to-cell signaling: Hormones and receptors. In Lodish H, et al. (eds): Molecular Cell Biology, 3rd ed. New York, WH Freeman and Co, 1995, pp 853–924.

2. Cell signalling. In Alberts B, et al. (eds): Molecular Biology of the Cell, 3rd ed. New York, Garland, 1994, pp 721–785.

3. Hemmings HC Jr. Cell signaling. In Hemmings HC Jr, Hopkins PM (eds): Foundations of Anesthesia: Basic and Clinical Sciences, London, Mosby, 2000, pp 21–36.

4. Venter JC, Adams MD, Myers EW, et al: The sequence of the human genome. Science 291:1304–1351, 2001.

5. Downward J: The ins and outs of signalling. Nature 411:759–762, 2001.

6. Carroll RC, Beattie EC, Von Zastrow M, Malenka RC: Role of AMPA receptor endocytosis in synaptic plasticity. Nat Rev Neurosci 2:315–324, 2001.

7. Hepler JR, Gilman AG: G proteins. Trends Biochem Sci 17:383–387, 1992.

8. Hamm HE, Gilchrist A: Heterotrimeric G proteins. Curr Opin Cell Biol 8:189–196, 1996.

9. Exton JH: Cell signalling through guanine-nucleotide-binding regulatory proteins and phospholipases. Eur J Biochem 243:10–20, 1997.

10. Coleman DE, Sprang SR: How G proteins work: a continuing story. Trends Biochem 21:41–44, 1996.

11. Yost CS: G proteins: Basic characteristics and clinical potential for the practice of anesthesia. Anesth Analg 77:822–834, 1993.

12. Yamakura T, Bertaccini E, Trudell JR, Harris RA: Anesthetics and ion channels: Molecular models and sites of action. Annu Rev Pharmacol Toxicol 41:23–51.

13. Jackson MB: Ligand-gated channels: postsynaptic receptors and drug targets. Adv Neurol 79:511–524, 1999.

14. Karlin A, Akabas MH: Toward a structural basis for the function of nicotinic acetylcholine receptors and their cousins. Neuron 15:1231–1244, 1995.

15. Jenkins A, Greenblatt EP, Faulkner HJ, et al: Evidence for a common binding cavity for three general anesthetics within the GABAA receptor. J Neurosci 2001;21:RC136.

16. Dingledine R, Borgas K, Bowie D, Traynelis SF: The glutamate receptor ion channels. Pharmacol Rev 51:7–61, 1999.

17. Harris RA, Mihic SJ, Dildy-Mayfield JE, Machu TK: Actions of anesthetics on ligand-gated ion channels: role of receptor subunit composition. FASEB J 9:1454–1462, 1995.

18. Hunter T: Protein kinases and phosphatases: The yin and yang of protein phosphorylation and signaling. Cell 80:225–236, 1995.

19. Van Der Geer P, Hunter T, Lindberg RA: Receptor protein tyrosine kinases and their signal transduction pathways. Annu Rev Cell Biol 10:251–337, 1994.

20. Schlessinger J: Cell signaling by receptor tyrosine kinases. Cell 103:211–225, 2000.

21. Blume-Jensen P, Hunter T: Oncogenic kinase signalling. Nature 411:355–365, 2001.

22. Pawson T, Scott JD: Signaling through scaffold, anchoring and adaptor proteins. Science 278:2075–2080, 1997.

23. Chang L, Karin M: Mammalian MAP kinase signalling cascades. Nature 410:37–40, 2001.

24. Nishida E, Gotoh Y: The MAP kinase cascade is essential for diverse signal transduction pathways. Trends Biochem Sci 18:128–130, 1993.

25. Hill CS, Treisman R: Transcriptional regulation by extracellular signals: mechanisms and specificity. Cell 80:199–211, 1995.

26. Hemmings HC Jr, Nairn AC, McGuinness TL, et al: Role of protein phosphorylation in neuronal signal transduction. FASEB J 3:1583–1592, 1989.

27. Brenman JE, Bredt DS: Synaptic signaling by nitric oxide. Curr Opin Neurobiol 7:374–378, 1997.

28. Moncada S, Higgs A: The L-arginine-nitric oxide pathway. N Engl J Med 329:2002–2012, 1993.

29. Berridge MJ, Lipp P, Bootman MD: The versatility and universality of calcium signalling. Nat Rev Mol Cell Biol 1:11–21, 2000.

30. Divecha N, Irvine RF: Phospholipid signaling. Cell 80:269–278, 1995.

31. Greengard P, Nairn AC, Girault JA, et al: The DARPP-32/protein phosphatase-1 cascade: A model for signal integration. Brain Res Rev 26:274–284, 1998.

3

Signal Transduction Mechanisms

Thomas McDowell, MD, PhD • Misha Perouansky, MD • Robert Pearce, MD, PhD

ION CHANNELS

Ion channels are integral membrane proteins that form an aqueous channel in the lipid bilayer through which charged particles can pass. There are many different types of ion channels, and they may be classified according to the factors that regulate channel opening and closing (gating), as well as the types of ions allowed to traverse the pore (selectivity). This chapter reviews the structure and function of the major classes of channels, focusing on those that are essential to neuronal and cardiac function and signaling. Many have at one time or another been investigated as a target for anesthetic action. These include the voltage-gated ion channels, which open and close in response to changes in the voltage across the cell membrane, and the ligand-gated ion channels, which open and close in response to changes in the presence of various extracellular ligands (e.g., neurotransmitters). Another type of ion channel that has only recently been identified and may be an important site of anesthetic action is the family of so-called background or baseline K^+ channels. These channels are not voltage-gated but are always open, and thus probably function primarily to maintain a negative membrane potential (see the section on voltage-gated potassium channels for discussion).

Basic Membrane Electrophysiology

Membrane Potential Is Determined by Ionic Conductances

Whether ions go into or out of the cell when a channel opens depends on both the membrane potential and the concentration gradient for that ion at the time the channel is open. During physiologic conditions, Na^+, Ca^{2+}, and K^+ ions generally flow down their respective concentration gradients. Thus when their respective channels are opened, Na^+ and Ca^{2+} ions flow into the cell, whereas K^+ ions flow out of the cell. However, Na^+ and Ca^{2+} ions will be repelled from entering the cell if the interior of the cell is very positively charged, whereas K^+ ions tend to be retained in the cell if it is very negatively charged. The membrane potential at which net flow for a particular ion through its channel is zero, and beyond which the direction of flow reverses, can be calculated using the Nernst equation,[1] which is based on thermodynamic principles and is shown in a simplified form as:

$$E_{ion} \approx \frac{60\,mV}{z_{ion}} \log \frac{[ion]_{extracellular}}{[ion]_{intracellular}}$$

In this equation, E_{ion} is the Nernst potential or reversal potential for the ion of interest, z_{ion} is the charge number for the ion, and the log term is the ratio of extracellular to intracellular concentrations of the ion. For the K^+ ion, for example, the ratio of extracellular to intracellular concentrations is approximately 5 mM/150 mM (= 0.033), making E_K about −90 mV. This means that at membrane potentials more positive than −90 mV, K^+ ions will flow out of the cell, whereas at potentials more negative than −90 mV, K^+ ions will flow into the cell. Conversely, the reversal potentials for Na^+ and Ca^{2+} are about +60 mV and +200 mV, respectively, because the concentrations of these ions are greater inside than outside the cell (especially Ca^{2+}, which has a resting intracellular concentration of about 100 nM).

The Nernst equation is used to determine the membrane potential at which no current will flow when the membrane is permeable to only one ion. Excitable cell membranes, however, are permeable to several different ions, mainly Na^+, Ca^{2+}, K^+, and Cl^-. In cells, the membrane potential at which no current flows is the resting membrane potential, and it can be estimated if the concentration gradients and resting conductances of the major permeant ions are known[2] by using the following equation:

$$E_m = \left[\left(\frac{g_{Na}}{g_{total}} \right) E_{Na} + \left(\frac{g_{Ca}}{g_{total}} \right) E_{Ca} + \left(\frac{g_k}{g_{total}} \right) E_K + \left(\frac{g_{Cl}}{g_{total}} \right) E_{Cl} \right]$$

E_m is the resting potential of the membrane, g stands for conductance (the reciprocal of resistance), g_{total} is the sum of all individual ionic conductances, and E_{Na}, E_{Ca}, and so on are the Nernst potentials for each permeant ion. The resting membrane potential is determined by the weighted sum of the Nernst potentials for all permeant ions, the weighting term being the conductance of each ion relative to the total conductance. Therefore, it is easy to see that the membrane potential will trend toward the Nernst potential for a particular ion when the conductance for that ion is large relative to other ionic conductances in the membrane. In normal neurons at rest, E_m is dominated by E_K and E_{Cl} because of the relatively large resting conductances for these ions, and the membrane is hyperpolarized at rest. When Na^+ and Ca^{2+} channels open, however, the membrane depolarizes toward the positive Nernst potentials for these ions.

Voltage-Gated Ion Channels

Three Types of Voltage-Gated Ion Channels

Voltage-gated channels are found in neurons, muscle, and endocrine cells. At normal resting membrane potentials (usually −60 to −80 mV), these channels are closed. When the membrane is depolarized (becomes less negative), the channels undergo a conformational change, which opens the pore of the channel allowing ions to pass through. The type of ion that is allowed to traverse the channel is determined by the structure of the pore and is used to classify the channel. The three main classes of voltage-gated channels are the Na^+, Ca^{2+}, and K^+ channels. Although they share some physical characteristics that determine their voltage sensitivity, other differences in their structures and ionic selectivities define their unique physiologic functions.

Opening and closing of individual ion channels are modeled as nearly instantaneous state transitions of the channel protein that are both voltage-dependent and time-dependent. In the most simple model, the channel can switch from the closed, nonconducting state (*C*) to the open, conducting state (*O*), and then either transition back to the closed state or to an inactivated, nonconducting state (*I*).

$$C \leftrightarrow O \rightarrow I$$

After the channel reaches the inactivated state, it cannot open again until the membrane is hyperpolarized, allowing a transition back to the closed state from which it can once again open. This is referred to as recovery from inactivation.

How Do Voltage-Gated Channels Affect Neuronal Activity and Signaling?

When a channel opens, ions flow passively according to the driving electrical and chemical gradients as described earlier. For Na^+ and K^+ channels, approximately 10^4 to 10^5 ions pass through a single channel each millisecond, and during an action potential, thousands of channels may open. This massive flux of ions, however, may represent only about 0.1% of the total number of ions inside a cell, so the concentration gradients for Na^+ and K^+ do not change much during periods of normal neuronal activity. Conversely, because of the ability of the cell membrane to separate and store electrical charge (the capacitance of the lipid bilayer is about 1 $\mu F/cm^2$), ionic shifts of this magnitude produce enormous changes in membrane potential. It is through these changes in membrane potential that information is coded and rapidly transferred from one part of the cell to another.

For example, consider a peripheral sensory neuron that responds to mechanical deformation of the skin. When the sensory terminal associated with the Ruffini ending in the skin is deformed, a generator potential is evoked in the nerve ending. This is a passive electrical response, in that the ionic shifts that produced the depolarization are short lived and the depolarization will dissipate as the ions travel through their aqueous environment to areas of lower potential energy. If, however, the depolarization reaches a critical threshold level, it will trigger an action potential, a series of complex voltage-dependent and time-dependent changes in ionic conductances. Voltage-gated Na^+ channels in the membrane open, which then produce a rapid depolarization that reaches a peak near the Nernst potential for Na^+. Ca^{2+} and K^+ channels may also be activated at this time. As Na^+ channels inactivate, the membrane potential returns to its resting level and other voltage-gated channels close or inactivate. The action potential is an active, regenerative, all-or-none response of constant magnitude and duration that does not dissipate over space or time. Deformation of the distal sensory nerve terminal, originally sensed as a generator potential, is converted by voltage-gated ion channels to an action potential, which can be propagated from the skin to the spinal cord, and from there to higher brain centers (via chemical synapses) where the skin deformation is sensed.

As described for Na^+ and K^+ channels, opening of voltage-gated Ca^{2+} channels also produces changes in membrane potential as charged Ca^{2+} ions enter the cell. However, Ca^{2+} channels also signal through a different mechanism. Because the intracellular Ca^{2+} concentration is normally maintained at very low levels (about 100 nM) compared with Na^+ (about 10 mM) and K^+ (about 150 mM) ions, the influx of even a small number of Ca^{2+} ions can transiently increase the intracellular Ca^{2+} concentration by several fold. This is particularly true in neuronal presynaptic terminals because of their small volume and high density of Ca^{2+} channels. Increases in intracellular Ca^{2+} can cause neurotransmitter release, open Ca^{2+}-activated ion channels, and regulate Ca^{2+}-dependent kinases and phosphatases.

General Structure of Voltage-Gated Ion Channels

The voltage-gated ion channels are protein complexes formed by the association of several individual subunits. The largest subunit of each channel is termed the α subunit ($α_1$ for the Ca^{2+} channel) (Fig. 3–1). The three-dimensional structure and function of the α subunits of the voltage-gated channels are strikingly similar, reflecting similarities in their voltage-dependent gating and high ionic conductance. If the α subunit of a voltage-gated ion channel is expressed in the absence of other subunits, it forms a channel with ionic selectivity and voltage-dependent behaviors that are similar to those of the native channel. The other subunits that associate with α subunits to form functional channels in vivo are much smaller proteins and are thought to stabilize the α subunit and modulate its function.

The α subunits of the Na^+ and Ca^{2+} channels were the first to be cloned and their primary amino acid sequences were the first to be deduced. These α subunits are large proteins containing four repeating homologous domains (I-IV) separated by long cytoplasmic loops, which allow the four domains to aggregate in the membrane, forming a central pore through which the ions pass (see Fig. 3–1). Each domain consists of six membrane-spanning α-helical segments (S1–S6) that anchor the protein in the membrane. The fourth transmembrane segment (S4) of each domain is considered to be the voltage sensor because it contains between five and eight positively charged amino acids. Movement of these positive charges during changes in transmembrane potential are thought to cause a screwlike rotation or twist in the α helical S4 segment, which produces conformational changes in the protein that ultimately lead to voltage-dependent gating of the channel.[3] The segment of the protein that connects the fifth and sixth transmembrane segments, sometimes called the H5 or P loop, forms part of the outer portion, or outer vestibule, of the pore. The amino acids within the P loop are important in determining the ionic selectivity of the channel. The overall structure of the pore-forming part of the voltage-gated K^+ channel is almost identical to that of the Na^+ and Ca^{2+} channels, the only exception

being that each of the four domains is a separate protein. K^+ channels are thus formed by the aggregation of four individual α subunits into either a homotetramer or, with different α subunits, a heterotetramer.

Individual Voltage-Gated Ion Channels

Na^+ Channels

The voltage-gated Na^+ channel is composed of three different subunits (see Chapter 30 for a detailed discussion). The α subunit is the largest subunit and contains both the pore region of the channel and the voltage sensor. Phosphorylation of the α subunit may alter its function in vivo. Several different genes encoding the Na^+ channel α subunit have been identified, as well as splice variants. These different subunits are preferentially expressed in different tissues or at different times of development.[4] The cytoplasmic linker between domains III and IV is responsible for inactivation of the Na^+ channel. After the channel opens, this segment of the protein is drawn to the inner surface of the channel like a "hinged lid," where it is thought to physically block ions from passing through the pore.[4,5]

In addition to the pore-forming α subunit, the Na^+ channel consists of two other accessory protein subunits. The α subunits of Na^+ channels isolated from rat brain are associated with two additional subunits: $β_1$ and $β_2$. These β subunits are each about one tenth of the mass of the α subunit and are anchored in the cell membrane through one transmembrane segment. They regulate the voltage-dependence and time-dependence of Na^+ current activation and inactivation.[4]

The effects of local anesthetics on Na^+ channel function is described in Chapter 30. General anesthetics, in contrast to local anesthetics, initially seemed to have very little effect on voltage-gated Na^+ channels (for reviews see Elliott and colleagues[6] and Richards[7]). More recent studies, however, have reexamined the effects of anesthetics on Na^+ channels from the central nervous system and found important effects at clinically relevant concentrations of both volatile and intravenous anesthetics.[8,9] Volatile anesthetics inhibit resting Na^+ channels but actually bind more strongly to the inactivated state of the channel, leading to a use-dependent block of Na^+ currents similar to that described for local anesthetics (see Fig. 3–1*B*; see also Chapter 29). The volatile anesthetic concentration at which 50% of the Na^+ current is inhibited was found to be equal to or even less than the concentrations corresponding to minimum alveolar concentration values for the anesthetics when the currents were elicited from the physiological holding potential of −60 mV.[9] At a potential of −60 mV, many more Na^+ channels are in the inactivated state than at more hyperpolarized potentials, thus increasing binding of volatile anesthetics and increasing their effect.

Ca^{2+} Channels

The voltage-gated Ca^{2+} channel is composed of five different subunits. The pore-forming and voltage-sensing portions

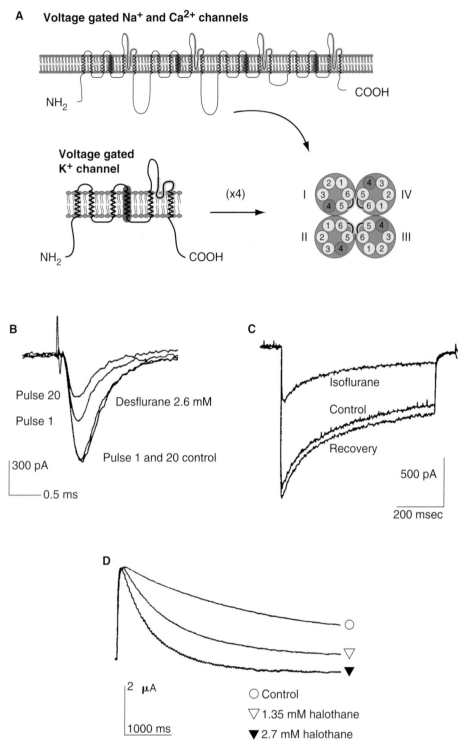

Figure 3–1. Structure of voltage-gated ion channels and the effects of anesthetics. *A,* Drawings of the main subunits of the voltage-gated ion channels are shown. The α subunit of the Na⁺ channel and the α_1 subunit of the Ca^{2+} channel have similar structures, shown schematically by the drawing at the top. A single protein is segregated into four repeating homologous domains (I-IV), each containing six membrane-spanning segments (S1–S6). The α subunit of the voltage-gated K⁺ channel *(A, bottom left)* contains only one domain of six membrane-spanning segments. In each domain of all three types of channels, the fourth transmembrane segment (shown in red) is highly charged and is the voltage sensor. The long extracellular loop between the fifth and sixth transmembrane segments (shown in yellow) forms the outer vestibule of the pore of the channel. In the membrane, four domains are thought to aggregate to form the main structure of the channel, as shown in an "end-on" view *(A, bottom right). B,* Currents through voltage-gated Na⁺ channels recorded from a Chinese hamster ovary cell stably transfected with the gene coding for rat brain IIA sodium channels. Twenty depolarizing voltage steps from –85 to 0mV were

Figure 3–1., cont'd. applied at a frequency of 5 Hz to elicit Na$^+$ currents. The large downward deflections represent inward ionic currents. In control conditions, Na$^+$ current activated and inactivated rapidly during the short depolarizations. The magnitude of the Na$^+$ current did not change after repetitive stimulation (compare pulse 1 and pulse 20). After exposing the cell to a solution containing desflurane (2.6 mM), the Na$^+$ current was immediately reduced (pulse 1) and decreased even more after repetitive stimulation (compare pulse 1 to pulse 20 in the presence of desflurane), indicating both tonic and phasic block of Na$^+$ channels. *C,* Currents through voltage-gated Ca^{2+} channels recorded from an isolated rat hippocampal pyramidal neuron in response to a depolarizing voltage step from –90 to –10 mV. Downward deflections in the traces indicate inward currents. The control current increased rapidly after the voltage step and decayed over time, representing inactivation of Ca^{2+} channels. Open channels closed rapidly at the end of the voltage step. Exposure of the cell to extracellular solution equilibrated with isoflurane 2.5% in the gas phase reduced the magnitude of the Ca^{2+} current evoked by the same voltage step. This inhibition was reversed after washout of anesthetic-containing solution (recovery). *D,* Currents through voltage-gated K$^+$ channels recorded from *Xenopus* oocytes injected with cRNA for the voltage gated K$^+$ channel K_v 2.1. The membrane potential was rapidly stepped from –50 mV to +50 mV at the beginning of the trace and held at +50 mV for 10 seconds. Upward deflections indicate outward membrane current. In control conditions, the K$^+$ current increased rapidly and showed a slow decay over the long depolarization, representing slow inactivation of these K$^+$ channels. Exposure of the cell to extracellular solution containing increasing concentrations of halothane (1.35 and 2.7 mM) did not change the early peak current but markedly accelerated the current inactivation. (*B,* From Rehberg B, Xiao YH, Duch DS: Central nervous system sodium channels are significantly suppressed at clinical concentrations of volatile anesthetics. Anesthesiology 84:1223–1233, 1996; *C,* From Study RE: Isoflurane inhibits multiple voltage-gated calcium currents in hippocampal pyramidal neurons. Anesthesiology 81:104–116, 1994; *D,* From Kulkarni RS, Zorn LJ, Anatharam V, et al: Inhibitory effects of ketamine and halothane on recombinant potassium channels from mammalian brain. Anesthesiology 84:900–909, 1996.)

---

of the voltage-gated Ca^{2+} channel are contained in the largest subunit: the α_1 subunit. Ten isoforms of the α_1 subunit exist. Each isoform generally correlates with one of the different types of Ca^{2+} channel current that historically have been distinguished by their biophysical properties and sensitivities to blockers and toxins.[4,10] Four different α_1 subunits form the large conductance, dihydropyridine-sensitive L-type Ca^{2+} channel: α_{1S}, α_{1C}, α_{1D}, and α_{1F}. The amino acid sequences of these four subunits are greater than 75% identical. All other Ca^{2+} channel α_1 subunits are less than 40% identical to α_{1S}, the first subunit cloned. The major differences lie in the cytoplasmic regions of the protein, with the membrane-spanning segments being conserved. These other subunits are termed α_{1A} (P/Q-type), α_{1B} (N-type), α_{1E} (R-type), and α_{1G}, α_{1H}, and α_{1I} (T-type).[4,10,11] Splice variants of these subunits also exist.

Four accessory subunits have been described. The β subunit of the Ca^{2+} channel, unlike that of the Na$^+$ channel, is an entirely cytoplasmic protein. It associates with the cytoplasmic linker between domains I and II of the α_1 subunit and contains sites that can be phosphorylated by many known kinases. The α_2 and δ subunits are separate proteins formed from a single gene product as a propeptide that are subsequently cleaved and linked together by a disulfide bond. The α_2 subunit is entirely extracellular, whereas the δ subunit contains a transmembrane segment that anchors the $\alpha_2\delta$ complex in the membrane. The β subunit, and to a lesser extent the $\alpha_2\delta$ subunits, modulate the gating of the α_1 subunit, usually by increasing the rates of activation and inactivation of the Ca^{2+} current. Multiple isoforms and splice variants of the β and $\alpha_2\delta$ subunits have been found. Finally, a γ subunit was first identified in skeletal muscle and its gene cloned, but it does not appear to be widely expressed in other tissues, suggesting that its role may be confined to excitation-contraction coupling.[4,11]

The α_{1A} and α_{1B} subunits of the P/Q-type and N-type Ca^{2+} channels, respectively, display two interesting structural features not found in most of the other α_1 subunits. The first is in the cytoplasmic loop linking domains I and II, which contains a site that interacts with the $\beta\gamma$ subunits of inhibitory GTP-binding proteins (G proteins).[12] This molecular interaction is responsible for the well-known inhibition of Ca^{2+} channels by agonists of G protein–coupled receptors (e.g., opioids, norepinephrine, baclofen). The other interesting feature of the α_{1A} and α_{1B} subunits is that the cytoplasmic linker between domains II and III interacts with the soluble *N*-ethylmaleimide-sensitive attachment factor receptor (SNARE) proteins syntaxin and SNAP-25, which are part of the cellular machinery involved in synaptic vesicle exocytosis and neurotransmitter release[13–15] (see also Chapter 9). This interaction may segregate Ca^{2+} channels to parts of the membrane where vesicle docking and release are occurring, allowing Ca^{2+} entry to be localized to these areas.

Most Ca^{2+} channels gate over the same range of voltages as Na$^+$ channels, although the rate of inactivation is much slower. Ca^{2+} channels prolong the duration of the action potential and provide Ca^{2+} entry during depolarization, an effect seen particularly in cardiac ventricular myocytes. T-type Ca^{2+} channels are somewhat unique in that they activate at more hyperpolarized membrane potentials and inactivate more quickly than other types of Ca^{2+} channels. These distinct biophysical properties allow the T-type channel to provide different functions, such as increasing the magnitude of low threshold potentials, neuronal pacemaking, and burst firing.[16]

The effects of general anesthetics on voltage-gated Ca^{2+} channels have been studied in a variety of tissues. Almost all anesthetics tested inhibit Ca^{2+} channels to some extent (see Fig. 3–1*C*). The volatile anesthetics (halothane, isoflurane, and enflurane) reduce Ca^{2+} currents in many types of neuronal tissue,[17–25] although the magnitude and concentration dependence of the effects are somewhat variable. The L-, N-, T-, P/Q-, and R-type channels have all been shown to be sensitive to the anesthetics. As with voltage-gated Na$^+$ channels, anesthetics appear to stabilize the inactivated state of Ca^{2+} channels, as reflected by increases in the rate of Ca^{2+} current inactivation, particularly for T-type current,[19–25] as well as hyperpolarizing shifts in the voltage dependence of inactivation of the current[20,21] and slowing of recovery from inactivation[21] by isoflurane. Further evidence comes from single channel recordings, in which open channel lifetimes were decreased and closed channel lifetimes were increased by halothane, suggesting stabilization of nonconducting (closed, inactivated, or both) states of the channel.[132]

K⁺ Channels

Four individual α subunit proteins aggregate in the cell membrane to create the pore-forming segment of the voltage-gated K⁺ channel (see Fig. 3–1*A*). The N-terminal portion of each protein is mobile in the cytoplasm and has been shown to be responsible for rapid "N-type" inactivation by blocking the pore in a "ball and chain" type of model. The N-terminal "ball" interacts with the small cytoplasmic linker between transmembrane segments 5 and 6 of the α subunit, where it prevents flow of K⁺ ions through the pore of the channel.[26] Only one of the four N-terminal regions is required to produce inactivation, although the rate of inactivation is four times slower if only one subunit retains its N-terminus.[5]

Hydrophilic β subunits associate with the α subunits in a 1:1 stoichiometry to form native K⁺ channels.[4,27] The β subunits of the K⁺ channel, like the β subunits of the Ca^{2+} channel, are thought to be entirely intracellular even though they have little sequence homology to the Ca^{2+} channel β subunits. K⁺ channel β subunits may increase the rates of activation and inactivation of currents through expressed α subunits.

The structure of the bacterial K⁺ channel KcsA has been deduced using x-ray crystallography.[28] The amino acid sequence of this channel is similar to that of voltage-gated K⁺ channel α subunits, although it contains only two transmembrane segments. The KcsA channel is shaped like an "inverted teepee," its narrowest external diameter on the cytoplasmic side. Conversely, the internal pore region is widest at the cytoplasmic end, forming a large water-filled cavity before becoming narrower at the selectivity filter, which is formed by the P loops at the extracellular end of the channel. These features of the pore explain how the K⁺ ion rapidly traverses the membrane in an energetically favorable manner while providing selective passage to K⁺ ions by excluding other cations.

As with Na⁺ and Ca^{2+} channels, voltage-gated K⁺ channels open in response to depolarization of the cell membrane. Historically, K⁺ channel currents have been classified according to their rates and voltage dependences of activation and inactivation. These biophysical attributes (i.e., how the channel responds to voltage over time) define the role that each K⁺ channel has in the cell. For example, delayed rectifier-type K⁺ channels activate rapidly and show little or no inactivation, whereas fast transient, or K_A channels, inactivate rapidly during a depolarization. Delayed rectifiers are found on nerve axons, where they keep axonal action potentials short so Na⁺ channels can recover from inactivation and initiate the next action potential as quickly as possible. Conversely, K_A channels are located at axon hillocks, dendrites, and other regions of the neuron where action potentials are generated. In these areas, passive membrane depolarizations produced by synaptic potentials and receptor potentials are converted to action potentials in a graded fashion, such that larger depolarizations are coded as a higher frequency of action potential firing. K_A channels contribute to this frequency modulation of passive electrical potentials. If K_A channels were not present, all depolarizations above the threshold for action potential generation would elicit the same high frequency of action potential firing, regardless of magnitude.[1]

Delayed rectifier-type K⁺ channels from the squid giant axon are inhibited by anesthetics, but only at high concentrations.[29,30] Interestingly, these normally sustained currents displayed rapid inactivation in the presence of anesthetics, as well as a depolarizing shift in the activation curve (see Fig. 3–1*D*). K_A currents recorded from ventricular myocytes also show enhanced inactivation, a prolongation of recovery from inactivation, and a hyperpolarizing shift in the inactivation curve.[31] These effects are all consistent with anesthetics stabilizing the inactivated state of K⁺ channels. More recent studies of anesthetic action on K⁺ channels have used cloned channels, which have the advantage that specific types of K⁺ channels can be examined in isolation. Both inactivating and noninactivating types of K⁺ channel clones have been shown to be inhibited by clinically appropriate concentrations of halothane[32] (see also Li and Correa[33]). Conversely, isoflurane has been shown to increase currents through a cloned voltage-gated K⁺ channel by increasing the probability of channel opening and stabilizing the open channel state.[33,34]

According to a recent review, more than 200 genes coding for K⁺ channels have been identified, and more than 50 of these are human genes.[35] All K⁺ channels share a highly conserved segment of amino acids within the outer segment of the pore region (e.g., the P loop from the S5–6 linker of the voltage-activated K⁺ channels) that defines the K⁺ selectivity of the channel. This "signature sequence" is incorporated into one of three main types of K⁺ channel structures (Fig. 3–2), thus forming what is commonly referred to as the three major classes of K⁺ channels.[5,27,35,36]

Channels with Six Transmembrane Segments and One Pore (6TM/1P)

K⁺ channels in this family include the voltage-gated channels from the Shaker, Shab, Shaw, and Shal lineage (K_v1–9), the human *ether-a-go-go* (hERG)-related K⁺ channels, K_vLQT channels, and Ca^{2+}-activated K⁺ channels. The α subunits of these channels are thought to form tetramers, and may or may not associate with β-subunits to form a native channel. These types of channels have been described in detail earlier.

Channels with Two Transmembrane Segments and One Pore (2TM/1P)

Channels with this simple structure include the inwardly rectifying K⁺ channels (K_{ir}) and adenosine triphosphate (ATP)-sensitive K⁺ channels (K_{ATP}). K_{ir} channels conduct K⁺ into the cell during hyperpolarization, but K⁺ efflux during depolarization is limited by intracellular Mg^{2+} and polyamines, which block the pore. These channels function primarily to maintain a hyperpolarized membrane potential. K_{ATP} channels are formed from a complex of four inwardly rectifying

A   Different classes of K⁺ channels

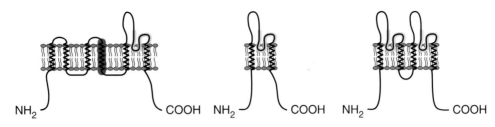

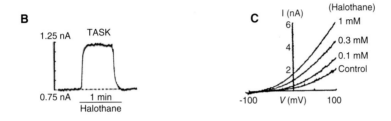

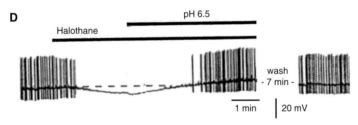

Figure 3–2. Structures of the main classes of K⁺ channels and the effects of anesthetics. *A,* Drawings of the three main classes of K⁺ selective channels are shown. They differ in the number of transmembrane (TM) segments and in the number of P loop (P) segments in each subunit. *A, Left to Right,* The 6TM/1P class of voltage-gated K⁺ channels (reproduced from Fig. 1*A* to facilitate comparison among the K⁺ channel classes); the 2TM/1P class (including K_{ir} and K_{ATP} channels); and the 4TM/2P class, also known as the two pore or tandem pore domain K⁺ channels. *B,* Membrane current measured at a holding potential of 0 mV in a COS cell transfected with DNA containing the human *TASK* gene. Application of halothane (1 mM) rapidly and reversibly increased outward currents, indicating activation of the TASK channel by halothane. *C,* Membrane current-voltage relations in a COS cell transfected with DNA containing the human *TREK-1* gene. Current was recorded during a rapid linear increase in membrane potential in the absence (control) and the presence of various concentrations of halothane in solution. Outward current is positive. Halothane increased currents through the TREK-1 channel. *D,* Membrane potential recorded from a rat locus ceruleus neuron in the presence of bicuculline and strychnine to block γ-aminobutyric acid type A receptor (GABA_A) and glycine receptors, respectively, in a brain slice preparation. These neurons contain mRNA for TASK-1.[43] Spontaneous action potential firing is seen at the beginning of the trace. Halothane (0.3 mM) hyperpolarized the membrane and inhibited action potential firing. Acidifying the extracellular solution (pH 6.5) reversed the hyperpolarization, as would be expected if the effect of halothane was caused by activation of the TASK-1 channel, which is inhibited by acidic solutions. (*B,C,* From Patel AJ, Honore E, Lesage, et al: Inhalational anesthetics activate two-pore-domain background K+ channels. Nat Neurosci 2:422–426, 1999; *D,* From Sirois JE, Lei Q, Talley EM, et al: The TASK-1 two-pore domain K+ channel is a molecular substrate for neuronal effects of inhalation anesthetics. J Neurosci 20:6347–6354, 2000.

K+ channel subunits and four sulfonylurea receptors. K_{ATP} channels close with increases in the intracellular ATP/adenosine diphosphate (ADP) ratio, thus coupling membrane potential and electrical excitability to the metabolic state of the cell. In pancreatic β-cells, inhibition of K_{ATP} channels causes insulin secretion. In myocardium and neuronal tissues, activation of K_{ATP} channels protects cells from ischemic, or hypoxic insults, or both. In vascular smooth muscle, K_{ATP} channel activation produces vasodilation and may mediate autoregulation in the coronary and cerebral circulations.[27,37]

Channels with Four Transmembrane Segments and Two Pores (4TM/2P)

Channels with four transmembrane segments and two pores are variously referred to as 4TM/2P, KCNK, K_{2P}, two pore domain, or tandem pore domain channels. To date, eight different channels in this family have been cloned in rodents and humans, and include TWIK (tandem of P domains in weak inward rectifier K^+ channels), TREK (TWIK-related K^+ channels), TASK (TWIK-related acid-sensitive K^+ channels), and TRAAK (TWIK-related arachidonic-acid-stimulated K^+ channels), which are expressed in a variety of mammalian tissues including neurons.[38] Tandem pore domain channels are always open and show little or no activation or inactivation. Their primary function seems to be maintenance of a hyperpolarized membrane potential by providing a constant background or baseline potassium "leak" conductance.

Tandem pore domain K^+ channels may be an important target for anesthetic action. In the early 1980s, Nicoll and Madison[39] reported that anesthetics produce an increase in K^+ conductance that caused hyperpolarization in a variety of neurons. Since then, reports of an increased leak conductance in the presence of anesthetics have continued, but only recently have tandem pore domain K^+ channels emerged as the likely molecular substrate for this effect (see Fig. 3–2*B* to *D*).[40-44] Volatile anesthetics activate TASK and TREK-1 channels, but not TRAAK channels, expressed in mammalian cells.[60,142,167] In rat hypoglossal motoneurons and locus ceruleus neurons, which both contain mRNA for TASK-1, anesthetics activate a potassium conductance with properties similar to those of expressed TASK-1.[44] Anesthetics hyperpolarize these neurons by up to 13 mV and inhibit their spontaneous electrical activity at clinically appropriate concentrations.[44]

Ligand-Gated Ion Channels

Ionotropic and Metabotropic Receptors

Neurotransmitters, hormones, and other small molecules released as intercellular messengers influence the activity of ion channels through two types of receptors. In the case of *ionotropic* receptors, such as the nicotinic acetylcholine receptor (nAChR) found at the neuromuscular junction, the transmitter binding site and the transmembrane ion channel are integral to a single protein (or protein complex, because most ion channels are formed as multimers of homologous or heterologous subunits). Binding of the transmitter directly alters the activity of the ion channel, allowing the flow of cations across the membrane for nAChR, which results in depolarization. Receptors that operate in this fashion are responsible for rapid synaptic transmission (over a time scale of milliseconds), although these may also display sustained or tonic activity. In the case of *metabotropic* receptors, such as the β-adrenergic receptor found in cardiac myocytes, the transmitter receptor (binding site) and the effector (calcium channels) are separate molecules. They are coupled through GTP-binding proteins (G proteins), either indirectly through cascades of intracellular signaling pathways, or more directly through membrane-delimited pathways where subunits of the G protein directly alters ion channel activity (see Chapter 2). The time course of action through metabotropic receptors is much slower than ionotropic receptors, typically operating over a time scale of seconds or even minutes, although in rare cases activation and deactivation occur as rapidly as 50 ms. G protein–coupled pathways are dealt with more extensively in Chapter 2, therefore the discussion in this chapter is limited primarily to ionotropic receptors. However, it should be noted that many of the ligand-gated as well as voltage-gated ion channels discussed in this chapter are subject to modulation through second messengers initiated by metabotropic receptors.

Three Families of Ionotropic Receptors

Just as voltage-gated channels are grouped into families on the basis of sequence similarities between the genes that encode different members, ligand-gated ion channels also have been grouped into three separate families based on sequence homology. The largest and most diverse family includes the nAChR, the ionotropic serotonin receptor (5-HT$_3$), the γ-aminobutyric acid type A receptor (GABA$_A$), and the glycine receptor. The N-terminus of each subunit of these receptors contains a characteristic 15-member loop that is formed by the disulfide linkage between a pair of cysteines, consequently recently this family has been referred to as the "Cys-loop" family.[45] Each of these receptors is a pentamer, composed of five homologous subunits, each with four transmembrane (TM) segments and an extracellular N-terminus segment that contains residues that form the neurotransmitter binding site (Fig. 3–3; see also Chapters 10, 24, and 25). Two of these receptors are cation-selective and excitatory (nAChR and 5-HT$_3$) and two are anion-selective and inhibitory (GABA$_A$ and glycine). The second family of receptors is activated by glutamate, the major excitatory neurotransmitter in the brain. Different combinations of subunits form channels that are activated by the selective ligands *N*-methyl-D-aspartate (NMDA), α-amino-3-hydroxy-5-methylisoxazole-4-propionic acid (AMPA), and kainate (KA). Each of these receptors is composed of four subunits, each of which has four transmembrane segments and a P loop that is structurally similar to that of voltage-activated channels. The third family of ionotropic receptors,

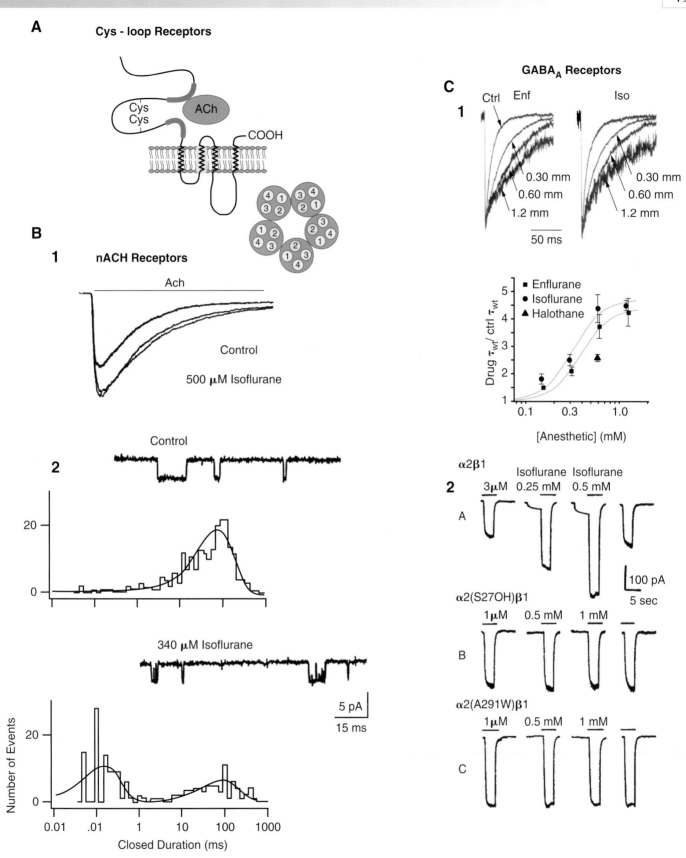

Figure 3–3. The Cys-loop receptor family of ligand-gated channels. Topology of Cys-loop receptors. *A,* Each subunit contains four membrane-spanning segments, designated TM1-TM4. The second segment, TM2 (shown in yellow), lines the pore of the channel. The transmitter-binding site (shown in red) is formed by several discontiguous loops formed by the large extracellular N-terminal domain. *B,* Functional receptors are composed of five subunits in a pseudosymmetrical arrangement. Ctrl, Control; Enf, enflurane; GABA_A, γ-aminobutyric acid type A receptor; Iso, isoflurane; nACh, nicotinic acetylcholine receptor.

termed P2X receptors, binds ATP in the extracellular space. Compared with the other two families much less is known about their structural and functional characteristics. Like the other ionotropic receptors, P2X receptors are multimers, but each subunit contains only two putative transmembrane domains. The number of subunits that combine to form a functional channel has not yet been determined, and may be as few as three or as many as six.

Cys-Loop Family (nAChR, GABA$_A$, Glycine, and 5-HT$_3$)

The transmitter binding sites for all receptors in this family are located at the interfaces between subunits,[46] and it is thought that at least two transmitter molecules are required to produce full channel activation, as reflected in Hill coefficients greater than one.[47,48] It has proved difficult to determine the precise stoichiometry and subunit composition of the majority of receptors in the brain, but it seems clear that the majority of receptors are heteromeric, composed of subunits from multiple classes, and even multiple subunits from a single class for some receptors[49,50] (see Chapters 10, 24, and 25 for further discussion of the Cys-loop family).

One TM2 segment from each subunit lines the ion-conducting pore of the channel, and the other TM segments are presumed to form rings around this central pore in contact with membrane lipids. Mutation of the channel-facing residues of TM2 leads to alterations in conductance and ion selectivity, and it has even been possible to change normally cation-selective channels to anion-selective channels and vice versa in chimeric receptors and through mutation of selected residues.[51-53] Whereas in the voltage-gated potassium channel the P loop located at the extracellular end of the channel confers charge selectivity, in the Cys-loop family an analogous coiled-loop structure that may serve a similar function is located at the cytoplasmic end of the channel.[52] The location of the "gate" appears to be close to the cytoplasmic end of the channel, but the mechanism by which ligand binding becomes transduced to channel gating remains unknown. In this chapter only the glycine and 5-HT$_3$ receptors of the Cys-loop family will be described; the other members are described in Chapters 10 (nAChR), 24 and 25 (GABA$_A$ receptor).

Glycine Receptors

Glycine receptors are closely related to GABA$_A$ receptors. They also are inhibitory receptors, selectively permeable to anions, and mediate rapid inhibitory synaptic transmission, primarily in the spinal cord. They are insensitive to bicuculline but inhibited by strychnine. Unlike GABA$_A$ receptors, which form functional receptors only as heteromers, glycine receptors are homomers of α subunits, of which several subtypes have been identified.[45]

Like GABA$_A$ receptors, the activity of glycine receptors is also enhanced by volatile anesthetics and alcohols.[54] This effect may play a role in the suppression of movement through a spinal action of these agents, but the inability to reverse anesthetic effects through spinal administration of glycine receptor antagonists suggests that this is not the entire mechanism by which movement is abolished by volatile agents.[55]

5-HT$_3$ Receptors

Many subtypes of serotonin (5-hydroxytryptophan or 5-HT) receptors exist, but with the exception of the ionotropic 5-HT$_3$ subtype all are metabotropic (G protein–coupled). Ionotropic 5-HT$_3$ receptors are excitatory, selectively permeable to cations, and may play a variety of roles in the central nervous system (CNS), including anxiolytic,[56] analgesic,[57] and emetic.[58] 5-HT$_3$ antagonists, such as ondansetron and dolasetron, have been widely used in the prevention and treatment of postoperative nausea and vomiting[59] and may also be useful in the treatment of inflammatory bowel syndrome.[60]

The P2X Receptor Family

ATP is used not only as a cellular fuel but also as a signaling molecule (see Khakh[61] for a recent review). Specialized receptors that respond to extracellular ATP, termed purinergic type 2 (P2) receptors to distinguish them from adenosine-sensitive purinergic type 1 (P1) receptors, exist as metabotropic (P2Y) and ionotropic (P2X) receptors. Seven different P2X receptor subunits have been identified to date. It is known that they combine to form homomultimers and heteromultimers, but the number of subunits that are required to form functional channels is not known. These subunits are structurally much simpler than the other ligand-gated channels, with only two transmembrane domains per subunit. A large cysteine-rich extracellular loop forms the ligand-binding domain. Channels are permeable to cations, but show little selectivity, with approximately equal permeability to Na^+ and K^+ and significant permeability to Ca^{2+}.

P2X receptors are found throughout the body and brain. In the smooth muscle of blood vessels and vas deferens they mediate constriction,[62] and in sensory neurons they may be involved in certain types of pain.[63] Because of the relatively recent identification of this family of receptors and the lack of subtype-specific antagonists, our understanding of the roles that are played by these receptors is limited. However, given their wide distribution it is clear that further research will uncover important roles.

Glutamate Receptor Family

Glutamate as a Neurotransmitter

Glutamate's role as an excitatory neurotransmitter is detailed in Chapter 9. In addition, glutamate and its receptors provide an important molecular interface for neuron-glia interaction–ionotropic and metabotropic glutamate receptors are widely expressed in various types of glial cells.[64] Glutamate released from neurons can activate these receptors and cause several effects including modulation of transmitter uptake into glial cells, thereby affecting synaptic transmission,[65] modulation of K^+ conductances within glial cells and consequent changes in the extracellular ion composition, and release of neuroactive substances from glia that can feedback and modulate synaptic transmission.[66]

Glutamic acid is found in very high levels in the CNS. Because it does not cross the blood–brain barrier, it must originate from local metabolism. It participates in intermediary glucose metabolism in addition to its role in intercellular communication and therefore shares with GABA the problem of dissociating neurotransmitter and metabolic roles. Glutamate is formed through two distinct pathways: either from glucose in the Krebs cycle and transamination of α-ketoglutarate or directly from glutamine. Inactivation of released glutamate is mainly through reuptake by dicarboxylic acid transporters, and enzymatic inactivation does not play a significant role. Glutamate also serves as the substrate source for glutamic acid decarboxylase, the GABA synthesizing enzyme (Fig. 3–4A).

Three Types of Ionotropic Glutamate Receptors

Glutamate acts through two types of receptors: metabotropic (mGluR) and ionotropic (iGluR) glutamate receptors. The ionotropic family comprises three classes of receptors based on agonist specificities: AMPA (formerly known as quisqualate), kainate, and NMDA receptors. The former two families were collectively referred to as non-NMDA receptors, because neither agonists nor antagonists clearly (until recently) distinguished between them. Cloning studies have demonstrated, however, that AMPA and kainate activate distinct receptor complexes (Fig. 3–4B).

The ionotropic glutamate receptors are tetrameric proteins—four subunits assemble to form a functional receptor-channel complex. Each subunit consists of a large extracellular N-terminus domain, three hydrophobic transmembrane segments (M1, M3, M4), and an intracellular C-terminus (Fig. 3–5). The pore region is formed by the amphipathic reentrant hairpin loop M2, similar in structure to the pore-forming region of K^+ channels. The ligand binds to two regions, one before M1, the other between M3 and M4.[67]

α-Amino-3-hydroxy-5-methylisoxazole-4-propionic Acid Receptors

AMPA receptors mediate fast excitatory transmission at most synapses in the CNS. The four subunits that are combined to form these receptors, GluR1-GluR4, are encoded by four closely related genes, and each subunit exists in two alternative splice variants: flip and flop. In the rodent embryonic brain, AMPA receptors are expressed predominantly as flip variants. Adult levels of the flop variant, which carries most of the excitatory transmission in the adult brain, are reached by the 14th postnatal day. AMPA receptors are either

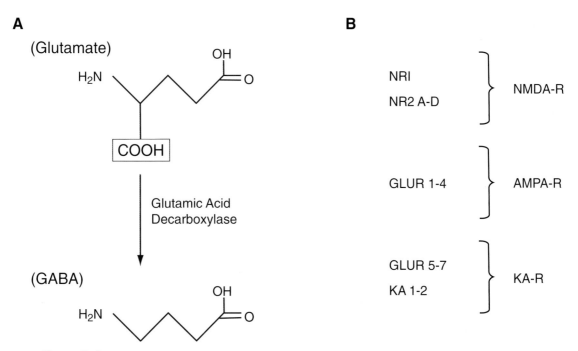

Figure 3–4. Glutamate in the central nervous system (CNS). *A,* L-glutamate ((S)-glutamate according to the official IUPAC nomenclature) has an acidic side chain that carries a negative charge at physiologic pH. In the CNS, it serves as the only substrate for the γ-aminobutyric acid (GABA) synthesizing enzyme glutamic acid decarboxylase. *B,* The ionotropic glutamate receptors are classified into three subtypes according to the most selective agonist available: N-methyl-D-aspartate (NMDA), α-amino-3-hydroxy-5-methylisoxazole-4-propionic acid (AMPA [formerly quisqualate]), and kainate (KA). Each subtype comprises several subunits and different splice variants exist for numerous subunits. Native receptors are likely to be heteromultimers.

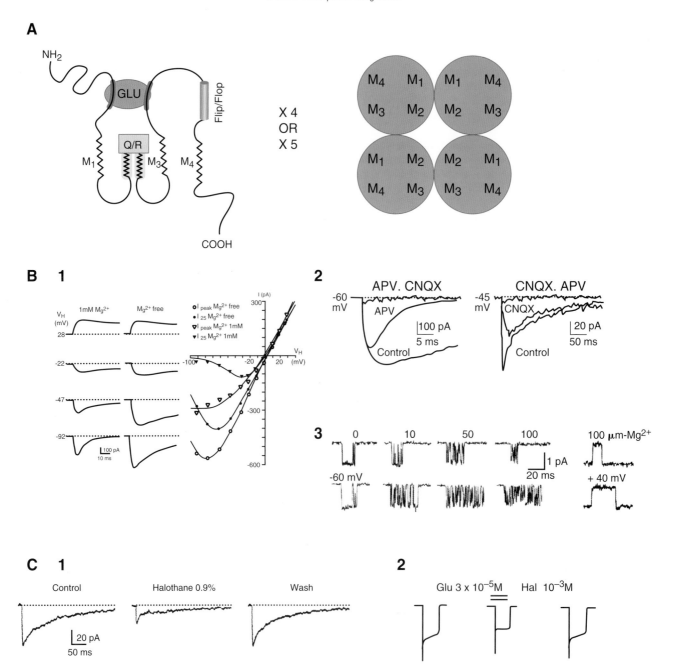

Figure 3–5. Glutamate receptors (GluR). *A,* Structure of GluR subunits. The three transmembrane domains (M1, M3, M4) and the pore-lining M2 loop are arranged as proposed by Hollmann et al.[117] The permeability determining Q/R site is positioned at the tip of the loop, facing the extracellular vestibule.[118] The box in the extracellular loop between M3 and M4 indicates the region where alternative splicing (flip/flop variants) occurs. Agonist binding properties are determined by two discontiguous segments located between the N-terminus and M1 and between M3 and M4. The subunit stoichiometry of glutamate receptors is not entirely clear: both tetrameric and pentameric structures have been proposed (for review see Dingledine[119]). Here, a heterotetrameric structure with the M2 loop lining the pore region is illustrated schematically. *B,* Basic physiology and pharmacology of glutamate receptor–mediated excitatory postsynaptic currents (glu-EPSCs). glu-EPSCs consist typically of a non-NMDA and an NMDA receptor–mediated component. *B1,* In Mg^{2+}-containing solution, glu-EPSCs have a fast time course at negative holding potentials, determined mainly by the non-NMDA receptor–mediated component. Depolarization of the holding potential removes the voltage-dependent block of the NMDA receptor channels by Mg^{2+} and recruits a slow glu-EPSC component. In Mg^{2+}-free saline, the slow, NMDA receptor–mediated component is present at all holding potentials. Plotting the current-voltage relationship of this glu-EPSC graphically illustrates these issues. The non-NMDA receptor–mediated component of the EPSC shows a linear current-voltage relationship across a wide range of voltages in the presence (*open triangles*) and absence (*open circles*) of Mg^{2+}. The NMDA receptor-mediated component, by contrast, displays a nonlinear behavior at voltages more negative than –20 mV

Figure 3–5, cont'd. in the presence of Mg^{2+} (*closed triangles*, negative slope conductance) that is rectified in nominally Mg^{2+}-free saline (*closed circles*). The nonlinearities of the I/V relationships in "Mg^{2+}-free" saline at negative holding potentials are probably caused by residual Mg^{2+}. *B2,* Selective antagonists were instrumental in delineating the physiologic roles of the glu-EPSC components. The slow, NMDA receptor–mediated component can be blocked by aminophosphonovaleric acid (APV), leaving the non-NMDA receptor–mediated component that is sensitive to 6-nitro-7-cyano-quinoxaline-2,3-dion (CNQX), which does not distinguish between α-amino-3-hydroxy-5-methylisoxazole-4-propionic acid (AMPA) and kainate receptors. Conversely, application of CNQX leaves a slow APV-sensitive component. *B3,* The Mg^{2+} block is further illustrated in two single channel recordings: long channel openings induced by NMDA are dose-dependently blocked by increasing Mg^{2+} concentrations at –60 mV, evidenced by increasing "flickering" of the channel. Flickering is absent at +40 mV. *C1,* EPSCs recorded from hippocampal CA1 pyramidal cells in acute mouse slices (from [214]). *C2,* Single channel recordings obtained from cultured mouse central neurons. (From Violet JM, Downie DL, Nakisa RC, et al: Differential sensitivities of mammalian neuronal and muscle nicotinic acetylcholine receptors to general anesthetics. Anesthesia 86:866–874, 1997.)

---

homomeric or heteromeric tetramers composed of these multiple subunits, which results in a marked functional diversity of the native receptors.

AMPA receptor channels are permeable to cations. Glutamate and AMPA elicit rapidly desensitizing responses in the AMPA receptor, whereas AMPA receptor-mediated responses to kainate do not desensitize.[68,69] The speed of desensitization depends on the subunit composition and on the splice variant (flip or flop) and can vary by more than an order of magnitude.[43,70]

Three different binding sites can be identified on AMPA receptors: a site that binds agonist (glutamate), a site that binds drugs that alter desensitization, and an intra-ion channel binding sites that binds blockers. The binding site for glutamate and competitive antagonists is formed by two discontiguous segments located between the N-terminal and M1 and between M3 and M4, respectively.[71] A separate site binds aniracetam (a pyrrolidine) and CTZ (cyclothiazide, a benzothiadiazine). Binding of these drugs removes desensitization in the flip variants.[72–74] A third binding site located near the intracellular entrance to the channel pore binds a variety of spider and wasp toxins, all of which act as channel blockers.

The AMPA receptor–mediated component of the glutamatergic excitatory postsynaptic current (EPSC) is characterized by its fast time course. As at other fast chemical synapses, this is the result of a brief (~1 ms) high concentration (~1 mM) transient of transmitter in the cleft.[75] Diffusion of transmitter away from the synaptic cleft appears to be very rapid (estimated time constant = 1.2 ms[75]), and deactivation rather than desensitization of receptors determines the time constant of EPSC decay.[76,77] At certain synapses, however, desensitization may be the determining factor.[78]

Typically, postsynaptic Ca^{2+} entry at a glutamatergic synapse takes place through NMDA receptor channels, with AMPA receptor-mediated depolarization of the postsynaptic membrane relieving the voltage-dependent block of NMDA receptor channels by Mg^{2+}. Recently, mice lacking the GluR2 subunit have been produced by gene targeting.[79] Despite the increased Ca^{2+} permeability and the ensuing physiologic changes in vitro, these mice survived into adulthood without obvious deficits except for reduced anesthetic drug requirements for certain anesthetic endpoints.[80,81]

Kainate Receptors

The kainate receptor family (KAR) comprises two groups of subunits (GluR5, GluR6, GluR7 and KA1, KA2), which differ in molecular size, percentage of sequence identity, affinity to kainate, and distribution throughout the CNS. Although AMPA and kainate receptor subunits can coexist in the same neuron,[79] they do not coassemble with each other.[82]

Our understanding of the physiologic role of KARs lags behind that of the other ionotropic glutamate receptors. The primary reason is that kainic acid, the agonist most frequently used to activate KARs, elicits large nondesensitizing currents at AMPA receptors and small desensitizing responses at native KARs, thereby obscuring kainate channel activity in native preparations. Conversely, AMPA activates certain KARs; hence the encompassing term non-NMDA receptors. Currently available KAR selective drugs are either difficult to use in the slice preparation (e.g., concanavalin A, a lectin that removes KAR desensitization[83,84]) or are selective for certain subunits (e.g., GluR5) with limited expression in the CNS,[85] making it difficult to assess the roles of specific subunit combinations in native receptors present at different sites in the CNS.

Despite these difficulties, a physiologic role for KARs has been demonstrated in rat hippocampus. Whereas rapid synaptic transmission does not seem to involve postsynaptic kainate receptors,[86] they do play an important role in modulation of transmitter release.[87] In the hippocampal CA3 region, release of GABA onto pyramidal cells and interneurons appears to be differentially regulated by kainate receptors. Functional native kainate receptors also have been demonstrated in dorsal root ganglion neurons.[88] Certain areas, e.g., the hippocampal CA3, show particularly high levels of kainate receptor expression.[89] It has been noted earlier that these areas are particularly susceptible to excitotoxic injury, and it has been proposed that kainate receptors may play a causal role.

N-methyl-D-aspartate Receptors

The NMDA receptor family comprises five subunits: the "fundamental" NR1 and the "modulatory" NR2A-NR2D. The NR1 subunit can form homomeric receptor channels with the basic NMDA receptor channel properties but small amplitude current responses.[90] NR2 subunits do not form functional receptors on their own but their coexpression with NR1 amplifies the current responses through the heteromeric receptors by several orders.[91] As for the other glutamate receptors, diversity is increased with alternative splicing—eight splice variants have been reported for the NR1 subunit.[91] In situ hybridization and immunohistochemistry have determined that the NR1 subunit is ubiquitous in the rodent brain. The NR2 subunits show distinct regional patterns and developmental changes in subunit expression.[92,93] NMDA receptor channels mediate excitatory neurotransmission in a way that is different from and complementary to the frequently colocalized AMPA receptors. AMPA receptors have a low affinity to glutamate, fast binding, and unbinding kinetics. NMDA receptors, by contrast, have high affinity to glutamate, prolonged binding, and repeated channel openings. The 10% to 90% rise time of NMDA receptor–gated currents is ~10 ms, which means that the AMPA receptor–mediated component of the synaptic current has mostly decayed before the NMDA component reaches its peak. The desensitization of NMDA receptors varies depending on the experimental conditions but is always significantly slower than the desensitization of AMPA receptors.[94–96] In contrast to AMPA receptors, a high permeability for Ca^{2+} is the rule rather than the exception for NMDA receptor channels. The Ca^{2+} permeability is characteristically combined with a voltage-dependent block of the channel by Mg^{2+}. Single channel studies have shown that the NMDA receptor channel has a conductance of 40–50 pS in saline containing no Mg^{2+}. Addition of Mg^{2+} causes the single channel currents to occur in bursts of short-lasting openings separated by brief closures, implicating a block of the open channel.[97,98] In addition, the degree of sensitivity to block by Mg^{2+} is determined by the type of NR2 subunit that forms the receptor-channel complex.[99,100] Glycine is an essential coagonist of glutamate at the NMDA receptor. It binds to the NR1 subunit at a region that corresponds to the glutamate recognition site at the NR2 subunits and has been termed the strychnine-insensitive glycine binding site. The ED_{50} of glycine is 0.1 to 0.7 μM.[101] D-serine and D-alanine are naturally occurring agonists at the glycine site. Considering that the extracellular concentration of D-serine in rodent frontal cortex is 6.5 μM, enough to saturate the glycine-binding site of the NMDA receptor, D-serine may also act as an endogenous coagonist.[102] In addition, drugs affecting the NMDA receptor can bind at the intra-ion channel binding site and at multiple modulatory sites, such as the redox, the H^+, the Zn^{2+}, and the polyamine binding sites.[103]

The NMDA receptor plays a special role in synaptic transmission. At resting membrane potential the channel is blocked by Mg^{2+} and current flows only if the neuronal membrane is depolarized when the Mg^{2+} block is relieved (see Fig. 3–5B). This depolarization is provided in the *post-natal* brain typically by AMPA receptors, which have been shown to colocalize at the same synapses.[104] In the *prenatal* brain, glutamatergic synapses may lack AMPA receptors. There, the depolarization necessary to remove the Mg^{2+} block can be provided by $GABA_A$ receptors, because of a more depolarized reversal potential for Cl^-.[105] Once current flows, extracellular Ca^{2+} enters the cell through the NMDA receptor channel. Once activated, NMDA receptor–mediated synaptic currents last for prolonged periods of time. Taken together, these properties enable the NMDA receptor channel to function as a "coincidence detector" of presynaptic activity and postsynaptic depolarization and,

through the injection of Ca^{2+}, to play a critical role in synaptogenesis and to initiate plastic changes in the strength of synaptic connections. Long-term potentiation (the strengthening of synaptic connections)[106–108] and long-term depression (the weakening of synaptic connections)[109,110] are changes that depend on the temporal pattern of synaptic activity and are mediated through glutamate receptors.

It is not surprising that the most important excitatory neurotransmitter system is also involved in important pathologic processes in the nervous system. Even though no pathogenic mutation has yet been demonstrated in a human glutamate receptor gene (mouse knockout mutations of these genes produce mild to severe neurologic symptoms), changes in the expression patterns of glutamate receptors seem to contribute to drug-induced behavioral adaptations, as evidenced by increased GluR1 levels in some parts of the brain that are found with chronic alcohol, cocaine, and morphine use. Mutations in GluR6 may influence the age of onset of Huntington disease. Better understood is the relationship between activation of the glutamatergic system during abnormal conditions or abnormal activation of the glutamatergic transmitter system leading to neuronal injury and cell death, collectively referred to as "excitotoxicity." Typical examples include focal and global ischemia, hypoglycemia and physical trauma, metabolic poisoning, drug abuse, certain food toxicities, and epilepsy. Glutamate, acting at its various receptors, induces neuronal death by (1) an increase in intracellular free Ca^{2+}, which activates a number of proteases, phospholipases, and endonucleases; (2) generation of free radicals that destroy cellular membranes; and (3) induction of apoptosis.[111] The ability of certain anesthetic agents to block the NMDA receptor has opened up the possibility that there are some anesthetics for which NMDA block contributes importantly to their anesthetic action. This class of anesthetic, exemplified by xenon,[112] nitrous oxide,[113] and ketamine,[114,115] reduce the efficacy of excitatory neurotransmission by "inhibiting" glutamate receptors. These anesthetic agents also have been used in pathologic settings in which the excitotoxic action of glutamate on NMDA receptors plays a prominent role.[116]

Summary

The great variety of ion channels present in excitable tissue endows cells with the potential for tremendous flexibility in integrating and transmitting information, transducing extracellular signals into cellular responses, and responding to changing environmental conditions. Many of the drugs that are used clinically act by modulating ion channel activity, in many cases acting on multiple types of channels to produce desirable actions as well as undesirable side effects. Traditional classification schemes based on pharmacologic characteristics are being supplemented or supplanted by schemes based on an emerging understanding of the underlying molecular components. In many cases these two approaches have become integrated, but in others there remains a separation that awaits fuller characterization of the pharmacologic properties of various gene products. It is hoped that more specific pharmacologic agents will result from our emerging understanding of the roles played by the various channels in normal function and in pathologic conditions.

References

1. Hille B: Ionic Channels of Excitable Membranes, 2nd ed. Sunderland, Mass, Sinauer Associates, 1992.
2. Hodgkin AL, Huxley AF: A quantitative description of membrane current and its application to conduction and excitation in nerve. J Physiol 117:500–544, 1952.
3. Glauner KS, Mannuzzu LM, Gandhi CS, Isacoff EY: Spectroscopic mapping of voltage sensor movement in the Shaker potassium channel. Nature 402:813–817, 1999.
4. Catterall WA: Structure and function of voltage-gated ion channels. Ann Rev Biochem 64:493–531, 1995.
5. Armstrong CM, Hille B: Voltage-gated ion channels and electrical excitability. Neuron 20:371–380, 1998.
6. Elliott JR, Elliott AA, Harper AA, et al: Effects of general anaesthetics on neuronal sodium and potassium channels. Gen Pharmacol 23:1005–1011, 1992.
7. Richards CD: The synaptic basis of general anaesthesia. Eur J Anaesthesiol 12:5–19, 1995.
8. Rehberg B, Duch DS: Suppression of central nervous system sodium channels by propofol. Anesthesiology 91:512–520, 1999.
9. Rehberg B, Xiao YH, Duch DS: Central nervous system sodium channels are significantly suppressed at clinical concentrations of volatile anesthetics. Anesthesiology 84:1223–1233, 1996.
10. Stotz SC, Zamponi GW: Structural determinants of fast inactivation of high voltage-activated Ca^{2+} channels. Trends Neurosci 24:176–181, 2001.
11. Perez-Reyes E, Schneider T: Calcium channels: structure, function, and classification. Drug Dev Res 33:295–318, 1994.
12. Dolphin AC: Mechanisms of modulation of voltage-dependent calcium channels by G proteins. J Physiol 506:3–11, 1998.
13. Rettig J, Sheng ZH, Kim DK, et al: Isoform-specific interaction of the alpha1A subunits of brain Ca^{2+} channels with the presynaptic proteins syntaxin and SNAP-25. Proc Natl Acad Sci USA 93:7363–7368, 1996.
14. Sheng ZH, Rettig J, Cook T, Catterall WA: Calcium-dependent interaction of N-type calcium channels with the synaptic core complex. Nature 379:451–454, 1996.
15. Sheng ZH, Rettig J, Takahashi M, Catterall WA: Identification of a syntaxin-binding site on N-type calcium channels. Neuron 13:1303–1313, 1994.
16. Huguenard JR: Low-threshold calcium currents in central nervous system neurons. Ann Rev Physiol 58:329–348, 1996.
17. McDowell TS, Pancrazio JJ, Lynch C: Volatile anesthetics reduce low-voltage-activated calcium currents in a thyroid C-cell line. Anesthesiology 85:1167–1175, 1996.
18. Hall AC, Lieb WR, Franks NP: Insensitivity of P-type calcium channels to inhalational and intravenous general anesthetics. Anesthesiology 81:117–123, 1994.
19. Herrington J, Stern RC, Evers AS, Lingle CJ: Halothane inhibits two components of calcium current in clonal (GH3) pituitary cells. J Neurosci 11:2226–2240, 1991.
20. Kamatchi GL, Chan CK, Snutch T, et al: Volatile anesthetic inhibition of neuronal Ca channel currents expressed in Xenopus oocytes. Brain Res 831:85–96, 1999.
21. Kameyama K, Aono K, Kitamura K: Isoflurane inhibits neuronal Ca^{2+} channels through enhancement of current inactivation. Br J Anesth 82:402–411, 1999.
22. Nikonorov IM, Blanck TJ, Recio-Pinto E: The effects of halothane on single human neuronal L-type calcium channels. Anesth Analg 86:885–895, 1998.
23. Study RE: Isoflurane inhibits multiple voltage-gated calcium currents in hippocampal pyramidal neurons. Anesthesiology 81:104–116, 1994.
24. Takenoshita M, Steinbach JH: Halothane blocks low-voltage-activated calcium current in rat sensory neurons. J Neurosci 11:1404–1412, 1991.
25. Todorovic SM, Perez-Reyes E, Lingle CJ: Anticonvulsants but not general anesthetics have differential blocking effects on different T-type current variants. Mol Pharmacol 58:98–108, 2000.
26. Zhou M, Morais-Cabral JH, Mann S, et al: Potassium channel receptor site for the inactivation gate and quaternary amine inhibitors. Nature 411:657–661, 2001.
27. Yost CS: Potassium channels: basic aspects, functional roles, and medical significance. Anesthesiology 90:1186–1203, 1999.
28. Doyle DA, Morais CJ, Pfuetzner RA, et al: The structure of the potassium channel: molecular basis of K+ conduction and selectivity. Science 280:69–77, 1998.
29. Haydon DA, Urban BW: The actions of some general anaesthetics on the potassium current of the squid giant axon. J Physiol 373:311–327, 1986.
30. Urban BW, Haydon DA: The actions of halogenated ethers on the ionic currents of the squid giant axon. Proc Royal Soc Lond B Biol Sci 231:13–26, 1987.
31. Davies LA, Hopkins PM, Boyett MR, Harrison SM: Effects of halothane on the transient outward K+ current in rat ventricular myocytes. Br J Pharmacol 131:223–230, 2000.
32. Zorn L, Kulkarni R, Anantharam V, et al: Halothane acts on many potassium channels, including a minimal potassium channel. Neurosci Lett 161:81–84, 1993.
33. Correa AM: Gating kinetics of Shaker K+ channels are differentially modified by general anesthetics. Am J Physiol 275:C1009–C1021, 1998.
34. Li J, Correa AM: Single-channel basis for conductance increase induced by isoflurane in Shaker H4 IR K+ channels. Am J Physiol Cell Physiol 280:C1130–C1139, 2001.
35. Shieh CC, Coghlan M, Sullivan JP, Gopalakrishnan M: Potassium channels: Molecular defects, diseases, and therapeutic opportunities. Pharm Rev 52:557–594, 2000.
36. Biggin PC, Roosild T, Choe S: Potassium channel structure: domain by domain. Curr Opin Struct Biol 10:456–461, 2000.
37. Kersten JR, Gross GJ, Pagel PS, Warltier DC: Activation of adenosine triphosphate-regulated potassium channels: mediation of cellular and organ protection. Anesthesiology 88:495–513, 1998.
38. Lesage F, Lazdunski M: Molecular and functional properties of two-pore-domain potassium channels. Am J Physiol Renal Fluid Electrolyte Physiol 279:F793–F801, 2000.
39. Nicoll RA, Madison DV: General anesthetics hyperpolarize neurons in the vertebrate central nervous system. Science 217:1055–1057, 1982.
40. Franks NP, Lieb WR: Background K+ channels: an important target for volatile anesthetics? Nat Neurosci 2:395–396, 1999.
41. Gray AT, Zhao BB, Kindler CH, et al: Volatile anesthetics activate the human tandem pore domain baseline K+ channel KCNK5. Anesthesiology 92:1722–1730, 2000.
42. Patel AJ, Honore E, Lesage F, et al: Inhalational anesthetics activate two-pore-domain background K+ channels. Nat Neurosci 2:422–426, 1999.
43. Perouansky M, Pearce RA: Is anesthesia caused by potentiation of synaptic or intrinsic inhibition? Recent insights into the mechanisms of volatile anesthetics. J Basic Clin Physiol Pharmacol 11:83–107, 2000.
44. Sirois JE, Lei Q, Talley EM, et al: The TASK-1 two-pore domain K+ channel is a molecular substrate for neuronal effects of inhalation anesthetics. J Neurosci 20:6347–6354, 2000.
45. Ortells MO, Lunt GG: Evolutionary history of the ligand-gated ion-channel superfamily of receptors [review]. Trends Neurosci 18:121–127, 1995.
46. Karlin A, Akabas MH: Toward a structural basis for the function of nicotinic acetylcholine receptors and their cousins. Neuron 15:1231–1244, 1995.
47. Corringer PJ, Le Novere N, Changeux JP: Nicotinic receptors at the amino acid level. Annu Rev Pharmacol Toxicol 40:431–458, 2000.
48. Smith GB, Olsen RW: Functional domains of GABAA receptors. Trends Pharmacol Sci 16:162–168, 1995.
49. Lukas RJ, Changeux JP, Le Novere N, et al: International Union of Pharmacology. XX. Current status of the nomenclature for nicotinic acetylcholine receptors and their subunits. Pharmacol Rev 51:397–401, 1999.
50. McKernan RM, Whiting PJ: Which GABA$_A$-receptor subtypes really occur in the brain? Trends Neurosci 19:139–143, 1996.

51. Galzi JL, Devillers-Thiery A, Hussy N, et al: Mutations in the channel domain of a neuronal nicotinic receptor convert ion selectivity from cationic to anionic. Nature 359:500–505, 1992.

52. Corringer PJ, Bertrand S, Galzi JL, et al: Mutational analysis of the charge selectivity filter of the α7 nicotinic acetylcholine receptor. Neuron 22:831–843, 1999.

53. Gunthorpe MJ, Lummis SC: Conversion of the ion selectivity of the 5-HT(3a) receptor from cationic to anionic reveals a conserved feature of the ligand-gated ion channel superfamily. J Biol Chem 276:10977–10983, 2001.

54. Mihic SJ, Ye Q, Wick MJ, et al: Sites of alcohol and volatile anaesthetic action on GABA(A) and glycine receptors. Nature 389:385–389, 1997.

55. Zhang Y, Wu S, Eger EI, Sonner JM: Neither GABA(A) nor strychnine-sensitive glycine receptors are the sole mediators of MAC for isoflurane. Anesth Analg 92:123–127, 2001.

56. Olivier B, van WI, Soudijn W: 5-HT³ receptor antagonists and anxiety: a preclinical and clinical review. Eur Neuropsychopharmacol 10:77–95, 2000.

57. Mason P: Central mechanisms of pain modulation. Curr Opin Neurobiol 9:436–441, 1999.

58. Hasler WL: Serotonin receptor physiology: relation to emesis. Dig Dis Sci 44:108S–113S, 1999.

59. Walton SM: Advances in use of the 5-HT3 receptor antagonists. Exp Opin Pharmacother 1:207–223, 2000.

60. Humphrey PP, Bountra C, Clayton N, Kozlowski K: Review article: the therapeutic potential of 5-HT3 receptor antagonists in the treatment of irritable bowel syndrome. Aliment Pharmacol Ther 13(Suppl 2):31–38, 1999.

61. Khakh BS: Molecular physiology of P2X receptors and ATP signaling at synapses. Nat Rev Neurosci 2:165–174, 2001.

62. Evans RJ, Surprenant A: Vasoconstriction of guinea-pig submucosal arterioles following sympathetic nerve stimulation is mediated by the release of ATP. Br J Pharmacol 106:242–249, 1992.

63. Burnstock G: Purine-mediated signaling in pain and visceral perception. Trends Pharmacol Sci 22:182–188, 2001.

64. Gallo V, Ghiani CA: Glutamate receptors in glia: new cells, new inputs and new functions. Trends Pharmacol Sci 21:252–258, 2000.

65. Bergles DE, Jahr CE: Synaptic activation of glutamate transporters in hippocampal astrocytes. Neuron 19:1297–1308, 1997.

66. Araque A, Parpura V, Sanzgiri RP, Haydon PG: Tripartite synapses: glia, the unacknowledged partner [review]. Trends Neurosci 22:208–215, 1999.

67. Wo ZG, Oswald RE: Unraveling the modular design of glutamate-gated ion channels [review]. Trends Neurosci 18:161–168, 1995.

68. Kiskin NI, Krishtal OA, Tsyndrenko AY, Akaike N: Are sulfhydryl groups essential for the glutamate-operated receptor-ionophore complex? Neurosci Lett 66:305–310, 1986.

69. Lesage F, Lazdunski M: Molecular and functional properties of two-pore-domain potassium channels. Am J Physiol Renal Fluid Electrolyte Physiol 279:F793–F801, 2000.

70. Mosbacher J, Schoepfer R, Monyer H, et al: A molecular determinant for submillisecond desensitization in glutamate receptors. Science 266:1059–1062, 1994.

71. Stern-Bach Y, Bettler B, Hartley M, et al: Agonist selectivity of glutamate receptors is specified by two domains structurally related to bacterial amino acid-binding proteins. Neuron 13:1345–1357, 1994.

72. Partin KM, Bowie D, Mayer ML: Structural determinants of allosteric regulation in alternatively spliced AMPA receptors. Neuron 14:833–843, 1995.

73. Partin KM, Fleck MW, Mayer ML: AMPA receptor flip/flop mutants affecting deactivation, desensitization, and modulation by cyclothiazide, aniracetam, and thiocyanate. J Neurosci 16:6634–6647, 1996.

74. Partin KM, Patneau DK, Mayer ML: Cyclothiazide differentially modulates desensitization of alpha-amino-3-hydroxy-5-methyl-4-isoxazolepropionic acid receptor splice variants. Mol Pharmacol 46:129–138, 1994.

75. Clements JD, Lester RA, Tong G, et al: The time course of glutamate in the synaptic cleft. Science 258:1498–1501, 1992.

76. Hestrin S: Activation and desensitization of glutamate-activated channels mediating fast excitatory synaptic currents in the visual cortex. Neuron 9:991–999, 1992.

77. Hestrin S: Different glutamate receptor channels mediate fast excitatory synaptic currents in inhibitory and excitatory cortical neurons. Neuron 11:1083–1091, 1993.

78. Barbour B, Keller BU, Llano I, Marty A: Prolonged presence of glutamate during excitatory synaptic transmission to cerebellar Purkinje cells. Neuron 12:1331–1343, 1994.

79. Jia Z, Agopyan N, Miu P, et al: Enhanced LTP in mice deficient in the AMPA receptor GluR2. Neuron 17:945–956, 1996.

80. Cheun JE, Yeh HH: Noradrenergic potentiation of cerebellar Purkinje cell responses to GABA: cyclic AMP as intracellular intermediary. Neuroscience 74:835–844, 1996.

81. Joo DT, Gong D, Sonner JM, et al: Blockade of AMPA receptors and volatile anesthetics: Reduced anesthetic requirements in GluR2 null mutant mice for loss of the righting reflex and antinociception but not minimum alveolar concentration. Anesthesiology 94:478–488, 2001.

82. Wenthold RJ, Trumpy VA, Zhu WS, Petralia RS: Biochemical and assembly properties of GluR6 and KA2, two members of the kainate receptor family, determined with subunit-specific antibodies. J Biol Chem 269:1332–1339, 1994.

83. Partin KM, Patneau DK, Winters CA, et al: Selective modulation of desensitization at AMPA versus kainate receptors by cyclothiazide and concanavalin A. Neuron 11:1069–1082, 1993.

84. Wong LA, Mayer ML: Differential modulation by cyclothiazide and concanavalin A of desensitization at native alpha-amino-3-hydroxy-5-methyl-4-isoxazolepropionic acid- and kainate-preferring glutamate receptors. Mol Pharmacol 44:504–510, 1993.

85. Wisden W, Seeburg PH: A complex mosaic of high-affinity kainate receptors in rat brain. J Neurosci 13:3582–3598, 1993.

86. Lerma J, Morales M, Vicente MA, Herreras O: Glutamate receptors of the kainate type and synaptic transmission. Trends Neurosci 20:9–12, 1997.

87. Frerking M, Nicoll RA: Synaptic kainate receptors. Curr Opin Neurobiol 10:342–351, 2000.

88. Huettner JE: Glutamate receptor channels in rat DRG neurons: activation by kainate and quisqualate and blockade of desensitization by Con A. Neuron 5:255–266, 1990.

89. Monaghan DT, Cotman CW: The distribution of [3H]kainic acid binding sites in rat CNS as determined by autoradiography. Brain Res 252:91–100, 1982.

90. Moriyoshi K, Masu M, Ishii T, et al: Molecular cloning and characterization of the rat NMDA receptor. Nature 354:31–37, 1991.

91. Mori H, Mishina M: Structure and function of the NMDA receptor channel [review]. Neuropharmacology 34:1219–1237, 1995.

92. Monyer H, Burnashev N, Laurie DJ, et al: Developmental and regional expression in the rat brain and functional properties of four NMDA receptors. Neuron 12:529–540, 1994.

93. Petralia RS, Wang YX, Wenthold RJ: Histological and ultrastructural localization of the kainate receptor subunits, KA2 and GluR6/7, in the rat nervous system using selective antipeptide antibodies. J Comp Neurol 349:85–110, 1994.

94. Benveniste M, Clements J, Vyklicky L Jr, Mayer ML: A kinetic analysis of the modulation of n-methyl-D-aspartic acid receptors by glycine in mouse cultured hippocampal neurones. J Physiol (Lond) 428:333–357, 1990.

95. Sather W, Johnson JW, Henderson G, Ascher P: Glycine-insensitive desensitization of NMDA responses in cultured mouse embryonic neurons. Neuron 4:725–731, 1990.

96. Vyklicky L, Benveniste M, Mayer ML: Modulation of N-methyl-D-aspartic acid receptor desensitization by glycine in mouse cultured hippocampal neurones. J Physiol 428:313–331, 1990.

97. Nowak L, Bregestovski P, Ascher P, et al: Magnesium gates glutamate-activated channels in mouse central neurones. Nature 307:462–465, 1984.

98. Ascher P, Nowak L: The role of divalent cations in the N-methyl-D-aspartate responses of mouse central neurones in culture. J Physiol 399:247–266, 1988.

99. Kutsuwada T, Kashiwabuchi N, Mori H, et al: Molecular diversity of the NMDA receptor channel. Nature 358:36–41, 1992.

100. Monyer H, Sprengel R, Schoepfer R, et al: Heteromeric NMDA receptors: molecular and functional distinction of subtypes. Science 256:1217–1221, 1992.

101. Johnson JW, Ascher P: Glycine potentiates the NMDA response in cultured mouse brain neurons. Nature 325:529–531, 1987.

102. Matsui T, Sekiguchi M, Hashimoto A, et al: Functional comparison of D-serine and glycine in rodents: the effect on cloned NMDA receptors and the extracellular concentration. J Neurochem 65:454–458, 1995.

103. Sucher NJ, Awobuluyi M, Choi YB, Lipton SA: NMDA receptors: from genes to channels. Trends Pharmacol Sci 17:348–355, 1996.

104. Jones KA, Baughman RW: Both NMDA and non-NMDA subtypes of glutamate receptors are concentrated at synapses on cerebral cortical neurons in culture. Neuron 7:593–603, 1991.

105. Ben-Ari Y, Khazipov R, Leinekugel X, et al: GABAA, NMDA and AMPA receptors: a developmentally regulated "menage a trios." Trends Neurosci 20:523–529, 1997.

106. Feldman DE, Nicoll RA, Malenka RC: Synaptic plasticity at thalamocortical synapses in developing rat somatosensory cortex: LTP, LTD, and silent synapses [review]. J Neurobiol 41:92–101, 1999.

107. Nicoll RA, Malenka RC: Expression mechanisms underlying NMDA receptor-dependent long-term potentiation [review]. Ann NY Acad Sci 868:515–525, 1999.

108. Tsien JZ: Linking Hebb's coincidence-detection to memory formation [review]. Curr Opin Neurobiol 10:266–273, 2000.

109. Kullmann DM, Asztely F, Walker MC: The role of mammalian ionotropic receptors in synaptic plasticity: LTP, LTD and epilepsy [review]. Cell Molecul Life Sci 57:1551–1561, 2000.

110. Manabe T: Two forms of hippocampal long-term depression, the counterpart of long-term potentiation [review]. Rev Neurosci 8:179–193, 1997.

111. Tanaka H, Grooms SY, Bennett MV, Zukin RS: The AMPAR subunit GluR2: still front and center-stage. Brain Res 886:190–207, 2000.

112. Franks NP, Dickinson R, de Sousa SL, et al: How does xenon produce anaesthesia? Nature 396:324, 1998.

113. Jevtovic-Todorovic V, Todorovic SM, Mennerick S, et al: Nitrous oxide (laughing gas) is an NMDA antagonist, neuroprotectant and neurotoxin. Nat Med 4:460–463, 1998.

114. Yamamura T, Harada K, Okamura A, Kemmotsu O: Is the site of action of ketamine anesthesia the N-methyl-D-aspartate receptor? Anesthesiology 72:704–710, 1990.

115. Krazowski MD, Harrison NL: General anaesthetic actions on ligand-gated ion channels. Cell Mol Life Sci 55:1278–1303, 1999.

116. Wilhelm S, Ma D, Maze M, Frank NP: Effect of xenon on in vitro and in vivo models of neuronal injury. Anesthesiology 96:1485–1491, 2002.

Principles of Drug Biotransformation

Evan D. Kharasch, MD, PhD

Basic Considerations
Pathways of Metabolism
Enzymes of Metabolism
   Phase I Enzymes
   Phase II Enzymes
Extrahepatic Metabolism
   Intestine

Kidney
Brain
Developmental Regulation
Transport Proteins
Interindividual Variability in Drug Metabolism

Biotransformation of drugs and xenobiotics is a complex and diverse field that has undergone explosive growth in the last decade because of the application of molecular biology and genetic techniques to a traditionally more chemically oriented discipline. From the perspective of new drug development, elucidation of biotransformation pathways and mechanisms has moved much earlier in the development timeline to terminate or modify compounds that may predispose toward undesirable responses, and regulatory agencies require more complete information about enzymes and pathways of metabolism and possible drug interactions. Information on the latter, which was traditionally painstakingly gathered over long periods of clinical use through reports of adverse drug reactions, is now prospectively determined from in vitro enzyme systems and clinical models of biotransformation. Known pathways of biotransformation are currently deliberately exploited in drug development to target routes or sites of metabolism, to develop prodrugs to permit routes of administration precluded by solubility characteristics of the active molecule, and to accelerate or retard rates of drug inactivation. Several recent reviews and textbooks provide a more comprehensive perspective on drug biotransformation.[1–6]

This chapter presents typical biotransformation reactions, pathways of drug biotransformation (phase I oxidation, hydrolysis, reduction, and dehydrogenation, and phase II glucuronidation, sulphation, acetylation, and glutathione conjugation), and the expression, activity, regulation, ontogeny, and genetics of hepatic biotransformation enzymes. The focus is directed exclusively toward the enzymes responsible for human drug biotransformation and does not address enzymes of biotransformation in animals, which often differ significantly, both qualitatively and quantitatively. In addition to hepatic metabolism, the increasingly recognized role of extrahepatic intestinal and renal biotransformation is discussed. Transport proteins, although not specifically catalyzing biotransformation, also are discussed because they are intimately involved with biotransformation and influence drug availability. Finally, the role of biotransformation in interindividual variability in metabolism and response are presented.

Basic Considerations

Therapeutic drugs tend to be relatively lipophilic. In general, biotransformation reactions convert compounds to more polar hydrophilic molecules that are more amenable to excretion through the kidney, or occasionally gastrointestinally. Traditionally, biotransformation reactions have been categorized as phase I and phase II reactions. The former are termed functionalization reactions, which introduce or uncover a functional group (hydroxyl, amine, acid) that moderately increases drug polarity and prepares it for a phase II reaction. The latter are conjugation reactions that covalently link the drug or metabolite with a highly polar molecule that renders the conjugate very water-soluble and thereby excreted. Phase I and II reactions can occur on the same molecule. Alternatively, other drugs may undergo only phase I or II reactions (the latter if a functional group is already present). Drugs may be eliminated unchanged, or as their phase I metabolites or as phase II conjugates. Biotransformation plays a prominent role in the disposition of numerous drugs used in anesthesia, including opioids (fentanyl, alfentanil, sufentanil, remifentanil, morphine, codeine, oxycodone, hydromorphone, dextromethorphan, meperidine, methadone, L-alpha acetylmethadol), benzodiazepines (midazolam, triazolam, diazepam, alprazolam), local anesthetics (lidocaine, bupivacaine, ropivacaine, procaine, chloroprocaine, cocaine), neuromuscular blockers (pancuronium, vecuronium, rocuronium, mivacurium, [cis]atracurium), and volatile anesthetics (particularly the more soluble ones).

Although typically considered mainly as a route of drug inactivation, phase I and II reactions can have several other consequences. Biotransformation can convert an active drug to an inactive metabolite, such as the metabolism of fentanyl to norfentanyl. It can also convert an active drug to a pharmacologically active metabolite. For example, the primary metabolite of midazolam, 1-hydroxymidazolam, possesses considerable pharmacologic activity and contributes to the apparent clinical effect of the parent drug, whereas 1-hydroxymidazolam-glucuronide has much less activity. Phase I or II reactions can convert an inactive prodrug to an active metabolite, such as the amide hydrolysis of the inactive precursor parexoxib to the active cyclooxygenase-2 selective inhibitor valdecoxib, or the oxidation of inactive codeine to the more active metabolite morphine and its subsequent conversion to the even more potent mu receptor agonist morphine-6-glucuronide. Phase I or II reactions also can convert a drug to a toxic metabolite, such as the *N*-demethylation of meperidine to normeperidine, which can cause seizures.

Pathways of Metabolism

Prominent pathways of phase I and II metabolism are shown in Figure 4-1. The various enzyme systems responsible for these reactions are detailed in the following section. Most phase I reactions are oxidations, which involve the initial insertion of a single oxygen atom. Oxygen remains on the drug molecule with hydroxylation and epoxidation reactions, and leaves on the alkyl group as the aldehyde with dealkylation reactions. Phase I oxidative reactions that are catalyzed by cytochrome P450 (CYP) include aromatic and aliphatic hydroxylation, *O*-dealkylation and *N*-dealkylation (*N*-demethylation is a subset), epoxidation, and oxidative deamination and dehalogenation. *N*-oxidation and *S*-oxidation are phase I reactions that may be catalyzed by either CYP or flavin-containing monooxygenase (FMO). Reductions are another type of phase I reaction, also catalyzed by CYP, often under anaerobic conditions. Some drugs may undergo both oxidation and reduction, depending on the oxygen tension. For example, halothane undergoes CYP-catalyzed (1) oxidation to a trifluoroacyl halide, which can subsequently react with liver proteins to form trifluoroacetylated protein neoantigens or with water to form trifluoroacetic acid; and (2) anaerobic reduction to a free radical, which gives rise to chlorodifluoroethylene and

chlorotrifluoroethane. Hydrolysis is a phase I reaction that is not catalyzed by CYP, but is catalyzed by esterases/amidases. Phase II conjugation reactions are depicted by reactions 15 through 18.

Enzymes of Metabolism

Phase I Enzymes

Cytochrome P450

The CYP system is a superfamily of membrane-bound heme proteins that catalyze the metabolism of endogenous and exogenous compounds. P450s are called mixed function oxidases or monooxygenases because they insert one atom of molecular oxygen into the substrate and one atom into water. However, P450s can also catalyze other reactions, such as reduction. There are more than 50 human P450s that have been identified, although only a small fraction are responsible for the majority of drug metabolism. The individual CYPs have evolved from a common ancestor protein and are classified according to their sequence evolution.[7–9] CYPs that share more than 40% sequence homology are grouped in a family (designated by an Arabic number, e.g., CYP2), those that share more than 55% homology are grouped in a subfamily (designated by a letter, e.g., CYP2A), and individual CYPs are identified by a third number (e.g., CYP2A6). Allelic variants are designated by an asterisk and number following the protein identifier (e.g., CYP2A6*1).[10] Seventeen CYP families and 42 subfamilies have been identified to date, with the majority of xenobiotics metabolized in humans by CYP1, CYP2 and CYP3 (particularly CYP2C, CYP2D6, and CYP3A); whereas the remainder are responsible for the synthesis or metabolism of endogenous compounds such as steroids, cholesterol, arachidonic acid, thromboxane, bile acids, prostacyclin, retinoic acid, and vitamin D. The hepatic CYPs responsible for most of human drug metabolism are shown in Figure 4–2. CYPs are predominantly microsomal enzymes, although there are also mitochondrial P450s. Microsomes are not a physiologic organelle, but rather correspond to the smooth endoplasmic reticulum. Microsomes are prepared by homogenizing tissue, removing mitochondria, nuclei, and debris with a low-speed centrifugation, and centrifuging the initial supernatant at $100,000\,g$ and resuspending the pellet. Other microsomal enzymes include glucuronosyltransferase and glutathione transferase.

The mixed function oxidase system involves several enzymes in addition to CYP, including the requisite participation of the flavoprotein nicotinamide adenine dinucleotide phosphate (NADPH)-CYP reductase, cytochrome b_5, and NADPH-cytochrome b_5 reductase. P450 contains a heme-bound iron at its active site. The typical oxidation reaction generally involves an initial hydroxylation, with NADPH providing two electrons to reduce one atom of molecular oxygen to water and insert the other into the substrate. The overall scheme is represented as:

$$RH + O_2 + NADPH + H^+ \rightarrow ROH + H_2O + NADP^+$$

Chapter 4 Principles of Drug Biotransformation

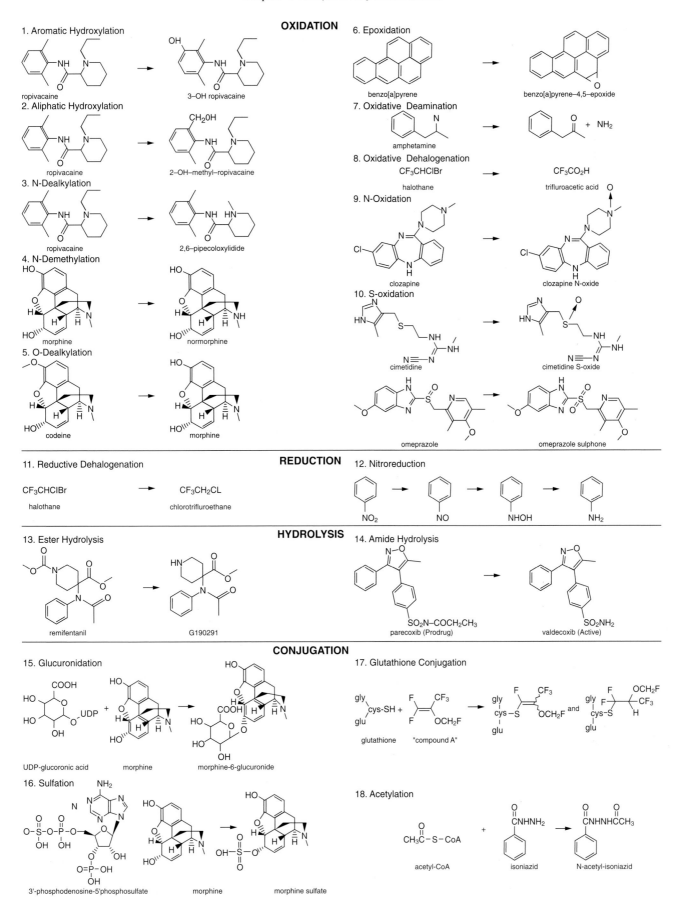

Figure 4–1. Major pathways of drug and xenobiotic biotransformation.

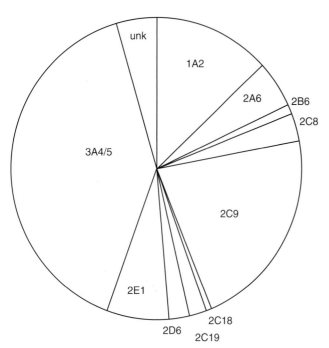

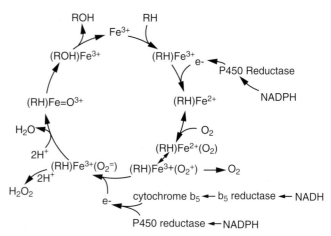

Figure 4–3. Conceptual scheme for the catalytic cycle of cytochrome P450. The iron represents the heme iron of P450 and R is the substrate. Also shown are sites at which uncoupling and release of activated oxygen can occur. NADH, NADPH, nicotinamide adenine dinucleotide phosphate.

Figure 4–2. Content of cytochrome P450 isoforms in human liver, based on immunoquantification. (Data from Levy RH, Thummel KI, Trager WF, et al: Metabolic Drug Interactions. Philadelphia, Lippincott Williams & Wilkins, 2000; Lasker JM, Waster MR, Aramsombatdee E, et al: Characterization of CYP2C19 and CYP2C9 from human liver: Respective roles in microsomal tolbutamide, S-mephenytoin, and omeprazole hydroxylations. Arch Biochem Biophys 353:16–28, 1998; and Shimada T, Yamazaki H, Mimura M, et al: Interindividual variations in human liver cytochrome P-450 enzymes involved in the oxidation of drugs, carcinogens, and toxic chemicals: Studies with liver microsomes of 30 Japanese and 30 Caucasians. J Pharmacol Exp Ther 270:414–423, 1994.)

where RH is the substrate and ROH is the oxidized metabolite. The catalytic cycle of the multienzyme pathway is shown in Figure 4–3.[11] Substrate binds to the resting oxidized (ferric) protein, followed by the acceptance of an electron from NADPH through the flavin mononucleotide– and flavin adenine dinucleotide–containing flavoprotein NADPH-CYP reductase, which reduces the heme iron to the ferrous state. This is followed by binding of molecular oxygen to form a ferrous-dioxygen complex. The next step is the acceptance of a second electron from NADPH through NADPH-CYP reductase or (depending on the exact CYP and substrate) from NADH through NADH-cytochrome b_5 reductase and cytochrome b_5. The exact structure of the resulting P450-oxygen-substrate complex(es) is not fully elucidated; however, the next step involves cleavage of the O—O bond to form the oxygenated substrate, water, and regenerate the oxidized (ferric) protein. An alternative pathway is for the P450-oxygen-substrate complex to liberate reduced activated dioxygen (as superoxide or peroxide) and unchanged substrate and regenerate the oxidized (ferric) protein. This is referred to as uncoupling electron transfer from substrate oxidation. In some cases, NADPH-CYP reductase itself can catalyze drug metabolism, such as nitro reduction or quinone reduction with consequent redox cycling (as with doxorubicin).

CYP isoforms can exhibit varying degrees of substrate specificity. Some, like CYP2E1, have a relatively small and restrictive active site and accept only structurally similar substrates. Others, like CYP3A, have an open and accommodating active site (indeed at least two active sites) and metabolize a large number and very diverse structural array of substrates (from halothane to cyclosporin). Similarly, substrates can exhibit a low degree of P450 isoform selectivity (antipyrine is metabolized by CYP1A2, CYP2A6, CYP2C9, CYP2C19, CYP2D6, CYP2E1, and CYP3A[12]) or a very high degree of isoform selectivity (alfentanil is metabolized predominantly by CYP3A4, and even the highly similar CYP3A5 does not appear to metabolize alfentanil[13,14]). Isoform selectivity can also exhibit an unusual oxygen dependence, as exemplified with halothane, which undergoes oxidation by CYP2E1 and CYP2A6, and reduction by CYP2A6 and CYP3A4.[15–17] CYPs can also exhibit regioselectivity, specifically oxidizing only one portion of a molecule. For example, CYP1A2 catalyzes ropivacaine 3-hydroxylation, whereas CYP3A4 catalyzes 4-hydroxylation, 2-methylhydroxylation, and *N*-dealkylation.[18,19]

Recently, there has been considerable emphasis on identifying the CYP isoforms responsible for metabolizing drugs and xenobiotics; indeed, this has become standard in drug development and is required by regulatory agencies. Both in vitro and in vivo reaction phenotyping are performed. Identification of a predominant CYP isoform in vitro is accomplished; (1) with human liver microsomes to determine which isoform-selective chemical inhibitors (mechanism-based inhibitors and competitive alternate substrates) and immunospecific inhibitory antibodies affect substrate metabolism; (2) by using a population of human liver microsomes to correlate the metabolism of a candidate substrate with either the protein content or catalytic activity of specific CYP isoforms (the former determined by immunoblotting and the latter is determined with known isoform-selective prototypic substrate probes); and (3) measuring substrate metabolism by individual cDNA-expressed CYP isoforms.[20] Although the latter approach allows evaluation of each isoform individually, it does not describe the relative contribution of each isoform to metabolism in the liver. Reaction phenotyping is optimally evaluated at therapeutic drug concentrations. When reactions are performed at high substrate concentrations, the results must be interpreted cautiously. The actual contribution of any individual isoform to overall microsomal metabolism will depend on the in vitro intrinsic clearance of the isoform/substrate pair (V_{max}/K_m), the relative content of that isoform in the liver (or other organ), and the substrate concentration in vivo. It is not uncommon for more than one CYP to catalyze a metabolic pathway. Often one pathway will be high-affinity (low K_m)/low-capacity (lower V_{max}) and the other or others will be low-affinity (high K_m)/high-capacity (higher V_{max}); the relative importance of these is again determined from the in vitro intrinsic clearance and the relative isoform contents. Occasionally, multiple CYPs may also have the same K_m. Identification of a predominant CYP isoform in vivo is accomplished using analogous methods.[8,21,22] Isoform-selective inducers (drugs that increase the expression and tissue content of enzyme) and inhibitors (often the same ones used in vitro) can be used to evaluate their effect on metabolism of the candidate drug. In a population of subjects, one can also correlate the metabolism of a candidate substrate with either the subjects' phenotype or genotype. The former is determined with known isoform-selective prototypic in vivo substrate probes, often the same ones used in vitro. The latter is accomplished using polymerase chain reaction, or restriction fragment length polymorphism analysis, or both. For each CYP isoform, prototypic in vitro and in vivo substrate and inhibitor probes have been identified.

CYP1A

The human CYP1A family consists of CYP1A1 and CYP1A2, which share only 68% sequence identity.[2,8,23,24] CYP1A2 is expressed almost exclusively in the liver, accounting for approximately 13% of total CYP, although low levels have been detected in brain and duodenum. In contrast, CYP1A1 is almost exclusively expressed extrahepatically, particularly in the lung. CYP1A1 metabolizes polycyclic aromatic hydrocarbons such as benzo[*a*]pyrene, and is highly inducible by these compounds. Indeed, CYP1A1 was one of the first CYPs shown to undergo induction and was originally termed the aryl hydrocarbon hydroxylase, with induction mediated by the aryl hydrocarbon hydroxylase receptor. CYP1A2 metabolizes the prototypic in vitro and in vivo substrates caffeine (*N*3-demethylation to paraxanthine) and phenacetin (*O*-demethylase) as well as clomipramine, imipramine, theophylline, lisofylline, olanzapine, tacrine, theophylline, (R)-warfarin, and toxic arylamines and nitrosamines. CYP1A2 catalyzes ropivacaine 3-hydroxylation.[18,19] Overall, CYP1A2 is responsible for metabolizing a small fraction of therapeutic drugs. CYP1A2 is the only CYP that is inducible by cigarette smoke and is also induced by charbroiled foods, cruciferous vegetables, and omeprazole (in high doses) (the former two containing high amounts of polycyclic aromatic hydrocarbons). Although there is considerable interindividual variability in hepatic CYP1A2 expression (>40-fold in various studies), there is no known genetic polymorphism. The prototype CYP1A2 inhibitors in vitro are furafylline and benzoflavone; however, because these are not available for clinical use, fluvoxamine has been used as an in vivo inhibitor probe. Other drugs including mexiletine, clozapine, theophylline and enoxacin have been reported to inhibit CYP1A. There is no effect of the menstrual cycle on human CYP1A2 activity.[25,26]

CYP2A

The expression and catalytic properties of CYP2A6 recently have been reviewed.[2,24,27–32] CYP2A6 accounts for approximately 5% (range 1–10%) of total human hepatic CYP. Extrahepatic CYP2A6 has only been found in human nasal mucosa (in small amounts) and lung. CYP2A6 metabolizes a small number of therapeutic drugs (coumarin, methoxyflurane, halothane, valproic acid) and a large number of environmental toxins (nicotine, cotinine, and numerous carcinogens and procarcinogens). It catalyzes both the aerobic oxidation and anaerobic reduction of halothane, and although it is the minor CYP isoform responsible for human halothane oxidation, nonetheless it may play a role in immune-based halothane hepatitis. The prototypic CYP2A6 substrate is coumarin. Coumarin 7-hydroxylation is catalyzed exclusively by CYP2A6, and this reaction is used as the highly selective in vitro and in vivo probe for CYP2A6 activity. Methoxsalen (8-methoxypsoralen) has been used as an inhibitory in vitro and in vivo CYP2A6 probe, however, it is not considered to be ideal because it may also inhibit other CYPs. Phenotyping studies have found a wide interindividual variability in CYP2A6 activity (coumarin 7-hydroxylation), and a few apparent poor or nonmetabolizers. It is now known that two allelic variants (CYP2A6*2 and CYP2A6*3) of the wild-type enzyme (CYP2A6*1), coding for defective enzyme, are responsible (in homozygotes) for the poor metabolizer phenotype. The incidence of these variants shows ethnic differences, with a greater incidence in Japanese. Little is known about the factors that regulate human CYP2A6 expression. There are, however, no apparent sex differences in CYP2A6 expression or activity. Two other members of the CYP2A gene family are CYP2A7, which has no known catalytic activity, and CYP2A13, which is found in human nasal mucosa, trachea, and lung. The latter enzyme has little coumarin 7-hydroxylase activity, but is very active toward toxins.

CYP2B

The human CYP2B family consists of CYP2B6 and CYP2B7, the former expressed primarily in liver and also in intestine, brain, and kidney, and the latter exclusively in lung.[8,33–37] CYP2B6 was initially considered to be expressed in only some individuals (~20%), in low levels in the liver (<0.2% of total CYP), and with much variability when it was expressed; thus it was not considered important in human drug biotransformation. This tenet has recently undergone major reconsideration, and it is now clear that CYP2B6 is expressed in greater amounts (up to 6% of total CYP), in all individuals, and metabolizes a considerable and diverse number of substrates. It is now apparent that its catalytic role was previously underappreciated. The prototype in vitro probes for human CYP2B6 are bupropion hydroxylation and S-mephenytoin N-demethylation. CYP2B6 also metabolizes antineoplastic agents (cyclophosphamide, ifosfamide), benzodiazepines (diazepam, temazepam, midazolam), and other drugs such as verapamil, lidocaine, clopidogrel, and tamoxifen. It was recently shown to be predominantly responsible for propofol hydroxylation and N-demethylation of both (R)- and (S)-ketamine.[38–40] In general, many substrates previously thought to be metabolized predominantly by CYP3A in microsomes are now recognized to be metabolized by both CYP2B and CYP3A. Because both isoforms are susceptible to induction by the same drugs (such as barbiturates), the potential for drug interactions with these CYP2B/CYP3A substrates is considerable. CYP2B6 has been reported as one of the most polymorphic CYPs, with several mutations occurring with high frequency, one of which results in CYP2B6 activity in heterozygotes and particularly homozygotes.[41] Thus both genetic variability and susceptibility to induction/inhibition account for the greater than 100-fold interindividual variability in CYP2B6 activity. Currently, neither an isoform-selective in vitro chemical inhibitor nor a selective in vivo probe have been identified. As these become available, the perceived role of CYP2B6 in human drug biotransformation may grow.

CYP2C

The human *CYP2C* gene family consists of *CYP2C8, CYP2C9, CYP2C18* and *CYP2C19,* which share greater than 82% sequence homology, and together account for approximately one fourth of total hepatic CYP.[2,22,42,43] CYP2C10 was another isoform initially reported, however, it is now known to be a cloning artifact. Together, the CYP2Cs are responsible for metabolizing approximately 15% to 20% of all therapeutic drugs, and hence are a major CYP class. The degree of interindividual variability in CYP2C activity (fivefold) is the lowest of the various CYPs.

CYP2C9 is the major CYP2C isoform in human liver. There is no one standard CYP2C9 in vivo probe, although metabolism of phenytoin, tolbutamide, diclofenac, and (S)-warfarin has been extensively used. Other CYP2C9 substrates include tienilic acid, fluoxetine, losartan, torsemide, and a large number of arylacetic and arylpropionic nonsteroidal anti-inflammatory drugs. CYP2C9 is inducible by antiepileptic drugs and rifampin. Suphaphenazole is the standard human CYP2C9 in vitro and in vivo inhibitor probe. Other inhibitors include fluconazole and some other azole antifungals, fluvastatin, trimethoprim, and several other sulfa drugs. Several variant CYP2C9 proteins with substantially decreased activity have been identified, which explains the small (0.2%) but known incidence of CYP2C9 poor metabolizers that are more sensitive to CYP2C9 substrates with low therapeutic index (i.e., warfarin).[44] The frequency of mutant alleles, which code for a protein with much less activity, occurs more commonly in whites (10–20%) than in Asians and African Americans (1–3%).

The prototypic CYP2C8 substrate is Taxol; other substrates include carbamazepine, troglitazone, rosiglitazone, zopiclone, and cerivastatin. CYP2C8 has the narrowest substrate specificity of the CYP2C isoforms, but there appears to be some overlap between CYP2C8 and CYP3A4.

CYP2C18 is expressed in low levels (<10% of CYP2C8 or CYP2C9) in human liver, and has yet to be purified; rather it has only been expressed from isolated DNA. CYP2C18 does not metabolize CYP2C9 or CYP2C19 substrates, and specific 2C18 substrates have not been identified.

CYP2C19 is a minor component, but has been extensively studied because of it is one of the early CYP isoforms for which a genetic polymorphism was identified. The prototype CYP2C19 substrate and in vitro and in vivo probe is S-mephenytoin hydroxylation, and the genetic variability was initially termed the mephenytoin polymorphism. More recently, omeprazole 5-hydroxylation and proguanil oxidation have also been used to probe CYP2C19 activity. Other substrates include barbiturates (R-mephobarbital, hexobarbital), citalopram, diazepam, and imipramine. There is no standard selective in vitro or in vivo inhibitor probe for CYP2C19. Individuals are classified as extensive (EM) or poor (PM) metabolizers of S-mephenytoin, and the incidence of PMs shows clear racial differences, with a frequency of 2% to 5% in whites, 2% in African Americans, 18% to 23% in Japanese, and 15% to 17% in Chinese. PM is caused by a mutation, inherited as an autosomal recessive trait, which causes a truncated inactive protein, hence PMs do not express CYP2C19. The CYP2C19 polymorphism accounts for interracial differences in the clinical disposition and dose requirements for diazepam, particularly PM homozygotes.[45] For example, the clearance of diazepam in PM is half that in EM, with dose requirements correspondingly less, and heterozygotes are intermediate. This is thought to account for lower diazepam dose requirements in Chinese. There is no known sex difference in CYP2C19 activity.[46]

CYP2D

CYP2D6, although accounting for only 2% to 5% of total human hepatic CYP protein, and the only member of the human CYP2D subfamily, nonetheless metabolizes approximately 25% of all therapeutic drugs and is one of the three most important human CYPs.[2,8,22,24,45,47–49] CYP2D6 is also of considerable historical significance because it was the first identified CYP genetic polymorphism. The antihypertensive debrisoquine caused orthostatic hypotension in a small fraction of individuals, which was linked to diminished metabolic elimination by the enzyme termed "debrisoquine hydroxylase" (CYP2D6). A similar pattern was seen with the drug sparteine, and the phenomenon was named the "debrisoquine/sparteine polymorphism." The prototype in vitro and in vivo substrate probe is now dextromethorphan (O-demethylation), because debrisoquine and sparteine are not available in the United States, and the standard in vitro and in vivo inhibitor probe is quinidine. CYP2D6 is not inducible by phenobarbital, and the effect of rifampin is unresolved. A representative sample of CYP2D6 substrates and inhibitors is listed in Table 4–1. The list is notable for a group of opioids that undergo both CYP2D6-mediated O-demethylation and CYP3A4-mediated N-demethylation (Fig. 4-4). Most pertinent is codeine, now accepted to be a prodrug that requires metabolic activation to morphine. The

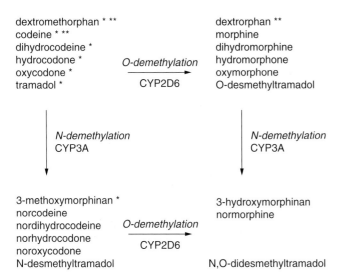

Figure 4–4. Role of CYP2D6 and CYP3A4 in the inactivation and bioactivation of opioids. Pathways known to be metabolized by CYP2D6 and CYP3A4 are indicated by (*) and (**), respectively.

TABLE 4–1.

Representative Human CYP2D6 Substrates and Inhibitors

Substrates

Opioids*: codeine,* dextromethorphan,*
    dihydrocodeine, hydrocodone, oxycodone, tramadol
Antipsychotics: haloperidol, risperidone, thioridazine,
    chlorpromazine
TCAs: amitriptyline, clomipramine, clozapine,
    desipramine, imipramine, nortriptyline, maprotiline,
    trazodone
Antiarrhythmics: encainide, flecainide, sparteine*
Beta-blockers: alprenolol, bufurolol,* labetalol,
    metoprolol, propranolol, timolol
SSRIs: fluoxetine, fluvoxamine, paroxetine, sertraline,
    citalopram, venlafaxine
Miscellaneous: debrisoquine,* selegiline, dolasetron,
    ondansetron, tropisetron, tamoxifen

Inhibitors

Quinidine,* cimetidine, haloperidol, SSRIs

---

*The most widely used human in vivo probes (selective substrates and inhibitors).
SSRIs, selective serotonin reuptake inhibitors.

genetic and drug interaction implications of codeine metabolism are discussed later.

The debrisoquine/sparteine phenotype is an autosomal recessive monogenic Mendelian trait. Populations are composed of EM (wild-type), PM, and ultrarapid metabolizers. The overall PM frequency is 7% to 8% in whites, 2% in

African Americans, and less than 1% in Asians. More than 20 mutant CYP2D6 alleles have been identified, and there is considerable racial diversity in their frequency. Most of the mutant alleles code for short and inactive proteins, and homozygotes are PM. However, some alleles that are particularly frequent in Asians code for a protein with reduced activity. Ultrarapid metabolizers are caused by gene duplication, with up to 13 copies. These individuals generally require substantially greater doses of CYP2D6 substrates, and also show ethnic variability (20% Ethiopian, 7% Spanish, 1% Scandinavian). There is even a spectrum of CYP2D6 activity within the EMs, because of the diversity of 2D6 alleles. Commercial assays are available that allow for accurate CYP2D6 genotyping. CYP2D6 activity is not effected by sex or the menstrual cycle.[46,50]

CYP2E1

The expression, regulation, and activity of CYP2E1 have been recently reviewed.[8,21,22,51,52] CYP2E1 comprises approximately 6% of total hepatic P450, with 6-fold to 20-fold interindividual variability. Although there are mutant CYP2E1 alleles, their frequency is low, there is no consensus that they code for altered enzyme activity, and they appear to be of no clinical significance. Although the amino acid sequence and catalytic activity of the CYP2E1 protein are markedly conserved among species, there are substantial species differences in CYP2E1 expression. In rats, CYP2E1 is found not only in the liver but also widely expressed extrahepatically, particularly in the kidney. In humans, CYP2E1 is expressed primarily in the liver; however, extrahepatic expression is largely absent (except in the brain), most notably the kidney. This difference has implications for interpreting animal models of CYP2E1-mediated biotransformation and toxicity. There are no apparent age or sex differences in human hepatic CYP2E1 expression.

CYP2E1 is of significant toxicologic importance. It metabolizes small molecular weight, often halogenated or volatile compounds, or both. The prototype in vitro substrate probe is chlorzoxazone hydroxylation, and the in vivo probe is chlorzoxazone plasma clearance. The standard in vivo inhibitor probe is disulfiram and, in vitro, its primary metabolite is diethyldithiocarbamate. CYP2E1 metabolizes a small number of therapeutic drugs, including isoniazid and acetaminophen, and is the primary enzyme oxidizing the volatile anesthetics halothane, enflurane, isoflurane, sevoflurane, desflurane (most likely), and methoxyflurane; although the latter is metabolized by several CYPs. CYP2E1 also metabolizes ethanol and other alcohols, aldehydes, alkanes, alkenes, ethers, aromatics, nitrosamines, and numerous halogenated hydrocarbons. Other CYP2E1 inhibitors include diallylsulfide and its metabolites (found in garlic), 4-methylpyrazole, and watercress. CYP2E1 is highly inducible, both by physiologic states and by numerous chemicals. Hepatic CYP2E1 activity is increased by obesity, ketosis, untreated diabetes, and numerous CYP2E1 substrates. Along with CYP2D6 and CYP3A4, CYP2E1 is one of the most important CYPs in anesthesia, because it mediates the hepatic and renal toxicity caused by the metabolic activation of volatile anesthetics.

CYP3A

The cytochrome P4503A family is the most clinically significant group of enzymes in human drug metabolism and has been extensively reviewed.[6,53–57] It is responsible for metabolizing more than half of all therapeutic drugs. The human CYP3A family is composed of CYP3A4, the polymorphically expressed CYP3A5, and the fetal form, CYP3A7. Early literature reported a CYP3A3; however, this is now known to be an allelic variant of CYP3A4. There is considerable genetic control of CYP3A activity.[58]

CYP3A4 is the most quantitatively abundant CYP in human liver, accounting for, on average, 30% of total hepatic CYP and as much as 60% in some livers. It is also the predominant CYP in human intestine. CYP3A4 exhibits the broadest substrate specificity of all CYPs and is remarkably susceptible to metabolic drug interactions, which alter the in vivo metabolism and clearance CYP3A substrates, often with profound clinical consequences (Table 4–2). CYP3A4 substrates range in size from halothane (a two carbon alkane, mw 197) to cyclosporine (mw 1201). CYP3A4 is the principal catalyst of *N*-demethylation reactions. Prototypic CYP3A4 in vitro substrate probes include testosterone 6ß-hydroxylation, midazolam, erythromycin, nifedipine, and cyclosporine. Because of the clinical importance of CYP3A4, there has been considerable interest in CYP3A4 in vivo probes.[22,59] Currently, erythromycin demethylation (specifically the erythromycin breath test, which measures exhaled $^{14}CO_2$ liberated by *N*-demethylation of radiolabeled drug) and especially midazolam systemic clearance are the most widely used, although alfentanil is gaining attention. Other probes, such as endogenous cortisol hydroxylation, lidocaine (serum concentrations of the primary metabolite monoethylglycinexylidide), and dapsone are no longer used. CYP3A4 activity is very susceptible to induction and inhibition. The prototype inducer is rifampin; however, barbiturates, phenytoin, carbamazepine, glucocorticoids, pregnane compounds, and herbals such as St. Johns wort also increase CYP3A4 content and activity several-fold. The prototype inhibitors are the noncompetitive, mechanism-based (suicide-substrate) macrolide antibiotic troleandomycin and the antifungal ketoconazole; however, others in the same drug classes also inhibit CYP3A4. Other drugs that are CYP3A4 substrates can act as competitive inhibitors. Although there is wide interindividual variability in CYP3A4 activity, there is no genetic polymorphism, and significant ethnic differences in activity have not been found. A few investigations have suggested greater CYP3A4 activity in women; however, this is not widely observed. Neither the menstrual cycle nor postmenopausal hormone replacement therapy in women affect CYP3A4 activity.[60,61]

CYP3A5 shares 84% sequence homology to CYP3A4. CYP3A5 metabolizes numerous but not all CYP3A4 substrates, and often, but not always, with diminished activity. Hepatic CYP3A5 is polymorphically expressed and traditionally has been thought to be present in only 25% of human livers and at levels much less than that of CYP3A4. Nevertheless, recent observations using more sensitive techniques now suggest that hepatic CYP3A5 expression is more frequent, occurs at a higher level, and is more contributory

TABLE 4–2.

Representative Human CYP3A Substrates, Inducers, and Inhibitors

Substrates
   Opioids: alfentanil,* fentanyl, sufentanil, methadone, L-alpha acetylmethadol, buprenorphine, codeine, dextromethorphan
   Benzodiazepines: midazolam,* triazolam, diazepam, alprazolam, temazepam
   Local anesthetics: lidocaine, bupivacaine, ropivacaine, cocaine
   Ca antagonists: verapamil, diltiazem, nifedipine, nicardipine, nimodipine, felodipine, amlodipine
   Immunosuppressants: cyclosporine, tacrolimus
   Miscellaneous: erythromycin,* tamoxifen, paclitaxel, ondansetron, granisetron, lovastatin, simvastatin, atorvastatin, cortisol, terfenadine, astemizole, quinidine, cisapride, lansoprazole, imipramine, amitriptyline, cyclophosphamide, dapsone, amiodarone, testosterone*

Inhibitors†
   Macrolides: troleandomycin,* erythromycin, clarithromycin ketoconazole,* miconazole, itraconazole, fluconazole, clotrimazole
   HIV drugs: indinavir, nelfinavir, ritonavir, saquinavir, amprenavir, nefazodone, delavirdine
   Miscellaneous: grapefruit juice, 3A4 substrates
Inducers
   Rifampin,* phenobarbital, phenytoin, carbamazepine, dexamethasone, nelfinavir, efavirenz

*The most widely used human in vivo probes (selective substrates and inhibitors).
†Many inhibitors and inducers are also substrates.

to the metabolism of certain CYP3A substrates than was previously appreciated. Indeed, CYP3A5 may account for more than half of the hepatic CYP3A protein in some individuals.[62] Unlike CYP3A4, CYP3A5 does show ethnic variability; it is expressed in 30% of whites, Japanese, and Mexicans, 40% of Chinese, and more than 50% of African Americans. Individuals expressing CYP3A5 along with CYP3A4 may have greater metabolism of CYP3A drugs. CYP3A5 is also polymorphically expressed in intestine, although levels are less than those of CYP3A4. CYP3A5 is the major CYP in human kidney.[63] Unlike the liver, in which CYP3A4 is ubiquitous and CYP3A5 is sometimes expressed, in the kidney, CYP3A5 is ubiquitous and CYP3A4 is expressed in only about 25% of subjects. Renal CYP3A may have a role in xenobiotic metabolism and the regulation of salt and water homeostasis.

CYP3A7 shares 88% sequence homology to CYP3A4. It is expressed exclusively in fetal liver, comprising 50% of total CYP. The metabolic capabilities of CYP3A7 are similar to those of CYP3A4 and CYP3A5.

Non-P450 Enzymes

Esterases

Ester/amide hydrolysis is an ubiquitous reaction catalyzed by a diverse array of enzymes in blood and tissue. Two major enzyme families catalyzing these reactions are carboxylesterases and cholinesterases.

Carboxylesterases (EC 3.1.1.1) are a family of predominantly microsomal and to a lesser extent lysosomal enzymes with wide tissue distribution.[64,65] Human carboxylesterase expression is greatest in the liver, and also occurs in the gastrointestinal tract, brain, and possibly blood. They have a very nonselective substrate specificity and also hydrolyze amides, thereby converting esters and amides to more water soluble acids, alcohols, and amines that are subsequently eliminated. Microsomal carboxylesterases are inducible by many of the compounds that induce microsomal CYP. Two broad-substrate human liver microsomal carboxylesterases have been isolated (hCE-1 and hCE-2).[66,67] For example, hCE-1 catalyzes the methylester hydrolysis of cocaine to benzoylecgonine, the hydrolysis of meperidine to meperidinic acid (the major route of metabolism), and the hydrolysis of heroin (3,6-diacetylmorphine) to 6-monoacetylmorphine, the active metabolite. hCE-2 also hydrolyzes heroin to 6-monoacetylmorphine and then to morphine. Liver microsomal esterase catalyzes the deamidation of the lidocaine metabolite monoethylglycinexylidide to 2,6-xylidine and ethylglycine.

Human cholinesterases include acetylcholinesterase (AChE, EC 3.1.1.7) and plasma cholinesterase (EC 3.1.1.8, also known as serum cholinesterase, pseudocholinesterase, butyrylcholine esterase, and nonspecific cholinesterase).[68,69] The major function of AChE is to hydrolyze acetylcholine at the neuromuscular junction, thereby terminating synaptic transmission. However, it is now known that there are two other AChE forms, which are located in erythrocytes and the brain. Plasma cholinesterase is widely distributed in plasma, as well as the liver and other tissues, and is of greater relevance to drug metabolism. The physiologic role of plasma cholinesterase is unknown. Plasma cholinesterase contains two active sites: the anionic site and the esteratic (catalytic) site at which ester hydrolysis actually occurs. Activity is mildly to moderately decreased by pregnancy, liver disease, renal failure (not attributable to dialysis), and cardiopulmonary bypass (due to hemodilution), and is markedly inhibited by echothiophate, organophosphate pesticides, and reversible inhibitors of AChE (neostigmine, edrophonium, physostigmine, pyridostigmine).

Plasma cholinesterase was one of the early enzymes for which pharmacogenetic variation was elucidated, based on observed heritable interindividual variability in the response to succinylcholine.[68] It is now known that a single autosomal locus is responsible for all the plasma cholinesterase variants. One method for evaluating plasma cholinesterase activity is with inhibition by dibucaine. The dibucaine number is the degree of inhibition (in percent); normal is 71 to 85, intermediate is about 60, and atypical is about 20. The activity of atypical cholinesterase is decreased by 70%, homozygotes are very sensitive to succinylcholine, and the frequency of this variant is about 2%. Another method for evaluating plasma cholinesterase activity is with inhibition by fluoride, which typically parallels dibucaine inhibition. A small number of patients (0.3%), however, express a fluoride-resistant enzyme whose activity is decreased by 60%, and who are moderately sensitive to succinylcholine. Patients with the silent variant (0.03%) have no enzyme activity. Molecular biologic techniques have recently identified several other plasma cholinesterase variants.

The prototype substrate for plasma cholinesterase is succinylcholine, which is successively hydrolyzed to succinylmonocholine and in turn to succinic acid. Hydrolysis is rapid, with 90% of a dose metabolized within 1 minute, thereby presystemic clearance is substantial and robust (a 70% reduction in enzyme activity only moderately prolongs neuromuscular blockade). Mivacurium is also hydrolyzed by plasma cholinesterase, at a rate 70% to 90% of that of succinylcholine. Patients with cholinesterase variants respond similarly to mivacurium and succinylcholine. A major route of cocaine metabolism is benzoyl ester hydrolysis by plasma cholinesterase to ecgonine methyl ester. The ester local anesthetics procaine and chloroprocaine (3 times faster than procaine) are metabolized by plasma cholinesterase. Heroin undergoes extensive deacetylation in blood to 6-monoacetylmorphine, and further hydrolysis to morphine. The former reaction is catalyzed rapidly by plasma cholinesterase and more slowly by erythrocyte AChE, although the latter reaction accounts for the majority of hydrolysis in vivo and only erythrocyte AChE can convert 6-monoacetylmorphine to morphine.

Other drugs, including esmolol and remifentanil, also undergo extensive biotransformation and inactivation in blood. However, their metabolism is catalyzed exclusively by erythrocyte AChE, and plasma cholinesterase has no catalytic activity.[70] Hence remifentanil elimination is not altered by pseudocholinesterase deficiency or by hepatic insufficiency.[71]

Flavin-Containing Monooxygenase

FMO is an NADPH-dependent microsomal flavoprotein enzyme that oxidizes nitrogen-, sulfur-, phosphorus-, and other heteroatom-containing compounds.[72,73] Currently, five FMO families have been identified. FMO1 is the major hepatic isoform in most animals used in experiments. FMO1 is the major form in human fetal liver and in human kidney, but is not appreciably expressed in adult human liver, where FMO3 is the predominant isoform. FMO1 is also expressed in human intestine. FMO5 is a lesser form in human liver. Cyclic and aliphatic tertiary amines are good substrates for FMO3, which converts the prototype substrate trimethylamine to a stable *N*-oxide. FMO3 also catalyzes the *N*-oxygenation or *S*-oxygenation of antipsychotics such as clozapine, several tricyclic antidepressants, H₂-antagonists such as cimetidine and ranitidine, amphetamine, methamphetamine, nicotine, and an important disulfiram metabolite. Most reactions that are catalyzed by FMO are also catalyzed by CYP; however, the relative importance of the two enzyme systems differs for various substrates. For example, *S*-oxidation of cimetidine and omeprazole (see Fig. 4–1) are catalyzed predominantly by FMO3 and CYP3A, respectively.

Others

Numerous other enzymes act on xenobiotics, but are quantitatively less important than those detailed earlier with respect to the metabolism of therapeutic drugs. These include the oxidoreductases xanthine oxidase-xanthine dehydrogenase, aldehyde oxidase, alcohol and aldehyde dehydrogenases, monoamine oxidase, and epoxide hydrolases.

Phase II Enzymes

There are several enzyme families including methyl and sulfotransferases, acetyl and acyltransferases, glucuronosyltransferases, and glutathione transferases that directly conjugate drugs or conjugate their oxidative metabolites.

Glucuronosyltransferase

The uridine diphosphate glucuronosyltransferases (UGTs) are a family of microsomal enzymes that catalyze the covalent addition of glucuronic acid to a variety of lipophilic endogenous and exogenous compounds containing phenolic, alcohol, amine, carboxyl, or sulfhydryl groups.[74–76] Glucuronides are more water-soluble than their parent compounds, circulate freely in plasma, and are rapidly excreted in bile or urine (depending on size). Because the intestine contains significant amounts of β-glucuronidase, which hydrolyzes glucuronides back to their parent compounds, the free compounds can be intestinally reabsorbed and transported to the liver to undergo reconjugation and re-excretion; this is referred to as enterohepatic recirculation. Glucuronides may be more or less pharmacologically active than their parent drugs. There are 15 human UGTs, broadly classified into the UGT1 (phenol/bilirubin) and UGT2 (steroid/bile) families. Humans express UGT1A1, UGT1A3, UGT1A4, and UGT1A6 through UGT1A10, which glucuronidate endogenous compounds such as bilirubin, bile acids, steroids, retinoids, thyroid hormones, and a considerable number of drugs (planar and bulky phenols, amines, anthraquinones, flavones). Humans also express UGT2A1, UGT2B4, UGT2B7, UGT2B15 and UGT2B17 subfamilies that glucuronidate bile acids, steroids, retinoids, fatty acids, and a small number of drugs. In general, UGT2B7 possesses the broadest substrate specificity among UGT2B isoforms. Although expressed predominantly in the liver, UGTs also have been found in human kidney, gastrointestinal tract, prostate, and brain. Glucuronidation is inducible by phenobarbital, phenytoin, carbamazepine, rifampin, and contraceptive steroids, and is inhibited by probenecid as well as other substrates that inhibit competitively.

Glucuronidation is an important biotransformation pathway for certain drugs used in anesthesia. Propofol glucuronidation by human liver and kidney UGT1A9[77] is the major route of systemic elimination. UGT2B7 glucuronidates a number of opioids and morphinans, such as morphine (both the 3- and 6-positions, with the former predominating), codeine, naloxone, nalorphine, buprenorphine, oxymorphone, and hydromorphone.[78,79] Morphine 6-glucuronidation is particularly important because this metabolite is much more potent than its parent drug; it is thought to play a significant role in morphine analgesia, and the finding of UGT2B7 in human brain suggests that in situ formation of this metabolite may play a role in analgesia.[80] The glucuronide of 1-hydroxymidazolam is pharmacologically active, circulates in high concentrations in plasma, is renally excreted, and is thought to underlie the prolonged effects of midazolam in patients with renal insufficiency when used for intensive care unit sedation.

Glutathione-*S*-transferase

Glutathione-*S*-transferases (GSTs) catalyze the reaction of the tripeptide glutathione (gly-Cys-glu) with the electrophilic carbon, nitrogen, or sulfur of a diverse array of drugs, pesticides, and environmental carcinogens and toxicants including haloalkanes, haloalkenes, epoxides, quinines, and aromatic halo and nitro compounds.[81–83] GSTs are primarily a defensive system for detoxification and protection against oxidative stress, and hence are abundantly and ubiquitously expressed in large amounts (as much as 4% of total hepatic cytosolic protein) in most tissues. There are two superfamilies of GSTs, a large number of cytosolic and a small number of membrane-bound microsomal GSTs. The human soluble cytosolic GSTs are classified into alpha, kappa, mu, pi, sigma, theta, zeta and omega classes (GSTA, GSTK, GSTM, GSTP, GSTS, GSTT, GSTZ, GSTO, respectively), with individual subfamilies in each class, and they are largely responsible for conjugating toxic xenobiotics and endobiotics. The microsomal GSTs are grouped together and are thought to be involved in arachidonic acid/prostaglandin and glutathione metabolism.

There is considerable polymorphism in GST expression, particularly GSTs A, M, P, T, and Z. Because of the importance of GST in detoxification, there has been extensive study of the association between GST expression and susceptibility to disease, particularly cancer and asthma, both as disease-causing and disease-modifying factors. For example, the GSTM1 *null* allele (50% of whites) and GSTT *null* allele (12–62%, varying between ethnic groups) are considered high risk for tobacco- and diet-associated cancers. The combination is linked to a poor response to chemotherapy of ovarian cancer, and an association between GSTP1 genotypes and atopic airway disease has been reported.

Bonding to the cysteine sulfur of GSH generally renders the resulting conjugates more water-soluble, less chemically reactive, and more rapidly eliminated. Nonetheless, for a small number of molecules such as haloalkanes and haloalkenes, GSH conjugation constitutes a mechanism for bioactivation and toxification, specifically nephrotoxicity.[84,85] These conjugates are excreted in bile and are cleaved sequentially in the bile duct and small intestine into corresponding cysteine conjugates, which may reenter the circulation. Cysteine conjugates may be *N*-acetylated to the corresponding *N*-acetylcysteine conjugate (also called a mercapturic acid). Mercapturates are nontoxic and are rapidly excreted in urine. Circulating glutathione and cysteine conjugates and mercapturic acids can be actively taken up by renal proximal tubular cells. There, the cysteine conjugates (and deacetylated mercapturates) may undergo bioactivation by cysteine conjugate ß-lyase to highly reactive intermediates that cause proximal tubular cell necrosis. This complex multiorgan, multienzyme pathway is often referred to as the ß-lyase pathway. The haloalkene "compound A," which results from sevoflurane degradation by carbon dioxide absorbents, undergoes metabolism by this complex pathway, both in animals and in humans.[86–89] Compound A nephrotoxicity in rats is attributed to glutathione- and β-lyase–dependent bioactivation.[90,91] The absence of compound A nephrotoxicity in humans has been ascribed to species differences in dose and relative biotransformation between detoxification (mercapturate formation) and toxification (β-lyase) pathways.[88,89]

N-acetyl-transferase

N-acetylation is a common phase II reaction for heterocyclic aromatic amines, arylamines hydrazines, and hydroxylamines. *N*-acetylation reactions can inactivate (isoniazid), create an active metabolite (*N*-acetylprocainamide), and bioactivate with toxic consequences (*N*-acetylation of arylamine carcinogens).[24,92–94] *O*-acetylation is also a bioactivating reaction. Both acetylations are catalyzed by the cytosolic enzyme *N*-acetyltransferase (NAT), which transfers the acetyl group from acetyl CoA. NAT is of great historical significance because it was the first drug metabolizing enzyme for which a genetic polymorphism was discovered. Isoniazid *N*-acetylation was observed to be diminished in some individuals, populations could be segregated into fast- and slow-acetylators, and pedigree studies showed this phenotype to be genetically linked. Slow acetylators show a greater therapeutic response than fast acetylators to several drugs (i.e., isoniazid, hydralazine, dapsone), and the latter group may require a greater dose. In contrast, slow acetylators may be more susceptible to the side effects of drugs that are mediated by acetylated metabolites. For example, slow acetylators have a greater incidence of isoniazid hepatotoxicity and a greater incidence of lupus-like syndrome after hydralazine or procainamide. Susceptibility to carcinogens has also been linked to genetic differences in NAT. There are two human *N*-acetyl-transferases, NAT1 and NAT2, with discrete but overlapping substrate specificities. NAT2 is expressed in liver and intestine, whereas NAT1 is more ubiquitously expressed. Although there are polymorphisms in NAT1, it is the genetic variability in NAT2 that is responsible for the slow-acetylator phenotype. The frequency of the alleles that code for proteins of lower NAT2 activity is genetically disparate, ranging from 50% to 60% in whites, 40% in African Americans, 20% in Chinese, to 8% in Japanese.

Sulfotransferase

Sulfotransferases, which are cytosolic, catalyze the transfer of a sulfate group from phosphoadenosine-phosphosulfate to numerous endogenous and a small number of exogenous compounds containing an amine, phenol, alcohol, or steroid functionalities.[95] Sulfation is an important pathway for the elimination of acetaminophen and of morphine in neonates.

Extrahepatic Metabolism

Intestine

Orally administered drugs traverse two organs of biotransformation, the small intestine and the liver, before reaching the systemic circulation. Although traditionally thought of as an organ of absorption, it is now clear that the small intestine also has considerable drug metabolizing activity, involving both phase I and phase II reactions.[5,96–98] Bioavailability, which is the fraction of administered drug that enters the systemic circulation, can be reduced by both intestinal and hepatic biotransformation (which act in series), referred to as first-pass, or presystemic metabolism. Almost all of the enzymes of biotransformation present in the liver are also present in the intestine, albeit at a smaller overall content. Principal enzymes include the P450s, glucuronosyltransferases, sulfotransferases, *N*-acetyl-transferase, glutathione transferases, esterases, and alcohol dehydrogenase. Unlike the liver in which there is uniform regional distribution of biotransformation activity, many of these enzymes are nonuniformly distributed in the intestine, with a decreasing content gradient from duodenum to jejunum and ileum, and a preferential expression at the apical portion of the intestinal villus.

Bioavailability (F) after oral administration is the product of the individual bioavailabilities in each successive organ, hence $F = f_{abs} \cdot F_G \cdot F_H = f_{abs} \cdot (1 - E_G) \cdot (1 - E_H)$, where f_{abs} is the fraction of drug absorbed across the gut lumen, F_G and F_H are the intestinal (gut) and hepatic bioavailabilities, respectively, and E_G and E_H are the intestinal and hepatic extraction ratios ($F = 1 - E$). The extraction ratio is the fraction of drug that escapes extraction (and metabolism) in each passage through the organ. First-pass metabolism can occur in the intestine, liver, or both organs. Intestinal extraction can range from less than 1% to more than 99%, but can be particularly important for drugs with high first-pass clearance and low oral bioavailability.[5] For drugs such as verapamil, midazolam, and cyclosporine with low oral bioavailabilities, once thought to be caused by hepatic first-pass extraction, it is now clear that intestinal first-pass extraction is quantitatively significant, particularly with respect to drug interactions (Table 4–3). Intestinal metabolism plays a relatively minor role in systemic drug elimination.

The CYP system is located throughout the gastrointestinal tract. The majority of P450 is in the small intestine, although small amounts of P450 are found in the esophagus, stomach and, colon. Total average intestinal P450 (20 pmol/mg microsomal protein) is less than in the liver (300 pmol/mg); however, the villus tip cells in which P450 predominates comprise a small fraction of intestinal protein,

TABLE 4–3.

Hepatic and Intestinal Metabolism and Drug Interactions

Drug	Pretreatment	f_{abs}	F_G*	F_H	Reference
S-Verapamil	none	16 – 6	47 – 14	38 – 8	150
	rifampin	0.7 – 0.4	8 – 11	8 – 9	
Midazolam	none	25 – 10	40 – 15	65 – 13	151
	ketoconazole	80 – 32	88 – 38	92 – 4	
Cyclosporine	none	22 – 5	30 – 8	75 – 7	152
	ketoconazole	56 – 12	65 – 11	86 – 4	

Results are mean ± SD.

*Actually $f_{abs} F_G$, because f_{abs} (the fraction of drug absorbed) is not independently measured.

so that localized concentrations are greater.[97] Only a limited number of P450 isoforms are expressed in human intestine.[5,99] CYP3A4 is the predominant isoform, and also accounts for most (>70%) of the total intestinal P450.[100] CYP3A5 is also expressed. The second most abundant isoforms are the CYP2C family, specifically CYP2C9 and CYP2C19.[101] CYP1A1 has also been detected, and some but not all investigators have detected CYP2D6. Total intestinal CYP2C content is approximately one-fifth that of CYP3A4.[97] Total intestinal CYP3A4 content is less than that in liver, and intestinal CYP3A4 expression is greater than in other extrahepatic organs; however, quantitative estimates vary.[5,97]

Human liver and intestinal CYP3A4 are identical proteins, and hepatic and intestinal metabolism of CYP3A4 substrates and effects of inhibitors are similar.[6,102,103] However, hepatic and intestinal CYP3A4 are independently regulated; the two enzymes are not coordinately expressed and are not necessarily similarly effected by drug interactions. Most hepatic CYP3A4 substrates are also metabolized by human intestinal cells, or microsomes, or both, and rates of intestinal microsomal metabolism (normalized for protein content) were 45% to 118% of those for hepatic microsomes and even greater than for hepatic microsomes when normalized to total CYP content (because CYP3A34 comprises a greater fraction of intestinal P450).[5,6,104] Thus microsomal intrinsic clearances are generally twofold to threefold greater in intestine than in liver.[5] In humans, in vivo, several CYP3A4 substrates (for example, cyclosporine, midazolam, nifedipine, verapamil, saquinavir) have been shown to undergo significant first-pass intestinal extraction and gut wall metabolism in vivo. The magnitude of such first-pass intestinal metabolism can be substantial; indeed, intestinal extraction ratios equal or exceed those in liver for cyclosporine, verapamil, saquinavir, and midazolam. Intestinal metabolism accounts for a significant portion of first-pass clearance of numerous orally administered CYP3A4 substrates.[5,98]

Kidney

Human kidneys are fully capable of oxidizing and conjugating drugs and endogenous substrates.[105] Kidneys express P450, glutathione peroxidase, glutathione reductase and glutathione transferases,[106–108] and aldo-keto reductases, flavin monooxygenases, esterases/amidases, glucuronyltransferases, N-acetyl-transferases, and cysteine conjugate-β-lyase.[105] Most of the extrahepatic glucuronidation in the body is thought to occur in the kidney. Total P450 content in the human kidney is approximately an order of magnitude less than in the liver.[109] CYP3A enzymes are the most abundant human renal P450s, with CYP3A5 ubiquitously expressed and accounting for 75% of CYP3A, and CYP3A4 more variably expressed.[63] Although total renal microsomal CYP3A content (per milligram protein) is two to three orders of magnitude less than that of liver, this is relative to total renal protein content. Considering that renal P450s are localized to the proximal tubule, the specific content of CYP3A in proximal tubular cells therefore approximates that in hepatocytes. Renal CYP3As are fully competent to metabolize hepatic CYP3A substrates and are thought to contribute significantly to the intrarenal metabolism of certain drugs and steroids, such as cortisol and methoxyflurane.[63,110] Human kidneys express only CYP3A4, CYP3A5, CYP4A, and CYP4F.[63,106,108,109,111] This is in contrast to rat kidneys, which express a considerable number of P450 isoforms. Renal CYP4As hydroxylate fatty acids such as arachidonic acid to hydroxyeicosatetraenoic acid, and may play a role in regulating renal salt and water balance and blood pressure.[112] Several renal P450s responsible for the metabolism of vitamin D analogs have been identified, although they are not known to metabolize drugs.[113]

Human and rat kidneys differ markedly in their expression of P450s and GSTs. A consistent and important finding is the absence of CYP2E1 in human kidneys,[108–111] particularly in comparison to human liver where it constitutes about

7% of total P450, and in rat kidneys where it is relatively highly expressed (10% of liver content).[114] This is important because CYP2E1 is the major isoform responsible for the metabolism of most volatile anesthetics. The ability of human kidneys to metabolize methoxyflurane but not sevoflurane, explained by the metabolism of the former by several P450s (including renal CYP3A) but the latter only by CYP2E1 (which is not present in human kidneys), is thought potentially to underlie the nephrotoxicity of methoxyflurane but not sevoflurane in humans, despite their similar hepatic metabolism.[110]

Brain

P450s from all three major families have been detected in human brain, although there are regioselective and isoform-selective differences in expression.[115,116] Cerebral P450 activity is low (>2 orders of magnitude less than liver), and most studies have used polymerase chain reaction to detect mRNA, although some have directly identified the proteins. A few studies have shown the ability of human brain to metabolize psychotropic drugs, and more have shown the ability of rat brain to metabolize a variety of drugs. In human brain, CYP1A1 and CYP2C8 are the most widely expressed isoforms, and CYP2D6, CYP2E1, CYP3A4 and CYP3A5 have been found in specific brain regions.

Developmental Regulation

Developmental aspects of drug metabolism have been recently reviewed.[54,117–120] The fetus is fully competent to metabolize hormones and drugs, and the liver is the main site of fetal biotransformation, catalyzing both phase I and phase II reactions. There are significant age-dependent differences in biotransformation. Neonatal biotransformation is much less than in infants and adults. Maturation of drug metabolizing enzymes, rather than changes in hepatic size or blood flow, is considered to be the major factor responsible for these changes. Fetal drug metabolism is unique because the more water-soluble metabolites produced by oxidation and conjugation do not readily cross the placenta back to the mother and may be swallowed and reabsorbed if excreted in urine, thereby prolonging fetal exposure. Changes in biotransformation occur primarily within the first year of life, with minimal changes in activity between childhood (<10 years) and adulthood (<60 years).[119]

Total hepatic CYP concentration at birth is approximately one third that of adults, and the individual CYP isoforms mature at different rates. Drugs with reduced clearance or metabolism in neonates include caffeine, diazepam, midazolam, fentanyl, nicotine, phenytoin, and theophylline.[120] CYP1A2 is absent in human fetal liver; however, expression and activity begin to increase in 8- to 28-day-old neonates, and reaches a plateau at adult levels of activity at 4 to 12 months of age.[117,120] This rate is slower than for other CYP isoforms. CYP1A1 is not expressed in adult human liver, but may be expressed in fetal liver.[118] CYP2A and CYP2B iso-

forms are not expressed in fetal liver, but do appear in infants and children. CYP2C protein and activity appear absent or negligible in human fetal liver, but increase rapidly after birth. Activity appears on the first postnatal day, increases substantially in neonates, and remains at about 40% of adult levels during the first year.[120] CYP2D6 activity is also absent or negligible at birth, but increases rapidly in the first week to levels that are, however, less than in adults.[117,120] Increases in CYP during the neonatal period (<4 weeks) are attributable primarily to CYP2C isoforms.[117] The presence of CYP2E1 in fetal liver is controversial, but expression does increase in infants and children.

CYP3A isoforms undergo the greatest and most complex pattern of maturation.[54] Figure 4–5A shows the age-dependent clearance of midazolam, a prototypic CYP3A

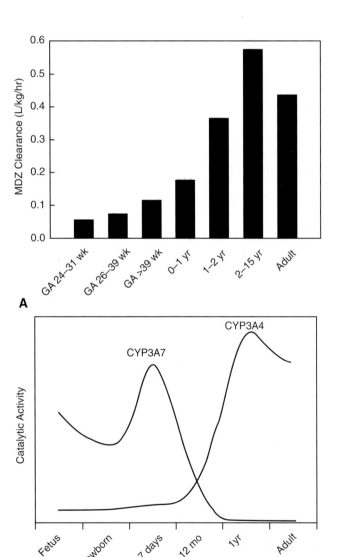

A

B

Figure 4–5. Developmental aspects of CYP3A activity. *A,* Clearance of the CYP3A4 probe midazolam (MDZ). GA, gestational age. *B,* CYP3A7 and CYP3A4 expression. (From de Wildt SN, Kearns GL, Leeder JS, et al: Cytochrome P450 3A: Ontogeny and drug disposition. Clin Pharmacokinet 37:485–505, 1999.)

probe. CYP3A7 is the major isoform present in human embryonic, fetal, and newborn liver, constituting on average about 30% of total hepatic CYP but occasionally as much as 50%. It is expressed in liver in early pregnancy, during embryogenesis, is greater at 20 than at 40 weeks, reaches a peak in the first week of life, and declines rapidly thereafter to less than 10% of newborn levels by 3 to 12 months (Fig. 4–5*B*). Fetal CYP3A4 expression is minimal, but increases immediately after birth, concomitant with the decline in CYP3A7, such that total hepatic CYP3A remains relatively constant. CYP3A4 activity reaches 30% to 50% of adult levels from 3 to 12 months. CYP3A7 is also expressed in the placenta and pregnant endometrium. Although CYP3A7 has 90% sequence similarity to CYP3A4, and metabolizes several 3A4 substrates, there are important quantitative differences; activity toward most substrates and some hormones is considerably less than for CYP3A4, whereas activity toward other hormones is greater.

Comparatively less is known about the developmental expression of phase II enzymes; the greatest amount of information available is for glucuronidation and sulfation.[118,120] Human fetal and neonatal hepatic glucuronidation is immature, with activity less than 10% to 30% of adult levels. UGT activity does not mature for several years into childhood. The clearance of morphine, which is extensively glucuronidated, increases with both gestational and postnatal age. Human fetal sulfotransferase activity, in contrast, is substantial, and some isoforms exhibit even greater activity than in adults. Whereas adults preferentially glucuronidate, neonates preferentially sulfate.

Transport Proteins

Although transmembrane transport proteins do not catalyze biotransformation per se, they nonetheless markedly affect drug bioavailability and can act in concert with intracellular drug metabolizing enzymes. These transport proteins are members of the large protein family known as ABC (adenosine triphosphate binding cassette) proteins.[121]

P-glycoprotein (P-gp) is a constitutively expressed, plasma membrane efflux pump that actively transports a structurally diverse array of compounds out of the interior of several cell types.[122–124] It is the first cloned and best-characterized ABC protein, and is also known as the multidrug resistance protein (MDR1) because cancer cell resistance was associated with this protein. P-gp is expressed on the apical (luminal) surface of epithelial cells, including the brush border of intestinal cells, hepatocyte biliary canalicular cell membranes, and the luminal surface of renal proximal tubular cells. In the gut, it actively pumps drugs from the intracellular milieu against a concentration gradient back into the intestinal lumen, actively countering intestinal drug absorption, and thereby limiting oral drug absorption and bioavailability. P-gp substrates include anti-cancer drugs, peptides, HIV protease inhibitors, and opioids.

The critical role of P-gp in determining drug pharmacokinetics and pharmacodynamics has been increasingly recognized.[122–124] For example, P-gp plays a significant role in the intestinal absorption, first-pass elimination, and

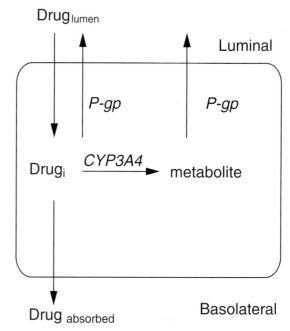

Figure 4–6. Concerted effect of CPY3A4 and P-gp on enterocyte drug metabolism and absorption.

bioavailability of cyclosporine, which had been previously attributed to intestinal CYP3A4-dependent metabolism.[125] Intestinal P-gp is colocalized with CYP3A4 in enterocytes, and the two systems are thought to act concertedly and synergistically to increase presystemic drug metabolism and decrease oral bioavailability (Fig. 4–6).[124,126] There is considerable overlap in the array of substrates metabolized by CYP3A and transported by P-gp. P-gp is thought to possibly increase drug exposure to enterocyte CYP3A4 and enhance metabolism through repeated cycles of absorption and efflux, and/or facilitate removal of CYP3A4-generated metabolites, which could otherwise cause product inhibition of parent drug metabolism (see Fig. 4–6). There is considerable interindividual variability in human P-gp intestinal expression, P-gp is inducible and inhibitable, and P-gp drug interactions in humans have been identified. For example, rifampin increased human intestinal P-gp content 3.5-fold[127] and decreased the bioavailability and plasma area under the concentration-time curve (AUC) of oral (but not intravenous [IV]) digoxin and cyclosporine.[128,129] Conversely, quinidine inhibition of P-gp increased plasma digoxin concentrations.[123]

P-gp is also expressed on the luminal surface of brain capillary endothelial cells, where it is an intrinsic part of the blood–brain barrier and limits central nervous system access of drugs. Thus P-gp can be a major determinant of drug pharmacodynamics.[123,130,131]

Of particular potential significance in anesthesia is that opioids are substrates for P-gp,[132] both in the intestine and the brain. Morphine, the best-characterized opioid, is extruded by brain capillary endothelial cells that comprise the blood–brain barrier, actively limiting morphine access to the central nervous system.[133–135] P-gp inhibition in mice in vivo increased the concentration of morphine in brain extracellular fluid, and increased the magnitude and duration of morphine antinociception.[134] In knockout mice lacking P-gp, brain extracellular fluid morphine concentrations were increased threefold to fourfold,[133] and morphine, methadone, and fentanyl analgesia were significantly increased.[136] Although P-gp is a major determinant of analgesic opioid central nervous system access and analgesia in animals, its role in humans is currently unknown. Nevertheless, a major role for P-gp in determining central nervous system access of the nonanalgesic opioid loperamide in humans was recently demonstrated.[137]

A second subfamily of ABC proteins are the multidrug resistance-associated proteins, also known as the multispecific organic anion transporter.[121,138] The first protein to be discovered in this family was MRP1, whose overexpression is responsible for the majority of non-P-gp—mediated multidrug resistance, and there are seven currently known MRPs. The MRPs are located on either the apical or luminal surface of epithelial cells. Substrates for MRPs include unconjugated organic anions and lipophilic compounds as their glutathione, glucuronide, or sulfate conjugates. Rifampin is known to induce human MRP2.[139] Because MRPs were only recently discovered, little is known about their clinical significance.

Interindividual Variability in Drug Metabolism

Interindividual variability in drug metabolism is a significant clinical issue that can markedly affect drug disposition and hence drug response. Variability can often result in greater than 100-fold ranges in the AUC and even render subjects nonresponsive to certain drugs. Causes of interindividual variability include genetics (sex, race, ethnicity, enzyme polymorphisms), age, environment (diet, smoking, ethanol, solvent or other xenobiotic exposure), disease, and drug interactions. Many of the genetic causes of variability have been addressed earlier.

Metabolic drug interactions are a major source of both interindividual and intraindividual variability in drug disposition, clinical response, and toxicity.[2,4,55] Such interactions are often hepatic, intestinal, or both. For example, troleandomycin inhibits hepatic and intestinal CYP3A, whereas grapefruit juice inhibits only intestinal CYP3A4.[140] Not only does genetic variability alter drug metabolism by influencing CYP expression, but such variability can also influence the type and magnitude of drug interactions. For example, for some CYP3A inhibitors, the susceptibility of polymorphic CYP3A5 differs from that of CYP3A4. Thus the level of CYP3A4 versus CYP3A5 expression influences the degree of inhibition.[103]

The kinetic consequences of enzyme inhibition and induction are dependent on the route of administration and the extraction ratios of the drug (Fig. 4–7).[141] For drugs that are administered intravenously, changes in hepatic metabolism (intrinsic clearance, CLint) will have little effect on the clearance and AUC of high-extraction drugs. This is because the efficiency of extraction is so great that hepatic blood flow is a more rate-limiting factor than metabolism. Conversely, the systemic clearance of low-extraction drugs is highly susceptible to even small changes in CLint, and the AUC

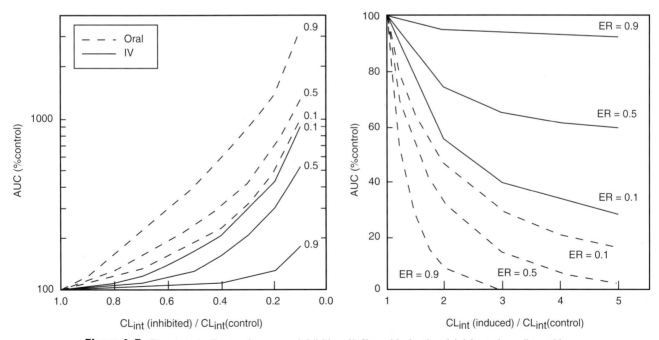

Figure 4–7. Simulated effects of enzyme inhibition (*left*) and induction (*right*) on drug disposition, and dependence on the extraction ratio (ER). The intrinsic clearance (CLint) is expressed as a ratio to that of the control clearance, and disposition is calculated as the area under the concentration-time curve (AUC) relative to control. Changes in hepatic and intestinal CLint were assumed to be equal. Results are shown for a high-, intermediate- and low-extraction drug. (From Lin JH, Lu AY: Interindividual variability in inhibition and induction of cytochrome P450 enzymes. Annu Rev Pharmacol Toxicol 41:535–567, 2001.)

Figure 4–8. Influence of CYP2D6 activity on codeine analgesia. *A,* Pharmacogenetic effects. Shown are the median of the peak changes in peak pain during the cold pressor test in extensive (EM) and poor (PM) metabolizers of sparteine who received placebo (*P*), codeine (*C*), or morphine (*M*). Plasma codeine concentrations were not different in PMs and EMs; however, morphine and morphine-6-glucuronide were undetectable in plasma of PMs. (From Poulsen L, Brøsen K, Arendt-Nielsen L, et al: Codeine and morphine in extensive and poor metabolizers of sparteine: Pharmacokinetics, analgesic effect, and side effects. Eur J Clin Pharmacol 51:292, 1996.) *B,* Drug interaction effects. Individual plasma and cerebrospinal fluid (CSF) concentrations of codeine and morphine in 17 patients 2 hours after 125 mg oral codeine without (■) or with (□) oral pretreatment with 200 mg quinidine. One patient was a PM of sparteine (*diagonal half-filled square*) and 16 were extensive metabolizers (■, □). (From Sindrup SH, Hofmann U, Asmussen J, et al: Impact of quinidine on plasma and cerebrospinal fluid concentrations of codeine and morphine after codeine intake. Eur J Clin Pharmacol 49:507, 1996.)

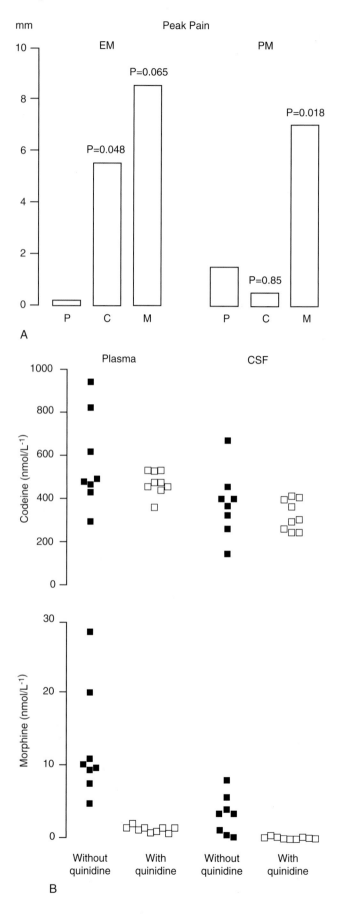

changes proportionately to the CLint. Hence, for example, after IV administration, the systemic clearance of the low-extraction opioid alfentanil is exquisitely sensitive to hepatic CYP induction and inhibition,[142] whereas clearance of the high-extraction opioids fentanyl and sufentanil is usually not affected.[143] For orally administered drugs, the changes in AUC with induction and inhibition will always be greater than those after IV administration, particularly for intermediate- and high-extraction drugs. In addition, the differences in the percentage change in the AUC after oral versus IV administration are greater for high- compared with low-extraction drugs. The extraction ratios of commonly used anesthetics are provided in Table 4-4.

TABLE 4–4.

Hepatic Extraction of Some Commonly Used Drugs

Low extraction (ER < 0.3)	Thiopental, diazepam, lorazepam, triazolam, theophylline, alfentanil, methadone
Intermediate extraction	Methohexital, midazolam, vecuronium, rocuronium, ropivacaine, mepivacaine, hydromorphone
High extraction (ER > 0.7)	Etomidate, propofol, ketamine, bupivacaine, lidocaine, metoprolol, propranolol, labetalol, fentanyl, sufentanil, remifentanil, meperidine, morphine, naloxone

ER, extraction ratio.

The role of biotransformation, pharmacogenetics, and drug interactions in interindividual variability in drug disposition and response is illustrated by codeine, a prodrug requiring CYP2D6-mediated metabolic activation (*O*-demethylation) to the mu agonist morphine, and even greater bioactivation to the more potent agonist morphine-6-glucuronide (reviewed by Wilcox and Owen[48]). CYP2D6-deficient individuals are PMs of codeine, have markedly diminished or absent morphine formation, and have minimal if any analgesia (Fig. 4–8*A*).[144] Conversely, individuals with CYP2D6 gene amplification, duplication (ultrarapid metabolizers), or both, have greater morphine formation from codeine than EMs and PMs. Ethnic variations attributable to codeine biotransformation have also been observed.[145] For example, Chinese produced less morphine from codeine, were less sensitive to the opioid effects of codeine, and therefore might experience reduced analgesia from codeine. The metabolic drug interaction with the CYP2D6 inhibitor quinidine markedly diminishes codeine bioactivation and morphine formation (Fig. 4–8*B*).[146] Interactions other than those at pathways of bioactivation or inactivation can also have metabolic consequence. For example, rifampin induction of CYP3A4 increased codeine *N*-demethylation (see Fig. 4–4), making less codeine available for *O*-demethylation, and thereby decreasing the formation of morphine.[147]

Summary

Biotransformation is a major determinant of drug disposition, bioavailability, clearance, clinical effect, and toxicity. Recent advances in molecular biology and genetics have markedly increased our understanding of the identity, expression, activity, regulation, ontogeny, and genetics of hepatic and extrahepatic biotransformation enzymes. CYP2C, CYP2D6, and CYP3A4/5 are the most clinically relevant human CYPs. Genetic polymorphisms in CYP2C9, CYP2C19, CYP2D6, and CYP3A5 are therapeutically significant, markedly affecting the ability to inactivate, eliminate, or bioactivate numerous drugs with therapeutic consequence. CYP1A, CYP2A6, and CYP2E1 metabolize a vast array of protoxins, and hence can modulate drug toxicity.[4,148] Identification of the role of these enzymes in anesthetic biotransformation has increased our understanding of fundamental mechanisms of interindividual variability in anesthetic disposition, clinical response, and toxicity. Genetic and phenotypic profiling of patients' biotransformation capabilities may permit more tailored therapies to maximize therapeutic benefit and minimize drug toxicity.[149]

References

1. Testa B: The metabolism of drugs and other xenobiotics. Biochemistry of redox reactions. San Diego, Academic Press, 1995.
2. Levy RH, Thummel KE, Trager WF, et al: Metabolic drug interactions. Philadelphia, Lippincott Williams & Wilkins, 2000.
3. Gibson GG, Skett P: Introduction to drug metabolism. Cheltenham, UK, Stanley Thornes Publishers, 1999.
4. Lin JH, Lu AY: Interindividual variability in inhibition and induction of cytochrome P450 enzymes. Annu Rev Pharmacol Toxicol 41:535–567, 2001.
5. Shen DD, Thummel KE, Kunze KL: Enzyme-catalyzed processes of first-pass hepatic and intestinal drug extraction. Adv Drug Deliv Rev 27:99–127, 1997.
6. Thummel KE, Wilkinson GR: In vitro and in vivo drug interactions involving human CYP3A. Annu Rev Pharmacol Toxicol 38:389–430, 1998.
7. Nelson DR, Koymans L, Kamataki T, et al: P450 superfamily: update on new sequences, gene mapping, accession numbers and nomenclature. Pharmacogenetics 6:1–42, 1996.
8. Smith G, Stubbins MJ, Harries LW, et al: Molecular genetics of the human cytochrome P450 monooxygenase superfamily. Xenobiotica 28:1129–1165, 1998.
9. Nelson DR: Cytochrome P450 and the individuality of species. Arch Biochem Biophys 369:1–10, 1999.
10. Nebert DW, Ingelman-Sundberg M, Daly AK: Genetic epidemiology of environmental toxicity and cancer susceptibility: Human allelic polymorphisms in drug-metabolizing enzyme genes, their functional importance, and nomenclature issues. Drug Metab Rev 31:467–487, 1999.
11. White RE, Coon MJ: Oxygen activation by cytochrome P-450. Ann Rev Biochem 49:315–356, 1980.
12. Sharer JE, Wrighton SA: Identification of the human hepatic cytochromes P450 involved in the *in vitro* oxidation of antipyrine. Drug Metab Dispos 24:487–494, 1996.
13. Labroo RB, Thummel KE, Kunze KL, et al: Catalytic role of cytochrome P4503A4 in multiple pathways of alfentanil metabolism. Drug Metab Dispos 23:490–496, 1995.
14. Guitton J, Buronfosse T, Désage M, et al: Possible involvement of multiple cytochrome P450s in fentanyl and sufentanil metabolism as opposed to alfentanil. Biochem Pharmacol 53:1613–1619, 1997.
15. Spracklin D, Thummel KE, Kharasch ED: Human reductive halothane metabolism in vitro is catalyzed by cytochrome P450 2A6 and 3A4. Drug Metab Dispos 24:976–983, 1996.
16. Spracklin D, Hankins DC, Fisher JM, et al: Cytochrome P450 2E1 is the principal catalyst of human oxidative halothane metabolism. J Pharmacol Exp Ther 281:400–411, 1997.
17. Spracklin D, Kharasch ED: Human halothane reduction *in vitro* by cytochrome P450 2A6 and 3A4: Identification of low and high K_m isoforms. Drug Metab Dispos 26:605–608, 1998.
18. Ekström G, Gunnarsson U-B: Ropivacaine, a new amide-type local anesthetic agent, is metabolized by cytochromes P450 1A and 3A in human liver microsomes. Drug Metab Dispos 24:955–961, 1996.
19. Oda Y, Furuichi K, Tanaka K, et al: Metabolism of a new local anesthetic, ropivacaine, by human hepatic cytochrome P450. Anesthesiology 82:214–820, 1995.
20. Clarke SE: *In vitro* assessment of human cytochrome P450. Xenobiotica 28:1167–1202, 1998.
21. Smith DA, Abel SM, Hyland R, et al: Human cytochrome P450s: Selectivity and measurement in vivo. Xenobiotica 28:1095–1128, 1998.
22. Streetman DS, Bertino JS Jr, Nafziger AN: Phenotyping of drug-metabolizing enzymes in adults: A review of in-vivo cytochrome P450 phenotyping probes. Pharmacogenetics 10:187–216, 2000.
23. Guengerich FP, Parikh A, Turesky RJ, et al: Inter-individual differences in the metabolism of environmental toxicants: Cytochrome P450 1A2 as a prototype. Mutat Res 428:115–124, 1999.
24. Wormhoudt LW, Commandeur JN, Vermeulen NP: Genetic polymorphisms of human *N*-acetyltransferase, cytochrome P450, glutathione-S-transferase, and epoxide hydrolase enzymes: Relevance to xenobiotic metabolism and toxicity. Crit Rev Toxicol 29:59–124, 1999.
25. Kashuba AD, Bertino Jr JS, Kearns GL, et al: Quantitation of three-month intraindividual variability and influence of sex and menstrual cycle phase on CYP1A2, *N*-acetyltransferase-2, and xanthine oxidase activity determined with caffeine phenotyping, Clin Pharmacol Ther 63:540–551, 1998.
26. Kamimori GH, Joubert A, Otterstetter R, et al: The effect of the menstrual cycle on the pharmacokinetics of caffeine in normal, healthy eumenorrheic females. Eur J Clin Pharmacol 55:445–449, 1999.
27. Honkakoski P, Negishi M: The structure, function, and regulation of cytochrome P450 2A enzymes. Drug Metab Rev 29:977–996, 1997.

28. Raunio H, Rautio A, Pelkonen O: The CYP2A subfamily: Function, expression and genetic polymorphism. IARC Sci Publ 148:197–207, 1999.

29. Lewis DF, Dickins M, Lake BG, et al: Molecular modelling of the human cytochrome P450 isoform CYP2A6 and investigations of CYP2A substrate selectivity. Toxicology 133:1–33, 1999.

30. Oscarson M, McLellan RA, Gullsten H, et al: Identification and characterization of novel polymorphisms in the CYP2A locus: Implications for nicotine metabolism. FEBS Lett 460:321–327, 1999.

31. Pelkonen O, Rautio A, Raunio H, et al: CYP2A6: A human coumarin 7-hydroxylase. Toxicology 144:139–147, 2000.

32. Su T, Bao Z, Zhang QY, et al: Human cytochrome P450 CYP2A13: Predominant expression in the respiratory tract and its high efficiency metabolic activation of a tobacco-specific carcinogen, 4-(methylnitrosamino)-1-(3-pyridyl)-1-butanone. Cancer Res 60:5074–5079, 2000.

33. Ekins S, Wrighton SA: The role of CYP2B6 in human xenobiotic metabolism. Drug Metab Rev 31:719–754, 1999.

34. Ekins S, Bravi G, Ring BJ, et al: Three-dimensional quantitative structure activity relationship analyses of substrates for CYP2B6. J Pharmacol Exp Ther 288:21–29, 1999.

35. Stresser DM, Kupfer D: Monospecific antipeptide antibody to cytochrome P-450 2B6. Drug Metab Dispos 27:517–525, 1999.

36. Gervot L, Rochat B, Gautier JC, et al: Human CYP2B6: Expression, inducibility and catalytic activities. Pharmacogenetics 9:295–306, 1999.

37. Hanna IH, Reed JR, Guengerich FP, et al: Expression of human cytochrome P450 2B6 in *Escherichia coli*: Characterization of catalytic activity and expression levels in human liver. Arch Biochem Biophys 376:206–216, 2000.

38. Oda Y, Hamaoka N, Hiroi T, et al: Involvement of human liver cytochrome P4502B6 in the metabolism of propofol. Br J Clin Pharmacol 51:281–285, 2001.

39. Court MH, Duan SX, Hesse LM, et al: Cytochrome P-450 2B6 is responsible for interindividual variability of propofol hydroxylation by human liver microsomes. Anesthesiology 94:110–119, 2001.

40. Yanagihara Y, Kariya S, Ohtani M, et al: Involvement of CYP2B6 in N-demethylation of ketamine in human liver microsomes. Drug Metab Dispos 29:887–890, 2001.

41. Lang T, Klein K, Fischer J, et al: Extensive genetic polymorphism in the human CYP2B6 gene with impact on expression and function in human liver. Pharmacogenetics 11:399–415, 2001.

42. Miners JO, Birkett DJ: Cytochrome P4502C9: An enzyme of major importance in drug metabolism. Br J Clin Pharmacol 45:525–538, 1998.

43. Lasker JM, Wester MR, Aramsombatdee E, et al: Characterization of CYP2C19 and CYP2C9 from human liver: Respective roles in microsomal tolbutamide, S-mephenytoin, and omeprazole hydroxylations. Arch Biochem Biophys 353:16–28, 1998.

44. Aithal GP, Day CP, Kesteven PJ, et al: Association of polymorphisms in the cytochrome P450 CYP2C9 with warfarin dose requirement and risk of bleeding complications. Lancet 353:717–719, 1999.

45. Bertilsson L: Geographical/interracial differences in polymorphic drug oxidation: Current state of knowledge of cytochromes P450 (CYP) 2D6 and 2C19. Clin Pharmacokinet 29:192–209, 1995.

46. Hägg S, Spigset O, Dahlqvist R: Influence of gender and oral contraceptives on CYP2D6 and CYP2C19 activity in healthy volunteers. Br J Clin Pharmacol 51:169–173, 2001.

47. Lundqvist E, Johansson I, Ingelman-Sundberg M: Genetic mechanisms for duplication and multiduplication of the human CYP2D6 gene and methods for detection of duplicated CYP2D6 genes. Gene 226:327–338, 1999.

48. Wilcox RA, Owen H: Variable cytochrome P450 2D6 expression and metabolism of codeine and other opioid prodrugs: Implications for the Australian anaesthetist. Anaesth Intensive Care 28:611–619, 2000.

49. Ramamoorthy Y, Tyndale RF, Sellers EM: Cytochrome P450 2D6.1 and cytochrome P450 2D6.10 differ in catalytic activity for multiple substrates. Pharmacogenetics 11:477–487, 2001.

50. Kashuba AD, Nafziger AN, Kearns GL, et al: Quantification of intraindividual variability and the influence of menstrual cycle phase on CYP2D6 activity as measured by dextromethorphan phenotyping. Pharmacogenetics 8:403–410, 1998.

51. Lieber CS: Cytochrome P-4502E1: Its physiological and pathological role. Physiol Rev 77:517–544, 1997.

52. Lewis DF, Bird MG, Dickins M, et al: Molecular modeling of human CYP2E1 by homology with the CYP102 haemoprotein domain: Investigation of the interactions of substrates and inhibitors within the putative active site of the human CYP2E1 isoform. Xenobiotica 30:1–25, 2000.

53. Guengerich FP: Cytochrome P-450 3A4: Regulation and role in drug metabolism. Annu Rev Pharmacol Toxicol 39:1–17, 1999.

54. de Wildt SN, Kearns GL, Leeder JS, et al: Cytochrome P450 3A: Ontogeny and drug disposition. Clin Pharmacokinet 37:485–505, 1999.

55. Dresser GK, Spence JD, Bailey DG: Pharmacokinetic-pharmacodynamic consequences and clinical relevance of cytochrome P450 3A4 inhibition. Clin Pharmacokinet 38:41–57, 2000.

56. Wrighton SA, Schuetz EG, Thummel KE, et al: The human CYP3A subfamily: Practical considerations. Drug Metab Rev 32:339–361, 2000.

57. Quattrochi LC, Guzelian PS: CYP3A regulation: From pharmacology to nuclear receptors. Drug Metab Dispos 29:615–622, 2001.

58. Özdemir V, Kalowa W, Tang BK, et al: Evaluation of the genetic component of variability in CYP3A4 activity: A repeated drug administration method. Pharmacogenetics 10:373–388, 2000.

59. Watkins PB: Noninvasive tests of CYP3A enzymes. Pharmacogenetics 4:171–184, 1994.

60. Kharasch ED, Russell M, Garton K, et al: Assessment of cytochrome P450 3A4 activity during the menstrual cycle using alfentanil as a noninvasive probe. Anesthesiology 87:26–35, 1997.

61. Gorski JC, Wang Z, Haehner-Daniels BD, et al: The effect of hormone replacement therapy on CYP3A activity. Clin Pharmacol Ther 68:412–417, 2000.

62. Kuehl P, Zhang J, Lin Y, et al: Sequence diversity in CYP3A promoters and characterization of the genetic basis of polymorphic CYP3A5 expression. Nat Genet 27:383–391, 2001.

63. Haehner BD, Gorski JC, Vandenbranden M, et al: Bimodal distribution of renal cytochrome P450 3A activity in humans. Mol Pharmacol 50:52–59, 1996.

64. Sone T, Wang CY: Microsomal amidases and carboxylesterases. In Guengerich FP (ed): Comprehensive Toxicology, New York, Pergamon, 265–281, 1999.

65. Satoh T, Hosokawa M: The mammalian carboxylesterases: From molecules to functions. Annu Rev Pharmacol Toxicol 38:257–288, 1998.

66. Pindel EV, Kedishvili NY, Abraham TL, et al: Purification and cloning of a broad substrate specificity human liver carboxylesterase that catalyzes the hydrolysis of cocaine and heroin. J Biol Chem 272:14769–14775, 1997.

67. Zhang J, Burnell JC, Dumaual N, et al: Binding and hydrolysis of meperidine by human liver carboxylesterase hCE-1. J Pharmacol Exp Ther 290:314–318, 1999.

68. Davis L, Britten JJ, Morgan M: Cholinesterase: Its significance in anaesthetic practice. Anaesthesia 52:244–260, 1997.

69. Salmon AY, Goren Z, Avissar Y, et al: Human erythrocyte but not brain acetylcholinesterase hydrolyses heroin to morphine. Clin Exp Pharmacol Physiol 26:596–600, 1999.

70. Manullang J, Egan TD: Remifentanil's effect is not prolonged in a patient with pseudocholinesterase deficiency. Anesth Analg 89:529–530, 1999.

71. Dershwitz M, Hoke JF, Rosow CE, et al: Pharmacokinetics and pharmacodynamics of remifentanil in volunteer subjects with severe liver disease. Anesthesiology 84:812–820, 1996.

72. Cashman JR: Human flavin-containing monooxygenase: Substrate specificity and role in drug metabolism. Curr Drug Metab 1:181–191, 2000.

73. Yeung CK, Lang DH, Thummel KE, et al: Immunoquantitation of FMO1 in human liver, kidney, and intestine. Drug Metab Dispos 28:1107–1111, 2000.

74. Tukey RH, Strassburg CP: Human UDP-glucuronosyltransferases: Metabolism, expression, and disease. Annu Rev Pharmacol Toxicol 40:581–616, 2000.

75. de Wildt SN, Kearns GL, Leeder JS, et al: Glucuronidation in humans: Pharmacogenetic and developmental aspects. Clin Pharmacokinet 36:439–452, 1999.

76. Miners JO, Mackenzie PI: Drug glucuronidation in humans. Pharmacol Ther 51:347–369, 1991.

77. Ethell BT, Beaumont K, Rance DJ, et al: Use of cloned and expressed human UDP-glucuronosyltransferases for the assessment of human drug conjugation and identification of potential drug interactions. Drug Metab Dispos 29:48–53, 2001.

78. Coffman BL, King CD, Rios GR, et al: The glucuronidation of opioids, other xenobiotics, and androgens by human UGT2B7Y(268) and UGT2B7H(268). Drug Metab Dispos 26:73–77, 1998.

79. Coffman BL, Rios GR, King CD, et al: Human UGT2B7 catalyzes morphine glucuronidation. Drug Metab Dispos 25:1–4, 1997.

80. King CD, Rios GR, Assouline JA, et al: Expression of UDP-glucuronosyltransferases (UGTs) 2B7 and 1A6 in the human brain and identification of 5-hydroxytryptamine as a substrate. Arch Biochem Biophys 365:156–162, 1999.

81. Armstrong RN: Structure, catalytic mechanism, and evolution of the glutathione transferases. Chem Res Toxicol 10:2–18, 1997.

82. Eaton DL, Bammler TK: Concise review of the glutathione S-transferases and their significance to toxicology. Toxicol Sci 49:156–164, 1999.

83. Hayes JD, Strange RC: Glutathione S-transferase polymorphisms and their biological consequences. Pharmacology 61:154–166, 2000.

84. Dekant W: Biotransformation and renal processing of nephrotoxic agents. Arch Toxicol Suppl 18:163–172, 1996.

85. Commandeur JNM, Stijntjes GL, Vermeulen NPE: Enzymes and transport systems involved in the formation and disposition of glutathione-S-conjugates. Pharm Rev 47:271–330, 1995.

86. Spracklin D, Kharasch ED: Evidence for the metabolism of fluoromethyl-2,2-difluoro-1-(trifluoromethyl)vinyl ether (Compound A), by cysteine conjugate β-lyase in rats. Chem Res Toxicol 9:696–702, 1996.

87. Iyer RA, Frink Jr EJ, Ebert TJ, et al: Cysteine conjugate β-lyase-dependent metabolism of compound A (2-[fluoromethoxy]-1,1,3,3,3-pentafluoro-1-propene) in human subjects anesthetized with sevoflurane and in rats given compound A. Anesthesiology 88:611–618, 1998.

88. Kharasch ED, Jubert C: Compound A uptake and metabolism to mercapturic acids and 3,3,3-trifluoro-2-fluoromethoxypropanoic acid during low-flow sevoflurane anesthesia: Biomarkers for exposure, risk assessment, and interspecies comparison. Anesthesiology 91:1267–1278, 1999.

89. Kharasch ED, Jubert C, Spracklin D, et al: Dose-dependent metabolism of fluoromethyl-2,2-difluoro-1-(trifluoromethyl)vinyl ether (Compound A), an anesthetic degradation product, to mercapturic acids and 3,3,3-trifluoro-2-fluoromethoxypropanoic acid in rats. Toxicol Appl Pharmacol 160:49–59, 1999.

90. Iyer RA, Baggs RB, Anders MW: Nephrotoxicity of the glutathione and cysteine S-conjugates of the sevoflurane degradation product 2-(fluoromethoxy)-1,1,3,3,3-pentafluoro-1-propene (compound A) in male Fischer 344 rats. J Pharmacol Exp Ther 283:1544–1551, 1997.

91. Kharasch ED, Garton K, Hankins D, et al: The role of glutathione and cysteine conjugates and renal cysteine conjugate _-lyase in compound A nephrotoxicity. Anesthesiology 83:A339, 1995.

92. Evans DAP: N-acetyltransferase. Pharmacol Ther 42:157–234, 1989.

93. Hein DW, Doll MA, Fretland AJ, et al: Molecular genetics and epidemiology of the NAT1 and NAT2 acetylation polymorphisms. Cancer Epidemiol Biomarkers Prev 9:29–42, 2000.

94. Upton A, Johnson N, Sandy J, et al: Arylamine N-acetyltransferases-of mice, men and microorganisms. Trends Pharmacol Sci 22:140–146, 2001.

95. Negishi M, Pedersen LG, Petrotchenko E, et al: Structure and function of sulfotransferases. Arch Biochem Biophys 390:149–157, 2001.

96. Krishna DR, Klotz U: Extrahepatic metabolism of drugs in humans. Clin Pharmacokinet 26:144–160, 1994.

97. Lin JH, Chiba M, Baillie TA: Is the role of the small intestine in first-pass metabolism overemphasized? Pharmacol Rev 51:135–158, 1999.

98. Hall SD, Thummel KE, Watkins PB, et al: Molecular and physical mechanisms of first-pass extraction. Drug Metab Dispos 27:161–166, 1999.

99. Zhang QY, Dunbar D, Ostrowska A, et al: Characterization of human small intestinal cytochromes P-450. Drug Metab Dispos 27:804–809, 1999.

100. de Waziers I, Cugnenc PH, Yang CS, et al: Cytochrome P-450 isoenzymes, epoxide hydrolase and glutathione transferases in rat and human hepatic and extrahepatic tissues. J Pharmacol Exp Ther 253:387–394, 1990.

101. Obach RS, Zhang QY, Dunbar D, et al: Metabolic characterization of the major human small intestinal cytochrome p450s. Drug Metab Dispos 29:347–352, 2001.

102. Lown KS, Ghosh M, Watkins PB: Sequences of intestinal and hepatic cytochrome P450 3A4 cDNAs are identical. Drug Metab Dispos 26:185–187, 1998.

103. Gibbs MA, Thummel KE, Shen DD, et al: Inhibition of cytochrome P-450 3A (CYP3A) in human intestinal and liver microsomes: Comparison of Ki values and impact of CYP3A5 expression. Drug Metab Dispos 27:180–187, 1999.

104. Paine MF, Khalighi M, Fisher JM, et al: Characterization of interintestinal and intraintestinal variations in human CYP3A-dependent metabolism. J Pharmacol Exp Ther 283:1552–1562, 1997.

105. Lohr JW, Willsky GR, Acara MA: Renal drug metabolism. Pharmacol Rev 50:107–141, 1998.

106. Schuetz EG, Schuetz JD, Grogan WM, et al: Expression of cytochrome-P450 3A in amphibian, rat, and human kidney. Arch Biochem Biophys 294:206–214, 1992.

107. Rodilla V, Benzie AA, Veitch JM, et al: Glutathione S-transferases in human renal cortex and neoplastic tissue: Enzymatic activity, isoenzyme profile and immunohistochemical localization. Xenobiotica 28:443–456, 1998.

108. Cummings BS, Lasker JM, Lash LH: Expression of glutathione-dependent enzymes and cytochrome P450s in freshly isolated and primary cultures of proximal tubular cells from human kidney. J Pharmacol Exp Ther 293:677–685, 2000.

109. Amet Y, Berthou F, Fournier G, et al: Cytochrome P450 4A and 2E1 expression in human kidney microsomes. Biochem Pharmacol 53:765–771, 1997.

110. Kharasch ED, Hankins DC, Thummel KE: Human kidney methoxyflurane and sevoflurane metabolism: Intrarenal fluoride production as a possible mechanism of methoxyflurane nephrotoxicity. Anesthesiology 82:689–699, 1995.

111. Lasker JM, Chen WB, Wolf I, et al: Formation of 20-hydroxy-eicosatetraenoic acid, a vasoactive and natriuretic eicosanoid, in human kidney: Role of CYP4F2 and CYP4A11. J Biol Chem 275:4118–4126, 2000.

112. Maier KG, Roman RJ: Cytochrome P450 metabolites of arachidonic acid in the control of renal function. Curr Opin Nephrol Hypertens 10:81–87, 2001.

113. Wikvall K: Cytochrome P450 enzymes in the bioactivation of vitamin D to its hormonal form. Int J Mol Med 7:201–209, 2001.

114. Cummings BS, Zangar RC, Novak RF, et al: Cellular distribution of cytochromes P-450 in the rat kidney. Drug Metab Dispos 27:542–548, 1999.

115. Voirol P, Jonzier-Perey M, Porchet F, et al: Cytochrome P-450 activities in human and rat brain microsomes. Brain Res 855:235–243, 2000.

116. McFadyen MCE, Melvin WT, Murray GI: Regional distribution of individual forms of cytochrome P450 mRNA in normal adult human brain. Biochem Pharmacol 62:207–212, 1998.

117. Hakkola J, Tanaka E, Pelkonen O: Developmental expression of cytochrome P450 enzymes in human liver. Pharmacol Toxicol 82:209–217, 1998.

118. Ring JA, Ghabrial H, Ching MS, et al: Fetal hepatic drug elimination. Pharmacol Ther 84:429–445, 1999.

119. Blanco JG, Harrison PL, Evans WE, et al: Human cytochrome P450 maximal activities in pediatric versus adult liver. Drug Metab Dispos 28:379–382, 2000.

120. Gow PJ, Ghabrial H, Smallwood RA, et al: Neonatal hepatic drug elimination. Pharmacol Toxicol 88:3–15, 2001.

121. Klein I, Sarkadi B, Varadi A: An inventory of the human ABC proteins. Biochim Biophys Acta 1461:237–262, 1999.

122. Ambudkar SV, Dey S, Hrycyna CA, et al: Biochemical, cellular, and pharmacological aspects of the multidrug transporter. Annu Rev Pharmacol Toxicol 39:361–398, 1999.

123. Fromm MF: P-glycoprotein: A defense mechanism limiting oral bioavailability and CNS accumulation of drugs. Int J Clin Pharmacol Ther 38:69–74, 2000.

124. Zhang Y, Benet LZ: The gut as a barrier to drug absorption: Combined role of cytochrome P450 3A and P-glycoprotein. Clin Pharmacokinet 40:159–168, 2001.

125. Lown KS, Mayo RR, Leichtman AB, et al: Role of intestinal P-glycoprotein (MDR1) in interpatient variation in the oral bioavailability of cyclosporine. Clin Pharmacol Ther 62:248–260, 1997.

126. Wacher VJ, Silverman JA, Zhang Y, et al: Role of P-glycoprotein and cytochrome P450 3A in limiting oral absorption of peptides and peptidomimetics. J Pharm Sci 87:1322–1330, 1998.

127. Schuetz EG, Schinkel AH, Relling MV, et al: P-glycoprotein: A major determinant of rifampicin-inducible expression of cytochrome P4503A in mice and humans. Proc Natl Acad Sci USA 93:4001–4005, 1996.

128. Hebert MF: Contributions of hepatic and intestinal metabolism and P-glycoprotein to cyclosporine and tacrolimus oral drug delivery. Adv Drug Delivery Rev 27:201–214, 1997.

129. Greiner B, Eichelbaum M, Fritz P, et al: The role of intestinal P-glycoprotein in the interaction of digoxin and rifampin. J Clin Invest 104:147–153, 1999.

130. Schinkel AH: P-Glycoprotein, a gatekeeper in the blood-brain barrier. Adv Drug Deliv Rev 36:179–194, 1999.

131. Tamai I, Tsuji A: Transporter-mediated permeation of drugs across the blood-brain barrier. J Pharm Sci 89:1371–1388, 2000.

132. Callaghan R, Riordan JR: Synthetic and natural opiates interact with P-glycoprotein in multidrug-resistant cells. J Biol Chem 268:16059–16064, 1993.

133. Xie R, Hammarlund-Udenaes M, de Boer AG, et al: The role of P-glycoprotein in blood-brain barrier transport of morphine: Transcortical microdialysis studies in *mdr1a^-/-* and *mdr1a^+/+* mice. Br J Pharmacol 128:563–568, 1999.

134. Letrent SP, Pollack GM, Brouwer KR, et al: Effects of a potent and specific P-glycoprotein inhibitor on the blood-brain barrier distribution and antinociceptive effect of morphine in the rat. Drug Metab Dispos 27:827–834, 1999.

135. Letrent SP, Polli JW, Humphreys JE, et al: P-glycoprotein-mediated transport of morphine in brain capillary endothelial cells. Biochem Pharmacol 58:951–957, 1999.

136. Thompson SJ, Koszdin KK, Bernards CM: Opiate-induced analgesia as increased and prolonged in mice lacking P-glycoprotein. Anesthesiology 92:1392–1399, 2000.

137. Sadeque AJ, Wandel C, He H, et al: Increased drug delivery to the brain by P-glycoprotein inhibition. Clin Pharmacol Ther 68:231–237, 2000.

138. Borst P, Evers R, Kool M, et al: A family of drug transporters: the multidrug resistance-associated proteins. J Natl Cancer Inst 92:1295–1302, 2000.

139. Fromm MF, Kauffmann HM, Fritz P, et al: The effect of rifampin treatment on intestinal expression of human MRP transporters. Am J Pathol 157:1575–1580, 2000.

140. Fuhr U: Drug interactions with grapefruit juice: Extent, probable mechanism and clinical relevance. Drug Saf 18:251–272, 1998.

141. Wilkinson GR, Shand DG: A physiologic approach to hepatic drug clearance. Clin Pharmacol Ther 18:377–390, 1975.

142. Kharasch ED, Russell M, Mautz D, et al: The role of cytochrome P450 3A4 in alfentanil clearance: Implications for interindividual variability in disposition and perioperative drug interactions. Anesthesiology 87:36–50, 1997.

143. Bartkowski RR, Goldberg ME, Huffnagle S, et al: Sufentanil disposition—is it affected by erythromycin administration? Anesthesiology 78:260–265, 1993.

144. Poulsen L, Brøsen K, Arendt-Nielsen L, et al: Codeine and morphine in extensive and poor metabolizers of sparteine: Pharmacokinetics, analgesic effect and side effects. Eur J Clin Pharmacol 51:289–295, 1996.

145. Caraco Y, Sheller J, Wood AJ: Impact of ethnic origin and quinidine coadministration on codeine's disposition and pharmacodynamic effects. J Pharmacol Exp Ther 290:413–422, 1999.

146. Sindrup SH, Hofmann U, Asmussen J, et al: Impact of quinidine on plasma and cerebrospinal fluid concentrations of codeine and morphine after codeine intake. Eur J Clin Pharmacol 49:503–509, 1996.

147. Caraco Y, Sheller J, Wood AJJ: Pharmacogenetic determinants of codeine induction by rifampin: The impact on codeine's respiratory, psychomotor and miotic effects. J Pharmacol Exp Ther 281:330–336, 1997.

148. Alvan G: Clinical consequences of polymorphic drug oxidation. Fundam Clin Pharmacol 5:209–228, 1991.

149. Alvan G, Bertilsson L, Dahl ML, et al: Moving toward genetic profiling in patient care: The scope and rationale of pharmacogenetic/ecogenetic investigation. Drug Metab Dispos 29:580–585, 2001.

150. Fromm MF, Busse D, Kroemer HK, et al: Differential induction of prehepatic and hepatic metabolism of verapamil by rifampin. Hepatology 24:796–801, 1996.

151. Tsunoda SM, Velez RL, von Moltke LL, et al: Differentiation of intestinal and hepatic cytochrome P450 3A activity with use of midazolam as an in vivo probe: Effect of ketoconazole. Clin Pharmacol Ther 66:461–471, 1999.

152. Gomez DY, Wacher VJ, Tomlanovich SJ, et al: The effects of ketoconazole on the intestinal metabolism and bioavailability of cyclosporine. Clin Pharmacol Ther 58:15–19, 1995.

5

Pharmacogenetics and Pharmacogenomics of Drug Action

Kirk Hogan, MD, JD

The principles of scientific investigation are currently taken for granted in clinical medicine and anesthesiology, but it is rewarding to consider that this was not always true. Before the introduction of ether, chloroform, and extracts of the poppy, foxglove, and belladonna, quantification of drug effect and hypothesis testing was not of proven benefit in comparison to therapeutics reliant on faith or inspiration. As Martin Pernick recounts in *A Calculus of Suffering: Pain, Professionalism, and Anesthesia in Nineteenth Century America,* it was the narrow, shifting margin between a life-saving and a lethal dose of these potent drugs that compelled practitioners to seek predictors of efficacy and toxicity in choosing a preferred agent and regimen for each patient.[1] In the mid-19th century, physical markers entered practice that abide as clinical mainstays including patient age, weight, coexisting disease, concurrent medications, nutritional status, and environmental exposures. These patient-specific characteristics, when coupled with dose-response profiles established in heterogeneous populations, established the foundations for empiricism in drug administration that continue to guide anesthetic practice at the turn of the 21st century.

By the late 1800s it had became apparent that the variances surrounding population means for drug responses were broad, pointing to unaccounted for contributors to such critical variables as time to onset, potency, and duration for most drugs used in the perioperative interval. A "trial and error" approach to selection and dosing, with counteracting drugs ready at hand, became the anesthesiologist's prag-

matic adaptation to wide and unpredictable heterogeneity in drug effect. The role of genetic factors was first recognized in identification of sex and ethnic background as components underlying interindividual differences in drug efficacy and toxicity,[1] but a half century was to pass before more sophisticated principles of genetics were brought to bear on problems confronting anesthesiologists and patients in their care. Even today, the instruments of pharmacogenetic assessment in anesthetic practice are remarkably blunt, consisting of no more than a family medical history box on the preoperative form to be checked after one or two questions.

History of Pharmacogenetics

The central role played by anesthetic agents and adjuvants in the genesis of scientific medicine has been recapitulated in the origin of the discipline of pharmacogenetics. In the 1880s, Freud reported interindividual differences in response to cocaine in laboratory animals, concomitant with the discovery by organic chemists that drugs are excreted from the body in changed form, and that variability in the relevant pathways obeys the laws of heredity described by Mendel.[2] In accord with Garrod's insight that genetically determined differences in biochemical processes could be the cause of adverse reaction after drug administration,[3] Kalow reported prolonged effects of succinylcholine in patients undergoing electroconvulsive therapy and deduced that the susceptibility arising from deficient activity of plasma cholinesterase was inherited as an autosomal recessive trait.[4,5] This observation in tandem with reports of primaquine-induced hemolysis associated with G-6-PD deficiency in soldiers during World War II[6] and peripheral neuropathy in slow acetylators of isoniazid[7] prompted Motulsky to lay the framework for recognition of heritable idiosyncrasies in efficacy and adverse drug reactions[8] and prompted Vogel to coin the term pharmacogenetics.[9] Coincident with these reports, in 1960, Denborough was the first to recognize malignant hyperthermia as distinct autosomal dominant disorder,[10] although it is certain that the condition engendered significant morbidity and mortality because potent anesthetic vapors were first used a century before.

Formal application of scientific methods to the identification and explanation of pharmacogenetic syndromes began with elucidation of a bimodal distribution for the metabolism of the experimental antihypertensive debrisoquine,[11] and the demonstration that the plasma half-life of dicumeral is similar in monozygotic twins, but varies widely in dizygotic twins, siblings, and the general population.[12] These findings lent support to the principle that occult genetic variation between individuals could lead without warning to life-threatening adverse drug reactions. The molecular basis for aberrancies in response to debrisoquine was shown in the 1970s to derive from isoforms of the hepatic cytochrome P450 enzyme CYP2D6.[13,14] Cloning and characterization of the gene encoding CYP2D6, and the first reports of causal mutations in its sequence, set the benchmark for dating the inception of the pharmacogenomic era.[15]

From a pharmacogenetic perspective the ensuing decade was marked by advances on three broad fronts. First, the number of pharmacokinetic and pharmacodynamic traits exhibiting clinically relevant variations accelerated sufficiently to require newly dedicated journals including *Pharmacogenetics*, *Pharmacogenomics*, *The American Journal of Pharmacogenomics*, and *The Pharmacogenomics Journal*. Second, epidemiologic evidence established that adverse drug reactions are severe, common, and growing causes of death, disability, and resource consumption in North America and Europe.[16–18] Because the reported complications occur during treatment with approved drug doses, thereby excluding intentional or accidental overdose, errors in administration, and noncompliance, up to 50% of mortality would be potentially preventable by a priori genomic drug susceptibility profiling.[19,20] Third, revolutionary technologies were introduced for detection of DNA sequence variations correlated with drug efficacy and toxicity. Anesthesiology, by virtue of its daily use of the most potent medications, is well-situated to take advantage of these strides and to enhance patient safety by rational selection of technique, agent, and dose based on individualized DNA signatures.

Pharmacogenetic Concepts

The term pharmacogenomics first entered scientific discourse in the early 1990s as amplification of human DNA fragments by polymerase chain reaction and direct DNA sequencing became robust and cost-effective.[21] Thereafter, pharmacogenomics came to refer generally to correlation of drug-specific traits with genome-wide DNA sequence variations, whereas pharmacogenetics connotes a sharper focus on traditional pedigree and population analysis of single gene effects.[22] In practice the two terms are interchangeable, both implying study of the influence of genetic diversity on drug response.

Until recently, measurement of the physical manifestations of a trait (the phenotype) was relatively straightforward, but accessing human DNA sequence variation (the genotype) was reserved for science fiction. With publication of the first "draft" human genome sequence,[23] and widespread availability of low cost, accurate molecular approaches, acquisition of genomic data is now facile such that the assembly of reliable phenotypic databases has become the bottleneck in pharmacogenomic research. For many investigators it came as a surprise that the number of discrete human genes ranges from only 30,000 to 35,000, perhaps because we appear to ourselves to be more complicated creatures than organisms with a greater gene count. This misconception is resolved by estimates that each human gene encodes a mean of 3 to 5 distinct proteins (many more for some), with limitless potential for genetic variation at each locus. DNA sequence variations, termed polymorphisms if they appear in greater than 1% of the population and mutations if in less than 1%, are staggering in frequency and in kind, ranging from single base pair substitutions to whole gene deletions and duplications. Contrary to early doctrine that most genetic changes would be deleterious, the preponderance of sequence alterations elicit no phenotypic effect whatsoever (i.e., those appearing in noncoding regions or as a redundant third base of a codon specifying an amino acid). Others, including single base changes, may be sufficient to kill in the presence of an environmental trigger (i.e., malignant hyperthermia).

Each nucleated human cell contains a genome composed of approximately 3 billion base pairs of DNA. Sorting through the 3 million polymorphisms unique to each human is motivated by the principle that a pharmacogenetic predictor will not change throughout life, and thus will need to be sought only once for each individual. Achieving this task is the central objective of bioinformatics, a silicon-based, web-enabled discipline that integrates clinical traits and outcomes with archived files of DNA sequence and its variations.[24,25] Virtually all of the traits considered in this chapter are monogenic, in which the great proportion of variability in a given trait between two individuals can be traced to the presence or absence of a causal mutation in a single gene. The existence of a monopharmacogenetic trait is established when DNA sequence variations within one gene correlate with segregation of the larger population into smaller groups (i.e., a bimodal distribution) on the basis of distinct drug effects. Hence most currently recognized pharmacogenetic traits reflect single gene defects, disclosed by the severity of their corresponding phenotypes.[26] More sophisticated bioinformatic models, enhanced computational capacity, and high throughput genotyping will be required to draw predictive correlations between drug responses and DNA sequence variations at more than one site in a gene or genes to predict susceptibilities characterized by polygenic, multifactorial inheritance.

Pharmacogenetic Phenotypes

Many drugs used by anesthesiologists exhibit significant interindividual variation in efficacy and toxicity, often in conformation to differences in drug or metabolite concentration in a given compartment (i.e., plasma or urine) for a given dose. Nonetheless, most pharmacogenetic susceptibilities go undetected in affected persons until a drug substrate for the impaired enzyme or target is administered. The search for genetic factors consonant with these observations must first address whether, in the setting of divergent responses to an identical dose, the cause is pharmacokinetic (compartment drug levels differ) or pharmacodynamic (compartment drug levels are identical). Pharmacokinetic polymorphisms that alter drug concentrations may be further subdivided into those that govern drug absorption, distribution, metabolism, or excretion (ADME). By far the most numerous and well-studied of these are polymorphisms in the genes encoding drug metabolizing enzymes (DMEs), accounting for up to 10- to 10,000-fold variations in drug activity.

Many pharmacogenetic classification schemes based on phenotype have been proffered.[27] In Table 5–1, a patient's genetic capacity to metabolize drug substrates is coordinated with predictors of inefficacy or toxicity. Normal or wild type individuals are termed extensive metabolizers (EM) with desired phenotypes after administration. Poor metabolizers (PM) are at risk for overdosage from accumulation of an active drug to potentially toxic levels, or therapeutic failure from impaired activation of a prodrug essential for clinical efficacy. PM status usually reflects an autosomal recessive mechanism of inheritance with two copies of the mutant allele, one from each parent, required to manifest the trait. Conversely, the increased drug metabolism of ultraextensive metabolizers (UEM) is most often observed as an autosomal dominant trait arising from gene duplication in one of the two parental alleles. Patients with UEM are in jeopardy for underdosage of an active ligand, and overdosage or toxicity if the drug effect relies on the presence of an active metabolite.

Not only may detection of genotypes incommensurate with dosing regimens predict inefficacy or toxicity, but they may also warn of potential drug-drug interactions if, for example, two drugs share a mutant pathway.[28] Drug interactions are a particularly common cause of adverse reactions during the polypharmacy characteristic of perioperative management. Patients awaiting surgery may be taking any prescribed, over-the-counter, or herbal remedy in addition to suspected and unsuspected drugs of abuse. In this context, fixed and discrete genomic data have the potential to anticipate the incidence and severity of untoward responses. For these reasons, as the number and predictive power of the pertinent genotypes expands, it will be increasingly important for anesthesiologists to acquire familiarity with the principles and practice of pharmacogenetics.[29]

Pharmacogenetic Genotypes

In aggregate, more than 60 pharmacogenetic differences of potential clinical relevance have been identified.[30] Proposed schemes to classify variations in drug response associated with specific DNA sequences are not mutually exclusive, and may be conveniently cross-referenced—i.e., by type of genetic alteration, by class or structure of protein, by phylogenetic relation, by mechanism of trait inheritance, or by functional role in drug response. For example, more than 20 DMEs have been genetically characterized in full with all coding and noncoding regions and boundaries sequenced, together with flanking regulatory regions. Many more have been isolated and copied ex vivo (i.e., cloned) in preparation for functional investigation and characterization (see www.sciencemag.org/feature/data/1044449.shl). Nearly every DME displays clinically relevant polymorphisms, with many additional variants producing no recognizable phenotype. Because each drug interacts with numerous carrier proteins, cell membrane transporters, metabolizing enzymes, receptors, and secondary messengers, and because most genes in outbred human populations are polymorphic, pharmacogenomic profiles will be essential to interpret variances around dose response sample means in subpopulations defined by shared stratification of risk. Consequently, control of the genomic contribution to heterogeneity in drug response will assist investigations of environmental factors by permitting exposed patients to be matched on the basis of shared genetic constitution.

TABLE 5–1.

Clinical Consequences as a Function of Pharmacogenetic Profiles for Patients Receiving Active Drugs and Drugs with Active or Toxic Metabolites

Genetic Profile	Active Drug	Active Metabolite	Toxic Metabolite
PM	Overdose	Underdose	Reduced toxicity
EM	Therapeutic	Therapeutic	No toxicity
UEM	Underdose	Overdose	Increased toxicity

PM, poor metabolizer; EM, extensive metabolizer; UEM, ultraextensive metabolizer.

Genotype-Phenotype Correlations

Whether pharmacogenomic data made available in advance of surgery is of any value to the caregiver or patient hinges on the extent to which the patient's genotype predicts changes in phenotype after administration of the drug in question. Currently, declarations of an association between a genotype and phenotype often elude the level of scrutiny that would ordinarily greet news of other newly proposed, nongenetic clinical correlations. But as pharmacogenomic data inevitably flow from the laboratory bench to the operating room, it will be crucial that practitioners adopt an attitude of skepticism. A quantifiable clinical drug response may be causally correlated with a DNA nucleotide change on the basis of statistical, inferential, and biologic-functional lines of evidence collectively referred as functional genomics.[31] Because each of these categoric criteria is subtle and vulnerable to error, the informed clinician will insist on a high degree of reproducibility and correspondence before weighing genomic data in management decisions. The prospect of abundant, novel genotype-phenotype correlations for anesthetic agents and adjuncts balances these concerns in exploiting the spectrum of inborn human diversity in drug treatment.

Genetic Pharmacokinetics

Since their presence was first suspected, it has been puzzling that genes encoding proteins responsible for drug ADME could not have evolved by exposure to modern pharmaceuticals. Rather, it is hypothesized that close chemical homologues expressed in ingested plants were rendered innocuous by these adaptations in our progenitors.[32] Why the genes responsible for transmission of pharmacokinetic defenses exhibit such a high degree of polymorphism is a second mystery. In part, the answer may reside in the loss of reproductive advantage of polymorphisms as environments and diets change with accumulation of neutral mutations, some of which may be deleterious in a novel environment (e.g., the operating room). Another possibility is that the extent of pharmacokinetic polymorphism reflects heterogeneity of the environments in which humans have evolved corresponding to varying allele frequencies in groups with distinct ethnic origins. In either case, for most ADME polymorphisms there are no phenotypes apparent on medical history or physical examination to warn caregivers in the absence of a challenge with the drug itself. This lack of easily detected phenotypic markers explains the delay in recognition of genetic correlates of drug responses as clinically important phenomena, and underscores the tremendous potential for growth of knowledge now that DNA-based technologies are widely available.

Absorption

Although only a small number of agents administered by anesthesiologists rely on absorption after oral dosing, unexpected complications during and immediately after surgery may nevertheless be elicited by patient-to-patient variations in absorptive capacity of narrow therapeutic ratio compounds. So, for example, the intracellular or tissue bioavailability and disposition of many drugs, e.g., digoxin, is influenced by functional polymorphisms in the human multidrug resistance gene (*MDR1*) with associated altered expression and activity of P-glycoprotein.[33,34] *MDR1* is part of the adenosine triphosphate—binding cassette protein superfamily whose members act as barriers to entry and as efflux pumps for drugs, metabolites, and exogenous substances in the intestine and other tissues.[35] Presence or absence of P-glycoprotein polymorphisms also plays a significant role in the first-pass elimination of cyclosporine by altering a rate-limiting step in absorption.[36]

Distribution: Drug Transporters

The functional genomic investigation of drug transporter polymorphisms is a young field with a strong likelihood for direct anesthetic implications in the near future. Currently, the most well-described polymorphism appears in the neuronal 5-hydroxytryptamine transporter, which regulates patient response to selective serotonin reuptake inhibitors.[37] The mutation, which consists of a 44-base pair insertion, resides in the promoter region of the gene responsible for increased transcription of DNA to mRNA in response to specific cellular triggers. Patients homozygous for the insertion exhibit an impaired response to selective serotonin reuptake inhibitors when compared with heterozygotes or homozygotes with the segment deleted.[38] Thus an autosomal recessive polymorphism in a noncoding region of the gene begets a negative impact on drug efficacy and is easily detectable in advance of drug administration.

Metabolism and Biotransformation

Extracellular Drug Metabolism

Plasma Cholinesterase

The circulating enzyme plasma cholinesterase, or butyrylcholinesterase, is responsible wholly or in part for the first-pass metabolism and elimination of a variety of anesthetic drugs sharing a vulnerable ester bond including succinylcholine, mivacurium, cocaine, and tetracaine.[2] Approximately 1 of 2500 patients are homozygous for the "atypical" mutation in which a glycine is substituted for an aspartate in the anionic binding site of the protein.[39] The mutation abolishes electrostatic interactions essential to drug substrate binding, prolonging duration of action. Approximately 1 of 100 whites are homozygous for a milder second polymorphism, the "K variant," with an overall allele frequency in both homozygotes and heterozygotes of 10% in whites compared with 17.5% frequency in Japanese populations.[40] In addition to the atypical and K variant polymorphisms, more than 20 rare mutations have been identified, with the possibility of compound heterozygotes—that is, distinct predisposing mutation from each parent, confirmed by direct sequencing.[41] A simple and accurate phenotypic test of butyrylcholinesterase activity was proposed by Morrow and Motulsky in 1968.[42] Its use never became routine, however, attesting to anesthesiologist's general preference for safety systems dependent on early warning rather than prevention.

Intracellular Drug Metabolism

Phase I: Cytochrome P450 Pharmacogenomics

Although more than 50 different CYP genes have been isolated,[43] (see http://www.imm.ki.se/CYPalleles), only 8 are known to be qualitatively important in human drug metabolism, with the preponderance of CYP activity generated by CYP2D6 and CYP3A4 isozymes. CYP nomenclature assigns each isozyme a gene family and subfamily on the basis of homology in amino acid composition. Thus CYP1A2 designates the second isoform of subfamily A in CYP family 1. To discriminate protein from genetic designations, gene names are italicized—e.g., CYP1A2 protein encoded by the *CYP1A2* gene.[44] It is not necessary for the protein and gene nomenclature to be identical, but reference to the gene will always be in italic.

All human CYP enzymes show interindividual genetic variability, often in correlation with substantial differences in metabolic capacity. Mutations in CYP-encoding genes inhibit enzyme function in many ways including inactivation, heightened activation, deletion, altered affinity, altered specificity, and instability. Because of their profound consequences for human health and disease management, research activity in this area is intense. A large number of drug metabolizing polymorphisms are known for which there is no associated phenotype. Similarly, for a subset of DMEs there is evidence for phenotypic heterogeneity before a molecular basis is found. Currently, it is reasonable to assume that all genetic changes causing all important phenotypic changes have yet to be disclosed for even one drug metabolizing isozyme. Several different CYP enzymes may participate in the metabolism of a single drug, and each CYP DME may contribute to the metabolism of many drugs. As a general principle, because of overlap in DME substrate specificity, greater than half of the total metabolism of a drug must pass through a particular mutant isozyme for an adverse effect to be observed. Although expression of CYP enzymes is primarily hepatic, polymorphisms may have consequences in expression of the identical isozyme in other tissues (e.g., intestinal CYP3A4 effects on cyclosporine availability).

CYP2D6

CYP2D6 is responsible for the phase I "functionalization" of nearly 25% of all drugs including analgesics, neuroleptics, antiarrhythmics, amide local anesthetics, antiemetics, beta-blockers, and tricyclic antidepressants. More than 80 genetic variants are catalogued (see http://drnelson.utmem.edu/CytochromeP450.html),[45] with 4 polymorphisms (*3,*4,*5,*6) accounting for more than 97% of the mutant alleles in whites; the remainder comprise "orphan" mutations in a small subset of families.[46] The CYP2D6*4 mutation is homozygous in 7% of whites, with genotyping 100% specific for identifying the autosomal recessive PM status. Summed with other *CYP2D6* mutations, up to 10% of whites are unable to obtain analgesia from dealkylation of codeine to morphine.[47] PM status appears in 2% or less in populations of Asian or African origin. The global distribution of UEMs, with polymorphic gene duplication (*CYP2D62XN*), is comparably inhomogeneous. Up to 30% of Ethiopian, 7% of Spanish, and 1.5% of Scandinavian samples demonstrate ultrarapid enzyme kinetics.[48] Most allelic variations of *CYP2D6* are loss of function mutations that produce a PM phenotype. In contrast to the general rule that ADME genotypes are silent in the absence of drug exposure, it has been suggested that CYP2D6 PM patients have a lower pain tolerance than patients with UEM because of a defect in synthesizing endogenous pain-modulating compounds.[49]

OTHER CYP POLYMORPHISMS

Comprising less than 0.2% of hepatic CYP enzymes, CYP2B6 has recently been shown to be responsible for the metabolism of ketamine[50] and propofol.[51] Functional *CYP2B6* genetic polymorphisms have been reported.[52] Therefore, soon it may be possible to correlate genetic changes with propofol kinetics in human tissue preparations and with the clinical occurrence of atypical propofol-associated complications (e.g., opisthotonus and rhabdomyolysis).[53,54]

Because patients with deficient activity of CYP2C9 have a predictably lower requirement for warfarin and higher risk for hemorrhage, *CYP2C9* genotyping in advance of administration has been advocated.[55] Amino acid substitutions Arg144Cys (CYP2C9*2)[56] and Iso359Leu (CYP2C9*3)[57] inhibit hydroxylation of warfarin, producing a greater than fivefold decline in metabolic activity in 5% of whites and Asians who are mutant CYP2C9 homozygotes.[58] Nonsteroidal analgesics, tetra-hydro-cannabinol, and phenytoin also rely on CYP2C9 for metabolic degradation and may compete with warfarin for limited bioactivity if coadministered.

CYP2C19 metabolizes omeprazole, diazepam, and propranolol. Increased sensitivity to these agents is observed in up to 5% of whites and 23% of Asians who are homozygotes for PM genotypes,[59] arising primarily from a shared mutation in exon 5. The mutant protein is enzymatically inert in the absence of a heme binding region, giving rise to overdosage in carriers of the mutant gene.

The gene encoding CYP2E1 is polymorphic (see Chapter 4), but no clearcut association with a clinical syndrome of relevance in perioperative care has been confirmed to date. In view of well-documented metabolism of isoflurane, desflurane, and other potent anesthetic agents mediated by CYP2E1,[60] the clinical significance of the mutant enzyme during and after exposure to these drugs clearly merits closer pharmacogenetic investigation.

Although it is the most abundant hepatic DME with up to 20-fold differences in expression found within a population,[61] no completely inactivating polymorphism has been found for *CYP3A4*. An allelic variant associated with altered nifedipine activity has been identified,[62] but despite 220-fold interindividual differences in isoform activity, the variances are unimodal, rather than the bimodal distributions characteristic of monogenic DME effects. Recently, a polymorphism (*3) has been discovered in intron 3 of the *CYP3A5* gene that generates a splice variant causing polymorphic CYP3A5 expression in humans.[63] This polymorphism influences overall CYP3A5 activity sharing CYP3A4 substrates in up to 30% of whites.

Phase II: Conjugation Transferases

Although the genes encoding Phase II conjugation DMEs are highly polymorphic, investigations of genotype-phenotype correlations have been confounded by limited substrate specificity and a less pronounced hereditary contribution to differences in bioactivity.[64] Despite lagging the genomic investigations of phase I reactions, several well-defined polymorphisms are prototypical of the maturing field. Hydralazine and procainamide rely on *N*-acetyltransferase (NAT2) for reducing hydrophilicity. The enzyme catalyzes transfer of an acetyl group from acetyl coenzyme A to target amines, generating a more soluble amide. Four allelic variants are known in association with slow acetylation and higher plasma concentrations.[65] Adverse drug reactions include peripheral neuropathy in slow acetylators induced by isoniazid in B_6-deficient patients, and toxicity from procainamide with delayed renal elimination of acetyl-procainamide in rapid acetylators.[66]

Thiopurine methyltransferase (TPMT) catalyzes the conjugation of the methyl group of *S*-adenosyl methionine to aromatic and heterocyclic sulfhydryl substrates.[67] Gene inactivating mutations result in therapeutic failure for 6-mercaptopurine and azathioprine used in the treatment of leukemia, rheumatoid arthritis, inflammatory bowel disease, multiple sclerosis, dermatologic disorders, and solid organ transplantation.[68] In turn, *S*-adenosyl methionine synthesis is contingent on adequate stores of active cobalamin,[69] which are depleted by exposure to nitrous oxide in clinically relevant inspired concentrations and durations. Mutations in genes encoding folate and homocysteine metabolism may concurrently depress levels of methyl moieties essential for neurotransmitter synthesis, myelination, and DNA assembly and repair.[70] TPMT-deficient patients are not only at risk for potentially fatal leukopenia, but failure of methylation shunts the parent compound through ancillary pathways to form toxic thioguanine nucleotide intermediaries.[71] TPMT activity is polymorphic in all populations investigated, with 90% of subjects exhibiting high activity, 10% with intermediate activity and 0.3% with no detectable activity.[72] Three alleles (TPMT*2, TPMT*3A, and TPMT*3C) underlie 95% of the intermediate and low activity phenotypes, producing enhanced proteolysis of the mutant enzyme.[73] Because patients carrying nonfunctional TPMT alleles experience serious toxic effects, pretesting patients who are candidates for these drugs is now routine in specialized centers.[28,75]

Genetic Pharmacodynamics

Drugs exert their actions through binding to specific macromolecular targets most often encoded by distinct genes. Given identical plasma concentrations, pharmacodynamic variation may originate as a result of DNA sequence changes in drug targets. Most drug targets consist of membrane receptors, enzymes, or ion channels serving as the cell's sensor elements to hormones, neurotransmitters, or other mediators (e.g., circulating cytokines). Functional genetic polymorphisms may be expressed in the effector molecules themselves, or in the intracellular second messenger pathways activated by association of a drug ligand with its target. Because these mechanisms fulfill essential cellular roles, nonsynonymous polymorphisms (i.e., those that alter the amino acid composition of a polypeptide) are less well tolerated than allelic variants of genes encoding pharmacokinetic proteins. Similarly, disease causing mutations in drug targets are more likely to produce severe or even lethal phenotypes, and thus are less widely perpetuated in a population compared with mutations that only become apparent on exposure to a drug. Variability surrounding the sample means of pharmacodynamic effects is typically large, reflecting the many molecular contributors to even the most narrowly delineated drug response. Investigations aimed at correlating interindividual differences in pharmacodynamic drug response to DNA sequence variations are further challenged by phenotypes that are much more diverse and difficult to quantify than distributions of drug and metabolite levels in relevant body fluids. Despite these obstacles to detection of genetic differences in pharmacodynamic effects, it is surprising that cognizance of the dramatic malignant hyperthermia (MH) phenotype took place only within the memory of living clinicians, or that reduced efficacy for β_2-agonists in a large subset of patients experiencing perioperative bronchospasm went unheeded until recently. The failure of pharmacodynamic syndromes to be identified with a frequency comparable to pharmacokinetic genetic predictors over the preceding three decades implies that many more of the former remain to be discovered.

Efficacy

Opioid Responsivity

In demonstrating that individuals of Chinese origin experience significantly greater ventilatory depression at identical plasma concentrations of morphine compared with whites, Zhou et al.[75] provided early evidence indicating that interethnic differences in pharmacokinetic capacity may be recapitulated in heritable pharmacodynamic effects. Differences in levels of υ-opioid receptor gene expression are associated with modified responses to painful stimuli and to analgesic drugs caused by a genetic polymorphism in the transcription regulating region.[76] An Ala118Gly transition results in a υ-receptor variant that binds β-endorphin with approximately three times greater affinity than the most common allelic isoform.[77] β-endorphin is consequently three times more potent in persons with the mutation. Lotsch et al. suggest that the Ala118Gly polymorphism confers protection from the sedative effects of morphine-6-glucuronide,[78] although it does not alter the potency of morphine.[79] A functional polymorphism, Ser268Pro, in the υ-receptor strongly impairs receptor signaling and is being investigated as a contributor to addiction.[80] Reviews of the genetic polymorphisms potentially associated with opioid dependence[81] and analgesia[82] are available.

Bronchodilation

Genetic polymorphisms of the β_2 adrenergic receptor (β_2-AR) predict responder and nonresponder phenotypes after administration of receptor-specific bronchodilatory agonists.[83] A polymorphism of the β_2-AR gene at DNA base 46 replacing an adenine with a guanine nucleotide (A46G) results in the substitution of glycine for arginine at the 16th amino acid residue of the drug target.[84] The amino acid substitution correlates with down-regulation of the β_2AR and loss of sensitivity to albuterol in homozygous patients representing 10% of the white population.[85,86] In a landmark study, FEV1 response to albuterol was shown to be greater than six times more effective in wild type Arg/Arg homozygotes than Gly/Gly homozygotes, even though plasma concentrations were identical.[87] Additional β_2-AR polymorphisms add power to the prediction of albuterol efficacy when examined by haplotype, i.e., small groups of coinherited polymorphisms.[88] This first demonstration that knowledge of polymorphisms en bloc improves trait predictability over assay of single polymorphisms is a likely paradigm for pharmacodynamic phenotypes in general.

Antibronchospastic effectiveness is also associated with polymorphisms in the 5-lipoxygenase (*ALOX5*) gene. Improvements in FEV1 elicited by ABT-761, a 5-lipoxygenase inhibitor that suppresses leukotriene production, depend on the presence of at least one allele carrying five tandem repeats of the Sp-1 binding motif in the 5' promoter region of *ALOX5*.[89] Genetic differences in the airway smooth muscle relaxation after inhalation of specific agonists exemplify the advantages to be gained by access to genomic information in advance of acute intervention,[90] and point out the deficiencies of the empiric "one dose fits all" approaches currently used.

Vasodilation and Vasoconstriction

Genetic factors underlying the diagnosis and therapy of cardiovascular disease of immediate relevance to anesthetic care are among the most well understood and intensively investigated in medicine.[91] For example, variable responses to angiotensin-converting enzyme (ACE) inhibitors as a function of an insertion/deletion (I/D) 287-bp DNA fragment *ACE* genotype are well recognized.[92,93] This common *ACE* polymorphism also determines responsivity to beta-blocker therapy in ACE inhibitor-treated patients with congestive heart failure.[94,95] Although both beta-blockers and ACE inhibitors are substrates for pharmacokinetic CYP2D6 inactivation, the drug interaction with the polymorphic ACE protein itself is an example of an enzymatic pharmacodynamic mechanism.

Toxicity

Anesthetic Myopathy Syndrome

Hereditary rhabdomyolysis associated with administration of volatile anesthetic agents and depolarizing muscle relaxants represents the paradigm of a pharmacodynamic toxic response.[96,97] Currently, the Malignant Hyperthermia Association of the United States (MHAUS) is notified of about 200 probable trigger events per year, with several deaths unfortunately part of a normal report. For more than 30 years after its elucidation as a clinical entity,[10] the syndrome was ascribed to a heterogenous inventory of underlying mechanisms including catechol excess, nonspecific membrane defects, and lipid theories. Fairhurst,[98] in drawing attention to the similarity between MH and toxicity of the sap of the ryana tree in Trinidadian rats, provided the first clue implicating a receptor-mediated phenomenon. The observation was accorded little attention until all porcine MH triggers, and a subset of human MH events, were linked to mutations in the skeletal muscle calcium release channel, which also came to be known as the ryanodine receptor (RYR1).[99,100] Recently, MH in the dog has been traced to a novel RYR1 mutation occurring in one of two "hotspot" regions encompassing many human mutations.[101] Similar to the human syndrome, but unlike the pig disorder, canine MH is inherited as an autosomal dominant trait, possibly in keeping with the outbred nature of canine and human populations. Currently, more than 20 *RYR1* polymorphisms have been found in patients manifesting the MH trait by clinical event or in vitro contracture test, each with varying degrees of causal certainty.[102,103] Mutation of a second locus in the skeletal muscle voltage-dependent calcium channel (*CACNA1S*, formerly *CACNL1A3*)[104] has been reported in five additional families worldwide since its first association with MH.[105,106] Linkage of various other chromosomal regions to MH in isolated human pedigrees has been reported, but no additional candidate genes or mutations have been forthcoming.[107]

To improve the genotype-phenotype correlation, and resolve the significant number of patients diagnosed as "MH equivocal" (MHE), a number of modifications of the in vitro contracture test have been proposed, with the addition of 4-chlorochresol appearing to hold the greatest promise.[108] Although this alteration segregates many equivocal muscle bundles into either MH susceptible or MH normal groups, it is premature to state whether the segregation is in fact correct (i.e., fully predictive of the clinical trigger phenotype), or to estimate the precise false equivocal rate. It is hoped that less invasive tests sufficiently sensitive to detect a single mutant *RYR1* copy may be developed in humans and model organisms, thereby sharpening phenotypic indicators for use in humans at risk.[109,110] Improved phenotypic and genotypic detection is particularly desired in view of growing recognition that MH-like events may occur in susceptible patients long after anesthesia,[111] or even in the absence of exposure to trigger drugs.[112,113]

Long QT Syndrome: Gene Specific Therapy

Inherited long QT syndrome (LQTS) denotes a cardiac dysrhythmia that predisposes to *torsades de pointes*, ventricular defibrillation, and sudden death. Mutations in five ion channels cause the preponderance of inherited LQTS. The molecular origin of LQTS can be traced to specific mutations in 50% of patients meeting clinical criteria for diagnosis of the disorder.[114] Of these, 50% have mutations in *KCNQ1* expressing the KvLQT1 α-subunit of the KvLQT1/minK channel conducting the slow (Iks) current.[115] Up to 40% of patients have mutations in the potassium channel gene *KCNH2*, which encodes the hERG (human *ether-a-go-go* related gene) α-subunit of the hERG/MiRP1 channel responsible for conducting the rapid component of the cardiac voltage-gated delayed rectifier K⁺ current.[116] Mutations in *KCNE1* (encoding the minK protein),[117] *KCNE2* (encoding the MiRP1 protein),[118] and *SCN5A* (encoding a cardiac sodium channel α-subunit)[119] account for the rest of known cases.

Many drugs commonly used in anesthetic practice interact with cardiac potassium currents causing either acquired LQTS or precipitating prolongation of the Q-T interval, ventricular dysrhythmia, and *torsades de pointes* in patients who may otherwise be presymptomatic.[120] These include sevoflurane and isoflurane,[121] atropine, glycopyrrolate,[122] succinylcholine, sodium thiopental, fentanyl, haloperidol, amiodarone, ketoconazole, class III antidysrhythmics, and nondepolarizing muscle relaxants.[123] Tailoring drug selection for treatment and prophylaxis to mutation analysis, termed gene specific therapy, has been advocated in the care of LQTS patients.[124] For example, patients with LQTS arising from *SCN5A* mutations are more responsive to sodium channel blockade with lidocaine or mexiletine, whereas shortening of the Q-T interval is observed in hERG-linked long Q-T patients with exogenous potassium or potassium channel agonists.[125]

Ethnicity

From the foregoing it is clear that interethnic variability characterizes many pharmacokinetic and pharmacodynamic responses investigated to date including those disrupting drug transporters, extracellular and intracellular metabolizing enzymes, and receptor and enzyme drug targets.[126] These may take the form of differences in the frequency of identical polymorphisms between two populations, differences in haplotype or genetic background, and entirely different mutations appearing in distinct populations.[127] With globalization of world economies, international travel, and intermarriage, geographic isolation of specific human genomes will become the exception rather than the rule. From the perspective of the anesthesiologist, ethnic variation in disease risk, disease incidence, and response to therapy will assume growing significance in the calculus of regimen, drug, and dose selection.[128] However, because external markers of ethnicity and self-report are unreliable predictors of genotype,[73] and because the range of differences in phenotype within a population typically exceed those observed between ethnic groups,[19] it will be crucial to base therapeutic decisions on direct assessment of genotype. Substitution of microsatellite DNA clusters for imprecise ethnic labels offers a promising "race-neutral" approach to the comparison of pharmacogenetic profiles between populations.[129]

Sex

Although human sex differences in drug response have long been recognized, it is unfortunate that this issue has not attracted more intensive pharmacogenomic research. When scientific attention has focused on patient sex, surprising and clinically relevant disparities in anesthetic practice emerge. Corrected for secondary sex-dependent effects such as body size and composition, significant differences between males and females have been reported in gastric absorption, a 40% more rapid clearance of drugs oxidized by CYP3A4 in females,[130] greater metabolic CYP2C19 and conjugation activity in males,[131] lower pain tolerance, greater opioid sensitivity, and heightened susceptibility to halothane toxicity and to adverse drug reactions among females generally.[132,133] Women awaken from propofol/alfentanil/nitrous oxide anesthesia 50% faster than males, and experience a threefold greater likelihood of awareness during general anesthesia.[134] Epistatic interactions, in which the effects of identical alleles in subjects grouped by sex or other trait vary under the influence of proteins expressed by loci elsewhere in the genome, are thought to account for the discordance. Thus sex-specific hormonal influences underlie a wide spectrum of phenotypic changes including those arising from a direct effect on gene transcription (e.g., altered CYP3A4 activity), as well as nongenomic indirect effects mediated by simultaneous hormone and drug receptor occupancy (e.g., increased potency of volatile agents during pregnancy). In turn, each of the enzymatic steps in steroid hormone synthetic pathways are regulated by the interplay of an ensemble of genes. Interrogation of multiple genetic sites for contributory variations to specific traits will render divergent genetic backgrounds amenable to quantitative investigations. Currently, few pharmacokinetic/pharmacodynamic investigations in humans control for the effects of menstrual cycle, menopause, menarche, pregnancy, and use of exogenous hormones for contraception or replacement therapy. As new clinical trials are designed, and as genomic profiling enters diagnostic and therapeutic trials, fuller consideration of sex as a significant variable will be crucial.

Pharmacogenetics in Anesthetic Practice

Will pharmacogenomic data have any clinical impact on a profession so apparently successful in meeting its objectives? Formal scrutiny of outcomes in contemporary anesthesiology belie overconfidence. The incidence of severe critical events and complications during anesthesia consistently exceeds 3% in prospective multicenter investigations, with more than half associated with genetic predispositions.[135] The source of complacency in the face of these statistics can be found in a discipline oriented toward early detection of complications once they have begun and skill in rescue, rather than focusing on risk stratification and prevention.[136] By corollary, no other medical specialty stands to gain more by the introduction of pharmacogenomics into the daily care of patients who may present with any coexisting disease, on every intercurrent medication, undergoing exposure to multiple anesthetic agents with inverted therapeutic ratios.[137]

During the preceding two decades human genomics has been enabled by a series of technical leaps, first with cloning and sequencing, followed by polymerase chain reaction amplification of DNA fragments *in vitro*. With technologies adopted from silicon industries including robotics, microfluidics, microarray (i.e., "gene chip") sorting, and internet-based bioinformatics, high throughput pharmacogenomic profiling will soon be feasible within clinical constraints of cost, efficiency, and precision.[138] Moreover, technologies have recently been introduced that enable direct detection of pharmacogenetic polymorphisms from unamplified genomic DNA templates, foregoing the time, cost, and potential contamination inherent to polymerase chain reaction-based methods.[139] Pharmacologic responses are most often polygenic traits determined by widely disparate genes encoding proteins participating in multiple pathways of drug metabolism, disposition, and target effectors. Underlying mutations may reflect a large repertoire of distinct molecular pathologies including alternate exon splicing, microsatellite expansions, gene deletions and duplications, and point mutations conferring truncation, protein instability, or functional amino acid substitutions. Automated multiplexed formats compressing years of conventional genotyping into a single operator day are now available to match the genetic heterogeneity and multiple genomic contributors to be encountered in prediction of complex pharmacogenomic phenotypes in advance of surgery.

Risks for loss of privacy, harms from unwarranted patient labeling, and discrimination in employment or insurance coverage drew attention from the first conception of human genome research. Today, it is acknowledged that although these risks persist, they may be tempered by legal and technical safeguards, e.g., fully informed consent and data encryption.[140] To the contrary, real risks to caregivers have been identified for legal liability and negligence should they administer drugs that are unsafe to patients who could be readily identified by perioperative genetic testing.[29,141,142] In a setting wherein the smallest possible differences in DNA sequence may predict life or death consequences, the immediate and direct benefit of pharmacogenomic profiling will outweigh theoretic and practical risks to patient and caregiver alike. For the clinician interested in tracking ethical, legal, and social issues pertinent to pharmacogenetics, as well as up to the minute syndrome and allele news, the Pharmacogenetics Research Network (http://www.nigms.nih.gov/pharmacogenetics/index.html) and Pharmacogenetics Knowledge Base (http://www.pharmgkb.org) are excellent resources.

Summary

Despite dogma accepted for more than a century that genetic factors are major determinants of variations in perioperative drug action between individuals and populations, technical limitations have precluded practitioners from incorporating heritable differences in drug choice and dose estimates. With introduction of technologies able to rapidly scan DNA sequence for causal alterations, together with a first composite draft of the human genome, the rate-limiting step to benefit from pharmacogenomic advances will now be clinicians skilled in the recognition of drug response outliers, and in testing novel genotype-phenotype correlations.

Today, the pharmacogenetic frontier is shifting from phase I to phase II pharmacokinetic effects, from drug metabolism to interindividual differences in pharmacodynamic responses, from monogenic to polygenic mechanisms, and from extreme to more subtle phenotypic correlates. As anesthetic drug administration evolves from empiric approaches of the past to regimens customized by patient genotype, greater safety will be assured, and autonomy will be restored to the care of our most vulnerable patients including the very old, the very young, and the very sick. In the alternative, the price to be paid for ignoring genetic diversity in human drug response will grow increasingly unacceptable.

References

1. Pernick MS: A calculus of suffering: Pain, professionalism, and anesthesia in nineteenth century America. New York, Columbia University Press, 1985.
2. Kalow W, Grant DM: Pharmacogenetics. In Scriver CR, et al (eds): The Metabolic and Molecular Bases of Inherited Disease, 8th ed. New York, McGraw-Hill, 2001.
3. Garrod AE: Inborn Errors of Metabolism. London, H. Frowde and Hodder & Stoughton, 1909.
4. Kalow W: Familial incidence of low pseudocholinesterase. Lancet 2:576, 1956.
5. Kalow W, Gunn DR: The relationship between dose of succinylcholine and duration of apnea in man. J Pharmacol Exp Ther 120:203, 1957.
6. Dern RJ, Beutler E, Alving AS: The hemolytic effect of primaquine. J Lab Clin Med 44:171, 1954
7. Evans DAP, McKusick VA: Genetic control of isoniazid in man. Br Med J 2:485, 1960.
8. Motulsky AG: Drug reactions, enzymes and biochemical genetics. JAMA 165:835, 1957.
9. Vogel F: Moderne Problem der Humangenetik. Ergeb Inn Med Kinderheilkd 12:65, 1959.
10. Denborough MA, Lovell RRH: Anaesthetic deaths in a family. Lancet 2:45, 1960.
11. Athanassiadis D, Cranston WI, Juel-Jensen BE, et al: Clinical observations on the effects of debrisoquine sulphate in patients with high blood pressure. BMJ 2:732, 1966.
12. Vessel ES: Genetic control of dicumarol levels in man. J Clin Invest 47:2657, 1968.
13. Mahgoub A, Idle JR, Dring LG, et al: Polymorphic hydroxylation of debrisoquine in man. Lancet 2:584, 1977.
14. Eichelbaum M, Spannbrucker N, Steinke B, et al: Defective N-oxidation of sparteine in man: A new pharmacogenetic defect. Eur J Clin Pharmacol 116:183, 1979.
15. Gonzalez FJ, Skoda RC, Kimuar S, et al: Characterization of the common genetic defect in humans deficient in debrisoquine metabolism. Nature 331:442, 1988.
16. Lazarou J, Pomeranz BH, Corey PN: Incidence of adverse drug reactions in hospitalized patients: A meta-analysis of prospective studies. JAMA 279:1200, 1998.
17. Chyka PA: How many deaths occur annually from adversed drug reactions in the United States? Am J Med 109:122, 2000.
18. White TJ, Arakelian A, Rho JP: Counting the costs of drug-related adverse events. Pharmacogenomics 15:445, 1999.
19. Alvan G, Bertilsson L, Dahl ML, et al: Moving toward genetic profiling in patient care: The scope and rationale of pharmacogenetic/ecogenetic investigation. Drug Metab Dispos 29:580, 2001.
20. Phillips KA, Veenstra DL, Oren E, et al: Potential role of pharmacogenomics in reducing adverse drug reactions: A systematic review. JAMA 286:2270, 2001.
21. Hogan K: Principles and techniques of molecular biology. In Hopkins P, Hemmings HC (eds): Basic and Applied Science for Anesthesia. New York, Mosby-Wolfe, 2000.

22. Rusnak JM, Kisabeth RM, Herbert DP, et al: Pharmacogenomics: A clinician's primer on emerging technologies for improved patient care. Mayo Clin Proc 76:299, 2001.

23. International Human Genome Sequencing Consortium: Initial sequencing and analysis of the human genome. Nature 409:860, 2001.

24. Altman RB, Klein TE: Challenges for biomedical informatics and pharmacogenomics. Ann Rev Pharmacol Toxicol 42:113, 2002.

25. Ligget SB: Pharmacogenetic applications of the Human Genome project. Nat Med 7:281, 2001.

26. Nebert DW: Extreme discordant phenotype methodology: An intuitive approach to clinical pharmacogenetics. Eur J Pharmacol 410:107, 2000.

27. Wolf CR, Smith G: Pharmacogenetics. Br Med Bull 55:366, 1999.

28. McLeod HL, Evans WE: Pharmacogenomics: Unlocking the human genome for better drug therapy. Annu Rev Pharmacol Toxicol 41:101, 2001.

29. Fagerlund TH, Braaten O: No pain relief from codeine? An introduction to pharmacogenomics. Acta Anaesthesiol Scand 45:140, 2001.

30. Nebert DQ: Pharmacogenetics and pharmacogenomics: Why is this relevant to the clinical geneticist? Clin Genet 56:247, 1999.

31. Hogan K: Genomics in perioperative critical care. In Murray MJ, Coursin DB, Pearl RG, Prough DS (eds): Critical Care Medicine: Perioperative Management. Philadelphia, Lippincott Williams & Wilkins, 2001.

32. Kalow W: Perspectives in pharmacogenetics. Arch Pathol Lab Med 125:77, 2001.

33. Fromm MF: P-glycoprotein: A defense mechanism limiting oral bioavailability and CNS accumulation of drugs. Int J Clin Pharmacol Ther 38:69, 2000.

34. Hoffmeyer S, Burk O, von Richter O, et al: Functional polymorphisms of the human multidrug-resistance gene: Multiple sequence variations and correlation of one allele with P-glycoprotein expression and activity *in vivo*. Proc Natl Acad Sci USA 97:34733, 2000.

35. Kerb R, Hoffmeyer S, Brinkmann U: ABC drug transporters: Hereditary polymorphisms and pharmacological impact in MDR1, MDRP1 and MRP2. Pharmacogenomics 2:51, 2001.

36. Lown KS, Mayo RR, Leichtman AB, et al: Role of intestinal P-glycoprotein (mdr-1) in interpatient variation in the oral bioavailability of cyclosporine. Clin Pharmacol Ther 62:248, 1997.

37. Lesch KP, Jatzke S, Meyer J, et al: Mosaicism for a serotonin transporter gene promoter-associated deletion: Decreased recombination in depression. J Neural Transm 106:1223, 1999.

38. Smeraldi E, Zanardi R, Benedetti F, et al: Polymorphism within the promoter of the serotonin transporter gene and antidepressant efficacy of fluvoxamine. Mol Psychiatry 3:508, 1998.

39. Pantuck EJ: Plasma cholinesterase: Gene and variations. Anesth Analg 77:380, 1993.

40. Maekawa M, Sudo K, Dey DC, et al: Genetic mutations of butyrylcholine esterase identified from phenotypic abnormalities in Japan. Clin Chem 43:927, 1997.

41. La Du BN: Butyrylcholinesterase variants and the new methods of molecular biology. Acta Anaesthesiologica Scand 39:139, 1995.

42. Morrow AC, Motulsky AG: Rapid screening method for the common atypical pseudocholinesterase variant. J Lab Clin Med 71:350, 1968.

43. Wolf CR, Smith G, Smith RL: Pharmacogenetics. Br Med J 320:987, 2000.

44. Nebert DW: Suggestions for the nomenclature of human alleles: Relevance to ecogenetics, pharmacogenetics and molecular epidemiology. Pharmacogenetics 10:279, 2000.

45. Daly AK, Brockmoller J, Broly F, et al: Nomenclature for human CYP2D6 alleles. Pharmacogenetics 6:193, 1996.

46. Marez D, Legrand M, Sabbagh N, et al: Polymorphism of the cytochrome P450 CYP2D6 gene in a European population: Characterization of 48 mutations and 53 alleles, their frequencies and evolution. Pharmacogenetics 7:193, 1996.

47. Sindrup SH, Brosen K: The pharmacogenetics of codeine hypoalgesia. Pharmacogenetics 5:335, 1995.

48. Aklillu E, Persson I, Bertilsson L et al: Frequent distribution of ultrarapid metabolizers of debrisoquine in an Ethiopian population carrying duplicated and multiduplicated functional CYP2D6 alleles. J Pharmacol Exp Ther 278:441, 1996.

49. Sindrup SH, Poulsen L, Brosen D, et al: Are poor metabolizers of sparteine/debrisoquine less pain tolerant than extensive metabolizers? Pain 53:335, 1993.

50. Yanagihara Y, Kariya S, Ohtani M, et al: Involvement of CYP2B6 in N-demethylation of ketamine in human liver microsomes. Drug Metab Dis 29:887, 2001.

51. Court MH, Duan SX, Hesse L, et al: Cytochrome P-450 2B6 is responsible for interindividual variability of propofol hydroxylation by human liver microsomes. Anesthesiology 94:110, 2001.

52. Lang T, Klein K, Fischer J, et al: Extensive genetic polymorphism in the human CYP2B6 gene with impact on expression and function in human liver. Pharmacogenetics 11:1, 2001.

53. Stelow EB, Johari VP, Smith SA, et al: Propofol-associated rhabdomyolysis with cardiac involvement in adults: Chemical and anatomic findings. Clin Chem 46:577, 2000.

54. Wolf A, Weir P, Segar P, et al: Impaired fatty acid oxidation in propofol infusion syndrome. Lancet 357:606, 2001.

55. Aithal GP, Day CP, Kesteven PJ, et al: Association of polymorphisms in the cytochrome P450 CYP2C9 with warfarin dose requirement and risk of bleeding complications. Lancet 353:717, 1999.

56. Rettie AE, Wienkers LC, Gonzalez FJ, et al: Impaired S-warfarin metabolism catalysed by the R144CC allelic variant of CYP2C9. Pharmacogenetics 4:39, 1994.

57. Haining RL, Hunter AP, Veronese ME, et al: Allelic variants of human cytochrome P450 2C9: Baculovirus-mediated expression, purification, structural characterization, substrate stereoselectivity, and prochiral selectivity of the wild type and I359L mutant forms. Arch Biochem Biophys 333:447, 1996.

58. Takahashi H, Echizen H: Pharmacogenetics of warfarin elimination and its clinical implications. Clin Pharmacokinet 40:587, 2001.

59. De Morais SM, Schweikl H, Blaisdell J, et al: Gene structure and upstream regulatory regions of human CYP2C19 and 2C18. Biochem Biophys Res Commun 194:194, 1993.

60. Lieber CS: Cytochrome P-450E1: Its physiological and pathological role. Physiol Rev 77:527, 1997.

61. Ozdemir V, Shear NH, Kalow W: What will be the role of pharmacogenetics in evaluating drug safety and minimizing adverse effects? Drug Safety 24:75, 2001.

62. Vessell ES: Advances in pharmacogenetics and pharmacogenomics. J Clin Pharmacol 40;930, 2000.

63. Kuehl P, Zhang J, Lin Y, et al: Sequence diversity in the *CYP3A* promoters and characterization of the genetic basis of polymorphic CYP3A5 expression. Nat Genet 27:383, 2001.

64. de Wildt SN, Kearns GL, Leeder JS, et al: Glucuronidation in humans. Clin Pharmacokinet 6:439, 1999.

65. Vastis KP, Weber WW, Bell DA, et al: Nomenclature for N-acetyltransferases. Pharmacogenetics 5:1, 1995.

66. Weber WW, Hein DW: N-acetylation pharmacogenetics. Pharmacol Rev 37:25, 1985.

67. Coulthard SA, Hall AG: Recent advances in the pharmacogenomics of thiopurine methyltransferase. Pharmacogenom J 1:254, 2001.

68. Black AJ, McLeod HL, Capell HA, et al: Thiopurine methyltransferase genotype predicts therapy-limiting severe toxicity from azathioprine. Ann Intern Med 129:716, 1998.

69. Rosenblatt DS, Fenton WA: Inherited disorders of folate and cobalamin transport and metabolism. In Scriver CR, et al (eds): The Metabolic and Molecular Basis of Inherited Disease, 8th ed. New York, McGraw-Hill, 2001.

70. Selzer RR, Rosenblatt DS, Laxova R, et al: Nitrous oxide and 5,10-methylenetetrahydrofolate reductase deficiency. Am J Hum Genet 71:429, 2002.

71. Vesell ES: Therapeutic lessons from pharmacogenetics. Ann Int Med 126:653, 1997.

72. Spire-Vayron de la Moureyre C, Debuysere H, Mastain B, et al: Genotypic and phenotypic analysis of the polymorphic thiopurine S-methyltransferase gene (*TPMT*) in a European population. Br J Pharmacol 125:879, 1998.

73. Hon YY, Fessing MY, Pui CH, et al: Polymorphism of the thiopurine S-methyl transferase gene in African Americans. Hum Mol Genet 8:371, 1999.

74. Tavadia SM, Mydlarski PR, Reis MD, et al: Screening for azathioprine toxicity: A pharmacoeconomic analysis based on a target case. J Am Acad Dermatol 42:628, 2000.

75. Zhou HH, Sheller JR, Nu H, et al: Ethnic differences in response to morphine. Clin Pharmacol Ther 54:507, 1993.

76. Uhl GR, Soar I, Wang Z: The mu opiate receptor as a candidate gene for pain: Polymorphisms, variations in expresssion, nociception, and opiate responses. Proc Natl Acad Sci USA 96:7752, 1999.

77. Bond C, LaForge KS, Tian M, et al: Single-nucleotide polymorphism in the human mu opioid receptor gene alteres beta-endorphin binding and activity: Possible implications for opiate addiction. Proc Natl Acad Sci USA 95;9608, 1998.

78. Lotsch J, Zimmerman M, Darimont J, et al: Does the A118G polymorphism at the υ-opioid receptor gene protect against morphine-6-glucuronide toxicity? Anesthesiology 97:814, 2002.

79. Lotsch J, Skarke C, Grosch S, et al: The polymorphism A118G of the human mu-opioid receptor gene decreases the pupil constrictory effect of morphine-6-glucuronide but not that of morphine. Pharmacogenetics 15:3, 2002.

80. Befort K, Fillol D, Decaillot FM, et al: A single-nucleotide polymorphic mutation in the mu-opioid receptor severely impairs receptor signalling. J Biol Chem 276:3130, 2001.

81. Lichtermann D, Franke P, Maier W, et al: Pharmacogenomics and addiction to opiates. Eur J Pharmacol 410:269, 2000.

82. Flores CM, Mogil JS: The pharmacogenetics of analgesia: Toward a genetically-based approach to pain management. Pharmacogenomics 2:177, 2001.

83. Ligget SB: The pharmacogenetics of beta2-adrenergic receptors: Relevance to asthma. J Allergy Clin Immunol 105:487, 2000.

84. Turki J, Pak J, Green SA, et al: Genetic polymorphisms of the beta-2-adrenergic receptor in nocturnal and nonocturnal asthma: Evidence that gly16 correlates with the nocturnal phenotype. J Clin Invest 95:1635, 1995.

85. Xie HG, Stein CM, Kim RB, et al: Frequency of functionally important beta-2 adrenoceptor polymorphisms varies markedly among African-American, Caucasian and Chinese individuals. Pharmacogenetics 9:511, 1999.

86. Martinez FD, Graves PE, Baldini M, et al: Association between genetic polymorphisms of the β2-adrenoreceptor and response to albuterol in children with and without a history of wheezing. J Clin Invest 100:3184, 1997.

87. Lima JJ, Thomason DB, Mohamed MHN, et al: Impact of genetic polymorphisms of the beta(2)adrenergic receptor on albuterol bronchodilator pharmacodynamics. Clin Pharmacol Ther 65:519, 1999.

88. Drysdale CM, McGraw DW, Stack CB, et al: Complex promoter and coding region β2-adrenergic receptor haplotyes alter receptor expression and predict in vivo responsiveness. Proc Natl Acad Sci USA 97:10483, 2000.

89. Drazen JM, Yandava CN, Dube L, et al: Pharmacogenetic association between the ALOX5 promoter genotype and the response to anti-asthma treatment. Nat Genet 22:168, 1999.

90. Palmer LJ, Silverman ES, Weiss ST, et al: Pharmacogenetics of asthma. Am J Resp Crit Care Med 165:861, 2002.

91. Nakagawa K, Ishizaki T: Therapeutic relevance of pharmacogenetic factors in cardiovascular medicine. Pharmacol Ther 86:1, 2000.

92. Nakano Y, Oshima T, Watanabe M, et al: Angiotensin I-converting enzyme gene polymorphism and acute response to captopril in essential hypertension. Am J Hypertens 10:1064, 1997.

93. Ueda S, Meredith PA, Morton JJ, et al: ADE (I/D) genotype as a predictor of the magnitude and duration of the response to an ACE inhibitor drug (enalaprilat) in humans. Circulation 98:2148, 1998.

94. O'Toole L, Stewart M, Padfield P, et al: Effect of the insertion/deletion polymorphism of the angiotensin-converting enzyme on response to angiotensin-converting enzyme inhibitors in patients with heart failure. J Cardiol Pharmacol 32:988, 1998.

95. McNamara DM, Holubkov R, Janosko K: Pharmacogenetic interactions between β-blocker therapy and the angiotensin-converting enzyme deletion polymorphism in patients with congestive heart failure. Circulation 103:1644, 2001.

96. Hogan K: The anesthetic myopathies and malignant hyperthermias. Curr Opin Neurol 11:469, 1998.

97. Schulte am Esch J, Scholz J, Wappler F: Malignant hyperthermia. Lengerich, Pabst Scientific Publishers, 2000.

98. Fairhurst AS, Hamamoto V, Macri J: Modification of ryanodine toxicity by dantrolene and halothane in a model of malignant hyperthermia. Anesthesiology 53:199, 1980.

99. MacLennan DH, Phillips MS: Malignant hyperthermia. Science 256:789,1992.

100. Hogan K, Couch F, Powers P, et al: A cysteine for arginine substitution (R614C) in the human skeletal muscle calcium release channel co-segregates with malignant hyperthermia. Anesth Analg 75:441, 1992.

101. Roberts, MC, Mickelson JR, Paterson EE, et al: Autosomal dominant canine malignant hyperthermia is caused by a mutation in the gene encoding the skeletal muscle calcium release channel (RYR1). Anesthesiology 95:716, 2001.

102. McCarthy TV, Quane KA, Lynch PJ: Ryanodine receptor mutations in malignant hyperthermia and central core disease. Hum Mutat 15:410, 2000.

103. Ruffert H, Olthoff D, Deutrich CD, et al: Mutation screening in the ryanodine receptor 1 gene (RYR1) in patients susceptible to malignant hyperthermia who show definite IVCT results: Identification of three novel mutations. Acta Anaesthesiol Scand 46:692, 2002.

104. Hogan K, Gregg RG, Powers PA: The structure of the gene encoding the human skeletal muscle α1 subunit of the dihydropyridine-sensitive L-type calcium channel (CACNL1A3). Genomics 31:392, 1996.

105. Monnier NV, Procaccio V, Stieglitz P, et al: Malignant hyperthermia susceptibility is associated with a mutation of the α1 subunit of the human dihydropyridine-sensitive L-type voltage dependent calcium-channel receptor in skeletal muscle. Am J Hum Genet 60:1316, 1997.

106. Stewart SL, Hogan K, Rosenberg H, et al: Identification of the Arg1086His mutation in the alpha subunit of the voltage-dependent calcium channel (CACNA1S) in a North American family with malignant hyperthermia. Clin Genet 59:178, 2001.

107. Jurkat-Rott KT, McCarthy TV, Lehmann-Horn F: Genetics and pathogenesis of malignant hyperthermia. Muscle Nerve 23:4, 2000.

108. Tegazzin V, Scutari E, Treves S, et al: Chlorocresol, an additive to commercial succinylcholine, induces contracture of human malignant hyperthermia-susceptible muscles via activation of the ryanodine receptor Ca2+ channel. Anesthesiology 84:1380, 1996.

109. Anetseder M, Hager M, Muller CR, et al: Diagnosis of susceptibility to malignant hyperthermia by use of a metabolic test. Lancet 359:1579, 2002.

110. Rosenberg H, Anognini JF, Muldoon S: Testing for malignant hyperthermia. Anesthesiology 96:232, 2002.

111. McKenney KA, Holman SJ: Delayed postoperative rhabdomyolysis in a patient subsequently diagnosed as malignant hyperthermia susceptible. Anesthesiology 96:674, 2002.

112. Wappler F, Fiege M, Markus S, et al: Evidence for susceptibility to malignant hyperthermia in patients with exercise-induced rhabdomyolysis. Anesthesiology 94:95, 2001.

113. Tobin J, Jason DR, Challa VR, et al: Malignant hyperthermia and apparent heat stroke. JAMA 286:168, 2001.

114. Larsen LA, Andersen PS, Kanters J, et al: Screening for mutations and polymorphisms in the genes *KCNH2* and *KCNE2* encoding the cardiac HERG/MiRP1 ion channel: Implications for acquired and congenital long Q-T syndrome. Clin Chem 47:1390, 2001.

115. Wang Q, Curran ME, Splawski I, et al: Positional cloning of a novel potassium channel gene: *KVLQT1* mutations cause cardiac arrhythmias. Nat Genet 12:17, 1996.

116. Priori SG, Barhanin J, Hauer RN, et al: Genetic and molecular basis of cardiac arrythmias: Impact on clinical management part III. Circulation 99:674, 1999.

117. Splawski I, Tristani-Firouzi M, Lehmann MH, et al: Mutations in the *hminK* gene cause long QT syndrome and suppress Iks function. Nat Genet 17:338, 1997.

118. Abbott GW, Sesti F, Splawski I, et al: MiRP1 forms Ikr potassium channels with HERG and is associated with cardiac arrythmia. Cell 97:175, 1999.

119. Curran ME: Potassium channels and human disease: Phenotypes to drug targets. Curr Opin Biotechnol 9:565, 1998.

120. Donger C, Denjoy I, Berthet M, et al: KVLQT1 C-terminal missense mutation causes a forme fruste long-QT syndrome. Circulation 96:2778, 1997.

121. Kleinsasser A, Loeckinger A, Lindner KH, et al: Reversing sevoflurane-associated Q-Tc prolongation by changing to propofol. Anaesthesia 56:248, 2001.

122. Pylem H, Bathen J, Spigseet O, et al: Ventricullar fibrillation related to reversal of the neuromuscular blockade in a patient with long QT syndrome. Acta Anaesthesiol Scand 43:352, 1999.

123. Saarnivaara L, Klemola UM, Lindgren L: QT interval of the ECG, heart rate and arterial pressure using five non-depolarizing muscle relaxants for intubation. Acta Anaesthesiol Scand 32:623, 1988.

124. Towbin JA, Wang Z, Li H: Genotype and severity of long QT syndrome. Drug Metab Dispos 29:574, 2001.

125. Geelen JLMC, Doevendans PA, Jongbloed RJE, et al: Molecular genetics of inherited long QT syndromes. Eur Heart J 19:1427, 1998.

126. Evans DAP, McLeod HL, Pritchard S, et al: Interethnic variability in human drug responses. Drug Metab Dispos 29:606, 2001.

127. Gaedigk A: Interethnic differences of drug metabolizing enzymes. Int J Clin Pharmacol Ther 38:61, 2000.

128. Wilcox RA, Owen H: Variable P450 2D6 expression and metabolism of codeine and other opioid prodrugs: Implications for the Australian anaesthetist. Anaesth Intensive Care 28:611, 2000.

129. Wilson JF, Weale ME, Smith AC, et al: Population genetic structure of variable drug response. Nat Genet 29:265, 2001.

130. Ciccone GK, Holdcroft A: Drugs and sex differences: A review of drugs relating to anaesthesia. Br J Anesth 82:255, 1999.

131. Tanaka E: Gender-related differences in pharmacokinetics and their clinical significance. J Clin Pharm Ther 24:339, 1999.

132. Martin G, Gan TJ: Gender difference: Hype or fact? Semin Anesth Perioper Med Pain 19:76, 2000.

133. Kest B, Sarton E, Dahan A: Gender differences in opioid-mediated analgesia: Animal and human studies. Anesthesiology 93:539, 2000.

134. Gan TJ, Glass PS, Sigl J, et al: Women emerge from general anesthesia with propofol/alfentanil/nitrous oxide faster than men. Anesthesiology 90;1283, 1999.

135. Bothner U, Georgieff M, Schwilk B: Building a large-scale perioperative anaesthesia outcome-tracking database: Methodology, implementation, and experiences from one provider within the German quality project. Br J Anaesth 85:271, 2000.

136. Sigurdsson GH, McAteer E: Morbidity and mortality associated with anesthesia. Acta Anaesthesiol Scand 40:1057, 1996.

137. Kennedy JM, van Rij AM, Spears GF, et al: Polypharmacy in a general surgical unit and consequences of drug withdrawl. Br J Clin Pharmacol 49:353, 2000.

138. Shi MM: Enabling large-scale pharmacogenetic studies by high-throughput mutation detection and genotyping technologies. Clin Chem 47:164, 2001.

139. Neville M, Selzer R, Aizenstein B, et al: Characterization of cytochrome P450 2D6 alleles using the Invader system. BioTechniques 32:S34, 2002.

140. Gostin LO, Hodge JG: Genetic privacy and the law: An end to genetics exceptionalism. Jurimetrics 40:21, 1999.

141. Reilly PR: Legal issues in genomic medicine. Nat Med 7:268, 2001.

142. Rothstein RA, Epps PG: Ethical and legal implications of pharmacogenomics. Nat Rev Genet 2:228, 2001.

6

Common Pharmacodynamic Drug Interactions in Anesthetic Practice

Talmage D. Egan, MD • Charles Minto, MBChB

Experimental Characterization of Anesthetic Drug
Interactions
   Additive, Synergistic, Antagonistic Interactions
   Isobologram
   Response Surfaces
   Interaction Models Used in Anesthesia

Prototype Examples of Pharmacodynamic
Anesthetic Interactions
   Volatile Anesthetics and Opioids
   Opioids and Propofol

Understanding drug interactions is a critical part of anesthetic practice. The modern concept of "balanced anesthesia" implies the use of multiple drugs to achieve the anesthetized state. As many as a dozen drugs might be administered during a typical anesthetic, which may include benzodiazepines, barbiturates and other sedative-hypnotics, opioid analgesics, neuromuscular blockers, other analgesic adjuncts, antibiotics, neuromuscular blockade reversal agents, sympathomimetics and autonomic nervous system blockers. The potential for drug interactions is therefore immense.

Anesthetic drug interactions can take several forms. Perhaps the simplest form of drug interaction in anesthesia is the physicochemical interaction. Physicochemical interactions occur when the physical properties of the interacting drugs are somehow incompatible; for example, the precipitation that occurs when certain neuromuscular blockers (e.g., pancuronium bromide) are injected into an intravenous line containing sodium thiopental (the precipitate is the conjugate salt of a weak acid and a weak base).[1] A second form is the pharmacokinetic interaction. Pharmacokinetic interactions occur when one drug somehow alters the disposition of another drug;[2] for example, the increased metabolism of neuromuscular blockers observed in patients who are taking anticonvulsants chronically.[3] The final and most important form of drug interaction in anesthesiology is pharmacodynamic. Pharmacodynamic interactions occur when one drug somehow augments or reduces the effect of another drug; for example, the minimum alveolar concentration (MAC) reduction when opioids are administered.

In anesthesiology, unlike most medical disciplines, pharmacodynamic drug interactions are frequently induced by design. Anesthesiologists take advantage of the pharmacodynamic synergy that results when two drugs with different mechanisms of action but similar therapeutic effects are combined. These synergistic combinations can be advantageous because the therapeutic goals of the anesthetic can often be achieved with less toxicity and faster recovery than when the individual drugs are used alone in greater doses.

In fact, except for specific, limited clinical circumstances wherein a volatile agent or propofol alone is acceptable approaches (e.g., a brief operation in a pediatric patient such as tympanostomy tubes), current anesthesia administration is at least a two-drug process. Opioids alone are not complete anesthetics because they cannot reliably produce unconsciousness.[4,5] Volatile anesthetics alone are inadequate unless the prestimulus hemodynamic variables are depressed to an unacceptable degree.[6,7] Modern anesthesia care is of necessity a multidrug exercise, and therefore mandates that practitioners become experts in manipulating pharmacodynamic anesthetic interactions.[8] From a strictly pharmacologic perspective, anesthesiology is the practice of pharmacologic synergism using central nervous system depressants.

The goals of this chapter are twofold. First, we'll review how anesthetic drug interactions are characterized experimentally with special focus on response surface methodology. Having built the theoretical foundation to understand the concept of pharmacodynamic synergism, we'll then briefly review the critical pharmacodynamic drug interactions in anesthesiology, focusing on (1) the interactions between volatile anesthetics and opioids and (2) the interaction between propofol and opioids.

Experimental Characterization of Anesthetic Drug Interactions

Additive, Synergistic, Antagonistic Interactions

The basic concepts of additive, synergistic, and antagonistic interactions are simple enough to understand. The term *additive interaction* is usually used in those cases in which the combined effect of two drugs (often acting by the same mechanism) is equal to that expected by simple addition; the term *synergistic interaction* is used when the combined effect of two drugs (often acting by a different mechanism) is greater than that expected by simple addition; and the term *antagonistic interaction* is used when the combined effect of two drugs is less than that expected by simple addition. However, the crux of the matter lies in how "that expected by simple addition" is defined.

Many authors define an *additive interaction* as one that obeys the simple effect addition model:

$$E_{AB} = E_A + E_B \qquad (1)$$

where the combined effect of two drugs (E_{AB}) is equal to the algebraic sum of their individual effects (E_A and E_B). Thus the "additive" concept is often explained through the simple equation $1 + 1 = 2$. With reference to this equation, the "synergy" concept is illustrated by $1 + 1 > 2$, and the "antagonism" concept is illustrated by $1 + 1 < 2$. Although the basic concepts of additive, synergistic, and antagonistic interactions may be clear from this explanation, the simple effect addition model has a major flaw. Imagine a sham experiment, in which a drug preparation is divided into two syringes; then the syringes are handled as if they contain different drugs ("drug A" and "drug B"). In the first phase of the experiment, 1 mg of "drug A" is given. This dose causes an effect, which is 5% of the maximum response. In the second phase of the experiment, 1 mg of "drug B" is given. This dose causes an effect that is also 5% of the maximum response. In the third phase, 1 mg of "drug A" is administered *together with* 1 mg of "drug B." What effect should occur if the interaction is additive? Will the combination cause a 10% effect, which is the algebraic sum of the individual effects (5% + 5%)? Actually, the combination causes

an effect equal to 50% of the maximum response. Should we conclude that the two drugs interact synergistically, because the effect of the combination is fivefold greater than expected from the algebraic sum of the individual effects? How is it possible to have a synergistic interaction when only one drug is being evaluated? Surely, by definition, one drug has "no interaction" with itself! Why didn't the effects add together as described by Equation 6.1.

The flaw with the simple effect addition model (Eq. 6.1) is that it presupposes that the relationship between drug dose and drug effect is linear, as illustrated in the left graph in Figure 6–1. It assumes that doubling the dose will double the effect. However, the hypothetical drug being investigated has a nonlinear relationship between dose and effect, as illustrated in the right graph in Figure 6–1, which shows that 1 mg causes an effect of 5% and 2 mg causes an effect of 50%. There is no synergy because the observed effect caused by 1 mg of "drug A" combined with 1 mg of "drug B" (the same drug) is the same as expected for the effect caused by a 2 mg bolus. Thus the simple effect addition model is only true if the dose-response relationship is linear. A more general definition of "no interaction" is required.

Isobologram

Synergism (and antagonism) can be defined as a greater (or lesser) pharmacologic effect for a two-drug combination than what would be predicted for "no interaction" based on what is known about the effects of each drug individually. Thus their definitions critically depend on the reference model for "no interaction."[9] We believe the best way to obtain a clear understanding of "no interaction" is by carrying out a thought experiment based on the sham combination of one drug with itself, as described earlier. Knowing that syringes A and B contain the same drug, we can describe an experiment to show that "drug A" and "drug B" have "no interaction" (i.e., they are additive). Imagine syringes A and B contain 2 mg of "drug A" and 2 mg of "drug B," respectively. We perform an experiment and find that 2 mg from syringe A causes 50% effect. We perform another experiment and find that 2 mg from syringe B also causes 50% effect. Clearly, 1 mg from syringe A together with 1 mg from syringe B will also cause 50% effect, because we are still giving 2 mg of our hypothetical drug. For the same reason,

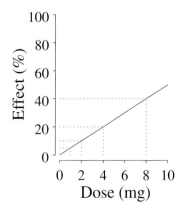
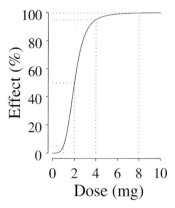

Figure 6–1. Linear and nonlinear dose-effect curves. Many authors define an *additive interaction* as one that obeys the simple effect addition model, where the combined effect of two drugs is equal to the algebraic sum of their individual effects (Eq. 6.1). This is only applicable if the dose-response (or concentration-response) relationship is linear (*left*). Often the relationship is nonlinear (*right*). *Left*, Doubling the dose doubles the effect. *Right*, Doubling the dose from 1 to 2 mg increases the effect from 5% to 50%. When the dose is doubled again, the effect increases from 50% to 95%. When the dose is doubled again, the effect only increases from 95% to 99.7%.

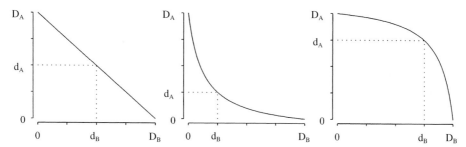

Figure 6–2. Isobolograms: additivity (*left*), synergy or supra-additivity (*middle*), antagonism or infra-additivity (*right*). D_A and D_B are isoeffective doses of two drugs when given alone. The administration of the two drugs as the combination (d_A, d_B) results in the same effect. If D_A and D_B are the doses causing 50% effect (the D_{50}), in each case the *line* represents the 50% isobole. When the drugs in combination are more effective than expected (synergy), smaller amounts are needed to produce the effect, and the combination (d_A, d_B) is shifted toward the origin (*middle*). Conversely, when the drugs in combination are less effective than expected (antagonism), greater amounts are needed to produce the effect, and the combination (d_A, d_B) is shifted away from the origin (*right*). *Left,* The equation for the *straight line* is given by $y = -D_A/D_B \cdot x + D_A$, where y is d_A and x is d_B, which is the same as the equation defining Loewe additivity (Eq. 6.2).

0.5 mg from syringe A together with 1.5 mg from syringe B, or 1.5 mg from syringe A together with 0.5 mg from syringe B, will also cause 50% effect. That we are using one or the other syringe (or some combination from the two syringes) to give the same total dose makes no difference to the observed effect. This is true regardless of the shape of the dose-response relationship.

There are two important models that deserve consideration as reference standards for "no interaction."[10] The first model is that of Loewe additivity, which is based on the idea that, by definition, a drug cannot interact with itself.[11] In other words, in the sham experiment in which a drug is combined with itself, the result will be Loewe additivity. The second model is Bliss independence, which is based on the idea of probabilistic independence—that is, two drugs act in such a manner that neither one interferes with the other, but each contributes to a common result.[12] We prefer the Loewe additivity model as the reference for "no interaction" because it yields the intuitively correct evaluation of the sham combination of one drug with itself, whereas the Bliss independence model does not.[10] All possible combinations of "drug A" and "drug B" that cause a specified effect will be described by the equation for Loewe additivity:[11]

$$\frac{d_A}{D_A} + \frac{d_B}{D_B} = 1 \qquad (2)$$

where D_A is the dose of "drug A" that causes the specified effect (e.g., 50% effect), D_B is the dose of "drug B" that causes the specified effect, and d_A and d_B are the doses of "drug A" and "drug B" in the various combinations that also cause specified effect.

When the dose of "drug A" is plotted on the *y*-axis and the dose of "drug B" is plotted on the *x*-axis, Equation 6.2 describes a straight line running from $D_{X,A}$ on the *y*-axis to $D_{X,B}$ on the *x*-axis. Such graphs (Fig. 6–2) are called isobolograms, and the lines on these graphs are called isoboles.

Isoboles show dose combinations that result in equal effect. If the isoboles are straight lines, the interaction is additive. If the isoboles bow toward the origin of the graph, the interaction is synergistic. If the isoboles bow away

from the origin of the graph, the interaction is antagonistic. Although an isobole clearly shows whether an interaction is additive, synergistic, or antagonistic, it is often only determined for a single level of drug effect. For example, in the anesthesia literature, a common approach has been to determine the 50% isobole for a specific endpoint, such as preventing movement in response to an incision. Although this isobole permits a statement to be made about whether there is any evidence of synergy or antagonism, it is not possible to make inferences about other levels of drug effect (e.g., the 95% isobole) that might be more clinically relevant. Although many different methods have been used for the analysis of drug interactions, the isobolographic method is the best validated for most applications.[13]

The focus on whether drug interactions can be reduced to simple descriptors, such as additive, synergistic, or antagonistic, may be too simplistic. Interactions have the potential to be very complex. For example, a drug combination can be synergistic in certain regions and antagonistic in others.[14] Rather than worry about which descriptor applies, the goal should be to characterize the response surface. From the surface one can identify the best combination to produce the desired therapeutic effect.

Response Surfaces

The name *response surface methodology* (RSM) has been given to the statistical methodology concerned with (1) the design of studies to estimate response surfaces, (2) the actual estimation of response surfaces, and (3) the interpretation of the results. Response surface methodology is generally used for two principal purposes: to provide a description of the response pattern *in the region of the observations studied*, and to assist in finding the region where the optimal response occurs (i.e., where the response is at a maximum or a minimum).

A response surface is a mathematical equation or the graph of that equation, which relates a dependent variable (such as a drug effect) to inputs (such as two drug

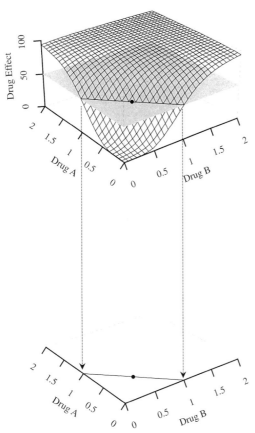

Figure 6–3. Response surface and isobologram. The "drug A" and "drug B" axes are labeled in units of the dose or concentration required to cause 50% of the maximum effect. *Top,* Response surface for two agonists with "no interaction" (i.e., additive interaction). The horizontal plane slices the surface at the 50% effect level. *Bottom,* Isobologram showing concentrations resulting in 50% effect. The isobologram is the two-dimensional representation of the three-dimensional response surface view. The *solid circle* in both panels shows the effect resulting from 0.5 units of "drug A" combined with 0.5 units of "drug B." The study of one point on the surface will reveal whether this point shows evidence of synergism or antagonism, but conveys little about the interaction at other levels of effect (the remainder of the response surface).

concentrations). Figure 6–3 shows that an isobole is obtained by making a horizontal slice through the response surface.

When two agonists differ only in their potency and there is "no interaction" between the two drugs, the surface is stretched tightly between the edges of drugs A and B, and the isobole's are straight lines. Figure 6–4 shows two response surfaces (and their 50% isoboles), which illustrate synergistic and antagonistic interactions between two agonists. Other interactions between full agonists, partial agonists, inverse agonists, and competitive antagonists can also be illustrated using response surface models.[15] When a response surface is viewed from above, a series of equally spaced horizontal slices will appear as a series of isoboles, in the same way that contour lines drawn on a map connect points of equal height. Where the gradient of the surface is steep the contour lines will be close together, and where the gradient of the surface is shallow the contour lines will be far apart.

A large variety of experimental designs have been developed for efficiently estimating response surfaces.[16] Examples for two drugs are illustrated in Figure 6–5.

The "ray" design studies the response (effect) for two drugs present in a number of fixed ratios. Each ratio can be considered as a single drug, which permits the analysis to be based on the same principles as that associated with single drug experiments. The "full factorial" design studies the response for all combinations of two drugs at a number of different doses ("fractional factorial" designs are also used).[17–19] When the interactions between three drugs are being investigated, the drugs should be (1) studied alone, (2) studied in three pairs, and (3) studied in the triple combination.[20]

In many experimental situations unrelated to drugs and anesthesia, response surfaces are used to determine optimal response conditions. For example, a company may wish to know which combination of two variables (e.g., charge rate and temperature) *maximizes* the expected life of power cells.[21] However, when the two variables are two drugs, the optimum combination is sometimes more difficult to define. For example, any relatively high dose combination of two agonists, which interact synergistically, will result in the maximum effect (see Fig. 6–4, *left surface*). However, if we are considering the interaction between an opioid and an hypnotic to maintain the state of general anesthesia, simply knowing that any high-dose combination works well is not particularly helpful. Determination of the optimum combination also requires that we consider the pharmacokinetic properties and side-effect profiles of the two drugs. We would like to have a combination somewhere up on the shoulder of the surface, where the desired intraoperative effect is achieved, hemodynamic side effects are minimal, and recovery from anesthesia is predictably rapid.

A description of methods used to estimate and evaluate a fitted response surface and of tests used to decide whether interaction effects are significant is beyond the scope of this chapter. However, the general strategy is outlined in Table 6–1, and a brief description of RSM is provided by Neter and colleagues,[21] as well as a full description by Box and Draper.[22]

Interaction Models Used in Anesthesia

Several investigators have modeled anesthetic drug interactions as extensions of the logistic regression model for a single drug.[23–26] We will now evaluate the models used in these important clinical studies according to the characteristics of an ideal pharmacodynamic interaction model suggested in Table 6–2.[15] In the logistic regression model for a single drug, the natural logarithm of the odds ratio (the logit) is modeled as a linear function of drug concentration (C):

$$\log it = \log(\text{odds ratio}) = \log\left(\frac{P}{1-P}\right) = \beta_0 + \beta_1 \cdot \log(C)$$

$$(3)$$

where P is probability of effect, and β_0 and β_1 are estimated parameters. Alternatively, the probability of effect can be expressed as:

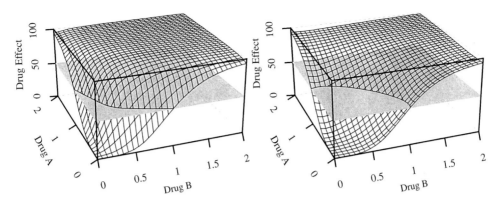

Figure 6–4. Synergistic and antagonistic interactions between two full agonists. The "drug A" and "drug B" axes are labeled in units of the dose or concentration required to cause 50% of the maximum effect. The maximum effect and the gradient of the concentration response relationship are the same for both drugs. *Left*, Synergism. The 50% isobole bows toward the origin and the surface is bulging upward (the effect is greater than expected). *Right*, Antagonism. The 50% isobole bows away from the origin and the surface is sagging downward (the effect is less than expected).

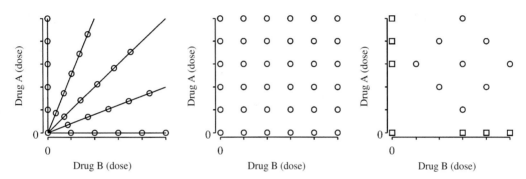

Figure 6–5. Graphic representation of various experimental designs for two drugs. Ray design (*left*), full factorial design (*middle*), and central composite design (*right*).[16] Each *circle* represents a dose (or concentration) combination that is investigated. The "central composite design" was developed to provide enough treatment combinations to permit the estimation of the parameters in a quadratic predictive model, while using fewer treatment groups than the full factorial design. This latter design would be useful to confirm that the optimum response occurred for the combination at the center of the 3 × 3 diamond.

$$P = \frac{e^{\beta_0 + \beta_1 \cdot \log(C)}}{1 + e^{\beta_0 + \beta_1 \cdot \log(C)}} \quad (4)$$

If $\beta_0 = -\gamma \cdot \log(C_{50})$ and $\beta_1 = \gamma$, then Equations 6.3 and 6.4 are algebraically equivalent to the more intuitive and familiar sigmoid relationship:

$$P = \frac{\left(\dfrac{C}{C_{50}}\right)^{\gamma}}{1 + \left(\dfrac{C}{C_{50}}\right)^{\gamma}} \quad (5)$$

where C_{50} is the drug concentration associated with a 50% probability of drug effect, and γ is the gradient of the concentration-response relationship.

This logistic model has been generalized to multiple drugs, either using the concentration or the natural log of the concentration. If concentration is used, the interaction between two drugs is modeled as:

$$\log\left(\frac{P}{1-P}\right) = \beta_0 + \beta_1 \cdot C_A + \beta_2 \cdot C_B \quad (6)$$

where P is the probability of effect; β, β_1, and β_2 are estimated parameters; and C_A and C_B are two drug concentrations. Solving Equation 6.6 for $P = 0.5$ yields the 50% isobole, given by the straight line:

$$\frac{C_A}{-\beta_0/\beta_1} + \frac{C_B}{-\beta_0/\beta_2} = 1 \quad (7)$$

where $-\beta_0/\beta_1 = C_{50,A}$ and $-\beta_0/\beta_2 = C_{50,B}$. Equation 6.6 has several limitations. If only one drug is present ($C_A = 0$), it can be shown that:

$$P = \frac{e^{\beta_0 + \beta_1 \cdot C_A}}{1 + e^{\beta_0 + \beta_1 \cdot C_A}} \quad (8)$$

which is inconsistent with the single drug model (Eq. 6.4) because C_A cannot be transformed to $\log(C_A)$, as required by

TABLE 6–1.

General Strategy for Assessment of Drug Interactions

1. Select the model for the concentration-response relationship for the individual drugs.

2. Select the model for the residual error (difference in observed and predicted effect).

3. Select the model for the response surface with interaction parameters.

4. Design the study.

5. Conduct the experiment.

6. Fit the response surface to all of the data at the same time, i.e., estimate the interaction parameters. If the fit is good, go to step 7. If not, consider going back through steps 1 to 5.

7. Interpretations and conclusions.

Adapted from Greco WR, Bravo G, Parsons JC: The search for synergy: A critical review from a response surface perspective. Pharmacol Rev 47:331–385, 1995.

TABLE 6–2.

Characteristics of an Ideal Pharmacodynamic Interaction Model

1. The interaction model is consistent with prior mathematical proofs (e.g., Loewe additivity; see Eq. 53.2).

2. The interaction model is equally valid for any measure of drug exposure, such as dose, plasma concentration, tissue concentration, or effect-site concentration.

3. The parameters of the interaction model can be accurately estimated from studies of reasonable size.

4. Interaction parameters provide flexibility in the concentration-response relationship of the interacting drugs, permitting assessment of additive, synergistic, and antagonistic interactions, and interactions when the interacting drugs differ in the gradient of the concentration effect relationship or the maximum effect of the drugs.

5. The interaction model predicts the effect over the entire clinical range of doses or concentrations for one, two, or three drugs.

6. The interaction model predicts no drug effect when no drugs are present.

7. If one of the drugs in the interaction model is not present, the model reduces to the correct model for the remaining drug(s).

Adapted from Minto CF, Schnider TW, Short TG, et al: Response surface model for anesthetic drug interactions. Anesthesiology 92:1603–1616, 2000.

the single drug model. Thus Equation 6.6 does not meet criteria 7 in Table 6–2. When both drugs are absent ($C_A = C_B = 0$), then:

$$P = \frac{e^{\beta_0}}{1 + e^{\beta_0}} \tag{9}$$

which predicts drug effect even when no drug is present (unless $\beta_0 = -\infty$), thus violating criteria 6 of Table 6–2. Although Equation 6.6 generates the correct linear isobole at the 50% level, for all other probabilities the isoboles are flawed, violating criteria 1 in Table 6–2.

An alternative approach for two drugs is to take the natural logarithm of the drug concentrations:[24,26]

$$\log\left(\frac{P}{1-P}\right) = \beta_0 + \beta_1 \cdot \log(C_A) + \beta_2 \cdot \log(C_B) \tag{10}$$

Solving for $P = 0.5$ yields the 50% isobole:

$$e^{\beta_0} \cdot C_A^{\beta_1} \cdot C_B^{\beta_2} = 1 \tag{11}$$

Equation 6.11 always suggests profound synergy, because it is the equation for an hyperbola. The isobole predicted in Equation 6.11 necessarily bends profoundly in the middle to reach infinity as it approaches each axis. One way of dealing with the problems of this model is to add an arbitrary constant to one or both drug concentrations.[24] This arbitrarily chosen constant has an enormous influence on the

other parameter estimates, but has no pharmacodynamic meaning, and even with this constant, Equation 6.11 is still an hyperbola.

We conclude that these extensions to the logistic regression model for a single drug are so beset with flaws that they should be abandoned.[15] An alternative approach, used for more than 50 years, is to model drug interactions based on pharmacological principles.[10] An example is provided by Greco and colleagues,[27] who adapted the guidelines of Berenbaum[28] and others to develop an interaction model for two drugs based on a sigmoidal E_{max} model and the following isobole constraint:

$$\frac{C_A}{C_{50,A}} + \frac{C_B}{C_{50,B}} + \alpha \cdot \frac{C_A}{C_{50,A}} \cdot \frac{C_B}{C_{50,B}} = 1 \tag{12}$$

This equation is one of five different isobole models illustrated by Machado and Robinson[29] based on a single "non-additivity parameter,". Such models can describe both synergy and antagonism depending on the value of α; positive values suggest synergy and negative values suggest antagonism. Although these isobole constraints enable objective statistical evaluation of drug interactions, they are relatively inflexible and cannot be used to model interactions that result in a maximum effect greater than either drug alone and cannot describe asymmetric isoboles. Thus this approach does not satisfy criteria 4 in Table 6–2.

Other more flexible approaches, each with their own limitations, have been described. These include the use of flexible parametric functions (splines) that are forced to obey certain constraints (e.g., a spline can be constrained to resemble an E_{max} model)[30] and the use of polynomial functions to connect the pharmacodynamic parameters of one drug to another.[15]

Before using any complex model, which relates two drug concentrations to a predicted drug effect, we advise that the response surface described by the model should be displayed graphically. The three-dimensional view of the response surface may provide important insights that are not immediately obvious from the equations.

Prototype Examples of Pharmacodynamic Anesthetic Interactions

Volatile Anesthetics and Opioids

Volatile anesthetic gases and injectable opioids used in combination constitute the pharmacologic basis of many modern anesthetics. In fact, isoflurane and fentanyl may well be the most commonly used anesthetic combination around the world. This opioid-volatile anesthetic combination has emerged as a popular anesthetic technique because of the appeal of its pharmacodynamic synergy and its pharmacokinetic responsiveness; the hemodynamic depression associated with high concentrations of volatile anesthetics and the slow return of spontaneous ventilation associated with high doses of opioid are both avoided.

Volatile anesthetic potency is measured in terms of MAC. Defined in humans as the expired concentration that prevents 50% of subjects from exhibiting purposeful movement to a skin incision (at normal body temperature and normal barometric pressure, among other stipulations), the MAC concept is one of the most unifying ideas in the clinical science of anesthesia.[31–34] It is widely applied in anesthesiology by both clinicians and investigators.

Although initially developed as a standardized means for comparing the potency of inhaled anesthetic gases, MAC has emerged as an important benchmark for clinicians in defining the appropriate concentration target for specific surgical procedures and anesthetic techniques; clinicians are accustomed to thinking in terms of what fraction or multiple of MAC is necessary to provide satisfactory anesthetic conditions for a given surgical procedure as part of a given anesthetic approach.[35] Clinicians come to understand intuitively the meaning of $\frac{1}{2}$ MAC or 1 MAC as it relates to the prevailing surgical stimulus and the other components of the anesthetic technique.

In the research domain, MAC reduction has become a common method for determining the potency of anesthetic adjuncts such as opioids.[23,24,26,36,37] Opioid-MAC reduction studies are conducted by assessing how a range of opioid concentration influences the MAC value. These MAC reduction studies, although initially devised to assess opioid potency, have dramatically improved our understanding of clinical opioid-volatile anesthetic interactions.[38,39]

Opioid-MAC reduction studies exhibit a general pattern irrespective of which opioid or volatile anesthetic is combined, as illustrated in the left graph of Figure 6–6, which depicts the relationship between fentanyl concentration and isoflurane MAC. With relatively low opioid levels (i.e., those associated with analgesia but minimal respiratory depression and sedation), MAC is reduced quite substantially. This trend of MAC reduction continues until a plateau is reached after which further increases in opioid concentration do not result in significant decreases in MAC. Whereas opioids can result in a substantial reduction in MAC (as much as 60–90%), they cannot completely eliminate the need for a volatile anesthetic. This "ceiling effect" has obvious implications in the clinical application of the volatile-opioid interaction.[4,5]

MAC reduction studies form the basis of our clinical understanding of opioid-volatile anesthetic interactions. The right graph in Figure 6–6 shows the response surface interaction of fentanyl and isoflurane using MAC as the effect measure.[24] The surface "bows" prominently toward the origin, indicating a considerable synergistic interaction.[15] The slope of the concentration-effect relationship for isoflurane (viewed from the right side of Fig. 6–6) steepens rapidly and shifts toward the origin as fentanyl concentrations increase. Note also that because the effect measure by definition has no meaning in the absence of the volatile anesthetic, the shape of the fentanyl curve is flat when the isoflurane concentration is zero.

Inspection of the right panel in Figure 6–6 reveals several important clinical pharmacology points when using these two drug classes in combination. For example, it is clear that there are numerous pairs of potential target concentrations for the two drug classes that result in similar pharmacodynamic synergy; that is, for any given fraction or multiple of MAC, there are numerous possible concentration pairs that achieve the same level of effect, ranging from high to low concentrations for both drugs. It is also clear that there is a large plateau area at the top of the response surface that represents the numerous concentration target pairs that produce maximal drug synergy. Within this nearly flat plateau area, the concentration pairs that are closer to the origin of the graph represent the clinically relevant pairs that minimize the concentration for both drugs, yet produce near maximal synergy. Conversely, the concentration pairs that are furthest from the origin within the maximal synergy plateau area represent the concentration pairs that maximize the concentration for both drugs (and would therefore presumably result in a greater incidence of undesired effects such as hemodynamic depression or prolonged recovery).

This volatile-opioid response surface represents a high resolution, detailed characterization of interaction between the two drugs. But how can this response surface information be applied clinically? How can the clinician choose an appropriate pair of target concentrations? Having chosen the

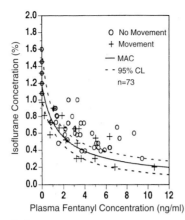 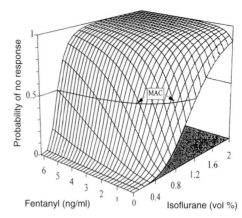

Figure 6–6. Example of the interaction between volatile anesthetics and opioids. *Left,* Depiction of the minimum alveolar concentration (MAC) reduction of isoflurane in humans by increasing concentrations of fentanyl; *solid line* represents isoflurane MAC and *dotted lines* represent the 95% confidence intervals (CI). *Right,* The same relationship among probability of no response, fentanyl concentration, and isoflurane concentration over the full range of response probability; this is the three-dimensional "response surface" representation of the two-dimensional relationship depicted in the left panel. (*Left,* From McEwan AI, Smith C, Dyar O, et al: Isoflurane minimum alveolar concentration reduction by fentanyl. Anesthesiology 78:864–869, 1993; *Right,* From Shafer SL. Principles of pharmacokinetics and pharmacodynamics. In Longnecker DE, Tinker JH, Morgan EG (eds): Principles and Practice of Anesthesiology, 2nd ed. St. Louis, Mosby, 1998, pp 1159–1210.)

concentration targets, how can the clinician then administer the drugs to hit the target concentrations?

By definition, targeting concentration pairs that produce 1 MAC will result in inadequate anesthesia in 50% of patients. An extension of this observation is that targeting concentration pairs that produce maximal drug synergy (i.e., concentration pairs on the maximal synergy plateau area far from the origin) may result in unacceptable hemodynamic depression or prolonged recovery. The optimal concentration pairs are typically found somewhere between the 50% effect level and the maximal effect level. Assuming that selecting target concentration pairs that result in lack of movement to incision for 95% of patients is a reasonable starting point, the clinician must then choose the appropriate ratio between the volatile anesthetic and the opioid because there is a range of opioid-volatile anesthetic ratios that will result in lack of response in 95% of patients.

The guiding principles in selecting the appropriate ratio between the opioid and the volatile anesthetic are intuitively straightforward, although the scientific evidence underpinning these choices is still insufficient and evolving. Ultimately, the clinician must identify the priorities of the case and select the opioid-volatile anesthetic ratio accordingly. These priorities may include pharmacodynamic, pharmacokinetic, and pharmacoeconomic considerations.

For example, for cases in which postoperative pain is likely to be a challenge, choosing a higher opioid target and a correspondingly lower volatile anesthetic target might be appropriate, thereby providing for a higher opioid level at the end of the anesthetic. Alternatively, if rapid recovery is a primary goal, relying on a higher level of volatile anesthetic that can be quickly exhaled at the end of the operation might be appropriate (depending on which volatile agent and opioid one is considering). When economic considerations are critical, it is possible to identify a concentration pair and the corresponding administration scheme that

minimizes drug acquisition costs (e.g., particularly if one of the drugs is proprietary and expensive and the other is generic and less expensive). It is important to recognize that these target concentration pairs simply represent starting points for initiating therapy. The clinician must assess patient response and adjust the drug administration scheme accordingly.

In clinical anesthesia, identifying the appropriate target concentrations is only part of the process. Having identified the targets, the clinician must then somehow administer the drugs to achieve the selected targets. In the case of volatile anesthetics, the use of an agent-specific vaporizer combined with an exhaled gas monitor represents a sophisticated solution to the problem. The clinician can target a specific concentration (partial pressure) in the blood with the vaporizer and can confirm that the target concentration has been achieved.[35]

For injectable opioids, unless one uses a target-controlled infusion system in which a microprocessor computes the appropriate infusion rates and reports a predicted drug concentration,[40-43] drug administration regimens that are intended to achieve concentrations that are close to the specified target must be devised based on population pharmacokinetic parameters. Most published opioid dosage schemes in package inserts and textbooks are formulated in this way. Knowledge about the drug's pharmacokinetics are combined with information about the concentration-effect relationship to develop drug dosage schemes that target concentrations within the appropriate therapeutic window.[44]

Opioids and Propofol

Since the introduction of propofol, a pharmacokinetically responsive intravenous sedative/hypnotic, total intravenous anesthesia has emerged internationally as a popular anesthetic technique.[45,46] Continuously infused propofol is typically combined with an injectable opioid such as fentanyl, sufentanil, or alfentanil administered either by continuous infusion or intermittent bolus injection. The advent of remifentanil, an ultra-short acting opioid, has further refined the possibilities for total intravenous anesthesia with propofol.[47,48] Propofol and remifentanil together represent a pharmacokinetically responsive intravenous anesthetic combination that was not possible before the development of these short-acting drugs.[49]

The pharmacodynamics of intravenous sedative/hypnotic agents such as propofol, thiopental, ketamine, and etomidate are typically characterized through the use of a sigmoidal "maximal effect (E_{max})" model.[50] Using an effect measure such as the processed electroencephalogram (EEG) or a clinically assessed sedation scale, these models estimate the concentrations that produce 50% of maximal effect, a potency parameter known as the EC_{50}. The EC_{50} is a clinical benchmark that allows the comparison of the various sedative/hypnotics in terms of the clinical concentrations (e.g., therapeutic windows) that are necessary for various anesthetic applications. Sigmoidal "maximum effect" models exist for the majority of the common intravenous sedative/hypnotics in anesthesia.[14,51–55]

The same basic study methodology is used to characterize the pharmacodynamics of the injectable opioids. Using the processed electroencephalogram (usually the spectral edge parameter) as the measure of opioid effect (or some other clinically oriented measure such as respiratory depression),[56] the EC_{50} for the opioids can be estimated as part of a sigmoidal "E_{max}" model.[49,57–59] The EC_{50} for the opioids can then be related to the concentrations necessary for various clinical applications. Recent work has shown that the therapeutic windows for the fentanyl congeners are a reproducibly constant fraction of the EEG EC_{50}, making it possible to forecast with confidence the therapeutic windows of any opioid once its EEG EC_{50} is known.[60]

Propofol-opioid interactions are characterized using "EC_{50}" reduction study methodology with a clinical effect measure such as hemodynamic or movement response to surgical stimuli. Like MAC reduction studies, propofol-opioid interaction studies exhibit a general pattern irrespective of the opioid that is used. Opioids produce a marked reduction in the level of propofol required (and vice versa); as the opioid concentration increases, the propofol requirement decreases asymptotically toward a non-zero minimum.

The left panel of Figure 6–7 shows the propofol and alfentanil concentrations necessary to prevent hemodynamic or movement response to intraabdominal surgical stimuli in 50% of patients, as reported by the pioneering work of Vuyk and colleagues.[61] This graph (Fig. 6–7, *left*) is typical of all propofol-opioid pharmacodynamic interactions no matter which effect is being studied.[62] Low concentrations of alfentanil dramatically reduce the need for propofol, but even

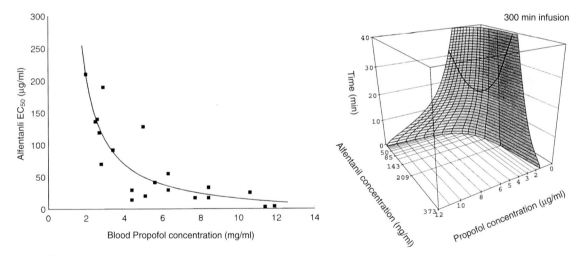

Figure 6–7. An example of the interaction between propofol and opioids. *Left*, Plasma alfentanil concentrations versus blood propofol concentrations associated with a 50% probability of no response to intraabdominal surgical stimuli, illustrating substantial pharmacodynamic synergy between the two drug classes. *Right*, Computer simulation of the effect site propofol and alfentanil concentrations versus time during the first 40 minutes after termination of target-controlled infusions of the two drugs to levels associated with a 50% probability of no response to surgical stimuli; the *bold line* superimposed on the concentration decay curves represents the concentration at which 50% of subjects are predicted to regain consciousness. The bold line parabolic minimum is the concentration target pair that produces equivalent pharmacodynamic synergy but more rapid recovery. The right panel is thus a clinically useful integration of drug-interaction pharmacodynamic data with pharmacokinetic information, permitting the rational selection of propofol-alfentanil targets (i.e., hypnotic{ts}:{ts}opioid ratios). (*Left*, From Vuyk J, Lim T, Engbers FH, et al: The pharmacodynamic interaction of propofol and alfentanil during lower abdominal surgery in women. Anesthesiology 83:8–22, 1995; *Right*, From Vuyk J, Mertens MJ, Olofsen E, et al: Propofol anesthesia and rational opioid selection: Determination of optimal EC50–EC95 propofol-opioid concentrations that assure adequate anesthesia and a rapid return of consciousness. Anesthesiology 87:1549–1562, 1997.)

very high concentrations of alfentanil cannot completely eliminate the need for propofol to maintain adequate anesthesia. The relationship is highly nonlinear, meaning that the dosage reduction of one drug produced by an increase in the other is not proportional, demonstrating the substantial pharmacodynamic synergy of the drug combination.[63] Experiments like these suggest that at high propofol concentrations, low-dose alfentanil is contributing primarily an analgesic effect to the overall anesthetized state, whereas at lower propofol concentrations, the higher alfentanil concentration required is also making important contributions to the hypnotic effect.[61] Similar findings have been reported by Kern and co-workers[64] for propofol and remifentanil using surrogate drug effect measures in volunteer subjects.

EC_{50} reduction studies form the basis of our clinical understanding of the propofol-opioid interaction. The right panel of Figure 6–7 is a computer simulation of effect-site propofol and alfentanil concentrations versus time during the first 40 minutes after termination of 300-minute, computer-controlled infusions targeted to concentrations designed to achieve a 50% probability of no response to surgical stimulation.[62] Based on response surface methodology, this simulation enables the rational selection of concentration target pairs for propofol and alfentanil (and other opioids as well). The bold line superimposed on the concentration decay curves in Figure 6–7 represents the concentration at which 50% of subjects are predicted to regain consciousness. The bold line is a parabolic curve identifying the concentration pair that optimizes predicted recovery time. According to the simulation, the concentration targets for propofol and alfentanil to minimize the time to return of consciousness after a 300-minute infusion while maintaining a 50% probability of no response to surgical stimuli intraoperatively are 3.4 μg/mL and 88.9 ng/mL, respectively.[62] The appropriate targets can be computed for any opioid, for any length infusion, and for any percentage probability of nonresponse.[62] The clinical application of these drug interaction models through the use of computer simulation constitutes a revolutionary advance in our understanding of intravenous anesthetic clinical behavior.[63]

The profound pharmacodynamic synergy of the propofol-opioid interaction is perhaps best illustrated by considering the pharmacodynamics of propofol when administered as the sole anesthetic. In the absence of opioids, the blood propofol concentration that is associated with loss of consciousness in 50% of patients is approximately 3.5 μg/mL,[65] whereas much higher concentrations (10–15 μg/mL) are necessary to suppress responses to surgical stimuli such as skin incision or intraabdominal manipulation.[61,66] In contrast, the lower limit of propofol's therapeutic window for adequate anesthesia in the presence of moderate concentrations of opioid adjuvants appears to be approximately 1 μg/mL, which represents a dramatic reduction compared with the levels necessary when propofol is administered alone.[61] Depending on the dosage of opioid used, the therapeutic range of propofol concentrations when using an opioid adjuvant is very large, necessitating a selection of the appropriate propofol:opioid ratio for any given anesthetic application.

The rational selection of the appropriate propofol:opioid ratio is in large part a function of opioid pharmacokinetics. Because the fentanyl congeners can be viewed as pharmacodynamic equals with important pharmacokinetic differences, the time to return of consciousness depends predominantly on the selected opioid (and also on the duration of infusion).[44,67,68] For the longer acting fentanyl congeners (i.e., alfentanil, sufentanil and fentanyl), a lower opioid concentration target and a higher propofol concentration target is prudent because the opioid pharmacokinetics are the rate-limiting step in the recovery process. Conversely, when the short-acting opioid remifentanil is combined with propofol, a lower propofol concentration is targeted because propofol's pharmacokinetic profile is the primary determinant of the time to regaining consciousness.[68]

Of course pharmacodynamic considerations also come into play when selecting the appropriate propofol:opioid ratio. In the hemodynamically compromised patient, for example, a higher opioid concentration target might help to promote hemodynamic stability.[69] In patients prone to nausea and vomiting after receiving opioids, a higher propofol concentration target might be prudent.[70]

Achieving the appropriate target concentrations when infusing propofol is perhaps more challenging than when administering inhalation anesthetics. In contrast to the inhaled anesthetics for which the clinician is accustomed to targeting a specific MAC-fraction or MAC-multiple with the use of a vaporizer, sedative/hypnotics are usually administered using calculator pumps. The clinician specifies an infusion rate rather than a concentration target. The clinician therefore thinks in terms of infusion rates and not target concentrations. A notable exception to this practice is the use of the Diprifusor (AstraZeneca, Waltham, Mass), a computer-controlled infusion device in which the clinician designates a propofol concentration target and the computer calculates the infusion rates that are necessary to hit the target based on the pharmacokinetics of propofol.[71,72] Through the use of computer simulation, it is possible to identify infusion rates that achieve specified concentration targets.[73]

References

1. Chambi D, Omoigui S: Precipitation of thiopental by some muscle relaxants. Anesth Analg 81:1112.
2. Wood M: Pharmacokinetic drug interactions in anaesthetic practice. Clin Pharmacokinet 21:285–307, 1991.
3. Alloul K, Whalley DG, Shutway F, et al: Pharmacokinetic origin of carbamazepine-induced resistance to vecuronium neuromuscular blockade in anesthetized patients. Anesthesiology 84:330–339, 1996.
4. Hug CC Jr: Does opioid "anesthesia" exist? Anesthesiology 73:1–4, 1990.
5. Wong KC: Narcotics are not expected to produce unconsciousness and amnesia. Anesth Analg, 62:625–6, 1983.
6. Zbinden AM, Petersen-Felix S, Thomson DA: Anesthetic depth defined using multiple noxious stimuli during isoflurane/oxygen anesthesia. II. Hemodynamic responses. Anesthesiology 80:261–267, 1994.
7. Zbinden AM, Maggiorini M, Petersen-Felix S, et al: Anesthetic depth defined using multiple noxious stimuli during isoflurane/oxygen anesthesia. I. Motor reactions. Anesthesiology 80:253–260, 1994.
8. Kissin I: General anesthetic action: an obsolete notion? Anesth Analg 76:215–218, 1993.
9. Berenbaum MC: Criteria for analyzing interactions between biologically active agents. Adv Cancer Res 35:269–335, 1981.
10. Greco WR, Bravo G, Parsons JC: The search for synergy: a critical review from a response surface perspective. Pharmacol Rev 47: 331–385, 1995.

11. Loewe S, Muischnek H: Effect of combinations: mathematical basis of problem. Arch Exp Pathol Pharmacol 114:313–326, 1926.

12. Bliss CI: The toxicity of poisons applied jointly. Ann Appl Biol 26:585–615, 1939.

13. Berenbaum MC: What is synergy? Pharmacol Rev 41:93–141, 1989.

14. Norberg L, Wahlstrom G: Anaesthetic effects of flurazepam alone and in combination with thiopental or hexobarbital evaluated with an EEG-threshold method in male rats. Arch Int Pharmacodyn Ther 292:45–57, 1988.

15. Minto CF, Schnider TW, Short TG, et al: Response surface model for anesthetic drug interactions. Anesthesiology 92:1603–1616, 2000.

16. Carter WH, Wampler GL, Stablein DM: Regression Analysis of Survival Data in Cancer Chemotherapy. New York, Marcel Dekker, 1983.

17. Kochar M, Guthrie R, Triscari J, et al: Matrix study of irbesartan with hydrochlorothiazide in mild-to-moderate hypertension. Am J Hypertens 12:797–805, 1999.

18. Scholze J, Zilles P, Compagnone D: Verapamil SR and trandolapril combination therapy in hypertension: A clinical trial of factorial design. German Hypertension Study Group. Br J Clin Pharmacol 45:491–495, 1998.

19. Pool JL, Cushman WC, Saini RK, et al: Use of the factorial design and quadratic response surface models to evaluate the fosinopril and hydrochlorothiazide combination therapy in hypertension. Am J Hypertens 10:117–123, 1997.

20. Short TG, Plummer JL, Chui PT: Hypnotic and anaesthetic interactions between midazolam, propofol and alfentanil. Br J Anaesth 69:162–167, 1992.

21. Neter J, Wasserman W, Kutner MH: Applied Linear Statistical Models, 3rd Ed.

22. Box GEP, Draper NR: Empirical Model-Building and Response Surfaces. New York, John Wiley & Sons, 1987.

23. Sebel PS, Glass PS, Fletcher JE, et al: Reduction of the MAC of desflurane with fentanyl. Anesthesiology 76:52–59, 1992.

24. McEwan AI, Smith C, Dyar O, et al: Isoflurane minimum alveolar concentration reduction by fentanyl. Anesthesiology 78:864–869, 1993.

25. Vuyk J, Engbers FH, Burm AG, et al: Pharmacodynamic interaction between propofol and alfentanil when given for induction of anesthesia. Anesthesiology 84:288–299, 1996.

26. Lang E, Kapila A, Shlugman D, et al: Reduction of isoflurane minimal alveolar concentration by remifentanil. Anesthesiology 85:721–728, 1996.

27. Greco WR, Park HS, Rustum YM: Application of a new approach for the quantitation of drug synergism to the combination of cis-diaminedichloroplatinum and 1-beta-D-arabinofuranosylcytosine. Cancer Res 50:5318–5327, 1990.

28. Berenbaum MC: Consequences of synergy between environmental carcinogens. Environ Res 38:310–318, 1985.

29. Machado SG, Robinson GA: A direct, general approach based on isobolograms for assessing the joint action of drugs in pre-clinical experiments. Stat Med 13:2289–2309, 1994.

30. Troconiz IF, Sheiner LB, Verotta D: Semiparametric models for antagonistic drug interactions. J Appl Physiol 76:2224–2233, 1994.

31. Eger EI 2nd, Saidman LJ, Brandstater B: Minimum alveolar anesthetic concentration: A standard of anesthetic potency. Anesthesiology 26:756–763, 1965.

32. Rampil IJ, Lockhart SH, Zwass MS, et al: Clinical characteristics of desflurane in surgical patients: Minimum alveolar concentration. Anesthesiology 74:429–433, 1991.

33. Stevens WD, Dolan WM, Gibbons RT, et al: Minimum alveolar concentrations (MAC) of isoflurane with and without nitrous oxide in patients of various ages. Anesthesiology 42:197–200, 1975.

34. Stoelting RK, Longnecker DE, Eger EI 2nd: Minimum alveolar concentrations in man on awakening from methoxyflurane, halothane, ether and fluroxene anesthesia: MAC awake. Anesthesiology 33:5–9, 1970.

35. Egan TD: Intravenous drug delivery systems: Toward an intravenous "vaporizer." J Clin Anesth 8(Suppl):8S–14S, 1996.

36. Westmoreland CL, Sebel PS, Gropper A: Fentanyl or alfentanil decreases the minimum alveolar anesthetic concentration of isoflurane in surgical patients. Anesth Analg 78:23–28, 1994.

37. Murphy MR, Hug CC Jr: The anesthetic potency of fentanyl in terms of its reduction of enflurane MAC. Anesthesiology 57:485–488, 1982.

38. Hall RI, Szlam F, Hug CC Jr: The enflurane-sparing effect of alfentanil in dogs. Anesth Analg 66:1287–1291, 1987.

39. Hall RI, Murphy MR, Hug CC Jr: The enflurane sparing effect of sufentanil in dogs. Anesthesiology 67:518–525, 1987.

40. Shafer SL, Siegel LC, Cooke JE, Scott JC: Testing computer-controlled infusion pumps by simulation. Anesthesiology 68:261–266, 1988.

41. Shafer SL, Varvel JR, Aziz N, Scott JC: Pharmacokinetics of fentanyl administered by computer-controlled infusion pump. Anesthesiology 73:1091–1102, 1990.

42. Shafer SL, Gregg KM: Algorithms to rapidly achieve and maintain stable drug concentrations at the site of drug effect with a computer-controlled infusion pump. J Pharmacokinet Biopharm 20:147–169, 1992.

43. Glass PS, Jacobs JR, Smith LR, et al: Pharmacokinetic model-driven infusion of fentanyl: Assessment of accuracy. Anesthesiology 73:1082–1090, 1990.

44. Shafer SL, Varvel JR: Pharmacokinetics, pharmacodynamics, and rational opioid selection. Anesthesiology 74:53–63, 1991.

45. Sebel PS, Lowdon JD: Propofol: a new intravenous anesthetic. Anesthesiology 71:260–277, 1989.

46. Smith I, White PF, Nathanson M, Gouldson R: Propofol. An update on its clinical use. Anesthesiology 81:1005–1043, 1994.

47. Epple J, Kubitz J, Schmidt H, et al: Comparative analysis of costs of total intravenous anaesthesia with propofol and remifentanil vs. balanced anaesthesia with isoflurane and fentanyl. Eur J Anaesthesiol 18:20–28, 2001.

48. Hogue CW Jr, Bowdle TA, O'Leary C, et al: A multicenter evaluation of total intravenous anesthesia with remifentanil and propofol for elective inpatient surgery. Anesth Analg 83:279–285, 1996.

49. Egan TD: Remifentanil pharmacokinetics and pharmacodynamics: a preliminary appraisal. Clin Pharmacokinet 29:80–94, 1995.

50. Campbell DB: The use of kinetic-dynamic interactions in the evaluation of drugs. Psychopharmacology (Berl) 100:433–450, 1990.

51. Arden JR, Holley FO, Stanski DR: Increased sensitivity to etomidate in the elderly: Initial distribution versus altered brain response. Anesthesiology 65:19–27, 1986.

52. Buhrer M, Maitre PO, Hung OR, et al: Thiopental pharmacodynamics. I. Defining the pseudo-steady-state serum concentration-EEG effect relationship. Anesthesiology 77:226–236, 1992.

53. Homer TD, Stanski DR: The effect of increasing age on thiopental disposition and anesthetic requirement. Anesthesiology 62:714–724, 1985.

54. Hung OR, Varvel JR, Shafer SL, Stanski DR: Thiopental pharmacodynamics. II. Quantitation of clinical and electroencephalographic depth of anesthesia. Anesthesiology 77:237–244, 1992.

55. Schuttler J, Stanski DR, White PF, et al: Pharmacodynamic modeling of the EEG effects of ketamine and its enantiomers in man. J Pharmacokinet Biopharm 15:241–253, 1987.

56. Levy WJ: Intraoperative EEG patterns: implications for EEG monitoring. Anesthesiology 60:430–434, 1984.

57. Scott JC, Ponganis KV, Stanski DR: EEG quantitation of narcotic effect: the comparative pharmacodynamics of fentanyl and alfentanil. Anesthesiology 62:234–241, 1985.

58. Scott JC, Stanski DR: Decreased fentanyl and alfentanil dose requirements with age: A simultaneous pharmacokinetic and pharmacodynamic evaluation. J Pharmacol Exp Ther 240:159–166, 1987.

59. Scott JC, Cooke JE, Stanski DR: Electroencephalographic quantitation of opioid effect: Comparative pharmacodynamics of fentanyl and sufentanil. Anesthesiology 74:34–42, 1991.

60. Egan TD, Muir KT, Hermann DJ, et al: The electroencephalogram (EEG) and clinical measures of opioid potency: Defining the EEG-clinical potency relationship ("fingerprint") with application to remifentanil. Int J Pharm Med 15:11–20, 2001.

61. Vuyk J, Lim T, Engbers FH, et al: The pharmacodynamic interaction of propofol and alfentanil during lower abdominal surgery in women. Anesthesiology 83:8–22, 1995.

62. Vuyk J: Pharmacokinetic and pharmacodynamic interactions between opioids and propofol. J Clin Anesth 9:23S–26S, 1997.

63. Stanski DR, Shafer SL: Quantifying anesthetic drug interaction: Implications for drug dosing [editorial; comment]. Anesthesiology 83:1–5, 1995.

64. Kern SE, Egan TE, White JL, Cluff M: Characterizing pharmacodynamic synergism between propofol and remifentanil in volunteers using response surfaces. Anesthesiology 91:A342, 1999.

65. Vuyk J, Engbers FH, Lemmens HJ, et al: Pharmacodynamics of propofol in female patients. Anesthesiology 77:3–9, 1992.

66. Smith C, McEwan AI, Jhaveri R, et al: The interaction of fentanyl on the Cp50 of propofol for loss of consciousness and skin incision. Anesthesiology 81:820–828; discussion 26A, 1994.

67. Mather LE: Pharmacokinetic and pharmacodynamic profiles of opioid analgesics: a sameness amongst equals [editorial]? Pain 43:3–6, 1990.

68. Vuyk J, Mertens MJ, Olofsen E, et al: Propofol anesthesia and rational opioid selection: Determination of optimal EC50–EC95 propofol-opioid concentrations that assure adequate anesthesia and a rapid return of consciousness. Anesthesiology 87:1549–1562, 1997.

69. Stanley TH, Webster LR: Anesthetic requirements and cardiovascular effects of fentanyl-oxygen and fentanyl-diazepam-oxygen anesthesia in man. Anesth Analg 57:411–416, 1978.

70. Borgeat A, Wilder-Smith OH, Saiah M, Rifat K: Subhypnotic doses of propofol possess direct antiemetic properties. Anesth Analg 74:539–541, 1992.

71. Short TG, Lim TA, Tam YH: Prospective evaluation of pharmacokinetic model-controlled infusion of propofol in adult patients. Br J Anaesth 76:313–315, 1996.

72. Arndt GA, Reiss WG, Bathke KA, et al: Computer-assisted continuous infusion for the delivery of target-controlled infusions of propofol during outpatient surgery. Pharmacotherapy 15:512–516, 1995.

73. Shafer SL, Stanski DR: Improving the clinical utility of anesthetic drug pharmacokinetics [editorial; comment]. Anesthesiology 76:327–330, 1992.

Pharmacoeconomics

Alex Macario, MD, MBA

This chapter provides a scientific foundation, as well as some practical pointers, for those delving into the discipline of pharmacoeconomics. The application of economics to pharmaceutical usage practice does not necessarily mean that less money should be spent, but rather that the use of resources might be better applied elsewhere. At some point, the extra money spent for small improvements in quality of medical care is not worthwhile. Economic study of drugs aims to identify appropriate usage, because money misspent could have been devoted to medical care that could achieve greater benefit.

Health care systems around the world are struggling to properly manage access, quality, and cost. The pharmaceutical industry is experiencing particular scrutiny because drug expenditures are increasing more rapidly than other medical costs.

Value for Money for New Pharmaceuticals

As drug costs increase, purchasers want proof of value for money.[1] Consequently, in the United States and internationally, the number of economic evaluation studies has increased. In 1970, a computer search using only the terms "drug" and "economics" revealed 68 published articles addressing cost-effectiveness. By 1990, this number had grown to 687.[2] Even herbal prescription medicines are undergoing pharmacoeconomic evaluations.[3]

Health care systems, regardless of their financing and delivery systems, employ a number of mechanisms to ration their finite health care resources. This is because health care is different from consumer goods, which rely on the marketplace to get allocated optimally (Table 7–1).

Health care resource allocations require systematic assessments of the value of health care products. This helps ensure that resources are allocated to preserve and restore the greatest amount of health as efficiently as possible (Table 7–2).

TABLE 7–1.

How Is Health Care Different from Consumer Goods?

- Suppliers may influence demand (i.e., new doctor in town increases the number of prescriptions written)

- Patients are cost unconscious because of insurance

- Patients are shielded from true cost of insurance (benefits are nontaxable)

- Uncertainty in the services needed to treat patients

- Information is lacking on what works (need outcomes research)

After decisions are made to allocate resources to health care (as opposed to other services such as education), resources need to be allocated within health care (e.g., preventive medicine or surgical care). Patients must make difficult decisions—for example, either expensive prescription drugs, better health insurance, or an airplane trip to a grandchild's graduation.

Including Economics in Medical Decision-Making

Physicians, as pharmaceutical decision makers, are aware of cost pressures. Most physicians (88%) agree that cost-effectiveness should be considered when weighing different courses of treatment.[4] Seventy-two percent of physicians also believe that patients and physicians alone should determine whether an intervention is "worth the cost." The majority of the physicians surveyed stated that the two greatest obstacles to cost-effective care are society's unwillingness "to acknowledge limited resources" and patients who hold "unrealistic expectations of medicine." Interestingly, just 24% of the respondents identified "physicians unaware of costs of medical interventions" as a major barrier to incorporating economics in clinical decision-making.

Hospital pharmacy managers are particularly interested in monitoring drugs that may cause morbidity if used inappropriately (e.g., chemotherapy agent), have a high cost per dose (e.g., thrombolytics), or draw pharmacoeconomic attention in a hospital setting because of their high usage. Anesthesia-related medications are in the last category[5] and are under constant surveillance because only a small number of medications have to be monitored to impact drug use and costs.

Although not overly expensive from a cost per dose perspective, anesthetic medications account for approximately 8% to 12% of a hospital's total drug expenditures because of their routine use in the large number of surgical patients anesthetized in hospital settings.[6,7]

Development of Pharmacoeconomics

Pharmacoeconomic research identifies, measures, and compares the costs (i.e., resources consumed) and the clinical, economic, and humanistic consequences of pharmaceutical products and services. Within the analytic framework of pharmacoeconomics are several research methods including decision analysis, technology assessment, cost-effectiveness analysis, and quality-of-life measurement.

Pharmacoeconomic evaluations inform decisions as to:

- Will the patient's quality of life be improved by a particular drug therapy?
- What is the cost per quality year of life extended by a drug?
- Which drugs should be included on the hospital formulary?
- Which drug delivery system is the best for a hospital?
- Which is the best drug for a particular patient or for a particular disease?

TABLE 7–2.

The Health Care Market Is Not "Efficient"

Patient (consumer) does not bargain with the doctor (supplier)	→	Consumer (patient) buys whatever the doctor says (at any price)
Employer (the ultimate payer) has no contact with the supplier	→	Supplier (doctor) supplies as much as he likes at any price
Insurer (intermediate payer) has no contact with the supplier	→	Insurer absorbs the excess cost and passes on to the employer

Prior to the 1980s, the word "pharmacoeconomics" did not exist as pharmaceuticals were evaluated for costs and effectiveness, but their assessment was considered as a subset of cost-effectiveness analysis,[8] which itself is a subset of medical technology assessment. In the United States, medical technology assessment was initially popularized by the Congressional Office of Technology Assessment in the mid-to-late 1970s.[9] Medical technology assessment was considered to be a broad policy analysis of the efficacy, the safety, and the social, ethical, and economic consequences of the introduction and use of a medical technology.

As examples of medical technology assessment, the Pharmaceutical Manufacturer's Association published on methodology and specific analyses of drugs, such as cimetidine for ulcer disease and beta-adrenoceptor blockers for postmyocardial infarction.[10,11] Then SmithKline's Cost-Benefit Program spawned one of the early economic assessments of a new drug by the pharmaceutical industry, which included a prospective clinical trial assessing the health-related, quality-of-life impact of captopril.[12]

Bootman's group introduced the concepts of cost-benefit and cost-effectiveness analyses and the term "pharmacoeconomics" in their study evaluating the outcomes of individualizing aminoglycoside dosages in severely burned patients with gram-negative septicemia.[13] Townsend described Post Marketing Drug Research and Development that reflected the need to develop pharmacoeconomic research.[14] By the 1990s, virtually all new major drugs had economic and health-related, quality-of life protocols built into phase III and phase IIIB clinical trials.

Role of Pharmacoeconomics in Drug Registration

The U.S. Food and Drug Administration (FDA) approved 53 new drugs in 1996, and 35 in 1999. The historical standard used by the FDA to determine whether information about the safety or effectiveness of a product (used in promotional communications) was false or misleading is the presence of "substantial evidence" established by "adequate and well-controlled trials," generally meant to be convincing evidence of efficacy in double-blind, placebo-controlled clinical trials.[15]

Because the FDA's role is to prevent ineffective or potentially harmful products from entering the marketplace, regulators primarily want to know whether a new drug is safe and effective. Hence the majority of protocols submitted to the FDA by the pharmaceutical industry are placebo-controlled efficacy/superiority trials. In addition, clinicians now require information regarding how much more effective a new therapy is for their patients than the existing treatment options. *The standard for economic analyses is "competent and reliable scientific evidence," not "substantial evidence from adequate and well-controlled trials."*

To address concerns that FDA regulation was limiting the development and dissemination of outcomes research, Congress included a section in the 1997 Food and Drug Administration Modernization Act. Congress amended Section 502(a) of the Federal Food, Drug and Cosmetic Act to change the standard to support promotional claims that comprise health care economic information (HCEI) and Drug Administration Modernization of 1997. The new

amendment, Section 114 of the FDA Modernization Act and Accountability Act ("FDAMA") (PL 105–115), amends the FDA's authority regarding regulation of promotional claims of the economic consequences of drugs. The new law specifies:

> . . . health care economic information provided to a formulary committee, or other similar entity, in the course of the committee or the entity carrying out its responsibilities for the selection of drugs for managed care for other similar organizations, shall not be considered to be false or misleading under this paragraph if the health care economic information directly relates to an indication approved under Section 505 OR UNDER section 351(a) of the Public Health Service Act for such drug and is based on competent and reliable scientific evidence."[16]

Thus the standard of *adequate and well-controlled trials* does not embrace economic analyses. For example, is there an adequate and well-controlled method of assigning costs from a payer database? Also, economic models require extrapolation from clinical events in well-controlled trials to longer term follow up (after the study is finished) or in non-protocol (uncontrolled) settings. For example, some studies include admission to a clinical research center, with its costs, that will be different than if the drug treatment occurred during routine office visits.

Differences in the price structures, treatment patterns, and provider incentives (along with social, political, and cultural perspectives) among health systems in different countries make generalizations of cost-effectiveness analyses performed in one country of questionable international relevance.

In some countries, including Australia[17,18] (which had the first guidelines [1991] required by the government payer), Canada[19], Finland, Norway[20] (beginning in January 2002) and Portugal, pharmacoeconomic studies are mandatory for pricing and reimbursement. These mandates require epidemiologic investigations to determine economic modeling and market size estimation. In Italy, pharmaceutical prices are set by comparing prices with other European Union countries. The level or reimbursement depends on the clinical importance assigned to the drug by the National Drugs Committee (Commissione Unica del Farmaco). In the Netherlands, a pharmaceutical company wishing to introduce a new drug is obliged to traverse two regulatory hurdles. First, the company must obtain registration to gain permission to enter the market. In this step, the main criteria are efficacy and safety. The second step is to be added to the list of drugs for which reimbursement can be sought. The main criteria for this step are related to pharmacoeconomics—interchangeability, effectiveness, safety, applicability, experience, feasibility, and costs.

Pharmacoeconomic analysis can quantify the additional cost and the additional benefit, but not a question in vacuo such as "is the drug worth the cost?"

When performing a pharmacoeconomic study, there are three different dimensions to consider.

1. Types of analysis: cost identification, cost-effectiveness, and cost-benefit

2. The context in which the analysis occurs: society, the patient, the payer, hospital, clinic, physician, or other health care provider
3. Types of costs that can be included: direct medical costs, direct nonmedical costs, indirect morbidity and mortality costs, and intangible costs.

The fundamental analytic concept relates to the incremental cost-effectiveness ratio (ICER) defined as:

$$ICER = (C2 - C1)/(E2 - E1)$$

where $C2$ and $E2$ are the cost and effectiveness of the new intervention being evaluated, and $C1$ and $E1$ are the cost and effectiveness of the standard therapy. Pharmacoeconomic studies may not have reached their full potential in medical decision-making, partly because of the reluctance of providers to be viewed as rationing pharmaceuticals based on economic considerations.

Costs

The price of a drug product is not equivalent to the cost of drug therapy because costs can be analyzed from different viewpoints—that of the patient, the provider, the payer, or society as a whole.[21] For example, the cost of a medical service to the payer (insurance company) equals the percentage of charges actually paid by the payer. However, the relevant cost to the patient is the out-of-pocket expense (not covered by insurance) plus other costs (e.g., inability to work) incurred due to illness. The cost of a medical service from society's point of view is the total cost to society of all the different components involved in providing that service, or the result of society having given up the opportunity to use those resources for some other purpose. A consensus study on economic analyses in health care recommended that costs be assessed from a societal perspective.[22] This facilitates comparison of studies.

The costs of disease and drug treatments can be divided into three types: direct, indirect, and intangible costs.

Direct Costs

Direct costs are the value of resources used to prevent, detect, and treat a health impairment. Medical resources are the services used to treat illness; they include hospital care, professional services, drugs, and supplies. The adjective "direct" indicates that there is an obvious matching of the expenditure with a patient. For example, an antibiotic administered to a patient is a direct medical cost because the antibiotic can be easily ascribed to the particular patient that received the medication.

An often posed question is whether to include only cause-specific costs or to include all costs in a pharmacoeconomic study. In a cancer treatment trial, for example, a pharmacoeconomist's goal could be measuring the cancer-related costs only, or measuring all the other costs of care as well.

Limiting measures to disease-specific costs has the advantage of reducing the variance of the cost data and may make the analysis more sensitive to small shifts in resources. Conversely, cause-specific costs may be handicapped if cancer treatment–related costs have been reduced, but other medical costs have increased.

Costs are not equal to charges because cost refers to the amount of money the facility has to spend (i.e., to buy pharmaceuticals), as well as the true cost of delivering care.[23] In contrast, charge refers to the amount of money the physician or the facility bills the insurance company for the pharmaceutical. Whereas facilities do know exactly what are the charges on the patient's facility bill, charge data may not reflect the true cost to the facility for providing care.

To determine costs, either a top-down or bottom-up approach can be used. In top-down methods, a cost-to-charge ratio (e.g., the Medicare ratio of cost to charges that all U.S. hospitals provide to the Health Care Finance Administration) is used. These ratios are then used to convert hospital billing data to average costs used for the pharmacoeconomic analysis. The biggest advantage of the cost-to-charge ratio method is that the data are commonly available and their use is well accepted.

Another top-down method uses Medicare diagnosis-related groups to classify episodes of care and to assign costs. Although simple and efficient, this method is limited because it does not account for any variations in care within a diagnosis-related group, and Health Care Finance Administration diagnosis-related group reimbursements may be less than true costs.

A third example of a "top-down" method is when hospitals use their own charge data and budgetary costs to compute their own hospital's overall cost-to-charge ratio (Table 7–3). In this example, the cost-to-charge ratio is 0.5. This means that if a hospital aims to compute the cost of administering a particular drug (or any other particular resource), the administrator will likely examine the patient charge (as it appears on the patient's hospital bill) for the drug and multiply that number by 0.50. This example illustrates the disadvantages of the top-down costing method, which includes an "averaging" effect that makes cost estimates for any particular item imprecise. Also, charges often reflect what the market forces of supply and demand will bear, and therefore do not necessarily maintain a constant relationship with costs (Table 7–4).[24] The differing cost-to-charge ratios are due to hospitals inflating the charges for services in one area (e.g., postanesthesia care unit) to invest in other nonreimbursed departments (i.e., medical records) or to pay for development of new clinical programs. The differing cost-to-charge ratios produce inaccurate cost estimates. For example, savings for choosing percutaneous transluminal coronary angioplasty procedures rather than coronary artery bypass graft surgery range from $1,935 to $10,087, depending on the type of cost measurement used.[25]

"Bottom-up" costing is a more precise way to measure costs because resources are tracked as care occurs.[26] One advantage of bottom-up costing is that total costs can be separated into fixed and variable components. Fixed costs (i.e., rental of building that houses the surgery suite) do not change in proportion to volume of activity.

TABLE 7–3.

Hypothetical Example of Cost-to-Charge Ratio

Hospital Budget

Expenses

Salaries	$200
Benefits	$62
Equipment	$212
Depreciation	$26
Total Costs	$500
Patient Charges	$1000

Cost-to-charge ratio = $500/$1000 = 0.50

TABLE 7–4.

Cost Ratios Vary by Hospital Departments

Hospital Department	Cost-to-Charge Ratio	Variable Cost/ Total Cost Ratio
Radiology	0.63	0.32
Postanesthesia care unit	0.54	0.33
Blood bank	0.53	0.73
Patient ward	0.52	0.38
Operating room	0.44	0.44
Pharmacy	0.41	0.70
Anesthesia	0.29	0.44

The majority of cost for providing hospital service is related to buildings, equipment, salaried or full-time hourly labor, and overhead, which are fixed over the short term. For inpatient surgical procedures, anesthesia costs account for about 6% of total hospital costs, with about half being vari-

able cost. Thus about 3% of total hospital costs are subject to the anesthesiologist's clinical decision-making and are potentially available for cost savings.

Tracking Costs Among Different Facilities

It is helpful to report units separately from assigning monetary values because monetary values can vary. In economic studies involving multiple hospitals, the methodologic question that arises is how to track costs (resources) among different hospitals.[27] For example, if one less antibiotic is administered at hospital X (because of some intervention) and that saves $40, then does saving a dose of the same antibiotic at hospital Y also save $40. There are two methods to address this.

Method 1: Based on resource counts
■ Count the resources
■ Obtain unit prices
■ Multiply the two to calculate the cost of the resource[28]

Method 2: Based on billing data
■ Obtain hospital bills on patients
■ Convert charges from bills to resource costs using cost-to-charge ratio

An attractive alternative is to report resource savings (e.g., antibiotic administration in our example) from an intervention as the number of units saved (e.g., number of antibiotic administrations) and not assign a monetary value to the resource. Alternatively, a service may reportedly consume, for example, $100 worth of pharmacist time per patient. A more precise method for reporting this resource would be as 4 hours of pharmacist time valued at $25 per hour.

Nonmedical resources are out-of-pocket expenses for goods and services outside the medical care sector. Transportation to the site of treatment, lodging for family during treatment, and hiring a person to help with home care are examples of nonmedical services.

Indirect Costs

Indirect costs are the value of production lost to society because of absence from work, disability, or death. In addition to direct medical and nonmedical costs, indirect costs also have substantial impact. Indirect costs are those that occur because of loss of life or livelihood and may result from morbidity or mortality. Because indirect costs do not directly influence expenditures for treating disease, they are not easily measurable.[29]

According to the "human capital" approach, indirect costs are estimated as the gross income (e.g., per capita average wages) lost during the time of absence from work. One of the limitations of this method is that people outside the labor force, such as students, homemakers, and the elderly, are discriminated against.

Intangible Costs

Intangible costs represent another category of costs and, like indirect costs, are difficult to measure. These are the costs of pain, suffering, grief, and the other nonfinancial outcomes of disease and medical care. Intangible costs relate to the non-monetary consequences that are difficult to measure. They are not usually included in economic evaluations, but they are captured indirectly through quality-of-life scales.

Skewness in Cost Data

A distinctive feature of cost data in health care is its asymmetrical distribution (skewed to the right) and large variance (Fig. 7–1).

The three measures of central tendency or "average" value of the distribution are mode, median, and mean. The high-cost patients will influence some measures of central tendency (the mean cost will be "increased" because of the right tail cases), but not others (medians). Also, the right skewness limits the power of parametric statistical tests; because the skewed distribution of cost data is often log-normal, the log-transformed cost data follow a normal distribution and can be analyzed with the parametric tests that are more commonly used.[30]

Discounting

Even when inflation has been taken into account, a cost or an outcome for today is not equivalent in value to the same cost or outcome in the future. Because people usually prefer to have something today instead of having it in the future, a future value must be discounted (typically at 3–7% per year) to the present value. For pharmaceuticals, time costs may be

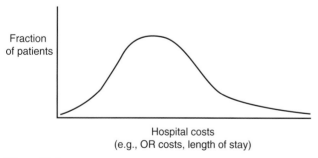

Figure 7–1. Cost data are right skewed. One important pharmacoeconomic issue is the proper statistical approach to the analysis of costs. Hospital costs plotted by frequency do not follow a normal distribution because data are positive. Clinical economists typically regard cost data as deterministic, i.e., having no variance. But patient-specific cost data are actually stochastic (random) and usually exhibit skewness at the high-cost end of the distribution. Causes of skewed (e.g., the right-sided tail) data include that the most severe cases may require substantially more resources.

relevant if drug therapy prevents a disease in the future. Certainly, the future benefits of drug therapies also need to be discounted.

Quality of Life

Health is more than repairing injury, alleviating pain, and eliminating illness. In 1948, the World Health Organization expanded the boundaries of health to include complete physical, mental, and social well-being. We now consider the impact of a disease and its treatment on a patient's daily life; therefore, information about physical and social functioning and mental well-being are also required to address pharmacoeconomic questions.[31]

Health-related quality of life (HR-QOL) data are commonly captured with standardized questionnaires, either by self-administration, telephone interview, personal interview, observation, or postal survey. Psychometrics, the science of testing questionnaires to measure attributes of individuals, is fundamental to this study.

Measurement of Health-Related Quality of Life

HR-QOL instruments can be either disease-specific (e.g., asthma[32]) or generic. Among the generic instruments available, the 36-Item Short Form (SF-36) health survey is one of the most widely used.[33] The SF-36 measures physical and mental health with 36 items and 8 multi-item scales: Physical Functioning, Role Functioning Physical, Bodily Pain, General Health, Vitality, Social Functioning, Role Functioning Emotional, and Mental Health.

Raw scores are linearly transformed to scales of 0 to 100, with 0 and 100 assigned to the lowest and highest possible value, respectively.[34] Higher transformed scores indicate better health. Two component summary scores, the physical dimension and the mental dimension, are computed.

The EuroQol© EQ-5D is another commonly used preference-weighted health state classification system used in clinical trials[35] (see the Appendix). Patients are classified into 1 of 243 (3^5) health states. These states can be assigned a preference or utility valuation by using scoring weights derived from general public responses to the instrument. It also contains a visual analogue scale for the elicitation of health state preference valuations made by patients experiencing the health states.

A third common method for measuring health state preferences is the Mark II Health Utility Index (HUI2) multiattribute utility function.[36] The HUI2 measures seven attributes of health status: sensation, mobility, emotion, cognition, self-care, pain, and fertility. This utility score is anchored by "perfect health" as the highest possible health state and "dead" as the lowest possible health state. The respondent completes a standardized 15-item questionnaire constructed specifically for the HUI2 that asks about their day-to-day health. A scoring algorithm applies utility weights to the respondents' health status as reported in the standardized questionnaire.

Internet sites exist that provide a guide to the choice of instruments for quality-of-life assessment in medicine.[37,37a]

Even though the multidimensional nature of HRQL is well accepted, the FDA has been presented with evidence from single-item questions to support claims. In general, an effect on a single item from an instrument will not provide credible evidence of a benefit. HRQL claims can be highly misleading unless they are accompanied by full disclosure of the meaning of the claim, the way the claim is supported, and the limitations of the claim.

Once quality of life has been quantified, for formal cost-effectiveness analyses, it needs to be converted to units that can be compared among different conditions. Utilities are numeric ratings of the desirability of health states that reflect a subject's preferences, on a linear scale from 0.00 (death) to 1.00 (perfect health). It may be that some states (e.g., recall with pain) are worse than death, which is not easily taken into account with the utility metric. Preference values for standardized health states are commonly obtained using valuation techniques such as the standard gamble, the time trade-off, or the visual analog scale.[38,39]

Visual analog scales are widely used for measuring health state preferences. These scales often consist of a single line on a page and require the respondent to locate his or her most preferred health state at one end of the line and least preferred health state at the other. The respondent then rates the desirability of each intermediate health state by placing it at some point on the line between these two endpoints.

In the standard gamble method, the object is to determine when a person is indifferent between living life for certain in some health condition and a gamble with probability, P, of a better outcome (typically life in excellent health) but with the possibility, $1 - P$, of a worse outcome (typically death) (Table 7–5).[40]

Quality-adjusted life years (QALYs) are now widely used in medical decision-making and health economics as a useful outcome measure that reflects both life expectancy and quality of life (Fig. 7–2). This single-score summary measure combines patient-perceived HR-QOL, patient preference (utility), and survival. However, utility scores are not always incorporated in clinical trials and outcomes research.

TABLE 7–5.

Examples of Utility Values for Different Conditions

Condition	Utility Value
Best attainable health	1
Side effects of beta-blockers	0.98
Symptoms of moderate prostatism	0.9
Disability after hip fracture	0.8
Severe angina	0.7
Severe congestive heart failure	0.6
Hospital kidney dialysis	0.5 (range 0.41–0.68)
Severe development disability (children)	0.4
Untreated depression	0.3
Above knee amputation	0.2
Death	0.0

QALYs include a length of time component (e.g., 1 year) and a quality of life component (i.e., utility). For example, 1 QALY for an individual in perfect health (utility = 1.0) for 1 year (QALY =1) is considered equivalent to 2 years in a health state with utility = 0.5 (QALY = 1).

For conditions in which quality-of-life weights (utilities) have not been previously studied, the Rosser classification of illness states, or Rosser index, can be used to form utilities for different health states.[41] The Rosser index has two dimensions, disability and distress, and 29 possible health states. The Rosser and Kind valuation matrix can be used to measure changes in health status.[42] This quality adjustment is combined with the life expectancy of patients (e.g., obtained from life table data from the National Center for Health Statistics, http://www.cdc.gov/nchs) to form QALYs.

For short-term morbidities, as might be appropriate for the patient recovering from anesthesia, a reduction in quality of life or disutility can be included. Disutilities (i.e., validated deductions from the utility value) can be obtained using the Quality of Well-Being classification system.[43] This system has established lists of scaled reductions in a patients quality of life or disutilities in four categories: mobility, physical activity, social activity, and symptom complexes.

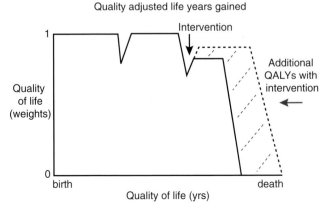

Figure 7–2. Quality-adjusted life years (QALYs) are calculated as the average number of additional years of life gained from any intervention multiplied by health state utilities measured at one point in time and then integrated over the remaining years of life.

Types of Economic Analyses

There are three different types of analysis: cost identification, cost-effectiveness, and cost-benefit. Cost-effectiveness analysis is the most widely accepted economic evaluation in health care because it measures benefit in patient-oriented terms (quality of life) and permits comparison between different interventions by standardizing the denominator.

Often, cost-effectiveness is not the product of the results of a pharmacoeconomic analysis that will impact a decision; rather, it is the process of structuring information in a systematic framework that brings to light the key uncertainties and the most important value trade-offs. Usually, a preliminary analysis is prepared based on the clinical evidence and resource use from clinical trials. If there is no significant outcome difference between the drug and its comparator, a cost-identification analysis is indicated. Conversely, if a significant outcome difference exists, a cost-effectiveness analysis is necessary to compute an incremental cost-effectiveness ratio.

Cost-Identification Analysis

Cost-identification analysis simply asks the question, "What is the cost?" By calculating the cost of delivering a drug, or computing the total cost of the medical services used to treat the condition for which drug is being used, the cost of alternative pharmaceutical choices can be determined. Cost-identification analysis is sometimes referred to as "cost-minimization analysis" because it is often used to identify the lowest cost of different available pharmaceutical strategies.

Cost-identification analysis assumes that the outcomes of the strategies are equivalent, so the goal becomes to find the least expensive way of achieving the outcome. For example, from society's perspective, the cost of a dose of succinylcholine equals the acquisition cost of the drug plus the cost of its adverse outcomes. The true cost per dose of succinylcholine from society's perspective was found to be more than 20 times the acquisition cost.[44] The authors also found that better knowledge of the incidence and consequences of anaphylactic or anaphylactoid reactions to succinylcholine was necessary.

As useful as cost-identification analysis may be in determining the cost of medical care or the financial burden of disease, it does not evaluate what these expenditures bring in terms of gains in health outcomes. Thus cost-identification analysis can guide medical practice only if a service has both lower cost and better or equal outcomes than its alternative.

Cost-Effectiveness Analysis

Cost-effectiveness analysis, on the other hand, incorporates both cost and effect. It measures the net cost of providing a service (expenditures − savings) as well as the outcomes obtained. The incremental cost-effectiveness ratio (ICER) is defined as

$$ICER = (C2 − C1)/(E2 − E1)$$

where $C2$ and $E2$ are the cost and effectiveness of the new intervention being evaluated, and $C1$ and $E1$ are the cost and effectiveness of the standard therapy. Outcomes are reported in a single unit of measurement, QALYs. The advantage of cost-effectiveness analysis is that it considers the possibility of improved outcomes in exchange for the use of more resources.

Notably, no medical intervention can be considered "cost-effective" in isolation, but must be compared with at least one other service. Decisions based on cost-effectiveness are always relative to the alternate choices, which may include nonmedical expenditures. Medical interventions are considered to be cost-effective when they produce health benefits at a cost comparable to that of other commonly accepted treatments.

A general guide is that interventions that produce 1 QALY (equivalent to 1 year of perfect health) for less than $50,000 are considered cost-effective, those that cost $50,000 to $100,000 per QALY are of questionable cost-effectiveness, and those greater than $100,000 per QALY are not considered cost-effective. A complete list of recently published cost-effectiveness studies is available[45] (Table 7–6).

In some instances, the cost-effectiveness of certain agents are dependent more on how patients value the treatments available for the disease (their preferences) than the cost of the pharmaceutical. For example, for some patients the treatment available for postoperative pain (e.g., opioid analgesia) is less appealing than the side effects (e.g., nausea) of the opioids.

Cost-Benefit Analysis

Cost-benefit analysis, a third type of economic assessment of pharmaceutical practice, forces an explicit decision about whether the cost is worth the benefit by quantifying benefit in dollar terms (estimated as the individual's maximum willingness to pay). Cost-benefit analysis was originally introduced as a tool for improving decision-making in situations in which markets fail (e.g., building of bridges or airports).

Because translating the value of health care (e.g., less pain and suffering a patient might experience) into monetary terms is tricky, cost-benefit studies are done less often. For example, if an analgesic provides pain relief but costs $20, a cost-benefit analysis would have the difficult methodologic challenge of placing a dollar value on analgesia.

Willingness to pay (WTP)

Contingent valuation involves asking individuals directly in a hypothetical survey the *maximum* amount they are WTP

TABLE 7–6.

Cost-Effectiveness of Life-Saving Interventions

Intervention	Cost/Life Year
Infant immunizations	≤$0
3 vessel cabg	$12,000
Heart transplant	$100,000
Estrogen for menopause (age > 50 yr)	$42,000
Dialysis for renal disease	$65,000
Kidney transplant	$29,000
Child restraint system in car	$73,000
Smoke detectors in home	$210,000
Motorcycle helmet laws	$2,000
Ban asbestos in roofing felt	$550,000
Ban chlorobenzilate pesticide (citrus)	$1,200,000

reassurance of normal fetal anatomy and growth) and $50 to avoid the minor side effects of intravenous contrast dye using nonionic agents. A disadvantage to WTP studies is that responses are affected by the subject's income level. Properly performed WTP studies are rare.[46]

In anesthesia care, many transient clinical anesthesia outcomes may occur with routine outpatient surgery and may be relevant to the anesthetic pharmacoeconomist. A mailed survey instrument to 56 anesthesiologists revealed that the items deemed to be most important to their patients were incisional pain, nausea, vomiting, preoperative anxiety, and discomfort from intravenous insertion.[47] Patients concurred as they rated from most undesirable to least undesirable (in order): vomiting, gagging on the tracheal tube, incisional pain, nausea, recall without pain, residual weakness, shivering, sore throat, and somnolence.[48]

Because these were the common side effects of anesthesia, 66 patients were surveyed to determine how much money they were willing to pay to prevent a given anesthesia outcome that hypothetically lasted for 6 hours after surgery.[49] Outcome descriptions were created using patients' own words. For example, nausea was described as: "You wake up and want to throw up, but cannot. Your mouth is dry and you are sweating. The nausea is associated with stomach spasms and dry heaving. You feel worse if you move." The entire survey may be viewed at the Stanford Medical School Department of Anesthesia Website (http://www.stanford.edu/~amaca/PostopPref). Patients were willing to the pay the most money to avoid pain, vomiting, and nausea (Table 7–7).

However, many noneconomists resist placing monetary values on the benefits of pain relief[50] or avoiding nausea.[51] Thus to be able to communicate with the health care community, alternative methods of evaluating benefits have been derived, the most prominent being QALYs.

to have the commodity in question, or the *minimum* amount they would be willing to accept in compensation to be deprived of it. Among the various theoretical measures that exist, WTP is a primary tool that health economists have for valuing the effect of acute conditions on patients.

For example, patients report a WTP of $1,200 for benefits of ultrasound in an uncomplicated pregnancy (e.g.,

Sensitivity Analyses

Sensitivity analyses are necessary to evaluate the impact of changing key variables.[52] The ranges of estimates for each parameter usually encompass the ranges reported in the clinical trials or the published literature. Probabilistic sensitivity analysis is particularly helpful in considering

TABLE 7–7.

Amounts (U.S. Dollars) Patients Are Willing to Pay to Avoid Given Outcome for 6 Hours

	Voiding	Hangover	Nausea	Nervousness	Shivering	Sore Throat	Vomiting	Cold	Pain
Mean	133	91	162	63	82	48	230	63	257
Median	60	50	100	27.5	50	15	100	30	110

TABLE 7–8.

Possible Study Designs

Modeling

- Retrospective, inexpensive, use secondary data

- Can determine if worthy under best case; if not, can reassess product development

Concurrent with clinical trial

- Protocol-induced demand is a negative

- Does protocol of trial reflect what will be done in the real world

Naturalistic

- Answer after product launched, may be costly

uncertainties in all probabilities, utilities, and costs simultaneously.[53]

Sources of Data for Pharmacoeconomic Studies

There are several possible designs for pharmacoeconomic studies (Table 7–8). The "naturalistic" trial is a randomized, prospective, cost-effectiveness clinical trial with minimal protocol requirements. In this type of study, the comparison arm(s) generally is usual care. The naturalistic trial is often the result of a collaborative effort between the pharmaceutical firm and a health system to satisfy the needs of both. For instance, the study may be specifically designed to determine the health and economic consequences of adding a new drug on formulary.

Another commonly performed study type for the FDA, the placebo-controlled trials, also may not be easily generalized. This is because there may be no head-to-head comparison to the existing standard of care. Because the only data available prior to the launch of a new product are preregistration efficacy data, prelaunch pharmacoeconomic modeling may err (relative to "real world" effectiveness) because of the (1) criteria used for study patient selection, (2) lack of physician experience with the new medication, and (3) patient motivation and compliance with the new treatment.

Trial-based economic studies have high internal validity, in that the differences among treatment groups are likely to be unbiased because of the randomized experimental design. However, they may have relatively low external validity (i.e., not be generalized), in that randomized controlled trials are often undertaken in conditions atypical of normal practice.

Modeling

Modeling must strike balance between necessary detail to reflect clinical real world and simplicity required for understanding.

Models are often used in cases in which relevant clinical trials have not been conducted or have excluded economic endpoints, for which trial results need to be extrapolated beyond the trial time horizon or from intermediate endpoints to final clinical outcomes, or where head-to-head comparisons between therapies are required but are lacking. Delaying decisions on new therapies until direct evidence on all relevant alternatives is not practical in the face of the cost of collecting such evidence and the potential forgone clinical benefits due to waiting. Models can organize and process available data in a quantitative framework.

Modeling entails building an experimental model that will "act like" (simulate) the system of interest (drug choice) in certain important respects (costs and side effects). In spite of its popularity in the physical, engineering, and management sciences, simulation is a relatively new technique in pharmacoeconomics. Modern high-speed computers provide the power to work through complicated structures unerringly, rapidly, and at a reasonable cost. Economic models become more robust by using realistic epidemiologic data on risk factors, treatment alternatives, and outcomes.

Simulation is especially useful for economic studies in which there is uncertainty. For example, in Monte-Carlo simulation it is assumed that the behavior of one or more factors can be represented by a probability distribution. Simulation models use random numbers to generate uncertain events by making random draws from a probability distribution. In a simulation model, the decisions of primary interest are input by the user, unlike an optimization model where the decisions of interest are produced by the model.

Advantages of simulation models include that they

1. Provide a means to deal with multiple uncertainties,
2. Can be run multiple times varying parameters to explore sensitivity effects,
3. Reproduce the amount of variability that actually occurs in the system being simulated (thus variability in the results of different simulations is intrinsically neither good nor bad), and
4. Explicitly identify and specify relationships of interest.

Because methodologic choices and inputs determine the output of models, modeling should structure the decision and its consequences over time for the time frames considered, assess the probability of the occurrence of each consequence in the model derived from appropriate expert panels, trials, and meta-analyses,[54] determine the costs associated with each treatment, determine the value of each possible outcome, and compare the cost-effectiveness of the treatments.

TABLE 7–9.

Unresolved Issues in Cost-Effectiveness Analyses

- Quality-adjusted life years (QALYs) neglect the tendency of human beings to cope with their ill health states and to place greater value on them as time passes.

- QALY-based systems tend to discriminate against those with shorter life expectancies (e.g., elderly people) because greater QALY benefits can be obtained by treating younger people and patients with longer life expectancies.

- QALYs do not easily value conditions with a high degree of patient distress.

- How to handle indirect costs value of time lost from work or leisure because of health problems or time spent receiving care is another unresolved issue.

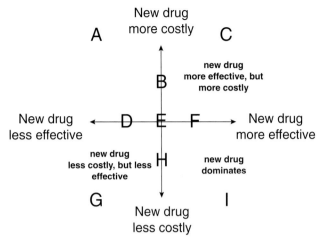

Figure 7–3. *y*-Axis is cost, and *x*-axis is effectiveness. Typically, with a new drug, the outcomes are better than those of "standard" care, otherwise the new therapy will not be introduced into the market. In most of these cases, the cost of the new agent is greater than the standard or comparison treatment. This situation (better outcomes and greater costs) calls for a cost-effectiveness analysis.

Limitations with the Use of Cost-Effectiveness Analysis

In theory, cost-effectiveness analysis allows all health interventions to be compared on similar terms. This allows one to move down the list until the cost-effectiveness ratio of the next intervention is "too high." However, this process is fraught by several limitations. First, for many diseases there are few adequate data on the effects of health interventions on patient survival and HR-QOL.[55] This means that cost-effectiveness estimates may be available for only a small proportion of the range of service options competing for priority. A second limitation is that the single point estimates of cost-effectiveness analyses may include uncertainty about the incremental cost-effectiveness. Ethical concerns also arise with the use of cost-effectiveness analysis[56] (Table 7–9).

Interpretation of Results

With the evaluation of any new drug for clinical use, two questions must be answered. First, is the therapy effective in improving clinically meaningful outcomes? If yes, the second question is: are those improved outcomes or extra benefits worth whatever extra costs they entail? Nine possibilities exist[57] (Fig. 7–3).

Situation A is a case of strong dominance: the existing drug is more effective ($P < 0.05$) and less costly ($P < 0.05$) than the new drug, making the existing drug the preferred agent (see Fig. 7–3). From an economist's view, such therapy is thus a dominant therapy—meaning that it should

be immediately adopted. Situation C arises when the new drug is both more effective ($P < 0.05$) and more costly ($P < 0.05$). The trade-off between costs and effects should then be quantified by the incremental cost-effectiveness ratio. Situation I occurs when a new drug treatment is less expensive and has improved effectiveness. An example of such a dominant therapy (i.e., greater quality-adjusted survival along with cost savings) is warfarin rather than aspirin for stroke prophylaxis in a 65-year-old patient (at high risk for stroke) with nonvalvular atrial fibrillation.[58] Situations B and H arise when the difference in effect is not statistically significant, but the difference in cost is significant. These situations lead to a cost minimization analysis. In Situations D and F, the cost difference is not significant, but the effect difference is significant. Situation E arises when no statistically significant difference in costs or effects is observed. Situation G refers to the very rare case in which there may be interest in a new drug that allows money to be saved, but only by sacrificing effectiveness.

Statistical Inference

There are two distinct approaches to statistical inference, namely frequentist and Bayesian. In the frequentist approach to inference, unknown parameters are not repeatable random things and therefore are not random variables. Instead they are fixed (unknown) quantities that do not have probability distributions and, as such, no probabilities can be attached to possible values of parameters.

In contrast, in a Bayesian framework, parameters are random variables and direct probabilistic statements can be made. The probability of a positive net (monetary) benefit against different threshold values to a health care provider of a unit increase in efficacy can be plotted.[59] Notably, the Bayesian model may produce results that are different from a simple analysis based on point estimates of probability and cost.

Quality of Design and Execution of Pharmacoeconomic Studies

Compliance

Pharmacoeconomic studies often are not compliant with guidelines as how to properly complete the studies.

In British Columbia, pharmaceutical manufacturers must present pharmacoeconomic evaluations compliant with Canadian guidelines (http://www.pharmacoeconomics. ubc.ca) along with submissions for their drug products. Guidelines typically reflect the appropriate type of study, the timing of the evaluation, the relevance of the comparator, the use of sensitivity and modeling analyses, and the reporting of results. Few cost comparison and budget-impact studies were found to be compliant with existing guidelines.[60] Interestingly, cost-effectiveness and cost-benefit analyses were more likely to be compliant with guidelines, which increased the likelihood that the new drug would be recommended for coverage (Table 7–10).

The nature of study problems encountered in pharmacoeconomic analyses used as a basis for reimbursement decisions was also studied in Australia from 1994 to 1997.[61] Of 326 submissions to the Pharmaceutical Benefits Scheme, 67% had significant methodologic problems and 31 had more than one problem. Of the 249 problems identified, 62% related to uncertainty in the estimates of comparative clinical efficacy, and 29% related clinical assumptions or cost estimates used in the economic models. There were 15 instances of disagreement over the choice of comparator, and serious calculation errors were found on 9 occasions. Overall, 159 problems (64%) were considered to be avoidable.

Conflict of Interest

Conflict of interests can occur if the pharmacoeconomic study is commercially sponsored.

The rational use of expensive new pharmaceuticals is necessary to control costs, but markets representing suppliers of technology and drugs benefit from increasing expenditures on technology. According to its annual report, Pfizer spent 39.2% of its revenues on marketing and administration in 1999.[62] Many doctors do indeed rely on pharmaceutical company representatives and promotional materials to learn about new drugs, and the public receives much of their information from direct-to-consumer advertising.[63]

A pharmaceutical company may perform an economic study for several reasons. The first reason is to determine early in a drug's development whether to continue. Second, economic analyses can be used to help find suitable price ranges for products. Third, the analyses can be used as a marketing tool directed to physicians and patients. Finally, health systems may require pharmacoeconomic evidence for formulary submissions. Thus the pharmaceutical industry has to fund the pharmacoeconomic analyses to provide formulary committees data supporting the claim that the new drugs (with higher prices) offer real value.

Health delivery systems may not engage in pharmacoeconomic research for several reasons, including insufficient in-house cost-effectiveness expertise, the view that using economic evaluations explicitly to withhold an intervention poses a public relations or litigation risk, and that sponsoring research is not in any single system's interest because it is difficult to keep the information proprietary, and thus to capture for itself the full return on the investment.

The research boundaries between academic medicine and for-profit industry are becoming more difficult to separate. Ties to industry are necessary to facilitate movement of new drugs and devices from the laboratory to the marketplace.[64] The term "technology transfer" received increased attention in 1980 with the Bayh-Dole Act.[65] This federal legislation encouraged academic institutions supported by federal grants to patent and license new products developed by their faculty members and to share royalties with the researchers. But why hasn't the U.S. government funded more pharmacoeconomic research? This may be because there is no natural home for such research, unlike in many European countries that maintain active, centralized, technology-assessment authority.

Researchers with ties to drug companies may be more likely to report results that are favorable to the products of those companies than researchers without such affiliations.[66] A study of official documents maintained by the University

TABLE 7–10.

Results of Reviews of the Manufacturers Submissions Reviewed by the British Columbia Pharmacoeconomic Initiative Scientific Committee between January 1996 and April 1999

Type of Analysis	Total Submitted	Acceptance
Cost comparison/ consequence	25	36%
Budget impact	29	7%
Cost minimization	11	27%
Cost effectiveness	14	36%
Cost utility/benefit	9	44%
Total	88	26%

of California at San Francisco Office of Research in 1999 found that 8% of faculty investigators reported personal financial ties (e.g., consulting fees, royalties, and equity) with sponsors of their research.[67] Most policies on conflict of interest in major research institutions in the United States lack specificity regarding the kinds of relationships with industry that are permitted or prohibited.[68]

The bias toward industry may affect judgments/assumptions made by the pharmacoeconomist. For example, therapeutic studies (in patients with multiple myeloma) funded by commercial organizations (n = 35) showed a greater trend toward higher quality than those supported solely by governmental or other nonprofit organizations (n = 95). A greater proportion of industry-sponsored studies compared innovative treatment to either placebo or no therapy than did studies sponsored by public resources (60% vs. 21%, $P < 0.001$). Trials supported solely or in part by commercial organizations new treatments were significantly favored over standard treatments (74% vs. 26%, $P = 0.004$).[69] It is not surprising then that journal editors are concerned with publishing biased articles and look with suspicion at commercially sponsored analyses.[70] Other biases may be at work as well.[71] For example, health plans that pay for pharmaceuticals may have a financial interest in not approving new drugs.

Debates about funding arrangements and the independence of investigators attract a lot of attention; but, interestingly, results from clinical trials, which are routinely funded by pharmaceutical manufacturers, are routinely accepted.

To minimize bias, the economic analyses must formally describe the research methods (e.g., criteria for inclusion and exclusion of studies), the assumptions, models, and possible biases. Transparency may be increased by making all evidence easily available to any critical reader (e.g., through the internet). The *New England Journal of Medicine* peer-review process policy statement considers high-quality cost-effectiveness analyses, including those supported by industry. However, manuscripts must adhere to certain conditions: (1) industry-funded research must be in the form of a grant to a not-for-profit entity—there would be no review if the author received a direct salary from or had an equity interest in the company, or was a member of an ongoing consultancy or board; (2) there must be assurances of each author's independence regarding issues of design, interpretation, publication, and access to data; and (3) manuscripts must include information about all data used and assumptions made, and the model must be straightforward and lucid.[72]

Conclusion

Economic evaluation is a useful conceptual framework to support evidence-based health care. However, it is not possible to specify the evaluative technique (e.g., should a cost minimization analysis be performed or should a cost-effectiveness analysis be performed) in advance (Fig. 7–4).

Whereas other developed nations sanction cost-effectiveness studies, the United States does not require

OUTCOME

		poorer	same	improved
	higher	no	no	YES
COST	equivalent	no	no	no
	lower	YES	no	no

Figure 7–4. When is cost-effectiveness analysis necessary? The key message is that the cost-effectiveness of pharmaceuticals requires clinical effectiveness and has to be considered relative and incremental to a reasonable standard of care.

these for licensing, reimbursement, or formulary listing of pharmaceuticals. Nevertheless, the actual use of pharmacoeconomic evaluations in real decision-making processes is unclear. This may be in part because of inappropriate representation of uncertainty in the results, comparison of the clinical trial population to the patients under consideration for treatment with the therapy, translation of the costs reported to the costs relevant to the perspective of the decision-maker, and translation of the clinical outcome measures to outcomes relevant to the length of treatment being proposed by the practitioner.

Certainly other factors besides economics are important in formulary decisions. Other considerations may include local market conditions (e.g., do patients demand the drug, do the physicians say they cannot practice without it), as well as the subjective values of the members of the formulary committees.

References

1. Fisher D, Macario A: Economics of anesthesia practice: A call to arms. Anesthesiology 86:1018–1019, 1997.
2. Eisenberg JM: Why a journal of pharmacoeconomics? Pharmacoeconomics 1:2–4, 1992.
3. De Smet PA, Bonsel G, Van der Kuy A, et al: Introduction to the pharmacoeconomics of herbal medicines. Pharmacoeconomics 18:1–7, 2000.
4. Ginsburg ME, Kravitz RL, Sandberg WA: MDs do not uniformly consider cost-effectiveness in care decisions. West J Med 173:390–394, 2000.
5. Watcha MF, White PF: Economics of anesthesia practice. Anesthesiology 86:1170–1196, 1997.
6. DeMonaco HJ, Shah AS: Economic considerations in the use of neuromuscular blocking drugs. J Clin Anesth 6:383–387, 1994.
7. White PF, White LD: Cost containment in the operating room: Who is responsible? [editorial]. J Clin Anesth 6:351–356, 1994.
8. Weinstein MC, Stason WB: Foundations of cost-effectiveness analysis for health and medical practices. N Engl J Med 296:716–721, 1977.
9. Office of Technology Assessment, U.S. Congress. Assessing the Efficacy and Safety of Medical Technology. Washington, DC, U.S. Government Printing Office, 1978.
10. Gewecke J, Weisbrod B: Clinical evaluation vs. economic evaluation: The case of a new drug. Med Care 20:821–830, 1982.
11. Pharmaceutical Manufacturers Association. Cost-Effectiveness of Pharmaceuticals. Report Series, 1982–1984. Washington, DC.

12. Croog SH, Levine S, Testa MA, et al: The effects of antihypertensive therapy on the quality of life. N Engl J Med 314:1657–1664, 1986.

13. Townsend RJ: Post marketing drug research and development: An industry clinical pharmacist's perspective. Am J Pharm Educ 50:480–482, 1986.

14. Townsend RJ: Postmarketing drug research and development. Drug Intell Clin Pharm 21:134–136, 1987.

15. Landow L: Current issues in clinical trial design: Superiority versus equivalency studies. Anesthesiology 92:1814–1820, 2000.

16. Public Law 105-89, Section 114, Food and Drug Administration Modernization and Accountability Act of 1997.

17. Australian Department of Health and Ageing on line: Available at: http://www.health.gov.au/haf/docs/pharmpac/gusubpac.htm. Accessed February 21, 2001.

18. Commonwealth Department of Human Services and Health. Guidelines for the Pharmaceutical Industry on Preparation of Submissions to the Pharmaceutical Benefits Advisory Committee. Canberra, Australia, Commonwealth Department of Human Services and Health, 1995.

19. Canadian Coordinating Office for Health Technology Assessment. Guidelines for Economic Evaluation of Pharmaceuticals: Canada. 2nd ed. Ottawa, Canada: Canadian Coordinating Office for Health Technology Assessment, 1997.

20. Website: www.slk.no/dok/la/Engretningslnov99.doc. Accessed February 21, 2001.

21. Eisenberg JM. Clinical economics. A guide to the economic analysis of clinical practices. JAMA. 1989 Nov 24;262(20): 2879–2886.

22. Russell LB, Gold MR, Siegel JE, Daniels N, Weinstein MC. The role of cost-effectiveness analysis in health and medicine. Panel on Cost-Effectiveness in Health and Medicine. JAMA. 1996 Oct 9;276(14):1172–1177.

23. Riley E, Cohen S, Macario A, et al: Spinal versus epidural anesthesia for cesarean section: Comparison of time efficiency, costs, charges, and complications. Anesth Analg 80:709–712, 1995.

24. Macario A, Vitez T, Dunn B, McDonald T: What does perioperative care really cost? Analysis of hospital costs and charges for inpatient surgical care. Anesthesiology 83:1138–1144, 1995.

25. Hlatky MA, Lipscomb J, Nelson C, et al: Resource use and cost of initial coronary revascularization. Coronary angioplasty versus coronary bypass surgery. Circulation 82(suppl 4):IV208–213, 1990.

26. Macario A, Vitez T, Dunn B, et al: Hospital costs and severity of illness in three types of elective surgery. Anesthesiology 86:92–100, 1997.

27. Macario A, Chang P, Stempel D, Brock-Utne J: A cost analysis of the laryngeal mask airway for adult elective outpatient surgery. Anesthesiology 83:250–257, 1995.

28. Macario A, Horne M, Goodman S, et al: The effect of a perioperative clinical pathway for knee replacement surgery on hospital costs. Anesth Analg 86:978–984, 1998.

29. Liljas B: How to calculate indirect costs in economic evaluations. Pharmacoeconomics 13(1 pt 1):1–7, 1998.

30. Zhou X, et al: Methods for comparison of cost data. Ann Intern Med 27(8S):752–756, 1997.

31. Sackett DL, Torrance GW: The utility of different health states as perceived by the general public. J Chronic Dis 31:697–704, 1978.

32. Juniper EF, Guyatt GH, Ferri PJ, et al: Measuring quality of life in asthma. Am Rev Respir Dis 147:832–838, 1993.

33. Ware Jr JE, Sherbourne JD: The MOS 36-Item Short-Form Health Survey (SF-36): I. Conceptual framework and item selection. Med Care 30:473–483, 1992.

34. Lundberg L, Johannesson M, Isacson DG, Borgquist L: The relationship between health-state utilities and the SF-12 in a general population. Med Decis Making 19:128–140, 1999.

35. The EuroQol Group. EuroQol-a new facility for the measurement of health-related quality of life. Health Policy 16:199–208, 1990.

36. Torrance GW, Feeny DH, Furlong WJ, et al: Multiattribute utility function for a comprehensive health status classification-Health Utilities Index 2. Med Care 34:702–722, 1996.

37. Rod O'Connor & Associates on line: Available at: http://www.rodoconnorassoc.com. Accessed May 1, 2001.

37a. Glamm DataService Group on line: Available at: http://www.glamm.com/ql/index.htm. Accessed April 3, 2001.

38. Froberg DG, Kane RL: Methodology for measuring health-state preferences. II. Scaling methods. J Clin Epidemiol 5:459–471, 1989.

39. Torrance GW: Social preferences for health states: An empirical evaluation of three measurement techniques. Socioecon Plann Sci 10:129–136, 1976.

40. Tengs TO, Wallace A: One thousand health-related quality-of-life estimates. Med Care 38:583–637, 2000.

41. Rosser R, Kind P: A scale of valuations of states of illness: Is there a social consensus? Int J Epidemiol 7:347–358, 1978.

42. Kind P, Rosser R, Williams A: Valuation of quality of life: Some psychometric evidence. In Jones-Lee MW (ed): The Value of Life and Safety. Amsterdam, North-Holland, 1982, p 159.

43. Kaplan RM, Anderson JP: The general health policy model: Update and applications. Health Serv Res 23:203–235, 1988.

44. Dexter F, Gan TJ, Naguib M, Lubarsky DA: Cost identification analysis for succinylcholine. Anesth Analg 92:693–699, 2001.

45. Harvard Center for Risk Analysis. Comprehensive league table of cost-utility analyses published through 1997, with ratios converted to 1998 U.S. dollars. Available at: http://www.hsph.harvard.edu/organizations/hcra/cuadatabase/comprehensive.pdf. Accessed June 5, 2001.

46. Diener A, O'Brien B, Gafni A: Health care contingent valuation studies: A review and classification of the literature. Health Econ 7:313–326, 1998.

47. Macario A, Weinger M, Truong P, Lee M: Which clinical anesthesia outcomes are both common and important to avoid? The perspective of a panel of expert anesthesiologists. Anesth Analg 88:1085–1091, 1999.

48. Macario A, Weinger M, Carney S, Kim A: Which clinical anesthesia outcomes are important to avoid? The perspective of patients. Anesth Analg 89:652–658, 1999.

49. Macario A, Vasanawala A: Improving quality of anesthesia care: Opportunities for the new decade. Can J Anesth 48:6–11, 2001.

50. Gaeta R, Macario A, Brodsky J, et al: Pain outcomes after thoracotomy: Lumbar epidural hydromorphone versus intrapleural bupivicaine. J Cardiothorac Vasc Anesth 9:534–537, 1995.

51. Macario A, Ronquillo R , Brose W, Gaeta R: Improved outcome with a continuous infusion of ondansetron for intractable nausea and vomiting. Anesth Analg 83:194–195, 1996

52. Mullahy J, Manning W: Valuing health care: costs, benefits, and effectiveness of pharmaceuticals and other medical technologies. In Sloan FA (ed): Statistical Issues in Cost-Effectiveness Analyses. New York, NY, Cambridge University Press, 1995, pp 149–184.

53. Doubilet P, Begg C, Weinstein M, et al: Probabilitic sensitivity analysis using Monte-Carlo simulation. Med Decis Making 5:157–177, 1985.

54. Berlin JA, Colditz GA: The role of meta-analysis in the regulatory process for foods, drugs, and devices. JAMA 281:830–834, 1999.

55. Ellis J, Mulligan I, Rowe J, et al: Inpatient general medicine is evidence based. Lancet 346:407–410, 1995.

56. Harris J: QALYfying the value of life. J Med Ethics 13:117–123, 1987.

57. Drummond MF, O'Brien B, Stoddart GL, et al: Methods for the Economic Evaluation of Health Care Programmes, 2nd ed. Oxford, Oxford University Press, 1997.

58. Gage BF, Cardinalli AB, Albers GW, Owens DK: Cost-effectiveness of warfarin and aspirin for prophylaxis of stroke in patients with nonvalvular atrial fibrillation. JAMA 274:1839–1845, 1995.

59. Van Hout BA, Al MJ, Gordon GS, Rutten F: Costs, effects and C/E ratios alongside a clinical trial. Health Econ 3:309–319, 1994.

60. Anis AH, Gagnon Y: Using economic evaluations to make formulary coverage decisions. So much for guidelines. Pharmacoeconomics 18:55–62, 2000.

61. Hill SR, Mitchell AS, Henry DA: Problems with the interpretation of pharmacoeconomic analyses: A review of submissions to the Australian Pharmaceutical Benefits Scheme. JAMA 283:2116–2121, 2000.

62. Annual report, 1999. New York: Pfizer, 1999.

63. Avorn J, Chen M, Hartley R: Scientific versus commercial sources of influence on the prescribing behavior of physicians. Am J Med 73:4–8, 1982.

64. Angell M. Is academic medicine for sale? N Engl J Med 342: 1516–1518, 2000.

65. University and Small Business Patent Procedures Act of 1980.

66. Bodenheimer T: Uneasy alliance: Clinical investigators and the pharmaceutical industry. N Engl J Med 342:1539–1544, 2000.

67. Boyd EA, Bero LA: Assessing faculty financial relationships with industry: A case study. JAMA 284:2209–2214, 2000.

68. Cho MK, Shohara R, Schissel A, Rennie D: Policies on faculty conflicts of interest at US universities. JAMA 284:2203–2208, 2000.

APPENDIX

EuroQol EQ-5D Health-Related Quality-of-Life Classification

Attribute	Level	Description
Mobility	1	No problems in walking
	2	Some problems in walking
	3	Confined to bed
Self-care	1	No problems with self-care
	2	Some problems with washing or dressing self
	3	Unable to wash or dress self
Usual activities	1	No problems with performing usual activities (e.g., work, study, housework, family or leisure activities)
	2	Some problems with performing usual activities
	3	Unable to perform usual activities
Pain/discomfort	1	No pain or discomfort
	2	Moderate pain or discomfort
	3	Extreme pain or discomfort
Anxiety/depression	1	Not anxious or depressed
	2	Moderately anxious or depressed
	3	Extremely anxious or depressed

69. Djulbegovic B, Lacevic M, Cantor A, et al: The uncertainty principle and industry-sponsored research. Lancet 356:635–638, 2000.

70. Rennie D, Luft H: Pharmacoeconomic analyses: Making them transparent, making them credible. JAMA 283:2158–2160, 2000.

71. Hillman AL, Eisenberg JM, Pauly MV, et al: Avoiding bias in the conduct and reporting of cost-effectiveness research sponsored by pharmaceutical. N Engl J Med 324:1362–1365, 1991.

72. Kassirer J, Angell M: The journal's policy on cost-effectiveness analyses. N Engl J Med 331:669–670, 1994.

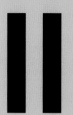

Physiologic Substrates of Drug Action

8

The Generation and Propagation of Action Potentials

Gary R. Strichartz, PhD

For a complex multicellular organism to function in a coordinated way, effective communication between individual cells is of crucial importance. Communication within cells or from cell to cell involves either chemical substances (such as hormones, transmitters, or second messengers) or electrical signals. Electrical signals are the language of the nervous system, but they are also generated in almost all cells in response to a variety of stimuli.

Action potentials are the hallmark of cellular excitability. In neurons, skeletal, cardiac, and smooth muscle, and most secretory cells action potentials are essential elements coupling stimuli to responses. Ionic currents passing through cellular plasma membranes are the dynamic roots of action potentials. Currents through ion channels, the "conductance" elements of cell membranes, and currents originating from active transport enzymes and exchange proteins, the "electrogenic pump" elements, are the sources of electricity that determine a cell's resting and action potentials.[1] Such ionic channels and pumps are frequently effected by drugs used in anesthesia, as the intended primary target or as incidental participants that contribute to therapeutic or side effects. Our understanding of the mechanisms of cellular excitability from the viewpoint of ion channels is therefore fundamental to an appreciation of the actions of anesthetic agents.

Importance of Ohm's Law: Definition of Terms

Electrical phenomena occur whenever charges (Q, measured in coulombs) of opposite sign are separated or can move independently. Any net flow of charges (or a change of charge with time, dQ/dt) is called a current (I), and is measured in amperes. In this discussion of cellular excitability, the magnitude of a current flowing between two points (e.g., from the extracellular to intracellular compartments) is determined by the potential difference (or "voltage," or "voltage difference") between the two points (V, measured in volts) and the resistance to current flow (R, measured in Ohms), as shown in the following equation:

$$I = V/R \quad \text{Ohm's Law} \tag{1a}$$

(If you are uncomfortable with electricity, try the hydraulic equivalent F = P/R. Here the potential difference corresponds to the pressure difference, P, and the current responds to the flow, F).

When Ohm's law is applied to biologic cell membranes, it is often easier to replace the electrical resistance by its reciprocal, the conductance, g, measured in reciprocal Ohms, or Siemens (S):

$$I = gV \quad \text{Ohm's Law} \quad (1b)$$

For simplicity, we will assume that all resistive elements in the cell membrane behave in an "ohmic way"—i.e., their current-voltage relationship (abbreviated as I–V) is described by Equation 8.1b: the I–V relation is linear, with a slope given by the conductance, g. This is shown graphically by the solid line in Figure 8–1A, which represents the transmembrane current (I) measured at different transmembrane potentials (V) in a hypothetical cell. Figure 8–1B shows the experimental arrangement. Two microelectrodes are inserted into the cell (glass microelectrodes have tip diameters of 0.1–0.5 microns and can penetrate into many cells, of 10–50 µm in diameter, without apparent damage to the membrane). One electrode is connected to a voltmeter to measure the transmembrane potential. The second microelectrode is hooked up to a tunable current source (e.g., a battery of variable output), which allows us to inject current into the cell and therefore to manipulate the membrane potential. The convention used in most current literature and in this chapter (see Figure 8–1A) is that the voltage is expressed as the difference between the intracellular and the extracellular potential (V = V_in − V_out). At negative values of

V, the cell is thought to be hyperpolarized, whereas at positive membrane potentials it is thought to be depolarized. Positive charge moving from inside to outside is called *outward current* and represented as an upward (positive) current, whereas *inward current* is shown as a negative current deflection.

Transmembrane Current Is Carried by Ion Channels

How does current actually flow through the cell membrane? Cell membranes are composed of a lipid bilayer with an hydrophobic center, which is practically totally impermeable to charged particles like small ions; a pure lipid bilayer presents an almost infinite resistance to ionic current flow.[2] For this reason, the presence of specialized membrane structures called ion channels was previously postulated. Now we know that ion channels are large, transmembrane protein molecules imbedded in the lipid bilayer. Each channel forms a relatively hydrophilic central pore that allows ions to cross from one side of the membrane to the other. Many different channel proteins exist and some of them will be considered in this chapter.[1] The two most important functional properties of ion channels are: (1) their ability to discriminate between different ions (channel selectivity), and (2) that the channels fluctuate between open (conducting and closed (nonconducting) states. This property is called channel *gating* and its importance will become obvious when we consider the factors that control it (see later).

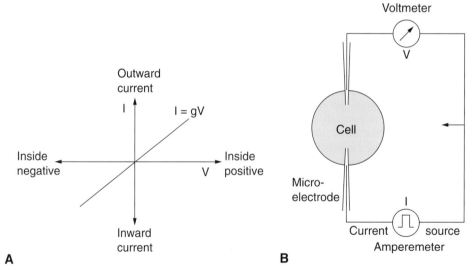

Figure 8–1. *A,* Graphic representation of Ohm's law. The conventions for directions of passive current flow (I; outward and inward) in response to voltage changes (V; depolarization and hyperpolarization, respectively) are used in all contemporary electrophysiology. The conductance (g, the reciprocal of resistance) is the slope of the I versus V line. In this chapter, all ionic I-V relations are assumed to obey Ohm's law; although, in reality, this relationship is not usually linear because of differences in permeant ion concentration, and thus the diffusion-limited conductances, between the inside and the outside of cells. *B,* Schematic diagram of the experimental arrangement for measuring a cell's electrical properties. The membrane potential difference between inside and outside the cell (V) is measured by the voltmeter coupled to one microelectrode, whereas the other microelectrode delivers current (I) across the membrane from a switchable, constant source. Both the voltmeter and the current source electrodes are connected at their opposite pole to a ground electrode (*open triangle*) in the extracellular solution.

Channel Selectivity: The Nernst Equation and the Resting Potential

The hypothetical I–V relation shown in Figure 8–1A does not apply to a real cell. It implies that in the absence of an externally applied current the potential difference across the membrane is zero. In contrast, when an experimenter actually inserts a microelectrode into a resting cell, a constant ("resting") potential of −80 to −90 mV is recorded (recall that this is defined as $V_{in} - V_{out}$). What is the basis for this resting potential?

As mentioned earlier, ion channels can be selective for a particular ion. The negative resting potential in most cells is caused by the fact that the resting membrane is primarily permeable to potassium ions (i.e., K channels are almost the only channels open at rest). The membrane potential develops because K^+ ions, which are 30 times more concentrated inside the cell, have diffused slightly to the outside, separating from their electrically neutralizing anions (thus leaving less positive charge inside) and forming the negative resting membrane potential.

The exact relation between concentration difference and membrane potential is given by the Nernst equation, which is derived below.

The extracellular and intracellular distribution of the main inorganic ions is:

	extracellular	intracellular
Na^+	145 mM	15 mM
K^+	5 mM	145 mM
Cl^-	150 mM	10 mM
Ca^{2+}	2 mM	0.0001 mM (!!)

We already know that ions cross membranes through channels, now we must consider WHY the ions move. Ion movement through channels is energetically *passive*—that is, ions move from a higher toward a lower level of free energy. The free energy of an ion is the sum of two components: *chemical* and *electrical*.

The chemical energy varies with ion concentration and temperature and has the following form:

$$\text{Chemical energy} = \mu_o + RT \ln[X]$$

where μ_o is the standard free energy of a 1 molar solution, R is the universal gas constant, T is the absolute temperature, and $[X]$ is the concentration of ion X. The chemical energy represents that random thermal motion tends to drive particles from regions where they are concentrated to regions where they are dilute. For the model cell considered earlier, this means that, for example, for K^+ ions there exists a chemical force driving K^+ efflux from the cell. The magnitude of this chemical energy gradient is simply the difference between the two free energies inside and outside of the membrane.

$$\text{Chemical energy gradient}$$
$$= \mu_o + RT \ln[X]_i - (\mu_o + RT \ln[X]_o)$$
$$= RT \ln([X]_i / [X]_o)$$

The electrical energy is proportional to the potential difference and has the following form:

$$\text{Electrical energy} = zFV \text{(per mole of ion)}$$

where V is the potential, F is the faraday constant (96,500 coulombs/mole), and z is the electrical charge (+1 for potassium). An ion will move toward a potential of opposite sign to its charge, thus a cation will be attracted to a region of negative potential. The electrical driving force is the difference between the electrical energies inside and outside.

$$\text{Electrical energy gradient} = zFV_{in} - zFV_{out}$$
$$= zF(V_{in} - V_{out})$$

The sum of the chemical and electrical energy gradients is called the electrochemical gradient. The transmembrane electrochemical gradient is the real driving force for ion movement through channels. This driving force vanishes when the sum of the chemical and electrical gradient equals zero, the equilibrium condition, because there is no longer a net transmembrane flux. At equilibrium, the force from the concentration gradient is exactly counterbalanced by the force from an electrical gradient:

$$RT \ln([K]_i / [K]_o) + zF(V_{in} - V_{out}) = 0$$

Rearranging yields the familiar *Nernst equation*:

$$V_x = V_{in} - V_{out} = (RT/zF) \ln([X]_o / [X]_I)$$
$$= (RT/zF) \ln(10) \log([X]_o / [X]_i) \qquad (2)$$

V_x is called the Nernst potential for ion X; it is the potential in which a membrane specifically permeable only to ion X would stabilize. With the physiologic extracellular and intracellular concentrations listed earlier, we can now calculate the Nernst potentials for the major ions. This will show at what value of the transmembrane potential the net driving force for a particular ion would vanish. At 37°C, the constant term RT/F ln (10) = 61 mV.

$$V_{Na} = 61 \log(145/15) = 60 \text{ mV}$$
$$V_K = 61 \log(5/145) = -89 \text{ mV}$$
$$V_{Cl} = 61 \log(150/10) = -72 \text{ mV}$$
$$V_{Ca} = 30.5 \log(2/.0001) = 131 \text{ mV}$$

Thus the measured value of the membrane resting potential in our cell (−80 to −90 mV) is very close to the Nernst potential for K^+ ions. It is as if the cell membrane was exclusively K-selective. This is confirmed by the fact that changes in extracellular K^+ lead to predictable changes in membrane potential, whereas changes in the other ions have little effect on the resting potential. The resting membrane behaves like a K^+-selective membrane because K^+ channels are the only channels conducting (open) during these conditions.

In reality, there are multiple types of K^+ channels that are sensitive to a variety of intracellular and extracellular stimuli.[3] For the basic explanations in this chapter we coarsely define the K^+ channels that contribute to the resting conductance as "leak channels," designated by "g_l." Those K^+ channels that open in response to depolarization, which may include several classes, are called "voltage-gated channels," and are generally designated in this chapter by "g_K" (see Figure 8–3).

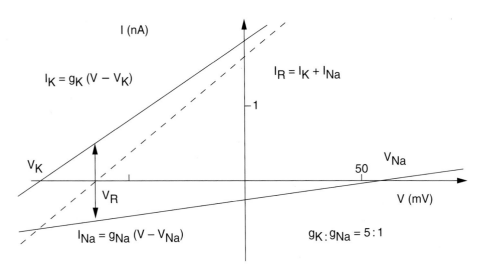

Figure 8–2. Current-voltage relations for theoretical K^+ and Na^+ currents through constant conductances in a "resting" membrane. Ohm's law now includes the Nernst potential for the permeant ion (V_{Na} or V_K) as an offset on the membrane potential (*x*-axis). *Broken line* represents the sum of K^+ and Na^+ currents at any membrane potential, with zero net current occurring at V_R, the resting potential. Changing the conductances g_K and g_{Na} will change the slopes of the I-V relations for the membrane and thus alter the value of V_R.

Figure 8–2. Current-voltage relations for theoretical K^+ and Na^+ currents through constant conductances in a "resting" membrane. Ohm's law now includes the Nernst potential for the permeant ion (V_{Na} or V_K) as an offset on the membrane potential (*x*-axis). *Broken line* represents the sum of K^+ and Na^+ currents at any membrane potential, with zero net current occurring at V_R, the resting potential. Changing the conductances g_K and g_{Na} will change the slopes of the I-V relations for the membrane and thus alter the value of V_R.

Notably, at the resting potential there exists a large inwardly directed electrochemical driving force for both Na^+ and Ca^{2+} ions. If Na^+ or Ca^{2+} channels, or both, were to open, this would lead to large inward currents that would depolarize the cell. Later it is shown that this is precisely the mechanism that leads to the generation of an action potential.

The Balance of Currents Determines the Potential

We can now return to our initial current-voltage relation and draw the correct relation for an open K^+ channel (Fig. 8–2). It will now intersect the current axis at V_K. Ohm's law still describes the I–V relation, but voltage offset (because of K^+ ions' asymmetric distribution) must be introduced, and Equation 8.1b becomes:

$$I_K = g_K(V - V_K) \qquad (3)$$

V-V_K is, of course, just the electrochemical driving force at any potential V. If K^+ channels are the only channels open, then as stated earlier the membrane potential will be V_K. However, if the cell membrane also has some other measurable conductance, then V will deviate from V_K. Let us assume, for instance, that the cell also has a measurable Na^+ conductance, with $g_{Na}:g_K = 1:5$.

$$I_{Na} = g_{Na}(V - V_{Na})$$

I_{Na} will be zero at V_{Na} (+60 mV) and have a slope of one fifth that of I_K (see Fig. 8–2). The resting potential, V_R, in this case will settle at a value between V_{Na} and V_K, where net K efflux (I_K) is exactly balanced by net Na influx (I_{Na}). This point can easily be determined graphically from Figure 8–2.

Since

$$I_{Na} = -I_K$$
$$g_{Na}(V_R - V_{Na}) = -g_K(V_R - V_K)$$

rearranging:

$$V_R = V_{Na}(g_k)/(g_k + g_{Na}) + V_K(g_K)/(g_K + g_{Na}) \qquad (8.4)$$

So V_R can have any value between V_{Na} and V_K. The actual value of V_R becomes a weighted average of the two Nernst potentials for Na^+ and K^+, where the weight is given by the relative conductances. In our example, with the above values for V_{Na}, V_K, and $g_{Na}:g_K$, $V_R = -64$ mV.

As expected, if $g_{Na} \gg g_K$, then $V_R = V_{Na}$

And, if $g_K \gg g_{Na}$, then $V_R = V_K$

This condition of constant V_R is one of "steady-state" but not of an equilibrium state. Because $V_R \neq V_{Na^+}$ or V_K, there is a net driving force on both ions and a unidirectional flux for Na^+ and for K^+, even though the net current is zero.

V will only stay constant as long as the ionic gradients do not change. If there was no independently operating, active transport system (see later) that maintains the ionic gradients, they would indeed run down. Thus although flux of ions through channels is a passive process, the metabolically requiring process of active transport is necessary to maintain the gradients that drive ions through channels.

Variable Conductances: The Generation of the Action Potential

When excitable cells are depolarized from their resting potential beyond a certain level (*threshold*), they respond with a relatively large, stereotyped potential change, the *action potential*. It is the action potential propagating away from the site of origin that constitutes impulse conduction in nerve, muscle, and heart. We will deal with impulse conduction later, in this section, we will just consider the ionic basis for the generation of the action potential. Figure 8–3 shows the typical configuration of a nerve action potential. An initial depolarization from the resting potential leads to a rapid depolarization, called the upstroke of the action potential. After the upstroke, the action potential peaks at a positive value, about +30 mV, and then repolarizes. In many cells repolarization is followed by an "undershoot" (afterhyperpolarization) of the membrane potential, which returns to its resting value a few milliseconds after the end of the action potential.

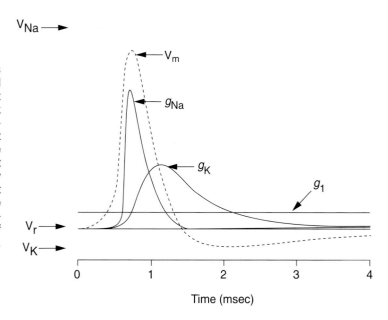

Figure 8–3. Conductance and potential changes during action potential (AP) propagation in a squid axon. The resting potential, V_r, is primarily dependent on the potential-independent and K^+-selective "leak conductance," g_1. Sodium conductance (g_{Na}) activated by depolarization, allows an inward Na^+ current that drives the rapidly depolarizing phase of the action potential, whereas the voltage-dependent potassium conductance (g_K) develops more slowly and, together with g_1, provides an outward K^+ current that reverses the AP and then hyperpolarizes the membrane for approximately 5 milliseconds. (Modified from Hodgkin Al, Huxley AF: The components of membrane conductance in the giant axon of Loligo. J Physiol (Lond) 116:473–496, 1952.)

We have seen that the resting membrane potential is determined by the relative conductances of the ion channels in the cell membrane. Fifty years ago, Hodgkin and Huxley concluded that the nerve action potential is generated by rapid conductance changes of Na^+ and K^+ channels. From Equation 8.4 it is clear that in the presence of Na^+ and K^+ channels[4-6] the membrane potential can swing between $V_K = -90$ mV and $V_{Na} = +60$ mV. At rest, total g_K (primarily from g_1)>>g_{Na}, and V is just slightly more positive than V_K. Upstroke and peak of the action potential are the result of a massive increase of g_{Na}, such that at the peak of the action potential the membrane potential approaches V_{Na} because now g_{Na}>>>$g_k + g_1$. Repolarization occurs because g_{Na} returns to its resting low level and voltage-dependent g_K increases. The resulting after-hyperpolarization marks the closest agreement between V and V_K, because at this time total $g_{K+}g_1$>>>g_{Na}. As g_K declines, total K^+ conductance returns to its resting level, g_1, and V depolarizes to the resting level. The time courses of the changes in g_{Na} and g_K underlying the generation of the nerve action potential are also shown in Figure 8–3.

Channel Gating Underlies Variable Conductance

As mentioned earlier, ion channels fluctuate between open and closed states, a process called channel gating. It is possible to measure the openings and closings of a single channel molecule directly using a method called "patch clamp." Figure 8–4 shows such a recording from a tiny "patch" of membrane, which contains just one K^+ channel. Current traces are shown at −20 and +20 mV. Current amplitudes are the same for every opening at one potential, but differ between these two potentials (because the electrochemical driving force differs). The other important difference between the two current traces is that the *channel is open more often at the positive potential.*[7] The fraction of time a channel spends in the open state is called the *open probability*, p_o (p_o ranges between 0 and 1).

p_o is voltage-dependent for many ion channels. The voltage-dependent change in p_o of Na^+ and K^+ channels underlies the conductance changes that produce the action potential. The voltage dependence of p_o for Na^+ channels is

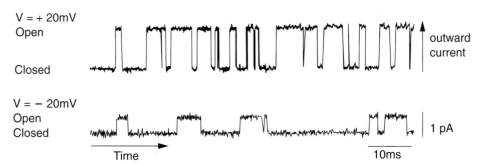

Figure 8–4. Records of a single K^+ channel showing discrete openings at two different membrane potentials. In the depolarized condition, at +20 mV, the open channel currents are larger ($V_m - V_K$ is greater) and the average closed times are briefer than in the hyperpolarized condition (−20 mV). This shows that the channel opens more frequently during the depolarized condition, but stays open for about the same time at either voltage. The average probability that the channel will be open (p_o) is $t_o/(t_o + t_c)$, where t_o is the mean open time and t_c is the mean closed time.

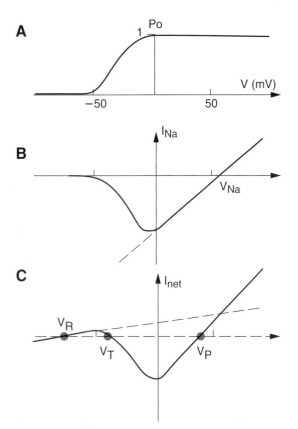

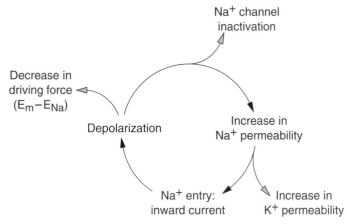

Figure 8–6. Factors that drive depolarization and repolarization of the action potential. Factors in the circle, and connected by *solid arrows,* drive the rising phase. An initial depolarization is the stimulus that opens Na$^+$ channels, increasing Na$^+$ conductance and leading to the inward Na$^+$ current that can further depolarize the membrane. Factors outside the circle (*open arrows*) decrease the depolarizing tendency. Inactivation of Na$^+$ channels limits the increase in Na$^+$ conductance, the opening of K$^+$ channels produces an outward current that opposes inward Na$^+$ current, and the lessening of the force driving on Na$^+$ influx, $V_m - V_{Na}$, directly reduces that current. During the initial, rising phase of the action potential, the factor in the circle dominates, and during the falling, repolarizing phase, the factors outside the circle are more important.

Figure 8–5. Voltage-dependent activation of Na$^+$ current. *A,* The mean probability of a Na$^+$ channel reaching the open state in response to a rapid depolarization is graphed as a sigmoidal curve. Few openings occur in response to many identical depolarizations negative to –50 mV; maximum openness is reached at about 0 mV and an open probability of 50% occurs near –20 mV for this prototypical Na$^+$ channel. For a large ensemble of channels (a typical sensory neuron soma, for example, might contain 10^4 Na$^+$ channels), the fraction of all channels that open in response to one single depolarization would also equal p_o. *B,* The product of voltage-dependent p_o and the I-V relation for an open channel (see I_{Na} line in Fig. 8–2) demonstrates the voltage-dependent activation of Na$^+$ current in an excitable cell. *C,* The sum of the voltage-dependent Na$^+$ current in (*B*) and the outward K$^+$ currents (see Fig. 8–2) reveals three points where net ionic current equals zero, the resting potential (V_R), the threshold potential (V_T), and the peak of the action potential (V_P). Note that V_R is near to (but less negative than) V_K and that V_P is near to (but less positive than) V_{Na}.

A depolarization that activates only K$^+$ channels generates an outward current that *repolarizes* the membrane and thus terminates itself (negative feedback), whereas a depolarization that activates Na$^+$ channels generates an inward current that, if sufficiently large, depolarizes the membrane and thus becomes *regenerative* through positive feedback between depolarization and further opening of Na$^+$ channels. This positive feedback leads to the explosive upstroke of the action potential, after the threshold is reached.

The last property of Na$^+$ channels necessary for the understanding of the action potential is *inactivation.*[5] The voltage-dependent increase of the opening probability of Na$^+$ channels is not maintained in time, but rapidly decays. When the membrane is depolarized rapidly but then held at positive potential, Na$^+$ channels open first but then enter a nonconducting "inactivated" state. The word "inactivated" means that as long as a Na$^+$ channel is in that state, it cannot be opened again by a subsequent or larger depolarization. The return of Na$^+$ channels from the inactivated to the resting (closed) state after repolarization largely determines the so-called *refractory period*—i.e., the minimal time required before the cell can be excited again to fire the next action potential. In nerve and muscle cells, this refractory period is short (a few milliseconds), but it is greatly prolonged (up to hundreds of milliseconds) in heart cells. Inactivation of Na$^+$ channels helps terminate the action potential. Reversal of inactivation requires membrane repolarization. Thus maintained depolarizations tend to drive Na$^+$ channels into the inactivated state and therefore render a cell inexcitable. (Large depolarizations will lead to inactivation after Na$^+$ channel opening, but smaller depolarizations, e.g., to –60 mV, can inactivate channels without their passage

shown in Figure 8–5A. Figure 8–5B shows the voltage dependence of the Na$^+$ current where we have now scaled the maximum conductance g$_{max}$ (conductance of an *open* Na$^+$ channel) with p_o to obtain $I_{Na} = g_{max} \, p_o \, (V - V_{Na})$. Figure 8–5C finally shows the *net* membrane current as the sum of the Na$^+$ channel properties and the conductance of the resting membrane (mainly g$_l$ channels, see Fig. 8–2). The net ionic membrane current has an "N-shaped" form with three intersects of the zero-current axis. Figure 8–5C is examined in greater detail later in the descriptions of the threshold for action potential generation. Here, let us just consider the strikingly different effects of an increase in the Na$^+$ or K$^+$ conductance on membrane depolarization (Fig. 8–6).

through the open state.[8]) The relative number of resting versus inactivated Na$^+$ channels decreases steeply between −80 and −40 mV, therefore steady depolarizations in this potential range will greatly reduce the excitability of a cell. An example of such a clinically important situation is that of elevated serum potassium levels. Of anesthetic relevance is the mechanism of inhibition of Na$^+$ channels by local anesthetic or class I antiarrhythmic drugs, which bind with relatively high affinity to inactivated channels and thereby stabilize this nonconducting state of the channel, reducing excitability even further.[9]

Active Ion Pumps Maintain Ion Gradients

To this point we have assumed that the ion gradients are not changed by the fluxes carried through ion channels during action potentials. Indeed, only a tiny fraction of the ions present on either side needs to cross the membrane to generate the required electrical signals. Nevertheless, particularly during maintained repetitive activity or prolonged (e.g., cardiac) depolarizations, the net gain in intracellular Na$^+$ and the loss of intracellular K$^+$ must be compensated. This is accomplished with a membrane transport protein called the Na$^+$ pump, or the Na$^+$/K$^+$ ATPase. This protein is an enzyme that transports Na$^+$ and K$^+$ ions *actively, against their electrochemical gradient*. This coupled Na$^+$ extrusion and K$^+$ uptake (three Na$^+$ ions are extruded for two K$^+$ ions taken up) requires energy, which the Na$^+$ pump obtains through hydrolysis of adenosine triphosphate to adenosine diphosphate and inorganic phosphate.[10] The Na$^+$ pump is present in all animal cells and has been estimated to consume as much as 60% of the basal metabolic energy. The steep chemical Na$^+$ gradient that the Na$^+$ pump creates and maintains is analogous to the energy stored in a battery. This battery is not only used for the generation of inward Na$^+$ current, but also at least partially provides the energy for the regulation of intracellular Ca^{2+} and protons through Na$^+$/Ca^{2+} and Na$^+$/H$^+$ exchangers, and it fuels the Na$^+$-coupled uptake of molecules such as glucose and amino acids.

Although the Na$^+$ pump is the most abundant active ion transporter in the plasma membrane, other ion pumps (e.g., Ca^{2+} pump) are also present and help maintain the ionic transmembrane gradients. Subcellular membranes with transport requirements differing widely from the plasma membrane also have different sets of passive (channels) and active (pumps) ion transport proteins. Examples include the membrane of the sarcoplasmic reticulum in muscle, with its very high density of Ca^{2+} pumps and Ca^{2+} release channels,[11] and mitochondrial membranes with the proton pumps that form an essential part of the energy transduction mechanism.

Ion Channels Are Formed by Transmembrane Proteins

All ion channels are composed of proteins that reside within the membrane and provide a pathway for ion permeation. Voltage-gated cation channels, such as the Na$^+$ and K$^+$ chan-

nels involved in the action potential, contain charged intramembrane segments that respond to the changing electrical force of a depolarization in ways that ultimately lead to channel opening (and, in some cases, inactivation). Figure 8–7 schematizes the structure of several types of K$^+$ channels (Fig. 8–7*A*) and a Na$^+$ channel (Fig. 8–7*B*), showing the major functional units.

Ionic pores that physically contact the permeating ions are formed by the "extracellular" loops of protein that connect transmembrane segments 5 and 6, the so-called P region. In K$^+$ channels, multiple subunits (usually 4) assemble to form a tetrameric channel and the four P regions, folding in toward the membrane, constitute the lining of the pore.[12]

Transmembrane segment 4 (S4) accounts for the major "gating" responsiveness, moving outward, or rotating, or both, during membrane depolarization and, by coupling to S5 and S6, leading to channel opening.[13,14] (The structure labeled K$_{ir}$ in Fig. 8–7*A* forms a channel that is gated by direct association with G proteins rather than by voltage, but it retains the distinctive K$^+$-selective pore.[15])

Sodium channels are homologous to the tetrameric K$^+$ channels, but the separate domains (I-IV) are covalently linked instead of reposing as separate subunits. Rapid inactivation of the Na$^+$ channel requires the movement of the cytoplasmic loop that connects homologous domains III and IV.[16] Many loci on Na$^+$ channels can be phosphorylated by selective kinases, providing a dynamic modulation of chemical gating by second messenger systems, activated by receptors for neurotransmitters, hormones, and ionic stimuli.[17]

Although most rapid physiologic functions of these ion channels occur from the major, α-subunits, associated β-subunits are important for the stability of channels in the membrane, anchoring them to cytoskeletal elements, or to extracellular basement membranes, or to both (see Figure 8–7*C*).[18]

The Nerve Impulse: Integrating the Membrane Properties

Previously we have discussed the conductive (resistance) properties of membranes through which ionic current flows. Now we introduce another electric element of membranes, the *capacitance*. Capacitance is simply the capability of an insulator to separate electric charge. The capacitance of the cell membrane resides specifically in the hydrophobic bilayer, which insulates the extracellular from the intracellular aqueous phase (Fig. 8–8). Capacitance (C, in farads) is defined as

$$C = Q/V \tag{5}$$

where Q is the amount of charge separated and V is the voltage difference across the capacitor. The physical properties of a membrane that determine its capacitance are the dielectric constant, ε, the membrane area, A, and the membrane thickness, d.

$$C = \varepsilon A/4\pi d \tag{6}$$

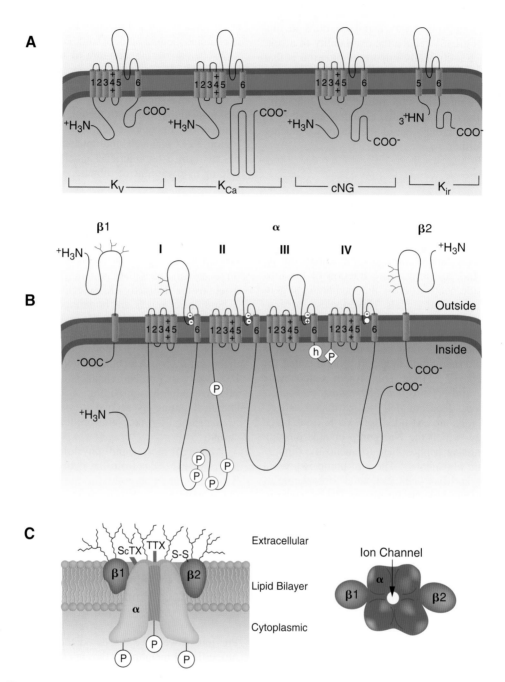

Figure 8–7. Molecular architecture of voltage-gated cation channels. *A,* Examples of K+ channels K_V, K_Ca, and cNG demonstrate the common feature of six membrane-spanning helices, with positively charged fourth segment (S4), of depolarization-activated channels, that are also sensitive to intracellular Ca2+ (K_Ca) or nucleotides (cNG). The fourth example is an inward rectifier channel, K_ir, which lacks the voltage-sensor S4 but maintains the K+ ion-selective P region that connects S5 and S6 and folds between them. In all cases it is believed that four of these subunits join noncovalently to form a functional tetrameric K+ channel. *B,* The analogous voltage-gated Na+ channel, shown as the major α-subunit and the two ancillary β-subunits. The α-subunit contains four homologous but nonidentical domains (I–IV), analogous to a heteromeric K+ channel with covalently (peptide)-bonded subunits. Voltage-sensitivity and ion (in this case, Na+) selectivity are conferred by the same parts as in K+ channels. Sites for phosphorylation, and corresponding modulation of channel gating, and shown by circled Ps on the intracellular loops, one of which (III-IV) is critical for channel inactivation. β-subunits anchor the α-structure to intracellular and, possibly, extracellular cellular skeletons and also can modify its gating and pharmacology. *C,* A cross-section (*left*) and end-on (*right*) view of a Na+ channel suggest how the four domains may organize themselves in the membrane to form a functional channel.

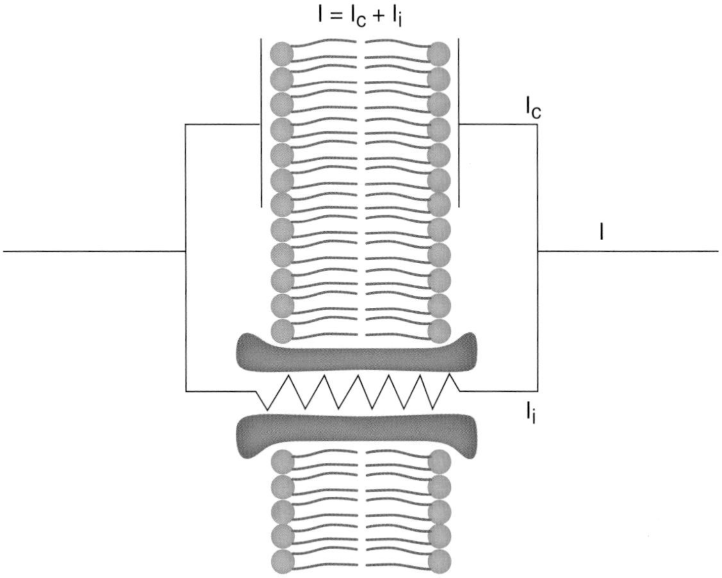

$$I = I_c + I_i$$

Figure 8–8. Schematic of a biologic membrane and its equivalent electrical circuit showing the pure identity of the lipid bilayer insulator with membrane capacitance, and of the ion channel with conductance (resistance). In reality, this identity is not so segregated; bilayers have weak conductance and channels have some capacitance properties.

The membrane capacitance is *proportional to the membrane area and inversely proportional to the membrane thickness*. All mammalian cell plasma membranes have about the same thickness and dielectric constant, and thus a specific membrane capacitance per area of 1 microfarad/cm^2.

Cell Capacitance and Metabolic Cost of an Action Potential

The capacitance property of a membrane determines the metabolic "cost" of an action potential, because from Equation 8.5 it becomes clear that the greater the capacitance, the more charge must be moved to generate the voltage of an action potential. The charge is supplied by an ionic current, and the greater the current, the more energy must be expended by the Na$^+$/K$^+$ ATPase to restore the ion gradients. Because the specific capacitance of a lipid bilayer is (μF/cm^2), we can calculate the number of Na$^+$ ions that must enter a cell to produce the typical depolarization of 100 mV associated with the action potential upstroke. Assume a spherical cell (e.g., a nerve cell body) with a diameter of 20 μm.

$$\text{Membrane area} = 4\pi r^2 = 1267\,\mu m^2$$
$$\text{Capacitance} = 1267\,\mu m^2 \times 1\mu F/cm^2 = 12.67\,pF$$
$$(1\,pF = 10^{-12}\,F)$$
$$\text{Charge} = 12.67\,pF \times 100\,mV$$
$$= 1.267 \times 10^{-12}\,\text{Coulombs (C)}.$$

Each Na$^+$ ion carries the elementary charge of 1.6×10^{-19} C, so

$$1.267 \times 10^{-12}\,C/1.6 \times 10^{-19}\,C/Na^+ \text{ ion}$$
$$= 7.91 \times 10^{-6}\,Na^+ \text{ ions/action potential}$$

Will this lead to a measurable increase of the intracellular Na$^+$ concentration? Our cell has a volume of $4/3\pi r^3 = 4187\,\mu m^3$.

At [Na]$_I$ = 15 mM, the cell contains

$$0.015\,\text{moles/liter } 6 \times 10^{23}\,\text{ions/mole} \times 4187 \times 10^{-15}\,\text{liter}$$
$$= 3.77 \times 10^{10}\,Na^+ \text{ ions/cell}$$

Therefore each action potential will increase [Na]$_i$ by approximately 0.05%, an increase that is not measurable chemically. After prolonged activity (i.e., hundreds of action potentials), [Na]$_i$ will start increasing and active pumping is required to maintain the transmembrane gradient. The relative change in ion concentration produced by each action potential also varies with the surface-to-volume ratio of a cell. Because in our example we have chosen a spherical cell (minimal surface/volume ratio), the relative Na$^+$ accumulation can be greater in cells of different geometries. Indeed, in small cylindrical axons of nonmyelinated C-fibers, with diameters 1 μm or less, as few as 5 to 10 action potentials can more than double [Na$^+$]$_{in}$ and stimulate the Na$^+$ pump, leading to an electrogenic outward pump current that, because of the high membrane resistance of such small axons, strongly hyperpolarizes the C-fibers for many seconds after repetitive activity, the so-called post-tetanic hyperpolarization.[19]

Cell Capacitance and the Membrane Reaction Time

Membranes cannot instantly change their voltages in response to sudden current changes. This is illustrated in Figure 8–9, where we use the experimental arrangement to look at the response to a constant current pulse injected by a microelectrode. This experimental arrangement is simple but qualitatively quite similar to the physiologic situation in which currents are produced in a cell by synaptic or sensory input.

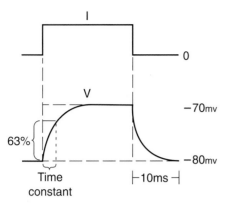

Figure 8–9. Passive response of a simple membrane. A capacitor and resistor arranged in parallel, as in the equivalent circuit of Figure 8–8, will show a slow change in potential (V) in response to the sudden application of a constant current (I). The change of V follows exponential kinetics with a membrane time constant (the time to reach I/e or 63% of complete change, in seconds) that is the product of membrane resistance (in ohms) and membrane capacitance (in farads).

Even though in Figure 8–9 the current applied across the membrane changes almost instantaneously, the voltage increases slowly to its new steady-state value. To understand this, we must represent the membrane by its two electric components (see Fig. 8–8): the bilayer capacitance and the ionic conductance. The slow increase of the membrane potential is caused by the fact that all of the initial current flows into the capacitance. Before we can get current to flow through the conductive element (e.g., a K^+ channel in the resting membrane), we must develop a voltage across it, which requires charging the membrane capacitance.

The speed of the voltage response is expressed by the rate of change of V, i.e., by dV/dt.

From Equation 8.5 and the definition of current (I = dQ/dt), we obtain

$$dV/dt_1 = 1/C_m \, (dQ/dt) = I_c/C_m \qquad (7)$$

where dV/dt_1 is the initial rate of potential change, when all current flow is into the membrane's capacitance, C_m (i.e., membrane current = capacitate current). As time passes, dV/dt declines because as soon as a transmembrane voltage develops, ionic current (I_i) starts flowing through the conductance, decreasing I_c. Eventually the capacitance is fully charged, capacitate current decreases to zero ($I_c = dV/dt = 0$), and V reaches a value that is just given by the ohmic drop (Ohm's law: V = RI) across the resistance of the membrane. The time course of the voltage change in response to a sudden current change is exponential. For a typical membrane the time it takes to reach 63% ("time constant") of the final steady value is about 5 milliseconds.

The important conclusion is that because of their electrical capacitance, excitable cells take a significant time to respond to stimuli. This represents a limitation on the speed of neuronal signaling. However, it also permits closely spaced, brief stimuli to be additive; if the membrane response to the first stimulus is not yet over by the time the second stimulus is delivered, then the second response will

be added on the remainder of the first one. Therefore input on the same cell membrane from more than one synapse can lead to summation, even if the inputs are separated by 5 to 10 milliseconds.

Subthreshold Responses Are Not Propagated

Voltage responses such as those shown in Figure 8–9 are called subthreshold, local, or passive responses. When they occur through synaptic or sensory input they are called excitatory postsynaptic potentials if they depolarize, or inhibitory postsynaptic potentials if they hyperpolarize the membrane. These *subthreshold responses are conducted with decrement*—i.e., their amplitude gets smaller with increasing distance from the point of origin. The reason for the decremental conduction is given (1) by the I–V relation of the membrane around the resting potential, and (2) by the resistive properties of cytoplasm and cell membrane. We have already examined the I–V relation of a nerve membrane in detail (see Fig. 8–5). Let's take a closer look now at the region around the resting potential (Fig. 8–10). We can see that small depolarizations will give rise to outward current (through K^+ channels), which will hyperpolarize the membrane as soon as the depolarizing stimulus stops. Thus depolarization in that region of the I–V produces current that antagonizes and reverses the depolarization. The only depolarizing current available for spatial spread is the one generated locally by the synaptic or sensory input in real life or the current injecting microelectrode in our experiment. The inward current density will therefore be highest at the site of current injection and will decay rapidly with distance. The most tractable case is that of a cable (e.g., an axon) with uniform cytoplasmic and membrane resistance.[20] In this case, injection of current at a particular point along the axon will lead to a voltage that decays exponentially with increasing distance from the point of current injection. This is shown in Figure 8–11. The distance at which the voltage difference has decayed to I/e is called λ, or the "space constant."

The space constant for this so-called electrotonic spread of a subthreshold depolarization depends entirely on the values of the cytoplasmic resistance and the membrane resistance. As shown schematically in Figure 8–11 (*top*), current at any point along the axon can either continue to flow axially (thereby spreading the potential difference spatially) or escape through the surface membrane. Both increased cytoplasmic resistance or decreased membrane resistance will favor current escape across the membrane and therefore shorten the distance over which the electrotonic potential spreads (shorter space constant). The cytoplasmic resistance is primarily influenced by the axon diameter. The resistance per unit length decreases with the cross-sectional area and thus with the square of the axon diameter. The resistance of the membrane close to the resting potential is determined primarily by the density of conducting channels (mainly K^+ channels, some Cl^- channels).

Typical values of space constants vary from 100 μm to several millimeters. As expected, particularly long space constants are achieved in nature by:

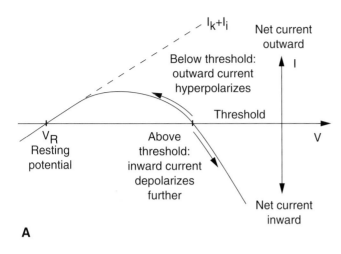

A

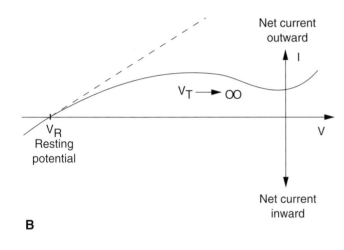

B

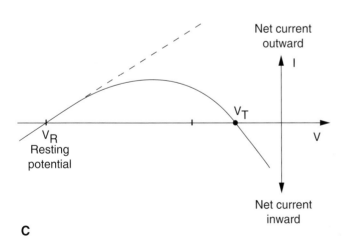

C

Figure 8–10. The current-voltage relationship around threshold for an excitable membrane. *A,* Stimulation by an external source depolarizes the resting membrane, resulting in ionic membrane currents that reverse from outward to inward at a "threshold" potential of V_T, with a negative slope. Crossing this point on the current-voltage relation results in the "unstable" situation diagrammed in Figure 8–6, the regenerative feedback cycle that marks the upstroke of the action potential. In contrast, passing through the zero current point at the resting potential, V_R, on a positively sloped I-V relation is a "stable" condition because the resulting currents lead the potential back to rather than away from V_R. *B,* Shortly after an action potential (AP) the Na^+ channels are more inactivated and the (voltage-gated) K^+ channels more activated than they are at rest. The resulting net current voltage relations at this time yield no point of instability to induce another AP; the membrane is in the *absolute refractory period*; $V_T = \infty$. *C,* Later after an AP the Na^+ channels are less inactivated and the K^+ (g_K) channels are less activated than in (*B*). Although the threshold is larger than at rest, a second AP can still be stimulated; the membrane is in the relative refractory period.

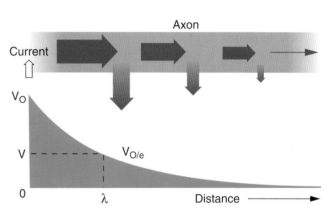

Figure 8–11. Current spread along a cylindric cell process. The passive spread of current away from its source (depolarizing or hyperpolarizing) is determined by the resistance to flow inside the cell (cytoplasmic) and the resistance to flow out from the cell (membrane). As the current density crossing the membrane decreases at increasing distance from the source (*left edge*), the (Ohmic) voltage change caused by that current also decreases.

axon of the barnacle photoreceptor. The high membrane resistance gives this axon a space constant of 1 to 2 cm despite its diameter of only about 20 μm. Distal dendrites of vertebrate neurons also have high membrane resistance, favoring the spread of postsynaptic currents to a zone of summation/integration.

■ *Adding outside insulation:* Myelin layers increase the effective membrane resistance in internodal regions of myelinated axons and therefore increase the space constant. Furthermore, the multiple wrapping of membranes around the axons of myelinated nerves constitutes a stack of many capacitors in a sequential configuration, a circumstance that greatly *reduces* the capacitance of the myelinated axon's internodal region. As a result, much less charge is required for the passive membrane depolarization of the internode, and depolarization occurs

■ *Large axon diameters:* The axial resistance decreases with the first power of the diameter. Therefore the space constant increases with the square root of the axon diameter. Squid giant axons have diameters of larger than 0.5 mm and space constants of 5 mm; very fine mammalian fibers may have space constants of 100 μm.

■ *Very high membrane resistance:* Some axonal membranes have very high resistances. An example is the much more rapidly than it would in an unmyelinated axon of the same diameter.[21]

Propagation of the Action Potential

Unlike electrotonic potentials, action potentials are conducted *without decrement*. Thus as synaptic or sensory input (or spontaneous pacemaker depolarization) reaches the firing threshold, an action potential originates and then travels at constant amplitude along the entire excitable membrane of the cell. Action potentials are the "units" of information transfer along the axons of nerve fibers and they also spread excitation in skeletal, cardiac, and smooth muscle. Even though there is considerable diversity between action potentials in different cells and different tissues, some of the fundamental properties of action potential initiation and propagation can be generalized.[6]

Let us further investigate the *threshold* for action potential initiation. We return to the I–V relation near threshold, and now include the voltage-dependent I_K as well as the leak and capacitate currents shown in Figure 8–10. The initial positive slope of the I–V relation from these outward, passive responses flattens with progressive depolarization and turns negative as we start activating Na$^+$ channels. The threshold, V_T, is marked by the point where the I–V curve crosses the zero current axis on its negative slope. The voltage range between the resting potential and this point is that of the electrotonic response, which corresponds to "subthreshold" depolarizations. Beyond this voltage range, more positive than the threshold potential, the net membrane current is now inward, which will depolarize the cell further; and it is this positive feedback between depolarization and further activation of inward current (see earlier) that produces the rapid upstroke of the action potential.

The presence of a threshold for the action potential explains why action potential excitation is referred to as "all or nothing." An observer with a microelectrode in an axon 5 cm downstream from the site of the excitatory input can only observe either of two things: if the input reaches threshold locally, a full-blown action potential after the appropriate conduction delay will be seen, whereas if the input does not reach threshold, the observer will not see any voltage change at all (the electrotonic subthreshold response will not spread that far from the site of origin). "All or nothing" also means that once threshold is reached, a stereotyped action potential is fired that is essentially independent of the strength of the initiating stimulus. This, of course, contrasts sharply with the electrotonic response that is a graded function of the excitatory input.

Dynamic Nature of Threshold

Threshold is a *condition of an excitable membrane*, not some absolute value of the membrane potential. Threshold is defined as that condition for which depolarization just produces a net inward current (see Fig. 8–10A); dynamic changes in voltage-gated channels make important contri-

butions to the threshold. The most obvious of these changes is the inactivation process of Na$^+$ channels; after an action potential some fraction of Na$^+$ channels are inactivated, effectively reducing the amount of the Na$^+$ current that can be generated by a stimulating depolarization. This effect shifts the threshold potential to more depolarized values; to infinity if no net inward current can be generated ($I_{Na} < I_{out}$), as in the *absolute refractory period* (see Fig. 8–10B), and to values larger than that from rest, in the *relative refractory period* (see Fig. 8–10C). Similarly, the shape of the stimulus will affect the threshold potential. Rapid, large depolarizations open Na$^+$ channels faster than their early inactivation or the slower opening of voltage-gated K$^+$ channels; slower developing depolarizations permit Na$^+$ inactivation to occur to a greater degree and K$^+$ channel activation to generate more of an outward current, both factors elevating the threshold and in some cases temporarily abolishing excitability. An apparent contradiction thus occurs, as small, persistent membrane depolarizations can actually be inhibitory rather than excitatory for impulse generation.

Metabolic conditions (acidosis, hypercarbia), drugs, and diseases all can alter threshold behavior. Although action potentials are qualitatively "all or nothing," the conditions for the transition between these states are rarely constant.

Action Potentials Are Conducted at the Same Amplitude

Propagation of the action potential without decrement occurs again because depolarization creates more depolarizing current, which gives the process its "regenerative" nature. All current flow must occur in loops, because the total charge moved must be conserved. Action potential propagation is driven by a loop of current with four limbs, illustrated in Figure 8–12, which include all the electrical elements in the cell membrane and cytoplasm that have been introduced in this chapter.

1. Na$^+$ entry, down its electrochemical gradient, through open Na$^+$ channels. V_{Na} is shown here with the electrical sign for a battery to indicate that it provides the driving force for the inward current.
2. Now there exists a spatial (longitudinal) potential difference along the axoplasm, between the region of Na$^+$ influx and an adjacent region at rest. This results in longitudinal current flow along the axoplasm.
3. The longitudinal current builds up charge on the membrane capacitance of the not yet active region. This membrane depolarizes.
4. The current loop is closed by longitudinal current flow in the extracellular fluid, opposite to the direction of propagation. Current at any point in the loop must be the same as at any other point. Because the effective resistance of the extracellular space is only a fraction of the intracellular resistance, the extracellular spatial voltage differences resulting from action potential conduction are much smaller than the corresponding

Figure 8–12. The cable properties of an axon shape the spread of depolarization during impulse propagation. In the excited region the inward Na^+ current enters the cell (process 1) where the action potential has depolarized the membrane. The difference in potential between this region and one still at rest results in longitudinal current flow inside the axon (process 2) that carries the charge to depolarize the resting membrane (mostly capacitate current for the initial depolarization; process 3). Laws of electricity require that current flow is returned to the site of original excitation along an extracellular path (process 4).

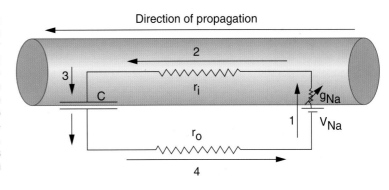

Direction of propagation

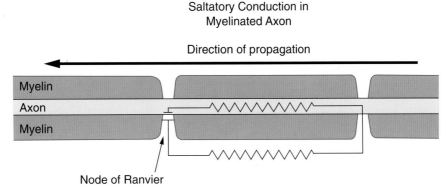

Saltatory Conduction in
Myelinated Axon

Direction of propagation

Figure 8–13. Impulse propagation in a myelinated nerve fiber. Excitation at the nonmyelinated nodes of Ranvier produces inward currents as in other excitable cells, but the heavily insulated myelinated internodes prevent ionic current from passing out through the local membrane and promote the spread of passive current much further and much faster than in a nonmyelinated axon of the same diameter. Propagation fails in demyelinated axons because of the increase of passive axonal membrane resulting from loss of myelin, loss of longitudinal current through the uninsulated internodal membrane that has no Na^+ channels, and the increase in membrane capacitance.

intracellular voltages (Ohm's law). Extracellular potentials resulting from the spatial spread of excitation can, however, be recorded and form the basis of such widely used diagnostic techniques as the electrocardiogram, electroencephalogram, electroretinogram, and so on.

Depolarization of the not yet active region (limb 3 of the above loop) leads to activation of Na^+ channels in that domain. This is apparent in Figure 8–3 as the earliest depolarization, a slow change that precedes by fractions of a millisecond the increase in g_{Na} and the corresponding rapid rise of the action potential. This region therefore becomes the new site of inward Na^+ current and the current loop travels further downstream. Conduction will proceed unimpaired as long as the newly excited region produces at least as much depolarizing current as was needed for its own depolarization. The ratio of the charge supplied in the "forward loop" of local circuit current from an active membrane region to the charge required to bring the resting membrane to threshold is called the "margin of safety" for conduction. This ratio is 5:10 for large myelinated axons (where both parameters can be directly measured), the same or larger for small, non-myelinated (C-) axons, but substantially less for the small, myelinated (Aγ-, Aδ,) peripheral axons (of the motor and sensory systems, respectively).

Factors Affecting Conduction Velocity

Membrane Capacitance

A lower capacitance means less charge separation during the action potential (Eq. 8.5). Less current must flow into the capacitance and more is available for longitudinal spread. Also, the membrane can be depolarized more rapidly (Eq. 8.8). The capacitance of a membrane can be decreased by making it thicker (Eq. 8.6). These principles are beautifully demonstrated in the myelinated axons. The large reduction of the membrane capacitance through the multiple layers of myelin greatly speeds up the spread of depolarization from one node of Ranvier to the next (internodal distance = 1–2 mm). This conduction is called "saltatory" (derived from Latin *saltare*, to jump). The pathophysiology of demyelinating diseases such as multiple sclerosis or Guillain-Barré syndrome is explained directly by the greatly impaired nerve conduction resulting from the loss of myelin.[22]

Conductance of the Resting Membrane

K^+ channels tend to electrically "shunt" the depolarization induced by the inward Na^+ current. Therefore a low resting conductance favors rapid conduction, again illustrated in the myelinated axon.

Na+ Channel Density

The bigger the Na+ current, the larger the inward current in the active zone, the forward loop local current, and the conduction velocity. Local anesthetics (e.g., lidocaine) block nerve conduction by specifically binding to Na+ channels and preventing them from opening.[23] Steady depolarization inactivates Na+ channels, so depolarized regions of excitable tissues will conduct much more slowly. Steady depolarization beyond ~ −50 mV will completely abolish Na+ channel-dependent conduction.

Conduction is not proportional, however, to the density of Na+ channels,[6,24] because the rapid rise of the action potential (and its brief duration) exceeds the response time for activation of Na+ channels; only a small fraction, about 20%, of these channels actually open during one impulse. This leaves most of the channels in reserve, such that partial reduction of Na+ channel density (e.g., by drugs, metabolic insufficiency [ischemia] or disease) to as low as 50% of normal, barely affects conduction. Below that level, however, conduction deficit is easily reached and impulse failure occurs at Na+ channel densities of 20% to 25% of control levels. As a result, functional losses during local anesthetic blockade are steeply dependent on dose of drug.

Axon Size

Bigger axons conduct faster.[25] The increased capacitance per unit length is swamped by the decreased axial resistance, which, as noted earlier, decreases with the square of the diameter. Conduction velocity for action potentials varies greatly in nature. As expected, the fastest conduction is found in myelinated axons of large diameter (10–20 μm, speed of conduction 80–120 m/sec), whereas small, nonmyelinated nerve fibers (e.g., C fibers, diameter 0.2–1.5 μm) conduct only at 0.5 to 2 m/sec.

Whereas conduction is uniform along the entire cylindrical region of nonmyelinated axons, nonuniform behavior is evident at places where axons branch.[26] Peripheral nerves branch multiple times at their distal terminals, whether for sensory endings or skeletal muscle innervation, and sensory fibers also branch in a complex anatomy after they enter the spinal cord. For distal branches, the "summation" behavior for spatially separate terminals that converge to a common axon may present a benefit, because graded, electrotonic "generator" currents that arise from sensory transduction at spatially separated terminals will be integrated at a convergence point where the capacitance and the membrane resistance of the common, proximal axon is lower less than that of the branches and, consequently, the resulting depolarization is both faster and higher. By the same reasoning, when impulses from a single axon encounter a branch point, as in the spinal cord, there may often be insufficient current from one invading impulse to raise both of the branches' membranes to threshold. Stimulation of only one branch by a single invading action potential will render it refractory, however (see earlier), so that a subsequent impulse may dis-tribute its current to stimulate the other branch. If you imagine a train of impulses traveling along one axon toward a spread of multiple branches, you can imagine the possibilities of "activity dependent" changes in the pattern of excitation distributed to all the nerve terminals. Add to this the dynamic responses caused by post-tetanic hyperpolarization of Na+-loaded small branches and you will begin to appreciate the complexities of axonal firing behavior that moderate information transmission in the nervous system. In summary, although axonal conduction is characterized at its simplest by an all or nothing, uniformly propagated wave, at its most complex it provides a highly modulated, dynamic process for shaping information transfer in the peripheral and, likely, the central nervous system.

References

1. Hille B: Ionic Channels in Excitable Membranes. Sunderland, Mass, Sinauer, 1991.
2. Robertson JD: Structure and Function of Subcellular Components. Cambridge, UK, Cambridge University Press, 1959.
3. Miller C: Annus mirabilis for potassium channels. Science 252:1092–1096, 1992.
4. Hodgkin AL, Huxley AF: Currents carried by sodium and potassium ions through the membrane of the giant axon of Loligo. J Physiol (Lond) 117:500–544, 1952.
5. Hodgkin AL, Huxley AF: The dual effect of membrane potential on sodium conductance in the giant axon of Loligo. J Physiol (Lond) 117:500–544, 1952.
6. Hodgkin AL, Huxley AF: The components of membrane conductance in the giant axon of Loligo. J Physiol (Lond) 116:473–496, 1952.
7. Baker OS, Larsson, HP, Mannuzzu LM et al: Three transmembrane conformations and sequence-dependent displacement of the S4 domain in shaker K+ channel gating. Neuron 20:1283–1294, 1998.
8. Vandenberg CA, Horn R: Inactivation viewed through single sodium channels. J Gen Physiol 84:535–564, 1984.
9. Hille B: Local anesthetics: Hydrophilic and hydrophobic pathways for the drug-receptor reaction. J Gen Physiol 69:497–515, 1977.
10. Glynn IM: Sodium and potassium movements in human red cells. J Physiol 134:278–310, 1956.
11. Franzini-Aemstrong C, Protasi F: Ryanodine receptors of striated muscle: A complex channel capable of multiple interactions. Physiol Rev 77:699–729, 1997.
12. Doyle DA, Cabral JM, Pfuetzner RA, et al: The structure of the potassium channel: Molecular basis of K+ conduction and selectivity. Science 280:69–77, 1998.
13. Stühmer W, Conti F, Suzuki H, et al: Structural parts involved in activation and inactivation of the sodium channel. Nature 339:597–603, 1989.
14. Cha A, Snyder GE, Selvin PR, et al: Atomic scale movement of the voltage-sensing region in a potassium channel measured via spectroscopy. Nature 402:809–813, 1999.
15. North RA: Drug receptors and the inhibition of nerve cells. Br J Pharmacol 98:13–28, 1989.
16. West JW, Patton DE, Scheuer T, et al: A cluster of hydrophobic amino acid residues required for fast sodium channel inactivation. Proc Natl Acad Sci USA 89:10910–10914, 1992.
17. Caterall WA: Structure and function of voltage-gated ion channels. Annu Rev Neurosci 65:493–531, 1995.
18. Isom L, De Jongh K, Patton DE, et al: Primary structure and functional expression of the β1-subunit of the rat brain sodium channel. Science 256:839–842, 1992.
19. Ritchie JM, Straub RW: The hyperpolarization which follows activity in mammalian non-myelinated nerve fibres. J Physiol 287:315–327, 1957.
20. Hodgkin AL, Rushton WAH: The electrical constants of a crustacean nerve fibre. Proc Roy Soc 133:97, 1946.

21. Huxley AF, Stampfli R: Evidence for saltatory conduction in peripheral myelinated nerve fibers. J Physiol (Lond) 108:315–339, 1949.

22. Rasminsky M, Sears TA: Internodal conduction in undissected demyelinated nerve fibres. J Physiol (Lond) 277:323–350, 1972.

23. Butterworth JF, Strichartz GR: Molecular mechanism of local anesthesia: A review. Anesthesiology 72:711–734, 1990.

24. Cohen IS, Atwell D, Strichartz G: The dependence of the maximum rate of rise of the action potential upstroke on membrane properties. Proc R Soc Lond (Biol) 214:85–98, 1981.

25. Jack JJB, Noble D, Tsien RW: Electric Current Flow in Excitable Cells. London, Oxford University Press, 1975.

26. Zhou L, Chiu SY: Computer model for action potential propagation through branch point in myelinated nerves. J Neurophysiol 85:197–210, 2001.

9

Synaptic Transmission

C. D. Richards, BSc, PhD • D. A. Richards, BSc, PhD • N. J. Emptage, BSc, PhD

Synapses are the main functional connections between the principal signaling elements of the nervous system: the neurons. To modify the activity of the nervous system—for example, during general anesthesia or the longer lasting changes that underlie learned behaviors—requires either some modification of synaptic physiology or of the excitability of the constituent neurons. Current evidence suggests that of these two alternatives, modulation of synaptic transmission is the more important. This chapter explores the mechanisms of synaptic transmission, emphasizing synaptic transmission in the mammalian central nervous system (CNS). A basic knowledge of nerve cell structure is assumed, but the chapter nevertheless begins with a brief overview of the main events of synaptic transmission. A more detailed discussion of the underlying processes then follow and the chapter ends with a discussion of synaptic plasticity—i.e., the ability of the nervous system to alter the strength of specific synaptic connections, which is the necessary condition for establishing specific memories.

Since the original description of the basic properties of synaptic transmission by Sherrington[1] in the early part of the 20th century, the detailed mechanisms that underpin synaptic transmission have gradually become clearer. In mammals, including humans, synapses generally operate by the secretion of a small quantity of a chemical (a neurotransmitter) from the nerve terminal. Such synapses are known as *chemical synapses* and their physiology forms the substance of this chapter. Some synapses operate by transmitting the electrical current generated by the action poten-

tial to the postsynaptic cell through gap junctions between adjacent neurons (electrical synaptic transmission). This type of synaptic transmission is rare in mammals but is important in some invertebrates (e.g., crayfish).[2] In annelids,[3,4] gap junctions exist in the longitudinal giant axons at the junction of the body segments. These junctions do not slow action potential propagation nor do they exhibit the one-way transmission characteristic of synapses. Similar nondirectional couplings are found between the horizontal cells of the retina that facilitate the lateral spread of activity and between the dendrites of some neurons.[5] Nevertheless, because the importance of electrical synapses in the activity of the mammalian CNS is uncertain, they are not discussed further in this chapter.

Systems Physiology

Structure of Chemical Synapses

When axons reach their target cells, they form small swellings known as *synaptic boutons*. In the CNS, a single axon frequently makes contact with a number of different target neurons as it courses though the tissue. Such synapses are known as *en passage synapses* and similar synaptic contacts also occur between autonomic nerves and their target cells.[6] In other cases, an axon branch ends in a small swelling called a *nerve terminal,* which contacts its target cell (Fig. 9–1). The classical example of this type of synaptic contact is the neuromuscular junction[7] (see Chapter 33). In this account, the terms synaptic bouton and nerve terminal will be used interchangeably as their function is identical. The synaptic bouton or nerve terminal together with the underlying membrane on the target cell constitute a synapse. The nerve terminal is the presynaptic component of the synapse that is usually closely attached to the target (or postsynaptic) cell leaving only a small gap of about 20 nm between the two elements. This small gap is known as the *synaptic cleft,* which electrically isolates the presynaptic and postsynaptic cells. The synaptic boutons contain mitochondria, cytoskeletal elements, and a large number of small vesicles known as *synaptic vesicles.* Under the electron microscope these may either appear as small, round membrane-delimited features lacking any electron dense material in their center (as is the case for the majority of synaptic contacts in the CNS), or they may contain electron dense material of some kind.[8] The latter are referred to as *dense-cored vesicles* and are typified by the noradrenergic nerve fibers of the sympathetic nervous system. The membrane immediately under the nerve terminal is called the *postsynaptic membrane* and it often contains electron-dense material that makes it appear thicker than the plasma membrane outside the synaptic region. This is known as the postsynaptic thickening. The postsynaptic membrane contains specific receptor molecules for the neurotransmitter released by the nerve terminal.

Main Stages of Chemical Transmission

The principal events during the operation of a chemical synapse are as follows: action potentials travel along the axon of the presynaptic neuron and invade the nerve terminals, which become depolarized. This depolarization opens voltage-gated calcium channels, allowing calcium ions to enter the nerve terminal. The consequential increase in free calcium triggers the secretion of a neurotransmitter (such as acetylcholine (ACh), glutamate, or γ-amino butyric acid [GABA]) from the nerve terminal into the synaptic cleft.

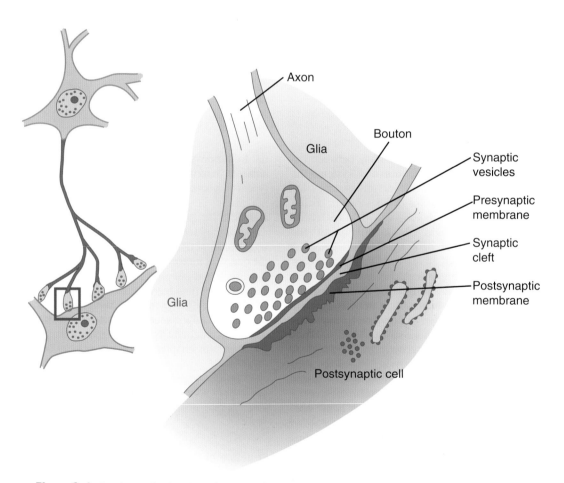

Figure 9–1. A schematic drawing of a central nervous system synapse. *Left,* Shown is a neuron making a number of synaptic contacts with the cell body of its target cell. *Right,* Enlargement of the area delimited by the square. The nerve terminal or bouton is shown ensheathed in glia and can be seen to possess a large number of synaptic vesicles and a number of mitochondria. The active zone is thickened, as is the postsynaptic membrane under the zone of synaptic contact. (From Brodal P: The Central Nervous System: Structure and Function. New York, Oxford University Press, 1992.)

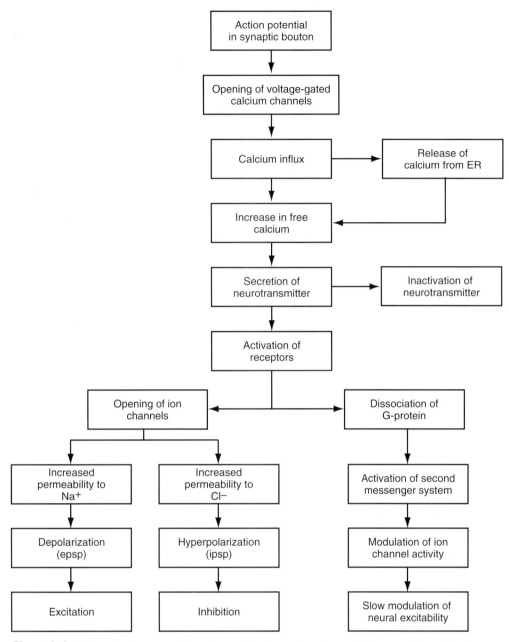

Figure 9–2. A flow chart summarizing the principal events of synaptic transmission. Postsynaptic events are summarized in bottom half of the figure, with fast synaptic transmission on the left and slow synaptic modulation through G protein activity on the right. epsp, excitatory postsynaptic potential; ipsp, inhibitory postsynaptic potential.

The neurotransmitter diffuses across the synaptic cleft and binds to specific receptor molecules on the postsynaptic membrane. As a result, ion channels open and change the permeability of the postsynaptic membrane, therefore modulating the excitability of the postsynaptic neuron. Action potentials in the presynaptic neuron may lead to excitation or to inhibition of the postsynaptic cells according to the type of synaptic contact. If the transmitter directly activates an ion channel, synaptic transmission is usually both rapid and short-lived. This type of transmission is called fast synaptic transmission and is typified by the action of ACh at the neuromuscular junction. If the neurotransmitter acti-

vates a G protein–linked receptor, the change in the postsynaptic cell is much slower in onset and lasts for much longer. An example is the excitatory action of noradrenaline (norepinephrine) on α_1-adrenoceptors in the peripheral blood vessels. The secreted neurotransmitter is removed from the synaptic cleft by diffusion, by enzymatic activity, or by uptake into the nerve terminals of surrounding glial cells. These events are summarized in Figure 9–2. From this bare outline it is clear that synaptic transmission can be divided into two main stages: presynaptic, which is concerned with the mechanisms involved in controlling the secretion of the neurotransmitter, and postsynaptic, which is concerned with the processes that occur in the postsynaptic cell after the secreted neurotransmitter has bound to its receptor.

To explain the mechanism of synaptic transmission in full requires us to answer to a number of key questions: What is the nature of the neurotransmitter at a particular synapse? How is it synthesized and stored? What is the mechanism by which the neurotransmitter is released into the synaptic cleft? How is the release process triggered? After a neurotransmitter has diffused across the synaptic cleft, how does it elicit its postsynaptic response? Is it a direct action on an ion channel or are its effects mediated through a G protein and second messenger system? If the latter, what specific mechanisms are involved? Finally, how is the action of the neurotransmitter terminated?

Chemical Identity of Neurotransmitters

To determine unequivocally the identity of the neurotransmitter responsible for synaptic transmission at a particular synapse is not a trivial matter. Any candidate must satisfy the following specific criteria:

1. The substance must either be synthesized and stored in the presynaptic nerve terminals or the nerve terminals must be capable of its rapid synthesis from available precursors.
2. The putative transmitter should be detectable in the extracellular fluid following a period of synaptic activation and should show the same dependence on extracellular calcium as the synaptic response.
3. The exogenous application of the putative neurotransmitter should mimic the normal postsynaptic effects of activation of the synapse under consideration.
4. Pharmacologic agents that modulate synaptic transmission should show similar effects on the action of the putative transmitter when it is applied artificially.
5. There must be a means of inactivating the released neurotransmitter.

Nerve cells use a variety of neurotransmitters that can be grouped into six main classes (Table 9–1):

1. Esters (e.g., ACh)
2. Monoamines (e.g., noradrenaline, dopamine, and serotonin)
3. Amino acids (e.g., glutamate and GABA)
4. Purines (e.g., adenosine and adenosine triphosphate [ATP])
5. Peptides (e.g., substance P and vasoactive intestinal polypeptide)
6. Inorganic gases (e.g., nitric oxide).

Dual Transmission

Some nerve terminals are known to contain two different kinds of neurotransmitter. As a result, both neurotransmitters may be released when such a nerve ending is activated.

This is called *cotransmission* or *dual transmission*. One example of dual transmission is shown by the parasympathetic nerves of the salivary glands, which release both ACh and vasoactive intestinal polypeptide when they are activated. In this case, the ACh acts on the acinar cells to increase secretion and the vasoactive intestinal polypeptide acts on the smooth muscle of the arterioles to increase the local blood flow.[9]

Cellular Physiology

Storage of Neurotransmitters in Synaptic Vesicles

Chemical analysis of nerve terminals isolated from the brain ("synaptosomes") has shown that they contain high concentrations of neurotransmitters. By careful subcellular fractionation, the synaptic vesicles can be separated from the other intracellular organelles of the nerve terminals, and analysis of their contents has shown that the vesicles contain almost all of the neurotransmitter present in the terminals.[10,11] It is therefore clear that some form of transport mechanism must exist to concentrate the neurotransmitter in the vesicles.

The mechanism responsible depends on the operation of two transporters. First, an ATP-dependent proton pump establishes a hydrogen ion gradient between the cytoplasm and the vesicle interior, then a second transport protein exploits this proton gradient to accumulate neurotransmitter in the vesicle.[12] Specific transport proteins have been characterized for the vesicular uptake of ACh, catecholamines (norepinephrine and dopamine), the excitatory amino acid glutamate, and the inhibitory amino acid GABA. The vesicular transport systems permit the accumulation of high concentrations of neurotransmitter in the vesicles. In cholinergic neurons, for example, the concentration of acetylcholine (ACh) in the synaptic vesicles is about 0.6^- M—over a thousand times more concentrated than the cytoplasm. It is unlikely that all this material is present in free solution within the vesicle. To reduce the effective osmotic gradient across the vesicle membrane, ACh is probably combined with some form of polyanionic matrix similar to the heparin-proteoglycan matrix of mast cells that binds histamine.[13] In addition to the neurotransmitter, the synaptic vesicles also contain ATP. The molar ratio of ATP/neurotransmitter varies from one neurotransmitter to another, being particularly high for the catecholamines in which the ratio is 1:3. The clear advantage of the vesicular storage of transmitter lies in the ready availability of neurotransmitter for release. In view of the high concentrations present in the vesicles, the discharge of a single vesicle in the synaptic cleft will increase the extracellular concentration of neurotransmitter to millimolar levels almost instantaneously.

Neurotransmitters secreted from synaptic vesicles are now often called classical neurotransmitters to distinguish them from substances that are synthesized as required. An example of this type of transmitter is nitric oxide,[14] which cannot be stored in vesicles because, as a gas, it would rapidly diffuse through the vesicle membrane.

TABLE 9–1.

Neurotransmitters and Their Receptors

Class of Compound	Specific Example	Receptor Types	Physiologic Role	Mechanism of Action
Ester	Acetylcholine	Nicotinic	Fast excitatory synaptic transmission especially at neuromuscular junction	Activates ion channels
		Muscarinic	Both excitatory and inhibitory slow synaptic transmission depending on tissue e.g., slowing of heart, smooth muscle relaxation in the gut	Acts via G protein
Monoamine	Noradrenaline	Various α and β adrenoceptors	Slow synaptic transmission in CNS and smooth muscle	Acts through G protein
	Serotonin (5-HT)	Various 5-HT receptors (e.g., 5-HT$_{1A}$, 5-HT$_{2A}$, etc.)	Slow synaptic transmission in CNS and periphery (smooth muscle and gut)	Acts through G protein
		5-HT$_3$	Fast excitatory synaptic transmission	Activates ion channels
	Dopamine	D1, D2 receptors	Slow synaptic transmission in CNS and periphery (blood vessels and gut)	Acts through G protein
Amino acid	Glutamate	AMPA	Fast excitatory synaptic transmission in CNS	Activates ion channels
		NMDA	Slow excitatory synaptic transmission in CNS	Activates ion channels
		Metabotropic	Neuromodulation	Acts through G protein
	GABA	GABA$_A$	Fast inhibitory synaptic transmission in CNS	Activates ion channels
		GABA$_B$	Slow inhibitory synaptic transmission in CNS	Acts through G protein
Purines	Adenosine	A$_1$ receptor	Neuromodulation	Acts through G protein
	ATP	P$_{2X}$ receptors	Fast excitatory synaptic transmission	Activates ion channels
		P$_{2Y}$ receptors	Neuromodulation	Acts through G proteins
Peptide	Substance P	NK$_1$	Slow excitation of smooth muscle and neurons in CNS	Acts through G protein
	Enkephalins	μ/δ-opioid	Slow synaptic signaling (reduction in excitability) Decrease in gut motility Promotes analgesia	Acts via G protein
	β-Endorphin	κ-opioid	Slow synaptic signaling analgesia	Acts through G protein
Inorganic gas	Nitric oxide	Guanylyl cyclase	Synaptic modulation	

AMPA, α-amino-3-hydroxy-5-methylisoxazole-4-propionic acid; ATP, adenosine triphosphate; CNS, central nervous system; GABA, γ-aminobutyric acid; GABA$_A$, γ-aminobutyric acid type A; GABA$_B$, γ-aminobutyric acid type B; NMDA, *N*-methyl-D-aspartate.

Biochemical and Molecular Mechanisms Underlying Synaptic Transmission

Mechanism of Transmitter Release

Under normal physiologic circumstances, the secretion of neurotransmitter at a particular synapse is triggered by the arrival of an action potential in the nerve terminal. This process is calcium-dependent both in peripheral synapses[15,16] and at synapses in the CNS.[17] The entry of calcium is triggered by a depolarization-induced opening of voltage-sensitive calcium channels located in the presynaptic bouton. These presynaptic calcium channels are subdivided into N, P/Q, and R channels (see later). Detailed analysis by Katz and his colleagues[18] of the synaptic events occurring at the frog neuromuscular junction showed that the neurotransmitter, in this case ACh, is spontaneously secreted at a low rate giving rise to small random depolarizations of about 1 mV in the muscle membrane. These small depolarizations are similar in time course to the main synaptic event, the endplate potential (or epp), and are called miniature endplate potentials (or mepps). Normally, the epp is very large and transmission between nerve and muscle is reliable. If, however, the extracellular calcium concentration in the solution bathing the motor endplate is reduced and the motor nerve is stimulated with a steady train of impulses, the epp will occasionally fail. During these conditions, the epp fluctuates in amplitude from stimulus to stimulus in multiples of the amplitude of the mepps. These findings led del Castillo and Katz[19] to suggest that each mepp is the result of the secretion of a small unit of neurotransmitter or "quantum."

Biochemical studies have shown that the amount of ACh in each vesicle is sufficient to account for the size of the mepps,[10,18] and the synaptic vesicles quickly became the likely candidates for the origin of the quanta. The idea developed that the presynaptic nerve terminal contained a large pool of vesicles from which there was a low probability that a single vesicle would be released. Depolarization of the motor nerve terminal by an action potential dramatically increased the chance of the nerve terminal secreting a quantum of transmitter and the simultaneous release of many quanta gives rise to the epp. Thus the epp depends on the size of the individual quanta, the number of vesicles available for release (i.e., the number of release sites), and the probability of a quantum being released at a particular site.

This model of synaptic transmission is now widely accepted and is, in many respects, similar to the processes occurring at the synapses of the CNS. An important difference between the neuromuscular junction and central synapses is the discovery that the nerve terminals of the CNS usually have just one release site. Because there is a finite probability that a particular release site is unable to respond to an action potential by secreting a synaptic vesicle, a CNS synapse is usually not activated by every action potential.[20–23] This differs from the neuromuscular junction where every action potential will result in an epp and cause contraction of the muscle fiber.

To summarize, the current vesicular theory of synaptic transmission proposes that the membrane of synaptic vesicles fuses with the plasma membrane of the nerve terminal (exocytosis) and, in so doing, they release their content of neurotransmitter into the synaptic cleft. Although usually considered a property of fast synapses, this process also occurs, albeit on a grander scale, in neuroendocrine cells. However, instead of small (40 nm in diameter) vesicles, the secretory structures are dense-cored granules (0.3–1.0 μm in diameter). Nevertheless, the fundamental linkage between exocytosis and secretion is the same, and the best direct evidence linking exocytosis with secretion comes from experiments on neuroendocrine cells and mast cells (see later).

Control of Vesicle Secretion

It should be clear that synaptic transmission depends on the nerve terminal releasing synaptic vesicles in an ordered fashion. In the nerve terminals of the CNS, it is generally assumed on the basis of evidence from electron microscopy that only one vesicle can be released per release site per action potential. The terminal itself holds many more than one vesicle, however, often close to a hundred. These vesicles must go through certain biochemical steps to prepare for exocytosis. Although the exact number of steps and their specific nature remains unclear, they are generally grouped into three. These are known as docking, priming, and fusion, and all are driven by interactions between proteins found both on the plasma membrane and the vesicle membrane (which form the so-called SNARE complex).

The proteins involved in vesicular exocytosis are conserved from yeast to man. They include three SNARE proteins, two of which, syntaxin and SNAP-25, are associated with the plasma membrane, and one, VAMP, with the vesicle membrane. The core SNARE complex also involves the ATPase NSF, its adapter protein SNAP, the *rab* family of monomeric G proteins, synaptotagmin (the calcium sensor protein), synaptophysin, complexin, and VAP33. The core SNARE complex appears to represent the minimum machinery for vesicle fusion.[24] The first step of exocytosis a vesicle must undergo is docking. As the name suggests, this reflects a linkage between the vesicle and the release machinery of the plasma membrane. Priming, an ATP-dependent process, is the next step in readying a vesicle for exocytosis. This reflects a partial assembly of the SNARE complex that can then support rapid exocytosis once it is triggered.[25] Both these steps can occur in advance of the stimulation by the action potential. The final step—fusion—is the exocytotic step. The vesicle moves the last few nanometers until it is in full contact with the plasma membrane, at which point the two membranes fuse together, creating an opening (the fusion pore) through which vesicle contents can diffuse out into the synaptic cleft. The trigger for vesicle fusion is thought to be the binding of calcium to synaptotagmin[26] (see later).

Calcium Regulation of Neurosecretion

After a vesicle has been primed, it is ready to be secreted, and the step between priming and fusion with the plasma membrane is regulated by the calcium concentration in the presynaptic terminal. In the cerebellum, pharmacologic evidence[27] indicates that several different types of calcium channels exist in the same cell type (cerebellar granule neurons). These are known as L, N, P/Q, and R channels. It is known that depolarization of the nerve terminal leads to the opening of voltage-gated calcium channels, but which of the subtypes of calcium channel are involved is known only for a few synapses. Initial studies on inhibitory postsynaptic potentials (ipsps; see later) in spinal neurons and excitatory postsynaptic potentials (epsps) in hippocampal neurons suggested that N and P type channels mediate synaptic transmission.[28] Using synaptosomes isolated from rat brain, Turner and Dunlap[29] have shown that at least three channel types contribute to the secretion of neurotransmitter. These are N, P, and a toxin-resistant channel (perhaps the R subtype described by Randall and Tsien[27]). In the hippocampus, synaptic transmission between CA3 and CA1 neurons is mediated by a combination of N-type calcium channels and Q-type channels.[30] N-type channels may even participate in the machinery for vesicle fusion discussed earlier.[31] What is striking is the absence of evidence implicating L-type and T-type channels in vesicle fusion, both of which contribute to the macroscopic calcium currents recorded from the cell body of neurons.[32,33]

A major problem for the role of calcium as the trigger for exocytosis is the need for rapid on and off rates to ensure that individual action potentials control secretion in a discrete manner. Moreover, the increase in free calcium must occur in about 0.5 milliseconds to account for the brevity of the synaptic delay at CNS synapses. The free calcium in the nerve terminal must therefore increase and decrease rapidly following the invasion of the nerve terminal by the action potential. Estimates made on synaptosomes suggest that the free calcium in the resting nerve terminal is about 80 nM,[34] but the control of transmitter secretion requires that the binding site that regulates the release of neurotransmitter must have a low affinity for calcium, in the micromolar region. (This requirement arises from the need to have fast on and off rates for calcium binding.) Thus the free calcium must increase more than 10-fold in about 0.5 milliseconds. Such a large and rapid increase in intracellular calcium can occur near to the open calcium channels,[35] which suggests that these channels must be associated with the secretory mechanism.

The calcium dependence of vesicle fusion presents a problem as mepps and their counterparts in the CNS (miniature epsps and ipsps) can occur in the absence of extracellular calcium. This apparent anomaly can be explained if calcium stored within the nerve terminal can also trigger vesicle fusion. Recent experiments suggest that this is indeed the case. Discharging the internal stores of calcium with ryanodine or by inhibiting the Ca-ATPase responsible for accumulating calcium into the endoplasmic reticulum reduces the number of miniature synaptic events by more than 50%. Moreover, inhibition of calcium release from the internal stores abolishes a form of short-term synaptic plasticity known as paired-pulse facilitation.[36]

Vesicle Cycling

This model of secretion implies that as vesicles fuse with the plasma membrane, the surface area of the secreting cell or nerve terminal should increase. This prediction has now been subject to direct experimental test using mast cells and chromaffin cells. Both of these cell types have dense-cored vesicles and, in the case of the mast cells from the beige mouse, these are few in number but are unusually large. If the hypothesis is correct, the surface area of the secreting cell should increase significantly when these cells undergo exocytosis. The surface area of a cell can be directly measured by its membrane capacitance; this fact was exploited by Breckenridge and Almers[37] to follow the degranulation of mast cells isolated from the beige mouse. They found that, as predicted, the capacitance increased as each granule fused with the plasma membrane. They also found that the capacitance increased in discrete steps, as expected if each step represented the fusion of one granule (Fig. 9–3A). Occasionally, they observed that the capacitance flickered before settling down to its new value. This was attributed to the processes involved in establishing the fusion pore (Fig. 9–3B,C). Subsequent experiments have combined membrane capacitance measurements with the detection of the secreted adrenaline by amperometry from chromaffin cells and have shown that the fusion of a single granule can be directly correlated with release of its contents as shown in Figure 9–4.[38]

The nature of the fusion pore remains a subject of debate, as does the fusion event itself. Is the pore made solely on membrane lipids (i.e., is it purely a product of two membranes coming together) or does it have a protein component? Do vesicles collapse into the plasma membrane (full fusion) or do they open a pore, stay attached for a limited time, and then pull directly back (the "kiss-and-run" model of exocytosis)? If the latter, how long do they remain attached before being internalized?

As the vesicular hypothesis has gained ground, a related concern has emerged. If each secretory event leads to the fusion of a membrane-bound organelle with the plasma membrane, then (as is shown by capacitance measurements) the surface area of the secreting cell must also increase. Consequently, some mechanism must be in place to counteract this. The opposite of exocytosis is *endocytosis*, the pinching off and internalization of regions of membrane. This occurs constitutively in most cells and is important for the internalization of certain receptors, and in epithelial cells for pathways of transcytosis. In neurosecretory cells, there must be an additional mode, because these cells undergo stimulated bursts of secretion. For example, resting membrane turnover is low in motor nerve terminals. However, intense stimulation can lead to a doubling of surface area that needs to be swiftly dealt with to maintain the structure of the synapse.

Data linking exocytosis and endocytosis first came from the electron-microscopic studies of Heuser and Reese[39] who showed evidence for vesicle fusion at sites directly opposed

A

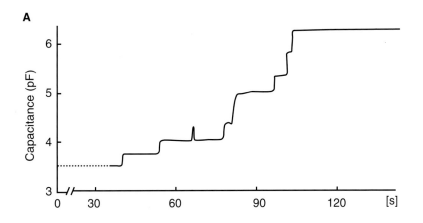

B

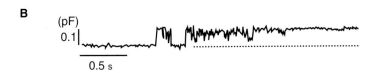

(pF)

0.1

0.5 s

C

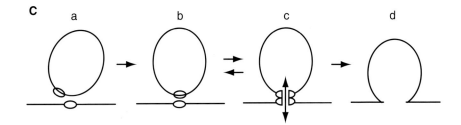

a   b   c   d

Figure 9–3. The membrane capacitance changes the accompanying exocytosis of granules from a mast cell. *A,* Stepwise increase in capacitance that follows the fusion of the individual granules. Each step corresponds to an increase in the area of the plasma membrane. *B,* Flickering of membrane capacitance between the initial and final states. *C,* Hypothetical scheme of the stages of fusion of a single granule. (Data from Breckenridge LJ, Almers W: Currents through the fusion pore that forms during exocytosis of a secretory vesicle. Nature (Lond) 328:814–817, 1987.)

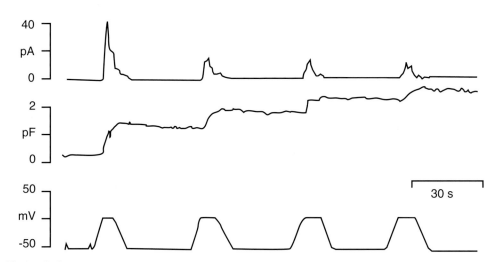

Figure 9–4. The release of catecholamines from bovine chromaffin cells. *Top,* Trace shows the time course of catecholamine release monitored by a carbon fiber microelectrode. *Middle,* Trace shows the accompanying increments in membrane capacitance. *Bottom,* Trace shows the stimulus pulses that evoke the secretory response. (Data from Chow RH, von Ruden L, Neher E: Delay in vesicle formation revealed by electrochemical monitoring of single secretory events in adrenal chromaffin cells. Nature (Lond) 356:60–63, 1992.)

to the postsynaptic folds (sites where nicotinic ACh receptors are densely clustered), whereas membrane budding was seen at more distant sites.

Pathways of Endocytosis

The conventional view of the vesicle cycle is that when synaptic vesicles fuse with the plasma membrane they collapse fully. This membrane is then retrieved through clathrin-mediated budding. Clathrin can mediate the internalization of small vesicle-like endosomes (essentially the same size as a secretory vesicle) or larger structures. Clathrin consists of three large and three small polypeptide chains, which come together to form a protein with a triskelion structure in which three bent chains radiate from a central region. This protein forms a latticework with its fellows on portions of the plasma membrane and participates in the inward budding of the plasma membrane to and from clathrin-coated pits. These inward buds can pinch off to form clathrin-coated vesicles (small endosomes) or form deeper invaginations that pinch off to form larger membrane structures known as cisternae (Fig. 9–5). Clathrin is only one of the proteins involved in this reaction and has special significance only in that it can be seen under the electron microscope. The precise function of the various proteins involved in clathrin-coat formation is not yet fully understood.

The biochemical description of endocytosis has probably been complicated by the diversity of endocytotic pathways. There is growing evidence that even in the same nerve terminal, different endocytotic pathways play a role. Originally proposed to explain electron micrographs of the embryonic *Drosophila* neuromuscular junction,[40] the proposal that different endocytotic pathways play a role has now been extended to other systems. Using low temperatures to slow endosome movement, Teng and colleagues[41] were able to see individual endocytotic structures at the level of the light microscope in fixed snake motor neurons. More recent studies have investigated this in living tissue. Richards and coworkers[42] found two endocytotic routes operating in parallel in frog motor nerve terminals, and Pyle and colleagues[43] had complementary findings in rat hippocampal boutons. The two pathways observed in frog differed both in speed of recycling (<2 minutes between initial release and release of a refilled vesicle, compared with 10–20 minutes) and ultrastructural intermediates (the slower route of internalization involved cisternae, whereas the fast routes appeared not to [see Fig. 9–5]). In both frog and hippocampal studies, rapid internalization was confined to vesicles within a "readily releasable pool"–i.e., a subset of vesicles that are preferentially recruited for release.

"Kiss-and-Run" or Full Collapse?

Ever since Ceccarelli and colleagues[44] challenged the interpretations of the work of Heuser and Reese[39] there has been a great deal of debate as to whether vesicles fully collapse into the plasma membrane and are retrieved perhaps elsewhere. The principal evidence to support "kiss-and-run" has come from studies in neuroendocrine cells. Capacitance recordings from small regions of membrane reveal "flickers" that correspond to transient fusion of granules with the plasma membrane giving rise to short-lived fusion pores. These are associated with release of granule contents[45] indicating that rapid (~50–100 milliseconds) reversal of fusion-pore formation does occur and does allow release of granule contents.

In the hippocampus, there is some evidence for "kiss-and-run" fusion, but it remains controversial because the methods are necessarily less direct (individual synaptic vesicles are far too small to detect through capacitance measurements). Two groups, using different approaches, have evidence that "kiss-and-run" may occur. Both groups have studied synaptic transmission using the fluorescent lipophilic dye, FM1–43, and its relatives. Synaptic vesicles can be labeled by stimulating in the presence of these dyes (they label all exposed membrane), and then the surface staining can be washed away to leave only internalized membrane fluorescent. When stimulated again, stained vesicles again undergo exocytosis, allowing the dye to wash away into the bathing solution. Klingauf and colleagues[46] found that the rate at which stained terminals lose fluorescence depends on the rate at which the dye departitions from the membrane. The critical difference was between FM2–10 and FM1–43, which departition with a $t_{1/2}$ of 0.5 and 2.5 seconds, respectively. They concluded that this

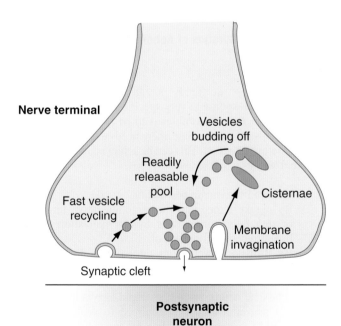

Figure 9–5. Postulated scheme for the recycling of vesicle membranes. Vesicles discharge their contents at the active zone shown in the middle. The vesicular membrane is retrieved by budding of the plasma membrane (far left). After intense stimulation there may be deep invaginations, which lead to the formation of cisternae from which vesicle membrane is recycled to the readily releasable pool.

indicated that vesicles can undergo endocytosis within about 1 second of exocytosis; this is far more rapidly than would be consistent with conventional clathrin-mediated endocytosis.

The second group studied release stimulated by hypertonic solution.[47] They found that stimulation with solutions of increasing hypertonicity led to a greater and greater dissociation between transmitter release (measured postsynaptically) and presynaptic loss of dye. They concluded that they were seeing extremely rapid endocytosis (of the order of 100 milliseconds) in a subset of vesicles, which internalized so rapidly that no dye was able to escape. The reason for the increasing divergence between dye loss and transmitter release was an increasing proportion of vesicles from which no dye escaped.

These results remain controversial because another group, using a very different approach, failed to see any endocytosis taking place with that sort of speed. By labeling an integral membrane protein found in synaptic vesicles with a fluorescent tag, Ryan and colleagues have been able to study vesicle trafficking without the complication of washing dyes on and off. By using a form of green fluorescent protein modified to enhance its pH sensitivity, they have been able to track the proportion of vesicle membrane externalized at all times during the vesicle cycle.[48] They found no sign that endocytosis can occur at the fast rates described earlier. As such, the "kiss-and-run" hypothesis is still controversial and many more experiments will need to be done to resolve this question.

Are Some Vesicles "More Equal" than Others?

The increasing evidence that vesicles reside in more than one pool raises the question of vesicle heterogeneity. The division of vesicles into readily releasable vesicles and reserve vesicles could indicate some structural components within the terminal, or a difference in the identity of vesicles. Readily releasable vesicles could be defined in terms of distance from their release site. Indeed, Schikorski and Stevens[49] have suggested that in hippocampal boutons, the readily releasable pool is the same as the pool of vesicles that can be seen to be morphologically docked in electron micrographs. This idea is appealing but cannot be universal because in frog motor nerve terminals, the number of docked vesicles is approximately a tenth the size of the readily releasable pool. In this preparation, there is no morphologic correlation apparent between readily releasable and reserve vesicles.[42] Indeed, there is some evidence that vesicles have a specific identity, so that vesicles from the readily releasable pool will always recycle within that pool, and vesicles from the reserve pool will always recycle back to the reserve pool. Thus recycling vesicles may carry an identifying mark such as a protein that interacts directly with one or other recycling pathway, a role that has been proposed for synapsin.[50] In chromaffin cells, removal of synaptotagmin IV appears to convert vesicles to a more releasable class.[51] In addition, two parallel pathways of exocytosis have been identified in melanotrophs, distinguished by the presence or absence of Ca^{2+}-dependent activator protein for secretion.[52] This supports the idea that the vesicle population is heterogeneous, at least to this extent. Interestingly, recent studies

on exocytosis in sea urchin eggs[53,54] have suggested that even the calcium-dependence of release varies from vesicle to vesicle.

Role of the Cytoskeleton

Nerve terminals contain a considerable number of cytoskeletal proteins, including both actin filaments and microtubules. Microtubules are principally thought to be involved in delivering newly synthesized proteins and other vesicle components to the presynaptic terminal. In contrast, many roles have been proposed for actin in secretion. In neuroendocrine cells, there is evidence that actin forms a barrier to the movement of secretory granules. This means that secretion involves the depolymerization of actin to allow the granule to move up to the plasma membrane.[55] In contrast, results from snake motor neurons suggest that actin filaments are required for vesicle mobilization. Depolymerization by treatment with latrunculin A caused an impairment of transmitter release characteristic of a blockade of release from the reserve pool.[56] Interestingly, similar results have been seen with the protein kinase inhibitor staurosporine,[57] suggesting that perhaps mobilization involves a protein kinase driven transportation process along an actin track. This is consistent with findings in hippocampal boutons,[58] where inhibition of myosin light chain kinase again blocks mobilization from the reserve pool.

What Limits the Duration of Action of a Neurotransmitter?

Neurotransmitters are highly potent chemical signals that are secreted in response to very specific stimuli. If the effect of a particular neurotransmitter is to be restricted to a particular synapse at a given time, there needs to be some means of terminating its action. This can be achieved in one of three different ways:

1. By rapid enzymatic destruction,
2. By uptake either into the secreting nerve terminals or into neighboring cells by internalization of the ligand/receptor complex, or
3. By diffusion away from the synapse followed by enzymatic destruction, uptake, or both.

For classical neurotransmitters, rapid enzymatic destruction of a neurotransmitter is confined to ACh, which is hydrolyzed to acetate and choline by acetylcholinesterase. The acetate and choline are not effective in stimulating the cholinergic receptors, but they may be taken up by the nerve terminal and resynthesized into new ACh.[59] Nitric oxide provides another example of a neurotransmitter that is rapidly inactivated. In this case it is inactivated by combination with the superoxide ion O_2^- to form nitrate. The levels of superoxide in the extracellular space are regulated by the enzyme superoxide dismutase.

The monoamines (such as norepinephrine) are inactivated by uptake into the nerve terminals where they may be reincorporated into synaptic vesicles for subsequent release.

This uptake is sodium-dependent and accounts for about 60% of the released catecholamine.[60] Any monoamine that is not removed by uptake into a nerve terminal is metabolized either by monoamine oxidase or by catechol *O*-methyltransferase. These enzymes are present in nerve terminals and in other tissues such as the liver, where they play a role in inactivating circulating epinephrine and other catecholamines. Glutamate and GABA released from the nerve terminals during synaptic transmission are rapidly taken up by the neighboring glia and, in the case of glutamate, recycled to the nerve terminals as glutamine where it is resynthesized into glutamate and stored in the presynaptic vesicles prior to release.[61]

Peptide neurotransmitters are thought to diffuse away from their site of action and become diluted in the extracellular fluid where they are destroyed by extracellular peptidases. The amino acids released in the process are taken up by the surrounding cells and enter the normal metabolic pathways.

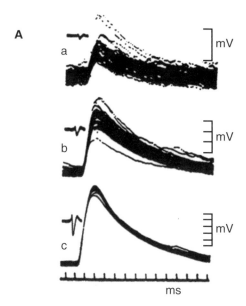

Fast Synaptic Transmission in the Central Nervous System

Recordings from neurons in the CNS reveal a constant traffic of synaptic activity. The observed synaptic potentials are of varying amplitude, duration, and polarity. Those that decrease the membrane potential (depolarizing potentials) are epsps, whereas those that increase the membrane potential (hyperpolarizing potentials) are ipsps. Epsps move the membrane potential toward the threshold for action potential generation. Indeed, if they are large enough they will trigger an action potential. In contrast, ipsps reduce the likelihood of an action potential occurring. Unlike action potentials, synaptic potentials sum with one another to provide a constantly changing membrane potential, and the balance between the activity of excitatory and inhibitory synapses of a neuron plays an important role in determining its level of excitability (i.e., the ease with which it can generate an action potential).

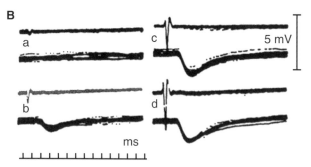

Figure 9–6. Excitatory postsynaptic potentials (*A*) and inhibitory postsynaptic potentials recorded from spinal motoneurons. In each series, as the stimulus strength increases, the amplitude of the synaptic response becomes greater. Note the different voltage calibrations for the excitatory postsynaptic potential traces and the variability of the response at low stimulus strengths. (Data from Eccles JC: The Physiology of Synapses. Berlin, Springer, 1964.)

Glutamate Receptors and Synaptic Excitation

Fast excitatory synaptic transmission occurs when a neurotransmitter (e.g., ACh or glutamate) is released from the presynaptic nerve ending and is able to bind to and open nonselective cation channels. The opening of these channels causes the postsynaptic cell to depolarize for a brief time resulting in an epsp. A single epsp occurring at a fast synapse reaches its peak value within 1 to 5 milliseconds of the arrival of the action potential in the nerve terminal and decays to nothing over the ensuing 20 to 50 milliseconds. In nerve cells, single epsps rarely exceed a few mV, although neurons may undergo large shifts in membrane potential during periods of intense excitation (Fig. 9–6*A*).

Why does activation of a nonselective cation channel lead to depolarization of the postsynaptic membrane? The membrane potential is determined by the distribution of ions across the plasma membrane and the permeability of the membrane to those ions. At rest, the membrane is much

more permeable to potassium than it is to sodium and the membrane potential is therefore close to the equilibrium potential for potassium, which is about −90 mV in nerve cells. If, however, the membrane was equally permeable to both sodium and potassium, the membrane potential would be zero. Consequently, when a neurotransmitter opens a nonselective cation channel in the postsynaptic membrane, the membrane potential in the region close to the receptor approaches zero—i.e., the postsynaptic cell depolarizes. The exact value of the depolarization will depend on how many channels have been opened.

The classical example of an excitatory synapse is the neuromuscular junction where ACh is released from the motor nerve endings onto the endplate region of the muscle. The ACh directly activates the nicotinic receptors resulting in the generation of the epp discussed earlier. The nicotinic receptor of the neuromuscular junction is distinct from the neuronal nicotinic receptor found in the CNS and autonomic ganglia. Nevertheless, molecular biology has revealed that there is considerable structural homology between them. The nicotinic receptor of the electroplax of *Torpedo* has been intensively studied and its sequence and three-dimensional structure are known.[62] The opening of the channel occurs as a consequence of the binding of ACh, which induces a conformational change. The ionic selectivity of the channel is determined by the sequence of amino acids in the region that forms the ion pore. Similar factors are thought to underlie the opening and permeability of other agonist-operated ion channels.

Within the CNS, the main excitatory neurotransmitter is glutamate, which activates a number of different types of receptor. Those responsible for fast excitatory synaptic transmission are known as *ionotropic receptors* and are grouped into *N*-methyl-D-aspartate (NMDA) and non-NMDA types according to the agonists that activate them. In addition, glutamate activates receptors linked to G proteins (see below) known as *metabotropic glutamate receptors*. The non-NMDA glutamate receptors are diverse in structure and are not structurally related to the nicotinic receptor.[63] Those non-NMDA channels that are activated by the chemical α-amino-3-hydroxy-5-methylisoxazolepropionic acid (AMPA) are widespread in the CNS and are responsible for most fast epsps. These synapses can be inhibited by specific antagonists of which CNQX is the best known. When they are activated by glutamate, the AMPA channels open and become permeable to small cations. This results in depolarization of the postsynaptic membrane and the generation of an epsp. The receptors rapidly inactivate so the response of these receptors is transient and the resulting epsp is of relatively short duration (10–50 milliseconds).

The NMDA receptors are activated by the agonist *N*-methyl-D-aspartic acid. As for the AMPA receptors, activation of NMDA receptors leads to depolarization of the postsynaptic cell and the generation of an epsp. The properties and time course of activation of NMDA receptors are, however, very different from those of the AMPA receptors. NMDA receptor channels are normally blocked by magnesium ions but this block is relieved by depolarization. It therefore appears that glutamate first activates AMPA receptors and, if the resulting epsp is sufficiently intense, the magnesium block of the NMDA receptors is relieved resulting in the opening of the NMDA channels. Activation of NMDA receptors is slow and the resulting current flow through the channel is prolonged. Unlike most AMPA receptor channels, the NMDA channels are very permeable to calcium ions and this property is important in synaptic plasticity (see later).

GABA$_A$ Receptors and ipsps

In the CNS, fast inhibitory synaptic transmission is mediated by GABA and glycine. Their receptors (GABA$_A$ and glycine receptors) are structurally related to the nicotinic ACh receptors with the important difference that the integral ion channels are permeable to chloride ions rather to small cations. The opening of these channels causes the

postsynaptic neuron to hyperpolarize resulting in an ipsp (see Fig. 9–6*B*). A single ipsp occurring at a fast synapse reaches its peak value within 1 to 5 milliseconds of the arrival of the action potential in the nerve terminal and decays to nothing within a few tens of milliseconds.

Why does the membrane hyperpolarize during an ipsp? As there is a small permeability of the membrane to sodium, the resting membrane potential is less than the equilibrium potential for potassium (about −70 mV compared with about −90 mV for the potassium equilibrium potential). The distribution of chloride ions across the plasma membrane, however, mirrors that of potassium so that the chloride equilibrium potential is about −90 mV. When an inhibitory neurotransmitter such as GABA opens chloride channels, the membrane potential adopts a more negative value that is closer to the equilibrium potential for chloride. The extent of the hyperpolarization will depend on how much the chloride permeability has increased relative to that of both potassium and sodium. Ipsps are generally small in amplitude (about 1–5 mV). Nevertheless, they tend to last for tens of milliseconds and play an important role in determining the membrane potential and therefore the excitability of neurons.

Presynaptic Inhibition

As illustrated in Figure 9–7, synapses may occur between a nerve terminal and the cell body of the postsynaptic cell (axosomatic synapses), between a nerve terminal and a dendrite on the postsynaptic cell (axodendritic synapses), and between a nerve terminal and the terminal region of another axon (axoaxonic synapses). Axoaxonic synapses are generally believed to be inhibitory, and activation of an axoaxonic synapse prevents an action potential invading the nerve terminal of the postsynaptic axon. This leads to a blockade of synaptic transmission at the effected synapse. This blockade is called *presynaptic inhibition* to distinguish it from the inhibition that results from an ipsp occurring in a postsynaptic neuron (*postsynaptic inhibition*). Unlike postsynaptic inhibition, which changes the membrane potential of the postsynaptic cell, presynaptic inhibition permits the selective blockade of a specific synaptic connection without altering the membrane potential of the postsynaptic neuron.

Current evidence suggests that GABA acts on GABA$_B$ receptors, which are coupled to a G protein that acts to reduce calcium channel activity in the presynaptic terminal. This would reduce the influx of calcium and therefore reduce or even block the secretion of neurotransmitter in response to an action potential. In addition, GABA$_B$ receptors activate a potassium channel that itself hyperpolarizes the presynaptic terminal. At other synapses (e.g., the varicosities of adrenergic nerve fibers), the released transmitter acts on presynaptic receptors to regulate the secretion of neurotransmitter by negative feedback.

Slow Synaptic Transmission

Fast synaptic transmission provides for rapid communication between neurons and, as we have seen, it depends on

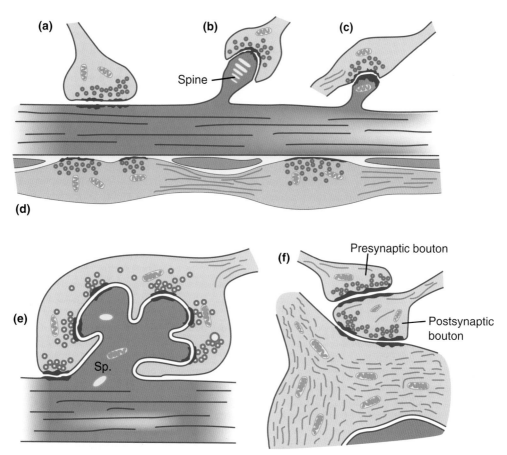

Figure 9–7. The principal kinds of synaptic contact made between neurons in the mammalian central nervous system. (*A*) Contact between an axon terminal and the main shaft of a dendrite. (*B*) Contact between a nerve ending and a dendritic spine. (*C*) En passage contact between an axon varicosity and a dendritic spine. (*D*) En passage boutons of an axon making contact with a dendrite. (*E*) A complex spine synapse and (*F*) an axoaxonic synapse (i.e., a synapse between two synaptic boutons).

the direct interaction between neurotransmitter and receptor to open the appropriate ion channels. In some situations, the excitability of neurons needs to be regulated over a period of seconds to minutes—for example during habituation to a constant but innocuous stimulus. This slow activation modulation of neuronal excitability is generally mediated by G protein–linked receptors which modulate the intracellular concentration of specific second messengers. Many neurotransmitters act on G protein linked–receptors (see Table 9–1) to produce slow synaptic responses that are of great importance for the control of such varied functions as the cardiac output, the caliber of blood vessels, and the secretion of hormones. Within the CNS, slow synaptic transmission may underlie changes of mood and the control of appetites, e.g., hunger and thirst. The activation of GABA_B receptors during presynaptic inhibition (see earlier) provides an example of the role of G protein–linked receptors in regulating the activity of ion channels.

The first electrophysiologic evidence for slow synaptic transmission came from studies of synaptic transmission in sympathetic ganglia. It was found that stimulation of the afferent fibers elicited prolonged epsps and ipsps according to cell type. These synaptic potentials lasted for many seconds and were found to have a different pharmacology to the fast synaptic events occurring in the same cells. More-

over, the ionic basis of the slow synaptic potentials was different from those of the faster variety. For example, the slow epsp in sympathetic postganglionic neurons was caused by the closure of potassium channels, therefore shifting the membrane potential closer to the equilibrium potential for sodium. The activity of these channels was regulated by muscarinic receptors and the underlying current was accordingly named the M-current.[64] In another type of sympathetic postganglionic neuron, a slow ipsp develops after afferent stimulation, in this case the hyperpolarization does not depend on the opening of chloride channels but on the opening of potassium channels.[65] In the heart, ACh released from the parasympathetic nerve endings activates a potassium channel (known as the GIRK1 channel) to slow the pacemaker potential. In this case the ion channel is directly activated by the βγ subunit of the G protein.[66] It is likely that some ion channels within the CNS will be activated in a similar way.[67]

Those neurotransmitters that activate G proteins linked to phospholipase C (e.g., M₁ muscarinic receptors and mGlu1 glutamate receptors) generate two potent second messengers: diacylglycerol and inositol 1,4,5 triphosphate. Both of which are able to modulate other biochemical events within the cell. Inositol 1,4,5 triphosphate acts to release calcium from intracellular stores, and the increase in intracellular calcium is able to modulate certain ion channels directly. For example, increasing intracellular calcium opens the large conductance potassium channel of neurons,[68,69] which would hyperpolarize the membrane potential.

To summarize, neurotransmitters not only directly activate ion channels to elicit epsps and ipsps, they can also activate receptors linked to second messenger systems. Activation of these receptors results in slower acting and more prolonged modulation of excitability that are observed as slow epsps or ipsps. These events occur as a result of several different processes. In some cases, the second messenger acts by regulating the phosphorylation of a specific ion channel; in others, it has a direct action on an ion channel. Finally, there is evidence that some G protein subunits can directly regulate certain ion channels.

Synaptic Plasticity

At many of the excitatory synapses within the mammalian brain the magnitude of the synaptic response is not fixed but can be modulated. They are said to show *plasticity*. The time over which this plasticity occurs ranges enormously. Some changes last for a few seconds, such as paired pulse facilitation (in which the second of a pair of synaptic responses is greater than the first), whereas other forms of plasticity may last for weeks. Long-lasting forms of plasticity have attracted an enormous amount of attention, as they are thought most likely to reflect the cellular basis of the behavioral changes that occur during development or during learning.

Much of what is known about the cellular and molecular basis of long-lasting changes in synaptic strength has been gathered from one brain region in particular, the hippocampus. One reason for this is its relatively simple anatomic organization, which makes this brain region amenable to electrophysiologic analysis. Moreover, it is also known that the hippocampus is essential for certain types of learning and memory. Thus it is believed that a detailed analysis of mechanisms that underlie plasticity in this brain region will provide an insight into the cellular basis of at least some forms of memory process.

The hippocampus comprises three major neuronal populations: the granule cells of the dentate gyrus and the pyramidal cells of regions CA3 and CA1 (Fig. 9–8A). Information flow through the hippocampal formation passes through each of these regions. Inputs onto the granule cells arise from the entorhinal cortex. The axonal projections from this cortical region form excitatory synapses with the dendrites of the granule cells. The axons of the granule cells are referred to as mossy fibers, which make excitatory synapses with CA3 pyramidal cells. The axons of CA3 pyramidal cells, the Schaffer collaterals, project to the CA1 pyramidal cells where they form excitatory connections. This comparatively simple neuronal architecture has come to be known as the "trisynaptic circuit." Each of the three sets of synaptic contacts within the trisynaptic circuit is able to support a long-lasting increase in synaptic strength following a short period of high-frequency stimulation. This phenomenon, first described by Bliss and Lømo in 1973,[70] has come to be known as *long-term potentiation* (LTP), and a

typical experiment shown in Figure 9–8. At first sight it would seem likely that the mechanisms that underlie LTP at different synaptic loci might be similar, in fact there are at least two forms of LTP. One form requires the activation of the NMDA receptor the other form does not. Each will be considered in turn.

NMDA Receptor–Dependent LTP

Part of the reason for the interest in LTP is that it shows a number of features thought to be important for learning. One of these, the lasting nature of the enhancement, is a crucial feature for any cellular substrate of memory. It is no surprise, therefore, that experiments to demonstrate the persistent nature of LTP, weeks in vivo, were conducted shortly after its initial description.[71] Other characteristics of LTP thought to be important for learning include synapse specificity, cooperativity, and associativity. *Synapse specificity* refers to that only synapses activated by high-frequency stimulation undergo LTP. Neighboring synapses, even on the same neuron, remain unpotentiated if not activated by the stimulus.[72–74] *Cooperativity* is a term introduced to describe that a certain minimum "threshold" number of synaptic inputs must be coactivated to induce LTP. High-frequency stimulation activating too few presynaptic fibers will fail to induce LTP.[75] *Associativity* refers to a situation in which even a small number presynaptic inputs, when stimulated at a high frequency, will show LTP if temporally associated with high-frequency stimulation of a larger group of inputs. Thus a weak input can be potentiated if associated with a strong input.[76]

To understand how these features of LTP arise, it is necessary to consider the role played by AMPA and NMDA receptors at the synapse. On binding glutamate, AMPA receptors become activated causing the neuron to depolarize. This depolarization relieves the voltage-dependent block of the NMDA receptor permitting the flow of current. The requirement for concurrent presynaptic (glutamate release) and postsynaptic (depolarization) activity has led the NMDA receptor to become known as the *coincidence detector* for LTP induction. How this feature of the receptor translates into specific properties of LTP is easily envisaged on considering the physiologic consequences of the high-frequency stimulus train used to induce LTP. High-frequency stimulation activates presynaptic fibers that release sufficient glutamate to ensure effective depolarization of the postsynaptic cell. The extent of the depolarization is directly related to the number of presynaptic fibers activated. If too few fibers are stimulated, or the high-frequency train is too short, then the depolarization may be insufficient to fully activate the NMDA receptor. Patterns of activity that enhance the magnitude of postsynaptic depolarization, such as cooperativity or associativity, will enhance NMDA receptor activation and are therefore more likely to induce LTP.

Probably the clearest indication of the crucial nature of the NMDA receptors involvement in the induction of LTP came with the demonstration that a selective NMDA receptor antagonist, AP5, blocks the induction of LTP.[77] AP5 now provides one of the most useful pharmacologic tools for the study of LTP.

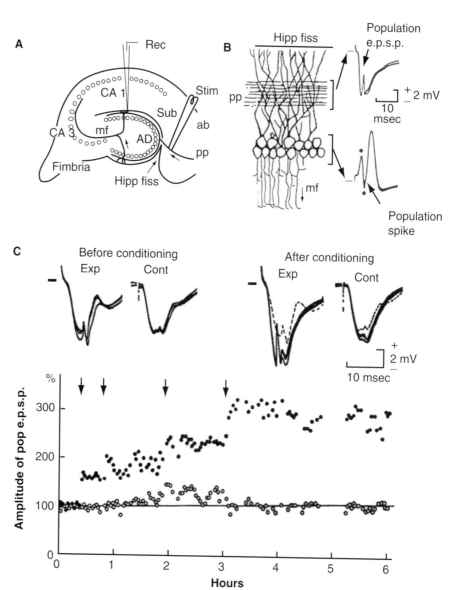

Figure 9–8. The hippocampus and long-term potentiation. *A,* Organization of the hippocampus of the rabbit (AD, dentate gyrus, CA1, CA3 pyramidal cell regions, mossy fibers [mf], subiculum [sub]). *B,* Cellular organization of the dentate gyrus and the synaptic activity that can be recorded after stimulation of the perforant path (pp). *C,* Shown is how the synaptic potentials can be potentiated after brief trains of high-frequency stimulation (*arrows*). Cont, control responses (*open circles*); Exp, responses recorded before and after delivery of the conditioning stimuli (*solid circles*). (Data from Bliss TV, Lømo T: Long-lasting potentiation of synaptic transmission in the dentate area of the anaesthetized rabbit following stimulation of the perforant path. J Physiol 232:331–356, 1973.)

Long-term Potentiation and Second Messengers

The high permeability of the NMDA receptor to Ca^{2+} gave a strong indication that an increase in intracellular Ca^{2+} was a key step in activating the signaling cascades that would ultimately give rise to LTP. The first demonstration of this came from Lynch et al.,[78] where it was shown that injecting the calcium chelator EGTA into the postsynaptic cell blocks LTP induction. This experiment illustrates that calcium is *necessary* for LTP induction; whether Ca^{2+} is *sufficient* to induce LTP is not, however, clear. In an attempt to address this issue, experiments were conducted with the photolabile caged Ca^{2+} compound nitr-5.[79] On being exposed to ultraviolet light, nitr-5 liberates Ca^{2+}. By preloading CA1 cells with nitr-5, it was possible to rapidly increase the level of intracellular Ca^{2+} by a brief flash of ultraviolet light. This approach revealed that LTP could be induced by an increase in intracellular Ca^{2+}, suggesting that Ca^{2+} is not simply necessary but also sufficient for LTP induction.

The critical role of the NMDA receptor and Ca^{2+} in the induction of LTP at Schaffer collateral-CA1 cell synapses is now widely agreed. The calcium-activated processes that follow are much less well understood. Many kinase pathways have been implicated, including roles for protein kinase A,[80] protein kinase C,[81] protein kinase G,[82] and tyrosine kinases.[83] Currently, however, one pathway in particular is thought to have a pivotal role. This incorporates the Ca^{2+}/calmodulin dependent protein kinase, CaM kinase II.[84,85] A number of the properties of this enzyme place it as an attractive candidate as the enzymatic target for the increase in intracellular calcium that accompanies LTP induction. First, the enzyme is found at extremely high levels within neurons, especially in the postsynaptic region of excitatory synapses. Second, the enzyme is activated by the calcium-binding protein calmodulin; it, therefore, has the capacity to sense increases in intracellular calcium. Third, the activity of the enzyme is regulated by autophosphorylation, permitting it to remain active after the calcium level has returned to basal levels. This feature of the enzyme is particularly attractive because it provides a mechanism by which a fleeting signal, the intracellular calcium rise, can be translated into a longer lasting biochemical change, and as such may represent the "molecular switch" for LTP.[86] Extensive experimental studies have implicated CaM kinase II in LTP. For example, the injection of selective inhibitors of CaM kinase II into individual CA1 pyramidal cells abolishes potentiation within 1 hour of the high-frequency stimulus being given.[87] Correspondingly, injection of preactivated CaM kinase II slowly potentiates the cells into which it is added.[88] Genetic approaches have also been used to examine the role of CaM kinase II. These experiments have included the generation of "knock-out" animals that do not express the alpha isoform of CaM kinase II, the isoform found at high levels in the hippocampus. In these animals stimuli that would normally induce LTP fail to do so. Finally, Fukunaga and colleagues[89,90] have shown that induction of LTP produces an increase in the level of CaM kinase II in the autophosphorylated state.

Locus for the Maintenance of Long-term Potentiation

A requirement for NMDA receptor activation, an increase in postsynaptic calcium, and a role for CaM kinase II strongly implicate the postsynaptic cell as the locus of expression for LTP. It is perhaps no surprise, therefore, that a number of appealing models have been proposed that extend this chain of events to produce a mechanism that results in the enhancement of the AMPA receptor function and thereby synaptic transmission. A number of these ideas have become firmly established as critical experimental observations are made. These include the demonstration that CaM kinase II can phosphorylate AMPA receptors[91] and that AMPA receptor–mediated responses are enhanced by CaM kinase II phosphorylation. The simplicity of such models adds to their appeal. There are, however, features of these models that do not adequately address all of what is known about LTP. For example, LTP lasts weeks in vivo, whereas a phosphorylation event is generally thought to be sustained for hours. LTP is also known to be blocked by inhibitors of transcription[92] and translation[93] results consistent with the long-lasting nature of LTP. Such observations require one to look beyond post-translational phosphorylation of AMPA receptors to understand the full complement of mechanisms that underlie LTP.

As enhancement of AMPA receptor function is just one of a number of mechanisms by which synaptic transmission might be enhanced, an examination of the locus of plasticity was conducted. The success of Katz in the statistical analysis of transmission at the neuromuscular junction precipitated attempts to perform a statistical analysis of transmitter release at hippocampal synapses. Unfortunately, the results are far from clear. During experimental conditions in which it was possible to monitor quantal release events, a number of investigations found that the induction of LTP was accompanied by a decrease in the number of failures of transmission.[94,95] This result is consistent with the idea that the probability of transmitter release increases with LTP; therefore LTP has a presynaptic expression mechanism. Subsequent experiments have also concluded that LTP has a presynaptic locus.[96–99] This view is not, however, universal. At least as many investigations have provided results consistent with a postsynaptic locus for LTP,[100,101] whereas some experiments indicate that both loci contribute.[102] The

basis of these contradictions appears to take a number of forms—technical limitations imposed by complex neuronal architecture and limitations imposed by an inadequate understanding of the mechanisms of synaptic transmission in the CNS (silent synapses are discussed later).

The difficulties inherent in using an electrophysiologic approach, in particular the interpretation of a statistical analysis, have precipitated interest in alternative strategies with which to examine the locus of expression of LTP. Optical approaches in particular have received much attention. The development of the dyes such as FM1–43[103] has provided a method by which the release of synaptic vesicles from the presynaptic terminal can be monitored both before and after the induction of LTP. A recent paper by Zakharenko et al.[104] describes how the unloading of the vesicular marker dye FM1–43 is accelerated after induction of LTP. This supports the notion that the maintenance of LTP has a presynaptic component. Emptage and colleagues[105] have also used an optical approach to monitor transmitter release at single synapses. Here, however, entry of calcium into dendritic spines provides the experimental assay. The approach of Emptage and colleagues yields information about both synaptic loci. The authors report that induction of LTP is accompanied both by an increase in the probability of transmitter release and an augmentation in the amplitude of the postsynaptic calcium transient. This result is interpreted as reflecting that LTP has both a presynaptic and a postsynaptic component.

Retrograde Messengers

Although several lines of evidence support the idea that LTP has a presynaptic component, that LTP induction is dependent on postsynaptic processes makes it necessary to consider the way in which the two synaptic loci communicate. Although a number of mechanisms can be envisaged, one popular idea is that a molecule is generated by the postsynaptic cell in response to LTP induction, this molecule diffuses in a retrograde manner across the synaptic cleft where it interacts with the biochemical pathways that regulate transmitter release. There are now a number of candidate "retrograde messenger" molecules including nitric oxide,[106] arachidonic acid,[107] carbon monoxide,[108] and platelet-activating factor.[109] Despite considerable effort, none of these molecules has been convincingly shown to be the retrograde messenger in LTP.[110]

Silent Synapses

A new difficulty in interpreting quantal analysis data was illustrated by the finding that NMDA and AMPA receptors are not always colocalized at a synapse. At some synapses within the CNS, NMDA receptors are found in isolation. Such synapses would be functionally inactive or "silent" at the cell resting membrane potential, as the voltage-dependent block by Mg^{2+} of the NMDA receptor would prevent current flow. To reveal the existence of such synapses, the cell membrane potential had to be experimentally manipulated (i.e., depolarized under voltage clamp conditions) to reveal synaptically elicited currents that were not evident at the cell resting membrane potential. These currents were shown to arise from the NMDA receptor as they are completely blocked by AP5. What has proved to be important about such synapses is that they can undergo an "unmasking" process following the induction of LTP—i.e., AMPA receptors are thought to be inserted into the synapse transforming it from a "silent" to an active form.[111,112] Evidence supporting activity-dependent trafficking of AMPA receptors came from the demonstration that the GluR1 subunit of the AMPA receptor can migrate to the cell membrane after induction of LTP.[113] The significance of these data for the debate about the relative importance of presynaptic and postsynaptic mechanisms in establishing LTP is clear. Unless it can be shown that a synaptic pathway contains no silent synapses, a decrease in the number of failures of synaptic transmission cannot be assumed to reflect a presynaptic increase in transmitter release.

Non-NMDA–Dependent Long-term Potentiation

Although the NMDA receptor plays a critical role in the generation of potentiation at many synapses within the CNS, there are some synapses capable of showing long-lasting potentiation in which the NMDA receptor appears to play little or no role. Within the hippocampus, one type of synapse, the mossy fiber synapses of the CA3 pyramidal cells show a form of LTP that is NMDA independent. The first clear indication for this came from data obtained by Harris and Cotman[114] that showed that the NMDA receptor antagonist AP5 did not block potentiation at the mossy fiber pathway. Furthermore, potentiation at these synapses does not require an increase in postsynaptic calcium, as calcium chelators such as BAPTA do not block potentiation.[115] Calcium does, however, appear to be the trigger for potentiation because it does not occur if the extracellular calcium is removed during inductive stimulation.[116] Thus calcium appears to be a trigger at the presynaptic mossy fiber terminal. Details of how the increase in presynaptic calcium serves to augment transmitter release are scant, although the protein kinase A second messenger cascade has been implicated.[117]

Long-term Depression

The increase in synaptic strength that accompanies LTP can be *saturated*—i.e., a point is reached in which the synaptic response can be augmented no further. During such conditions, the encoding of new information by the brain might be compromised. Indeed, experimental evidence exists to support this view.[118] An important feature of normal brain function might therefore include a process by which synapses can be selectively weakened. An activity-dependent mechanism able to achieve this has been described at the Schaffer collateral-CA1 cell synapses and is referred to as long-term depression (LTD). LTD reduces synaptic efficacy after a sustained period (10–15 minutes) of low-frequency synaptic stimulation.[119] Experiments examining the cellular processes that underlie LTD have revealed that it shares features in common with LTP. Specifically, it is dependent on the activation of the NMDA receptor and requires calcium. The amplitude and temporal characteristics of the calcium increase are, however, different from those required to induce LTP, and it is these differences that are thought to permit the neurons to discriminate between LTP- and LTD-inducing stimuli. The biochemical processes that underlie LTD are to a degree opposite from those for LTP. For example, it has been shown that calcium-dependent phosphatases, enzymes that dephosphorylate proteins, are essential for LTD induction.[120] However, experiments exploring the mechanisms of LTD, like LTP, still have some way to go before the full complement of downstream processes and cellular targets are revealed.

Although a great deal is known about the mechanisms of plasticity in the mammalian brain, much remains unknown. Questions still persist about the locus of change that accompanies NMDA receptor–dependent LTP; the nature, or indeed existence, of the retrograde messenger(s); and the mechanisms by which LTP is maintained for periods extending to weeks. There is also no indication as to why different synapses have mechanistically different processes underlying the change in efficacy. Perhaps most important of all is the question of whether the synaptic mechanisms described thus far really are the processes by which the brain develops memories. Many features of these processes are highly suggestive of this possibility, but definitive experiments still must be conducted.

Current and Potential Targets of Drug Action in Synaptic Transmission

Given the complexity of the processes involved in synaptic transmission, there are many current and potential targets for drug action; these are exemplified nonexhaustively.

Synthesis of Neurotransmitter

The concentration of functional neurotransmitter can be reduced by inhibition of the rate-limiting enzymes responsible for their synthesis or by introducing a "false" substrate. Tyrosine is converted into dihydroxyphenylalanine by tyrosine hydroxylase, the rate-limiting enzyme in the synthesis of catecholamines. Competitive inhibition of this enzyme by alpha-methyl-para-tyrosine has been used in the treatment of pheochromocytoma. Alpha-methyl-dihydroxyphenylalanine (Aldomet, Merck, Whitehouse Station, NJ) has been used in the treatment of hypertension through its action as a "false" neurotransmitter after it is converted to alpha-methyl-norepinephrine, which has almost no affinity for the alpha-1 adrenoceptor but relatively high affinity for the autoinhibitory alpha-2 adrenoceptor (see also Chapter 34).

Storage of Neurotransmitter

Influx of neurotransmitter into the storage vesicles is an energy-dependent process. Therefore perturbations of the neuron's energy supply may result in a less stored neurotransmitter.

Vesicle Secretion

Vesicle secretion can be interrupted by calcium entry blockers (see Chapter 39), ephedrine (see Chapter 34), and amphetamine (see Chapter 34).

Vesicle Cycling and Endocytosis

Currently, there are no useful therapeutic agents that target vesicle cycling and endocytosis.

Re-uptake

Several antidepressant agents (tricyclic antidepressants, serotonin-specific re-uptake inhibitors) as well as drugs of abuse (cocaine, "ecstasy") inhibit the re-uptake of neurotransmitters (see Chapter 34).

Biotransformation of Neurotransmitter

The monoamine oxidase inhibitor class of antidepressants act by interrupting the biotransformation of neurotransmitter (see Chapter 34). These will have the effect of enhancing neurotransmission.

Neurotransmitter Receptor Antagonists

Neurotransmitter receptor antagonists are addressed in Chapter 34.

Conclusion

The complex process of synaptic transmission is being unraveled for many mammalian systems. It is possible that these processes may vary depending on the neurotransmitter involved and will require a systematic examination for each type of neuronal pathway.

References

1. Sherrington CS: The Integrative Action of the Nervous System. New Haven, Yale University Press, 1906.
2. Furshpan EJ, Potter DD: Transmission at the giant synapses of the crayfish. J Physiol 145:289–325, 1959.
3. Rushton WAH: Action potentials from the isolated nerve cord of the earthworm. Proc R Soc B 132:423–437, 1945.
4. Kao CY, Grundfest H: Postsynaptic electrogenesis in septate giant axons. 1. Earthworm medium giant axon. J Neurophysiol 20:553–573, 1957.
5. Borst A, Engelhaaf M: Dendritic processing of synaptic information by sensory interneurons. Trends Neurosci 17:257–263, 1994.
6. Peters A, Palay SL, Webster HD: The Fine Structure of the Nervous

System: Neurons and Their Supporting Cells, 3rd ed. New York, Oxford University Press, 1991.
7. Birks R, Huxley HE, Katz B: The fine structure of the neuromuscular junction of the frog. J Physiol 150:134–144, 1960.
8. Lundberg JM, Hokfelt T: Coexistence of peptides and classical neurotransmitters. Trends Neurosci 6:325–332, 1983.
9. Lundberg JM, Anggard A, Fahrenkrug J, et al: Co-release of VIP and acetylcholine in relation to blood flow and salivary secretion in cat submandibular salivary gland. Acta Physiol Scand 115:525–528, 1982.
10. Whittaker VP: The isolation and characterization of acetylcholine containing particles from brain. Biochem J 72:694–706, 1959.
11. Whittaker VP, Michaelson IA, Kirkland RJA: The separation of synaptic vesicles from nerve-ending particles ('synaptosomes'). Biochem J 90:293–303, 1964.
12. Liu YJ, Edwards RH: The role of vesicular transport proteins in synaptic transmission and neural degeneration. Ann Rev Neurosci 20:125–156, 1997.
13. Rahamimoff R, Fernandez JM: Pre- and post-fusion regulation of transmitter release. Neuron 18:17–27, 1997.
14. Dawson TM, Snyder SH: Gases as biological messengers: Nitric oxide and carbon monoxide in the brain. J Neurosci 14:5147–5159, 1994.
15. del Castillo J, Engbak L: The nature of the neuromuscular block produced by magnesium. J Physiol 124:370–384, 1954.
16. Hutter OF, Kostial K: Effect of magnesium and calcium ions on the release of acetylcholine. J Physiol 124:234–241, 1954.
17. Richards CD, Sercombe R: Calcium, magnesium and the electrical activity of guinea-pig olfactory cortex in vitro. J Physiol 211:571–584, 1970.
18. Katz B: The release of neural transmitter substances. Liverpool, UK, Liverpool University Press, 1969.
19. del Castillo J, and Katz B: Quantal components of the end plate potential. J Physiol 124:560–573, 1954.
20. Redman S: Quantal analysis of synaptic potentials in neurons of the central nervous system. Physiol Rev 70:165–198, 1990.
21. Isaacson JS, Walmsley B: Counting quanta: Direct measurements of transmitter release at a central synapse. Neuron 15:875–884, 1995.
22. Korn H, Faber DS: Quantal analysis and synaptic efficacy in the CNS. Trends Neurosci 14:439–445, 1991.
23. Emptage NJ, Bliss TVP, Fine A: Single synaptic events evoke NMDA receptor-mediated release of calcium from internal stores in hippocampal dendritic spines. Neuron 22:115–124, 2000.
24. Weber T, Zemelman BV, McNew JA, et al: SNAREpins: Minimal machinery for membrane fusion. Cell 92:759–772, 1998.
25. Chen YA, Scales SJ, Scheller RH: Sequential SNARE assembly underlies priming and triggering of exocytosis. Neuron 30:161–170, 2001.
26. Fernandez-Chacon R, Konigstorfer A, Gerber SH, et al: Synaptotagmin I functions as a calcium regulator of release probability. Nature (Lond) 410:41–49, 2001.
27. Randall A, Tsien RW: Pharmacological dissection of multiple types of Ca^{2+} channel currents in rat cerebellar granule neurons. J Neurosci 15:2995–3012, 1995.
28. Takahashi T, Momiyama A: Different types of calcium channels mediate central synaptic transmission. Nature 366:156–158, 1993.
29. Turner TJ, Dunlap K: Pharmacological characterization of presynaptic calcium channels using subsecond biochemical measurements of synaptosomal neurosecretion. Neuropharmacology 34:1469–1478, 1995.
30. Wheeler DB, Randall A, Tsien RW: Roles of N-type and Q-type Ca^{2+} channels in supporting hippocampal synaptic transmission. Science 264:107–111, 1994.
31. Degtiar VE, Scheller RH, Tsien RW: Syntaxin modulation of slow inactivation of N-type calcium channels. J Neurosci 20:4355–4367, 2000.
32. Nowycky MC, Fox AP, Tsien RW: Three types of neuronal calcium-channel with different calcium agonist sensitivity. Nature 316:440–443, 1985.
33. Bean BP: Classes of calcium channels in vertebrate cells. Ann Rev Physiol 51:367–384, 1989.
34. Richards CD, Metcalfe JC, Smith GA, Hesketh TR: Free calcium levels and pH in synaptosomes during transmitter release. Biochim Biophys Acta 803:215–220, 1984.
35. Zucker RS, Fogelson AL: Relationship between transmitter release

and presynaptic calcium influx when calcium enters through discrete channels. Proc Natl Acad Sci USA 83:3032–3036, 1986.

36. Emptage NJ, Reid C, Fine A: Calcium stores in hippocampal synaptic boutons mediate short-term plasticity, store operated Ca^{2+} entry and spontaneous release. Neuron 29:197–208, 2001.

37. Breckenridge LJ, Almers W: Currents through the fusion pore that forms during exocytosis of a secretory vesicle. Nature (Lond) 328:814–817, 1987.

38. Chow RH, von Ruden L, Neher E: Delay in vesicle formation revealed by electrochemical monitoring of single secretory events in adrenal chromaffin cells. Nature (Lond) 356:60–63, 1992.

39. Heuser JE, Reese TS: Structural changes after transmitter release at the frog neuromuscular junction. J Cell Biol 88:564–580, 1981.

40. Koenig JH, Ikeda K: Synaptic vesicles have two distinct recycling pathways. J Cell Biol 135:797–808, 1996.

41. Teng HB, Cole JC, Roberts RL, Wilkinson RS: Endocytic active zones: Hot spots for endocytosis in vertebrate neuromuscular terminals. J Neurosci 19:4855–4866, 1999.

42. Richards DA, Guatimosim C, Betz WJ: Two endocytic recycling routes selectively fill two vesicle pools in frog motor nerve terminals. Neuron 27:551–559, 2000.

43. Pyle JL, Kavalali ET, Choi S, Tsien RW: Visualization of synaptic activity in hippocampal slices with FM1-43 enabled by fluorescent quenching. Neuron 24:803–808, 2000.

44. Ceccarelli B, Hurlbut WP, Iezzi N: Effect of alpha latrotoxin on the frog neuromuscular junction at low temperature. J Physiol 402:195–217, 1988.

45. Ales E, Tabares L, Poyato JM, et al: High calcium concentrations shift the mode of exocytosis to the kiss-and-run mechanism. Nat Cell Biol 1:40–44, 1999.

46. Klingauf J, Kavalali ET, Tsien RW: Kinetics of fast endocytosis at hippocampal synapses. Nature 394:581–585, 1998.

47. Stevens CF, Williams JH: "Kiss and run" exocytosis at hippocampal synapses. Proc Natl Acad Sci USA 97:12828–12833, 2000.

48. Sankaranarayanan S, Ryan TA: Calcium accelerates endocytosis of vSNAREs at hippocampal synapses. Nat Neurosci 4:129–136, 2001.

49. Schikorski T, Stevens CF: Quantitative ultrastructural analysis of hippocampal excitatory synapses. J Neurosci 17:5858–5867, 1997.

50. Pieribone VA, Shupliakov O, Brodin L, et al: Distinct pools of synaptic vesicles in neurotransmitter release. Nature 375:493–497, 1995.

51. Eaton BA, Haugwitz M, Lau D, Moore HPH: Biogenesis of regulated exocytotic carriers in neuroendocrine cells. J Neurosci 20:7334–7344, 2000.

52. Rupnik M, Kreft M, Sikdar SK, et al: Rapid regulated dense-core vesicle exocytosis requires the CAPS protein. Proc Natl Acad Sci USA 97:5627–5632, 2000.

53. Blank PS, Cho MS, Vogel SS, et al: Submaximal responses in calcium-triggered exocytosis are explained by differences in the calcium sensitivity of individual secretory vesicles. J Gen Physiol 112:559–567, 1998.

54. Blank PS, Vogel SS, Cho MS, et al: The calcium sensitivity of individual secretory vesicles is invariant with the rate of calcium delivery. J Gen Physiol 112:569–576, 1998.

55. Oheim M, Stuhmer W: Tracking chromaffin granules on their way through the actin cortex. Eur J Biophys Lett 29:67–89, 2000.

56. Cole JC, Villa BR, Wilkinson RS: Disruption of actin impedes transmitter release in snake motor terminals. J Physiol 525:579–586, 2000.

57. Becherer U, Guatimosim C, Betz WJ: Effects of staurosporine on exocytosis and endocytosis at frog motor nerve terminals. J Neurosci 21:782–787, 2001.

58. Ryan TA: Inhibitors of myosin light chain kinase block synaptic vesicle pool mobilization during actin potential firing. J Neurosci 19:1317–1223, 1999.

59. Birks R, MacIntosh FC: Acetylcholine metabolism at nerve endings. Br Med Bull 13:157–161, 1957.

60. Iversen LL: Uptake mechanisms for neurotransmitter amines. Biochem Pharmacol 23:1927–1935, 1974.

61. Bradford HF, Ward HK, Thomas AJ: Glutamine–a major substrate for nerve endings. J Neurochem 30:1453–1459, 1978.

62. Unwin N: The Croonian Lecture 2000. Nicotinic acetylcholine receptor and the structural basis of fast synaptic transmission. Philos Trans R Soc Lond B Biol Sci 355:1813–1829, 2000.

63. Hollman M, Heinemann S: Cloned glutamate receptors. Ann Rev Neurosci 17:31–108, 1994.

64. Brown DA, Adams P: Muscarinic suppression of a novel voltage-sensitive K$^+$ current in a vertebrate neuron. Nature 283:673–676, 1980.

65. Horn JP, Dodd J: Mono-synaptic muscarinic activation of K$^+$ conductance underlies the slow inhibitory postsynaptic potential in sympathetic ganglia. Nature 292:625–627, 1981.

66. Logothetis DE, Kurachi Y, Galper J, et al: The beta-subunit and gamma-subunit of GTP-binding proteins activate the muscarinic K$^+$ channel in the heart. Nature 325:321–326, 1987.

67. North RA: Drug receptors and the inhibition of nerve cells. Br J Pharmacol 98:13–28, 1989.

68. Smart TG: Single calcium-activated potassium channels recorded from cultured rat sympathetic neurons. J Physiol 389:337–360, 1989.

69. Wann KT, Richards CD: Properties of single calcium-activated potassium channels of large conductance in rat hippocampal neurons in culture. Eur J Neurosci 6:607–617, 1994.

70. Bliss TV, Lømo T: Long-lasting potentiation of synaptic transmission in the dentate area of the anaesthetized rabbit following stimulation of the perforant path. J Physiol 232:331–356, 1973.

71. Bliss TV, Gardner-Medwin AR: Long-lasting potentiation of synaptic transmission in the dentate area of the unanaesthetized rabbit following stimulation of the perforant path. J Physiol 232:357–374, 1973.

72. Engert F, Bonhoeffer T: Synapse specificity of long-term potentiation breaks down at short distances. Nature 388:279–284, 1997.

73. Schuman EM, Madison DV: Locally distributed synaptic potentiation in the hippocampus. Science 263:532–536, 1994.

74. Andersen P, Sundberg SH, Sveen O, Wigstrom H: Specific long-lasting potentiation of synaptic transmission in hippocampal slices. Nature 266:736–737, 1977.

75. McNaughton BL, Douglas RM, Goddard GV: Synaptic enhancement in fascia dentata: Cooperativity among coactive afferents. Brain Res 157:277–293, 1978.

76. Barrionuevo G, Brown TH: Associative long-term potentiation in hippocampal slices. Proc Natl Acad Sci USA 80:7347–7351, 1983.

77. Collingridge GL, Kehl SJ, McLennan H: Excitatory amino acids in synaptic transmission in the Schaffer collateral-commissural pathway of the rat hippocampus. J Physiol 334:33–46, 1983.

78. Lynch G, Larson J, Kelso S, et al: Intracellular injections of EGTA block induction of hippocampal long-term potentiation. Nature 305:719–721, 1983.

79. Malenka RC, Kauer JA, Zucker RS, Nicoll RA: Postsynaptic calcium is sufficient for potentiation of hippocampal synaptic transmission. Science 242:81–84, 1988.

80. Frey U, Huang YY, Kandel ER: Effects of cAMP simulate a late stage of LTP in hippocampal CA1 neurons. Science 260:1661–1664, 1993.

81. Reymann KG, Brodemann R, Kase H, Matthies H: Inhibitors of calmodulin and protein kinase C block different phases of hippocampal long-term potentiation. Brain Res 461:388–392, 1988.

82. Zhuo M, Hu Y, Schultz C, et al: Role of guanylyl cyclase and cGMP-dependent protein kinase in long-term potentiation. Nature 368:635–639, 1994.

83. O'Dell TJ, Kandel ER, Grant SG: Long-term potentiation in the hippocampus is blocked by tyrosine kinase inhibitors. Nature 353:558–560, 1991.

84. Malinow R, Schulman H, Tsien RW: Inhibition of postsynaptic PKC or CaMKII blocks induction but not expression of LTP. Science 245:862–866, 1989.

85. Malenka RC, Kauer JA, Perkel DJ, et al: An essential role for postsynaptic calmodulin and protein kinase activity in long-term potentiation. Nature 340:554–557, 1989.

86. Miller SG, Kennedy MB: Regulation of brain type II Ca2+/calmodulin-dependent protein kinase by autophosphorylation: A Ca^{2+}-triggered molecular switch. Cell 44:861–870, 1986.

87. Barria A, Muller D, Derkach V, et al: Regulatory phosphorylation of AMPA-type glutamate receptors by CaM-KII during long term potentiation. Science 276:2001–2001, 1997.

88. Lledo PM, Hjelmstad GO, Mukherji S, et al: Calcium/calmodulin-dependent kinase II and long-term potentiation enhance synaptic transmission by the same mechanism. Proc Natl Acad Sci USA 92:11175–11179, 1995.

89. Fukunaga K, Muller D, Miyamoto E: Increased phosphorylation of Ca2+/calmodulin-dependent protein kinase II and its endogenous substrates in the induction of long-term potentiation. J Biol Chem 270:6119–6124, 1995.

90. Fukunaga K, Muller D, Miyamoto E: Increased phosphorylation of Ca2+/calmodulin-dependent protein kinase II and its endogenous substrates in the induction of long-term potentiation. J Biol Chem 270:6119–6124, 1995.

91. Barria A, Derkach V, Soderling T: Identification of the CA^{2+}/calmodulin-dependent protein kinase II regulatory phosphorylation site in the alpha-amino-3-hydroxyl-5-methyl-4-isoxazole-propionate-type glutamate receptor. J Biol Chem 272:32727–32730, 1997.

92. Nguyen PV, Abel T, Kandel ER: Requirement of a critical period of transcription for induction of a late phase of LTP. Science 265:1104–1107, 1994.

93. Frey U, Krug M, Reymann KG, Matthies H: Anisomycin, an inhibitor of protein synthesis, blocks late phases of LTP phenomena in the hippocampal CA1 region in vitro. Brain Res 452:57–65, 1988.

94. Malinow R, Tsien RW: Presynaptic enhancement shown by whole-cell recordings of long-term potentiation in hippocampal slices. Nature 346:177–180, 1990.

95. Bekkers JM, Stevens CF: Presynaptic mechanism for long-term potentiation in the hippocampus. Nature 346:724–729, 1990.

96. Stevens CF, Wang Y: Changes in reliability of synaptic function as a mechanism for plasticity. Nature 371:704–707, 1994.

97. Malgaroli A, Ting AE, Wendland B, et al: Presynaptic component of long-term potentiation visualized at individual hippocampal synapses. Science 268:1624–1628, 1995.

98. Bolshakov VY, Siegelbaum SA: Regulation of hippocampal transmitter release during development and long-term potentiation. Science 269:1730–1734, 1995.

99. Larkman A, Hannay T, Stratford K, Jack J: Presynaptic release probability influences the locus of long-term potentiation. Nature 360:70–73, 1992.

100. Foster TC, McNaughton BL: Long-term enhancement of CA1 synaptic transmission is due to increased quantal size, not quantal content. Hippocampus 1:79–91, 1991.

101. Manabe T, Renner P, Nicoll RA: Postsynaptic contribution to long-term potentiation revealed by the analysis of miniature synaptic currents. Nature 355:50–55, 1992.

102. Kullmann DM, Nicoll RA: Long-term potentiation is associated with increases in quantal content and quantal amplitude. Nature 357:240–244, 1992.

103. Betz WJ, Bewick GS: Optical analysis of synaptic vesicle recycling at the frog neuromuscular junction. Science 255:200–203, 1992.

104. Zakharenko SS, Zablow L, Siegelbaum SA: Visualization of changes in presynaptic function during long-term synaptic plasticity. Nat Neurosci 7:711–717, 2001.

105. Emptage NJ, Reid CA, Fine A, Bliss TVP: Optical quantal analysis of LTP at single hippocampal synapses (In preparation), 2001.

106. Schuman EM, Madison DV: A requirement for the intercellular messenger nitric oxide in long-term potentiation. Science 254:1503–1506, 1991.

107. Williams JH, Errington ML, Lynch MA, Bliss TV: Arachidonic acid induces a long-term activity-dependent enhancement of synaptic transmission in the hippocampus. Nature 341:739–742, 1989.

108. Stevens CF, Wang Y: Reversal of long-term potentiation by inhibitors of haem oxygenase. Nature 364:147–149, 1993.

109. Kato K, Clark GD, Bazan NG, Zorumski CF: Platelet-activating factor as a potential retrograde messenger in CA1 hippocampal long-term potentiation. Nature 367:175–179, 1994.

110. Williams JH, Li YG, Nayak A, et al: The suppression of long-term potentiation in rat hippocampus by inhibitors of nitric oxide synthase is temperature and age dependent. Neuron 11:877–884, 1993.

111. Liao D, Hessler NA, Malinow R: Activation of postsynaptically silent synapses during pairing-induced LTP in CA1 region of hippocampal slice. Nature 375:400–404, 1995.

112. Nicoll RA, Malenka RC: Contrasting properties of two forms of long-term potentiation in the hippocampus. Nature 377:115–118, 1995.

113. Shi SH, Hayashi Y, Petralia RS, et al: Rapid spine delivery and redistribution of AMPA receptors after synaptic NMDA receptor activation. Science 284:1811–1816, 1999.

114. Harris EW, Cotman CW: Long-term potentiation of guinea pig mossy fiber responses is not blocked by N-methyl D-aspartate antagonists. Neurosci Lett 70:132–137, 1986.

115. Zalutsky RA, Nicoll RA: Comparison of two forms of long-term potentiation in single hippocampal neurons. Science 248:1619–1624, 1990.

116. Castillo PE, Weisskopf MG, Nicoll RA: The role of Ca^{2+} channels in hippocampal mossy fiber synaptic transmission and long-term potentiation. Neuron 12:261–269, 1994.

117. Weisskopf MG, Castillo PE, Zalutsky RA, Nicoll RA: Mediation of hippocampal mossy fiber long-term potentiation by cyclic AMP. Science 265:1878–1882, 1994.

118. Barnes CA, Jung MW, McNaughton BL, et al: LTP saturation and spatial learning disruption: Effects of task variables and saturation levels. J Neurosci 14:5793–5806, 1994.

119. Dudek SM, Bear MF: Homosynaptic long-term depression in area CA1 of hippocampus and effects of N-methyl-D-aspartate receptor blockade. Proc Natl Acad Sci USA 89:4363–4367, 1992.

120. Mulkey RM, Herron CE, Malenka RC: An essential role for protein phosphatases in hippocampal long-term depression. Science 261:1051–1055, 1993.

10

Neuromuscular Function

Joe Henry Steinbach, PhD • Ling-Gang Wu, MD

The major known actions of clinically used agents on motor function take place at the final synapse in the motor pathway: the synapse between the motor neuron and the muscle fiber. This chapter reviews the cellular structure and function of this synapse, and the role of each key molecule on synaptic transmission at this synapse. Various clinically used agents including anesthetics affect synaptic transmission in different aspects. Their potential molecular targets are briefly discussed in this chapter.

Structure and Function of the Neuromuscular Junction

Structure

The cell bodies of motor neurons are located in the ventral horn of the spinal cord or brain stem. The axon of the motor neuron innervates the muscle at a specialized region of the muscle membrane called the *endplate*, the neuromuscular junction (NMJ), or the neuromuscular synapse (Fig. 10–1). A myelinated axon extends from the cell body to the muscle. Inside the muscle, each axon branches to innervate between 10 and several hundred separate muscle fibers (the motor unit). At the region where the motor axon approaches the muscle fiber, the axon loses its myelin sheath and terminates on a single muscle fiber at the NMJ (Fig. 10–1). The ends of the fine branches form multiple expansions or varicosities, called synaptic boutons, from which the motor neuron releases its transmitter. Each bouton is positioned over a junctional fold, a deep depression in the surface of the postsynaptic muscle fiber that contains the transmitter receptors (Fig. 10–1). The transmitter released by the axon terminal is acetylcholine (ACh, see "Presynaptic Release Mechanisms"), and the receptor on the muscle membrane is the nicotinic type of ACh receptor (AChR; see "Postsynaptic Aspects"). The presynaptic and the postsynaptic membranes are separated by a synaptic cleft approximately 50 nm wide (Fig. 10–1). Within the cleft is a basement membrane composed of collagen and other extracellular matrix proteins. The enzyme acetylcholinesterase (AChE), which rapidly hydrolyzes ACh, is anchored to the collagen fibrils of the basement membranes (see "Cleft Aspects").

Function

The NMJ must produce very reliable and very rapid excitation of the muscle fiber in response to a presynaptic action potential. As schematically summarized in Figure 10–2, **157**

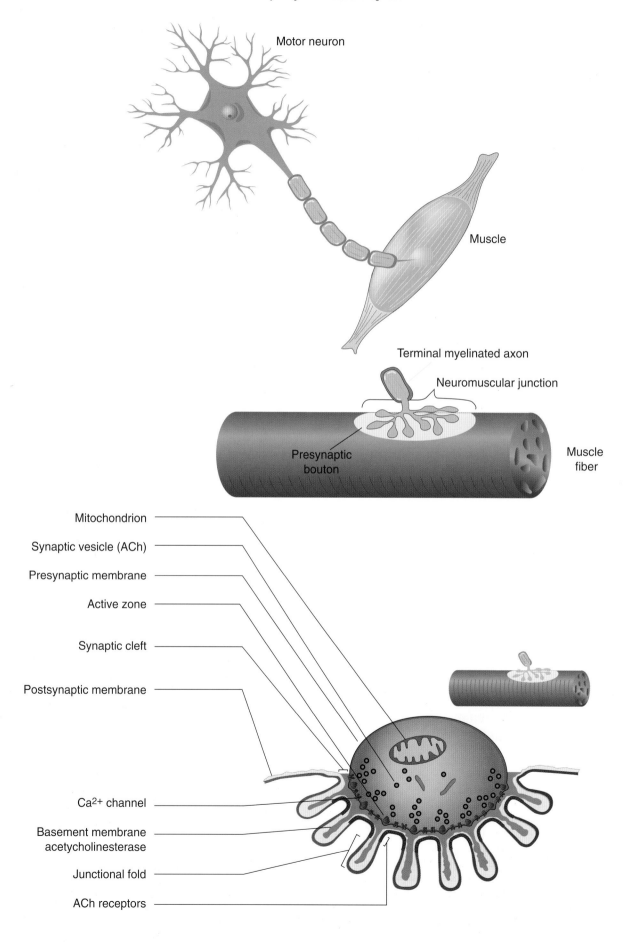

Motor neuron

Muscle

Terminal myelinated axon

Neuromuscular junction

Presynaptic bouton

Muscle fiber

Mitochondrion

Synaptic vesicle (ACh)

Presynaptic membrane

Active zone

Synaptic cleft

Postsynaptic membrane

Ca2+ channel

Basement membrane acetycholinesterase

Junctional fold

ACh receptors

Figure 10–1. The structure of a neuromuscular junction. The muscle fiber is innervated by a motor neuron originated from the spinal cord. At the muscle, the motor axon ramifies into several fine branches. Each branch forms multiple swellings called presynaptic boutons, which are covered by a thin layer of Schwann cells. The boutons lie over a specialized region of the muscle fiber membrane, the endplate, and are separated from the muscle membrane by a 50-nm synaptic cleft. Each presynaptic bouton contains mitochondria and synaptic vesicles. Synaptic vesicles are clustered around active zones, where the acetylcholine (ACh) transmitter is released. Immediately under each bouton in the endplate are several junctional folds, which contain a high density of ACh receptors at their crests. The muscle fiber is covered by a layer of connective tissue, the basement membrane (or basal lamina), consisting of collagen and glycoproteins. Both the presynaptic terminal and the muscle fiber secrete proteins into the basement membrane, including the enzyme acetylcholinesterase, which inactivates the ACh released from the presynaptic terminal by breaking it down into acetate and choline. The basement membrane also organizes the synapse by aligning the presynaptic active zones with the postsynaptic junctional folds.

there is minimal synaptic delay at the NMJ. The presynaptic action potential invades the axon terminal and activates voltage-dependent Ca^{2+}-selective channels. The increased intracellular Ca^{2+} concentration induces fusion of synaptic vesicles with the plasma membrane and release of the ACh into the cleft. The cleft ACh binds to postsynaptic AChR, and the channel of the receptor rapidly opens. A net inward flux of cations flows through the channels, producing a postsynaptic depolarization. This depolarization activates voltage-dependent Na^+-selective channels, leading to an action potential, which propagates along the muscle fiber. Finally, the action potential induces Ca^{2+} release from the sarcoplasmic reticulum that, in turn, produces muscle contraction.

The rapidity and reliability of transmission is particularly remarkable when considering that the muscle fiber is a large cell that has a low input impedance—in other words, it takes a lot of membrane current (and hence, activation of many AChRs) to excite the muscle fiber. However, it is also critical that the excitation is terminated rapidly, so that the fiber can both follow nerve activity at relatively high frequencies and so that the muscle does not show repetitive activity in response to a single presynaptic action potential.

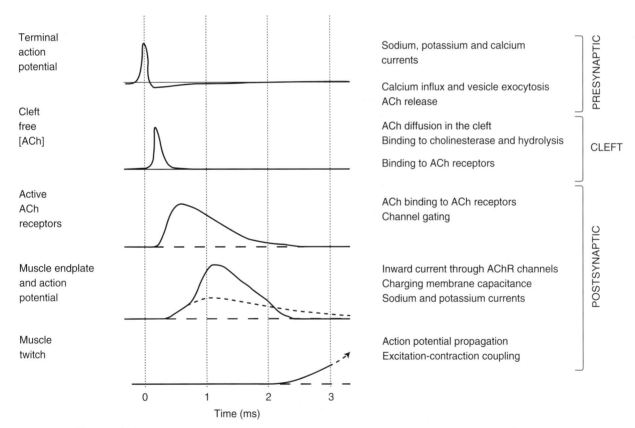

Figure 10–2. A summary of the timing of events during neuromuscular transmission, appropriate for a mammalian neuromuscular junction at 37° C. The horizontal scale shows time (in milliseconds), starting at the peak of the action potential in the presynaptic terminal (top row). Each row shows a different phenomenon: the top shows the presynaptic action potential, the second shows the relative cleft-free acetylcholine concentration, the third shows the relative activation of postsynaptic acetylcholine (ACh) receptors, the fourth shows the muscle membrane potential (and, in a *dashed line*, the endplate potential that would be observed if the action potential were blocked), whereas the final row shows the resulting twitch (which is mostly after the events shown). The third column lists some of the major molecules or processes that affect the time course shown. These topics are explored in greater detail in the text.

Presynaptic Release Mechanisms

Generation of an Action Potential

To activate voltage-gated Ca^{2+} channels, the plasma membrane of the axon and the nerve terminal use voltage-gated Na^+ and K^+ channels. An action potential is produced by rapid influx of Na^+ through Na^+ channels followed by rapid efflux of K^+ through K^+ channels[1,2] (Fig. 10–3). The Na^+ channels are responsible for depolarization or the rise of the action potential, whereas the K^+ channels are responsible for repolarization or the decay of the action potential. The half-width of a typical action potential is less than 1 millisecond and depolarizes the terminal by about 110 mV.[3] Such a brief but large depolarization activates voltage-gated Ca^{2+} channels. The amplitude and duration of the action potential determine the number of Ca^{2+} channels being opened and their opening time. Consequently, modulation of Na^+ or K^+ channels may affect the Ca^{2+} influx during an action potential and therefore alter transmitter release evoked by an action potential.

Ca²⁺ Influx Triggers Vesicle Fusion

There are many types of voltage-gated Ca^{2+} channels, including L, N, P/Q, R, and T type, with specific biophysi-

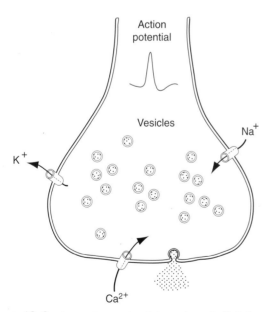

Figure 10–3. An action potential evokes Ca^{2+} influx and transmitter release. An action potential is generated by rapid Na^+ influx followed by rapid K^+ efflux. The action potential, which lasts for about 1 millisecond, activates the voltage-gated Ca^{2+} channels. The influx of Ca^{2+} through open Ca^{2+} channels triggers fusion of vesicles with the plasma membrane at the active zone. After vesicle fusion, transmitter molecules diffuse out of the fused vesicles. The dimension is not drawn to be proportional to the real structure.

cal and pharmacologic properties and different physiologic functions.[4] The distinct properties of these channel types are determined by the identity of their pore-forming subunit (termed the $\alpha 1$-subunit), which is encoded by a family of related genes. Ca^{2+} channels also have associated subunits (termed $\alpha 2$, β, γ, δ) that modify the properties of the channel formed by the $\alpha 1$-subunits. Depending on the species, the nerve terminal of the endplate may predominantly contain P/Q or N type Ca^{2+} channels.[5–7] The Ca^{2+} channels located in the terminal of the mammalian NMJ are P/Q type.[6,7]

There is a large inward electrochemical driving force on Ca^{2+}. The extracellular Ca^{2+} concentration is normally four orders of magnitude greater than the intracellular concentration—therefore opening of voltage-gated Ca^{2+} channels would result in a large Ca^{2+} influx. One striking feature of transmitter release at synapses is its steep and nonlinear dependence on Ca^{2+} influx—a twofold increase in Ca^{2+} influx can increase transmitter release up to 16-fold.[8–11] This relationship indicates that at some site, called the Ca^{2+} sensor, the binding of up to four Ca^{2+} ions is required to trigger release.

Available evidence suggests that Ca^{2+} channels are highly localized at or near active zones where transmitter release occurs.[3,12–15] Opening of these channels provides a high, local increase in Ca^{2+} concentration at the site of transmitter release during the action potential. During an action potential, the Ca^{2+} concentration at the active zone can increase 100-fold to 1000-fold (from the resting level of about 100 nM to 10–100 μM) within a few hundred microseconds.[16–19] This large and rapid Ca^{2+} transient is required for the rapid synchronous release of transmitter. The Ca^{2+} sensor responsible for transmitter release may have a relatively low affinity for Ca^{2+}, with a K_d ranging between 10 and 100 μM.[17–19] Because of the relatively low affinity Ca^{2+} sensor, release may only take place in a narrow region surrounding Ca^{2+} channels, where the Ca^{2+} concentration is sufficient to trigger release.[20] The requirement for a high concentration of Ca^{2+} also ensures that release will be rapidly terminated on repolarization. The delay between Ca^{2+} influx and transmitter release is extremely short (approximately 0.2 milliseconds).[3,21,22]

Quantal Transmitter Release

Transmitter is released in quantal units. Fatt and Katz first observed small spontaneous postsynaptic potentials, called miniature endplate potentials (mepps), at the frog NMJ.[23] The size of these mepps is relatively fixed, about 0.5 mV. Each mepp is caused by release of about 7000 to 12,000 ACh molecules from a single vesicle.[24] During an action potential, the Ca^{2+} influx triggers fusion between the synaptic vesicle membrane and the plasma membrane. A fusion pore spans these two membranes.[25] The pore rapidly dilates, and transmitter inside the vesicle rapidly diffuses across the synaptic cleft to act on its postsynaptic receptors. The opening of postsynaptic receptors generates an epp (see "Postsynaptic Aspects").

In addition to acting on the postsynaptic receptors, ACh may also act on nicotinic ACh autoreceptors on motor nerve terminals, which may depolarize the nerve terminal and increase the intracellular Ca^{2+} level.[26–29] These actions may result in facilitation of ACh release during subsequent action potential stimulation. Consequently, inhibition of presynaptic AChRs by the muscle relaxant drug tubocurarine may block facilitation of release during a train of presynaptic firing. This mechanism, together with the well-characterized inhibitory effect of tubocurarine on the postsynaptic AChR, may contribute to muscle relaxation during administration of tubocurarine.

An action potential triggers fusion of about 300 vesicles at a frog NMJ.[30] A smaller number of released vesicles is observed in mammalian NMJs. For example, an action potential releases about 40 vesicles in rat diaphragm.[31] During an action potential, each active zone releases about one vesicle. In each active zone, tens of vesicles are attached to the plasma membrane. These vesicles are called docked vesicles. They are believed to be immediately available for release.[32,33] The number of vesicles released from each active zone during an action potential depends on the number of immediately releasable vesicles (releasable pool size) and the mean release probability of each releasable vesicle. Modulation of either of these two parameters may change the epp size.

Cycling of Synaptic Vesicles

In various physiologic conditions, the motor nerve may fire (generate action potentials) repetitively. Continued repetitive firing inevitably causes depletion of the releasable pool, which results in depression of the epp evoked by presynaptic action potentials. To maintain synaptic transmission during repetitive firing, vesicles in a pool not adjacent to the active zone plasma membrane (called the reserve pool) must move to those empty docking sites and become available for release. This process is called vesicle mobilization.[34] The rate of mobilization might be facilitated during repetitive firing, possibly mediated by an increase of the intracellular Ca^{2+} concentration.[35–38]

During prolonged repetitive firing, vesicles in the reserve pool will eventually be depleted if there is no replenishment of vesicles. To continue supplying vesicles, the vesicle membrane that is fused with the plasma membrane is retrieved and recycled, generating new synaptic vesicles[39,40] (Fig. 10–4). The rate of membrane retrieval (endocytosis) may be critical for maintaining transmitter release during prolonged repetitive action potential stimulation.[41] The time constant of endocytosis is increased as the intensity of stimulation is increased.[42,43] There appear to be at least two temporally distinct types of endocytosis. Slow endocytosis (time constant of tens of seconds to minutes) is believed to be mediated by clathrin-coated pits.[44] In the 1970s, it was hypothesized that vesicles bud from the plasma membrane and then fuse together to form an endosome, a type of internal membrane compartment[39] (Fig. 10–4). After processing, new synaptic vesicles bud off the endosome, completing the recycling process. Recent studies suggest that endosomes are generated by endocytosis of a large plasma membrane invagination, a process called macropinocytosis.[45] Slow endocytosis may be important at normal to high rates of release. A fast form of endocytosis (time constant of 1–2

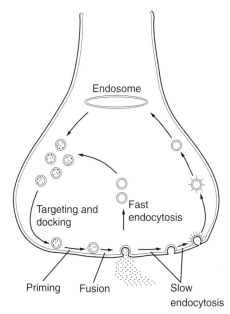

Figure 10–4. Cycling of synaptic vesicles at nerve terminals. Vesicles are targeted to the active zone and then dock at the active zone. The docked vesicles become primed so that they can undergo exocytosis. In response to an increase in Ca^{2+}, vesicles undergo fusion and release their contents. The fused vesicle membrane is taken into the interior of the cell by endocytosis. Endocytosis can be slow or fast. The slow endocytosis is believed to be mediated by clathrin-coated pits. It was hypothesized that endocytosed vesicles fuse with the endosome, an internal membrane compartment (see the report by Heuser and Reese[39]). After processing, new synaptic vesicles bud off the endosome, completing the recycling process. Fast endocytosis is believed to occur at the same site where exocytosis occurs and is not mediated through clathrin-coated pits. Vesicles endocytosed through the fast process may join the pool of vesicles for targeting and docking or priming.

seconds) is thought to involve release of transmitter through the transient opening and closing of the fusion pore without full membrane fusion.[46] The advantage of such "kiss-and-run" release is that it rapidly recycles the vesicle for subsequent release because it requires only closure of the fusion pore. Fast endocytosis might predominate at lower to normal release rates.

Proteins Involved in Vesicle Fusion

The molecular mechanisms that drives vesicles to cluster near synapses, to dock at active zones, to fuse with the membrane in response to Ca^{2+} influx, and to recycle has been intensively studied in the past decade.[47] Proteins have been identified that are thought to (1) restrain the vesicles so as to prevent their accidental mobilization, (2) target the freed vesicles to the active zone, (3) dock the targeted vesicles at the active zone and prime them for fusion, (4) allow fusion and exocytosis, and (5) retrieve the fused membrane by endocytosis (Fig. 10–5). Synapsin I is thought to anchor vesicles that are away from active zones to a network

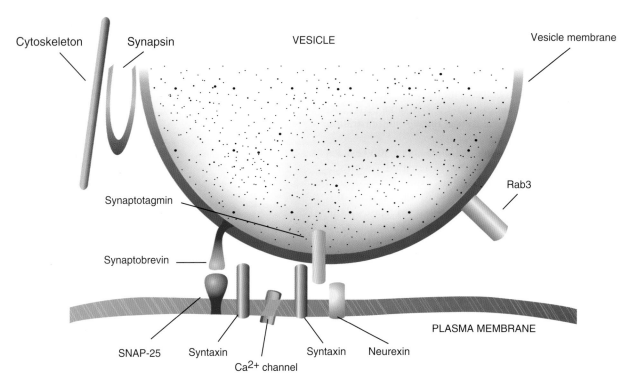

Figure 10–5. Some characterized vesicle proteins and their postulated localization and function. Synapsins are vesicle-associated proteins that are thought to mediate interaction between the synaptic vesicle and the cytoskeletal elements of the nerve terminal. The Rab proteins appear to be involved in vesicle trafficking within the cell and also in targeting of vesicles within the nerve terminal. The docking and fusion of vesicles appear to involve interactions between vesicle proteins and proteins of the nerve terminal plasma membrane: synaptobrevin (VAMP) and synaptotagmin (p65) on the vesicle membrane, and SNAP-25, syntaxins, and neurexins on the nerve terminal membrane.

of cytoskeletal filaments.[48–50] When the nerve terminal is depolarized and Ca^{2+} enters, synapsin is thought to become phosphorylated by Ca^{2+}/calmodulin-dependent protein kinase. Phosphorylation frees the vesicles from the cytoskeletal constraint, allowing them to move into the active zone.

The targeting of synaptic vesicles to docking sites for release is thought to be carried out by Rab3A and Rab3C, two members of a class of small proteins, related to the *ras* proto-oncogene superfamily, that bind GTP and hydrolyze it to GDP and inorganic phosphate.[51] Following the targeting of a vesicle to its release site, a complex set of interactions occurs between proteins in the synaptic vesicle membrane and proteins in the presynaptic membrane. Such interactions are thought to complete the docking of vesicles and to prime them so they are ready to undergo fusion in response to Ca^{2+} influx. One prominent hypothesis for this complex interaction is called the SNARE hypothesis.[52,53] According to this hypothesis, specific integral proteins in the vesicle membrane including synaptobrevin (or VAMP) bind to specific receptor proteins in the presynaptic membrane, including syntaxin and SNAP-25.

Synaptotagmin (or p65) is an integral membrane protein of the synaptic vesicle thought to be the Ca^{2+} sensor for transmitter release.[54–57] Synaptotagmin contains two domains (the C2 domains) homologous to the regulatory region of protein kinase C. The C2 domains bind to phos-

pholipids in a Ca^{2+}-dependent manner. This property suggests that synaptotagmin might insert into the presynaptic phospholipid bilayer in response to Ca^{2+} influx, thus serving as the Ca^{2+} sensor for exocytosis. Only a few proteins critical for transmitter release have been discussed in this chapter. There are many other vesicle proteins that may be involved in transmitter release.[47] How these proteins interact with each other and control transmitter release is currently being intensively studied. A clearer picture regarding the function of each protein in control of transmitter release may emerge in the near future.

Summary

An action potential, generated by rapid Na^+ influx and K^+ efflux, activates Ca^{2+} channels. The Ca^{2+} influx through Ca^{2+} channels triggers vesicle fusion and transmitter release. Vesicle mobilization and recycling ensures sufficient supply of vesicles for release. These processes may be the sites where anesthetics act. For example, local anesthetic agents stop sensation by blocking conduction of nerve impulses, an effect achieved by blocking Na^+ channels.[58] Volatile anesthetics may activate K^+ channels and inhibit Ca^{2+} channels, which may contribute to their inhibitory effect on transmitter release.[59–65] Genetic evidence suggests that volatile anesthetics may modulate transmitter release by interaction with syntaxin, a membrane protein that interacts with vesicle proteins and Ca^{2+} channels.[66] Vesicle mobilization and recycling process might also be targets for anesthetics, although this issue has not been studied.

Cleft Aspects

Acetylcholinesterase

The synaptic cleft provides the delimited volume in which released ACh diffuses to the AChR on the postsynaptic membrane. The major macromolecular component of the cleft, in the context of neuromuscular transmission, is AChE. AChE at the NMJ is a large complex, comprising four catalytic subunits bound to a long collagenous "tail" that serves to anchor AChE to the extracellular matrix in the cleft.[67]

Physical Dimensions

The synaptic cleft is about 50 nm across. The very small volume of the cleft means that the local concentrations of critical molecules can be very high. For example, there are about 2000 AChE active sites per square micrometer at the NMJ.[68] If this number is uniformly distributed through the volume of the cleft, the concentration of active sites is about 60 μM. Similarly, the density of AChR in the postsynaptic membrane is about 10,000 per square micrometer.[68] If these receptors were uniformly distributed, the concentration of binding sites (two on each receptor) would be about 600 μM.

The small dimensions also can result in rapid processes. Because the diffusion constant for ACh is approximately $1 \times 10^{-5}\,cm^2\,s^{-1}$, it will take only about 1 microsecond for ACh released at the presynaptic membrane to equilibrate across the cleft. It is also true that the concentration of ACh in the cleft reaches a very high level. The estimated number of ACh molecules in a vesicle is 5,000 to 10,000 (see earlier). When this number of molecules is rapidly released, the concentration in the cleft is likely to approach 1 mM for a brief period.[68,69] There are three basic events that a free ACh molecule can experience: it can continue to diffuse in the cleft, it can bind to cholinesterase (and be degraded), or it can bind to a postsynaptic AChR (and participate in activation). Free diffusion is important immediately after release, because the binding sites on AChE and AChR are saturated by the high local ACh concentration. However, the high concentrations of sites means that the free ACh is rapidly bound and immobilized (see Fig. 10–2); for example, a disk of radius 0.4 μm contains about 10,000 binding sites on AChR and 1,000 on AChE.

Muscle excitation follows after binding of ACh to the AChR, and is discussed in the next section. Binding of ACh to AChE results in cleavage of ACh to acetate and choline.

This reaction is rapid, with an association rate of about $2 \times 10^8\,M^{-1}\,s^{-1}$ and a dissociation constant of about 50 μM.[67] The catalytic rate for AChE is about $10^4\,s^{-1}$, corresponding to an average time between binding of ACh and hydrolysis of 100 microseconds.[67] Choline is, in general, a very weak activator of the AChR and therefore the hydrolysis products are inactive. Choline, in turn, is cleared from the synaptic cleft by diffusion and by a high-affinity uptake transporter, which is located on the presynaptic nerve membrane. It should be noted, however, that at least one of the mutations of the AChR that is found in congenital myasthenic syndrome has a significantly greater likelihood of being activated by choline.[70] Accordingly, choline may serve as a long-lasting activator at NMJ in some patients.

After the initial high concentration, there is a slow release of ACh from AChR with closed channels. Because the release is not synchronized, the concentration stays low and AChE hydrolyzes the free ACh.

Acetylcholinesterase Inhibition

AChE is clearly an essential component of the NMJ. Indeed, the toxicity of anticholinesterases (including some pesticides and nerve gases) is due in part to muscle paralysis.[71] The mechanism(s) by which paralysis is produced is still somewhat controversial, and it may be that different mechanisms are relatively more important at different times after intoxication or in different species. However, all of the processes are initiated by the fact that the ACh in the cleft is not degraded. In this case, the postsynaptic receptors are exposed to high concentrations of ACh for a longer period of time. In addition, the ACh can diffuse from the synaptic cleft and reach portions of the nerve terminal axon that normally would not be exposed to ACh during neuromuscular transmission.

There are likely to be at least two postsynaptic and two presynaptic processes involved. On the postsynaptic side, the first is prolonged depolarization of the muscle fiber in response to trains of nerve action potentials.[72,73] Prolonged depolarization initially produces multiple action potentials in the muscle fiber in response to a single nerve action potential, and can enhance the twitch. However, prolonged depolarization results in inactivation of voltage-gated sodium channels in the muscle fiber near the NMJ, and a resulting failure of action potential generation. A second action is desensitization of the AChR,[73] as a result of the continued presence of ACh. Desensitization is a process in which AChRs bind ACh, but enter a state in which each has a closed channel and is refractory to activation (see "Receptor Desensitization").

On the presynaptic side, a common observation is the presence of repetitive action potentials in the motor axons.[74,75] This repetitive activity apparently reflects depolarization of the axon as a result of the activation of nicotinic receptors that are located on the terminal axon, although not immediately at the nerve terminal. Prolonged depolarization could produce sodium channel inactivation and failure of the action potential to invade the terminal, resulting in reduced release of ACh. The final proposed mechanism involves a second type of presynaptic nicotinic receptor that, when activated, provides a positive feedback mechanism that normally enhances release of ACh (see "Cycling of Synaptic Vesicles"). The prolonged presence of ACh could desensitize these receptors, which could result in a more rapid decrement in transmitter release during trains of nerve action potentials.

Longer inhibition of cholinesterase activity results in characteristic degeneration of the NMJ. The fragmentation probably results from excessive entry of Ca^{2+} into the postjunctional volume of the muscle fiber.[76]

A rare congenital muscular disorder is associated with very low (or absent) AChE activity at the NMJ. Individuals with this disorder show muscle weakness and fatigability, and many die at young ages. The NMJs are smaller than usual, and show evidence of disorganization.[77] It is fascinating that the disorder does not appear to reflect a mutation in the gene encoding the AChE enzyme. Instead, all the affected individuals show mutations in the gene encoding a large extracellular molecule (collagen Q) that serves to anchor AChE in the synaptic cleft.[77–79] Transgenic mice have been produced with either the collagen Q gene[80] or the AChE gene[81] deleted. Both deletions result in a great increase in mortality—when the cholinesterase gene is knocked out, no animals survived past 3 weeks, whereas when the collagen Q gene was knocked out, only 50% survived after 3 weeks and only 10% lived to adulthood. That the loss of AChE activity was not immediately lethal was surprising to both groups of researchers, given the effects of acute inhibition of cholinesterase activity. Various possible compensating mechanisms may operate, including a low residual activity of either AChE or butyrylcholinesterase in the cleft.[80,81] The animals that lacked AChE activity also showed numerous developmental abnormalities, which might reflect a role for AChE as a neurotrophic factor more generally in the nervous system.[82,83] The structure of the NMJ was normal in the mice without AChE, which was unexpected based on the effects of long-term anticholinesterase treatment (see earlier). In contrast, animals in which ColQ had been genetically removed showed simpler junctions with a reduction in the functional area of the NMJ, reflecting both a smaller size and an increased number of glial processes interposed between the nerve terminal and the muscle fiber.[80]

The physiologic processes underlying interactions between neuromuscular blocking agents and anticholinesterase drugs will be explored later (see "Neuromuscular Transmission and Functional Consequences of Drug Action").

Postsynaptic Aspects

Muscle Nicotinic Acetylcholine Receptors

Langley[84] first postulated the idea of a "receptive substance" on the muscle fiber, localized to the site of nerve contact. Subsequent physiologic studies demonstrated that the muscle response consisted of a depolarization caused by an increase in membrane conductance.[85] The channel is selective for cations over anions but relatively weakly selective among monovalent cations.[86] Divalent cations, most notably calcium ions, also are permeant through the channel.[87,88] Channel gating is dependent on membrane potential (at positive membrane potentials the channel closes more rapidly),[89,90] but the voltage dependence is weak.

The muscle nicotinic AChR is a member of an extended gene family that includes neuronal nicotinic receptors, and receptors for γ-aminobutyric acid ($GABA_A$ and $GABA_C$ receptors), glycine, and serotonin ($5\text{-}HT_3$ receptors).[91,92] It is intriguing that the physiologic role for neuronal nicotinic receptors appears to be the modulation of transmitter release (see earlier).[93–95] All of the receptors in this gene family have a similar overall structure (see summary in Figure 10–6). Each complete receptor is composed of five subunits, arranged in a donut with the gated ion channel in the middle. The nicotinic receptor at the adult NMJ is composed of two copies of the α-subunit, one β-subunit, one δ-subunit, and one ε-subunit. The receptor found early in fetal development and after denervation has a γ-subunit replacing the ε-subunit.[96]

Each subunit of the AChR is predicted to have four membrane-spanning regions (M1–M4). The pore of the ion channel is thought to be formed by the M2 region of each of the five subunits constituting a single receptor. The receptor has a relatively large extension into the extracellular space, with a tapering funnel leading down to the mouth of the ion channel proper.[97,98] There is a smaller extension into the cytoplasm, which probably interacts with the cytoplasmic proteins required to concentrate the receptors in the postsynaptic membrane.[99] The amino-terminal domains of the various subunits form the extracellular portion of the receptor and contain the bindings sites for ACh. These binding sites (two on each AChR) recognize ACh and other agonists, as well as competitive antagonists. The binding sites are located at the interfaces between subunits; for the adult AChR, one binding site is located between an α-subunit and the ε-subunit, and the other between an α-subunit and the δ-subunit.[100] The crystal structure of a related ACh-binding protein suggests that the ACh binding sites are located about half of the way down the interface from the extracellular space.[98] The crystal structure is also fascinating in that it demonstrates how the protein folds bring together residues widely separated along the primary sequence of the protein to form the ACh binding site.[101]

The second major identified pharmacologic site is located within the pore of the ion channel and is the site at which noncompetitive "channel-blocking" drugs act. These drugs are thought to enter an open channel and basically plug the hole, preventing ion movement.[90] Many of the mutations that have been found to affect the gating of the channel occur in the membrane-spanning regions; the largest number have been found in M2, but examples in all the regions are known[101,102] (see Fig. 10–6).

Receptor Activation

The postsynaptic receptor is specialized for rapidly detecting and responding to high concentrations of ACh in the cleft. The basic scheme for receptor activation is shown in Figure 10–7. Almost all receptors with open channels have

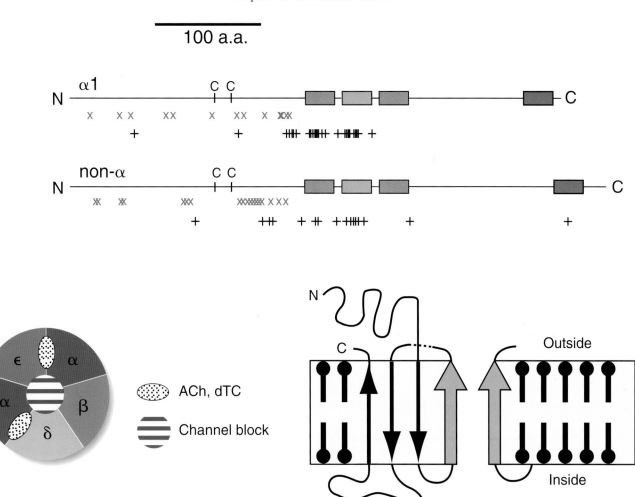

Figure 10–6. A summary of the structure of the muscle nicotinic receptor. *Top,* Schematic summaries of the primary sequences of the α- and non-α (β, δ, γ and ε)-subunits. The amino terminus of the protein is shown to the left. *Bottom right,* The amino terminus is located extracellularly, followed by three membrane-spanning regions. The second membrane-spanning region (shown as orange) forms a major part of the channel lining for the receptor. There is a relatively long cytoplasmic loop between the third and fourth membrane-spanning regions, then a final membrane-spanning region and a short, extracellular carboxy-terminal sequence. A number of residues have been identified that contribute to binding sites for nicotinic agonists and competitive antagonists (x), as well as residues that, when mutated, affect channel gating (+). In addition to the residues involved in binding agonists, a number of residues in the second membrane-spanning regions (orange segment, residues not shown) are involved in binding noncompetitive antagonists. *Bottom left,* Schematic view of the receptor (as viewed face-on from the outside of the membrane). The receptor is a pentamer of subunits, and the binding sites for ACh are formed at intersubunit interfaces (α/δ and α/ε). The site for noncompetitive blockers ("channel block") is formed from residues contributed by all five subunits, and is in the ion channel.

two ACh molecules bound. The channel can open without any bound ACh, or with only one ACh molecule bound.[103,104] However, with normal receptors (i.e., receptors that are neither mutated nor chemically modified) the opening rates for unliganded or partially liganded receptors are very low and the closing rates are very high, therefore the contributions of these open receptors are physiologically negligible. The most recent estimates indicate that the association rate for ACh binding to the resting state of the receptor is similar for the two sites (at the αε and αδ interfaces) and are large, about $10^8 M^{-1} sec^{-1}$; the dissociation rate is also large, about

$10,000 sec^{-1}$.[105,106] The channel opening rate is even larger than the dissociation rate, about $60,000 sec^{-1}$.[107] On the average, then, after the second ACh molecule binds it is more likely that the channel will open rather than that ACh will dissociate. The channel opens, on the average, within 10 microseconds after the second ACh binds. The channel closing rate is about $2000 sec^{-1}$,[105,106] therefore a channel remains open only about 0.5 millisecond. An active receptor does not produce a single opening, but rather makes a "burst" of activity,[108,109] which contains an average of five or so openings (the number is determined by the ratio of the

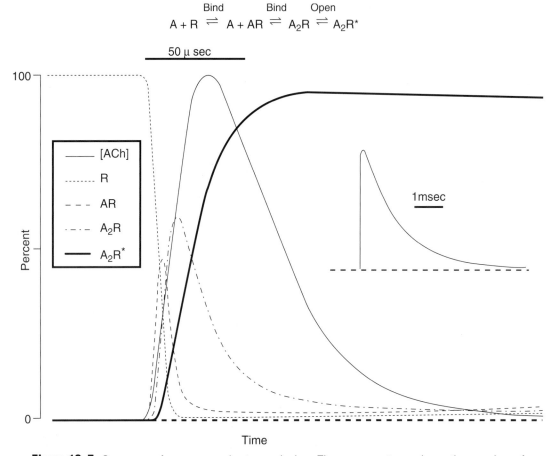

Figure 10–7. Summary of neuromuscular transmission. Figure presents a schematic overview of receptor activation during transmission. The top line shows a kinetic scheme for receptor activation: an acetylcholine receptor (AChR) with a closed channel (R) binds two ACh molecules (A) to form the diliganded receptor with a closed channel (A_2R). The channel then opens (A_2R^*). *Bottom*, Traces show a calculated time course for the various states shown. It is assumed that the free ACh concentration in the cleft rises and falls as shown by the *thin solid line* (peak concentration of 500 µM). The other lines show the various receptor states, as percentage of the total receptors exposed to that concentration of ACh. The resting receptors (R; *dotted line*) diminish rapidly; monoliganded receptors (AR; *dashed line*) increase, but then decrease as the second site is occupied. Diliganded receptors with closed channels increase rapidly (A_2R; *dash-dot line*), but diminish in number as the channels open. Finally, the active receptors (A_2R^*; *thick solid line*) increase with a short lag following A_2R, and then stay highly prevalent because of the relatively slow receptor burst duration. *Inset*, The time course of the predicted A_2R^* state, at a slower resolution. The rates used to simulate these traces were chosen to be representative of the measured rates (see text) and were: association rate for ACh, $2 \times 10^9 \, M^{-1}s^{-1}$; dissociation rate for ACh, $2 \times 10^4 \, s^{-1}$; channel opening rate, $6 \times 10^4 \, s^{-1}$; channel closing rate, $2 \times 10^3 \, s^{-1}$. The association and dissociation rates give an estimated microscopic dissociation constant of $2 \times 10^{-5} \, M$.

opening rate to the dissociation rate). The closings within the burst are brief, only about 10 microseconds in duration; therefore a burst functionally resembles a single, longer opening. The burst is terminated when one ACh molecule dissociates from the receptor. During transmission at a normal junction, an AChR gets only one chance to become active, by binding ACh during the initial high concentration transient. Because the burst lasts about 1 millisecond, the free ACh concentration in the cleft has already declined to a low level by the end of the burst. Accordingly, the rate for rebinding ACh molecules and initiating a second burst is negligible.

The adult ($\alpha_2\beta\delta\epsilon$) and fetal ($\alpha_2\beta\delta\gamma$) receptors have characteristic physiologic differences—the fetal receptor has a

longer burst duration (threefold to sixfold) and a lower single channel conductance (about 60% of the adult receptor conductance).[96] There are some additional pharmacologic differences,[110] which might have some consequences in particular circumstances. The remainder of this chapter concentrates on the properties of the adult AChR and NMJ.

Receptor Desensitization

AChR can become desensitized.[111,112] If ACh or another agonist is present for a long time (approximately 1 second or longer), the receptor enters a different conformation in which it binds ACh with a high affinity but no longer is activatable.[113] Data indicate that there are at least two distinguishable desensitized states[114–116]; the states can be distinguished because one is faster to develop and recover than the other. It also is likely that desensitization preferentially develops from receptors with open channels,[117] although there is evidence that some receptors with no or one bound ACh molecule can desensitize.[118,119] Currently, there is no evidence that desensitization plays a role in normal transmission,[120] although it seems quite possible that desensitization plays a role in some phases of neuromuscular block by depolarizing blocking drugs (see later) and anticholinesterase agents.

Mechanisms and Sites of Action for Drugs on the Muscle Acetylcholine Receptors

Noncompetitive Inhibitors

There are a variety of noncompetitive inhibitors of the AChR, including local anesthetics, nondepolarizing blocking agents, and even ACh itself. The primary mechanism for noncompetitive block is open channel block, as briefly described earlier. In physiologic experiments, these drugs reduce the duration of channel openings.[90] The simplest explanation for this effect is that the drugs actually plug the channel and so prevent ion movement. This simple view has gained some support from biochemical studies that have shown that some photoactivatable noncompetitive drugs can be chemically linked to portions of the receptor that are thought to line the ion channel after irradiation in the appropriate conditions.[121] Finally, in an elegant set of experiments, a series of mutations were made in a set of amino acid residues in this region of the receptor and it was shown that changes were made in the action of a local anesthetic on the mutated receptor.[122,123] This convergent set of experiments has identified one pharmacologic site as the actual channel, and one mechanism of action to be occlusion of the channel.

Many cholinergic drugs, including ACh and carbamylcholine,[124,125] d-tubocurarine,[126] metocurine,[127] decamethonium,[128] and succinylcholine,[129] are able to block channels by this mechanism. As a rule, however, this action is not of physiologic significance. For example, d-tubocurarine actually has a higher affinity as a noncompetitive blocker for the receptors at the frog NMJ than as a competitive antagonist.[126] However, the neuromuscular blockade that results in paralysis is almost entirely caused by its actions as a competitive antagonist.[126,130] This apparent contradiction is explained by the fact that noncompetitive blockers act only after the channel has opened, and under normal conditions the channel opens for such a brief time that the noncompetitive block cannot reach equilibrium.[126] Conversely, the competitive action is established during the long periods between episodes of neuromuscular transmission.

There are still some significant areas of uncertainty in terms of the actions of noncompetitive blockers. The first question is whether there are multiple mechanisms of noncompetitive inhibition. For example, some drugs have been found to enhance development of desensitization,[131,132] and

some inhibiting drugs apparently bind to regions of the receptor far from the pore.[133] There are also several questions with regard to the better-characterized noncompetitive blockers. Is the physical mechanism simple occlusion of the ion channel by the blocker, or is there a conformational change in the protein that closes the channel?[90] Do some blockers act on both closed and open channels (as has been suggested for isoflurane)?[134] The final question is: can the channel close around a noncompetitive blocker and produce a long-lived "trapped block"? Trapping has been found to occur for some drugs acting on the muscle AChR,[135] but the overall importance of trapping is not known.

Nondepolarizing Competitive Blocking Drugs

The most venerable nondepolarizing blocking drug (NDB) is d-tubocurarine. Almost 150 years ago, it was suggested that the paralyzing action of d-tubocurarine was caused by a block of muscle excitability, rather than an action on the nerve.[136] The greatest advance in understanding the structure of the receptor, and in understanding the interactions of drugs with the ACh binding site, came with the realization that some paralyzing snake venoms contained a toxin that bound essentially irreversibly to the AChR and prevented ACh from binding.[137–139] The use of snake α-neurotoxins as high-affinity ligands for the ACh binding sites on the AChR has been exploited to define the interactions of many drugs with these sites.

In the 1980s it was shown that there are two sites on each receptor that would bind an α-neurotoxin, and that an agonist or an NDB could occupy either of the sites. However, the two sites had different affinities for most NDBs.[140,141] The affinities could differ by up to 100-fold (for metocurine), or as little as 10-fold (for pancuronium).[130,141] Subsequent biochemical work has shown that the site formed at the interface between the α- and δ-subunits has the lower affinity, and the αε (or αγ) site has the higher affinity.[100,142] Careful comparisons of the occupancy of sites by NDBs and block of receptor activation have shown that occupancy of one or both sites results in functional block of adult receptors.[130,143] Accordingly, direct measurement of the inhibition of activation of AChR shows a half-blocking concentration of NDB, which is close to the affinity for the high affinity site. It has been suggested[144] that some NDBs might show functional synergy in block because the two sites on the AChR had opposite selectivities for some NDBs. However, the data indicate that this is not correct, and that the αδ site has low affinity for NDBs,[130] with the exception of a peptide toxin (α cenotoxin M1).[145]

One possible complication in understanding the actions of NDBs has been the suggestion that these drugs, although they bind with high affinity, have rapid dissociation rates (possibly >1000 sec⁻¹).[146] If an NDB had an average binding time of less than 1 millisecond, then there would likely be a competitive interaction between the NDB and the high cleft ACh concentrations. This would mean that the equilibrium occupancy measurements would not be the appropriate parameters to use in understanding block of transmission. However, recent experiments have found that the dissociation rates from mammalian (mouse) receptors are slow—about 30 sec⁻¹ for d-tubocurarine and about

4 sec^{-1} for pancuronium.[147–149] This dissociation rate is sufficiently slow that no competition would occur during normal transmission.

The relationship between the occupancy of sites on the AChR by an NDB and block of twitch is nonlinear, as discussed in "Neuromuscular Transmission and Functional Consequences of Drug Action."[150] A critical point is that block of the twitch requires occupancy of more than 90% of the ACh binding sites on the AChR, and indeed the concentrations of NDBs required to block twitch are 10-fold or more greater than the concentrations necessary to block activation by 50% or to occupy half of the high-affinity binding sites.[130]

Depolarizing Blocking Drugs

The depolarizing blocking drugs succinylcholine and decamethonium act as weak activators of the muscle AChR.[129,151] They produce depolarization of the muscle, can desensitize the receptor after prolonged exposure, and can also block the channel.[129,151] However, the mechanism by which they produce paralysis is still debated.[152] The same basic postsynaptic and presynaptic mechanisms have been proposed as in the case of anticholinesterases (see earlier), with the exogenous depolarizing blocking drug acting as an agonist on postsynaptic or presynaptic nicotinic receptors.

Neuromuscular Transmission and Functional Consequences of Drug Action

We have emphasized that during neuromuscular transmission there is a high concentration of ACh in the cleft, for a brief time. There is also a high density of binding sites, on both the AChR and AChE. Accordingly, the released ACh does not have the opportunity to diffuse any great distance, and the contents of each vesicle act only very locally. For example, the response to the exocytosis of a single vesicle produces a miniature endplate current with peak amplitude corresponding to the opening of about 1,000 channels. This number of receptors is within a disk of radius less than 0.2 micrometer. Even though a number of quanta are released during normal transmission (about 50 to 100), the release sites are relatively widely separated compared with the diffusion distance, and only a small fraction of the available AChR are involved. Accordingly, the response to the many vesicles released following an action potential can be thought of in terms of a simple summation of the response to 50 or 100 separate quantal releases.[153] A number of experimental studies and theoretic calculations have indicated that most of the ACh that is released actually is captured by AChR (50% to 80%),[154–157] which occurs in a small disk of postsynaptic membrane.

These considerations, and others, led to the idea that transmission occurs in a "saturated disk"—a small region of postsynaptic membrane in which most receptors bind two ACh molecules, with a relatively small annulus of partially occupied receptors.[68,153,157,158] As mentioned earlier, the ion channel opens for most receptors that have bound two molecules of ACh, but not for receptors that have bound only

one, therefore the disk of activated receptors is sharply delineated.

Transmission at the NMJ has a large safety factor—block of a twitch evoked by nerve stimulation requires a high concentration of blocking agent.[159–161] The safety factor arises from several basic mechanisms. One is that there is a nonlinear relationship between the activated conductance and the resulting membrane depolarization, so that a larger fraction of the endplate current must be blocked to produce a similar relative reduction in endplate potential. One simple way to think about the necessary number of open channels is to compare the resting input conductance of a muscle fiber to the activatable conductance. A typical muscle fiber might have an input resistance of 500,000 Ohms (or a conductance of 2×10^{-6} Siemens).[162] An adult AChR has a single channel conductance of about 60×10^{-12} Siemens; and for simplicity we will assume that the reversal potential for current through the channel is 0 mV. At steady-state, to depolarize the muscle fiber from a resting potential of −70 mV to a threshold for action potential generation of −50 mV, it would be necessary to activate only about 13,000 AChRs. In contrast, there are about 50,000 to 100,000 AChR channels open at the peak of the evoked response (see earlier), giving a safety factor of threefold to sixfold. It is also clear that there is a large excess of AChR available—only 0.5% to 1% of the total receptors are involved in producing a typical EPC, and only 0.1% of the receptors are required to produce an EPC that reaches threshold.

The final origin for the large safety factor arises from the properties of the "saturated disk" model for transmission. Experiments and theoretic calculations[157,163,164] have shown that the block of the evoked endplate current is not a linear function of the amount of block of the postsynaptic AChR. Instead, when only a small fraction of the receptors are blocked there is even less block of the EPC. This phenomenon arises because the released ACh can diffuse a little further to encounter an unblocked receptor; that some of the binding sites are already occupied by blocker means that ACh is then free to diffuse further and encounter more receptors. To reduce the EPC to 30% of normal, about 90% of the AChR need to be rendered inactive.[150]

This last consideration is thought to underlie the ability of anticholinesterase agents to reverse the block produced by nondepolarizing blocking agents. The released ACh can diffuse further, to encounter more available AChR, when it is not bound and hydrolyzed by AChE. It is also possible that the longer persistence of ACh in the cleft might result in more competition between ACh and blocker (depending on the dissociation rate for the blocker).

There is a possibility that the same mechanism could allow an antiesterase to reverse a block produced by desensitization of receptors by a depolarizing blocking agent. Greater diffusion of ACh could allow it to encounter a sufficient number of nondesensitized receptors to permit the re-establishment of transmission.

References

1. Hodgkin AL, Huxley AF: Currents carried by sodium and potassium ions through the membrane of the giant axon of loligo. J Physiol (Lond) 116:449–472, 1952.

2. Hodgkin AL, Huxley AF: The components of membrane conductance in the giant axon of loligo. J Physiol (Lond) 116:473–496, 1952.

3. Borst JGG, Sakmann B: Calcium influx and transmitter release in a fast CNS synapse. Nature 383:431–434, 1996.

4. Dunlap K, Luebke JI, Turner TJ: Exocytotic Ca^{2+} channels in mammalian central neurons. Trends Neurosci 18:89–98, 1995.

5. Kerr LM, Yoshikami D: A venom peptide with a novel presynaptic blocking action. Nature 308:282–284, 1984.

6. Uchitel OD, Protti DA, Sanchez V, et al: P-type voltage-dependent calcium channel mediates presynaptic calcium influx and transmitter release in mammalian synapses. Proc Natl Acad Sci USA 89:3330–3333, 1992.

7. Katz E, Ferro PA, Weisz G, Uchitel OD: Calcium channels involved in synaptic transmission at the mature and regenerating mouse neuromuscular junction. J Physiol 497:687–697, 1996.

8. Dodge FA, Rahamimoff R: Co-operative action of calcium ions in transmitter release at the neuromuscular junction. J Physiol 193:419–432, 1967.

9. Augustine GJ, Charlton MP, Smith SJ: Calcium entry and transmitter release at voltage-clamped nerve terminals of squid. J Physiol 369:163–181, 1985.

10. Landò L, Zucker RS: Ca^{2+} Cooperativity in neurosecretion measured using photolabile Ca^{2+} chelators. J Neurophysiol 72:825–830, 1994.

11. Wu LG, Saggau P: Presynaptic calcium is increased during normal synaptic transmission and paired-pulse facilitation, but not in long-term potentiation in area CA1 of hippocampus. J Neurosci 14:645–654, 1994.

12. Robitaille R, Adler EM, Charlton MP: Strategic location of calcium channels at transmitter release sites of frog neuromuscular synapses. Neuron 5:773–779, 1990.

13. Adler EM, Augustine GJ, Duffy SN, Charlton MP: Alien intracellular calcium chelators attenuate neurotransmitter release at the squid giant synapse. J Neurosci 11:1496–1507, 1991.

14. Stanley EF: Single calcium channels and acetylcholine release at a presynaptic nerve terminal. Neuron 11:1007–1011, 1993.

15. Wu LG, Westenbroek RE, Borst JGG, et al: Calcium channel types with distinct presynaptic localization couple differentially to transmitter release in single calyx-type synapses. J Neuorsci 19:726–736, 1999.

16. Llinás RR, Sugimori M, Silver RB: Microdomains of high calcium concentration in a presynaptic terminal. Science 256:677–679, 1992.

17. Heidelberger R, Heinemann C, Neher E, Matthews G: Calcium dependence of the rate of exocytosis in a synaptic terminal. Nature 371:513–515, 1994.

18. Bollmann JH, Sakmann B, Borst JG: Calcium sensitivity of glutamate release in a calyx-type terminal. Science 289:953–957, 2000.

19. Schneggenburger R, Neher E: Intracellular calcium dependence of transmitter release rates at a fast central synapse. Nature 406:889–893, 2000.

20. Neher E: Vesicle pools and Ca^{2+} microdomains: New tools for understanding their roles in neurotransmitter release. Neuron 20:389–399, 1998.

21. Hubbard JI, Schmidt RF: An electrophysiological investigation of mammalian motor nerve terminals. J Physiol 166:145–167, 1963.

22. Llinás RR, Steinberg IZ, Walton K: Relationship between presynaptic calcium current and postsynaptic potential in squid giant synapse. Biophys J 33:323–352, 1981.

23. Fatt P, Katz B: Spontaneous subthreshold activity at motor nerve endings. J Physiol 117:109–128, 1952.

24. Van der Kloot W: The regulation of quantal size. Prog Neurobiol 36:93–130, 1991.

25. Breckenridge LJ, Almers W: Currents through the fusion pore that forms during exocytosis of a secretory vesicle. Nature 328:814–817, 1987.

26. Wessler I: Control of transmitter release from the motor nerve by presynaptic nicotinic and muscarinic autoreceptors. Trends Pharmacol Sci 10:110–114, 1989.

27. Wessler I, Apel C, Garmsen M, Klein A: Effects of nicotine receptor agonists on acetylcholine release from the isolated motor nerve, small intestine and trachea of rats and guinea-pigs. Clin Invest 70:182–189, 1992.

28. Tsuneki H, Kimura I, Dezaki K, et al: Immunohistochemical localization of neuronal nicotinic receptor subtypes at the pre- and postjunctional sites in mouse diaphragm muscle. Neurosci Lett 196:13–16, 1995.

29. Tian L, Prior C, Dempster J, Marshall IG: Hexamethonium- and methyllycaconitine-induced changes in acetylcholine release from rat motor nerve terminals. Br J Pharmacol 122:1025–1034, 1997.

30. Van der Kloot W, Molgó J: Quantal acetylcholine release at the vertebrate neuromuscular junction. Physiol Rev 74:899–991, 1994.

31. Glavinovic MI: Voltage clamping of unparalysed cut rat diaphragm for study of transmitter release. J Physiol 290:467–480, 1979.

32. Schikorski T, Stevens CF: Quantitative ultrastructural analysis of hippocampal excitatory synapses. J Neuorsci 17:5858–5867, 1997.

33. Schikorski T, Stevens CF: Quantitative fine-structural analysis of olfactory cortical synapses. Proc Natl Acad Sci USA 96:4107–4112, 1999.

34. Zucker RS: Short-term synaptic plasticity. Annu Rev Neurosci 12:13–31, 1989.

35. Kusano K, Landau EM: Depression and recovery of transmission at the squid giant synapse. J Physiol 245:13–32, 1975.

36. Dittman JS, Regehr WG: Calcium dependence and recovery kinetics of presynaptic depression at the climbing fiber to purkinje cell synapse. J Neurosci 18:6147–6162, 1998.

37. Wang L-Y, Kaczmarek LK: High-frequency firing helps replenish the readily releasable pool of synaptic vesicles. Nature 394:384–388, 1998.

38. Wu LG, Borst JGG: The reduced release probability of releasable vesicles during recovery from short-term synaptic depression. Neuron 23:821–832, 1999.

39. Heuser JE, Reese TS: Evidence for recycling of synaptic vesicle membrane during transmitter release at the frog neuromuscular junction. J Cell Biol 57:315–344, 1973.

40. Ceccarelli B, Hurlbut WP, Mauro A: Turnover of transmitter and synaptic vesicles at the frog neuromuscular junction. J Cell Biol 57:499–524, 1973.

41. Wu LG, Betz WJ: Kinetics of synaptic depression and vesicle recycling after tetanic stimulation of frog motor nerve terminals. Biophys J 74:3003–3009, 1998.

42. Von Gersdorff H, Matthews G: Dynamics of synaptic vesicle fusion and membrane retrieval in synaptic terminals. Nature 367:735–739, 1994.

43. Wu LG, Betz WJ: Nerve activity but not intracellular calcium determines the time course of endocytosis at the frog neuromuscular junction. Neuron 17:769–779, 1996.

44. Schmid SL, McNiven MA, De Camilli P: Dynamin and its partners: A progress report. Curr Opin Cell Biol 10:504–512, 1998.

45. Wilkinson RS, Cole JC: Resolving the Heuser-Ceccarelli debate. Trends Neurosci 24:195–197, 2001.

46. Meldolesi J, Ceccarelli B: Exocytosis and membrane recycling. Phil Trans R Soc Lond B 296:55–65, 1981.

47. Fernandez-Chacon R, Sudhof TC: Genetics of synaptic vesicle function: Toward the complete functional anatomy of an organelle. Annu Rev Physiol 61:753–776, 1999.

48. Rosahl TW, Geppert M, Spillane D, et al: Short-term synaptic plasticity is altered in mice lacking synapsin I. Cell 75:661–670, 1993.

49. Rosahl TW, Spillane D, Missler M, et al: Essential functions of synapsins I and II in synaptic vesicle regulation. Nature 375:488–493, 1995.

50. Ryan TR, Li L, Chin L-S, et al: Synaptic vesicle recycling in synapsin I knock-out mice. J Cell Biol 134:1219–1227, 1996.

51. Geppert M, Sudhof TC: RAB3 and synaptotagmin: The yin and yang of synaptic membrane fusion. Annu Rev Neurosci 21:75–95, 1998.

52. Hanson PI, Heuser JE, Jahn R: Neurotransmitter release—four years of SNARE complexes. Curr Opin Neurobiol 7:310–315, 1997.

53. Jahn R, Sudhof TC: Membrane fusion and exocytosis. Annu Rev Biochem 68:863–911, 1999.

54. Littleton JT, Stern M, Schulze K, et al: Mutational analysis of Drosophila synaptotagmin demonstrates its essential role in Ca^{2+}-activated neurotransmitter release. Cell 74:1125–1134, 1993.

55. Geppert M, Goda Y, Hammer RE, et al: Synaptotagmin I: A major Ca^{2+} sensor for transmitter release at a central synapse. Cell 79:717–727, 1994.

56. DiAntonio A, Parfitt KD, Schwarz TL: Synaptic transmission persists in synaptotagmin mutants of Drosophila. Cell 73:1281–1290, 1993.

57. Nonet ML, Grundahl K, Meyer BJ, et al: Synaptic function is impaired but not eliminated in C. elegans mutants lacking synaptotagmin. Cell 73:1291–1305, 1993.

58. Moorman JR: Sodium channels. In Yaksh C, Lynch C, Zapol WM, et al (eds): Anesthesia: Biologic Foundations. Philadelphia, Lippincott-Raven, 1997, pp 145–162.

59. Franks NP, Lieb WR: Volatile general anaesthetics activate a novel neuronal K+ current. Nature 333:662–664, 1988.

60. Patel AJ, Honore E, Lesage F, et al: Inhalational anesthetics activate two-pore-domain background K+ channels. Nat Neurosci 2:422–426, 1999.

61. Ries CR, Puil E: Mechanism of anesthesia revealed by shunting actions of isoflurane on thalamocortical neurons. J Neurophysiol 81:1795–1801, 1999.

62. Ries CR, Puil E: Ionic mechanism of isoflurane's actions on thalamocortical neurons. J Neurophysiol 81:1802–1809, 1999.

63. Takenoshita M, Steinbach JH: Halothane blocks low-voltage-activated calcium current in rat sensory neurons. J Neurosci 11:1404–1412, 1991.

64. Hall AC, Lieb WR, Franks NP: Insensitivity of P-type calcium channels to inhalational and intravenous general anesthetics. Anesthesiology 81:117–123, 1994.

65. Study RE: Isoflurane inhibits multiple voltage-gated calcium currents in hippocampal pyramidal neurons. Anesthesiology 81:104–116, 1994.

66. van Swinderen B, Saifee O, Shebester L, et al: A neomorphic syntaxin mutation blocks volatile-anesthetic action in Caenorhabditis elegans. Proc Natl Acad Sci USA 96:2479–2484, 1999.

67. Taylor P, Radic Z. The cholinesterases: From genes to proteins. Annu Rev Pharmacol Toxicol 34:281–320, 1994.

68. Salpeter MM: Vertebrate neuromuscular junctions: General morphology, molecular organization, and functional consequences. In Salpeter MM (ed): The Vertebrate Neuromuscular Junction. New York, Alan R. Liss, 1987, pp 1–54.

69. Steinbach JH, Stevens CF: Neuromuscular transmission. In Llinas R, Precht W (eds): Frog Neurobiology. Berlin, Springer-Verlag, 1976, pp 33–91.

70. Zhou M, Engel AG, Auerbach A: Serum choline activates mutant acetylcholine receptors that cause slow channel congenital myasthenic syndromes. Proc Natl Acad Sci USA 96:10466–10471, 1999.

71. Karalliedde L: Organophosphorus poisoning and anaesthesia. Anaesthesia 54:1073–1088, 1999.

72. Maselli RA, Soliven BC: Analysis of the organophosphate-induced electromyographic response to repetitive nerve stimulation: paradoxical response to edrophonium and D-tubocurarine [see comments]. Muscle Nerve 14:1182–1188, 1991.

73. Maselli RA, Leung C: Analysis of anticholinesterase-induced neuromuscular transmission failure. Muscle Nerve 16:548–553, 1993.

74. Clark AL, Hobbiger F, Terrar DA: Nature of the anticholinesterase-induced repetitive response of rat and mouse striated muscle to single nerve stimuli. J Physiol 349:157–166, 1984.

75. Besser R, Vogt T, Gutmann L, et al: Impaired neuromuscular transmission during partial inhibition of acetylcholinesterase: The role of stimulus-induced antidromic backfiring in the generation of the decrement-increment phenomenon. Muscle Nerve 15:1072–1080, 1992.

76. Leonard JP, Salpeter MM: Agonist-induced myopathy at the neuromuscular junction is mediated by calcium. J Cell Biol 82:811–819, 1979.

77. Ohno K, Engel AG, Brengman JM, et al. The spectrum of mutations causing end-plate acetylcholinesterase deficiency. Ann Neurol 47:162–170, 2000.

78. Donger C, Krejci E, Serradell AP, et al: Mutation in the human acetylcholinesterase-associated collagen gene, COLQ, is responsible for congenital myasthenic syndrome with end-plate acetylcholinesterase deficiency (Type Ic). Am J Hum Genet 63:967–975, 1998.

79. Ohno K, Brengman J, Tsujino A, Engel AG: Human endplate acetylcholinesterase deficiency caused by mutations in the collagen-like tail subunit (ColQ) of the asymmetric enzyme. Proc Natl Acad Sci USA 95:9654–9659, 1998.

80. Feng G, Krejci E, Molgo J, et al: Genetic analysis of collagen Q: Roles in acetylcholinesterase and butyrylcholinesterase assembly and in synaptic structure and function. J Cell Biol 144:1349–1360, 1999.

81. Xie W, Stribley JA, Chatonnet A, et al: Postnatal developmental delay and supersensitivity to organophosphate in gene-targeted mice lacking acetylcholinesterase. J Pharmacol Exp Ther 293:896–902, 2000.

82. Layer PG, Willbold E: Novel functions of cholinesterases in development, physiology and disease. Prog Histochem Cytochem 29:1–94, 1995.

83. Holmes C, Jones SA, Budd TC, Greenfield SA: Non-cholinergic, trophic action of recombinant acetylcholinesterase on mid-brain dopaminergic neurons. J Neurosci Res 49:207–218, 1997.

84. Langley JN: Nerve endings and special excitable substances in cells. Proc R Soc Lond B Biol Sci 78:170–195, 1906.

85. Fatt P, Katz B: An analysis of the end-plate potential recorded with an intra-cellular electrode. J Physiol 115:320–370, 1951.

86. Takeuchi A, Takeuchi N: On the permeability of end-plate membrane during the action of transmitter. J Physiol 154:52–67, 1960.

87. Takeuchi N: Effects of calcium on the conductance change of the end-plate membrane during the action of transmitter. J Physiol 167:141–155, 1963.

88. Decker ER, Dani JA: Calcium permeability of the nicotinic acetylcholine receptor: The single-channel calcium influx is significant. J Neurosci 10:3413–3420, 1990.

89. Magleby KL, Stevens CF: A quantitative description of end-plate currents. J Physiol 223:173–197, 1972.

90. Neher E, Steinbach JH: Local anaesthetics transiently block currents through single acetylcholine-receptor channels. J Physiol 277:153–176, 1978.

91. Ortells MO, Lunt GG: Evolutionary history of the ligand-gated ion-channel superfamily of receptors. Trends Neurosci 18:121–127, 1995.

92. Lindstrom J: The structures of neuronal nicotinic receptors. In Clementi F, Fornasari D, Gotti C (eds): Handbook of. Berlin, Springer-Verlag, 2000, pp 101–162.

93. Wonnacott S: Presynaptic nicotinic ACh receptors. Trends Neurosci 20:92–98, 1997.

94. Jones S, Sudweeks S, Yakel JL: Nicotinic receptors in the brain: Correlating physiology with function. Trends Neurosci 22:555–561, 1999.

95. Vizi ES, Lendvai B: Modulatory role of presynaptic nicotinic receptors in synaptic and non-synaptic chemical communication in the central nervous system. Brain Res Brain Res Rev 30:219–235, 1999.

96. Mishina M, Takai T, Imoto K, et al: Molecular distinction between fetal and adult forms of muscle acetylcholine receptor. Nature 321:406–411, 1986.

97. Miyazawa A, Fujiyoshi Y, Stowell M, Unwin N: Nicotinic acetylcholine receptor at 4.6 angstrom resolution: Transverse tunnels in the channel wall. J Mol Biol 288:765–786, 1999.

98. Brejc K, van Dijk WJ, Klaassen RV, et al: Crystal structure of an ACh-binding protein reveals the ligand-binding domain of nicotinic receptors. Nature 411:269–276, 2001.

99. Sanes JR, Lichtman JW: Development of the vertebrate neuromuscular junction. Annu Rev Neurosci 22:389–442, 1999.

100. Blount P, Merlie JP: Molecular basis of the two nonequivalent ligand binding sites of the muscle nicotinic acetylcholine receptor. Neuron 3:349–357, 1989.

101. Corringer PJ, Le NN, Changeux JP: Nicotinic receptors at the amino acid level. Annu Rev Pharmacol Toxicol 40:431–458, 2000.

102. Engel AG, Ohno K, Sine SM: Congenital myasthenic syndromes: recent advances. Arch Neurol 56:163–167, 1999.

103. Jackson MB: Kinetics of unliganded acetylcholine receptor channel gating. Biophys J 49:663–672, 1986.

104. Jackson MB: Dependence of acetylcholine receptor channel kinetics on agonist concentration in cultured mouse muscle fibres. J Physiol 397:555–583, 1988.

105. Akk G, Sine S, Auerbach A: Binding sites contribute unequally to the gating of mouse nicotinic alpha-d200n acetylcholine receptors. J Physiol 496:185–196, 1996.

106. Ohno K, Wang HL, Milone M, et al: Congenital myasthenic syndrome caused by decreased agonist binding affinity due to a mutation in the acetylcholine receptor epsilon subunit. Neuron 17:157–170, 1996.

107. Maconochie DJ, Steinbach JH: The channel opening rate of adult- and fetal-type mouse muscle nicotinic receptors activated by acetylcholine. J Physiol 506:53–72, 1998.

108. Colquhoun D, Sakmann B: Fluctuations in the microsecond time range of the current through single acetylcholine receptor ion channels. Nature 294:464–466, 1981.

109. Colquhoun D, Hawkes AG: On the stochastic properties of bursts of single ion channel openings and clusters of bursts. Philos Trans R Soc Lond B Biol Sci 300:1–59, 1982.

110. Kopta C, Steinbach JH: Comparison of mammalian adult and fetal nicotinic acetylcholine receptors stably expressed in fibroblasts. J Neurosci 14:3922–3933, 1994.

111. Thesleff S: The mode of neuromuscular block caused by acetylcholine, nicotine, decamethonium and succinylcholine. Acta Physiol Scand 34:218–231, 1955.

112. Katz B, Thesleff S: A study of the 'desensitization' produced by acetylcholine at the motor end-plate. J Physiol 138:63–80, 1957.

113. Heidemann T, Changeux JP: Structural and functional properties of the acetylcholine receptor protein in its purified and membrane-bound states. Annu Rev Biochem 47:317–357, 1978.

114. Feltz A, Trautmann A: Desensitization at the frog neuromuscular junction: A biphasic process. J Physiol 322:257–272, 1982.

115. Chesnut TJ: Two-component desensitization at the neuromuscular junction of the frog. J Physiol 336:229–241, 1983.

116. Paradiso K, Brehm P: Long-term desensitization of nicotinic acetylcholine receptors is regulated via protein kinase A-mediated phosphorylation. J Neurosci 18:9227–9237, 1998.

117. Auerbach A, Akk G: Desensitization of mouse nicotinic acetylcholine receptor channels. A two-gate mechanism. J Gen Physiol 112:181–197, 1998.

118. Boyd ND, Cohen JB: Kinetics of binding of [3H]acetylcholine and [3H]carbamoylcholine to Torpedo postsynaptic membranes: slow conformational transitions of the cholinergic receptor. Biochemistry 19:5344–5353, 1980.

119. Pennefather P, Quastel DM: Fast desensitization of the nicotinic receptor at the mouse neuromuscular junction. Br J Pharmacol 77:395–404, 1982.

120. Magleby KL, Pallotta BS: A study of desensitization of acetylcholine receptors using nerve-released transmitter in the frog. J Physiol 316:225–250, 1981.

121. White BH, Cohen JB: Agonist-induced changes in the structure of the acetylcholine receptor M2 regions revealed by photoincorporation of an uncharged nicotinic noncompetitive antagonist. J Biol Chem 267:15770–15783, 1992.

122. Leonard RJ, Labarca CG, Charnet P, et al: Evidence that the M2 membrane-spanning region lines the ion channel pore of the nicotinic receptor. Science 242:1578–1581, 1988.

123. Charnet P, Labarca C, Leonard RJ, et al: An open-channel blocker interacts with adjacent turns of alpha-helices in the nicotinic acetylcholine receptor. Neuron 4:87–95, 1990.

124. Sine SM, Steinbach JH: Agonists block currents through acetylcholine receptor channels. Biophys J 46:277–284, 1984.

125. Ogden DC, Colquhoun D: Ion channel block by acetylcholine, carbachol and suberyldicholine at the frog neuromuscular junction. Proc R Soc Lond B Biol Sci 225:329–355, 1985.

126. Colquhoun D, Dreyer F, Sheridan RE: The actions of tubocurarine at the frog neuromuscular junction. J Physiol 293:247–284, 1979.

127. Sine SM, Steinbach JH: Acetylcholine receptor activation by a site-selective ligand: Nature of brief open and closed states in BC3H-1 cells. J Physiol 370:357–379, 1986.

128. Adams PR, Sakmann B: Decamethonium both opens and blocks end plate channels. Proc Natl Acad Sci USA 75:2994–2998, 1978.

129. Marshall CG, Ogden DC, Colquhoun D: The actions of suxamethonium (succinyldicholine) as an agonist and channel blocker at the nicotinic receptor of frog muscle. J Physiol 428:155–174, 1990.

130. Fletcher GH, Steinbach JH: Ability of nondepolarizing neuromuscular blocking drugs to act as partial agonists at fetal and adult mouse muscle nicotinic receptors. Mol Pharmacol 49:938–947, 1996.

131. Galzi JL, Revah F, Bouet F, et al: Allosteric transitions of the acetylcholine receptor probed at the amino acid level with a photolabile cholinergic ligand. Proc Natl Acad Sci USA 88:5051–5055, 1991.

132. Pedersen SE, Sharp SD, Liu WS, Cohen JB: Structure of the noncompetitive antagonist-binding site of the Torpedo nicotinic acetylcholine receptor. [3H]meproadifen mustard reacts selectively with alpha-subunit Glu-262. J Biol Chem 267:10489–10499, 1992.

133. Blanton MP, Xie Y, Dangott LJ, Cohen JB: The steroid promegestone is noncompetitive antagonist of the Torpedo nicotinic acetylcholine receptor that interacts with the lipid-protein interface. Mol Pharmacol 55:269–278, 1999.

134. Dilger JP, Brett RS, Lesko LA: Effects of isoflurane on acetylcholine receptor channels. 1. Single-channel currents. Mol Pharmacol 41:127–133, 1992.

135. Neely A, Lingle CJ: Trapping of an open-channel blocker at the frog neuromuscular acetylcholine channel. Biophys J 50:981–986, 1986.

136. Thomas KB: Curare. Philadelphia, JB Lippincott, 1963.

137. Changeux J-P, Kasai M, Lee C-Y: Use of a snake venom toxin to characterize the cholinergic receptor protein. Proc Natl Acad Sci USA 67:1241–1247, 1970.

138. Miledi R, Potter LT: Acetylcholine receptors in muscle fibres. Nature 233:599–603, 1971.

139. Patrick J, Heinemann SF, Lindstrom J, et al: Appearance of acetylcholine receptors during differentiation of a myogenic cell line. Proc Natl Acad Sci USA 69:2762–2766, 1972.

140. Neubig R, Cohen JB: Equilibrium binding of [3H]tubocurarine and [3H]acetylcholine by Torpedo postsynaptic membranes: stoichiometry and ligand interactions. Biochemistry 18:5464–5475, 1980.

141. Sine SM, Taylor P: Relationship between reversible antagonist occupancy and the functional capacity of the acetylcholine receptor. J Biol Chem 256:6692–6699, 1981.

142. Sine SM, Claudio T: gamma- and delta-Subunits regulate the affinity and the cooperativity of ligand binding to the acetylcholine receptor. J Biol Chem 266:19369–19377, 1991.

143. Steinbach JH, Chen Q: Antagonist and partial agonist actions of d-tubocurarine at mammalian muscle acetylcholine receptors. J Neurosci 15:230–240, 1995.

144. Waud BE, Waud DR: Quantitative examination of the interaction of competitive neuromuscular blocking agents on the indirectly elicited muscle twitch. Anesthesiology 61:420–427, 1984.

145. Sine SM, Kreienkamp HJ, Bren N, et al: Molecular dissection of subunit interfaces in the acetylcholine receptor: Identification of determinants of alpha-conotoxin m1 selectivity. Neuron 15:205–211, 1995.

146. Colquhoun D, Sheridan RE: The effect of tubocurarine competition on the kinetics of agonist action on the nicotinic receptor. Br J Pharmacol 75:77–86, 1982.

147. Maconochie DJ, Steinbach JH. Unpublished observations.

148. Roper JF, Bradley RJ, Dilger JP: Kinetics of the inhibition of ach receptor channels by D-tubocurarine. Biophys J 64:A323, 1993.

149. Demazumder D, Dilger JP: A mathematical technique for determining the kinetics of competitive antagonism in the presence of agonist at the nicotinic acetylcholine receptor. Biophys J 80:463a, 2001.

150. Lingle CJ, Steinbach JH: Neuromuscular blocking agents. Int Anesthesiol Clin 26:288–301, 1988.

151. Liu Y, Dilger JP: Decamethonium is a partial agonist at the nicotinic acetylcholine receptor. Synapse 13:57–62, 1993.

152. Feldman S, Hood J: Depolarizing neuromuscular block–a presynaptic mechanism? Acta Anaesthesiol Scand 38:535–541, 1994.

153. Hartzell HC, Kuffler SW, Yoshikami D: Post-synaptic potentiation: Interaction between quanta of acetylcholine at the skeletal neuromuscular synapse. J Physiol 251:437–463, 1975.

154. Katz B, Miledi R: The binding of acetylcholine to receptors and its removal from the synaptic cleft. J Physiol 231:549–574, 1973.

155. Colquhoun D, Large WA, Rang HP: An analysis of the action of a false transmitter at the neuromuscular junction. J Physiol 266:361–395, 1977.

156. Land BR, Salpeter EE, Salpeter MM: Acetylcholine receptor site density affects the rising phase of miniature endplate currents. Proc Natl Acad Sci USA 77:3736–3740, 1980.

157. Pennefather P, Quastel DM: Relation between subsynaptic receptor blockade and response to quantal transmitter at the mouse neuromuscular junction. J Gen Physiol 78:313–344, 1981.

158. Fertuck HC, Salpeter MM: Quantitation of junctional and extrajunctional acetylcholine receptors by electron microscope autoradiography after ^{125}I-alpha-bungarotoxin binding at mouse neuromuscular junctions. J Cell Biol 69:144–158, 1976.

159. Paton WD, Waud DR: The margin of safety of neuromuscular transmission. J Physiol 191:59–90, 1967.

160. Waud BE, Waud DR: The margin of safety of neuromuscular transmission in the muscle of the diaphragm. Anesthesiology 37:417–422, 1972.

161. Waud DR, Waud BE: In vitro measurement of margin of safety of neuromuscular transmission. Am J Physiol 229:1632–1634, 1975.

162. Albuquerque EX, Thesleff S: A comparative study of membrane properties of innervated and chronically denervated fast and slow skeletal muscles of the rat. Acta Physiol Scand 73:471–480, 1968.

163. Albuquerque EX, Barnard EA, Jansson SE, Wieckowski J: Occupancy of the cholinergic receptors in relation to changes in the endplate potential. Life Sci 12:545–552, 1973.

164. Wathey JC, Nass MM, Lester HA: Numerical reconstruction of the quantal event at nicotinic synapses. Biophys J 27:145–164, 1979.

11

Sensory Processing

Mark A. Schumacher, MD, PhD • Helge Eilers, MD

PERIPHERAL NOCICEPTORS

Physicians of ancient times faced a clinical dilemma that remains true today. How does one relieve a patient's pain and suffering without doing additional harm? Although modern pain management has led the way in refining our use of opioid analgesics and developing exciting techniques of concurrent neural blockade, current therapies often remain inadequate to control severe debilitating pain. Unwanted side effects including central nervous system depression and risk for addiction limit the ability to manage acute and chronic pain states even if adequate pain relief has been achieved. The persistent activation of peripheral sensory neurons that transduce painful stimuli has been identified as a critical factor in the maintenance of pain. If these nociceptive pathways could be identified and selectively blocked, it could provide an elegant alternative to centrally acting analgesics. Our understanding of the molecular neurobiology of nociceptor function is advancing rapidly. Emerging from this intensive investigation is a framework of new strategies to block the signaling of painful sensations at their origins—at the peripheral terminals of primary afferent nociceptors.

The study of pain transduction began with the observations of Sherrington[1] who believed that the experience of pain was based on nerves that responded to specific types of noxious stimuli that cause tissue damage. Through the study of protective reflexes in experimental animal models, Sherrington introduced the concept of "nociceptive nerves" and later the term *nociceptor* to describe what is now referred to as primary afferent nociceptors.[1] This chapter focuses on recent findings that begin to describe the molecular mechanisms of nociceptive *transduction*—the process of converting a noxious stimulus into an electrochemical potential. In addition, those factors that modify the sensitivity of peripheral pain transduction are briefly discussed.

Systems Physiology

Nociceptors represent the portion of the peripheral nervous system that is specialized for the detection of noxious stimuli. This portion of the peripheral nervous system is further distinguished anatomically and functionally to include primary afferent neurons that innervate cutaneous tissues as skin (somatic) and those that innervate internal organs (visceral). One of the principal benefits provided by nociceptors is their rapid detection of impending or actual tissue injury. Nociceptors can accomplish this by being a part of an integrated system. The simplest model of a "pain pathway" begins with peripheral nociceptive terminals that function to detect multiple noxious stimuli (transduction), the relay of these signals to the central nervous system through the conduction of action potentials (transmission), and finally their interpretation as a harmful or unpleasant experience (perception).[2]

Organ Physiology

Somatic

In the peripheral nervous system, somatosensory detection of tissue damaging stimuli (thermal, mechanical, chemical) occurs at the peripheral terminals of primary afferent nociceptors whose cell bodies reside primarily in the trigeminal (V) and dorsal root ganglia (DRG). In addition, cranial nerves V (innervation of the majority of the face, conjunctiva, mouth, and dura mater) and cranial nerves VII, IX, and X (innervation of the skin of the external ear, and mucous membranes of the larynx and pharynx) also participate in nociception.[3] Likewise, nerve terminals derived from nociceptors residing in spinal DRG (cervical, thoracic, and lumbar) innervate the somatotopic dermatomes of the skin and underlying tissue. Nociceptors derived from DRG then send central processes to laminae I, II, and V of the dorsal horn of the spinal cord. After synaptic connection with second order dorsal horn neurons, nociceptive information is then relayed to the brain.

Visceral

Painful visceral stimuli are transmitted to the central nervous system in a more complex manner than is found for the detection of noxious somatic stimuli. Nociceptive innervation is confounded by the various routes that visceral nociceptive processes take from DRG to their peripheral targets. In many cases, peripheral nociceptive processes combine with sympathetic nerves—e.g., visceral afferents that are responsible for cardiac pain or extrinsic innervation of small and large intestines. There, primary afferent processes are found within both sympathetic and parasympathetic nerves (see review by Cervero[4]). Vagal afferents provide a second source of visceral innervation from cell bodies located within the nodose (inferior vagal) ganglion. Despite this dual innervation, afferents involved with the transduction of painful visceral stimuli (ischemia, stretch, distension) are primarily derived from the DRG.[4] Vagal afferents also play a role in pain transduction; however, their function may be more global in nature, providing feedback loops to the brain and neuroendocrine systems resulting in systemic pain modulation and associated perceptions of nausea or malaise.[5]

Cellular Physiology

Somatic Nociceptors

Historically, detection of noxious stimuli of the skin and underlying deep tissues (somatic) has been divided into three modalities: noxious *thermal*, *mechanical*, and *chemical*. The behavioral and physiologic responses following the application of one of these three painful modalities has served as the cornerstone for a classification scheme of nociceptors. Within this framework, the threshold for evoking the sensation of pain has been determined in human volunteer subjects with certain external forces applied to the skin, such as noxious thermal stimuli (temperatures $\geq$43–45° C) or intense mechanical stimuli. Criteria for detection of noxious chemical stimuli have also been applied and rely on the sensation of pain in response to certain compounds such as capsaicin, the pungent principal ingredient in hot chili peppers. Using these noxious stimuli in animal models, nociceptive reflexes and electrophysiologic current responses have served to correlate human pain thresholds to the activation of a subpopulation of primary afferent neurons that transduce noxious stimuli—nociceptors.[2]

Nociceptors have been further classified based on their axon diameter conduction velocity (CV), degree of myelination, and more recently, cross-sectional area of neuronal soma. The axons of primary afferent neurons fall into three distinct groups: Aß (large diameter 6–22 μm, heavily myelinated with fast conduction velocities (CV) of 33–75 m/sec), Aδ (diameter 2–5 μm, thinly myelinated with CVs 5–30 m/sec), and C fibers (diameter 0.3–3 μm, unmyelinated with CV of 0.5–2 m/sec).[6] CV and DRG neuron diameter have also been correlated resulting in primary afferent neurons with small-diameter/cross-sectional areas correlating with C and Aδ fiber type nociceptors. Those with a large-diameter/cross-sectional area correlated with Aß afferents that transduce non-nociceptive sensations.[7] Correlation of nociceptor fiber type with modality of activation has resulted in additional subclasses. Primary afferent neurons activated by multiple noxious stimuli are referred to as "polymodal nociceptors."[8] Included in this category are C fiber type mechanoheat nociceptors and at least two types of A fiber type nociceptors: mechanoheat type I (high heat threshold >49° C) and mechanoheat type II (heat threshold ~43° C).[2] Finally, high-threshold mechanonociceptors that fail to respond to thermal stimuli have been characterized for both C and A fiber types as well as for nociceptors that respond only to noxious chemical stimuli. Despite this elegant classification of nociceptor subtypes, discharge patterns of polymodal nociceptors do not correlate with stimulus-induced pain sensation.[9] Therefore, central processing of nociceptor impulses must be required for the discrimination of painful sensations. From the point of view of understanding the molecular basis of pain transduction, one use of the classification schemes summarized here is as physiologic "fingerprints" to help determine precisely what type of ion channels and receptors define a nociceptor. This strategy has facilitated the isolation and characterization of several "nociceptor specific" ion channels that are candidate transducers of noxious stimuli and hence targets for analgesic drug action (see later).

Visceral Nociceptors

The notion that visceral nociceptors exist as an independent class of primary afferent neurons when compared with their somatic counterparts remains a point of much discussion and intensive investigation.[10] Not all aspects of physiology are easily translated from somatic to visceral nociceptors. A case in point is the gastrointestinal system. Passing through the esophagus into the stomach, there is a proportionate decrease in the ability to detect noxious thermal stimuli, where, at the cardiac portion of the stomach, only extremes of temperature can be discerned. Beyond this point, only extremes of distension and muscular contraction can be perceived. Even more remarkable is that the entire length of the small intestine is insensitive to touch, thermal stimuli, cutting, burning, or clamping under normal conditions.[4] However, during conditions of inflammation, these same tissues are found to be sensitive to thermal, mechanical, and chemical stimuli.[11] The existence of so-called silent or sleeping nociceptors has been invoked in an attempt to explain these observations[12] (see "Nociceptor Neurotransmission and Modulation" for detailed discussion).

Biochemical and Molecular Mechanism

Mounting evidence exists that ion channels selectively expressed in nociceptors function as the transducers of noxious thermal, mechanical, and chemical stimuli.[13] This is based on recent electrophysiologic investigations that have demonstrated inward current responses to noxious heat (I_{heat})[14–17] and mechanical stimuli (I_{mech}) in cultured sensory neurons.[18] Surprisingly, in the search to identify the molecular mechanism underlying chemical (capsaicin)-induced activation of nociceptors, a new family of nociceptive-

specific receptors/ion channels has been revealed. Considerable detail has been afforded to the description of the vanilloid (capsaicin) receptor because it appears to represent an archetype for a broader family of ion channels that transduce virtually all modalities of painful stimuli. In addition to vanilloid receptors, other ion channels have been isolated and characterized that may function in peripheral pain transduction. These are discussed and summarized in Table 11–1.

Vanilloid Receptors

Nociceptors are activated by capsaicin and produce a sensation of burning pain. Capsaicin, the principal pungent component in hot chili peppers, selectively activates a subset of primary afferent nociceptors. Structurally, capsaicin contains a homovanillic acid group that is important for its pungent activity; therefore, capsaicin and its related derivatives are usually referred to as "vanilloid compounds." In mammals, exposure to capsaicin produces excitation of nociceptors with secondary release of inflammatory and vasoactive peptides.[19] In humans, intradermal injection of capsaicin produces immediate burning pain, similar to that reported with noxious thermal stimuli or in certain painful neuropathies.[2] Although initial applications of capsaicin are painful, paradoxically, repeated application of capsaicin in emollient creams has been used as a topical analgesic producing a desensitization or destruction of nociceptive terminals.[20] Therefore, capsaicin has the property of both

TABLE 11–1.

Candidate Nociceptive Transducers

Modality	Stimulus	Ion Channel	
Thermal	$T \geq 43\text{–}45\ °C$	I_{Heat}	Nonselective cation channel
	$T \geq 43\text{–}45\ °C$	VR1	Vanilloid receptor subtype 1
	$T \geq 53\ °C$	VRL1	Vanilloid receptor-like protein 1
Mechanical	**Force**	I_{Mech}	Nonselective cation channel
	Cell Stretch (Hypotonic)	VROAC	Vanilloid receptor-like protein osmotically activated channel
Chemical	**Vanilloids** (Capsacin, RTX)	VR1	Vanilloid receptor subtype 1
	H⁺ (pH 7.0–7.4)	ASIC3	Acid-sensing ion channel
	H⁺ (pH < 6.3)	VR1	Vanilloid receptor subtype 1
	ATP	$P2X_3$	ATP-gated ion channel

ATP, adenosine triphosphate; RTX, resiniferatoxin.

exciting and inactivating vanilloid sensitive neurons. In addition to the nociceptive response, capsaicin can also evoke a wide range of other physiologic responses depending on the route of delivery. These include effects on the pulmonary (apnea), cardiovascular (bradycardia), and thermoregulatory (hypothermia) systems.[21]

Capsaicin acts through a membrane-associated receptor. Before the isolation of cDNA encoding a functional vanilloid (capsaicin) receptor, evidence that the effects of capsaicin may be mediated by a receptor began with measuring the dose-dependent effects of capsaicin and its analogues on protective eye wiping behavior in the rat. Subsequently, dose-response experiments measuring calcium influx and current responses in cultured sensory neurons were completed.[22] Resiniferatoxin (RTX), a diterpene derived from the latex of the plant Euphorbia resinifera, was found to share structural similarity to capsaicin by containing a vanilloid moiety. Both capsaicin and RTX induced a dose-dependent influx of calcium in cultured sensory neurons. RTX has an apparent nanomolar binding affinity in DRG membranes and was used as a high-affinity radioligand for the characterization of purported vanilloid binding sites.[23] The existence of specific vanilloid binding sites was further substantiated with the development of capsazepine, an inactive capsaicin analog that competitively inhibits the activation and binding of capsaicin and RTX. Several comprehensive reviews have been published encapsulating vanilloid receptor biology.[21,23]

The vanilloid (capsaicin) receptor is an ion channel that is activated *in vitro* by multiple painful stimuli. With the isolation of a cDNA clone encoding a capsaicin-activated ion channel,[24] the hypothesis that vanilloid compounds activate nociceptors through a protein receptor site has been demonstrated. Vanilloid receptor type-1 (VR1) is proposed to encode a nonselective cation channel expressed predominantly in small-diameter neurons of DRG and trigeminal ganglion. It is activated by capsaicin and RTX in a dose-dependent manner and is inhibited by both capsazepine and ruthenium red, a noncompetitive inhibitor of vanilloid receptor activation. Its structure (Fig. 11–1) most resembles that of members of the store-operated calcium channel family, although its activation is independent of intracellular calcium stores. Dose-response experiments confirmed that RTX is more potent than capsaicin in the activation of VR1, and that activation of the receptor requires the binding of more than one agonist molecule.[22,24]

Evidence for a family of vanilloid receptors. Receptor heterogeneity has become the rule rather than the exception in understanding how cell surface receptors mediate diverse biologic functions. During the past decade, differences in vanilloid efficacy, binding affinities, and degree of cooperativity have been published from numerous laboratories.[23] Differences in RTX desensitization have also supported the receptor subtype hypothesis. Electrophysiologic evidence for receptor divergence has provided even stronger evidence for a family of vanilloid receptors. Individual small-diameter neurons derived from DRG trigeminal ganglia were found to produce a complex set of current responses. Some sensory neurons respond only to capsaicin, whereas others respond to both capsaicin and RTX.[25] Although a search for other receptor subunits that express vanilloid sensitivity has been underway for several years, no such cDNA

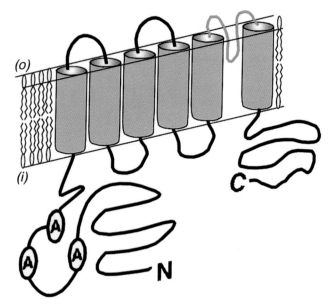

Figure 11–1. Vanilloid receptor subtype-1 (VR1) protein topology model. VR1 is distinguished by six transmembrane spanning regions flanked by two intracellular domains: (*N*) amino-terminal and (*C*) carboxyl-terminal. The N-terminal domain includes three ankyrin (*A*) repeats. A pore loop domain (shown in *gray*) is predicted between the fifth and sixth transmembrane spanning region. It is hypothesized that at least four such subunits assemble to form a functional ion channel.

have been isolated to date. Alternately, heterogeneous vanilloid physiology and pharmacology may arise from tissue-specific post-translational modification or coassembly with other subunits (see later).

Ion channels, whether they are voltage-gated potassium channels or members of a ligand-gated ion channel family (e.g., postsynaptic nicotinic cholinergic receptors), are predominantly multisubunit protein complexes. Depending on the cell type, stage of development, or presence of pathology, the composition of the individual subunits may diverge. Drawing on these examples, it could be expected that vanilloid receptors as typified by VR1 also form functional heteromers in sensory neurons. Evidence for a heteromeric complex constituting a functional vanilloid receptor has recently been reported.[26] Potential candidates include recently described vanilloid receptor variants that include VR5sv, a vanilloid receptor splice variant that diverges from VR1 through the loss of the majority of its N-terminal intracellular domain and ankyrin repeat elements.[27] Functional expression of VR.5sv in Xenopus oocytes and mammalian cells showed no sensitivity to capsaicin, the potent vanilloid RTX, hydrogen ions (pH 6.2), or noxious thermal stimuli (≥45° C).[27] Because VR.5sv is otherwise identical to VR1 throughout its transmembrane spanning domains and C-terminal intracellular region, these results support the hypothesis that the N-terminal intracellular domain is essential for the formation of functional receptors activated by vanilloid compounds and noxious thermal stimuli.[27] Furthermore, these observations are consistent with electrophysiologic studies of heterologously expressed VR1 demonstrating that the site of capsaicin activation is on the intracellular surface of the channel.[28] Because VR5sv is expressed in relatively equal abundance with VR1 in brain subregions[27] and shares an identical transmembrane domain structure, potential heteromeric complexes may occur and perform functions that are independent of vanilloid activation or the detection of noxious stimuli.

The role of vanilloid receptors in the detection of noxious thermal stimuli. One of the most intriguing observations resulting from the isolation of VR1 is its ability to be activated in vitro by temperature increases into the noxious range ($\geq 43°$ C).[24] This suggests that it could serve as a transducer of noxious thermal stimuli in vivo. However, VR1 expresses some but not all the properties that have been described for thermal activation of sensory neurons in vitro.[14,15] Therefore it is reasonable to consider that multiple pathways exist that transduce noxious thermal stimuli. This idea has gained additional support based on studies of VR1-deficient mice that exhibited nearly normal behavioral responses to noxious thermal stimuli, although thermal hyperalgesia was completely abolished.[29,30] Experiments with cultured DRG neurons have shown that capsaicin-induced current responses can be observed independently from thermally induced channel activation. If VR1 is not the primary transducer for noxious thermal stimuli during normal conditions, it is probable that other pathways or channels are involved. Thus far, a vanilloid receptor homologue, vanilloid receptor-like protein-1 (VRL1), has been isolated and characterized that exhibits a high threshold for heat ($I_{heat} \geq 53°$ C) in vitro and is expressed in the medium-diameter sensory neurons of DRG and trigeminal ganglia.[31] However, VRL1 is absent in small-diameter sensory neurons and is widely expressed in non-neuronal tissues. Determining the physiologic role of VRL1 in the transduction of noxious thermal stimuli will likely be achieved through in vivo studies of genetically altered mice or through its down-regulation by antisense strategies.

Protons modulate and directly activate VR1. Protons (H^+), as found in excess during acidic conditions (low pH), have been shown to potentiate both the vanilloid and noxious thermal response of VR1 through direct activation of VR1 in vitro.[24,32] Moreover, an extracellular site essential for proton-induced activation of VR1 has been identified and apparently differs from the sites that mediate capsaicin and heat activation.[33,34] Although the detection of "mild" acidic conditions, pH 7.0 to 7.4, may be mediated by a family of acid-sensing sodium channels,[35] the ability of hydrogen ions to potentiate or directly activate VR1-induced currents suggests a nociceptive role during pathophysiologic conditions of ischemia or infection.[32] Additional behavioral studies should help determine the degree to which VR1 participates in vivo to proton-mediated nociception.[29,30]

Activation of VR1 during conditions of inflammation. Tissue injury results in a complex series of local and systemic responses that have been shown to modulate nociceptor activation. Of the multiple inflammatory products that have been characterized, several have been recently identified to directly activate VR1. Anandamide, the endogenous ligand for the cannabinoid receptor, activates VR1 and is a full agonist for the human orthologue of VR1.[36] Products of the lipoxygenase pathway of arachidonic acid, 12-(S)-hydroperoxyeicosatetraenoic acid (12-(S)-HPETE) and leukotriene B4, have also been found to activate VR1 in vitro.[37] Most recently, activation of protein kinase C (PKC), as occurs through the action of bradykinin (BK), has been shown to activate VR1.[38]

Vanilloid receptors and noxious mechanical transduction. The molecular basis underlying the transduction of noxious mechanical stimuli in mammalian sensory neurons is unknown. Our current understanding is based largely on the electrophysiologic characterization of channels activated during hypotonic/hypobaric conditions that produce cell stretch (stretch-activated channels).[39] However, the isolation and characterization of an ion channel that directs a whole-cell current response to mechanical stretch has been elusive. Another type of noxious mechanical stimuli is cell shrinkage following exposure to hypertonic conditions. Hypertonic stimuli have been demonstrated to selectively activate small-diameter (C fiber type) nociceptive neurons in animals and to produce pain in humans. Previous investigations on how cell shrinkage results in inward current responses revealed a class of mechanically gated nonselective cation channels known as "stretch-inactivated channels" (SICs).[39] Activation of SICs can result in membrane depolarization and has been studied in several cell types including snail neurons, cardiac myocytes, skeletal muscle, and in hypothalamic magnocellular cells that serve as central osmoreceptors.[39] Recent efforts to clone mechanosensitive channels (from rat kidney) resulted in the isolation of an SIC that was reported to direct whole-cell inward current responses to hypertonic conditions (cell shrinkage). Additional experiments are ongoing to confirm these findings because SIC does not appear to be a simple splice variant of the vanilloid receptor gene.[40]

A second osmotically activated channel homologous to vanilloid receptors (VR/OAC) has been reported. VR/OAC shares homology with members of the TRP superfamily of calcium channels, VR1, VR5sv, and VRL1, but is not a splice variant of VR1 because it has been localized to chromosome 12 rather than 17 in humans.[41] Although VR/OAC is insensitive to vanilloid compounds, Anandamide, and noxious thermal stimuli, it is activated during hypotonic (cell stretch) conditions with a large single channel conductance.[41] Interestingly, both VR/OAC and SIC share a nearly identical C-terminal intracellular domain that may direct channel sensitivity to mechanical stimuli.[41] Although VR/OAC was reported to be expressed in the medium-diameter sensory neurons of DRG and trigeminal ganglion neurons, a subsequently cloned orthologue, VRL2, was not found to be expressed in sensory ganglion. Given the emerging nature of this area of investigation, additional confirmation is anticipated that directly links these vanilloid receptor variants with nociceptor transduction of noxious mechanical stimuli.

Toward a molecular model of nociceptor sensitization. Mechanical and thermal hyperalgesia can produce significant pain and morbidity, whether as a consequence of a surgical procedure or as the result of a chronic inflammatory process. Moreover, mechanical stimuli that initially had evoked little or no response can produce strong activation of nociceptors after exposure to inflammatory mediators. This implies that certain mechanosensitive elements remain relatively silent until costimulated with both an inflammatory event and noxious stimulus. Members of this emerging vanilloid receptor family appear to be serendipitous targets of both inflammatory mediators and noxious stimuli. Based on the recent functional studies of VR1 in vitro and in vivo, evidence for the development of a model describing peripheral nociceptor sensitization at the molecular level may be at hand.

Vanilloid receptor gene. Although vanilloid receptors and their variants are currently recognized as important elements in the transduction of pain and hyperalgesia, very little is known about what controls their level of expression during normal or pathologic conditions.[24,29,30,32] Just as it has been essential to understand what ligands or conditions directly activate VR1 and its variants, an equally important goal is to determine what factors control the quantity, subtype, or both, of vanilloid receptor expression in nociceptors. Progress in understanding the biology of vanilloid receptors has been advanced with the isolation of four independent cDNAs encoding human VR1.[42–45] This work has revealed important pharmacologic differences between rat and human VR1.[44] Moreover, the genomic organization of the human vanilloid receptor gene has been determined[40] and serves as a starting point in understanding the regulation of vanilloid receptor expression and linkage to human disease.

Acid-Sensing Ion Channels

Tissue acidosis resulting from ischemia, inflammation, and infection is a potentially life-threatening condition. Ischemia resulting from coronary artery insufficiency can produce a tissue acidosis to approximately pH 6.7 and the pH of an abscess has been reported to be as low as pH 5.0. Although acidic conditions (pH < 7.0) produce the sensation of pain and activate sensory neurons in culture, only in the past few years have the molecular targets of proton (H^+)-induced nociceptor activation been characterized. As previously mentioned, at the forefront of these discoveries has been the observation (described earlier) that VR1 is both modulated and directly activated by protons at a pH < 6.3.[24,32] However, an independent subfamily of epithelial sodium channels related to the degenerins and activated by protons in a range that represents less severe acidic conditions has been described. These acid-sensing ion channels (ASICs) are sodium selective, calcium permeable, and have a simple structure of two membrane spanning domains. Of the growing number of subtypes (at least five), two ASIC subtypes are predominantly expressed in sensory neurons, ASIC1b (ASIC-beta) and ASIC3 (DRASIC).[35] Of particular interest is ASIC3, which has been recently implicated as responsible for mediating the acid-gated current in cardiac ischemic-sensing neurons. Although multiple mediators of ischemic pain have been proposed including adenosine, adenosine triphosphate (ATP), BK, and histamine, proton-induced currents appear to be the predominant driving force for primary cardiac nociceptor activation. Currently, there is no selective pharmacologic means to block ASICs, and the investigation of their individual contribution to the mediation of somatic and visceral pain may require behavioral testing of genetically altered, ASIC-deficient mice. Alternate strategies may involve the study of endogenous compounds such as neuropeptides FF and FMRF that are capable of modulating ASIC-mediated, acid-evoked currents in sensory neurons.

Adenosine Triphosphate and Ionotropic Channels

The hypothesis that ATP plays an important role in the synaptic transmission of sensory neurons began with the early observations of Holton and Holton.[46] Although it was known that ATP facilitated neurotransmission within the dorsal horn of the spinal cord, the observation that ATP induced pain in a human blister-based model created interest in understanding how ATP could directly activate sensory neurons. Moreover, cellular activation in response to ATP revealed that one or more "fast" ATP-gated channels may exist in various tissues, including small-diameter sensory neurons. Furthermore, it is plausible that ATP released from cells functions as a signal of tissue injury. Since the initial cloning of the first two ATP-gated channels, $P2X_1$ and $P2X_2$, a total of seven such channels have been described.[47] Of importance is the ATP-gated channel subtype $P2X_3$, which is predominantly expressed in small-diameter sensory neurons and is proposed to mediate ATP-induced activation of nociceptors through either homomultimers of $P2X_3$ channel subunits or more likely as a $P2X_{2/3}$ heteromultimer of $P2X_2$ and $P2X_3$ subunits.[48] Electrophysiologic and behavioral studies of genetically altered $P2X_3$-deficient mice have established a direct link between this channel subunit and nociceptor activation in vivo.[49,50] $P2X_3$-deficient mice lose the rapidly desensitizing ATP-induced currents in DRG neurons, reduce the sustained ATP-induced currents in vagal ganglion neurons, and have a reduced pain/behavior-related response to injected ATP. Although there is no evidence to link the $P2X_3$ receptor subunits to the acute transduction of noxious thermal or mechanical stimuli, it may play a role in enhancing thermal or mechanical transduction, or both, during inflammatory or pathophysiologic conditions.[51] $P2X_3$ may also subserve other mechanosensory roles in control of urinary bladder volume because $P2X_3$-deficient mice exhibit marked urinary bladder hyporeflexia.[47,50]

Nociceptor Neurotransmission and Modulation

In contrast to the various ion channels described earlier that are directly gated by noxious stimuli, there are a number of receptors and ion channels expressed in nociceptors that are not directly activated by noxious stimuli. Nociceptors also provide for the detection of pathophysiologic conditions in tissues that could lead to irreversible cellular injury or possibly death. Therefore, nociceptors have the ability to adjust their sensitivity following repetitive noxious stimuli or tissue injury. *Sensitization* encompasses an increase in spontaneous nociceptor activity, a decreased threshold for activation, and an increase in action potential firing after suprathreshold stimuli.[2] During these circumstances, prolonged nociceptor activation may be warranted to ensure protective behavioral responses. Together with plasticity changes in the dorsal horn of the spinal cord, sensitization of nociceptors contribute to hyperalgesia. Nociceptor modulation is complex and multiple pathways exist both to detect noxious stimuli and to modulate transducing element sensitivity. During conditions of tissue injury and inflammation, this complexity increases (Fig. 11–2). Because a comprehensive review of each modulatory pathway is prohibitive, we have chosen to emphasize receptor/channel systems that have the most compelling evidence to affect peripheral ion channels mediating pain transduction.

Action Potential Generation

After the initial step of transducing noxious stimuli into a depolarizing current, nociceptors use voltage-gated sodium channels (VGSCs) to propagate this signal to the dorsal horn of the spinal cord. Sodium influx through VGSCs is responsible for the generation and propagation of action potentials. VGSCs are classified based on their sensitivity to

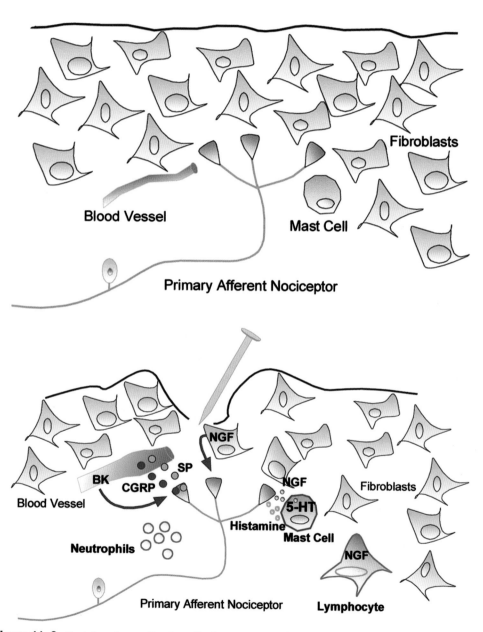

Figure 11–2. Peripheral sensitization. During normal conditions (*upper panel*), nociceptive terminals derived from C and Aδ fibers are interposed with skin fibroblasts, mast cells, and the microvasculature. Following injury or inflammation (*lower panel*), nociceptor terminals depolarize releasing neuropeptides substance P (SP) and calcitonin gene-related peptide (CGRP), which produces vascular leak and edema. Bradykinin (BK) cleaved from circulating kallikreins and nerve growth factor (NGF) produced by fibroblasts both activate and sensitize nociceptor terminals. NGF produces additional sensitization through the degranulation of mast cells containing serotonin (5-HT) and histamine. NGF and cytokines are associated with the accumulation of neutrophils and lymphocytes that participate in the maintenance of sensitization: hyperalgesia.

tetrodotoxin (TTX) and there is evidence that sodium currents in small-diameter neurons of C and Aδ fibers are predominantly carried by a TTX-resistant (TTX-r) sodium channel (SNS/PN3, now $Na_v1.8$).[52] Multiple subunits of this large ion channel family are expressed in the DRG (for review see Baker and Wood[53]). Inflammatory mediators like serotonin (5-HT) and PGE_2 have been shown to increase TTX-r currents in dissociated sensory neurons, and thereby could contribute to the development of hyperalgesia.[54] The finding that SNS-null mutant mice have a significantly greater threshold for noxious mechanical stimuli and delayed development of inflammatory hyperalgesia further supports the importance of TTX-r sodium channels in pain transduction and development of neuropathic and inflammatory pain.

Nociceptor Neurotransmission

The excitatory neurotransmitter released from the central terminals of nociceptors is glutamate. There is evidence for the expression of at least two types of ionotropic glutamate receptors in primary afferent sensory neurons of the DRG.[55] Non-*N*-methyl-D-aspartate (NMDA) kainate receptors are associated predominantly with C fiber type small-diameter neurons. NMDA receptors are not exclusively associated with small-diameter neurons.[55] In fact, there is evidence that NMDA receptors may be predominately expressed in larger diameter sensory neurons. Pharmacologic studies in skin-nerve preparations of the rat have demonstrated glutamate-evoked excitation of Aδ and C fibers but not Aβ fibers. Glutamate can also produce a thermal sensitization.[56] These results confirm earlier behavioral studies of the role of glutamate receptors in the peripheral modulation of pain sensation. In addition to the ionotropic glutamate receptors, the presence of two group I metabotropic receptors (mGluR1 and mGluR5) on peripheral unmyelinated afferents has been reported. These G protein–coupled receptors signal through inositol 1,4,5-triphosphate/diacylglycerol pathways. Like their ionotropic counterparts, mGluR1 and mGluR5 appear to modulate peripheral nociceptors by participating in peripheral sensitization.

Bradykinin

BK, a naturally occurring inflammatory nonapeptide, has been shown to directly activate nociceptors and to produce nociceptor sensitization through several mechanisms.[57] The effects of BK are believed to be mediated through two receptor subtypes: B_1 and B_2. The B_2 receptor is widely expressed being responsible for the majority of BK-induced effects including those in nociceptors. In contrast, the B_1 subtype is expressed in smaller abundance and has a greater affinity for the BK metabolite, Des [Arg^9] BK. B_1 receptors are up-regulated during conditions of injury/inflammation and have been shown to contribute to inflammatory hyperalgesia.[58] Nevertheless, BK activation of nociceptors was eliminated in B_2-deficient mice, reaffirming the role of the B_2 receptor as the predominant target for BK action on nociceptors.[59]

Nociceptor activation by BK has been previously linked to the activation of PKC. Moreover, at least three potential pathways have been described that could link BK to VR1 activation in nociceptors: (1) BK activation of phospholipase A2 with subsequent metabolism of arachidonic acid into products of the lipoxygenase pathway,[37] (2) BK-mediated production of diacylglycerol and inositol 1,4,5-triphosphate with subsequent activation of PKC,[38] and (3) BK-induced release of VR1 from phosphatidylinositol-4, 5-biphosphate–mediated inhibition.[60]

Protein Kinase C

Activated forms of PKC are associated with the phosphorylation of selective domains of receptors and ion channels.[61] Activation of PKC produces C-fiber type nociceptor depolarization. Multiple isozymes of PKC have been identified and their role in mediating pain transduction is emerging. Of these, the epsilon isozyme of protein kinase C (PKCε) has been implicated in nociceptor function because it may mediate a component of nerve growth factor (NGF)-mediated hyperalgesia.[62] Furthermore, PKCε mutant mice have reduced mechanical and thermal hyperalgesia but have normal baseline thresholds for noxious stimuli.[62]

Peptide Growth Factors and Receptors

NGF is best known for its action on the developing nervous system where it is essential for the early survival of the central and peripheral nervous system. However, it has increasingly been shown to be an important link between inflammation, nerve injury, and the development of pain.[63] NGF has been found to be synthesized and secreted by a wide variety of tissues including Schwann cells located within sensory ganglion and within epidermal fibroblasts. Subsequently, additional NGF family members have been isolated and characterized. Termed "neurotrophins," they include the related peptides, brain-derived neurotrophic factor, NT-3, and NT-4/5. As a peptide family, they all have been implicated in the regulation of nociceptive transduction and pain. The biologic effects of neurotrophins are believed to occur through binding to either a high- or low-affinity receptor. *High-affinity* class receptors contain a cytoplasmic tyrosine kinase (Trk) domain and are conventionally referred to as TrkA, TrkB, or TrkC. NGF binds primarily to the "TrkA" receptor. The TrkA-mediated phosphorylation then propagates the NGF signal locally–at the cell membrane/nerve terminal or, after internalization, into the nucleus where it affects transcriptional control. Activation of Trk receptors can have both rapid and delayed effects, presumably from protein modifications of transmembrane receptors/ion channels and a change in transcriptional control resulting in the increase or decrease of mRNA-encoding elements of nociceptive transduction.

Somatic nociceptors require TrkA activation during and after development. Within the DRG, TrkA expression is restricted to a subset of small-diameter primary afferent neurons (the role of TrkA expression on other cell types in close association with nociceptors will be discussed later). In genetic knockout mice, in which the gene for TrkA has been disrupted, virtually all TrkA receptor–deficient mice have lost their small-diameter nociceptive neurons and are also profoundly hypoalgesic. Moreover, NGF appears to continue to play a fundamental role beyond the developmental period in the maintenance of a subpopulation of nociceptors. For example, immunization of adult rats with NGF produces anti-NGF antibodies and subsequent hypoalgesia. Other neurotrophins such as glial-derived neurotrophic factor (GDNF) is currently being explored as an important factor in the maintenance of the adult phenotype of both peptidergic and non-peptidergic nociceptors.

NGF plays a dynamic role in maintaining the function of nociceptors. Although neurotrophins play a critical role in sensory neuron development, adult sensory neurons do not require neurotrophins for their survival. Rather, they appear to play an essential role in the regulation of "normal" properties of pain transduction. Steady-state synthesis and release of NGF in the local environment of nociceptive terminals may regulate the expression of specialized peptides, receptors, and ion channels that help define a sensory neuron as a nociceptor. NGF has been shown to positively regulate both the mRNA and peptide content of substance P (SP) and calcitonin gene-related peptide (CGRP) in cultured sensory neurons. Furthermore, NGF enhances functional recovery of nociceptive terminals injured by capsaicin treatment by restoring neuropeptide content. In addition, TTX-r sodium channel ($Na_v1.8$) expression in small-diameter sensory neurons is dependent on the level of target-derived neurotrophic factors.[64] This is demonstrated by the ability of NGF to prevent the down-regulation of sodium channel expression ($Na_v1.8$) that normally follows axotomy.[64] Capsaicin activity in cultured sensory neurons requires the presence of NGF. Recent studies have suggested that a decrease in target-derived neurotrophins in vitro and in vivo may be responsible for the concomitant decrease in mRNA encoding VR1.[65] Non-neurotrophin growth factors also have been found to regulate VR1. GDNF regulates VR1 and SP levels in cultured sensory neurons and may regulate both peptidergic and nonpeptidergic nociceptors. Evidence that NGF can also regulate additional nociceptive elements including the BK B_2 subtype receptor and a VGSC expressed preferentially in small-diameter sensory neurons is emerging.

NGF may be a critical link between peripheral inflammation and hyperalgesia. Inflammation is associated with local and systemic changes. Peripheral changes include inflammatory cell migration, cytokine release, edema, erythema, pain, and hyperalgesia. Increasing evidence exists that NGF plays an essential role in peripheral inflammatory pain. Although NGF-induced changes in pain threshold are associated with thermal and mechanical hyperalgesia, the mechanism(s) to explain these changes remain poorly understood because of several confounding circumstances: (1) other inflammatory mediators may play similar roles in conjunction with NGF to activate or positively modulate nociceptors, (2) there is a complex of neurotrophins (NGF, brain-derived neurotrophic factor, NT-4/5) and non-neurotrophin growth factors such as GDNF that may be released during inflammatory conditions and act on overlapping populations of nociceptors.[63] SP and CGRP are two

of a number of neuropeptides released from nociceptors terminals in response to an inflammatory stimulus.

Although no single factor is acting alone, there is significant evidence to support the idea that NGF has a primary role in the development of inflammatory pain and hyperalgesia through its action on nociceptors. Included in this evidence are the following:

1. In experimental models of inflammation, concentrations of NGF increase within the tissue and parallel the development of behavioral signs of pain and hyperalgesia.
2. NGF produces both early (within minutes) and delayed (hours to days) increases in pain and hyperalgesia.
3. NGF produces both mechanical and thermal hyperalgesia. Human studies also corroborate a role for NGF in peripheral pain transduction. Intradermal injection of NGF in human volunteer subjects induces thermal hyperalgesia and mechanical allodynia at the site of injection, beginning as early as 3 hours and lasting up to 21 days.[66] Patients with congenital insensitivity to pain with anhydrosis have an absence of reaction to noxious stimuli and have recently been shown to contain mutations within the gene that encodes the NGF-TrkA receptor.

What controls the production of NGF during inflammation? One important candidate is the production of interleukin 1B (IL-1B), a cytokine that is produced by activated macrophages, B lymphocytes, and endothelial cells. Use of IgG-Trk fusion protein and anti-NGF antibodies to block inflammatory models of thermal and mechanical hyperalgesia has helped to confirm this hypothesis. Notable is the finding that blockade of hyperalgesia occurs with continued evidence of erythema and edema.[67]

NGF can modulate nociceptors through associated cell types. Mast cells, containing an abundant source of histamine and 5-HT, are found adjacent to nociceptive terminals. NGF-mediated mast cell degranulation may contribute to the acute phase of hyperalgesia through the release of 5-HT acting on multiple 5-HT receptor subtypes. However, a mast cell–independent mechanism is also activated by NGF and participates in the maintenance of hyperalgesia because decreased thermal thresholds continued to develop despite prior mast cell depletion. White blood cell subtypes, such as neutrophils and lymphocytes, are attracted to sites of injury and inflammation and have also been shown to participate in NGF-mediated hyperalgesia. In addition, the sympathetic nervous system contributes to certain chronic pain states and peripheral inflammatory hyperalgesia.

Neuropeptides

The most well-studied peptide in primary afferent nociceptors is SP, a member of a family of tachykinins that is widely expressed throughout the body (see review by Hokfelt and colleagues[68]). Despite intensive efforts, a specific physiologic class of nociceptors has not been distinguished by the presence or absence of SP. A similar conclusion can be made for other neuropeptides such as CGRP, somatostatin, and others. However, neuropeptides exert important physiologic effects when released from nociceptor central and peripheral terminals. Peripheral actions of SP release include vasodilation and increased vascular permeability that are hallmarks of neurogenic inflammation. Centrally, SP release serves as a neuromodulator, producing excitation and facilitation of synaptic transmission of second order dorsal horn neurons that relay nociceptive transmission. Another peptide, CGRP, is selectively expressed in the central terminals of primary afferent nociceptors that innervate superficial layers of the dorsal horn. CGRP functions to potentiate the actions of SP and can both activate and facilitate dorsal horn neurotransmission. Although apparently linked to the inflammatory response, genetic knockout mice lacking either SP or its receptor (NK1) develop hyperalgesia normally and appear not to have a direct effect on the initial step of the transduction of noxious stimuli. However, knockout mice exhibited other deficiencies, such as intensity-coding of noxious stimuli, development of neurogenic edema, and certain pain behaviors.[69–71]

Fatty Acid Metabolites

Nociceptors are sensitized by a wide range of inflammatory products of arachidonic acid (AA) metabolism. These include certain products of the cyclooxygenase pathway (PGE_2, PGI_2) that are known to exert their biologic action through G protein–coupled receptors and more recently isoprostanes, compounds that are formed by nonenzymatic peroxidation of AA such as 8-iso PGE_2 and 8-iso $PGF2_\alpha$. Alternately, AA is metabolized through the lipoxygenase pathway, producing a multitude of products including 8R and leukotriene B4, and 15-S-di HETE that have been shown to sensitize nociceptors. Although lipoxygenase products have a wide range of biologic activities and their receptor targets remain largely uncharacterized, 12-(S)-hydroperoxyeicosatetraenoic acid and leukotriene B4 have been recently shown to directly activate the nociceptive cation channel VR1.[37]

Other Mediators of Nociceptor Sensitization

Histamine released from mast cells is another inflammatory mediator capable of sensitizing nociceptors. It appears that it acts in conjunction with other factors as NGF, BK, and PGE_2 (see review by Shu and Mendell[63]).

Calcium channels. Voltage-sensitive calcium channels are important for the regulation of the intracellular calcium concentration that serves as a second messenger. Experiments on DRG neurons isolated from control and nerve-injured rats suggest that suppression of calcium channel activity after nerve injury leads to an increased excitability that can contribute to hyperalgesia.[72]

Alpha-2 adrenoceptors. During normal conditions, sympathetic stimulation and norepinephrine injection do not activate peripheral nociceptors. There is recent evidence that alpha-2 receptors in peripheral sensory neurons are involved

in the modulation of noxious thermal stimuli leading to thermal hyperalgesia.[73]

Adenosine, acting through A2 receptors, has also been reported to directly sensitize nociceptors.[74]

Nitric oxide may positively modulate nociceptor activation because subcutaneous injection of nitric oxide precursors produced pain in humans, and evidence of neural nitric oxide synthase has been localized to small-diameter sensory neurons and is associated with PGE_2-mediated hyperalgesia.[75]

Peripheral Opioid Peptides and Analgesics

The action of opioid analgesics to block transmission of nociceptive impulses at the level of the spinal cord has been widely accepted and has propelled spinal and epidural opioid use in clinical pain management (see Yaksh[76] for review; see also Chapter 27). Potential targets of opioid analgesics include the central and peripheral terminals of primary afferent nociceptors. Acting primarily through mu subtype receptors, peripherally injected opioids can produce analgesia in inflamed or injured tissue but have no similar effect in normal tissue. This observation has led to their clinical use following knee surgery.[77] Advancement of this paradigm includes the finding of endogenous opioid peptides delivered to the site of inflammation by immune cells and the development of peripherally acting opioid analgesics as loperamide.

Current and Potential Targets of Drug Actions

How do we selectively block peripheral pain transduction? Current approaches to pain management use a broad range of pharmacologic agents and techniques to deliver potentially harmful agents (e.g., opioid analgesics, local anesthetics) to discrete neuronal targets to produce a more restricted and desired therapeutic effect. Understanding how to target pain transducing receptors and ion channels that are selectively expressed in nociceptors could improve the therapeutic window between pain relief and harmful side effects.

Potential therapeutic targets currently include:

- VR1, because of its predominant expression in nociceptors and evidence of activation by products of inflammation
- ASICs that mediate the pain associated with ischemia, as occurs in refractory angina
- Isozymes of PKC that either directly activate nociceptive ion channels or positively modulate the transducers of noxious stimuli as I_{heat} and I_{mech}
- TrkA, the high-affinity receptor for NGF that mediates nociceptor sensitization
- $Na_v1.8$ (SNS/PN3), a TTX-r subtype of sodium channel responsible for the transmission of nociceptive signaling to the spinal cord.

These examples represent general classes of potential targets (transduction, modulation, and transmission) that if selectively blocked, could offer a novel approach to pain management (Fig. 11–3). However, as with any critically important system, pain transduction appears to have multiple (possibly redundant) pathways to ensure detection of tissue damaging stimuli. In combination with the multitude of human diseases, identifying effective "therapeutic targets" may appear to be an overwhelming task. Therefore future strategies using peripheral targets for pain management may require a combination of therapeutic agents that block both primary pain transducing channels and their modulatory pathways.

Conclusions

Despite tremendous advances in our understanding of nociceptor function, the identities of the receptors/channels that transduce noxious mechanical and thermal stimuli remain elusive. If these transducing elements are related to the vanilloid receptor family, then progress may be rapid and their identification forthcoming. However, isolating additional channels activated by mechanical or thermal stimuli is only one part of a complex story. Although VR1 is activated by thermal stimuli in vitro, its role in vivo may be primarily to mediate thermal hyperalgesia. Therefore VR1 may represent a molecular model of nociceptor sensitization in which the action of both an *inflammatory mediator* and a *noxious stimulus* are required for nociceptor activation. Nociceptive ion channels functioning in this manner may serve to signal ongoing tissue injury and inflammation rather than acute noxious stimuli. A similar mechanism may underlie mechanical hyperalgesia. Given the diversity of inflammatory products previously discussed, finding a single pathway or receptor that will block peripheral pain transduction is unlikely. However, understanding nociceptive transduction at the molecular level should one day provide a means to treat painful conditions with fewer side effects and identify patients predisposed to the development of chronic pain.

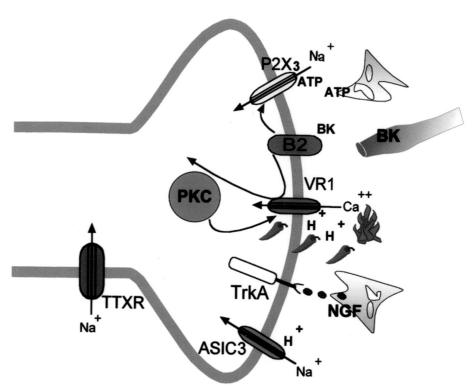

Figure 11–3. Nociceptive transduction. Hypothetical nociceptor terminal containing multiple ion channels sensitive to noxious stimuli. Vanilloid receptor subtype 1 (VR1) is activated at an intracellular site by capsaicin (pepper), noxious heat, and extracellular protons (H^+). Activation of VR1 by thermal stimuli in vivo probably requires the additional action of inflammatory mediators. Bradykinin (BK) acting through B_2 receptors has been proposed to activate VR1 through stimulation of protein kinase C (PKC), formation of lipoxygenase products, or release of bound phosphoinositides (see text). Both BK and protons also modulate VR1, decreasing its threshold of activation. Nerve growth factor (NGF) produced from fibroblasts binds to its high-affinity receptor tyrosine kinase type A (TrkA) and participates in nociceptor sensitization through its action on VR1 and tetrodotoxin-resistant (TTX-r sodium channels). Adenosine triphosphate (ATP) released from damaged cells directly activates $P2X_3$ and is also positively modulated by BK. Acid-sensing ion channel subtype 3 (ASIC3) detects acidic conditions that might occur during conditions of ischemia.

References

1. Sherrington CS: The Integrative Action of the Nervous System. New York, C. Scribner's Sons, 1906.
2. Fields HL: Pain Syndromes in Neurology, London, Butterworths-Heinemann, 1990.
3. Carpenter MB: Core Text of Neuroanatomy, 3rd ed. Baltimore, Williams & Wilkins, 1985.
4. Cervero F: Sensory innervation of the viscera: Peripheral basis of visceral pain. Physiol Rev 74:95–138, 1994.
5. Janig W, Khasar SG, Levine JD, et al: The role of vagal visceral afferents in the control of nociception. Prog Brain Res 122:273–287, 2000.
6. Burgess PR, Perl ER: Cutaneous mechanoreceptors and nociceptors. In Iggo A (ed): Handbook of Sensory Physiology: Somatosensory System. Berlin, Springer-Verlag, 1973.
7. Harper AA, Lawson SN: Conduction velocity is related to morphological cell type in rat dorsal root ganglion neurones. J Physiol (Lond) 359:31–46, 1985.
8. Bessou P, Perl ER: Response of cutaneous sensory units with unmyelinated fibers to noxious stimuli. J Neurophysiol 32:1025–1043, 1969.
9. Adriaensen H, Gybels J, Handwerker HO, et al: Nociceptor discharges and sensations due to prolonged noxious mechanical stimulation—a paradox. Hum Neurobiol 3:53–58, 1984.
10. McMahon SB: Are there fundamental differences in the peripheral mechanisms of visceral and somatic pain? Behav Brain Sci 20:381–391; discussion 435–513, 1997.
11. Cervero F, Janig W: Visceral nociceptors: a new world order? Trends Neurosci 15:374–378, 1992.
12. McMahon SB, Koltzenburg M: Novel classes of nociceptors: Beyond Sherrington. Trends Neurosci 13:199–201, 1990.
13. McCleskey EW, Gold MS: Ion channels of nociception. Annu Rev Physiol 61:835–856, 1999.
14. Cesare P, McNaughton P: A novel heat-activated current in nociceptive neurons and its sensitization by bradykinin. Proc Natl Acad Sci USA 93:15435–15439, 1996.
15. Reichling DB, Levine JD: Heat transduction in rat sensory neurons by calcium-dependent activation of a cation channel. Proc Natl Acad Sci USA 94:7006–7011, 1997.
16. Cesare P, Moriondo A, Vellani V, et al: Ion channels gated by heat. Proc Natl Acad Sci USA 96:7658–7663, 1999.
17. Reichling DB, Levine JD: In hot pursuit of the elusive heat transducers. Neuron 26:555–558, 2000.
18. McCarter GC, Reichling DB, Levine JD: Mechanical transduction by rat dorsal root ganglion neurons in vitro. Neurosci Lett 273:179–182, 1999.
19. Levine JD, Fields HL, Basbaum AI: Peptides and the primary afferent nociceptor. J Neurosci 13:2273–2286, 1993.
20. Robbins WR, Staats PS, Levine J, et al: Treatment of intractable pain with topical large-dose capsaicin: Preliminary report. Anesth Analg 86:579–583, 1998.
21. Buck SH, Burks TF: The neuropharmacology of capsaicin: Review of some recent observations. Pharmacol Rev 38:179–226, 1986.
22. Oh U, Hwang SW, Kim D: Capsaicin activates a nonselective cation channel in cultured neonatal rat dorsal root ganglion neurons. J Neurosci 16:1659–1667, 1996.
23. Szallasi A, Blumberg PM: Vanilloid (Capsaicin) receptors and mechanisms. Pharmacol Rev 51:159–212, 1999.
24. Caterina MJ, Schumacher MA, Tominaga M, et al: The capsaicin receptor: A heat-activated ion channel in the pain pathway. Nature 389:816–824, 1997.
25. Petersen M, Lamotte RH, Klusch A, et al: Multiple capsaicin-evoked currents in isolated rat sensory neurons. Neuroscience 75:495–505, 1996.
26. Kedei N, Szabo T, Lile JD, et al: Analysis of the native quaternary structure of vanilloid receptor 1. J Biol Chem 276:28613–28619, 2001.
27. Schumacher MA, Moff I, Sudangunta SP, et al: Molecular cloning of an N-terminal splice variant of the capsaicin receptor. Loss of N-terminal domain suggests functional divergence among capsaicin receptor subtypes. J Biol Chem 275:2756–2762, 2000.
28. Jung J, Hwang SW, Kwak J, et al: Capsaicin binds to the intracellular domain of the capsaicin-activated ion channel. J Neurosci 19:529–538, 1999.

29. Caterina MJ, Leffler A, Malmberg AB, et al: Impaired nociception and pain sensation in mice lacking the capsaicin receptor. Science 288:306–313, 2000.
30. Davis JB, Gray J, Gunthorpe MJ, et al: Vanilloid receptor-1 is essential for inflammatory thermal hyperalgesia. Nature 405:183–187, 2000.
31. Caterina MJ, Rosen TA, Tominaga M, et al: A capsaicin-receptor homologue with a high threshold for noxious heat. Nature 398:436–441, 1999.
32. Tominaga M, Caterina MJ, Malmberg AB, et al: The cloned capsaicin receptor integrates multiple pain-producing stimuli. Neuron 21:531–543, 1998.
33. Jordt SE, Tominaga M, Julius D: Acid potentiation of the capsaicin receptor determined by a key extracellular site. Proc Natl Acad Sci USA 97:8134–8139, 2000.
34. Welch JM, Simon SA, Reinhart PH: The activation mechanism of rat vanilloid receptor 1 by capsaicin involves the pore domain and differs from the activation by either acid or heat. Proc Natl Acad Sci USA 97:13889–13894, 2000.
35. Waldmann R, Lazdunski M: H^+ gated cation channels: Neuronal acid sensors in the NaC/DEG family of ion channels. Curr Opin Neurobiol 8:418–424, 1998.
36. Smart D, Gunthorpe MJ, Jerman JC, et al: The endogenous lipid anandamide is a full agonist at the human vanilloid receptor (hVR1). Br J Pharmacol 129:227–230, 2000.
37. Hwang SW, Cho H, Kwak J, et al: Direct activation of capsaicin receptors by products of lipoxygenases: Endogenous capsaicin-like substances. Proc Natl Acad Sci USA 97:6155–6160, 2000.
38. Premkumar LS, Ahern GP: Induction of vanilloid receptor channel activity by protein kinase C. Nature 408:985–990, 2000.
39. Sackin H: Mechanosensitive channels. Annu Rev Physiol 57:333–353, 1995.
40. Xue Q, Yu Y, Trilk SL, et al. The genomic organization of the gene encoding the vanilloid receptor: Evidence for multiple splice variants. Genomics 76:14–20, 2001.
41. Liedtke W, Choe Y, Marti-Renom MA, et al: Vanilloid receptor-related osmotically activated channel (VR-OAC), a candidate vertebrate osmoreceptor. Cell 103:525–535, 2000.
42. Cortright DN, Crandall M, Sanchez JF, et al: The tissue distribution and functional characterization of human VR1. Biochem Biophys Res Commun 281:1183–1189, 2001.
43. Hayes P, Meadows HJ, Gunthorpe MJ, et al: Cloning and functional expression of a human orthologue of rat vanilloid receptor-1. Pain 88:205–215, 2000.
44. McIntyre P, McLatchie LM, Chambers A, et al: Pharmacological differences between the human and rat vanilloid receptor 1 (VR1). Br J Pharmacol 132:1084–1094, 2001.
45. Wiemann S, Weil B, Wellenreuther R, et al: Toward a catalog of human genes and proteins: Sequencing and analysis of 500 novel complete protein coding human cDNAs. Genome Res 11:422–435, 2001.
46. Holton FA, Holton P: The capillary dilator substances in dry powders of spinal roots: A possible role of adenosine triphosphate in chemical transmission from nerve endings. J Physiol (Lond) 126:124–140, 1954.
47. Burnstock G: Purine-mediated signalling in pain and visceral perception. Trends Pharmacol Sci 22:182–188, 2001.
48. Brake A, Schumacher M, Julius D: ATP receptors in sickness, pain and death. Chem Biol 3:229–232, 1996.
49. Souslova V, Cesare P, Ding Y, et al: Warm-coding deficits and aberrant inflammatory pain in mice lacking P2X3 receptors. Nature 407:1015–1017, 2000.
50. Cockayne DA, Hamilton SG, Zhu QM, et al: Urinary bladder hyporeflexia and reduced pain-related behaviour in P2X3-deficient mice. Nature 407:1011–1015, 2000.
51. Paukert M, Osteroth R, Geisler HS, et al: Inflammatory mediators potentiate ATP-gated channels through the P2X3 subunit. J Biol Chem 276:21077–21082, 2001.
52. Akopian AN, Sivilotti L, Wood JN: A tetrodotoxin-resistant voltage-gated sodium channel expressed by sensory neurons. Nature 379:257–262, 1996.
53. Baker MD, Wood JN: Involvement of Na^+ channels in pain pathways. Trends Pharmacol Sci 22:27–31, 2001.
54. Gold MS: Inflammatory mediator-induced modulation of TTX-R INa: An underlying mechanism of inflammatory hyperalgesia. Proc West Pharmacol Soc 42:111–112, 1999.
55. Huettner JE: Glutamate receptor channels in rat DRG neurons: Activation by kainate and quisqualate and blockade of desensitization by Con A. Neuron 5:255–266, 1990.

56. Du J, Koltzenburg M, Carlton SM: Glutamate-induced excitation and sensitization of nociceptors in rat glabrous skin. Pain 89:187–198, 2001.

57. Burgess GM, Mullaney I, McNeill M, et al: Second messengers involved in the mechanism of action of bradykinin in sensory neurons in culture. J Neurosci 9:3314–3325, 1989.

58. Rupniak NM, Boyce S, Webb JK, et al: Effects of the bradykinin B1 receptor antagonist des-Arg9[Leu8]bradykinin and genetic disruption of the B2 receptor on nociception in rats and mice. Pain 71:89–97, 1997.

59. Seabrook GR, Bowery BJ, Heavens R, et al: Expression of B1 and B2 bradykinin receptor mRNA and their functional roles in sympathetic ganglia and sensory dorsal root ganglia neurones from wild-type and B2 receptor knockout mice. Neuropharmacology 36:1009–1017, 1997.

60. Chuang H, Prescott ED, Kong H, et al: Bradykinin and nerve growth factor release the capsaicin receptor from ^{PtdIns4,5_2}-mediated inhibition. Nature 411:957–962, 2001.

61. Huganir RL, Greengard P: Regulation of neurotransmitter receptor desensitization by protein phosphorylation. Neuron 5:555–567, 1990.

62. Khasar SG, Lin YH, Martin A, et al: A novel nociceptor signaling pathway revealed in protein kinase C epsilon mutant mice. Neuron 24:253–260, 1999.

63. Shu XQ, Mendell LM: Neurotrophins and hyperalgesia. Proc Natl Acad Sci USA 96:7693–7696, 1999.

64. Dib-Hajj SD, Black JA, Cummins TR, et al: Rescue of alpha-SNS sodium channel expression in small dorsal root ganglion neurons after axotomy by nerve growth factor in vivo. J Neurophysiol 79:2668–2676, 1998.

65. Michael GJ, Priestley JV: Differential expression of the mRNA for the vanilloid receptor subtype 1 in cells of the adult rat dorsal root and nodose ganglia and its downregulation by axotomy. J Neurosci 19:1844–1854, 1999.

66. Dyck PJ, Peroutka S, Rask C, et al: Intradermal recombinant human nerve growth factor induces pressure allodynia and lowered heat-pain threshold in humans. Neurology 48:501–505, 1997.

67. McMahon SB, Bennett DL, Priestley JV, et al: The biological effects of endogenous nerve growth factor on adult sensory neurons revealed by a trkA-IgG fusion molecule. Nat Med 1:774–780, 1995.

68. Hokfelt T, Pernow B, Wahren J: Substance P: A pioneer amongst neuropeptides. J Intern Med 249:27–40, 2001.

69. De Felipe C, Herrero JF, O'Brien JA, et al: Altered nociception, analgesia and aggression in mice lacking the receptor for substance P. Nature 392:394–397, 1998.

70. Cao YQ, Mantyh PW, Carlson EJ, et al: Primary afferent tachykinins are required to experience moderate to intense pain. Nature 392: 390–394, 1998.

71. Zimmer A, Zimmer AM, Baffi J, et al: Hypoalgesia in mice with a targeted deletion of the tachykinin 1 gene. Proc Natl Acad Sci USA 95:2630–2635, 1998.

72. Abdulla FA, Smith PA: Axotomy reduces the effect of analgesic opioids yet increases the effect of nociception on dorsal root ganglion neurons. J Neurosci 18:9685–9694, 1998.

73. Kingery WS, Guo TZ, Davies MF, et al: The alpha(2A) adrenoceptor and the sympathetic postganglionic neuron contribute to the development of neuropathic heat hyperalgesia in mice. Pain 85:345–358, 2000.

74. Taiwo YO, Levine JD: Direct cutaneous hyperalgesia induced by adenosine. Neuroscience 38:757–762, 1990.

75. Aley KO, McCarter G, Levine JD: Nitric oxide signaling in pain and nociceptor sensitization in the rat. J Neurosci 18:7008–7014, 1998.

76. Yaksh TL: Spinal systems and pain processing: Development of novel analgesic drugs with mechanistically defined models. Trends Pharmacol Sci 20:329–337, 1999.

77. Stein C, Comisel K, Haimerl E, et al: Analgesic effect of intraarticular morphine after arthroscopic knee surgery. N Engl J Med 325: 1123–1126, 1991.

12

Sensory Processing

Istvan Nagy, MD, PhD

PRIMARY AFFERENT NEURON/DORSAL ROOT GANGLIA

Heterogeneity of Primary Sensory Neurons
  Morphologic Heterogeneity
  Neurochemical Heterogeneity

Physiologic Heterogeneity
Pharmacologic Heterogeneity

Primary afferent or primary sensory neurons that connect the peripheral tissues, such as skin, viscera, joints, and muscles, to the central nervous system (CNS) are pseudounipolar neurons with a spherical perikaryon, peripheral and central processes, and peripheral and central terminals. Detailed accounts on the neurobiology of the peripheral (see Chapter 11) and central terminals (see Chapter 13) are found elsewhere in this textbook; therefore, this chapter concentrates exclusively on primary sensory neurons as whole cells.

The majority of the perikarya of primary sensory neurons are located in dorsal root ganglia (DRG). Based on this location, these cells are also called dorsal root ganglion neurons. The perikarya of the somatosensory and viscerosensory fibers of cranial nerves V, VII, IX, and X, which provide sensory innervation to the face, oral cavity, cranial dura, and the majority of organs in the respiratory and gastrointestinal system, are in the trigeminal, geniculate, superior and inferior glossopharyngeal, intracranial jugular, and nodose ganglia. Primary sensory neurons originating from teeth, periodontium, hard palate, capsule of the temporomandibular joint, and muscle spindles and Golgi organs of masticatory muscles are in the mesencephalic nucleus of the trigeminal nerve.

Morphologic and physiologic heterogeneity of primary sensory neurons have been known for almost 100 years. Using DRG sections, Cajal[1] found that the perikarya of primary sensory neurons were either large light or small dark cells. The processes of primary sensory neurons also form two groups: the group of fast-conducting myelinated and the group of slow-conducting unmyelinated fibers. Gasser and Edinger[2] found that although the fast-conducting myelinated (A-type) fibers could be activated by low-intensity innocuous stimuli, the slow-conducting unmyelinated (C-type) fibers are activated by high-intensity noxious stimuli.

According to the classical definition, the functions of primary sensory neurons are to detect peripheral innocuous and noxious stimuli, generate action potentials, transmit them from the periphery to the CNS, and release transmitters in the CNS. This definition implies that primary sensory neurons are probably heterogeneous but simple and static cells, which express only transducers, ion-channels, and transmitter release machinery necessary for stimulus detection, action potential generation and transmission, and transmitter release. However, a large number of membrane-bound molecules may change the responsiveness of primary sensory neurons; therefore, primary sensory neurons not only transmit but also process the sensory information. This processing starts at the peripheral terminals.

The classical description of primary sensory neurons also suggests that they are static cells, but it has recently been shown that peripheral pathologic events such as chronic inflammation or physical or metabolic nerve injuries can induce post-translational and transcriptional changes in them. As a result, the phenotype of primary sensory neurons is changed, which alters their excitability.[3] (For more information regarding pathologic event-induced changes, refer to some recently published reviews on these topics.[3–7])

This chapter describes the morphologic, neurochemical, physiologic, and pharmacologic characteristics of primary sensory neurons that enable the processing of sensory information.

Heterogeneity of Primary Sensory Neurons

Morphologic Heterogeneity

Morphologically, the processes and the perikarya of primary sensory neurons form two subpopulations. The diameter of the processes in humans varies between 0.1 and 12 μm. Primary sensory fibers thicker than 1 μm are surrounded by a myelin sheet. Among the myelinated fibers, thicker fibers (5–10 μm) have a thicker myelin sheet than thin fibers (1–5 μm). Furthermore, the thicker myelin sheets correlate with longer distance between the nodes of Ranvier, where neighboring myelin sheets meet and saltatory action potential transmission occurs. At the periphery, myelinated and unmyelinated fibers can terminate both in encapsulated and nonencapsulated endings; however, at their termini in the spinal cord, myelinated and unmyelinated fibers are differentially located. Most of the unmyelinated fibers terminate in the most superficial laminae (lamina I and II), whereas thick myelinated fibers in physiologic conditions never enter those areas.[8] Thin myelinated fibers terminate predominantly in lamina I.

In humans, the diameter of the perikarya of primary sensory neurons varies between 20 and 100 μm. Based on the cross-sectional area, primary sensory neurons distribute into two separate subpopulations: a group of small and a group of large cells.[9] Using background staining with toluidin blue, the small cells appear dark whereas large cells appear light.[1] About 60% of the total neuronal population in sensory ganglia belong to the subpopulation of small dark cells.

Neurochemical Heterogeneity

Markers of the Three Major Subpopulations

Immunohistochemical and histochemical staining differentiate three major subpopulations of primary sensory neurons. An antibody (RT97) raised against the 145- and 200-kD subunits of neurofilaments stains about 40% of the neurons.[10] About half of the remaining 60% of the cells contains neuropeptides, such as substance P (SP), calcitonin gene-related peptide (CGRP), or somatostatin, whereas the other half of the cells produces specific enzymes, such as fluoride-resistant acid phosphatase (FRAP) or bind lectins, such as the *Bandeiraea simplicifolia* isolectin B4 (IB4).[11–13] Size analyses of the different subpopulations reveal that the RT97 immunopositive cells are the large light cells, whereas the peptidergic and fluoride-resistant acid phosphatase positive/IB4-binding cells are the small dark ones. Terminals of peptidergic and nonpeptidergic small cells appear to be spatially segregated both at the periphery and within the spinal cord. Recent results suggest that the wall of viscera contains more peptidergic than IB4-positive fibers, whereas somatic tissues are more likely to be innervated by IB4-binding than peptidergic fibers.[14,15] In the spinal cord, peptidergic fibers terminate in lamina I and outer lamina II, whereas IB4-binding fibers terminate in inner lamina II.[16] Furthermore, spinal terminals of IB4-binding fibers are involved in the formation of special synaptic arrangements, called synaptic glomeruli, in which a primary afferent terminal is surrounded by a number of postsynaptic dendrites and presynaptic inhibitory axon terminals, whereas peptidergic terminals are not involved in such arrangements.[17] These findings suggest that the function of peptidergic and IB4-binding small cells must be different.

Neurotransmitters in Primary Sensory Neurons

Although all primary sensory neurons use glutamate as the principal neurotransmitter, neurons can be further differentiated by the additonal neurotransmitters that they release. Peptidergic cells use neuropeptides, and the majority of the peptidergic cells contain CGRP and tachykinins.[18] Smaller numbers of peptidergic cells also contain other peptides, such as somatostatin, bombesin, or vasointestinal polypeptide. Peptidergic cells also use the brain-derived neurotrophic factor (BDNF) as a neuromodulator.[19] Some of the primary sensory neurons produce and release cytokines, which form a large and diverse group of polypeptides also produced by different other cells, such as immune and Schwann cells.[20,21] Subpopulations of DRG cells produce different cytokines. Large and medium size cells produce IL-1, whereas small cells produce tumor necrosis factor-alpha (TNF-α), IL-2, IL-6, and leukemia inhibitory factor. Whereas glutamate, neuropeptides, and BDNF are involved in synaptic transmission, the role of cytokines is not known.

Physiologic Heterogeneity

Conduction Velocity and Sensitivity of Primary Afferent Fibers to Different Stimulus Modalities

Based on the conduction velocity (CV) of action potentials, four major types of primary afferent fibers can be distinguished: Aα-fibers (CV: 80–120 m/sec), Aβ-fibers (CV: 30–70 m/sec), Aδ-fibers (CV: 5–30 m/sec), and C-fibers (CV: 0.6–2 m/sec). CV of action potentials depends on the thickness of the fibers (thicker fibers correlate with faster CV), the thickness of the myelin sheet (thicker myelin sheets also correlate with faster CV), and the distance between the nodes of Ranvier (CV increases with increasing distance between nodes of Ranvier); thus Aα- and Aβ-fibers are thick fibers with thick myelin sheet, Aδ-fibers are thin fibers with thin myelin sheet, and C-fibers are thin fibers with no myelin sheet.

Different primary afferent fibers are sensitive to mechanical, thermal and/or chemical stimuli, and the intensity of the stimulus. As mentioned, Gasser and Edinger[2] showed unequivocally that in physiologic conditions most fibers sensitive to innocuous stimuli belong to the subpopulation of fast-conducting myelinated fibers (non-nociceptive Aα- and Aβ-fibers), whereas noxious stimulus-sensitive fibers belong to the subpopulations of slow-conducting, thinly myelinated or unmyelinated fibers (nociceptive Aδ- and C-fibers). Table 12–1 shows the types of primary

TABLE 12–1.

Major Types of Primary Sensory Fibers

Type of Fiber	Conduction Velocity (m/sec)	Function of Fiber
Aα	80–120	Muscle spindle afferent Golgi organ afferent
Aβ	30–70	G-hair, rapidly adapting innocuous mechano-sensitive Rapidly adapting nonhair innocuous mechano-sensitive Slowly-adapting innocuous mechano-sensitive
Aδ	5–25	D-hair, rapidly adapting innocuous mechano-sensitive Slowly adapting innocuous mechano-sensitive Innocuous cold-sensitive Noxious mechano-heat-sensitive Noxious mechano-cold-sensitive Noxious mechano-sensitive
C	0.6–2	Slowly-conducting innocuous mechano-sensitive Noxious mechano-sensitive Noxious mechano-cold-sensitive Noxious mechano-heat-sensitive Noxious mechano-heat-cold-sensitive Noxious heat-sensitive "Silent" nociceptor

afferent fibers based on their CV and sensitivity. Whereas Aα-fibers originate from muscle spindles and Golgi organs in tendons and are sensitive to muscle and tendon stretching, other fibers either originate from sensory organs in the skin or as free endings in the skin or wall of different organs and are sensitive to different stimulus modalities, such as touch, pressure, heat, cold, and chemicals. Notably, although non-nociceptive fibers are sensitive to one stimulus modality (e.g., mechanical or warm stimulation), most nociceptive fibers can be activated by more than one modality (e.g.,) mechano-cold-heat nociceptor. Moreover, essentially all nociceptive primary afferent fibers are sensitive to different exogenous, or endogenous chemical agents, or both, a few of which are listed in Chapter 11 (for more detailed information see Nagy and Rice[6] and Kress and Reeh[22]). Based on this multiple sensitivity, nociceptive primary sensory fibers are also referred to as polymodal nociceptors. One type of C-fibers, the "silent" fibers, do not respond to any physical (mechanical or thermal) stimulation during physiologic con-

ditions. However, after sensitization, exposure to different inflammatory mediators[22] induces response to different stimuli (see reports by Woolf and Costigan[3] and Nagy and Rice[6]).

The sensitivity of the primary afferents depends on the transducer(s) and receptor(s) they express. There are different molecules for transducing physical stimuli, such as noxious and innocuous heat, cold, and mechanical stimuli, and chemical stimuli. The majority of chemical excitation of primary afferents is produced by different neurotransmitters and modulators, and the effects of these agents are mediated by the respective receptors that are also expressed elsewhere in the human body. The type of receptors and the subpopulation of primary sensory neurons in which they are expressed is discussed later in this chapter.

Currently, detailed information exists only about the molecules involved in noxious heat and pH transduction. Limited information exists about the possible warm, innocuous cold, and innocuous and noxious mechanotransducers. Nothing is known about the noxious cold transducer(s).

Transducers

Noxious Heat Transduction

Both of the currently known noxious heat transducers have been recently cloned.[23,24] One is the vanilloid receptor 1 (VR1; see Chapter 11 for a detailed account of the molecular characteristics of VR1). As described in Chapter 11, VR1 is a "polymodal" transducer sensitive to noxious heat (>~45° C) vanilloids, such as capsaicin, the pungent ingredient of the chili pepper, and proton (<~pH6.5).[24,25] The involvement of VR1 in noxious heat transduction is shown by recordings of noxious heat-activated currents in VR1-injected or transfected non-neuronal cells and by the loss of the noxious heat-induced currents in primary sensory neurons taken from mice in which the gene encoding VR1 had been deleted.[25,26]

VR1 is expressed in about 40% of the total primary sensory neuronal population and all VR1-expressing cells belong to the subpopulation of small cells.[15] Approximately half of the VR1-expressing primary sensory neurons contain CGRP, whereas the other half bind IB4. At the periphery, VR1 is expressed by subpopulations of both visceral and somatic primary afferent fibers.[14,15] In the spinal cord, as it could be expected, most of VR1 immunopositivity can be seen in lamina I and II where most peptidergic and IB4-binding primary sensory fibers terminate.[15] Based on the heat threshold of VR1 and its expression by peptidergic and IB4-binding primary sensory neurons, it has been proposed that VR1 is the noxious heat transducer in type 2 noxious heat-sensitive primary sensory fibers.[27]

The other known noxious heat transducer is the vanilloid receptor-like protein 1 (VRL-1), which, although being an homologue of VR1, is not sensitive to any vanilloids.[23] VRL-1, which is also a nonselective cationic channel, responds to noxious heat only greater than 50° C.[27] About a sixth of the total neuronal primary sensory neuronal population express VRL-1 and have a medium or large diameter.[23,27] Less than 10% of the VRL-1–expressing primary sensory neurons express SP or bind IB4; however, about 80% of VRL-1 immunopositive cells express RT97, which is a marker for myelinated neurons (see earlier).[10,23] In the spinal cord, VRL-1–expressing fibers terminate in lamina I, which is the main termination area of Aδ-fibers.[23] The heat threshold of VRL-1 and its expression by cells with Aδ-fibers indicates that VRL-1 is responsible for noxious heat transduction in type 1 noxious heat-sensitive primary sensory fibers.[27]

Non-noxious Thermotransduction

Recently, two ion channels—the heat-activated background K$^+$ channel (TREK-1) and the adenosine triphosphate (ATP)-gated ion channel P2X$_3$—have been suggested to be involved in thermotransdution in the physiologic temperature range.[28,29] TREK-1 activates at about 25° C, and its activity increases up to about 42° C. Further increase of the temperature reduces the activity of TREK-1. TREK-1 is expressed by a subpopulation of small- and medium-sized primary sensory neurons. TREK-1 is a potassium channel, so its activity stabilizes the membrane and reduces action potential generation. Thus TREK-1 could be a non-noxious cold transducer. Another possibility is that TREK-1 is a background channel important for fine-tuning the temperature sensitivity of noxious heat-sensitive primary sensory neurons.

Suto and Gotoh[30] have recently found that exposure of primary sensory neurons to non-noxious cold (>20° C) increases Ca^{++} influx in a subpopulation of cells. This finding indicates that there must be another non-noxious cold transducer in addition to TREK-1.

The P2X$_3$ receptor is a member of the ATP-sensitive ion channel family and is expressed selectively by about one third of the total primary sensory neuronal population.[31,32] Virtually all P2X$_3$-expressing primary sensory neurons belong to the subpopulation of IB4-binding small cells.[31] Accordingly, P2X$_3$ immunoreactivity in the spinal cord can be seen in inner lamina II. It has been reported recently that mice in which the gene encoding the P2X$_3$ receptor had been deleted have warm-coding deficits[29] indicating that P2X$_3$ is involved in mediating warm sensation. The temperature range in which P2X$_3$ receptors are active has been shown to be between 30° C and 45° C.[29]

Mechanotransduction

The limited information on mechanotransduction in vertebrates, including human vertebrates, are derived either from data obtained in *Caenorhabditis elegans* or from mice in which certain genes had been deleted. In *C. elegans,* mutations revealed the existence of 15 genes, called *mec* genes, encoding MEC proteins, which could be involved in mechanotransduction.[33] Deletion of any of the *mec* genes results in altered mechanosensation in *C. elegans*. To date, homologues of two MEC proteins have been found in vertebrates, stromatin, and brain sodium channel 1 (BNC1),[34,35] which could be involved in mechanotransduction. Stromatin is expressed by all primary sensory neurons, whereas BNC1 is expressed by subpopulations of both small and large cells.

However, large cells show a greater intensity of BNC1 immunostaining indicating that these cells express more BNC1 proteins than small cells. Primary afferent fibers from mice lacking BNC1 show reduced responses in low-threshold, rapidly-adapting mechanosensitive fibers. In the skin, BNC1 is expressed in nerve endings running around hair follicles, the movement of which activates rapidly-adapting mechanoreceptors. These findings suggest that BNC1 is a non-noxious mechanotransducer.

BNC1 belongs to the denegerin/epithelial sodium channel superfamily, which also comprises the so-called acid-sensing ion channels (ASICs).[36] One type of the ASICs that is expressed exclusively in DRG neurons is called dorsal root ASIC (DRASIC); it has been recently shown to be involved in mechanotransduction. DRASIC is expressed both by small and large primary sensory neurons and in sensory organs, such as Meissner corpuscles, hair folliculus' lanceolate endings and Merkel cell-neurite complexes, and in free nerve endings in the skin.[37] In DRASIC knockout, mice the non-noxious, mechanical stimulation–evoked activity of rapidly adapting mechanoceptors is increased, whereas the noxious mechanical stimulation-evoked activity of slowly-conducting myelinated mechanonociceptors is decreased.[37] These findings indicate that DRASIC could be a part of molecule complexes involved in mechanotransduction.

Another molecule that could be involved in non-noxious mechanotransduction is the ATP receptor P2Y$_1$. When P2Y$_1$ cDNA is injected to oocytes, they become mechanosensitive.[38] P2Y$_1$ receptor expression has been demonstrated on large DRG cells.[38]

Biophysical Properties

Based on electrophysiologic properties, two major types of primary sensory neurons can be distinguished. The first type of cells produces fast action potentials with a small afterhyperpolarization, whereas the other type of cells produces slow action potentials with a plateau on the falling phase and a large afterhyperpolarization.[39,40] Whereas the first type of cells has fast-conducting Aβ-fibers, the second type of cells has slow-conducting Aδ- or C-fibers.[39] Both Na$^+$ and Ca^{++} are involved in the generation of somatic action potentials in the second type of cells, whereas only Na$^+$ is involved in the generation of somatic action potentials in the first type of neurons.[40,41] The plateau phase in the second type of cells is produced by Ca^{++} currents.[39] Harper and Lawson[41] combined intracellular electrophysiologic recordings with intracellular dye injection and found a strong correlation between the physiologic and morphologic parameters of primary sensory neurons; thus fast somatic action potentials are produced by large cells with fast-conducting Aβ-fibers, whereas slow somatic action potentials are produced by small cells with slow-conducting Aδ- and C-fibers. These findings were particularly important because they confirmed previous suggestions that small primary sensory neurons are nociceptive cells that give rise to high-threshold, slow-conducting Aδ- and C-fibers, whereas large cells are non-nociceptive cells that give rise to low-threshold, fast-conducting Aβ-fibers. As Na$^+$ and Ca^{++} currents are involved in the generation of action potentials, these findings also suggest that voltage-gated Na^+ and Ca^{++} channels must be different on the two types of primary sensory neurons.

Voltage-Gated Na^+ Channels

Among the ten known voltage-gated Na^+ channels, six are expressed in primary sensory neurons: $Na_v1.1$, $Na_v1.6$, $Na_v1.7$, $Na_v1.8$, $Na_v1.9$, and Na_x.[42,43] Four of these ($Na_v1.1$, $Na_v1.7$, $Na_v1.9$, Na_x) are uniquely expressed by these cells, whereas the other two are also expressed elsewhere in the nervous system.[43] Both the biophysical and pharmacologic properties of the six channels are different.[42–45] Regarding the biophysical parameters, some of the channels, such as the $Na_v1.6$, have fast kinetics, some of the others, such as the $Na_v1.8$, have slow kinetics.[43–45] Moreover, the activation and inactivation parameters are also different.[43–45] Pharmacologically, the channels can be classified as tetrodotoxin (TTX)-sensitive and TTX-resistant channels.[42–47] TTX-sensitivity correlates with some of the biophysical properties of the channels, e.g., TTX-resistant channels have slower kinetics than the TTX-sensitive ones.[43–45] Each DRG neuron expresses multiple Na^+ channels, and it has been found that the combination of the different types of channels characterizes the different subpopulations.[42,43,45] The two TTX-resistant sodium channels are preferentially expressed by the small nociceptive subpopulation of primary sensory neurons.[42–47] This preferential expression of TTX-resistant sodium channels on nociceptive cells partially explains the long action potential duration in these cells.

Voltage-Gated Ca^{++} Channels

Voltage-gated Ca^{++} channels expressed by neurons are usually characterized as high voltage–activated, such as the N-, L-, R-, P-, and Q-type channels, and low voltage–activated, such as the T-type channels.[48] Similar to the voltage-gated Na^+ channels, the biophysical and pharmacologic properties of the distinct voltage-gated Ca^{++} channels are different, and primary sensory neurons express multiple voltage-gated Ca^{++} channels. As mentioned earlier, only small nociceptive primary sensory neurons exhibit the plateau phase or "hump" on the falling phase of their action potentials, which is produced by the activation of voltage-gated Ca^{++} channels.[40] These findings indicate that different subpopulations of primary sensory neurons should express different combinations of voltage-gated Ca^{++} channels. Indeed, Scroggs and Fox[49,50] found that although both nociceptive and non-nociceptive primary sensory neurons express L- and N-type channels, the P/Q- and T-type channels are expressed predominantly by non-nociceptive and nociceptive cells, respectively.

Pharmacologic Heterogeneity

As mentioned in the introduction, in the last two decades a large number of ionotropic-, metabotropic-, Trk-, and Trk-linked receptors are expressed by primary sensory neurons. All of the known receptors are expressed by the perikarya, central and peripheral processes, and terminals. Some of the receptors have direct excitatory or inhibitory effect on primary sensory neurons, whereas the activity of others induces changes in the intracellular second messenger system resulting in altered excitability of the cell. Each cell expresses multiple receptors, and different subpopulations of primary sensory neurons seem to express distinct sets of receptors. The endogenous ligands of the receptors expressed by primary sensory neurons are released either by the sensory neurons themselves (e.g., glutamate or SP), from the terminals of descending neurons within the spinal cord, or from different peripheral cells. The net result of the combined actions of receptors determines the characteristics of action potential generation (at the peripheral terminals), action potential propagation (within the fiber), and transmitter release (at the central terminals). The existence of these excitatory and inhibitory receptors on primary afferent neurons enable us to modify the activity of the cells by exogenously applied ligands.

Receptors for Amino Acids

Glutamate Receptors

Subcutaneous injection of glutamate induces pain, which indicates that some of the excitatory glutamate receptors are expressed by nociceptive primary afferent fibers.[51] Glutamate acts on two major types of receptors: the ionotropic and metabotropic glutamate receptors (mGluRs). Receptors from both types have been shown to be expressed and to be functional on primary sensory neurons.

Pharmacologic studies show that subpopulations of primary sensory fibers and neurons can be activated by glutamate or selective agonists of 3 ionotropic glutamate receptors: α-amino-3-hydroxy-5-methyl-4-isoxazolepropionic acid (AMPA), kainate, and N-methyl-D-aspartate (NMDA) receptors.[52,53] Immunohistochemical staining using antibodies raised against the different subunits of the AMPA, kainate, or NMDA receptors confirmed that about half of the myelinated and 20% of the unmyelinated cutaneous primary afferent fibers express these receptors. Although in glabrous skin each type of the receptors is equally expressed, in hairy skin NMDA receptor predominates on both the myelinated and unmyelinated fibers. At the periphery, glutamate is released during inflammatory conditions and by activating the peripheral terminals of primary sensory fibers it contributes to the development of inflammatory pain. In the spinal cord, glutamate acting on NMDA receptors expressed by the terminals of nociceptive primary sensory neurons induces release of SP and BDNF[54,55]; glutamate acting on kainate receptors will inhibit release of these transmitters.[56]

Among the eight currently known mGluRs, at least three—mGluR4, mGluR5 and mGluR7—are expressed by primary sensory neurons.[57–59] Excitatory mGluR5 is expressed by small cells[58]; inhibitory mGluR4 and mGluR7 are expressed by small and medium cells and by virtually all DRG cells, respectively.[59] Activation of mGluR5 at the periphery contributes to the development of hyperalgesia in pathologic conditions. mGluR4 and mGluR7 on spinal terminals may serve as autoreceptors.

γ-Aminobutyric Acid Receptors

Application of the inhibitory amino acid, γ-aminobutyric acid (GABA), to primary sensory neurons produces either GABA$_A$ receptor-mediated depolarization, or GABA$_B$ receptor-mediated reduction of voltage-gated Ca^{++} currents, or both.[60,61] These effects reduce the synaptic transmission between primary and secondary sensory neurons in the spinal cord. The GABA$_A$ receptor-induced inhibition is produced through the so-called primary afferent depolarization. This chloride current-produced depolarization reduces the amplitude of action potentials entering the terminals by producing membrane shunt. The membrane shunt reduces the membrane potential below the threshold of the sodium channels; thus the number of open sodium channels is decreased. Conversely, the GABA$_B$ receptor-mediated inhibition reduces transmitter release by reducing the amount of Ca^{++} entering the cell. The GABA$_A$ receptor-mediated responses are larger in cells with Aβ-fibers than in cells with Aδ- or C-fibers,[62] indicating that the density of GABA$_A$ receptor on non-nociceptive cells is greater than on nociceptive cells. However, GABA$_A$ and GABA$_B$ receptors are coexpressed on nociceptive neurons as activation of either of the receptors induces responses in cells with Aδ- or C-fibers.[63] Recent findings indicate that about 10% of the primary sensory neurons with unmyelinated fibers innervating the skin expresses GABA$_A$ receptor,[64] whereas a larger number of nociceptive, such as capsaicin-sensitive cells, expresses the GABA$_B$ receptor (I. Nagy, unpublished observation).[65] In agreement with these findings, GABA$_B$ but not GABA$_A$ receptor activation reduces the SP release from nociceptive primary sensory neurons. Interestingly, peripheral application of GABA, through GABA$_A$ receptor activation, induces nociception.[64]

Receptors for Small Peptides

Neuropeptide Receptors

Application of SP (the endogenous ligand of the neurokinin [NK] receptors) or CGRP activates a subpopulation of DRG cells. The SP-responding cells have either Aβ-, Aδ- or C-fibers,[66] whereas the CGRP-responding cells belong to the small subpopulation.[67] The SP-evoked depolarization of DRG cells can only be partially reduced by the NK1 receptor antagonist suggesting that other NK.[66,68] The NK1 receptor is expressed by about 30% of DRG cells, a third of which also express SP. The NK3 receptor is expressed on capsaicin-sensitive nociceptive neurons, half of which produce SP.[68] Currently, there are no published data on the coexpression of NK1 and NK3 receptors. SP activates both the NK1 and NK3 receptors with different potencies, thus some of these receptors may serve as autoreceptors. In contrast to the NK1 and NK3 receptors, the CGRP receptor(s) is expressed exclusively on CGRP-producing DRG neurons[67]; thus probably all of these receptors are autoreceptors. It is assumed that neuropeptides, released from the peripheral and central terminals of the peptidergic cells, induce further transmitter release through these autoreceptors.[66–68]

Opioid Receptors

The antinociceptive effect of opioids is produced in part by opioid receptors expressed by nociceptive primary sensory neurons. All three classic opioid receptors—δ–, μ–, and κ-receptors—are expressed by nociceptive and non-nociceptive subpopulations of primary sensory neurons, although different subpopulations express the receptors in different patterns.[69,70] Whereas almost all peptidergic cells express the μ-receptor, only a few express the δ-receptor. The κ-receptors seem to be exclusively expressed by visceral nociceptive cells.[71] Opioid receptors reduce the activity of, and the transmitter release from, primary sensory neurons by reducing the high voltage–activated Ca^{++} currents and increasing the K$^+$ current. However, although in micromolar concentrations opioids have antinociceptive action in low nanomolar concentration, they activate primary sensory neurons, which is mediated by the reduction in K$^+$ currents.[72]

The function of the recently identified opioid, nociceptin and its receptor, the opioid receptor-like receptor 1, has not been established. In the peripheral nervous system, opioid receptor-like receptor 1 is expressed on capsaicin-sensitive neurons,[73] which suggests that nociceptin induces transmitter release from capsaicin-sensitive primary sensory neurons. However, it also reduces voltage-gated Ca^{++} currents.

Cholecystokinin Receptors

The octapeptide, cholecystokinin (CCK), may be an endogenous opioid antagonist.[74] CCK activates two receptors, the CCK$_A$ and CCK$_B$ receptors, among which the CCK$_B$ receptor seems to be a functional antagonist of opioid action.[75] The CCK$_B$ receptor has been shown to be expressed by a subpopulation of primary sensory neurons, the majority of which are capsaicin sensitive.[75] Activation of the CCK$_B$ receptor reverses the opioid receptor activation-induced reduction in voltage-gated Ca^{++} currents.[76]

Bradykinin Receptors

Bradykinin is an inflammatory mediator involved in "neurogenic inflammation,"[22] whereby primary sensory neurons induces and/or promote the development of inflammation. One of the key processes in neurogenic inflammation is the formation and release of inflammatory mediators, such as bradykinin, nerve growth factor, cytokines, prostaglandins, purines, protons, histamine, and serotonin. Bradykinin is produced from inactive precursors in response to tissue injury. Bradykinin induces pain, indicating that bradykinin receptors are expressed by some nociceptive primary sensory neurons. There are two known subtypes of bradykinin receptors, B$_1$ and B$_2$, and both are G protein–coupled receptors. Bradykinin acts predominantly on the B$_2$ receptor, whereas the B$_1$ receptor is activated by bradykinin metabolites such as des-Arg^9 bradykinin. Both receptors have been shown to be expressed on a subpopulation of primary sensory neurons, most of which belong to the small and medium cells. The pattern of spinal terminations of the B$_2$ receptor-expressing primary afferent fibers and the coexpression of the B_1 receptors with CGRP and IB4-binding sites in DRGs suggest that both receptors are expressed by peptidergic and by nonpeptidergic nociceptive cells.[77,78] A large number of bradykinin-responsive cells are capsaicin sensitive. The expression of the B_1 receptor is greatly enhanced by a cytokine-driven process during inflammation, and the concentration of the B_1 receptor endogenous agonist, des-Arg[9]-bradykinin, is also increased in inflammation. Based on these results, it has been suggested that B_2 receptor activation is involved in acute, whereas B_1 receptor activation is involved in chronic noxious stimulation-induced activation of nociceptive primary sensory neurons. Activation of bradykinin receptors induces inward currents in primary sensory neurons. However, it also induces the activation of different second messenger pathways, which has been suggested to be important in the regulation of VR1. According to a recent hypothesis, the bradykinin-induced burning pain sensation is produced by bradykinin receptor-induced post-translational change in VR1; thus the post-translational modification reduces the temperature threshold of VR1 causing it to open at body temperature, thereby resulting in burning pain.[79]

Receptors for Large Peptides

Receptors for Growth Factors

Growth factors such as the neurotrophins (NTs), glial cell-derived neurotrophic factors (GDNFs), and the ciliary neurotrophic factor are produced in a variety of peripheral tissues and cells of the nervous system. Members of two groups of growth factors—the NT nerve growth factor (NGF), BDNF, NT3, and NT4/5, and the member of the GDNF family, GDNF—exert effects on primary sensory neurons. These effects include regulation and promotion of proliferation and differentiation of primary sensory neurons in embryonic life, and regulation and maintenance of the function of different types of DRG cells after birth.[80] Growth factor receptors are expressed, and responses to them are produced by different subpopulations of primary sensory neurons. In adults, at least five growth factor receptors—the low-affinity NGF receptor p75, the high-affinity NGF receptor TrkA, the high-affinity BDNF/NT4/5 receptor TrkB, the high-affinity NT3 receptor TrkC, and the GDNF receptor family α 1 (GFRα1)/RET complex—are expressed in a morphologically, functionally, and neurochemically specialized manner.[81] TrkA and GFRα1/RET receptors are expressed by about 40% of the total neuronal DRG population, whereas TrkB and TrkC receptors are expressed by about 30% and 10% of the cells, respectively. Ten to 15% of the neurons coexpress TrkA and GFRα1/RET, whereas about 5% to 10% of the cells coexpress TrkA and TrkB. Most of the TrkA- and GFRα1/RET receptor-expressing neurons are nociceptive belonging to the peptidergic and IB4-binding subpopulations, respectively. Conversely, most of the TrkB and TrkC receptor-expressing cells belong to the large, non-nociceptive subpopulation of primary sensory neurons. The low-affinity p75 receptor, which binds all NTs with equal affinity, is expressed in virtually all Trk receptor-expressing neurons.

NGF acting on TrkA receptor is a major inflammatory mediator. The NGF-induced post-translational and transcriptional changes include regulation of the responsiveness of VR1 and voltage-gated sodium channels[82,83]; production of neurotransmitters and neuromodulators, such as SP and BDNF[19]; and voltage-gated ion-channels, such as $Na_v1.8$.[84] GDNF regulates the expression of VR1 and $Na_v1.9$ in IB4-binding DRG cells.[85,86] BDNF acting on TrkB receptor-expressing cells regulates the normal low-threshold, slowly adapting mechanosensitivity of the neurons. NT3 seems to be involved in the regulation of neurons with proprioceptive function.[80]

Cytokine Receptors

Subpopulations of primary sensory neurons respond to different cytokines.[21,22,87–89] The cytokine-induced responses of DRG cells involve direct opening of ion channels (e.g., produced by TNF-α or IL-1), induction of transcriptional changes (e.g., produced by leukemia inhibitory factor), promotion of differentiation and survival (e.g., produced by IL-6), or regulation of regeneration (e.g., produced by IL-6). Cytokine receptors are Trk-coupled receptors, which partly share intracellular pathways with Trk receptors. At least six types of cytokine receptors are expressed by different subpopulations of primary sensory neurons. It is believed that the activity of some of these receptors may play an important role in the development of neuropathic pain.

Receptors for Phospholipid Derivatives

Prostanoid Receptors

Subpopulations of primary sensory neurons respond to prostaglandin E2 and prostacyclin with a change in their cyclin adenosine monophosphate level and their pronociceptive effect suggests that they are expressed by the nociceptive cells.[90] Prostanoids, by acting through PKA-mediated phosphorylation sensitize primary sensory neurons. For example, prostaglandin E2 increases the TTX-resistant Na currents in nociceptive DRG cells.[91]

Cannabinoid Receptors

Exogenous and endogenous cannabinoids (CB) activate the CB1 and CB2 receptors, among which the CB1 receptor has been shown to be expressed by primary sensory neurons.[92,93] Recent findings suggest that there is a relationship between the inhibitory CB1 and the excitatory VR1 receptors, which share the endogenous ligand Anandamide (see Chapter 29 for a detailed discussion).[94]

Receptors for Nucleotides

Purine Receptors

Subpopulations of primary sensory neurons respond to both adenosine and ATP,[31,32] the latter coming from a wide range of cells, including sympathetic neurons, Merkel cells, vascular and visceral epithelial cells, and tumor cells. The source of adenosine may be from biotransformation of ATP or release from neurons such as capsaicin-sensitive DRG cells.[95] Both adenosine and ATP injected into peripheral tissues induce pain, whereas adenosine injected intrathecally produces antinociception. It has been suggested that although the excitatory effect of adenosine is mediated by A2 receptors, A1 receptors are responsible for the inhibitory effect of adenosine.[96] It seems that both the excitatory and inhibitory effect of adenosine can be produced on capsaicin-sensitive neurons, suggesting that the A1 and A2 receptor expression may be different at the peripheral and central terminals of the cells. Interestingly, adenosine acting through the A1 receptor reduces both the transmitter release from the central terminals of, and the GABA-induced currents in, DRG cells indicating that adenosine has a major modulatory effect on the activity of primary sensory neurons.[97] ATP activates the ionotropic P2X and the G protein–coupled P2Y receptors.

Receptors for Protons

Vanilloid Receptor 1

The pH of the extracellular fluid is decreased in different pathologic conditions such as inflammation or hypoxia. Subcutaneous injection of low pH solution or accumulation of acids, e.g., in the stomach or muscles, induces burning pain sensation. Acidic solutions induce inward currents in subpopulations of primary sensory neurons, including nociceptive cells.[98,99] Molecules responsive to low pH in primary sensory neurons form two major groups. One of the groups currently contains only one molecule, VR1,[24,98] which is a polymodal transducer responsive to noxious heat, low pH, and chemical agents (see earlier), such as vanilloids and the endogenous CB1 receptor agonist, anandamide.[94] Because VR1 is expressed only by nociceptive cells, its activation by protons results in pain.

Members of the ASIC Subfamily

ASICs are involved in proton-evoked responses in primary sensory neurons.[36] Some of the ASIC molecules are expressed not only by small nociceptive cells but also by larger, presumably non-nociceptive, primary sensory neurons indicating that either protons also activate non-nociceptive neurons, or ASIC molecules assembling with other membrane proteins are involved in other functions such as mechanotransduction.[36]

Receptors for Other Chemicals

Acetylcholine Receptors

Both types of acetylcholine receptors, the ionotropic nicotinic and the metabotropic muscarinic receptors, are expressed on primary sensory neurons. In agreement with the functional data, both the nicotinic and muscarinic receptors are preferentially expressed on nociceptive cells. Recent results show that the activation of acetylcholine receptors induces desensitization not only to mechanical but also to noxious heat stimuli, and that the desensitization is mediated by the muscarinic type of receptors.[100,101] Intradermal injection of the nicotinic receptor agonist, epibatidine, a poison from the Ecuadorian arrow frog, reduces the noxious stimulation-induced activity of dorsal horn neurons, thus producing antinociception.[102] The mechanisms underlying this peripheral nicotinic receptor-mediated antinociception is not understood.

Catecholamine Receptors

Both epinephrine and norepinephrine induces complex compound action potential changes in peripheral nerves, indicating that both α and β receptors are expressed by primary sensory neurons.[103] Selective activation of the receptors produces α_2 adrenoceptor-mediated hyperpolarization, α_1 adrenoceptor-mediated fast, and β_2 receptor-mediated slow depolarization both in peripheral nerves and in the perikarya of primary sensory neurons.[103,104] In agreement with these findings, α_2 adrenoceptor activation reduces transmitter release from primary sensory neurons.[105] Among the α_2 adrenoceptors, the α_{2C} subtype is expressed by almost all neurons, α_{2A} is expressed by only about 20%, and α_{2B} is expressed in only a small number of the neurons.[106] The different subtypes seem to distribute in different subpopulations of the DRG cells—α_{2A} is predominantly expressed by medium cells, α_{2B} is present in small cells, and α_{2C} is expressed primarily in small and medium CGRP-containing neurons. Whereas the α_2 receptor is inhibitory in nature, the α_1 and β_2 are excitatory. The finding that nociceptive DRG cells can be sensitized by β_2 activation suggests that this type of adrenergic receptor is expressed by nociceptive primary sensory neurons.[104] The cell types expressing the α_1 adrenoceptors are not known. It has been shown that the α_1 and β_2 adrenoceptors play an important role in the development of inflammatory and neuropathic pain.[104,107] As in peripheral nerve injury, newly formed sympathetic baskets surround the perikarya of primary sensory neurons,[108] it is believed that changes in α_1 and β_2 adrenoceptor expression in neuropathy may be particularly important.

Histamine Receptors

Histamine, as an inflammatory mediator, plays an important role in the development of neurogenic inflammation.[22] Histamine is released from mast cells in response to stimulation by SP released from the peripheral terminals of nociceptive cells. Histamine, depending on the concentration, induces itch or pain, which suggests that histamine receptors are expressed by nociceptive primary sensory neurons. Indeed, electrophysiologic recordings show that primary afferent fibers with a CV less than 10 m/sec can be activated by histamine. Up to 80% of these fibers, especially those of visceral origin, are sensitive to histamine. The histamine-induced excitation in primary sensory neurons is mediated by the H1 receptor.[109–111]

5-HT Receptors

Serotonin (5-HT) is released from mast cells at the periphery and is an inflammatory mediator that activates a subpopulation of presumably nociceptive primary afferents. More than one subtype of 5-HT receptor is expressed by primary afferent neurons,[112] and these receptor subtypes mediate both excitatory (5-HT2A) and inhibitory (5-HT3) effects.[113] Some of the C-type cells express both the 5-HT3 and 5-HT1A receptors[114] and are involved in the descending pain control in the spinal dorsal horn.

Conclusions

Although primary sensory neurons are generally divided into three major subpopulations—non-nociceptive cells, IB4-binding, and peptidergic nociceptive neurons—notably, there are overlapping subpopulations and each subpopulation could be further divided into several smaller overlapping groups. Moreover, the characteristics of primary sensory neurons, depending on the activity of the cells, are subject to changes during pathologic conditions such as peripheral inflammation or physical or metabolic nerve injury. Detailed descriptions on the possible mechanisms and consequences of such inflammation- or neuropathy-induced phenotypic changes are available elsewhere.[3–7] The description in this chapter demonstrates that primary sensory neurons are far from being simple action potential generating and conducting cells. Instead, they are complex neurons, which actively participate in sensory processing. At their peripheral endings, the activity of a large number of molecules, such as transducers, ion channels, and receptors, determines whether a particular stimulation induces action potential generation. Similarly, at the spinal terminals, the activity of the numerous receptors determines whether a particular action potential invades the terminals and induces transmitter release. The activity-induced phenotypic changes result in altered processing characteristics, which play a major role in the development of pathologic sensations such as chronic pain. The altered processing characteristics of primary sensory neurons in inflammation and neuropathy are comprehensively discussed in the literature.[3–7]

References

1. Cajal RS: Histologie du Systeme Nerveux de l'Homme et des Vertebres, Paris, Malonie. 1909.
2. Gasser HS, Edinger J: The role played by the sizes of the constituent fibers of a nerve trunk in determining the form of its action potential wave. Am J Physiol 80:522–547, 1927.
3. Woolf CJ, Costigan M: Transcriptional and posttranslational plasticity and the generation of inflammatory pain. Proc Natl Acad Sci USA 96:7723–7730, 1996.
4. Urban L, Nagy I, Bevan SJ: Chronic neuropathic pain—pathomechanism and pharmacology. Drug Develop Res (in press).
5. Millan MJ: The induction of pain: An integrative review. Prog Neurobiol 57:1–164, 1999.
6. Nagy I, Rice AS: Changes in nociceptive neurons during the development of inflammatory hyperalgesia. In Rice, Warfield, Justins, Eccleston (eds): Textbook of Clinical Pain Management. Arnold, London (in press).
7. Woolf CJ, Mannion RJ: Neuropathic pain: Aetiology, symptoms, mechanisms, and management. Lancet 353:1959–1964, 1999.
8. Woolf CJ, Shortland P, Coggeshall RE: Peripheral nerve injury triggers central sprouting of myelinated afferents. Nature 355:75–78, 1992.
9. Lawson SN: The postnatal development of large light and small dark neurons in mouse dorsal root ganglia: A statistical analysis of cell numbers and size. J Neurocytol 8:275–294, 1979.
10. Perry MJ, Lawson SN, Robertson J: Neurofilament immunoreactivity in populations of rat primary afferent neurones: A quantitative study of phosphorylated and non-phosphorylated subunits. J Neurocytol 20:746–758, 1991.
11. Knyihar E, Csillik B: Representation of cutaneous afferents by fluoride-resistant acid phosphatase (FRAP)-active terminals in the rat substantia gelatinosa rolandi. Acta Neurol Scand 53:217–225, 1976.
12. Price J: An immunohistochemical and quantitative examination of dorsal root ganglion neuronal subpopulations. J Neurosci 5:2051–2059, 1985.
13. Silverman JD, Kruger L: Lectin and neuropeptide labeling of separate populations of dorsal root ganglion neurons and associated "nociceptor" thin axons in rat testis and cornea whole-mount preparations. Somatosens Res 5:259–267, 1988.
14. Avelino A, Cruz C, Nagy I, et al: Vanilloid receptor 1 expression in the rat urinary tract. Neuroscience 109:787–798, 2002.
15. Guo A, Vulchanova L, Wang et al: Immunocytochemical localization of the vanilloid receptor 1 (VR1): Relationship to neuropeptides, the P2X3 purinireceptor and IB4 binding sites. Eur J Neurosci 11:946–958, 1999.
16. Averil S, McMahon SB, Clary DO, et al: Immunocytochemical localization of trkA receptors in chemically identified subgroups of adult rat sensory neurons. Eur J Neurosci 7:1484–1494, 1995.
17. Coimbra A, Sodre-Borges BP, Magalhaes MM: The substantia gelatinosa Rolandi of the rat. Fine structure, cytochemistry (acid phosphatase) and changes after dorsal root section. J Neurocytol 3:199–217, 1974.
18. Battaglia G, Rustioni A: Coexistence of glutamate and substance P in dorsal root ganglion neurons in the rat and monkey. J Comp Neurol 277:302–312, 1988.
19. Mannion RJ, Costogan M, Decostred I, et al: Neurotrophins: Peripherally and centrally acting modulators of tactile stimulus-induced inflammatory pain hypersensitivity. Proc Natl Acad Sci USA 96:9385–9390, 1999.
20. Copray JC, Mantingh I, Brouwer N, et al: Expression of interleukin-1 beat in rat dorsal root ganglia. J Neuroimmunol 118:203–211, 2001.
21. Gadient RA, Otten U: Postnatal expression of interleukin-6 (IL-6) and IL-6 receptor (IL-6R) mRNAs in rat sympathetic and sensory ganglia. Brain Res 724:41–46, 1996.
22. Kress M, Reeh P: Chemical excitation and sensitization in nociceptors. In Belmonte C, Cervero F (eds): Neurobiology of Nociceptors. Oxford, Oxford University Press, 1996, pp 258–298.
23. Caterina MJ, Rosen TA, Tominaga M, et al: A capsaicin-receptor homologue with a high threshold for noxious heat. Nature 398:436–441, 1999.
24. Caterina MJ, Schumacher MA, Tominaga M, et al: The capsaicin receptor: A heat-activated ion channel in the pain pathway. Nature 389:816–824.
25. Nagy I, Rang HP: Similarities and differences between the responses of rat sensory neurons to noxious heat and capsaicin. J Neurosci 19:10647–10655, 1999.
26. Caterina MJ, Leffler A, Malmberg AB, et al: Impaired nociception and pain sensation in mice lacking the capsaicin receptor. Science 288:306–313, 2000.
27. Nagy I, Rang HP: Noxious heat activates all capsaicin-sensitive and also a subpopulation of capsaicin-insensitive dorsal root ganglion neurons. Neuroscience 88:995–997, 1999.
28. Maingret F, Lauritzen I, Patel AJ, et al: TREK-1 is a heat-activated background K(+) channel. EMBO J 19:2483–2491, 2000.
29. Souslova V, Cesare P, Ding Y, et al: Warm-coding deficits and aberrant inflammatory pain in mice lacking P2X3 receptors. Nature 407:1015–1017, 2000.
30. Suto K, Gotoh H: Calcium signaling in cold cells studied in cultured dorsal root ganglion neurons. Neuroscience 92:1131–1135, 1999.

31. Burnstock G: P2X receptors in sensory neurones. Br J Anaesth 84:476–488, 2000.

32. Bradbury EJ, Burnstock G, McMahon SB: The expression of P2X3 purinoreceptors in sensory neurons: Effects of axotomy and glial-derived neurotrophic factor. Mol Cell Neurosci 12:256–268, 1998.

33. Garcia-Anoveros J, Corey DP: The molecules of mechanosensation. Annu Rev Neurosci 20:567–594, 1997.

34. Price MP, Lewin GR, McIlwrath SB, et al: The mammalian sodium channel BNC1 is required for normal touch sensation. Nature 407:1007–1011, 2000.

35. Mannsfeldt AG, Carroll P, Stucky CL, et al: Stomatin, a MEC-2 like protein, is expressed by mammalian sensory neurons. Mol Cell Neurosci 13:391–404, 1999.

36. Waldmann R, Champigny G, Lingueglia E, et al: H⁺-gated cation channels. Ann NY Acad Sci 868:67–76, 1999.

37. Price MP, McIlwrath SL, Xie J, et al: The DRASIC cation channel contributes to the detection of cutaneous touch and acid stimuli in mice. Neuron 32:1071–1083, 2001.

38. Nakamura F, Strittmatter SM: P2Y1 purinergic receptors in sensory neurons: Contribution to touch induced impulse generation. Proc Natl Acad Sci USA 93:10465–10470, 1996.

39. Gorke K, Pierau FK: Spike potentials and membrane properties of dorsal root ganglion cells in pigeons. Pflugers Arch 386:21–28, 1980.

40. Scott BS, Edwards BA: Electric membrane properties of adult mouse DRG neurons and the effect of culture duration. J Neurobiol 11:291–301, 1980.

41. Harper AA, Lawson SN: Electrical properties of dorsal root ganglion neurones with different peripheral nerve conduction velocities. J Physiol 359:47–63, 1985.

42. Goldin AL: Resurgence of sodium channel research. Annu Rev Physiol 63:871–894, 2001.

43. Waxman SG, Cummins TR, Dib-Haj S, et al: Sodium channels, excitability of primary sensory neurons, and the molecular basis of pain. Muscle Nerve 22:1177–1187, 1999.

44. Dietrich PS, McGivern JG, Delgado SG, et al: Functional analysis of a voltage-gated sodium channel and its splice variant from rat dorsal root ganglia. J Neurochem 70:2262–2272, 1998.

45. Cummins TR, Dib-Hajj SD, Black JA, et al: A novel persistent tetrodotoxin-resistant sodium current in SNS-null and wild-type small primary sensory neurons. J Neurosci 19:RC43, 1999.

46. Dib-Hajj SD, Tyrell L, Black JA, et al: NaN, a novel voltage-gated Na channel, is expressed preferentially in peripheral sensory neurons and down-regulated after axotomy. Proc Natl Acad Sci USA 95:8963–8968, 1998.

47. Sangemeswaran L, Delgado SG, Fish LM, et al: Structure and function of a novel voltage-gated, tetrodotoxin-resistant sodium channel specific to sensory neurons. J Biol Chem 271:5953–5656, 1996.

48. Dolphin AC: Voltage-dependent calcium channels and their modulation by neurotransmitters and G proteins. Exp Physiol 80:1–36, 1995.

49. Scroggs RS, Fox AP: Calcium current variation between acutely isolated adult rat dorsal root ganglion neurons of different size. J Physiol 445:639–658, 1992.

50. Scroggs RS, Fox AP: Multiple Ca2+ currents elicited by action potential waveforms in acutely isolated adult rat dorsal root ganglion neurons. J Neurosci 12:1789–1801, 1992.

51. Zhou S, Bonasera L, Carlton SM: Peripheral administration of NMDA, AMPA or KA results in pain behaviors in rats. Neuroreport 7:895–900, 1996.

52. Huettner JE: Glutamate receptor channels in rat DRG neurons: Activation by kainate and quisqualate and blockade of desensitization by Con A. Neuron 5:255–266, 1990.

53. Carlton SM, Hargett GL, Coggeshall RE: Localization and activation of glutamate receptors in unmyelinated axons of rat glabrous skin. Neurosci Lett 197:25–28, 1995.

54. Lever IJ, Bradbury EJ, Cunningham JR, et al: Brain-derived neurotrophic factor is released in the dorsal horn by distinctive patterns of afferent fiber stimulation. J Neurosci 21:4469–4477, 2001.

56. Liu H, Mantyh PW, Basbaum AJ: NMDA-receptor regulation of substance P release from primary afferent nociceptors. Nature 386:721–724, 1997.

56. Kerchner GA, Wilding TJ, Li P, et al: Presynaptic kainate receptors regulate spinal sensory transmission. J Neurosci 21:59–66, 2001.

57. Azuke JI, Murga M, Fernandez-Capetillo O, et al: Immunoreactivity for the group III metabotropic glutamate receptor subtype mGluR4a in the superficial laminae of the rat spinal dorsal horn. J Comp Neurol 430:448–457, 2001.

58. Valerio A, Rizzonelli P, Paterlini M, et al: mGluR5 metabotropic glutamate receptor distribution in rat and human spinal cord: A developmental study. Neurosci Res 28:49–57, 1997.

59. Li JL, Ohisi H, Kaneko T, et al: Immunohistochemical localization of a metabotropic glutamate receptor, mGluR7, in ganglion neurons of the rat; with special reference to the presence in glutamatergic ganglion neurons. Neurosci Lett 204:9–12, 1996.

60. Leonard JP, Wickelgren WO: Prolongation of calcium action potentials by gamma-aminobutyric acid in primary sensory neurones of lamprey. J Physiol 375:481–497, 1986.

61. Gallagher JP, Higashi H, Nishi S: Characterization and ionic basis of GABA-induced depolarizations recorded in vitro from cat primary afferent neurones. J Physiol 275:263–282, 1978.

62. Desamenien M, Santangelo F, Loeffler JP, et al: Comparative study of GABA-mediated depolarizations of lumbar A delta and C primary afferent neurones of the rat. Exp Brain Res 54:521–528, 1984.

63. Desamenien M, Feltz P, Occhipinti G, et al: Coexistence of GABAA and GABAB receptors on A delta and C primary afferents. Br J Pharmacol 81:327–333, 1984.

64. Carlton SM, Zhou S, Coggeshall RE: Peripheral GABA(A) receptors: Evidence for peripheral primary afferent depolarization. Neuroscience 93:713–722, 1999.

65. Tower S, Princivalle A, Billinton A, et al: GABAB receptor protein and mRNA distribution in rat spinal cord and dorsal root ganglia. Eur J Neurosci 12:3201–3210, 2000.

66. Szucs P, Polgar E, Spigemam I, et al: Neurokinin-1 receptor expression in dorsal root ganglion neurons of young rats. J Periph Nerv Sys 4:270–278, 1999.

67. Segond von Banchet GG, Pastor A, Biskup C, et al: Localization of functional calcitonin gene-related peptide binding sites in a subpopulation of cultured dorsal root ganglion neurons. Neuroscience 110:131–145, 2002.

68. Schmid G, Carita F, Bonanno G, et al: NK-3 receptors mediate enhancement of substance P release from capsaicin-sensitive spinal cord afferent terminals. Br J Pharmacol 125:621–626, 1998.

69. Wang H, Wessendorf MW: Equal proportions of small and large DRG neurons express opioid receptor mRNAs. J Comp Neurol 429:590–600, 2001.

70. Minami M, Maekawa K, Yabuuchi K, et al: Double in situ hybridization study on coexistence of mu-, delta-, and kappa-opioid receptor mRNAs with preprotachykinin A mRNA in the rat dorsal root ganglia. Brain Res Mol Brain Res 30:203–210, 1996.

71. Su X, Wachtel RE, Gebhart GF: Inhibition of calcium currents in rat colon sensory neurons by K- but not mu- or delta-opioids. J Neurophysiol 80:3112–3119, 1998.

72. Crain SM, Shen K-F: Acute thermal hyperalgesia elicited by low-dose morphine in normal mice is blocked by ultra-low-dose naltrexone, unmasking potent opioid analgesia. Brain Res 888:75–82, 2001.

73. Minami T, Okuda-Asithika E, Mori H, et al: Characterization of nociceptin/orphanin FQ-induced pain responses in conscious mice: neonatal capsaicin treatment and N-methyl-D-aspartate receptor GluRepsilon subunit knockout mice. Neuroscience 97:133–142, 2000.

74. Ghilardi JR, Allen CJ, Vigna SR, et al: Trigeminal and dorsal root ganglion neurons express CCK receptor binding sites in the rat, rabbit, and monkey: Possible site of opiate-CCK analgesic interactions. J Neurosci 12:4854–4866, 1992.

75. Schafer M, Zhou L, Stein C: Cholecystokinin inhibits peripheral opioid analgesia in inflamed tissue. Neuroscience 82:603–611, 1998.

76. Liu NJ, Xu T, Xu C, et al: Cholecystokinin octapeptide reverses mu-opioid-receptor-mediated inhibition of calcium current in rat dorsal root ganglion neurons. J Pharmacol Exp Ther 275:1293–1299, 1995.

77. Lopes P, Kar S, Chretien L, et al: Quantitative autoradiographic localization of [¹²⁵I-Tyr⁸] brodykinin receptor binding sites in the rat spinal cord: Effects of neonatal capsaicin, noradrenergic deafferentation, dorsal rhizotomy and peripheral axotomy. Neuroscience 68:867–881, 1995.

78. Ma Q-P: The expression of bradykinin B1 receptors on primary sensory neurons that give rise to small calibre sciatic nerve fibers in rats. Neuroscience 107:665–673, 2001.

79. Reeh PW, Petho G: Nociceptor excitation by thermal sensitization—a hypothesis. Prog Brain Res 29:39–50, 2000.

80. Ernfors P: Local and target-derived actions of neurotrophins during peripheral nervous system development. Cell Mol Life Sci 58:1036–1044, 2001.

81. Butte MJ: Neurotrophic factor structures reveal clues to evolution, binding, specificity and receptor activation. Cell Mol Life Sci 58:1003–1013.

82. Shu XQ, Mendell LM: Neurotrophins and hyperalgesia. Proc Natl Acad Sci USA 96:7693–7696, 1999.

83. Hilborn MD, Vaillancourt RR, Rane SG: Growth factor receptor tyrosine kinases acutely regulate neuronal sodium channels through the src signaling pathway. J Neurosci 18:590–600, 1998.

84. Fjell J, Cummins TR, Dib-Hajj SD, et al: Differential role of GDNF and NGF in the maintenance of two TTX-resistant sodium channels in adult DRG neurons. Brain Res Mol Brain Res 67:267–282, 1999.

85. Cummins TR, Black JA, Dib-Hajj SD, et al: TI: Glial-derived neurotrophic factor upregulates expression of functional SNS and NaN sodium channels and their currents in axotomized dorsal root ganglion neurons. J Neurosci 20:8754–8761, 2000.

86. Ogun-Muyiwa P, Helliwell R, McIntyre P, et al: Glial cell line derived neurotrophic factor (GDNF) regulates VR1 and substance P in cultured sensory neurons. Neuroreport 10:2107–2111, 1999.

87. Rothwell NJ, Luheshi G, Toulmond S: Cytokines and their receptors in the central nervous system: Physiology, pharmacology and pathology. Pharmacol Ther 69:85–95, 1996.

88. Zhong J, Dietzel ID, Wahle P, et al: Sensory impairments and delayed regeneration of sensory axons in interleukin-6-deficient mice. J Neurosci 19:4305–4313, 1999.

89. Pollock J, McFarlane SM, Connel MC, et al: TNF-alpha receptors simultaneously activate Ca(2+) mobilization and stress kinases in cultured sensory neurons. Neuropharmacology 42:93–106, 2002.

90. Vanegas H, Schaible H-G: Prostaglandins and cyclooxygenases in the spinal cord. Prog Neurobiol 64:327–363, 2001.

91. England S, Bevan S, Docherty RJ: PGE2 modulates the tetrodotoxin-resistant sodium current in neonatal rat dorsal root ganglion neurones via the cyclic AMP-protein kinase A cascade. J Physiol 495:429–440, 1996.

92. Ahluwalia J, Urban L, Capogna M, et al: Cannabinoid 1 receptors are expressed in nociceptive primary sensory neurons. Neuroscience 100:685–688, 2000.

93. Ahluwalia J, Urban L, Bevan SJ, et al: Cannabinoid 1 receptors are expressed by nerve growth factor- and glial cell-derived neurotrophic factor-responsive primary sensory neurones. Neuroscience 110:747–753, 2002.

94. Zygmunt PM, Petersson J, Andersson DA, et al: Vanilloid receptors on sensory nerves mediate the vasodilator action of anandamide. Nature 400:452–457, 1999.

95. Sweeney MI, White TD, Sawynok J: Morphine, capsaicin and K+ release purins from capsaicin-sensitive primary afferent nerve terminals in the spinal cord. J Pharmacol Exp Ther 248:447–454, 1989.

96. Burnstock G, Wood JN: Purinergic receptors: Their role in nociception and primary afferent neurotransmission. Curr Opin Neurobiol 6:526–532, 1996.

97. Hu HZ, Li ZW: Modulation by adenosine of GABA-activated current in rat dorsal root ganglion neurons. J Physiol 501:67–75, 1997.

98. Tominaga M, Caterina MJ, Melmberg AB, et al: The cloned capsaicin receptor integrates multiple pain-producing stimuli. Neuron 21:531–543, 1998.

99. Bevan S, Gepetti P: Protons: Small stimulants of capsaicin-sensitive sensory nerves. Trends Neurosci 17:509–512, 1994.

100. Steen KH, Reeh PW: Actions of cholinergic agonists on sensory nerve endings in rat skin, in vitro. J Neurophysiol 70:397–405, 1993.

101. Bernardini N, Sauer SK, Haberberger R, et al: Excitatory nicotinic and desensitising muscarinic (M2) effects on C-nociceptors in isolated rat skin. J Neurosci 21:3295–3302, 2001.

102. Bannon AW, Decker MW, Holladat MW, et al: Broad-spectrum, non-opioid analgesic activity by selective modulation of neuronal nicotinic acetylcholine receptors. Science 279:77–81, 1998.

103. Wohlberg CJ, Hackman JC, Ryan GP, et al: Epinephrine- and norepinephrine-evoked potential changes of frog primary afferent terminals: Pharmacological characterization of alpha and beta components. Brain Res 327:289–301, 1985.

104. Khasar SG, McCarter G, Levine JD: Epinephrine produces a beta-adrenergic receptor-mediated mechanical hyperalgesia and in vitro sensitization of rat nociceptors. J Neurophysiol 81:1104–1112, 1999.

105. Averbeck B, Reeh PW, Michaelis M: Modulation of CGRP and PGE2 release from isolated rat skin by alpha-adrenoceptors and kappa-opioid-receptors. Neuroreport 12:2097–2100, 2001.

106. Shi TS, Winzer-Serhan U, Leslie F, Hokfelt T: Distribution and regulation of α_2-adrenoceptors in rat dorsal root ganglia. Pain 84:319–330, 2000.

107. Lee YH, Ryu TG, Park SJ, et al: Alpha1-adrenoceptors involvement in painful diabetic neuropathy: A role in allodynia. Neuroreport 11:1417–1420, 2000.

108. McLachlan EM, Janig W, Devor M, et al: Peripheral nerve injury triggers noradrenergic sprouting within dorsal root ganglia. Nature 363:543–546, 1993.

109. Koda H, Minagawa M, Si-Hong L, et al: H1-receptor-mediated excitation and facilitation of the heat response by histamine in canine visceral polymodal receptors studied in vitro. J Neurophysiol 76:1396–1404, 1996.

110. Amann R, Schuligoi R, Lanz I, et al: Histamine-induced edema in the rat paw–effect of capsaicin denervation and a CGRP receptor antagonist. Eur J Pharmacol 279:227–231, 1995.

111. Kashiba H, Fukui H, Senba E: Histamine H1 receptor mRNA is expressed in capsaicin-insensitive sensory neurons with neuropeptide Y-immunoreactivity in guinea pigs. Brain Res 901:85–93, 2001.

112. Khasabov SG, Lopez-Garcia JA, King AE: Serotonin-induced population primary afferent depolarization in vitro: The effects of neonatal capsaicin treatment. Brain Res 782:339–342, 1998.

113. Tokunaga A, Saika M, Senba E: 5-HT2A receptor subtype is involved in the thermal hyperalgesic mechanism of serotonin in the periphery. Pain 76:349–355, 1998.

114. Todorovic S, Anderson EG: Serotonin preferentially hyperpolarizes capsaicin-sensitive C-type sensory neurons by activating 5-HT1A receptors. Brain Res 585:212–218, 1992.

13

Sensory Processing

Jerry Collins, MD

SPINAL CORD

This chapter focuses on hypotheses yet to be tested more than on ones that have survived critical scientific scrutiny, because the large number of currently unanswered questions about anesthetic actions on spinal sensory processing.

In two of the earliest publications about general anesthetic actions on spinal sensory neurons, the authors proposed that spinal actions of general anesthetics may contribute to the production of anesthesia.[1,2] In the ensuing decades, we have come full circle. It was recently proposed, based on new experimental data, that anesthetic actions at the level of the spinal cord, by blunting noxious inputs to the cortex and thalamus, may indirectly contribute to anesthetic endpoints such as amnesia and loss of consciousness.[3]

If it was apparent in 1967 that spinal anesthetic actions could be important, why is that question still being asked? And is there any evidence to support the hypothesis that spinal sites of drug actions are important? These are the first two questions addressed in this chapter, in part because each answer is closely related.

In the late 1960s and early 1970s, several laboratories worked to better understand drug effects on sensory processing within the spinal cord. An initial emphasis was placed on drugs that would be expected to block pain signals. In those early studies, general anesthetics were the focus until it was reported, by three different laboratories, that opioids also appeared to be able to block spinal sensory processing of information arising from a noxious peripheral stimulus.[4–6] With a subsequent report by Yaksh and Rudy[7] that analgesia could be produced by direct spinal actions of opioids, and subsequent reports of human efficacy of

perispinal opioid analgesia, research focused almost exclusively on spinal opioid actions, at the expense of spinal actions of general anesthetics. The resulting understanding of the physiology and pharmacology of spinal opioid actions has provided a fertile ground for renewed interest in the spinal actions of general anesthetics.

The question of how important a drug effect could be on spinal sensory processing is well answered by the clinical use of perispinal opioid analgesia. Before the introduction of this pain-relieving technique, a caregiver might administer a local anesthetic near the spinal cord or administer an opioid systemically. Although both methods are capable of producing clinically effective analgesia in many settings, each is associated with specific and, at times, limiting side effects that can be attributed to lack of specificity. A perispinally administered local anesthetic, while producing analgesia, also blocks other sensations (the area is numb), blocks motor output (the patient can't be mobilized), and may block or significantly reduce sympathetic outflow (the patient is susceptible to orthostatic hypotension). Perispinal opioids block pain and nothing else. The anatomic location of the drug action, because of selected receptors, makes it possible for a specific effect to be produced. The anatomy and physiology of spinal sensory neurons provides a unique target for pharmacologic action of general anesthetics (see later).

A comparison of the efficacy of perispinal versus systemic opioid administration for the production of analgesia provides insights into the importance of drug actions on spinal sensory processing. Although systemic opioids do **199** produce analgesia, they are also associated with central nervous system (CNS) depression, especially at higher doses sometimes needed to provide adequate pain relief. With systemic opioids, it is not uncommon for the patient to state that the pain is still present but it is weak. With perispinal opioid administration, it is much more common to hear that the pain is gone. By acting at a level distal to the region of the CNS that involves the effective component of pain, perispinal opioid administration can be much more selective for the pain signal itself.

That a large proportion of primary afferent sensory input has its first synapse within the spinal dorsal horn (and its homologue the trigeminal system for cranial sensory input) means that it is an ideal target for pharmacologic actions on spinal sensory processing. This chapter begins here to focus on our current understanding of the role that spinal actions of general anesthetics may play through actions on spinal sensory processing.

Systems Physiology

Dorsal Horn

In the early 1950s Rexed described a laminar organization of cell bodies within the spinal cord.[8,9] In Rexed's original description, the spinal cord was divided into 10 different laminae based on cytoarchitectonic detail. This chapter focuses on the sections of the spinal cord referred to as the spinal dorsal horn, Rexed laminae I–VI, an area of the spinal cord rich in synaptic connections between primary afferents and second order neurons.

In early studies of the spinal dorsal horn it was assumed that laminae were composed of cell types associated with a particular form of sensory input. As examples, lamina IV was thought to process only information from low threshold (LT) neurons, lamina V only information about noxious input, and lamina VI only information about joint position and proprioception. That assumption was proven to be incorrect, but older literature presents laminae as if they had predetermined physiologic functions.

Figure 13–1 depicts the organization of the spinal dorsal horn. There are three basic elements within the spinal dorsal horn that contribute to and/or regulate spinal sensory processing: primary afferents synapse on second order spinal sensory neurons; spinal sensory neurons give rise to tracts that communicate information to motor neurons (reflex responses) and to supraspinal sensory neurons (sensations and perceptions); propriospinal and descending modulatory systems influence the activity of primary afferent terminals, or second order neurons, or both.[10–12]

Anatomy

A brief comment about anatomy will enable us to identify likely sites of action for general anesthetics. As early as 1952 it was proposed that synaptic transmission, not axonal con-

duction, is the likely site of general anesthetic inhibition of spinal sensory pathways,[13,14] an assumption that is still considered to be valid.[15] Although this chapter focuses on the synapse primarily, it is important to remember that branching points on axons may be more sensitive to drug effects than currently appreciated.[16] It is also important to recognize that nonvoltage-dependent (e.g., biochemical) processes within a neuron may also be seen in the future as anesthetic targets for this disruption of information transmission.[17] Future studies may reveal drug sensitivities that do not rely on the presence of synapses or voltages.

If the synapse is the primary site of action for general anesthetics, then the spinal dorsal horn provides a unique opportunity for anesthetic modulation of sensory input. The first synapse for a great number of primary afferents, from tissues throughout the body, occurs within the spinal dorsal horn. Those primary afferents range in size from the largest of the myelinated A-fibers to the smallest unmyelinated C-fibers. They are associated with receptors in most tissues in the body and are responsible for conveying information about sensations like cutaneous touch, temperature, pain, visceral sensations, muscle and joint sensations, and proprioception.[11,12,18–23]

Certainly not all primary afferents make an initial synapse in the spinal dorsal horn. Fibers rising in the lemniscal pathway, for example, do not synapse with a second order neuron until they reach the dorsal column nuclei. However, it is clear that a significant proportion of an animal's sensory input about both the external and internal environment is processed initially at a synapse between a primary afferent and a second order neuron within the spinal dorsal horn (Fig. 13–2). If a general anesthetic could impede or block the synaptic transmission at that site, or the subsequent integration of information by the sensory neuron, then upstream systems would be disconnected from both the external and internal environment. For our purposes it is sufficient to postulate that general anesthetics either directly or indirectly decrease the efficacy of excitatory mechanisms or increase the efficacy of inhibitory mechanisms within the synapse. These actions can be either presynaptic or postsynaptic and are likely to include combinations of all of those mentioned earlier.

Another way to use spinal cord anatomy to identify possible anesthetic sites of action is to examine the output from the dorsal horn to the rest of the body. One of the more obvious outputs is to motor neurons in the ventral horn. With the exception of monosynaptic reflexes that involve a direct connection between primary afferents and motor neurons, all other spinal reflex pathways are derived from second order neurons that have received primary afferent input within the dorsal horn. This is of particular relevance to anesthetics because a cardinal action of general anesthesia (immobility in the presence of the noxious peripheral stimulus) has been shown to depend almost exclusively on spinal actions (see later).

Reflexes

When discussing reflexes, it is also important to comment briefly on the cardiovascular reflexes that are associated with

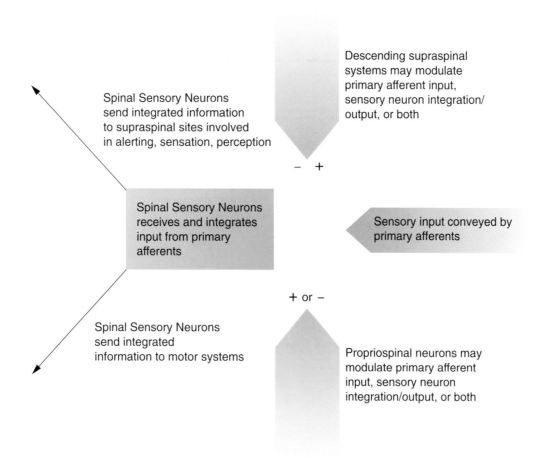

Spinal Sensory Neurons
send integrated information
to supraspinal sites involved
in alerting, sensation, perception

Descending supraspinal
systems may modulate
primary afferent input,
sensory neuron integration/
output, or both

− +

Spinal Sensory Neurons
receives and integrates
input from primary
afferents

Sensory input conveyed by
primary afferents

Spinal Sensory Neurons
send integrated
information to motor systems

+ or −

Propriospinal neurons may
modulate primary afferent
input, sensory neuron
integration/output, or both

Figure 13–1. Diagram representing information flow through the spinal dorsal horn. Synapses between primary afferents and second order neurons in the spinal dorsal horn are the site of information transfer from the peripheral nervous system to the central nervous system. This important center of sensory integration is influenced by propriospinal and descending supraspinal systems. Integrated information is then forwarded to motor systems involved in reflex responses and to supraspinal sites involved in sensation and perception.

primary afferent input and also their sensitivity to general anesthetic actions. That general anesthetic effect may also be postulated to be caused by, at least in part, anesthetic actions on reflexes that use synaptic inputs within the spinal dorsal horn.

Ascending Pathways

In addition to motor responses to primary afferent input, it is apparent that major ascending spinal pathways are derived from second order neurons within the spinal dorsal horn. As shown in Figure 13–3, information about multiple sensations are transmitted by those pathways.[11,12,20] If general anesthetics can disrupt the information transmission between the primary afferents and the second order neurons that give rise to the pathways shown in Figure 13–3, it is likely that the sensory modalities represented in the figure will be altered by general anesthetic actions within the spinal dorsal horn.

Descending Modulatory Systems

As depicted in Figure 13–1, the spinal dorsal horn includes modulatory neurons that are either of propriospinal origin or are derived from descending supraspinal modulatory systems. During normal circumstances, these systems may decrease or increase the activity of spinal dorsal horn neurons and thus modulate spinal sensory transmission. Therefore, anesthetic effects could also influence spinal sensory transmission. Willis and Coggeshall[11] listed the following sites within the CNS as sources of either excitatory (medullary reticular formation, regions of the cerebral cortex) or inhibitory (nucleus raphe magnus, medullary reticular formation, periaqueductal gray) modulation of spinothalamic tract neurons, the source of a major output tract arising from the spinal dorsal horn. Anesthetic effects on these modulatory systems could either result from an action on synapses within the spinal cord or from anesthetic effects on cells or origin within the supraspinal nuclei.

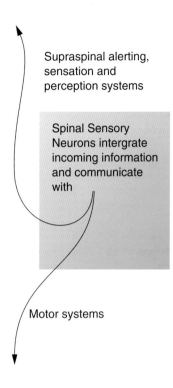

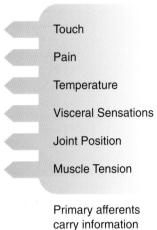

Supraspinal alerting, sensation and perception systems

Spinal Sensory Neurons intergrate incoming information and communicate with

Touch

Pain

Temperature

Visceral Sensations

Joint Position

Muscle Tension

Motor systems

Primary afferents carry information about the above to synapse with spinal sensory neurons

Figure 13–2. Diagram representing the nature of the sensory input that is conveyed to neurons in the spinal dorsal horn. The transfer of information between the peripheral and central nervous system that occurs within the spinal dorsal horn is essential to an organism's ability to monitor both the external and internal environment. *Right,* Multiple sensations could be influenced if general anesthetics altered that information transfer.

Organ Physiology

Figure 13–4 depicts the four classes of spinal dorsal horn neurons that are thought to subserve spinal sensory transmission. The first class of neurons depicted are the LT neurons. LT neurons respond maximally to low-intensity (usually mechanical) stimulation of peripheral receptive fields of primary afferents synapsing on them. A high-intensity mechanical stimulus may also activate them, but the maximum firing rate does not go any higher than that seen with low-intensity stimuli impinge on the receptive fields.

The second class of neurons depicted in Figure 13–4 is high threshold (HT) neurons. These neurons respond only when the peripheral receptive fields of primary afferents synapsing on them are exposed to stimuli of sufficient intensity (mechanical, thermal, chemical, electrical) that tissue damage is likely to occur. They do not respond to low-intensity receptive field stimulation.

The third class incorporates features from the first two. This class is referred to as multireceptive (MR). (They have also been referred to as wide dynamic range [WDR] neurons.) These will typically respond weakly to low-intensity stimuli and demonstrate an increasing response to increasing intensities of stimuli until a maximum response is elicited by high-intensity noxious stimuli. Of importance, they also respond to both noxious and non-noxious input from visceral structures.

The final class of neurons depicted in Figure 13–4 is made up of those neurons that responded exclusively to joint position and muscle tension. This response is elicited both by non-noxious and noxious stimuli from those sources.

Cellular Physiology

The following statements about general anesthetic effects on spinal sensory neurons do not include an exhaustive review of all of the relevant literature. This section cites selected studies that reflect the current status of our understanding of such effects. An emphasis has been placed on inhibition of neuronal activity, although increased excitation may also result from anesthetic effects (see earlier). The emphasis on inhibitory effects is due to the preponderance of studies that show such effects of general anesthetics.

In spite of the relatively small number of studies of anesthetic effects on spinal sensory neurons, there exists an adequate amount of data that indicate that spinal sensory processing is inhibited by general anesthetics. This was apparent in early studies,[2,24–30] even though the physiologic responses of the neurons were not well tested and it was, therefore, not possible to place the neurons in the appropriate categories. However, as reviewed by deJong and colleagues,[30] it was apparent from initial studies that general anesthetics are capable of inhibiting responses of spinal dorsal horn neurons to both non-noxious and noxious receptive field stimulation.

Low Threshold Neurons

General anesthetics are capable of depressing the response of spinal LT neurons to low-intensity stimulation of their peripheral receptive fields. Halothane, in both acute rat and chronic cat preparations,[31,32] reduced both the number of

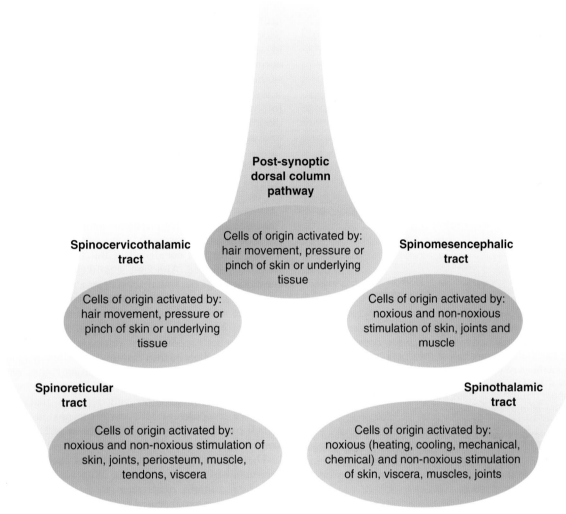

Figure 13–3. Diagram representing ascending fiber tracts with cells of origin in the spinal dorsal horn. The types of stimuli typically associated with activation of cells of origin of each tract are listed. Anesthetic-induced disruption of information transmission within those systems could degrade sensations and perceptions associated with each of the forms of stimulation listed.

action potentials elicited by receptive field stimulation and the receptive field area on the skin from which responses could be elicited. This effect was shown to be dose-dependent and independent of supraspinal modulatory systems. (This independence from supraspinal systems is similar to more recently reported spinal actions of general anesthetics producing immobility in the presence of a noxious stimulus.[33–36]) However, Herrero and Headley[37] reported that halothane increased the receptive field size in sheep rather than decreasing it. That suggests possible species differences and possible excitatory effects.

Xenon[38] and halothane[32,37] both have been shown to depress WDR neuronal responses to both non-noxious and noxious peripheral receptive field stimulation. As with LT neurons, both the number of action potentials and the receptive field area from which activity could be elicited was reduced in rats and cats. However, in sheep, although the number of action potentials was reduced, the receptive field area was not altered.[37] Halothane depression of responses of WDR neurons to noxious visceral stimuli (colorectal distension) have also been observed (Collins and colleagues, unpublished observations).

Wide Dynamic Range Neurons

The response of WDR neurons in rats, cats, and sheep has been reported to be depressed by general anesthetics.

HT Neurons/Proprioceptive Neurons

Limited unpublished work in our laboratory demonstrated that halothane depresses HT and proprioceptive neuronal

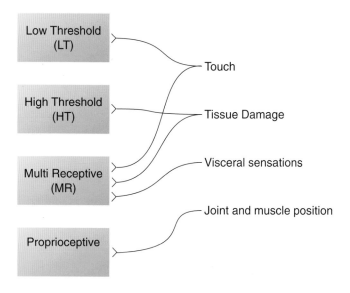

Types of spinal
sensory neurons

Types of
sensory input

Figure 13–4. Diagram representing the four classes of spinal dorsal horn sensory neurons. Spinal dorsal horn sensory neurons have been divided into four classes based on their responses to natural stimulation of their peripheral receptive fields. This simplified diagram suggests that there is a class of neurons that responds exclusively to low-intensity stimuli (low threshold neurons), a class that responds exclusively to high-intensity stimuli (high threshold neurons), and a class that responds to stimuli of varying intensity as well as to visceral stimulation (multi receptive neurons). In addition to those three there is also a class that responds exclusively to joint and muscle position (proprioceptive neurons). Activity in each of these classes of neurons may be influenced by general anesthetics.

responses to natural stimulation of their peripheral receptive field.

Targets for Anesthetic Action

Consciousness

Two separate lines of evidence suggest that anesthetic depression of spinal sensory processing is not due simply to a loss of consciousness. The first evidence comes from studies that demonstrated that anesthetic induced immobility in the presence of a noxious stimulus[33–36] and anesthetic depression of LT neurons[31] is the result of spinal not supraspinal effects. If we assume that consciousness is primarily a supraspinal construct then the absence of supraspinal contributions makes it unlikely that changes in consciousness, by themselves, are responsible for the observed anesthetic depression of spinal sensory processing.

A second and more direct experiment compared differences between the effects of rapid eye movement (REM)

sleep and general anesthesia (propofol) on the neuronal activity of spinal sensory neurons.[39] During REM sleep, when sleep effects on LT neurons were maximum, the neurons demonstrated a greatly increased response to peripheral receptive field stimulation. This was in contrast to spinal motor neurons that are profoundly depressed during REM sleep. When the effects of propofol were studied on the same LT neurons, depression, not excitation, was observed. This opposite effect of REM sleep and propofol sleep (anesthesia) in the same neurons suggests that anesthetic depression of spinal sensory neurons is not simply due to drug induced loss of consciousness.

Spinal Level

The generalizability of anesthetic actions on spinal sensory processing is unknown both because not all drugs have been tested and because not all cells within the spinal dorsal horn have been studied. Although it is likely that most general anesthetics depress spinal sensory processing, there is evidence suggesting that at least one drug does not depress all classes of sensory neurons in the spinal dorsal horn. In one of the early studies of anesthetic spinal actions, Conseiller and colleagues[28] reported that ketamine depressed neuronal responses to high-intensity stimuli, but not responses to low-intensity stimuli. However, neuronal types were not described. We repeated those experiments in an intact, awake animal preparation and reported that ketamine depressed responses of MR neurons to noxious peripheral stimuli but did not depress the response of LT neurons to low-intensity receptive field stimulation.[40]

These results point out an important cautionary note in our studies of anesthetic effects. With ketamine and other drugs, e.g., nitrous oxide (see later), there are important exceptions to what appeared to be general rules. Currently, although it is easy to attempt to produce broad generalizations to cover all anesthetic effects, we should be cautioned to recognize that it is quite likely that as we gain a better understanding of anesthetic sites and mechanisms of action, there will be specific effects and sites of action associated with specific drugs that cannot be broadly generalized across all general anesthetics.

Descending Modulatory Pathways

So far this chapter has focused on drug effects that are mediated directly on spinal sensory neurons. However, Figure 13–1 indicates that the modulatory systems derived either from propriospinal or supraspinal systems could also be targets of anesthetic action that could, in turn, influence spinal sensory neurons. In early studies, deJong and colleagues[26] reported that nitrous oxide could only depress noxiously evoked activity in the spinal cord of intact animals. If the cord was transected, no such depression was observed. Recently, Maze and colleagues[41] extended those early observations and demonstrated that spinal analgesic actions of nitrous oxide result from activation of descending adrenergic systems that are capable of depressing responses of spinal dorsal horn neurons to noxious peripheral stimuli. Those studies not only demonstrate an anesthetic action that is dependent on a supraspinal system, but also provide additional evidence of difference among drugs. As mentioned earlier, other general anesthetics have been shown to produce spinal analgesia in the absence of supraspinal actions.[33-36]

Work of deJong and colleagues and Maze and colleagues demonstrates that, for at least one anesthetic, the depression of spinal sensory neurons is caused by an action on supraspinal systems rather than by a direct action on the spinal cord itself.

A Simple System?

A review of the material presented so far in this chapter suggests a rather simple pharmacology and physiology by which general anesthetics could alter spinal sensory processing. That system is represented in Figure 13–5 where the processing of a pain message from the periphery is depicted. In the absence of an anesthetic, a tissue damaging stimulus sends an action potential down the C-fiber primary afferent to synapse on a spinal dorsal horn MR or HT neuron. In turn, that neuron sends axons up ascending fiber tracks to result in the sensation of pain and out to motor neurons to cause a reflex withdrawal from the source of the tissue injury. In the presence of a general anesthetic, the system is blocked either directly at the synapse (see Fig. 13–5, number 1) or because of anesthetic effects on modulatory systems (see Fig. 13–5, number 2). The validity of this hypothetical model is apparent from the huge literature associated with spinal opioid analgesia as first reported by Yaksh and Rudy.[7] The placement of an opioid at location 1 in Figure 13–5 will block the pain sensation and the reflex withdrawal. Can we assume that general anesthetics do the same? Unfortunately, the current answer is no, because of a series of unanswered questions about anesthetic actions within the spinal dorsal horn.

The first question relates to the amount of depression necessary to completely block information transmission. The remainder of this chapter focuses on the sensation of pain, recognizing that similar processes are likely to be associated with other sensory modalities that are integrated by the spinal dorsal horn.

If, as shown in Figure 13–5, noxious input from primary afferents activates second order neurons, to what degree must that activation be reduced before the message is no longer perceived as painful—i.e., how much of a change in stimulus-evoked activity is associated with a detectable change in behavior or sensation? Namiki and colleagues[42] studied the effects of halothane on noxiously evoked activity of MR neurons in decerebrate, spinal cord–transected cats. They reported that one MAC (minimum alveolar concentration at which 50% of a population does not move in the presence of a surgical stimulus) of halothane reduced the mean response of the population of neurons to 60% of the control value and that 1.5 MAC caused a reduction to 80% of the control response to noxious thermal stimulation of the neurons' peripheral receptive field. Is a 60% reduction adequate to block pain processing at the level of the spinal dorsal horn or is it necessary to have an 80% reduction? Unfortunately, we do not yet know the answer to that question. In the absence of an understanding of the relationship between neuronal activity and behavior, we are limited in our ability to predict the physiologic impact of pharmacologic depression of spinal sensory neurons.

The impact of our lack of understanding of the relationship between neuronal activity and behavior becomes even more apparent because of work by Rampil and colleagues[33,35] and Antognini and colleagues.[34,36] In a series of elegant studies, those two laboratories provided convincing evidence that immobility in the presence of a noxious stimulus is mainly caused by general anesthetic actions at the level of the spinal cord, with little or no involvement of supraspinal sites. Anesthetic-induced immobility in the presence of a noxious stimulus is the cardinal sign for the determination of MAC. In one of the early papers on MAC[43] the authors state the following: "We believe that in none of these

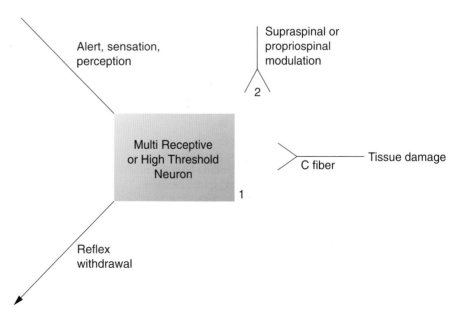

Figure 13–5. Diagram representing sites of action at which general anesthetics could later spinal sensory of information about tissue damage. This simplified diagram emphasizes two potential sites of action. Action at site *1,* the synapse between the primary afferent and the second order neuron, could alter the C fiber's ability to send the message, could alter the multi receptive or high threshold neuron's ability to respond to the message or could alter both. In all instances, the information about tissue damage could be modified. In a similar fashion, anesthetic actions at site *2* could alter information flow through the spinal dorsal horn.

or the subsequent studies did any dog suffer pain on application of these noxious stimuli. This belief is based on published and unpublished observations in man at similar depths of anesthesia." Although not frequently stated, it is assumed that the absence of a coordinated motor response to a noxious stimulus means the absence of the sensation of pain.

If immobility is caused by spinal anesthetic actions, can we assume that the depression of spinal dorsal horn neurons blocks the pain message and therefore produces immobility? Until recently that seemed like a valid assumption. However, Cheng and Kendig[44] have provided evidence that inhalation anesthetics depress the response of spinal motor neurons elicited by direct application of excitatory neurotransmitters. With that publication, the research community was forced to acknowledge that at least a portion of spinally mediated, anesthetic-induced immobility could be caused by a direct action on motor neurons rather than on the blockage of the pain signal at the level of the sensory neurons. Previous investigators reported that the response of spinal motor neurons was more sensitive to depression by pentobarbital than were spinal sensory neurons[45] and that barbiturate depression of spinal motor neurons was not always accompanied by depression of spinal sensory neurons.[6,7] Currently, we know that general anesthetics depress spinal sensory neurons, but we have no clear understanding of the impact that depression has on the behavior of the animal.

The absence of a clear understanding of the importance of general anesthetic pharmacology at the level of spinal sensory neurons is compounded by our lack of understanding of spinal dorsal horn physiology and pharmacology. Earlier in this chapter the four types of spinal sensory neurons were briefly reviewed. Maintaining our focus on pain transmission, it is clear that both MR and HT neurons are capable of transmitting information about pain. Until recently it was assumed that the MR neurons were responsible for conveying pain messages to motor neurons and therefore were the only class of spinal sensory neurons involved in the reflex responses elicited by a painful stimulus. However, Morgan[47,48] has provided data suggesting that populations of both HT and MR neurons participate in noxiously evoked motor reflexes. To the best of our knowledge there are no studies that provide information about general anesthetic effects on spinal sensory neurons that are intercalated between primary afferents carrying pain messages and motor output. Is it possible that those subpopulations are insensitive to general anesthetics and that immobility is exclusively due to anesthetic depression of motor neurons?

We face a similar dearth of information about spinal sensory neurons that contribute information through ascending fiber tracts. Although we know that ascending fiber tracts conveying pain information originate in spinal sensory interneurons, there is no information about anesthetic effects on those specific neurons. It is possible that separate populations of interneurons participate in information transmission for sensory versus motor functions.[49] We have no way of knowing if the populations of neurons involved in sensory functions are sensitive to general anesthetic depression at the level of the spinal dorsal horn.

Conclusion

At best, our current state of knowledge about anesthetic effects on spinal sensory processing allows us to develop several testable hypotheses that provide reasonable explanations for ways in which general anesthetic actions at the level of the spinal sensory neuron could disrupt sensory transmission throughout the body. Given that most general anesthetics depress all four classes of spinal sensory neurons, to varying degrees, it is reasonable to hypothesize that the upstream systems responsible for motor output, alerting, perception, and sensation of the stimuli will receive less information about the stimulus event in the presence of anesthesia than they would have in the absence of anesthesia. That hypothesis, if it is proven correct, will then provide a reasonable mechanism by which spinal actions of general anesthetics could reduce or eliminate the motor response to a stimulus as well as reduce or eliminate the associated painful sensation. If we broaden this to all the other forms of stimuli, it becomes quite apparent that anesthetic action on spinal sensory neurons is likely to play an important role in reducing afferent input and therefore contributing to the general state of anesthesia resulting from the administration of these drugs.

Acknowledgment
The authors are supported by grants from the National Institutes of Health-National Institute of General Medical Sciences (NIH-NIGMS).

References

1. Wall PD: The mechanisms of general anesthesia. Anesthesiology 28:46–53, 1967.
2. deJong RH, Wagman IH: Block of afferent impulses in the dorsal horn of monkey: A possible mechanism of anesthesia. Exp Neurol 20:352–358, 1968.
3. Antognini JF, Carstens E, Sudo M, et al: Isoflurane depresses electroencephalographic and medial thalamic responses to noxious stimulation via an indirect spinal action. Anesth Analg 91:1282–1288, 2000.
4. Besson JM, Wyon-Maillard MC, Benoist JM, et al: Effects of phenoperidine on lamina V cells in the cat dorsal horn. J Pharm Exp Ther 187:239–245, 1973.
5. Calvillo O, Henry JL, Neuman RS: Effects of morphine and naloxone on dorsal horn neurons in the cat. Can J Physiol Pharmacol 52:1207–1211, 1974.
6. Kitahata LM, Kosaka Y, Taub A, et al: Lamina-specific suppression of dorsal horn unit activity by morphine sulfate. Anesthesiology 41:39–48, 1974.
7. Yaksh TL, Rudy TA: Analgesia mediated by a direct spinal action of narcotics. Science 192:1357–1358, 1976.
8. Rexed B: The cytoarchitectonic organization of the spinal cord in the rat. J Comp Neurol 96:415–466, 1952.
9. Rexed B: The cytoarchitectonic organization of the spinal cord in the cat. J Comp Neurol 100:297–380, 1954.
10. Dubner R, Bennett GS: Spinal and trigeminal mechanisms of nociception. Ann Rev Neurosci 6:381–418, 1983.
11. Willis WD, Coggeshall RE: Sensory Mechanisms of the Spinal Cord, 2nd ed. New York, Plenum, 1991.

12. Davidoff RA: Handbook of the Spinal Cord, Vol. 2-3, Anatomy and Physiology. New York, Marcel Dekker, 1987.

13. Larrabee MG, Holaday DA: Depression of transmission through sympathetic ganglia during general anesthesia. J Pharm Exp Ther 105:400–448, 1952.

14. Larabee MG, Pasternck JM: Selective action of anesthetics on synapses and axons in mammalian sympathetic ganglia. J Neurophysiol 15:91–114, 1952.

15. Franks NP, Lieb WR: Molecular and cellular mechanisms of general anesthesia. Nature 367:607–614, 1994.

16. Waikar SS, Thalhammer JG, Raymond SA, et al: Mechanoreceptive afferents exhibit functionally-specific activity dependent changes in conduction velocity. Brain Res 721:91–100, 1996.

17. Katz PS, Clemens S: Biochemical networks in nervous systems: Expanding neuronal information capacity beyond voltage signals. Trends Neurosci 24:18–25, 2001.

18. Light AR, Perl ER: Spinal termination of functionally identified primary afferent neurons with slowly conducting myelinated fibers. J Comp Neurol 186:133–150, 1979.

19. Cervero F, Iggo A: The substantiagelatinosa of the spinal cord: A critical review. Brain 103:717–772, 1980.

20. Brown AG: Organization in the spinal cord: The anatomy and physiology of identified neurons. Berlin, Springer-Verlag, 1981.

21. Craig AD, Mense S: The distribution of afferent fibers from the gastrocnemius-soleus muscle in the dorsal horn of the cat, as revealed by the transport of horseradish peroxidase. Neurosci Lett 41:233–238, 1983.

22. Craig AD, Heppelmann B, Schaible HG: Projection of the medial and posterior articular nerves of the cat's knee to the spinal cord. J Comp Neurol 266:279–288, 1988.

23. Sugiura Y, Teruci N, Hosoya Y: Differences in distribution of central terminals between visceral and somatic unmyelinated primary afferent fibers. J Neurophysiol 62:834–840, 1989.

24. Wall PD: The laminar organization of dorsal horn and effects of descending impulses. J Physiol 188:403–423, 1967.

25. deJong RH, Robles R, Morikawa K: Actions of halothane and nitrous oxide on dorsal horn neurons ('the spinal gate'). Anesthesiology 31:205–212, 1969.

26. deJong RH, Robles R, Heavner JE: Suppression of impulse transmission in the cat's dorsal horn by inhalation anesthetics. Anesthesiology 32:440–445, 1970.

27. Kitahata LM, Taub A, Sato I: Lamina-specific suppression and facilitation of dorsal horn unit activity by nitrous oxide and by hyperventilation. J Pharmacol Exp Ther 176:101–108, 1971.

28. Conseiller C, Benoist JM, Hamann KF, et al: Effects of ketamine (C1581) on cell response to coetaneous stimulations in laminae IV and V in the cat's dorsal horn. Eur J Pharmacol 18:346–353, 1972.

29. Kitahata L, Taub A, Yosaka Y: Lamina-specific suppression of dorsal horn unit activity by ketamine hydrochloride. Anesthesiology 38:4–11, 1973.

30. Heavner JE: Jamming spinal sensory input: Effects of anesthetic and analgesic drugs in the spinal cord dorsal horn. Pain 1:239–255, 1975.

31. Yamamori Y, Kishikawa K, Collins JG: Halothane effects on low-threshold receptive field size of rat spinal dorsal horn neurons appear to be independent of supraspinal modulatory systems. Brain Res 702:162–168, 1995.

32. Ota K, Yanagidani T, Kishikawa K, et al: Cutaneous responsiveness of lumbar spinal dorsal horn neurons is reduced by general anesthesia: An effect dependent in part on $GABA_A$ mechanisms. J Neurophysiol 80:1383–1390, 1998.

33. Rampil IS, Mason P, Singh H: Anesthetic potency (MAC) is independent of forebrain structures in the rat. Anesthesiology 78:707–712, 1993.

34. Antognini JF, Schwartz K: Exaggerated anesthetic requirements in the preferentially anesthetized brain. Anesthesiology 79:1244–1249, 1993.

35. Rampil IJ: Anesthetic potency is not altered after hypothermic spinal cord transection in rats. Anesthesiology 80:606–610, 1994.

36. Antognini JF: The relationship among brain, spinal cord and anesthetic requirements. Med Hypotheses 48:83–87, 1997.

37. Herrero JF, Headley PM: Cutaneous responsiveness of lumbar spinal neurons in awake and halothane-anesthetized sheep. J Neurophysiol 74:1549–1562, 1995.

38. Miyazaki Y, Adache T, Utsumi J, et al: Xenon has greater inhibitory effects on spinal dorsal horn neurons than nitrous oxide in spinal cord transected cats. Anesth Analg 88:893–897, 1999.

39. Kishikawa K, Uchida H, Yamamori Y, et al: Low-threshold neuronal activity of spinal dorsal horn neurons increases during REM sleep in cats: Comparison with effects of anesthesia. J Neurophys 74:743–769, 1995.

40. Collins JG: Effects of ketamine on low threshold tactile sensory input are not dependent upon a spinal site of action. Anesth Analg 65:1123–1129, 1986.

41. Zhang C, Davies MF, Guo T-Z, et al: The analgesic action of nitrous oxide is dependent on the release of norepinephrine in the dorsal horn of the spinal cord. Anesthesiology 91:1401–1407, 1999.

42. Namiki A, Collins JG, Kitahata LM, et al: Effects of halothane on spinal neuronal responses to graded noxious heat stimulation in the cat. Anesthesiology 53:475–480, 1980.

43. Eger EI II, Saidman LJ, Brandstater B: Minimum alveolar anesthetic concentration: A standard of anesthetic potency. Anesthesiology 26:756–763, 1965.

44. Cheng G, Kendig JJ: Enflurane directly depresses glutamate AMPA and NMDA currents in mouse spinal cord motor neurons independent of actions on $GABA_A$ or glycine receptors. Anesthesiology 93:1075–1084, 2000.

45. Paik KS, Nam SC, Chung JM: Different classes of cat spinal neurons display differential sensitivity to sodium pentobarbital. Neurosci Res 23:107–115, 1989.

46. Carstens E, Campbell IG: Responses of motor units during the hind limb flexion withdrawal reflex evoked by noxious skin heating: Phasic and prolonged suppression by midbrain stimulation and comparison with simultaneously recorded dorsal horn units. Pain 48:215–226, 1992.

47. Morgan M: Paradoxical inhibition of nociceptive neurons in the dorsal horn of the rat spinal cord during a nociceptive hind limb reflex. Neuroscience 88:489–498, 1999.

48. Morgan M: Direct comparison of heat-evoked activity of nociceptive neurons in the dorsal horn with the hindlimb withdrawal reflex in the rat. J Neurophysiol 79:174–180, 1998.

49. Jasmin L, Carstens E, Bashaum AI: Interneurons presynoptic to rat tail-flick motorneurons as mapped by transneuronal transport of pseudorabies virus: Few have long ascending collaterals. Neuroscience 76:859–876, 1997.

14

AUTONOMIC FUNCTION

Jonathan Moss, MD, PhD • David Glick, MD

Systems Physiology
Organ Physiology
Cellular Physiology
Cholinergic

Biochemical Mechanisms
G Proteins
Assessment of Autonomic Function
Autonomic Failure and Hyperactivity

The autonomic nervous system (ANS) maintains cardiovascular, gastrointestinal, and thermal homeostasis. It controls an organism's maintenance functions and its responses to homeostatic challenges. The ANS is divided into sympathetic, parasympathetic, and enteric branches. The sympathetic nervous system (SNS) responds to challenges by increasing heart rate, blood pressure, and cardiac output, dilating the bronchial tree, and shunting blood away from the viscera and toward the muscles involved in the response to the challenge. The parasympathetic nervous system (PNS) acts primarily to conserve energy and to support the function of the endocrine, digestive, and urogenital systems. An additional branch of the ANS, the enteric nervous system (ENS), has recently come into prominence.

Understanding the ANS is central to contemporary anesthetic practice for several reasons. Anesthesiologists must understand the interaction of anesthetics with the involuntary control system to avoid triggering adverse effects. In addition, disease states may impair autonomic function and alter expected responses to surgery, anesthesia, or other stresses. Finally, the stress response itself can have both positive and negative effects that directly impact clinical care.

Systems Physiology

Each branch of the ANS exhibits a different anatomic motif, which is recapitulated on a cellular and molecular level. The underlying theme of the SNS is an *amplification* response, whereas that of the PNS is a *discrete* and narrowly *targeted* response. The ENS is arranged nontopographically, which is appropriate for the viscera, and relies on the mechanism of chemical coding to differentiate among nerves subserving different functions.

It was Claude Bernard who initially proposed the theory of chemical synaptic transmission, but it was not until 1899 that epinephrine was first synthesized. Subsequently, it was demonstrated that epinephrine, when administered exogenously, had the same effect as electrical stimulation of postganglionic neurons leading to some organs. Sir Henry Dale isolated choline and studied acetylcholine (ACh) in animals. The subsequent demonstration by Julius Axelrod that norepinephrine (NE) was the primary neurotransmitter involved in sympathetic postganglionic transmission earned him the Nobel Prize.

Nerves are classified by the chemical transmitters they contain. Nerves that contain ACh are cholinergic. Nerves that contain NE (noradrenaline) or epinephrine (adrenaline) are called adrenergic. Cholinergic neurons may be either nicotinic or muscarinic, depending on the receptors they activate. Almost 100 years ago, nicotine was found to act on ganglionic and skeletal muscle synapses, on nerve membranes, and on sensory endings. The drugs that act on those parts of the cholinergic system are called nicotinic drugs. Nicotinic drugs affect ganglionic or neuromuscular transmission. Muscarinic neurons activate the PNS. Muscarine, a chemical isolated from mushrooms, mimics the actions of direct nerve stimulation. Agonists and antagonists for these systems play an important role in contemporary anesthetic practice.

The third branch of the ANS, the ENS, often contains neither noradrenaline nor ACh. Understanding nonadrenergic, noncholinergic (NANC) neurons is necessary for understanding the ENS.[1]

The underlying organizational scheme of the SNS and PNS is given in Figure 14–1. The SNS modulates the activity of vascular and uterine smooth muscle, cardiac muscle, and glands. Aside from transmitters for a few anatomically unusual sympathetic neurons (e.g., sweat glands), the major transmitter of the SNS is NE. Activation of the SNS and the adrenal gland (which releases both NE and epinephrine)

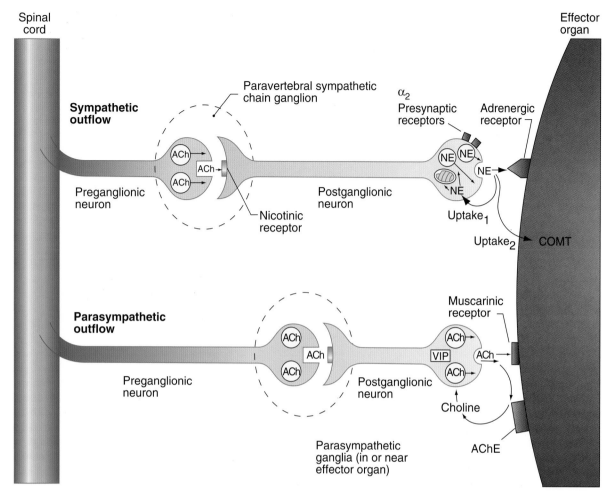

Figure 14–1. Schematic representation of the sympathetic and parasympathetic nervous systems from the spinal cord to effector organs. ACh, acetylcholine; AChE, acetylcholinesterase; COMT, catechol-o-methyl transferase; NE, norepinephrine; VIP, vasoactive intestinal protein.

results in a robust series of coordinated activities designed to maintain homeostasis and protect an organism from internal and external challenges. Sympathomimetic drugs mimic the actions of the SNS and sympatholytic drugs attenuate these actions. Systemic administration of sympathomimetic drugs constricts blood vessels, which increases blood pressure, whereas administration of sympatholytic drugs decreases blood pressure. Epinephrine and other sympathomimetic drugs also have inotropic and chronotropic effects on cardiac muscle and are often useful when treating shock. Epinephrine decreases bronchial and uterine smooth muscle tone so it is useful as a bronchodilator and to arrest uterine contractions. The release of renin, mediated through a β2 receptor in the kidney, potentiates many of the effects of NE.

The motif of the SNS is amplification, which occurs at molecular, tissue, and cellular levels. The stimulus that activates the SNS may emerge from several challenges to homeostasis including alterations in blood volume or blood sugar. The SNS originates from the spinal cord from the first thoracic through the second or third lumbar segments (Fig. 14–2). The preganglionic sympathetic neurons have cell bodies within the horns of the spinal gray matter. Nerve fibers extend from these cell bodies to three types of ganglia:

the paired sympathetic ganglia, various unpaired distal plexuses, and terminal (or collateral) ganglia near the target organ. The preganglionic fibers leave the cord within the anterior nerve roots, they join the spinal nerve trunks, and then they enter the ganglion through the white or myelinated ramus. Postsynaptic fibers re-enter the spinal nerve through the gray (unmyelinated) ramus and then innervate effectors of blood vessels in the skeletal muscle, skin, and sweat glands. Sympathetic innervation to the trunk and limbs is carried by the spinal nerves.

Although commonly thought of as one-to-one connections, the autonomic ganglia are organized anatomically to permit a systematized response. The functional imperative of the sympathetic ganglia is amplification. Sympathetic preganglionic fibers are short and lie close to the central nervous system. Their distribution is diffuse and capable of amplification. In fact, at each of these ganglia there is up to 7000-fold amplification. Thus the goal of a rapid, magnified response is served by these ganglia. Many autonomic reflexes are inhibited by supraspinal feedback, which is lost after spinal cord transection. As a result, in paraplegic patients small stimuli can evoke exaggerated sympathetic discharges. In addition to the paired ganglia, the sympathetic distribution to the head and neck arrives through the three

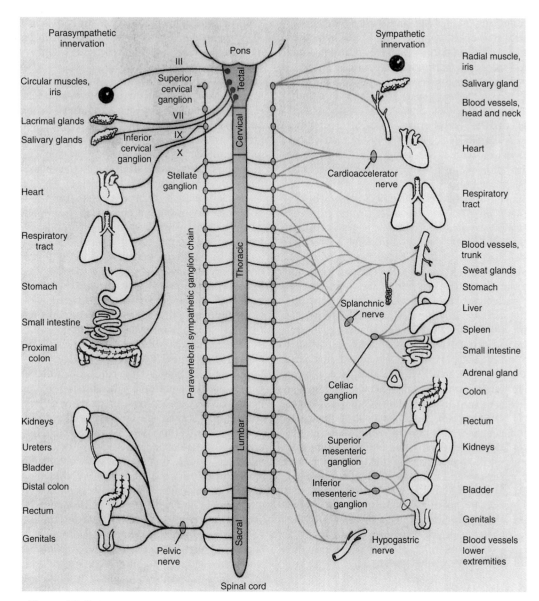

Figure 14–2. Schematic representation of the autonomic nervous system depicting the functional innervation of peripheral effector organs and the anatomic origin of peripheral autonomic nerves from the spinal cord. Although both paravertebral sympathetic ganglia chains are presented, the sympathetic innervation to the peripheral effector organs is shown only on the *right,* whereas the parasympathetic innervation of peripheral effector organs is depicted on the *left.* Roman numerals on nerves originating in the tectal region of the brain stem refer to the cranial nerves that provide parasympathetic outflow to the effector organs of the head, neck, and trunk. (From Ruffolo R: Physiology and biochemistry of the peripheral autonomic nervous system. In Wingard L, Brody T, Larner J, et al (eds): Human Pharmacology: Molecular-to-Clinical. St. Louis, Mosby–Year Book, 1991, p 77.)

ganglia of the cervical sympathetic chain. Although these ganglia are fused anatomically they still demonstrate a profound ability to amplify nervous responses. The unpaired paravertebral ganglia, in the abdomen and pelvis anterior to the vertebral column, include the celiac, superior mesenteric, and inferior mesenteric ganglia. The celiac ganglion, innervated by T5 to T12, innervates the spleen, liver, kidney, pancreas, small bowel, and proximal colon. Many preganglionic fibers from T5 to T12 pass through the paired paravertebral ganglia to form the splanchnic nerves. Most of these fibers do not synapse until they reach the celiac gan-

glion. Other fibers innervate the adrenal medulla. The superior mesenteric ganglion innervates the distal colon, whereas the inferior mesenteric ganglion subserves the rectum, bladder, and genitals. The adrenal gland, which is rich in both NE and epinephrine, has its primary neuron within the organ itself.

Unlike the response of the SNS, the response of the PNS is highly selective. The PNS emerges from the craniosacral outflow (see Fig. 14–2). The ganglia of the PNS are in close proximity to, or within, the innervated organ (see Fig. 14–1). Of all parasympathetic nerves, the vagus is unquestionably the most important, carrying up to 75% of the parasympathetic traffic. It supplies the heart, tracheo-bronchial tree, liver, spleen, kidney, and the gastrointestinal tract except for the distal colon (see Fig. 14–2). The pre-ganglionic fibers of the vagus nerve are long and its post-ganglionic fibers are short. This arrangement permits targeted and discrete functional responses. Most vagal fibers do not synapse until they arrive at small ganglia on or about the thoracic or abdominal viscera. Usually the parasympathetic nerves synapse with a one-to-one ratio of nerve to effector cell; occasionally, as in Auerbach plexus, there can be significant amplification.

The third branch of the ANS is the ENS. *An important difference between the ENS and the other two branches of the ANS is its degree of local autonomy.* The ENS contains as many nerve cells as the spinal cord. This system of neurons and their supporting cells is located within the walls of the gastrointestinal (GI) tract. They derive from the neural crest and migrate to the GI tract along the vagus nerve. Although the gut is notably influenced by sympathetic and parasympathetic activity, it is the ENS through the myenteric and submucous plexi that regulates digestive activity. Thus digestion and peristalsis can go on after spinal cord transection or during spinal anesthesia, albeit with impaired sphincter function. Unlike the SNS and PNS, which have topographic representation conferring selective action, the ENS uses a pattern of chemical coding for its functional organization. This system is highly dependent on the combination of amines and peptides that constitute the NANC neurons that control the function of the ENS. Although ACh is the principal excitatory trigger of the nonsphincteric portion of the ENS, causing muscle contraction, evidence has emerged that the NANC neurons, particularly the inhibitory vasoactive intestinal protein-nitric oxide (VIP-NO) neurons, play an important role. The importance of the NO-containing NANC neurons has been emphasized in digestion and in sexual function.

Organ Physiology

To predict the action of various drugs, the interaction of the SNS and PNS in different organs must be understood. Imbalances between the parasympathetic and SNS play important roles in many disease states. Pharmacologic blockade of either system can unmask preexisting activity of the other. Thus administration of atropine blocks the resting muscarinic state of the parasympathetically dominated heart, and unopposed sympathetic tone then causes tachycardia.

Almost all organs exhibit dual innervation, with sympathetic and parasympathetic inputs frequently mediating opposing effects. In nearly every instance, one branch dominates and provides the "resting tone" for that organ[2] (Table 14–1). For example, sympathetic stimulation acts on the heart to increase rate and strength of contraction and to enhance conduction through the atrioventricular node, whereas parasympathetic stimulation tends to decrease rate and contractility and to slow conduction through the node. The SNS is dominant in arterioles and veins, whereas the PNS dominates in the GI tract, urinary tract, and salivary glands. Certain organs such as the spleen and piloerector muscles are almost exclusively innervated by the SNS, but this is the exception.

The β_2 effects on smooth muscle elicit bronchial smooth muscle relaxation and decrease the tone and contractions of the gut and gravid uterus. The effects on the bladder are mixed. α_1 stimulation causes constriction of prostatic smooth muscle and urinary sphincters, whereas β activation relaxes the detrusor muscle of the bladder. In the eye, epinephrine causes mydriasis through α_1 receptors on the radial papillary dilator muscle of the iris.

In addition to the effects of epinephrine on regional blood flow, there are also important metabolic effects. Epinephrine increases blood sugar both by α_2 inhibition of insulin secretion and by stimulating the breakdown of glycogen to glucose in the liver and muscles through activation of the phosphorylase. Epinephrine also increases free fatty acids by activating lipase, which cleaves triglycerides. Epinephrine and the other naturally occurring catecholamines (dopamine and NE) can also have effects on organs distant from the sites of their synaptic release, but because they are polar molecules they do not easily penetrate the blood–brain barrier.

Epinephrine activates the cardiac β_1 adrenoceptors resulting in positive inotropic and chronotropic responses, the latter by direct action on pacemaker cells. However, because epinephrine accelerates the rate of myocardial relaxation, diastolic filling time may be increased. The net result of increased heart rate and a more forceful contraction is increased cardiac output. The electrophysiologic effects of epinephrine on the pacemaker are more complex. They include increasing conduction velocity and decreasing the refractory period in the Bundle of His and in Purkinje fibers, as well as activation of ectopic pacemaker cells. Premature ventricular contraction and even ventricular fibrillation can occur. Although the net result of epinephrine administration is to increase blood pressure, there are important differences in regional blood flow. In blood vessels, epinephrine can act either as a vasoconstrictor or vasodilator depending on the relative balance of α_1 or β_2 receptors. At low doses, epinephrine causes a relaxation of vascular smooth muscle of the hepatic and mesenteric vasculature through β_2 receptor activation. In other vascular beds, particularly renal and cutaneous vessels, the α_1 receptors predominate, and epinephrine causes intense vasoconstriction.

In addition to their well understood effects on the heart, lungs, and blood vessels, catecholamines also exert important effects by mobilizing glucose in response to hypoglycemia or stress. Overall, SNS stimulation increases the glycogenolysis in liver and muscle and liberates free fatty acids from adipose tissue by activation of β adrenoceptors. In neonates, epinephrine helps maintain body temperature through exothermic breakdown of brown fat, in part by β_3 receptors. β Receptor stimulation increases glucagon and insulin secretion, whereas α_2 receptor activation suppresses insulin secretion and inhibits lipolysis. In the plasma, epinephrine regulates short-term changes in potassium homeostasis. Exogenously administered or endogenously released epinephrine stimulates the β_2 receptors of red cells activating adenylate cyclase and sodium potassium adenosine triphosphatase, driving potassium into cells. This leads

TABLE 14–1.

Responses Elicited in Effector Organs by Stimulation of Sympathetic and Parasympathetic Nerves

Effector Organ	Adrenergic Response	Receptor Involved	Cholinergic Response	Dominant Response (A or C)
Heart				
Rate of contraction	Increase	β_1	Decrease	C
Force of contraction	Increase	β_1	Decrease	C
Blood vessels				
Arteries (most)	Vasoconstriction	α_1		A
Skeletal muscle	Vasodilation	β_2		A
Veins	Vasoconstriction	α_2		A
Bronchial tree	Bronchodilation	β_2	Bronchoconstriction	C
Splenic capsule	Contraction	α_1		A
Uterus	Contraction	α_1	Variable	A
Vas deferens	Contraction	α_1		A
Prostatic capsule	Contraction	α_1		A
Gastrointestinal tract	Relaxation	α_2	Contraction	C
Eye				
Radial muscle, iris	Contraction (mydriasis)	α_1		A
Circular muscle, iris			Contraction (miosis)	C
Ciliary muscle	Relaxation	β	Contraction (accommodation)	C
Kidney	Renin secretion	β_1		A
Urinary bladder				
Detrusor	Relaxation	β	Contraction	C
Trigone and sphincter	Contraction	α_1	Relaxation	A, C
Ureter	Contraction	α_1	Relaxation	A
Insulin release from pancreas	Decrease	α_2		A
Fat cells	Lipolysis	β_1		A
Liver glycogenolysis	Increase	α_1		A
Hair follicles, smooth muscle	Contraction (piloerection)	α_1		A
Nasal secretion			Increase	C
Salivary glands	Increase secretion	α_1	Increase secretion	C
Sweat glands	Increase secretion	α_1	Increase secretion	C

A, adrenergic; C, cholinergic.
From Ruffolo R: Physiology and biochemistry of the peripheral autonomic nervous system. In Wingard L, Brody T, Larner J, et al: Human Pharmacology: Molecular-to-Clinical. St. Louis, Mosby–Year Book, 1991, p 531.

to a reduction in serum potassium concentration. β Adrenergic blockade inhibits this potassium shift.[3-5]

In contrast to the amplified and diffuse discharge in the SNS, activation of the PNS is tonic. The muscarinic effects are marked by vasodilation and decreased heart rate. The vasodilatory effects of ACh depend on the integrity of the vascular endothelium because muscarinic receptors on the endothelium cause the release of NO, an endothelium-derived relaxant factor.[6,7] If the endothelium is damaged, receptor activation by ACh can provoke paradoxical vasoconstriction. In the heart, ACh decreases the rate of contraction, the velocity of conduction through the sinoatrial and atrioventricular nodes, and contractility. The decrease in nodal conduction may account for the complete heart block after administration of large amounts of cholinergic agents. In the ventricle, ACh decreases automaticity and increases the fibrillation threshold. In addition, ACh can inhibit the release of NE when muscarinic receptors residing on the presynaptic terminals are stimulated. Thus the effect of ACh on the heart results from its presynaptic inhibition of NE release from sympathetic nerve endings as well as its postsynaptic opposition of the effects of catecholamines on the myocardium. Additional effects of ACh include smooth muscle constriction (including constriction of the smooth muscle of the bronchial wall). In the GI and GU tracts, there is constriction of the smooth muscle of the walls but relaxation of the sphincters. Parasympathetic input into the endocrine system causes the release of secretions from tracheobronchial, salivary, and digestive glands.

The baroreflex provides the vital link among branches of the ANS that influence cardiovascular function. The baroreflex allows the body to maintain a relatively constant blood pressure in the face of internal and external events that would otherwise push the blood pressure to extraphysiologic extremes. The baroreflex is mediated through the ANS and functions both centrally and peripherally. The central effects are predominantly controlled by the PNS. High blood pressure results in increased vagal tone and a compensatory slowing of the heart rate. Conversely, a decrease in blood pressure leads to a decrease in vagal activity and a higher heart rate. The peripheral components of the baroreflex are tied to vascular smooth muscle tone, and it is the SNS that determines this component of systemic blood pressure. Low blood pressure leads to increased sympathetic outflow and increased vascular tone, whereas elevated blood pressure leads to reflex relaxation of the vascular smooth muscle. A diminution in the sensitivity of the components of the baroreflex can result in less narrowly controlled blood pressure, especially during acute systemic stresses (e.g., anesthetic induction and surgical stimulation).

Cellular Physiology

The processes of neurotransmitter synthesis, storage, release, inactivation, and receptor activation are repeated in the different branches of the ANS.

NE is synthesized from tyrosine, which is actively transported into the varicosity of the preganglionic sympathetic nerve terminal. The rate-limiting step in the conversion of tyrosine to NE and epinephrine in the adrenal medulla depends on the enzyme tyrosine hydroxylase. High levels of NE inhibit tyrosine hydroxylase, whereas low levels stimulate the enzyme. During chronic stress, there is evidence for induction of this enzyme. Tyrosine hydroxylase is exquisitely dependent on the presence of molecular oxygen. As a result, hypoxemia may significantly reduce NE synthesis.

An adrenergic response results when the nerve potential arrives at the varicosity, a fine beadlike specialization of the neuroeffector junction. Small amounts of calcium are translocated across the membrane and cause fusion of the NE-containing vesicle with the cell membrane. Notably, NE is not alone within the sympathetic nerve vesicle. Recent studies have documented the importance of adenosine triphosphate (ATP) and neuropeptide Y (NPY) as cotransmitters and neuromodulators.[8-12]

The dominant mechanism of release is exocytosis (Fig. 14–3), in which the vesicles merge with the membrane of the cell and expel their contents. Proof for exocytosis is derived from elegant experiments in which nerve stimulation caused release of the biosynthetic enzyme dopamine-beta-hydroxylase and NE in the same proportions that are contained within the vesicles.[13] The detailed mechanism by which docking and fusion occurs is only partially understood, but it appears to be a highly differentiated process in which a series of soluble binding proteins—SNAP (soluble NSF [*N*-ethyl maleimide sensitive factor] attachment proteins) and SNARE (soluble NSF receptors)—interact.[14,15] In vesicular docking and release, a subpopulation of vesicles is tethered to the active zone of the prejunctional neuron. Some of these vesicles, called readily releasable vesicles, are primed for fusion in response to Ca++ influx. Vesicular fusion is mediated by a coordinated series of actions by the synaptic vesicular protein synaptobrevin/vesicle-associated membrane protein (VAMP) and two plasma membrane proteins, syntaxin and SNAP25 (the binding site of botulinus toxin). These proteins form a complex that mediates vesicular fusion. A series of proteins called complexins are the key molecules in initiating exocytosis, possibly acting in direct concert with calcium sensors.[16] Exocytosis accounts for the majority of NE release although continuous leakage from the cytoplasm into the neuroeffector junction also occurs. NE leakage from storage vesicles into the axoplasm actually exceeds leakage into the presynaptic cleft by 100-fold and presynaptic reuptake by 10-fold, which explains the initial hypertensive effect of drugs (such as reserpine) that cause release of neurotransmitter from this compartment.[17]

Another hypothesis of vesicular release termed "kiss and run" has been proposed by Stevens and Williams.[18] This mechanism is thought to account for less than 15% of the total release of NE. Studies from cultured hippocampal cells have elucidated the nature of pools of synaptic vesicles. It is currently believed that there is a resting pool of 180 vesicles and a recycling pool of approximately 25 vesicles, of which only 5 to 8 are in the readily releasable subset.[19] This results in a small active pool and a large inactive reserve pool.[15] New data suggest the presence of an additional vesicular pool cycle.[18] After exocytosis, the fusion pores seal rapidly and the vesicles immediately refill with transmitters, this is the so-called kiss and run subset.[20] Therefore, the readily releasable pool of vesicles appears to consists of two

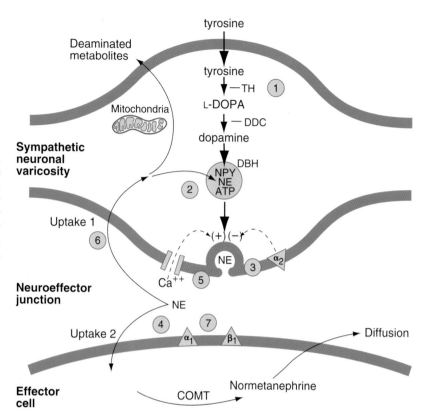

Figure 14–3. Norepinephrine synthesis, release, reuptake, and metabolism at the sympathetic postganglionic synapse. ATP, adenosine triphosphate; COMT, catechol-O-methyl transferase; DBH, dopamine-beta-hydroxylase; DDC, dopamine decarboxylase; MAO, monoamine oxidase; NE, norepinephrine; NPY, neuropeptide Y; TH, tyrosine hydroxylase.

separate populations. The majority of these vesicles participate in traditional exocytosis, whereas 15% participate in the kiss and run mechanism.

The structure of the adrenergic vesicle has been studied by electron microscopy and other techniques. NE is stored in large dense core vesicles, although NE itself does not contribute to the dense core. The dense core is formed by other binding proteins. In the adrenal gland, NE and epinephrine are stored in and secreted from separate chromaffin cell subtypes. In addition to NE, these vesicles also contain calcium, NPY, and ATP. Depending on the nature and frequency of the stimuli received at the presynaptic nerve-ending, ATP is selectively released to cause an immediate postsynaptic effect through purinoreceptors.[12] Synaptic vesicles are heterogenous and exist within functionally defined compartments. There is an actively recycling population of synaptic vesicles (estimated at 10%) and a reserve population (90%) that is resistant to depletion and is mobilized only after intensive or prolonged stimulation. Newly synthesized or recently taken up transmitter is preferentially incorporated into the actively recycling vesicles and is therefore the first to be released on stimulation. Thus drugs such as ephedrine, which are taken up into the presynaptic terminal and cause vesicular fusion and NE release, initially liberate newly synthesized or newly taken up amine. Approximately 1% of NE in a neuron is released from the varicosity with each nerve stimulation.

After nerve stimulation, NE is removed rapidly from the synaptic cleft. The reuptake into the presynaptic terminal, uptake-1, represents the first and most important step in the inactivation of released NE. Approximately 75% of the released NE is transported into the storage vesicle for reuse.

Specific uptake mechanisms have been elucidated.[21] Drugs such as cocaine and tricyclic antidepressants are potent antagonists of the uptake pump and increase the amount of NE within the cleft. The transporter is extremely efficient, but it is not entirely specific; therefore many false transmitters that may be clinically important can be taken up into the presynaptic terminal. Tyramine, which is contained within many foods, is such an agent. In addition, drugs that mimic NE may be taken up into the presynaptic terminal and packaged as false transmitters. Ephedrine and bretylium act in this fashion.

There are important differences in the adrenergic function of the peripheral blood vessels and the heart. The heart has the highest rate of reuptake and the lowest rate of synthesis of NE. The converse is true of the blood vessels. Therefore, drugs that selectively affect reuptake have a greater effect on cardiac function, whereas drugs that affect biosynthesis of NE act predominantly on blood vessels.

Approximately 75% of NE is taken up into the presynaptic varicosity by the high-affinity, specialized uptake-1 system. An additional mechanism (uptake-2) involves a less potent and less specific uptake of NE into postjunctional tissues. The NE that escapes both reuptake mechanisms spills over into plasma. Metabolism of this plasma-borne NE occurs in the blood, liver, kidney,[22] and in the lungs, where up to 25% of the NE is removed (except when pulmonary hypertension is present).[23] The metabolism of NE involves the mitochondrial enzyme monoamine oxidase and the cytoplasmic enzyme catechol-o-methyltransferase (COMT). These enzymes metabolize NE and epinephrine as well as several of the sympathomimetic drugs. The metabolic endproduct of the inactivation of these amines is vanil-

Part II Physiologic Substrates of Drug Action

lylmandelic acid, which is excreted in the urine. As a result, urinary vanillylmandelic acid levels can be used to identify patients with catecholamine-secreting tumors. COMT is present in abundance in the liver, where it metabolizes circulating catecholamines. Drug-induced inhibition of monoamine oxidase (MAO) is surprisingly well tolerated, but this stability belies that amine metabolism is fundamentally changed. Anesthesiologists must be attuned to these changes as they may present as life-threatening events.

Release of NE in the neuroeffector junction stimulates adrenergic receptors. Adrenergic receptors have been classi-

fied as α_1, α_2, and β. Each class has three major subtypes (Fig. 14–4). Justification for this classification scheme is derived from the pharmacologic analysis of drug affinity patterns, differences in signal transduction mechanisms, and primary structural differences in the receptors.[24] In general, the receptors in cardiac tissue are β_1, and those acting on smooth muscle and exocrine glands are β_2. β_2 receptors can respond to NE, but they are primarily stimulated by epinephrine released from the adrenal gland. Excess NE within the cleft binds to presynaptic α_2 receptors, inhibiting the release of additional NE. In clinical practice, agonists and

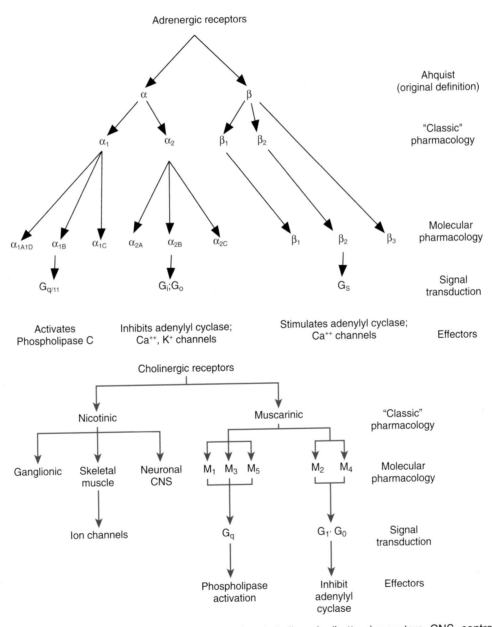

Figure 14–4. Classification of adrenergic *(top)* and cholinergic *(bottom)* receptors. CNS, central nervous system. (*Top,* From Moss J, Renz CL: The autonomic nervous system. In Miller RD (ed): Anesthesia, 5th ed. Philadelphia, Churchill Livingstone, vol 1, 2000, p 540.)

antagonists are available for α_1, α_2, β_1, and β_2 receptors. Although α_1 and α_2 receptors are differentiated on the basis of their pharmacologic characteristics, it is generally true that α_1 receptors are expressed postsynaptically, whereas α_2 receptors are expressed presynaptically or in non-neuronal tissues. The ability to discriminate between subtypes of α receptors has proven to be clinically useful because it has permitted the development of therapies for postural hypotension and benign prostatic hypertrophy (α_{1A}). The recent development of *dexmedetomidine* takes advantage of relative selectivity for the α_2 subtype, and the β_3 receptor has been recognized as a potential therapeutic target for cardiovascular drugs.[25]

Cholinergic

Much of our knowledge of the role of ACh in the PNS is derived from studies of the neuromuscular junction, which demonstrates prototypical nicotinic transmission. ACh is synthesized intraneuronally from acetyl coenzyme A and choline. Choline is present in diet or liberated into the bloodstream through the liver. It is transported as a phospholipid and taken up by a high-affinity transport system. The transport process appears to be the rate-limiting step for determining ACh levels, although there is some evidence suggesting that precursor availability (i.e., diet or hepatic function) can affect ACh levels, particularly during periods of rapid firing of cholinergic neurons. Once choline is taken up, it is synthesized into ACh by the enzyme choline acetyltransferase (Fig. 14–5).

ACh coexists with VIP in parasympathetic nerves. Unlike the sympathetic system, where NPY, ATP, and NE are contained within the same vesicle, ACh and VIP are stored in separate vesicles within the presynaptic muscarinic terminal and are released differentially depending on the frequency of stimulation. VIP is thought to act at high-frequency stimulation to augment the effects of ACh.[9,26,27]

Drawing on studies of the neuromuscular junction, it is believed that the presynaptic cholinergic neuron releases its contents largely by the process of exocytosis (as described earlier). Unlike the dense core vesicles that are the ultrastructural hallmark of adrenergic neurons, cholinergic neurons contain smaller (30 nm) clear vesicles, each of which may contain as many as 10,000 molecules of ACh. The motif of nicotinic receptor activation and reuptake is one of summation rather than amplification because each synaptic cleft adjoins a single postsynaptic neuron.

Most of the ACh released into the neuroeffector junction is hydrolyzed by acetylcholinesterase, a membrane-bound enzyme that is present in all cholinergic synapses. This exceptionally efficient enzyme is also present in red blood cells. The acetylcholinesterase regenerates choline, most of which is taken up into the presynaptic terminal and repackaged. A second enzyme, butyrylcholinesterase (sometimes called plasma cholinesterase or pseudocholinesterase), is a soluble enzyme that is synthesized in the liver and is found in plasma and in abundance in the placenta. It appears that the driving force for the perpetuation of this isoenzyme resides in its relative resistance to solanaceous glycoalkaloids, which are present as natural insecticides in potatoes, tomatoes, and eggplant.[28] Its role in normal physiology is unknown, but individuals who are genetically incapable of synthesizing this enzyme are otherwise phenotypically normal.

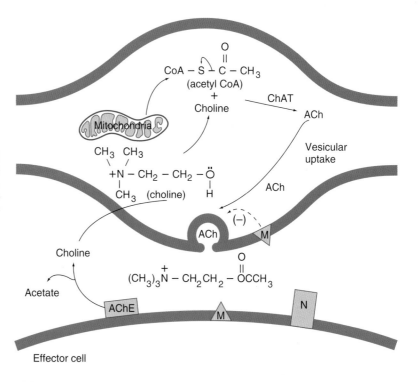

Figure 14–5. Synthesis, release, and metabolism of acetylcholine (ACh) at the parasympathetic postganglionic synapse. AChE, acetylcholinesterase; ChAT, choline acetyltransferase; CoA, coenzyme A; M, muscarinic; N, nicotinic.

Biochemical Mechanisms

The biochemical and molecular mechanisms underlying both parasympathetic and sympathetic nervous function are well understood. It is at this level that most drugs exert important pharmacologic activity.

As noted earlier, NE is synthesized from the aromatic amino acid tyrosine and is converted to dopamine by aromatic amino acid decarboxylase (Fig. 14–6). Although Parkinson disease has for years been viewed as a central dopamine-mediated neuropathy leading to motor dysfunction, recent data suggest a systemic defect. Patients with Parkinson disease may initially have symptoms of autonomic failure and may be clinically indistinguishable from patients with multiple system atrophy syndrome or patients with primary autonomic failure. All of these patients can have orthostatic hypotension, and the correct diagnosis often cannot be made until postmortem examinations are performed.[29]

Imaging procedures have demonstrated decreased neuronal uptake, release, turnover, and synthesis of NE in the myocardium of patients with Parkinson disease. This indicates a nearly complete loss of sympathetic terminal innervation in the hearts of patients with Parkinson-associated autonomic dysfunction. Additional imaging studies demonstrated the destruction of postganglionic cardiac sympathetic function in Parkinson disease. Sympathetic denervation of the heart was even present in 50% of patients with Parkinson disease with no clinical signs of autonomic failure on provocative testing. This fits the pathologic model of this disease because it disables the long axon nerves by means of cytoskeletal damage and leaves the short axon nerves (e.g., the sympathetic preganglionic neurons) undamaged.[29]

In addition to its role in the basal ganglia, dopamine can and does act as a neurotransmitter in other cells, particularly in the viscera and kidney. However, in most adrenergic neurons, dopamine is biotransformed by monoamine oxidase enzyme or converted to NE within the dense core vesicles by dopamine β hydroxylase. In the adrenal medulla, there is a further conversion of about 85% of the NE to epinephrine.

The NE that is released into the neuroeffector junction acts on postsynaptic α and β adrenergic receptors either alone or in concert with neuromodulators such as NPY. β adrenergic receptors were among the first receptors to be identified and characterized,[30] and are one of a superfamily of receptors that have seven helices woven through the cellular membrane (Fig. 14–7). The intracellular terminus can modulate the function of the β receptor and its subsequent

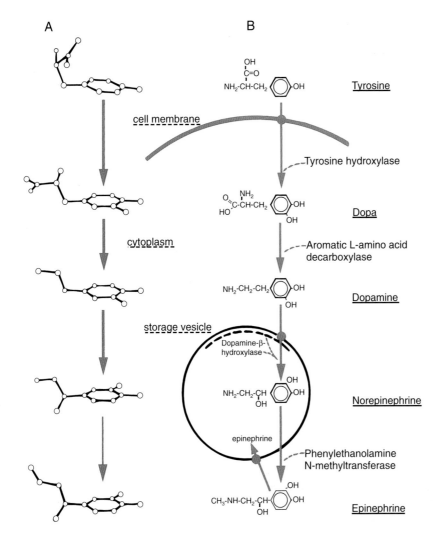

Figure 14–6. Biosynthesis of norepinephrine and epinephrine in sympathetic nerve terminal (and adrenal medulla). *A,* Perspective view of molecules. *B,* Enzymatic processes. (Modified from Tollenaerè JP: Atlas of the Three-Dimensional Structure of Drugs. Amsterdam, Elsevier North Holland, 1979, as modified by Vanhoutte PM: Adrenergic neuroeffector interaction in the blood vessel wall. Fed Proc 37:181, 1978.)

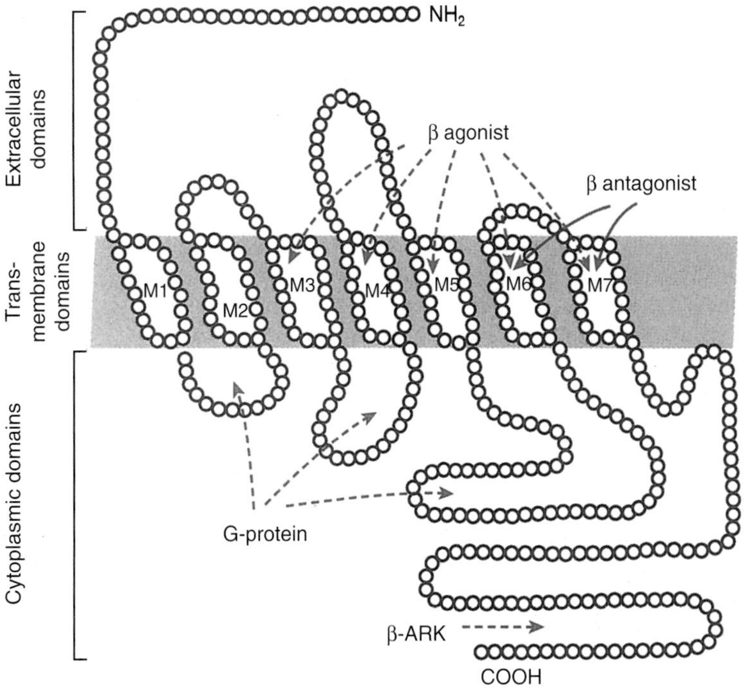

Figure 14–7. Molecular structure of the β-adrenergic receptor. Note the three domains. The transmembrane domains act as a ligand-binding pocket. Cytoplasmic domains can interact with G proteins and kinases, such as β adrenergic receptor kinase (β-ARK). The latter can phosphorylate and desensitize the receptor. (Modified from Opie L: Receptors and signal transduction. In Opie LH (ed): The Heart: Physiology and Metabolism. New York, Raven Press, 1991.)

interaction with G proteins through kinases.[31] The β receptor has mechanistic and structural similarities with muscarinic but not nicotinic receptors, primarily in the transmembrane domains. In fact, both muscarinic and β receptors are coupled through adenylate cyclase to G proteins and both can initiate the opening of ion channels. β receptors are further divided into β_1, β_2, and β_3 subtypes, all of which increase cyclic adenosine monophosphate (cAMP) through adenylate cyclase and G protein mediators.

β adrenergic receptors are not fixed but change significantly in response to the amount of NE present in the synaptic cleft or in plasma. Clinically, and at the cellular level, responses to many hormones and neurotransmitters wane rapidly despite continuous exposure to adrenergic agonists.[32] This phenomenon, termed desensitization, has been particularly well studied for the stimulation of cAMP levels by plasma membrane β-adrenergic receptors.[33] Mechanisms postulated for desensitization include uncoupling, sequestration, and down-regulation initiated by phosphorylation. The molecular mechanisms underlying *rapid* β adrenergic receptor desensitization do not appear to require internalization of the receptors, but rather an alteration in the functioning of β receptors themselves, which uncouples the receptors from the stimulatory G_s protein. Agonist-induced desensitization involves phosphorylation of G protein–coupled receptors by two classes of serine-threonine kinases (GPKs). One of these initiates receptor-specific or homologous desensitization. The other works through second messenger–dependent kinases, thus mediating a general cellular hyporesponsiveness, termed heterologous desensitization. Ultimately, an inhibitory arrestin protein binds to the phosphorylated receptor, causing desensitization by blocking signal transduction. Because GPKs only phosphorylate receptors in the activated state, there has been an attempt to use transient β-blockade in states of receptor desensitization such as congestive heart failure (CHF) or cardiopulmonary

bypass to block desensitization and to give a receptor "holiday."[34–36] Regeneration of a functional β adrenergic receptor is contingent on sequestration of the receptor with dephosphorylation and recycling. Recent work has suggested that the arrestins contribute to desensitization not only by uncoupling signal transduction but also by contributing to the process of receptor internalization.[36,37] Down-regulation is different from these rapid mechanisms of desensitization because it occurs after hours of exposure to an agonist (as in chronic stress or CHF), and receptors are not merely internalized but destroyed. New receptors must be synthesized before return to a baseline state is possible. These remarkable changes in receptor activity provide a physiologic explanation for why sudden discontinuation of chronic β adrenergic receptor blockade causes rebound tachycardia and increases the incidence of myocardial infarction and ischemia.[38]

The best studied example of a change in receptor number involves chronic CHF. Traditionally, β_1 receptors were thought to be isolated to cardiac muscle and β_2 receptors were believed to be restricted to vascular and bronchial smooth muscle. The β_2 receptor population in cardiac muscle is actually quite sizable, accounting for 15% of the β receptors in the ventricles and 30% to 40% in the atria.[39] These receptors may play a compensatory role in CHF. When the failing heart is depleted of catecholamines, plasma levels of catecholamines are markedly increased to maintain systemic vascular resistance. This leads to a decrease in β receptors in the heart, which explains why administration of β agonists in this syndrome is largely ineffective. Interestingly, although β_1 receptor density is markedly decreased, β_2 density remains unchanged.[40,41] Thus β_2 receptors account for 60% of the inotropic response in CHF.[42] β_3 receptors are relatively refractory to desensitization because they lack cytoplasmic phosphorylation sites; as a result, they may also play a part in the compensatory response.[25]

In addition to α and β receptors there are also dopamine receptors. Although dopamine in higher doses acts on both α and β receptors, Goldberg and Rajfer[43] demonstrated conclusively that distinct dopamine receptors exist and are physiologically important. Although five dopamine receptors have been cloned, only dopamine 1 (D1) and dopamine 2 (D2) subtypes are of physiologic importance.[44] D1 receptors are postsynaptic and mediate vasodilation, whereas presynaptic dopamine receptors inhibit the release of NE and dopamine. Certain drugs such as fenoldopam act as direct D1 agonists and are important in selective vasodilation of renal and mesenteric beds. The D2 receptors are presynaptic and central D2 receptors are targeted by butyrophenones.

G Proteins

After adrenergic receptor stimulation, the extracellular signal is transformed into an intracellular signal by a process known as signal transduction, in which the α_1 and β receptors are coupled to G proteins.[45] Although thorough discussions of receptor/effector coupling and signal transduction are found elsewhere (see Chapter 2), a brief discussion is included in this chapter. Activated G proteins modulate either the synthesis or availability of intracellular cytoplasmic messengers,[46] and ultimately the activation of protein kinases and phosphorylation of target proteins. The G protein consists of three subunits (α, β, γ) and has a remarkable potential for amplification, which is consistent with the motif of the SNS. Of the three subunits, the α-subunit is the most variable and determines the activity of the protein (G_s [stimulatory], G_o [inhibitory], or G_{q11}). Each class of adrenergic receptor couples to a different major subfamily of G proteins, which are in turn linked to different effectors. On receptor activation, the α-subunit is cleared and binds to the effector, initiating a series of intracellular events by activation of second messengers. The briefest encounter of β adrenergic receptors with epinephrine and NE results in up to a 400-fold increase in intracellular cAMP. The number of G protein molecules greatly exceeds the number of β adrenergic receptors. The relative abundance of G proteins results in amplification of receptor agonist at the signal transduction step. In addition, the stoichiometry requires that it is the receptor concentration and ultimately adenylate cyclase activity that limits the response to catecholamines. The physiologic relevance of these proteins is all the more important because many of the tools pharmacologists use for dissecting signal transduction are associated with diseases of great severity including pertussis, cholera, and botulism.

The links between stimulus and response are different in nicotinic and muscarinic receptors. The ACh that is released can affect nicotinic receptors at either the neuromuscular junction or within the ganglia or muscarinic receptors. Much is known about the nicotinic receptors from the neuromuscular junction, but the nicotinic subtype present in the ganglia are structurally different. ACh receptors of the nicotinic type belong to the superfamily of ligand-gated ion channels, which includes glutamate and glycine receptors.

The nicotinic receptors are heteropentameric membrane proteins that form nonselective cation channels. There are two α-subunits and one each of β, ϵ, or δ.[47] The α-subunits present the binding sites for ACh or nicotinic antagonists. In humans, a γ-subunit present at birth is replaced by the ϵ-subunit within the first 2 weeks of life. This change in structure converts the receptor from one with low conductance and long duration of opening to a receptor with high conductance and brief duration of opening.[48,49] When ACh occupies both α-subunits, the channel opens. If only one site is occupied, the channel remains closed and there is no flow of ions or change in electrical potential. The motif of a targeted response is recapitulated in synaptic electrophysiology, as the postjunctional action of several vesicles appears to be necessary to initiate a response. Furthermore, unlike adrenergic receptors that react instantly to changes in catecholamine levels through phosphorylation of the receptor, changes to nicotinic receptor number and function take days.[49]

In contrast to the ion-gated nicotinic receptors, muscarinic receptors belong to the superfamily of G protein–coupled receptors and are more homologous to adrenergic receptors than to nicotinic receptors. Five muscarinic receptors are known. Receptors in the muscarinic series are coupled to a second messenger system such as cyclic nucleotides or phosphoinositides, which are in turn coupled to ion channels. The nature of the response is determined by the specific cation involved. The M_2 and M_3 receptors are particularly important because they have been identified in the airway smooth muscle of many species. The M_3 receptor also mediates contractile and secretory response. Muscarinic receptors exhibit different signal transduction mechanisms. Odd numbered receptors (M_1, M_3, M_5) work predominantly through the hydrolysis of phosphoinositide and release of intracellular calcium, whereas even numbered receptors (M_2, M_4) work primarily through the G_i proteins to regulate adenylate cyclase.[50] The M_2 receptors in cardiac pacemaker cells oppose the increased contractility caused by β-adrenergic stimulation and activate potassium channels through G_i, causing hyperpolarization and decreasing heart rate. In addition to their role in the heart, M_2 and M_4 receptors act through G_o to inhibit presynaptic neuronal calcium channels, which modulate neurotransmitter release. Like the other G protein–coupled receptors, the response of the muscarinic system is sluggish. No response may be seen from seconds to minutes following the application of ACh; offset is also prolonged and outlives the presence of the agonist.

Assessment of Autonomic Function

Because of the increased operative risk for patients with autonomic dysfunction that may occur with aging and diabetes,[51] the diagnosis of autonomic neuropathy is extremely important. Five evocative tests of cardiovascular function have been developed to evaluate autonomic function in patients with diabetes.[52] The tests include heart rate responses to the Valsalva maneuver, standing up, and deep breathing, and blood pressure responses to standing up and sustained handgrip. The tests, involving changes in heart rate, measure injury to the parasympathetic system and precede changes in the measures of blood pressure that reflect sympathetic injury. Early autonomic dysfunction is defined as a single abnormal or two borderline abnormal results on the tests involving changes in heart rate. Definite involvement comes when two of the tests of changes in heart rate are abnormal. Severe dysfunction is defined as abnormalities in the blood pressure assessments. The application of these standards requires that the investigator understand both the proper techniques for performing the five tests and the expected results in patients without autonomic neuropathy (Table 14–2). The simplicity and effectiveness of this clinical assessment has also led to its use in the evaluation of patients with nondiabetic causes of autonomic dysfunction.

In addition to clinical tests of autonomic function, sensitive and reliable techniques for measurement of plasma NE and epinephrine have been available for three decades; however, the interpretation of such data is confounded by other influences. Plasma epinephrine levels (normally 100–400 pg/mL) reflect adrenal release but vary consider-

ably with psychological and physical stress. Evidence from animal studies suggests that NE levels in plasma can be increased by direct sympathetic stimulation. Plasma NE levels (normally 100–400 pg/mL) reflect both sympathetic and adrenal activity. Unlike plasma epinephrine levels, plasma NE levels reflect spillover from neuroeffector junctions, which may represent 10% to 20% of total sympathetic release and may vary among the regional organ beds. Thus although marked increases in plasma catecholamines may be significant, isolated levels less than 1000 pg must be interpreted with caution.

Autonomic Failure and Hyperactivity

Failure of the ANS, such as in aging or diabetes, can be associated with increased morbidity and mortality rates.[51] The common clinical manifestations of autonomic dysfunction in the elderly are orthostatic hypotension, postprandial

TABLE 14–2.

Clinical Assessment of the Autonomic Nervous System

Clinical Examination	Technique	Normal Value
Parasympathetic HR response to Valsalva	The seated subject blows into a mouthpiece (maintaining a pressure of 40 mm Hg) for 15 seconds. The Valsalva ratio is the ratio of the longest R-R interval (which comes shortly after the release) to the shortest R-R interval (which occurs during the maneuver).	Ratio of >1.21
HR response to standing	HR is measured as the subject moves from a resting supine position to standing. Normal tachycardic response is maximal around the 15th beat following rising. A relative bradycardia follows that is most marked around the 30th beat after standing. The response to standing is expressed as the "30:15" ratio and is the ratio of the longest R-R interval around the 30th beat to the shortest R-R interval around the 15th beat.	Ratio of >1.04
HR response to deep breathing	The subject takes six deep breaths in 1 minute. The maximum and minimum hear rates during each cycle are measured and the mean of the differences (maximum HR − minimum HR) during three successive breathing cycles is taken as the maximum − minimum HR.	Mean difference >15 bpm
Sympathetic BP response to standing	The subject moves from resting supine to standing and the standing SBP is subtracted from the supine SBP.	Difference <10 mm Hg
BP response to sustained handgrip	The subject maintains a handgrip of 30% of maximal squeeze for up to 5 minutes. The blood pressure is measured every minute, and the initial DBP is subtracted from the DBP just prior to release.	Difference >16 mm Hg

BP, blood pressure; bpm, beats per minute; DBP, diastolic blood pressure; HR, heart rate; SBP, systolic blood pressure.

hypotension, hypothermia, and heat stroke. These presentations are all consequences of the limited ability of elderly patients to adapt to stresses with normal, autonomic-mediated vasoconstriction and vasodilation. These alterations may require modifications in the anesthetic management of these patients.

The decrement in autonomic function with aging is not the result of lower neurotransmitter levels or fewer postjunctional receptors but of fewer prejunctional terminals. Plasma epinephrine levels are normal in the elderly as are the number of β adrenergic receptors, and NE levels actually increase with age (independent of age-related hypertension). The increase in plasma NE levels is the result of both an increase in NE appearance and a decrease in NE clearance,[53] suggesting that *the primary physiologic deficit is in the reuptake mechanism.* Clinically, there is a marked attenuation of physiologic response to β adrenergic stimulation in the elderly. Exogenous β adrenergic agonists have a less profound effect on heart rate, left ventricular ejection fraction, cardiac output, and vasodilation in the healthy elderly.[54] The decreased response to adrenergic stimulation in the elderly appears to be the result of decreased affinity (not number) of the β receptors and decreases in the coupling of the G_s protein and the adenylate cyclase unit.[54]

Aside from direct effects on autonomic function, aging also has been associated with decreased levels of plasma renin, angiotensin II, and aldosterone and increased levels of atrial natriuretic factor, all of which increase salt wasting and predispose to hypovolemia. Unfortunately, hypovolemia can be devastating in these patients whose cardiac output is particularly preload dependent because of the relatively diminished compensatory autonomic response seen in the elderly.

Another example of autonomic failure occurs in patients with diabetes. Diabetic autonomic neuropathy is the most common form of autonomic neuropathy and is the most extensively investigated. It occurs in 20% to 40% of all insulin-dependent patients with diabetes. Common manifestations of diabetic autonomic neuropathy include impotence, postural hypotension, gastroparesis, diarrhea, and sweating abnormalities. When impotence or diarrhea is the sole manifestation, there is little effect on survival; however, with postural hypotension or gastroparesis, 5-year mortality rates are greater than 50%.[55]

The symptoms associated with diabetic autonomic neuropathy confer an increased risk during anesthesia and surgery by both direct and secondary mechanisms. Gastroparesis increases the risk for aspiration. Systemic injury to the *vasa vasorum* in patients with postural hypotension increases the risk for hemodynamic instability and cardiovascular collapse in the perioperative period. Even in seemingly minor surgery, diabetic autonomic neuropathy can lead to significant complications. In a series of ophthalmologic procedures requiring general anesthesia, patients with diabetes with autonomic neuropathy had a significantly greater drop in blood pressure with induction and a greater need for vasopressors than patients with diabetes without autonomic dysfunction.[56] Furthermore, Page and Watkins[57] reported five cases of unexpected cardiorespiratory arrest in young patients with diabetes, all of whom had symptoms of autonomic neuropathy. In a large prospective study of diabetic autonomic neuropathy using the five evocative clinical tests discussed earlier, parasympathetic dysfunction preceded

sympathetic failure in 96% of the patients followed.[58] This battery of autonomic tests identifies patients with autonomic neuropathy and is highly predictive both of mortality[55] and perioperative risk.[51]

Although autonomic failure presents a challenge for anesthesiologists, there is increasing evidence that chronic sympathetic stimulation may also increase morbidity and mortality rates. Evaluation of catecholamine-containing tumors and attempts to attenuate the surgical stress response confirm the risks for chronic sympathetic stimulation. One such tumor is a pheochromocytoma. Pheochromocytoma is characterized by an explosive, unpredictable, and uncontrolled release of catecholamines. Even relatively minor stress can trigger 100- or 1000-fold increases in plasma catecholamine levels. Symptoms are excessive sweating, headaches, hypertension, orthostatic hypotension, glucose intolerance, polycythemia, weight loss, and psychiatric disturbances. Up to 1% of patients with hypertension have pheochromocytomas. Ten percent of the tumors are extra-adrenal, 10% are bilateral, 10% are malignant, and 10% are familial. Pheochromocytomas are of particular concern to anesthesiologists because 25% to 50% of all in-hospital deaths in patients with pheochromocytomas occur during induction or other stressful perioperative events. In early series, perioperative mortality rates for surgical removal of pheochromocytomas were 40% to 60%. The current mortality rate is 0% to 6%. The improvement in survival has been attributed to the routine use of α-blockade for 2 months before surgery.[59] It is important not to give beta-blockers to these patients until they are adequately α-blocked because unopposed beta-blockade can lead to vascular smooth muscle contraction and can actually worsen hypertensive crises. Chronic increases in circulating catecholamines have a profound effect on the potency of the SNS. Several series[60-62] of patients before and after surgical resection of pheochromocytomas have shown a marked increase in sympathetic tone relative to vagal tone after the catecholamine-secreting tumor was removed.

Decreased sympathetic nerve activity at the peroneal nerve in patients with pheochromocytoma normalizes after tumor removal.[63] Furthermore, iobenguane sulfate I 123 uptake has been correlated with cardiac sympathetic activity, and both Agostini et al.[64] and Izumi et al.[65] have demonstrated lower than normal uptake of isotope in the hearts of patients with pheochromocytomas. Uptake returns to normal after the pheochromocytoma is removed.

Although these tumors lead to pathologic increases in circulating catecholamines, even physiologic responses that lead to sustained ANS hyperactivity can increase morbidity and mortality rates. Surgical stress, particularly associated with major surgeries, results in profound metabolic and endocrine responses. The combination of autonomic, hormonal, and catabolic changes that accompany surgery has been termed the "surgical stress response."[66] The extent of this response depends on the preoperative condition of the patient, the magnitude of the operation, and the surgical and anesthetic techniques. Despite the widespread clinical intuition that attenuation of the stress response is of benefit, there has been a long-standing debate as to whether such a strategy affects outcomes. The weight of current evidence suggests that treatment of the acute stress response may be of limited value, *but a comprehensive anesthetic plan that focuses on attenuation of the stress response during the entire perioperative period may influence morbidity and mortality rates.* Evidence for this is derived from several important studies.

Evidence has shown that the stress response for surgery is not only acute, but begins before surgery and extends well into the postoperative period. Psychological stress with transport into the operating room can itself be significant.[67] In addition, after surgery, there is a prolonged increase of plasma catecholamines that has been associated with hemodynamic alterations.[68] This appears not only to be caused by postoperative pain, but is a response to the surgical intervention itself. Psychological stress appears to be largely mediated by the release of epinephrine from the adrenal glands, whereas physical stress involves sympathoadrenal release of NE and epinephrine.[69]

Three separate lines of evidence suggest that attenuation of the surgical stress response can lead to improved outcomes. In a series of studies, interruption of the sympathetic response to surgery markedly reduced surgical stress intraoperatively and postoperatively.[70] Use of continuous thoracic epidural infusions of local anesthetics minimized the increase in plasma catecholamines, cortisol, and glucagon and improved outcome. This improved outcome was independent of a decrease in pain perception as patients receiving other methods of pain relief (including nonsteroidal anti-inflammatory drugs and opioids) did not exhibit similar reductions in metabolic and endocrine responses to surgery.[70] Continuation of epidural infusions well into the postoperative period was regarded as essential to improving outcome. Although many potentially detrimental effects were blocked, the patients' inflammatory and immunologic responses, which are necessary for infection control and wound healing, appeared to be unaffected. Using similar techniques and other stress-reducing maneuvers, faster and more complete recoveries were achieved in elderly patients undergoing colon resections.[71]

A separate line of evidence supporting the hypothesis that long-term attenuation of the stress response alters outcome comes from the pediatric literature. When neonates with complex congenital heart disease underwent cardiac surgery, those who received high-dose sufentanil infusions intraoperatively and for the first 24 hours after surgery to reduce the stress response had lower beta endorphin, NE, epinephrine, glucagon, aldosterone, and cortisol levels compared with control subjects.[72] The mortality rate in the opiate group was significantly lower than in the study or historical control subjects. Thus anesthetic techniques can have profound effects on the metabolic and endocrine responses to surgery, and effective management of these reflexes can alter outcomes.

A third line of evidence that has proved to be compelling involves the results from the multicenter study of the perioperative ischemia research group.[73] Surgical patients were randomized to receive either atenolol or placebo before and after surgery (until their discharge from the hospital) and were followed over 2 years. The overall mortality rate was significantly less in the atenolol group and persisted at the 2-year follow-up. Survival rates 2 years after surgery were 68% in the placebo group and 83% in the atenolol group. This study demonstrated conclusively that perioperative β-blockade could significantly improve outcomes even 2 years

after the "stressful" episode. There is little or no evidence demonstrating that treatment of acute events could lead to such a dramatic change in outcome.

In addition to the panoply of pharmacologic interventions available to clinicians, acute changes in intravascular volume, ventilatory status, and choice and depth of anesthetics influence autonomic function. Both hypercapnia and hypoxia can independently increase plasma catecholamines through the release of NE from sympathetic nerves. The relationship between hypoxia and autonomic excitation can be chronic as well as acute. Hypoxic episodes in patients with obstructive sleep apnea are common and lead to a reflex tachypnea and tachycardia.[74]

Although current evidence suggests that long-term sympathetic hyperactivity contributes to changes in outcome, there are compelling data for a direct effect of anesthetics in blocking adrenergic release and the associated tachycardia and hypertension in vitro and in vivo.[75,76] Most general anesthetics reduce stress-induced sympathoadrenal discharge, but certain anesthetics, such as desflurane, can cause paradoxical increases in sympathetic activity.[77,78] Rapid increases in desflurane concentration increase sympathetic nerve activity, plasma NE concentrations, and tachycardia and hypertension. *Taken as a whole, however, these various lines of evidence suggest that anesthetics or adjuvants that can interfere with the stress response in the perioperative period can markedly improve morbidity and mortality rates.* Newer anesthetic drugs such as the α_2 agonists, which can also target presynaptic receptors to block the stress response, could influence outcome in the same fashion.

Because of its central importance in homeostasis, the ANS has long been studied for potential therapeutic intervention at virtually every biochemical and cellular site. A primary clinical goal has been to develop drugs that target the synthesis, storage, release, and reuptake of NE. Drugs such as a methyltyrosine inhibit tyrosine hydroxylase and have been used in management of pheochromocytomas. Carbidopa, which is derived from methyldopa but does not cross the blood–brain barrier, is used with L-dopa in Parkinson disease to inhibit the amino acid decarboxylase enzyme. The development of reserpine, which prevents vesicular reuptake of NE, was the first of these important drugs.

There has been an interest in uptake inhibitors by the psychiatric community. Correlation between mood and amine availability in the synaptic cleft underlies the basis of modern psychopharmacology.[79] Cocaine and tricyclic antidepressants specifically block the NE transporter of the uptake-1 system. In addition, other drugs such as guanethidine or methyldopa are used as false transmitters to increase the available amine in the cleft. Guanethidine depletes NE in the presynaptic terminal, whereas α methyldopa is taken up and converted to α-methylnorepinephrine, which displaces NE from the vesicle but exerts minimal biologic activity.

In addition to drugs that target vesicular and synaptic uptake and release, there are many drugs that inhibit the MAO enzyme. The role of this enzyme in catabolizing monoamines (catecholamines, serotonin) has long been recognized, but it was not until the euphoria associated with the antituberculosis drug iproniazid was appreciated that highly potent and specific MAO inhibitors were developed.

Although still useful as antidepressants, their interactions with certain drugs (notably meperidine) and foods (those containing tyramine-like aged cheeses and wine) has limited their use. In patients who are taking MAO inhibitors, tyramine that is ingested is not catabolized and remains at high levels in plasma. Tyramine is then taken up by sympathetic nerve terminals as a "false transmitter" and is converted to octopamine, which is biologically inactive. Thus many patients taking MAO inhibitors have symptoms of autonomic failure such as orthostatic hypotension. Perhaps of greater consequence, if foods high in tyramine are ingested by patients taking MAO inhibitors, there is the potential for massive displacement of NE into the cleft and for a life-threatening hypertensive crisis.

Although virtually every component of sympathetic, and to a lesser extent, parasympathetic function has been accessed pharmacologically, the areas of most intensive interest have been receptor ligands. The appreciation that certain receptor subtypes may play unique roles in autonomic function has led to the development of super-selective agonists and antagonists. This has already achieved clinical use with the introduction of dexmedetomidine, a selective α_2 agonist, as a sedative-analgesic for intensive care unit use.[80] A greater understanding of the regional distribution of receptor subtypes in the vasculature,[81] brain,[82,83] and spinal cord will permit targeting by new autonomic agonist and antagonist drugs.

Although the development of selective antagonists has already achieved clinical usage, there has also been renewed interest in the mechanisms of receptor regeneration and coupling. Recent observations that β receptors may be uncoupled from G proteins during cardiopulmonary bypass[84] suggest that the linkage between receptor and G protein may be a target. An increased understanding of the molecular mechanisms of receptor desensitization[85,86] may provide another useful target for drug development. Another approach, recognizing a possible immunologic role in entities such as cardiomyopathy,[87,88] in which antibodies to both β and muscarinic receptors have been identified, suggests an immunologic strategy may be developed. The recognition of the importance of cotransmission and neuromodulation in autonomic function provides yet another potential therapeutic target.[89] Finally, the possibility of genetic strategies using adenovirus transfection to modulate autonomic function or address functionally important polymorphisms may ultimately prove to be clinically useful as well.

References

1. Burnstock G: Autonomic neuromuscular junctions: Current developments and future directions. J Anat 146:1, 1986.
2. Ruffolo R: Physiology and biochemistry of the peripheral autonomic nervous system. In Wingard L, Brody T, Larner J, et al (eds): Human Pharmacology: Molecular-to-Clinical. St. Louis, Mosby, 1991.
3. Kharasch ED, Bowdle TA: Hypokalemia before induction of anesthesia and prevention by beta-2 adrenoceptor antagonism. Anesth Analg 72:216, 1991.
4. Williams ME, Gervino EV, Rosa RM, et al: Catecholamine modulation of rapid potassium shifts during exercise. N Engl J Med 312:823, 1985.
5. Struthers AD, Reid JL: The role of adrenal medullary catecholamines in potassium homoeostasis. Clin Sci 66:377, 1984.
6. Furchgott RF, Zawadzki JV: The obligatory role of endothelial cells in the relaxation of arterial smooth muscle by acetylcholine. Nature 288:373, 1980.
7. Johns RA: EDRF/nitric oxide. The endogenous nitrovasodilator and a new cellular messenger. Anesthesiology 75:927, 1991.
8. Von Kügelgen I, Starke K: Noradrenaline-ATP co-transmission in the sympathetic nervous system. Trends Pharmacol Sci 12:319, 1991.
9. Burnstock G: Local mechanisms of blood flow control by perivascular nerves and endothelium. J Hypertens Suppl 8:S95, 1990.
10. Jacobson KA, Trivedi BK, Churchill PC, Williams M: Novel therapeutics acting via purine receptors. Biochem Pharmacol 41:1399, 1991.
11. Walker P, Grouzmann E, Burnier M, Waeber B: The role of neuropeptide Y in cardiovascular regulation. Trends Pharmacol Sci 12:111, 1991.
12. Lincoln J, Burnstock G: Neural-endothelial interactions in control of local blood flow. In Warren J (ed): The Endothelium: An Introduction to Current Research. New York, Wiley-Liss, 1990.
13. Weinshilboum RM, Thoa NB, Johnson DG, et al: Proportional release of norepinephrine and dopamine-hydroxylase from sympathetic nerves. Science 174:1349, 1971.
14. Jahn R, Sudhof TC: Membrane fusion and exocytosis. Annu Rev Biochem 68:863, 1999.
15. Sudhof TC: The synaptic vesicle cycle revisited. Neuron 28:317, 2000.
16. Reim K, Mansour M, Varoqueaux F, et al: Complexins regulate a late step in Ca2+-dependent neurotransmitter release. Cell 104:71, 2001.
17. Eisenhofer G: In vivo kinetics of catecholamines. J Auton Pharmacol 14:7, 1994.
18. Stevens CF, Williams JH: "Kiss and run" exocytosis at hippocampal synapses. Proc Natl Acad Sci USA 97:12828, 2000.
19. Murthy VN, Stevens CF: Reversal of synaptic vesicle docking at central synapses. Nat Neurosci 2:503, 1999.
20. Pyle JL, Kavalali ET, Piedras-Renteria ES, Tsien RW: Rapid reuse of readily releasable pool vesicles at hippocampal synapses. Neuron 28:221, 2000.
21. Pacholczyk T, Blakely RD, Amara SG: Expression cloning of a cocaine-and antidepressant-sensitive human noradrenaline transporter. Nature 350:350, 1991.
22. Kopin IJ: False neurochemical transmitters and the mechanism of sympathetic blockade by monoamine oxidase inhibitors. J Pharmacol Exp Ther 147:186, 1965.
23. Sole MJ, Drobac M, Schwartz L, et al: The extraction of circulating catecholamines by the lungs in normal man and in patients with pulmonary hypertension. Circulation 60:160, 1979.
24. Lawhead RG, Blaxall HS, Bylund DB: α_2A is the predominant α_2-adrenergic receptor subtype in human spinal cord. Anesthesiology 77:983, 1992.
25. Gauthier C, Langin D, Balligand J-L: β_3-Adrenoceptors in the cardiovascular system. Trends Pharmacol Sci 21:426, 2000.
26. Bloom SR, Edwards AV: Vasoactive intestinal peptide in relation to atropine resistant vasodilatation in the submaxillary gland of the cat. J Physiol 300:41, 1980.
27. Lundberg JM: Evidence for coexistence of vasoactive intestinal polypeptide (VIP) and acetylcholine in neurons of cat exocrine glands: Morphological, biochemical and functional studies. Acta Physiol Scand Suppl 496:1, 1981.
28. McGehee DS, Krasowski MD, Fung DL, et al: Cholinesterase inhibition by potato glycoalkaloids slows mivacurium metabolism. Anesthesiology 93:510, 2000.
29. Braak H, Braak E: Pathoanatomy of Parkinson's disease. J Neurol 247:II3, 2000.
30. Lefkowitz RJ: The superfamily of heptahelical receptors. Nat Cell Biol 2:E133, 2000.
31. Raymond JR, Hnatowich M, Lefkowitz RJ, Caron MG: Adrenergic receptors: Models for regulation of signal transduction processes. Hypertension 15:119, 1990.
32. Insel PA: Adrenergic receptors—evolving concepts and clinical implications. N Engl J Med 334:580, 1996.
33. Hausdorff WP, Caron MG, Lefkowitz RJ: Turning off the signal: Desensitization of β-adrenergic receptor function. FASEB J 4:2881, 1990.
34. Hirst GD, Bramich NJ, Edwards FR, Klemm M: Transmission at autonomic neuroeffector junctions. Trends Neurosci 15:40, 1992.
35. Michel MC, Kenny B, Schwinn DA: Classification of β_1-adrenoceptor subtypes. Naunyn Schmiedebergs Arch Pharmacol 352:1, 1995.
36. Menard L, Ferguson SS, Zhang J, et al: Synergistic regulation of β_2-adrenergic receptor sequestration: Intracellular complement of β-

adrenergic receptor kinase and β-arrestin determine kinetics of internalization. Mol Pharmacol 51:800, 1997.

37. Ferguson SS, Barak LS, Zhang J, Caron MG: G-protein-coupled receptor regulation: Role of G-protein-coupled receptor kinases and arrestins. Can J Physiol Pharmacol 74:1095, 1996.

38. Nattel S, Rangno RE, Van Loon G: Mechanism of propranolol withdrawal phenomena. Circulation 59:1158, 1979.

39. Vanhees L, Aubert A, Fagard R, et al: Influence of β1- versus β2-adrenoceptor blockade on left ventricular function in humans. J Cardiovasc Pharmacol 8:1086, 1986.

40. Brodde OE: The functional importance of β1 and β2 adrenoceptors in the human heart. Am J Cardiol 62:24C, 1988.

41. Lefkowitz RJ, Rockman HA, Koch WJ: Catecholamines, cardiac beta-adrenergic receptors, and heart failure. Circulation 101:1634, 2000.

42. Opie L: Ventricular overload and heart failure. In Opie LH (ed): The Heart: Physiology and Metabolism, 2nd ed. New York, Raven Press, 1991.

43. Goldberg LI, Rajfer SI: Dopamine receptors: Applications in clinical cardiology. Circulation 72:245, 1985.

44. Missale C, Nash SR, Robinson SW, et al: Dopamine receptors: From structure to function. Physiol Rev 78:189, 1998.

45. Linder ME, Gilman AG: G proteins. Sci Am 267:56, 1992.

46. Simonds WF: G protein regulation of adenylate cyclase. Trends Pharmacol Sci 20:66, 1999.

47. Standaert F: Donuts and holes: Molecules and muscle relaxants. In Katz RL (ed): Muscle Relaxants: Basic and Clinical Aspects. Orlando, FL, Grune and Stratton, 1984.

48. Martinou JC, Falls DL, Fischbach GD, Merlie JP: Acetylcholine receptor-inducing activity stimulates expression of the β-subunit gene of the muscle acetylcholine receptor. Proc Natl Acad Sci USA 88:7669, 1991.

49. Martyn JA, White DA, Gronert GA, et al: Up-and-down regulation of skeletal muscle acetylcholine receptors. Effects on neuromuscular blockers. Anesthesiology 76:822, 1992.

50. Hosey MM: Diversity of structure, signaling and regulation within the family of muscarinic cholinergic receptors. FASEB J 6:845, 1992.

51. Charlson ME, MacKenzie CR, Gold JP: Preoperative autonomic function abnormalities in patients with diabetes mellitus and patients with hypertension. J Am Coll Surg 179:1, 1994.

52. Ewing DJ, Martyn CN, Young RJ, Clarke BF: The value of cardiovascular autonomic function tests: 10 years experience in diabetes. Diabetes Care 8:491, 1985.

53. Veith RC, Featherstone JA, Linares OA, Halter JB: Age differences in plasma norepinephrine kinetics in humans. J Gerontol 41:319, 1986.

54. Lakatta EG: Deficient neuroendocrine regulation of the cardiovascular system with advancing age in healthy humans. Circulation 87:631, 1993.

55. Ewing DJ, Campbell IW, Clarke BF: The natural history of diabetic autonomic neuropathy. Q J Med 49:95, 1980.

56. Burgos LG, Ebert TJ, Asiddao C, et al: Increased intraoperative cardiovascular morbidity in diabetics with autonomic neuropathy. Anesthesiology 70:591, 1989.

57. Page MM, Watkins PJ: Cardiorespiratory arrest and diabetic autonomic neuropathy. Lancet 1:14, 1978.

58. Ewing DJ, Clarke BF: Diagnosis and management of diabetic autonomic neuropathy. Br Med J 285:916, 1982.

59. Roizen MF, Schreider BD, Hassan SZ: Anesthesia for patients with pheochromocytoma. Anesthesiol Clin North Am 5:269, 1987.

60. Stein PK, Rottman JN, Hall AF, Kleiger RE: Heart rate variability in a case of pheochromocytoma. Clin Auton Res 6:41, 1996.

61. Dabrowska B, Dabrowski A, Pruszczyk P, et al: Heart rate variability in pheochromocytoma. J Cardiol 76:1202, 1995.

62. Munakata M, Aihara A, Imai Y, et al: Altered sympathetic and vagal modulations of the cardiovascular system in patients with pheochromocytoma: Their relations to orthostatic hypotension. Am J Hypertens 12:572, 1999.

63. Grassi G, Seravalle G, Turri C, Mancia G: Sympathetic nerve traffic responses to surgical removal of pheochromocytoma. Hypertension 34:461, 1999.

64. Agostini D, Darlas Y, Filmont JE, et al: The reversibility of cardiac neuronal function after removal of a pheochromocytoma: An I-123 MIBG Scintigraphic Study. Clin Nucl Med 24:514, 1999.

65. Izumi C, Himura Y, Konishi T: Abnormal cardiac sympathetic nerve function in a patient with pheochromocytoma. An analysis using 123I metaiodobenzylguanidine scintigraphy. Int J Cardiol 50:189, 1995.

66. Selye H: Forty years of stress research: Principal remaining problems and misconceptions. Can Med Assoc J 115:53, 1976.

67. Moss J, Donlon JV, McGoldrick DE, et al: Perioperative anxiety: Difference in the adrenergic response to local and general anesthesia. In Belmaker RH, Sandler M, Dahlstrom A (eds): Progress in Catecholamine Research, Part C: Clinical Aspects. New York, Alan Liss, 1988.

68. Breslow MJ, Jordan DA, Christopherson R, et al: Epidural morphine decreases postoperative hypertension by attenuating sympathetic nervous system hyperactivity. JAMA 261:3577, 1989.

69. Dimsdale JE, Moss J: Plasma catecholamines in stress and exercise. JAMA 243:340, 1980.

70. Kehlet H: Manipulation of the metabolic response in clinical practice. World J Surg 24:690, 2000.

71. Bardram L, Funch-Jensen P, Jensen P, et al: Recovery after laparoscopic colonic surgery with epidural analgesia, and early oral nutrition and mobilization. Lancet 345:763, 1995.

72. Anand KJS, Hickey PR: Halothane-morphine compared with high-dose sufentanil for anesthesia and postoperative analgesia in neonatal cardiac surgery. N Engl J Med 326:1, 1992.

73. Mangano DT, Layug EL, Wallace A, Tateo I: Effect of atenolol on mortality and cardiovascular morbidity after noncardiac surgery. N Engl J Med 335:1713, 1996.

74. Zwillich CW: Sleep apnoea and autonomic function. Thorax 53:S20, 1998.

75. Roizen MF, Horrigan RW, Frazer BM: Anesthetic doses blocking adrenergic (stress) and cardiovascular responses to incision-MAC BAR. Anesthesiology 54:390, 1981.

76. Roizen MF, Moss J, Muldoon S: The effects of anesthesia, anesthetic adjuvant drugs, and surgery on plasma norepinephrine. In Lake CR, Zeigler MG (eds): Norepinephrine: Clinical Neuroscience, Vol 4. Baltimore, Williams & Wilkins, 1984.

77. Ebert TJ, Perez F, Uhrich TD, Deshur MA: Desflurane-mediated sympathetic activation occurs in humans despite preventing hypotension and baroreceptor unloading. Anesthesiology 88:1227, 1998.

78. Muzi M, Ebert TJ, Hope WG, et al: Site(s) mediating sympathetic activation with desflurane. Anesthesiology 85:737, 1996.

79. Schildkraut JJ: Neuropsychopharmacology and the affective disorders. (First of three parts). N Engl J Med 281:197, 1969.

80. Kamibayashi T, Maze M: Clinical uses of alpha2-adrenergic agonists. Anesthesiology 93:1345, 2000.

81. Rudner XL, Berkowitz DE, Booth JV, et al: Subtype specific regulation of human vascular alpha(1)-adrenergic receptors by vessel bed and age. Circulation 100:2336, 1999.

82. Lakhlani PP, MacMillan LB, Guo TZ, et al: Substitution of a mutant alpha2a-adrenergic receptor via "hit and run" gene targeting reveals the role of this subtype in sedative, analgesic, and anesthetic-sparing responses in vivo. Proc Natl Acad Sci USA 94:9950, 1997.

83. Maze M, Fujinaga M: Alpha2 adrenoceptors in pain modulation: Which subtype should be targeted to produce analgesia? Anesthesiology 92:934, 2000.

84. Gerhardt MA, Booth JV, Chestnut LC, et al: Acute myocardial beta-adrenergic receptor dysfunction after cardiopulmonary bypass in patients with cardiac valve disease. Duke Heart Center Perioperative Desensitization Group. Circulation 98:II275, 1998.

85. McDonald PH, Chow CW, Miller WE, et al: Beta-arrestin 2: A receptor-regulated MAPK scaffold for the activation of JNK3. Science 290:1574, 2000.

86. Bohn LM, Gainetdinov RR, Lin FT, et al: Mu-opioid receptor desensitization by beta-arrestin-2 determines morphine tolerance but not dependence. Nature 408:720, 2000.

87. Wallukat G, Muller J, Podlowski S, et al: Agonist-like beta-adrenoceptor antibodies in heart failure. Am J Cardiol 83:75H, 1999.

88. Wallukat G, Nissen E, Morwinski R, Muller J: Autoantibodies against the beta- and muscarinic receptors in cardiomyopathy. Herz 25:261, 2000.

89. Sneddon P, Westfall TD, Todorov LD, et al: Modulation of purinergic neurotransmission. Prog Brain Res 120:11, 1999.

15

Neural Substrates for Behavior

Laura Nelson, PhD • Mervyn Maze, MB, ChB

CONSCIOUSNESS

Identification of the neural correlates of consciousness is a vexing problem. Philosophers continue to wrestle with the plausibility of correlating the behavioral state with specific neural substrates and have expressed doubt whether the actions of individual neurons can explain such an abstraction as consciousness.[1] Neuroscientists, however, believe that consciousness is a phenomenon necessarily correlated with neuronal actions that can be explained by current neurobiology rather than untestable metaphysical theories, and they grapple with determining the precise identity and role of these correlates.

This chapter focuses on current knowledge regarding the neural correlates of level of consciousness (i.e., awake, asleep) as distinguished from the neural correlates of specific phenomenal content (i.e., the redness of red or the painfulness of pain) for two reasons. First, level of consciousness (i.e., being conscious or not) is arguably more fundamental because it precludes and enables conscious experiences (i.e., being conscious of something or not).

Second, an understanding of the neural correlates of the three naturally occurring cardinal states of consciousness—wakefulness, non–rapid eye movement (NREM) sleep, and rapid eye movement (REM) sleep—is of far greater value to the anesthesiologist who represents the exogenous manipulator of the level of consciousness.

Endogenous sleep and the hypnotic/sedative component of anesthesia share a key fundamental property: both create a similar loss of response to external stimuli. A growing body of evidence indicates that they may be transduced by related mechanisms. The mechanisms of anesthesia are relatively unclear, but the mechanisms of sleep/wake regulation are better understood. Sleep is not a simple, uniform suspension of activity, as was assumed for centuries, but rather it is a multifaceted and highly organized pattern of diverse physiologic variables. It is characterized by a complex pattern of neuronal activity in hypothalamic and thalamocortical systems.

Systems Physiology

In addition to the central nervous system (see "Brain and Cellular Physiology" and "Biochemical and Molecular Mechanisms Underlying Cellular Physiology"), specific physiologic changes accompany sleep in nearly every other bodily system; therefore only a brief overview of the systems physiology of sleep is provided in this chapter, which focuses to a greater degree on those issues most relevant to clinical anesthesia.

Central Nervous System

Neurons in many anatomically discrete regions of the brain exhibit changes in activity related to the states of sleep and wakefulness. Briefly, (see "Brain and Cellular Physiology" for a detailed discussion), during NREM sleep, most neurons in the brain exhibit a reduced mean discharge rate, and the overall level of neuronal metabolism is decreased. In contrast, during the tonic aspect of REM sleep, the mean firing rate in many regions increases compared with NREM or wakefulness, thus refuting the myth that brain rests during sleep, and during the phasic aspect of REM some regions, particularly the visual system, exhibits marked increases in neuronal firing rate (for review of the visual system during REM sleep see Callaway and colleagues[2]).

Autonomic Nervous System

During NREM sleep, sympathetic nervous activity is at a level roughly equivalent to that during relaxed wakefulness, but parasympathetic activity is increased, indicating a slight predominance of parasympathetic over sympathetic drives. During tonic REM sleep, the level of sympathetic activity decreases, therefore the imbalance swings further toward parasympathetic activation. Phasic REM sleep induces increases in both sympathetic and parasympathetic activity, sometimes to favor sympathetic activation.[3]

Cardiovascular System

During NREM sleep, compared with resting wakefulness, systemic blood pressure is decreased slightly and exhibits reduced variability, cardiac output is reduced, and the vessels that supply resistance to the circulatory system are actively vasodilated. Regional cerebral blood flow studies in cats have shown that only a few brain areas receive greater blood flow during NREM sleep than during relaxed wakefulness. During tonic REM sleep, blood pressure remains at the NREM level, most vessels remain dilated (bar striated skeletal muscles), and most brain areas show markedly increased blood flow (i.e., 50–200% above the waking level); but during phasic REM sleep, blood pressure is highly variable (occasionally increasing by 30% above resting level), vasoconstriction is generalized (which may be mechanistically related to greatly increased blood pressure during phasic REM), and short transient further increases in blood flow perfuse most brain regions (for a review of cardiovascular physiology across sleep states see Franzini[4]).

Endocrine System

Secretions of several endocrine systems appear to be directly linked to sleep state or circadian factors (for a review of endocrine physiology across sleep states see Cauter[5]). Growth hormone secretion peaks within minutes of the onset of stage 3 and 4 NREM sleep (known as slow wave sleep), prolactin secretion increases 30 to 90 minutes after the sleep onset to reach maximal levels in early morning, and plasma cortisol levels peak toward the end of sleep periods but sleep onset has an inhibitory effect on cortisol release. In adolescents, the release of gonadotropins, leuteinizing hormone, and follicle-stimulating hormone occur only during sleep. Thyrotropin stimulating hormone (TSH) release reaches a peak at the end of the waking day and declines across the sleep period. Circadian melatonin release at night from the pineal gland is influenced by light but not sleep, and its release patterns adjust slowly, taking 10 to 12 days to adjust to a reverse in the light/dark schedule. Melatonin receptors have been localized to the suprachiasmatic nucleus in the hypothalamus, a region strongly implicated as the mammalian circadian pacemaker, and melatonin is thought to function in part as a hormonal transducer of the light/dark signal. Some reports indicate that endogenous melatonin can induce drowsiness in humans, but there is no evidence that endogenous melatonin release is involved in sleep processes. Interruptions in nighttime sleep are associated with increased cortisol and TSH concentrations, and it has been noted that sleep loss and diminishing sleep quality correlate with disturbances of hormonal secretion.

Respiratory System

During NREM sleep there is 13% to 15% decrease in minute ventilation and a corresponding decrease in alveolar ventilation such that $PaCO_2$ increases and PaO_2 decreases. The onset of sleep removes (1) behavioral activity driving breathing, and (2) the tonic cortical state-related, nonmetabolic drive that stimulates breathing during wakefulness. Sleep also increases resistance to inspiratory airflow caused by decreased skeletal muscle tone in the upper airway dilator muscles, resulting in decreased ventilation during sleep. During NREM sleep, breathing is automatic and normally very regular, under chemical and mechanical feedback control dependent on levels of CO_2 in the arterial blood (to the extent that breathing ceases below the apneic threshold level of CO_2). In contrast, the greatest degree of respiratory irregularity occurs during phasic REM sleep, when breathing appears much less mediated by chemical feedback control and is modulated instead by some higher cortical drive (for a review of respiratory physiology across sleep states see Kreiger[6]).

Immune System

Unfortunately, few studies of the relationship of infection to sleep have been performed in humans. Animal experiments indicate that (1) large changes in sleep patterns occur during infection, (2) sleep changes are a key sign of infectious disease, (3) sleep changes are adaptive and may play a role in nonspecific host defenses, and (4) in animals, extreme sleep deprivation leads to increased mortality. The proximate cause of death in sleep-deprived rats is bloodstream infection by systemic invasion of opportunistic facultative anaerobic bacteria generally ascribed to gut origin, such as *Klebsiella pneumoniae, Staphylococcus aureus, Streptococcus agalactiae,* and *Corynebacterium jejeikum,*[7] all of which are organisms that do not cause life-threatening primary bacteremia unless the host is immunocompromised.

Renal System

Kidney functions increased by sleep state include a sleep-related increase in plasma aldosterone levels, an increase in prolactin secretion (see "Endocrine System"), and increased parathyroid hormone release during sleep (affecting calcium excretion). Renal plasma flow, glomerular filtration rate, filtration fraction, and the excretion of sodium, chloride, potassium, and calcium are reduced during sleep. During NREM sleep, urine excretion is reduced and more concentrated urine than during wakefulness and during REM sleep urine excretion is further reduced and concentrated.

Thermoregulatory Systems

Brain temperature is generally decreased during NREM sleep and occasionally increases above the waking level during REM sleep (for a review of thermoregulatory physiology across sleep states see Glotzbach and Heller[8]). The brain is slightly warmer than blood (by 0.2–0.6° C), but changes in brain temperature correlate with changes in temperature of the blood supplying the brain. Body temperature is lower during NREM sleep and shivering is initiated at a lower temperature than during wakefulness. Furthermore, sweating can occur even in the waking thermoneutral range. During REM sleep, however, body temperature is not regulated and the body tends toward ambient conditions. Newborns spend up to 50% of sleep time in REM, and thus are at particular risk for catastrophic thermal events while sleeping.

Brain and Cellular Physiology

It has been known for more than 40 years that the ascending reticular activating system in the brain stem releases excitatory neurotransmitters into the thalamus, which projects widely through cerebral cortex to promote wakeful-

ness; only recently it has been revealed that brain stem reticular neurons project onto the hypothalamic nuclei, which promote wakefulness by similarly releasing excitatory neurotransmitters throughout the cortex and are of key importance in regulating sleep/wake states.

Wakefulness

The arousal-promoting circuitry of the brain is known as the ascending reticular activating system, which consists of two branches of projections from the caudal midbrain and rostral pons area to the thalamus and hypothalamus (Fig. 15–1). The thalamic branch originates from the cholinergic pedunculopontine and laterodorsal tegmental nuclei (PPTg and LDTg)[9] and projects through the paramedian midbrain reticular formation and diencephalon to the thalamus, including the intralaminar nuclei,[10] thalamic relay nuclei, and the reticular nucleus. Cholinergic modulation, which is known to be crucial in activating thalamocortical neurotransmission,[11] has a key role in regulating thalamic activity. The PPTg and LDTg neurons fire rapidly both during wakefulness when a low-voltage, fast activity cortical electroencephalogram (EEG) activity is observed and during REM sleep when REM and a loss of tonic muscle tone accompany a similar EEG to wakefulness (Table 15–1). During both wakefulness and to a lesser degree during REM sleep, a release of tonic monoamine inhibition allows the PPTg and LDTg to fire rapidly. In contrast, during NREM sleep, EEG waves are larger and PPTg and LDTg neurons are inactive.

The hypothalamic branch of the ascending arousal system originates in the caudal midbrain and rostral pons and includes projections from the noradrenergic locus ceruleus (LC), serotonergic dorsal and median raphe nuclei, and parabrachial nucleus and projects through the lateral hypothalamus, where it is joined by histaminergic projections from the tuberomamillary nucleus (TMN) and by orexin- (or hypocretin-) and melanin-concentrating, hormone-containing projections from the lateral hypothalamus, as well as cholinergic projections from the basal forebrain cholinergic nuclei. All of these pathways diffusely innervate the cortex and release neurotransmitters of arousal. In contrast to cholinergic arousal pathways (see earlier in this section), neurons in the monoaminergic cell groups in these pathways (i.e., from the LC, raphe nuclei, and the TMN) fire rapidly during wakefulness, very infrequently during NREM, and virtually not at all during REM sleep.[12,13] These differences in firing rates across sleep and wake states of consciousness in the cholinergic and monoaminergic ascending arousal systems are believed to modulate the generation of these different behavioral states.[14]

Non–Rapid Eye Movement Sleep

NREM sleep is an actively generated state, involving anatomically discrete supraspinal pathways in the hypothalamus and brainstem. Its mechanisms are currently being

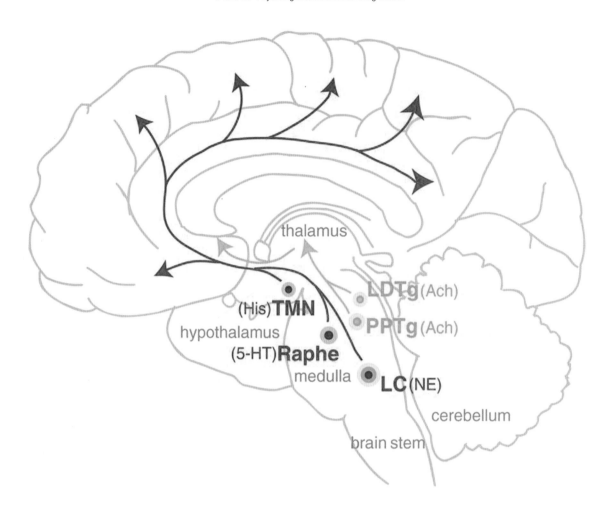

Figure 15–1. The neural substrates of wakefulness. This sagittal cartoon illustrates that projections from the brain stem through the hypothalamus (red) or thalamus (orange) into the cortex and forebrain form the two branches of the ascending arousal system. Monoaminergic (red) projections from the pontine noradrenergic locus ceruleus (LC), midbrain serotonergic raphe nuclei, and hypothalamic histaminergic tuberomamillary nucleus (TMN) diffusely innervate the forebrain areas and regulate cortical and hypothalamic activity to promote arousal. Similarly, cholinergic (orange) projections from the pedunculopontine and laterodorsal tegmental nuclei innervate the thalamus and forebrain to modulate wakefulness. NE, norepinephrine.

characterized. It has also been long known that both electrical and chemical stimulation of the basal forebrain produces NREM sleep, and that the anterior hypothalamus is the most active area in the induction of NREM sleep. Recent investigations have described "sleep-promoting"[15] neurons in this region and the adjacent basal forebrain, specifically in the ventrolateral preoptic nucleus (VLPO), which are under inhibitory control by norepinephrine and serotonin[16,17] and discharge maximally during sleep while remaining relatively inactive during wakefulness. VLPO neurons, which form a dense cluster just lateral to the optic chiasm (the VLPO cluster; important for NREM sleep) and a diffuse population of cells extending medially and dorsally from this cluster (the extended VLPO; more important for REM sleep[18]), are defined by three characteristics: they (1) are uniquely sleep-active (show c-Fos expression during sleep);[15] (2) contain the colocalized (80%) inhibitory neurotransmitters γ-aminobutyric acid (GABA) and galanin

across species, whereas surrounding neurons contain GABA only[19,20]; and (3) project to the arousal-promoting[21] TMN.[19] VLPO neurons also extend inhibitory projections to all of the other wake-active ascending monoaminergic, cholinergic, and orexinergic arousal-promoting sites in the brain; the noradrenergic LC, serotonergic dorsal raphe (DR), cholinergic PPTg and LDTg, and the orexinergic perifornical area (PeF) in the lateral hypothalamic area[19]; these VLPO neuronal projections inhibit their release of arousal-promoting neurotransmitters into the cortex, forebrain, and subcortical areas (Fig. 15–2).

A decrease in firing of the noradrenergic neurons in the LC of the pons releases the LC's tonic inhibition of GABAergic VLPO neurons, which are then activated and release GABA and galanin into LC, TMN, and other arousal-promoting centers.[19] At the level of the LC, this has an inhibitory effect, further decreasing firing in the LC, and therefore further decreasing norepinephrine's tonic inhibi-

TABLE 15–1.

EEG, EMG, and EOG Characteristics of Wakefulness, NREM and REM Sleep States

Sleep State	EEG	EMG	EOG
Wakefulness	Desynchronized activation (10–30 mV low voltage, 16–25 Hz fast activity) alternates with alpha activity (sinusoidal, 20–40 mV voltage, 8–12 Hz activity)	High or moderate, depending on degree of muscle tension	REMs abundant or scarce, depending on amount of visual scanning
NREM stage 1	Decreased alpha activity, little activation, mostly low voltage, mixed frequency activity (at 3–7 Hz)	Moderate to low	REMs absent, slow rolling eye movements
NREM stage 2	Background of low voltage, mixed frequency activity, bursts of distinctive 12 to 14 Hz sinusoidal waves ("sleep spindles") appear	Moderate to low	Eye movements rare
NREM stage 3 (SWS)	High amplitude (>75 mV), slow frequency (0.5–2 Hz) delta waves appear	Moderate to low	Eye movements rare
NREM stage 4 (SWS)	Delta waves dominate the EEG trace	Moderate to low	Eye movements rare
REM	Reverts to a low voltage, mixed frequency pattern similar to stage 1	Small muscle twitches against virtually silent background	Bursts of prominent REMs appear

EEG, electroencephalogram; EMG, electromyogram; EOG, electro-oculogram; NREM, non–rapid eye movement; REM, rapid eye movement; SWS, slow wave sleep.

tion of the VLPO neurons. At the level of the TMN, descending projections from the VLPO release GABA and galanin.[19] This inhibition of the TMN by the VLPO is believed to play a key role in causing sleep.

The inhibition of the TMN (as well as the LC, dorsal raphe, perifornical area, and LDTg/PPTg) by GABA and galanin believed to be released by VLPO neurons[22] is believed to play a key role in causing NREM sleep. Galanin and GABA are observed in the TMN, and GABA type A (GABA_A) inhibitory postsynaptic potentials in the TMN region are observed when the VLPO is stimulated.[23] Discrete bilateral lesions induced by microinjection of the nonspecific excitotoxin ibotenic acid into the VLPO induce persistent insomnia in rats.[24] This may be explained by that GABA-mediated anesthetic drugs are believed to act by inhibiting the wake-active (c-Fos-immunoreactive during wakefulness) TMN. Discrete injections of GABA_A receptor agonist muscimol cause sedation and at higher doses hypnosis, and potentiate the hypnotic effects of anesthetic agents; direct injections of anesthetic agents induce sedation, and of GABA_A receptor antagonist gabazine attenuate the hypnotic effect of anesthetics.[25]

Other pathways may also be involved in the generation of NREM sleep. Earlier it was suggested that there are two main hypnogenic centers involved in the generation of NREM sleep: the preoptic area (VLPO) and the nucleus of the solitary tract (NTS) in the medulla.[26] Subsequent research demonstrated that low frequency stimulation of the vagoaortic nerve or of the NTS produces a slow wave EEG, distension of the carotid sinus (an NTS stimulus) induces behavioral sleep, discharge of certain NTS neurons, which are hypothesized to be reciprocally interconnected with cells in the midbrain EEG arousal region, increases during NREM sleep, and inactivation of the lower brain stem, particularly the NTS, induces a marked arousal. However, a causal involvement of NTS in NREM sleep has not been definitively established, and available evidence suggests that it is a far weaker NREM sleep-promoting center than the VLPO.

Rapid Eye Movement Sleep

The neuronal pathways mediating REM sleep are also currently being characterized (Fig. 15–3); much of what is known stems from four types of animal experiments (for review see Siegel[27]). First, transection studies have determined that the pons is sufficient to generate much of the

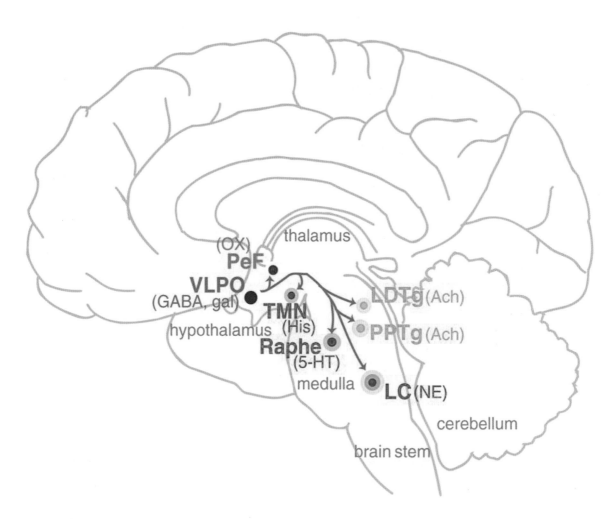

Figure 15–2. Efferent projections from ventrolateral preoptic nucleus (VLPO). Figure illustrates the efferent sleep-promoting (purple) projections from the VLPO. VLPO is uniquely active during sleep and is believed to release inhibitory γ-aminobutyric acid (GABA) and galanin onto the cell bodies and proximal dendrites of the monoaminergic (red) and cholinergic (orange) nuclei of the ascending arousal system and the orexinergic (green) perifornical area (PeF) in the lateral hypothalamus. The ensuing dwindling of release of the neurotransmitters of arousal into the forebrain and cortex is thought to be responsible for the induction of loss of consciousness. 5-HT, serotonin; His, histamine; LC, locus ceruleus; NE, norepinephrine; OX, orexin; TMN, tuberomamillary nucleus. (Adapted from Saper CB, Chou TC, Scammell TE: The sleep switch: Hypothalamic control of sleep and wakefulness. Trends Neurosci 24:726–731, 2001.)

phenomenology of REM sleep. These experiments demonstrated that when the midbrain is transected to separate the brain stem from the diencephalon and telencephalon such that the pons is connected only to midbrain and forebrain structures (and transected from the medulla and spinal cord), defining signs of REM sleep (atonia, REMs, REM-like activation of the reticular formation) are seen in rostral structures. Similarly, when the pons is connected to the medulla and spinal cord only, signs of REM sleep are observed in caudal structures and desynchronized EEG closely resembles that of wakefulness observed in rostral structures. In addition, when the junction between spinal cord and medulla is transected, rostral brain areas (medulla, pons, midbrain) show signs of REM sleep. Considered together, these find-

ings lead to the conclusion that the pons and caudal midbrain are both necessary and sufficient to generate the basic phenomena of REM sleep.

Second, the discrete destruction of very small loci of the brain stem in an otherwise healthy brain can permanently prevent REM sleep. Discrete neuronal lesioning studies have identified a small area of the lateral pontine tegmentum corresponding to lateral portions of the pontine reticular nucleus oralis (PnO), which projects to the PPTg, and the region immediately ventral to the LC that is required for the descending components of normal REM sleep (atonia and possibly eye movements), but not the ascending components (periods of EEG desynchronization). These lesions block both the atonia of REM sleep and the expression of motor

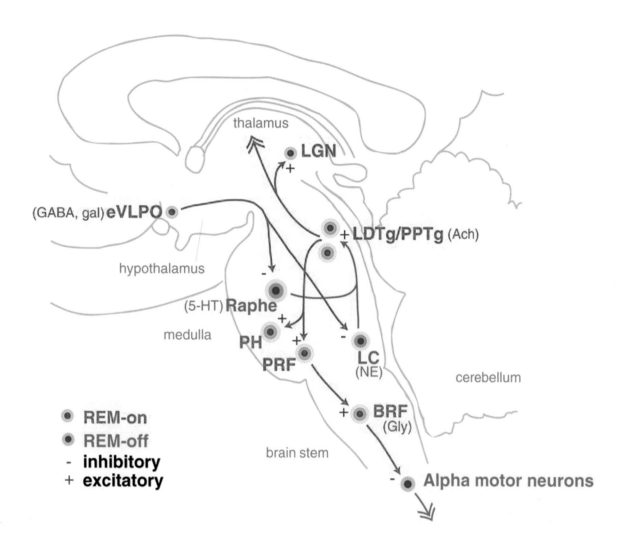

Figure 15–3. The neural substrates of rapid eye movement (REM) sleep. "REM-on" (red) cholinergic neurons in the pedunculopontine and laterodorsal tegmental nuclei (PPTg and LDTg) are active during REM sleep and innervate the thalamus and cortex to modulate the characteristic electroencephalogram (EEG) synchronization of REM sleep; the pontine reticular formation (PRF), thalamic lateral geniculate nucleus (LGN), medullary prepositus hypoglossi nucleus (PH), all of which are involved in the generation of pontine-geniculo-occipital (PGO) waves that herald the onset of REM; and the glycinergic brain stem reticular formation (BRF) that acts to inhibit alpha motor neurons to create skeletal muscle atonia. Muscle atonia is further enhanced by a reduction of serotonergic and noradrenergic input from the "REM-off" (blue) raphe nuclei and locus ceruleus (LC), which are tonically active during wakefulness, markedly less active during non-REM (NREM), and virtually silent during REM sleep. Although it is known that orexin-deficient mice, dogs, and humans demonstrate narcolepsy, a disorder characterized by inappropriate transitions into REM or partial REM sleep, the critical role of orexin in normal REM regulation is not yet fully understood. It is known that orexin neurons innervate to the sleep-promoting extended and cluster ventrolateral preoptic nucleus (eVLPO and VLPO; where coordination between NREM to REM transitions may be modulated), the monoaminergic arousal-promoting centers including the LC, tuberomamillary nucleus (TMN), and raphe nuclei, as well as the REM modulating PPTg and LDTg. 5-HT, serotonin; ACh, acetylcholine; Gly, glycine; NE, norepinephrine.

activity during REM sleep (likely by damaging areas that control locomotion). Similar lesions of the nearby noradrenergic LC, but not the PnO, do not block REM sleep, suggesting that a tiny and anatomically discrete population of neurons can recruit the massive changes in brain activity seen during REM sleep. In cats, lesions of the LDTg block REM sleep. PnO neurons modulate the atonia of REM sleep through excitatory innervation of the lower brain stem and then through projections that postsynaptically inhibit motor neurons in the spinal cord.

Third, in vivo electrophysiology studies have localized a subpopulation of large cholinergic PPTg neurons at the mesopontine junction that are selectively active during REM sleep. These neurons project to both the thalamus (responsible for phasic pontine-geniculo-occipital wave excitation and EEG desynchronizations of REM) and the pontine reticular formation (responsible for the atonia of REM). Single unit recording studies reveal that this subpopulation of PPTg neurons discharge at a high rate throughout REM sleep, have little or no activity during NREM sleep, and are generally silent during wakefulness (another subpopulation of PPTg/LDTg neurons are wake-active). There are three major groups of "REM-on" cells: region that the lesions described earlier encompassed; the PPTg, the PnO of the pontine reticular formation; and a population of glycinergic neurons in the medial medullary reticular formation.

During REM sleep, noradrenergic cells of the LC and serotonergic cells of the raphe nuclei, which project to the LDTg/PPTg[28] where they are believed to inhibit cholinergic neurons, fire rapidly during wakefulness, markedly less so during NREM and very minimally or are completely silent during REM sleep.[29,30] Thus inhibition of noradrenergic and serotonergic neurons by GABAergic inputs from the extended VLPO are thought to promote REM sleep.[18]

Finally, pharmacologic studies have provided further information. Administration of physostigmine (an anticholinesterase agent that increases acetylcholine [ACh] at the synapse) precipitates REM sleep during an ongoing period of NREM sleep and enhances the phasic periods of REM sleep, whereas blocking muscarinic ACh receptors (AChRs) inhibit the appearance of REM sleep and reduce phasic periods. Discrete microinjections of the cholinergic agonist carbachol into the medial pontine reticular formation (which is receives projections from the PPTg) induces REM sleep in cats and rats. REM sleep can also be induced by microinjecting ACh into the PnO, and glutamate injection into the PPTg increases REM sleep. These results suggest that pontine cholinoceptive neurons (1) act on other reticular neurons to excite ascending circuits and (2) inhibit sensory and motor transmission. Noradrenergic neurons of the LC appear to act in a reciprocal manner to the cholinergic neurons, being selectively active during wakefulness (for review see Jones[31]).

Switching Between Sleep and Wake States

Switching between these sleep and wake states is thought to be controlled by a reciprocal relationship of mutual inhibition between the activities of neurons in the VLPO and the major monoamine areas (TMN, LC, and midbrain raphe nuclei) of the ascending reticular arousal system[14] (Fig. 15–4). The VLPO innervates the arousal system and inhibits activity during sleep, and the nuclei of the ascending arousal system inhibit the VLPO during wakefulness (Fig. 15–5) (see "Wakefulness" and Non–Rapid Eye Movement Sleep"). Therefore when the firing rate of the VLPO is high during sleep, it inhibits the monoaminergic arousal nuclei and thereby further disinhibits or activates its own firing; and

when the monoaminergic neurons fire rapidly during wakefulness, they act to inhibit the VLPO and disinhibit, or further activate, their own firing.

Saper and colleagues[14] report that this reciprocal relationship tends toward two stable firing patterns (sleep or wake) and away from intermediate transition states (and drew comparisons to the bistable circuit known to electrical engineers as a "flip-flop"; i.e., when one side is firing rapidly, there is a "resistance" to "switching" such that it occurs infrequently but rapidly), so that only large-scale influences such as circadian drive to sleep or a sufficient degree of sleep drive or deprivation exerts pressure on the circuit until it reaches a critical threshold and the firing patterns reverse rapidly.[14] When the firing of the sleep-promoting VLPO side of the circuit is weakened by ablation of the VLPO, the circuit is destabilized and animals experience insomnia plus an increased drive to sleep, which may bring the circuit balance closer to the transition state.[24] A destabilizing deficit on the waking side of this sleep switch induces the inappropriate abrupt transitions from wakefulness to sleep (particularly REM or fragments of REM sleep, such as cataplexy or the loss of muscle tone while awake) seen in the sleep disorder narcolepsy.

Saper and colleagues[14] further hypothesized that the recently discovered orexin-containing (also known as hypocretin; see "Orexin Receptors") neurons in the perifornical area of the lateral hypothalamus act as a stabilizing "finger" helping to hold the sleep switch pointing toward wakefulness and prevent switching to sleep. Dysfunction of this "finger," and the consequent susceptibility to sudden and inappropriate transitions, is seen in narcolepsy, which is characterized by an orexinergic deficiency.[32] The TMN, LC, and raphe nuclei all receive input from orexinergic neurons, contain orexin receptors, and inhibit REM sleep,[33] so that the inappropriate transitions into REM or fragments of REM sleep experienced with narcolepsy may be modulated by the weakening of the sleep switch reinforcement "finger." Specifically, the absence of excitatory orexin input is hypothesized to weaken the arousal system's inhibition of the extended VLPO (which is thought to modulate REM, whereas the VLPO cluster modulates NREM sleep[18]), allowing more frequent transitions into REM[14] (see Fig. 15–4).

Biochemical and Molecular Mechanisms Underlying Cellular Physiology

The gap between our current understanding of the mechanisms of sleep and its functions may be bridged by elucidating its molecular basis. Currently, many of the neuronal substrates, neurochemical messengers, and regulatory processes involved in sleep are known (see earlier), but molecular correlates of consciousness states are less clear. Several avenues of investigation are underway, but none are yet conclusive. The next section of this chapter discusses the fruits of the major research approaches in understanding the molecular genetics of sleep states.

A

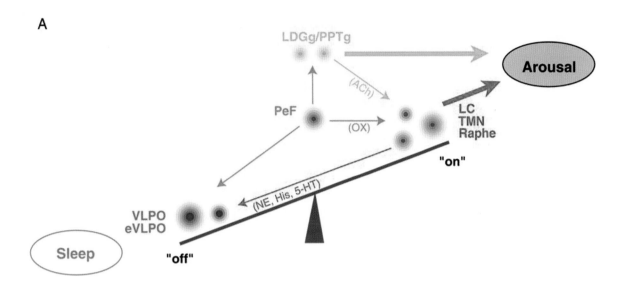

B

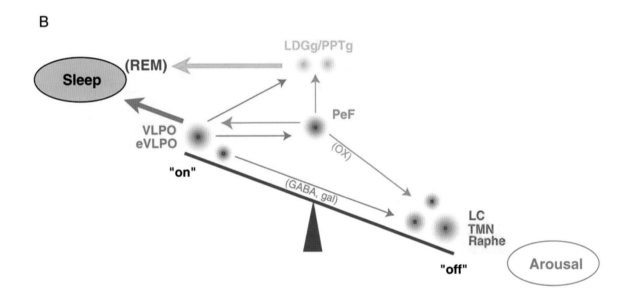

Figure 15–4. The "sleep switch." Saper and colleagues[14] postulated that a reciprocal relationship of mutual inhibition between the galanin- and GABAergic sleep-promoting (purple) ventrolateral preoptic nucleus (VLPO) and the monoaminergic arousal-promoting (red) locus ceruleus (LC), tuberomamillary nucleus (TMN), and raphe nuclei modulates transitions among sleep states such that intermediate states are disallowed. The monoaminergic LC, TMN, and raphe nuclei promote wakefulness activating the cortex and forebrain while inhibiting the sleep-promoting VLPO. During NREM sleep, the VPLO core inhibits the TMN and the eVLPO inhibits the LC and raphe nuclei (which further disinhibits, or activates, the VLPO and stabilizes the VLPO's sleep promotion). During REM sleep, the eVLPO is thought to disinhibit the REM-active cholinergic (orange) pedunculopontine and laterodorsal tegmental nuclei (PPTg and LDTg) and inhibit the LC and raphe nuclei, whereas the VLPO core inhibits the TMN. Orexin (OX)-containing neurons (green) in the perifornical area (PeF) of the lateral hypothalamic area (LHA) innervate all the sleep- and wake-promoting nuclei and are thought to stabilize the sleep switch by further activating the monoaminergic arousal-promoting nuclei and cholinergic REM-promoting nuclei and possibly further inhibiting VLPO by presynaptic action. 5-HT, serotonin; GABA, γ-aminobutyric acid; His, histamine; NE, norepinephrine. (Adapted from Saper CB, Chou TC, Scammell TE: The sleep switch: Hypothalamic control of sleep and wakefulness. Trends Neurosci 24:726–731, 2001.)

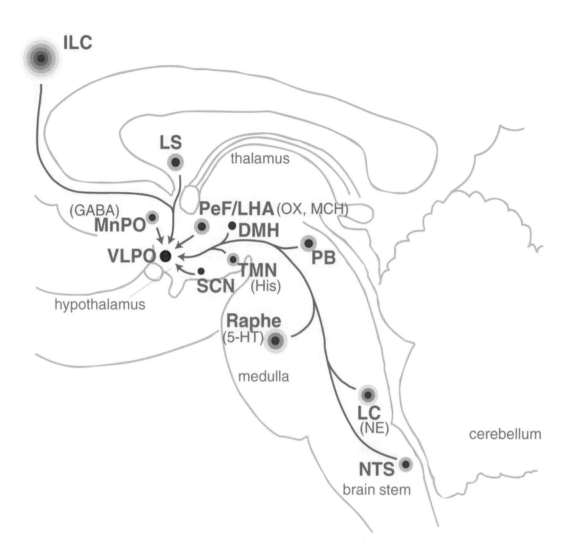

Figure 15–5. Afferent projections to ventrolateral preoptic nucleus (VLPO). Chou et al.[17] described the efferent projections to the VLPO (purple) after conducting extensive anterograde and retrograde tracing studies in the rat, and sleep-promoting pathways are believed to be similar in humans (see Gaus and colleagues[20]). The VLPO is innervated by the monoaminergic arousal-promoting tuberomamillary nucleus (TMN), raphe nuclei, locus ceruleus (LC), the median preoptic nucleus (MnPO; also believed to be sleep promoting), and the lateral hypothalamus including orexinergic neurons in the perifornical area (PeF). Other hypothalamic projections from the dorsomedial hypothalamic nucleus (DMH) and suprachiasmatic nucleus (SCN) also reach VLPO. In addition, VLPO receives projections from autonomic areas such as the infralimbic cortex (ILC) and parabrachial nucleus (PB) and limbic areas such as the lateral septum (LS). 5-HT, serotonin; GABA, γ-aminobutyric acid; His, histamine; LHA, lateral hypothalamic area; NE, norepinephrine; NTS, nucleus of the solitary tract.

Gene Expression During Sleep Deprivation

One approach is to study gene expression in sleep-deprived animals, assuming that because sleep drive and intensity are homeostatically modulated, sleep deprivation leads to a change in expression of genes encoding protein products essential for sleep regulation. The first limitation of this approach is correlative gene expression (the expression of many genes varies with consciousness state without being actively involved in regulating consciousness state), but this can be overcome by confirming the involvement of identified genes by using "loss-of-function" and "gain-of-function" experiments. Second, the extreme complexity of mammalian brain mRNA populations may impose a technical limitation, although recent advances in gene expression profiling has facilitated the identification of orexin and cortistatin.[34–36]

Candidate Genes

A second strategy that examines candidate genes selected based on prior implication in sleep by way of sleep physiology or pharmacology studies has shown the differential expression of tyrosine hydroxylase, growth hormone–releasing hormone, IL-1β, somatostatin, and brain-derived neurotrophic factor to be potentially involved in sleep regulation (for review see Tafti and Franken[37]). The obvious limitation of this approach is that it precludes the discovery of truly novel sleep genes.

The standout success story of this approach was the "coincidental" discovery of orexin's involvement in sleep. As mentioned earlier, the orexin A and B peptides (also termed hypocretin 1 and 2) and their orexin 1 and 2 receptors were identified in 1998.[35,36] In rapid succession (i) mutations in the orexin 2 receptor were identified through linkage analysis and positional cloning as causal in canine narcolepsy;[38] (ii) a targeted deletion in the prepro-orexin (synthe-tic precursor to orexin) gene was associated with murine narcolepsy;[32] (iii) narcoleptic humans were reported to have undetectable levels of orexin in the cerebrospinal fluid and a markedly reduced number of hypothalamic orexinergic neurons,[39] and, (iv) an orexin-deficient transgenic mouse (possessing a narcoleptic, hypophagic, and obese phenotype) was created by inserting a transgene construct consisting of human prepro-orexin gene ligated to a truncated cell death inducing ataxin-3 gene, which when expressed leads to cell death of orexinergic neurons by apoptosis at roughly 3 weeks of age (4–15 week range).[40] This evidence, beginning with the candidate gene study, causally implicates orexin in narcolepsy and, together with further research, in sleep regulation (for review see Sakurai[41] and Sutcliffe[42]).

Genome-Wide Screening by Mutagenesis

Other investigators use a third strategy of genome-wide searching and mapping experiments with no *a priori* assumptions on the gene systems involved in hopes of discovering new "sleep genes." Linkage disequilibrium between closely localized genes can be exploited to determine cosegregation of traits, and consequently the large chromosomal pieces that are transmitted as individual units. Following this type of gene segregation requires that they are polymorphic (include nucleotide variation from individual to individual) or, as powerful substitutes, contain highly polymorphic elements (i.e., restriction fragment length polymorphisms, simple sequence length polymorphisms, single nucleotide polymorphisms, and so on), which are mostly found in noncoding genetic material. Two major approaches are used to do this: mutagenesis and quantitative trait loci (QTL) analysis. In the former, a mutagen (e.g., N-ethyl-N-nitrosurea) is used to mutate the whole genome followed by high-throughput screening of all mutant offspring to detect a major effect on a given phenotype (either dominant or recessive mutations can be detected), followed by candidate gene or positional cloning approaches used for identification, and finally functional analysis can be assessed by gain or loss of function. *Clock*, one of the key mammalian circadian clock genes was discovered this way.[43]

Quantitative Trait Loci Analysis

QTL can be powerfully used for the genetic dissection of complex traits (mutagenesis screens can miss small-effect sequence variations that can turn out to be important for some key aspect of the phenotype; for review see Flint and Mott[44]). This strategy, which does not map a gene but rather a genetic effect in a large chromosomal area that may contain a single major gene or many genes with small effects, was used to better understand the complex circadian behavior of mice. Although much of the circadian timekeeping molecular machinery was first identified by mutagenesis and direct molecular techniques, the genes identified this way have not been able to explain the complex circadian behavioral subtleties observed, such as differences in 24-hour amount of sleep between inbred mouse strains, which are likely accounted for by complex interactions among many genes. Shimomura and colleagues[45] intercrossed two inbred mouse strains with a 1-hour difference in free-running wake times (BALB/c and C57BL/6) to discover several new nonallelic loci with epistatic interactions potentially mediating this subtlety of circadian behavior. Other groups performed similar experiments on the offspring of these intercrossed inbred mice and reported that the QTL for the amount of REM sleep in the light period is on chromosome 1,[46] and also estimated that 40% to 60% of the variance in all sleep amounts can be accounted for by the additive effects of 6 to 15 genes.

Future Approaches

Although we are far from an understanding of the molecular basis of sleep states, the earlier approaches to understanding the molecular basis of consciousness states have revealed several important lessons: (1) many genes are involved in the regulation of consciousness states, (2) relevant QTLs may be interacting with each other; (3) even when a major QTL is identified for a given sleep parameter, its effect may vary from one genetic background of inbred mice to another by the action of unrelated modifier genes; (4) identifying a QTL is only the first step; the next step is to map the QTL down to the smallest chromosomal region feasible for candidate gene analysis, followed by the very difficult identification of functional sequence variants by quantitative trait nucleotide (QTN) analysis, then mutation, classical homologous recombination (knockout), or serial nested chromosomal deletions, then systemic crosses between QTL alleles and mutants to identify the function of a given QTN, followed by high-throughput genotyping technologies, gene translation, and post-translational protein analysis to identify which of these selected QTNs are involved in gene regulation and which are mutations actually affecting protein function. Indeed, advances in high-resolution QTL mapping and high-throughput genotyping and phenotyping techniques, the availability of the whole mouse genome for several inbred mouse strains, and enormous genetic and genomic resources are needed to better identify the underlying molecular mechanisms of consciousness states.

Current and Potential Targets of Drug Action

Anesthetic and hypnotic agents influence a variety of targets, and a wide range of drugs influence sleep states, or the sleep cycle, or both. This chapter describes current and potential targets of pharmacologic action to alter consciousness level.

γ-Aminobutyric Acid Type A Receptor

Inhibitory $GABA_A$ receptors, which are composed of multivariant pentameric combinations of two α ($α_1$-$α_6$), two β ($β_1$-$β_3$), and one γ ($γ_1$-$γ_3$), δ, or ε subunit assembled to form a GABA-gated chloride channel, play a key role in sleep and are believed to be one of the primary targets of general anesthetic agents. GABA-containing neurons are located throughout the brain, including the brain stem, thalamus, hypothalamus, basal forebrain, and cortex, and GABA is released into the cerebral cortex in the highest concentration during NREM sleep. Clinically relevant concentrations of anesthetics (e.g., barbiturates, etomidate, propofol, neuroactive steroids, benzodiazepines, and volatile anesthetics) markedly enhance $GABA_A$ receptor–mediated chloride current or GABAergic neurotransmission in neurons in vivo and in a variety of recombinant expression systems in vitro[47] to ultimately enhance chloride ion flow, resulting in hyperpolarization and decreased cell firing.

"GABAergic" general anesthetics are far more effective at enhancing the actions of GABA at its $GABA_A$ receptors than they are at directly activating the receptors in the absence of GABA (e.g., propofol is more effective enhancing the action of endogenous GABA at the $GABA_A$ receptors than it is as a direct activator[48]). The direct connection between the activation of $GABA_A$ receptors and the hypnotic response is supported by the fact that the $GABA_A$ receptor agonist muscimol and the GABAergic anesthetic agents propofol and pentobarbital transduce their hypnotic effects via acting on $GABA_A$ receptors in regionally discrete anatomic sites within an endogenous NREM sleep-promoting pathway: the VLPO and TMN[25] (Fig. 15–6).

Benzodiazepines interact with all the benzodiazepine-sensitive α subunits ($α_1$, $α_2$, $α_3$, and $α_5$) with the classical high-affinity stereospecific benzodiazepine binding site located between the α and $γ_2$ subunits. It is known that a knockin point mutation (histidine to arginine at position 101) introduced into the murine $α_1$ subunit (which contributes to 60% of $GABA_A$ receptors in the brain) gene renders homomeric $α_1$ $GABA_A$ receptors insensitive to benzodiazepine agents in vitro, and in vivo these $α_1$ (H101R) mice are insensitive to the sedative and amnestic but not anxiolytic actions of benzodiazepines. This suggests that the multiple actions of benzodiazepines can be molecularly distinguished; the sedative action appears to be mediated by $α_1$ $GABA_A$ receptors,[49] and the anxiolytic action is mediated by $α_2$, $α_4$, and $α_5$ $GABA_A$ receptors.[50]

One clinical application of this observation is zaleplon (CL284,846), the pyrazolopyrimidine hypnotic agent developed for the treatment of insomnia, which binds preferentially to $GABA_A$ receptors containing the $α_1$ subunit 8- to 20-fold stronger than to $α_2$, $α_3$, and $α_5$ subunit-containing receptors, as well as to those containing the $γ_3$ subunit (although the contribution of $γ_3$ subunit-mediated action is unclear).[51] Other agents have been developed for their anxiolytic effects with a distinct lack of effect on $α_1$ subunits, including L-838,417, SL65.1498, pagoclone, pazinaclone, and PNY-101017. Pharmacologic analysis in animal models in which particular $GABA_A$ receptor subunits are either inactivated (knockout strategy) or point-mutated (knockin strategy), as described earlier, is expected to lead further $GABA_A$ receptor subtype-targeted drugs with selective therapeutic action in the near future.

$α_2$ Adrenoceptor

One of the highest densities of G protein–coupled $α_2$ adrenoceptor has been detected in the LC,[52] the predominant noradrenergic nucleus in the brain and an important modulator of vigilance.[53] Hypnotic and sedative effects of $α_2$ adrenoceptor activation have been attributed to the LC,[54] which densely innervates and tonically inhibits the sleep-active VLPO during wakefulness. When a selective $α_2$ adrenoceptor agonist (e.g., dexmedetomidine, clonidine, or xylazine) binds to an $α_2$ adrenoceptor in the LC, transmembrane signaling is thought to activate an inwardly rectifying potassium channel allowing for a K^+ efflux and to inhibit voltage-gated Ca^{2+} channels. The resulting hyperpolarization decreases the firing rate in LC projections.[55] From an anesthetic viewpoint, hyperpolarization of noradrenergic neurons in the LC appears to be a key factor in the mechanism of action of dexmedetomidine and other $α_2$ adrenoceptor agonist.[54,56] Relative to its effects on the $α_1$ adrenoceptor, dexmedetomidine is eight times more specific for the $α_2$ adrenoceptor than clonidine, the next most selective $α_2$ adrenoceptor agonist (action at the $α_1$ adrenoceptor counteracts action at the $α_2$ adrenoceptor).

Future refinement of drugs targeting the $α_2$ adrenoceptor may yield a pharmacologic sedation with more of the restorative features of endogenous sedation. It is hypothesized that the decrease in firing of noradrenergic neurons in the LC results in a loss of consciousness by converging on an endogenous sleep pathway upstream of that where putatively GABAergic agents influence these pathways[25,57] (see Fig. 15–6). Qualitative observations by nursing staff indicate that dexmedetomidine induces a clinically effective sedation that is uniquely arousable (as is natural sleep), an effect not observed with any other clinically available sedatives.[58] Recent data from a functional magnetic resonance imaging study in healthy volunteers seemed to confirm that the blood oxygen level–dependent signal, which positively correlates with local brain activity, changes during

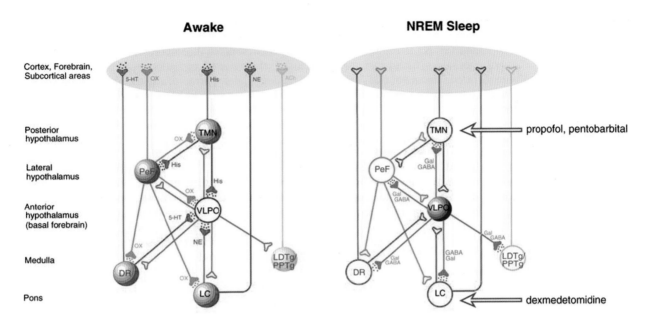

Figure 15–6. GABAergic and α2 adrenergic anesthetic agents converge on endogenous sleep pathways to exert their hypnotic effects. A schematic summarizing the monoaminergic (red) and cholinergic (orange) and galanin- and GABAergic (purple) neural substrates of arousal (*left*) and non–rapid eye movement (NREM) sleep (*right*). Wakefulness is promoted by the release of the arousal-promoting monoamine (red) neurotransmitters norepinephrine (NE), serotonin (5-HT), and histamine (His) in the locus ceruleus (LC), raphe nuclei, and tuberomamillary nucleus (TMN), respectively, as well as acetylcholine (ACh; orange) from the pedunculopontine and laterodorsal tegmental nuclei (PPTg and LDTg) into the forebrain and cortex. During NREM sleep, the sleep-active galanin- and GABAergic ventrolateral preoptic nucleus (VLPO; purple) inhibits the ascending arousal system to induce loss of consciousness. It is believed that the α2 adrenergic agonist dexmedetomidine converges on this endogenous sleep circuitry at the level of the LC to exert its sedative effects (see Nelson and Colleagues[57]), whereas putatively "GABAergic" agents such as pentobarbital and propofol converge further downstream at the level of the TMN (see Nelson and coworkers[25]). DR, dorsal raphe; GABA, γ-aminobutyric acid; Gal, galanin; OX, orexin; PeF, perifornical area. (Adapted from Nelson LE, Guo TZ, Lu J, et al: The sedative component of anesthesia is mediated by GABA_A receptors in an endogenous sleep pathway. Nat Neurosci 5:979–984, 2002.)

dexmedetomidine-induced sedation in a manner similar to that during natural sleep and is markedly different from midazolam sedation.[59]

N-methyl-D-aspartate Receptor

Another class of anesthetics targets the excitatory *N*-methyl-D-aspartate (NMDA) subtype of glutamate receptors, where they act antagonistically to reduce the efficacy of excitatory neurotransmission. Examples include ketamine,[60] nitrous oxide (laughing gas),[61] and the inert gas xenon[62] during normobaric conditions (where other inert gases can also induce hypnosis, although only at high concentrations during hyperbaric conditions). Glutamate is an arousal-promoting excitatory amino acid that also is maximally released into the cortex, forebrain, and brain stem during wakefulness. Glutamatergic neurons likely also modulate the ascending reticular activating system. Glutamate receptor agonists induce prolonged central excitation and cortical activation, whereas antagonists such as NMDA receptor antagonists have hypnotic properties.

Nicotinic Acetylcholine Receptor

Anesthetics act on both nicotinic and muscarinic AChRs, although effects at the excitatory nicotinic variety are regarded as more important. Nicotinic AChRs, like glycine and GABA_A receptors, consist of five subunits: α (containing the principal component of the ACh binding site, characterized by two neighboring cysteines at positions 192 and 193 in *T. electroplaque*), β, γ, δ, and ε. Central neuronal nicotinic AChRs are more diverse, more sensitive to anesthetics (with the exception of the α_7 subunit), and better understood than their peripheral and neuromuscular junction counterparts. Currently, 12 subunits have been cloned in the vertebrate nervous system (α_2-α_10 and β_2-β_4).[63]

Interestingly, all of the more polar anesthetic agents act on AChRs and the inhibitory GABA_A and glycine receptors, although the less polar agents, act on ACh and NMDA receptors. Furthermore, a molluscan ACh-binding protein has been crystallized, with a highly homologous sequence with the N-terminal and pretransmembrane domain 1 portion of the α subunit, supporting the hypothesis that agonist binding sites are located at interfaces between subunits. Clinically relevant concentrations of volatile anesthetics and ketamine potently inhibit both muscular and neuronal nicotinic ACh receptors, and competitive inhibition, open channel block, allosteric mechanisms, and increased desensitization have all been reported. The major $\alpha_4\beta_2$ brain receptor and $\alpha_3\beta_4$ ganglionic receptor are inhibited by subanesthetic concentrations of volatile agents, and $\alpha_3\beta_4$ is inhibited by similar doses of ketamine, whereas α_7-type are unaffected.[64] Barbiturates and intravenous anesthetic agents also inhibit these receptors, but only at suprasurgical concentrations, indicating that nicotinic AChRs are likely a secondary target. Further research (for a review of current research see Tassonyi[65]) is necessary to determine the importance of nicotinic AChRs as targets for future anesthetic and hypnotic agents.

Glycine Receptor

Glycine receptors, which are responsible for the majority of inhibitory neurotransmission in the brain stem and spinal cord, are also potentiated by volatile anesthetic agents and alcohols.[66] They are a part of the same superfamily of ligand-gated ion channels as serotonin-3, $GABA_A$, and nicotinic AChRs. Studies of chimeric glycine/ρ subunits (ρ [ρ_1-ρ_3] subunits that characterize $GABA_C$ receptors are insensitive to both anesthetics and alcohols) identified two key regions—Ser267 and Ala288—in the membrane-spanning domains of the glycine α_1 subunit that contribute to the potentiating effects of ethanol and enflurane. Furthermore, mutation of the corresponding amino acids in the GABA α_2 subunit similarly rendered $GABA_A$ receptors insensitive to the effects of ethanol and enflurane, but not by intravenous agents[47,66]; and a similar decrement in potentiation with the substitution of Ser267 with larger amino acids revealed the possibility of a binding pocket at this site.[67,68]

Two-Pore Domain Potassium Channels

Most voltage-gated and G protein–coupled receptors are relatively insensitive to general anesthetics at clinically relevant concentrations. One of the first exceptions reported indicated that a potassium conductance in molluscan neurons is sensitive to clinically relevant concentrations of halothane.[69] In vertebrates, this channel is a member of a family of widely distributed two-pore domain potassium channels that are not activated by voltage but rather act as background currents to maintain cellular resting potential—TWIK-1 and TWIK-2 (two-pore, weakly inward-rectifying potassium channel); TREK-1 and TREK-2 (TWIK-related potassium channel); TASK-1, TASK-2, and TASK-3 (TWIK-related, acid-sensitive, potassium channel); and TRAAK (TWIK-related, arachidonic acid-sensitive, potassium channel).

Recent cloning of these background potassium channels has generated strong evidence that they may be of importance in the pharmacology of volatile anesthetics. In particular, TASK-1, TASK-2, and TASK-3 are all found throughout the brain and are activated by halothane.[70,71] Both TASK-1 and TASK-3 are expressed in serotonergic raphe neurons,[72] which may be relevant to the hypnotic actions of anesthetics, given the important role of the raphe in endogenous sleep/wake regulation (see "Brain and Cellular Physiology"). Furthermore, anesthetic activation and neurotransmitter binding at TASK-1 and TASK-3 require the same region at the interface of the final transmembrane domain and the cytoplasmic C-terminus.[73] TREK-1 and TREK-2 also have a broad distribution in the central nervous system and are sensitive to halothane, isoflurane, diethyl ether, and chloroform, whereas TRAAK channels are insensitive to anesthetics, and TWIK channels, the originally identified member of this family, have not yet been investigated for anesthetic action. Further pharmacologic studies of genetically modified mice are needed to elucidate the importance of the two-pore domain potassium channels as targets for hypnotic and anesthetic drugs.

Orexin Receptors

As recently as 1998, while screening for ligands for orphan G protein–coupled receptors Sakurai and colleagues[36] identified two peptides, which they named "Orexin A" and "Orexin B" because they promoted feeding; simultaneously, de Lecea and coworkers[35] reported their discovery of two hypothalamus-specific mRNA coding for the same two peptides, which they termed "hypocretins" because of their sequence similarities to secretin. Orexin/hypocretin knockout mice express a narcoleptic phenotype,[32] canine narcolepsy is attributed to mutations in the gene for the orexin 2 receptor,[38] and an absence of orexin in the hypothalamus and cerebrospinal fluid of humans with narcolepsy is observed.[39]

The precise role of orexin in endogenous regulation of sleep states is still being characterized, but orexin 1 or orexin 2 receptors are potential future targets for hypnotic agents. Orexinergic neurons also innervate the monoaminergic and cholinergic nuclei of the ascending arousal system,[74] and they act to further increase firing during wakefulness.[75–77] The LC is rich in orexin 1 receptors; orexin 2 receptors are found in the TMN and basal forebrain, and both are present in the midbrain raphe nuclei and pontine reticular formation.[33] Conversely, orexin-containing neurons also innervate the VLPO region, and although VLPO neurons do not bear orexin receptors,[33] discrete injection of orexin into the VLPO area increases wakefulness and decreases both REM and NREM sleep,[78] possibly by presynaptic actions on monoaminergic or cholinergic axons. Orexin neurons are wake-active (synthesize c-Fos protein, a common surrogate marker of neuronal activation), which correlates with amount of wakefulness (whether natural or artificially induced by sleep deprivation or pharmacologic stimulants such as modafinil or amphetamine).[79]

Other Potential Targets

Pharmacologic agents with a variety of other targets influence sleep and wake states and may provide insight into future hypnotic and anesthetic drug targets. Some examples of potential targets of hypnotic, sedative, or adjuvant agents are discussed later in this chapter.

Most nonprescription hypnotics act by antagonizing the histamine receptor, which have some moderate sleep-enhancing properties but frequently also have significant anticholinergic properties limiting their usefulness, particularly in the elderly. As described earlier (see "Wakefulness"), the primary neuronal source of the arousal-promoting neurotransmitter histamine is the TMN in the posterior hypothalamus.

Pharmacologic agents such as amphetamine and cocaine potentiate the release of catecholamines including dopamine and enhance and prolong wakefulness, whereas catecholamine-depleting drugs induce a decrease in cortical activation and may increase sleep. Dextroamphetamine and pemoline enhance dopaminergic and catecholaminergic activity, increase sleep latency, decrease total sleep time, and greatly reduce REM sleep. The REM sleep reduction effect results from increased wakefulness, in marked contrast to the actions of drugs that primarily alter noradrenergic or serotonergic activity. Large REM sleep reduction occurs regardless of changes in total sleep or wakefulness.

Adenosine promotes sleep, adenosine receptor antagonists such as caffeine have stimulant properties, and adenosine agonists promote sleep, although none are currently used in the clinical setting. Considerable evidence indicates that adenosine may be an endogenous sleep promoter, but the mechanisms remain unclear. However, it is not known whether adenosine is released by specific adenosinergic neurons or by all active neurons in the metabolite form of adenosine triphosphate. A general decrease in neuronal adenosine triphosphate as brain activity slows could potentially explain the phenomenon of fatigue in addition to contributing to sleep onset. It may also reduce REM, particularly in the later part of the night. The well-known adenosine receptor antagonist caffeine induces wakefulness and reduces sleep, and systemic or intracerebroventricular administration of the highly selective adenosine A2A receptor agonist 2-(4-(2-carboxyethyl)phenylethylamine) adenosine-5′-N-ethylcarboxamideadenosine (CGS21680) induces increases in both REM and NREM sleep, and increases c-Fos expression in the sleep-promoting VLPO, whereas decreasing it in wake-promoting TMN.[80]

A wide variety of peptides—for example, thyrotropin-releasing factor, corticotropin-releasing factor, and vasoactive intestinal peptide—are contained in neurons believed to promote the maintenance of cortical activation and wakefulness when they are released into synaptic spaces or the cerebrospinal fluid. Other peptides and hormones such as in epinephrine, histamine, adrenocorticotropin hormone, and TSH act at sites outside the blood–brain barrier to elicit and potentiate wakefulness and arousal when they circulate in the blood. Other substances that can cross the blood–brain barrier, such as the glucocorticoids, can also promote wakefulness, likely by acting on specific receptors.[14]

Endogenous sleep-enhancing compounds have been detected in circulating blood and CSF including delta-sleep inducing peptide, arginine vasotocin, the adrenal steroid tetrahydrodeoxycorticosterone, cholecystokinin, and muramyl dipeptide. The lymphokine IL-1 increases NREM sleep through the prostaglandin D2 receptor,[81] suggesting a relationship between the immune system and consciousness. Other "sleep substances" isolated from the cerebrospinal fluid include opiate peptides, alpha-acetyl-melanocyte stimulating hormone, and somatostatin, which colocalize with smaller neurotransmitters and act as neuromodulators, may have a role in facilitating sleep onset. Substances released into the blood, such as insulin, cholecystokinin, prostaglandins, interleukins, growth hormone, and prolactin also have NREM sleep-promoting activities and could represent future targets for hypnotic or adjuvant agents.

Conclusion

In conclusion, the networks of neural substrates mediating endogenous regulation of consciousness level are complex. Much research has focused on understanding the neural correlates of wakefulness, NREM sleep, REM sleep, and transitions between them, but a molecular basis for these behavioral alterations is only beginning to emerge. The mechanisms governing pharmacologic modulation of consciousness level are less clear, but share a common key feature with endogenous sleep—a loss of response to external stimuli. Indeed, new lines of investigation suggest that sleep and anesthesia may be transduced by similar mechanisms. We can hope to identify better therapeutically selective hypnotic drug targets by further clarifying how and where these mechanisms overlap.

References

1. Chalmers DJ: The Conscious Mind: In Search of a Fundamental Theory. Oxford University Press, Oxford, 1996.
2. Callaway CW, Lydic R, Baghdoyan HA, Hobson JA: Pontogeniculooccipital waves: Spontaneous visual system activity during rapid eye movement sleep. Cell Mol Neurobiol 7:105–149, 1987.
3. Verrier RL, Harper RM, Hobson JA: In Kryger MH, Roth T, Dement WC (eds): Principles and Practice of Sleep Medicine, 3rd ed. Philadelphia, WB Saunders, 2000, pp 179–192.
4. Franzini C: In Kryger MH, Roth T, Dement WC (eds): Principles and Practice of Sleep Medicine, 3rd ed. Philadelphia: WB Saunders, 2000, pp 193–205.
5. Cauter EV: In Kryger MH, Roth T, Dement WC (eds): Principles and Practice of Sleep Medicine, 3rd ed. Philadelphia: WB Saunders, 2000, pp 266–288.
6. Kreiger J: In Kryger MH, Roth T, Dement WC (eds): Principles and Practice of Sleep Medicine, 3rd ed. Philadelphia: WB Saunders, 2000, pp 229–241.
7. Everson CA, Toth LA: Systemic bacterial invasion induced by sleep deprivation. Am J Physiol Regul Integr Comp Physiol 278:R905–916, 2000.
8. Glotzbach SF, Heller HC: In Kryger MH, Roth T, Dement WC (eds): Principles and Practice of Sleep Medicine, 3rd ed. Philadelphia, WB Saunders, 2000.
9. Hallanger AE, Wainer BH: Ascending projections from the pedunculopontine tegmental nucleus and the adjacent mesopontine tegmentum in the rat. J Comp Neurol 274:483–515, 1988.
10. Herkenham M: Laminar organization of thalamic projections to the rat neocortex. Science 207:532–535, 1980.
11. Steriade M, McCormick DA, Sejnowski TJ: Thalamocortical oscillations in the sleeping and aroused brain. Science 262:679–685, 1993.

12. Aston-Jones G, Chiang C, Alexinsky T: Discharge of noradrenergic locus coeruleus neurons in behaving rats and monkeys suggests a role in vigilance. Prog Brain Res 88:501–520, 1991.

13. Steininger TL, Alam MN, Gong H, et al: Sleep-waking discharge of neurons in the posterior lateral hypothalamus of the albino rat. Brain Res 840:138–147, 1999.

14. Saper CB, Chou TC, Scammell TE: The sleep switch: Hypothalamic control of sleep and wakefulness. Trends Neurosci 24:726–731, 2001.

15. Sherin JE, Shiromani PJ, McCarley RW, Saper CB: Activation of ventrolateral preoptic neurons during sleep. Science 271:216–219, 1996.

16. Gallopin T, Fort P, Eggermann E, et al: Identification of sleep-promoting neurons in vitro. Nature 404:992–995, 2000.

17. Chou TC, Bjorkum AA, Gaus SE, et al: Afferents to the ventrolateral preoptic nucleus. J Neurosci 22:977–990, 2002.

18. Lu J, Bjorkum AA, Xu M, et al: Selective activation of the extended ventrolateral preoptic nucleus during rapid eye movement sleep. J Neurosci 22:4568–4576, 2002.

19. Sherin JE, Elmquist JK, Torrealba F, Saper CB: Innervation of histaminergic tuberomammillary neurons by GABAergic and galaninergic neurons in the ventrolateral preoptic nucleus of the rat. J Neurosci 18:4705–4721, 1998.

20. Gaus SE, Strecker RE, Tate BA, et al: Ventrolateral preoptic nucleus contains sleep-active, galaninergic neurons in multiple mammalian species. Neuroscience 115:285–294, 2002.

21. Lin JS, Sakai K, Jouvet M: Evidence for histaminergic arousal mechanisms in the hypothalamus of cat. Neuropharmacology 27:111–122, 1988.

22. Steininger TL, Gong H, McGinty D, Szymusiak R: Subregional organization of preoptic area/anterior hypothalamic projections to arousal-related monoaminergic cell groups. J Comp Neurol 429:638–653, 2001.

23. Yang QZ, Hatton GI: Electrophysiology of excitatory and inhibitory afferents to rat histaminergic tuberomammillary nucleus neurons from hypothalamic and forebrain sites. Brain Res 773:162–172, 1997.

24. Lu J, Greco MA, Shiromani P, Saper CB: Effect of lesions of the ventrolateral preoptic nucleus on NREM and REM sleep. J Neurosci 20:3830–3842, 2000.

25. Nelson LE, Guo TZ, Lu J, et al: The sedative component of anesthesia is mediated by GABA$_A$ receptors in an endogenous sleep pathway. Nat Neurosci 5:979–984, 2002.

26. Bremer F: Cerebral hypnogenic centers. Ann Neurol 2:1–6, 1977.

27. Siegel JM: In Kryger MH, Roth T, Dement WC (eds): Principles and Practice of Sleep Medicine, 3rd ed. Philadelphia, WB Saunders, Philadelphia, 2000.

28. Semba K, Fibiger HC: Afferent connections of the laterodorsal and the pedunculopontine tegmental nuclei in the rat: A retro- and anterograde transport and immunohistochemical study. J Comp Neurol 323:387–410, 1992.

29. Aston-Jones G, Bloom FE: Nonrepinephrine-containing locus coeruleus neurons in behaving rats exhibit pronounced responses to non-noxious environmental stimuli. J Neurosci 1:887–900, 1981.

30. McGinty DJ, Harper RM: Dorsal raphe neurons: Depression of firing during sleep in cats. Brain Res 101:569–575, 1976.

31. Jones BE: Paradoxical sleep and its chemical/structural substrates in the brain. Neuroscience 40:637–656, 1991.

32. Chemelli RM, Willie JT, Sinton CM, et al: Narcolepsy in orexin knockout mice: Molecular genetics of sleep regulation. Cell 98:437–451, 1999.

33. Marcus JN, Aschkenasi CJ, Lee CE, et al: Differential expression of orexin receptors 1 and 2 in the rat brain. J Comp Neurol 435:6–25, 2001.

34. de Lecea L, Criado JR, Prospero-Garcia O, et al: A cortical neuropeptide with neuronal depressant and sleep-modulating properties. Nature 381:242–245, 1996.

35. de Lecea L, et al: The hypocretins: Hypothalamus-specific peptides with neuroexcitatory activity. Proc Natl Acad Sci USA 95:322–327, 1998.

36. Sakurai T, et al: Orexins and orexin receptors: A family of hypothalamic neuropeptides and G protein-coupled receptors that regulate feeding behavior. Cell 92:573–585, 1998.

37. Tafti M, Franken P: Invited review: Genetic dissection of sleep. J Appl Physiol 92:1339–1347, 2002.

38. Lin L, et al: The sleep disorder canine narcolepsy is caused by a mutation in the hypocretin (orexin) receptor 2 gene. Cell 98:365–376, 1999.

39. Peyron C, et al: A mutation in a case of early onset narcolepsy and a generalized absence of hypocretin peptides in human narcoleptic brains. Nat Med 6:991–997, 2000.

40. Hara J, et al: Genetic ablation of orexin neurons in mice results in narcolepsy, hypophagia, and obesity. Neuron 30:345–354, 2001.

41. Sakurai T: Roles of orexins in regulation of feeding and wakefulness. Neuroreport 13:987–995, 2002.

42. Sutcliffe JG, de Lecea L: The hypocretins: Setting the arousal threshold. Nat Rev Neurosci 3:339–349, 2002.

43. Vitaterna MH, et al: Mutagenesis and mapping of a mouse gene, Clock, essential for circadian behavior. Science 264:719–725, 1994.

44. Flint J, Mott R: Finding the molecular basis of quantitative traits: Successes and pitfalls. Nat Rev Genet 2:437–445, 2001.

45. Shimomura K, et al: Genome-wide epistatic interaction analysis reveals complex genetic determinants of circadian behavior in mice. Genome Res 11:959–980, 2001.

46. Tafti M, Chollet D, Valatx JL, Franken P: Quantitative trait loci approach to the genetics of sleep in recombinant inbred mice. J Sleep Res 8(suppl 1):37–43, 1999.

47. Mihic SJ, et al: Sites of alcohol and volatile anaesthetic action on GABA(A) and glycine receptors. Nature 389:385–389, 1997.

48. Adodra S, Hales TG: Potentiation, activation and blockade of GABAA receptors of clonal murine hypothalamic GT1-7 neurones by propofol. Br J Pharmacol 115:953–960, 1995.

49. Rudolph U, et al: Benzodiazepine actions mediated by specific gamma-aminobutyric acid(A) receptor subtypes. Nature 401:796–800, 1999.

50. Low K, et al: Molecular and neuronal substrate for the selective attenuation of anxiety. Science 290:131–134, 2000.

51. Sanger DJ, Morel E, Perrault G: Comparison of the pharmacological profiles of the hypnotic drugs, zaleplon and zolpidem. Eur J Pharmacol 313:35–42, 1996.

52. MacDonald E, Scheinin M: Distribution and pharmacology of alpha 2-adrenoceptors in the central nervous system. J Physiol Pharmacol 46:241–258, 1995.

53. Aston-Jones G, Rajkowski J, Kubiak P, Alexinsky T: Locus coeruleus neurons in monkey are selectively activated by attended cues in a vigilance task. J Neurosci 14:4467–4480, 1994.

54. Correa-Sales C, Rabin BC, Maze M: A hypnotic response to dexmedetomidine, an alpha 2 agonist, is mediated in the locus coeruleus in rats. Anesthesiology 76:948–952, 1992.

55. Williams JT, Henderson G, North RA: Characterization of alpha 2-adrenoceptors which increase potassium conductance in rat locus coeruleus neurones. Neuroscience 14:95–101, 1985.

56. Nacif-Coelho C, Correa-Sales C, Chang LL, Maze M: Perturbation of ion channel conductance alters the hypnotic response to the alpha 2-adrenergic agonist dexmedetomidine in the locus coeruleus of the rat. Anesthesiology 81:1527–1534, 1994.

57. Nelson LE, Lu J, Guo T, et al: The α_2-adrenoceptor agonist dexmedetomidine converges on an endogenous sleep pathway to produce its hypnotic response. Anesthesiology 98:428–438, 2003.

58. Venn RM, et al: Preliminary UK experience of dexmedetomidine, a novel agent for postoperative sedation in the intensive care unit. Anaesthesia 54:1136–1142, 1999.

59. Jones MEP, Coull JT, Egan,TD, Maze M: Are subjects more easily aroused during sedation with the alpha(2) agonist, dexmedetomdine? Br J Pharmacol 86:324P, 2002.

60. Anis NA, Berry SC, Burton NR, Lodge D: The dissociative anaesthetics, ketamine and phencyclidine, selectively reduce excitation of central mammalian neurones by N-methyl-aspartate. Br J Pharmacol 79:565–575, 1983.

61. Jevtovic-Todorovic V, et al: Nitrous oxide (laughing gas) is an NMDA antagonist, neuroprotectant and neurotoxin. Nat Med 4:460–463, 1998.

62. Franks NP, Dickinson R, de Sousa SL, et al: How does xenon produce anaesthesia? Nature 396:324, 1998.

63. McGehee DS, Role LW: Physiological diversity of nicotinic acetylcholine receptors expressed by vertebrate neurons. Annu Rev Physiol 57:521–546, 1995.

64. Violet JM, Downie DL, Nakisa RC, et al: Differential sensitivities of mammalian neuronal and muscle nicotinic acetylcholine receptors to general anesthetics. Anesthesiology 86:866–874, 1997.

65. Tassonyi E, Charpantier E, Muller D, et al: The role of nicotinic acetylcholine receptors in the mechanisms of anesthesia. Brain Res Bull 57:133–150, 2002.

66. Downie DL, Hall AC, Lieb WR, Franks NP: Effects of inhalational general anaesthetics on native glycine receptors in rat medullary

neurones and recombinant glycine receptors in Xenopus oocytes. Br J Pharmacol 118:493–502, 1996.

67. Koltchine VV, et al: Agonist gating and isoflurane potentiation in the human gamma-aminobutyric acid type A receptor determined by the volume of a second transmembrane domain residue. Mol Pharmacol 56:1087–1093, 1999.

68. Beckstead MJ, Phelan R, Mihic SJ: Antagonism of inhalant and volatile anesthetic enhancement of glycine receptor function. J Biol Chem 276:24959–24964, 2001.

69. Franks NP, Lieb WR: Volatile general anaesthetics activate a novel neuronal K+ current. Nature 333:662–664, 1988.

70. Patel AJ, et al: Inhalational anesthetics activate two-pore-domain background K+ channels. Nat Neurosci 2:422–426, 1999.

71. Meadows HJ, Randall AD: Functional characterization of human TASK-3, an acid-sensitive two-pore domain potassium channel. Neuropharmacology 40:551–559, 2001.

72. Washburn CP, Sirois JE, Talley EM, et al: Serotonergic raphe neurons express TASK channel transcripts and a TASK-like pH- and halothane-sensitive K+ conductance. J Neurosci 22:1256–1265, 2002.

73. Talley EM, Bayliss DA: Modulation of TASK-1 (Kcnk3) and TASK-3 (Kcnk9) potassium channels: volatile anesthetics and neurotransmitters share a molecular site of action. J Biol Chem 277:17733–17742, 2002.

74. Peyron C, et al: Neurons containing hypocretin (orexin) project to multiple neuronal systems. J Neurosci 18:9996–10015, 1998.

75. Hagan JJ, et al: Orexin A activates locus coeruleus cell firing and increases arousal in the rat. Proc Natl Acad Sci USA 96:10911–10916, 1999.

76. Brown RE, Sergeeva O, Eriksson KS, Haas HL: Orexin A excites serotonergic neurons in the dorsal raphe nucleus of the rat. Neuropharmacology 40:457–459, 2001.

77. Eriksson KS, Sergeeva O, Brown RE, Haas HL: Orexin/hypocretin excites the histaminergic neurons of the tuberomammillary nucleus. J Neurosci 21:9273–9279, 2001.

78. Methippara MM, Alam MN, Szymusiak R, McGinty D: Effects of lateral preoptic area application of orexin-A on sleep-wakefulness. Neuroreport 11:3423–3426, 2000.

79. Estabrooke IV, et al: Fos expression in orexin neurons varies with behavioral state. J Neurosci 21:1656–1662, 2001.

80. Scammell TE, et al: An adenosine A2a agonist increases sleep and induces Fos in ventrolateral preoptic neurons. Neuroscience 107:653–663, 2001.

81. Terao A, Matsumura H, Saito M: Interleukin-1 induces slow-wave sleep at the prostaglandin D2-sensitive sleep-promoting zone in the rat brain. J Neurosci 18:6599–6607, 1998.

16

Neural Substrates for Behavior

Pierre Fiset, MD • M. Catherine Bushnell, PhD

PAIN

The control of pain transmission, whether achieved through general and regional anesthesia or with other pharmacological techniques, is the "raison d'être" of the anesthesiologist. The development of modern anesthesiology techniques and advances in pharmacology have allowed the performance of complex surgical procedures, and sophisticated approaches to the problems of postoperative acute and "chronic pain syndromes." These have resulted in a marked improvement in our patients' quality of life.

Although we often refer to pain as a sensation, it is probably better described as a multidimensional experience.[1] There are certain qualities of somatosensations that are almost exclusively associated with pain, such as stinging, pricking, burning, and aching. However, pain also encompasses an unpleasant emotional experience. It is because of this dimension that the adjective "painful" is sometimes applied to emotional experiences, in the absence of sensory stimulation. Pain has a strong motivational component, evoking both withdrawal reflexes and highly organized avoidance and escape behavior. It is the motivational aspect of pain that is probably its primary function, and without it the organism will not survive. The importance of pain to the health and integrity of the organism is illustrated by the rare syndrome of congenital insensitivity to pain. These individ-uals lack small diameter primary afferent fibers that transmit information about tissue-damaging stimuli. People with this syndrome frequently injure themselves and are unaware of internal injury or disease when the sole symptom is pain.

The multidimensional aspect of pain is reflected by the various responses resulting from the balance between central nervous system (CNS) depression by anesthetic drugs and surgical stimuli. Conscious and unconscious responses under general anesthesia are expressed over a range: from the primitive, reflex-like increases in blood pressure and pulse rate, lacrimation and sweating, as well as reflex movements to the highly organized and emotionally charged phenomenon of intraoperative awareness.[2]

This chapter discusses our current knowledge of the neural substrates for pain perception. First, the pathways involved in the transmission of pain from the dorsal columns to cortical structures, as well as the descending modulatory pathways are reviewed. These constitute the basic framework needed to understand the multidimensional aspects of pain.

However, the whole physiologic picture changes when, after nerve injury, chronic inflammation, or tissue destruction, pain becomes a chronic process. Some specific changes occur at different levels of the classical pathways to the extent that pain then becomes a syndrome in its own right, a "disease" that does not anymore subserve the behavioral and motivational purposes related to self-protection. Typically, pain then becomes much more difficult to alleviate. Thus in the second part of this chapter, the physiologic changes induced in the context of peripheral and central sensitization as well as neuropathic pain will be detailed.

Pain Pathways

From the Periphery to the Dorsal Horn

In previous chapters, the topics of peripheral nociceptors, primary afferent neurons, and dorsal horn physiology have been addressed. In summary, pain is transmitted by free ending nerve receptors present in the skin, muscles, joints, viscera, and vasculature and conveyed to the dorsal horn by small myelinated Aδ (rapid, early response) and unmyelinated C fibers (dull, more delayed response).[3] These are activated by high-intensity stimulation (mechanical, heat, and cold) that sometimes travels as a specific modality, but also in a polymodal fashion through a single fiber. Some C fibers, in addition to their afferent function, also convey efferent impulses (antidromic transmission) that mediate neurogenic inflammation, a phenomenon responsible for the immediate flaring response elicited by tissue injury. Nociceptive Aδ and C fibers travel from the periphery through spinal and trigeminal primary afferent nerves toward their cell body located in the dorsal root ganglia.[3] As shown in Figure 16–1, Aδ fibers form their first synapse in the dorsal horn of the spinal cord, in Rexed's laminae I, IIo, III, V, VI, and X, whereas the C fibers synapse in laminae I, Iio, and V. Branches of the non-nociceptive Aδ fibers synapse in laminae III, IV, and V.[4]

Nociceptive primary afferents innervating the viscera enter the spinal cord along with somatic nociceptive primary afferents and converge onto neurons in laminae I and V.[5] It appears that visceral sensations are mediated through convergent viscerosomatic dorsal horn neurons. This convergence could explain the phenomenon of *referred pain* first described by Head,[6] in which pain arising from deep tissue is felt in a body region remote from the site of pathology. A familiar example of referred pain is the pain of myocardial infarction, in which many patients report pain not only in the chest and upper abdomen, but also along the ulnar aspect of the left arm. However, the *postsynaptic dorsal column pathway* may have a specific role to play in the transmission of visceral pain[7] (see later).

Nociceptive second-order projection neurons are located mainly in laminae I and V. The small receptive fields and specific response properties of lamina I neurons render them suitable to signal the location and characteristics of noxious stimuli. Lamina V wide dynamic range neurons are less specialized for transmitting specific information about pain, but their discharge frequencies exquisitely code the intensity of noxious stimuli. From the dorsal horn, neurons transmitting nociceptive information project through a series of different

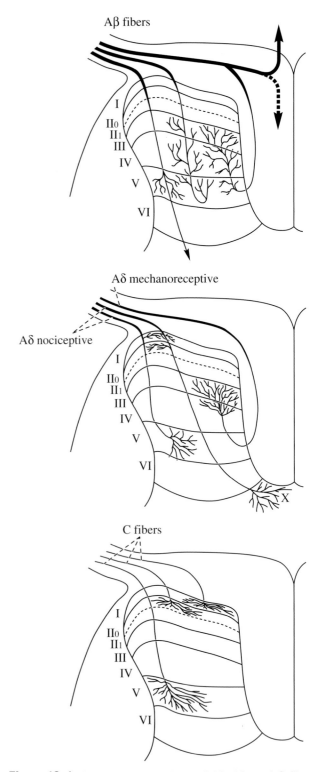

Figure 16–1. Synaptic connections of Aβ, Aδ, and C fibers in the dorsal horn. Aβ fibers do not project to lamina IIo in normal circumstances. However, in some patients with chronic neuropathic pain, sprouting of Aδ terminal endings occurs, and somatosensory and non-noxious mechanical information is conveyed in areas usually exclusively reserved to pain perception, contributing to the phenomena of allodynia and hyperalgesia. (From Coderre TJ, Bushnell MC: Psychobiology of pain. In Gallagher M, Nelson RJ (eds): Comprehensive Handbook of Psychology, vol 3. New York, John Wiley & Sons, 2001, adapted from Bonica JJ: The Management of Pain, Philadelphia, Lea & Febiger, 1990.)

pathways to higher centers in the brain stem, thalamus, and cerebral cortex to initiate a number of specific responses related to the autonomic, affective-motivational, and sensory-discriminative aspects of pain perception.

Neurotransmission of Pain

Two main classes of neurotransmitters are associated with primary afferent nociceptive transmission in the dorsal horn: the *excitatory amino acids* (EAAs), primarily glutamate, and the *neurokinin peptides* (NK), primarily substance P[8,9] (Fig. 16–2). These compounds are present in dorsal root ganglion cells, primary afferent fibers, and terminals in the dorsal horn, and their intrathecal administration in the spinal cord produces nocifensive behavior in animals and excitation of nociceptive dorsal horn neurons. The postsynaptic sites of action of the EAAs on spinal cord neurons include both *N*-methyl-D-aspartate (NMDA) and non-NMDA receptors,[10] but the NMDA receptors are more likely involved in nociceptive transmission. Three neurokinin receptor types are found in the spinal cord: NK1, NK2, and NK3. The NK1 and NK2 receptors are proposed to activate nociceptive transmission pathways, whereas NK3 receptors are thought to activate pain modulation pathways.

Ascending Pathways

The classification adopted in this chapter has been proposed by Willis and Westlund.[11]

Pathways Ascending in the Anterolateral Quadrant

Four different pathways projecting to different areas of the CNS ascend in the anterolateral aspect of the spinal cord. This diversity of targets and pathways illustrates the multidimensional nature of pain perception.

Spinothalamic Tract

The most widely studied and best known pathway is the spinothalamic tract (Fig. 16–3). It is formed mainly from cells located in the laminae I, IV, V, and VI,[12,13] with some others originating from lamina X. Fibers cross the midline at or near the level of their origin and ascend in the anterolateral aspect of the spinal cord. They are organized somatotopically and synapse in the lateral and medial thalamus. Lateral projections are made mainly of cells from laminae I and V, whereas medial ones come from collaterals from the laterally projecting fibers as well as specific fibers originating from the deep dorsal horn and ventral horn.[12] The spinothalamic tract conveys information related to pain, cold, warmth, and touch, which is suggested by results from the surgical procedure anterolateral cordotomy that is performed to relieve pain. Most spinothalamic cells have receptive fields on a restricted area of the contralateral part of the body. Many spinothalamic fibers terminate in a somatotopic

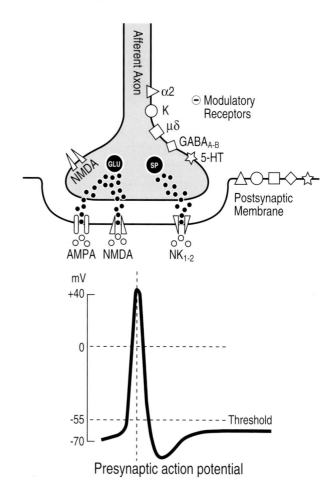

Figure 16–2. The major neurotransmitters involved in pain transmission in the dorsal horn. Presynaptic depolarization induces the liberation of glutamate (GLU) and substance P (SP). Glutamate binds to α-amino-3-hydroxy-5-methylisoxazole-4-propionic acid (AMPA) and *N*-methyl-D-aspartate (NMDA) receptors, and substance P to NK$_1$ (neurokinin) and NK$_2$ receptors, causing Ca^{++} influx and depolarizing of the postsynaptic membrane. Multiple intracellular pathways are then activated. NMDA receptors can also be found on the presynaptic membranes where their activation enhances further glutamate liberation. Neuromodulators are found on the presynaptic and postsynaptic membranes. Activation of opioid (μ and δ), γ-aminobutyric acid (GABA$_B$), alpha adrenergic (α$_2$), and serotoninergic (5-HT) receptors decreases the activation of the dorsal horn synapse in two ways. Presynaptic activation decreases the liberation of pain transmitters into the synaptic cleft. Postsynaptic activation induces a state of hyperpolarization of the postsynaptic membrane, making it less likely to undergo depolarization by a given quantum of agonist. Serotonin also possesses some excitatory properties.

fashion in the ventroposterior (VP) thalamic nucleus, which also receives the main output of tactile information from the dorsal column nuclei. Other spinothalamic fibers terminate in the posterior thalamus. A nucleus in the posterior thalamus has recently been identified that receives specific pain and temperature information from lamina I of the dorsal horn.[14] Spinothalamic fibers also terminate in medial thalamic intralaminar nuclei.

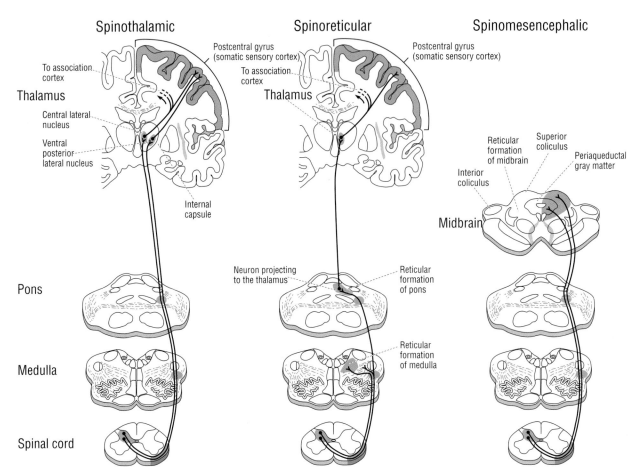

Figure 16–3. Nociceptive information is relayed from the spinal cord to the brain through several pathways, including the spinothalamic tract (*left*), the spinomesencephalic tract (*middle*), and the spinoreticular tract (*right*). (From Kendel ER, Schwartz JH, Jessel IM: Principles of Neural Science, 4th ed. New York, McGraw-Hill, 2000, pp 482–486.)

Spinomesencephalic Tract

Cells of origin of this tract are also located in laminae I, IV-VI, and X. Fibers decussate locally and ascend in the lateral funiculus,[11,15,16] which may be left untouched during an anterior cordotomy, allowing pain to persist or recur. They project to a series of midbrain nuclei, including the periaqueductal gray (PAG), nucleus cuneiformis, and superior colliculus.[3,17,18] These cells have complex receptive fields and respond to noxious and innocuous stimuli. The spinomesencephalic tract may serve multiple functions: it may serve to initiate aversive behavior and play a role in orientation relative to the stimulus. It may also activate the descending analgesia system through its connections to the PAG, and thus underlie the clinical phenomenon of counterirritation by which one noxious stimulus reduces the pain provoked by another.

Spinoreticular Tracts

These cells respond to noxious stimuli and one of their primary functional roles is to signal homeostatic changes to the brain stem autonomic centers. Through their connections to higher centers, information is relayed to trigger motiva-tional and affective responses. The cell bodies of spinoreticular neurons are located in the deep layers of the dorsal horn and in laminae VII and VIII of the ventral horn[3,19] and send fibers that decussate and ascend in the lateral funiculus. Their targets are several nuclei of the reticular formation of the medulla and the pons. Some spinoreticular neurons terminate on cells involved in descending pain modulation pathways. Other spinoreticular neurons make up the spinoreticulothalamic tract, which terminates in medial thalamic nuclei, along with spinothalamic neurons described earlier.

Spinolimbic Tracts

Other pathways support the affective-motivational aspect of pain through direct activation of the limbic system. Direct spinohypothalamic[20] and spinoparabrachiaoamygdalar[21,22] pathways originating from cells located in the deep dorsal horn in the grey matter surrounding the central canal travel in the contralateral funiculus. The spinopontoamygdaloid system originates in laminae I and V of the dorsal horn, ascending in the dorsolateral funiculus, and synapsing in the parabrachial area of the pons before reaching the amygdaloid complex. Bernard and Besson, who have studied the pathway extensively, suggest that this system normally is involved in the fear and memory of pain, as well as behavioral and autonomic reactions to noxious events, such as vocalization, flight, freezing, pupil dilation, and cardiorespiratory responses.[21]

Pathways in the Dorsal Quadrant

Spinocervicothalamic Pathway

Fibers of the spinocervicothalamic pathway originate from laminae III and IV and ascend ipsilaterally to synapse in the lateral cervical nuclei located in the white matter of CI and C2 segments.[3] From there they decussate in the medial lemniscus and reach the ventroposterolateral (VPL) thalamus.[23] Although its functional role is not precisely known, this is another potential route for the noxious information to reach the lateral thalamus. Although this pathway is well developed in cats, it appears to be less important in primates.

Postsynaptic Dorsal Column Pathway

Clinical as well as some recent laboratory reports suggest that pelvic visceral pain might reach the thalamus through the postsynaptic dorsal column pathway. Its cells, found in lamina III, activate a projection neuron located in lamina X.[24] The axon is then sent posteriorly near the midline of the dorsal column to synapse in the nucleus gracilis. From there another projection ends in the contralateral VPL of the thalamus. This system responds to mechanical and chemical irritation of the viscera, and may not have a role in perception of cutaneous pain.[7,25]

The Thalamus

Although some of the nociceptive afferent traffic reaches the higher brain centers through other pathways, most of the information is relayed first to thalamic nuclei directly by the spinothalamic and indirectly by the spinoreticular and spinomesencephalic tracts. These nuclei include the VPL and ventroposteromedial (VPM) nuclei, ventromedial aspect of the posterior (VM$_{PO}$) thalamus, and the ventrocaudal portion of the medial dorsal (MD$_{vc}$), and parafascicular (Pf) nuclei of the medial thalamus.[26] The somatotopic organization and projection to cortical and subcortical structures suggest a different role for nociceptive nuclei in the lateral and medial thalamus. The role definition is further refined by the response pattern of neuron populations to some very specific aspects of pain processing—localization, modality determination, and intensity discrimination, as well as affective-motivational aspects.

Lateral Thalamus

Dense projections from dorsal horn nuclei terminate in the VPL and projections from the trigeminal equivalent of the dorsal horn (trigeminal nucleus caudalis) terminate in VPM. Neurons in the VP thalamus (VPL and VPM) are somatotopically organized, and have restricted receptive fields[26] (for an extensive description see Lenz and Dougherty[27]). Moreover, the size of the field does not change with behavioral state or after repeated stimulation, indicating that these neurons are involved in the localization of pain and temperature and are not greatly influenced by emotional/motivational behavior.[26,28] Conversely, many of these neurons seem to be of the wide dynamic range type, meaning that they respond in a graded fashion to touch, pressure, pinch, and noxious heat. The lack of specificity of these neurons suggests that modality discrimination is probably performed by other cell populations. Finally, VP thalamic neurons are exquisitely sensitive to the intensity of the stimulus. In some experimental conditions, it has been shown that there is a significant correlation between the neuronal response to a small change in noxious heat intensity and a monkey's ability to detect the temperature steps.[29] Most of the evidence suggests that VPM and VPL cells project to the primary somatosensory cortex (SI), reinforcing their role in pain localization.[30,31]

Medial Thalamus

The spinothalamic tract sends collateral as well as direct projections to the medially located MD$_{VC}$ nucleus and to the Pf nucleus.[29] These cells have large receptive fields and little somatotopic organization. Determination of their response to precise pain modalities has helped define the role of this projection system in affective-motivational behavior. It has been reported that there are much less wide dynamic range neurons in medial thalamic nuclei, and that the response to a certain type of pain (modality specificity), such as noxious heat or pinch, can be specific. Moreover, the response characteristics of these cells are highly variable, being influenced by the behavioral states.[26,28]

There is evidence showing that MD$_{VC}$/Pf neurons project to the anterior cingulate cortex,[32,33] and that those from the VM$_{PO}$ thalamus project to the rostral insular cortex. Connectivity to these limbic system centers suggests that activity in the medial thalamus may be important for the affective-motivational aspect of pain.

Cortical Projections

The multidimensional aspect of pain perception is best illustrated by the cortical centers involved in pain processing (Fig. 16–4). Early neurosurgical experiments failed to determine the existence of a single cortical pain center, and it is now known that different regions play a specific role in the experience of pain in relation to the sensory-discriminative, affective-motivational, and autonomic aspects. These regions include the primary and secondary sensory cortices, the cingulate and insular cortices, and the amygdala.[34–37] Neuroanatomic studies on connectivity and pathways have mapped out the circuitry of the system, and brain imaging experiments have greatly improved our understanding of the functional aspects of pain processing.

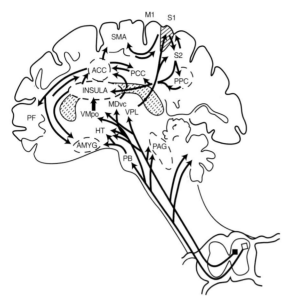

Figure 16–4. Diagram of supraspinal nociceptive pathways. Information is conveyed from the dorsal horn of the spinal cord to the periaqueductal gray (PAG), parabrachial nucleus (PB) of the pons, and several thalamic nuclei. Nociceptive neurons in parabrachial nucleus (PB) project to the amygdala (AMYG), those in ventroposterolateral (VPL) thalamus project to SI and SII cortices, those in ventrocaudal portion of the medial dorsal (MD$_{vc}$) project to ACC and those in ventromedial aspect of the posterior (VM$_{PO}$) project to insula. These cortical areas in turn form complex cortico/cortical connections. ACC, ; PCC, ; PF, parafascicular; PPC, ; SMA, supplemental motor area. (From Price DD: Psychological and neural mechanisms of the affective dimension of pain. Science 288:1769–1772, 2000.)

pain perception. These studies are based on changes in hemodynamic parameters, such as regional cerebral blood flow, during the performance of a task that reflects changes in synaptic activity. Figure 16–5 shows functional magnetic resonance imaging data of pain-evoked activation in SI, SII, ACC, and insula.[38] It has been shown that attentional modulation can selectively influence primary sensory cortical processing, so much that it could well be a source of variability in the reports on the role of SI in pain perception.[39] In addition, studies of hypnotic suggestions for reinterpretation of sensations reveal that cognitive states can lead to selective modulation of pain effect without altering pain intensity—when only pain effect is changed, pain-related activity in the ACC is modulated, whereas when perceived pain sensation is changed, pain-related activity in SI is modulated.[40–42]

From this pattern of anatomic organization, it is possible to understand how our reaction to pain takes shape.[1] The first type of response relates to activation of structures in the medullary and midbrain reticular formation, superior colliculus, central gray, amygdala, hypothalamus, and specific medial thalamic nuclei. These are involved in the rudimentary aspects of autonomic system activation, escape, motor orientation, arousal, and fear during the early phase of pain.[20]

A second type of response relates to the perceptual and cognitive aspects of pain processing and results from the activation of somatosensory cortices. The intensity, quality, and nature of pain are determined, and the integration with other sensory modalities through posterior parietal projections refines the definition of the context.[43,44]

Finally, the convergence of direct and indirect input to the ACC is the substrate for the third response: affective-motivational. At that level, under the influence of attention,

As indicated earlier, both sensory and limbic cortical areas receive direct thalamocortical nociceptive input (see Fig. 16–4). The primary (SI) and secondary (SII) sensory cortices receive nociceptive input from the VP thalamus (VPM and VPL). Anterior cingulate cortex receives a nociceptive input from medial thalamic nuclei, including MD$_{vc}$, and insular cortex receives input from VM$_{PO}$ thalamus. Once this nociceptive information reaches the cortex, there are many cortico/cortical connections that could lead to widespread dissemination of nociceptive information (see Fig. 16–4). For example, there are connections from SI and SII to posterior parietal areas through the posterior cingulate cortex and to the insular area. From there connections are sent to the ACC, amygdala, perirhinal cortex, and hippocampus. There are also connections from the ACC to the supplemental motor area and prefrontal cortex. Notably, some pathways that bypass the thalamus, including the spinohypothalamic and spinoparabrachioamygdaloid pathways project nociceptive information from the dorsal horn to limbic structures. The existence of this converging, dual projection system to cortical centers involved in the sensory, affective, and motivational aspects of pain illustrates both the complexity of the pain experience and the diverse influences that can modify the experience of pain.[1]

Human functional brain imaging using positron emission tomography and functional magnetic resonance imaging has greatly enhanced our understanding of the factors affecting

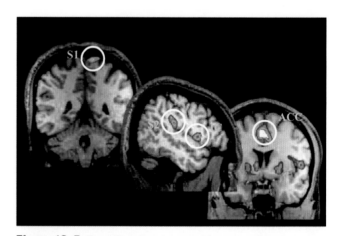

Figure 16–5. Functional and anatomic magnetic resonance imaging of a single subject exposed to a painful heat stimulus (3 × 3 cm thermode on the left leg; 46° C). Ten 9-second noxious heat stimuli and ten 9-second neutral warm stimuli (36° C) were presented sequentially with 9-second interstimulus intervals. The *circled* color-coded areas represent regions that show a significantly greater activation during the noxious heat than during the warm stimuli. *Left, Right,* Coronal slices; *middle,* sagittal slice. (From Bushnell MC, Duncan GH, Ha B, et al: Noninvasive brain imaging during experimental and clinical pain. In Proceedings of the 8th World Congress on Pain. Seattle, IASP Press, 2000, pp 485–495.)

emotions, and past experience, painful sensations are integrated into a highly organized behavioral state directed toward self-protection.[41,45]

Modulation of Pain

Many factors, including pharmacologic treatments, environmental influences, and cognitive state, influence pain perception. After hundreds of years of use, opiates are still one of the best means of pain control. We now know that opiates bind to endogenous opiate-like receptors in the brain, spinal cord, and primary afferent fibers, and thus activate both local inhibitory circuits and descending pain modulatory pathways.

Descending Modulatory Pathways

After the stimulation of a number of medullary nuclei, nociceptive dorsal horn neurons are inhibited[46] (Fig. 16–6). The PAG is one of the main nuclei implicated. When it is stimulated, antinociception is induced through direct[47] and indirect projections to the spinal cord through different neurotransmitter systems. Microinjection of morphine into the PAG also produces significant analgesia, and endogenous opiate-like substances (enkephalin and endorphins) are released in this region. Serotoninergic modulation happens through excitatory connections sent from the PAG to the nucleus raphe magnus and other medullary serotonergic nuclei, which then sends inhibitory projections to the dorsal horn. The PAG also projects to the locus ceruleus and other nuclei of the parabrachial area to activate noradrenergic projections to all regions of the spinal cord and to mediate antinociception.[48]

Stimulation of another nucleus, the anterior pretectal, also results in long-lasting antinociception[49]; however, the descending pathway and neurotransmitters involved are still undetermined. Other areas of the CNS are involved in antinociception. Stimulation of the VP thalamus causes a reduction of pain in patients suffering from neuropathic pain syndromes such as facial anesthesia dolorosa, postherpetic neuralgia, and the thalamic syndrome.[50] This could occur through antidromic activation of the spinothalamic tract and its connections to the PAG or nucleus raphe magnus.[51] Alternatively, a cortical inhibitory mechanism resulting in a decrease of the response to innocuous stimulation could also be a cause.

Ascending Modulatory Pathways

Both tactile and thermal afferent stimulation has inhibitory influences on pain perception. The basis of the gate control theory[52] is that Aδ fiber stimulation activates interneurons in the dorsal horn that inhibit the activity of nociceptive transmission neurons. The details of this theory have not been completely substantiated, but divergent evidence shows that activation of low-threshold tactile pathways inhibits pain.

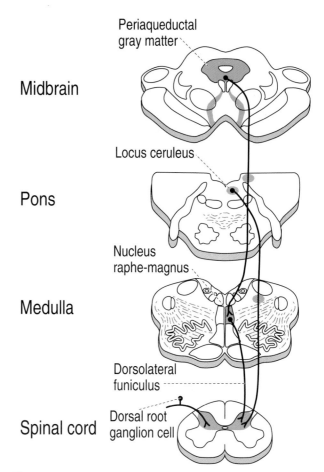

Figure 16–6. Descending pain modulatory pathways that modulate dorsal horn nociceptive activity include projections from the periaqueductal gray to nucleus raphe magnus and other medullary serotonergic nuclei, as well as noradrenergic projections from the locus ceruleus and other nuclei of the parabrachial area.

This inhibition is the basis of transcutaneous electrical nerve stimulation, as well as spinal cord stimulation and thalamic stimulation for pain control. Similarly, several types of evidence show that activation of thermal pathways with cold leads to pain inhibition. It is the interruption of activity in these pathways that may lead to pain associated with lesions of the CNS, such as thalamic pain syndrome.[53]

Cognitive Modulation of Pain

Both clinical and experimental evidence show that cognitive state alters pain perception. Stress-produced analgesia is a common phenomenon in humans and animals. More subtle factors, such as attentional state or meaning attributed to the pain, also are shown to modify pain perception. These factors are important for many cognitive manipulations, such as hypnosis, behavioral modification, relaxation training, biofeedback, operant conditioning, and cognitive-behavioral therapy. Human brain imaging studies reveal a clear neurophysiologic basis for cognitive modulation of pain. Figure 16–7 shows that when attention is directed away from a painful stimulus, there is reduced pain percep-

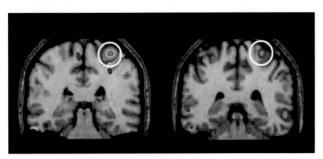

Figure 16–7. Pain-related activity when attention was directed to a painful heat stimulus (*left*) or to an auditory stimulus (*right*). Images illustrate, for each attentional state, positron emission tomography (PET) data recorded during the presentation of a painfully hot stimulus (46.5–48.5° C), compared with those recorded during the presentation of a warm stimulus (32–38° C). PET data, averaged across nine subjects, are illustrated against a magnetic resonance imaging scan from one subject. A direct comparison of the activity in the two attentional conditions revealed a significantly larger pain-evoked activation in SI cortex when the subjects were paying attention to the painful stimulus than when they received pain while attending to the auditory stimulus. (From Bushnell MC, Duncan GH, Ha B, et al: Noninvasive brain imaging during experimental and clinical pain. In Proceedings of the 8th World Congress on Pain. Seattle, IASP Press, 2000, pp 485–495.)

tion and an associated decrease in pain-evoked activity in the SI cortex.[38,39] The circuitry underlying cognitive modulation of pain is unknown and probably involves multiple modulatory systems in the brain.

Pain as a Dynamic Process

After the initial perception and transmission of pain, a series of mechanisms come into play if tissue damage has occurred. The net result is postinjury pain hypersensitivity, which is characterized by a reduction in the intensity of the stimulus necessary to initiate pain. This can be caused by an increase in the sensitivity of peripheral nociceptors, a phenomenon called peripheral sensitization. Alternatively, central sensitization results from a change in dorsal horn physiology caused by persistent pain. Clinically, sensitization is expressed by an exaggerated responsiveness to noxious stimuli, called hyperalgesia, sometimes with a spread of hypersensitivity to noninjured tissue, named secondary hyperalgesia. Allodynia occurs when pain is felt during the administration of a non-noxious stimulus, such as brushing or lightly touching the skin.

Peripheral Sensitization

Immediately after tissue injury, a cocktail of inflammatory mediators and other chemicals are liberated by damaged tissues and sympathetic nerve endings in the vicinity of the high-threshold nociceptors. These include histamine,

bradykinin, K^+, H^+, prostaglandins, purines, cytokines, leukotrienes, nerve growth factor, neuropeptides, serotonin, and norepinephrine.[54,55] This causes an increase in the sensitivity of Aδ and C fibers enabling low-intensity stimuli to cause pain. In addition, thermal sensitivity is also changed in the immediate vicinity of the wound. Inhibition of prostaglandin production by nonsteroidal anti-inflammatory drugs is thought to play a major role in the prevention of peripheral sensitization in the perioperative period.[56]

Central Sensitization

In the context of inflammatory injury resulting from surgical trauma, ongoing firing of C fibers induces a change in the response pattern of dorsal horn neurons, called central sensitization. This is characterized by an increase in the size of the receptive fields of nociceptive dorsal neurons, an increase in the magnitude and duration of suprathreshold stimuli, and a reduction in threshold that allows a response to non-nociceptive input (such as light pressure) in neurons originally depolarized only by nociceptive stimuli.[57] This is dependent on neurochemical, cellular, and molecular events in the dorsal horn neurons. Persistent C fiber input results in a summation of potentials that generates a progressively increasing and long-lasting depolarization in dorsal horn neurons through the activation of NMDA and glutamate receptors and also possibly of tachykinin receptors by substance P and neurokinin.[58,59] This triggers a change in the level of second messenger protein kinase activation and a positive feedback effect on NMDA receptors that increases their efficacy. Second messengers can also alter gene expression of certain proteins (dynorphin, preproenkephalin) by activating immediate-early gene products, switching on or off particular genes.[57] The clinical consequence of this process is hypersensitivity to pain (or hyperalgesia) mediated by Aδ and C fibers, but also allodynia mediated by Aβ fibers normally conducting only non-nociceptive inputs.

Preemptive Analgesia

Characterization of central sensitization with its dependence on ongoing peripheral neuronal firing has triggered novel ideas in relation to therapeutic approaches to pain. The concept of preemptive analgesia was introduced by Wall in 1988[60] as a way to alleviate pain in the perioperative period. Wall proposed that if nociceptive afferent inputs or their effect on dorsal horn neurons could be efficiently blocked before the start of tissue injury, the process of central sensitization would be halted or at least delayed, windup of the dorsal horn response would be decreased, and the magnitude of postoperative pain would be decreased through a decrease of hypersensitivity. Initial animal studies tended to support the hypothesis that preinjury administration of analgesics or anesthetics decreased behavioral nociceptive responses to a greater extent than did postinjury treatment (reviewed by Woolf and Chong[57]).

The multiplicity of biologic targets able to mediate the modulation of pain transmission allows for the use of many different preemptive therapeutic regimens in animal and humans, alone or in combination. Parenteral opioids inhibit presynaptic neurotransmitter release and hyperpolarize dorsal horn nociceptive neurons.[61] They also increase the activity of inhibitory descending pathways through their action on PAG. Local anesthetics block neural transmission along afferent axons and can be administered anywhere from the periphery to the intrathecal space to prevent dorsal horn activation. Blockade of NMDA receptors by ketamine (or similar compounds) acts on one of the pivotal mechanisms involved in central sensitization. Finally, nonsteroidal anti-inflammatory drugs, by blocking the production of inflammatory mediators, can decrease the magnitude of primary sensitization, thereby decreasing afferent input.[56]

Some initial human studies seemed promising, but they were followed by others with equivocal and even negative results.[62] In fact, the apparent lack of effect found in certain studies is probably related to the conceptual approach on which they are based.[63,64] The efficacy of postoperative analgesia is dependent on the extent by which afferent impulses are controlled during the whole perioperative period. During surgery, nociceptive transmission is initiated with surgical incision, and comprehensive preemptive strategies should start before that event. However, high intensity nociceptive transmission is maintained during surgery in relation to deeper structure lesioning and the secondary inflammatory response. In the immediate postoperative period, intense nociceptive input persists in relation to nerve damage and peripheral sensitization. It is therefore not surprising that strategies aimed only at comparing preincisional and postincisional treatment fail to demonstrate an effect on postoperative outcome variables. A comprehensive approach based on administration of analgesia over the whole period of intensive nociceptive transmission would certainly be maximally effective, but should probably then be labeled as perioperative analgesia.[64]

Concerning the definition of preemptive analgesia, much of the confusion and current debate are related to the timing of its administration, the nature of perioperative events likely to induce central sensitization, and the study design to be adopted to validate positive results. That viewpoint is illustrated by Katz[64] in his interpretation of a study where epidural ketamine was given before versus after the surgical incision. Both groups showed a similar use of opioids after surgery. Some might interpret this "negative" result as a proof that ketamine has no preemptive effect, but Katz suggests that a different study design might reveal that the preemptive effect of ketamine is present, but that it is not dependent on whether it is used before or after incision.

Neuropathic Pain

Types of Neuropathic Pain

Chronic intractable pain is commonly associated with a variety of injuries to the peripheral nervous system, CNS, or both. Neuropathic pain of peripheral origin includes such syndromes as diabetic neuropathy, postherpetic neuropathy, trigeminal neuralgia, phantom limb pain, and complex regional pain syndrome.[65-67] Neuropathic pain of predominantly central origin is associated with a variety of pathologic conditions, including multiple sclerosis, spinal cord injury, hemispherectomy, and stroke.[68-71] Despite the wide variety of peripheral nervous system and CNS tissue damage that can lead to neuropathic pain, there are surprising similarities in symptoms across syndromes. Virtually all neuropathic pain syndromes are characterized by spontaneous ongoing pain, hyperalgesia (increased sensitivity to normally painful stimuli), and tactile and thermal allodynia (pain evoked by normally nonpainful stimuli, such as lightly brushing or cooling the skin).[72]

Peripheral Neuropathic Pain

The specific causes of these various types of neuropathic pain are not well understood, but accumulating evidence suggests multiple and varied underlying mechanisms. For peripheral neuropathies, there is evidence suggesting that some symptoms can be accounted for either by the sensitization of primary afferent fibers normally responsive to noxious stimuli (Aδ or C fibers) or by the formation of neuromas that could also cause activation of primary afferent nociceptive fibers.[73] In neuropathic pain of peripheral origin, such as diabetic neuropathy, some patients have minimal sensory loss in the painful area but have severe allodynia, whereas others show the opposite greater sensory loss but a variable degree of allodynia. Fields and Rowbotham[73] propose that the main source of pain observed in patients with neuropathic pain with preserved sensation comes from aberrant primary afferent nociceptor activity ("irritable nociceptor"), whereas the pain seen in patients with impaired thermosensory and nociceptor function comes from an alteration of CNS activity ("deafferentation-type pain"). Changes in the CNS could involve structural reorganization, whereby previously nonexistent connections form between Aδ fibers and nociceptive neurons in the spinal cord[74] or could result from an interruption of thermal, or tactile, or both pathways that normally inhibit pain transmission.[52,53,75] Consistent with this latter possibility are positron emission tomography studies showing a thalamic hypoperfusion in patients with neuropathic pain.[76]

Central Neuropathic Pain

Central neuropathic pain (CNP) is defined as pain caused by CNS damage along the spinothalamocortical pathway.[77] Investigators have proposed varied explanations for the pathophysiology underlying this syndrome, including: (1) aberrant bursting of nociceptive neurons in the thalamus or elsewhere,[78,79] (2) up-regulation or down-regulation of receptors for neurotransmitters, including GABAergic inhibition[80] and noradrenergic systems,[71] and (3) disinhibition of pain by damage to endogenous pain modulatory pathways.[53] Although clinical features of central pain are similar to those of peripheral neuropathic pain (PNP), there are a number of differences. First, emotional or physical stress exacerbates CNP in up to 50% of cases[71]; this phenomenon is seldom reported for PNP. Similarly, cold-evoked allodynia and exacerbation of ongoing pain in a cool environment is a much more common feature of CNP than PNP.[71,81] Bowsher[71] has also reported movement allodynia in 22% of patients with CNP. The most common description of the spontaneous pain of CNP is burning or scalding, with the second most common description being aching or throbbing. Although both of these symptoms are sometimes seen in PNP, they are more prevalent for CNP. Almost all patients with CNP have a deficit of pinprick, thermal sensation, or both (both subserved primarily by Aδ primary afferent fibers), whereas only some patients with PNP have such a deficit (see earlier).[71,81] Because in patients with CNP there is no peripheral nerve damage, the sensory deficit most likely arises from a disturbance of central processing of information arising from these inputs.

Cellular and Molecular Changes in the Peripheral Nociceptive System

Nerve injury initially induces a host of reactions involving inflammatory substances. Longer lasting modifications of neuronal physiology include a decrease in availability of growth factors that normally regulate concentrations of neuropeptide transmitters. This results in a disruption in communication between the cell body and its target (nerve ending) with a possible profound change in the sensory neuron phenotype. Another possible effect of nerve damage is a dedifferentiation of Schwann cell resulting in a decrease in production of myelin and growth factors, and a modification of sodium channel expression. These effects disrupt the equilibrium between the neuron and its environment and can initiate profound changes in sensory function.[72,82]

Spontaneous pain can result from a proliferation of sodium channels in injured axons. There are two types of sodium channels that can be differentiated by their response to tetrodotoxin, a toxin extracted from the pufferfish. Tetrodotoxin-sensitive channels are found in all sensory neurons, whereas the tetrodotoxin-insensitive type is found only on nociceptor neurons. The accumulation of the latter could be responsible for hyperexcitability and ectopic action potential discharge in C and Aβ fibers, both injured and uninjured.[83]

After nerve injury, proliferation of α-adrenoreceptors in both injured and intact neurons or sprouting of sympathetic neurons into the dorsal root ganglion has been described and could provide a mechanistic explanation for sympathetically mediated pain.[84]

Neuropathic Pain Induces Changes in the Dorsal Horn

Neuropathic pain results, at least partially, from ongoing firing of C fibers that induces central sensitization. The pivotal role of NMDA receptors in this mechanism offers interesting therapeutic opportunities. However, the dorsal horn undergoes more profound neurochemical and plastic changes that further complicate the pathophysiology.

It has been suggested that peripheral nerve injury reduces the inhibitory control of dorsal horn neurons as a consequence of reduced γ-aminobutyric acid (GABA) concentrations and down-regulation of GABA and opioid receptors. This mechanism would exert its effects presynaptically on primary sensory neurons and postsynaptically on dorsal horn neurons. It could allow for spontaneous firing of dorsal horn neurons and could be a cause of stimulus-independent pain.[72]

One of the most striking plastic change occurs in lamina II of the dorsal horn, which usually receives only nociceptive information from C fibers. Peripheral nerve damage to C fibers induces sprouting of Aβ (non-nociceptive) fibers into lamina II[85] that starts to receive non-nociceptive information that could be misinterpreted as nociceptive and contributing to the persistence of allodynia.

Other changes in the dorsal horn physiology are related to substance P. It has been suggested by Mantyh and colleagues[86] that SP is only released during conditions in which severe pain would be produced. This is true of somatic and visceral tissue, and multiple modalities are effective. This group also reported that in a rodent model of cancer pain there was a profound induction of glial cells throughout the ipsilateral dorsal horn. Moreover, light palpation of the painful area provoked an immediate withdrawal response (indicating mechanical allodynia), accompanied by a dramatic increase in the number of receptors that internalized substance P receptors, offering another possible mechanistic explanation for mechanical allodynia.

Treatment

The characterization of neurobiologic changes occurring in neuropathic pain provides the clinician with potential targets and a rationale for treatment. Antidepressants are used for membrane stabilization through sodium channel blockade but can also exert their action through a modulation of serotoninergic and noradrenergic descending inhibitory pathways. In addition, their cortical action might influence the effective aspects of pain perception. Antiepileptics, such as carbamazepine and gabapentin, are used for their membrane stabilization properties. Carbamazepine is especially useful in trigeminal neuralgia. Another promising path is offered with antagonists of NMDA receptors that show an enhanced activity profile in the context of central sensitization. Ketamine is the only typical drug of this type currently available clinically, and its side effect pattern limits its use. However, this treatment modality will be used more widely when newer, safer agents become available. Dextromethorphan also acts as a weak NMDA blocker, but has a low affinity for the receptor. Levodopa has been used in some clinical trials for its effects on dopaminergic pathways, and capsaicin has been shown to effect substance P release and has been used with some success in diverse peripheral neuropathic syndromes. Finally, modulation of the postsynaptic response can be achieved by hyperpolarization of the dorsal horn cell through the activation of $GABA_B$ and μ-opioid receptors with baclofen and narcotics (see Sindrup and Jensen[87]).

Although the multiplicity of targets offers a potential opportunity for alternative or complementary drug therapy, it is also a reflection of the elusive nature of pain. The symptomatology can materialize using so many routes that the clinician is more than occasionally faced with failure, even if a multiple drug regimen is used. This was eloquently illustrated in recent review on the efficacy of pharmacologic treatments of neuropathic pain using numbers needed to treat to obtain one patient with more than 50% pain relief. The reported numbers needed to treat are rarely less than two, a reflection of our inability to offer proper treatment to a majority of patients.[87]

Moreover, even if our understanding of the physiopathology of pain has progressed significantly, we know little about pain-induced cortical plasticity or about the influence of affective and emotional states on pain perception. Although depression, fatigue, demotivation, and altered activity pattern is very often found in the context of chronic pain,[88] it is often impossible to determine whether the pain or the emotional/motivational status is the cause or the consequence in the persistence of the symptomatology.

Finally, pain is reported, analyzed, and rated using sophisticated questionnaires, scales, and behavioral measures. Intensity and unpleasantness are useful correlates of perceptive and affective/motivational aspects of pain and are used for the determination of treatment efficacy. However, these sophisticated measures remain subjective, and by nature are susceptible to bias in reporting and interpretation. Until the advent of an objective biologic tool allowing reliable measurement of the amount of pain that is transmitted or perceived by a given patient, a number of cases will exist for which functional solutions will be hard to find.

References

1. Price DD: Psychological and neural mechanisms of the affective dimension of pain. Science 288:1769–1772, 2000.
2. Sandin RH, Enlund G, Samuelsson P, Lennmarken C: Awareness during anesthesia: A prospective case study. Lancet 355:707–711, 2001.
3. Willis WD, Coggeshall RE: Sensory mechanisms of the spinal cord. New York, Plenum Press, 1991.
4. Rexed B: The cytoarchitectonic organization of the spinal cord in the cat. J Comp Neurol 96:415–495, 1952.
5. Cervero F: Visceral nociception: Peripheral and central aspects of visceral nociceptive systems. Phil Trans R Soc Lond B Biol Sci 308:325–337, 1985.
6. Head H: On disturbances of sensation with special reference to the pain of visceral disease. Brain 16:1132, 1893.
7. Al-Chaer ED, Lawand NB, Westlund KN, Willis WD: Pelvic visceral input into the nucleus gracilis is largely mediated by the postsynaptic dorsal column pathway. J Neurophysiol 76:2675–2690, 1996.
8. Schneider SP, Perl ER: Selective excitation of neurons in the mammalian spinal dorsal horn by aspartate and glutamate in vitro: Correlation with location and excitatory input. Brain Res 360:339–343, 1985.
9. Dray A, Urban L, Dickenson A: Pharmacology of chronic pain. Trends Pharmacol Sci 15:190–197, 1994.
10. Watkins JC, Evans RH: Excitatory amino acid transmitters. Annu Rev Pharmacol Toxicol 21:165–204, 1981.
11. Willis WD, Westlund KN: Neuroanatomy of the pain system and of the pathways that modulate pain. J Clin Neurophysiol 14:2–31, 1997.
12. Willis WD, Kenshalo DR, Leonard RB: The cells of origin of the primate spinothalamic tract. J Comp Neurol 188:543–574, 1979.
13. Apkarian AV, Hodge CJ: Primate spinothalamic pathways: I. A quantitative study of the cells of origin of the spinothalamic pathways. J Comp Neurol 288:447–473, 1989.
14. Craig AD, Bushnell MC, Zhang E-T, Blomqvist A: A specific thalamic nucleus for pain and temperature sensation in macaques and humans. Nature 372:770–773, 1994.
15. Trevino DL: The origin and projections of a spinal nociceptive and thermoceptive pathway. In Zotterman Y (ed): Sensory function of the skin in primates, with a special reference to man. New York, Pergamon Press, 1976, pp 367–376.
16. Mantyh PW: The ascending input to the midbrain periaqueductal gray of the primate. J Comp Neurol 211:50–64, 2001.
17. Mehler WR: The anatomy of the so-called "pain tract" in man: An analysis of the course and distribution of the ascending fibers of the fasciculus anterolateralis. In French JD, Porter RW, (eds): Basic Research in Paraplegia. Springfield, Ill., Charles C Thomas, 1962, pp 26–55.
18. Kerr FWL: The ventral spinothalamic tract and other ascending systems of the ventral funiculus of the spinal cord. J Comp Neurol 159:335–356, 2001.
19. Kevetter GA, Haber LH, Yezierski RP, et al: Cells of origin of the spinoreticular tract in the monkey. J Comp Neurol 207:61–74, 2001.
20. Burstein R, Cliffer KD, Giesler GJ: Cells of origin of the spinohypothalamic tract in the rat. J Comp Neurol 291:329–344, 1990.
21. Bernard JF, Besson JM: The spino(trigemino)pontoamygdaloid pathway: Electrophysiological evidence for an involvement in pain processes. J Neurophysiol 63:473–490, 1990.
22. Ménétrey D, de Pommery J: Origins of the spinal ascending pathways that reach central areas involved in visceroception and visceronociception in the rat. Eur J Neurosci 3:249–259, 1991.
23. Ha H: Cervicothalamic tract in the Rhesus monkey. Exp Neurol 33:205–212, 1971.
24. Rustioni A, Hayes NL, O'Neill S: Dorsal column nuclei and ascending spinal afferents in macaques. Brain 102:95–125, 1979.
25. Al-Chaer ED, Lawand NB, Westlund KN, Willis WD: Visceral nociceptive input into the ventral posterolateral nucleus of the thalamus: A new function for the dorsal column pathway. J Neurophysiol 76:2661–2674, 1996.
26. Bushnell MC, Duncan GH: Sensory and affective aspects of pain perception: Is medial thalamus restricted to emotional issues? Exp Brain Res 78:415–418, 1989.
27. Lenz FA, Dougherty PM: Pain processing in the human thalamus. In Steriade M, Jones EG, McCormick DA (eds): Thalamus: Experimental and Clinical Aspects. Amsterdam, Elsevier, 1997, pp 617–651.
28. Bushnell MC, Duncan GH, Tremblay N: Thalamic VPM nucleus in the behaving monkey. I. Multimodal and discriminative properties of the thermosensitive neurons. J Neurophysiol 69:739–752, 1993.
29. Bushnell MC: Thalamic processing of sensory-discriminative and affective-motivational dimensions of pain. In Besson JM, Guilbaud G, Ollat H (eds): Forebrain areas involved in pain processing. Paris, John Libbey Eurotext, 1995, pp 63–77.
30. Rausell E, Jones EG: Chemically distinct compartments of the thalamic VPM nucleus in monkeys relay principal and spinal trigeminal pathways to different layers of the somatosensory cortex. J Neurosci 11:226–237, 1991.
31. Rausell E, Bae CS, Viñuela A, et al: Calbindin and parvalbumin cells in monkey VPL thalamic nucleus: Distribution, laminar cortical projections, and relations to spinothalamic terminations. J Neurosci 12:4068–4111, 1992.
32. Musil SY, Olson CR: Organization of cortical and subcortical projections to anterior cingulate cortex in the cat. J Comp Neurol 272:203–218, 1988.
33. Vogt BA, Pandya DN, Rosene DL: Cingulate cortex of the rhesus monkey: I. Cytoarchitecture and thalamic afferents. J Comp Neurol 262:256–270, 1987.
34. Talbot JD, Marret S, Evans AC, et al: Multiple representations of pain in human cerebral cortex. Science 251:1355–1357, 1991.
35. Coghill RC, Talbot JD, Evans AC, et al: Distributed processing of pain and vibration by the human brain. J Neurosci 14:4095–4108, 1994.

36. Casey KL, Minoshima S, Berger KL, et al: Positron emission tomographic analysis of cerebral structures activated specifically by repetitive noxious heat stimuli. J Neurophysiol 71:802–807, 1994.

37. Jones AKP, Brown WJ, Friston KJ, et al: Cortical and subcortical localization of response to pain in man using positron emission tomography. Proc R Soc Lond B Biol Sci 244:39–44, 1991.

38. Bushnell MC, Duncan GH, Ha B, et al: Non-invasive brain imaging during experimental and clinical pain. In Proceedings of the 8th World Congress on Pain. Seattle, IASP Press, 2000, pp 485–495.

39. Bushnell MC, Duncan GH, Hofbauer RK, et al: Pain perception: Is there a role for primary somatosensory cortex? Proc Natl Acad Sci USA 96:7705–7709, 1999.

40. Rainville P, Carrier B, Hofbauer RK, et al: Dissociation of sensory and affective dimensions of pain using hypnotic modulation. Pain 82:159–171, 1999.

41. Rainville P, Duncan GH, Price DD, et al: Pain affect encoded in human anterior cingulate but not somatosensory cortex. Science 277:968–971, 1997.

42. Hofbauer RK, Rainville P, Duncan GH, Bushnell MC: Cortical representation of the sensory dimension of pain. J Neurophysiol 86:402–411, 2001.

43. Friedman DP, Murray EA, O'Neill JB, Mishkin M: Cortical connections of the somatosensory fields of the lateral sulcus of macaques: Evidence for a corticolimbic pathway for touch. J Comp Neurol 252:323–347, 1986.

44. Vogt BA, Rosene DL, Pandya DN: Thalamic and cortical afferents differentiate anterior from posterior cingulate cortex in the monkey. Science 204:205–207, 1979.

45. Tolle TR, Kaufman T, Seismeier T, et al: Region-specific encoding of sensory and affective components of pain in the human brain: a positron emission tomography correlation analysis. Ann Neurol 45:40–47, 1999.

46. Basbaum AI, Fields HL: Endogenous pain control systems: Brainstem spinal pathways and endorphin circuitry. Ann Rev Neurosci 7:309–338, 2001.

47. Carsten E, Yokota T, Zimmermann M: Inhibition of spinal neuronal responses to noxious skin heating by stimulation of mesencephalic periaqueductal gray in the cat. J Neurophysiol 42:558–568, 1979.

48. Cameron AA, Khan IA, Westlund KN, Willis WD: The efferent projections of the periaqueductal gray in the rat: A *Phaseolus vulgaris*-leucoagglutinin study. II. Descending projections. J Comp Neurol 351:585–601, 1995.

49. Rees H, Roberts MHT: The antinociceptive effects of stimulating the pretectal nucleus of the rat. Pain 25:83–93, 1986.

50. Gerhart KD, Yezierski RP, Fang ZR: Inhibition of primate spinothalamic tract neurons by stimulation in ventral posterior lateral (VPL$_c$) thalamic nucleus: Possible mechanisms. J Neurophysiol 49:406–423, 1983.

51. Tsubokawa T, Yamamoto T, Katayama Y, Noriyaso N: Clinical results and physiological basis of thalamic relay nucleus stimulation for relief of intractable pain with morphine tolerance. Appl Neurophysiol 45:143–155, 1982.

52. Melzak R, Wall P: Pain mechanisms: A new theory. Science 150:971–979, 1965.

53. Craig AD, Bushnell MC: The thermal grill illusion: Unmasking the burn of cold pain. Science 265:252–255, 1994.

54. Treede R-D, Meyer RA, Raja SN, Campbell JN: Peripheral and central mechanisms of cutaneous hyperalgesia. Prog Neurobiol 38:397–421, 1992.

55. Rang HP, Bevan S, Dray A: Chemical activation of nociceptive peripheral neurons. Br Med Bull 47:534–538, 1991.

56. Dahl JB, Kehlet H: Non-steroidal anti-inflammatory drugs: Rationale for use in severe postoperative pain. Br J Anaesth 66:703–712, 1991.

57. Woolf CJ, Chong M-S: Preemptive analgesia: Treating postoperative pain by preventing the establishment of central sensitization. Anesth Analg 77:362–379, 1993.

58. Thompson SWN, King AE, Woolf CJ: Activity-dependent changes in rat ventral horn neurons in vitro; Summation of prolonged afferent evoked postsynaptic depolarizations produce a D-2-amino-5-phosphonovaleric acid sensitive windup. Eur J Neurosci 2:638–649, 1990.

59. Nagy I, Maggi CA, Dray A, et al: The role of neurokinin and N-methyl-D-aspartate receptors in synaptic transmission from capsaicin-sensitive primary afferents in the rat spinal cord in vitro. Neuroscience 52:1029–1037, 1993.

60. Wall PD: The prevention of postoperative pain. Pain 33:289–290, 1988.

61. Dickenson AH: Mechanisms of the analgesic actions of opiates and opioids. Br Med Bull 47:690–702, 1991.

62. Kissin I: Preemptive analgesia. Why its effect is not always obvious. Anesthesiology 84:1015–1019, 1996.

63. Taylor BK, Brennan TJ: Preemptive analgesia: Moving beyond conventional strategies and confusing terminology. J Pain 1:77–84, 2000.

64. Katz J: Preemptive analgesia: Where do we go from here? J Pain 1:89–92, 2000.

65. Flor H, Elbert T, Knecht S, et al: Phantom-limb pain as a perceptual correlate of cortical reorganization following arm amputation. Nature 375:482–484, 1995.

66. Price DD, Bennett GJ, Rafii A: Psychophysical observations on patients with neuropathic pain relieved by a sympathetic block. Pain 36:273–288, 2000.

67. Rowbotham MC, Fields HL: The relationship of pain, allodynia and thermal sensation in post-herpetic neuralgia. Brain 119:347–354, 1996.

68. Andersen G, Vestergaard K, Ingeman-Nielsen M, Jensen TS: Incidence of central post-stroke pain. Pain 61:187–193, 1995.

69. Bogousslavsky J, Regli F, Uske A: Thalamic infarcts: Clinical syndromes, etiology and prognosis. Neurology 38:837–848, 1988.

70. Boivie J, Leijon G: Clinical findings in patients with central poststroke pain. In Casey KL (eds): Pain and the Central Nervous System Disease: The Central Pain Syndrome. New York, Raven Press, 1991.

71. Bowsher D: Central pain: Clinical and physiological characteristics. J Neurol Neurosurg Psychiatry 61:62–69, 1996.

72. Woolf CJ, Mannion RJ: Neuropathic pain: Aetiology, symptoms, mechanisms and management. Lancet 353:1959–1964, 1999.

73. Fields HL, Rowbotham M: Postherpetic neuralgia: Irritable nociceptors and deafferentation. Neurobiol Dis 5:209–227, 1998.

74. Woolf CJ: The pathophysiology of peripheral neuropathic pain: Abnormal peripheral input and abnormal central processing. Acta Neurochir Suppl 58:125–130, 1993.

75. Duncan GH, Kupers RC, Marchand S, et al: Stimulation of human thalamus for pain relief: Possible modulatory circuits revealed by positron emission tomography. J Neurophysiol 80:3326–3330, 1998.

76. Iadarola J, Max MB, Berman KF, et al: Unilateral decrease in thalamic activity observed with positron emission tomography in patients with chronic neuropathic pain. Pain 63:55–64, 1995.

77. Casey KL: Pain and Central Nervous System Disease: The Central Pain Syndrome. New York, Raven Press, 1991.

78. Jeanmonod D, Magnin M, Morel A: Thalamus and neurogenic pain: Physiological, anatomical and clinical data. Neuroreport 4:475–478, 1993.

79. Lenz FA: The thalamus and central pain syndromes: Human and animal studies, pain and central nervous system disease. In Casey KL (ed): Pain and Central Nervous System Disease: The Central Pain Syndrome. New York, Raven Press, 1991.

80. Canavero S, Bonicalzi V: The neurochemistry of central pain: Evidence from clinical studies, hypothesis and therapeutic implications. Pain 74:109–114, 1998.

81. Boivie J, Leijon G, Johansson I: Central post-stroke pain: A study of the mechanisms through analyses of the sensory abnormalities. Pain 37:173–185, 1989.

82. Coderre TJ, Katz J, Vaccarino AL, Melzack R: Contribution of central neuroplasticity to pathological pain: Review of clinical and experimental evidence. Pain 52:259–285, 1993.

83. Novakovic SD, Tzoumaka E, McGivern JG, et al: Distribution of the tetrodotoxin-resistant sodium channel PN3 in rat sensory neurons in normal and neuropathic conditions. J Neurosci 18:2174–2187, 1998.

84. McLachlan EM, Janig W, Devor M, Michaelis M: Peripheral nerve injury triggers noradrenergic sprouting within the dorsal root ganglia. Nature 363:543–546, 1993.

85. Woolf CJ, Shortland P, Coggeshall RE: Peripheral nerve injury triggers central sprouting of myelinated afferents. Nature 355:75–78, 1992.

86. Schwei MJ, Honoré P, Rogers SD, et al: Neurochemical and cellular reorganization of the spinal cord in a murine model of bone cancer. J Neurosci 19:10886–10897, 1999.

87. Sindrup SH, Jensen TS: Efficacy of pharmacological treatments of neuropathic pain: An update and effect related to mechanism of drug action. Pain 83:389–400, 1999.

88. Ashbum MA, Staats PS: Management of chronic pain. Lancet 353:1865–1869, 1999.

17

Cardiac Rhythm

Jeffrey R. Balser, MD, PhD

Cardiac arrhythmias are one of the leading causes of morbidity and mortality in the industrialized world, and remain a significant complication in the period surrounding surgery and anesthesia. At the same time, existing antiarrhythmic drug therapies are plagued by poor efficacy and specificity, as well as toxicities that include genesis of new (and sometimes lethal) cardiac arrhythmias. Fortunately, our molecular understanding of the cardiac rhythm is expanding exponentially alongside recent advances toward defining the human genome. These developments have advanced the pace of investigation aimed at defining new molecular targets for manipulating the cardiac rhythm, with the promise of new and improved antiarrhythmic therapies. This chapter mirrors the companion chapters in this textbook, following a reductionist approach that first examines the electrophysiology of the heart at an organ and multicellular level, followed by a detailed discussion of the molecular targets that underlie the cardiac action potential in individual myocardial cells. This discussion on molecular targets serves as a mechanistic scaffold for Chapter 35, where the molecular pharmacology of specific antiarrhythmic agents is presented in detail.

Systems Physiology

Neural Control of the Heart Rhythm

Our information on the neural innervation and control of cardiac rhythm derives largely from canine models, which clarify that both sympathetic efferent fibers and vagal fibers course throughout the atria and ventricles. Vagal postganglionic neurons in the atrium and the sinoatrial (SA) and atrioventricular (AV) nodes underlie the parasympathetic effects on the heart rhythm. Parasympathetic stimulation causes release of acetylcholine, which alters the rhythmic firing of the SA and AV nodal cells through two complementary mechanisms.[1] First, through the inhibitory (guanine) regulatory protein G_i, adenyl cyclase activity is reduced, cyclic adenosine monophosphate (cAMP) concentrations decrease, and the phosphorylation of cardiac ion channels by cAMP-dependent protein kinase is attenuated. As such, the activity of L-type calcium (Ca^{2+}) channels

257

responsible for depolarization and excitation of SA and AV nodal tissue is depressed (see "Ca^{2+} channels [I$_{Ca}$]"). Second, adenosine stimulates potassium channels (see "Cardiac Inward Rectifiers") that hyperpolarize the SA and AV nodal cell membranes, driving the cells further away from their firing threshold. These combined actions cause the SA node firing rate to slow, and also produce AV nodal blockade; moreover, selective vagal denervation of the atria, SA, and AV nodes reduces minute-to-minute heart rate variability, and eliminates heart rate-baroreflex sensitivity. Notably, efferent vagal fibers that innervate the ventricular chambers travel separately, and as such, reflex-mediated autonomic changes in the SA node firing rate are not necessarily manifest in the ventricles.[2]

The sympathetic nervous system stimulates both heart rate and contractility through sympathetic efferent fibers that course through the superficial epicardium of the atria and ventricles, as well as the SA and AV nodes. Catecholamines, released from the sympathetic nerve terminal (or administered systemically) bind to β1 adrenergic receptors, which in turn activate stimulatory guanine regulatory proteins (G$_s$) that activate adenyl cyclase, increasing intracellular cAMP, and activating cAMP-dependent protein kinase.[1] This in turn augments the activity of L-type Ca^{2+} channels in the SA and AV nodes, increasing the rate of firing by these nodal cells. At the same time, the increased Ca^{2+} channel activity in the ventricular myocytes leads to a higher intracellular Ca^{2+} concentration, with greater excitation-contraction coupling, and a positive inotropic effect.

Organ Physiology

Conduction Pathway

Our understanding of how drugs may be used to intervene in particular cardiac arrhythmias, and how these agents modify the configuration of the electrocardiogram (ECG), is largely based on the structure and physiology of the cardiac conduction pathway. The cardiac impulse normally arises in the SA node, and passes through the atria to enter the AV node. Impulses that successfully navigate the AV node enter the specialized conduction system that includes the His bundle, the major bundle branches, and the arborizing Pürkinje fiber network; this system spreads the impulse into the ventricular myocardium. Agents or conditions that impede conduction from the sinus node to (or through) the AV node prolong the interval from the P wave (which represents atrial systole) to the QRS complex (which represents ventricular systole), manifest as the "PR" interval on the ECG (Fig. 17–1). Conversely, conditions that prolong or modify conduction through the specialized conduction system usually lengthen the QRS complex, and sometimes slur the upstroke (R wave) of this complex (see "Accessory Pathways" below).

Although the mechanistic details of each supraventricular arrhythmia are beyond the scope of this chapter, the role of the conduction system in arrhythmogenesis is nicely exemplified by the rhythm-specific action of adenosine (Table 17–1), which transiently blocks conduction within

TABLE 17–1.

The Response of Commons Supraventricular Tachyarrhythmias to Intravenous Adenosine

Rhythm	Mechanism	Adenosine Response
AV nodal reentry	Reentry within AV node	Termination
AV reciprocating tachycardias (orthodromic and antidromic)	Reentry involving AV node and accessory pathway (WPW)	Termination
Intra-atrial reentry	Re-entry in the atrium	Transiently slows ventricular response
Atrial flutter/fibrillation	Re-entry in the atrium	Transiently slows ventricular response
Other atrial tachycardias	1. Abnormal automaticity 2. cAMP-mediated triggered activity	1. Transient suppression of the tachycardia 2. Termination
AV junctional rhythms	Variable	Variable
Ventricular arrhythmias	Re-entry or automaticity	No response

AV, atrioventricular; cAMP, cyclic adenosine monophosphate; WPW, Wolff-Parkinson-White syndrome.
Adapted from Balser JR: Perioperative management of arrhythmias. In Barash PG, Fleisher LA, Prough DS (eds): Problems in Anesthesia. Philadelphia, Lippincott-Raven, 1998, p 201.

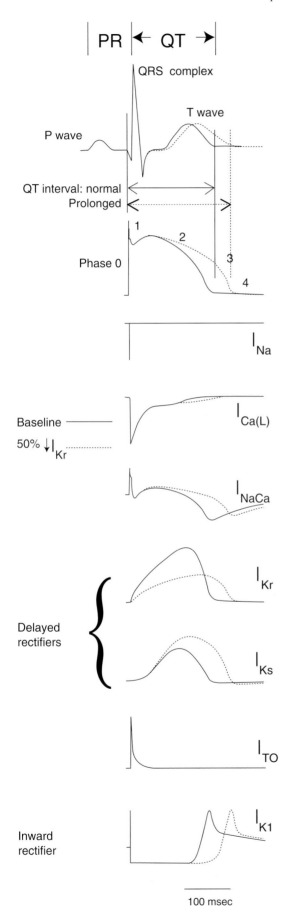

Figure 17–1. The action potential in ventricular muscle and its temporal relationship with the surface electrocardiogram. The PR interval indicates the time required for conduction of the impulse through the atrium and the atrioventricular node. The duration of the QRS complex is related to the rate of upstroke of the action potential, which partly determines the rate of impulse conduction through the ventricular myocardium. The QT interval is related to the duration of the action potential (the refractory period). The phases of the action potential are indicated, as are the major ionic currents that flow during each phase (*below*). The individual ionic currents were computed using the Luo-Rudy formalism.[203] *Solid lines* represent the baseline, and *dotted lines* represent the computation when I_{Kr} is reduced by 50%. Note that this change not only prolongs action potential duration (APD) (as expected), but also generates changes in the time course of I_{Ca-L}, I_{Ks}, and the sodium-calcium exchange current, each one of which thus also modulates the effect of reduced I_{Kr} on the APD. The amplitudes of the currents are not drawn to scale. (From Roden DM, Balser JR, Geroge A, et al: Cardiac ion channels. Annu Rev Physiol 64:431–475, 2002.)

the AV node. This characteristic feature makes adenosine a choice agent for terminating supraventricular tachycardia (SVT) that originates in the AV node (or involve the AV node in a reentrant pathway).[3] Conversely, rhythms that originate in atrial tissue above the AV node, including atrial flutter or fibrillation, as well as paroxysmal rhythms stimulated by unopposed catecholamines, respond to adenosine only with transient slowing of the ventricular response rate, because the passage of impulses from the atrium to the ventricle through the AV node is slowed. Junctional tachycardia, common during the surgical period, arises in the specialized conduction system, and may convert to sinus rhythm in response to adenosine only if it originates very close to the AV node, but is otherwise unresponsive. Ventricular arrhythmias usually exhibit no response to adenosine, because these rhythms originate in tissues distal to the AV node.

Reentrant Arrhythmias

Reentry is a mechanism that may precipitate a wide variety of supraventricular and ventricular arrhythmias, and implies the existence of a pathologic circus movement of electrical impulses around an anatomic loop, or around a "functional" loop generated by pathologic conductions that transiently block conduction through a segment of myocardium (i.e., ischemia). Fibrillation, in either the atrium or ventricle, is believed to involve multiple coexistent reentrant circuits of the functional type. A classic form of anatomic reentry elicits paroxysmal supraventricular tachycardia (PSVT), and derives from reentrant circuits through abnormal accessory pathways (congenital electrical connections between the atrium and ventricle that bypass the AV node). During sinus rhythm, forward (antegrade) conduction through the accessory pathway may produce ventricular pre-excitation on the ECG (known as Wolff-Parkinson-White syndrome, or WPW) with a short PR interval (<0.12 seconds), a slurred

QRS upstroke (delta wave), and a wide QRS complex. The QRS complex is modified because ventricular excitation, normally facilitated by the spread of impulses through the specialized conduction system and Pürkinje network, is "bypassed" by pre-excitation through the accessory bundle.

During PSVT, when the conduction circuit is antegrade through the AV node and retrograde through the accessory bundle, the QRS complex will be narrow; however, in 5% to 10% of cases the conduction is antegrade through the accessory bundle, producing a wide QRS complex that may be confused with ventricular tachycardia. Normally, PSVT does not provoke a marked deterioration in hemodynamic status. However, 10% to 35% of patients with Wolff-Parkinson-White syndrome eventually develop atrial fibrillation (AF), and an episode of PSVT sometimes precipitates AF. In this case, the rapid rate of atrial excitation (>300 impulses/min), normally transmitted to the ventricle after considerable "filtering" by the AV nodal system, may instead be transmitted to the ventricle through the accessory bundle at a rapid rate. The danger of inducing ventricular fibrillation in this scenario is exacerbated by treatment with classic AV nodal blocking agents (digoxin, Ca^{2+} channel blockers, beta-blockers, adenosine) because they reduce the accessory bundle refractory period. Intravenous procainamide, which slows conduction over the accessory bundle, is often the drug of choice for treating AF in this condition.

Our understanding of functional reentry and its pharmacologic termination by ion channel current suppression is far less complete. Drugs may terminate reentry through at least two mechanisms. Agents that suppress currents responsible for initiation of the cardiac action potential, such as the sodium (Na^+) current (see Fig. 17–1), may slow or block conduction in a reentrant pathway, and thus terminate an arrhythmia. Alternatively, interventions that prolong the cardiac action potential, such as potassium channel blockade (see Fig. 17–1), in turn prolong the refractory period of cells in a reentrant circuit, and thus "block" impulse propagation through the circuit. In clinical trials, agents operating through the latter mechanism have proven to be more successful in suppressing fibrillation in both the atrium[4] and ventricle.[5] Additional mechanisms are now under investigation that involve reentry between cell layers, and depend on layer-specific differences in cellular electrophysiology that are discussed here in greater detail.

Cellular Physiology

Cardiac Action Potential

The earlier discussion alludes to the fact that the effects of conditions and interventions on the surface ECG can be predicted from their effects on the cardiac action potential, which in turn result from their ensemble effects on any number of ionic currents (see Fig. 17–1). The action potential represents the time-varying transmembrane potential of the myocardial cell during the cardiac cycle. As such, the ECG can be viewed as the ensemble average of the action potentials arising from all myocardial cells, and is biased

toward the activity of the left ventricle because of its greater overall mass. The trajectory of the cardiac action potential is divided into five distinct phases, which reflect changes in the predominant ionic current flowing during the cardiac cycle (see Fig. 17–1). The current responsible for "phase 0," the initial period of the action potential, propagates impulses through cardiac tissue. In the atria and the ventricles, the impulse is initiated by sodium current (I_{Na}) through Na^+ channels. Hence drugs that suppress Na^+ current (the local anesthetic-type drugs, such as lidocaine) slow myocardial conduction and prolong the QRS complex (ventricle) and the P wave (atrium). In AV and SA nodal cells (not shown in Fig. 17–1), phase 0 is actually produced by Ca^{2+} current through L-type Ca^{2+} channels, and not through Na^+ current. Hence drugs that suppress Ca^{2+} current indirectly or directly (beta-blockers and Ca^{2+} channel blockers, respectively) slow the heart rate by acting on the SA node, and also prolong the PR interval by slowing conduction through the AV node. The latter effect renders the AV node a more efficient "filter" for preventing rapid trains of atrial beats from passing into the ventricle; hence the rationale for AV nodal blockade during SVT.

The later phases of the action potential (1, 2, and 3; see Fig. 17–1) inscribe repolarization. Although an electrophysiologic curiosity for years, the early "notch" of repolarization during phase 1 is induced by the transient outward current (I_{to}) and seems to be present to varying degrees in the different cell layers (greater in epicardium than endocardium). This gradient between layers may have proarrhythmic implications during conditions that modify the Na^+ current during phase 0 (see "Layer-Specific Electrophysiology and Arrhythmias" for detailed discussion). The long plateau (phase 2) is maintained by Ca^{2+} current and is terminated (phase 3) by a number of K^+ currents. Hence the QT interval on the ECG reflects the length of the action potential and is determined by a delicate balance between these and many other smaller inward and outward currents. Drugs that reduce Ca^{2+} current tend to abbreviate the action potential plateau, shorten the QT, and reduce the inward movement of Ca^{2+} into the cardiac cell (hence the negative inotropic effect). Conversely, agents that block outward K^+ current prolong the action potential and the QT interval on the ECG. Notably, electrophysiologic behavior of all the voltage-gated ion channels is linked to the configuration of the cardiac action potential; hence when an intervention modifies the time-varying behavior of a single ion channel (i.e., K^+ channel blockade), the behavior of all other time-varying ionic currents is modified (see Fig. 17–1). In K^+ channel blockade and QT prolongation, these complex effects on the other ionic currents may be either therapeutic or arrhythmogenic (see discussion in "Automaticity and Arrhythmias").

Layer-Specific Electrophysiology and Arrhythmias

Clinical trials have shown that suppression of I_{Na} during conditions of ischemia may exacerbate ventricular arrhythmias.[6] An inherited idiopathic ventricular arrhythmia, the "Brugada Syndrome,"[7] provides a model system for understanding how Na^+ channel blockade and layer-specific differences in cellular electrophysiology may interact to generate arrhythmias through "functional" reentry. Patients with the Brugada syndrome have an abnormal ECG pattern that includes ST-segment elevation in the right precordial leads (resembling an ischemic pattern, Fig. 17–2) and a right bundle branch block. These patients experience unanticipated cardiac arrest caused by ventricular fibrillation. It was recently shown that a kindred of patients with the Brugada syndrome carry mutations in the gene encoding the cardiac Na^+ channel (*SCN5A* on chromosome 3; see Tables 17–2 and 17–3) that leads in some cases to a loss of Na^+ current during phase 0 of the action potential.[8] Moreover, treatment of these patients with sodium channel blockers (procainamide, flecainide) worsens the ST-segment elevation.

Mechanistic insight into how a loss of Na^+ channel function (either genetic or pharmacologic) may induce reentry between cell layers and ventricular fibrillation predates the Brugada syndrome-Na^+ channel linkage studies (see Fig. 17–2).[9,10] In short, the duration of the epicardial myocardial cell action potential is more "sensitive" to a reduction in I_{Na} than is the endocardial action potential. In the epicardium, a prominent transient outward potassium current (I_{to}; see Fig. 17–1) counterbalances I_{Na} during the earliest phases of the action potential; hence any misadventure that reduces Na^+ current (ischemia,[11] "class I" antiarrhythmic drugs,[12,13] or Na^+ channel mutations[12]) can trigger "all or none" repolarization in the epicardium, grotesquely shrinking the duration of the epicardial action potential. This condition creates a temporal imbalance between endocardial and epicardial repolarization, and such heterogeneity across the right ventricular outflow tract may engender reentry and thus explain the ECG pattern and arrhythmic manifestations of the Brugada syndrome.[12] It has been proposed that this mechanism may underlie the proarrhythmic toxicity of

potent Na^+ channel blockers in large-scale clinical trials, such as the Cardiac Arrhythmias Suppression Trial (CAST),[6] particularly because outcome in that trial was exaggerated by ischemia, a condition also linked to Na^+ current depression.

Automaticity and Arrhythmias

Automaticity refers to abnormal depolarization of atrial or ventricular muscle cells during periods of the action potential normally characterized by repolarization (see Fig. 17–1, phases 2 or 3) or rest (see Fig. 17–1, phase 4). A pathologic process such as ischemia may cause a gradual increase in the rate of phase 4 depolarization and may induce the ventricular tachycardias seen in the days after myocardial infarction.[14] More striking depolarizations that occur during phase 2 or 3 (early afterdepolarization, or EAD) or phase 4 (delayed afterdepolarization, or DAD) are known as *triggered automaticity*. Studies during the past decade have identified some of the key molecular substrates that underlie triggered automaticity.

K^+ channel blockade prolongs the duration of the action potential, and thus prolongs the QT interval on the ECG (see Fig. 17–1). In addition to pharmacologic reduction of K^+ current, low serum potassium ion (K^+) concentrations, hypomagnesemia, and slow heart rates all synergistically prolong the action potential. As a consequence of the sustained period required for full action potential repolarization, the time-dependent behavior of many ionic currents is modified (per Fig. 17–1). Specifically, the L-type Ca^{2+} currents have sufficient opportunity to "reactivate" during the latest phase of the action potential and may precipitate formation of EADs in vitro (Fig. 17–3, *top*).[15] These EADs may in turn precipitate the polymorphic ventricular tachycardia (Fig. 17–3, *bottom*) known as "torsade de pointes."[16] Recent studies have revealed inherited mutations in a number of cardiac ion channels that cause action potential prolongation. These mutations (see "Biochemical and Molecular Mechanisms Underlying Cellular Physiology" for detailed discussion; see also Table 17–3) are responsible for the congenital long QT (LQT) syndrome, inherited conditions where the QT interval is abnormally prolonged and the risk for sudden death from torsade de pointes is increased.[17] Hence the proarrhythmic aspects of QT-prolongation with drug therapy appear to be "acquired" analogues of the same basic molecular mechanisms operative in forms of the congenital LQT syndrome.[18]

DADs are a less understood form of triggered automaticity that are most common during conditions of intracellular calcium ion (Ca^{2+}) overload. Although many conditions induce intracellular Ca^{2+} overload, commonly recognized clinical entities are digitalis toxicity, excess catecholamine states (exercise, acute myocardial infarction, perioperative stress), and heart failure.[19] Digitalis toxicity produces Ca^{2+} overload indirectly; Na^+ overload is induced by direct inhibition of the Na^+-K^+ pump, and high intracellular Na^+ inhibits the normal Ca^{2+} extrusion from the cell by the Na^+-Ca^{2+} exchanger.[20] Catecholamines induce Ca^{2+} overload directly by increasing I_{Ca} through L-type Ca^{2+} channels,[21] which are up-regulated through protein kinase A

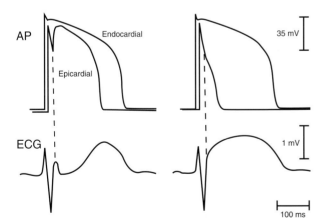

Figure 17–2. Hypothesized linkage between distinct epicardial and endocardial action potential (AP) morphologies in the right ventricular outflow tract and the Brugada electrocardiogram (ECG) phenotype. Epicardial and endocardial action potential morphologies are shown during normal conditions (*left*) and during conditions in which the Na^+ current in the epicardium is markedly reduced (*right*). Loss of I_{Na} may drastically shorten the epicardial AP duration, augmenting transmural heterogeneity and allowing ST-segment elevation in the surface ECG. (From Alings M, Wilde A: "Brugada" syndrome: Clinical data and suggested pathophysiological mechanism. Circulation 99:666–673, 1999.)

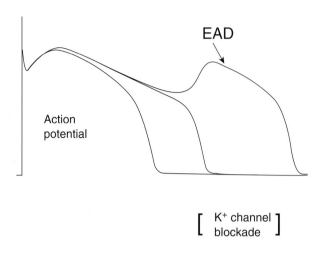

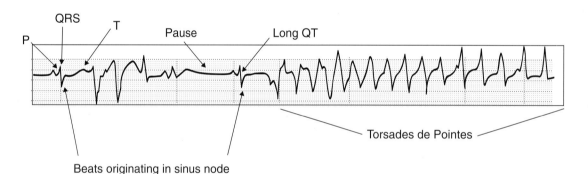

Figure 17–3. Early afterdepolarizations (EAD) and torsades de pointes. *Top,* On exposure to a K⁺-channel blocker, or with a reduction in extracellular potassium, the cardiac action potential gradually lengthens until an EAD is formed. These waveforms were generated using the Luo-Rudy formalism with incremental K⁺ current reduction[203] (Courtesy of Dr. Prakash Viswanathan, Vanderbilt University School of Medicine). The EAD, a form of triggered automaticity, is believed to precipitate polymorphic ventricular tachycardia. *Bottom,* The torsades de pointes arrhythmia that occurs in congenital long QT syndrome or on challenge with drugs that prolong the QT interval. The changes in cardiac cycle lengths before the initiation of the arrhythmia are typical and are consistent with suggested roles for EADs during the initiation and maintenance of the arrhythmia. (*Bottom,* From Roden DM, Balser JR, George AL, et al: Cardiac ion channels. Annu Rev Physiol 64:431–475, 2002.)

(PKA) through cardiac β₁ receptor stimulation.[22] In heart failure, a disruption of Ca²⁺ homeostasis may result from altered expression of a number of signaling molecules, including increased expression of the Ca²⁺/calmodulin-dependent protein kinase (CaMK).[23] Arrhythmias provoked by DADs should therefore be responsive to maneuvers aimed at lowering intracellular Ca²⁺, such as Ca²⁺ channel blockade.[24] Moreover, recent studies suggest that CaMK stimulates Ca²⁺ channel activity[25] and facilitates both EAD and DAD formation when the action potential is prolonged,[26,27] suggesting CaMK may prove to be a valuable drug target for managing triggered arrhythmias.

Cell-to-Cell Coupling and Gap Junctions

In addition to the ionic currents that inscribe the cardiac action potential, rapid propagation of the electrical wave front through cardiac muscle requires low resistance connections between individual cardiac myocytes. This is accomplished by specialized membrane protein complexes that form contacts between adjacent cells, creating conduits for intercellular passage of ions and other small molecules. The portion of this complex contributed by each cell is assembled from six connexins, small subunits that assemble into a hemichannel (a connexon) that spans the cell membrane. The end-to-end connection between the hexameric connexons in two adjacent cells occurs in the extracellular "gap" between myocytes, hence the term "gap junction." Hydropathy analysis predicts a structure for connexins that includes four hydrophobic domains and two extracellular loops, with intracellular N- and C-termini. Studies of the principal cardiac connexin isoform, α1 (termed Cx43), show that the gap junction function is regulated by intracellular pH, binding of hormones, intracellular Ca^{2+}, neurotransmitters, and phosphorylation by various kinases.[28] Hence the gap junction may either serve as an arrhythmogenic precipitant (during acidosis) or as a potential pharmacologic target.

Many cardiac connexin isoforms have been cloned, and their functional properties and distribution in the heart are distinctive.[28] Cx37 has the highest membrane conductance and the greatest voltage sensitivity, whereas Cx43 has the lowest conductivity. Cx40 and Cx43 have been localized in nodal tissues and the conduction system (Pürkinje fibers), whereas Cx45 is concentrated in the atrial and ventricular chambers. Expression also appears to be layer-specific, with Cx37 and Cx40 localizing to the endocardium, the endothelial cells, and blood vessels. These differences in distribution and functional behavior may partly underlie the marked differences in the rate of propagation of action potentials in various myocardial regions, such as the specialized conducting tissues (rapid) and the working myocardium (slow).

Biochemical and Molecular Mechanisms Underlying Cellular Physiology

Cardiac Ion Channels: General Characteristics of Structure and Function

The voltage-gated ion channels are primarily responsible for the maintenance of cardiac rhythm. These porelike molecules "sense" the transmembrane voltage, and open and close in a cyclical manner as the membrane field continually changes. Ionic current recordings from single and multiple ion channels through the "patch-clamp"[29] provided our first direct measurements of cardiac ion channel function. With the subsequent cloning of individual ion channel genes, it has been possible to begin to link ion channel structure to function. The Na^+ channel, first cloned from electric eel,[30] has a predicted structure that includes four homologous domains (I–IV), each containing six membrane-spanning segments (Fig. 17–4). This architecture is preserved in both the cardiac Na^+ and Ca^{2+} channels. In contrast, many of the voltage-gated cardiac K^+ channels are homologous to a single domain of the Na^+ or Ca^{2+} channel, and assemble as tetramers to generate the pore-forming structure. In addition, a number of smaller "β subunits" coassemble with these pore-forming "α" subunits and modulate key elements of ion channel function.

A number of approaches have been used to discern the structure-function relationships in cloned, voltage-gated ion channels. The principal approach has been to use site-directed mutagenesis to modify individual amino acid residues in the primary channel sequence, and then to assess the effects of these structure-altering mutations on gating function using patch-clamp methods. More recently, the methods of structural biology have begun to provide high-resolution three-dimensional structures of ion channels, such as the bacterial inward rectifier K^+ channel KcsA.[31] These defined structures of noncardiac channels serve as powerful anchors for hypotheses regarding structure and function in the homologous cardiac ion channels.

The ion channel structure must serve two primary, interrelated functions. First, the ion channel must provide a "path" for selective permeation of a particular ion species through the cell membrane (so-called permeation). Second, the channel must "gate" such that the permeation pathway is opened or closed during particular phases of the cardiac cycle, depending on the transmembrane voltage.[32] It is now apparent that the permeation pathway involves both external and internal segments. The loop connecting the 5th and 6th membrane spanning α helices (S5 and S6; see Fig. 17–4) reenters the membrane to form the P-loop, a structure that lines the outer pore.[33–35] The pore region of virtually all K^+-selective channels includes a signature GXG (GYG, GFG, or GLG) motif that forms the selectivity filter, i.e., the region of the pore that allows the channel to discriminate among cations and selectively pass K^+. In contrast, mutagenesis studies indicate that the selectivity filter of Na^+ and Ca^{2+} channels is formed by a ring of four amino acids, each contributed by one P-loop from each of the four domains. In Ca^{2+} channels, this ring is made up of four glutamates at the same sequence-aligned position in each P-loop. In contrast, the selectivity filter in the Na^+ channel is generated by four different amino acids at these positions (D-E-K-A); notably, mutagenesis of the lysine (K) in the domain III P-loop renders Na^+ channels permeant to Ca^{2+}.[36] At the same time, studies of the K_{csA} structure[31] indicate that the four S6 segments form a teepee-like structure that forms the inner lining of the pore, and mutagenesis studies support a similar model of an S6 inner lining for both the Na^+ and Ca^{2+} channels.

Voltage-sensitive gating (Fig. 17–5) requires that ion channels open and close in response to the changing transmembrane field. In nearly all voltage-gated cardiac ion channels, the fourth membrane spanning segment (S4) of each six-membrane spanning domain includes a positive charge, arginine or lysine, at every third residue. This structural motif defines a "voltage sensor,"[37] and cysteine scanning mutagenesis experiments have shown that the S4 sensor couples the changing membrane potential to the rest of the channel structure by moving within a water-filled "canaliculus" in response to the voltage gradient (see Fig. 17–5).[38] On depolarization, the S4 segments move outward relative to the channel pore, and this initiates opening of the permeation pathway (so-called *activation* gating). In addition, many ion channels display the characteristic of *inactivation* gating, time-dependent entry into a nonconducting state during sustained depolarization. Inactivation provides a convenient means to terminate the flow of ionic current before the cell membrane fully repolarizes; hence the hallmark of inactivation is a slow decline of activated current during a sustained depolarization. Depolarization-induced inactivation, although delayed in time relative to pore

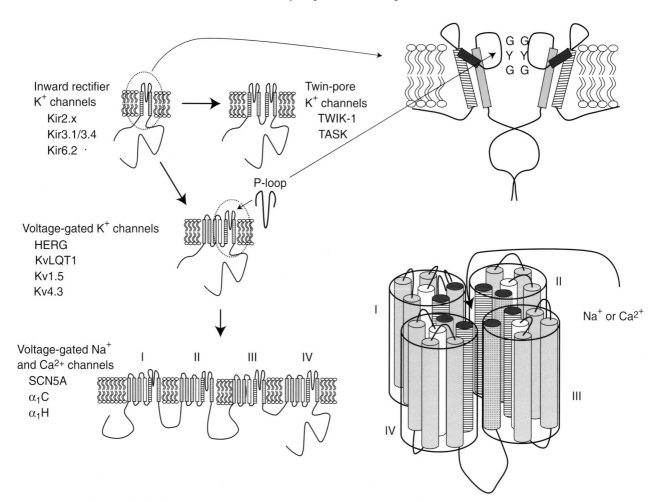

Figure 17–4. The topology of the voltage-gated ion channels in heart, presented from an "evolutionary view" of ion channel phylogeny. The inward rectifiers include only the pore region between the two membrane-spanning segments (*shaded*), and are presumably the most primitive ion channel structure. In this structure, a "P-loop" connecting the two transmembrane segments dips into the membrane and lines the outer pore. This P-loop structure is maintained in the voltage-gated K⁺ channels, which also include four additional transmembrane segments (S1-S4). The S4 transmembrane segment contains positively charged amino acids that "sense" the membrane potential (*unshaded segment*) and allow voltage-dependent gating. Gene duplication of the inward rectifier structure may also have led to the "twin pore" channels (TWIK, TASK). Voltage-gated Na⁺ and Ca²⁺ channels are assembled as four homologous domains (I–IV) that resemble the voltage-gated K⁺ channel. In the case of Na⁺, K⁺, and Ca²⁺ channels, these linear amino acid sequences assemble as tetrameric three-dimensional structures with four-fold symmetry to generate ion-permeant pores (*heavy arrow*), indicated at the *bottom right* (the P-loops are omitted for clarity). (From Roden DM, Balser JR, George AL, et al: Cardiac ion channels. Annu Rev Physiol 64:431–475, 2002.)

opening, is nonetheless initiated by the same S4 segment outward motion as activation gating.[39,40] Notably, multiple types of inactivation with varying time courses (fast, intermediate, slow) are manifest in cardiac ion channels, and a single ion channel may even enter more than one inactivated state during the cardiac cycle. Two general mechanisms of inactivation have been proposed (see Fig. 17–5): the original "ball-and-chain" model for one type of inactivation,[41] termed N-type inactivation, involves motion of a portion of the channel (often the N-terminus) to occlude the pore from inside the channel.[42,43] The other type of inactivation, termed C-type, usually proceeds more slowly than N-type, and involves a more complex rearrangement of residues in or

near the outer pore permeation pathway (P-loops), analogous to closing the shutter on a camera.[44,45] In this latter case, it becomes clear that the same amino acid residues may at once control features of both ion permeation and voltage-sensitive gating.

Cardiac Ion Channels: Specific Features of Structure and Function

With the completion of the human genome project, the identification of genes and gene products that comprise the

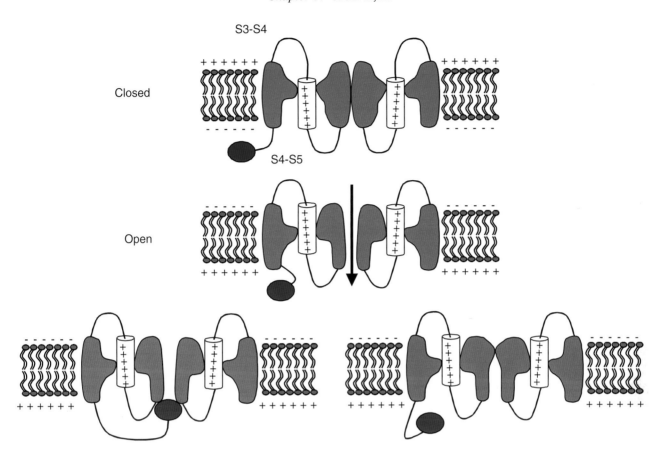

Figure 17–5. Schematic view of voltage-dependent gating in ion channels. Channels in the closed state are impermeant to cations. Channel opening ("activation") involves outward movement of the voltage sensor (S4) within a water-accessible crevice in the protein complex; this outward motion initiates a protein rearrangement that opens the channel, the details of which remain undefined. Outward motion of the S4 segment also initiates channel inactivation, which again renders the channel impermeant. Two major types of inactivation are shown: N-type (ball-and-chain) involves block of the intracellular end of the pore, whereas C-type inactivation involves an outer pore rearrangement that may constrict the permeation pathway. Inactivation can occur on multiple time scales, and may be rapid or slow compared with channel opening. (From Roden DM, Balser JR, George AL, et al: Cardiac ion channels. Annu Rev Physiol 64:431–475, 2002.)

cardiac ion channels is proceeding at a breathtaking pace. Table 17–2 indicates the genes identified to date[46] and their various protein products. Table 17–2 is organized to identify the gene products that underlie pharmacologically distinct ionic currents in heart, many of which are illustrated in Figure 17–1. In some cases, α subunits (pore-forming) and a number of associated β subunits are listed; notably, some β subunits may be associated with multiple α subunits (i.e., minK/I_{sK}). Studies are only now clarifying the key functional manifestations of these α and β subunit interrelationships, and the details of Table 17–2 should dramatically expand during the next decade.

Exciting insights into the linkages between cardiac rhythm, ion channel structure, and the genetic code have emerged from the study of monogenetic cardiac arrhythmia syndromes (Table 17–3). These include several varieties of the LQT syndrome, the idiopathic ventricular fibrillation syndromes, and genetic syndromes of conduction disease. These are discussed, with the relevant ion channels, in

"Channel Dysfunction in Disease." Although these syndromes affect only small segments of the general population, it is clear that the mechanisms they reveal are fundamentally related to common acquired arrhythmia syndromes. For example, the inherited LQT syndrome is a model for drug-induced QT prolongation that provokes torsades de pointes, whereas Brugada syndrome mutations may shed light on the mechanism of ischemia-induced reentry and ventricular tachycardia.

Na⁺ Channel (I_Na)

Structure and Function

The *SCN5A* gene on chromosome 3p21 encodes the cardiac Na⁺ channel α subunit, a 2016 amino acid polypeptide

TABLE 17–2.

Genes Encoding Cardiac Ion Channel α and β Subunits

Current	α Subunits		β Subunits	
	Gene	Human Chromosomal Location	Gene	Human Chromosomal Location
Inward Currents				
I_{Na}	SCN5A	3p21	β_1 (SCN1B) β_2 (SCN2B)	19q13.1–q13.2 11q23
I_{Ca-L}	α_1C (CACNL1A1)	12pter-p13.2	β_1 (CACNB1) β_2 (CACNB2) $\alpha_2\delta$ (CACNA2D1)	17q21–q22 10p12 7q21-22
I_{Ca-T}	α_1H (CACNA1H)	16p13.3		
Outward Currents				
I_{Ks}	KvLQT1 (KCNQ1)	11p15.5	minK/IsK (KCNE1)	21q22.12
I_{Kr}	HERG (KCNH2)	7q36-q36	minK/IsK (KCNE1) MiRP1 (KCNE2)	21q22.12 21q22.12
I_{Kur}	Kv1.5 (KCNA5)		Kvβ1 (KCNAB1) Kvβ2 (KCNAB2 ??)	3q26.1 1p36.3
I_{K1}	Kir2.1 (KCNJ2) Kir2.2 (KCNJ12)	17q 17p11.1		
I_{K-Ach}	GIRK1, Kir3.1 (KCNJ3) + GIRK4, Kir3.4 (KCNJ5)	2q24.1 11q24		
I_{K-ATP}	Kir6.2, BIR (KCNJ11)	11p15.1	SUR2 (ABCC9)	12p12.1
I_{TO}	Kv4.3 (KCND3) Kv1.4 (KCNA4)	1p13.2 11p14		
I_f, I_h (pacemaker current)	BCNG2, HCN2 HCN4	19p13.3 15q24-q25		
I_{Kp}	TWIK1 (KCNK1) CFTR (ABCC7) KvLQT1 (KCNQ1)	1q42-q43 7q31.2 11p15.5	MiRP1 (KCNE2)	21q22.12

"Common" names (usually first assigned) are given first, with the currently-designated gene name in parentheses. Information obtained from NCBI website (http://www.ncbi.nlm.nih.gov/), including LocusLink and OMIM, as well the Human Genome Nomenclature database (http://www.gene.ucl.ac.uk/nomenclature/).

From Roden DM, Balser JR, George AL, et al: Cardiac ion channels. Annu Rev Physiol 64:431–475, 2002.

TABLE 17–3.

Monogenic Cardiac Arrhythmia Syndromes Listed with Their Identified Genetic Substrates

	Disease Gene	Inheritance	Functional Consequences of Mutations	Key Clinical Features
Long QT Syndromes*↑				
LQT1	*KvLQT1 (KCNQ1)*	Autosomal dominant	$\downarrow I_{Ks}$	TdP with exertion or emotional stress; often beta-blocker responsive
LQT2	*HERG (KCNH2)*	Autosomal dominant	$\downarrow I_{Kr}$	TdP with stress, at rest, or with abrupt auditory stimulus
LQT3	*SCN5A*	Autosomal dominant	$\uparrow$plateau I_{Na}	Syncope/death at rest/sleep
LQT4	Unknown	Autosomal dominant	—	Bradycardia, atrial fibrillation
LQT5	*MinK/IsK (KCNE1)*	Autosomal dominant	$\downarrow I_{Ks}$	
LQT6	*MiRP1 (KCNE2)*	Autosomal dominant	$\downarrow I_{Kr}$	
JLN1	*KvLQT1 (KCNQ1)*	Autosomal recessive	$\downarrow\downarrow I_{Ks}$	Congenital deafness, severe arrhythmia symptoms in childhood
JLN2	*MinK/IsK (KCNE1)*	Autosomal recessive	$\downarrow\downarrow I_{Ks}$	Congenital deafness, severe arrhythmia symptoms in childhood
Idiopathic Ventricular Fibrillation (IVF) syndromes				
Brugada syndrome*	*SCN5A*	Autosomal dominant	$\uparrow I_{Na}$	Normal QT; right precordial ECG abnormalities; sudden death due to VF
Catecholamine-triggered VT with short QT	Cardiac ryanodine release channel (*RYR2*)	Autosomal dominant	Unknown; altered ($\uparrow$) $[Ca^{2+}]_i$ likely	Normal/short QT; bidirectional VT, polymorphic VT and VF with stress
Polymorphic VT with short QT	Unknown	Autosomal recessive		
Familial conduction system disease	*SCN5A*	Autosomal dominant	Multiple Na^+ channel gating defects (see text)	Atrioventricular block, often at a young age
Andersen syndrome	*Kir2.1 (KCNJ2)*			Bidirectional VT

*Indicates linkage has been reported to further loci, at which disease genes have not yet been identified.
↑The Romano-Ward syndrome describes the autosomal dominant forms of LQTS (LQT1–6), and Jervell-Lange-Nielsen syndrome (JLN), the autosomal recessive form with congenital deafness.
TdP, torsades de pointes; VF, ventricular fibrillation; VT, ventricular tachycardia.
From Roden DM, Balser JR, Geroge AL, et al: Cardiac ion channels. Annu Rev Physiol 64:431–475, 2002.

whose heterologous expression in *Xenopus* oocytes or mammalian cells recapitulates cardiac I_{Na}.[47] At least two ancillary subunits, β_1 and β_2, can be coimmunoprecipitated with brain Na$^+$ channel α subunits.[48] Although a role for β_2 in the heart is uncertain, most experimentalists find β_1 coexpression with wild-type or mutant *SCN5A* increases current amplitude, suggesting a potential role for β_1 in trafficking the α subunit to the cell membrane.[49] In addition, the β_1 subunit may have subtle functional effects on cardiac Na$^+$ channel inactivation gating.[49,50]

Mutation of three adjacent hydrophobic (isoleucine-phenylalanine-methionine, or IFM) residues in the cytoplasmic linker connecting domains III and IV disrupts the most rapid Na$^+$ channel inactivation gating process ("fast inactivation").[51] It is thus tempting to view the III–IV linker as a "lid" that closes over the inner vestibule (an N-type inactivation mechanism), and, in this context, the IFM motif as a "latch" that holds the inactivation gate shut. Nonetheless, peptide-binding studies suggest that inactivation may not involve simple occlusive block of the inner mouth of the pore[52]; rather, the III–IV linker may bind to a site on the channel that allosterically regulates or mediates pore closure. In either scheme, a number of modulatory or "docking" sites for fast inactivation have been identified near the cytoplasmic end of the pore, including the S4–S5 linker intracellular loops and residues in the cytoplasmic portion of the S6 segment.[53]

Channels that open and then rapidly inactivate can be reopened after even brief hyperpolarization that allows the channel to reassume the closed ("activatable") conformation. However, after prolonged depolarization, recovery does not occur with brief hyperpolarization, indicating the presence of other (slow) inactivated states.[54] Several lines of evidence suggest that this may be a form of C-type inactivation (see Fig. 17–5).[55] In particular, Na$^+$ channels engineered to include cysteine in P-loops of multiple domains can be shown to generate disulfide bonds during prolonged, but not brief, depolarization, indicating that the structural rearrangements required to enter slower inactivated states involve motion in the pore-lining segments.[56]

Regulation of I_{Na}

In vivo experiments show that chronic therapy with Na$^+$ channel blockers increases Na$^+$ channel synthesis.[57] Conversely, in experimental models of AF (where rapid rates are induced by pacing), Na$^+$ currents are depressed.[58] A silencing element, termed REST, is widely expressed in extraneuronal tissues and is responsible for suppression of neuronal Na$^+$ channel expression in extraneuronal tissues.[59] However, the molecular basis for regulated cardiac Na$^+$ channel expression during drug therapy or in arrhythmia models remains largely unexplored. The cardiac channel undergoes extensive post-translational modification, including glycosylation and phosphorylation, which modifies channel trafficking to the cell membrane, as well as channel gating function.[60,61] Protein kinase C (PKC) phosphorylates a highly conserved serine residue in the Na$^+$ channel III–IV linker,[62] whereas there are a number of PKA consensus sites in the I–II linker.[63,64]

Cardiac Na$^+$ Channel Dysfunction in Disease

Mutations in *SCN5A* cause the LQT3 variant of the LQT syndrome (see Table 17–3),[65] an autosomal dominant disorder in which patients exhibit prolonged ECG QT intervals and are at risk for the polymorphic ventricular tachycardia torsades de pointes. A common mechanism is failure of fast inactivation gating, a so-called gain of function resulting in a population of channels that exhibit recurrent openings throughout the action potential plateau.[66,67] The small net depolarizing "pedestal" of current through these channels is sufficient to upset the balance between inward and outward currents in the action potential plateau, and hence prolong action potential duration, and consequently, the QT interval. The first such defect to be described was a 9-nucleotide deletion, resulting in deletion of three amino acids (ΔKPQ) in the III–IV linker of the channel.[66] This finding is consistent with the prominent role of this region in normal fast inactivation.[51] The next two mutations to be described, R1644H and N1325S, are both located in cytoplasmic S4–S5 linkers (see Fig. 17–4), supporting a role for these regions as docking sites for the inactivation "lid."[67,68] However, further studies in more kindreds have shown that mutations in other regions of the channel protein also result in defective inactivation.[55] This, in turn, reinforces the notion that primary sequence changes can exert prominent allosteric effects on distant regions of this large channel protein.

Inherited mutations in *SCN5A* that cause a marked loss of I_{Na} (in contrast to LQT3 gain of function) cause a form of idiopathic ventricular fibrillation known as Brugada syndrome (see Table 17–3).[8,55] Patients with Brugada syndrome experience sudden death in the absence of any detectable heart disease (and a normal QT interval), but do display an unusual electrocardiographic feature, J-point elevation in the right precordial leads (see Fig. 17–2).[7] Some Brugada syndrome mutations result in a highly truncated, and therefore nonfunctional protein, whereas others augment the inactivation gating processes (either fast or slow) to yield a loss of I_{Na}. At least one mutation, insertion of a glutamate at position 1795 in the Na$^+$ channel C terminus (1795insD), produces gain of function defects in fast inactivation and loss of function defects in slow inactivation and results in both the LQT3 and Brugada syndrome phenotypes in the same carrier.[69] Thus inherited mutations have provided important insights into how structure and function in this large protein relate to arrhythmia phenotypes in the whole heart.

A third phenotype associated with Na$^+$ channel mutations is conduction system disease (see Table 17–3).[70] One such mutation, G514C in the I–II linker, was identified in a Dutch family and has been studied in detail.[71] The voltage dependence of channel activation was shifted in a manner that would reduce I_{Na} (and therefore might be associated with the Brugada phenotype). However, the voltage dependence of G514C inactivation was also shifted in a manner that would cause a gain of function. Computational modeling of these complex effects indicated a slight net overall reduction in channel function that produced conduction slowing, but it was not sufficient to elicit action potential heterogeneities associated with LQT3 or the Brugada syndrome. Hence a small degree of loss of function is sufficient to provoke isolated cardiac conduction disease, whereas a more substantial loss of Na$^+$ channel function seems to provoke more lethal tachyarrhythmias.

The Brugada phenotype may provide insight into the proarrhythmic effects of potent Na$^+$ channel blockade in the CAST,[6] where investigators reported that treatment with the potent Na$^+$ channel blocking drugs flecainide and encainide enhanced mortality (likely caused by arrhythmias) in patients convalescing from acute myocardial infarction. Analysis of the CAST database indicated that the group at greatest risk for an increase in drug-associated mortality was those patients at greatest risk for recurrent myocardial ischemia. Since CAST, studies have identified a reduction in Na$^+$ channel function in cardiac cells isolated from the ischemic border zone surrounding a cardiac infarct.[72] Hence the clinical observation that flecainide worsens the Brugada syndrome ECG phenotype may suggest a link between loss of Na$^+$ channel function (caused by either ischemia or genetic predisposition) and proarrhythmic susceptibility to potent Na$^+$ channel blocking agents. Moreover, determining the extent to which DNA variants in *SCN5A* (or other ion channels) may produce little or no baseline clinical phenotype but nevertheless increase an individual patient's risk for ventricular arrhythmias on exposure to a range of stressors, including myocardial ischemia or drugs, is a critical future direction of arrhythmia research.

Ca^{2+} Channels (I$_{Ca}$)

Structure and Function

The major Ca^{2+} channels in cardiac muscle are the L-type and T-type. The L-type Ca^{2+} channel contributes inward current to sustain the characteristically prolonged action potentials in heart (in contrast to nerve). The Ca^{2+} ions introduced into the cell act as the trigger for excitation-contraction coupling, triggering the release of myofilament-activating Ca^{2+} from sarcoplasmic reticulum stores by opening the sarcoplasmic reticulum Ca^{2+} release channel (also known as the ryanodine receptor). Whereas L-type channels are found throughout cardiac muscle, T-type channels play a role in determining automaticity, and are thus localized to sinus node, AV node, atrium, and the specialized conducting system, and are thought to be absent from normal ventricle. Calcium channels are assembled from a number of distinct α- and β-subunits. These include α_1C, which encodes the L-type α-subunit,[73] and α_{1H}, which encodes the T-type.[74] Two major L-type Ca^{2+} channel ancillary subunits have been identified. The β subunits are intracellular, and increase Ca^{2+} current, modify activation and inactivation gating,[75,76] enhance prepulse facilitation,[77] and may be involved in channel trafficking. The other major Ca^{2+} channel ancillary subunit is a large polypeptide generated by expression of a single gene, with two protein products (α_2 and δ subunits) that are linked by a disulfide bridge.[78] The α_2 protein is extracellular, whereas the δ subunit includes a single membrane spanning segment and an extracellular domain that links to (and anchors) the α_2 subunit. The $\alpha_2\delta$ subunit may increase cell surface α_1 subunit expression.

As mentioned earlier, a highly conserved glutamate in each of the four P-loops generates a "ring" in the pore that confers Ca^{2+} selectivity over Na$^+$.[79] Multiple Ca^{2+} binding sites may be present within the permeation pathway, with repulsion between adjacent Ca^{2+} ions facilitating high ionic throughput.[80] That barium currents through L-type Ca^{2+} channels consistently inactivate much more slowly than do calcium currents, as well as experiments with flash release of caged Ca^{2+},[81] indicate that Ca^{2+} channel inactivation is partly mediated by the intracellular Ca^{2+} ion. The intracellular Ca^{2+} sensor, while complex, involves an "EF-hand"-containing domain in the intracellular C-terminus of the channel,[82] as well as two calmodulin-binding domains located nearby on the C-terminus[83,84]; the mechanism involves calmodulin binding of Ca^{2+} rather than direct interaction of Ca^{2+} with the channel protein. Another unique feature of L-type Ca^{2+} channel behavior is "facilitation," whereby Ca^{2+} currents increase in size on repeated, closely coupled activating pulses. Calmodulin may also act as the Ca^{2+} sensor for facilitation; this may occur through direct binding to the Ca^{2+} channel α subunit C-terminus, or through activation of the Ca^{2+}/calmodulin-dependent protein kinase CaMK II.

Regulation of Ca^{2+} Channels

Ca^{2+} channels are heavily regulated by adrenergic pathways through the action of protein kinases. Kinase phosphorylation places the Ca^{2+} channels into distinct gating "modes," described in single-channel experiments. Sweeps displaying mode 0 gating have rare brief openings, whereas those showing mode 1 gating show frequent brief openings. Mode 2 is characterized by long openings and is promoted by either PKA or CaMK-mediated phosphorylation.[85,86] Hence β-adrenergic stimulation markedly increases I$_{Ca}$ through the traditional Gs-related second messenger pathway,[87] causing a lengthening of action potential duration and a positive inotropic effect in cardiac muscle. Of the multiple consensus PKA sites in the L-type Ca^{2+} channel, S1928 in the C-terminus appears to be functionally important.[88] Cardiac channel-specific A-kinase anchoring proteins appear to be crucial for mediating these PKA effects.[89,90] Ca^{2+} channels can also be PKC-phosphorylated, but the significance for cardiac rhythm is not clear.

Cardiac Ca^{2+} Channel Dysfunction in Disease

Alternatively spliced forms of both the L- and the T-type Ca^{2+} channel have been described in cardiac preparations, and differences in both drug sensitivity and isoform expression in heart failure have been described.[91–93] Both L-type Ca^{2+} channels and Na$^+$ channels are reduced in number in atrial myocytes from animals with AF, and it is believed that these changes perpetuate the arrhythmia.[94] Conversely, L-type Ca^{2+} channels have been implicated as a carrier of arrhythmogenic inward current. Prolongation of the action potential increases the amplitude of the intracellular Ca^{2+} transient, activating CaMK (and thus enhancing L-type Ca^{2+} current and other arrhythmogenic inward currents), and thereby promoting arrhythmogenic EADs and DADs (see Fig. 17–3).[95,96] Ca^{2+}-channel blockers inhibit arrhythmogenic EADs during these conditions,[97] as does CaMK inhibition.[98] In animal models of hypertrophy,[99] the amplitude of the T-type Ca^{2+} current is increased, reminiscent of the electrophysiologic phenotype observed in fetal cells (which exhibit large T-type currents), perhaps representing reversion to the fetal phenotype.

Transient Outward Current, I_{TO}

Structure and Function

The I_{TO} current (see Fig. 17–1) is present in most, but not all, human ventricular epicardial and atrial cells, and is generated by a number of channels with "transient outward" gating properties that include rapid inactivation. One of the first K^+ channels cloned from human heart, Kv1.4, displays inactivation gating superficially typical of I_{TO} in heterologous expression systems. However, human I_{TO} recovers from inactivation between stimuli much more rapidly than does Kv1.4-mediated current,[100] and Kv1.4 mRNA and protein have been difficult to detect in human heart. By contrast, heterologous expression of Kv4.3 results in a transient outward current with rapid recovery from inactivation, and could thus contribute a rapid repolarization "notch" in phase 1 (see Fig. 17–1), even at rapid heart rates. Kv4.3 also displays drug sensitivity similar to human I_{TO}, reinforcing the idea that it is a reasonable candidate for human I_{TO}. There is a gradient of Kv4 subunit expression across the ventricular wall in rat, corresponding to the larger I_{TO} in epicardium[101]; it is proposed that an analogous Kv4.3 gradient is present in humans. Whereas human endocardium does not generally display a prominent phase 1 notch during stimulation of physiologic rates, a small I_{TO} with slow kinetics of recovery from inactivation can be recorded, and suggests that Kv1.4 may mediate I_{TO} in the human endocardium (versus Kv4 in epicardium). Recently identified function-modifying subunits, termed Kv channel-interacting proteins, are present in heart and brain and modulate Kv4-mediated currents, although the extent to which they modulate cardiac I_{TO} is under investigation. Kv channel-interacting proteins appear to interact with Kv4 N-termini, and may act as Ca^{2+} sensors.[102] In some species, a calcium-activated I_{TO} (termed I_{TO2}) can be recorded, and may be carried by K^+ or by Cl^-.[103,104]

I_{TO} Dysfunction in Disease

A common finding in human heart failure is action potential prolongation, an effect that has been attributed in part to reduction of I_{TO}.[105] The extent of reduction of I_{TO} and reduction in abundance of mRNA transcripts encoding Kv4.3 in human heart failure correlate, suggesting heart failure reduces Kv4 channel expression.[106] The mechanisms underlying this transcriptional regulation have not been elucidated, although action potential prolongation and consequent "triggered" arrhythmias (EADs; see Fig. 17–3) as a mechanism for sudden death during heart failure is a

hypothesis under active investigation. Moreover, as discussed previously, the gradient in I_{TO} expression across the right ventricular free wall forms the basis of a leading hypothesis for the ECG manifestations of the Brugada syndrome (see Fig. 17–2), and may also form the basis for the proarrhythmic manifestations of Na^+ channel blockade.

Delayed Rectifier K^+ Currents

In contrast to I_{TO}, which activates rapidly during the cardiac action potential, these K^+ currents activate after some delay (see Fig. 17–1), and play a greater role in later phases of the action potential. There are three principle delayed rectifier currents (I_{Kr}, I_{Ks}, and I_{Kur}) that represent distinct gene products and are distinguishable in human heart by their kinetics of activation and deactivation, as well as their distinctive pharmacologic sensitivities.

Rapid Delayed Rectifier Current, I_{Kr}

Structure and Function

The gene *HERG* encodes a six membrane spanning α subunit (see Fig. 17–4) underlying the current I_{Kr} (see Fig. 17–1) and is expressed abundantly in heart. In addition, there is accumulating evidence that the *HERG* gene product is associated with subunits that modify its function. In mouse atrial tumor (AT1) cells, antisense suppression of the single-transmembrane domain membrane protein minK (see Table 17–2), encoded by the gene *KCNE2*, reduces I_{Kr},[107] and coexpression of *minK* with *HERG* in heterologous systems increases I_{Kr} compared with *HERG* alone.[108] The *minK*-related gene *KCNE2* (also termed *MiRP1*) has also been implicated as a HERG interactor. When *MiRP1* and *HERG* are coexpressed, the unitary conductance of the HERG channel is reduced, and I_{Kr} gating and the rate of onset of drug block are both accelerated, which is consistent with the experimentally observed characteristics of I_{Kr} in native myocytes.[109] At the same time, the extent of *KCNE1* expression in human heart is controversial, and the role of *MiRP1* mutations on I_{Kr} pharmacology (see later) thus remains somewhat uncertain.

Close inspection of I_{Kr} currents on membrane depolarization yields a number of unusual features. Whereas depolarization causes activation and opening of the channel, the measured current decreases markedly as depolarization potential is made more positive—i.e., the current displays striking "inward rectification." In brief, this results from an unusual C-type inactivation process (see Fig. 17–5) that develops rapidly and predominates when the channel is strongly depolarized.[110,111] Studies have examined the time course of I_{Kr} current during a cardiac action potential,[112,113] and at maintained positive potentials (such as during the action potential plateau) inactivation is favored over channel opening, so that little outward current is generated to oppose the inward I_{Ca}. However, on sudden repolarization (i.e., phase 3 of the action potential; see Fig. 17–1), I_{Kr} rapidly recovers from inactivation (before closure), therefore a large outward current is generated that not only repolarizes the cell, but also "protects" the myocyte from a spurious proarrhythmic depolarization (i.e., an EAD or DAD; see Fig. 17–3) before the action potential fully terminates and the inward currents (I_{Na}, I_{Ca}) have recovered. Hence pharmacologic blockade of I_{Kr} is the most common cause of drug-induced QT prolongation with torsades de pointes.

Paradoxically, increasing the serum K^+ concentration has a salutary effect on the QT interval in patients with pharmacologic suppression of I_{Kr}.[114] Although it follows that raising extracellular K^+ also increases the amplitude of current through channels encoded by *HERG*,[115] both results are contrary to what is expected by simple Nernstian considerations based on the concentration gradient, given intracellular K^+ concentrations are ~30-fold greater than extracellular. However, recent studies have shown that when extracellular K^+ is entirely removed, the extracellular Na^+ normally present in serum serves as a potent blocker of outward I_{Kr}, with an IC_{50} of only 3.1 mM. Hence extracellular K^+ normally competes with extracellular Na^+ to relieve I_{Kr} block, and increases in serum K^+ over the therapeutic (3–6 mM) range increase I_{Kr} by additionally protecting the channel from serum Na^+.[116]

I_{Kr} Dysfunction in Disease

Mutations in *HERG* cause the LQT2 variety of the congenital LQT syndrome (see Table 17–3), just as drugs that block I_{Kr} evoke the acquired form of the disease. I_{Kr} suppression, caused by either drugs or mutations, tends to prolong the cardiac action potential with "reverse use dependence" (i.e., greatest action potential prolongation at slow rates), and patients are thus at greatest risk for torsades de pointes arrhythmias during bradycardia.[117] A mechanism for this rate dependence may arise from the observation that the counterpart of I_{Kr}, termed I_{Ks} (see later), deactivates more slowly and incompletely at rapid heart rates. Hence I_{Ks} current accumulates at rapid heart rates and becomes larger than I_{Kr}, whereas at slow rates, I_{Kr} is a relatively more important component of repolarizing current. Hence I_{Kr} block produces marked prolongation of action potentials, and the QT interval, at slow rates or after along diastolic interval.[118]

Although certain clinical risk factors can be identified, the development of excess QT prolongation and torsades de pointes during exposure to many I_{Kr}-blocking drugs is infrequent and remains largely unpredictable. Similarly, patients with inherited forms of the LQT syndrome are life-long mutation carriers, yet have relatively rare arrhythmia events. It is postulated that risk factors, including genetic predisposition, drug exposure, hypokalemia, and so on, come together in an individual patient to culminate in torsades de pointes. Thus patients who develop excess QT prolongation on drug exposure may be viewed as having a "subclinical" genetic defect that slightly impedes repolarization, causing a reduction in "repolarization reserve."[119] Only when repolarization reserve is sufficiently impaired (by the addition of drug therapy) does torsades de pointes occur. This hypothesis is supported by reports of patients with inherited ion channel mutations who only present after drug challenge. These reports implicate two distinct mechanisms. First, increased sensitivity of the *HERG* channel complex to drug

block. This has been noted primarily in patients with mutations in the MiRP1 subunit (see Table 17–2), who have normal baseline ECGs but develop torsades de pointes on exposure to I_{Kr} blockers.[120] Second, reduction of I_{Ks} or another repolarizing current that is well-tolerated until the superposition of I_{Kr} block.[121–124] These findings suggest the possibility of genetic screening for patients susceptible to drug-induced arrhythmias.

Slow Delayed Rectifier I_{Ks}

Structure and Function

In cardiac myocytes, long depolarizing pulses also give rise to a slowly activating outward current, termed I_{Ks} for I_K slow (see Fig. 17–1). Expression of *KvLQT1* (see Table 17–2), the disease gene in the LQT1 variant of the inherited LQT syndrome (see Table 16–3), gives rise to rapidly activating, slowly deactivating current that does not have a readily identifiable correlate in cardiac myocytes. Conversely, coexpression of *minK* and *KvLQT1* recapitulates I_{Ks}, indicating the coassembly of these two products produces the I_{Ks} current in cardiac myocytes.[125,126] KvLQT1 retains the molecular architecture of the typical pore-forming subunit of a voltage-gated K^+ channel (see Fig. 17–4), and accessibility data are consistent with the idea that minK resides in a crevice that is not part of the pore, but nevertheless influences movement of the minK-KvLQT1 channel complex during gating.[127]

Regulation of I_{Ks}

The action potential in the ventricle shortens with adrenergic stimulation, even controlling for heart rate. Because I_{Ca} increases with adrenergic stimulation (an effect that would prolong action potentials), a counterbalancing increase in outward K^+ current must also occur, and likely involves I_{Ks}. In most studies, I_{Ks} amplitude is increased by adrenergic stimulation as well as by increases in intracellular Ca^{2+} or by PKC stimulation,[128] and a consensus PKC phosphorylation site is present in the C-terminus of human minK. Although regulatory elements have not been identified in the *KvLQT1* gene,[129] a recent report suggested that target residues for the PKA effect may reside in the C-terminus, possibly reflecting a physical association between the *KvLQT1* subunit and elements of the signaling pathway.[130] Further, coexpression of an A-kinase anchoring protein with *KvLQT1* + *minK* has been shown necessary for the I_{Ks} response to PKA stimulation.[131]

I_{Ks} Dysfunction in Disease

Autosomal dominant mutations in *KvLQT1* or *minK* evoke (respectively) the LQT1 or LQT5 varieties of the LQT syndrome (see Table 17–3). Pharmacologic I_{Ks} block tends to produce homogeneous action potential prolongation in ventricular tissue; however, β-adrenergic agonists such as isoproterenol evoke marked heterogeneities of action potential duration and arrhythmias. This experimental finding is consistent with the sensitivity of I_{Ks} to adrenergic stimulation (described earlier), and with the observation that arrhythmias in LQT1 and LQT5 patients with inherited *KvLQT1* or *minK* mutations almost always arise during periods of adrenergic stress.[132] Examination of currents generated by heterologous expression of KvLQT1 and minK channels with inherited mutations in widely divergent areas of the protein results in a wide variety of defects that lead to a reduction in I_{Ks} current, including altered channel gating[133] or failure of the mutant channel to traffic to the cell surface.[134,135]

The rare Jervell-Lange-Nielson (JLN) variant of the LQT syndrome (see Table 17–3) associated with congenital deafness arises in children who inherit abnormal *KvLQT1* or *minK* alleles from both parents.[136,137] The KvLQT1-minK complex is responsible for endolymph secretion in the inner ear, and its absence in patients with JLN results in collapse of the endolymphatic space. This situation arises through consanguinity (i.e., the child inherits alleles each encoding the same abnormal protein) or occasionally by chance (in which case the child inherits alleles that encode different abnormal proteins). Thus both parents are obligate gene carriers for LQT1 or LQT5. Although QT intervals are generally normal in these parents, it is now recognized that occasional cases of sudden unexpected death, presumably caused by LQT-related arrhythmias, can occur in the parents, an observation that has obvious implications for family screening (and preoperative assessment) of a patient with JLN.[137]

Ultra-Rapid Delayed Rectifier, I_{Kur}

Structure and Function

This current activates even more rapidly than I_{Kr} (hence the designation I_{Kur}, for ultrarapid), and exhibits little inactivation during sustained depolarization. Heterologous expression of the Kv1.5 channel subunit results in a current with gating kinetics essentially identical to I_{Kur},[138,139] and native I_{Kur} and heterologously expressed Kv1.5 are both sensitive to quinidine and to 4-aminopyridine, suggesting Kv1.5 is the major protein substituent of I_{Kur}. In addition, multiple members of the Kvβ1 subunit family (see Table 17–2) have been cloned[140,141] and coexpression of these with Kv1.5 accelerates inactivation, making the channel appear more like I_{TO}. The C-termini of Kvβ1 subunits are highly homologous and interact with the α subunit in this locus.[142] These β-subunits appear to be almost exclusively cytosolic and may mediate inactivation of the Kv1.5 subunit through an N-type ball-and-chain mechanism (see Fig. 17–5), whereby the β subunit acts as the ball.[143] The crystal structure of Kvβ has been solved and is homologous to oxidoreductase enzymes; therefore it is proposed that Kvβ subunits couple the cell redox state to K+ channel function.[144,145]

I_{Kur} Regulation and Dysfunction in Disease

In animal models, Kv1.5 current is up-regulated by endogenous or exogenous glucocorticoids[146] as well as thyroid hormone.[147] Kv1.5 also contains SH3 domains that interact with tyrosine kinase, and are tyrosine phosphorylated in human heart.[148] In addition, Kv1.5 has been reported to target to lipid rafts,[149,150] specific membrane regions enriched in certain subtypes of lipids (i.e., cholesterol) that may allow localization of Kv1.5 channels in the vicinity of signaling molecules and substrates within the cell. Moreover, adaptor proteins (ZIP1 and ZIP2) may generate a physical link between the Kvα/β complex and protein kinases.[151] In this context, it is believed that Kvβ1 alters sensitivity of Kv1.5 to phosphorylation by PKC or PKA.[152,153] Although largely characterized in heterologous systems, the extent to which these biochemical associations are operative in the heart (vs. other tissues in which Kv1.5 resides) is under investigation.

Because Kv1.5 is abundant in human atrium but is absent from normal human ventricle, maneuvers that reduce Kv1.5 would be expected to prolong atrial action potentials and yet not prolong repolarization in the ventricle, thus avoiding QT prolongation and the risk for inducing torsade de pointes. Efforts to produce such a "chamber-specific" antiarrhythmic drug (targeted at AF) are ongoing, although Kv1.5 expression in extracardiac tissues may elicit side effects with this strategy. Notably, in chronic AF, Kv1.5 mRNA and protein (like other ion currents, including I_{Ca-L} and I_{Na}) are down-regulated,[154] which may limit the effectiveness of this approach.

Cardiac Inward Rectifiers

Structure and Function

These K+ channels (I_{K1}, I_{K-ATP}, I_{K-Ach}), encoded by the K_{ir} superfamily (see Fig. 17–4), are notable for the absence of a charged, S4 segment (see Fig. 17–5), and therefore exhibit less intrinsic voltage-dependent gating. Nonetheless, as their "inward rectifier" name implies, these K+ channels pass inward current in preference to outward current, and are primarily operative at hyperpolarized (rather than depolarized) potentials near the cell resting potential (the potassium equilibrium potential, ~−85 mV). Hence K_{ir} channels play a key role in "setting" the myocyte resting potential. The inward rectification of these channels usually reflects block of outward current by intracellular constituents. For I_{K1}, Mg^{2+} alone appears sufficient,[155,156] whereas for other members of this group, polyamines (such as spermidine) have been implicated as further mediators of rectification.[157–159]

The inward rectifier current I_{K1} likely represents expression of members of the Kir2.x family (see Table 17–2).[160] The acetylcholine-gated channel (I_{K-Ach}) is recapitulated by coexpression of Kir3.1 and Kir3.4 (also termed GIRK1 and GIRK4),[161] whereas the adenosine triphosphate (ATP)-inhibited channel (I_{K-ATP}) results from coexpression of a Kir6 channel with an ancillary protein, the sulfonylurea receptor (SUR).[162] I_{K-ATP} channels are widespread and diverse in character, but the cardiac channel is recapitulated by coexpression of Kir6.2 with SUR2. SUR2 is a member of the ATP-binding-cassette superfamily that includes the cystic fibrosis transport regulator (CFTR). Members of this family share a common structural motif, consisting of putative 12 membrane spanning segments and two intracellular ATP binding cassettes.

Kir Channel Regulation and Dysfunction in Disease

In addition to maintenance of the resting membrane potential, evidence supporting a role for Kir2.1/I_{K1} in the terminal phase of cardiac repolarization has come from the linkage of mutations in Kir2.1 with Andersen syndrome (see Table 17-3), a neuromuscular disease whose manifestations include unusual forms of ventricular tachycardia.[163] Acetylcholine activates I_{K-Ach} through a G protein–delineated pathway,[164] and activation of this channel is partly responsible for bradycardia and slowing of AV conduction seen with vagal stimulation. ATP-sensitive K^+ channels provide a link between the metabolic state of the cell and electrophysiologic activity. Several drugs activate these channels, but are not cardiac-specific ("K^+ channel openers" such as nicorandil or pinacidil); cardiac-specific agents, on the horizon, may be useful to protect the myocardium against the deleterious effects of ischemia (including arrhythmias). ATP-sensitive channels are expressed not only on the cell surface, but also in mitochondria, where they may be attractive targets for cardioprotection.[165]

Pacemaker Current

The cardiac rhythm, a sine qua non characteristic of the heart, is generated in sinus node cells by an inward current that continually depolarizes the cell toward its firing threshold during phase 4 of the action potential. Unlike other cardiac ionic currents activated by depolarization, this hyperpolarization-activated pacemaker current[166] has been termed funny (I_f) or hyperpolarization-activated (I_h). The pacemaker channel superfamily includes cyclic nucleotide binding domains in its C-terminus, and it follows that pacemaker activity is regulated in vivo by cyclic nucleotide-related (i.e., adrenergic) signaling pathways. Four members of this superfamily (HCN1, HCN2, and HCN4) have been found in mouse heart,[167–170] and heterologous expression of these channels results in a hyperpolarization-activated current that, like I_h, displays only very weak selectivity for K^+ over Na^+ (and with a reversal potential of $-35\,mV$). Although HCN channels display the typical six-membrane segment spanning architecture of voltage-gated K^+ channels, the mechanisms for their unusual hyperpolarization-activated gating and lack of selectivity have not been fully determined, and might involve sequence differences in the S4 sensor and the selectivity filter regions of the pore.[171]

The zebrafish mutant "Smo" contains a mutation in a single I_h gene and displays marked heart rate slowing, but only partial loss of the I_h current (specifically, a fast kinetic component), suggesting the total I_h current may represent the ensemble current from several different gene products.[172] In addition to pacemaker cells, I_h current can be elicited by excessive hyperpolarization in ventricular muscle cells,[173] suggesting that altered regulation of this current could underlie ventricular arrhythmias during pathologic conditions. The molecular basis of regulation of I_h by intracellu-

lar signaling systems has not been elucidated, nor have mechanisms to modify I_h function in bradyarrhythmias using pharmacologic agents, although this strategy may hold future promise as the molecular basis of I_h becomes further defined.

Background Current

In addition to currents that exhibit time- and voltage-dependent gating properties, voltage clamp studies of heart cells reveal additional currents that do not exhibit gating characteristics, known generally as "background" currents. At least three types of ion channels may underlie background currents in heart. I_{Kp} (for plateau) is a time-independent current, originally identified in guinea pig cardiomyocytes.[174,175] It has been suggested that expression of the twin-pore K^+ channel, known as TWIK1, may underlie I_{Kp}.[176] Some data suggest that CFTR channels may also underlie background current, because CFTR transcripts can be identified in heart.[177] More generally, studies have identified chloride channels activated by changes in cell volume, as well as intracellular Ca^{2+}.[178] Finally, recent studies have shown that coexpression of *KvLQT1* with *KCNE2* (*MiRP1*) produces a background current,[179] although the question of the extent of *MiRP1* expression in heart and its localization are unresolved. Moreover, whether any background currents are appropriate targets for drug therapy is unknown.

Current and Potential Targets of Drug Action

Emerging View of a Common Ion Channel Drug Receptor

The pharmacologic principles that underlie control of the cardiac rhythm (antiarrhythmic therapy) are necessarily complex, given the vast array of ion channels, receptors, and signaling pathways involved. The general principles that underlie antiarrhythmic therapy are discussed in detail in Chapter 35. This chapter focuses on the molecular mechanism whereby most antiarrhythmic compounds modulate the cardiac rhythm—i.e., suppression of ionic current through binding to voltage-gated ion channels. The ability to clone and mutagenize specific amino acid residues in channel proteins has revolutionized our approach to defining and characterizing the drug receptors and is leading toward a surprising "common view" of the mechanism whereby drugs block ion channels in multiple classes.

The first insights into the putative drug receptor in voltage-gated ion channels were provided by studies of tetraethylammonium (TEA) and the larger quaternary ammonium (QA) derivatives (Fig. 17-6) on delayed rectifier K^+ channels in squid axons.[180] These studies showed that low concentrations of QA blocked the channel from inside the cell, and that the affinity increased as the hydrophobicity (length of the QA compound carbon tail) of the com-

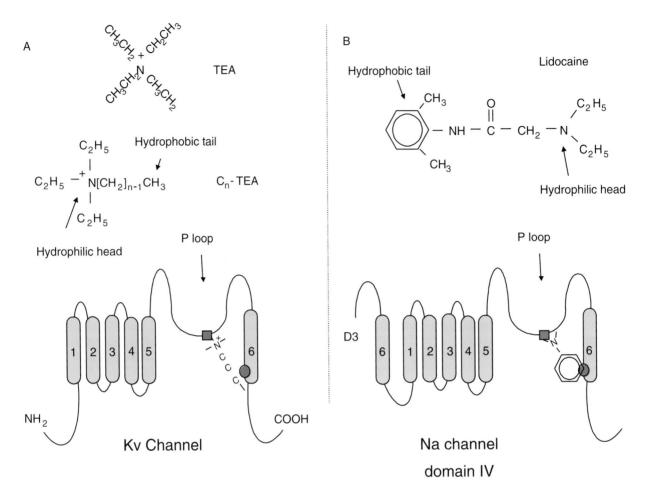

Figure 17–6. Voltage-gated K$^+$ and Na$^+$ channels have analogous bidomain drug receptor motifs. *A,* The structure of tetraethylammonium (TEA) and the longer-chain TEA derivatives (Cn-TEA) are shown (*top*). Mutations in the S6 domain (*green circle*) of the Kv channel have prominent effects on the affinity of long-chain QA derivatives (*bottom*). Conversely, mutation in the P-loop (*green square*) reduces binding of TEA and short-chain QA derivatives. *B,* The structure of lidocaine, a local anesthetic molecule, is shown with its hydrophobic aromatic tail and hydrophilic amino head group, separated by an amide linkage (*top*). *B,* Mutation of residues in the S6 segment of the domain IV critically determines local anesthetic binding (*bottom*). In addition, residues that determine cation selectivity in the P loops also modify local anesthetic block (see text). (From Balser JR, George AL: Pharmacology of ion channels. In Rose MR, Griggs RC (eds): Channelopathies of the Nervous System. Boston, Butterworth-Heinemann, 2001, pp 23–48.)

pound increased. Moreover, internal blockade by TEA suppressed outward current through the channel to a much greater degree than inward current, and increasing the inward flux of K$^+$ ions through the channel sped the rate of dissociation of TEA from its receptor, as if the K$^+$ ions "knocked off" the drug. These directional effects were best explained by a hydrophobic drug receptor that lies within the pore, in a vestibule on the internal side of a narrow selectivity "filter."

Later studies that used site-specific modification of ion channel amino acid residues satisfied these predictions and mapped the locus of the K$^+$ channel QA receptor to amino acid residues residing in the inner pore. Consistent with the two functional ends of QA compounds, two regions of the K$^+$ channel influence drug binding from inside the channel.[181] The P-loop (see Fig. 17–1) primarily influences internal TEA binding, but has less effect on longer (more

hydrophobic) QA derivatives. Conversely, the binding affinity of long QA derivatives is determined by the hydrophobicity of amino acid residues lining the pore in the S6 segment. The picture that emerges is a bidomain receptor, with a hydrophilic binding interaction between the charged amino head of the QA compound and the P-loop, and a hydrophobic interaction between the QA alkyl tail and hydrophobic amino acids in the S6 region (see Fig. 17–6). S6 amino acid residues have been shown to be important in the binding of a number of K$^+$ channel blockers including 4-aminopyridine[182] and quinidine.[183] It has been noted that binding of the hydrophobic tail of QA derivatives to S6 residues seems to reduce the interaction of the polar amino head with the P-loop, suggesting a "tension" between binding at the two sites that might be modulated by changing the physical separation between the charged head and alkyl tail.[181]

A striking parallel exists between QA binding in K⁺ channels and binding of the local anesthetic class of antiarrhythmic molecules to their target, the voltage-gated Na⁺ channel. These compounds contain an ionizable amino head group and a hydrophobic tail, much like the QA compounds (see Fig. 17–6). An intrapore binding site for these molecules is well supported by evidence that the charged derivatives (e.g., QX-314) move deeply (50–70%) into the pore from the cytoplasmic side.[184,185] Specific aromatic hydrophobic residues in the S6 segments of domains I and IV line the inner pore of the channel and figure critically in block (Fig. 17–7).[186–188] Analogous sites in domain IV, S6 of L-type Ca^{2+} channels, have been linked to both dihydropyridine and phenylalkylamine block of Ca^{2+} current.[189,190] At the same time, studies have shown that the polar head of the compound is repelled by positively charged residues in the Na⁺ channel P-region, near the selectivity filter, suggesting that this region normally restricts extracellular access to (and escape from) the intrapore binding site.[191] Notably, antiarrhythmic drug blockade of Na⁺ channels increases markedly during depolarization, while the channels are mainly inactivated.[192,193] This "use-dependent" block[194] may be related to gating-dependent conformational changes that secondarily increase the "affinity" of the drug receptor. For example, mutation of residues in either the III-IV linker fast inactivation gate (see Fig. 17–7) or the P-loop modify the N-type and C-type Na⁺ channel inactivation processes, respectively,[51,195] and these modifications also markedly reduce use-dependent Na⁺ channel blockade.[196–198] Moreover, recent studies suggest that drug binding to both K⁺ and Na⁺ channels "stabilize" C-type inactivated conformation of the channel, and thus contribute to use-dependent current reduction partly through an allosteric mechanism.[199,200]

The prominent role of the *HERG* gene, and the I_{Kr} channel, in the proarrhythmic effects of drugs on the cardiac rhythm warrants some additional comment. I_{Kr} channels are blocked by a myriad of agents, both antiarrhythmics and "noncardiovascular" drugs that share the potential to produce marked QT prolongation and torsades de pointes. The recognition that HERG is "promiscuous" in its ability to be blocked by drugs from various classes has important implications for drug development, it has driven investigation into structural determinants of HERG block. Drug binding to HERG subunits occurs in the S6 region (analogous to Fig. 17–7), but is nearly irreversible, a finding that has been attributed to the channel closing during diastole with the drug trapped in its receptor within the pore.[201] In addition, structural modeling, based on the sequence analogy between HERG and the KcsA K⁺ channel crystal structure, reveals two unusual features of the HERG inner vestibule.[202] Most K⁺ channel primary sequences include two highly conserved proline residues in the S6 segment that are predicted to "kink" the segment and limit the size of the inner vestibule. The absence of such prolines in *HERG* may enlarge the inner vestibule, allowing relatively bulky drugs to enter. Second, the *HERG* S6 sequence has two aromatic residues predicted to face the inner pore, whereas other K⁺ channels have none or one (i.e., KvLQT1). Alanine mutagenesis of these residues markedly decreases drug block, suggesting that one or more of the eight aromatic residues lining the tetrameric pore can provide a high-affinity site for π-bonding interactions with aromatic groups on putative blocking drugs. It is hoped that these evolving structural insights will allow in silico screening of candidate molecules to eliminate proarrhythmic agents during the drug development process.

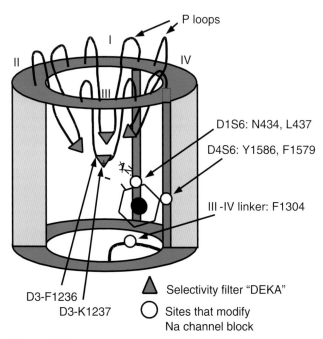

Figure 17–7. Highly schematic view of the Na⁺ channel pore, lined by the four homologous domains (I–IV), with a lidocaine analogue residing in the pore. The outer pore is formed by the P-loops, whereas the S6 segments line the inner pore. P-loop selectivity filter residues bridge the outer and inner pore regions (*triangles*). Residues in the selectivity filter (i.e., K1237) and the domain I and IV S6 segments interact with Na⁺ channel-blocking antiarrhythmic drugs (see text). Residues in the figure are numbered according to the original sequence of the rat skeletal muscle Na⁺ channel isoform.[204] D1S6 refers to domain I, S6, and so on. (Adapted from Balser JR: Structure and function of the cardiac sodium channel. Cardiovasc Res 42:327–338, 1999.)

Conclusion

The large number of genes in Table 17–2 comprising the existing substrate for the cardiac rhythm suggest a myriad of potential targets for antiarrhythmic therapy. However, as Chapter 35 discusses, the number of molecular targets currently exploited by existing antiarrhythmic therapies is relatively limited. Hence a major challenge is to not only expand the "arrhythmonome," genes encoding proteins that modulate cardiac excitability, but also to greatly extend our structural and functional understanding of those gene products already identified. Through an active synergy between the methods of new gene identification and the emerging technologies for high-resolution determination of protein structure and function, exciting targets for antiarrhythmic therapy are likely to be identified during the next decade. It is hoped that these new compounds will greatly improve the specificity and efficacy of antiarrhythmic therapy in both perioperative and nonsurgical settings.

Acknowledgment

Salary support was provided by the Established Investigator Award of the American Heart Association and the National Institutes of Health (R01 GM56307 and P01 HL46681).

References

1. Norris JF, Zipes DP: Electrophysiology of the slow channel. In Podrid PJ, Kowey PR (eds): Cardiac Arrhythmia: Mechanisms, Diagnosis, and Management. Baltimore, Williams & Wilkins, 1995.

2. Schwartz PJ, Zipes DP: Autonomic modulation of cardiac arrhythmias. In Zipes DP, Jalife JS (eds): Cardiac Electrophysiology: From Cell to Bedside, 3rd ed. Philadelphia, WB Saunders, 2000.

3. Engelstein ED, Lippman N, Stein KM, et al: Mechanism-specific effects of adenosine on atrial tachycardia. Circulation 89:2645, 1994.

4. Roden DM: Ibutilide and the treatment of atrial arrhythmias. Circulation 94:1499, 1996.

5. Mason JW: A comparison of seven antiarrhythmic drugs in patients with ventricular tachyarrhythmias: Electrophysiologic Study versus Electrocardiographic Monitoring Investigators. N Engl J Med 329:452, 1993.

6. Echt DS, Liebson PR, Mitchell LB, et al: Mortality and morbidity in patients receiving encainide, flecainide, or placebo. N Engl J Med 324:781, 1991.

7. Brugada P, Brugada J: Right bundle branch block, persistent ST segment elevation and sudden cardiac death: A distinct clinical and electrocardiographic syndrome. A multicenter report. J Am Coll Cardiol 20:1391, 1992.

8. Chen Q, Kirsch GE, Zhang D, et al: Genetic basis and molecular mechanism for idiopathic ventricular fibrillation. Nature 392:293, 1998.

9. Krishnan SC, Antzelevitch C: Flecainide-induced arrhythmia in canine ventricular epicardium. Phase 2 reentry? Circulation 87:562, 1993.

10. Krishnan SC, Antzelevitch C: Sodium channel block produces opposite electrophysiological effects in canine ventricular epicardium and endocardium. Circ Res 69:277, 1991.

11. Lukas A, Antzelevitch C: Differences in the electrophysiological response of canine ventricular epicardium and endocardium to ischemia: role of the transient outward current. Circulation 88:2903, 1993.

12. Alings M, Wilde A: "Brugada" syndrome: Clinical data and suggested pathophysiological mechanism. Circulation 99:666, 1999.

13. Roden DM, Wilde AA: Drug-induced J point elevation: A marker for genetic risk of sudden death or ECG curiosity? J Cardiovasc Electrophysiol 10:219, 1999.

14. Zipes DP: Cardiac electrophysiology: Promises and contributions. J Am Coll Cardiol 13:1329, 1989.

15. Roden DM, Hoffman BF: Action potential prolongation and induction of abnormal automaticity by low quinidine concentrations in canine Purkinje fibers. Relationship to potassium and cycle length. Circ Res 56:857, 1985.

16. Roden DM, Woosley RL, Primm K: Incidence of clinical features of the quinidine associated long QT syndrome: Implications for patient care. Am Heart J 111:1088, 1986.

17. Priori SG, Barhanin J, Hauer RN, et al: Genetic and molecular basis of cardiac arrhythmias: Impact on clinical management parts I and II. Circulation 99:518, 1999.

18. Sanguinetti MC, Jiang C, Curran ME, et al: A mechanistic link between an inherited and an acquired cardiac arrhythmia: HERG encodes the I_{Kr} potassium channel. Cell 81:299, 1995.

19. Beuckelmann DJ, Nabauer M, Erdmann E: Intracellular calcium handling in isolated ventricular myocytes from patients with terminal heart failure [see comments]. Circulation 85:1046, 1992.

20. Wit AL: Triggered activity. In Podrid PJ, Kowey PR (eds): Cardiac Arrhythmia: Mechanisms, Diagnosis, and Management. Baltimore, Williams & Wilkins, 1995.

21. Reuter H: Localization of beta adrenergic receptors, and effects of noradrenaline and cyclic nucleotides on action potentials, ion currents and tension in mammalian cardiac muscle. J Physiol 242:429, 1974.

22. Kameyama M, Hoffmann F, Trautwein W: On the mechanism of β-adrenergic regulation of the Ca^{2+} channel in the guinea-pig heart. Pflugers Arch 405:285, 1985.

23. Hoch B, Meyer R, Hetzer R, et al: Identification and expression of δ−isoforms of the multifunctional Ca^{2+}/calmodulin-dependent protein kinase in failing and nonfailing human myocardium. Circ Res 84:713, 1999.

24. Task Force of the Working Group on Arrhythmias of the European Society of Cardiology: The Sicilian Gambit: A new approach to the classification of antiarrhythmic drugs based on their actions on arrhythmogenic mechanisms. Circulation 84:1831, 1991.

25. Dzhura I, Wu Y, Colbran RJ, et al: Calmodulin kinase determines calcium-dependent facilitation of L-type calcium channels. Nat Cell Biol 2:173, 2000.

26. Wu Y, MacMillan LB, McNeill RB, et al: CaM kinase augments cardiac L-type Ca^{2+} current: A cellular mechanism for long QT arrhythmias. Am J Physiol 276:H2168, 1999.

27. Wu Y, Roden DM, Anderson ME: Calmodulin kinase inhibition prevents development of the arrhythmogenic transient inward current. Circ Res 84:906, 1999.

28. Yeager M: Molecular biology and structure of cardiac gap junction intercellular channels. In Zipes DP, Jalife JS: Cardiac Electrophysiology: From Cell to Bedside, 3rd ed. Philadelphia, WB Saunders, 2000.

29. Hamill OP, Marty A, Neher E, et al: Improved patch-clamp techniques for high-resolution current recording form cells and cell-free membrane patches. Pflügers Arch 391:85, 1981.

30. Noda M, Shimizu S, Tanabe T, et al: Primary structure of *Electrophorus electricus* sodium channel deduced from cDNA sequence. Nature 312:121, 1984.

31. Doyle DA, Cabral JM, Pfuetzner RA, et al: The structure of the potassium channel: Molecular basis of K+ conduction and selectivity. Science 280:69, 1998.

32. Hodgkin AL, Huxley AF: A quantitative description of membrane current and its application to conduction and excitation in nerve. J Physiol 117:500, 1952.

33. MacKinnon R, Yellen G: Mutations affecting TEA blockade and ion permeation in voltage-activated K+ channels. Science 250:276, 1990.

34. Yellen G, Jurman ME, Abramson T, et al: Mutations affecting internal TEA blockade identify the probable pore-forming region of a K+ channel. Science 251:939, 1991.

35. Yool AJ, Schwarz TL: Alteration of ionic selectivity of a K+ channel by mutation of the H5 region. Nature 349:700, 1991.

36. Heinemann SH, Terlau H, Stühmer W, et al: Calcium channel characteristics conferred on the sodium channel by single mutations. Nature 356:441, 1992.

37. Stühmer W, Conti F, Suzuki H, et al: Structural parts involved in activation and inactivation of the sodium channel. Nature 339:597, 1989.

38. Yang N, George AL, Horn R: Molecular basis of charge movement in voltage-gated sodium channels. Neuron 16:113, 1996.

39. Mitrovic N, George AL Jr, Horn R: Independent versus coupled inactivation in sodium channels: Role of the domain 2 S4 segment. J Gen Physiol 111:451, 1998.

40. Cha A, Ruben PC, George AL Jr, et al: Voltage sensors in domains III and IV, but not I and II, are immobilized by Na+ channel fast inactivation. Neuron 22:73, 1999.

41. Armstrong CM, Bezanilla F: Inactivation of the sodium channel. II. Gating current experiments. J Gen Physiol 70:567, 1977.

42. Zagotta WN, Hoshi T, Aldrich RW: Restoration of inactivation in mutants of Shaker potassium channels by a peptide derived from ShB. Science 250:568, 1990.

43. Hoshi T, Zagotta WN, Aldrich RW: Biophysical and molecular mechanisms of Shaker potassium channel inactivation. Science 250:533, 1990.

44. Hoshi T, Zagotta WN, Aldrich RW: Two types of inactivation in *Shaker* K+ channels: Effects of alterations in the carboxy-terminal region. Neuron 7:547, 1991.

45. Liu Y, Jurman ME, Yellen G: Dynamic rearrangement of the outer mouth of a K+ channel during gating. Neuron 16:859, 1996.

46. Roden DM, Balser JR, George AL, et al: Cardiac ion channels. Annu Rev Physiol 64:431, 2002.
47. Gellens ME, George AL, Chen L, et al: Primary structure and functional expression of the human cardiac tetrodotoxin-insensitive voltage-dependent sodium channel. Proc Natl Acad Sci USA 89:554, 1992.
48. Isom LL, Dejongh KS, Catterall WA: Auxiliary subunits of voltage-gated ion channels. Neuron 12:1183, 1994.
49. Nuss HB, Chiamvimonvat N, Perez-Garcia MT, et al: Functional association of the β_1 subunit with human cardiac (hH1) and rat skeletal muscle (μ1) sodium channel α subunits expressed in *Xenopus* oocytes. J Gen Physiol 106:1171, 1995.
50. An RH, Wang XL, Kerem B, et al: Novel LQT-3 mutation affects Na$^+$ channel activity through interactions between alpha- and beta1-subunits. Circ Res 83:141, 1998.
51. West J, Patton D, Scheuer T, et al: A cluster of hydrophobic amino acid residues required for fast Na$^+$-channel inactivation. Proc Natl Acad Sci USA 89:10910, 1992.
52. Tang L, Kallen RG, Horn R: Role of an S4-S5 linker in sodium channel inactivation probed by mutagenesis and a peptide blocker. J Gen Physiol 108:89, 1996.
53. Balser JR: Structure and function of the cardiac sodium channels. Cardiovasc Res 42:327, 1999.
54. Rudy B: Slow inactivation of the sodium conductance in squid giant axons: Pronase resistance. J Physiol 238:1, 1978.
55. Balser JR: The cardiac sodium channel. J Mol Cell Cardiol 33:599, 2001.
56. Benitah JP, Chen Z, Balser J, et al: Molecular dynamics of the sodium channel pore vary with gating: Interactions between P-segment motions and inactivation. J Neurosci 19:1577, 1999.
57. Taouis M, Sheldon RS, Duff HJ: Upregulation of the rat cardiac sodium channel by in vivo treatment with a class I antiarrhythmic drug. J Clin Invest 88:375, 1991.
58. Yue L, Melnyk P, Gaspo R, et al: Molecular mechanisms underlying ionic remodeling in a dog model of atrial fibrillation. Circ Res 84:776, 1999.
59. Chong JA, Tapia-Ramirez J, Kim S, et al: REST: A mammalian silencer protein that restricts sodium channel gene expression to neurons. Cell 80:949, 1995.
60. Murphy BJ, Rogers J, Perdichizzi AP, et al: cAMP-dependent phosphorylation of two sites in the alpha subunit of the cardiac sodium channel. J Biol Chem 271:28837, 1996.
61. Qu YS, Rogers JC, Tanada TN, et al: Phosphorylation of S1505 in the cardiac Na$^+$ channel inactivation gate is required for modulation by protein kinase C. J Gen Physiol 108:375, 1996.
62. Li M, West JW, Numann R, et al: Convergent regulation of sodium channels by protein kinase C and cAMP-dependent protein kinase. Science 261:1439, 1993.
63. Smith RD, Goldin AL: Potentiation of rat brain sodium channel currents by PKA in Xenopus oocytes involves the I-II linker. Am J Physiol Cell Physiol 278:C638, 2000.
64. Zhou J, Yi J, Hu N, et al: Activation of protein kinase A modulates trafficking of the human cardiac sodium channel in Xenopus oocytes. Circ Res 87:33, 2000.
65. Wang Q, Shen J, Splawski I, et al: *SCN5A* mutations associated with an inherited cardiac arrhythmia, long QT syndrome. Cell 80:805, 1995.
66. Bennett PB, Yazawa K, Naomasa M, et al: Molecular mechanism for an inherited cardiac arrhythmia. Nature 376:683, 1995.
67. Dumaine R, Wang Q, Keating MT, et al: Multiple mechanisms of Na$^+$ channel-linked long-QT syndrome. Circ Res 78:916, 1996.
68. Wang DW, Yazawa K, George AL, et al: Characterization of human cardiac Na$^+$ channel mutations in the congenital long QT syndrome. Proc Natl Acad Sci USA 93:13200, 1996.
69. Veldkamp MW, Viswanathan PC, Bezzina C, et al: Two distinct congenital arrhythmias evoked by a multidysfunctional Na$^+$ channel. Circ Res 86:E91, 2000.
70. Schott JJ, Alshinawi C, Kyndt F, et al: Cardiac conduction defects associate with mutations in SCN5A. Nat Genet 23:20, 1999.
71. Tan HL, Bink-Boelkens MTE, Bezzina CR, et al: A sodium channel mutation causes isolated cardiac conduction disease. Nature 409:1043, 2001.
72. Pu J, Boyden PA: Alterations of Na$^+$ currents in myocytes from epicardial border zone of the infarcted heart: A possible ionic mechanism for reduced excitability and postrepolarization refractoriness. Circ Res 81:110, 1997.
73. Schultz D, Mikala G, Yatani A, et al: Cloning, chromosomal localization, and functional expression of the alpha 1 subunit of the L-type voltage-dependent calcium channel from normal human heart. Proc Natl Acad Sci USA 90:6228, 1993.
74. Perez-Reyes E, Cribbs LL, Daud A, et al: Molecular characterization of a neuronal low-voltage-activated T-type calcium channel. Nature 391:896, 1998.
75. Chien AJ, Zhao X, Shirokov RE, et al: Roles of a membrane-localized beta subunit in the formation and targeting of functional L-type Ca^{2+} channels. J Biol Chem 270:30036, 1995.
76. Perez-Reyes E, Castellano A, Kim HS, et al: Cloning and expression of a cardiac/brain beta subunit of the L-type calcium channel. J Biol Chem 267:1792, 1992.
77. Cens T, Mangoni ME, Richard S, et al: Coexpression of the beta2 subunit does not induce voltage-dependent facilitation of the class C L-type Ca^{2+} channel. Pflugers Arch 431:771, 1996.
78. De Jongh KS, Warner C, Catterall WA: Subunits of purified calcium channels. Alpha 2 and delta are encoded by the same gene. J Biol Chem 265:14738, 1990.
79. Yang J, Ellinor PT, Sather WA, et al: Molecular determinants of Ca^{2+} selectivity and ion permeation in L-type Ca^{2+} channels. Nature 366:158, 1993.
80. Hess P, Tsien RW: Mechanism of ion permeation through calcium channels. Nature 309:453, 1984.
81. Hadley RW, Lederer WJ: Ca^{2+} and voltage inactivate Ca^{2+} channels in guinea-pig ventricular myocytes through independent mechanisms. J Physiol 444:257, 1991.
82. de Leon M, Wang Y, Jones L, et al: Essential Ca^{2+}-binding motif for Ca^{2+}-sensitive inactivation of L- type Ca^{2+} channels. Science 270:1502, 1995.
83. Zuhlke RD, Pitt GS, Deisseroth K, et al: Calmodulin supports both inactivation and facilitation of L-type calcium channels. Nature 399:159, 1999.
84. Peterson BZ, Lee JS, Mulle JG, et al: Critical determinants of Ca^{2+}-dependent inactivation within an EF- hand motif of L-type Ca^{2+} channels. Biophys J 78:1906, 2000.
85. Yue DT, Herzig S, Marban E: Beta-adrenergic stimulation of calcium channels occurs by potentiation of high-activity gating modes. Proc Natl Acad Sci USA 87:753, 1990.
86. Dzhura I, Wu Y, Colbran RJ, et al: Calmodulin kinase determines calcium-dependent facilitation of L-type calcium channels. Nat Cell Biol 2:173, 2000.
87. Hartzell HC, Mery PF, Fischmeister R, et al: Sympathetic regulation of cardiac calcium current is due exclusively to cAMP-dependent phosphorylation. Nature 351:573, 1991.
88. Perets T, Blumenstein Y, Shistik E, et al: A potential site of functional modulation by protein kinase A in the cardiac Ca^{2+} channel alpha 1C subunit. FEBS Lett 384:189, 1996.
89. Gao T, Yatani A, Dell'Acqua ML, et al: cAMP-dependent regulation of cardiac L-type Ca^{2+} channels requires membrane targeting of PKA and phosphorylation of channel subunits. Neuron 19:185, 1997.
90. Gray PC, Scott JD, Catterall WA: Regulation of ion channels by cAMP-dependent protein kinase and A-kinase anchoring proteins. Curr Opin Neurobiol 8:330, 1998.
91. Welling A, Ludwig A, Zimmer S, et al: Alternatively spliced IS6 segments of the alpha 1C gene determine the tissue-specific dihydropyridine sensitivity of cardiac and vascular smooth muscle L-type Ca^{2+} channel. Circ Res 81:526, 1997.
92. Soldatov NM, Bouron A, Reuter H: Different voltage-dependent inhibition by dihydropyridines of human Ca^{2+} channel splice variants. J Biol Chem 270:10540, 1995.
93. Yang Y, Chen X, Margulies K, et al: L-type Ca^{2+} channel alpha 1c subunit isoform switching in failing human ventricular myocardium. J Mol Cell Cardiol 32:973, 2000.
94. Yue L, Melnyk P, Gaspo R, et al: Molecular mechanisms underlying ionic remodeling in a dog model of atrial fibrillation. Circ Res 84:776, 1999.
95. Anderson ME, Braun AP, Schulman H, et al: Multifunctional Ca^{2+}/calmodulin-dependent protein kinase mediates Ca^{2+}-induced enhancement of the L-type Ca^{2+} current in rabbit ventricular myocytes. Circ Res 75:854, 1994.
96. Wu Y, Roden DM, Anderson ME: Calmodulin kinase inhibition pre-

vents development of the arrhythmogenic transient inward current. Circ Res 84:906, 1999.

97. Marban E, Robinson SW, Weir WG: Mechanisms of arrhythmogenic delayed and early afterdepolarizations and triggered activity in vivo. J Clin Invest 78:1185, 1986.

98. Mazur A, Roden DM, Anderson ME: Systemic administration of calmodulin antagonist W-7 or protein kinase A inhibitor H-8 prevents torsades de pointes in rabbits. Circulation 100:2437, 1999.

99. Nuss HB, Houser SR: T-type Ca^{2+} current is expressed in hypertrophied adult feline left ventricular myocytes. Circ Res 73:777, 1993.

100. Po SS, Snyders DJ, Baker R, et al: Functional expression of an inactivating potassium channel cloned from human heart. Circ Res 71:732, 1992.

101. Dixon JE, McKinnon D: Quantitative analysis of potassium channel mRNA expression in atrial and ventricular muscle of rats. Circ Res 75:252, 1994.

102. An WF, Bowlby MR, Betty M, et al: Modulation of A-type potassium channels by a family of calcium sensors. Nature 403:553, 2000.

103. Tseng GN, Hoffman BF: Two components of transient outward current in canine ventricular myocytes. Circ Res 64:633, 1989.

104. Zygmunt AC, Gibbons WR: Calcium-activated chloride current in rabbit ventricular mycoytes. Circ Res 68:424, 1991.

105. Beuckelmann DJ, Näbauer M, Erdmann E: Alterations of K^+ currents in isolated human ventricular myocytes from patients with terminal heart failure. Circ Res 73:379, 1993.

106. Kaab S, Dixon J, Duc J, et al: Molecular basis of transient outward potassium current downregulation in human heart failure: A decrease in Kv4.3 mRNA correlates with a reduction in current density. Circulation 98:1383, 1998.

107. Yang T, Kupershmidt S, Roden DM: Anti-minK antisense decreases the amplitude of the rapidly-activating cardiac delayed rectifier K^+ current. Circ Res 77:1246, 1995.

108. McDonald TV, Yu Z, Ming Z, et al: A minK-HERG complex regulates the cardiac potassium current I(Kr). Nature 388:289, 1997.

109. Abbott GW, Sesti F, Splawski I, et al: MiRP1 forms I_{Kr} potassium channels with HERG and is associated with cardiac arrhythmia. Cell 97:175, 1999.

110. Shibasaki T: Conductance and kinetics of delayed rectifier potassium channels in nodal cells of the rabbit heart. J Physiol (Lond) 387:227, 1987.

111. Smith PL, Baukrowitz T, Yellen G: The inward rectification mechanism of the *HERG* cardiac potassium channel. Nature 379:833, 1996.

112. Viswanathan PC, Shaw RM, Rudy Y: Effects of IKr and IKs heterogeneity on action potential duration and its rate dependence: A simulation study. Circulation 99:2466, 1999.

113. Zhou Z, Gong Q, Ye B, et al: Properties of HERG channels stably expressed in HEK 293 cells studied at physiological temperature. Biophys J 74:230, 1998.

114. Choy AM, Lang CC, Chomsky DM, et al: Normalization of acquired QT prolongation in humans by intravenous potassium. Circulation 96:2149, 1997.

115. Sanguinetti MC, Jiang C, Curran ME, et al: A mechanistic link between an inherited and an acquired cardiac arrhythmia: HERG encodes the I_{Kr} potassium channel. Cell 81:299, 1995.

116. Numaguchi H, Johnson JP Jr, Petersen CI, et al: A sensitive mechanism for cation modulation of potassium current. Nat Neurosci 3:429, 2000.

117. Hondeghem LM, Snyders DJ: Class III Antiarrhythmic agents have a lot of potential, but a long way to go: Reduced effectiveness and dangers of reverse use-dependence. Circulation 81:686, 1990.

118. Jurkiewicz NK, Sanguinetti MC: Rate-dependent prolongation of cardiac action potentials by a methanesulfonanilide class III antiarrhythmic agent: Specific block of rapidly activating delayed rectifier K^+ current by dofetilide. Circ Res 72:75, 1993.

119. Roden DM: Taking the idio out of idiosyncratic-predicting torsades de pointes. Pacing Clin Electrophysiol 21:1029, 1998.

120. Sesti F, Abbott GW, Wei J, et al: A common polymorphism associated with antibiotic-induced cardiac arrhythmia. Proc Natl Acad Sci USA 97:10613, 2000.

121. Donger C, Denjoy I, Berthet M, et al: KVLQT1 C-terminal missense mutation causes a forme fruste long-QT syndrome. Circulation 96:2778, 1997.

122. Yang P, Wei J, Murray KT, et al: Frequency of ion channel mutations and polymorphisms in a large population of patients with drug-

associated Long QT Syndrome. PACE North American Society for Pacing and Electrophysiology, 2001.

123. Napolitano C, Schwartz PJ, Brown AM, et al: Evidence for a cardiac ion channel mutation underlying drug-induced QT prolongation and life-threatening arrhythmias. J Cardiovasc Electrophysiol 11:691, 2000.

124. Piippo K, Holmstrom S, Swan H, et al: Effect of the antimalarial drug halofantrine in the long QT syndrome due to a mutation of the cardiac sodium channel gene SCN5A. Am J Cardiol 87:909, 2001.

125. Sanguinetti MC, Curran ME, Zou A, et al: Coassembly of KvLQT1 and *minK* (IsK) proteins to form cardiac I_{Ks} potassium channel. Nature 384:80, 1996.

126. Barhanin J, Lesage F, Guillemare E, et al: KvLQT1 and IsK (*minK*) proteins associate to form the I_{Ks} cardiac potassium current. Nature 384:78, 1996.

127. Tapper AR, George AL Jr: The KVLQT1 S6 transmembrane segment is a structural requirement for minK-mediated gating modulation. Biophys J 80:192a, 2001.

128. Tohse N: Calcium-sensitive delayed rectifier potassium current in guinea pig ventricular cells. Am J Physiol 258:H1200, 1990.

129. Wang Q, Curran ME, Splawski I, et al: Positional cloning of a novel potassium channel gene: *KVLQT1* mutations cause cardiac arrhythmias. Nat Genet 12:17, 1996.

130. Motoike HK, Marx SO, Reiken S, et al: Modulation of the cardiac delayed rectifier K^+ channel (IKS) by macromolecular signaling complex. Biophys J 80:507A, 2001.

131. Potet F, Scott JD, Mohammad-Panah R, et al: AKAP proteins anchor cAMP-dependent protein kinase to KvLQT1/IsK channel complex. Am J Physiol Heart Circ Physiol 280:H2038, 2001.

132. Schwartz PJ, Priori SG, Spazzolini C, et al: Genotype-phenotype correlation in the long-QT syndrome: Gene-specific triggers for life-threatening arrhythmias. Circulation 103:89, 2001.

133. Bianchi L, Priori SG, Napolitano C, et al: Mechanisms of I(Ks) suppression in LQT1 mutants. Am J Physiol Heart Circ Physiol 279:H3003, 2000.

134. Schmitt N, Schwarz M, Peretz A, et al: A recessive C-terminal Jervell and Lange-Nielsen mutation of the KCNQ1 channel impairs subunit assembly. EMBO J 19:332, 2000.

135. Bianchi L, Shen Z, Dennis AT, et al: Cellular dysfunction of LQT5-minK mutants: Abnormalities of IKs, IKr and trafficking in long QT syndrome. Hum Mol Genet 8:1499, 1999.

136. Schulze-Bahr E, Wang Q, Wedekind H, et al: KCNE1 mutations cause Jervell and Lange-Nielsen syndrome. Nat Genet 17:267, 1997.

137. Splawski I, Timothy KW, Vincent GM, et al: Molecular basis of the long QT syndrome associated with deafness. N Engl J Med 336:1562, 1997.

138. Snyders DJ, Tamkun MM, Bennett PB: A rapidly-activating and slowly-inactivating potassium channel cloned from human heart. J Gen Physiol 101:513, 1993.

139. Fedida D, Wible B, Wang Z, et al: Identity of a novel delayed rectifier current from human heart with a cloned K^+ channel current. Circ Res 73:210, 1993.

140. England SK, Uebele VN, Kodali J, et al: A novel K^+ channel Beta-subunit (hKvbeta1.3) is produced via alternative mRNA splicings. J Biol Chem 270:28531, 1995.

141. England SK, Uebele VN, Shear H, et al: Characterization of a voltage-gated K^+ channel beta subunit expressed in human heart. Proc Natl Acad Sci USA 92:6309, 1995.

142. Wang Z, Kiehn J, Yang Q, et al: Comparison of binding and block produced by alternatively spliced Kvbeta1 subunits. J Biol Chem 271:28311, 1996.

143. Wissmann R, Baukrowitz T, Kalbacher H, et al: NMR structure and functional characteristics of the hydrophilic N terminus of the potassium channel beta-subunit Kvbeta1.1. J Biol Chem 274:35521, 1999.

144. Doyle DA, Cabral JM, Pfuetzner RA, et al: The structure of the potassium channel—molecular basis of K^+ conduction and selectivity. Science 280:69, 1998.

145. Bahring R, Milligan CJ, Vardanyan V, et al: Coupling of voltage-dependent potassium channel inactivation and oxidoreductase active site of Kvbeta subunits. J Biol Chem 276:22923, 2001.

146. Levitan ES, Hershman KM, Sherman TG, et al: Dexamethasone and stress upregulate Kv1.5 K^+ channel gene expression in rat ventricular myocytes. Neuropharmacology 35:1001, 1996.

147. Nishiyama A, Kambe F, Kamiya K, et al: Effects of thyroid status on expression of voltage-gated potassium channels in rat left ventricle. Cardiovasc Res 40:343, 1998.

148. Sobko A, Peretz A, Attali B: Constitutive activation of delayed-rectifier potassium channels by a Src family tyrosine kinase in Schwann cells. EMBO J 17:4723, 1998.

149. Martens JR, Navarro-Polanco R, Coppock EA, et al: Differential targeting of Shaker-like potassium channels to lipid rafts. J Biol Chem 275:7443, 2000.

150. Martens JR, Sakamoto N, Sullivan SA, et al: Isoform-specific localization of voltage-gated K$^+$ channels to distinct lipid raft populations: Targeting of Kv1.5 to caveolae. J Biol Chem 276:8409, 2001.

151. Gong J, Xu J, Bezanilla M, et al: Differential stimulation of PKC phosphorylation of potassium channels by ZIP1 and ZIP2. Science 285:1565, 1999.

152. Kwak YG, Hu N, Wei J, et al: Protein kinase A phosphorylation alters Kvbeta1.3 subunit-mediated inactivation of the Kv1.5 potassium channel. J Biol Chem 274:13928, 1999.

153. Murray KT, Hu N, England SK, et al: Coexpression of a beta subunit enhances the effect of a phorbol ester on the Kv1.5 channel. Circulation 94:I-473, 1996.

154. Van Wagoner DR, Pond AL, McCarthy PM, et al: Outward K$^+$ current densities and Kv1.5 expression are reduced in chronic human atrial fibrillation. Circ Res 80:772, 1997.

155. Matsuda H, Saigusa A, Irisawa H: Ohmic conductance through the inwardly rectifying K$^+$ channel and blocking by internal Mg^{2+}. Nature 325:156, 1987.

156. Vandenberg CA: Inward rectification of a potassium channel in cardiac ventricular cells depends on internal magnesium ions. Proc Natl Acad Sci USA 84:2560, 1987.

157. Lopatin AN, Makhina EN, Nichols CG: Potassium channel block by cytoplasmic polyamines as the mechanism of intrinsic rectification. Nature 372:366, 1994.

158. Fakler B, Braendle U, Glowatzki E, et al: Strong voltage-dependent inward rectification of inward rectifier K$^+$ channels is caused by intracellular spermine. Cell 80:149, 1995.

159. Ficker E, Taglialatela M, Wible BA, et al: Spermine and spermidine as gating molecules for inward rectifier K$^+$ channels. Science 266:1068, 1994.

160. Wible BA, De Biasi M, Majumder K, et al: Cloning and functional expression of an inwardly rectifying K$^+$ channel from human atrium. Circ Res 76:343, 1995.

161. Krapivinsky G, Gordon EA, Wickman K, et al: The G-protein-gated atrial K$^+$ channel I$_{KACh}$ is a heteromultimer of two inwardly rectifying K$^+$-channel proteins. Nature 374:135, 1995.

162. Inagaki N, Gonoi T, Clement JP, et al: Reconstitution of I$_{KATP}$: An inward rectifier subunit plus the sulfonylurea receptor. Science 270:1166, 1995.

163. Plaster NM, Tawil R, Tristani-Firouzi M, et al: Mutations in Kir2.1 cause the developmental and episodic electrical phenotypes of Andersen's Syndrome. Cell 105:511–519, 2001.

164. Kurachi Y, Nakajima T, Sugimoto T: Acetylcholine activation of K$^+$ channels in cell-free membrane of atrial cells. Am J Physiol 251:H681, 1986.

165. Sato T, Sasaki N, Seharaseyon J, et al: Selective pharmacological agents implicate mitochondrial but not sarcolemmal K(ATP) channels in ischemic cardioprotection. Circulation 101:2418, 2000.

166. DiFrancesco D: Pacemaker mechanisms in cardiac tissue. Annu Rev Physiol 55:455, 1993.

167. Ludwig A, Zong X, Jeglitsch M, et al: A family of hyperpolarization-activated mammalian cation channels. Nature 393:587, 1998.

168. Santoro B, Liu DT, Yao H, et al: Identification of a gene encoding a hyperpolarization-activated pacemaker channel of brain. Cell 93:717, 1998.

169. Moroni A, Gorza L, Beltrame M, et al: Hyperpolarization-activated cyclic nucleotide-gated channel 1 is a molecular determinant of the cardiac pacemaker current I(f). J Biol Chem 276:29233, 2001.

170. Shi W, Wymore R, Yu H, et al: Distribution and prevalence of hyperpolarization-activated cation channel (HCN) mRNA expression in cardiac tissues. Circ Res 85:e1, 1999.

171. Miller AG, Aldrich RW: Conversion of a delayed rectifier K$^+$ channel to a voltage-gated inward rectifier K$^+$ channel by three amino acid substitutions. Neuron 16:853, 1996.

172. Baker K, Warren KS, Yellen G, et al: Defective "pacemaker" current (I$_h$) in a zebrafish mutant with a slow heart rate. Proc Natl Acad Sci USA 94:4554, 1997.

173. Yu H, Chang F, Cohen IS: Pacemaker current exists in ventricular myocytes. Circ Res 72:232, 1993.

174. Backx PH, Marban E: Background potassium current active during the plateau of the action potential in guinea pig ventricular myocytes. Circ Res 72:890, 1993.

175. Yue DT, Marban E: A novel cardiac potassium channel that is active and conductive at depolarized potentials. Pflügers Arch 413:127, 1988.

176. Lesage F, Guillemare E, Fink M, et al: TWIK-1, a ubiquitous human weakly inward rectifying K$^+$ channel with a novel structure. EMBO J 15:1004, 1996.

177. Levesque PC, Hart PJ, Hume JR, et al: Expression of cystic fibrosis transmembrane regulator Cl$^-$ channels in heart. Circ Res 71:1002, 1992.

178. Hume JR, Duan D, Collier ML, et al: Anion transport in heart. Physiol Rev 80:31, 2000.

179. Tinel N, Diochot S, Borsotto M, et al: KCNE2 confers background current characteristics to the cardiac KCNQ1 potassium channel. EMBO J 19:6326, 2000.

180. Armstrong CM: Ionic pores, gates, and gating currents. Q Rev Biophys 7:179, 1975.

181. Choi KL, Mossman C, Aube J, et al: The internal quaternary ammonium receptor site of *Shaker* potassium channels. Neuron 10:533, 1993.

182. Kirsch GE, Shieh CC, Drewe JA, et al: Segmental exchanges define 4-aminopyridine binding and the inner mouth of K$^+$ pores. Neuron 11:503, 1993.

183. Yeola SW, Rich TC, Uebele VN, et al: Molecular analysis of a binding site for quinidine in a human cardiac delayed rectifier K$^+$ channel: Role of S6 in antiarrhythmic drug binding. Circ Res 78:1105, 1996.

184. Gingrich KJ, Beardsley D, Yue DT: Ultra-deep blockade of Na$^+$ channels by a quaternary ammonium ion: Catalysis by a transition-intermediate state? J Physiol 471:319, 1993.

185. Strichartz GR: The inhibition of sodium currents in myelinated nerve by quarternary derivatives of lidocaine. J Gen Physiol 62:37, 1973.

186. Ragsdale DS, McPhee JC, Scheuer T, et al: Molecular determinants of state-dependent block of Na$^+$ channels by local anesthetics. Science 265:1724, 1994.

187. Ragsdale DS, McPhee JC, Scheuer T, et al: Common molecular determinants of local anesthetic, antiarrhythmic, and anticonvulsant block of voltage-gated Na$^+$ channels. Proc Natl Acad Sci USA 93:9270, 1996.

188. Nau C, Wang SY, Strichartz GR, et al: Point mutations at N434 in D1-S6 of mu1 Na$^+$ channels modulate binding affinity and stereoselectivity of local anesthetic enantiomers. Mol Pharmacol 56:404, 1999.

189. Hockermann GH, Johnson BD, Scheuer T, et al: Molecular determinants of high affinity phenylalkylamine block of L-type calcium channels. J Biol Chem 270:22119, 1995.

190. Schuster A, Lacinova L, Klugbauer N, et al: The IVS6 segment of the L-type calcium channel is critical for the action of dihydropyridines and phenylalkylamines. EMBO J 15:2365, 1996.

191. Sunami A, Dudley SC Jr, Fozzard HA: Sodium channel selectivity filter regulates antiarrhythmic drug binding. Proc Natl Acad Sci USA 94:14126, 1997.

192. Hille B: Local anesthetics: hydrophilic and hydrophobic pathways for the drug-receptor reaction. J Gen Physiol 69:497, 1977.

193. Hondeghem LM, Katzung BG: Time- and voltage-dependent interactions of the antiarrhythmic drugs with cardiac sodium channels. Biochim Biophys Acta 472:373, 1977.

194. Courtney KR: Mechanism of frequency-dependent inhibition of sodium currents in the frog myelinated nerve by the lidocaine derivative gea 968. J Pharm Exp Ther 195:225, 1975.

195. Balser JR, Nuss HB, Chiamvimonvat N, et al: External pore residue mediates slow inactivation in µ1 rat skeletal muscle sodium channels. J Physiol 494:431, 1996.

196. Bennett PB, Valenzuela C, Li-Qiong C, et al: On the molecular nature of the lidocaine receptor of cardiac Na$^+$ channels. Circ Res 77:584, 1995.

197. Kambouris N, Hastings L, Stepanovic S, et al: Mechanistic link between local anesthetic action and inactivation gating probed by outer pore mutations in the rat µ1 sodium channel. J Physiol 512:693, 1998.

198. Chen Z, Ong B-H, Kambouris NG, et al: Lidocaine induces a slow inactivated state in rat skeletal muscle sodium channels. J Physiol 524:37, 2000.

199. Baukrowitz T, Yellen G: Use-dependent blockers and exit rate of the last ion from the multi-ion pore of a K$^+$ channel. Science 271:653, 1996.

200. Ong BH, Tomaselli GF, Balser JR: A structural rearrangement in the sodium channel pore linked to slow inactivation and use dependence. J Gen Physiol 116:653, 2000.

201. Mitcheson JS, Chen J, Sanguinetti MC: Trapping of a methanesulfonanilide by closure of the HERG potassium channel activation gate. J Gen Physiol 115:229, 2000.

202. Mitcheson JS, Chen J, Lin M, et al: A structural basis for drug-induced long QT syndrome. Proc Natl Acad Sci USA 97:12329, 2000.

203. Luo CH, Rudy Y: A dynamic model of the cardiac ventricular action potential. II. Afterdepolarizations, triggered activity, and potentiation. Circ Res 74:1097, 1994.

204. Trimmer JS, Cooperman SS, Tomiko SA, et al: Primary structure and functional expression of a mammalian skeletal muscle sodium channel. Neuron 3:33, 1989.

18

Myocardial Performance

Pierre Foëx, DM, MA • Helen Higham, MB, ChB

The heart can be considered as both a muscle and a pump. As a pump, it must be able to deliver oxygen and fuels to, and remove carbon dioxide and metabolic byproducts from, the tissues. It must also allow for the transport of hormones, vasoactive and immune substances, as well as a large number of metabolic mediators. Because the heart is coupled to two circulations, its performance is, to an extent, determined by the characteristics of these circulations. During normal physiologic conditions, the systemic circulation plays a dominant role in the function of the heart by modifying its venous return and its resistance to ejection through changes in vasomotor tone reflecting changes in metabolic requirements.

System Physiology

Cardiac Cycle

Before mechanical activity begins, an electrical signal is delivered by a specialized conduction system to the myocardium. This system controls the heart rate and responds to a variety of influences, notably sympathetic and parasympathetic stimulation. It provides a sequence of activation that maximizes efficient contraction and filling, while initiating the biochemical processes that underlie contraction. The conduction system cells have the property of undergoing spontaneous depolarization, thereby functioning as pacemakers. The sinus node has the fastest rate of spontaneous depolarization, and therefore provides the normal initiation of contraction.

Activity of the conduction system and spread of electrical impulses through the myocardium form, at body surface, is the signal described as the electrocardiogram (ECG). At cellular level, electrical excitation consists of transmission of membrane depolarization followed by repolarization—the action potential that is propagated through the myocardium. The action potential arises in the sinoatrial node and spreads to the atria causing atrial contraction. Impulses in the atrial conduction system converge on the atrioventricular node and more distally reach the His bundle. Conduction is slow in the atrioventricular node such that there is a delay between atrial and ventricular contraction.

The His bundle gives rise to intraventricular fascicles, the right and left bundles; the latter is divided into left anterior and left posterior fascicles. Depolarization of the atria accounts for the P waves, whereas depolarization of the ventricles accounts for the QRS complex of the ECG. Within the myocardium, the action potential spreads from myocytes to myocytes through the intercalated disks.

The mechanical cycle, conventionally, begins at end-diastole just before activation of the ventricle causes a rapid increase in intraventricular pressure (Fig. 18–1). As pressure in the ventricles exceeds atrial pressure, the atrioventricular valves close. When ventricular pressures exceed aortic and pulmonary pressures, the aortic and pulmonary valves open and ejection begins. Before ejection starts, ventricular con-

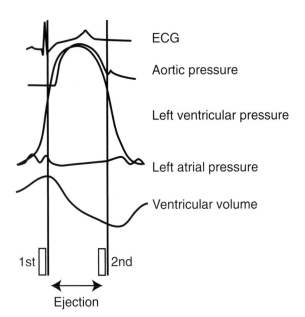

Figure 18–1. Schematic representation of the temporal relationships of electrical, mechanical, and auditory events of the cardiac cycle. ECG, electrocardiogram.

tractions are isovolumic. During ejection, ventricular, aortic, and pulmonary artery pressures increase and decrease together. Ejection stops when aortic and pulmonary pressures exceed their respective ventricular pressures causing the aortic and pulmonary valves to close; these events are marked by dicrotic notches. Whereas in the left ventricle there is a rapid decrease in pressure before the mitral valve opens, representing isovolumic relaxation, the low pulmonary artery pressure in respect of the right atrial pressure makes isovolumic relaxation almost nonexistent in the right ventricle.[1] Opening of the atrioventricular valves allows ventricular filling to begin. The initial rapid filling phase is followed by slow filling, and a complete halt (diastasis) before atrial contraction completes the ventricular filling.

Whereas systolic pressures between left and right ventricle differ because of differences in ventricular wall thickness and in resistance to ejection, diastolic filling pressures are fairly similar. However, as the thicker left ventricular wall is less distensible than the thinner right ventricular wall, diastolic pressure is usually slightly greater in the left than in the right ventricle.

The Heart Attached to the Circulation

Vascular Systems

The heart is at the center of two series-coupled vascular circuits: the pulmonary and the systemic vascular beds. The elasticity of the larger arteries and the resistance to flow of the peripheral vessels reduce the changes in arterial and pulmonary pressures in respect of the changes in ventricular pressures, i.e., the changes in pulse pressures are much smaller than the changes in ventricular pressures.

The large arteries offer little resistance to flow. They are distensible and damp the pulsatile output of the ventricles; their elasticity allows systolic storage and diastolic propulsion of blood flow between cardiac contractions. As blood reaches small arteries, flow is relatively steady throughout the cardiac cycle in the systemic but not in the pulmonary circulation where it remains pulsatile. As arteries subdivide, the proportion of elastic fibers decreases and the walls become thinner. In the systemic circulation, the media of the arterioles consist predominantly of smooth muscle with a rich nerve supply. The caliber of arterioles determines the distribution of blood flow throughout the body and allows arterial pressure to be maintained within relatively narrow limits in the face of even large changes in cardiac output. In pulmonary circulation, large changes in cardiac output are accommodated by recruitment of capillaries.

The systemic precapillary resistance vessels consisting of small arteries and arterioles offer the greater part of the total resistance to flow. Small changes in their diameter cause large changes in their resistance. Even though at each branching the combined cross-sectional area of the branches exceeds that of the stem, the resistance offered to flow increases because the radius of each branch is smaller than that of the stem. This is because resistance (R) is inversely proportional to the cross-sectional area of the vessel multiplied by the square of its radius:

$$R = 8 | \, L/\pi r^2 . r^2$$

Where $|$ is the fluid viscosity, L is the length of the vessel, and r is its radius.

The precapillary sphincters determine the size of the capillary exchange area by altering the number of open capillaries.

The capillary exchange vessels form a dense network with a large cross-sectional area, a large surface limited by a single layer of endothelial cells, and a short length. The average dimensions of systemic capillaries are: radius = 3 μm; length = 750 μm; cross-sectional area = 30 μm²; and surface area = 15,000 μm². At rest, 25% to 35% of the capillaries are open, and the effective total surface area is between 250 and 350 m². The pulmonary capillaries are wider (4 μm) and shorter (350 μm) than the systemic capillaries; their total effective surface area is approximately 60 m² at rest, increasing to 90 m² in heavy exercise.[2,3] The average transit time through the lung capillaries is approximately 1 second decreasing to 0.35 second with heavy exercise.

As the heart is coupled with both the systemic and the pulmonary circulations, its ability to generate blood flow depends on the intrinsic characteristics of its fibers (see later) and the functional state of the greater and lesser circulations. These determine both the venous return to the ventricles (the preload) and the dynamic load imposed on its ejection (the afterload). The level of activity of all tissues and organs, through local regulation, determines their blood flow and the total cardiac output. As this, in turn, determines venous return, the preload of the right ventricle is a function of metabolic demands unless extraneous factors alter the size of the capacitance vessels. The pulmonary circulation passively adapts to accommodate the cardiac output with little change in pressure unless the pulmonary vasculature is diseased giving rise to pulmonary hypertension. Thus during normal circumstances, the preload of the left ventricle is the same as that of the right ventricle. When metabolic demands increase, resistance to left ventricular ejection is reduced and ejection is facilitated.

Vascular resistance is generally used as an index of vascular tone. Vascular resistance is the relationship between mean pressure and mean flow assuming a nonpulsatile circulation. However, pressure and flow are pulsatile, especially in the pulmonary circulation. Thus the concept of impedance, the dynamic relationship between pressure and flow, is more appropriate. It includes a mean term representing mean pressure and mean flow, and pulsatile terms, the impedance moduli for different harmonics of the fundamental frequency (the heart rate), and the phase angles between pressure and flow.[4] In normal systemic circulation, the static component of the impedance spectrum (i.e., systemic vascular resistance) is large with respect to the oscillatory components. However, in pulmonary circulation, the static term (pulmonary vascular resistance) is much smaller and oscillatory components cannot be ignored as they contribute significantly to the load opposing right ventricular ejection.

Cardiac Pump Function

The effect of changes in preload on cardiac pump function have been characterized by Starling[5] and later by Sarnoff[6] and can be described in terms of ventricular function curves. An increase in the filling of the ventricles causes a curvilinear increase in stroke volume, stroke work, and cardiac output (Fig. 18–2). This relationship is steeper for the thick-walled left ventricle than for the thin-walled right ventricle.

Ventricular function is also influenced by the afterload: a reduction in outflow resistance allows the heart to eject a larger stroke volume. In the presence of cardiac muscle dysfunction, an increased afterload causes larger reductions of stroke volume and cardiac output than in the healthy heart.

In the healthy heart, increases in resistance cause a decrease in ejection that is limited by the presence of a homeometric mechanism: an increase in outflow resistance initially reduces ejection, this in turn increases diastolic wall tension so that the preload increases for the next contraction. This effect allows output to be relatively well maintained in the face of rising afterload, unless the heart is damaged. Beat-to-beat variations in loading of the heart related to normal function such as respiration require fine tuning of the stroke volume produced by each side of the heart because any mismatch of left- and right-sided stroke volumes cannot be tolerated.

In the intact circulation, the dynamic characteristics of the cardiac pump are best described in terms of pressure-volume relationships (Fig. 18–3A). If ventricular pressure is plotted against ventricular volume, each cardiac cycle can

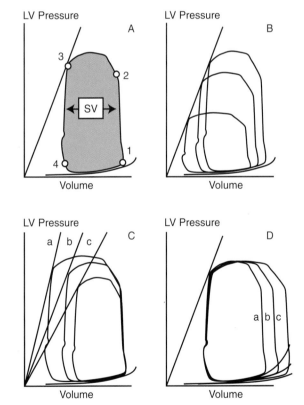

Figure 18–3. Each cardiac cycle can be represented by a pressure-volume loop. *A,* Mitral valve closure (*1*), aortic valve opening (*2*), aortic valve closure (*3*), mitral valve opening (*4*). The end-diastolic (*a*) and the end-systolic (*b*) pressure-volume relationships represent the boundaries for the loops. *B,* Effect of changes in vascular resistance on the pressure-volume loop. *C,* Increases (*a*)/decreases (*c*) in contractility make the end-systolic pressure volume relationship steeper or shallower. *D,* Effect of changes in ventricular compliance allowing the end-diastolic volume to become larger (increased compliance; *a*) or smaller (reduced compliance; *c*). LV, left ventricle.

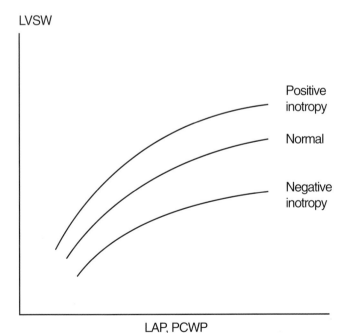

Figure 18–2. Diagram representing the relationship between left ventricular stroke work (LVSW) and filling pressures, left atrial pressure (LAP) and pulmonary capillary wedge pressure (PCWP). Ventricular function curves are shifted upward or downward by increases/decreases in contractility.

be represented by a pressure-volume loop. Isovolumic contraction, ejection, isovolumic relaxation, and ventricular filling constitute the four segments of the loop and are delineated for the left ventricle, in succession, by mitral valve closure, aortic valve opening, aortic valve closure, and mitral valve opening. The width of the pressure-volume loop represents the stroke volume and its area represents the stroke work. The end-diastolic pressure-volume coordinates form part of the end-diastolic pressure-volume relationship or ventricular compliance, whereas the end-systolic pressure-volume coordinates form part of the end-systolic pressure-volume relationship or maximum ventricular elastance (Fig. 18–3B).[7,8] Irrespective of preload and afterload, all ventricular pressure-volume loops are bounded by these relationships unless contractility is increased (maximum elastance increases) or decreased (maximum elastance decreases) (Fig. 18–3C). Similarly, a decrease in compliance shifts the end-diastolic pressure-volume relationship upward, whereas an increase in compliance shifts it downward (Fig. 18–3D).

Changes in contractility and in compliance, although best described in terms of instantaneous pressure-volume relationships, are also reflected in the ventricular function curve. Increases in contractility shift the ventricular function curve upward, whereas decreases shift it downward. When compliance is altered, the filling volume, i.e., the true preload, is altered. Therefore, the curve is also shifted upward by an increase in compliance and downward by a decrease in compliance. Finally, increases and decreases in resistance shift the ventricular function curve downward and upward, respectively (Fig. 18–4). The curvilinearity of the ventricular function curves is characteristic of the stroke volume-filling pressure relationship. When stroke volume is plotted against end-diastolic ventricular volume, the relationship is linear. This reflects the curvilinear relationship between end-diastolic pressure and volume.

Another way of representing changes in contractility is the preload recruitable stroke work. In this approach, the area of pressure-volume loops (the stroke work) is plotted against left ventricular end-diastolic volume.[9] The values form a straight line, the slope of which is an index of contractility. The slope becomes steeper with positive inotropy and flatter with negative inotropy.

Cardiac function can also be assessed in terms of the relationship between stroke volume and end-diastolic volume: the ejection fraction. Because the stroke volume (the width of the pressure-volume loop) depends on preload, afterload, contractility, and compliance, the ejection fraction is not a pure index of contractility.[10] Contractility and preload have proportional direct effects on the ejection fraction, whereas afterload and compliance have inverse effects.

The determinants of cardiac pump function are influenced by the activity of the autonomic nervous system. α_1-Adrenoceptor stimulation decreases venous compliance, thereby increasing venous return; it also increases systemic vascular tone and myocardial contractility, in part by sensitizing the contractile proteins to calcium. β_1-Adrenoceptor stimulation increases contractility and heart rate, whereas β_2-adrenoceptor stimulation increases contractility and heart rate and decreases vascular tone.

Coronary Circulation

Unlike other organs and tissues, the heart has to provide its own perfusion while supplying blood flow to the whole body. This imposes considerable metabolic demands on the heart muscle and therefore on the coronary circulation. Yet perfusion is impeded by the high extravascular compressive forces resulting from the development of wall tension during ventricular systole. Because of the mechanical constraints imposed on the coronary circulation, oxygen extraction approaches 70% at rest.[11] This means that increases in myocardial oxygen consumption (mVO_2) must be met by commensurate increases in coronary blood flow, because there is little scope for an increase in extraction. Consequently, there is a linear relationship between coronary blood flow and myocardial oxygen consumption.[12]

The large epicardial branches of the left and right coronary arteries give rise to smaller branches. These penetrate the myocardium at right angle and divide in an extensive network of small arteries and arterioles that, in turn, give rise to an extremely dense capillary network. The intercapillary distance is approximately 10 to 14 μm and there is one capillary for each cardiac fiber. Thus the distance between capillaries and sites of oxygen utilization is only a few micrometers. Control of subepicardial and subendocardial vessels allows the transmural distribution of blood flow to vary to adjust oxygen supply to local demands. There are intercoronary and intracoronary collateral vessels. These vessels may play an important role in the presence of coronary artery lesions, limiting the extent of ischemia and preventing cell death.[13]

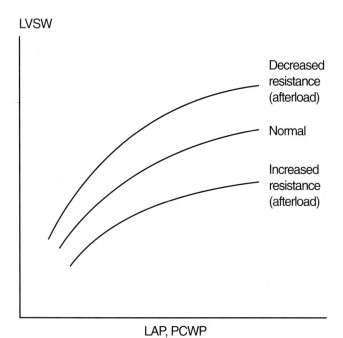

Figure 18–4. Diagram representing the relationship between cardiac work (stroke work) and filling pressures. Ventricular function curves are shifted upward by increases and downward by reductions in vascular resistance. LVSW, left ventricular stroke work.

The endothelium of the coronary circulation plays an important role because it is capable of releasing endothelium-dependent vasoactive substances. Shear stress, pulsatile flow, and hypoxia stimulate the production of prostacyclin, a potent coronary vasodilator.[14] Similarly, shear stress, hypoxia, and acetylcholine stimulate constitutive nitric oxide synthase (NOS), thereby increasing the production and release of NO, resulting in cyclic guanosine monophosphate–mediated coronary vasodilatation. Endothelium-dependent vasoconstrictors such as endothelins, thromboxane A2, and angiotensin are also released under the influence of endogenous and exogenous substances, or stimuli, or both.[15,16] An imbalance between vasodilators and vasoconstrictors can develop in advanced coronary artery disease, especially a reduced release of NO and an increased synthesis of endothelins. The latter cause vasoconstriction and facilitate platelet adhesion. These changes increase the risk for thrombosis and smooth muscle proliferation.

Regulation of Myocardial Perfusion

The major determinant of coronary vascular resistance is intramyocardial pressure. During systole, lateral shearing forces may completely abolish flow to certain regions of the myocardium.[17] In the wall of the left ventricle, systolic extravascular compression is so pronounced that only 20% to 30% of flow occurs during systole, and 70% to 80% during diastole. In the wall of the right ventricle, because the compressive forces are much lower than in the left ventricle, flow occurs during both systole and diastole. The distribution of flow is not uniform.[18] Because of greater metabolic requirements, subendocardial flow exceeds subepicardial flow by approximately 10%. This is possible because there is a greater degree of vasodilatation at the subendocardium; but, as a consequence, the subendocardium is very sensitive to a reduction in coronary perfusion pressure, and coronary flow reserve is smaller than in the subepicardium.

The coronary perfusion pressure is the difference between the upstream and downstream pressures. The upstream pressure is the pressure at the aortic root, whereas the downstream pressure is difficult to define.[19] It can be taken as the coronary sinus pressure or the left ventricular end-diastolic pressure. However, the pressure-flow relationship during a long diastole suggests that flow becomes zero at a pressure that is greater than the left ventricular end-diastolic pressure, the so-called critical closing pressure.[20]

The coronary flow reserve is the difference between locally regulated flow and flow when the coronary arteries are maximally dilated.[21] The coronary flow reserve varies with the coronary perfusion pressure and is reduced in the presence of coronary artery lesions.

Autoregulation of Coronary Blood Flow

Autoregulation is the intrinsic ability of the heart to maintain constant coronary flow in the face of wide changes in coronary perfusion pressure.[22] It is observed in experimental studies where the coronary circulation is perfused independently. In the intact heart, increases in coronary perfusion pressure result from greater systemic and left ventricular pressures, and are therefore associated with increased metabolic demands (Fig. 18–5). Autoregulation may be the result of myogenic mechanisms and of changes in metabolic mediators.

Metabolic Control

Metabolic control of coronary blood flow results from local mechanisms that are capable of adjusting coronary blood flow to match metabolic demands. Metabolic demands are the sum of basal metabolism (25–5%), wall tension (30%), external work (10–15%), activation processes (10–15%), and electrical activity (1%).[23] The major determinants of wall tension and external work are heart rate, systolic pressure, ventricular diastolic pressure, and contractility. The precise mechanisms of the coupling of blood flow and metabolic demands are not fully elucidated. They include local PO_2, PCO_2, pH, K^+, Ca^{2+}, osmolality, and adenosine.[24] Adenosine is a potent coronary vasodilator. It is postulated that a reduction in cellular oxygen partial pressure causes an increase in the synthesis and release of adenosine. Adenosine, in turn, acts on the vascular smooth muscle causing coronary vasodilatation. However, adenosine does not appear to be the primary mediator of the close coupling of oxygen demand and supply. Adenosine triphosphate (ATP)-sensitive K^+ channels (K^+_{ATP} channels), by contrast, appear to play a major role. Opening of the K^+_{ATP} channels results in hyperpolarization of the cell membrane. This closes the calcium channels. As cytosolic Ca^{2+} decreases, vascular smooth muscle relaxes. K^+_{ATP} channels are opened by receptor activation (adenosine, acetylcholine) or by metabolic

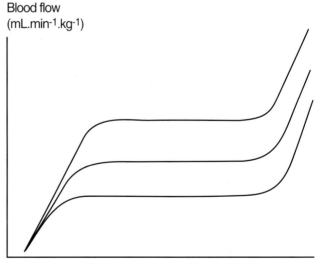

Blood flow
$(mL.min^{-1}.kg^{-1})$

Perfusion pressure (mm Hg)

Figure 18–5. The relationship between blood flow and perfusion may exhibit autoregulation. In the coronary circulation, as metabolic requirements vary where there is a change in coronary perfusion pressure, the autoregulation curve cannot be unique. The autoregulation curve is shifted upward by increases and downward by decreases in oxygen consumption.

factors (decreased ATP caused by hypoxia or ischemia).[25] Blockade of K^+_{ATP} channels increases coronary vascular resistance and reduces coronary blood flow.[26]

Other substances including prostaglandins and NO alter coronary vascular resistance. Recently, NO has been shown to play a role in the normal control of coronary blood flow.[27]

Neurogenic Control

Both sympathetic and parasympathetic nerves supply the heart. Autonomic innervation can influence coronary blood flow. Cholinergic stimulation causes coronary vasodilatation that is mediated by the release of NO by the endothelium of the vessels.[28]

Adrenergic stimulation increases metabolic demands by increasing heart rate and contractility (β_1 stimulation) and arterial pressure (α_1 stimulation). This results in increases in oxygen consumption that, in turn, increase coronary blood flow because the vasoconstriction caused by α_1-adrenoceptor stimulation is overshadowed by local metabolic regulation. However, in the case of hypoperfusion, local and neurogenic regulation may compete, the latter opposing the metabolic vasodilatation. If the endothelium is damaged, α_1-mediated vasoconstriction is enhanced.[29]

Organ and Cellular Physiology

The behavior of the heart as a pump is the result of the characteristics of the heart fibers that form the heart muscle.

Cardiac Cell

Myocytes are branched filament-like structures 10 to 20 μm in diameter and 50 to 100 μm in length. They are attached to one another at intercalated disks. Approximately every 2 μm in their longitudinal axis, transverse tubules (T tubules) penetrate the cells and facilitate their activation because they are regions of ion fluxes. Ion fluxes in and out of the myocytes are controlled by pumps and channels in the sarcolemma and in the membranes of the sarcoplasmic reticulum (SR) and the mitochondria.

Cardiac cells include three systems: (1) sarcolemmal excitation system participating in the spread of conduction and in the initiation of intracellular events responsible for contraction; (2) an intracellular excitation-contraction coupling system that converts an amplified electrical signal into a chemical signal; and finally, (3) a contractile system within which cross-bridges between actin and myosin are formed.

The basic contractile functional unit is the sarcomere. Each sarcomere is composed of two bundles of longitudinal filaments. The thick filaments consist of about 300 individual molecules of myosin, approximately 1.6 μm in length and 10 to 15 μm in width. They are placed in the center of the sarcomeres' length. Each molecule of myosin has a

bilobed head.[30] Half of these are oriented toward one end of the sarcomere and half toward the other end. Sets of three heads are rotated about 40 degrees in relation to their predecessors, at a distance of 14.3 nm. This is essential as each filament of myosin is surrounded by six filaments of actin.

The thin filaments are composed of actin, tropomyosin (Tm), and troponin (Tn). The length of actin molecules is approximately 1 μm; they interdigitate with the myosin filaments at one end, whereas they are attached to the Z-line at the other end. Actin monomers are arranged in a double helix to form the core of the thin filament[31,32]; Tm is adsorbed longitudinally along the thin filament. Troponins C, I, and T (TnC, TnI, and TnT) are adsorbed on Tm. The combined Tm-Tn complex is responsible for the ability of calcium ions to act as a switch for the initiation of cross-bridge formation. They are 1 μm in length and 5.7 nm in width. Tn complexes are placed at intervals of 38 nm. TnC, the binding site for calcium, is part of a complex that includes TnI (the inhibitory protein for the interaction of actin and myosin) and TnT, which links the Tn complex to Tm. Tns are released when the myocardium is damaged. TnT and TnI are controlled by different genes in cardiac and skeletal muscle. They can be differentiated and used as markers of cardiac injury.[33–35]

With activation, calcium ions bind to TnC and cause a rearrangement of the Tn complex with strong binding of TnI to TnC rather than to Tm. This, in turn, alters the position of Tm on actin and releases the inhibition of actin-myosin interaction (Fig. 18–6). The binding of calcium to Tn causes the process of cross-bridge formation to spread down the thin filament; strong binding encourages additional filament activation.[36] During most physiologic conditions, systolic calcium concentration does not achieve a level resulting in maximum force or shortening. Although the myosin head is strongly bound to actin, energy released from hydrolysis of ATP causes the myosin head to rotate, resulting in an oarlike motion. In the absence of restraining forces, cross-bridges

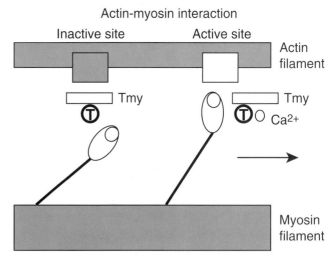

Figure 18–6. Diagram representing the interaction between actin and myosin filaments. As an interaction site on the actin filament becomes active, the lateral projections of myosin are elongated and the heads rotate. Tmy, tropomyosin; T, troponins.

propel the filaments at maximum speed with no force development (unloaded shortening). If an external load opposes shortening, cross-bridge motion is slowed allowing for force to be developed.

At diastolic calcium concentration, cross-bridges exist as a truly detached or blocked state and a weakly attached state that does not produce force. The latter may be closed or open, depending on the position of Tm on actin.[37]

Myocytes are capable of increasing the number, and changing the arrangement, of sarcomeres in response to physiologic or pathologic changes in demands. An increase in sarcomeres in series increases the capacity for shortening, whereas an increase in parallel increases that for force generation.

Excitation System

The excitation system consists of a transient local depolarizing inward sodium current that raises the transmembrane potential from −80 to −90 mV to slightly positive values followed by a repolarizing current. With respect to contraction, the most important component of the action potential is the slow inward calcium current through voltage-sensitive, L-type, calcium channels. Potassium efflux repolarizes the cell (Fig. 18–7). L-type calcium channels are concentrated in the transverse tubules that are in close proximity to the SR membrane-associated ryanodine receptor calcium release channels (Fig. 18–8). The sodium-calcium exchanger moves calcium ions out of the cell against its concentration gradient while using energy from the sodium gradient to move one sodium ion into the cell.

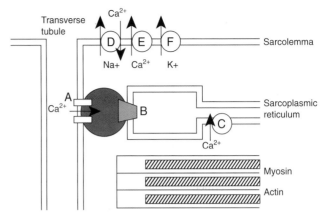

Figure 18–8. Diagram representing channels and pumps in the vicinity of transverse tubules. (*A*) A L-type Ca^{2+} channel; (*B*) a sarcolemmal ryanodine receptor; (*C*) a sarcoplasmic Ca^{2+} pump; (*D*) a Na^+-Ca^{2+} exchange pump; (*E*) a Ca^{2+} pump; and (*F*) a K^+ pump. The *hatched* area is the dyad. (Modified from Katz AM: Physiology of the Heart, 2nd ed. New York, Raven, 1992.)

The SR is longitudinally oriented and encircles the contractile filaments at 1 to 2 μm spacing. It contains a large store of calcium ions, the bulk of which is associated with binding proteins such as calsequestrin. The action potential depolarizes the cell membrane in the region where T tubules are in close proximity of subsarcolemmal cisternae (the dyad); this opens the gate of L-type calcium channels, allowing calcium ions to cross the sarcolemma into the gap region of the dyad (Fig. 18–8). Nearby ryanodine calcium release channels are activated by this local increase in calcium concentration, resulting in the rapid release of much larger amounts of calcium ions from the cisternae of the SR into the cytoplasm.[38,39] As a result of this amplifying system, calcium concentration increases from 0.1 to 1–10 μmol (peak of the calcium transient). The increase in calcium concentration is very transient because calcium binds to contractile proteins and is removed by both the sodium-calcium exchanger and by the sarcoplasmic calcium ATPase (SERCA2).[40] This is a membrane spanning protein of the SR that uses energy from ATP hydrolysis to pump calcium ions back into the SR. The activity of SERCA2 is self-regulating such that its speed increases in proportion to free calcium concentration. It is also regulated by phospholamban, a key modulator of cardiac responses to adrenergic signaling.[41] As an example, β_1-adrenergic stimulation activates the cyclic adenosine monophosphate (cAMP)-dependent protein kinase A (PKA) resulting in the phosphorylation of phospholamban. As phospholamban is phosphorylated, its inhibitory effect on SERCA2 is reduced resulting in increased calcium cycling and increased rate and force of contraction.

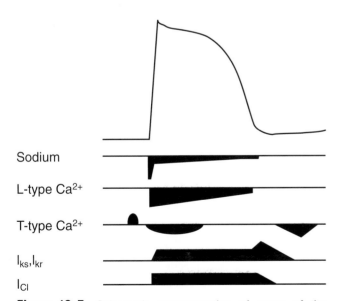

Figure 18–7. Schematic representation of some of the sodium, calcium, and potassium ion fluxes responsible for the action potential of cardiac cells. For each ion, inward fluxes are denoted by an area under the line; conversely, outward fluxes are represented by areas above the respective line (Redrawn from Snyders DJ: Structure and function of cardiac potassium channels. Cardiovas Res 42:377–390, 1999.)

Cardiac Contraction

After depolarization, the thick and thin filaments slide past each other[42,43] in an oarlike motion, as hydrolysis of ATP supplies the energy to the process of contraction.[42,43] This motion is possible because of the lateral projections of the myosin filaments with their articulated head attached to an arm that is capable of sustaining tension. Abduction of the arms brings the heads closer to the actin filaments, thus allowing cross-bridges to form at the level of new active sites on the actin molecules. Head rotation pulls on the arm and causes the actin filaments to move relative to the myosin filament.[44] As the actin filaments of each unit are attached to those of adjacent units, this motion results in force development and shortening. The formation of a cross-bridge represents the consumption of one molecule of ATP. The total force developed is a function of the number of cross-bridges. The rate of change of force depends on the number of cross-bridges formed by unit time. As the formation of each cross-bridge consumes one molecule of ATP, both increased force development and increased rate of force development (i.e., increased contractility) contribute directly to the energy requirement of contraction. Once calcium is removed from the Tn-Tm complex, the active sites are blocked, the cross-bridges separate, and relaxation and resting state ensue.

A change in cytosolic calcium concentrations is central to the interaction of actin and myosin. Calcium concentration increases to a peak (contraction) before it decreases again (relaxation occurs). As calcium binds with TnC molecules, the total length of actin available for the formation of cross-bridges increases. There are several sites for calcium on the TnC molecule, and one of them is responsible for conformational changes in the distant region of the molecule promoting contraction.[45] In addition to initiating the contractile cycle, calcium alters the kinetics of cross-bridge formation, altering the myosin ATPase activity, thereby increasing contractility.[46]

Although calcium entry through calcium channels contributes to an increase in myoplasmic calcium, the major contributor to the peak of calcium concentration is the triggered release of calcium from the SR. Similarly, the major determinant of the decline in myoplasmic concentration is an energy-dependent re-uptake of calcium by the SR.

Cardiac Mechanics

Most of the knowledge relating to cardiac mechanics derives from observations made in two experimental models: isometric and isotonic contractions (Fig. 18–9). For isometric contractions, a small length of cardiac muscle (often papillary muscles) is attached to a fixed point and to a force transducer such that contraction occurs without shortening. For isotonic contractions, a length of muscle is attached to a fixed point and is allowed to shorten as it lifts a predetermined weight, the afterload. Thus there is both force development and shortening. As the weight is set, the contraction is isotonic. Experiments with isolated heart muscle are effected at an experimentally determined rate of stimulation; the initial length of the muscle is controlled and there are no humoral or neural influences, thus observations reflect the characteristics of the cardiac muscle itself.

During isometric contractions, from a set resting length (and its associated resting tension) representing the true preload, the muscle develops its active tension. The active tension increases with increases in resting length and tension

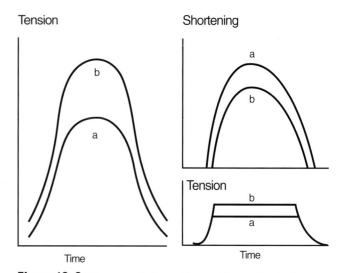

Figure 18–9. Representation of isometric and isotonic contractions. For isotonic contractions, two sets of traces indicate lower (*a*) and higher (*b*) developed tension. As more tension is developed, there is less shortening.

and then declines after passing a peak. The influence of the preload on the active tension is the expression of Starling's law of the heart.[5] Studies of isolated cardiac fibers have shown that the maximum active force occurs for a sarcomere length of 2.2 μm.[47] This length is optimal for the formation of cross-bridges. Below that length the overlap of actin and myosin is too extensive and fewer cross-bridges are formed. Recently, an alternative view has been put forward: at short sarcomere lengths, actin and myosin are farther apart and this is the cause of reduced cross-bridge formation.[48] Beyond the optimal length, the overlap of actin and myosin is reduced and force development is inhibited. This traditional view is now challenged as the pericellular collagen and connecting filaments within the cardiac cells confer a high resting stiffness that opposes myofibrils overstretching. However, the degree of actin-myosin overlap (a pure function of the resting length) may not be the critical factor in Starling's law of the heart.[49] Length-dependent mechanisms may play an important role by increasing the sensitivity of the myofilaments to calcium. If calcium sensitivity is a major factor, the effects of preload changes on muscle performance may not be very different from the effects of inotropic interventions.

The heart muscle is sensitive to calcium and to a large number of hormones and drugs that increase its contractility at constant preload and rate of contraction. Positive inotropic interventions, for a given preload, increase the active force the muscle can develop; conversely, drugs with negative inotropy (halogenated anesthetics, calcium channel antagonists) decrease the active force. Generally inotropic interventions cause their effect through an increase in myoplasmic calcium, and less frequently by increasing the sensitivity of the contractile apparatus to calcium. Though changes in contractility are characteristic of cardiac muscle, it is difficult to dissociate them from changes in preload because of the length-dependence of calcium fluxes and calcium sensitivity. Irrespective of their common mechanisms, the effects of positive inotropic interventions are additive to the effects of increasing the preload.

During isotonic contractions, once enough force has developed, the weight (i.e., the afterload) is lifted and shortening occurs. The extent of shortening and its velocity are inversely related to the afterload. Many indices of contractility derive from the relationship between velocity of shortening and the tension (or force) developed during isotonic contractions (Fig. 18–10*A,B*). It has been shown that extrapolation of the velocity-force relationship to zero force yields a value termed maximum velocity of shortening (Vmax), which is unchanged by alterations of the preload. By contrast, positive inotropic interventions increase Vmax, velocity of shortening and developed tension.[50,51]

In the intact heart, the maximum velocity of circumferential shortening, the maximum rate of pressure development of the ventricles, the peak power of the left ventricle, and the acceleration of the blood in the aorta relate closely to the maximum velocity of shortening. These variables are used as indices of contractility. However, they are influenced by the loading conditions of the ventricle. This is not the case for maximum elastance, which is preload and afterload independent.

Control of Contractility

Intrinsic control systems in the myocardium include the length-dependent activation and the force-frequency relation. Increases in the rate of stimulation augment the speed of contraction and relaxation and enhance the strength of contraction. This allows the stroke volume to be maintained even though less time is available for filling and emptying the ventricles. As frequency increases, there is more rapid calcium cycling. Calcium entry increases as there is more frequent opening of L-type calcium channels, at the same time the calcium pump of the SR speeds up and SERCA2 activity increases.

Extrinsic control systems result mostly from adrenergic and cholinergic neural discharge and circulating catecholamines. Agonist binding to β_1- and β_2-adrenoceptors on the surface of the cell membrane results in an interaction between a G protein and guanidine triphosphate that activates adenylate cyclase. This enzyme, at the cytoplasmic side of the receptor, activates the conversion of ATP into cAMP. In turn, cAMP activates PKA, which phosphorylates the L-type calcium channels, altering their gating such that calcium entry is facilitated. PKA also phosphorylates TnI resulting in decreased affinity of calcium for TnC. This facilitates relaxation.

NO is produced by endothelial cells and by the myocytes themselves.[52] NOS3 is calcium-sensitive and is activated by levels of intracellular calcium achieved during normal contractions. NO has a negative inotropic effect mediated by cGMP possibly resulting in myofilament desensitization to calcium and a blunting of the responses to catecholamines.[53] Inflammatory cytokines enhance NOS3, and through increased NO synthesis depress cardiac function.[54]

α_1-Adrenergic agonists, endothelin-1, and angiotensin II influence myocyte function through activation of phospholipase, inositol triphosphate (IP$_3$), and diacylglycerol. IP$_3$ increases the release of intracellular calcium, whereas increases in diacylglycerol may phosphorylate calcium channels and the sarcolemmal Na^+-H^+ exchanger.

Diastolic Ventricular Function

Immediately after the peak of left ventricular pressure has been reached relaxation dominates over contraction, even though ejection continues on a reduced scale. When aortic pressure, determined by the volume ejected and the impedance of the systemic circulation, exceeds ventricular pressure, the aortic valve closes. Its elastic recoil is responsible for the dicrotic notch of the aortic pressure wave-form. As the mitral valve is also closed, the initial phase of ventricular relaxation is isovolumic. When the ventricular pressure becomes lower than the atrial pressure, the mitral valve opens and ventricular filling begins. The early filling is rapid and becomes slower in the later phase of diastole. Atrial contraction may contribute as much as 25% of total ventricular filling.

The duration of diastole depends on the heart rate. Over a wide range of rates, the duration of systole varies within relatively narrow limits, typically from 300 to 200 milliseconds for large changes in heart rate. Conversely, the duration of diastole decreases substantially from 500 to 125 milliseconds as heart rate increases from 75 to 180 beats/min. The effect of heart rate on the duration of diastole ultimately limits both ventricular filling and coronary perfusion.

Diastole is not a passive phenomenon: it is an active process that uses approximately 15% of the energy of the cardiac cycle.[55] Thus in conditions such as hypertensive heart disease, cardiomyopathies, and myocardial ischemia, the diastolic characteristics of the ventricles may be affected earlier than their systolic properties.[56]

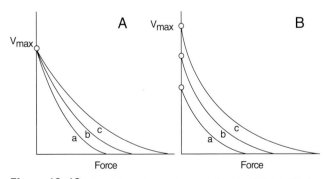

Figure 18–10. *A,* Extrapolation to zero force of the velocity of shortening versus developed force relationship yields a constant value (V$_{max}$) when preload is decreased (less force is developed) or increased (more force is developed). *B,* Extrapolation to zero force of the velocity of shortening versus developed force relationship yields increased or decreased value for V$_{max}$ as a result of positive or negative inotropic interventions.

Evaluation of Diastolic Function

Isovolumic relaxation is the term used for the pressure decline in the ventricles. It can be described as an exponential function and is expressed as a time constant (τ). Several equations are used for this analysis. The most frequently used is:

$$P(t) = P_0 \, e^{-t/\tau}$$
$$\ln P = \ln P_0^{-t/\tau}$$

Where P is left ventricular pressure, P_0 is the left ventricular pressure at peak negative dP/dt, and t is time.[57]

The time constant of isovolumic relaxation (τ) depends on load, inactivation, homogeneity of relaxation in the whole ventricle, and coronary blood flow.[58] A high load forces the fibers to relax more quickly when the active process subsides. Relaxation is further facilitated by the diastolic engorgement of the coronary vessels because this causes a relative increase in wall thickness, intramyocardial pressure, and therefore total diastolic load.[59] Conversely, inhomogeneity of relaxation resulting from dyssynchrony increases the time constant of isovolumic relaxation. This is particularly prominent in acute myocardial ischemia because ischemic segments show paradoxic early diastolic thickening and shortening, thus impairing the pattern of pressure decline.[60]

Ventricular filling results from the elongation of sarcomeres that follow the dissociation of the cross-bridges between actin and myosin. The efficiency of filling is reduced when the end-systolic volume is increased (ventricular dilatation), cross-bridges do not dissociate, or fibrosis develops in the myocardium. The early filling phase reflects the velocity of flow through the atrioventricular valves.

Contraction of the atria increases the pressure gradient across the atrioventricular valves. The peristaltic nature of atrial contraction and the geometry of the venoatrial junctions minimize the backward transmission of pressure, especially into the pulmonary veins.[61] The Frank-Starling mechanism operates in the left atrium.[62] The contribution of atrial systole is increased in hypertrophic cardiomyopathies, in the presence of myocardial infarction, and in the elderly.[63,64]

In the presence of mitral or tricuspid valve disease, large differences in rapid filling and its relationship with late filling occur. Indeed, the pattern of flow through the atrioventricular valves, recorded by ultrasonography, is used to determine the severity of mitral or tricuspid disease.[65]

Ventricular compliance, or its reciprocal, ventricular stiffness, can be estimated from the relationship between pressure and volume at end-diastole over a wide range of end-diastolic volumes obtained during a fluid challenge. Alternatively, ventricular stiffness can be estimated by analyzing the instantaneous relationship between pressure and volume during individual diastoles. The relationship is a function of the ability of the ventricle to relax to accommodate the venous return.[66] If ventricular stiffness is acutely or chronically increased, ventricular filling may be impaired such that hypovolemia and hypervolemia cause large changes in end-diastolic ventricular pressure and in cardiac output. With increased ventricular stiffness, hypervolemia may cause pulmonary edema, whereas hypovolemia may cause an exaggerated reduction of cardiac output.

Diastolic stiffness may be structural (ventricular hypertrophy, fibrosis) or functional (hypoxia, ischemia, altered diastolic handling of calcium). In many cardiopathies,

increased ventricular stiffness is the first manifestation of the disease, especially in hypertrophic cardiomyopathies, hypertensive heart disease, and acute myocardial ischemia.[67] This is often reflected in a high pulmonary artery occluded pressure (PAOP, PCWP). Episodes of regional myocardial ischemia may cause stiffening of both the ischemic and remote well-perfused myocardium.[68] Therefore, regional ischemia may result in a global increase in ventricular stiffness that facilitates the development of acute diastolic ventricular failure, i.e., acute pulmonary edema.

Molecular Mechanisms Underlying Cellular Physiology

Structure and Function of the Cardiac Sodium Channels

Voltage-gated sodium channels are transmembrane proteins responsible for the rapid upstroke of the cardiac action potential, and for rapid impulse conduction in the cardiac tissue.[69] Na^+ channels are dynamic molecules that change their structural conformation in response to transmembrane electric fields. Sodium channels have been cloned and sequenced. Two processes are linked: gating and permeation.

The sodium channel consists of a principal α-subunit composed of four homologous domains (I–IV), each containing six transmembrane (S1–S6) segments; the four domains are attached to one another (Fig. 18–11). Residues between the fifth and sixth transmembrane segments line the pore (P-loop). In each domain, the P-loop is unique; this is at variance with the similarity of P-loops in potassium channels. In Na^+ and Ca^{2+} channels, the P-loop asymmetries are critically linked to the unique permeation characteristics of the channels.[70] It is still unclear how residues on P-loops, forming the putative selectivity filter, permit selective flux of Na^+ over other cations by a factor of 100:1 and, at the same time, allow throughput rates approaching 10^8 ions/sec. Possible explanations include: (1) a water-filled cavity and hydrophobic lining that minimizes the distance over which the cation interacts with the channel, and (2) a relatively short selectivity filter that supports multi-ion occupancy.

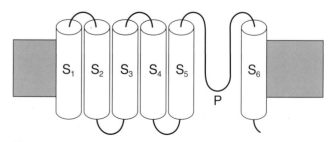

Figure 18–11. Schematic representation of one domain of the tetramer of an ion channel showing six transmembrane segments (S1 to S6) and the P loop. The latter forms part of the ion channel itself.

Hodgkin and Huxley[71] propose that Na^+ channels exist in various conformational states in the process of opening (activation), and a distinct conformation is entered when the channels shut (inactivation). The activation and inactivation gates were postulated to have intrinsic voltage dependence. However, the Na^+ channel gating processes are better understood as complex allosteric interactions among structural domains. Site-directed mutations have implicated specific regions of the Na^+ channel in gating. The linker between domains II–IV may be regarded as a "lid" that closes over the inner vestibule, causing the state of inactivation. The S4 segment in each domain underlies activation, the voltage-dependent gating process responsible for channel opening. Recent evidence, based on mutagenesis experiments in the outer S4 segment of domain IV, shows activation and inactivation to be functionally coupled. Mutations in the cardiac Na^+ channel gene (SCN5A) modify inactivation by rendering it less stable, generating a small nonactivating plateau of inward current during repolarization. This prolongs the QT interval, making it possible for fatal ventricular arrhythmias.

Auxiliary β-subunits are important modulators of Na^+ channel gating. The human β_1-subunit is widely expressed in skeletal muscle, heart, and neuronal tissue; its exact role in heart muscle is not fully understood.[72,73]

Neuronal isoforms of Na^+ channels have a large intracellular linker between domains I and II that contain five sites for cAMP-dependent PKA. Conversely, the cardiac Na^+ channels have only two sites in the same linker. When stimulated by PKA, cardiac Na^+ channel gating remains unchanged, but the whole cell conductance increases. Protein kinase C (PKC) also modulates the Na^+ channel, reducing the maximal conductance and altering gating. The site of action for PKC appears to reside in the domain III-IV linker.[74,75]

Structure and Function of Cardiac Potassium Channels

Cardiac K^+ selective channels carry outward currents and either set the resting potential near the K^+ equilibrium potential or repolarize the cell. The long duration of the cardiac action potential results from the coordinated action of multiple ionic conductances that activate and inactivate on different time scales. Potassium currents are involved in nearly all phases. Whereas the upstroke of the action potential is caused by an inward sodium current, the partial early repolarization is caused by outward potassium flux through rapidly activating and inactivating K^+ channels. The extent of the early repolarization affects the time course of other voltage-gated currents, thereby controlling the action potential duration. The plateau phase is supported mainly by a Ca^{2+} influx that slowly declines as L-type Ca^{2+} channels inactivate and by activating Na^+ current. Repolarization depends on K^+ efflux through several voltage-gated potassium channels. Inwardly rectifying K^+ channels maintain or modulate the resting potential; these channels carry no current during the plateau phase. There is a considerable diversity of K^+ channel subunits with more than 60 cloned.[76]

Like other ion channels, K^+ channels have a central pore through which ions flow down their electrochemical gradient, a selectivity filter, and a gating structure. Ion gating may be determined by electrical, chemical, or mechanical forces; their behavior can be modified by intracellular processes, toxins, or drugs. A single conformational change allows permeation of up to 10^8 ions/sec.

Voltage-Gated K^+ Channels

The encoded protein contains six membrane spanning segments. Four α-subunits assembled in a tetrameric structure are needed to create a functional K^+ channel. The ion conduction pathway (P-region) occurs between the S5 and S6 segments with contributions of S6 and the S4-S5 linker. The S5-S6 sections face each other, creating the central pore. The narrow P region dictates the K^+ selectivity. The S4-S5 linker forms the receptor for inactivation.[76]

The major component of the voltage sensor for gating resides in the S4 segment. Depolarization of the membrane causes an outward movement of S4, which, in turn, induces further conformational changes that open the channel.[77] After initial activation, some K^+ channels inactivate during maintained depolarization. N- and C-type inactivation are associated with different molecular domains.[78,79]

Inward Rectifier K^+ Channels

These K^+ channels have only two membrane-spanning segments (M1, M2) and an intervening P-loop. These channels lack the voltage-dependent gating. The M1-P-M2 section of the K^+ inward rectifier channel (K_{ir}) confers ion conducting characteristics, which suggest that the voltage-gated channels evolved from the simpler K_{ir} structure. X-ray analysis has shown cloned K^+ channels to contain four identical subunits, each of which has two transmembrane α-helices and an intervening P-domain.[80] The subunits create an inverted cone. The selectivity filter fills the wider base on the extracellular face. The overall length of the pore is 45Å; its width is between 6 and 12Å.

Although heterologous expression of the pore-forming α-subunits does not disrupt the generation of functional K^+ channels, an expanding family of functional alternating β-subunits has been identified.[81] Among the more than 12 cardiac K^+ currents, two types of voltage-gated channels play a major role in determining repolarization: transient outward (I_{TO}) and delayed rectifier (I_K) currents.[82] The latter has two components including the rapidly activating current (I_{KR}) and the slowly activating current (I_{KS}). The former (I_{KR}) is blocked by flecainide. A time-independent K^+ channel (I_{KP}) and a rapidly activating K^+ current (I_{KUR}) also have been described. The Kv4 channels are major contributors to the cardiac transient outward current.

Parasympathetic stimulation slows the heart rate by activation of muscarinic receptors. This reduces the hyperpolarization-activated cation current (I_f) in pacemaking tissue and opens muscarinic K^+ channels (K_{ACH}) in the sinoatrial node and in the atrium. Muscarinic K^+ channels are inwardly rectifying K^+ channels coupled directly to a G protein.

Finally, ATP-regulated K^+ channels (K_{ATP}) link the membrane potential to the metabolic status of the cell in that K_{ATP} channels are inhibited by physiologic intracellular ATP levels, but open when the ATP levels decrease. These channels play an important role in myocardial ischemia, act as regulators of smooth muscle tone, and are involved in insulin secretion.[83]

The pacemaker current results from the slow activation of nonselective cation current at the end of the action potential contributing to diastolic depolarization and spontaneous pacemaking activity in the sinoatrial node. cAMP directly modulates this current and enhances heart rate by shifting its activation toward depolarization. This channel belongs to the family of cyclic nucleotide-gated channels.

Regulation of K^+ Channels

Many voltage-gated K^+ channels contain multiple sites for PKA- and PKC-mediated phosphorylation. K^+ channels can also be regulated at the transcriptional, or translational level, or both. Glucocorticoids and thyroid hormone appear to alter channel expression.

Potassium channels are down-regulated in cardiac disease. In patients with the congenital long T syndrome, the K^+ currents are typically reduced by 50% or more, leading to prolonged action potentials predisposing to arrhythmias.[84] Similarly, in myocytes from hypertrophied and failing hearts, the action potential duration is increased, and significant reductions of I_{KA} and I_{TO} have been observed.[85]

Structure and Function of Calcium Channels

The cardiac voltage-gated calcium channels are classified into transient (T-type), long-lasting (L-type), and Purkinje cell (P) currents. T-type channels are low-voltage activated, whereas L- and P-type are high voltage activated. The voltage-gated calcium channels (L-type; Fig. 18–12) are modulated by cAMP-dependent PKA through certain G proteins.[86]

The T channels open at a more negative voltage (−70 to −60 mV), have short bursts of opening, and do not interact with conventional calcium antagonist drugs. The T channels probably account for the earlier phase of the entry of calcium into the cell. This may give them a special role in the early electrical depolarization of the sinoatrial node, and hence of the initiation of the heart beat. By contrast, the L-type channels are activated at −40 to −30 mV with peak calcium influx at 0 to +10 mV. The amount of calcium entering the myocytes during the plateau phase of the action potential is far less than the amount required for initiating contraction; it serves as a trigger for the release of calcium by the SR through ryanodine channels.

The sarcolemmal L channels are the standard calcium channels found in the myocardium. They are also the channels that are involved in calcium-induced calcium release. They are subject to inhibition by the calcium antagonist drugs.

Eight different α_1-subunit genes have been identified. The high selectivity for calcium over sodium is conferred by a group of glutamate residues forming a high-affinity calcium binding site.[87] Different splice variants of the same gene encode the L-type calcium channel of the heart (α_{1Ca}) and smooth muscle (α_{1Cb}), whereas the main subunit of the L-type calcium channel of skeletal muscle (α_{1S}) is encoded by another gene.[88,89]

The α_1-subunits form functional channels by themselves; however, α_2, β, and δ subunits also exist. Coexpression of any of the four β-subunits increases both the number of channel complexes inserted into the membrane and the current amplitude. The type of β-subunits determines the current characteristics.[90,91]

Two distinct classes of channels mediate the release of calcium from intracellular stores. They are sensitive to IP_3 or ryanodine. Ryanodine receptors are large proteins with a molecular mass of approximately 565 kD.[92] They release calcium from the SR or the endoplasmic reticulum. Calcium release from the cardiac SR is triggered by calcium influx through the fast-acting T-type channels and is maintained by L-type channels.

Pharmacologic agents that either enhance (L-type Ca^{2+} channel agonists, β-adrenergic receptor agonists) or reduce L-type channel current (Ca^{2+} channel blockers) directly influence the amount of calcium released by the SR, thereby altering both the excitation-contraction coupling and myocardial contractile performance. Abundance and functional state of L-type calcium channels play a role in the development of cardiac failure.

Structure and Function of Anion Channels

Initially, six different types of sarcolemmal chloride currents were identified in cardiac cells. Anion channels have also been identified in internal membranes. Anion channels, in addition to transport and exchange proteins, mediate a variety of functions in the cardiac cell. Activation of anion channels can alter the resting membrane potential, regulate

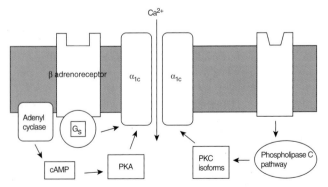

Figure 18–12. Diagram representing an L-type calcium channel and its relationship with β-adrenoreceptors and receptors linked with phospholipase C. cAMP, cyclic adenosine monophosphate; PKA, protein kinase A; PKC, protein kinase C.

chloride activity, pH, volume homeostasis, and the transport of osmotically active substances. Anion transport may also alter immunologic responses, cell migration, proliferation, and differentiation, and possibly apoptosis.[93]

Sarcolemmal Chloride Channels

Chloride channels regulated by cAMP-dependent protein kinase have been identified in cardiac cells. These channels are activated by β-adrenergic agonists. The CFTR chloride channel (CTFR CCl⁻) is composed of 1480 amino acids organized into two 6-transmembrane spanning domains, two nucleotide binding domains, and one large regulatory (R) domain. The highly charged R domain may represent a blocking particle that keeps the channel closed until it becomes phosphorylated. The ion conduction pathway may relate to residues M1, M5, M6, and M12 of the transmembrane spanning domains.[94] Activation of the channel requires both phosphorylation of the R domain and binding of ATP to the nucleotide-binding domain.

The coupling of β-adrenergic receptors and muscarinic receptors to the regulation of chloride channels involves G proteins. In the absence of agonists, the PKA-dependent chloride channels do not appear to be active. Although activation of chloride channels may be predicted to shorten the action potential duration, the relevance of these channels is still unclear.

From Genes to Channels

The electrophysiologic properties of cardiac tissue are well recognized and are expressed as action potentials and propagation that vary in different specific regions of the heart. Understanding the fundamental mechanisms of these differences has been greatly advanced by the cloning of genes in which expression results in production of ion channels and other important proteins. The new information also allows a greater understanding of the electrophysiologic changes observed in heart failure, atrial fibrillation, and myocardial ischemia.[95]

Expression of ion channel genes, or the function of their protein products, is altered in disease. Genes encoding for the major structural proteins (α-subunits) have been identified, although more may soon be cloned. For the sodium and calcium channels α-subunits are large molecules that are capable of forming functional ion channels. Potassium channels assemble as multimers of α-subunits (dimers or tetramers); there are also heterometric potassium channel complexes.[96] The latter have different properties from those with homeometric assembly. The α-subunit of chloride channels differ from that of Na⁺, Ca²⁺, or K⁺ channels.[97] The functional implications are that coexpression of different α-subunits results in currents that resemble more closely native tissue currents than currents from isoforms alone. Multiple chloride currents have been described in the heart; they are activated or modulated by cAMP, PKC, elevated intracellular calcium, or stretch. Also important are the connexons, the structures responsible for the gap junctions. Connexon

isoforms have been described in heart tissue. Alteration in their expression may explain some of the disorders of conduction velocity seen in heart disease.[98]

Beat-to-Beat Modulation

Transcription and translation are relatively "long-term" processes (hours to days), yet channel function can be modulated on a beat-to-beat basis. This may occur because of changes in [H⁺] or [K⁺] or by phosphorylation of channel proteins. As an example, β-adrenoceptor stimulation results in a cascade of intracellular events (G protein, adenylcyclase, cAMP, activation of PKA). This leads to stimulation of L-type calcium channels. These channels exhibit longer and later openings than in the nonstimulated state, probably caused by phosphorylation of key residues on the channel protein, mediated by PKA.[99] Activation of PKC may also cause phosphorylation of important molecules of the channels. For these regulatory events to occur, kinases and channel protein complexes must be in close apposition. This association results from the presence of anchoring proteins containing a specific protein binding site (PDZ domain).[100]

Current and Potential Targets of Drug Action

There are many actual and potential targets for the action on drugs on the heart and the circulation. These include a direct effect on the contractile apparatus itself, both in the myocytes and in the vascular smooth muscle (e.g., calcium ions), or a sensitization of the contractile apparatus (calcium sensitizers). The interaction of actin and myosin in cardiac and smooth muscle is increased by any agent capable of increasing the intracellular concentration of calcium. Such an increase may be brought about by increased entry through ion-specific channels at the cell membrane or at the SR (triggered release). Many types of receptors, especially β- and α-adrenoceptors, enhance calcium entry through a mechanism involving cAMP or inositol phosphate, to cite only two mediators. Activation of receptors for glucagon, angiotensin, endothelins, and many other autocoids can also increase calcium entry into cardiac or vascular smooth muscle cells, thus altering contractile performance and vascular tone. A direct effect on ion pumps, such as the Na⁺/K⁺ATPase, may also alter calcium entry by modifying the availability of another ion, in this case Na⁺. Alterations in the extent of synthesis of mediators by the endothelium play an important role in the control of vascular tone, involving NO, prostanoids, and endothelins. Over and above drugs with direct actions on cardiac myocytes and vascular smooth muscle, many drugs act through the control mechanisms of the circulation, altering the level of sympathetic or parasympathetic activity, or the transmission of impulses in the autonomic nervous system. Drugs acting centrally on α_2 or imidazoline I_1 receptors exert important effects on the heart and the circulation protecting against sympathetic overactivity and reducing blood pressure. Complex effects on the circulation also result from drugs that alter the activity of the renin-angiotensin-aldosterone system.

References

1. Myhre ES, Slinker BK, LeWinter MM: Absence of right ventricular isovolumic relaxation in open-chest anesthetized dogs. Am J Physiol 263:H1587–H1590, 1992.
2. Weibel ER: Morphological basis of alveolar-capillary gas exchange. Physiol Rev 53:419–495, 1973.
3. Gil J, Bachofen H, Gehr P, Weibel ER: Alveolar volume-surface area relation in air- and saline-filled lungs fixed by vascular perfusion. J Appl Physiol 47:990–1001, 1979.
4. Noble MI: Left ventricular load, arterial impedance and their interrelationship. Cardiovasc Res 13:183–198, 1979.
5. Starling EK: The Linacre lecture on the Law of the Heart, given at Cambridge, 1915. London, Longmans, 1918.
6. Sarnoff SJ, Case RB, Berglund E, Sarnoff L: Ventricular function: I. Starling's law of the heart studied by means of simultaneous right and left ventricular function curves in the dog. Circulation 9:706–718, 1954.
7. Suga H, Sagawa K, Shoukas AA: Load independence of the instantaneous pressure-volume ratio of the canine left ventricle and effects of epinephrine and heart rate on the ratio. Circ Res 32:314–322, 1973.
8. Suga H: Left ventricular time-varying pressure-volume ratio in systole as an index of myocardial inotropism. Jpn Heart J 12:153–160, 1971.
9. Glower DD, Spratt JA, Snow ND, et al: Linearity of the Frank-Starling relationship in the intact heart: The concept of preload recruitable stroke work. Circulation 71:994–1009, 1985.
10. Robotham JL, Takata M, Berman M, Harasawa Y: Ejection fraction revisited. Anesthesiology 74:172–183, 1991.
11. Weiss HR: Effect of coronary artery occlusion on regional arterial and venous O2 saturation, O2 extraction, blood flow, and O2 consumption in the dog heart. Circ Res 47:400–407, 1980.
12. Khouri EMN, Gregg DE, Rayford CR: Effect of exercise on cardiac output, left coronary blood flow and myocardial metabolism in the unanesthetized dog. Circ Res 17:427–437, 1965.
13. Fujita M, Sasayama S, Ohno A, et al: Importance of angina for development of collateral circulation. Br Heart J 57:139–143, 1987.
14. Moncada S, Vane JR: Pharmacology and endogenous roles of prostaglandin endoperoxides, thromboxane A2, and prostacyclin. Pharmacol Rev 30:293–331, 1978.
15. Rubanyi G: Endothelium, platelets, and coronary vasospasm. Coron Artery Dis 1:645, 1990.
16. Rubanyi GM: Endothelium-derived relaxing and contracting factors. J Cell Biochem 46:27–36, 1991.
17. Downey JM, Kirk ES: Distribution of the coronary blood flow across the canine heart wall during systole. Circ Res 34:251–257, 1974.
18. Rovai D, L'Abbate A, Lombardi M, et al: Nonuniformity of the transmural distribution of coronary blood flow during the cardiac cycle. In vivo documentation by contrast echocardiography. Circulation 79:179–187, 1989.
19. Klocke FJ, Mates RE, Canty JM Jr, Ellis AK: Coronary pressure-flow relationships. Controversial issues and probable implications. Circ Res 56:310–323, 1985.
20. Bellamy RF: Diastolic coronary artery pressure-flow relations in the dog. Circ Res 43:92–101, 1978.
21. Gould KL, Lipscomb K, Hamilton GW: Physiologic basis for assessing critical coronary stenosis. Instantaneous flow response and regional distribution during coronary hyperemia as measures of coronary flow reserve. Am J Cardiol 33:87–94, 1974.
22. Marcus ML: Autoregulation in the coronary circulation. In Marcus ML (ed): The Coronary Circulation in Health and Disease. New York, McGraw-Hill, 1983, pp 93–112.
23. Gibbs CL, Chapman JB: Cardiac emergencies. In Berne RM (ed): The Cardiovascular System. Bethesda, American Physiological Society, 1979, pp 775–804.
24. Feigl EO: Coronary physiology. Physiol Rev 63:1–205, 1983.
25. Nichols CG, Lederer WJ: Adenosine triphosphate-sensitive potassium channels in the cardiovascular system. Am J Physiol 261:H1675–H1686, 1991.
26. Ishibashi Y, Duncker DJ, Zhang J, Bache RJ: ATP-sensitive K+ channels, adenosine, and nitric oxide-mediated mechanisms account for coronary vasodilation during exercise. Circ Res 82:346–359, 1998.
27. Feliciano L, Henning RJ: Coronary artery blood flow: Physiologic and pathophysiologic regulation. Clin Cardiol 22:775–786, 1999.
28. Ludmer PL, Selwyn AP, Shook TL, et al: Paradoxical vasoconstriction induced by acetylcholine in atherosclerotic coronary arteries. N Engl J Med 315:1046–1051, 1986.
29. Bassenge E, Heusch G: Endothelial and neuro-humoral control of coronary blood flow in health and disease. Rev Physiol Biochem Pharmacol 116:77–165, 1990.
30. Spudich JA: How molecular motors work. Nature 372:515–518, 1994.
31. Holmes KC, Popp D, Gebhard W, Kabsch W: Atomic model of the actin filament. Nature 347:44–49, 1990.
32. Tobacman LS: Thin filament-mediated regulation of cardiac contraction. Annu Rev Physiol 58:447–481, 1996.
33. Coudrey L: The troponins. Arch Intern Med 158:1173–1180, 1998.
34. Lopez Jimenez F, Goldman L, Sacks DB, et al: Prognostic value of cardiac troponin T after noncardiac surgery: 6-month follow-up data. J Am Coll Cardiol 29:1241–1245, 1997.
35. Metzler H, Gries M, Rehak P, et al: Perioperative myocardial cell injury: The role of troponins. Br J Anaesth 78:386–390, 1997.
36. Kress M, Huxley HE, Faruqi AR, Hendrix J: Structural changes during activation of frog muscle studied by time-resolved x-ray diffraction. J Mol Biol 188:325–342, 1986.
37. McKillop DF, Geeves MA: Regulation of the interaction between actin and myosin subfragment 1: Evidence for three states of the thin filament. Biophys J 65:693–701, 1993.
38. Anderson K, Lai FA, Liu QY, et al: Structural and functional characterization of the purified cardiac ryanodine receptor-Ca2+ release channel complex. J Biol Chem 264:1329–1335, 1989.
39. Sitsapesan R, Williams AJ: Gating of the native and purified cardiac SR Ca(2+)-release channel with monovalent cations as permeant species. Biophys J 67:1484–1494, 1994.
40. Schatzmann HJ: The calcium pump of the surface membrane and of the sarcoplasmic reticulum. Annu Rev Physiol 51:473–485, 1989.
41. Koss KL, Kranias EG: Phospholamban: A prominent regulator of myocardial contractility. Circ Res 79:1059–1063, 1996.
42. Huxley AF, Niedergerke R: Structural changes in muscle during contraction. Nature 173:971–973, 1954.
43. Huxley HE, Hanson J: Changes in cross-striation of muscle during contraction and stretch and their structural interpretation. Nature 173:973–976, 1954.
44. Pollack GH, Krueger JW: Sarcomere dynamics in intact cardiac muscle. Eur J Cardiol 4(Suppl):53–65, 1976.
45. Babu A, Scordilis SP, Sonnenblick EH, Gulati J: The control of myocardial contraction with skeletal fast muscle troponin C. J Biol Chem 262:5815–5822, 1987.
46. Brenner BM, Troy JL, Ballermann BJ: Endothelium-dependent vascular responses. Mediators and mechanisms. J Clin Invest 84:1373–1378, 1989.
47. Spiro D, Sonnenblick EH: Comparison of the ultrastructural basis of the contractile process in heart and skeletal muscle. Circ Res 14:14–37, 1964.
48. McDonald KS, Moss RL: Osmotic compression of single cardiac myocytes eliminates the reduction in Ca2+ sensitivity of tension at short sarcomere length. Circ Res 77:199–205, 1995.
49. Lakatta EG: Starling's law of the heart is explained by an intimate interaction of muscle length and myofilament calcium activation. J Am Coll Cardiol 10:1157–1164, 1987.
50. Hill AV: Heat of shortening and dynamic constants of muscle. Proc R Soc London Biol 126:136–195, 1938.
51. Abbott BC, Mommaerts WFHM: A study of inotropic mechanisms in the papillary muscle preparation. J Gen Physiol 42:553–551, 1959.
52. Kelly RA, Balligand JL, Smith TW: Nitric oxide and cardiac function. Circ Res 79:363–380, 1996.
53. Kaye DM, Wiviott SD, Balligand JL, et al: Frequency-dependent activation of a constitutive nitric oxide synthase and regulation of contractile function in adult rat ventricular myocytes. Circ Res 78:217–224, 1996.
54. Haque R, Kan H, Finkel MS: Effects of cytokines and nitric oxide on myocardial E-C coupling. Basic Res Cardiol 93(Suppl 1): 86–94, 1998.
55. Langer GA: Ion fluxes in cardiac excitation and contraction and their relation to myocardial contractility. Physiol Rev 48:708–757, 1968.
56. Van de Werf F, Boel A, Geboers J, et al: Diastolic properties of the left ventricle in normal adults and in patients with third heart sounds. Circulation 69:1070–1078, 1984.

57. Weiss JL, Frederiksen JW, Weisfeldt ML: Hemodynamic determinants of the time-course of fall in canine left ventricular pressure. J Clin Invest 58:751–760, 1976.
58. Brutsaert DL, Rademakers FE, Sys SU: Triple control of relaxation: Implications in cardiac disease. Circulation 69:190–196, 1984.
59. Brutsaert DL, Rademakers FE, Sys SU, et al: Analysis of relaxation in the evaluation of ventricular function of the heart. Prog Cardiovasc Dis 28:143–163, 1985.
60. Doyle RL, Foex P, Ryder WA, Jones LA: Differences in ischaemic dysfunction after gradual and abrupt coronary occlusion: Effects on isovolumic relaxation. Cardiovasc Res 21:507–514, 1987.
61. Little WC, Downes TR: Clinical evaluation of left ventricular diastolic performance. Prog Cardiovasc Dis 32:273–290, 1990.
62. Kagawa K, Arakawa M, Miwa H, et al: Left atrial function during left ventricular diastole evaluated by left atrial angiography and left ventriculography. J Cardiol 24: 317–325, 1994.
63. Arora RR, Machac J, Goldman ME, et al: Atrial kinetics and left ventricular diastolic filling in the healthy elderly. J Am Coll Cardiol 9:1255–1260, 1987.
64. Bonow RO, Frederick TM, Bacharach SL, et al: Atrial systole and left ventricular filling in hypertrophic cardiomyopathy: Effect of verapamil. Am J Cardiol 51:1386–1391, 1983.
65. Samstad SO, Rossvoll O, Torp HG, et al: Cross-sectional early mitral flow-velocity profiles from color Doppler in patients with mitral valve disease. Circulation 86:748–755, 1992.
66. Katz AM: Influence of altered inotropy and lusitropy on ventricular pressure-volume loops. J Am Coll Cardiol 11:438–445, 1988.
67. Nonogi H, Hess OM, Bortone AS, et al: Left ventricular pressure-length relation during exercise-induced ischemia. J Am Coll Cardiol 13:1062–1070, 1989.
68. Marsch SC, Wanigasekera VA, Ryder WA, et al: Graded myocardial ischemia is associated with a decrease in diastolic distensibility of the remote nonischemic myocardium in the anesthetized dog. J Am Coll Cardiol 22:899–906, 1993.
69. Balser JR: Structure and function of the cardiac sodium channels. Cardiovasc Res 42:327–338, 1999.
70. Fozzard HA, Hanck DA: Structure and function of voltage-dependent sodium channels: Comparison of brain II and cardiac isoforms. Physiol Rev 76:887–926, 1996.
71. Hodgkin A, Huxley A: A quantitative description of membrane current and its application to conduction and excitation in nerve. J Physiol 117:500–544, 1952.
72. Hartshorne RP, Messner DJ, Coppersmith JC, Catterall WA: The saxitoxin receptor of the sodium channel from rat brain. Evidence for two nonidentical beta subunits. J Biol Chem 257:13888–13891, 1982.
73. Isom LL, Scheuer T, Brownstein AB, et al: Functional co-expression of the beta 1 and type IIA alpha subunits of sodium channels in a mammalian cell line. J Biol Chem 270:3306–3312, 1995.
74. Li M, West JW, Lai Y, et al: Functional modulation of brain sodium channels by cAMP-dependent phosphorylation. Neuron 8:1151–1159, 1992.
75. Qu Y, Rogers JC, Tanada TN, et al: Phosphorylation of S1505 in the cardiac Na+ channel inactivation gate is required for modulation by protein kinase C. J Gen Physiol 108:375–379, 1996.
76. Snyders DJ: Structure and function of cardiac potassium channels. Cardiovasc Res 42:377–390, 1999.
77. Choi KL, Mossman C, Aube J, Yellen G: The internal quaternary ammonium receptor site of Shaker potassium channels. Neuron 10:533–541, 1993.
78. Hoshi T, Zagotta WN, Aldrich RW: Biophysical and molecular mechanisms of Shaker potassium channel inactivation. Science 250:533–538, 1990.

79. Hoshi T, Zagotta WN, Aldrich RW: Two types of inactivation in Shaker K+ channels: Effects of alterations in the carboxy-terminal region. Neuron 7:547–556, 1991.
80. Doyle DA, Morais Cabral J, Pfuetzner RA, et al: The structure of the potassium channel: Molecular basis of K+ conduction and selectivity: Science 280:69–77, 1998.
81. Rettig J, Heinemann SH, Wunder F, et al: Inactivation properties of voltage-gated K+ channels altered by presence of beta-subunit. Nature 369:289–294, 1994.
82. Barry DM, Nerbonne JM: Myocardial potassium channels: Electrophysiological and molecular diversity. Annu Rev Physiol 58:363–394, 1996.
83. Inagaki N, Gonoi T, Clement JP, et al: Reconstitution of IKATP: an inward rectifier subunit plus the sulfonylurea receptor [see comments]. Science 270:1166–1170, 1995.
84. Keating MT, Sanguinetti MC: Pathophysiology of ion channel mutations. Curr Opin Genet Dev 6:326–333, 1996.
85. Beuckelmann DJ, Nabauer M, Erdmann E: Alterations of K+ currents in isolated human ventricular myocytes from patients with terminal heart failure. Circ Res 73:379–385, 1993.
86. Lehmann Horn F, Jurkat Rott K: Voltage-gated ion channels and hereditary disease. Physiol Rev 79:1317–1372, 1999.
87. Yang J, Ellinor PT, Sather WA, et al: Molecular determinants of Ca2+ selectivity and ion permeation in L-type Ca2+ channels [see comments]. Nature 366:158–161, 1993.
88. Beam KG, Adams BA, Niidome T, et al: Function of a truncated dihydropyridine receptor as both voltage sensor and calcium channel. Nature 360:169–171, 1992.
89. De Jongh KS, Warner C, Colvin AA, Catterall WA: Characterization of the two size forms of the alpha 1 subunit of skeletal muscle L-type calcium channels. Proc Natl Acad Sci USA 88:10778–10782, 1991.
90. Lacerda AE, Kim HS, Ruth P, et al: Normalization of current kinetics by interaction between the alpha 1 and beta subunits of the skeletal muscle dihydropyridine-sensitive Ca2+ channel. Nature 352:527–530, 1991.
91. Singer D, Biel M, Lotan I, et al: The roles of the subunits in the function of the calcium channel. Science 253:1553–1557, 1991.
92. Fontaine B, Vale Santos J, Jurkat Rott K, et al: Mapping of the hypokalaemic periodic paralysis (HypoPP) locus to chromosome 1q31-32 in three European families. Nat Genet 6:267–272, 1994.
93. Hume JR, Duan D, Collier ML, et al: Anion transport in heart. Physiol Rev 80:31–81, 2000.
94. Higgins CF: The ABC of channel regulation. Cell 82:693–696, 1995.
95. Roden DM, Kupershmidt S: From genes to channels: Normal mechanisms. Cardiovasc Res 42:318–326, 1999.
96. Ketchum KA, Joiner WJ, Sellers AJ, et al: A new family of outwardly rectifying potassium channel proteins with two pore domains in tandem. Nature 376:690–695, 1995.
97. Foskett JK: ClC and CFTR chloride channel gating. Annu Rev Physiol 60:689–717, 1998.
98. Peters NS, Coromilas J, Severs NJ, Wit AL: Disturbed connexin43 gap junction distribution correlates with the location of reentrant circuits in the epicardial border zone of healing canine infarcts that cause ventricular tachycardia. Circulation 95:988–996, 1997.
99. Yue DT, Herzig S, Marban E: Beta-adrenergic stimulation of calcium channels occurs by potentiation of high-activity gating modes. Proc Natl Acad Sci USA 87:753–757, 1990.
100. Tsunoda S, Sierralta J, Sun Y, et al: A multivalent PDZ-domain protein assembles signalling complexes in a G-protein-coupled cascade. Nature 388:243–249, 1997.

19

Vascular Reactivity

Isao Tsuneyoshi, MD • Takashi Akata, MD, PhD • Walter A. Boyle, MD

The vascular system refers to the system of conduits whose primary function is to carry blood, nutrients, and humoral signals, and remove metabolic waste for cells throughout the body. This function is dependent on the performance of the cardiac pump, but the role of the vascular system is far from passive. The blood vessels are made of living tissue and vascular reactivity, which refers to the active contraction and relaxation of vascular smooth muscle (VSM), is of vital importance to the maintenance of adequate perfusion pressures throughout the system, and is the primary determinant for the specific distribution of flow to the various organ systems. For this purpose, the vascular system is divided functionally into the large conductance vessels that are generally static but have important capacitance functions, and the vast network of small resistance vessels where vascular diameter is dynamically adjusted in response to changes in perfusion pressure and the metabolic demands of the individual parenchymal tissues. VSM contractile function in small resistance arteries and veins is primarily regulated by a myogenic mechanism(s) that is intrinsic to VSM itself, as well as endothelium-dependent vasodilatory mechanisms that are influenced by flow and locally produced metabolic factors. Together, these intrinsic mechanisms result in what is collectively referred to as autoregulation—a process whereby blood supply to individual organs and cells is adjusted for physiologic demands over a wide range of perfusion pressures. The capillary bed generally plays no direct role in vascular reactivity per se, but the single layer of vascular endothelial cells, where exchange of nutrients and metabolic products with the tissue occurs, is in close contact with the parenchymal cells and is ideally positioned to sense and transduce important mechanical and metabolic signals to upstream endothelial and VSM cells. Extrinsic control of VSM through neuronal or humoral mechanisms may also come into play, particularly during conditions when blood pressure is low or the organism is threatened, and these mechanisms may result in vasoconstriction and marked decreases in flow to certain "nonessential" vascular beds. Although such decreases in flow occur unrelated to changes in metabolic demand, thereby overriding local autoregulation and potentially inducing tissue ischemia, compensatory reduction in metabolic demands in these beds also occurs, and counterregulatory processes mediated by metabolic and endothelial factors can effectively blunt or even eliminate the effects of extrinsic vasoconstrictors under such circumstances. Thus minimal metabolic demands and organ integrity can be preserved even during the most physiologically demanding circumstances. Nevertheless, a number of **297** pathophysiologic processes can affect the functioning of vascular tissue, thereby disrupting the local autoregulatory processes as well as the responses to extrinsic neuronal and humoral mechanisms. During such conditions, the vascular system may operate outside the physiologic range and impair the ability of the organism to respond appropriately, with serious, even mortal, consequences.[1]

Although the importance of vascular reactivity has been long appreciated, the discovery by Furchgott and Zawadzki in 1980 of an endothelium-derived relaxing factor (EDRF)[2] has resulted in a dramatic evolution in our understanding of the importance of the vascular endothelium. Indeed, although the endothelium's role in vascular reactivity received comparatively little attention before 1980, it has subsequently become a major focus. As a result, it is now apparent that endothelium-derived relaxing and contracting factors are involved in virtually all important adjustments in blood flow,[3] and altered release of these endothelium-derived factors appears to have a pivotal role in pathophysiologic changes of vascular reactivity that occur in systemic and pulmonary hypertension, atherosclerosis, diabetes mellitus, and coronary artery disease.[4–8] In addition, it is now clear that vascular endothelial cells are directly and actively involved in controlling thrombosis and platelet activation, as well as in the mobilization and activation of circulating immune cells.[9–11] Thus it is now evident that maintaining the functional integrity of endothelium is critical in the effective regulation of blood pressure and organ blood flow, as well as in control of both the coagulation and inflammatory responses.[12]

More recently, it has also become evident that vascular endothelial cells play a key role in neovascularization or angiogenesis, both sensing the angiogenic stimuli and responding with the initial formation of endothelium-lined tubes and extracellular matrix (ECM).[13] This process has long been of interest in wound healing, but it has only recently been appreciated that unwanted angiogenesis associated with diabetic retinopathy, chronic inflammatory diseases, and particularly tumor growth could potentially be controlled by targeting specific endothelial markers.[14] Indeed, it is now evident that perturbations in the vascular endothelium appear to be either directly or indirectly involved in the pathophysiology of almost every disease process. Appreciation of the pivotal importance of the endothelium in these processes and the interplay between VSM and the vascular endothelium has provided new insights into physiology and the pathophysiology of a number of conditions. Recent advances aimed at clarifying the smooth muscle and endothelium-derived factors, receptors, and signaling mechanisms involved in these processes offer potentially important new strategies for treating a wide variety (cardiovascular, inflammatory, infectious, or oncologic) of pathologic conditions.

This chapter provides an overview of many of the basic functions of the cellular and extracellular components of the vascular system, focusing on the intrinsic and extrinsic mechanisms involved in control of vascular reactivity, and also provides an overview of biochemical and molecular mechanisms involved in smooth muscle contraction and relaxation. The involvement of the vascular endothelium in coagulation, inflammation, and angiogenesis is discussed briefly.

Vascular System Components

The vascular wall is an active and integrated organ made up of VSM and endothelial cells and ECM components. It is not a static organ; the components dynamically change shape and size, or reorganize in response to physiologic and pathologic stimuli. In the mature vascular system, all three elements play vital and distinct roles that serve structural and functional requirements of the system and the organism. The VSM is arranged circumferentially so that contraction and relaxation produce diameter changes that translate directly to changes in resistance that serve to control local blood flow and perfusion pressure. The single layer of endothelial cells lining the lumen of the vessel are positioned to sense changes in flow as well as locally released and circulating signals, with elaboration of factors capable of effecting an appropriate response from the adjacent VSM. Release of factors by the endothelium, as well as expression of endothelial cell receptors and glycoproteins (GPs) on the luminal side are actively involved in control of platelet activation, the coagulation cascade, and mobilization and activation of immune cells. The ECM elaborated by the endothelial and VSM cells provides an organized but appropriately pliable stratum that binds integrin molecules expressed on the contact surfaces of both of these cells. The ECM composition and organization is thus critical for providing the distensibility of the vessel as well as the ability to sense and respond to mechanical stimuli such as stretch. In addition, the ECM provides a highly thrombogenic surface in the event that matrix is inadvertently exposed by endothelial or vascular damage, and matrix proteins provide the template for interaction with endothelial cell integrin molecules during angiogenesis. Changes in matrix components and structure appear to be part of the pathophysiologic process for a number of vascular diseases and genetic defects, resulting in altered matrix composition that can result in significant vascular wall pathology.

Vascular Endothelium

The entire circulatory system is lined with a single layer of vascular endothelial cells. These cells cover an estimated surface area of $3000\,m^2$ while having a mass less than $1\,kg$ in the healthy adult. The endothelium lining the resistance vessels and capillaries represents the majority of the cell mass, where exposure of a relatively large endothelial surface to a small volume of blood (up to $5000\,cm^2/mL$) facilitates the exchange of nutrients and metabolic products.[15] By contrast, large arteries and veins contain most of the blood volume, but provide exposure to only a few square meters of endothelium ($<10\,cm^2/mL$). Although previously considered merely a nonthrombogenic surface and permeability barrier, it is now clear that endothelial cell function is profoundly important for maintenance of vascular integrity and function.[15] As discussed later, endothelium-derived relaxing and contracting factors have a prominent role in the control of vascular reactivity. The release of vasoactive factors by the endothelium appears to be a component of the response profile to virtually all metabolic, physical, neuronal, and humoral stimuli that affect VSM tone.

Coagulation and Inflammation

The importance of the endothelium in preventing local thrombosis and platelet aggregation has long been appreciated, and several endothelium-dependent mechanisms involved in these actions have been elucidated. Endothelium-derived nitric oxide (NO) and prostacyclin (PGI_2) increase cyclic nucleotide concentrations in circulating platelets, thereby inhibiting platelet activation or adhesion to the vascular wall. As discussed later, endothelium-derived factors are potent vasodilators and also serve to attenuate the vasoconstrictor and platelet-activating effects of thromboxane A_2 (TxA_2), the major cyclo-oxygenase (COX) product of activated platelets.[15] In addition, expression of an adenosine diphosphatase by endothelial cells hydrolyzes and thereby neutralizes locally produced adenosine diphosphate, another potent platelet agonist.[16] Endothelial cells synthesize and express heparan sulfate proteoglycans, which bind and potentiate the activity of antithrombin III (ATIII) and the tissue factor pathway inhibitor (TFPI). ATIII is the main inhibitor of thrombin and activated factor X, and TFPI inhibits the tissue factor-activated factor VII complex.[12,16–18] Thrombomodulin (TM), the thrombin receptor expressed on the surface of quiescent endothelial cells, binds thrombin and changes substrate specificity such that thrombin no longer converts fibrinogen to fibrin, or activates factor V; but bound to TM, thrombin binds and activates circulating protein C, which in the presence of its cofactor, protein S, enzymatically inactivates activated factors V and VIII. This action also prevents thrombin-induced platelet activation. In addition, the endothelium is a source of tissue plasminogen activator (tPA), which activates the fibrinolytic system.[16,18,19] In addition to mechanisms that favor inhibition of coagulation and platelet activation during most physiologic conditions,[16,18] endothelial cells synthesize and secrete procoagulant factors including von Willebrand factor (vWF), an important clotting cofactor, and plasminogen activator inhibitor-1 (a tPA inhibitor).[16,18,20–22] The relative contribution of these anticoagulatant and procoagulant mechanisms varies among the different vascular beds, which presumably accounts for the fact that specific deficiencies in each of these mechanisms produce stereotypical site-specific coagulation abnormalities.[18]

Whereas the normally quiescent endothelium thus elaborates important factors and binding GPs to inhibit thrombogenesis and prevent attachment and activation of platelets to the luminal surface, endothelial cells activated by factors from damaged tissue or inflammatory cells also synthesize and elaborate a variety of adhesion molecules that promote coagulation as well as attachment and activation of both platelets and white blood cells.[10–12,16,23] There is involution and loss of surface proteoglycans and TM under such circumstances, and the endothelial surface becomes prothrombogenic.[16,18,24–26] Endothelial injury or stimulation of endothelial cells with thrombin, bradykinin (BK), or histamine induces the endothelial cells to translocate the contents of their storage granules (Weibel-Palade bodies) containing vWF and P-selectin to the membrane surface.[11,23,26] The exposed P-selectin interacts with circulating white cells and platelets, inducing rolling along the membrane surface that facilitates contact of these cells with activator molecules, including platelet-activating factor (PAF), vWF, and exposed ECM proteins.[11,23,26] In platelets, GPIa/IIa binds with collagen, and GPIb/IX with vWF in the matrix or on the endothelial surface, causing firm attachment and activation, with resulting expression of the surface integrin receptor for fibrinogen, GPIIb/IIIa. Fibrinogen has multiple high-affinity GPIIb/IIIa binding sites, and the symmetric dumbbell structure of fibrinogen allows it to bind adjacent activated platelets to induce aggregation.[10,26] The binding of fibrinogen in exposed matrix provides for further stabilization of the platelet plug, which serves as a surface for assembly of other coagulation factors including thrombin, which is no longer bound to endothelial TM or protein C.[18] The platelet aggregate thus serves to catalyze the formation of an occlusive thrombus.[10,26]

More prolonged stimulation of the endothelial cells, as occurs with exposure to inflammatory mediators such as tumor necrosis factor-α or IL-1 produces an endothelial response that, unlike the immediate expression of stored P-selectin and PAF, requires transcription and de novo protein synthesis.[11,16,23] Activated endothelial cells in this paradigm begin expressing the endothelial cell specific E-selectin, which further promotes leukocyte rolling, as well as IL-8 and adhesion molecules of the immunoglobulin superfamily, including intracellular adhesion molecule 1 and 2 (ICAM-1, ICAM-2) and vascular cell adhesion molecule-1.[11,23,26] IL-8, locally produced tissue factor, and cytokines promote white cell activation that results in expression of β_1 and β_2 integrin receptors on the surface of these cells, which bind endothelial vascular cell adhesion molecule-1 and the ICAMs, respectively.[11] Leukocyte diapedesis between endothelial cells to the inflamed tissue is facilitated by the immunoglobulin superfamily protein platelet-endothelial cell adhesion molecule-1 located at the lateral endothelial borders.[11,23,26]

From the foregoing discussion, it is evident that the endothelium plays a crucial role in the response to injury and inflammation, exhibiting active expression of effector molecules that serve to direct platelets, coagulation factors, and inflammatory cells to the appropriate site. The prothrombotic mechanisms result in containment of the injury or infection and loss of blood from the intravascular space. The second phase of the endothelial response, involving protein synthesis and expression of immunoglobulin superfamily proteins, is more specifically intended to activate the inflammatory response, which is then self-perpetuating until the stimulus decays and the stimulus for endothelial adhesion molecule expression is terminated.[11] The endothelial response to inflammation and injury is of considerable interest in vascular biology because it is clear that most chronic inflammatory conditions involve endothelial activation. Better understanding of the mechanism(s) of endothelial activation could lead to novel approaches to controlling chronic inflammation such as antiadhesion therapy.[11] It is clear that ongoing and excessive activation of endothelial cells in chronic inflammation can lead to endothelial damage and a vicious cycle of uncontrolled activation of circulating inflammatory cells, further endothelial cell damage, and disseminated intravascular coagulation.[18,24] Indeed, recent evidence places the endothelium at the center of control of coagulation and inflammation cascades in the systemic inflammatory response and adult respiratory distress syndromes (ARDS).[16,23,27] Moreover, while therapeutic trials aimed at curtailing the inflammatory responses in the systemic inflammatory response and ARDS have failed to produce improved outcomes, recent therapies aimed at preventing activation of prothrombotic elements at the endothelial surface have produced some promising results in patients with severe sepsis. Although such approaches may seem antithetical, the crosstalk between the inflammatory and coagulation cascades at the level of the vascular endothelium provides the basis for some of the unforeseen benefits from such treatments. As some investigators have recently demonstrated,[28] thrombin-activated protein C, which is decreased in patients with severe sepsis, suppresses cytokine-induced expression of NFκB, as well as the NFκB-regulated downstream inflammatory responses. In addition, activated protein C appears to up-regulate antiapoptotic and down-regulate proapoptotic gene expression in cultured human endothelial cells.[28] Such studies provide evidence for the importance of mechanisms involving inflammatory and coagulation interactions at the endothelial surface and have important implications in the treatment of a broad range of diseases including atherosclerosis, ARDS, vasculitis, allograft rejection, and sickle cell disease, in which endothelial cell activation and inflammation play a prominent role.[6,12,18,28]

Angiogenesis

Angiogenesis, or the formation of a new vascular network out of pre-existing vessels, begins with proliferation of endothelial cells and the formation of new endothelium-lined capillaries. The importance of angiogenesis in healing, growth, and increasing vascular supply in response to tissue hypoxia or ischemia, has long been appreciated. However, until recently, little was known about the mechanisms that initiate and control this process.[13,29,30] Intensified interest over the last several years—largely because of interest in tumor angiogenesis—has led to identification of a number of endogenous proangiogenic and antiangiogenic signaling molecules and pathways that appear to act in concert to control the "angiogenic switch" in endothelial cells.[13,29,30] As tissues grow, local tissue hypoxia appears to be one of the principal driving forces for angiogenesis. Hypoxia during both physiologic and pathologic conditions activates hypoxia-inducible transcription factors that induce expression of proangiogenic growth factors including vascular endothelial growth factor (VEGF), platelet-derived growth factor (PDGF), and angiopoietin.[13,29,30] These growth factors induce local endothelial cells to secrete matrix metalloproteinases (MMP), which degrade the ECM, and endothelial cells then actively migrate into the interstitial space.[13,29,30] The resulting increased vascular permeability also results in interstitial accumulation of plasma proteins and the formation of a provisional fibrin-rich matrix into which the replicating endothelial cells grow. The endothelial cell sprouts from the original vessel thereby continue to grow in the direction of the hypoxic stimulus, forming new vascular channels that interconnect to the established circulation. The process continues until the proangiogenic stimulus is withdrawn and the angiogenic balance then favors antiangiogenic mechanisms.[13,30]

In addition to hypoxia-inducible transcription factor–induced expression of tissue-derived growth factors, cytokines derived from white cells and platelets—including PDGF, basic fibroblast growth factor, transforming growth factor-β, and tumor necrosis factor-α—as well as proteins associated with activation of the coagulation cascade including thrombin and plasmin and factors expressed by activated endothelial cells—including NO, PGI$_2$, tPA, plasminogen activator inhibitor-1 and E-selectin—have all been demonstrated to have angiogenic activity.[13,29,30] Thus endothelial activation with concurrent activation of the coagulation and inflammatory cascades (such as occurs with tissue injury or infection) appears to be an important stimulus for angiogenesis during wound healing and inflammation. Conversely, the angiogenic factors derived from activated white cells, platelets, and endothelial cells may also contribute to unwanted angiogenesis or neovascularization such as occurs in a number of chronic inflammatory diseases.[29]

Once angiogenesis is initiated, the replicating endothelial cells express a unique complement of integrins—most notably the $\alpha_V\beta_3$ integrin—on the cell surface that must acquire contact with their matrix protein ligand(s), or the angiogenic switch is turned "off" and the endothelial cells undergo apoptosis.[31] In addition, a number of endogenous antiangiogenic molecules have been identified, most notably endostatin and angiostatin, which are peptide cleavage products of vascular-specific collagen XVIII and plasminogen, respectively. These factors inhibit endothelial proliferation and thus may be important in controlling angiogenesis during physiologic or pathologic conditions.[13,29]

Recently, trials have been initiated to assess the efficacy of growth factors such as VEGF and fibroblast growth factor-β to augment angiogenesis in ischemic tissues.[29,30] In addition, a number of antiangiogenic therapy trials for the treatment of solid tumors are also ongoing. VEGF antibodies to block growth factor signaling, matrix metalloproteinase inhibitors to inhibit matrix degradation, anti-$\alpha_V\beta_3$ integrin antibodies to induce endothelial cell apoptosis, as well as the endogenous angiogenesis inhibitors endostatin and angiostatin, have all shown promise in treating tumors in animals; human trials are underway.[29,30] Other bold and exciting antiangiogenic strategies on the horizon will potentially use the unique cellular markers of dividing endothelial cells (including $\alpha_V\beta_3$ integrin, E-selectin, and peptides containing the RGD (arginine-glycine-asparagine amino acid recognition sequence common to VSM and endothelial integrins) as homing probes to target the tumor vasculature with cytotoxic or immunogenic agents.[29,31,32] The unwanted angiogenesis that occurs in vascular malformations, diabetic retinopathy, and chronic inflammatory conditions may also represent potential targets for antiangiogenic therapies.[29,30] Indeed, it has even been proposed that angiogenesis in adipose tissue could be a potential target to treat massive obesity.[29]

Vascular Smooth Muscle

The VSM cells are the fundamental machinery of the vascular system. VSM actively contracts and relaxes to produce changes in blood vessel diameter that are responsible for both physiologic adjustments and pathologic changes in hemodynamics and blood flow. VSM has thus evolved with a complex repertoire of contractile proteins, ion channels, agonist receptor and signal transduction systems that permit VSM to carry out its specialized functions.[33] Signaling pathways and ion channels linked to integrins and cytoskeletal proteins have imparted on the VSM the capacity for intrinsic "autoregulatory" responses to changes in pressure that are then modulated by local metabolic and endothelial cell factors, as well as by external neuronal and humoral signals. Ultimately, the diverse inputs are integrated at the level of the VSM that adjusts microvessel diameter to ensure that the blood flow demands of both the individual tissues and the organism are met.

Contractile Proteins

VSM has contractile machinery and regulatory mechanisms that differ considerably from those found and used in cardiac and skeletal muscle. The principal cytoskeletal and contractile protein in VSM is smooth muscle-specific α-actin, which is the single most abundant protein in these cells— making up 70% of the total actin and 40% of the total cellular protein. With the exception of transient expression in cardiac and skeletal muscle during development, α-actin is exclusively expressed in adult smooth muscle, which may also contain varying amounts of smooth muscle γ-actin and nonmuscle β-actin and γ-actin.[34] Globular actin monomers (G-actin) polymerize to form actin filaments (F-actin) that are anchored in the plasma membrane at focal adhesion points or focal contacts on the ventral surface, and to diffuse integral membrane protein sites at the apical surface and the nuclear membrane. The points of contact are generally multiprotein structures that include specific actin-binding proteins and the intracellular domains of the integrins. This complex thereby provides a direct link between the actin filaments and the ECM proteins.[35] Myosin II, or the "myosin motor" is the other major contractile protein expressed in VSM, which is composed of two heavy chains, two functional light chains, and two regulatory light chains. Myosin heavy chains bind actin at their N-terminus; and following phosphorylation at the serine 19 residue of the myosin regulatory light chain (MLC), the N-terminal myosin head displays adenosine triphosphatase (ATPase) ("motor") activity. Actin and myosin filaments in VSM are generally oriented parallel to the long axis or circumferentially in intact vessels. Thus activation of the myosin ATPase results in force generation and decreased luminal diameter (vasoconstriction) as myosin moves along the actin filaments.[35] Further details regarding the cellular mechanisms that control MLC phosphorylation and activation of the contractile machinery in VSM are provided in the subsequent section detailing contractile mechanisms.

Gap Junctions

VSM gap junctions provide direct cell-to-cell electrical connectivity, thereby allowing VSM to function as a syncytium, with synchronized contraction and relaxation of adjacent cells.[36] Gap junctions in VSM are composed of connexin (Cx) proteins that form an intercellular passage allowing diffusion of small molecules less than 1 kD. This includes ions such as Ca^{2+} and K^+, and small second messenger molecules such as the phosphoinositides and cyclic nucleotides, which are important regulators of contraction and relaxation. The connexin gene family is now known to contain 12 or more members, 3 of which—Cx37, Cx40 and Cx43—have been isolated from vascular tissue.[37,38] The connexin distribution is also dependent on the type of vessel. For example, Cx43 is expressed abundantly in large conductance vessels compared with more limited expression in small resistance vessels.[39] Gap junctions also appear to be responsible for communication between smooth muscle and endothelial cells, allowing electrical coupling and direct transfer of endothelium-dependent vasodilatory signals, including hyperpolarization, to adjacent VSM.[40,41]

Extracellular Matrix

VSM and vascular endothelial cells produce an extracellular matrix consisting of collagen, elastin, laminin, fibronectin, vitronectin, proteoglycans, and a number of other less abundant components. These ECM proteins are ligands for the integrin "receptors," a group of heterodimeric transmembrane proteins consisting of α- and β-subunits that are expressed on VSM and endothelial cells.[42] The extracellular domains of the integrins recognize specific RGD (arginine-glycine-aspartic acid) peptide motifs present in matrix components, and integrin/matrix interactions serve to organize the vessel wall, determining cellular polarity and position, as well as assembly of the matrix.[25,43] The intracellular domains of integrins are attached to the actin cytoskeleton, providing a mechanical link between the ECM and the cytoskeleton.[35] Vascular cells scattered throughout the media can thereby function as a syncytium, even in the absence of direct contact, and changes in wall tension may thereby be transduced to effector proteins including stretch-sensitive membrane ion channels and the kinases involved in chemical and mechanical transduction pathways. Such mechanisms are fundamental to the development of myogenic tone and are of great importance in autoregulation of blood flow during changes in transmural pressure. Matrix components are also important ligands for adhesion molecules in nonvascular cells, as discussed earlier. In addition, collagen and vWF in the ECM exposed after endothelial injury bind platelet GPIa/IIa and GPIb/IX, respectively, resulting in platelet activation, expression of the platelet fibrinogen receptor, $\alpha_{IIb}\beta_3$ integrin (GPIIb/IIIa), formation of a platelet plug, activation of the coagulation cascade, and vascular occlusion.[10] Prevention of such matrix/platelet interactions with anticoagulation and GPIIb/IIIa antagonists has proven clinically useful with arteriosclerotic plaque rupture or after angioplasty-induced vascular injury.[10]

Genetic modifications of matrix or integrin composition may be associated with significant vascular abnormalities, and vascular diseases are conversely associated with alterations in the composition of the ECM and the integrins expressed. Mice lacking fibronectin or $\alpha_5\beta_1$ integrin (a fibronectin receptor) have severe defects in vasculogenesis and die early in gestation; whereas those lacking collagen I or the α_v integrin subunit die from vascular complications just before or after birth.[25] Similarly, genetic abnormalities in matrix protein expression or structure are associated with vascular abnormalities in humans. Both Marfan syndrome, which is caused by mutations in the matrix protein fibrillin, and Ehlers-Danlos syndrome (type IV), which is caused by mutations in type III collagen, are associated with altered vessel structure and premature rupture of large vessels.[25,44] Conversely, abnormalities in the expression of elastin are associated with vascular thickening and subaortic stenosis.[45] In atherosclerotic disease or after vascular injury during angioplasty, there is up-regulation of $\alpha_v\beta_3$ integrin expression on VSM cells, which appears to mediate migration of these cells into the neointima; and there is increased production of matrix proteins that fill the neointima, including the $\alpha_v\beta_3$ integrin ligand osteopontin.[6,25] Similar to the endothelial cell proliferation that occurs with vasculogenesis, in which there is also up-regulation of $\alpha_v\beta_3$ integrin, proangiogenic growth factors (including PDGF, transforming growth factor-β, and others) generated by the inflammatory response appear to be important in driving both VSM proliferation and increased production of matrix proteins.[6,25,29]

Control of Vascular Tone

Vascular contraction and relaxation are highly regulated by intrinsic "autoregulatory" mechanisms involving myogenic vasoconstriction—developed in response to intravascular pressure—and counterbalancing release of EDRFs in response to flow (Fig. 19–1). Together these mechanisms ensure that perfusion is relatively constant over a wide range of blood pressures and provide appropriate "fine-tuning" based on the adequacy of tissue oxygen delivery and removal of metabolic products (i.e., tissue PO_2, PCO_2, lactate, pH^+, and so on). The importance of the endothelium in the autoregulation of flow is now appreciated, and impaired endothelium-dependent relaxation leads to unopposed myogenic vasoconstriction, increased resistance, and decreased organ perfusion. Endothelial dysfunction, with release of the potent endothelium-dependent constricting factor endothelin 1, appears to contribute to the pathogenesis of cardiac failure—a situation in which the cardiac pump is unable to sustain adequate organ flow against increased systemic resistance.[46] Extrinsic neurohumoral mechanisms, involv-

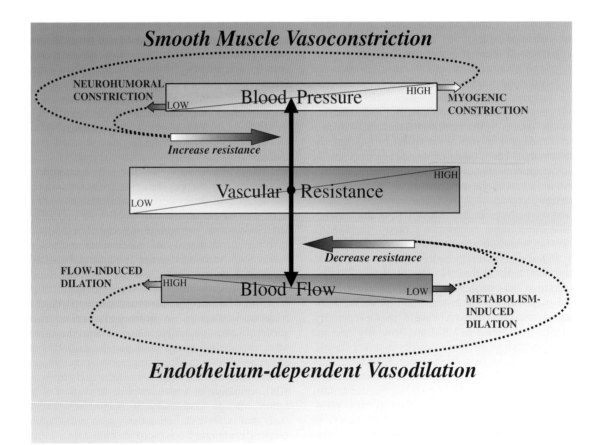

Figure 19–1. Ohm's Law describes the relationships among pressure, resistance, and flow as shown in the diagram where *blood pressure* is directly proportional to and *blood flow* is indirectly proportional to *vascular resistance*. In addition, vascular resistance and thereby pressure and flow are set by myogenic vasoconstriction, which is countered by flow and metabolism-induced vasodilation. During conditions in which blood pressure is low or threatened, neurohumoral constriction may also come into play. In the absence of endothelium-dependent vasodilation, myogenic vasoconstriction would generate a positive feedback loop potentially leading to vasospasm that is unresponsive to flow or metabolic changes.

ing sympathetic nervous system output, production of angiotensin II (Ang II), and vasopressin release, which are largely regulated by baroreflexes, make significant contributions to vascular tone only during conditions in which venous or arterial pressures are low, or when other sensory neural inputs suggest a threat. These neurohumoral mechanisms can lead to widespread vasoconstriction that overrides local control mechanisms, particularly in "nonessential" vascular beds such as those supplying the mesentery, skin, and skeletal muscle. The potent constricting effects of neurohumoral mediators, however, continue to be integrated by local intrinsic mechanisms to ensure that minimal flow necessary for tissue preservation is maintained while the overall demands of the organism—in terms of blood pressure control and perfusion of critical organs—are met.

The interplay of local intrinsic and extrinsic neurohumoral mechanisms is of greatest importance during extreme physiologic conditions such as those seen after severe trauma or hemorrhage. During these circumstances, sensory and baroreflex afferents evoke the "fright, fight, flight" response and increased sympathetic nervous system output. In the vascular system, the result is α-adrenergic–induced vasoconstriction, which both recruits volume from capacitance veins, and constricts resistance arteries supplying the densely innervated mesenteric, skeletal muscle, and cutaneous vascular beds. Blood flow is thereby redistributed away from these latter beds to ensure adequate perfusion or flow reserve for critical organs such as heart and brain, which are largely spared. Renal blood flow is also decreased, although juxtaglomerular apparatus-induced secretion of renin, and the resulting increase in Ang II levels, produces efferent arteriolar constriction that relatively preserves glomerular filtration—the major physiologic function of renal blood flow. Baroreflex-mediated release of vasopressin from the posterior pituitary potentiates adrenergic vasoconstriction with little effect on the renal bed; although massive vasopressin release, such as occurs in severe hemorrhage, may produce levels of vasopressin sufficient to produce coronary artery constriction, which would appear to threaten the viability of the entire organism. The heart is protected, however, by release of endothelium-dependent relaxing factors and vasodilatory metabolites that assure that blood flow is optimally distributed according to metabolic demand, and myocardial work is maintained.[47] Moreover, the vasopressin-induced vasoconstriction does not affect the maximal coronary vasodilatory reserve in response to hypoxia.[48] Thus even during the most extreme conditions, extrinsic vasoconstrictor mechanisms are able to ensure adequate delivery of oxygen to critical tissues, whereas intrinsic control mechanisms continue to ensure that minimal tissue perfusion is not compromised. Coexisting pathologic conditions, particularly those in which endothelium-dependent vasodilatory mechanisms are impaired, however, can lead to unopposed vasoconstriction leading to tissue ischemia and injury, with potentially fatal consequences.

Myogenic Mechanisms

Vascular transmural pressure or stretch of VSM generates a rapid and sustained contraction that is independent of endothelial function or any neurohumoral influence. Previously thought to be mediated by metabolic or local tissue factors, it is now clear that the myogenic response is fundamental to the smooth muscle itself as a response to increased load or stretch.[49,50] The VSM myogenic response is considered to be largely responsible for the phenomenon of autoregulation of blood flow and capillary hydrostatic pressure, which are well-maintained at a relatively constant level over a wide range of perfusion pressures. Of equal or greater importance, myogenic contraction provides basal vascular tone that can then be decreased as needed in response to decreased perfusion pressure, increased metabolic demand, or other physiologic vasodilatory stimuli. In addition, it has been noted that myogenic VSM contraction increases the sensitivity of VSM to vasoconstricting agonists, and these agonists enhance myogenic contraction as well. The intrinsic myogenic response thus provides for both vasodilatory and vasoconstricting reserve, broadening the dynamic range of blood flow responses in both directions.

Numerous studies indicate that myogenic contraction is dependent of both membrane depolarization and Ca^{2+} influx (Fig. 19–2).[49,50] The resulting increased intracellular Ca^{2+} concentration ($[Ca^{2+}]_i$) thereby activates the Ca^{2+}/calmodulin/myosin light chain kinase (MLCK) mechanism (see later). In addition, investigation of the Ca^{2+} sensitization/desensitization mechanisms that have been shown to be involved in responses to vascular agonists suggests that these mechanisms also contribute to the myogenic response.[50] These include the classic mechanism involving heterotrimeric G protein-induced activation of phospholipase C (PLC) and protein kinase C (PKC)–induced sensitization, as well as mechanisms involving small G proteins, such RhoGTPase, and their downstream kinases (e.g., Rho kinase). PKC and/or protein tyrosine kinase (PTK)-induced activation of downstream mitogen-activated protein kinases (MAPKs) and phosphorylation of thin filament modulators such as caldesmon may also be involved.[49,50]

The genesis of the membrane depolarizing action of mechanical stretch is not entirely clear, but it appears to involve mechanosensitive (MS) ion channels that may be either activated (nonselective cation or Cl^-) or inhibited (K^+) by stretch-sensitive processes. Nonselective cation channels are probably the most widely observed, although volume-sensitive Cl^- channels may also be activated by stretch. K^+ channels, including the large conductance Ca^{2+}-activated K^+ (BK) channels, which are ubiquitous in VSM, may be inhibited by stretch-dependent processes.[50] The membrane depolarizing action of these MS channels activates voltage-dependent Ca^{2+} (VDC) channels (L-type) in VSM, which produces increased Ca^{2+} influx that in turn activates the contractile machinery. VDC channels in some vessels, such as cerebral arterioles, may themselves be sensitive to stretch. However, whereas VDC channel blockers abolish the stretch-induced $[Ca^{2+}]_i$ increases and contraction, the membrane depolarizing action of stretch persists.[51]

There has been considerable recent interest in identification of stretch- or tension-sensing mechanism(s) whereby changes in pressure and other mechanical stimuli are transduced to the MS channels or signaling pathways involved in myogenic constriction and flow-induced vasodilation (see later).[49] The current view suggests that ECM/integrin interactions may be the primary sensing structure that converts

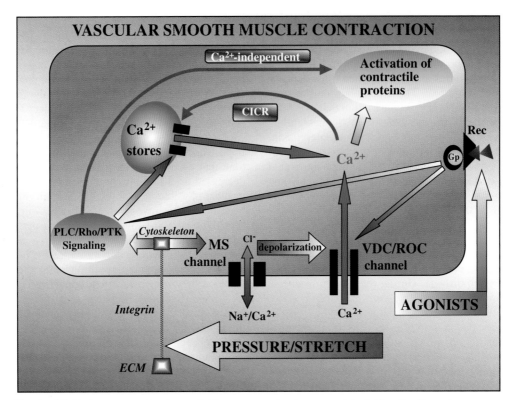

Figure 19–2. Basic mechanisms linking myogenic (pressure/stretch) stimuli and vasoconstrictor agonists to activation of contractile proteins in vascular smooth muscle cells (VSM). Integrins anchor the VSM to the extracellular matrix (ECM) and provide a physical link to VSM cytoskeleton-associated mechanosensitive (MS) channels and signaling pathways involving phospholipase C (PLC), small G proteins (e.g., Rho), and protein tyrosine kinase (PTK). Activation of MS channels results in membrane depolarization and activation of voltage-dependent calcium (VDC) channels. Agonists use receptor (Rec)-associated heterotrimeric G proteins to activate these same signaling pathways, as well as VDC and receptor-operated calcium (ROC) channels. CICR, Ca^{2+}-induced Ca^{2+} release.

changes in tension or wall stress to altered intracellular signaling (Figure 19–2). This model of "outside-in" signaling is supported by the association of integrins with a number of signaling proteins with effects on VSM contraction including PLC, RhoGTPase, and PTKs. Moreover, the integrin/signaling protein complexes are "clustered," by the multivalent ECM proteins, with contractile and cytoskeletal proteins at focal adhesion points in VSM cells.[49] As discussed earlier, cytoskeletal/contractile proteins anchored at focal adhesion points provide a mechanical link between matrix/integrin interactions and the actin cytoskeleton/contractile apparatus. In a somewhat analogous model, so-called tensegrity (based on the term coined by R. Buckminster Fuller to describe the structural rigidity of the geodesic dome), the rigid cytoskeletal structure is positioned as the primary sensing element, whereby cytoskeleton deformation by mechanical stimuli is telegraphed to focal adhesions and transducing elements located throughout the cell ("inside-out" signaling). Transduction by the cytoskeleton may thereby involve MS or VDC channels, as well as signal transduction pathways clustered at focal adhesions, which are mechanically coupled to the cytoskeleton.[49,50]

The sensing and transduction mechanisms involved in the myogenic response thus appear likely to involve complex interactions among matrix-integrin-effector elements localized at the focal adhesion structure. Further evidence supporting this concept is that the downstream targets of matrix-integrin-effector coupling that have been shown to modulate contractile protein function, including MAPK and Rho kinase, which are activated by integrin-associated PTKs and RhoGTPase, respectively, that are themselves anchored in cytoskeletal/contractile protein "scaffolds" linked to integrins.[49,52]

Endothelial Mechanisms

The vascular endothelium, located at the interface between blood flow and the vessel wall, is ideally positioned to detect changes in vascular flow and blood-borne biochemical or neurohumoral signals. Blood flow in arteries is generally laminar; however, the vessel geometry near branches, bifurcations, and curved regions promotes flow separation and vortex formation. At such locations, shear stresses can fluctuate greatly in magnitude and direction over short distances. When endothelial cells are subjected to shear stress or mechanical stretching, a diverse set of responses are generated that lead to changes in both the structural and functional properties of the cells.[53]

Indeed, sensing flow and responses to "shear stress" have recently been recognized as one of the most important physiologic functions of the endothelium. Laminar flow results in elaboration of endothelium-dependent relaxing factors, most notably NO and PGI_2, which inhibit contraction of adjacent VSM as well as activation and attachment of circulating platelets and inflammatory cells (Fig. 19–3). The flow-induced, endothelium-dependent relaxation thereby offsets the myogenic constriction generated during the cardiac cycle caused by pressure, and thus ensures that organ blood flow is well maintained.[54] Normal laminar flow also prevents endothelial cell activation, which would otherwise lead to expression of adhesion molecules and activation of transcription factors involved in smooth muscle proliferation and atherogenesis.[55]

The mechanism of mechanotransduction in endothelial cells has been of considerable interest. Endothelial cells are anchored to the ECM, and ECM-integrin-cytoskeleton-effector pathways described for the myogenic response are also involved in endothelium-dependent responses to mechanical stimuli.[56] ECM/integrin signaling with RGD peptides or β_3 integrin antibodies results in attenuation of endothelium-dependent vasodilatory responses to flow.[57] As in VSM, mechanotransduction and signaling in endothelial cells also involves activation of cytoskeleton-linked MS channels, MAPKs, and PLC. In contrast to VSM, however, the resulting increases in $[Ca^{2+}]_i$ in endothelial cells lead to activation of NO synthase (NOS) and COX, and result in relaxation, not contraction, of adjacent VSM. Mechanotransduction by endothelial cells is also responsible for suppressing expression of a number of surface receptors and transcription factors involved in cellular proliferation and activation of the immune response.[55,56,58]

The endothelium also appears to be important in coupling of metabolic demands and organ blood flow, or metabolic autoregulation.[59] Hypoxia results in increased production

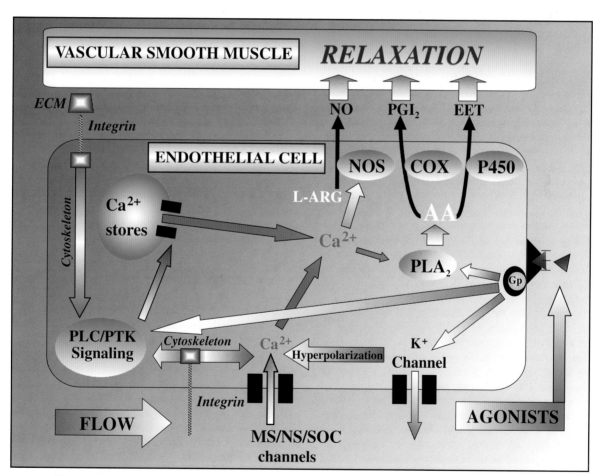

Figure 19–3. Activation of endothelium-dependent relaxation mechanisms in response to flow is initiated by activation of mechanosensitive (MS) channels and extracellular matrix (ECM)/integrin/cytoskeleton signaling. Activation by agonists involves receptor-coupled heterotrimeric G protein–induced activation of phospholipase C (PLC) and K^+ channels, as well as activation of phospholipase A_2 (PLA_2), which is critical to agonist-induced relaxation. In both cases, the net result is increased release and influx of Ca^{2+}, activation of nitric oxide synthase (NOS), and increased NO production, as well as increased release of vasodilatory and hyperpolarizing products of arachidonic acid (AA) metabolism, produced by the cyclo-oxygenase (COX) and the cytochrome P450 monooxygenase (P450) pathways. EET, epoxyeicosatrienoic acids; PTK, protein tyrosine kinase.

of endothelium-dependent vasodilators, and inhibition of endothelium-dependent relaxation results in loss of the normal vasodilatory response to hypoxia.[60] In the physiologic situation, the small arterioles controlling local blood flow lie upstream of the parenchymal tissue they supply. To increase flow, it is thus necessary to sense hypoxic stimuli arising in the parenchymal tissue and to propagate the relaxing signal retrograde. The capillary endothelial cells are clearly positioned to accomplish both hypoxia-induced activation of ATP-gated potassium (K_{ATP}) channels and retrograde propagation of endothelial cell hyperpolarization through gap channels, which may be critical for optimal vasodilatory responses to hypoxia.[61] Hyperpolarization results in endothelial release of NO, PGI_2, and endothelium-dependent hyperpolarizing factor with relaxation of adjacent VSM. The resulting increases in distal flow would be further propagated retrograde to more proximal supply vessels through flow-induced dilation. Electrotonic spread of hyperpolarization to smooth muscle through myoendothelial gap junctions may also contribute to smooth muscle relaxation in response to tissue hypoxia.[62]

Nitric Oxide

Mechanical stimuli and endothelial receptor agonists result in EDRF release, first described by Furchgott and Zawadzki in 1980, which is now synonymous with NO.[2] NO is a heterodiatomic molecule synthesized from the terminal guanidino nitrogen atom(s) of L-arginine, by NOS which converts L-arginine to L-citrulline and NO through a 5-electron oxidation. Three main NOS isoforms have been isolated, although only the constitutive endothelial NOS isoform, eNOS or NOS III,[63] is present in vascular endothelial cells. eNOS is activated on binding Ca^{2+}-calmodulin, generated by endothelial stimuli that increase $[Ca^{2+}]_i$. There is also an inducible isoform, iNOS or NOS II, which is expressed in VSM and endothelial cells after transcriptional induction by pathologic stimuli, most notably infectious and inflammatory mediators. Unlike eNOS, iNOS is tonically active independent of Ca^{2+} concentration.[64]

Once generated in the endothelial cell, the amphophilic NO molecule is capable of rapidly crossing membranes where it binds the heme moiety of guanyl cyclase and activates that enzyme in the adjacent smooth muscle cells. The resulting increased production of cyclic 3′,5′-guanosine monophosphate (cGMP) from guanosine 5′-triphosphate results in cGMP-dependent protein kinase (PKG)–mediated smooth muscle relaxation.[65] PKG-mediated phosphorylation of Ca^{2+} channels and transporters, as well as proteins involved in control of myosin phosphorylation, appear to be involved in the vasodilatory action of EDRF. In addition, NO itself may activate K^+ channels, producing hyperpolarization and decreased Ca^{2+} influx, independent of cGMP or PKG.[66]

Prostacyclin

Flow and endothelial agonists also result in activation of phospholipase A2 (PLA_2) and elaboration of vasodilatory COX products, most notably PGI_2 and prostaglandin E_2

(PGE_2). In addition, recent evidence strongly suggests that PLA_2-derived arachidonic acid itself, not a metabolite, is important for agonist-induced activation of eNOS and agonist-induced endothelium-dependent relaxation.[67] Unlike NO, the actions of the prostanoids are mediated by activation of adenylate cyclase in VSM,[19] with resulting increases in the intracellular concentration of cyclic 3′,5′-adenosine monophosphate (cAMP) and activation of cAMP-dependent protein kinase A (PKA). However, the vasorelaxing effects of cAMP in VSM appear to be largely related to the ability of cAMP to activate the considerably more abundant PKG in these cells. Thus, activation of PKG appears to be a point of convergence for endothelium-dependent vasodilators that activate either adenylate or guanylate cyclase.[68,69]

As with the NOS enzyme family, there are both constitutive and inducible COX isoforms (COX-1 and COX-2, respectively), although only COX-1 is expressed at substantial levels in most endothelial cells.[70] Many of the same stimuli that result in expression of NOS II also induce expression of COX-2 in both endothelial and VSM cells.[71] Vasoconstrictor COX products such as $PGF_{2\alpha}$, PGH, and the potent constrictor TxA_2, may also be produced under certain conditions.[72] In addition to COX products, arachidonic acid metabolism through the cytochrome P450 monooxygenase pathway appears to result in production of vasodilatory epoxyeicosatrienoic acids (EETs), which may account for endothelium-dependent hyperpolarizing factor activity in some systems.[73,74] The 5′-lipoxygenase pathway leads to the production of the leukotrienes (LTA_4, LIB_4, LTC_4 and LTD_4) from arachidonic acid, which have diverse biologic activities including both VSM contracting and relaxing effects.[75] However, the role of the 5′-lipoxygenase products, as well as the lysophospholipid products of PLA_2, such as PAF, in agonist or flow-induced, endothelium-dependent relaxation or constriction is unclear.

Endothelium-Derived Hyperpolarizing Factor

Endothelium-derived hyperpolarizing factor (EDHF) activity persists in the presence of both NOS and COX inhibitors. However, the molecular identity of EDHF remains unclear. EDHF release is associated with activation of membrane K^+ channels in adjacent VSM, resulting in both hyperpolarization, relaxation, and resistance to agonist-induced depolarization.[76,77] EDHF responses are inhibited by application of the K^+ channel blockers, apamin and charybdotoxin, although coapplication of both toxins is necessary to completely block EDHF responses.[76] Thus, it has been proposed that both the apamin-sensitive small conductance Ca^{2+}-sensitive K^+ channels (SK_{Ca}) and the charybdotoxin-sensitive intermediate and large conductance Ca^{2+}-sensitive K^+ channels (IK_{Ca} and BK_{Ca}, respectively) are involved in EDHF activity or responses.[77] In both porcine and bovine coronary arteries, the EETs products of cytochrome P450 monooxygenase metabolism of PLA_2-derived arachidonic acid appear to function as EDHF.[73,78] However, cytochrome P450 inhibitors do not inhibit EDHF activity in other systems, and the molecular nature of EDHF in some systems remains uncertain.

Endothelins

It has recently become clear that the endothelium may also elaborate vasoconstrictor substances during certain conditions. The best known of these— the endothelins—are a family of three related peptides, of 21 amino acids each, that are potent endothelium-derived VSM constrictors.[79,80] The three peptides are the products of separate genes (*ET-1, ET-2,* and *ET-3*) of which *ET-1* and *ET-2* exhibit the closest structural similarity.[79,81] There are specific high-affinity smooth muscle binding sites for the *ETs*: the ET_A receptor has a high affinity for *ET-1*, whereas the ET_B receptor has approximately equal affinity for all three *ETs*. As with other potent vasoconstrictors, *ETs* vasoconstricting action is exerted largely through PLC activation resulting in increases in $[Ca^{2+}]_i$ and PKC activation, which sensitizes the contractile proteins to Ca^{2+}.[80] In addition, *ETs* may also act on endothelial *ET* receptors and induce release of NO or PGI_2, thereby acting as an autacoid to modulate the constrictor actions of *ET*; conversely endothelial production of *ET*-1 is inhibited by NO and nitrovasodilators.[82] Although the role of *ETs* remains unclear, their existence is of considerable interest in conditions associated with endothelial dysfunction. *ET* release and *ET*-induced vasoconstriction and mitogenesis have been implicated in the pathophysiology of a variety of diseases including atherosclerosis, hypertension, coronary endothelial dysfunction, diabetic vascular disease, and cerebral vasospasm following subarachnoid hemorrhage.[83–85] It has also been noted that *ET*-1 concentrations are elevated in patients with Raynaud disease and coronary vasospasm, in which it has been proposed that dysregulation of endothelial function leads to an excess of endothelium-derived *ETs* that contribute to pathologic vasoconstriction.[86,87]

Neuronal Mechanisms

Sympathetic Nervous System

Vascular tissue is extensively innervated by sympathetic (adrenergic) nerves, stimulation of which produces increases in vascular resistance and decreases in vascular compliance. Norepinephrine (NE) is the principal neurotransmitter released, and the vasoconstrictor effect of NE is largely mediated by activation of smooth muscle α_1 adrenoceptors. The mechanism of the action involves activation of PLC, which results in increases in smooth muscle $[Ca^{2+}]_i$ from inositol 1,4,5-trisphosphate (IP_3)-sensitive intracellular stores and activation of contractile proteins. Sensitization of the contractile proteins to Ca^{2+} induced by activation of PKC, and a membrane depolarizing action in which voltage-dependent sarcolemmal Ca^{2+} channels are activated, are also important in α_1 adrenoreceptor-mediated constriction.[50] In some vessels, smooth muscle α_2 receptors also appear to mediate vasoconstriction by activation of Ca^{2+} channels; although in most beds, presynaptic α_2 adrenoceptors produce presynaptic inhibition of NE release, and endothelial cell α_2 adrenoceptors induce $[Ca^{2+}]_i$ increases resulting in activation of eNOS and NO-dependent vasodilation.[88,89] Smooth muscle and endothelial cell β receptors, generally of the β_2 receptor subtype, also mediate vasodilation in coronary and skeletal muscle beds.

Sympathetic nerve terminals also contain neuropeptide Y (NPY), a 36-amino acid peptide that produces smooth muscle contraction similar to that produced by NE. NPY and NE appear to act synergistically to produce vasoconstriction on sympathetic nerve stimulation. NPY may also serve to regulate catecholamine release.[90] Sympathetic nerve terminals also contain ATP as well as small quantities of adenosine diphosphate, AMP, and adenosine, which are coreleased with NE and NPY. These compounds interact with specific endothelial and smooth muscle purinergic receptors producing dual effects on isolated vessels, causing concentration-dependent contraction at resting tension, while inducing relaxation of precontracted vessels.[91] As with NPY, coreleased ATP inhibits NE release presynaptically,[92] and both ATP and NPY may account for nonadrenergic, noncholinergic (NANC) effects of nerve stimulation observed in the presence of adrenergic and cholinergic receptor blockade.[93]

The systemic circulation is influenced by central reflex control mechanisms that are also mediated largely by alterations in sympathetic tone. Stimulation of the hypothalamic integrative areas involved in defense reactions causes increased sympathetic nerve activity, increases in vascular resistance, and decreases in vascular compliance.[94,95] Stimulation of chemoreceptors in the carotid or aortic bodies also increases peripheral vascular resistance and decreases vascular compliance[95]; and stimulation of baroreceptors in the carotid sinus or aortic arch elicited by elevations in blood pressure induces reflex vasodilation through a decrease in sympathetic outflow and activation of sympathetic vasodilator nerves.[96,97]

Parasympathetic Nervous System

The vascular system is innervated with parasympathetic cholinergic nerves, although not nearly as extensively as in the heart and the airways. Moreover, in contrast to airway smooth muscle, where vagal stimulation results in contraction, activation of vascular endothelial cell muscarinic (M_3) receptors results in activation of PLC, Ca^{2+} release from IP_3-sensitive stores, and hyperpolarization-induced Ca^{2+} influx, which result in activation of eNOS, NO release, and cGMP-dependent relaxation of VSM.[98] Cholinergic stimulation induces a contractile response in some vascular beds because of activation of smooth muscle M_1 or M_2 receptors, or both, which induce activation of PLC in VSM; but this generally only occurs when the endothelium is removed or damaged.[99] Moreover, whereas the presence of endothelial muscarinic receptors is widespread in the vascular system, cholinergic innervation is sparse, and the functional significance of cholinergic mechanisms in control of VSM tone is uncertain.

Nonadrenergic, Noncholinergic Nerves

NANC mechanisms are in many cases related to cotransmitter release from sympathetic or cholinergic neurons, although transmitter release from distinct NANC sensory neural pathways is evident in some preparations. NANC-dependent vasodilating responses have been identified involving vasoactive intestinal polypeptide (VIP), substance P, and calcitonin gene-related product (CGRP).[100] VIP, an octacosapeptide structurally related to secretin and glucagon, acts directly on smooth muscle, producing increases in cAMP and vascular relaxation.[101] Immunohistochemical studies indicate that VIP immunoreactivity is associated with parasympathetic cholinergic nerves and VIP may thus function largely as a cotransmitter with acetylcholine. Substance P has dual effects on VSM including a direct vascular contracting effect mediated by COX products and an endothelium-dependent relaxing effect mediated by both NO- and EDHF-dependent mechanisms.[102] CGRP, which is often colocalized with substance P in sensory neurons, is released during stimulation of the vagus nerve and on stimulation of perivascular nerves of large arteries such as the main pulmonary arteries. CGRP is a potent vasodilator[103] that acts through specific receptors to activate adenylate cyclase in VSM producing cAMP-dependent relaxation. In addition, CGRP activates eNOS in endothelial cells, producing a cGMP-dependent vasodilatory response.[104]

Humoral Mechanisms

Circulating mediators produce profound effects on vascular tone, although the importance of these mechanisms usually comes into play only during extreme physiologic conditions when blood pressure is threatened. Nevertheless, these mediators can be essential to appropriate redistribution of blood flow that allows the organism to adapt to and thereby survive extreme insults such as severe hemorrhage. In general, the renin-angiotensin system product, Ang II, and the posterior pituitary hormone, arginine vasopressin (AVP), are the most important and best studied of the humoral mediators; although a number of other compounds including BK, histamine, and PAF can also have important effects on blood flow. Notably, the effects of these humoral mediators on vascular tone vary considerably depending on the vascular bed. In general, the potent constrictors Ang II and AVP have little effect on essential vascular beds such as the cerebral and coronary beds, whereas constriction produced by these agents can profoundly decrease flow in the mesenteric, cutaneous, and, in the case of Ang II, renal beds.

Angiotensin II

Ang II is an octapeptide produced by the action of angiotensin-converting enzyme on the vasoinactive circulating form, Ang I, which is itself formed by the action of renin on circulating angiotensinogen. Ang II is thus the vasoactive endproduct of the renin-angiotensin system, which produces direct VSM constriction caused by activation of PLC, Ca^{2+} release, activation of PKC, and Ca^{2+} influx, as described earlier for NE (see Fig. 19–2). In addition, Ang II induces release of the potent endothelium-dependent vasoconstrictor, endothelin-1, in some beds. Ang II is

also involved in regulation of plasma volume through aldosterone-regulated sodium excretion, and Ang II can itself stimulate central sympathetic output and thirst responses, as well as smooth muscle cell growth, cell migration, and ECM deposition.[105] Ang II interacts with VSM AT_1 receptors; AT_1 receptor antagonists thus both decrease blood pressure and induce regression of structural and functional abnormalities of the vascular wall in subjects with hypertension.[106]

Arginine Vasopressin

AVP is a circulating neuropeptide hormone released from the posterior pituitary that, in addition to its well-known action as antidiuretic hormone, is a potent vasoconstrictor.[107] The vasoconstrictor action of AVP is mediated by interaction with smooth muscle V_1 receptors that activate PLC, resulting in release of Ca^{2+} from IP_3-sensitive intracellular stores, activation of PKC, and Ca^{2+} influx through VDCs.[108] AVP produces little effect on renal blood flow.

Atrial Natriuretic Peptide

Atrial natriuretic peptide (ANP) is a 28-amino acid peptide synthesized in the atrium and released into the systemic circulation in response to atrial dilation, such as occurs with fluid overload and heart failure. Although ANP has a wide range of biologic effects including natriuresis and inhibition of renin and aldosterone secretion,[109] the role of ANP in the physiologic control of vascular tone is uncertain. ANP acts on specific ANP receptors in VSM to activate the particulate, membrane-associated, guanylate cyclase, thereby producing NO and endothelium-independent, but cGMP-dependent relaxation.

Platelet and White Cell Factors

Activated platelets release vasoconstricting prostanoids, mainly TxA_2 and serotonin (5-HT), which act on specific VSM receptors to produce vasoconstriction. This is physiologically important in stemming ongoing hemorrhage. In addition, the lysophospholipid PAF is coreleased with the vasoconstricting prostanoids from membrane phospholipids and acts on endothelial PAF receptors, stimulating the production of vasodilatory prostaglandins and NO. In this manner, PAF serves to limit the potent vasoconstricting effects of TxA_2 and 5-HT in areas where the endothelium remains intact.[110] Similarly, activation of kallikrein by the clotting cascade results in the conversion of kininogen to BK, another potent endothelium-dependent vasodilator that acts on B_2 kinin receptors to release NO, PGI_2, and EDHF from vascular endothelial cells.[111] BK has also been reported to stimulate afferent vagal C fibers, inducing release of vasodilatory neuropeptides from NANC neurons.[112]

Histamine released by activated circulating mast cells generally causes vasodilation caused by stimulation of H_2

receptors on VSM, which increase intracellular cAMP concentration, as well as H_1 receptors of vascular endothelium, which activate PLC. This then induces release of both NO and PGI_2 producing endothelium-dependent relaxation of adjacent VSM.[113,114] Histamine can also cause vasoconstriction mediated by H_1 receptors on VSM.[113]

Control Mechanisms in Specific Vascular Beds

Although the general principles of vascular contraction and relaxation apply to the entire vascular system, as do the intrinsic and extrinsic mechanisms whereby the vascular system is regulated, each vascular bed is unique. The mechanisms in individual vascular beds are thus adapted to meet the special requirements imposed by the function of the specific organ supplied. Some of the general principles that govern vascular reactivity in these individual beds are described briefly in this section.

Cerebral Circulation

The cerebral bed is unique in that brain blood flow needs to be maintained at a constant level over the physiologic range of perfusion pressures. In addition, cerebral blood flow needs to be coupled to metabolic demands, even in situations in which there is profound stress or when blood pressure is threatened. The ability of cerebral blood flow to be maintained over a wide range of perfusion pressures results from autoregulatory changes in cerebrovascular resistance primarily involving the myogenic mechanism, which is modulated by endothelium-dependent relaxation and the effects of metabolic factors that serve to modulate myogenic responses and couple metabolic activity to blood flow.[157] A number of factors including adenosine, adenosine diphosphate, and H^+ ion have been proposed to provide this metabolic coupling, and all appear to contribute. In addition, recent findings indicate that neuronally-produced NO is a critical factor in mediating the increases in regional brain blood flow during increases in metabolic activity.[116] Hypercapnia and hypoxia are also potent stimuli for vasodilation in the cerebral circulation, and these responses are mediated in part by increased neuronal NO formation, as well as by neuronal release of adenosine and activation of ATP-sensitive K^+ channels in smooth muscle and endothelial cells.[117,118] Although cerebral blood vessels do have dense innervation from sympathetic nerves, parasympathetic fibers, and the trigeminal nerve, sympathetic nerve stimulation has little effect on cerebral blood flow. The endothelial blood–brain barrier limits access of many humoral vasoconstrictor substances, particularly circulating vasoactive peptides such as Ang II and AVP. In some cases, however, humoral stimuli such as Ang II and vasopressin have access to receptors in areas of the brain located outside the blood–brain barrier. Such signals can thereby provide additional feedback to the brain that may further augment sympathetic output and other central nervous system–mediated responses.

Pulmonary Circulation

The adult pulmonary circulation is a low-pressure, low-resistance circuit that accommodates the entire cardiac output at less than 20% of the pressure and resistance of the systemic circulation. Consistent with this, pulmonary arteries have a much thinner smooth muscle layer than systemic arteries. In addition, although the pulmonary circulation is innervated by sympathetic, parasympathetic, and NANC nerves, these influences and humoral mediators usually have relatively minor direct effects. Passive or secondary effects on cardiac output, left atrial pressure, airway and interstitial pressure, gravitational force, and vascular obstruction or recruitment are the most important determinants of total and regional pulmonary resistance and perfusion. Given the primary importance of the lung in gas exchange, it is not surprising that oxygen tension is the dominant influence on pulmonary vascular resistance. It has long been appreciated that oxygen is a pulmonary vasodilator, and that hypoxic pulmonary vasoconstriction (HPV) is a physiologic response whereby circulating blood is diverted away from hypoxic alveoli, thus optimizing the matching of perfusion and ventilation to maximize arterial oxygenation. In contrast, hypoxia in systemic arterial beds usually results in vasodilation, thus indicating the unique nature of HPV. However, despite more than four decades of investigation, the mechanism of HPV remains unclear. Endothelial NO appeared to be an ideal candidate for the HPV modulator molecule, particularly because NO production is dependent on molecular oxygen. However, inhibition of NOS and decreased NO production do not account for the gain in the HPV response. Recent evidence supports the involvement of oxygen-sensitive cation channels that open in response to hypoxia, leading to smooth muscle depolarization, Ca^{2+} entry, and smooth muscle contraction.[119] Pulmonary vascular endothelial cells may also play an important role by synthesizing PGI_2, and endothelial cells are important in metabolism of a number of circulating vasoactive substances including NE and 5-HT.[120] Pulmonary endothelial cells contain angiotensin-converting enzyme, which catalyzes formation of Ang II and degrades BK, and endopeptidases, which degrade enkephalin and other peptides, including tachykinins.[121,122]

Coronary Circulation

The coronary circulation has obvious critical importance to the organism, and the coronary circulation is uniquely adapted to prevent any limitation of coronary perfusion even during periods of extreme physiologic stress.[123] Perfusion pressure and the myogenic mechanism are major determinants of blood flow in the coronary circulation. However, the ventricular myocardium generates sufficient pressure during systole to nearly stop coronary inflow. Thus most coronary flow, particularly that to the subendocardium, occurs during diastole, and flow is driven by the diastolic blood pressure rather than systolic or mean arterial pressure.[123] As in cerebral circulation, blood flow and oxygen delivery are tightly coupled to metabolic activity in the coronary circulation, and there is substantial vasodilatory reserve. Thus any reduction of oxygen delivery, such as occurs with decreases in perfusion pressure, hypoxia, or hemodilution, results in compensatory coronary vasodilation.[123] Hypercapnia increases coronary blood flow, whereas hypocapnia results in mild to moderate decreases in coronary flow.[124] Coronary vessels are innervated by both parasympathetic and sympathetic nerves that mediate endothelium-dependent coronary vasodilation and endothelium-independent α adrenoreceptor–mediated constriction.[125] However, experimental evidence indicates that the overall effect of sympathetic nerve stimulation on coronary vessels in vivo is vasodilation caused by activation of β adrenergic receptors, which increase myocardial metabolic demand and thereby produce metabolic vasodilation.[125] Thus although α receptor coronary vasoconstriction and metabolic vasodilation would appear to be in competition during periods associated with high sympathetic tone, the balance favors maintenance of coronary perfusion, and metabolic autoregulation is not significantly disrupted. Indeed, myocardial hypoxia is a potent stimulus for coronary vasodilation and the coronary constrictor effects of potent coronary constricting agonists such as vasopressin are eliminated by hypoxia in normal hearts.[48] However, the vascular endothelium is critically important to maintaining the balance between the constricting effects of vascular agonists and metabolic autoregulation, and this balance is significantly disrupted by endothelial damage or dysfunction.

Splanchnic Circulation

The splanchnic circulation is most notable for its dense innervation by sympathetic nerves and modulation by neural and humoral influences. Indeed, constriction of the small splanchnic and mesenteric arteries can be important to vascular resistance and maintenance of blood pressure during conditions in which blood pressure is threatened. Unlike cerebral and coronary flow, splanchnic blood flow can be profoundly decreased by α adrenergic- and vasopressin-induced vasoconstriction, resulting in a substantial shift of blood flow to the more vital cerebral and coronary circulations. Nevertheless, there are physiologic limits to the ability of the organism to sustain prolonged decreases in mesenteric flow. Several reports have suggested that inadequate oxygen delivery to splanchnic organs can impair liver and intestinal mucosal barrier function leading to the translocation of bacterial products, the development of the systemic inflammatory response syndrome, multiple organ dysfunction and failure, and a high mortality rate.[126]

Renal Circulation

The renal bed is unique in that it receives 20% of the cardiac output, but most of this is directed at glomerular ultrafiltration rather than the metabolic function or needs of renal tissue. Thus microcirculatory regulation in the renal bed has additional importance in maintaining the interstitial environment for glomerular ultrafiltration, reabsorption of fluid into the peritubular capillaries, and maintenance of the medullary concentration gradient. Myogenic mechanisms play a major role in maintaining flow at a relatively constant level, although renal microvascular resistance is also influenced by a complex interplay of locally produced prostanoids, NO, adenosine, and the so-called tubuloglomerular feedback mechanism that modulates afferent arteriolar resistance to maintain delivery of solutes to the distal tubule. The renal bed is unique in having a postcapillary efferent arteriole that is highly regulated by the renin angiotensin system.

Cutaneous Circulation

The skin and subcutaneous tissues are highly innervated by sympathetic nerves and are substantially influenced by circulating humoral vasoactive substances. Adequate cutaneous circulation is maintained by local metabolic and myogenic autoregulation. The blood supply to skin consists of a blanket of capillaries, which are particularly important in temperature regulation and the formation of sweat. Decreases or increases in external temperature produce local vasoconstriction or vasodilation, respectively, whereas changes in hypothalamic temperature are associated with modulation of cutaneous tone mediated by changes in sympathetic nervous system activity and, during extreme conditions, release of vasopressin. The cutaneous circulation is an important first line of defense in the recognition of and response to foreign materials or mechanically inflicted trauma. Acute cutaneous inflammation is characterized by the release of a variety of vasoactive inflammatory mediators, including histamine and PGE_2, which have an initial transient vasoconstricting action, followed by dilation and enhanced vascular permeability that gives rise to extravasation of plasma protein and tissue edema designed to clear the offending agent.[127]

Contraction and Relaxation Mechanisms

Molecular Mechanisms of Smooth Muscle Contraction

Whether responding to neural, humoral, local, or mechanical stimuli, an increase in intracellular free Ca^{2+} concentration ($[Ca^{2+}]_i$) is the major determinant of VSM tone (Fig. 19–4). During basal conditions, Ca^{2+} influx in VSM is low despite a 10,000-fold concentration gradient across the sarcolemma, and $[Ca^{2+}]_i$ is maintained in the 50 to 100 nM range. Vasoconstricting agonists increase VSM $[Ca^{2+}]_i$ rapidly with a threshold for contraction of approximately 150 mM. Maximal contraction is achieved at $[Ca^{2+}]_i$ in the 1 to 5 μM range. The mechanisms responsible for the increases in $[Ca^{2+}]_i$ include both Ca^{2+} influx through sarcolemmal Ca^{2+} channels and Ca^{2+} release from intracellular stores.[128] Release of Ca^{2+} from intracellular stores in VSM is mediated by a Ca^{2+}-induced Ca^{2+} release (CICR) mechanism, and by an IP$_3$-induced Ca^{2+} release (IICR) mechanism. The CICR channels are synonymous with sarcoplasmic reticulum ryanodine receptors, which are activated by increases in cytosolic $[Ca^{2+}]_i$. Activation of IICR channels generally involves agonist-induced increases in PLC activ-

Activation of contractile proteins

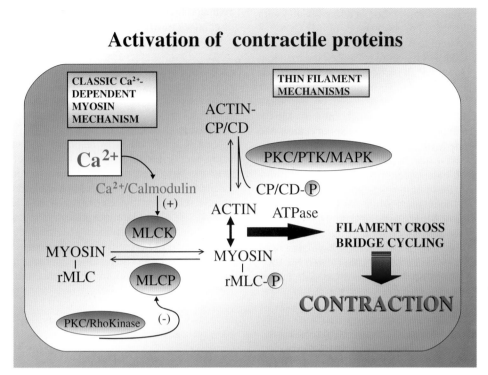

Figure 19–4. Contraction of vascular smooth muscle is dependent on the association of actin and myosin to activate the actomyosin adenosine triphosphatase (ATPase), which induces cross-bridge cycling, filament movement, and contraction. The classic mechanism involves Ca^{2+}-induced activation of myosin light chain kinase (MLCK) and phosphorylation of the regulatory myosin light chain (rMLC). Ca^{2+} sensitization mechanisms involve inhibition of myosin light chain phosphatase (MLCP) by agonist- or myogenic-induced activation of protein kinase C (PKC) or the small G protein Rho kinase. Phosphorylation of the thin filament associated proteins caldesmon (CD) or calponin (CP) by the PKC, protein tyrosine kinase/mitogen-activated protein kinase pathways (PTK/MAPK), results in dissociation from actin and removal of CD- or CP-induced inhibition of actin/myosin interaction.

ity resulting in IP_3 release from membrane phospholipids.[129,130] The observation that both stores are depleted by agonists that are selective for either CICR or IICR channels suggests that the CICR and IICR receptors are most likely present on the same physical stores in VSM.[130] Influx of Ca^{2+} from the extracellular space occurs largely through voltage-dependent sarcolemmal Ca^{2+} channels, although receptor-operated Ca^{2+} channels (ROCs), Ca^{2+} release-activated Ca^{2+} channels, and Na^+/Ca^{2+} exchange may also contribute to agonist-induced $[Ca^{2+}]_i$ increases.[128,130] Voltage-dependent sarcolemmal Ca^{2+} channels are opened by membrane depolarization induced by a variety of stimuli including NE. Other agonists such as ATP, which is notably colocalized with NE in sympathetic nerve terminals, can also induce Ca^{2+} influx by activating ROCs in the absence of membrane depolarization.[130]

Increases in VSM $[Ca^{2+}]_i$ bring about contraction by inducing an ATP-dependent cyclic interaction of myosin thick filaments and actin thin filaments resulting in the formation of actomyosin crossbridges.[131] The biochemical sequence of events leading to the formation of actomyosin crossbridges and initial force development in smooth muscle differs considerably from other muscle types (see Fig. 19–4).[132] Smooth muscle does not contain troponin, the Ca^{2+} sensor protein that binds Ca^{2+} and activates the contractile

apparatus through interaction with tropomyosin in thin filaments of striated muscle. Rather, the actin/myosin interaction in smooth muscle is initiated by phosphorylation of the serine 19 residue of the 20 kD regulatory MLC_{20} subunit.[132] MLC_{20} phosphorylation is mediated by MLCK. The Ca^{2+} dependence of contraction in smooth muscle results from the dependence of MLCK activity on binding to Ca^{2+}-calmodulin complex formed after increases in $[Ca^{2+}]_i$.[133,134] Phosphorylated MLC_{20} results in activation of the actomyosin-associated ATPase, resulting in crossbridge cycling and contraction.[134] When agonist is withdrawn, $[Ca^{2+}]_i$, the concentration of the Ca^{2+}-calmodulin complex, and MLCK activity are reduced, MLC_{20} is dephosphorylated by a specific myosin light chain phosphatase (MLCP), and smooth muscle relaxes.

In addition to the well-understood role $[Ca^{2+}]_i$ increases play in the contractile responses to stimuli, the amplitude of contraction in VSM is not always proportional to $[Ca^{2+}]_i$.[128] This is particularly evident during sustained contractions in response to physiologic agonists, where contraction may be well maintained, whereas $[Ca^{2+}]_i$ has decreased to a value that may be only minimally elevated above baseline.[135] The increases in the relative amount of contraction for a given $[Ca^{2+}]_i$ is referred to as Ca^{2+} sensitization. In permeabilized VSM, treatments with agonist that activate heterometric G proteins produce increased contraction at a fixed [Ca^{2+}] with parallel increases in the phosphorylation of MLC$_{20}$.[136,137] Indeed, it is now apparent that the activities of both MLCK and MLCP can be modified by cellular kinases independent of changes in [Ca^{2+}]$_i$. MLCP, in particular, is a point of convergence for regulation by a number of physiologic agonists that activate PKC and the kinase activated by the small molecular weight G protein, Rho, which inhibits MLCP activity, and thereby maintains MLC$_{20}$ phosphorylation and contraction independent of [Ca^{2+}]$_i$.[131,132,137–139] Mechanisms of Ca^{2+} sensitization have also been described in which contraction is maintained independent of [Ca^{2+}]$_i$ or MLC phosphorylation. Among these is the so-called latch state, in which contraction is maintained while MLC phosphorylation decreases. [Ca^{2+}]$_i$ or MLC phosphorylation-independent mechanisms involving phosphorylation of the thin filament regulatory proteins calponin and caldesmon have also been described. These proteins may be phosphorylated by PKC or the PKC/MAPK pathways leading to dissociation from

actin and increased actomyosin ATPase activity independent of changes in MLC$_{20}$ phosphorylation.[140]

Molecular Mechanisms of Smooth Muscle Relaxation

Vascular relaxation occurs on withdrawal of vasoconstricting agonist[134,188] as well as in response to a number of vasodilating agents that effectively reverse the effects of vasoconstrictors by independent receptor and biochemical mechanisms (Fig. 19–5). These vasodilators produce smooth muscle relaxation by decreasing [Ca^{2+}]$_i$ and Ca^{2+} sensitivity.[128,132,135,140,141] β adrenoceptor agonists, and the vasodilating prostanoids act at their specific receptors to activate heterotrimeric G protein (G$_s$) that result in the activation of adenylate cyclase. The resulting increase in the intracellular levels of cAMP results in VSM relaxation through cAMP-

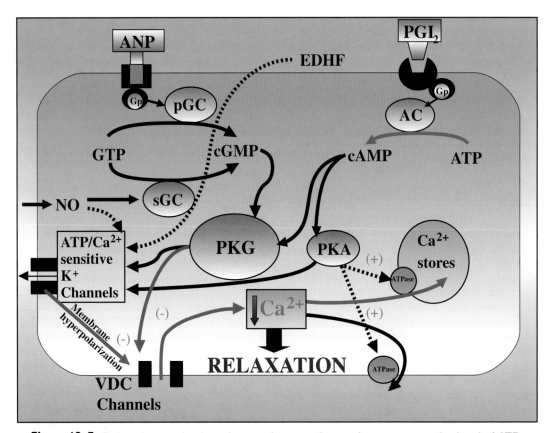

Figure 19–5. Relaxation mechanisms in vascular smooth muscle converge at the level of ATP- and Ca^{2+}-gated K$^+$ channels, although evidence suggests that each effector—nitric oxide (NO), endothelium-dependent hyperpolarizing factor, protein kinase A (PKA), and protein kinase G (PKG)—affect distinct classes of channels with different pharmacologic sensitivities. The result is membrane hyperpolarization, closure of voltage-dependent Ca^{2+} (VDC) channels, decreased Ca^{2+}, and relaxation. NO activates soluble guanylate cyclase (sGC), whereas atrial natriuretic peptide (ANP) activates membrane-associated particulate guanylate cyclase (pGC). Vasodilatory prostanoids such as prostacyclin (PGI$_2$) activate adenylate cyclase (AC) and PKA, which may also accelerate Ca^{2+} clearance, but cyclic adenosine monophosphate (cAMP) may also activate the more abundant PKG in most vascular smooth muscle cells thereby producing cross-talk between these two pathways.

dependent protein kinase (PKA)-induced phosphorylation of specific protein targets including MLCK. MLCK is also phosphorylated by other kinases including PKC, cGMP-dependent protein kinase (PKG), and Ca^{2+}-CAM-dependent protein kinase II (CAMKII), but only the PKA and CAMKII sites on MLCK are in the region of the Ca^{2+}-CAM binding domain, where phosphorylation results in reduced affinity for Ca^{2+}-CAM and decreased Ca^{2+} sensitivity.[142] Caffeine and other inhibitors of phosphodiesterase have vasorelaxant effects that are also mediated by increases in cAMP in smooth muscle. In addition to a Ca^{2+} desensitization mechanism, increases in cAMP also increase the extrusion of Ca^{2+} from the cell or reuptake into the SR, thereby producing relaxation related to a decrease in $[Ca^{2+}]_i$.[128]

ANP and the nitrosodilators including NO or EDRF produce vasodilation by increasing intracellular cGMP. ANP activates the membrane-bound particulate fraction of guanylate cyclase, whereas endogenous NO and NO donor compounds, including the organic nitrates and sodium nitroprusside, activate the soluble fraction. The resulting activation of the cGMP-dependent protein kinase (PKG), results in phosphorylation of specific targets that mediate vasodilation.[143] PKG-induced phosphorylation of Ca^{2+} channels results in decreased Ca^{2+} influx, whereas increased PKG activity also mediates increased MLCP activity, thereby accelerating dephosphorylation of MLC_{20} and decreasing contraction for a given $[Ca^{2+}]_i$ (i.e., Ca^{2+} desensitization).[143] Interestingly, unlike many tissues where cAMP and cGMP have opposing actions, both cyclic nucleotides mediate relaxation in VSM by decreasing $[Ca^{2+}]_i$ and by producing Ca^{2+} desensitization. However, smooth muscle is particularly rich in content of PKG compared with PKA, and considerable recent data suggest that cAMP-induced activation of PKG represents a major mechanism for cAMP-dependent relaxation in VSM, and a major point of cross-talk between these two signaling pathways.[68,69]

Ion Channels Involved in Vascular Smooth Muscle Contraction and Relaxation

VSM is an excitable tissue in which the principal trigger for agonist-induced contraction involves $[Ca^{2+}]_i$ increases, caused in large part by activation of sarcolemmal VDCs. As such, the membrane potential (Vm) is an important determinant of the contractile state. In the relaxed state, VSM membrane potential is maintained at –45 to –75 mV by Ca^{2+}- and ATP-activated, voltage-dependent K^+ channels.[134,144] In addition, a series of sarcolemmal and sarcoplasmic reticulum pumps and transporters contribute significantly to Ca^{2+} clearance after agonist stimulation and maintenance of the physiologic transmembrane ionic gradients.[145]

The main current involved in membrane depolarization and action potential generation in VSM is Ca^{2+} current passing through VDCs.[128] VDCs of the L type (long lasting; or high-voltage activated; 20- to 28-pS channel conductance) are thought to represent the main pathway for Ca^{2+} entry in VSM. L-type VDCs are activated at relatively high membrane potential and are sensitive to dihydropyridine-type Ca^{2+} channel blockers. T-type Ca^{2+} channels (transient;

or low-voltage activated; 7- to 15-pS channel conductance) with rapid inactivation and resistance to dihydropyridine derivatives have also been identified in some types of VSM, although T-type channels are normally inactivated at the depolarized potential (–30 to 10 mV) seen in contracted VSM.[128] Their role is thus presumably limited to the initial depolarizing inward current and $[Ca^{2+}]_i$ increases. L-type channels are also inactivated by membrane depolarization; however, the overlap of the activation and inactivation curves of L-type channels appear capable of generating the "window currents" necessary to maintain Ca^{2+} entry for sustained contraction in VSM.[128] It is clear that sustained agonist-induced contraction of VSM is dependent on Ca^{2+} currents through L-type channels. The precise mechanism, whereby vasoconstrictors enhance currents through L-type Ca^{2+} channels, however, is not well defined. There is some evidence that vasoconstrictors modulate Ca^{2+} currents through GTP-binding proteins. Alternatively, membrane depolarization may occur through activation of nonselective cation channels or inhibition of K^+ channels and may produce voltage-dependent activation of L-type channels in VSM.[128] As mentioned earlier, certain agonists also appear to activate ROCs that may play some role in generating inward Ca^{2+} currents that contribute to both $[Ca^{2+}]_i$ increases and membrane depolarization with these agonists. Voltage-activated sodium ion (Na^+) channels are also present in VSM. Recent studies suggest that the rapidly activating inward Na^+ currents through these channels can account for a significant part of the action potential in certain types of phasically active VSM.[130] Finally, MS ion channels activated by stretch can depolarize the VSM membrane, increasing Ca^+ entry into the cell and contraction.[147–149]

The dense distribution (up to 15,000/cell) and large conductance (200–300 pS) of the maxi-K^+ or BK channels suggests the importance of these channels in VSM.[150] Activity of BK channels is inhibited by tetraethylammonium, charybdotoxin, and iberiotoxin;[151] and studies using these inhibitors suggest BK channels are important determinants of hyperpolarizing responses to β adrenergic agonists, cAMP, CGRP, and 11,12-EEA, a P450 metabolic product of arachidonic acid with purported EDHF activity.[152–155] Recent studies also suggest that reactive oxygen species such as hydrogen peroxide, oxidizing agents, and oxidized glutathione produce vascular relaxation by activation of calcium-activated potassium channels.[156] Both delayed rectifier-type potassium channels and inward rectifier potassium channels are also present in VSM and contribute to maintenance of membrane potential. In addition, the hyperpolarizing actions of nitrosodilators and EDHF result from activation of ATP-sensitive K^+ channels characterized by their activation by the synthetic compounds cromakalim and aprikalim, and inhibition by the sulfonylurea drugs such as glibenclamide. Recent data also suggest that ATP-sensitive K^+ channels play a role in the hyperpolarizing and relaxing effects of a number of other endogenous vasodilator substances including EDHF, VIP, CGRP, and adenosine.[157,158] As their name implies, ATP induces physiologic inhibition of these channels, which are then activated when cellular high-energy phosphate stores are depleted, such as occurs during tissue hypoxemia; the resulting hyperpolarization and vascular relaxation promotes increased blood flow and oxygen supply.

The Vascular System as a Rich Target for Drug Action

The variety of molecular target(s) involved in vascular function is evident from the large number of pharmacologic agents that affect vascular function. The potential importance of these targets is suggested by the involvement of the vascular system in a number of highly prevalent disease states. This section reviews some of the general principles that have emerged from studies over the last several years regarding the physiology and pharmacology of the vascular system, followed by a brief description of some common pharmacologic agents and disease states that affect the vascular system.

In general, the molecular physiology and pharmacology of the vascular system follows a pattern similar to that of other excitable tissues with a limited number of agonists exhibiting diverse functions that depend on the specific receptor subtypes, and agonist redundancy such that a number of different agonists converge at the level of the G proteins, or effector molecules, or both, to produce similar cellular responses. The agonists epinephrine and NE, for example, have both vasoconstricting and vasodilating actions depending on whether α_1 or β_2 adrenergic receptors are present in the target tissue. These receptors are in turn coupled to specific G proteins that activate either PLC or adenylate cyclase, respectively, in VSM cells. Conversely, activation of α_1 adrenoreceptors, V_1 vasopressin, AT_1 angiotensin, or ET_A endothelin receptors in the presence of their respective agonists converge at the level of the same G proteins to activate PLC, thereby producing vasoconstriction by similar downstream mechanisms.

The feature of pluripotent agonists has several important implications. First, desired actions of a given agonist can generally be isolated from undesired actions using synthetic agonists or antagonists. Phenylephrine is often used for its "pure" α_1 agonist action—e.g., to avoid β adrenergic–mediated effects in patients with coronary artery disease. However, phenylephrine suffers from poor receptor efficacy, which limits it potency; and a similar result might also be achieved—without the issue of limited potency—by using the native α_1 agonist, NE, combined with a β receptor antagonist. Conversely, synthetic agonists for a given receptor subtype also often have limited agonist efficacy at the other receptor subtypes activated by the native agonist. For example, the synthetic α_2 adrenergic agonist dexmedetomidine also binds α_1 receptors, albeit with poor receptor efficacy. Thus dexmedetomidine has little undesired vasoconstricting activity, but it can compete with endogenous or exogenously administered α_1 agonists. Dexmedetomidine can thereby act as an α_1 antagonist and produce resistance to administration of α_1 agonists or hypotension in situations in which cardiovascular homeostasis is reliant on high sympathetic tone.[159]

The redundancy in the vascular system has several important implications. First, it is evident that no particular system is essential and that the effects of exogenously administered agonists or antagonists will be countered by compensatory increases in the activity of competing systems. An attempt to block endothelium-dependent relaxation with NOS inhibitors results in increases in the "redundant" production of vasodilatory prostanoids and EDHF, which converge on the same vasodilatory effector molecules in the adjacent VSM cells. Indeed, when any one of these systems is blocked by NOS, COX, or P450 inhibitors, the other system(s) assume greater importance, such that block of endothelium-dependent vasodilation may only be observed in the presence of inhibitors of all three systems. Moreover, this redundancy can obscure which system(s) are most important in the normal physiologic situation. Similarly, when trying to block vasoconstrictor mechanisms in treating severe hypertension, compensatory increases in other systems may make it necessary to block activity of adrenergic-, vasopressin-, and angiotensin-dependent vasoconstrictor mechanisms. This is particularly true if the vasoconstriction is driven by baroreflexes, such as occurs when trying to induce hypotension with nitroprusside. Increases in circulating catecholamines, vasopressin, and Ang II during these conditions produce tachyphylaxis, increasing the nitroprusside dose requirements and the potential for nitroprusside toxicity. Conversely, therapies directed distal to the point where the constrictor mechanisms converge, at the level of sarcolemmal Ca^{2+} channels, for example, can produce a desired effect with a single agent. Finally, the redundancy in the system may also allow the use of multiple points of attack, both before and after the point of convergence. For example, both NO and PGI_2 may be useful for the treatment of pulmonary hypertension by different upstream mechanisms involving cGMP and cAMP, respectively. Synergistic action may thus be predicted at the point of convergence, activation of PKG.[68,69] Indeed, attacking another point before the convergence, at the level of the phosphodiesterase that metabolizes cAMP and cGMP, may even provide additional efficacy.[160]

Another recurring theme in the vascular system is the modulating or competing roles of VSM and the vascular endothelium. There are numerous examples where receptors for agonists have been identified on both VSM and vascular endothelial cells where identical transduction and effector systems in the two cells produce competing contracting and relaxing effects. Thus while the observed effect of a given agonist may depend on which of the two competing effects is dominant in the particular vascular bed or circumstance, the balance between VSM and endothelial function is important to produce the desired physiologic effect. The effects of the α_1 adrenergic agonists, for example, are significantly modulated by an endothelium-dependent vasodilating action such that α_1 agonist–induced vasoconstriction is markedly potentiated on removal of the endothelium. Conversely, agonists such as acetylcholine, BK, 5-HT, and histamine, which activate endothelial cell receptors and generally produce endothelium-dependent vasodilation, produce vasoconstriction when the endothelium is damaged or removed because of unopposed activation of VSM receptors. Even the potent vasoconstricting effect of the endothelium-derived constrictor endothelin has autocoid effects on the endothelium resulting in increased NO production; and endothelial (or exogenous) NO limits endothelin release. The basis for the different responses to agonist in VSM and endothelial cells results from the fact that increases in $[Ca^{2+}]_i$ produce opposing effects in VSM and endothelial cells. $[Ca^{2+}]_i$ increases in VSM activate the Ca^{2+}/CAM-dependent MLCK, thereby producing contraction, whereas endothelial cell $[Ca^{2+}]_i$ increases result in activation of Ca^{2+}/CAM-dependent NOS and NO-dependent relaxation of adjacent VSM. Myoendothelial gap junctions observed in some vascular systems may also participate in coordination between effects in VSM and adjacent endothelial cells. Such connections could allow for Ca^{2+} exchange between adjacent cells such that vasoconstricting agonists produce competing endothelium-dependent relaxation even in the absence of endothelial cell receptors. In contrast, however, changes in membrane potential have opposing effects on mobilization of extracellular Ca^{2+} in VSM and endothelial cells. Ca^{2+} influx occurs through VDCs in VSM, whereas in endothelial cells Ca^{2+} influx occurs through voltage-independent nonselective cation channels. Thus hyperpolarization of the endothelial membrane results in increased Ca^{2+} influx because Vm is further from the positive Ca^{2+} equilibration potential.

Pharmacologic Agents with Prominent Vascular Actions

Several major classes of existing pharmacologic agents have major actions on the vascular system. Most of these are discussed in this chapter. Particularly important are the organic nitrates, sodium nitroprusside, calcium channel blockers, PGE1, and PGI$_2$ (see Chapters 36 and 39), and the adrenergic agonists and antagonist (see Chapters 34 and 37). Because the focus of the text is anesthetic pharmacology, the vascular actions of anesthetic agents are briefly discussed here in greater detail.

Inhalational Anesthetics

Inhalational anesthetics have multiple, often competing, actions on VSM and vascular endothelial cells. These agents produce a transient increase in VSM $[Ca^{2+}]_i$ and a transient contraction related to release of Ca^{2+} from ryanodine-sensitive intracellular stores.[161,162] In permeabilized arteries, inhalational anesthetics also decrease Ca^{2+} uptake by the SR, and enhance caffeine-induced Ca^{2+} release from the SR.[163,164] In addition, even in ryanodine-treated arteries, some anesthetics appear to have a slowly developing sustained contraction, which may be related in part to a Ca^{2+}-sensitizing action.[161] Inhalational anesthetics also may inhibit both NO- and EDHF-mediated, endothelium-dependent vasorelaxation, which may enhance contractile responses to agonists in an endothelium-dependent manner.[165,166]

Nevertheless, although inhalational anesthetics may produce vasoconstriction during certain circumstances, they are best known as potent smooth muscle relaxants and vasodilators due to a direct smooth muscle relaxing action.[161,162,167] In some studies, this appears to be caused by an effect on agonist-induced increases in VSM $[Ca^{2+}]_i$,[167] due to a blocking effect on Ca^{2+} channels.[168] However, more recent data indicate that inhalational anesthetics decrease not only $[Ca^{2+}]_i$ but Ca^{2+} sensitivity as well.[169,170]

Intravenous Anesthetics

Propofol is a widely used intravenous anesthetic agent with rapid onset, short duration of action, and rapid elimination. Induction and maintenance of anesthesia with propofol is, however, usually accompanied by mild to moderate hypotension, caused in large part by a vasodilating action. In isolated vessels, propofol inhibits agonist-induced contractions that involve both a Ca^{2+} channel blocking and a Ca^{2+} desensitizing action.[171,172] Like volatile anesthetics, propofol has also been reported to attenuate endothelium-dependent relaxation.[173] However, other investigators have reported that propofol-induced vasodilation is partly inhibited by indomethacin and inhibitors of NOS, suggesting the vasorelaxing effect of propofol may be in part endothelium-dependent.[174]

Midazolam, a benzodiazepine agonist, is widely used to produce amnesia and hypnosis, and for the induction of general anesthesia. Midazolam produces hypotension, particularly in combination with narcotics or during cardiopulmonary bypass, which is caused by a vasodilating action. This action appears to be related to a direct VSM relaxing action mediated by inhibition of Ca^{2+} influx through the L-type Ca^{2+} channels in VSM,[175] and by an endothelium-dependent mechanism.[176]

Ketamine is widely used in patients with cardiovascular instability because of its cardiovascular stimulation, which results in both vasoconstriction and cardiac inotropy. The stimulatory effects of ketamine are, however, indirect and are ascribed to its sympathomimetic action, which is related in large part to inhibition by ketamine of neuronal uptake of catecholamines by sympathetic nerve endings.[177] The direct effect of ketamine on VSM is a relaxing action, which can contribute to hypotension in patients who are critically ill or chronically depleted of catecholamines. The mechanisms underlying the vasodilating effects of ketamine involve inhibition of both Ca^{2+} influx through the VDCs and agonist-induced Ca^{2+} release from intracellular stores.[178] The latter action of ketamine appears to be related to inhibition of PLC leading to decreased production of the intracellular second messenger IP$_3$.[179] Ketamine has recently been reported to inhibit agonist-induced, endothelium-dependent relaxation in isolated pulmonary arteries.[180]

Disease States with Important Vascular System Involvement

Atherosclerosis

Endothelial injury and activation is an early initiating event in the development of atherosclerotic lesions. Products of smoking, homocystinemia, glycosylation endproducts, bacterial toxins, and shear stress contribute to the oxidation of lipoproteins—particularly lysophosphatidylcholine derived from oxidation of phosphatidylcholine (lecithin) in LDL, which has been implicated in the initial endothelial injury. The early injury is characterized by impaired endothelium-dependent signal transduction and relaxation and by expression of leukocyte adhesion molecules such as ICAM-1 on the surface of endothelial cells.[181] The mobilization of activated leukocytes into the early lesion results in further oxidation of membrane phospholipids and further impairment of endothelial relaxation and endothelial cell damage. Small areas of desquamated endothelium, with exposure of matrix proteins, contributes to the generation of thrombi and activated platelets and white cells, which contribute factors that lead to a vicious cycle of ongoing inflammation. Growth of the atherosclerotic plaque, and thickening of the intima and media lead to progressive vessel narrowing, with further impairment of vasodilatory reserve that will eventually lead to critical stenosis and ischemia in the distal tissue. As discussed earlier, hypoxia-induced angiogenesis may compensate to some degree with neovascularization, but plaque rupture, as occurs most notably in unstable coronary syndromes, is a catastrophic event that does not require the presence of critical stenosis.[182] A large matrix surface is exposed with plaque rupture, which is a potent stimulus for thrombosis and activation of platelets. Thrombin, platelet-derived TxA_2, and 5-HT produce local VSM contraction and formation of an intravascular thrombus that leads to profound tissue hypoxia and cell death.

Hypertension

Impairment of endothelial-dependent relaxation is a relatively constant feature observed in blood vessels from experimental animals and humans with hypertension.[183] Although the direct involvement of this impairment in the pathogenesis of hypertension is unclear, it clearly contributes to exaggerated vasoconstrictor responses and labile hypertension, which is also mirrored in abnormal responses to circulating platelets and inflammatory cells. As in the development of atheromatous lesions, these latter effects facilitate vascular remodeling that may contribute to sustained increases in vascular resistance and may also promote the development of atherosclerosis.[183] A number of potential mechanisms to account for the endothelial dysfunction have been identified. Local application of superoxide dismutase or deferoxamine restores vasodilator responses to acetylcholine toward normal, suggesting that increased production of reactive oxygen species may be involved in NO inactivation.[184] In addition there may be increased endothelium-dependent release of contracting factors including endothelin and vasoconstricting prostanoid products of COX-1,[185] which is abnormally expressed in VSM in spontaneously hypertensive rats.[186] Relaxation of arteries in response to activators of ATP-sensitive potassium channels is also impaired in hypertension, and there may be compensatory increases in the activity of calcium-dependent potassium channels.[187]

Diabetes

Diabetes, like both hypertension and atherosclerosis is also associated with endothelial dysfunction.[188] As with these other cardiovascular diseases, the mechanisms underlining the endothelial injury and its role in the pathogenesis of diabetic vascular complications are not completely understood.[7,188,189] As in subjects with hypertension, endothelium-

dependent relaxation may be impaired by excess generation of reactive oxygen species that destroy NO and catalyze the production of vasoconstrictor prostanoids.[188,189] Impairment of endothelium-dependent relaxation in diabetic subjects may also be caused by increased production of endothelium-dependent contracting factors.[190] Conversely, COX-1 levels are decreased, not increased, in aortas from diabetic animals, and diabetes mellitus does not result in the generalized impairment of vasodilator mechanisms observed in hypertension.[191]

Ischemia/Reperfusion

Tissue injury during periods of ischemia or hypoxia is of obvious considerable importance in medicine. Ischemia/hypoxia and reperfusion/reoxygenation have major effects on vascular tissue that may contribute to parenchymal tissue injury. First, severe hypoxia limits the ability of the vascular endothelium to produce both NO and PGI_2, which are both dependent on molecular oxygen, and indeed release of endothelium-dependent contracting factors may be increased after a period of ischemia.[192] Thus vasodilatory reserve both during and after a period of ischemia or hypoxia may be limited. Vascular endothelium also produces hydroxyl radical through the NOS pathway in response to ischemia/reperfusion that may in part neutralize endothelium-produced NO, and may also result in formation of peroxynitrite, which may produce tissue injury.[193] The endothelium may thus contribute to the increased production of damaging reactive oxygen species during ischemia and reperfusion.[194] Ischemia/reperfusion injury is also associated with expression of endothelial cell adhesion molecules, such as ICAM-1, which directs the accumulation of free radical–producing neutrophils into ischemic tissue.[195]

Septic Shock

Recent evidence places the vascular system, and vascular endothelium in particular, at the center of pathogenesis of septic shock and sepsis-induced tissue injury. Vascular reactivity is severely impaired in septic shock, vascular resistance is reduced, and blood pressure may be low and difficult to increase even with potent vasoconstrictors.[23,196] Some vascular beds are inappropriately dilated, whereas others are constricted, and blood flow is often severely maldistributed.[196] As discussed earlier, the endothelium plays a critical role with the expression of selectins and adhesion molecules which direct the activation and tissue accumulation of neutrophils and platelets and the development of coagulation disorders in septic shock.[12,16,24] Neutrophils in turn release cytokines and reactive oxygen species that further activate the endothelium and damage parenchymal cells.[16,27,196] Inflammatory mediators induce expression of NOS, which produces the large amount of NO that is the basis for the life-threatening hypotension.[197,198] In addition, iNOS-produced NO combines with the white cell-derived superoxide ion to form the extremely reactive peroxynitrite, which is capable of producing tissue damage.

Summary

The various cellular and noncellular elements of the vascular system are critically involved in virtually every function of the organism; the organism's ability to adapt to changing physiologic circumstances is absolutely dependent on appropriate modulation of vascular function. The vascular system is also involved in nearly all pathologic processes, whether cardiovascular, inflammatory, or oncologic. The importance of the vascular endothelium and particularly vascular endothelial relaxing mechanism in coupling of flow to metabolism, in directing cellular traffic throughout the system, and in the pathogenesis of disease has received particular attention in recent years. The vascular system contains a diverse and intricate set of membrane receptors and signaling pathways, messenger molecules, and effector proteins, including a complex array of contractile proteins and ion channels, which serve the unique function of this tissue and constitute the current and future targets of pharmacologic agents.

References

1. Guyton AC, Hall JE (eds): Overview of the circulation: Medical physics of pressure, flow, and resistance. In Textbook of Medical Physiology. Philadelphia, WB Saunders, 2000, pp 144–151.
2. Furchgott RF, Zawadzki JV: The obligatory role of endothelial cells in the relaxation of arterial smooth muscle by acetylcholine. Nature 288:373–376, 1980.
3. Alexander RW, Dzau VJ: Vascular biology: The past 50 years. Circulation 102(20 Suppl 4):IV112–116, 2000.
4. Panza JA, Quyyumi AA, Brush JE Jr, Epstein SE: Abnormal endothelium-dependent vascular relaxation in patients with essential hypertension. N Engl J Med 323:22–27, 1990.
5. Chen YF, Oparil S: Endothelial dysfunction in the pulmonary vascular bed. Am J Med Sci 320:223–232, 2000.
6. Ross R: Atherosclerosis—an inflammatory disease. N Eng J Med 340:115–126, 1999.
7. Johnstone MT, Creager SJ, Scales KM, et al: Impaired endothelium-dependent vasodilation in patients with insulin-dependent diabetes mellitus. Circulation 88:2510–2516, 1993.
8. Cannan CR, Mathew V, Lerman A: New insight into coronary endothelial dysfunction: Role of endothelin. J Lab Clin Med 131:300–305, 1998.
9. Vallet B, Wiel E: Endothelial cell dysfunction and coagulation. Crit Care Med 29(7 Suppl):S36–41, 2001.
10. Fitzgerald DJ: Vascular biology of thrombosis: The role of platelet-vessel wall adhesion. Neurology 57(5 Suppl 2):S1–4, 2001.
11. Harlan JM, Winn RK: Leukocyte-endothelial interactions: Clinical trials of anti-adhesion therapy. Crit Care Med 30(5 Suppl):S214–219, 2002.
12. Levi M, ten Cate H, van der Poll T: Endothelium: Interface between coagulation and inflammation. Crit Care Med 30(5 Suppl):S220–224, 2002.
13. Griffioen AW, Barendsz-Janson AF, Mayo KH, Hillen HF: Angiogenesis, a target for tumor therapy. J Lab Clin Med 132:363–368, 1998.
14. Folkman J, Browder T, Palmblad J: Angiogenesis research: Guidelines for translation to clinical application. Thrombosis Haemost 86:23–33, 2001.
15. Van Hinsbergh VWM: The endothelium: Vascular control of haemostasis. Eur J Obstet Gynecol Reprod Biol 95:198–201, 2001.
16. Hack CE, Zeerleder S: The endothelium in sepsis: Source of and a target for inflammation. Crit Care Med 29(7 Suppl):S21–27, 2001.
17. Marcum JA, McKenney JB, Rosenberg RD: Acceleration of thrombin-antithrombin complex formation in rat hindquarters via heparin like molecules bound to the endothelium. J Clin Invest 74:341–350, 1984.
18. Aird WC: Vascular bed-specific hemostasis: Role of endothelium in sepsis pathogenesis. Crit Care Med 29(7 Suppl):S28–34; discussion S34–35, 2001.
19. Siegel G, Schnalke F, Stock G, Grote J: Prostacyclin, endothelium-derived relaxing factor and vasodilatation. Adv Prostaglandin Thromboxane Leukot Res 19:267–270, 1989.
20. Jaffe EA, Hoyer LW, Nachman RL: Synthesis of von Willebrand factor by cultured human endothelial cells. Proc Natl Acad Sci USA 71:1906–1909, 1974.
21. Loskutoff DJ, Edgington TE: Synthesis of a fibrinolytic activator and inhibitor by endothelial cells. Proc Natl Acad Sci USA 74:3903–3907, 1977.
22. van Mourik JA, Lawrence DA, Loskutoff DJ: Purification of an inhibitor of plasminogen activator (anti-activator) synthesized by endothelial cells. J Biol Chem 259:14914–14921, 1984.
23. Zimmerman GA, Albertine KH, Carveth HJ, et al: Endothelial activation in ARDS. Chest 116(1 Suppl):18S–24S, 1999.
24. Van Hoozen BE, Albertson TE: Endothelial cell dysfunction: A potential new approach for the treatment of sepsis. Crit Care Med 27:2836–2838, 1999.
25. Ruoslahti E, Engvall E: Integrins and vascular extracellular matrix assembly. J Clin Invest 99:1149–1152, 1997.
26. Frenette PS, Wagner DD: Adhesion molecules—Part II: Blood vessels and blood cells. N Engl J Med 335:43–45, 1996.
27. Hinshaw LB: Sepsis/septic shock: participation of the microcirculation: an abbreviated review. Crit Care Med 24:1072–1078, 1996.
28. Joyce DE, Gelbert L, Ciaccia A, DeHoff B, and Grinnell BW: Gene expression profile of anti-thrombotic protein C defines new mechanisms modulating inflammation and apoptosis. J Biol Chem 276:11199–11203, 2001.
29. Carmeliet P, Jain, RK: Angiogenesis in cancer and other diseases. Nature 407:249–257, 2000.
30. Folkman J: Angiogenesis and angiogenesis inhibition: an overview. Exs 79:1–8, 1997.
31. Bischoff J: Cell adhesion and angiogenesis. J Clin Invest 99:373–376, 1997.
32. Schnitzer JE: Vascular targeting as a strategy for cancer therapy. N Engl J Med 339:472–474, 1998.
33. Kuriyama H, Kitamura K, Itoh T, Inoue R: Physiological features of visceral smooth muscle cells, with special reference to receptors and ion channels. Physiol Rev 78:811–920, 1998.
34. Fatigati V, Murphy RA: Actin and tropomyosin variants in smooth muscles. Dependence on tissue type. J Biol Chem 259:14383–14388, 1984.
35. Carpenter CL: Actin cytoskeleton and cell signaling. Crit Care Med 28(4 S):N94–99, 2000.
36. Christ GJ, Spray DC, el-Sabban M, Moore LK, Brink PR: Gap junctions in vascular tissues. Evaluating the role of intercellular communication in the modulation of vasomotor tone. Circ Res 79:631–646, 1996.
37. Larson DM, Haudenaschild CC, Beyer EC: Gap junction messenger RNA expression by vascular wall cells. Circ Res 66:1074–1080, 1990.
38. Reed KE, Westphale EM, Larson DM, Wang HZ, Veenstra RD, Beyer EC: Molecular cloning and functional expression of human connexin37, an endothelial cell gap protein. J Clin Invest 91:997–1004, 1993.
39. Hong T, Hill CE: Restricted expression of the gap junctional protein connexin43 in the arterial system of the rat. J Anat 192:583–593, 1998.
40. Emerson GG, Segal SS: Electrical coupling between endothelial cells and smooth muscle cells in hamster feed arteries: role in vasomotor control. Circ Res 87:474–479, 2000.
41. Sandow SL, Tare M, Coleman HA, Hill CE, Parkington HC: Involvement of myoendothelial gap junctions in the actions of endothelium-derived hyperpolarizing factor. Circ Res 90:1108–1113, 2002.

42. Hynes RO: Integrins: versatility, modulation, and signaling in cell adhesion. Cell 69:11–25, 1992.

43. Ruoslahti E: RGD and other recognition sequences for integrins. Ann Rev Cell Dev Biol 12:697–715, 1996.

44. Dietz HD, Pyeritz RE: Mutations in the human gene for fibrillin-1 (FBN1) in the Marfan syndrome and related disorders. Hum Mol Genet 4:799–809, 1995.

45. Li DY, Faury G, Taylor D, Davis EC, Boyle WA, Mecham RP, Stenze P, Boak B, Keating MT: Novel arterial pathology in mice and humans hemizygous for elastin. J Clin Invest 102:1783–1787, 1998.

46. Teerlink JR: The role of endothelium in the pathogenesis of heart failure. Current Cardiology Reports 4(3):206–212, 2002.

47. Boyle WA, Segel L: Direct effects of vasopressin on the heart and reversal with a vascular antagonist. Am J Physiol 251:H734–H741, 1986.

48. Boyle WA, Segel L: Attenuation of vasopressin-mediated coronary constriction and myocardial depression in the hypoxic heart. Circ Res 66:710–721, 1990.

49. Davis MJ, Wu X, Nurkiewicz TR, Kawasaki J, Davis GE, Hill MA, Meininger GA: Integrins and mechanotransduction of the vascular myogenic response. Am J Physiol 280:H1427–H1433, 2001.

50. Davis MJ, Hill MA: Signaling mechanisms underlying the vascular myogenic response. Physiol Rev 79:387–423, 1999.

51. Knot HJ, Nelson MT: Regulation of membrane potential and diameter by voltage-dependent K^+ channels in rabbit myogenic cerebral arteries. Am J Physiol 269:H348–H355, 1995.

52. Hall A: Rho GTPases and the actin cytoskeleton. Science 279:509–514, 1998.

53. Davies PF, Tripathi SC: Mechanical stress mechanisms and the cell. An endothelial paradigm. Circ Res 72:239–245, 1993.

54. Bevan JA: Shear stress, the endothelium and the balance between flow-induced contraction and dilation in animals and man. Int J Microcir 17:248–256, 1997.

55. Barakat AI, Davies PF: Mechanisms of shear stress transmission and transduction in endothelial cells. CHEST 114:58S–63S, 1998.

56. Ali MH, Schumacker PT: Endothelial responses to mechanical stress: Where is the mechanosensor? Crit Care Med 30(5):S198–S206, 2002.

57. Muller JM, Chilliam WM, Davies MJ. Integrin signaling transduces shear stress-dependent vasodilation of coronary arterioles. Circ Res 80:320–326, 1998.

58. Nerem RM, Alexander W, Chappell DC, Medford RM, Varner SE, Taylor R: The study of the influence of flow on vascular endothelial biology. AM J Med Sci 316(3):169–175, 1998.

59. Benoit V: Endothelial cell dysfunction and abnormal tissue perfusion. Crit Care Med 30(5):S229–S234, 2002.

60. Pohl U, Busse R: Hypoxia stimulates release of endothelium-derived relaxant factor. Am J Physiol 256:H1595–H1600, 1989.

61. Daut J, Maier-Rudolph W, Von Beckerath N, et al.: Hypoxic dilation of coronary arteries is mediated by ATP-sensitive potassium channels. Science 247:1341–1344, 1990.

62. Emerson GG, Segal SS: Electrical activation of endothelium evokes vasodilation and hyperpolarization along hamster feed arteries. Am J Physiol 280:H160–H167, 2001.

63. Forstermann U, Schmidt HHHW, Pollock JS, Sheng H, Mitchell JA, Warner TD, Nakane M, Murad F: Isoforms of nitric oxide synthase. Characterization and purification from different cell types. Biochem Pharmacol 42:1849–1857, 1991.

64. Xie Q, Cho HI, Calaycay J, Mumford RA, Swiderek KM, Lee TD, Ding A, Troso T, Nathan C: Cloning and characterization of inducible nitric oxide synthase from mouse macrophages. Science 256:225–228, 1992.

65. Moncada S, Palmer RMJ, Higgs EA: Nitric oxide: Physiology, pathophysiology, and pharmacology. Pharmacol Rev 43:109–142, 1991.

66. Bolotina VA, Najibi S, Palacino JJ, Pagano PJ, Cohen RA: Nitric oxide directly activates calcium-dependent potassium channels in vascular smooth muscle cells. Nature 368:850–853, 1994.

67. Seegers HC, Gross RW, Boyle WA: Calcium-independent phospholipase A2-derived arachidonic acid is essential for endothelium-dependent relaxation by acetylcholine. J Pharmacol Exp Ther 302:918–923, 2002.

68. Kawada T, Toyosato A, Islam O, Yoshida Y, Imai S: cGMP-kinase mediates cGMP- and cAMP-induces Ca^{2+} desensitization of skinned rat artery. Eur J Pharmacol 323:75–82, 1997.

69. White RE, Kryman JP, El-Mowafy AM, Han G, Carrier GO: cAMP-dependent vasodilators cross-activate the cGMP-dependent protein kinase to stimulate BK_{Ca} channel activity in coronary artery smooth muscle cells. Circ Res 86:897–905, 2000.

70. Smith WL, Garavito RM, DeWitt DL: Prostaglandin endoperoxide H synthases (cyclooxygenases)-1 and -2. J Biol Chem 271:33157–33160, 1996.

71. Wu KK: Inducible cyclooxygenase and nitric oxide synthase. Adv Pharmacol 33:179–207, 1995.

72. Selig WM, Noonan TC, Kern DF, Malik AB: Pulmonary microvascular responses to arachidonic acid in isolated perfused guinea pig lung. J Appl Physiol 60:1972–1979, 1986.

73. Hecker M, Bara AT, Bauersachs J, Busse R: Characterization of endothelium-derived hyperpolarizing factor as a cytochrome P450-derived arachidonic acid metabolite in mammals. J Physiol 481:407–414, 1994.

74. Fisslthaler B, Popp R, Kiss L, Potente M, Harder DR, Fleming I, Busse R: Cytochrome P450 2C is an EDHF synthase in coronary arteries. Nature 401:493–497, 1999.

75. McLeod JD, Piper PJ: Effect of removing the endothelium on the vascular responses induced by leukotrienes C4 and D4 in guinea–pig isolated heart. Eur J Pharmacol 212:67–72, 1992.

76. Zygmunt PM, Hogestatt ED: Role of potassium channels in endothelium-dependent relaxation resistant to nitroarginine in the rat hepatic artery. Br J Pharmacol 117:1600–1606, 1996.

77. Edwards G, Weston AH: EDHF — are there gaps in the pathway? J Physiol 531:299, 2001.

78. Rosolowsky M, Campbell WB: Role of PGI2 and epoxyeicosatrienoic acids in relaxation of bovine coronary arteries to arachidonic acid. Am J Physiol 264:H327–H335, 1993.

79. Yanagisawa M, Kurihara H, Kimura S, Tomobe Y, Kobayashi M, Mitsui Y, Yazaki Y, Goto K, Masaki T: A novel potent vasoconstrictor peptide produced by vascular endothelial cells. Nature 332:411–415, 1988.

80. Haynes WG, Webb DJ: The endothelin family of peptides: local hormones with diverse roles in health and disease? Clin Sci (Colch) 84:485–500, 1993.

81. Inoue A, Yanagisawa M, Kimura S, Kasuya Y, Miyauchi T, Goto K, Masaki T: The human endothelin family: three structurally and pharmacologically distinct isopeptides predicted by three separate genes. Proc Natl Acad Sci U S A 86:2863–2867, 1989.

82. Boulanger C, Luscher TF: Release of endothelin from the porcine aorta. Inhibition by endothelium-derived nitric oxide. J Clin Invest 85:587–590, 1990.

83. Best PJM, Lerman A: Endothelin in cardiovascular disease: From atherosclerosis to heart failure. J Cardiovasc Pharmacol 35(S2):S61–S63, 2000.

84. Zimmermann M, Seifert V: Endothelin and subarachnoid hemorrhage: An overview. Neurosurgery 43(4):863–875, 1998.

85. Hopfner RL, Gopalakrishnan V: Endothelin: emerging role in diabetic vascular complications. Diabetologia 42(12):1383–1394, 1999.

86. Zamora MR, O'Brien RF, Rutherford RB, Weil JV: Serum endothelin-1 concentrations and cold provocation in primary Raynaud's phenomenon. Lancet 336:1144–1147, 1990.

87. Stewart JT, Nisbet JA, Davies MJ: Plasma endothelin in coronary venous blood from patients with either stable or unstable angina. Br Heart J 66:7–9, 1991.

88. Guimaraes S, Moura D: Vascular adrenoceptors: an update. Pharmacol Rev 53:319–356, 2001.

89. Starke K, Gothert M, Kilbinger H: Modulation of neurotransmitter release by presynaptic autoreceptors. Physiol Rev 69:864–989, 1989.

90. Franco-Cereceda A, Lundberg JM, Dahlof C: Neuropeptide Y and sympathetic control of heart contractility and coronary vascular tone. Acta Physiol Scand 124:361–369, 1985.

91. Liu SF, McCormack DG, Evans TW, Barnes PJ: Characterization and distribution of P2-purinoceptor subtypes in rat pulmonary vessels. J Pharmacol Exp Ther 251:1204–1210, 1989.

92. von Kugelgen I, Starke K: Noradrenaline-ATP co-transmission in the sympathetic nervous system. Trends Pharmacol Sci 12:319–324, 1991.

93. Liu SF, Crawley DE, Evans TW, Barnes PJ: Endothelium-dependent nonadrenergic, noncholinergic neural relaxation in guinea pig pulmonary artery. J Pharmacol Exp Ther 260:541–548, 1992.

94. Anderson FL, Brown AM: Pulmonary vasoconstriction elicited by stimulation of the hypothalamic integrative area for the defense reaction. Circ Res 21:747–756, 1967.

95. Harris MC: Effects of chemoreceptor and baroreceptor stimulation

on the discharge of hypothalamic supraoptic neurones in rats. J Endocrinol 82:115–125, 1979.

96. Kendrick JE, Matson GL, Lalley PM: Central interaction between the baroreceptor reflexes from the carotid sinus and aortic arch. Am J Physiol 236:H127–H133, 1979.

97. Hilz MJ, Stemper B, Neundorfer B: [Physiology and methods for studying the baroreceptor reflex]. Fortschr Neurol Psychiatr 68:37–47, 2000.

98. McMahon TJ, Hood JS, Kadowitz PJ: Pulmonary vasodilator response to vagal stimulation is blocked by N omega-nitro-L-arginine methyl ester in the cat. Circ Res 70:364–369, 1992.

99. el-Kashef HA, Hofman WF, Ehrhart IC, Catravas JD: Multiple muscarinic receptor subtypes in the canine pulmonary circulation. J Appl Physiol 71:2032–2043, 1991.

100. Inoue T, Kannan MS: Nonadrenergic and noncholinergic excitatory neurotransmission in rat intrapulmonary artery. Am J Physiol 254:H1142–H1148, 1988.

101. Itoh T, Sasaguri T, Makita Y, Kanmura Y, Kuriyama H: Mechanisms of vasodilation induced by vasoactive intestinal polypeptide in rabbit mesenteric artery. Am J Physiol 249:H231–H240, 1985.

102. Tanaka Y, Kaneko H, Tanaka H, Shigenobu K: Pharmacologic characteristics of non-prostanoid, non-nitric oxide mediated and endothelium-dependent relaxation of guinea-pig aorta in response to substance P. Res Commun Mol Pathol Pharmacol 103:65–81, 1999.

103. McCormack DG, Mak JC, Coupe MO, Barnes PJ: Calcitonin gene-related peptide vasodilation of human pulmonary vessels. J Appl Physiol 67:1265–1270, 1989.

104. Marshall I: Mechanism of vascular relaxation by the calcitonin gene-related peptide. Ann N Y Acad Sci 657:204–215, 1992.

105. Touyz RM, Schiffrin EL: Signal transduction mechanisms mediating the physiological and pathophysiological actions of angiotensin II in vascular smooth muscle cells. Pharmacol Rev 52:639–672, 2000.

106. Schiffrin EL, Park JB, Intengan HD, Touyz RM: Correction of arterial structure and endothelial dysfunction in human essential hypertension by the angiotensin receptor antagonist losartan. Circulation 101:1653–1659, 2000.

107. Laszlo FA, Laszlo F, Jr., De Wied D: Pharmacology and clinical perspectives of vasopressin antagonists. Pharmacol Rev 43:73–108, 1991.

108. Nemenoff RA: Vasopressin signaling pathways in vascular smooth muscle. Front Biosci 3:D194–D207, 1998.

109. Koller KJ, Lowe DG, Bennett GL, Minamino N, Kangawa K, Matsuo H, Goeddel DV: Selective activation of the B natriuretic peptide receptor by C-type natriuretic peptide (CNP). Science 252:120–123, 1991.

110. Yamanaka S, Miura K, Yukimura T, Okumura M, Yamamoto K: Putative mechanism of hypotensive action of platelet-activating factor in dogs. Circ Res 70:893–901, 1992.

111. Schini VB, Boulanger C, Regoli D, Vanhoutte PM: Bradykinin stimulates the production of cyclic GMP via activation of B2 kinin receptors in cultured porcine aortic endothelial cells. J Pharmacol Exp Ther 252:581–585, 1990.

112. Kaufman MP, Coleridge HM, Coleridge JC, Baker DG: Bradykinin stimulates afferent vagal C-fibers in intrapulmonary airways of dogs. J Appl Physiol 48:511–517, 1980.

113. Marshall I: Characterization and distribution of histamine H1- and H2-receptors in precapillary vessels. J Cardiovasc Pharmacol 6:S587–S597, 1984.

114. Abacioglu N, Ercan ZS, Kanzik L, Zengil H, Demiryurek T, Turker RK: Endothelium-dependent relaxing effect of histamine on the isolated guinea-pig main pulmonary artery strips. Agents Actions 22:30–35, 1987.

115. Paulson OB, Strandgaard S, Edvinsson L: Cerebral autoregulation. Cerebrovasc Brain Metab Rev 2:161–192, 1990.

116. Fabricius M, Akgoren N, Lauritzen M: Arginine-nitric oxide pathway and cerebrovascular regulation in cortical spreading depression. Am J Physiol 269:H23–H29, 1995.

117. Faraci FM, Breese KR, Heistad DD: Cerebral vasodilation during hypercapnia. Role of glibenclamide- sensitive potassium channels and nitric oxide. Stroke 25:1679–1683, 1994.

118. Fredricks KT, Liu Y, Rusch NJ, Lombard JH: Role of endothelium and arterial K+ channels in mediating hypoxic dilation of middle cerebral arteries. Am J Physiol 267:H580–H586, 1994.

119. Post JM, Hume JR, Archer SL, Weir EK: Direct role for potassium channel inhibition in hypoxic pulmonary vasoconstriction. Am J Physiol 262:C882–C890, 1992.

120. Said SI: Metabolic functions of the pulmonary circulation. Circ Res 50:325–333, 1982.

121. Johnson AR, Erdos EG: Metabolism of vasoactive peptides by human endothelial cells in culture. Angiotensin I converting enzyme (kininase II) and angiotensinase. J Clin Invest 59:684–695, 1977.

122. Erdos EG, Johnson AR, Boyden NT: Hydrolysis of enkephalin by cultured human endothelial cells and by purified peptidyl dipeptidase. Biochem Pharmacol 27:843–848, 1978.

123. Feigl EO: Coronary physiology. Physiol Rev 63:1–205, 1983.

124. von Beckerath N, Cyrys S, Dischner A, Daut J: Hypoxic vasodilatation in isolated, perfused guinea-pig heart: an analysis of the underlying mechanisms. J Physiol 442:297–319, 1991.

125. Ross G: Adrenergic responses of the coronary vessels. Circ Res 39:461–465, 1976.

126. Gibson PR, Dudley FJ: Ischemic hepatitis: clinical features, diagnosis and prognosis. Aust N Z J Med 14:822–825, 1984.

127. Bouclier M, Cavey D, Kail N, Hensby C: Experimental models in skin pharmacology. Pharmacol Rev 42:127–154, 1990.

128. Kuriyama H, Kitamura K, Itoh T, Inoue R: Physiological features of visceral smooth muscle cells, with special reference to receptors and ion channels. Physiol Rev 78:811–920, 1998.

129. Berridge MJ: Inositol trisphosphate and calcium signalling. Nature 361:315–325, 1993.

130. Kuriyama H, Kitamura K, Nabata H: Pharmacological and physiological significance of ion channels and factors that modulate them in vascular tissues. Pharmacol Rev 47:387–573, 1995.

131. Somlyo AP, Somlyo AV: Signal transduction and regulation in smooth muscle. Nature 372:231–236, 1994.

132. Savineau JP, Marthan R: Modulation of the calcium sensitivity of the smooth muscle contractile apparatus: molecular mechanisms, pharmacological and pathophysiological implications. Fundam Clin Pharmacol 11:289–299, 1997.

133. Ikebe M, Hartshorne DJ, Elzinga M: Phosphorylation of the 20,000-dalton light chain of smooth muscle myosin by the calcium-activated, phospholipid-dependent protein kinase. Phosphorylation sites and effects of phosphorylation. J Biol Chem 262:9569–9573, 1987.

134. Horowitz A, Menice CB, Laporte R, Morgan KG: Mechanisms of smooth muscle contraction. Physiol Rev 76:967–1003, 1996.

135. Itoh T, Kajikuri J, Kuriyama H: Characteristic features of noradrenaline-induced Ca^{2+} mobilization and tension in arterial smooth muscle of the rabbit. J Physiol 457:297–314, 1992.

136. Kitazawa T, Gaylinn BD, Denney GH, Somlyo AP: G-protein-mediated Ca^{2+} sensitization of smooth muscle contraction through myosin light chain phosphorylation. J Biol Chem 266:1708–1715, 1991.

137. Kitazawa T, Masuo M, Somlyo AP: G protein-mediated inhibition of myosin light-chain phosphatase in vascular smooth muscle. Proc Natl Acad Sci U S A 88:9307–9310, 1991.

138. Gong MC, Iizuka K, Nixon G, Browne JP, Hall A, Eccleston JF, Sugai M, Kobayashi S, Somlyo AV, Somlyo AP: Role of guanine nucleotide-binding proteins—ras-family or trimeric proteins or both—in Ca^{2+} sensitization of smooth muscle. Proc Natl Acad Sci U S A 93:1340–1345, 1996.

139. Noda M, Yasuda-Fukazawa C, Moriishi K, Kato T, Okuda T, Kurokawa K, Takuwa Y: Involvement of rho in GTP gamma S-induced enhancement of phosphorylation of 20 kDa myosin light chain in vascular smooth muscle cells: inhibition of phosphatase activity. FEBS Lett 367:246–250, 1995.

140. Allen BG, Walsh MP: The biochemical basis of the regulation of smooth-muscle contraction. Trends Biochem Sci 19:362–368, 1994.

141. Abe A, Karaki H: Mechanisms underlying the inhibitory effect of dibutyryl cyclic AMP in vascular smooth muscle. Eur J Pharmacol 211:305–311, 1992.

142. Kamm KE, Stull JT: Regulation of smooth muscle contractile elements by second messengers. Annu Rev Physiol 51:299–313, 1989.

143. Karaki H, Ozaki H, Hori M, Mitsui-Saito M, Amano K, Harada K, Miyamoto S, Nakazawa H, Won KJ, Sato K: Calcium movements, distribution, and functions in smooth muscle. Pharmacol Rev 49:157–230, 1997.

144. Nelson MT, Quayle JM: Physiological roles and properties of potassium channels in arterial smooth muscle. Am J Physiol 268:C799–C822, 1995.

145. O'Donnell ME, Owen, NE: Regulation of Ion Pumps and Carriers in Vascular Smooth Muscle. Physio Rev 74:683–711, 1994.

146. Nelson MT, Patlak JB, Worley JF, Standen NB: Calcium channels,

potassium channels, and voltage dependence of arterial smooth muscle tone. Am J Physiol 259:C3–C18, 1990.

147. Harder DR, Madden JA, Dawson C: Hypoxic induction of Ca²⁺-dependent action potentials in small pulmonary arteries of the cat. J Appl Physiol 59:1389–1393, 1985.

148. Lansman JB, Hallam TJ, Rink TJ: Single stretch-activated ion channels in vascular endothelial cells as mechanotransducers? Nature 325:811–813, 1987.
    Christensen O: Mediation of cell volume regulation by Ca²⁺ influx through stretch-activated channels. Nature 330:66–68, 1987.

149. Kirber MT, Walsh JV, Jr., Singer JJ: Stretch-activated ion channels in smooth muscle: a mechanism for the initiation of stretch-induced contraction. Pflugers Arch 412:339–345, 1988.

150. Brayden JE, Nelson MT: Regulation of arterial tone by activation of calcium-dependent potassium channels. Science 256:532–535, 1992.

151. McCobb DP, Fowler NL, Featherstone T, Lingle CJ, Saito M, Krause JE, Salkoff L: A human calcium-activated potassium channel gene expressed in vascular smooth muscle. Am J Physiol 269:H767–H777, 1995.

152. Hong KW, Yoo SE, Yu SS, Lee JY, Rhim BY: Pharmacological coupling and functional role for CGRP receptors in the vasodilation of rat pial arterioles. Am J Physiol 270:H317–H323, 1996.

153. Lang MG, Paterno R, Faraci FM, Heistad DD: Mechanisms of adrenomedullin-induced dilatation of cerebral arterioles. Stroke 28:181–185, 1997.

154. White RE, Kryman JP, El-Mowafy AM, Han G, Carrier GO: cAMP-dependent vasodilators cross-activate the cGMP-dependent protein kinase to stimulate BK(Ca) channel activity in coronary artery smooth muscle cells. Circ Res 86:897–905, 2000.

155. Gebremedhin D, Ma YH, Falck JR, Roman RJ, VanRollins M, Harder DR: Mechanism of action of cerebral epoxyeicosatrienoic acids on cerebral arterial smooth muscle. Am J Physiol 263:H519–H525, 1992.

156. Park MK, Lee SH, Lee SJ, Ho WK, Earm YE: Different modulation of Ca-activated K channels by the intracellular redox potential in pulmonary and ear arterial smooth muscle cells of the rabbit. Pflugers Arch 430:308–314, 1995.

157. Kleppisch T, Nelson MT: ATP-sensitive K⁺ currents in cerebral arterial smooth muscle: pharmacological and hormonal modulation. Am J Physiol 269:H1634–H1640, 1995.

158. Standen NB, Quayle JM, Davies NW, Brayden JE, Huang Y, Nelson MT: Hyperpolarizing vasodilators activate ATP-sensitive K⁺ channels in arterial smooth muscle. Science 245:177–180, 1989.

159. Junichirou H, Tsuneyoshi I, Kayai R, Hidaka T, Boyle WA: Dual alpha2-adrenergic agonist and alpha1-adrenergic antagonist actions of dexmedetomidine on human isolated endothelium-denuded gastro-epiplotic arteries. Anest Analg 94:1434–1440, 2002.

160. Ghofrani HA, Wiedemann R, Rose F, Olschewski H, Schermuly RT, Weissmann N, Seeger W, Grimminger F: Combination therapy with oral sildenafil and inhaled iloprost for severe pulmonary hypertension. Annals of Internal Medicine. 136(7):515–522, 2002.

161. Kakuyama M, Hatano Y, Nakamura K, Toda H, Terasako K, Nishiwada M, Mori K: Halothane and enflurane constrict canine mesenteric arteries by releasing Ca²⁺ from intracellular Ca²⁺ stores. Anesthesiology 80:1120–1127, 1994.

162. Boyle WA, Maher GM: Endothelium-independent vasoconstricting and vasodilating actions of halothane on rat mesenteric resistance blood vessels. Anesthesiology 82:221–235, 1995.

163. Su JY, Chang YI, Tang LJ: Mechanisms of action of enflurane on vascular smooth muscle. Comparison of rabbit aorta and femoral artery. Anesthesiology 81:700–709, 1994.

164. Akata T, Boyle WA: Dual actions of halothane on intracellular calcium stores of vascular smooth muscle. Anesthesiology 84:580–595, 1996.

165. Akata T, Nakashima M, Kodama K, Boyle WA, 3rd, Takahashi S: Effects of volatile anesthetics on acetylcholine-induced relaxation in the rabbit mesenteric resistance artery. Anesthesiology 82:188–204, 1995.

166. Izumi K, Akata T, Takahashi S: The action of sevoflurane on vascular smooth muscle of isolated mesenteric resistance arteries (part 1): role of endothelium. Anesthesiology 92:1426–1440, 2000.

167. Tsuchida H, Namba H, Yamakage M, Fujita S, Notsuki E, Namiki A: Effects of halothane and isoflurane on cytosolic calcium ion concentrations and contraction in the vascular smooth muscle of the rat aorta. Anesthesiology 78:531–540, 1993.

168. Buljubasic N, Rusch NJ, Marijic J, Kampine JP, Bosnjak ZJ: Effects of halothane and isoflurane on calcium and potassium channel currents in canine coronary arterial cells. Anesthesiology 76:990–998, 1992.

169. Akata T and Boyle WA: Effects of volatile anesthetics on contractile proteins in small splanchnic resistance arteries. Anesthesiology 82:700–712, 1995.

170. Akata T, Izumi K, Nakashima M: The action of sevoflurane on vascular smooth muscle of isolated mesenteric resistance arteries (part 2): mechanisms of endothelium-independent vasorelaxation. Anesthesiology 92:1441–1453, 2000.

171. Chang KS, Davis RF: Propofol produces endothelium-independent vasodilation and may act as a Ca²⁺ channel blocker. Anesth Analg 76:24–32, 1993.

172. Imura N, Shiraishi Y, Katsuya H, Itoh T: Effect of propofol on norepinephrine-induced increases in [Ca²⁺]ᵢ and force in smooth muscle of the rabbit mesenteric resistance artery. Anesthesiology 88:1566–1578, 1998.

173. Yamashita A, Kajikuri J, Ohashi M, Kanmura Y, Itoh T: Inhibitory effects of propofol on acetylcholine-induced, endothelium-dependent relaxation and prostacyclin synthesis in rabbit mesenteric resistance arteries. Anesthesiology 91:1080–1089, 1999.

174. Gacar N, Gok S, Kalyoncu NI, Ozen I, Soykan N, Akturk G: The effect of edothelium on the response to propofol on bovine coronary artery rings. Acta Anaesthesiol Scand 39:1080–1083, 1995.

175. Shiraishi Y, Ohashi M, Kanmura Y, Yamaguchi S, Yoshimura N, Itoh T: Possible mechanisms underlying the midazolam-induced relaxation of the noradrenaline-contraction in rabbit mesenteric resistance artery. Br J Pharmacol 121:1155–1163, 1997.

176. Chang KS, Feng MG, Davis RF: Midazolam produces vasodilation by mixed endothelium-dependent and -independent mechanisms. Anesth Analg 78:710–717, 1994.

177. Wong DH, Jenkins LC: An experimental study of the mechanism of action of ketamine on the central nervous system. Can Anaesth Soc J 21:57–67, 1974.

178. Kanmura Y, Yoshitake J, Casteels R: Ketamine-induced relaxation in intact and skinned smooth muscles of the rabbit ear artery. Br J Pharmacol 97:591–597, 1989.

179. Kanmura Y, Kajikuri J, Itoh T, Yoshitake J: Effects of ketamine on contraction and synthesis of inositol 1,4,5-trisphosphate in smooth muscle of the rabbit mesenteric artery. Anesthesiology 79:571–579, 1993.

180. Ogawa K, Tanaka S, Murray P: Inhibitory effects of etomidate and ketamine on endothelium-dependent relaxation in canine pulmonary artery. Anesthesiology 94:668–677, 2001.

181. Cybulsky MI, Gimbrone MA, Jr.: Endothelial expression of a mononuclear leukocyte adhesion molecule during atherogenesis. Science 251:788–791, 1991.

182. Ambrose JA, Tannenbaum MA, Alexopoulos D, Hjemdahl-Monsen CE, Leavy J, Weiss M, Borrico S, Gorlin R, Fuster V: Angiographic progression of coronary artery disease and the development of myocardial infarction. J Am Coll Cardiol 12:56–62, 1988.

183. Mombouli J-V, Vanhoutte PM: Endothelial dysfunction: from physiology to therapy. J Mol Cell Cardiol 31:61–74, 1999.

184. generation and reversal of acetylcholine-induced cerebral arteriolar dilation after acute hypertension. Circ Res 57:781–787, 1985.

185. Mayhan WG: Role of prostaglandin H2-thromboxane A2 in responses of cerebral arterioles during chronic hypertension. Am J Physiol 262:H539–H543, 1992.

186. Ge T, Hughes H, Junquero DC, Wu KK, Vanhoutte PM, Boulanger CM: Endothelium-dependent contractions are associated with both augmented expression of prostaglandin H synthase-1 and hypersensitivity to prostaglandin H2 in the SHR aorta. Circ Res 76:1003–1010, 1995.

187. Takaba H, Nagao T, Ibayashi S, Kitazono T, Fujii K, Fujishima M: Altered cerebrovascular response to a potassium channel opener in hypertensive rats. Hypertension 28:143–146, 1996.

188. Diederich D, Skopec J, Diederich A, Dai FX: Endothelial dysfunction in mesenteric resistance arteries of diabetic rats: role of free radicals. Am J Physiol 266:H1153–H1161, 1994.

189. Hattori Y, Kawasaki H, Abe K, Kanno M: Superoxide dismutase recovers altered endothelium-dependent relaxation in diabetic rat aorta. Am J Physiol 261:H1086–H1094, 1991.

190. Tesfamariam B: Free radicals in diabetic endothelial cell dysfunction. Free Radic Biol Med 16:383–391, 1994.

191. Mayhan WG: Impairment of endothelium-dependent dilatation of

the basilar artery during diabetes mellitus. Brain Res 580:297–302, 1992.

192. Brunner F: Interaction of nitric oxide and endothelin-1 in ischemia/reperfusion injury of rat heart. J Mol Cell Cardiol 29:2363–2374, 1997.

193. Villa LM, Salas E, Darley-Usmar VM, Radomski MW, Moncada S: Peroxynitrite induces both vasodilatation and impaired vascular relaxation in the isolated perfused rat heart. Proc Natl Acad Sci U S A 91:12383–12387, 1994.

194. Zweier JL, Kuppusamy P, Lutty GA: Measurement of endothelial cell free radical generation: evidence for a central mechanism of free radical injury in post-ischemic tissues. Proc Natl Acad Sci U S A 85:4046–4050, 1988.

195. Kukielka GL, Hawkins HK, Michael L, Manning AM, Youker K, Lane C, Entman ML, Smith CW, Anderson DC: Regulation of intercellular adhesion molecule-1 (ICAM-1) in ischemic and reperfused canine myocardium. J Clin Invest 92:1504–1516, 1993.

196. Parrillo JE: Pathogenetic mechanisms of septic shock. N Engl J Med 328:1471–1477, 1993.

197. Tsuneyoshi I, Kanmura Y, Yoshimura N: Nitric oxide as a mediator of reduced arterial responsiveness in septic patients. Crit Care Med 24:1083–1086, 1996.

198. Boyle WA, Parvathaneni LS, Bourlier V, Sauter C, Laubach VE, and Cobb JP: iNOS gene expression modulates microvascular responsiveness in endotoxin-challenged mice. Circ Res 87:18–24, 2000.

20

Lung Function

Andrew Lumb, MB, BS, FRCA • Albert Dahan, MD, PhD • Denham S. Ward, MD, PhD

Ventilation
   Respiratory Muscles
   Respiratory Epithelium
   Control of Airway Diameter
   The Alveolus
Oxygenation
   Systems and Organ Physiology

Control of Breathing
   Hypoxia
   Hypercapnia
   Pain

To accomplish the task of the primary purpose of the lung, namely that of oxygenation of the venous blood and removal of carbon dioxide, the lung behaves in an integrated fashion with other organ systems. It requires an external pump (the chest wall and muscles) and a central neural controller in addition to the gas exchanger. Each of these elements has functions other than the exchange of gases and are susceptible to alterations in function both by intended drug effects and by side effects. In particular, the need for a brainstem controller to generate the basic respiratory rhythm means that many centrally acting drugs will affect respiration. The large surface area of the gas-conducting and gas-exchanging regions of the lung that are exposed to the external environment provides many opportunities for additional interactions. Modern physiology covers not only the macroscopic functions but also the cellular and subcellular functions of the organ. The first section of this chapter discusses the respiratory muscles and the airways that conduct air to the gas-exchanging regions of the lung. The second section details the exchange of gas from the air to and from the blood and how perfusion is matched to ventilation. Finally, the last section describes the ventilatory controller that responds to hypoxemia and acidemia (hypercapnia) to increase ventilation and hence gas exchange.

Ventilation

Pulmonary ventilation is achieved by the contraction of several inspiratory muscles to bring about expansion of the chest cavity, i.e., drawing air into the lungs. In so doing, the muscles must overcome both the inherent elasticity of the respiratory system and the resistance encountered by gas flowing into the lungs. The inherent elasticity results from a combination of elastin in the lungs and chest wall along with the surface forces of the alveoli, whereas the resistance arises from that produced by deformation of the thoracic tissues as well as frictional resistance to gas flow in the airways. Expiration is then usually an entirely passive process, with the elasticity of the respiratory system returning the lungs to their resting position of functional residual capacity (FRC). In the supine position, the weight of the abdominal contents assist passive expiration by pushing the diaphragm in a cephalad direction; but in the upright position or when hyperventilating, the internal intercostals and abdominal muscles contract to assist expiration.

Respiratory Muscles

Activation of the inspiratory neuron group of the respiratory center in the medulla leads to contraction of many muscle groups. To enable gas to flow into the lungs, a negative pressure must be generated between the alveoli and the mouth, and this small subatmospheric pressure in the mouth and pharynx promotes collapse of the upper airway and, if unopposed, airway obstruction. To overcome this, many of the pharyngeal dilator muscles show both tonic activity and inspiratory phasic contraction to maintain airway patency. This pharyngeal dilation during inspiration is reinforced by reflex stimulation of mechanoreceptors in the larynx and pharynx, which respond to subatmospheric pressure and cause rapid (<50 milliseconds) further contraction of pharyngeal dilators. There is similar phasic activity in the laryngeal muscles, resulting in abduction of the vocal cords during inspiration and adduction during early expiration, which is believed to act as a "brake" on exhalation to reduce alveolar collapse.[1]

The external, and parasternal portion of the internal, intercostal muscles along with the diaphragm are the main inspiratory muscles when at rest, with the scalene muscles and many other accessory muscles around the upper chest and neck only contributing during hyperventilation. The internal intercostals and all of the abdominal wall muscles make up the expiratory muscles and are generally only active when standing or when minute ventilation is several times normal. Many of the respiratory muscles have multiple other functions, such as maintenance of posture, coughing, sneezing, speech, and so on, each of which must be performed alongside their role in breathing.

Control of Respiratory Muscle

Respiratory muscles are controlled in the same way as other skeletal muscles. The intercostal muscles and the diaphragm contain muscle spindles innervated by gamma efferent fibers, whereas the bulk of the fibers are supplied by alpha motor neurons. Stimulation of gamma efferents leads to contraction of the muscle spindle fibers followed by a spinal reflex activation of the alpha motoneurons and muscle contraction. This "servo" mechanism allows fine control of muscle activity such that the respiratory center can send impulses to the gamma efferents requiring a certain degree of shortening of the respiratory muscle (and therefore tidal volume) and allow the spinal reflex to control how much contraction is required of the whole muscle.

Muscle Fiber Subtypes

Unlike many other skeletal muscles, respiratory muscle contains a mixture of both type I (slow twitch fatigue–resistant) and type II (fast twitch fatigable) fibers.[2] This finding is consistent with the diverse requirements placed on respiratory muscles. The type I fibers are believed to predominate for breathing and posture, which do not require fast responses and need to be fatigue-resistant, whereas type II fibers contribute to contraction during active locomotion and expulsive efforts such as coughing and sneezing when fatigue is less important. Differing fiber types correspond to different isoforms of the myosin chains, which are encoded in separate families of genes on human chromosomes 14 and 17.[3] Mechanical signals are able to influence the relative expression of fast and slow isoforms of myosin, and therefore influence the functional properties of the muscle. In animals this has been demonstrated in the diaphragm, where increased respiratory resistance or endurance training changes the expression of myosin heavy chains to more fatigue-resistant subtypes.[3,4]

Respiratory Epithelium

The respiratory tract is lined with ciliated epithelium until the terminal bronchioles where the cilia disappear and the cells progressively flatten as they merge with the alveolar epithelial cells. Along with goblet cells, airway epithelial cells are responsible for producing and controlling the constituents of the liquid lining of the airway. This lining has several important functions such as humidification of inspired gas, acting as a chemical barrier to inhaled irritants, capture and clearance of particles, and the first line of defense against airborne pathogens.

Airway Surface Liquid

The fluid lining the airway is produced by the submucosal glands and goblet cells with epithelial cells being mostly involved in controlling the water and electrolyte content of the fluid as it ascends the respiratory tract. The fluid is now known to form two distinct layers—a sol or liquid layer in which the cilia beat with a gel or mucous layer above, which the tips of the cilia grip and move along.[5] Mucins, which form the gel layer, are produced by goblet cells that are present only in small amounts in the normal healthy airway. However, preformed mucin is discharged rapidly by goblet cells in response to a wide range of stimuli including irritant gases (e.g., tobacco smoke), inflammatory mediators, proteinases, and biophysical stress on the cells.[6] Goblet cell hypersecretion and hyperplasia characterize many chronic respiratory diseases, in particular chronic obstructive pulmonary disease and asthma. Mucin production originates from several different genes,[7] and animal studies have shown increased production of mucin mRNA in response to airway endotoxin,[8] indicating de novo synthesis during pulmonary infection. Attempts to reduce the mucous hypersecretion associated with airways disease have involved either direct mucolysis—e.g., with *N*-acetylcysteine to cause thiol reduction of the glycoproteins in mucin—or suppression of mucin production by glucocorticoids that reduce inflammatory mediators[9] and directly suppress mucin gene expression.[10]

J Receptors

Named after their anatomic site, juxtapulmonary capillary receptors are present throughout the respiratory tract, including the alveoli. J receptors consist of C-fiber nerve endings and are nociceptive receptors that respond to inhaled irritants, increased interstitial fluid, and a variety of inflammatory mediators.[11] Stimulation leads to both respiratory effects (apnea or rapid shallow breathing, bronchoconstriction, stimulation of mucous secretion) and cardiovascular changes (bradycardia and hypotension). J receptors are implicated in the clinical presentation of many pulmonary diseases, including the tachypnea seen with pulmonary embolism and edema.

Control of Airway Diameter

Airway diameter, and therefore the resistance to gas flow, is closely related to lung volume. For laminar flow through a straight tube, flow rate is related to the fourth power of the radius of the tube,[12] therefore the relationship between lung volume and airways resistance is hyperbolic (Fig. 20–1). Figure 20–1 shows that at FRC resistance is already minimal and further lung expansion has only a small effect on airway resistance.

In airways disease, bronchospasm, increased production of airway lining fluid, and mucosal edema all contribute to increased pulmonary resistance. However, from a pharmacologic standpoint, it is the contribution played by airway smooth muscle that offers the greatest therapeutic challenge.

Control of Bronchial Smooth Muscle

A summary of the physiologic control of bronchial smooth muscle is shown in Figure 20–2.

Neural Control

In spite of its dominant role in many systems, the sympathetic nervous system is believed to make no contribution to the control of bronchial smooth muscle in humans. Those adrenergic fibers present in the human lung are normally in close proximity to vessels and glands rather than bronchial muscle.[13]

In contrast, the parasympathetic system is highly functional in humans.[14] Parasympathetic fibers run with the vagus nerve and release acetylcholine (ACh) to activate muscarinic ACh receptors of the M_3 subtype. Stimulation of

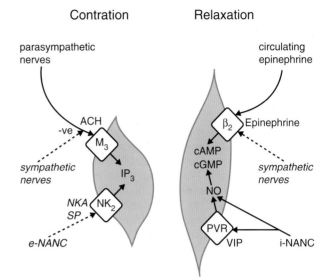

Figure 20–2. Summary of physiologic control of bronchial smooth muscle. Systems shown with dashed lines do not have a proven physiologic role in humans but are well described in animals. ACh, acetylcholine; cAMP, cyclic adenosine monophosphate; cGMP, cyclic guanosine monophosphate; CGRP, calcitonin gene-related peptide; eNANC, excitatory nonadrenergic noncholinergic; iNANC, inhibitory nonadrenergic noncholinergic; IP_3, inositol triphosphate; NKA, neurokinin A; NO, nitric oxide; SP, substance P; VIP, vasoactive intestinal polypeptide.

preganglionic M_2 ACh receptors exerts a negative feedback on ACh release to limit the response. These preganglionic receptors are important in airways disease. For example, viral respiratory infections inhibit M_2 receptor gene expression and inactivate existing receptors, causing an exaggerated bronchoconstrictor response to normal vagal stimuli.[15]

A further system of neurologic control of airway diameter by the autonomic nervous system (See Chapter 14) is the nonadrenergic noncholinergic system (NANC), which is further divided into inhibitory (iNANC) and excitatory (eNANC) pathways.[16,17] The iNANC nerves are colocalized with parasympathetic nerves and have vasoactive intestinal polypeptide and nitric oxide (NO) as neurotransmitters. eNANC responses are believed to originate from sensory C-fibers in the airway releasing neuropeptides in response to nociceptive stimulation. The role of the NANC systems in humans remains controversial. The iNANC system is the only neural-mediated bronchodilator in humans, and may be responsible for the normal diurnal variations seen in bronchial muscle tone,[18] whereas the eNANC system seems to be primarily involved in mediating bronchoconstriction from inflammatory mediators.

Humoral Control

There are abundant β_2 adrenoreceptors in bronchial smooth muscle in humans. The absence of sympathetic innervation indicates that these receptors respond only to circulating catecholamines, particularly epinephrine, and are vital for a

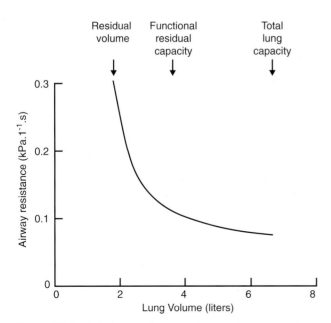

Figure 20–1. Relationship between lung volume and airway resistance in a healthy upright subject.

normal bronchodilator response during exercise and other "stress response" situations. The mechanism of the bronchodilator action of β_2 adrenoreceptors and M_3 ACh receptors is described in detail later.

Local Cellular Effects

Inhalation of foreign bodies, chemical irritants, or cold air causes bronchoconstriction through a reflex pathway involving afferents from J receptors and efferents through the parasympathetic or eNANC systems. These reflex pathways are responsible for bronchoconstriction seen with airway or lung inflammation and are present in healthy subjects, but are usually "hyper-responsive" in patients with asthma. This enhanced bronchoconstrictor response is particularly intense during and after viral invasion of the respiratory tract.[15,19]

Bronchoconstriction in Airway Disease

Mast cells are found in large numbers throughout the respiratory epithelium and may be activated by physical stimulation (e.g., coughing) or in response to allergens and infection through immunoglobulin E (IgE), complement fractions, and cytokines. In addition to inflammatory mediators, mast cells also release a range of cytokines that are responsible for chemotaxis and activation of other inflammatory cells including eosinophils, neutrophils, macrophages, and lymphocytes, all of which amplify the inflammatory response. A further source of proinflammatory

mediators are the eNANC nerves described earlier. These C-fiber nerve endings release several mediators, but the tachykinins in particular are believed to play a role in bronchial hyper-responsiveness.[20] A summary of inflammatory mediators affecting bronchial smooth muscle is shown in Table 20–1.

This complex cascade of proinflammatory cells and mediators provides a huge source of potential therapeutic approaches[21]; although currently, steroids are the mainstay of asthma treatment. Glucocorticoids reduce airway inflammation by modulating the production of most of the proteins involved. Production of proinflammatory cytokines (e.g., interleukin [IL]-1β, IL-6, and IL-11), bronchoconstrictor receptors (e.g., neurokinin receptors), and inflammatory enzymes (e.g., cyclooxygenase-2) are all suppressed, whereas anti-inflammatory cytokine and bronchodilator receptor (β_2-adrenoceptor) production is stimulated.[22] Glucocorticoid receptors (GRs) are present in the cytoplasm of almost all cells and consist of a single protein of approximately 800 amino acids bound, in its central portion, to 2 zinc atoms. The molecular mechanism of GR activation is well described.[9,22] Binding to agonists occurs in the cytoplasm and induces a conformational change to the GR that allows it to pass through the nuclear membrane. Within the nucleus, DNA transcription is modified either by binding directly to specific DNA sequences, by reduction of mRNA activity, or by interaction with other transcription factors to suppress gene expression. In the last of these mechanisms, the reliance of activated GR on other gene transcription proteins is believed to explain individual variations in steroid responsiveness.[9]

TABLE 20–1.

Mediators Involved in Alteration of Bronchial Smooth Muscle Tone During Airway Inflammation

| Source | Bronchoconstriction | | Bronchodilatation | |
	Mediator	Receptor	Mediator	Receptor
Mast cells and other proinflammatory cells	Histamine	H_1	Prostaglandin E_2	EP
	Prostaglandin D_2	TP	Prostacyclin (PGI$_2$)	EP
	Prostaglandin $F_{2\alpha}$	TP		
	Leukotrienes C_4 D_4 E_4	CysLT$_1$		
	PAF	PAF		
	Bradykinin	B_2		
C-fibers (e-NANC)	Substance P	NK$_2$		
	Neurokinin A	NK$_2$		
	CGRP	CGRP		
Endothelial and epithelial cells	Endothelin	ET$_B$		

CGRP, calcitonin gene-related peptide; e-NANC, excitatory nonadrenergic noncholinergic; EP, Prostaglandin E receptor; PAF, platelet activating factor; TP, Thromboxane receptor.
Adapted from Thirstrup S: Control of airway smooth muscle tone. I. Electrophysiology and contractile mediators. Respir Med 94:328–336, 2000; Barnes PJ: Pharmacology of airway smooth muscle. Am J Respir Crit Care Med 158:S123–S132, 1998.

Receptor Signaling Pathways in Airway Smooth Muscle

Bronchoconstriction

Stimulation of the ACh receptor activates a guanosine triphosphate–binding regulatory protein (G protein), characterized as G_q, which in turn activates phospholipase C to catalyze the formation of inositol triphosphate (IP_3) (see Fig. 20–2). Next, IP_3 binds to sarcoplasmic reticulum receptors causing release of calcium from intracellular stores. The elevation of intracellular calcium activates myosin light chain kinase, which phosphorylates part of the myosin chain to activate myosin adenosine triphosphatase to initiate cross-bridging between actin and myosin.[21] IP_3 is converted into the inactive inositol diphosphate by IP_3 kinase. Tachykinin, histamine, and leukotriene receptors responsible for bronchoconstriction from other mediators (see Table 20–1) act by a similar mechanism, being linked to G protein-phospholipase C complexes, which lead to IP_3 formation.[20]

Bronchodilatation

A similar series of interactions between membrane-bound proteins produces relaxation of airway smooth muscle. Stimulation of the β_2 adrenoreceptor activates a G_s protein, which in turn activates adenylate cyclase to convert adenosine triphosphate to cyclic adenosine monophosphate (cAMP).[23] cAMP causes relaxation of the muscle cell by inhibition of calcium release from intracellular stores and probably also activates protein kinase A to phosphorylate some of the regulatory proteins involved in the actin/myosin interaction. cAMP is hydrolyzed by the intracellular enzyme phosphodiesterase (PDE), of which seven subgroups have now been identified. Subgroups PDE3 and PDE4 are present in airway smooth muscle and are active against cAMP, but the PDE inhibitors currently used in asthma such as theophylline are nonspecific for these subgroups.[21]

Currently, it is believed that there are many molecular interactions between these two opposing signaling pathways. Activation of phospholipase C by protein G_q also liberates intracellular diacylglycerol, which activates another membrane-bound enzyme protein kinase C. This enzyme is able to phosphorylate a variety of proteins including G proteins and the β_2 receptor itself, causing uncoupling of the receptor from the G protein and down-regulation of the transduction pathway.[21,23] Similar mechanisms are involved in desensitization of the receptor with frequent stimulation when a variety of intracellular protein kinase enzymes phosphorylate the receptor at a specific location[23,24] (Fig. 20–3).

Molecular Basis of β_2 Receptor Activity

The molecular basis of the functional characteristics of the β adrenoceptor are now clearly elucidated.[23,25,26] It contains 413 amino acids and has seven transmembrane helices (see Fig. 20–3). The agonist binding site is within this hydrophobic core of the protein within the lipid bilayer of the cell membrane. This affects the interaction of drugs at

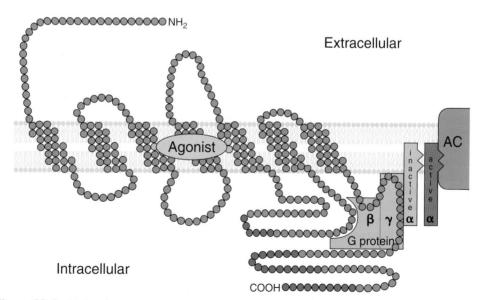

Figure 20–3. Molecular mechanisms of β_2 adrenoreceptor stimulation. The receptor exists in active and inactive states according to whether the α-subunit of the G protein is bound to adenyl cyclase (AC). The agonist binds to three amino acid residues on the third and fifth transmembrane domains (orange) and stabilizes the receptor G protein complex in the activated state. The intracellular C-terminal region of the protein (dark green) is the area susceptible to phosphorylation by intracellular kinases causing inactivation of the receptor and down-regulation. (Modified from Johnson M: The β_2-adrenoceptor. Am J Respir Crit Care Med 158:S146-S153, 1998; Thirstrup S: Control of airway smooth muscle tone: II. Pharmacology of relaxation. Respir Med 94:519–528, 2000; Aranson R, Rau JL: The evolution of beta- agonists. Respir Care Clin N Am 5:479–519, 1999.)

the binding site in that more lipophilic drugs form a depot in the lipid bilayer from which they can repeatedly interact with the binding site of the receptor, producing a much longer duration of action than hydrophilic drugs. Receptors exist in either activated or inactivated form, the former state occurring when the third intracellular loop (see Fig. 20–3) is bound to guanosine triphosphate and the α-subunit of the G protein. β_2 receptor agonists probably do not induce a significant conformational change in the protein structure but simply stabilize the active form allowing this to predominate.

Two β_2 adrenoceptor genes are present in humans, with a total of nine polymorphisms described,[27] giving rise to a large number of possible phenotypes. Studies of these phenotypes are at an early stage, but some genetic differences have been shown to be associated with worse nocturnal decreases in peak flow and varying degrees of receptor desensitization by β_2 agonists.[23]

The Alveolus

In the respiratory bronchioles (i.e., those that have alveoli in their walls), gas flow progressively changes from tidal flow to simple diffusion until in the alveoli; movement of gases is completely by diffusion. The barrier to gas diffusion between alveolus and pulmonary capillary is, of necessity, very thin (≈ 0.5 μm). To reach hemoglobin within a red blood cell (RBC), O_2 must diffuse through the alveolar lining fluid, epithelial cell, basement membrane, endothelial cell, a variable depth of plasma, the RBC membrane, and some RBC intracellular fluid.[12] To minimize this diffusion path, particularly in plasma, RBCs are a similar size to the lumen of the pulmonary capillary and change shape as they pass through the pulmonary capillary, therefore bringing the RBC wall in close contact with the endothelial cell. The significance of this shape change has been demonstrated by the observation that drugs (such as salicylates) that increase the deformability of RBCs can increase diffusing capacity.[28] In spite of these considerable barriers, diffusion is rapid with hemoglobin becoming fully saturated in about 0.25 second, less than half the estimated normal capillary transit time of 0.8 second, and reduced diffusion alone is rarely a cause of hypoxia.[12]

The very thin alveolar wall required for diffusion lacks structural strength, in particular the ability to resist alveolar collapse from surface tension, and surfactant in the alveolar lining fluid is therefore crucial for the structural integrity of the alveoli.[29] Furthermore, the molecular structure of surfactant is such that its ability to alter surface tension varies with the size of the alveolus, maintaining alveolar stability throughout the whole range of lung volumes required for normal breathing. Loss of surfactant function is implicated in the pathophysiology of many lung diseases, particularly respiratory distress syndrome in neonates, and replacement with exogenous surfactant is currently a recognized therapy.[30]

Oxygenation

Oxygenation has long been recognized as an important clinical problem, as epitomized in the quote attributed to J. S. Haldane by Joseph Barcroft in his "Presidential Address on Anoxaemia" (*Lancet*, Sept. 4, 1920, pp 485–489): "Anoxaemia not only stops the machine, it wrecks the machinery." The impairment of gas exchange by general anesthesia has also been noted.[31,32] However, because the ability of the lungs to oxygenate blood in the pulmonary artery depends on so many interacting systemic and local factors, the mechanisms behind this impairment have been difficult to determine. For more than 50 years, the importance of matching ventilation and perfusion in the lung to efficiently transfer O_2 has been appreciated; our knowledge of the changes in the distribution of ventilation/perfusion ratios ($\dot{V}_A/\dot{Q}$) throughout the lung under anesthesia and with disease has increased.

Routine blood gas analysis and now the near-universal application of pulse oximetry has shown how common is transient decreases in oxygenation during and after surgery.[33,34] Such easy measurement of arterial saturation has also demonstrated how readily in most clinical situations the use of supplemental O_2 in the perioperative period prevents such desaturations. Thus for practical clinical purposes, the use of supplemental O_2 is the safest, most readily available treatment for the usual impairment of oxygenation. However, with lung disease, and in particular with adult respiratory distress syndrome, adequate oxygenation may become impossible even with 100% O_2. The mainstay of treatment for this impaired oxygenation is one of the various modes of mechanical ventilation,[35] but new pharmacologic approaches are being developed.[36]

Systems and Organ Physiology

The transportation of O_2 from the environment to the mitochondria down its partial pressure gradient has been termed the O_2 cascade.[37] A large decrease in partial pressure occurs in the lung, where the inspired O_2 is diluted with water vapor and alveolar CO_2 before diffusing from the alveolar space into pulmonary capillaries. The decrease in Po_2 from inspired to alveolar gas is described by the alveolar air equation and accounts for the dilution of the inspired tidal volume with CO_2 and for the difference between inspired and expired volume from the difference in O_2 consumption and CO_2 production (usually expressed as a ratio or respiratory quotient).[38]

Oxygen diffuses passively from the alveolar space down its partial pressure or gradient into the pulmonary capillary. The lung structure is complex, with capillaries from a single arteriole branching to several alveolar structures; thus in the wall of a single alveolus are multiple capillaries. The structure of the gas-exchanging units in the lung has been compared to a multilevel parking structure with air spaces separated by plates and posts containing the capillary blood (see Mania[39] for an interesting discussion of the comparative anatomy of gas exchanges in different species).

Although O_2 diffusion is relatively slow (compared with CO_2), ordinarily the transit time across the pulmonary capillary is sufficient for equilibrium between the PO_2 in the alveolus and the capillaries surrounding it. Physiologically, it is only during conditions of severe stress, such as exercise (increased cardiac output and thus shortened pulmonary capillary transient time), or at altitude (decreased inspired O_2) that a substantial difference between alveolar and capillary PO_2 may occur.[40] Only rarely is there sufficient disease on the alveolar capillary membrane to cause a diffusion block, and there is no evidence that anesthesia interferes with this diffusion process.

Although in a quantity of alveolar air the amount of O_2 is directly proportional to its partial pressure, this is not true for the amount of O_2 contained in a quantity of blood. In blood, the amount of O_2 depends on the hemoglobin concentration and the shape and position of the hemoglobin dissociation curve. Thus the amount of O_2 transferred to the blood depends on these factors as well as on the content of O_2 in the blood (mixed venous) entering the gas-exchanging region. Whereas the rate of diffusion is directly related to the partial pressure gradient, the increase in PO_2 is a nonlinear function of the amount of O_2 transferred.

Although not immediately obvious, the major determinant of the final equilibrium PO_2 in the alveolar capillary unit is the ventilation perfusion ratio of the unit.[41] If there is relatively little ventilation in relation to perfusion, the equilibrium will be at a partial pressure closer to the PO_2 in the blood entering the unit, whereas if there is a relatively large ventilation, the equilibrium will be a value closer to the alveolar gas. Of course, this conceptual model is extremely simplified from the spatial and temporal reality in the lung, where there are multiple blood pulmonary transit times within a single breath and where the gas-exchanging region is anatomically complex. The best summary of these systemic factors determining gas exchange was perfected by Fenn and colleagues in the O_2-CO_2 diagram.[42] This diagram (Fig. 20-4) shows all possible PO_2 and PCO_2 values within a lung unit with a given inspired gas composition and mixed venous blood composition for the range of $\dot{V}_A/\dot{Q}$ ratios. Because of the shape of the dissociation curves, mixing blood from units of different $\dot{V}_A/\dot{Q}$ ratios will tend to provide an arithmetic average for CO_2 (because of the approximately linear CO_2 partial pressure-to-content relationship); thus areas with high CO_2 (low $\dot{V}_A/\dot{Q}$) tend to be averaged out by blood from areas with low CO_2 (high $\dot{V}_A/\dot{Q}$). However, because of the nonlinear shape of the O_2-hemoglobin dissociation curve, this is not true for O_2; blood with low PO_2 (areas of low $\dot{V}_A/\dot{Q}$) will not be averaged out by blood from areas with a high $\dot{V}_A/\dot{Q}$. Thus a broadening of the $\dot{V}_A/\dot{Q}$ distribution (rather than a sharp peak around a single mean value) will result in a decrease in the resulting PaO_2.

The Fenn diagram also clearly illustrates the important roles played by the inspired and mixed venous PO_2 as the anchoring points for the curve. Although the Fenn diagram has led to the common clinical use of a three-compartment model (shunt, dead-space, and ideal alveolus), the complete curve readily shows the central role played by the range of $\dot{V}_A/\dot{Q}$ matching in the lung. The total amount of venous admixture can be expressed as the difference between the calculated alveolar O_2 partial pressure (using the alveolar air equation) and the measured arterial partial pressure (A-aO_2). Although the A-aO_2 difference in an awake, upright healthy subject is quite small (about 2–3 mm Hg),[43] there are many factors contributing to the increase commonly seen under anesthesia.

The distribution of $\dot{V}_A/\dot{Q}$ ratios in the lung are affected by mechanical, gravitational, and physiologic factors. Under anesthesia, these factors are often modified from the awake state and can account for the observed widening of the A-aO_2. Mechanical factors included compression of the lung and pulmonary vasculature, as well as changes in the regional lung volumes and ventilation, by intrinsic (e.g., airway positive pressure) or extrinsic (e.g., abdominal

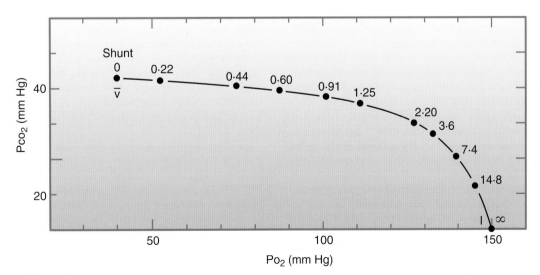

Figure 20-4. CO_2-O_2 diagram showing the possible combinations of PCO_2 and PO_2 for a gas-exchanging lung unit. The curve is anchored on the left by the values in the mixed venous blood ($\bar{v}$) and on the right by the inspired gas (*I*). The ventilation perfusion ratio ($\dot{V}_A/\dot{Q}$) for the unit determines the equilibrium values. Illustrative $\dot{V}_A/\dot{Q}$ ratios are shown on the curve, ranging from shunt, $\dot{V}_A/\dot{Q} = 0$, to dead-space, $\dot{V}_A/\dot{Q} = \infty$.

contents pressing on the diaphragm) factors. Because the pulmonary artery pressure is low, the relative perfusion of lung regions will be determined by the hydrostatic pressure gradient. In a healthy upright subject, this gradient results in lower perfusion to the lung apices. When the patient is supine, this gradient is reduced but still exists in the anteroposterior direction. Similarly, the lateral decubitus position results in greater perfusion to the dependent lung. The main physiologic autoregulation is the adjustment of regional blood flow in the lung through active vasoconstriction of small pulmonary arteries caused by alveolar and mixed venous hypoxia, or hypoxic pulmonary vasoconstriction (HPV)[44] (see later for discussion of the cellular mechanisms for HPV).

Two mechanisms have long been thought to play the primary roles in the development of increased venous admixture under anesthesia: atelectasis[45] and airway closure.[46] The actual collapse of the air-exchanging units with atelectasis would contribute to shunt, whereas airway closure may contribute to low $\dot{V}_A/\dot{Q}$ regions.[47] Both of these mechanisms are most likely a consequence of the consistent reduction in FRC found with anesthesia (in the supine position) with either spontaneous or mechanical ventilation.[48,49] Many factors contribute to this reduction in FRC, but the mechanism is related to alterations in the magnitude, pattern, and distribution of ventilatory drive to the respiratory muscles (e.g., reduction in diaphragmatic tonic activity). These alterations change the shape of the chest wall because of gravitational and elastic forces resulting in atelectasis, decreases in alveolar gas volume (without frank atelectasis), and changes in thoracic blood volume.[50] The relative contribution of these factors (e.g., cephalad movement of the diaphragm, changes in thoracic blood volume, and so on) has been controversial, and the results have varied depending on the investigation.[48,49] When these regions of $\dot{V}_A/\dot{Q}$ mismatch develop, HPV works to decrease perfusion to frankly atelectatic areas and to redirect perfusion to areas of higher $\dot{V}_A/\dot{Q}$. Inhalational anesthetics decrease the HPV response, but their other systemic effects (e.g., decreased cardiac output, decreased pulmonary artery pressure, and changes in mixed venous PO_2) change their total contribution to the increase in venous admixture.[51,52]

Although atelectasis has long been postulated[31] to be one of the important causes of the increased shunt observed during anesthesia, it has not been possible to demonstrate this atelectasis on plain radiographs. However, using computed tomography, Hedenstierna and colleagues have been able to demonstrate radiographic densities that are presumed to be compression atelectasis.[45,47] The volume of this atelectasis correlates with the increase in A-aO_2[49] and shunt[53] found during anesthesia.

Hedenstierna and colleagues used both single photon emission computerized tomography and multiple inert gas elimination in the same subjects.[54] They found that the increase and location of the shunt correlated with the atelectatic areas in the dependent lung regions. Considerable $\dot{V}_A/\dot{Q}$ mismatch also developed because of preferential perfusion of the dorsal regions and ventilation of the ventral regions.

The reduction in FRC may also permit some small airways to close during a portion of the complete respiratory cycle, with the effect of reducing ventilation to these units. If they are closed for a long enough time (depending on the O_2 concentration), these areas may actually become atelectatic because of absorption of the O_2.[55] Although airway closure certainly occurs during the respiratory cycle, its relative contribution to gas exchange impairment has been controversial.[46] However, Hedenstierna and colleagues have estimated that atelectasis and airway closure together may explain up to 75% of the increased A-aO_2 with anesthesia.[47]

A special circumstance of extreme $\dot{V}_A/\dot{Q}$ mismatching occurs during anesthesia for thoracic surgery when selective ventilation of one lung is accomplished with a double lumen endotracheal tube. Here, there is clearly a large increase in the shunt from perfusion of the unventilated lung. For most thoracic procedures, the patient is placed in the lateral decubitus position with the nondependent lung unventilated. In this position, gravitational effects result in a greater proportion of the perfusion going to the dependent, ventilated lung. The ability of small pulmonary arteries to contract with alveolar hypoxia permits physiologic adjustment of blood flow to the ventilated lung. HPV may be able to reduce blood flow to the unventilated lung by as much as 50%.

Because inhalational anesthetics have been shown to reduce HPV[56] in vitro, there has been considerable controversy about their relative role in increasing venous admixture, particularly in the setting of one-lung ventilation.[57] However, clinically it would seem that the use of inhalational anesthetics during one-lung ventilation does not play a major role in the development of hypoxemia[58] and that accepted clinical techniques, such as using a fraction of inspired oxygen (FIO_2) of 1.0, nonventilated lung continuous positive airway pressure and ventilated lung positive end-expiratory pressure, can most often provide for adequate oxygenation.[59]

NO, an endothelium-derived vasodilator, has received considerable interest as a possible treatment for adult respiratory distress syndrome as well as other conditions associated with high pulmonary artery pressure, or $\dot{V}_A/\dot{Q}$ mismatch, or both.[60,61] Giving NO by inhalational, ventilated units of the lung will vasodilate and potentially increase their perfusion. However, this increase in perfusion to partially ventilated areas may be too great and may result in a worsening of the mismatch. Inhaled NO is able to reverse HPV,[62] but HPV is dependent on both alveolar and mixed venous PO_2, and inhaled NO actually may gain access to relatively underventilated areas.[63,64]

Cellular Physiology

The cellular mechanism underlying the constriction of small muscular pulmonary arteries has attracted interest because of the importance of HPV in maintaining oxygenation when there is $\dot{V}_A/\dot{Q}$ mismatch and because of its role in the development of chronic pulmonary artery hypertension, as well as because of the more general problem of the molecular mechanisms of O_2-mediated signal transduction (e.g., carotid body hypoxic chemosensitivity). The vasoconstriction from hypoxia is primarily in the small pulmonary arteries, but there is also constriction in other small pulmonary vessels.[65] Although it is alveolar hypoxia that is the primary stimulus, decreases in mixed venous O_2 will also cause general pulmonary artery vasoconstriction that can overcome the more regional response.[66]

HPV occurs rapidly (within seconds), but the full response occurs in two phases. The initial phase is localized solely in the vascular smooth muscle and does not require the vascular endothelium. This constriction peaks quickly and then declines while phase 2 develops.[67,68] The sustained phase 2 response, which gradually increases over several minutes, however, does require constrictor factors derived from the endothelium.[69] These endothelium-derived factors include both vasodilators and constrictors, but they appear to be modulators of the response and not instigators of HPV.[67] There have been several good recent reviews of the mechanisms of HPV.[70–72]

Recently, there has been interest in the role of voltage-gated K^+ channels in pulmonary artery smooth muscle as an important element in O_2 sensing and transduction.[73,74] A current hypothesis is that hypoxia inhibits K^+ channels, resulting in depolarization of the smooth muscle cell. There are several classes of K^+ channels, but the voltage-gated K_v channels appear to be the ones most likely to be involved.[75] These channels have four α-subunits and may be associated with accessory β-subunits. Either monomeric or heteromeric channels can be formed from α-subunit isomers, but not all are functional or sensitive to O_2. Some forms require an accessory β-subunit to confer O_2 sensitivity. The actual coupling of the hypoxic signal to the closing of the K^+ channel may involve a heme protein that contains an NADPH oxidase-generating reactive O_2 species; but there is also evidence against this and there are several other current theories.[75,76] The hypoxic-induced closure of the K^+ channel causes depolarization, which results in the activation of voltage-gated Ca^{2+} channels. The entry of Ca^{2+} into the cell then triggers muscle contraction.[77–79] Figure 20–5 illustrates the possible cellular mechanisms for HPV. However, there is also evidence that hypoxia releases Ca^{2+} from intracellu-

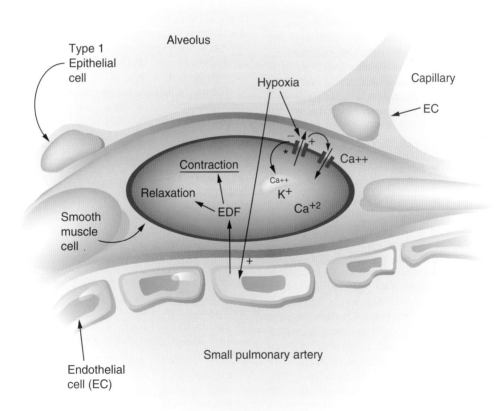

Figure 20–5. Illustration of possible mechanism for hypoxic pulmonary vasoconstriction (HPV). Alveolar hypoxia (or mixed venous hypoxemia, not illustrated) inhibits K^+ channels and hence efflux of K^+ in the small pulmonary artery smooth muscle cells. This inhibition causes depolarization and opening of voltage-dependent Ca^{2+} channels (represented by the *arrow* between the K^+ and the Ca^{2+} channels). The resulting increase in intracellular Ca^{2+} causes myosin light chain phosphorylation resulting in contraction of the smooth muscle cell. Hypoxia also acts on endothelial cells resulting in release of endothelial-derived factors (EDF) that sustain the contraction but also modulate the contraction by either inhibition or potentiation of HPV.

lar stores without the presence of endothelium. A recent study by Dipp et al.[69] indicated that HPV may not require the opening of plasmalemma voltage-gated Ca^{2+} channels. Both these mechanisms may be part of the total response making up HPV.[68]

Interestingly, O_2-sensitive K^+ channels may also be involved in the chemosensitivity of the carotid body[80]; this chemosensitivity is markedly depressed by inhalational anesthetics as is HPV. There could be a common mechanism of action of inhalational anesthetics on the K^+ channels in the carotid body type 1 glomus cells and the pulmonary smooth muscle.

Control of Breathing

To maintain cellular CO_2, O_2, and H^+ homeostasis during all sorts of activity and emotional states, the human body makes use of two ventilatory control systems: the chemical control of breathing and the behavioral control of breathing.[81] Chemical control of breathing indicates that ventilation is critically dependent on arterial and brain tissue PO_2, PCO_2, and pH and involves two sets of chemoreceptors: the peripheral chemoreceptors located in the carotid bodies at the bifurcation of the carotid artery, and the central chemoreceptors located in the ventral medulla. The peripheral chemoreceptors cause an increase in afferent input to the respiratory centers in the brain stem when perfused with hypoxic, hypercapnic, or acidotic arterial blood; the central chemoreceptors are sensitive to brain tissue hypercapnia and acidosis. Whereas hypoxia, hypercapnia, and acidosis cause brisk ventilatory responses, hyperoxia, hypocapnia, and alkalosis have variable depressant effects on respiration depending on the circumstances; for example, when hypocapnic, behavioral control, at least in the awake state, prevents the occurrence of hypopnea/apnea and irregular breathing. The efferent pathways involved constitute spinal respiratory motoneurons, phrenic nerves, intercostal nerves, neuromuscular junctions, the diaphragm, intercostals muscles, lungs, and airways. Pure chemical control of breathing is operable predominantly during non–rapid eye movement sleep and anesthesia. Otherwise, behavioral control of breathing is active. This control system receives input from different sites (e.g., cortical and subcortical regions, hypothalamus, proprioceptors, nociceptors) and affects respiration either by direct control of respiratory motoneurons (i.e., corticospinal control of respiration) or by modulation of respiratory centers in the brain stem through the reticular system.[82] Behavioral control may inhibit, override, or enhance chemical control, optimizing breathing to our needs (allowing respiratory adaptations so we can exercise, sleep and dream, eat, sing, play a musical instrument, dive, and so on). However, the behavioral control system is second in command and chemical control will eventually determine the pattern of breathing without any voluntary action able to suppress breathing activity. An example of the latter is the diver who has lost all O_2 reserves. When sufficiently asphyxic (i.e., the combination of hypoxia and hypercapnia), the chemical control system will force the diver to breathe even if this causes inhalation of water.

Hypoxia

Ventilatory Response to Short-Term Hypoxia

Because the O_2 reserves in the body are limited (lasting no longer than 3 minutes), when hypoxic, the body responds within seconds with an increase in ventilation directed at an increase in O_2 uptake and restoration of the O_2 level in the body. These compensatory ventilatory adjustments originate at the peripheral chemoreceptors of the carotid bodies.[83] The magnitude of the acute hypoxic ventilatory response depends on the depth of hypoxia, and is highly variable among humans. Experimental studies indicate that the slope of the linear relationship between ventilation and isocapnic (i.e., endtidal CO_2 kept constant throughout the hypoxic exposure) hypoxia in terms of arterial hemoglobin-O_2 saturation (S_pO_2) varies between 0.2 and 3.0 L/min per percent desaturation among subjects.[84] When isocapnia is not maintained (i.e., poikilocapnia), the ventilatory response is much smaller (0 to 0.5 L/min per % desaturation). Note that neonates lack a well-developed hyperventilatory response to hypoxia.

The O_2 sensing in the peripheral chemoreceptors is a complex process that is not well understood. Chemoreceptor tissue is composed of two cell types: type I (glomus) and type II cells. Type I cells are of neural origin and are most probably the site of O_2 sensing and cause the release of neurotransmitters (e.g., ACh, substance P, norepinephrine, dopamine, enkephalins) in response to hypoxia.[85] These neurotransmitters activate, either directly or indirectly through other carotid body cells (glomus cells interconnect through gap junctions), the sinus nerve, which connects the carotid bodies to the brain. Type II are supportive cells resembling glial cells. There are two main hypotheses for the O_2 sensing/neurotransmitters release mechanism. The first hypothesis suggests the involvement of glomus cell mitochondrial or nonmitochondrial heme-containing enzymes. The enzymatic activity of these enzymes depends on O_2 availability.[85] The other hypothesis suggests the involvement of K^+ channels.[6] Hypoxia and acidosis inhibit outward potassium currents and increases the membrane potential. Interestingly, it was recently shown that 1.5% halothane (a profound depressant of the ventilatory response to hypoxia at the carotid bodies)[87] increased O_2-sensitive K^+ current in TASK-1 background K^+ channels of type I glomus cells.[86] It is possible that both mechanisms are operational although at different levels of hypoxia.

Ventilatory Response to Sustained Hypoxia

When hypoxia persists from more than 2 to 5 minutes, there is a slow decline in ventilation (hypoxic ventilatory decline [HVD]). A new steady-state is reached after 15 to 20 minutes (time constant of the ventilatory roll-off is 3 to 4 minutes),[87,88] with ventilation still 25% greater than normoxic baseline. In adults, HVD takes away about 40% to 60% of the hypoxic drive of the carotid bodies. Because this mechanism is operable in neonates and they possess little to no peripheral hypoxic drive, neonates may respond with severe hypoventilation and possibly even apnea to hypoxia.[89] The mechanism(s) and site(s) of generation of HVD in awake humans remain poorly understood. There are several possibilities: (1) an exclusive peripheral mechanism (e.g., adaptation of the carotid bodies); (2) a selective effect of central hypoxia; or (3) the central modulation of the peripheral drive from the carotid bodies into HVD. Recent animal and human studies indicate that the second and third factors are responsible for the development of HVD. During mild hypoxia, a hypoxia-induced increase in brain blood flow causes the washout of acid metabolites (CO_2, H^+, or both) from the brain compartment and consequently a reduction of CO_2 drive of the central chemoreceptors.[90] In awake humans, there is a decrease in the gradient between jugular venous and arterial P_{CO_2} of ~2 torr,[91] which, taking into account the slope of the hypercapnic ventilatory response (see later), may be sufficient for 15% to 30% of HVD. At deeper levels of hypoxia (S_pO_2 60–85%), the central accumulation of inhibitory neuromodulators/transmitters such as adenosine, γ-aminobutyric acid (GABA), or dopamine during central hypoxia may cause a net inhibitory effect on the respiratory neuronal pool in the brain stem.[89] The relatively slow turnover of these substances after the relief of hypoxia may explain the persistent reduction of hypoxic ventilatory responses after 20-minute hypoxic exposures (Fig. 20–6, *middle*), which needs at least 1 hour to wane.[92–94] Interestingly, in awake humans, central hypoxia in the absence of a hypoxic drive from the carotid bodies (either caused by infusion of low-dose dopamine, which silences the carotid bodies, or by bilateral removal of the carotid bodies; Fig. 20–6, *bottom*) is unable to generate HVD.[94–96] This indicates that the increased peripheral input during hypoxia activated the buildup of inhibitory agents in the central nervous system. Animal studies show that carotid body stimulation caused by hypoxia or hypercapnia causes the increase of glutamate (a stimulatory neurotransmitter) in respiratory centers in the central nervous system.[97–99] Glutamate serves as the precursor of GABA and conversion of glutamate into GABA during sustained hypoxia may cause a net inhibitory effect on ventilation (i.e., HVD). This mechanism not only explains the lack of HVD in carotid body resected subjects but also the observation that the magnitude of HVD is proportional to the magnitude of the acute ventilatory response to hypoxia. During deep hypoxia ($S_pO_2 <$ 50%), the acute lack of O_2 because of an impaired O_2 flux (at mild and moderate hypoxia the O_2 flux is often maintained or only modestly effected) may cause direct neuronal dysfunction or the intracellular accumulation of acid metabolites (e.g., lactic acid) and consequently hypoventilation.[89]

Ventilatory Response to Hyperoxia

High inspired concentrations of O_2 cause an initial small reduction in ventilation caused by depression (but not silencing) of the carotid bodies. The magnitude of depression of the carotid bodies by hyperoxia is variable and may range from no depression in some persons to 70% depression in others.[100,101] Next, ventilation increases slowly. The magnitude of hyperoxia-induced ventilatory stimulation is dependent on the O_2 concentration and may be as great as 20 to 30 L/min during isocapnic conditions, but significantly less

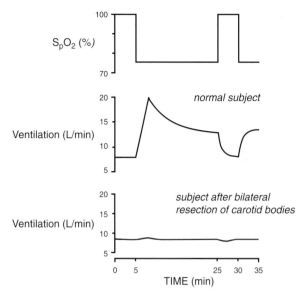

Figure 20–6. Influence of two bouts of hypoxia in a healthy (normal) subject (*middle*) and a subject 2 years after bilateral removal of the carotid bodies (*bottom*). *Top,* The two hypoxic events. Initially, the subjects breath 5 minutes of a normoxic gas mixture, followed by 20 minutes of hypoxia (S_pO_2 75%), 5 minutes of normoxia, and the reintroduction of hypoxia (S_pO_2 75%). The healthy subject shows a biphasic ventilatory response: an initial increase caused by activation of the peripheral chemoreceptors is followed by a slow ventilatory decline caused by the development of central hypoxic depression. A steady-state in ventilation is reached after ~15 minutes. Reintroduction of hypoxia causes a second ventilatory response that is about 50% of the first response. The subject after bilateral removal of both carotid bodies shows the absence of an acute hyperventilatory response and consequently absence of a slow ventilatory decline. Afferent input from the carotid bodies is needed for the central development of hypoxic depression of ventilation.

during poikilocapnic conditions (as exists in perioperative patients).[102] The mechanism of hyperoxic hyperventilation is the central release of excitatory agents during hyperoxia (glutamate, NO, or both).[103,104]

Anesthetics, Analgesics, and the Ventilatory Response to Hypoxia

Because anesthetics and analgesics act at specific receptors in the peripheral and central nervous system and integrity of the ventilatory control system is dependent on many of these receptors and their endogenous ligands, it is not surprising that agents commonly used to induce anesthesia and analgesia may affect ventilation and the ventilatory responses to acute and sustained hypoxia. Already at subanesthetic doses, inhalational anesthetics (halothane, enflurane, isoflurane, sevoflurane, and desflurane: 0.05–0.2 minimum alveolar concentration)[84,87,105–109] and intravenous anesthetics (propofol: 500–1500 ng/mL blood concentration)[110] reduce the magnitude of the acute response to hypoxia, whereas halothane, propofol, and midazolam enhance the magnitude of the slow ventilatory decline during sustained hypoxia.[105,110,111] Recent studies indicate that high-dose inhalational anesthetics cause a reduction in respiratory drive of expiratory neurons in the brain stem through reduction of glutamatergic excitatory mechanisms and enhancement of GABAergic inhibition.[112] Furthermore, anesthetic concentrations of halothane affect TASK-1 background K^+ channels in the central nervous system and carotid bodies (see earlier).[86] The mechanism of carotid body depression from low-dose inhalational anesthetics remains unknown but is probably related to anesthetic action at background K^+ channels in the cell membrane of type I glomus cells.[86]

In humans, opioids affect the hypoxic drive from the carotid bodies through sex-dependent mechanisms.[113,114] This is not surprising taking into account that opioid receptors and endogenous opioid peptides are found in high concentrations in areas of the central and peripheral nervous system that play a role in the control of breathing, and the observation of sex differences in opioid analgesia.[115–118] In humans, morphine tends to be the more potent analgesic and respiratory depressant in women, an observation related to morphine's pharmacodynamics and not its pharmacokinetics.[113,114,118] Recent studies in μ-opioid receptor knockout mice indicate the involvement of non–μ-opioid receptors in the modulation of respiratory frequency and the μ-opioid receptor as molecular site of morphine respiratory and antinociceptive effects.[119]

The loss or severe reduction of the hypoxic drive from the carotid bodies is clinically important. Recurrent hypoxic events are common in the perioperative period, especially during the first few postoperative nights.[120] This is partly because of a reduced ventilatory drive from analgesic and residual anesthetics and partly because of upper airway obstruction. The arousal needed to overcome upper airway obstruction is partly mediated and dependent on effective functioning of the peripheral chemoreceptors at the carotid bodies.[121] In comparison to healthy subjects, patients under anesthesia (or just after anesthesia) require much deeper levels of hypoxia to activate the carotid bodies (compare animal data).[122,123] This may be especially important in patients with a history of nightly upper airway obstructions (e.g., obese patients, patients with obstructive sleep apnea, the elderly). Deep hypoxic events may be an important cause of postoperative morbidity and mortality.

Hypercapnia

Ventilatory Response to Carbon Dioxide

The ventilatory response to inhaled CO_2 (hypercapnic ventilatory response [HCVR]) is a sensitive tool to examine the effects of drugs on ventilatory control. At CO_2 levels above resting, there is a linear relationship between CO_2 and ventilation with a slope of 0.3 to 3.0 L/min per torr increase in endtidal PCO_2 among tested volunteer subjects.[88,100] Below resting values, the response curve is flat because of behavioral control influences not allowing hypopnea or apnea even at extreme hypocapnia (i.e., the *wakefulness drive*; Fig. 20–7). There are various techniques to determine the slope of the HCVR. Non–steady-state methods, such as Read's rebreathing technique, use the rebreathing of CO_2 from a 6- to 8 L-bag filled with O_2 and 7% CO_2.[124] Although this tech-

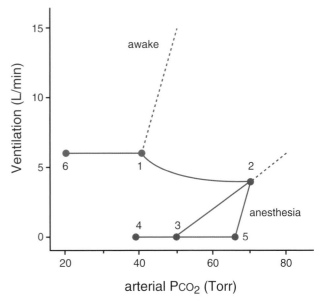

Figure 20–7. Influence of hypocapnia on ventilation in the awake state (red) and during anesthesia-induced loss of consciousness (blue). *1,* Awake; *2,* just after induction of general anesthesia; *3,* initial hypocapnia during anesthesia = apneic threshold; *4,* further hypocapnia; *5,* point at which ventilation resumes during/after anesthesia; *6,* hypocapnia awake. *Dotted lines* depict the effect of added CO_2 on ventilation in awake (red) and anesthetized (blue) patients. Note that the slope of the hypercapnic ventilatory response (HCVR) during anesthesia is depressed relative to the awake state. Induction of anesthesia and recovery will cause the following sequence: 1—2—3—4—5—2—1. The effect of hypocapnia in the awake state (i.e., the *wakefulness drive* or the dog leg of the HCVR) is represented by the line from *1* to *6.*

nique is easy to use its results are often hard to interpret.[88,125] More reliable are steady-state and dynamic endtidal CO_2-forcing (DEF) techniques.[88,100] The former technique uses the inhalation of fixed endtidal or inspired concentrations of CO_2. Next, an appreciable amount of time is allowed to elapse before ventilation reaches a steady-state that may be between 5 minutes (in case of inhalation of a fixed endtidal concentration) and 20 to 40 minutes (in case of inhalation of a fixed inspired concentration) and one measurement point is taken. Three to five data points are needed for a reliable estimate of the slope of the HCVR. The DEF technique uses rapid increases and decreases in endtidal PCO_2 and the simultaneous measurement of breath-to-breath ventilation. Using a mathematic model of the ventilatory control system, it gives a reliable assessment of the steady-state CO_2 sensitivity and estimates of the CO_2 sensitivities of the peripheral and central chemoreceptors.[87,88,95,100] Using DEF, it was observed that about 30% of the ventilatory drive from CO_2 originates at the carotid bodies, whereas 70% is of central origin, and it was also observed that there is a synergistic O_2-CO_2 interaction at the carotid bodies (hypoxia augments the slope of the peripheral ventilatory CO_2 response).[100] Other factors that influence the peripheral and central components of the HCVR are given in Table 20–2.

Anesthesia-induced loss of consciousness results in the loss of the flat part of the HCVR and a severe reduction of

TABLE 20–2.

Factors Affecting Peripheral and Central Ventilatory Carbon Dioxide Sensitivity

Independent Factor	Peripheral CO_2 Response	Central CO_2 Response
FiO$_2$		
Hypoxia	↑	=
Hyperoxia	↓	=
Disease		
Hypothyroidism	↓	↓
Fever	=	↓
Artificial ventilation	↓	↓
Carotid body resection	↓	↓
Drugs		
Dopamine	↓	=
Almitrine	↑	=
Opioids (e.g., morphine)	↓*	↓
Tramadol†	=	↓
Low dose inhalational	↓	=
Anesthetics‡		
High dose inhalational anesthetics	↓	↓
Nitrous oxide	=	=
Benzodiazepines	=	↓
Low and high dose propofol	↓	↓
Ketamine†	↓	↓

↓, indicates a decrease in ventilatory CO_2 sensitivity; ↑, indicates an increase in ventilatory CO_2 sensitivity.
*Sex-dependent effect with more depression in women relative to men.
†Partially dependent on activation of μ-opioid receptors.
‡Less than 0.3 minimum alveolar concentration.

the slope of the HCVR. Now, hypocapnia (induced by the anesthesiologist or caused by anxiety-related hyperventilation) will cause immediate apnea (see Fig. 20–7). Apnea occurs at arterial PCO$_2$ levels below the so-called apneic threshold. Note PCO$_2$ values much greater than the apneic threshold are needed to restart respiratory activity (Fig. 20–2).[126] The delay in the postoperative initiation of respiration is often related to the relative hypocapnia induced by mechanical ventilation during general anesthesia. This hypocapnia is relative to the right-shifted CO$_2$ response curve and right-shifted apneic threshold (see Fig. 20–7).

Pain

Noxious stimulation modulates the ventilatory control system. Pain and surgical stimulation act as respiratory stim-ulants in the awake, sedated, and anesthetized states, causing a chemoreflex-independent tonic drive.[127–129] In other words, pain is unable to reverse *anesthetic*-induced impairment of chemoreflex-related responses. However, from a clinical viewpoint, all that matters is whether a patient maintains an adequate minute ventilation. Because pain increases ventilatory drive it may be able to offset the anesthetic-induced loss of chemoreceptor drive. The respiratory effects of the pharmacologic treatment of patients with acute or chronic pain should therefore always be viewed as the balance between the stimulatory effects of pain and the depressant effects of the agents used to treat pain. For example, the removal of pain by regional anesthesia may be dangerous for patients with acute pain initially treated with opioids. Indeed, there are several reports showing profound and life-threatening respiratory depression when regional anesthesia causes the relief of pain in patients treated with opioids.[130] That is, patients in pain tolerate larger doses of opioids than those without pain.

References

1. Kuna ST, Insalaco G, Woodson GE: Thyroarytenoid muscle activity during wakefulness and sleep in normal adults. J Appl Physiol 65:1332, 1988.
2. Mizuno M: Human respiratory muscles: Fibre morphology and capillary supply. Eur Respir J 4:587, 1991.
3. Gea JG. Myosin gene expression in the respiratory muscles. Eur Respir J 10:2404, 1997.
4. Powers SK, Coombes J, Demirel H: Exercise training-induced changes in respiratory muscles. Sports Med 24:120, 1997.
5. Widdicombe JH, Widdicombe JG: Regulation of human airway surface liquid. Respir Physiol 99:3, 1995.
6. Rogers DF: Airway goblet cells: Responsive and adaptable frontline defenders. Eur Respir J 7:1690, 1994.
7. King M, Rubin BK: Mucous controlling agents: Past and present. Respir Care Clin N Am 5:575, 1999.
8. Steiger DJ, Bajaj L, Omori H, et al: Endotoxin induces mucin gene activation in rat airways. Am Rev Respir Dis 147S:A437, 1993.
9. Barnes PJ: Molecular mechanisms of glucocorticoid action in asthma. Pulm Pharmacol Ther 10:3, 1997.
10. Kai H, Yoshitake K, Hisatsune A, et al: Dexamethasone suppresses mucus production and MUC-2 and MUC-5AC gene expression by NCI-H292 cells. Am J Physiol 271:L484, 1996.
11. Widdicombe JG: Afferent receptors in the airways and cough. Respir Physiol 114:5, 1998.
12. Lumb AB: Nunn's Applied Respiratory Physiology, 5th ed. Oxford: Butterworth-Heinemann, 2000.
13. Thirstrup S: Control of airway smooth muscle tone. I: Electrophysiology and contractile mediators. Respir Med 94:328, 2000.
14. Fryer AD, Jacoby DB: Muscarinic receptors and control of airway smooth muscle. Am J Respir Crit Care Med 158:S154, 1998.
15. Jacoby DB, Fryer AD: Interaction of viral infections with muscarinic receptors. Clin Exp Allergy 29(Suppl 2):59, 1999.
16. Widdicombe JG: Autonomic regulation. i-NANC/e-NANC. Am J Respir Crit Care Med 158:S171, 1998.
17. van der Velden VHJ, Hulsmann AR: Autonomic function of human airways: Structure, function, and pathophysiology in asthma. Neuroimmunomodulation 6:145, 1999.
18. Mackay TW, Fitzpatrick MF, Douglas NJ: Non-adrenergic, non-cholinergic nervous system and overnight airway calibre in asthmatic and normal subjects. Lancet 338:1289, 1991.
19. Folkerts G, Busse WW, Nijkamp FP, et al: Virus-induced airway hyperresponsiveness and asthma. Am J Respir Crit Care Med 157:1708, 1998.

20. Reynolds PN, Holmes MD, Scicchitano R: Role of tachykinins in bronchial hyper-reponsiveness. Clin Exp Pharmacol Physiol 24:273, 1997.

21. Barnes PJ: Pharmacology of airway smooth muscle. Am J Respir Crit Care Med 158:S123, 1998.

22. van der Velden VHJ: Glucocorticoids: Mechanisms of action and anti-inflammatory potential in asthma. Mediators Inflamm 7:229, 1998.

23. Johnson M: The β-adrenoceptor. Am J Respir Crit Care Med 158:S146, 1998.

24. McGraw DW, Liggett SB: Heterogeneity in β-adrenergic receptor kinase expression in the lung accounts for cell-specific desensitization of the β2-adrenergic receptor. J Biol Chem 272:7338, 1997.

25. Thirstrup S: Control of airway smooth muscle tone: II. Pharmacology of relaxation. Respir Med 94:519, 2000.

26. Aranson R, Rau JL: The evolution of beta-agonists. Respir Care Clin N Am 5:479, 1999.

27. Reishaus E, Innis M, MacIntyre N, et al: Mutations in the gene encoding for the β2-adrenergic receptor in normal and asthmatic subjects. Am J Respir Cell Mol Biol 8:334, 1993.

28. Betticher DC, Reinhart WH, Geiser J: Effect of RBC shape and deformability on pulmonary O_2 diffusing capacity and resistance to flow in rabbit lungs. J Appl Physiol 78:778, 1995.

29. Hamm H, Kroegel C, Hohlfeld J: Surfactant: A review of its functions and relevance in adult respiratory disorders. Respir Med 90:251, 1996.

30. Rodriguez RJ, Martin RJ: Exogenous surfactant therapy in newborns. Respir Care Clin N Am 5:595, 1999.

31. Bendixen HH, Hedley-Whyte J, Laver MB: Impaired oxygenation in surgical patients during general anesthesia with controlled ventilation. N Engl J Med 269:991, 1963.

32. Nunn JF, Bergman NA, Coleman AJ, et al: Factors influencing the arterial oxygen tension during anaesthesia with artificial ventilation. Br J Anaesth 37:898, 1965.

33. Möller JT, Johannessen NW, Espersen K, et al: Randomized evaluation of pulse oximetry in 20,802 patients: II. Perioperative events and postoperative complications. Anesthesiology 78:445, 1993.

34. Möller JT, Wittrup M, Johansen SH: Hypoxemia in the postanesthesia care unit: An observer study. Anesthesiology 73:890, 1990.

35. Tobin MJ: Advances in mechanical ventilation. N Engl J Med 344:1986, 2001.

36. Bigatello LM, Zapol WM: New approaches to acute lung injury. Br J Anaesth 77:99, 1996.

37. Treacher DF, Leach RM: Oxygen transport-1: Basic principles. Br Med J 317:1302, 1998.

38. Lumb AB: Nunn's Applied Respiratory Physiology, 5th ed. Oxford, Butterworth-Heinemann, 2000.

39. Mania JN: Comparative respiratory morphology: Themes and principles in the design and construction of the gas exchangers. Anat Rec 261:25, 2000.

40. West JB, Hackett PH, Maret KH, et al: Pulmonary gas exchange on the summit of Mount Everest. J Appl Physiol 55:678, 1983.

41. West JB, Wagner PD: Pulmonary gas exchange. Am J Respir Crit Care Med 157:S82, 1998.

42. Fenn WO, Otis AB, Rahn H: A theoretical study of the composition of the alveolar air at altitude. Am J Physiol 146:653, 1946.

43. Whipp B, Wasserman K: Alveolar-arterial gas tension differences during graded exercise. J Appl Physiol 27:361, 1969.

44. Marshall C, Marshall B: Site and sensitivity for stimulation of hypoxic pulmonary vasoconstriction. J Appl Physiol 55:711, 1983.

45. Brismar B, Hedenstierna G, Lundquist H, et al: Pulmonary densities during anesthesia with muscular relaxation—a proposal of atelectasis. Anesthesiology 62:422, 1985.

46. Wahba RM: Airway closure and intraoperative hypoxaemia: Twenty-five years later. Can J Anaesth 43:1144, 1996.

47. Rothen HU, Sporre B, Engberg G, et al: Airway closure, atelectasis and gas exchange during general anaesthesia. Br J Anaesth 81:681, 1998.

48. Hedenstierna G, Strandberg A, Brismar B, et al: Functional residual capacity, thoracoabdominal dimensions, and central blood volume during general anesthesia with muscle paralysis and mechanical ventilation. Anesthesiology 62:247, 1985.

49. Warner DO, Warner MA, Ritman EL: Atelectasis and chest wall shape during halothane anesthesia. Anesthesiology 85:49, 1996.

50. Nunn JF: Effects of anaesthesia on respiration. Br J Anaesth 65:54, 1990.

51. Domino KB, Borowec L, Alexander CM, et al: Influence of isoflurane on hypoxic pulmonary vasoconstriction in dogs. Anesthesiology 64:423, 1986.

52. Eisenkraft JB: Effects of anaesthetics on the pulmonary circulation. Br J Anaesth 65:63, 1990.

53. Gunnarsson L, Strandberg A, Brismar B, et al: Atelectasis and gas exchange impairment during enflurane/nitrous oxide anaesthesia. Acta Anaesthesiol Scand 33:629, 1989.

54. Tokics L, Hedenstierna G, Svensson L, et al: V/Q distribution and correlation to atelectasis in anesthetized paralyzed humans. J Appl Physiol 81:1822, 1996.

55. Dantzker DR, Wagner PD, West JB: Instability of lung units with low VA/Q ratios during O2 breathing. J Appl Physiol 38:886, 1975.

56. Marshall C, Lindgren L, Marshall BE: Effects of halothane, enflurane, and isoflurane on hypoxic pulmonary vasoconstriction in rat lungs in vitro. Anesthesiology 60:304, 1984.

57. Benumof JL: Isoflurane anesthesia and arterial oxygenation during one-lung ventilation. Anesthesiology 64:419, 1986.

58. Benumof JL, Augustine SD, Gibbons JA: Halothane and isoflurane only slightly impair arterial oxygenation during one-lung ventilation in patients undergoing thoracotomy. Anesthesiology 67:910, 1987.

59. Conacher ID: 2000—time to apply Occam's razor to failure of hypoxic pulmonary vasoconstriction during one lung ventilation. Br J Anaesth 84:434, 2000.

60. Steudel W, Hurford WE, Zapol WM: Inhaled nitric oxide: Basic biology and clinical applications. Anesthesiology 91:1090, 1999.

61. Ullrich R, Bloch KD, Ichinose F, et al: Hypoxic pulmonary blood flow redistribution and arterial oxygenation in endotoxin-challenged NOS2-deficient mice. J Clin Invest 104:1421, 1999.

62. Frostell CG, Blomqvist H, Hedenstierna G, et al: Inhaled nitric oxide selectively reverses human hypoxic pulmonary vasoconstriction without causing systemic vasodilation. Anesthesiology 78:427, 1993.

63. Marshall BE, Marshall C: The influence of nitric oxide in adult respiratory distress syndrome when Pv(O2) is varied. Anesthesiology 86:1228, 1997.

64. Benzing A, Mols G, Brieschal T, et al: Hypoxic pulmonary vasoconstriction in nonventilated lung areas contributes to differences in hemodynamic and gas exchange responses to inhalation of nitric oxide. Anesthesiology 86:1254, 1997.

65. Hillier SC, Graham JA, Hanger CC, et al: Hypoxic vasoconstriction in pulmonary arterioles and venules. J Appl Physiol 82:1084, 1997.

66. Pellett AA, Cairo JM, Levitzky MG: Hypoxemia and hypoxic pulmonary vasoconstriction: Autonomic nervous system versus mixed venous PO2. Respir Physiol 109:249, 1997.

67. Ward JP, Robertson TP: The role of the endothelium in hypoxic pulmonary vasoconstriction. Exp Physiol 80:793, 1995.

68. Weissmann N, Grimminger F, Olschewski A, et al: Hypoxic pulmonary vasoconstriction: A multifactorial response? Am J Physiol Lung Cell Mol Physiol 281:L314, 2001.

69. Dipp M, Nye PC, Evans AM: Hypoxic release of calcium from the sarcoplasmic reticulum of pulmonary artery smooth muscle. Am J Physiol Lung Cell Mol Physiol 281:L318, 2001.

70. Weir EK, Archer SL: The mechanism of acute hypoxic pulmonary vasoconstriction: The tale of two channels. FASEB J 9:183, 1995.

71. Ward JP, Aaronson PI: Mechanisms of hypoxic pulmonary vasoconstriction: Can anyone be right? Respir Physiol 115:261, 1999.

72. Dumas JP, Bardou M, Goirand F, et al: Hypoxic pulmonary vasoconstriction. Gen Pharmacol 33:289, 1999.

73. Osipenko ON, Tate RJ, Gurney AM: Potential role for kv3.1b channels as oxygen sensors. Circ Res 86:534, 2000.

74. Perez-Garcia MT, Lopez-Lopez JR: Are Kv channels the essence of O2 sensing? Circ Res 86:490, 2000.

75. Coppock EA, Martens JR, Tamkun MM: Molecular basis of hypoxia-induced pulmonary vasoconstriction: Role of voltage-gated K+ channels. Am J Physiol Lung Cell Mol Physiol 281:L1, 2001.

76. Archer SL, Weir EK, Reeve HL, et al: Molecular identification of O2 sensors and O2-sensitive potassium channels in the pulmonary circulation. Adv Exp Med Biol 475:219, 2000.

77. Barman SA: Potassium channels modulate hypoxic pulmonary vasoconstriction. Am J Physiol 275:L64, 1998.

78. McCulloch KM, Osipenko ON, Gurney AM: Oxygen-sensing potassium currents in pulmonary artery. Gen Pharmacol 32:403, 1999.

79. Post JM, Hume JR, Archer SL, et al: Direct role for potassium channel inhibition in hypoxic pulmonary vasoconstriction. Am J Physiol 262:C882, 1992.

80. Gonzalez C, Lopez-Lopez JR, Obeso A, et al: Cellular mechanisms of oxygen chemoreception in the carotid body. Respir Physiol 102:137, 1995.

81. von Euler C: Brain stem mechanisms for generation and control of breathing pattern. In Fishman AP, Cherniack NS, Widdicombe JG, Geiger SR (eds): Handbook of Physiology, vol II, Control of Breathing. Bethesda, American Physiological Society, 1986.

82. Orem J, Trotter RH: Behavioral control of breathing. News Physiol Sci 9:228, 1994.

83. Vizek M, Picket CK, Weil JV: Biphasic ventilatory response of adult cats to sustained hypoxia has central origin. J Appl Physiol 63:1659, 1987.

84. Dahan A, Sarton E, van den Elsen M, et al: Ventilatory response to hypoxia: Influence of subanesthetic desflurane. Anesthesiology 85:60, 1996.

85. Prabhakar NR: Oxygen sensing by the carotid body chemoreceptors. J Appl Physiol 88:2287, 2000.

86. Buckler KJ, Williams BA, Honore E: An oxygen-, acid- and anaesthetic-sensitive TASK-like background potassium channel in rat arterial chemoreceptor cells. J Physiol 525:135, 2000.

87. Dahan A, van den Elsen E, Berkenbosch A, et al: Effects of subanesthetic halothane on the ventilatory responses to hypercapnia and acute hypoxia in healthy volunteers. Anesthesiology 80:727, 1994.

88. Dahan A: The ventilatory response to carbon dioxide and oxygen in man: Methods and implications [PhD thesis]. Leiden, Leiden University, 1990.

89. Neubauer JA, Melton JE, Edelman NH: Modulation of respiration during brain hypoxia. J Appl Physiol 68:441, 1990.

90. Ward DS, Berkenbosch A, DeGoede J, et al: Dynamics of the ventilatory response to central hypoxia in cats. J Appl Physiol 68:1107, 1990.

91. Suzuki A, Nishimura M, Yamamoto K, et al: No effect of brain blood flow on ventilatory depression during sustained hypoxia. J Appl Physiol 68:1674, 1989.

92. Easton PA, Slykerman LJ, Anthonisen NR: Recovery of the ventilatory response to hypoxia in normal adults. J Appl Physiol 64:521, 1988.

93. Berkenbosch A, Dahan A, DeGoede J, et al: The ventilatory response to CO2 of the peripheral and central chemoreflex loop before and after sustained hypoxia in man. J Physiol 456:71, 1992.

94. Dahan A, Ward DS, van den Elsen M, et al: Influence of reduced carotid body drive during sustained hypoxia on hypoxic depression of ventilation in humans. J Appl Physiol 81:565, 1996.

95. Fatemian M, Dahan A, Meinesz S, et al: Modelling the ventilatory response to variations in endtidal PO2 inpatients who have undergone bilateral carotid body resection. In Poon CS, Kazemi H, (eds): Frontiers in Modeling and Control of Breathing: Integration at Molecular, Cellular and Systems Levels. Dordrecht, Kluwer Academic/Plenum, 2001.

96. Kimura H, Tanaka M, Nagano K, et al: Possible role of the carotid body responsible for the hypoxic ventilatory decline in awake humans. In Dahan A, Teppema L, van Beek H (eds): Physiology and Pharmacology of Cardio-Respiratory Control. Dordrecht, Kluwer Academic Publishers, 1998.

97. Ang RC, Hoop B, Kazemi H: Role of glutamate as the central neurotransmitter in the hypoxic ventilatory response. J Appl Physiol 71:1480, 1992.

98. Chitravanashi VC, Sapru HN: NMDA as well as non-NMDA receptors in phrenic nucleus mediate respiratory effects of carotid chemoreflex. Am J Physiol 272:R302, 1997.

99. Ohtake PJ, Torres PJ, Gozal YM, et al: NMDA receptors mediate peripheral chemoreceptor afferent input in the conscious rat. J Appl Physiol 84:853, 1998.

100. Dahan A, DeGoede J, Berkenbosch A, et al: The influence of oxygen on the ventilatory response to carbon dioxide in man. J Physiol 428:485, 1989.

101. Pedersen MEF, Fatemian M, Robbins PA: Identification of fast and slow ventilatory responses to carbon dioxide under hypoxic and hyperoxic conditions in humans. J Physiol 521:273, 1999.

102. Becker H, Polo O, McNamara G, et al: Ventilatory response to isocapnic hyperoxia. J Appl Physiol 78:696, 1995.

103. Honda Y: Effect of prior O2 breathing on ventilatory response to sustained hypoxia in adult humans. J Appl Physiol 81:1627, 1996.

104. Gozal D: Potentiation of hypoxic ventilatory response to sustained hypoxia in adult humans. J Appl Physiol 85:129, 1998.

105. Dahan A, van den Elsen M, Berkenbosch A, et al: Influence of a subanesthetic concentration of halothane on the ventilatory response to step changes into and out of sustained isocapnic hypoxia in healthy volunteers. Anesthesiology 81:850, 1994.

106. van den Elsen M, Dahan A, DeGoede J, et al: Influences of subanesthetic isoflurane on ventilatory control in humans. Anesthesiology 83:478, 1995.

107. Sarton E, Dahan A, Teppema L, et al: Acute pain and central nervous system arousal do not restore impaired hypoxic ventilatory response during sevoflurane sedation. Anesthesiology 85:295, 1996.

108. Sarton E, van der Wal M, Nieuwenhuijs D, et al: Sevoflurane-induced reduction of hypoxic drive is sex-independent. Anesthesiology 90:1288, 1999.

109. Nagyova B, Dorrington KL, Robbins PA: Effect of low-dose enflurane on the ventilatory response to hypoxia in humans. Br J Anaesth 72:509, 1994.

110. Nieuwenhuijs D, Sarton E, Teppema L, Dahan A: Propofol for monitored anesthesia care: Implications on hypoxic control of cardiorespiratory responses. Anesthesiology 92:46, 2000.

111. Dahan A, Ward DS: Influence of i.v. midazolam on the ventilatory response to sustained hypoxia in man. Br J Anaesth 66:454, 1991.

112. Stuth EAE, Krolo M, Stucke AG: Effects of halothane on excitatory neurotransmission to medullary neurons in a decerebrate dog model. Anesthesiology 93:1474, 2000.

113. Dahan A, Sarton E, Teppema L, et al: Sex-related differences in the influence of morphine on ventilatory control in humans. Anesthesiology 88:903, 1998.

114. Sarton E, Teppema L, Dahan A: Sex differences in morphine-induced ventilatory depression reside within the peripheral chemoreflex loop. Anesthesiology 90:1329, 1999.

115. McQueen JS, Ribeiro JA: Inhibitory actions of methionine-enkephalin and morphine on the cat carotid chemoreceptor. Br J Pharmacol 71:297, 1980.

116. Shook JE, Watkins WD, Camporesi EM: Differential roles of opioid receptors in respiration, respiratory disease and opiate-induced respiratory depression. Am Rev Respir Dis 142:895, 1990.

117. Gray PA, Rekling JC, Bocchiaro CM, Feldman JL: Modulation of respiratory frequency by peptidergic input to rhythmogenic neurons in the preBötzinger complex. Science 286:156, 1999.

118. Sarton E, Olofsen E, Romberg R, et al: Sex differences in morphine analgesia. Anesthesiology 93:1245, 2000.

119. Dahan A, Sarton E, Teppema L, et al: Anesthetic potency and influence of morphine and sevoflurane on respiration in mu-opioid receptor knockout mice. Anesthesiology, 94:824, 2001.

120. Stone JG, Cozne KA, Wald A: Nocturnal oxygenation during patient-controled analgesia. Anesth Analg 89:104, 1999.

121. Parisi RA, Santiago TV, Edelman NH: Genioglossal and diaphragmatic EMG responses to hypoxia during sleep. Am Rev Respir Dis 138:610, 1988.

122. Ponte J, Sadler CL: Effect of halothane, enflurane and isoflurane on carotid body chemoreceptor activity in the rabbit and the cat. Br J Anaesth 62:33, 1989.

123. Koh SO, Severinghaus JW: Effect of halothane on hypoxic and hypercapnic ventilatory responses of goats. Br J Anaesth 65:713, 1990.

124. Berkenbosch A, Bovill JG, Dahan A, et al: The ventilatory CO2 sensitivities from Read's rebreathing method and the steady-state method are not equal in man. J Physiol 411:367, 1989.

125. Dahan A, Berkenbosch A, DeGoede J, et al: On a pseudo-rebreathing technique to assess the ventilatory response to carbon dioxide in man. J Physiol 423:615, 1990.

126. Nishino T, Kochi T: Effects of surgical stimulation on the apneic threshold for carbon dioxide during anaesthesia with sevoflurane. Br J Anaesth 73:583, 1994.

127. Lam AM, Clement JL, Knill RL: Surgical stimulation does not enhance ventilatory chemoreflexes during enflurane anesthesia in man. Can Anaesth Soc J 27:22, 1980.

128. Rosenberg M, Tobias B, Bourke DL, et al: Respiratory responses to surgical stimulation during enflurane anesthesia. Anesthesiology 52:163, 1983.

129. Sarton E, Dahan A, Teppema L, et al: Acute pain and central nervous system arousal do not restore impaired hypoxic response during sevoflurane sedation. Anesthesiology 85:295, 1996.

130. Hanks GW, Twycross RG, Lloyd JW: Unexpected complications of successful nerve block. Anaesthesia 36:35, 1981.

21

Renal Physiology

Robert Sladen, MBChB, MRCP(UK), FRCP(C)

The kidney is a remarkable organ, the primary defender of the internal milieu, and it lends itself well to an exploration of its physiology from a systemic to molecular level. At the systemic level, this involves an interpretation of the complex "yin and yang" of the opposing processes that regulate vasomotor tone and salt and water metabolism in the renal response to hypovolemia and hypervolemia. At the organ level, a description of the functional anatomy and physiology of the nephron reveals how the kidney is able to mediate these systemic responses. Next, the function of the tubule is highlighted by an outline of the specialized biochemistry of the different types of tubular cell. This physiologic background provides the context for a discussion of current and potential targets of drug action in the kidney, with particular reference to diuretic agents and drugs that might protect the kidney from ischemic or nephrotoxic injury.

Kidney as Defender of the Internal Milieu

The kidney plays an extraordinarily important role in regulating blood pressure, salt, and water homeostasis.[1] Although it is highly metabolically active and receives 20% of the total cardiac output, it extracts relatively little oxygen, therefore the renal arteriovenous oxygen difference $[(a - v)O_2]$ is only 1.5 mL/dL. The primary control mechanism involves complex interactions between opposing reflex systems (Fig. 21–1).[2] A series of vasoconstrictor, salt-retaining systems protect against hypovolemia, hypotension, and hyponatremia. These include the sympathoadrenal axis, the renin-

angiotensin-aldosterone system, and arginine vasopressin (AVP). Opposing these are vasodilator, salt-excreting systems that protect against hypervolemia, hypertension, and hypernatremia, consisting of the prostaglandins, atrial natriuretic peptide (ANP), and endogenous dopamine.

Vasoconstrictor, Salt-Retaining Systems

Sympathoadrenal System

Sympathoadrenal effects are mediated by circulating epinephrine and the release of norepinephrine from sympathetic nerve endings derived from the T12-L4 segments of the spinal cord. Low levels of sympathetic discharge preferentially constrict the efferent arteriole, whereas high levels constrict the afferent arteriole as well. In the afferent arteriole, epinephrine acts on β receptors that promote renin release and the formation of angiotensin II. Sympathetic nerve fibers supply the afferent arteriole (also releasing renin) and the proximal tubule, medullary thick ascending limb of Henle (mTAL) and collecting duct, where they enhance sodium reabsorption.

Renin-Angiotensin System

Angiotensinogen, a glycoprotein synthesized by the liver, enters the afferent arteriole where it is cleaved by renin to angiotensin I, a decapeptide, which is further cleaved by ACE to angiotensin II, an octapeptide (Fig. 21–2).[3] Similar

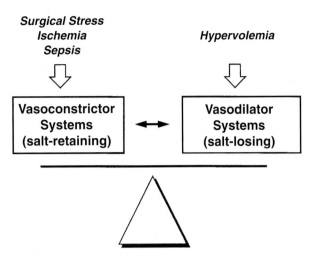

Figure 21-1. Regulating mechanisms in salt and water homeostasis. Neurohormonal regulation of renal function. There is a balance between those systems promoting renal vasoconstriction and sodium retention versus those systems promoting renal vasodilation and sodium excretion. Surgical stress, ischemia, and sepsis tip the balance in favor of vasoconstriction and sodium retention. Hypervolemia (or the induction of atrial stretch) tips the balance in favor of vasodilation and sodium excretion. (From Sladen RN: Renal physiology. In Miller RD (ed): Anesthesia, 5th ed. Philadelphia, Churchill Livingstone, 2000, p 677.)

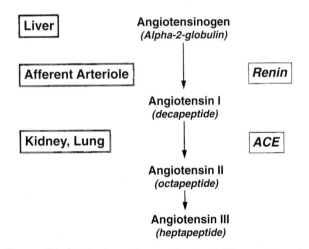

Figure 21-2. Angiotensin synthesis. ACE, angiotensin-coverting enzyme. (From Sladen RN: Renal physiology. In Miller RD (ed): Anesthesia, 5th ed. Philadelphia, Churchill Livingstone, 2000, p 678.)

to catecholamines, low levels of angiotensin II cause preferential efferent arteriolar constriction, whereas high levels constrict the afferent arteriole and the mesangial cells of the glomerulus.

Minute concentrations of angiotensin II are found in the general circulation, but it contributes considerably to systemic arteriolar tone as evidenced by the pronounced antihypertensive effect of drugs that inhibit ACE or antagonize the angiotensin II receptor. In addition, angiotensin II promotes salt and water retention by stimulating the release of aldosterone secretion from the adrenal cortex, stimulating

the release of AVP by the posterior pituitary, and enhancing sodium reabsorption in the proximal tubule.[1]

Aldosterone

Aldosterone is a steroid hormone produced by the zona glomerulosa of the adrenal cortex and is released under the influence of adrenocorticotrophic hormone and angiotensin II. It acts at the distal tubule to cause sodium reabsorption and potassium loss. Its release and actions are opposed by ANP.

Arginine Vasopressin

AVP, previously known as antidiuretic hormone, is a nonapeptide synthesized in the supraoptic and paraventricular nuclei of the anterior hypothalamus and is stored in the posterior pituitary gland prior to its release into the systemic circulation. Hypothalamic osmoreceptors respond to increases in serum osmolality of more than 1% greater than normal and thereby maintain serum osmolality within a narrow range (280–290 mOsm/kg). At a plasma level of only 1 to 5 pg/mL, its antidiuretic action is mediated by specific V_2 receptors in the collecting ducts that induce water reabsorption and a decreased flow of concentrated urine.[4]

Osmotic stimuli to the release of AVP are overridden by intravascular hypovolemia (through venous stretch receptors), arterial hypotension (through carotid baroreceptors), and psychic stress (through cortical input). This may result in water retention and hypo-osmolality, i.e., a syndrome of inappropriate antidiuretic hormone secretion (ADH).[5]

In shock, severe arterial hypotension stimulates the release of AVP to plasma levels of 10 to 100 pg/mL or greater. At these concentrations, AVP acts predominantly on the V_1 receptor, which induces vasoconstriction. This appears to be an important compensatory response in maintaining blood pressure. In sepsis, activation of inducible nitric oxide synthase and release of massive amounts of nitric oxide causes profound vasodilation refractory to norepinephrine.[6] AVP opposes the actions of nitric oxide by inhibiting the formation of cyclic guanosine monophosphate (cGMP), which mediates its vasodilator effect. It also restores membrane polarity by closing potassium–adenosine triphosphate (ATP) channels.[6] When AVP stores become depleted, plasma AVP levels decrease and the profound hypotension characteristic of septic shock ensues. These patients are exquisitely sensitive to the administration of exogenous AVP, which promptly restores normal blood pressure.[4]

Vasodilator, Salt-Losing Systems

Prostaglandins

The kidney produces several vasodilator prostaglandins (PGD_2 and PGE_2) and prostacyclin (PGI_2). The key enzyme in their synthesis from arachidonic acid is phospholipase A_2, which resides in the lipid layer of the cell membrane and is stimulated by norepinephrine, angiotensin II, and AVP. Thus the same factors that induce vasoconstriction and salt retention during the stress response also activate prostaglandins, which promote vasodilation and salt excretion.[7] The prostaglandins also provide endogenous renal protection in conditions of stress by maintaining perfusion to the oligemic renal medulla.[8]

Atrial Natriuretic Peptide

ANP is actually one of a series of peptides with potent vasodilator and natriuretic activity.[3,9,10] ANP is synthesized in specialized atrial myocytes and is released in response to atrial stretch. It acts on a G protein phospholipase C–linked receptor coupled with guanylate cyclase to form cGMP, which induces afferent arteriolar vasodilation and inhibits sodium absorption in the medullary portion of the collecting duct.[11]

ANP reverses the vasoconstrictor effects of norepinephrine (competitively) and angiotensin II (noncompetitively). It inhibits renin release from the afferent arteriole and angiotensin-induced aldosterone release, as well as the salt-retaining action of aldosterone itself. It suppresses posterior pituitary release of AVP and its action on the V_2 receptor in the collecting duct, promoting diuresis.

The importance of atrial pressure elevation and the release of endogenous ANP is illustrated by the relative preservation of renal blood flow and urine output in animal models of cardiogenic shock compared with hemorrhagic shock.[12] It also explains the decline in natriuresis observed after mitral valve replacement and acute reduction of previously elevated left atrial pressure.[13]

Endogenous Dopamine

Dopamine is produced in renal tubular cells and acts as an autocrine (i.e., intracellular) and paracrine (i.e., transcellular) factor that inhibits the activity of the primary sodium pump, Na^+, K^+-ATPase, as well as other sodium influx pathways.[14] Dopamine and ANP oppose the salt-retaining actions of norepinephrine and angiotensin II. Holtbäck and colleagues have suggested that ANP acts through the renal dopamine system by recruitment of silent DA-1 receptors from the interior of the cell toward the plasma membrane.[14] The natriuretic effect of endogenous dopamine becomes most prominent with a high salt diet and appears to play an important role in the maintenance of sodium homeostasis and normal blood pressure.

Responses to Altered Intravascular Volume

Hypovolemia

Hypovolemia provokes reflex responses through volume receptors in the atria and great veins, baroreceptors in aortic arch, carotid sinuses, and afferent arterioles. When extracellular volume is contracted, the initial response is a decrease in glomerular filtration rate (GFR) and the filtered sodium load. In the proximal tubule, sympathetic activity and angiotensin II increase sodium reabsorption from about 66% to 80% of the total filtered. In the mTAL, distal tubule, and collecting duct, aldosterone and AVP also increase sodium reabsorption. Release of AVP and activation of V_2 receptors causes avid reabsorption of water in the collecting duct, therefore urine becomes highly concentrated (>600 mOsm/kg) with virtually no sodium (<10 mEq/L). This is a classic prerenal syndrome, indicating intact tubular function and a perfectly appropriate response to intravascular hypovolemia. Although it can be overcome by inappropriate diuretic therapy (see later), tubular salt and water retention may persist in severe dehydration despite the administration of "low dose" dopamine.[15]

Hypervolemia

Reflex decreases in sympathetic and angiotensin II activity and the release of ANP promote an increase in renal blood flow, GFR, and the filtered sodium load. In the proximal tubule, sodium reabsorption decreases from 66% to 50% of the total filtered. At the same time, decreased aldosterone and AVP limit sodium reabsorption in the mTAL, distal tubule, and collecting duct. The absence of AVP (and the presence of ANP) impairs water absorption at the collecting duct, therefore dilute urine (300 mOsm/kg) with abundant sodium (80 mEq/L) is produced.

This urine profile (low osmolality, high urine sodium) may also be encountered in hypovolemia if loop diuretics have been given that depress tubular resorptive capacity. It is pathognomonic of oliguric acute tubular necrosis (ATN), where it indicates complete loss of the normal ability of the tubules to conserve sodium and water in the face of intravascular hypovolemia.

Physiology of the Kidney

The kidneys contain approximately 2×10^6 nephrons, each of which consists of a glomerulus and a tubule emptying into a collecting duct. Urine is formed by the combination of glomerular ultrafiltration and tubular reabsorption and secretion. The glomerulus, a highly convoluted tuft of capillary loops, is supplied by the afferent arteriole and drained by the efferent arteriole (Fig. 21–3). In juxtamedullary nephrons, the efferent arteriole in turn drains into vasa recta, which line the loops of Henle that dive down into the medulla and create the countercurrent system.

Glomerular Filtration

Filtrate Formation

Glomerular filtrate requires passage through three distinct layers, which are size-selective and charge-selective.[16] The fenestrated capillary endothelium restricts the passage of cells only, the basement membrane filters plasma proteins,

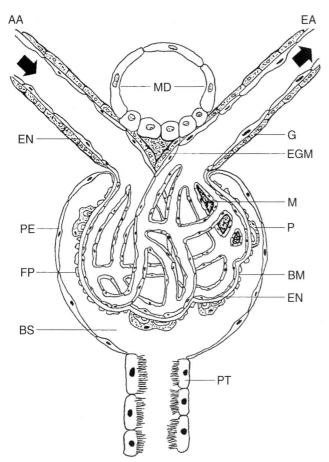

Figure 21–3. The renal corpuscle. AA, afferent arteriole; BM, basement membrane; BS, Bowman speace; EA, efferent arteriole; EGM, extraglomerular mesangial cells between the afferent and efferent arterioles; EN, endothelial cell; G, granular cell of the afferent and efferent arterioles; FP, foot processes of the podocyte; M, mesangial cells between capillaries; MD, macula densa; P, podocyte cell body (visceral cell layer); PE, parietal epithelium; PT, proximal trubule cell. (Modified from Koushanpour E, Kriz W: Renal Physiology: Principles, Structure, and Function, 2nd ed. New York, Springer-Verlag, 1986.)

and the epithelial podocytes regulate pore size. Molecules with a radius less than 18Å (e.g., water, sodium, urea, glucose, inulin) are freely filtered, whereas those greater than 36Å (e.g., hemoglobin, albumin) are not. Filtration of molecules 18 to 36Å depends on their electrical charge. In the glomerulus, negatively charged glycoproteins retard the passage of other negatively charged proteins, therefore cations are filtered but anions are not. In glomerulonephritis, negatively charged glycoproteins are destroyed, polyanionic proteins are filtered, and proteinuria ensues.

GFR depends on the permeability of the filtration barrier; and the net difference between the hydrostatic forces pushing fluid into Bowman's space and the osmotic forces keeping fluid in the plasma:

$$GFR = K_{UF}[(P_{GC} - P_{BS}) - (\Pi_{GC} - \Pi_{BS})].$$

K_{UF} is the ultrafiltration coefficient, which reflects capillary permeability and glomerular surface area. P_{GC} is the glomerular hydrostatic pressure, determined by the renal arterial pressure. Π_{GC} is the plasma oncotic pressure: it is decreased by increased renal plasma flow, which washes out osmotically effective molecules. P_{BS} and Π_{BS} reflect the hydrostatic and oncotic pressure in Bowman's space, which oppose the plasma pressures.

An important regulating system for GFR is the juxtaglomerular apparatus, which consists of the afferent and efferent arterioles and the macula densa, a modified portion of the loop of Henle interposed between the two.

The afferent arterioles contain renin-producing granular cells and baroreceptors and are innervated by sympathetic fibers. Renin is released by arterial hypotension, sympathetic stimulation, or both, and triggers salt and water retention. The cells of the macula densa are chemoreceptors. When the tubular chloride concentration is increased, renin-angiotensin elaboration is enhanced and arteriolar constriction ensues, which decreases GFR (tubuloglomerular feedback). This could be a protective mechanism to prevent polyuria and dehydration in ATN referred to as "acute renal success."[17]

Regulation of Glomerular Filtration

Extrinsic Regulation

The GFR is largely determined by the glomerular filtration pressure (GFP), which depends on the balance between afferent and efferent arteriolar tone (Fig. 21–4).

A low level of sympathetic discharge and angiotensin II activation (e.g., mild hypovolemia, anesthetic induction, positive pressure ventilation) causes preferential efferent arteriolar constriction, which increases filtration fraction and preserves the GFR. This differential effect may be explained by increased nitric oxide activity in the afferent arteriole, which confers relative resistance to vasoconstriction.[18] Preferential efferent arteriolar constriction may be abolished by ACE inhibitors (e.g., captopril, enalapril, lisinopril) or

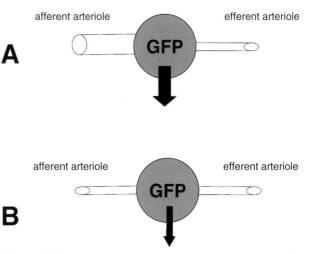

Figure 21–4. Afferent versus efferent arteriolar tone. (From Sladen RN, Landry D: Anesthesiol Clin North America;18:794, 2000.)

angiotensin II receptor blockers (e.g., losartin) and may result in deteriorating GFR.

Intense sympathoadrenal and angiotensin II activation (e.g., severe hypovolemia, sepsis, shock) also constricts the afferent arteriole, decreases filtration fraction, and worsens GFR already attenuated by renal hypoperfusion.[19] In addition, the glomerular mesangial cells contain actin fibers that constrict in response to norepinephrine, angiotensin II, and endothelin through a G protein–coupled phospholipase C receptor.[20] This decreases glomerular surface area and further decreases GFR.

It is noteworthy that even at higher levels AVP provides more selective vasoconstriction in the efferent arteriole[21] and is more likely to preserve GFP and GFR than norepinephrine or angiotensin II.

Intrinsic Regulation (Autoregulation)

Renal autoregulation implies that the kidney intrinsically maintains its blood flow, GFR, solute, and water regulation independently of wide fluctuations of mean arterial pressure.[22] There are two theories of autoregulation. One holds that the resistance of the preglomerular afferent arteriole increases as arterial pressure increases, and vice versa (myogenic response). The other theory is based on tubuloglomerular feedback: increased arterial blood pressure enhances delivery of chloride to the macula densa, which triggers renin-angiotensin activation, afferent arteriolar constriction, and decreases renal blood flow and GFR.[16]

Endogenous nitric oxide formation may play a role in both mechanisms.[18] Regardless, it is noteworthy that urine flow rate is not autoregulated—it is subject to the peritubular hydrostatic pressure and decreases with hypotension.

Although it is not abolished by most anesthetic agents, autoregulation appears to be impaired in severe sepsis[23] possibly because of the generation of massive amounts of endogenous nitric oxide.[18] It is almost certainly lost in acute renal failure[24] and perhaps during cardiopulmonary bypass.[25] In these situations, renal blood flow is much more dependent on renal perfusion pressure, is acutely decreased during hypotension, and is restored by vasoconstrictor therapy.

Tubular Structure and Function

The renal tubule comprises four distinct segments: the proximal tubule; the loop of Henle (which includes the pars recta, descending and ascending thin limb segments, and the mTAL); the distal tubule, and the collecting duct (Fig. 21–5). The last courses through the cortex, outer medulla, and inner medulla before entering the renal pelvis at the papilla. The more numerous outer cortical nephrons have short loops of Henle and receive about 85% of the renal blood flow. The juxtamedullary nephrons, which receive less than 10% of the renal blood flow, have long loops of Henle. These dive deeply into the inner medulla together with the vasa recta and are responsible for the countercurrent

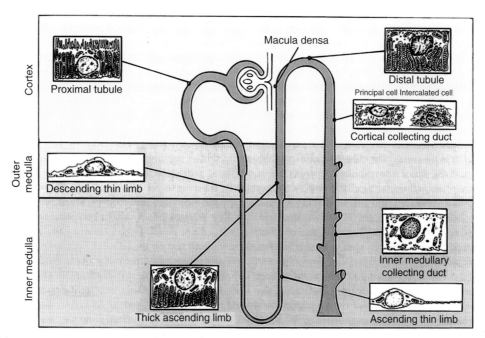

Figure 21–5. Tubular structure and function. Structure/function relationships in the renal tubule. The most metabolically active components of the tubule are the proximal tubule, the thick ascending loop of Henle, and the first part of the distal tubule. Their cells are large, and on the capillary surface (basolateral membrane) there are many invaginations rich in mitochondria. The cells of the proximal tubule have a brush border on the luminal surface (apical cell membrane), whereas the cells of the descending and thin ascending loops of Henle are flattened, with few mitochondria. The second part of the distal tubule and collecting duct are intermediate in nature. The intercalated cells of the distal tubule have many mitochondria, the principal cells have few. (From Berne RM, Levy MN (eds): Physiology, 4th ed. St. Louis, Mosby, 1998, p 680.)

mechanism that generates medullary hypertonicity and creates the concentrating ability of the kidney.

Tubular Reabsorption and Secretion

Each day the glomeruli produce 180 L ultrafiltrate, of which the tubules reabsorb 99% of the salt and water. Many other filtered substances are completely reabsorbed, but some have a maximum rate of tubular reabsorption (T_{max}). For glucose, the T_{max} is 375 mg/dL, greater rates result in glycosuria in direct proportion to the filtered load.

Proximal Tubule

The first part of the proximal tubule reabsorbs about 100% of the filtered glucose, lactate, and amino acids, as well as some phosphate.[16] About two thirds of the filtered water, chloride, and potassium are also reabsorbed, then coupled with, and strongly influenced by sodium absorption. The proximal tubule is also an important site of secretion of many endogenous anions (bile salts, urate), cations (creatinine, dopamine), and drugs (diuretics, penicillin, probenecid, cimetidine). Organic ions compete for protein transport systems. For example, probenecid impairs tubular secretion of penicillin and prolongs its action. In chronic renal insufficiency, excess organic acids compete for secretor proteins with drugs such as furosemide and confer "resistance" to loop diuretics.

Medullary Thick Ascending Limb

The mTAL reabsorbs about 20% of filtered sodium, chloride, potassium, and bicarbonate, but does so in an oligemic milieu. The medulla receives only 6% of the renal blood flow, extracts a large proportion of oxygen, and the tissue PO_2 is just 8 mm Hg. Severe hypoxia may develop rapidly despite "adequate" total renal blood flow. Because it is metabolically active, the mTAL is particularly vulnerable to nephrotoxin-mediated ischemic injury.[26] Endogenous vasoactive compounds normally direct blood flow to the medulla. Adenosine induces cortical vasoconstriction, whereas in the juxtamedullary zone prostaglandins and nitric oxide promote vasodilation. Prostaglandin inhibitors such as nonsteroidal anti-inflammatory agents can thus cause medullary ischemia.

The initial response to renal hypoperfusion is increased active sodium chloride absorption in the mTAL, which increases oxygen consumption (VO_2) in the face of decreased oxygen delivery (DO_2). When ATP stores become depleted, active sodium chloride reabsorption winds down. This increases the chloride concentration in tubular fluid reaching the macula densa, resulting in angiotensin release and afferent arteriolar constriction (tubuloglomerular feedback). The resultant decrease in GFR benefits renal oxygen balance by decreasing solute reabsorption and mTAL VO_2.[27] Thus it is theoretically possible that by inhibiting active sodium reabsorption in the mTAL, loop diuretics or dopaminergic (DA) agents might alleviate ischemic or nephrotoxic insults to the tubules.[28]

Countercurrent Mechanism and Osmotic Equilibrium

Urinary concentrating ability is reflected by the ability to generate a high urine/plasma osmolar ratio (up to 5:1) in the presence of dehydration and intravascular hypovolemia. It is dependent on the development of a hypertonic medullary interstitium, which is created by the countercurrent multiplier effect of the loop of Henle, in which solute is separated from water (the single effect). The mTAL actively reabsorbs sodium from the lumen but is impermeable to water, which becomes trapped so that as the tubular fluid ascends in the mTAL it becomes more and more dilute. By the end of this "diluting segment," tubular fluid osmolality has decreased to less than $150 \, mOsm/kg \, H_2O$. This in turn results in increased sodium chloride concentration and osmolality in the medullary interstitium. The descending loop of Henle is permeable to water, which diffuses out along the osmotic gradient so that the tubular fluid becomes maximally concentrated at the inferior pole of the loop.

The vasa recta are a continuation of the efferent arteriole and are closely applied to the loops of Henle. They maintain this condition by removing water and adding solute as they pass through the medullary interstitium. A standing osmotic gradient is set up between the cortex (300 mOsm/kg), juxtamedullary zone (600 mOsm/kg), and deep medulla (1200 mOsm/kg). This process is enhanced by the passive recycling of urea, which diffuses out of the inner medullary collecting duct into the interstitium and then into the distal loop of Henle.

Finally, AVP released from the posterior pituitary acts on V_2 receptors in the distal tubule and collecting ducts and enhances their permeability to water, which is reabsorbed, resulting in an antidiuresis.

Urinary concentrating ability can be abolished by diuretics, especially osmotic diuretics (i.e., mannitol), which "wash out" the hypertonic medulla, potentially resulting in severe intravascular hypovolemia and renal injury. Concentrating ability is highly dependent on normal tubular function, and loss of concentrating ability (i.e., urine to plasma osmolar ratio of 1:1) is an early sign of acute tubular injury.

Physiology and Biochemistry of the Tubular Cell

General Characteristics

Each tubular cell has an apical (luminal) cell membrane with adjoining tight junctions, and a basolateral cell membrane, which interfaces with the peritubular capillary (Fig. 21–6). There are many protein-based active transport systems, of which the most important is the sodium/potassium adenosine triphosphatase (Na/K ATPase) pump on the basolateral membrane. This pumps sodium out of the tubular cell into the blood against a concentration and an electrical gradient in exchange for potassium. Intracellular sodium concentration is decreased, which passively draws sodium from the tubular lumen into the cell. The transport of virtually all solutes is coupled to that of sodium. Active transport

Figure 21–6. The tubular cell. This is an idealized schematic of the major mechanisms of secretion and reabsorption, one or more of which is used by various segments of the tubule. The energy-requiring Na-K-ATPase pump in the basolateral cell membrane (*1*) is ubiquitous and pumps sodium out into the interstitium against its concentration gradient and maintains a low intracellular concentration. This favors inward movement of sodium from the tubular lumen, facilitated by a sodium chloride symporter system on the apical cell membrane (*2*). In the medullary thick ascending loop of Henle (mTAL), this is the primary inhibitory site of action of loop diuretics. In the proximal tubule, a sodium-H⁺ antiporter system on the apical cell membrane (*3*) aids sodium reabsorption and extrudes H⁺, thereby promoting reaction of water with carbon dioxide to form H⁺ and bicarbonate ion under the influence of carbonic anhydrase (CA). Bicarbonate diffuses out into the capillary. Sodium reabsorption is thereby coupled to H⁺ loss and bicarbonate reabsorption. The transport proteins create a positive charge in the lumen, which drives ions such as sodium, calcium, potassium, and magnesium passively through the tight junctions by paracellular diffusion. (From Berne RM, Levy MN (eds): Physiology, 4th ed. St. Louis, Mosby, 1998, p 701.)

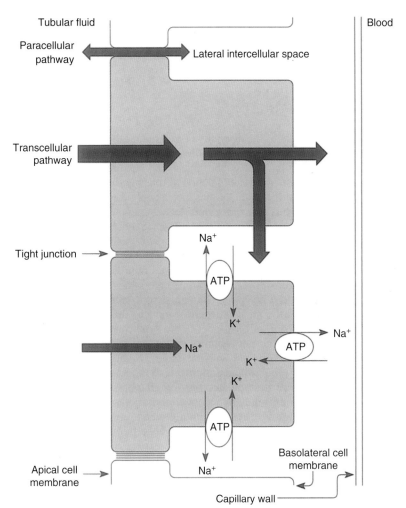

systems move solutes in the same direction (symporter) or in opposite directions (antiporter). Solutes are transported by both active and passive mechanisms, but water always diffuses passively along an osmotic gradient.

Specialized Cell Types and Receptors

Proximal Tubule

The proximal tubule is a potent site for sodium absorption, which draws with it about two thirds of the filtered water, chloride, and potassium.[11] The sodium/symporter systems also couple the reabsorption of filtered glucose, lactate, amino acids, and phosphate. Sodium is absorbed across the cell by a sodium/hydrogen and chloride/base antiporter system in the apical cell membrane, where it is pumped into the interstitial space by the sodium/potassium ATPase pump. This increases interstitial osmolality and also draws water across.

A sodium/hydrogen antiporter system extrudes hydrogen ion into the tubule in exchange for bicarbonate. With the absorption of organic anions and bicarbonate in the first part

of the proximal tubule, the downstream concentration of chloride increases and promotes passage of chloride into the cell along its concentration gradient. The tubular fluid thus becomes positively charged relative to blood, and the electrical gradient further promotes the movement of sodium from the tubular fluid into the cell.

Medullary Thick Ascending Loop of Henle

In the mTAL, sodium is actively drawn in from the tubular fluid at the apical membrane, along with chloride and potassium, by a symporter protein system—the major site of action of loop diuretics that inhibit sodium chloride reabsorption in the mTAL. The potent sodium absorptive capacity of the mTAL is also driven by a sodium/potassium ATPase pump in the cell basolateral membrane, which draws more sodium from the tubular lumen by passive diffusion along its concentration gradient.

Loss of urinary concentrating ability is an early and singular manifestation of ATN. It is primarily caused by the breakdown of the energy-requiring, sodium/potassium ATPase pump in the mTAL. This prevents any enhancement of tubular reabsorption of sodium in response to hypovolemia. Medullary hypertonicity is lost, and water returns to the tubular lumen, resulting in formation of small amounts of dilute (hypo-osmolar) urine with a high-sodium concentration (>80 mEq/L).

Distal Tubule and Collecting Duct

The proximal segment of the distal tubule is structurally and functionally similar to the mTAL. Sodium and chloride are actively drawn into the cell at the apical cell membrane by a symporter system—the site of action of thiazide diuretics. In the last part of the distal tubule, specialized principal cells reabsorb sodium and water and secrete potassium, driven by a sodium/potassium ATPase pump. Specialized intercalated cells secrete hydrogen ion and reabsorb bicarbonate.

The actions of the aldosterone on the distal tubular cell are illustrated in Figure 21–7. Aldosterone enters the cytoplasm and attaches to a receptor. The aldosterone/receptor complex migrates to the nucleus where it induces the formation of mRNA. Here, mRNA induces the synthesis of a protein that enhances the permeability of the apical (i.e., luminal) membrane to sodium and potassium. Sodium is reabsorbed from the tubular fluid and travels to the basolateral membrane, where it stimulates the sodium/potassium ATPase pump. The intracellular concentration of potassium increases, and it follows its concentration gradient out into the lumen. The net effect is increased sodium absorption and potassium excretion. If aldosterone secretion is excessively stimulated (e.g., by intravascular hypovolemia), this culminates in hypokalemic metabolic alkalosis ("contraction alkalosis").

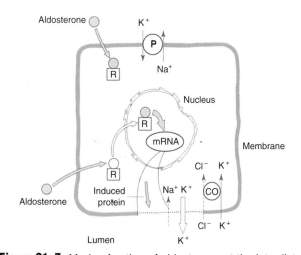

Figure 21–7. Mode of action of aldosterone at the late distal tubule. Cl⁻, chloride; CO, cotransporter (= symporter); K⁺, potassium; mRNA, messenger ribonucleic acid; Na⁺, sodium; P, sodium-potassium adenosine triphosphatase pump; R, receptor. (From Wingard LB, Brody TM, Larner J, Schwartz A: Diuretics: Drugs that increase excretion of water and electrolytes. In Wingard LB, Brody TM, Larner J, Schwartz A (eds): Human Pharmacology: Molecular-to-Clinical. London, Wolfe Publishing, 1991, p 249.)

Current and Potential Targets of Drug Action

Glomerulus: Efferent Arteriolar Constriction

Vasopressin Receptors

AVP is the endogenous hormone that controls the renal antidiuretic response to dehydration, hence the name ADH. This nonapeptide is synthesized in the supraoptic and paraventricular nuclei of the anterior hypothalamus and is stored in the posterior pituitary gland. Osmoreceptors in the hypothalamus respond to minute increases in serum osmolality—as small as 1% greater than normal. Consequently, AVP is released from storage vesicles in the posterior pituitary, and through a plasma range of only 1 to 5 pg/mL maintains serum osmolality within the narrow range of 280 to 290 mOsm/kg. In the distal tubule and collecting ducts, AVP stimulates specific vasopressin$_2$ (V$_2$) receptors. After activation of cyclic adenosine monophosphate, intracellular conduits are formed that allow water reabsorption and a decreased flow of concentrated urine.[4]

Antidiuresis is also triggered by hypovolemia and arterial hypotension. Activation of stretch receptors in the atria and great veins, or baroreceptors in the aortic arch and carotid sinuses and psychic stress all cause release of AVP. As a consequence of "nonosmotic" stimulation of the V$_2$ receptor, water retention and hypo-osmolality may culminate in the syndrome of inappropriate secretion of ADH.[5]

Severe arterial hypotension encountered in various forms of vasodilated shock (e.g., septic shock) stimulates the release of AVP to much higher plasma levels—10 to 100 pg/mL or greater. At these concentrations, AVP acts predominantly on the V$_1$ receptor present in vascular smooth muscle and induces intense vasoconstriction. This is particularly beneficial to the kidney because AVP preferentially constricts the efferent arteriole.[21] This preserves GFP and GFR in the face of decreased renal perfusion pressure or flow. In contrast, high levels of catecholamines and angiotensin II constrict both the afferent and efferent arteriole and worsen GFP.

A remarkable vasopressor response to low levels of infused AVP was first observed by Landry and colleagues[29] in patients with vasodilated shock and oliguria refractory to infused catecholamines. Vasodilated shock—i.e., severe arterial hypotension, low systemic vascular resistance, and elevated cardiac index—is pathognomonic of sepsis, but also may be encountered with high-dose milrinone for severe ventricular failure and in the contact inflammatory response to cardiopulmonary bypass or placement of a ventricular assist device, or both. In all these situations, AVP infusion (1–6 units/hr) consistently increases systemic blood pressure, decreases catecholamine requirement, and in some cases markedly improves urinary flow without increasing pulmonary vascular resistance.[29–34]

Profound vasodilation refractory to norepinephrine is characteristic of septic shock and is largely related to massive generation of nitric oxide by inducible nitric oxide synthase in activated macrophages.[6] Infusion of AVP is able to provide effective vasoconstriction because it opposes the actions of nitric oxide and inhibits cGMP formation. In vascular smooth muscle cells, AVP restores membrane polarity, closes potassium/ATP channels, and opens calcium channels.[6] It also restores vascular responsiveness to catecholamines. Landry and colleagues[35] also observed that plasma AVP levels are remarkably low in septic shock (about 3 pg/mL), probably because of sustained baroreceptor-mediated AVP release during the initial hypotensive stages of sepsis. "Hypersensitivity" to AVP infusion is explained by restoration of plasma AVP levels to those appropriate for the response to severe hypotension.

Renal Tubule and Diuretic Agents

Renal Tubule—Osmotic Diuresis

Osmotic diuretics are small molecules that increase tubular flow by drawing water into the renal tubule and include mannitol, urea, isosorbide, and glycerol. The archetype is mannitol, an "inert" sugar that is not metabolized, is largely confined to the blood, and is directly excreted by the kidneys.[36] It prevents water (but not sodium) reabsorption in all segments of the tubule that are freely permeable to water—that is, the proximal tubule, the descending loop of Henle and the collecting duct. A marked tubular diuresis occurs without natriuresis.

Infusion of mannitol may provide protection against renal ischemic and nephrotoxic insults by several mechanisms. Mannitol enhances blood flow to the oligemic renal medulla by activating vasodilator intrarenal prostaglandins, notably prostacyclin (PGI$_2$).[37] Increased tubular flow rate in the ischemic proximal tubule attenuates tubular obstruction by cellular debris[38] and tubular injury by myoglobin.[39] Expansion of the intravascular volume stretches the atria and liberates ANP, further increasing renal blood flow and diuresis. It also increases ventricular preload, cardiac output, renal blood flow, transglomerular pressure gradient, and GFR. Mannitol appears to protect against ischemic reperfusion injury by scavenging free radicals (although this has been disputed in myoglobinuria[39]) and by preventing endothelial swelling in the vessels of the inner medulla. This avoids red cell aggregation and the so-called "no-reflow" phenomenon when microcirculatory perfusion is restored.

Notably, osmotic diuresis "washes out" the countercurrent system that creates medullary hypertonicity, resulting in a loss of urinary concentrating ability that may last for several hours. During this time the kidney is unable to respond appropriately to dehydration and an obligate diuresis continues. Injudicious mannitol diuresis without adequate fluid replacement may exacerbate intravascular hypovolemia and renal injury.[40]

Proximal Tubule—Carbonic Anhydrase Inhibition

The proximal tubule is an important site for the conservation of bicarbonate by the kidney. It does this through carbonic anhydrase, a family of five zinc-containing isoenzymes that are produced in the luminal brush border of the proximal tubular cell. Carbonic anhydrase catalyzes the reversible combination of water and carbon dioxide to form carbonic acid, which serves as a source of hydrogen ion that is exchanged for filtered bicarbonate.

Administration of a carbonic anhydrase inhibitor such as acetazolamide blocks bicarbonate reabsorption, resulting in diuresis and obligatory bicarbonate loss. However, sodium excretion (natriuresis) is not enhanced, and the fractional excretion of sodium remains low—approximately 3% to 5%.[36] There are several reasons for this. Although the proximal tubule is the major site for sodium reabsorption in the nephron, most of the sodium that escapes is reabsorbed more distally, especially at the mTAL. In addition, only a portion of the proximal tubule is affected by carbonic anhydrase inhibition, and acetazolamide administration itself decreases the GFR.

Acetazolamide is usually indicated in the management of persistent metabolic alkalosis uncorrected by potassium chloride replacement, especially if it inhibits respiratory drive. It is important to first exclude "contraction alkalosis" (hypokalemic metabolic alkalosis) induced by hypovolemia and aldosterone secretion, which will be exacerbated by further diuretic therapy. In rhabdomyolysis and myoglobinuria, the primary intervention includes aggressive maintenance of intravascular volume and high tubular flow with fluid and mannitol administration. Urinary alkalization (urinary pH > 6.0), accomplished by the addition of sodium bicarbonate (25 mEq/L) to the intravenous fluid, retards the conversion of myoglobin to toxic ferrihematin and decreases the risk for tubular injury.[41] Administration of acetazolamide may be considered if metabolic alkalosis develops and myoglobinuria persists.

Loop of Henle—Medullary Thick Ascending Limb of Henle Blockade

Loop diuretics such as furosemide, bumetanide, torasemide, and ethacrynic acid are the most potent saliuretic agents available and generate the highest fractional excretion of sodium (Fig. 21–8). They act at the mTAL, where up to 25% of all sodium reabsorption occurs, and there is very limited capability for compensatory reabsorption distal to this.[36] To reach the mTAL these agents are far less dependent on the GFR than on active secretion by an organic acid secretory pump in the straight segment of the proximal tubule.[42] In the mTAL, cells their major action is to inhibit the sodium/potassium chloride symporter situated at the luminal membrane and, to a lesser extent, the sodium/potassium ATPase pump at the basolateral cell membrane (see Fig. 21–6). Loop diuretics also block the reabsorption of magnesium, calcium, and uric acid. Inhibition of these active transport pumps decreases mTAL oxygen requirement, and it has been suggested that loop diuretics may provide renal protection by favoring tubular oxygen balance during ischemia.[26]

Loop diuretics also have specific vasodilator effects. Furosemide-induced renal cortical dilation may attenuate ischemic and nephrotoxic insults through inhibition of the tubuloglomerular feedback that invokes cortical vasoconstriction. Although this is consistently demonstrated in

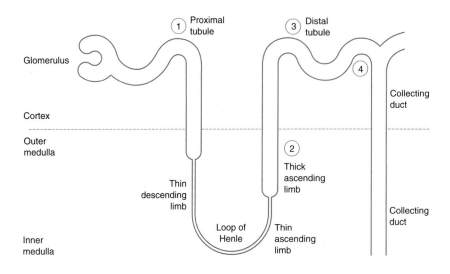

Site	Segment	Sodium reabsorption (%)	Diuretic effects of blockade
1	Proximal tubule	60–70	Relatively weak – sodium can be reabsorbed distally
2	Medullary thick ascending loop of Henle	15–25	Potent – important site for sodium reabsorption with relatively few distal sites
3	Early distal tubule	5–8	Less potent – less important site for sodium reabsorption
4	Late distal tubule, collecting ducts	<3	Relatively weak – little sodium reabsorption

Figure 21–8. Sites of action of diuretics. mTAL, medullary thick ascending loop of Henle; Na, sodium. (Modified from Warnock DG: Diuretic agents. In Katzung BG (ed): Basic and Clinical Pharmacology, 5th ed. East Norwalk, Conn., Appleton & Lange, 1992, p 212.)

animal models, in clinical practice loop diuretics are usually given to treat oliguria—i.e., they are administered *after* a renal insult, not before. Intravenous injection of larger doses induces systemic venodilation that can decrease excessive cardiac preload and relieve acute pulmonary edema or congestive cardiac failure.

Prophylactic administration of loop diuretics is most appropriate in the pigment nephropathies—intravascular hemolysis or rhabdomyolysis—if there is an inadequate diuretic response to aggressive fluid replacement and osmotic agents. High tubular flow "washes out" nephrotoxic pigments and cellular debris and prevents tubular obstruction and damage.

Administration of large doses of furosemide, with or without dopamine, has achieved some success in generating increased urinary output in patients with incipient or early established oliguric renal failure.[43,44] So-called "conversion" of oliguric to nonoliguric renal failure[45] does not appear to alter the outcome once dialysis becomes necessary,[46] and a response to diuresis most likely reflects a lesser degree of intrinsic renal injury. Nonetheless, in these patients, increased urine flow does facilitate fluid management and nutritional support and tends to slow the onset of hyperkalemia and metabolic acidosis.

Loop diuretics should be administered only in the context of normal or increased intravascular volume. Acute hypo-

volemia may be a consequence of inappropriate administration of loop diuretics to "make urine" in hypovolemic states. Diuretic-induced dehydration and hypotension further exacerbates ischemic injury and concentrates nephrotoxins in the tubules. Excessive ongoing diuresis can induce hypokalemic metabolic alkalosis and supraventricular arrhythmias.[47] High doses (>1 g/day) of furosemide are ototoxic; strategies to avoid this are enumerated later in this chapter.

Loop Diuretic Resistance

Resistance to loop diuretic therapy may be encountered in a wide variety of circumstances. The most common is acute tolerance, known as the "braking phenomenon." Decreased diuretic response to repeated diuretic doses is induced by reflex salt and water retention in the face of a contracted extracellular volume and can be overcome by simple fluid repletion.[48] Chronic tolerance occurs with long-term administration of loop diuretics and is characterized by gradually increasing dose requirement. It occurs because tubular epithelial cells of the distal tubule undergo hypertrophy and increase their capacity for both active and passive sodium reabsorption. It can be overcome by concomitant administration of a thiazide diuretic, which may also actually

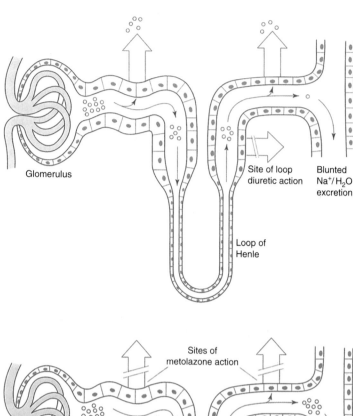

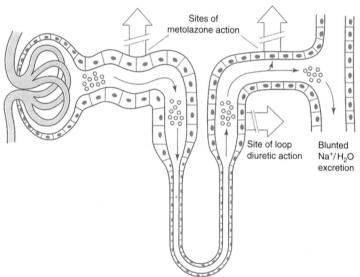

Figure 21-9. Dual segment blockade. *Top,* The exaggerated sodium reabsorption that occurs at the proximal and distal tubules in diuretic resistant states (congestive heart failure, cirrhosis, nephropathy). This blunts the responsiveness to loop diuretics at the medullary thick ascending loop of Henle (mTAL). *Bottom,* The application of segmental nephron blockade by the addition of metolazone, which blocks sodium reabsorption at the proximal and distal tubule, to a loop diuretic, which blocks sodium reabsorption at the mTAL. (From Sica DA, Gehr TW: Diuretic combinations in refractory oedema states: Pharmacokinetic-pharmacodynamic relationships. Clin Pharmacokinet 30:231, 1996.)

prevent distal tubule hypertrophy.[49] This strategy, known as dual segment blockade, is also extremely effective in overcoming diuretic resistance in oliguria associated with renal insufficiency and low GFR (Fig. 21–9).

Diuretic resistance may also be caused by altered pharmacokinetics (i.e., decreased diuretic delivery to the luminal border of the tubule) or pharmacodynamics (i.e., a decreased sodium excretory response to a given concentration of drug in the urine). Diuretic delivery to the tubule is decreased in severe hypoalbuminemia because loop diuretics are highly protein bound[50] and is decreased in renal insufficiency because secretion of accumulated endogenous organic acids competes with loop diuretics at the proximal tubule.[42] In disease states notorious for refractory edema, such as renal insufficiency, congestive heart failure, and hepatic cirrhosis, the effective intravascular volume is markedly decreased. This triggers avid sodium reabsorption at the proximal

tubule and much less sodium is available for diuretic action at the mTAL and distal tubule.[51] Pharmacodynamic resistance is characteristic of liver failure for reasons not completely understood.

Strategies for overcoming diuretic resistance are summarized in Table 21–1.

Distal Tubule Blockade

Thiazide diuretics block sodium reabsorption at a symporter system in the luminal membrane of cells of the early part of the distal tubule. Because only 15% of the glomerular filtrate reaches this segment and only 5% to 8% of tubular sodium reabsorption occurs here, thiazides have less potent diuretic and natriuretic properties than the loop diuretics.[36]

TABLE 21–1.

Strategies for Overcoming Diuretic Resistance

■ Restore normal hemodynamics (CO, RBF, perfusion pressure)

■ Administer higher doses of diuretic agents; e.g., furosemide 80–120 mg, bumetanide 2.5–5 mg IV (doses of furosemide = 240 mg IV induce venodilation and increase the risk for ototoxicity)

■ Concomitant administration of human albumin: useful in hypoalbuminemia, albumin is necessary for furosemide delivery to the tubules

■ Continuous diuretic infusion: maintains tubular drug concentration just above diuretic threshold, avoids evanescent peaks (and potential toxic effects) associated with bolus dosing; e.g., furosemide 40 mg IV load, followed by 2–10 mg/hr infusion (requires close monitoring to avoid hypovolemia, electrolyte imbalance)

■ Segmental nephron blockade (loop diuretic + thiazide): loop diuretic blocks Na^+ reabsorption at mTAL, thiazide blocks compensatory reabsorption downstream at DT; e.g., bumetanide 5 mg IV + metolazone 5 mg PO (metolazone, a thiazide-type diuretic, has unpredictable GI absorption and should be administered at least 1 hour before the parenteral loop diuretic)

CO, carbon monoxide; GI, gastrointestinal; IV, intravenous; mTAL, medullary thick ascending limb of Henle; PO, per os (by mouth); RBF, renal blood flow.

So-called "potassium-sparing" diuretics such as triamterene and amiloride inhibit sodium transport in the remote distal tubule and collecting duct. They have weak diuretic activity because less than 5% of filtered sodium is reabsorbed in these segments. These agents are used in combination with loop diuretics or thiazides to augment diuresis and restrict potassium loss; they are not available for parenteral injection and are seldom used in the perioperative period. Because of their propensity to induce hyperkalemia they should be discontinued in critically ill patients at risk for renal insufficiency or acute renal failure.

Aldosterone Antagonism

Competitive aldosterone antagonism at its sites of synthesis in the distal tubule is provided by a unique agent: spironolactone. This agent is useful in reversing sodium retention and potassium excretion in edematous prerenal states characterized by excessive aldosterone secretion such as liver failure and congestive heart failure. The drug is a synthetic steroid analog that binds to cytoplasmic mineralocorticoid receptors and prevents the aldosterone/receptor complex from translocating to the cell nucleus (see Figure 21–7). This explains why its onset of action takes 2 to 4 days for full potency. In the presence of acute renal insufficiency or failure there is a danger of hyperkalemia because although the drug itself is rapidly metabolized, its effects on aldosterone transport last for 48 to 72 hours after it is discontinued.

Diuretic and Vascular Receptors

Dopaminergic Receptors

DA receptors are currently classified into two subtypes: DA_1 receptors, which stimulate adenylate cyclase and phospholipase C and the formation of cyclic adenosine monophosphate, and DA_2 receptors, which do not.[52] Several subtypes have been characterized by molecular cloning.

In the renal and splanchnic vasculature, DA_1 receptors directly mediate vasodilation and increase renal blood flow and GFR.[53] When a nonselective agent such as dopamine is administered, these changes may be difficult to distinguish from those induced by its β adrenergic effects on cardiac output. However, dopamine-induced natriuresis can occur independently of increases in renal blood flow, and GFR and can be inhibited by selective DA_1 antagonists. This response is provided by DA_1 receptors located in the renal tubule, predominantly in the proximal tubule and mTAL.[54] Stimulation of DA_1 receptors inhibits the sodium/hydrogen antiporter system at the luminal membrane and the sodium/potassium ATPase pump at the basolateral membrane.[52] Thus DA_1 activation results in inhibition of sodium reabsorption and promotes diuresis.[55,56]

In the renal vasculature, DA_2 receptors indirectly mediate vasodilation by inhibiting the release of norepinephrine from the presynaptic terminal of postganglionic sympathetic nerves (i.e., similar to the presynaptic α_2 receptor). However, stimulation of DA_2 receptors does not increase renal blood flow or GFR.

In the kidney, dopamine is synthesized in tubular cells from L-dopa taken up from the tubular lumen. It exerts autocrine (intracellular) and paracrine (transcellular) inhibition of the sodium/potassium ATPase pump.[14] It also opposes the antinatriuretic effects of norepinephrine and angiotensin II and may mediate some of the actions of ANP. There is considerable evidence that endogenous dopamine plays an important role in the regulation of normal sodium homeostasis and blood pressure, and that abnormalities of the system can lead to hypertension when salt intake is excessive.[56,57]

Based on the receptor subtypes, DA agonists and antagonists may be categorized as selective or nonselective agents (Table 21–2). Dopamine and dopexamine are nonselective DA agents. Fenoldopam is a selective DA_1 agonist. Haloperidol,[58] chlorpromazine, and metoclopramide[59] are used in studies as nonselective DA antagonists, but there are few clinical data on their ability to inhibit dopamine-induced diuresis.

TABLE 21–2.

Dopaminergic Agonists and Antagonists

Receptor	Agonist	Antagonist
DA₁, DA₂	Dopamine	Haloperidol, chlorpromazine, metoclopromide
DA₁	Fenoldopam	SCH 23390
DA₂	Bromocriptine	Domperidone

Dopamine is a nonselective dopaminergic agonist; haloperidol, chlorpromazine, and metoclopromide are nonselective dopaminergic antagonists (the clinical importance of this property is not known). Fenoldopam is a selective dopamine-1 (DA₁) receptor agonist that shows promise as a vasodilator agent that preserves renal blood flow. Bromocriptine is a selective dopamine-2 (DA₂) receptor agonist used in Parkinson disease to enhance central dopaminergic activity. SCH 23390 and domperidone are selective DA₁ and DA₂ receptor antagonists.
Source: From Sladen RN: Renal physiology. In Miller RD (ed): Anesthesia, 5th ed. Philadelphia, Churchill Livingstone, 2000, p 683.

Dopamine

Dopamine is a mixed DA₁ and DA₂ agonist in the low-dose range (1–3 µg/kg per minute). It may enhance renal function by several mechanisms. Dopamine's renal vasodilator action increases renal blood flow and blocks the renal vasoconstrictor effects of norepinephrine.[60] Its β₁-mediated inotropic effect increases cardiac output and thereby renal blood flow and renal perfusion pressure. Stimulation of tubular DA₁ receptors evokes saliuresis. Dopamine could protect the renal tubules from ischemia by suppressing the sodium pump, decreasing oxygen consumption, and increasing tubular flow. However, there are relatively few data that suggest that prophylactic administration of low-dose dopamine protects the kidney from injury.[61–64]

There are several limitations to an agent with nonselective activity. At moderate doses (3–10 µg/kg per minute), the β₁ adrenergic effect of dopamine may induce unwanted tachycardia, and at doses greater than 10 µg/kg per minute, its α adrenergic effect causes progressive renal vasoconstriction. Moreover, the pharmacodynamic effect of dopamine is unpredictable because of a wide (up to 27-fold) interindividual variability in its pharmacokinetics.[65] In a study with healthy volunteers, MacGregor and colleagues found that in some individuals, infusion of "low-dose" dopamine resulted in plasma levels in the α adrenergic range.[66]

Fenoldopam

Given the above, a selective DA₁ agonist such as the dopamine analog fenoldopam has potential pharmacologic advantages over dopamine in attenuating renal dysfunction.

As a DA₁ agonist it provides renal and splanchnic vasodilation and has a tubular natriuretic effect. It has no effect on DA₂, β, or α adrenoreceptors.[67] When administered by intravenous infusion at 0.1 to 0.5 µg/kg per minute, it has a rapid onset and offset of effect with an elimination half-life (t₍₁/₂₎) of 10 minutes. Its pharmacokinetic profile is predictable and it has a dose-dependent effect in increasing renal blood flow.[59] At low doses it can increase renal blood flow without affecting blood pressure, and at higher doses it decreases blood pressure but still maintains renal perfusion.[68,69] In laboratory studies, fenoldopam relaxes norepinephrine-induced arterial vasoconstriction, reverses cyclosporine-induced nephrotoxicity,[70] and prevents radiocontrast-induced renal cortical constriction.[71] Fenoldopam also attenuates the prerenal response to aortic cross-clamping and acute hypovolemia.[72,73] However, its role in perioperative renal protection has not yet been established by prospective clinical trials.

Atrial Natriuretic Peptide

ANP is one of a family of endogenous peptides that have a characteristic enhancing effect on renal hemodynamics and sodium excretion in response to volume loading.[9,10] Others in its class include brain natriuretic peptide, C-type natriuretic peptide, and urodilatin (produced in the kidney itself), all of which have a similar core of 25 to 28 amino acids.

ANP is synthesized in electron-dense granules in atrial myocytes in response to atrial distension. It has a potent vasodilator effect mediated through the activation of guanylate cyclase and formation of cGMP. As discussed earlier, its intrarenal actions may be mediated in part through the endogenous dopamine system. There is evidence that ANP recruits silent DA₁ receptors from the interior of the cell toward the plasma membrane.[14] ANP antagonizes the renal vasoconstrictor and salt- and water-retaining effects of norepinephrine, angiotensin II, aldosterone, and vasopressin[3] and it induces a prompt, sustained increase in GFR with natriuresis. This occurs even when arterial pressure is decreased, suggesting that ANP evokes afferent arteriolar dilation with efferent arteriolar constriction.

There is considerable evidence that exogenously administered ANP, with or without dopamine, acts as a "rescue agent" in animal models of established ischemic or nephrotoxic ATN.[74–76] However, it has not been effective in preventing radiocontrast nephropathy in patients.[77] Initial multicenter clinical studies in patients with established ATN suggested that an ANP congener, anaritide, decreased dialysis requirement in oliguric, but not nonoliguric acute renal failure.[78] It was postulated that hypotension induced by anaritide may have caused nephron injury (or prevented recovery) in patients with the nonoliguric (i.e., less severe) form of acute renal failure. Moreover, a subsequent study of patients with oliguric renal failure was not able to confirm any advantage for the administration of anaritide.[79]

When ANP is administered exogenously it acts as a potent venous and arterial vasodilator and decreases cardiac preload and afterload. In 2001, nesiritide, a human recombinant natriuretic peptide, was approved by the Food and Drug Administration for the intravenous treatment of acutely decompensated congestive heart failure.[80,81]

Diuresis may occur because of its direct natriuretic action, increased cardiac output, or decreased aldosterone levels. However, at greater doses, it may induce hypotension that can worsen renal function in patients dependent on the renin-angiotensin system to sustain renal perfusion pressure, an adverse effect analogous to that encountered with ACE inhibitors or angiotensin II receptor antagonists. Urodilatin lacks the systemic vasodilator effects of ANP and appears to be a more potent diuretic agent.[82] There are a number of anecdotal reports of favorable effects on renal function after cardiac surgery and cardiac and liver transplantation. These await confirmation by large prospective clinical studies.[83-86]

Cellular Receptors—Cytoprotection

Calcium Channels

Blockade of calcium channels provides potentially important cytoprotection against ischemic reperfusion injury. By preventing intracellular calcium influx and the conversion of xanthine dehydrogenase to xanthine oxidase (dependent on the calcium/calmodulin complex), calcium channel blockers may decrease the accumulation of oxygen free radicals. There is also evidence that these agents confer protection by attenuating reflow-induced vasoconstriction after ischemia, inhibiting angiotensin-induced constriction in the glomerulus and by decreasing circulating IL-2 receptors that promote cell injury.[87]

There is some evidence from small clinical studies that calcium channel blockers attenuate renal injury from a number of nephrotoxic agents, including cyclosporine A,[88] cisplatinum, and radiocontrast dyes.[89] The calcium channel blocker, diltiazem, has shown an additional unexpected benefit in renal transplantation in that it impairs cyclosporine A metabolism. This results in greater plasma cyclosporine A levels with fewer episodes of early acute rejection, but with less risk for cyclosporine A nephrotoxicity.[90]

The vasodilator effects of calcium channel blockers also impact renal function. Control of hypertension by diltiazem and nifedipine has been shown to promote natriuresis and increase renal blood flow and GFR.[91] In contrast, calcium blockers may overcome renal autoregulation and worsen renal function when they induce hypotension. For example, administration of nifedipine to patients with renal insufficiency caused nonoliguric renal failure that improved when the drug was discontinued.[92]

Adenosine Receptors

Ischemic preconditioning is a well-known phenomenon in cardiac muscle, whereby a series of short-lived sublethal ischemic events confers profound resistance to subsequent, more severe ischemic insults.[93] The key mediator of cytoprotection and increased cellular resistance to ischemia is adenosine, the endogenous degradation product of ATP. More recently, Lee and Emala[94,95] have demonstrated in an in vivo rat model of acute renal failure that ischemic preconditioning also occurs in the kidney and appears to be mediated by the adenosine receptor.

Adenosine plays an essential role in regulating intrarenal distribution of blood flow, renin release and electrolyte transport. Currently, four subtypes of adenosine receptors have been described: A_1, A_{2a}, A_{2b}, and A_3.[96] The A_1 and A_{2a} receptors may together potentially protect against renal ischemic reperfusion injury by enhancing renal oxygen balance. Stimulation of the A_1 receptor induces renal cortical vasoconstriction, which decreases GFR. This decreases renal oxygen consumption and promotes distribution of blood flow to the oligemic medulla. Stimulation of the A_{2a} adenosine receptor increases medullary renal blood flow and oxygen delivery. The two receptors are mutually antagonistic with regard to renin release, diuresis, and natriuresis—the A_1 receptor inhibits them, whereas the A_{2a} receptor does the opposite.

In Lee and Emala's in vivo model of ARF described earlier,[94,95] sharp differences have emerged regarding the role of adenosine receptor subtypes in ischemic reperfusion injury. Preischemic administration of adenosine (i.e., nonselective receptor stimulation) and selective A_1 adenosine receptor activation provides significant renal protection against global renal injury. In contrast, selective A_3 receptor activation actually worsens ischemic injury. Selective A_{2a} adenosine receptor stimulation has the greatest renal protective effects, even if delayed until the early reperfusion period after termination of renal ischemia.

These findings appear to support the pharmacologic development of a safe, specific A_{2a} adenosine receptor agonist, which could provide effective protection against renal ischemic injury. However, as pointed out by Lee and Sladen,[97] success in animal models does not necessarily translate into clinical efficacy in patients.

Conclusions

Through its regulation of vasomotor tone and salt and water homeostasis, the kidney provides remarkable control of the internal milieu. It does this through a complex interaction between glomerulus and tubule, and the specialized cells of these structures. It swiftly responds to changes in intravascular volume and coordinates a finely tuned mechanism of neurohormonal interactions that protect against hypovolemia or hypervolemia. Through antidiuresis or diuresis, the urine may be concentrated or diluted over a 500% range of osmolality. There exist many targets for current and potential drug action. Of these, those that allow us to manipulate urinary flow—diuretic agents—are the most established, predictable, and reliable in their ability to provide the desired effect. The most challenging realm remains the search for agents that consistently protect the kidney against ischemic or nephrotoxic injury. Although diuretics may attenuate renal injury by preventing tubular obstruction by ischemic cells or nephrotoxic debris, increased urine flow does not necessarily represent improved renal outcome. Agents that enhance renal blood flow and diuresis—DA agonists and ANPs—have shown great promise in animal studies, but clinical validation has not yet been forthcoming. Of agents that confer cytoprotection, the calcium channel blockers appear to have a role in protection against nephrotoxic injury, and specific A_{2a} adenosine receptor agonists offer the hope that success in animal studies finally may be translated to effectiveness in humans.

References

1. Levens NR, Peach MJ, Carey RM: Role of the intrarenal renin-angiotensin system in the control of renal function. Circ Res 48: 157–167, 1981.

2. Sladen RN, Landry D: Renal blood flow regulation, autoregulation, and vasomotor nephropathy. Anesthesiol Clin North America 18:791–807, ix, 2000.

3. Ballerman BJ, Zeidel ML, Gunning ME, Brenner BM: Vasoactive peptides and the kidney. In Brenner BM, Rector FCJ (eds): The Kidney, 4th ed. Philadelphia, WB Saunders, 1991, pp 510–583.

4. Landry DW: Vasopressin deficiency and hypersensitivity in vasodilatory shock: Discovery of a new clinical syndrome. P & S Medical Review 3:3–7, 1996.

5. Bartter FC, Schwartz WB: The syndrome of inappropriate secretion of antidiuretic hormone. Am J Med 42:790–806, 1967.

6. Landry DW, Oliver JA: The pathogenesis of vasodilatory shock. N Engl J Med 345:588–595, 2001.

7. Gerber JG, Olsen RD, Nies AS: Interrelationship between prostaglandins and renin release. Kidney Int 19:816–821, 1981.

8. Garella S, Matarese RA: Renal effects of prostaglandins and clinical adverse effects of nonsteroidal anti-inflammatory agents. Medicine 63:165–181, 1984.

9. de Bold AJ, Borenstein HB, Veress AT, Sonnenberg H: A rapid and potent natriuretic response to intravenous injection of atrial myocardial extract in rats. Life Sci 28:89–94, 1981.

10. Laragh J: Atrial natriuretic hormone, the renin-angiotensin axis, and blood-pressure electrolyte homeostasis. N Engl J Med 313:1330–1340, 1985.

11. Stanton BA, Koeppen BM: Control of body fluid osmolality and volume. In Berne RM, Levy MN (eds): Physiology, 3rd ed. St Louis, Mosby Year-Book, 1993, pp 754–783.

12. Gorfinkel HJ, Szidon JP, Hirsch LJ, et al: Renal performance in experimental cardiogenic shock. Am J Physiol 222:1260–1268, 1972.

13. Shannon RP, Libby E, Elahi D, et al: Impact of acute reduction in chronically elevated left atrial pressure on sodium and water excretion. Ann Thorac Surg 46:430–437, 1988.

14. Holtbäck U, Kruse MS, Brismar H, Aperia A: Intrarenal dopamine coordinates the effect of antinatriuretic and natriuretic factors. Acta Physiol Scand 168:215–218, 2000.

15. Bryan AG, Bolsin SN, Vianna PTG, Haloush H: Modification of the diuretic and natriuretic effects of a dopamine infusion by fluid loading in preoperative cardiac surgical patients. J Cardiothorac Vasc Anesth 9:158–163, 1995.

16. Stanton BA, Koeppen BM: Elements of renal function. In Berne RM, Levy MN (eds): Physiology, 3rd ed. St Louis, Mosby Year-Book, 1993, pp 719–753.

17. Thurau K, Boylan JW: Acute renal success: The unexpected logic of oliguria in acute renal failure. Am J Med 61:308–315, 1976.

18. Ito S, Carretero OA, Abe K: Nitric oxide in the regulation of renal blood flow. New Horiz 3:615–623, 1995.

19. Schrier RW: Effects of the adrenergic nervous system and catecholamines on systemic and renal hemodynamics, sodium and water excretion and renin secretion. Kidney Int 6:291–306, 1974.

20. Maddox DA, Brenner BM: Glomerular ultrafiltration. In Brenner BM, Rector FCJ (eds): The Kidney, 4th ed. Philadelphia, WB Saunders, 1992, pp 215–231.

21. Edwards RM, Rizna W, Kinter LB: Renal microvascular effects of vasopressin and vasopressin antagonist. Am J Physiol 256:F526–534, 1989.

22. Shipley RE, Study RS: Changes in renal blood flow, extraction of inulin, glomerular filtration rate, tissue pressure and urine flow with acute alterations of renal artery pressure. Am J Physiol 167:676–688, 1951.

23. Desjars PH, Pinaud M, Bugnon D, et al: Norepinephrine has no deleterious renal effects in human septic shock. Crit Care Med 17:426–429, 1989.

24. Kelleher SP, Robinette JB, Miller F, Conger JD: Effect of hemorrhagic reduction in blood pressure on recovery from acute renal failure. Kidney Int 31:725–730, 1987.

25. Mackay JH, Feerick AE, Woodson LC, et al: Increasing organ blood flow during cardiopulmonary bypass in pigs: Comparison of dopamine and perfusion pressure. Crit Care Med 23:1090–1098, 1995.

26. Brezis M, Rosen S: Hypoxia of the renal medulla: Its implications for disease. N Engl J Med 332:647–655, 1995.

27. Brezis M, Rosen S, Epstein F: The pathophysiologic implications of medullary hypoxia. Am J Kidney Dis 13:253–258, 1989.

28. Gelman S: Preserving renal function during surgery. Anesth Analg 74(suppl 1):88–92, 1992.

29. Landry DW, Levin HR, Gallant EM, et al: Vasopressin pressor hypersensitivity in vasodilatory septic shock. Crit Care Med 25:1279–1282, 1997.

30. Tsuneyoshi I, Yamada H, Kakihana Y, et al: Hemodynamic and metabolic effects of low-dose vasopressin infusions in vasodilatory septic shock. Crit Care Med 29:487–493, 2001.

31. Holmes CL, Walley KR, Chittock DR, et al: The effects of vasopressin on hemodynamics and renal function in severe septic shock: A case series. Intensive Care Med 27:1416–1421, 2001.

32. Gazmuri RJ, Shakeri SA: Low-dose vasopressin for reversing vasodilation during septic shock. Crit Care Med 29:673–675, 2001.

33. Morales DL, Gregg D, Helman DN, et al: Arginine vasopressin in the treatment of 50 patients with postcardiotomy vasodilatory shock. Ann Thorac Surg 69:102–106, 2000.

34. Argenziano M, Choudri AF, Oz MC, et al: A prospective randomized trial of arginine vasopressin in the treatment of vasodilatory shock after left ventricular assist device placement. Circulation 96(suppl II): II286–290, 1997.

35. Landry DW, Levin HR, Gallant EM, et al: Vasopressin deficiency contributes to the vasodilation of septic shock. Circulation 95:1122–1125, 1997.

36. Puschett JB: Pharmacological classification and renal actions of diuretics. Cardiology 84(suppl 2):4–13, 1994.

37. Johnston PA, Bernard DB, Perrin NS, Levinsky NS: Prostaglandins mediate the vasodilatory effect of mannitol in the hypoperfused rat kidney. J Clin Invest 68:127–133, 1981.

38. Mason J: The pathophysiology of ischemic acute renal failure. A new hypothesis about the initiation phase. Ren Physiol 9:129–147, 1986.

39. Zager RA, Foerder C, Bredl C: The influence of mannitol on myoglobinuric acute renal failure: Functional, biochemical, and morphological assessments. J Am Soc Nephrol 2:848–855, 1991.

40. Gubern JM, Martinez-Rodenas F, Sitges-Serra A: Use of mannitol as a measure to prevent postoperative renal failure in patients with obstructive jaundice. Am J Surg 159:444–445, 1990.

41. Clyne DH, Kant KS, Pesce AJ, Pollack VE: Nephrotoxicity of low molecular weight serum proteins. Physicochemical interactions between myoglobin, hemoglobin, Bence-Jones protein and Tamm-Horsfall mucoprotein. Curr Prob Clin Biochem 9:299, 1979.

42. Rose HJ, O'Malley K, Pruitt AW: Depression of renal clearance of furosemide in man by azotemia. Clin Pharmacol Ther 21:141–146, 1976.

43. Lindner A: Synergism of dopamine and furosemide in diuretic-resistant, oliguric acute renal failure. Nephron 33:121–126, 1983.

44. Memoli B, Libetta C, Conte G, Andreucci VE: Loop diuretics and renal vasodilators in acute renal failure. Nephrol Dial Transplant 4:168–171, 1994.

45. Anderson R, Linas S, Berns A, et al: Nonoliguric acute renal failure. N Engl J Med 296:1134–1137, 1977.

46. Brown C, Ogg C, Cameron J: High dose furosemide in acute renal failure: A controlled trial. Clin Nephrol 15:90–96, 1981.

47. Wilson NJ, Adderley RJ, McEniery JA: Supraventricular tachycardia associated with continuous furosemide infusion. Can J Anaesth 38: 502–505, 1991.

48. Sjostrom PA, Odlind BG, Beermann BA, et al: On the mechanism of acute tolerance to furosemide diuresis. Scand J Urol Nephrol 22:133–140, 1988.

49. Sica DA, Gehr TW: Diuretic combinations in refractory oedema states: Pharmacokinetic-pharmacodynamic relationships. Clin Pharmacokinet 30:229–249, 1996.

50. Inoue M, Okajima K, Itoh K, et al: Mechanism of furosemide resistance in analbuminemic rats and hypoalbuminemic patients. Kidney Int 32:198–203, 1987.

51. Brater DC: Diuretic resistance: Mechanisms and therapeutic strategies. Cardiology 84(suppl 2):57–67, 1994.

52. Olsen NV: Effects of dopamine on renal haemodynamics tubular function and sodium excretion in normal humans. Dan Med Bull 45:282–297, 1998.

53. Goldberg L, Rajfer S: Dopamine receptors: Applications in clinical cardiology. Circulation 72:245–248, 1985.

54. Bello-Reuss E, Higashi Y, Kaneda Y: Dopamine decreases fluid reabsorption in straight portions of rabbit proximal tubule. Am J Physiol 242:F634–F640, 1982.

55. Olsen NV, Olsen MH, Bonde J, et al: Dopamine natriuresis in salt-repleted, water-loaded humans: A dose-response study. Br J Clin Pharmacol 43:509–520, 1997.

56. Lokhandwala MF, Amenta F: Anatomical distribution and function of dopamine receptors in the kidney. FASEB J 5:3023–3030, 1991.

57. Aperia A: Dopamine action and metabolism in the kidney. Curr Opin Nephrol Hypertens 3:39–45, 1994.

58. Armstrong DK, Dasta JF, Reilley TF, Tallman RDJ: Effect of haloperidol on dopamine-induced increase in renal blood flow. Drug Intell Clin Pharm 20:543–546, 1986.

59. Allison NL, Dubb JW, Ziemniak JA, et al: The effect of fenoldopam, a dopaminergic agonist, on renal hemodynamics. Clin Pharmacol Ther 41:282–288, 1987.

60. Schaer GL, Fink MP, Parrillo JE: Norepinephrine alone versus norepinephrine plus low-dose dopamine: Enhanced renal blood flow with combination pressor therapy. Crit Care Med 13:492–496, 1985.

61. O'Hara Jr JF: Low-dose "renal" dopamine. Anesthesiol Clin North America 18:835–851, ix, 2000.

62. Lassnigg A, Donner E, Grubhofer G, et al: Lack of renoprotective effects of dopamine and furosemide during cardiac surgery. J Am Soc Nephrol 11:97–104, 2000.

63. Vincent JL: Renal effects of dopamine: Can our dream ever come true? Crit Care Med 22:5–6, 1994.

64. Thompson BT, Cockrill BA: Renal-dose dopamine: A siren song? Lancet 344:7–8, 1994.

65. Bailey JM: Dopamine: One size does not fit all. Anesthesiology 92:303–305, 2000.

66. MacGregor DA, Smith TE, Prielipp RC, et al: Pharmacokinetics of dopamine in healthy male subjects. Anesthesiology 92:338–346, 2000.

67. Garwood S: New pharmacologic options for renal preservation. Anesthesiol Clin North Am 18:753–771, 2000.

68. Nichols AJ, Ruffolo RR Jr, Brooks DP: The pharmacology of fenoldopam. Am J Hypertens 3(6 pt 2):116S–119S, 1990.

69. Panacek EA, Bednarczyk EM, Dunbar LM, et al: Randomized, prospective trial of fenoldopam vs sodium nitroprusside in the treatment of acute severe hypertension. Fenoldopam Study Group. Acad Emerg Med 2:959–965, 1995.

70. Brooks DP, Drutz DJ, Ruffolo RRJ: Prevention and complete reversal of cyclosporine A-induced renal vasoconstriction and nephrotoxicity in the rat by fenoldopam. J Pharmacol Exp Ther 254:375–379, 1990.

71. Bakris GL, Lass NA, Glock D: Renal hemodynamics in radiocontrast medium-induced renal dysfunction: A role for dopamine-1 receptors. Kidney Int 56:206–210, 1999.

72. Halpenny M, Markos F, Snow HM, et al: The effects of fenoldopam on renal blood flow and tubular function during aortic cross-clamping in anaesthetized dogs. Eur J Anaesthesiol 17:491–498, 2000.

73. Halpenny M, Markos F, Snow HM, et al: Effects of prophylactic fenoldopam infusion on renal blood flow and renal tubular function during acute hypovolemia in anesthetized dogs. Crit Care Med 29:855–860, 2001.

74. Atanasova I, Girchev R, Dimitrov D, et al: Atrial natriuretic peptide and dopamine in a dog model of acute renal ischemia. Acta Physiol Hung 82:75–85, 1994.

75. Conger JD, Falk SA, Hammond WS: Atrial natriuretic peptide and dopamine in established acute renal failure in the rat. Kidney Int 40:21–28, 1991.

76. Seki G, Suzuki K, Nonaka T, et al: Effects of atrial natriuretic peptide on glycerol induced acute renal failure in the rat. Jpn Heart J 33:383–393, 1992.

77. Kurnik BR, Allgren RL, Genter FC, et al: Prospective study of atrial natriuretic peptide for the prevention of radiocontrast-induced nephropathy. Am J Kidney Dis 31:674–680, 1998.

78. Allgren RL, Marbury TC, Rahman SN, et al: Anaritide in acute tubular necrosis. N Engl J Med 336:828–834, 1997.

79. Lewis J, Salem MM, Chertow GM, et al: Atrial natriuretic factor in oliguric acute renal failure. Anaritide Acute Renal Failure Study Group. Am J Kidney Dis 36:767–774, 2000.

80. Mills RM, LeJemtel TH, Horton DP, et al: Sustained hemodynamic effects of an infusion of nesiritide (human b-type natriuretic peptide) in heart failure: A randomized, double-blind, placebo-controlled clinical trial. Natrecor Study Group. J Am Coll Cardiol 34:155–162, 1999.

81. Colucci WS: Nesiritide for the treatment of decompensated heart failure. J Card Fail 7:92–100, 2001.

82. Hildebrandt DA, Mizelle HL, Brands MW, Hall JE: Comparison of renal actions of urodilatin and atrial natriuretic peptide. Am J Physiol 262:R395–399, 1992.

83. Cedidi C, Kusz ER, Meyer M, et al: Treatment of acute postoperative renal failure after liver and heart transplantation by urodilatin. Clin Invest 71:435–436, 1993.

84. Cedidi C, Meyer M, Kuse ER, et al: Urodilatin: A new approach for the treatment of therapy-resistant acute renal failure after liver transplantation. Eur J Clin Invest 24:632–639, 1994.

85. Hummel M, Kuhn M, Dub A, et al: Urodilatin: A new peptide with beneficial effects in the postoperative care of cardiac transplant patients. Clin Invest 70:674–682, 1992.

86. Wiebe K, Meyer M, Wahlers T, et al: Acute renal failure following cardiac surgery is reversed by administration of Urodilatin (INN: Ularitide). Eur J Med Res 1:259–265, 1996.

87. Neumayer HH, Gellert J, Luft FC: Calcium antagonists and renal protection. Ren Fail 15:353–358, 1993.

88. Wagner K, Albrecht S, Neumayer H-H: Prevention of post-transplant acute tubular necrosis by the calcium antagonist diltiazem: A prospective, randomized study. Am J Nephrol 7:287–291, 1987.

89. Neumayer HH, Junge W, Kufner A, Wenning A: Prevention of radiocontrast-media-induced nephrotoxicity by the calcium channel blocker nitrendipine: A prospective randomized clinical trial. Nephrol Dial Transplant 4:1030–1036, 1989.

90. Neumayer HH, Kunzendorf U, Schreiber M: Protective effects of calcium antagonists in human renal transplantation. Kidney Int 36(suppl):87–93, 1992.

91. Bauer J, Sunderrajan S, Reams G: Effects of calcium entry blockers on renin-angiotensin-aldosterone system, renal function and hemodynamics, salt and water excretion and body fluid composition. Am J Cardiol 56:62H-67H, 1985.

92. Diamond J, Cheung J, Fang L: Nifedipine-induced renal dysfunction. Am J Med 77:905–909, 1984.

93. Murry CE, Jennings RB, Reimer KA: Preconditioning with ischemia: A delay of lethal cell injury in ischemic myocardium. Circulation 74:1124–1136, 1986.

94. Lee HT, Emala CW: Protective effects of renal ischemic preconditioning and adenosine pretreatment: Role of A(1) and A(3) receptors. Am J Physiol Renal Physiol 278:F380–387, 2000.

95. Lee HT, Emala CW: Protein kinase C and G(i/o) proteins are involved in adenosine- and ischemic-preconditioning-mediated renal protection. J Am Soc Nephrol 12:233–240, 2001.

96. Fozard JR, Hannon JP: Adenosine receptor ligands: Potential as therapeutic agents in asthma and COPD. Pulm Pharmacol Ther 12:111–114, 1999.

97. Lee HT, Sladen RN: Perioperative renal protection. In: Murray MJ, Coursin DB, Pearl RG, Prough DS (eds): Critical Care Medicine: Perioperative Management, 2nd ed. New York, Raven Press, 2001.

22

Liver Physiology

Rupert Negus, MA, MB, BS, MRCD, PhD • John Summerfield, MD, FRCD

At 1200 to 1500 g the liver is the largest discrete organ in the body. It is central to the metabolism of carbohydrate, protein, and fats and is the main organ responsible for detoxification, both of endogenously produced metabolites and exogenous compounds. The liver plays a major role in protein synthesis, particularly albumin, in the clotting factors, and in other members of the acute phase response. This chapter describes the essential elements of liver physiology, with reference to those aspects that may be amenable to modification by conventional drug therapy. However, the immunologic functions of the liver are not detailed. Recently, it has been recognized that hemopoietic stem cells can differentiate into hepatocytes.[1] This raises the exciting possibility of gene therapy—e.g., using ex vivo transfection strategies that may overcome the problems that have been encountered to date with targeting genes to specific cell types. Treating inherited disorders of metabolism that have been identified as being due to single gene defects is now a possibility and will pave the way to treating conditions that may be caused by multiple gene defects.

Systems Physiology

Measurement of hepatic blood flow: A variety of techniques can be used to estimate hepatic blood flow, including indicator dilution techniques, dye or radioactive clearance techniques, constant infusion techniques, single injection methods, inert gas washout, Echo-Doppler and allied techniques, and oral or intravenous pharmacokinetics.

Indicator dilution techniques require the cannulation of one of the major vessels supplying the liver and are therefore too invasive for routine clinical use. However, this method does have the advantage that it is not dependent on hepatic function. This relies on the Fick principle[2] and requires peripheral access to provide the infusion, a peripheral arterial catheter and a catheter in the hepatic vein. The best indicator dye is indocyanine green, because its uptake is preserved in liver disease.[3] More recently, flow has been assessed by magnetic resonance angiography,[4] which may ultimately supersede the older invasive techniques.

Blood flow during physiologic conditions: During normal conditions, the liver receives 20% to 25% of the cardiac output at rest. The liver is unusual in receiving a blood supply from both the hepatic artery and the portal vein. The hepatic artery is a branch of the coeliac axis and supplies intrahepatic branches, which enter the liver sinusoids adjacent to the portal tracts[5,6]; although in humans direct arterioportal anastomoses are not seen. During resting conditions, the portal vein supplies about two thirds of the flow, this blood being derived from the splanchnic circulation. Assessments of liver blood supply during surgery indicate that 35% of the blood flow but 50% of hepatic oxygen requirements are met by the hepatic artery.[7] The branches of both the hepatic artery and the portal vein reach the liver lobules by way of the portal tracts. From these blood flows toward the central vein through the liver sinusoids, with blood being separated from the hepatocytes by a specialized endothelium, which contains relatively large holes. Between the sinusoid and the hepatocytes lies the space of Disse, which therefore can be accessed directly by plasma, but not the cellular elements of blood. It is here that the uptake of macromolecules in the blood, derived from both the systemic and splanchnic circulation, occurs.

Microcirculation within the liver: A liver lobule is recognized by its hexagonal structure; the central vein runs through the center. At the angles of the lobule margins are the portal tracts. Rappaport[8] redescribed hepatic architecture in functional terms as the acinus. Because blood arrives in the portal tracts both by way of the branches of the portal vein and the hepatic artery, an oxygen gradient is set up whereby the least oxygenated blood is found around the tributaries of the hepatic vein (Fig. 22–1). Considerations of the physical properties of oxygen and tissues led to a value of about 150 to 200 μm[9], calculated as the effective diffusion distance of oxygen from its source; this has been confirmed more recently by direct measurements in living tissues.[10] The distance between a portal tract and the draining hepatic vein in the human liver is about 500 μm. Thus it may be expected that certain parts of the hepatic lobule exist at low oxygen tensions. This may not only have implications in disease states, because the regions adjacent to the hepatic veins usually suffer most from viral, toxic, or anoxic injury, but it may also have functional implications that are not yet fully understood, because there exists a family of hypoxically regulated transcription factors; the best characterized factor is hypoxia inducible factor 1, which controls the expression of genes involved in cellular metabolism such as the glucose transporters and also those involved in regeneration and repair such as vascular endothelial growth factor.[11]

Hepatocyte function and blood flow: There is increasing evidence that the relationship of a hepatocyte to the blood supply may be critical in determining its function. It has been known for some time that periportal hepatocytes contain higher levels of rate-limiting enzymes involved in glycogen breakdown and gluconeogenesis, whereas hepatocytes around the hepatic venules have higher levels of enzymes involved in glycolysis and lipogenesis.[12]

Kupffer cell function and blood flow: In addition to endothelial cells, the liver sinusoids are lined by numerous resident macrophages known as Kupffer cells. These cells are derived from the circulating monocytes, because in liver transplantation, the donor liver rapidly becomes populated by host macrophages.[13] A variety of factors, including members of the chemokine family, promote macrophage migration.[14] In addition, there are also cytokines that inhibit macrophage migration, such as migration inhibition factor.[15] More recently the role of oxygen tension in the movement of these cells has been investigated and it has been found that low oxygen tension reversibly inhibits macrophage movement without interfering with phagocytic function.[16] These cells could therefore be used to deliver therapeutic genes to specific targets.

Adaptation to changes in blood flow: Given the high flow of blood to the liver it is perhaps not surprising that any increase in the demand for oxygen is met by an increase in oxygen extraction rather than an increase in blood flow.[17] However, flow in the hepatic artery does change in response to changes in flow in the portal vein, a reduction in portal vein flow being met by an increase in hepatic arterial flow[18] of anywhere between 22% and 100%[19]; although even these increases may not be enough to restore total hepatic blood flow. The mechanisms by which hepatic arterial flow are regulated are not fully understood, but may be mediated by adenosine.[20] However, unlike the hepatic artery, resistance in the portal vein appears to be passively dependent on flow and is not dependent on hepatic arterial flow.[21] Portal venous flow is largely dependent on flow in the splanchnic bed. Thus the increase in splanchnic flow that results from eating results in increased portal venous flow.[22]

Blood flow in disease states: A wide variety of disorders may affect hepatic blood flow. These may be conveniently divided into disorders of hepatic arterial flow, disorders of

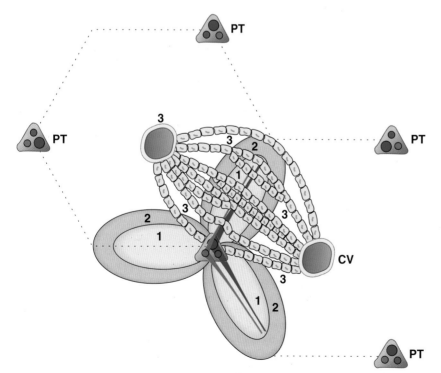

Figure 22–1. The microcirculation of the liver acinus. Hepatocytes fall into three zones according to their distance from the arteriolar blood supply (*1, 2,* and *3*). Varying oxygenation across these zones probably in part determines hepatocyte function by differential gene expression of hypoxically regulated genes. CV, central venule; PT, portal tract.

hepatic venous flow, and disturbed flow in the portal vein (Table 22–1).

The most frequently seen derangement of liver blood flow encountered clinically is cirrhosis caused most frequently by alcohol and hepatitis C. The primary event in cirrhosis is obstruction to portal venous flow. Blood is therefore diverted into collateral channels; some bypass hepatocytes altogether and flow into the hepatic veins by way of porto-hepatic anastomoses. Because of the fibrotic process, hepatic veins are displaced and ultimately regenerating nodules of hepatocytes become divorced from their portal blood supply, being supplied directly by the hepatic artery. More than 30% of the blood supply to the liver can bypass functioning liver tissue in cirrhosis. The obstruction to blood flow is probably a combination of distortion of blood vessels by regenerating nodules and collagen deposition in the space of Disse,[23] leading directly to increases in sinusoidal resistance. With cirrhosis there is probably a compensatory increase in hepatic artery pressure to supply blood to the liver in the face of increased sinusoidal resistance.

The major hemodynamic consequences of portal hypertension from any cause are ascites formation and esophageal varices. To form varices, a portal venous pressure gradient of 12 mm Hg or greater is required, but the absolute pressure is not a good predictor of subsequent bleeding.[24] The portal venous pressure gradient is the difference between the "wedged" hepatic venous pressure (sinusoidal pressure) and the "free" hepatic venous pressure.[25] The mortality rate associated with bleeding esophageal varices remains high, and 50% of patients may die as a direct result of their first variceal bleed.

Biochemical and Molecular Mechanisms Underlying Cellular Physiology

Bilirubin Metabolism

Bilirubin is a linear tetrapyrrole derived from the breakdown of a variety of haem-containing proteins, especially the cytochromes and hemoglobin. Cytochromes are found embedded in the inner mitochondrial membrane where they form part of the respiratory chain. All cytochromes are bound to an iron-containing haem group. Hemoglobin is the other major heme-containing molecule and is the major oxygen-carrying molecule in higher animals.

Heme is broken down by the action of heme oxygenase and nicotinamide adenine dinucleotide phosphate (NADPH)-cytochrome P450. Heme oxygenase is in the endoplasmic reticulum, whereas NADPH-cytochrome P450 is a microsomal enzyme. The action of these enzymes results in the formation of biliverdin IXα by the oxidation of heme at specific α-CH bridges (Fig. 22–2). Biliverdin IXα is in turn converted to bilirubin IXα by a cytosolic biliverdin IXα reductase.[26] Heme oxygenase is ubiquitous to all tissues, but is found in particularly high amounts in the spleen, the major site of breakdown of red blood cells.

Like heme oxygenase, biliverdin IXα reductase is present in almost all mammalian tissues, with high concentrations found in spleen, liver, and kidney. Radiolabeled bilirubin studies have given estimates of bilirubin production of 250 to 350 mg/day. One gram of haem yields 36.2 mg bilirubin.

Most bilirubin (80–85%) is derived from hemoglobin, which is broken down by the reticuloendothelial system, particularly in the spleen, and the remainder is derived from the breakdown of other haem-containing proteins. Bilirubin is then released from its sites of production into the plasma, where it binds albumin with high affinity ($K_a = 108$/mole). Because of their large size, these bilirubin-albumin conjugates cannot undergo glomerular filtration and are therefore retained in the circulation until the liver extracts them. During normal physiologic conditions, albumin binding of bilirubin prevents the concentration of free bilirubin from increasing, when it would otherwise diffuse into and bind to tissue components as in disease states leading to excess unconjugated bilirubin, such as hemolysis. Bilirubin trans-

TABLE 22–1.

Disease-Causing Disorders of Hepatic Blood Flow

Disorders of the hepatic artery
—Disorders causing occlusion

Ischemic cholangitis following transplantation
Polyarteritis nodosa
Trauma
Intrahepatic cytotoxic therapy

Disorders of the hepatic veins
—Disorders causing hepatic venous obstruction (Budd-Chiari syndrome)

Myeloproliferative disease
Systemic lupus erythematosus
Lupus anticoagulant
Paroxysmal nocturnal hemoglobinuria
Anticoagulant factor deficiency
Behçet disease
Pregnancy
Trauma
Malignant infiltration
Right atrial myxoma
Veno-occlusive disease
Unknown

Disorders of the portal venous system
—Portal venous hypertension

Schistosomiasis
Congenital hepatic fibrosis
Myeloproliferative disorders
Systemic mastocytosis
Primary biliary cirrhosis
Noncirrhotic portal hypertension
Cirrhosis

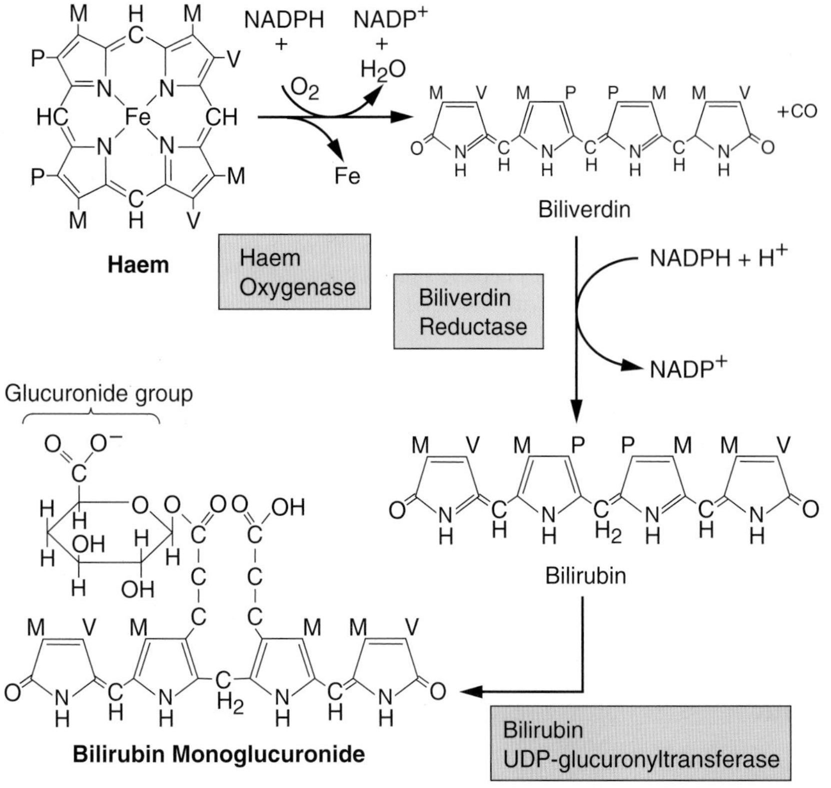

Figure 22–2. The metabolism of haem to bilirubin. Heme oxygenase is located in the endoplasmic reticulum of all tissues and in the presence of molecular oxygen and nicotinamide adenine dinucleotide phosphate (NADPH) oxidizes the α-CH bridge of heme to produce biliverdin. This is subsequently reduced to bilirubin, which is esterified within the liver by conjugation to glycosyl groups, thereby rendering bilirubin water soluble. M, methyl; P, propionate; UDP, uridine diphosphate; V, vinyl.

port into hepatocytes occurs through a specific membrane organic anion transporter system.[27] Once within the hepatocyte, bilirubin is actively transported to the endoplasmic reticulum for conjugation and then to the bile canaliculus for excretion in the bile.

Bilirubin conjugation (or esterification) occurs by reaction with glycosyl groups derived from various activated cytosolic sugars, such as uridine diphosphate-xylose (UDP-xylose), UDP-glucose, and UDP-glucuronic acid, itself derived from glucose. Conjugation yields diesters such as diglucuronides, and these are the principal bilirubin esters that are excreted in humans.[28] The process of esterification occurs on the endoplasmic reticulum and is catalyzed by UDP-glucuronyltransferase. The role of these enzymes in esterification extends beyond bilirubin to other potential toxins that require conjugation for detoxification and subsequent excretion through a "xenobiotic" response. These include opiates, phenols, steroids, bile acids, catecholamines, and thyroid hormones.

Conjugated bilirubin reaches the membrane through an active process involving a canalicular multispecific organic anion transporter (cMOAT).[29] This complex has adenosine triphosphatase (ATPase) activity, and a mutation in the human *cMOAT* gene is responsible for Dubin-Johnson syndrome.[30] The flow of bile in part is regulated by storage and release from the gallbladder. Once in the gut, conjugated bilirubin passes to the large intestine where it is deconjugated and reduced as a result of bacterial action. This results in the formation of urobilinogens that can undergo intestinal absorption, reconjugation, and resecretion in bile. A small amount of urobilinogen is normally excreted in urine and this is enhanced in hemolytic states.[31]

Carbohydrate and Fat Metabolism

The liver can be considered to be the seat of carbohydrate metabolism, regulating the production and storage of glucose according to metabolic demands. Sugars of all types are absorbed in the small intestine. The naturally occurring hexose sugars (containing 6 carbon atoms each)—glucose (the most prevalent), fructose, and galactose—are released by the digestion of complex carbohydrates and are actively transported by carrier systems located in the brush border of enterocytes.[32] They are carried in the portal blood flow to the liver where they are transported into the liver by active carrier-mediated systems, such as the glucose transporter family of proteins.[33] Glucose uptake is controlled by the autonomic nervous system and intestinal hormones, which both regulate insulin release.[34,35] Once within the hepatocyte, it may undergo glycolysis through the Embden-Meyerhof pathway to yield pyruvate and lactate or undergo polymerization to be stored as glycogen.[36] The net energy gain from this glycolysis is three molecules of adenosine triphosphate (ATP). Pyruvic acid may subsequently enter the citric acid cycle by conversion to acetic acid with the loss of 1 molecule of CO_2. For every molecule of acetic acid that enters the cycle, 8 atoms of hydrogen are liberated that enter the respiratory chain and eventually combine with molecular oxygen to form water. The citric acid cycle generates 12 molecules of ATP for every molecule of acetic acid and is therefore much more efficient than glycolysis in the release of energy. Pyruvic acid may also be used to generate glucose and can be formed from the metabolism of amino acids and fat. This molecule therefore holds a central place in metabolism (Fig. 22–3). The other hexose sugars, fructose and galactose, can also enter the Embden-Meyerhof pathway; fructose is converted to glyceraldehyde and dihydroxyacetone phosphate, and galactose is converted to uridine diphosphoglucose, which can then be converted to glucose through the formation of glycogen.

If energy is abundant, it can be stored as glycogen in the liver. This process is regulated by the concentration of blood glucose, which determines the activity of phosphorylase *a,* an enzyme involved in the degradation of glycogen.[37] Glycogen is a polymer of glucose and is formed after the conversion of glucose to glucose-1-phosphate by hexokinase and ATP and then to uridine diphosphate glucose by the reaction of glucose-1-phosphate with uridine triphosphate, catalyzed by glycogen synthase. Conversely, glucose can be released from glycogen by its breakdown, a process known as glycogenolysis. This reaction depends on the phosphorylation of glycogen to split off a molecule of glucose-1-phosphate, which can be converted to glucose-6-phosphate by phosphoglucomutase and thereby re-enter the glycolytic pathway. In the liver, an alternative pathway exists for the oxidation of sugars. This is the hexose monophosphate shunt. Glucose-6-phosphate is oxidized to phosphogluconic acid, which then undergoes oxidative decarboxylation to release H atoms and to form pentose phosphates. The latter may be used in nucleotide formation or may be reconverted to glucose.

Lipid Metabolism

Lipids are the water-insoluble cellular molecules that are soluble in organic solvents. They include the fatty acids, triglycerides, phospholipids, glycolipids, steroids including cholesterol, and the isoprenoids. Among the most important are the triglycerides, which are formed from the esterification of glycerol with three molecules of fatty acid. The fatty acids have the general formula $CH_3(CH_2)_nCOOH$ and include palmitic ($CH_3(CH_2)_{14}COOH$) and stearic acid ($CH_3(CH_2)_{16}COOH$). Fatty acids that contain double bonds are known as unsaturated, e.g., oleic acid: $CH_3(CH_2)_7CH=CH(CH_2)_7COOH$. Phospholipids, sphingomyelins, and cerebrosides are more complex molecules formed from fatty acids (Table 22–2). The latter two groups are particularly important in the function of neurons. Other lipids include cholesterol, cholesterol esters, steroid hormones, and the fat-soluble vitamins.

Fat may be derived either from dietary sources or by synthesis from acetic acid, which as discussed earlier can be generated from hexose sugars. Dietary fat is absorbed in the small intestine and after lipolysis by pancreatic lipase[38] and bile salts. The main role of bile salts is to produce micelles,[39]

TABLE 22–2.

The Major Components of the Compound Lipids

Compound	Components
Phospholipid	Glycerol, 2 molecules fatty acid, phosphate, nitrogen-containing base (e.g., choline)
Sphingomyelin	Fatty acid, phosphate, choline, complex base (sphingosine)
Cerebrosides	Galactose, fatty acid, sphingosine

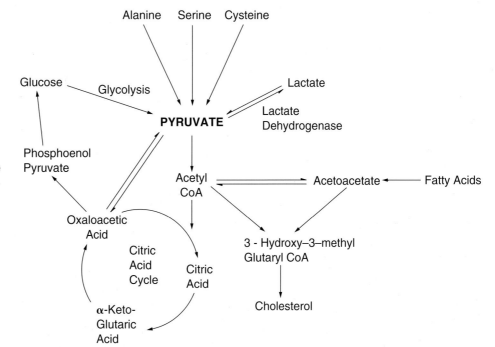

Figure 22–3. The central role of pyruvate in metabolism. CoA, coenzyme A.

which are able to solubilize polar lipids such as triglycerides, and thereby facilitate the action of pancreatic lipases and esterases in promoting absorption of dietary fats across enterocyte apical membranes. Bile salts, fatty acids, cholesterol, phospholipids, and triglycerides form polymolecular aggregates within the bowel lumen known as micelles, which are then absorbed across the intestinal brush border.[40] Within the enterocytes, monoglycerides and fatty acids containing more than 14 carbon atoms are re-esterified to triglycerides. Collections of triglyceride are coated with β-lipoprotein to form chylomicrons. Short chain fatty acids—i.e., those with less than 14 carbon atoms—are transported as free fatty acids in the bloodstream bound to albumin. Transport of triglycerides to and from the liver occurs within lipoproteins. These are complexes containing phospholipid, cholesterol, and structural components called apoproteins. Apoproteins are amphipathic, containing both hydrophilic and hydrophobic regions, the latter enabling them to bind to phospholipids. A variety of apoproteins have been characterized. Different apoproteins tend to be associated with different classes of lipoprotein. For instance, the major apoprotein in chylomicrons is C-III, whereas that found in very low density lipoprotein (VLDL) and low density lipoprotein (LDL) is B-100 and A-1 in high density lipoprotein (HDL).

After absorption, fat may be either metabolized to yield energy or stored as triglyceride in fat deposits. The extraction of triglycerides from chylomicrons is by the activity of lipoprotein lipase, an extracellular lipase that is attached to the endothelial lining of capillaries by heparan sulphate. The liver takes up the remnant chylomicrons, where cholesterol is extracted. This is the exogenous pathway. In the endogenous pathway, triglyceride is supplied to the tissues by the liver. It is transported as VLDL, in which it is packaged with cholesterol, cholesterolester, phospholipid apolipoprotein B-100, C apoproteins, and apolipoprotein E. Once again, the action of lipoprotein lipase allows the release of free fatty acids, which may be taken up by adipocytes for storage or oxidized within body tissues as an energy source. Because VLDL contains cholesterol, this becomes the main component of these particles after the removal of triglycerides. But the removal of triglyceride also alters the density of these particles that therefore become known as LDL. LDL is then removed from the circulation mainly within the liver by hepatocytes that bear a LDL surface receptor. Fat is very rich in energy, 1 g yielding 38 kJ heat, compared with 16.7 kJ from the breakdown of 1 g glucose. Because fat may make up to 10% of total body weight in an adult, this may represent 7 kg, which translates into approximately 3800 kJ/kg, or more than a month of energy reserve.

Cholesterol and the Enterohepatic Circulation

Cholesterol not only forms a key component of the cell wall and intracellular organelles, but it is also associated with the transport of fatty acids and triglyceride. Unlike the particles in which triglyceride is transported to peripheral tissues, cholesterol transport from the periphery to the liver occurs as HDL. Once it has reached the liver, cholesterol can be excreted in the bile in association with bile acids. However,

unlike the bile acids, more than 97% of which are reabsorbed in the terminal ileum, only 50% of cholesterol is reabsorbed. Thus the formation of HDLs represents a major route of cholesterol excretion. Cholesterol itself is mainly synthesized in the tissues from acetate, in a reaction catalyzed by β-hydroxy-β-methyglutaryl coenzyme A (HMG CoA) reductase. There is evidence that biliary cholesterol excretion may depend on dietary cholesterol,[41] but the exact mechanism remains unknown. Certainly bile salts and phospholipids are important in increasing the solubility of cholesterol in water.[42]

The primary bile acids, cholate and chenodeoxycholate, are themselves produced from cholesterol. In a reaction catalyzed by colonic bacteria the primary bile acids are converted to deoxycholic and lithocholic acids. Bile acids are conjugated in the liver with the amino acids glycine or taurine, which prevents absorption in the biliary tree and the majority of the small intestine, but allows reabsorption in the terminal ileum. Bile salts are actively excreted into the bile by a transport-mediated process that relies on a 100-KD glycoprotein[43] and is helped by an intracellular negative potential of about −35 mV. As described earlier, bile salts are intimately involved with the absorption of dietary fats. Once absorbed, bile salts return to the liver through the portal vein where they are taken up by hepatocytes in a sodium-coupled transport system (Fig. 22–4). The enterohepatic circulation

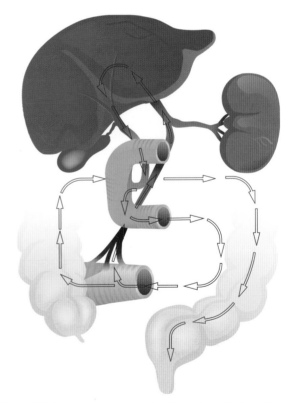

Figure 22–4. The enterohepatic circulation of bile salts. Bile salts produced in the liver consist primarily of cholic and chenodeoxycholic acid derived from cholesterol. These enter the small bowel through the bile duct and pass through to the terminal ileum, where most are reabsorbed in micelles associated with cholesterol and phospholipids. Some pass through to the large bowel, where they undergo 7α-dehydroxylation by colonic bacteria to produce deoxycholic and some lithocholic acid.

results in bile acids being absorbed and excreted up to five times a day. Fractional absorptions differ, therefore the different bile acids have different synthesis and turnover rates. In cholestatic syndromes, bile acids enter the urine by both active transport and passive diffusion.[44]

Protein Metabolism

Short peptide sequences and amino acids are delivered to the liver after active uptake from the lumen of the small intestine by enterocytes. The liver synthesizes a variety of proteins (Table 22–3), including albumin and the clotting factors. The liver is also largely responsible for the oxidative deamination of amino acids that are no longer required, a process that liberates energy and generates urea.

Albumin, the most abundant serum protein, is largely responsible for maintaining plasma oncotic pressure and, as described earlier, also has an important transport role. Normally the liver synthesizes about 10 g albumin per day[45] and has a relatively long half-life of 22 days; therefore serum albumin is not always significantly diminished in fulminant acute hepatic failure. Albumin synthesis can also be switched off by the action of cytokines such as IL-1 in sepsis

TABLE 22–3.

The Major Proteins Synthesized by the Liver

Transport proteins	Albumin
	Ceruloplasmin
	Transferrin
	Ferritin
Acute phase proteins	Fibrinogen
	α_1-Antitrypsin
	C-reactive protein
	Serum amyloid A
Coagulation factors	Prothrombin (factor II)
	Proconvertin (factor VII)
	Stuart-Prower factor (factor X)
Anticoagulant factors	Antithrombin III
	Proteins S and C
	Heparin cofactor II
Other proteins	α-Fetoprotein
	α_2-Macroglobulin
	α_1-Antichymotrypsin
	Complement components: C_1, C_3, C_6
	Hemopexin
	Haptoglobin

syndromes.[46] Ceruloplasmin and transferrin are also transport proteins, responsible for the carriage of copper and iron, respectively. Reduced levels of ceruloplasmin are seen in Wilson disease,[47] in which there is accumulation of excess copper in hepatocytes, which eventually leads to liver failure. Hemopexin is a protein that can bind free haem in plasma. The liver mainly removes haem/hemopexin complexes. α_1-Antitrypsin deficiencies may result in liver and pulmonary disease. Its normal function is to inhibit the action of trypsin and other serum proteases. Mutations in the gene for α_1-antitrypsin lead to accumulation of abnormally folded, insoluble α_1-antitrypsin the liver,[48] although exactly how this causes liver damage is unclear.

The hepatocyte is the major site for synthesis of all the coagulation factors with the exception of von Willebrand factor and factor VIIIC. The proteins produced include the vitamin K-dependent factors II (prothrombin), VII (stable factor), IX (Christmas factor), and X (Stuart-Prower factor), the vitamin K-independent factor V (labile factor), factor VIII (antihemophilic factor), factors XI (plasma thromboplastin antecedent) and XII (Hageman factor), fibrinogen, and fibrin-stabilizing factor XIII (fibrin-stabilizing factor). Because the half-life of these clotting factors, particularly factor VII ($t_{1/2}$ = 100–300 minutes) is short, the coagulation cascade is particularly sensitive to acute hepatocellular damage. Vitamin K is found in two forms, K_1 and K_2. Vitamin K_1 is derived from plants and is the major dietary source of this vitamin. Because uptake is dependent on bile salts, it frequently becomes deficient in cholestatic states. K_2 is largely produced by colonic *Escherichia coli*, and alone is insufficient to provide dietary needs. Vitamin K is required for the post-translational modification of several of the clotting factors that contain a number of glutamic acid residues in their amino terminal regions. Vitamin K is a cofactor for a carboxylase that converts these residues to γ-carboxylic acid. Several anticoagulant factors also rely on vitamin K. These include antithrombin III, protein S, and protein C. The administration of vitamin K will usually restore prothrombin levels when vitamin K deficiency is caused by bile salt malabsorption as occurs in cholestasis, but may also help in hepatocellular necrosis because there is frequently an element of failure of bile salt secretion.

Oxidative deamination leads to the breakdown of surplus amino acids, once again with the release of energy. Deamination may also be coupled with the transfer of an amino group from one amino acid to another, so-called transamination. Surplus ammonia, which is not used for transamination, is extremely toxic and is therefore converted into urea for excretion by the kidneys. Urea formation only occurs in the liver.[49] The reaction does not proceed directly, but requires ornithine that is recycled. Ornithine initially combines with CO_2 and NH_3 to give citrulline. Citrulline combines with a second molecule of NH_3 to give arginine and arginine is hydrolyzed by arginase to yield water, ornithine, and urea (Fig. 22–5). The kidney then excretes urea. There is some proximal tubular reabsorption as a consequence of sodium reabsorption. Serum urea levels are usually held constant between 2.5 and 7.5 mmol/L, but because of the way it is synthesized and subsequently handled, urea concentrations are altered in a number of conditions. In starvation, urea levels initially diminish because of reduced

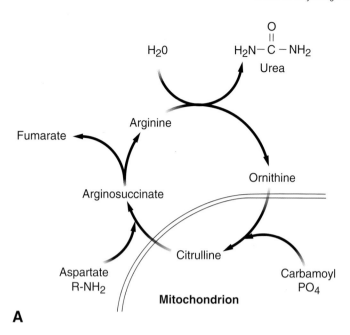

B

Figure 22–5. Kreb's urea cycle. *A,* NH_2 group-derived amino acids are combined with water to produce urea. *B,* The conversion of arginine to ornithine with the production of urea.

dietary intake. However, in prolonged starvation, when other body energy stores are exhausted, muscle and other proteins are broken down and urea levels increase. Any form of renal impairment leading to a reduction in the excretion of urea causes urea levels to increase. A large protein meal will cause urea levels to increase. This is particularly true after a large gastrointestinal hemorrhage. However, in hepatocellular failure, urea production is reduced and serum urea levels decrease.

Portal Hypertension

Currently, the standard therapies for esophageal varices include pharmacologic agents to decrease portal venous pressure to prevent bleeding, and drugs and endoscopic or surgical procedures to deal with bleeding once it has occurred. This may be sufficient by itself in patients whose varices have not yet bled. The mainstay of prophylaxis to prevent bleeding is propranolol.[50] Nitrates can be used in those unable to tolerate beta-blockers. In the event of variceal bleeding, various drugs have been used in an attempt to decrease portal venous pressure. These include both vasoconstrictors and vasodilators. Amongst the vasoconstrictors, vasopressin and terlipressin[51] are effective and have been used in clinical practice for some time. However, both can cause coronary vasoconstriction and must be used with caution in patients with ischemic heart disease. Somatostatin and its analogues such as octreotide are also useful and may be superior.[52] These act on vascular smooth muscle to increase the resistance in the splanchnic bed and therefore to reduce flow. Endoscopic therapy is recommended even if bleeding is controlled pharmacologically.[53]

Hyperlipidemia

Hyperlipidemia and in particular high levels of serum HDL is a major risk factor for atherosclerotic heart disease.[54,55] Lesions resembling those seen in human coronary atherosclerosis can be induced in primates by feeding with a high fat, high cholesterol diet; and in heterozygous familial hypercholesterolemia, severe atherosclerotic lesions develop in association with elevated LDL levels.[56] A variety of drugs are now available that help to reduce the level of serum cholesterol. The first group that showed promise in clinical practice was those that bind bile salts, thereby preventing cholesterol from re-entering the circulation as part of the enterohepatic circulation. Such bile acid-sequestering agents include cholestyramine and colestipol. However, these may exacerbate hypertriglyceridemia. Another group of drugs in current use are the fibrates, e.g., bezafibrate and gemfibrozil. Fibrates activate a transcription factor named peroxisome proliferator-activated receptor α.[57] They act by reducing VLDL cholesterol and are not very effective at decreasing LDL cholesterol. Most recently has been the introduction of a class of HMG CoA reductase inhibitors collectively known as statins. Statins have been show to successfully reduce the likelihood of coronary events in two large trials,[58,59] although the number of subjects needed for treatment to prevent a single clinical event is large. It may be sensible to target those with elevated serum LDL cholesterol levels greater than 160 mg/dL.[60]

Inborn Errors of Metabolism

Because of its central place in metabolism and the large number of enzymes involved, there are many single gene defects that result in aberrations of metabolism. These inborn errors of metabolism affect carbohydrate, fat, and protein synthesis. In addition, the liver may also be primarily responsible for disorders of haem metabolism.

The glycogenoses: Ten major forms of glycogen storage disease have been recognized (0-IX). Of these, eight involve the liver and may also involve other organs. The remaining two are restricted to muscle (Table 22–4). As described earlier, glycogen is a polymer of glucose. It has a highly branched structure with about 12 glucose residues between each branch. The branched formation allows for more compact storage. Glycogen is abundant in liver and muscle, but can be formed by any tissue. A variety of enzymes are involved in the formation and degradation of glycogen. Glycogen synthetase adds glucose residues to the growing chain and branching enzyme catalyzes branch formation. Conversely, phosphorylase catalyzes the cleavage of glucose from the ends of chains until a branch point is reached where debranching enzyme acts. Glycogen is both stored and metabolized within the cytosol, but can also be broken down within lysosomes by the action of α-1,4 glucosidase.

Other than type II glycogen storage disease that results from a defect in α-1,4 glucosidase, all the glycogenoses result in abnormal storage of cytosolic glycogen. All of these conditions are rare, having a combined incidence of about 1:60,000, and all are inherited in an autosomal recessive fashion with the exception of IXb, which is sex-linked recessive. The main forms to affect the liver are types I, III, and IV. One of the main clinical manifestations of those forms of glycogen storage disease that predominantly affect the liver is hepatomegaly. In type I disease, hepatomegaly is present at birth, and in the others appears within the first few months of life. Types III, VI, and IX give rise to mild disease and the prognosis is usually good. In type I disease, hypoglycemia is a particular problem and has to be overcome by regular glucose feeds. In this condition, the brain adapts to by using β-hydroxybutyrate and acetoacetate as energy sources. Because type II disease represents a problem with lysosomal glycogen storage, organ involvement is widespread and cardiac enlargement is frequently a prominent feature. Patients usually survive only to the second or third decade.

Because these diseases are brought about by single enzyme defects, it should be possible to treat them by replac-

TABLE 22–4.

Classification of the Glycogenoses

Type	Name	Enzyme Defect	Main Site of Glycogen Storage
0	—	Glycogen synthetase	Liver
I	von Gierke disease	Glucose-6-phosphatase	Liver, kidney, gut
II	Pompe's disease	Lysosomal α-1,4 glucosidase	Liver, muscle, myocardium
IIIa	Forbes disease	Amylo-1,6 glucosidase	Liver, muscle
IIIb	Cori disease	Debranching enzyme	Liver
IV	Andersen disease	Amylo-1,4,1,6 transglucosidase	Liver
V	McArdle	Muscle phosphorylase	Muscle
VI	Hers disease	Liver phosphorylase	Liver
VII	Tauri	Phosphofructokinase	Muscle
VIII	—	Phosphorylase activation	Liver, brain
IXa	—	Phosphorylase kinase	Liver, muscle
IXb	—	Phosphorylase kinase	Liver, muscle
X	—	Phosphorylase kinase	Liver, muscle
XIa	—	Not known	Liver, kidney

ing the missing enzyme. Liver transplantation has been used with success in type I disease[61] and type IV disease. Both of these types may be complicated by the development of hepatic adenomas and subsequent hepatocellular carcinoma. Transplantation ideally should be performed before malignant transformation has occurred. Recently, four of six patients suffering from hemophilia A responded to transplantation of autologous dermal fibroblasts transfected with plasmids containing factor VIII sequences.[62] This approach may become clinically important in patients suffering from the glycogenoses.

Other inborn errors of sugar metabolism include hereditary fructose intolerance, caused by a mutation in the gene for aldose B[63] and galactosemia in which hepatocytes and red blood cells lack galactose-1-phosphate-uridyl transferase. Hereditary fructose intolerance results in fructose intoxication caused by cytoplasmic accumulation of fructose-1-phosphate.[64] Treatment is with fructose and sucrose avoidance. Galactosemia causes tissue accumulation of galactose-1-phosphate.[65] The prognosis is poor, with cirrhosis and portal hypertension occurring in those who survive the first few weeks of life. Avoidance of milk, however, greatly improves the prognosis and may allow development to adult life.

Disorders of fat metabolism: Hyperlipidemias are common. They may result from genetic abnormalities or arise secondary to other diseases particularly simple obesity and diabetes. Primary hyperlipidemias are known to occur as a result of defects in the enzymes that process lipids, such as lipase, defects in lipoprotein receptors, defects in the lipoproteins themselves, and others in which the defect has not yet been characterized. The main form of hyperlipidemia for which the liver is primarily responsible is familial hypercholesterolemia.

Absence of the cell surface LDL receptor results in an increase in total plasma cholesterol. Sixty percent of LDL receptors are found in the liver. Because of the increase in plasma cholesterol, cholesterol is laid down in the tissues resulting in cutaneous xanthomata and premature vascular disease. Hypercholesterolemia is also a feature of primary biliary cirrhosis, an autoimmune condition characterized by the presence of antimitochondrial antibodies, which results in the progressive destruction of intrahepatic bile dusts. Increased levels of LDL occur in primary biliary cirrhosis, but the mechanism underlying this is not certain.

Disorders of amino acid metabolism: Given the central role that the liver plays in the metabolism of proteins, it is not surprising that abnormalities of amino acid metabolism can occur leading to disease. One of the best recognized of these is hereditary tyrosinemia, an autosomal recessive condition characterized by lack of the enzyme that normally catalyzes the last step of tyrosine degradation. The condition is diagnosed by finding elevated levels of plasma and urinary tyrosine, phenylalanine, and methionine. The prognosis is related to the age at presentation, being better the longer symptoms take to develop. Treatment is avoidance of aromatic amino acids and methionine, but this does not appear to prevent the development of hepatocellular carcinoma that can complicate up to 40% of cases of hereditary tyrosinemia. Liver transplantation is a therapeutic option that can be used.[66] As discussed earlier, single gene defects may also be amenable to gene therapy approaches.

Summary

This chapter has presented a brief overview of the physiologic functions of the liver and has commented on some diseases that arise when normal regulatory systems fail. The emphasis on metabolism reflects the central role that the liver plays in performing and co-ordinating these processes. Given the large number of enzymes and other regulatory proteins involved, it is not surprising that a large number of potential therapeutic targets are available, only a handful of which are currently exploited. With increasing knowledge of the human genome, it is to be expected that not only will our understanding of normal liver physiology improve, but so too will our ability to identify novel therapeutic strategies and targets.

References

1. Alison MR, Poulsom R, Jeffery R, et al: Hepatocytes from non-hepatic adult stem cells. Nature 406:257, 2000.
2. Bradley SE, Ingelfinger FJ, Bradley GP, et al: The estimation of hepatic blood flow in man. J Clin Invest 24:890, 1945.
3. Lebrec D, Blanchet L, Lacroix S: Measurement of hepatic blood flow in the rat using fractional clearance of indocyanine green and colloidal radiogold. Pflugers Archiv 391:353, 1981.
4. Manfredi R, Scarano E, Pedicelli A, et al: Functional radiology of the liver: Magnetic resonance imaging. Rays 22:295, 1997.
5. Charnsangavej C, Chuang VP, Wallace S, et al: Angiographic classification of hepatic arterial collaterals. Radiology 144:485, 1982.
6. Oikawa H, Masuda T, Yashima A, et al: Blood-flow route from the hepatic artery and portal vein to the sinusoid in normal human liver observed by confocal laser scanning microscopy. Anal Quant Cytol Histol 21:255, 1999.
7. Tygstrup N, Winker K, Mellemgaard K, et al: Determination of the arterial blood flow and oxygen supply in man by clamping the hepatic artery during surgery. J Clin Invest 41:447, 1962.
8. Rappaport AM: Hepatic blood flow: Morphologic aspects and physiologic regulation. Int Rev Physiol 21:1, 1980.
9. Tannock IF: The relation between cell proliferation and the vascular system in a transplanted mouse mammary tumour. Br J Cancer 22:258, 1968.
10. Helmlinger G, Yuan F, Dellian M, et al: Interstitial pH and pO2 gradients in solid tumors in vivo: High-resolution measurements reveal a lack of correlation. Nat Med 3:177, 1997.
11. Pugh CW, Chang GW, Cockman M, et al: Regulation of gene expression by oxygen levels in mammalian cells. Adv Nephrol Necker Hosp 29:191, 1999.
12. Jungermann K, Katz N: Functional specialization of different hepatocyte populations. Physiol Rev 69:708, 1989.
13. Steinhoff G, Wonigeit K, Sorg C, et al: Patterns of macrophage immigration and differentiation in human liver grafts. Transplant Proc 21:398, 1989.
14. Negus RP: The chemokines: Cytokines that direct leukocyte migration. J R Soc Med 89:312, 1996.
15. David JR: Delayed type hypersensitivity in vitro: Its mediation by cell free sustances formed by lymphoid cell-antigen interaction. Proc Natl Acad Sci USA 56:72, 1966.
16. Turner L, Scotton C, Negus R, et al: Hypoxia inhibits macrophage migration. Eur J Immunol 29:2280, 1999.
17. Lautt WW: Hepatic vasculature: A conceptual review. Gastroenterology 73:1163, 1977.
18. Greenway CV, Oshiro G: Intrahepatic distribution of portal and hepatic arterial blood flows in anaesthetized cats and dogs and the effects of portal occlusion, raised venous pressure and histamine. J Physiol 227:473, 1972.

19. Groszmann RJ, Blei AT, Kniaz JL, et al: Portal pressure reduction induced by partial mechanical obstruction of the superior mesenteric artery in the anesthetized dog. Gastroenterology 75:187, 1978.

20. Lautt WW, Legare DJ, d'Almeida MS: Adenosine as putative regulator of hepatic arterial flow (the buffer response). Am J Physiol 248:H331, 1985.

21. Hanson KM, Johnson PC: Local control of hepatic arterial and portal venous flow in the dog. Am J Physiol 211:712, 1966.

22. Hopkinson BR, Schenk WG Jr: The electromagnetic measurement of liver blood flow and cardiac output in conscious dogs during feeding and exercise. Surgery 63:970, 1968.

23. Loreal O, Clement B, Schuppan D, et al: Distribution and cellular origin of collagen VI during development and in cirrhosis. Gastroenterology 102:980, 1992.

24. Lebrec D, de Fleury P, Rueff B: Portal hypertension, size of esophageal varices and risk of gastrointestinal bleeding in alcoholic cirrhosis. Gastroenterology 79:1139, 1980.

25. Groszmann RJ, Glickman M, Blei AT, et al: Wedged and free hepatic venous pressure measured with a balloon catheter. Gastroenterology 76:253, 1979.

26. Maines MD, Polevoda BV, Huang TJ, et al: Human biliverdin IX alpha reductase is a zinc-metalloprotein. Characterization of purified and Escherichia coli expressed enzymes. Eur J Biochem 235:372, 1996.

27. Tiribelli C, Ostrow JD: New concepts in bilirubin chemistry, transport and metabolism: Report of the Second International Bilirubin Workshop, April 9-11, 1992, Trieste, Italy. Hepatology 17:715, 1993.

28. Fevery J, Van de Vijver M, Michiels R, et al: Comparison in different species of biliary bilirubin-IX alpha conjugates with the activities of hepatic and renal bilirubin-IX alpha-uridine diphosphate glycosyltransferases. Biochem J 164:737, 1977.

29. Kitamura T, Jansen P, Hardenbrook C, et al: Defective ATP-dependent bile canalicular transport of organic anions in mutant (TR-) rats with conjugated hyperbilirubinemia. Proc Natl Acad Sci USA 87:3557, 1990.

30. Paulusma CC, Kool M, Bosma PJ, et al: A mutation in the human canalicular multispecific organic anion transporter gene causes the Dubin-Johnson syndrome. Hepatology 25:1539, 1997.

31. Bernstein RB: Comparison of serum clearance and urinary excretion of mesobilirubinogen-H 3 in control subjects and patients with liver disease. Gastroenterology 61:733, 1971.

32. Stevens BR, Kaunitz JD, Wright EM: Intestinal transport of amino acids and sugars: Advances using membrane vesicles [Review]. Ann Rev Physiol 46:417, 1984.

33. Silverman M: Structure and function of hexose transporters. Ann Rev Biochem 60:757, 1991.

34. Xue C, Aspelund G, Sritharan KC, et al: Isolated hepatic cholinergic denervation impairs glucose and glycogen metabolism. J Surg Res 90:19, 2000.

35. Kreymann B, Williams G, Ghatei MA, et al: Glucagon-like peptide-1 7-36: A physiological incretin in man. Lancet 2:1300, 1987.

36. Pilkis SJ, Granner DK: Molecular physiology of the regulation of hepatic gluconeogenesis and glycolysis. Ann Rev Physiol 54:885, 1992.

37. Roach PJ: Control of glycogen synthase by hierarchil protein phosphorylation. FASEB J 4:2961, 1990.

38. Blow D: Enzymology. Lipases reach the surface [letter; comment]. Nature 351:444, 1991.

39. Almgren M: Mixed micelles and other structures in the solubilization of bilayer lipid membranes by surfactants [Review]. Biochim Biophys Acta 1508:146, 2000.

40. Compassi S, Werder M, Boffelli D, et al: Cholesteryl ester absorption by small intestinal brush border membrane is protein-mediated. Biochemistry 34:16473, 1995.

41. Sehayek E, Ono JG, Shefer S, et al: Biliary cholesterol excretion: A novel mechanism that regulates dietary cholesterol absorption. Proc Natl Acad Sci USA 95:10194, 1998.

42. Carey MC, Small DM: The physical chemistry of cholesterol solubility in bile. Relationship to gallstone formation and dissolution in man. J Clin Invest 61:998, 1978.

43. Hofmann AF: Bile acid secretion, bile flow and biliary lipid secretion in humans. Hepatology 12:17S; discussion 22S, 1990.

44. Summerfield JA, Cullen J, Barnes S, et al: Evidence for renal control of urinary excretion of bile acids and bile acid sulphates in the cholestatic syndrome. Clin Sci Mol Med 52:51, 1977.

45. Caso G, Scalfi L, Marra M, et al: Albumin synthesis is diminished in men consuming a predominantly vegetarian diet. J Nutr 130:528, 2000.

46. Ballmer PE, McNurlan MA, Grant I, et al: Down-regulation of albumin synthesis in the rat by human recombinant interleukin-1 beta or turpentine and the response to nutrients. JPEN J Parenter Enteral Nutr 19:266, 1995.

47. Bearn AG: Wilson's Disease: An inborn error of metabolism with multiple manifestations. Am J Med 22:747, 1957.

48. Lomas DA: Loop-sheet polymerization: The structural basis of Z alpha 1-antitrypsin accumulation in the liver. Clin Sci (Lond) 86:489, 1994.

49. Bollman JL, Mann FC, Magath TB: Studies on the physiology of the liver on deamination XV. Effect of total removal of the liver on deamination. Am J Physiol 78:258, 1926.

50. Grace ND: Nonsurgical treatment of variceal bleeding. Curr Treat Options Gastroenterol 2:104, 1999.

51. Goulis J, Burroughs AK: Role of vasoactive drugs in the treatment of bleeding oesophageal varices. Digestion 60(Suppl 3):25, 1999.

52. Corley DA, Cello JP, Adkisson W, et al: Octreotide for acute esophageal variceal bleeding: A meta-analysis. Gastroenterology 120:946, 2001.

53. Seewald S, Seitz U, Yang AM, et al: Variceal bleeding and portal hypertension: Still a therapeutic challenge? Endoscopy 33:126, 2001.

54. Keys A: Alpha lipoprotein (HDL) cholesterol in the serum and the risk of coronary heart disease and death. Lancet 2:603, 1980.

55. Assmann G, Schulte H, Funke H, et al: The emergence of triglycerides as a significant independent risk factor in coronary artery disease. Eur Heart J 19(Suppl M):M8, 1998.

56. Sprecher DL, Schaefer EJ, Kent KM, et al: Cardiovascular features of homozygous familial hypercholesterolemia: Analysis of 16 patients. Am J Cardiol 54:20, 1984.

57. Neve BP, Fruchart JC, Staels B: Role of the peroxisome proliferatoractivated receptors (PPAR) in atherosclerosis [Review]. Biochem Pharmacol 60:1245, 2000.

58. Downs JR, Clearfield M, Weis S, et al: Primary prevention of acute coronary events with lovastatin in men and women with average cholesterol levels: Results of AFCAPS/TexCAPS. Air Force/Texas Coronary Atherosclerosis Prevention Study. JAMA 279:1615, 1998.

59. Shepherd J, Cobbe SM, Ford I, et al: Prevention of coronary heart disease with pravastatin in men with hypercholesterolemia. West of Scotland Coronary Prevention Study Group. N Engl J Med 333:1301, 1995.

60. Anonymous: Summary of the second report of the National Cholesterol Education Program (NCEP) Expert Panel on Detection, Evaluation, and Treatment of High Blood Cholesterol in Adults (Adult Treatment Panel II) [letter; comment]. JAMA 269:3015, 1993.

61. Coire CI, Qizilbash AH, Castelli MF: Hepatic adenomata in type Ia glycogen storage disease. Arch Pathol Lab Med 111:166, 1987.

62. Roth DA, Tawa NE, O'Brien, JM, et al: Nonviral transfer of the gene encoding coagulation factor VIII in patients with severe hemophilia A. N Engl J Med 344:1735, 2001.

63. Cross NC, de Franchis R, Sebastio G, et al: Molecular analysis of aldolase B genes in hereditary fructose intolerance. Lancet 335:306, 1990.

64. Froesch ER, Wolf HP, Baitsch H, et al: Hereditary fructose intolerance: An inborn defect of hepatic fructose-1-phosphate splitting aldolase. Am J Med 34:151, 1963.

65. Gitzelmann R: Galactose-1-phosphate in the pathophysiology of galactosemia. Eur J Pediatr 154:S45, 1995.

66. Freese DK, Snover DC, Sharp HL, et al: Chronic rejection after liver transplantation: A study of clinical, histopathological and immunological features. Hepatology 13:882, 1991.

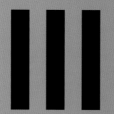

Pharmacologic Basis
of Clinical Practice

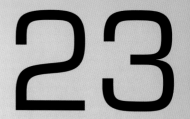

Inhalational Anesthetics

Alex S. Evers, MD • Donald D. Koblin, MD, PhD

The inhaled anesthetics are a class of drugs that are administered as gases and that produce a state referred to as general anesthesia. Until the mid-nineteenth century, surgical procedures were performed on a limited basis because there were no safe and effective anesthetic agents. Between 1842 and 1847 it was demonstrated that inhalation of diethyl ether (by Crawford Long and W.T.G. Morton), nitrous oxide (by Horace Wells), or chloroform (by J.Y. Simpson) could produce general anesthesia. The inhaled anesthetics were rapidly incorporated into clinical practice and, coupled with the subsequent discovery of aseptic technique, spawned the development of surgery. Both chloroform and diethyl ether had major limitations including flammability, unfavorable pharmacokinetics (slow onset and slow recovery), and adverse side effects. This led to a continuous search for better-inhaled anesthetics (see "Properties of the Ideal Inhaled Anesthetic"). Halothane, a halogenated alkane was introduced in the 1950s, providing the first nonflammable, potent inhaled agent. Subsequently, a series of halogenated short-chain ethers have been introduced with improved pharmacokinetic and side effect profiles; isoflurane, sevoflurane, and desflurane are the agents currently in clinical use. The structures of the clinically used inhaled anesthetics are illustrated in Figure 23–1.

Despite their clinical importance, the mechanism of action of the inhaled anesthetics remains one of the unsolved

Clinically Used Inhalational Anesthetics

Non-Halogenated Anesthetics

Nitrous oxide   Xenon

Halogenated Alkanes

Halothane

Halogenated Ethers

Isoflurane   Desflurane

Sevoflurane   Enflurane

Figure 23–1. Chemical structures of inhaled anesthetics currently in clinical use or likely to be in use in the future (xenon). Xe, xenon.

mysteries of pharmacology. The difficulty in understanding the mechanisms of anesthetic action is partially attributable to the fact that a wide variety of structurally unrelated gases can produce anesthesia. This led to the notion that there are no structure/activity relationships for inhaled anesthetics and that all gases produce anesthesia by a common mechanism based on physical properties of the gases (the Unitary Theory of Anesthesia). The recent demonstration that there are relationships between the molecular structure and anesthetic activity of gases[1,2] indicates that inhaled anesthetics must act through specific interactions with target molecules (presumably proteins) in the central nervous system. This has led to a concerted effort to identify the molecular and neuroanatomic loci of inhaled anesthetic action. This chapter reviews the results of these efforts using a reduc-

tionist approach, proceeding from behavior to anatomy to cellular physiology to molecular biology.

Although all inhaled anesthetics produce an apparently similar anesthetic state, the drugs are quite dissimilar in their pharmacokinetics and in their secondary actions (side effects) on other organ systems. This is important because the inhaled anesthetics are among the most dangerous pharmacologic agents used (therapeutic indices of 2–4). The selection of specific inhaled anesthetics is aimed at minimizing toxicity and is based on the pharmacokinetic properties and on the secondary effects of the various drugs, in the context of the individual patient's age, pathophysiology, and medication use. The second part of this chapter explores the clinical use of inhaled anesthetics focusing on pharmacokinetics and side effect profiles of the various agents.

MECHANISMS OF ACTION

To understand the mechanisms of anesthetic action it is essential to precisely define anesthesia. General anesthesia is commonly defined as *a reversible depression of the central nervous system sufficient to permit surgery to be performed without movement, obvious distress, or recall*. It has long been apparent that this global definition of anesthesia is inadequate, because different inhaled anesthetics produce different patterns of effects. For example, nitrous oxide (N_2O) is a potent analgesic at concentrations at which it produces minimal sedation. In contrast, analgesia is more closely associated with unconsciousness with the halogenated ethers and alkanes. An alternative way of defining general anesthesia is as a collection of component behaviors, including sedation, immobilization in response to noxious stimulation, amnesia, analgesia, and attenuation of autonomic responses to noxious stimulation. The discovery that some of the components of anesthesia are produced in specific loci in the central nervous system (see later) suggests that each of the various components of anesthesia could have a unique mechanism of action.

Anatomic Localization of Inhaled Anesthetic Action

Inhaled anesthetics could, in principle, produce their various behavioral effects via actions in the cerebral cortex, brain stem, spinal cord or peripheral nervous system. At only 2 minimum alveolar concentration (MAC; see "Clinical Measurements of Anesthetic Potency") isoflurane can produce electrical silence in the brain,[3] showing that virtually any neuron is a plausible target for anesthetic action. Interestingly, at anesthetic concentrations at and below MAC, the inhaled anesthetics are quite selective in their effects on various neuronal pathways. For example, neither halothane nor N_2O produces any inhibition of mechanosensor

responses or C fiber conduction in cats[4] and actually sensitizes peripheral nociceptors in monkeys.[5] This indicates that the peripheral nervous system is unlikely to be involved in the actions of the inhaled anesthetics. Similarly, studies in cerebral cortex have shown that specific neuronal circuits show markedly different sensitivity to inhaled anesthetic agents.[6,7] These data have prompted detailed efforts to find specific anatomic regions responsible for specific components of anesthesia.

The endpoint most frequently used to measure anesthetic potency is MAC, the alveolar concentration of an inhaled anesthetic at which there is no purposeful response to a noxious stimulus. Studies in rats have shown that neither cervical spinal cord transection[8] nor decerebration[9] alters MAC. This suggests that anesthetic inhibition of motor response to a noxious stimulus results from anesthetic action in the spinal cord. This hypothesis was confirmed by Antognini, who isolated the brain circulation of goats and selectively perfused either the brain or the rest of the body with isoflurane. He found that isoflurane MAC was 1.2 volume % when the whole body was exposed to isoflurane, 2.9% when only the brain was exposed to isoflurane, and 0.8% when only the body (including spinal cord) was exposed to isoflurane.[10,11] These results indicate that inhibition of purposeful response to noxious stimulus is a spinal cord effect and that anesthetic actions on brain may actually sensitize the cord to noxious stimuli. The effects of isoflurane on the spinal cord are due, at least in part, to direct inhibition of spinal motor neuron excitability.[12,13] The demonstration that MAC for isoflurane is produced through action on the spinal cord has not yet been extended to other halogenated anesthetics or N_2O.

Analgesia is another important component of general anesthesia. Recent studies by Maze and colleagues have demonstrated that N_2O produces analgesia through actions on opioidergic neurons in the periaqueductal gray matter in the brain stem.[14,15] These neurons project to the dorsal horn of the spinal cord where they act through α_{2B} adrenergic receptors to inhibit nociception.[16,17] A circuit diagram showing the pathways involved in N_2O analgesia is shown in Figure 23–2. There is no evidence that other inhalational anesthetics produce analgesia through this pathway. Indeed, even the analgesic effects of the α_2 adrenergic agonist, dexmedetomidine (see Chapter 28), are produced through different α_2 adrenergic receptors (α_{2A} rather than α_{2B}) in spinal cord.

The anatomic loci at which inhaled anesthetics produce other components of anesthesia, such as unconsciousness or amnesia, remain undefined. It seems likely that the amnesic effects of the inhaled anesthetics are produced, at least in part, by actions in the hippocampus. Synaptic transmission in the hippocampus is inhibited by all of the halogenated anesthetics,[18] and the hippocampus is important in memory

formation. The anatomic loci at which inhaled anesthetics produce unconsciousness is also unknown. The halogenated anesthetics have been shown to depress the excitability of thalamocortical neurons.[19] This suggests the thalamus as a potential locus for the sedative effects of inhaled anesthetics because blockade of thalamocortical communication would produce unconsciousness.

Physiologic Actions of Inhaled Anesthetics

In principle, anesthetics could produce their effects on central nervous system function by either reducing neuronal excitability or by altering synaptic function. Reduced excitability could result from neuronal hyperpolarization, which would inhibit neuronal automaticity, pattern genera-

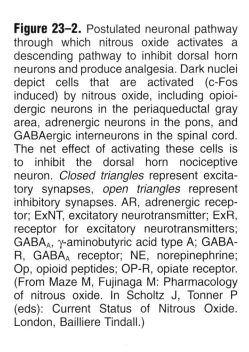

Figure 23–2. Postulated neuronal pathway through which nitrous oxide activates a descending pathway to inhibit dorsal horn neurons and produce analgesia. Dark nuclei depict cells that are activated (c-Fos induced) by nitrous oxide, including opioidergic neurons in the periaqueductal gray area, adrenergic neurons in the pons, and GABAergic interneurons in the spinal cord. The net effect of activating these cells is to inhibit the dorsal horn nociceptive neuron. *Closed triangles* represent excitatory synapses, *open triangles* represent inhibitory synapses. AR, adrenergic receptor; ExNT, excitatory neurotransmitter; ExR, receptor for excitatory neurotransmitters; GABA$_A$, γ-aminobutyric acid type A; GABA-R, GABA$_A$ receptor; NE, norepinephrine; Op, opioid peptides; OP-R, opiate receptor. (From Maze M, Fujinaga M: Pharmacology of nitrous oxide. In Scholtz J, Tonner P (eds): Current Status of Nitrous Oxide. London, Bailliere Tindall.)

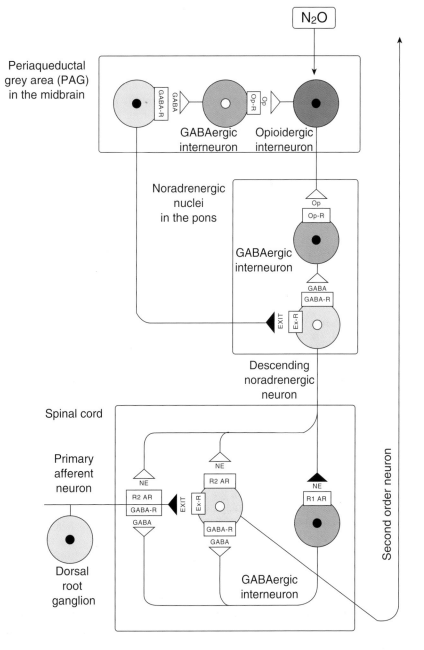

tion, and action potential generation. Inhibition of voltage-gated ion channels could also reduce neuronal excitability by preventing action potential generation and propagation. With regard to synaptic function, anesthetics could act either by enhancing inhibitory synaptic function or by reducing excitatory synaptic function. Furthermore, the effects of anesthetics could be either presynaptic or postsynaptic. Current evidence indicates that inhaled anesthetics are heterogeneous in their physiologic actions, with different agents affecting different physiologic processes. The actions of inhaled anesthetics on cellular neurophysiology are explored in the following section.

Effects on Neuronal Excitability

There is strong evidence that a variety of inhaled anesthetics can hyperpolarize both cortical and spinal neurons.[20,21] There is a rough correlation between the ability of an agent to hyperpolarize neurons and its potency as an anesthetic. Although the magnitude of the neuronal hyperpolarization produced by inhaled agents is small, it is enough to inhibit the *initiation* of an action potential either at a postsynaptic site or in a spontaneously firing neuron. Indeed, in the invertebrate, *Lymnaea stagnalis* (the great pond snail), halothane selectively hyperpolarizes a subpopulation of neurons producing a reduction in their spontaneous rate of firing (Fig.

23–3*A*).[22] Similarly, isoflurane hyperpolarizes thalamocortical neurons, leading to an inhibition of tonic firing of action potentials.[19]

The halothane-induced hyperpolarization observed in snail neurons results from activation of a "background potassium channel," originally designated as the anesthetic potassium current ($I_{K(an)}$).[23] Activation of a similar potassium current is responsible for isoflurane hyperpolarization of thalamocortical neurons.[24] Recently, a family of "background potassium channels" has been described with a unique structure consisting of two pore domains in tandem with four transmembrane-spanning segments (2P/4TM; see Fig. 23–3*C,D*). The 2P/4TM channels are important in regulating resting membrane potential, can be modulated by chemical second messengers, and appear to be the vertebrate homologs of $I_{K(an)}$. Studies by Yost originally showed that one member of this family, TOK1, can be activated by inhaled agents.[25] Subsequent detailed studies by Lazdunski and colleagues have shown that various inhaled agents differentially modulate the various members of the 2P/4TM family (see Fig. 23–3*B,D*). For example, TREK-1 (TWIK-related K⁺ channels) channels are activated by clinical concentrations of chloroform, diethyl ether, halothane, and isoflurane; TRAAK (TWIK-related arachidonic acid-stimulated K⁺ channels) channels are insensitive to all inhaled anesthetics; and TASK (TWIK-related acid-sensitive K⁺ channels) channels are activated by halothane and isoflurane, inhibited by diethyl ether, and unaffected by chloroform.[26] They have also shown that specific portions of the 2P/4TM channel protein are required for anesthetic action, suggesting the existence of anesthetic binding site(s) on the channel protein.

Inhaled anesthetics do not appear to have significant effects on the generation or propagation of action potentials. This is consistent with findings from the 1950s that synaptic function, rather than axonal propagation, is the major locus for anesthetic action.[27] There is no evidence indicating that anesthetics alter the threshold potential of a neuron for action potential generation. Similarly, most evidence indicates that clinically relevant concentrations of anesthetics do not alter the function of the voltage-gated channels involved in action potential generation.[28] Thus neuronal hyperpolarization through activation of potassium channels appears to be the major effect of inhaled anesthetics on neuronal excitability. Although the role of neuronal hyperpolarization in the various components of anesthesia is not defined, this is a plausible mechanism by which inhaled anesthetics could produce some components of the anesthetic state.

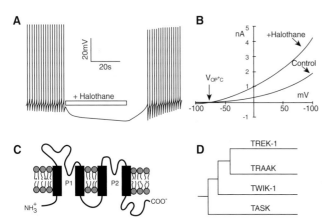

Figure 23–3. Inhaled anesthetics activate background K⁺ channels. (*A*) Halothane (400 μM) reversibly hyperpolarizes a pacemaker neuron from *Lymnaea stagnalis* to a potential below that needed to trigger an action potential by activating anesthetic potassium channel. (*B*) Halothane (300 μM) causes a large increase in activity of human recombinant TREK-1 cells expressed in COS cells. (*C*) Predicted membrane topology of a subunit of the family of the mammalian background K⁺ channels. There are four transmembrane segments and two pore-forming domains in tandem (2P/4TM). (*D*) Phylogenetic tree of the mammalian 2P/4TM family. Some but not all of these channels are activated by inhaled anesthetics. TASK, TWIK-related acid-sensitive K⁺ channels; TRAAK, TWIK-related arachidonic-acid-stimulated K⁺ channels; TREK, TWIK-related K⁺ channels; TWIK, tandem of P domains in weak inward rectifier K⁺ channels. (From Franks NP, Lieb WR: Background K⁺ channels: An important target for volatile anesthetics? Nat Neurosci 2:395, 1999.)

Effects on Synaptic Function

The effects of inhaled anesthetics on synaptic function are heterogeneous, varying as a function of both the agent and the synapse being studied. Enhancement[6,29] and reduction[7,30-34] of both excitatory and inhibitory synaptic transmission by inhaled agents have been documented. This multitude of effects suggests that various inhaled anesthetics may act at different molecular targets, and that a given anesthetic may affect more than one aspect of synaptic function. The multitude of observed effects is also consistent with the large variation in synaptic structure, function (i.e., efficacy), and chemistry (neurotransmitters, modulators) extant in the nervous system. Despite the complexity described earlier, there is substantial agreement about some of the major effects of inhaled anesthetics on synaptic function.

There is widespread agreement that the halogenated inhalation anesthetics enhance inhibitory synaptic transmission.[35,36] This has been best studied in synapses at which γ-aminobutyric acid (GABA, the major inhibitory neurotransmitter in brain) is the predominant neurotransmitter (Fig. 23–4A,C). These studies show that halogenated inhaled anesthetics prolong the duration of the inhibitory postsynaptic current (IPSC) while either reducing or having no effect on the IPSC amplitude (see Fig. 23–4B).[37] Inhaled anesthetics also enhance the currents elicited by exogenous application of GABA, indicating that the anesthetic effect is postsynaptic and is probably the result of direct anesthetic action on the GABA$_A$ receptor protein[38,39] (see Chapter 3 for a discussion of ligand-gated ion channels and Chapter 9 for a discussion of inhibitory synaptic transmission).

Electrophysiologic studies examining the actions of halogenated inhaled anesthetics on GABA$_A$ receptors indicate that the anesthetics do not affect the conductance of the ion channel.[40] Rather, they produce a change in the conformation of GABA$_A$ receptors that increases the affinity of the receptor for GABA, shifting the GABA concentration-response curve to the left.[38] This enhancement of GABA effectiveness is referred to as potentiation and produces the observed increase in IPSC duration, because higher affinity binding of GABA slows the dissociation of GABA from postsynaptic GABA$_A$ channels (see Fig. 23–4B). Inhaled anesthetics would not be expected to increase the amplitude of a GABAergic IPSP, because synaptically-released GABA probably reaches saturating concentrations in the synapse. Higher concentrations of inhaled anesthetics can produce

additional effects, either directly activating or blocking GABA$_A$ channels.[41] Blocking of GABA$_A$ receptor ion channels by high concentrations of inhaled anesthetics may explain the decreased IPSC amplitude sometimes observed during anesthetic administration.

Glycine is another important inhibitory neurotransmitter, particularly in the spinal cord and brain stem. Whereas the actions of inhaled anesthetics on glycinergic synapses have not been as widely studied as on GABAergic synapses, there is strong evidence that clinical concentrations of inhaled anesthetics potentiate glycine-activated currents in intact neurons[38] and in cloned glycine receptors expressed in oocytes.[42] The inhaled anesthetics appear to produce their enhancing effect by increasing the affinity of the receptor for glycine,[43] analogous to their effect on GABA$_A$ receptors.

In stark contrast to the robust effects of the halogenated alkanes and ethers on inhibitory neurotransmitter receptors, there is a subset of inhaled anesthetics that do not appear to have any effect on GABA$_A$ receptor function. This was first demonstrated for N$_2$O.[44,45] It has subsequently been shown that xenon (Xe)[46,47] and cyclopropane[48] are virtually devoid of effect on currents mediated by the GABA$_A$ receptor. Although it has not been definitively proven, it is likely that the actions of halogenated inhaled anesthetics on GABAergic and glycinergic inhibitory neurotransmission are important in producing some of the components of anesthesia. That N$_2$O, Xe, and cyclopropane do not affect inhibitory neurotransmission suggests that these anesthetics may constitute a distinct group with a completely different mechanism of action.

Inhaled anesthetics have also been shown to inhibit excitatory neurotransmission in some central nervous system synapses.[7,30,31,49] The major excitatory neurotransmitter in the central nervous system is glutamate and there are three categories of postsynaptic glutamate receptors: α-amino-3-hydroxy-5-methylisoxazole-4-propionic acid (AMPA),

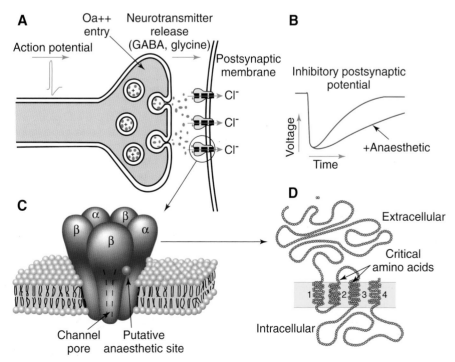

Figure 23–4. Inhaled anesthetics enhance inhibitory neurotransmission by potentiating the actions of γ-aminobutyric acid (GABA) and glycine at GABA$_A$ (GABA type A) and glycine receptors. (*A*) GABA and glycine are released at inhibitory synapses and bind to GABA$_A$ and glycine receptors. This allows chloride ions to enter the postsynaptic neuron. (*B*) Inhaled anesthetics prolong the opening of ion channels (GABA$_A$ and glycine receptors), enhancing postsynaptic inhibition. (*C,D*) GABA$_A$ and glycine receptors are pentamers of closely related subunits. The membrane topology of a single subunit is shown in *D*. The *red balls* illustrate the putative sites of isoflurane action. (From Franks NP, Lieb WR: Inhibitory synapses. Anaesthetics set their sites on ion channels. Nature 380:334, 1997.)

kainate, and *N*-methyl-D-aspartate (NMDA) receptors (see Chapter 9 for a detailed discussion). The bulk of experimental evidence indicates that all three types of glutamate receptors are insensitive to clinical concentrations of the halogenated inhaled anesthetics.[38,50] Studies using cloned and expressed glutamate receptor subunits show that agonist responses of AMPA receptors (glutamate receptor 3 subunit) are inhibited by halogenated anesthetics, whereas agonist responses of kainate receptors (glutamate receptor 6 subunit) are enhanced.[51] However, these effects of halogenated anesthetics are observed only at concentrations significantly above the clinical range.

N_2O has recently been shown to be an inhibitor of excitatory postsynaptic currents.[44] This effect is produced by selective inhibition of glutamate-stimulated currents mediated by the NMDA receptor; N_2O has minimal effects on currents mediated by AMPA or kainate receptors.[45] These data suggest that N_2O acts through a different mechanism than the halogenated inhaled agents; it blocks NMDA-type glutamate receptors and does not affect $GABA_A$ receptors. Recently, both Xe[46,47] and cyclopropane[48] have also been shown to selectively block currents mediated by the NMDA receptor. These data suggest that N_2O, Xe, and cyclopropane constitute a family of inhaled agents with different sites and mechanisms of action than the ethers and halogenated alkanes that act, at least in part, through actions on $GABA_A$ receptors. It remains undefined which components of anesthesia are mediated by inhibition of NMDA-type glutamate receptors.

In addition to effecting postsynaptic neurotransmitter receptors, there is substantial evidence from brain slice preparations[52,53] and from synaptosomes[54] that halogenated alkanes and ether anesthetics can act presynaptically to inhibit release of excitatory and inhibitory neurotransmitters. Inhibition of neurotransmitter release may explain how these drugs can inhibit inhibitory synaptic transmission.[32-34] Inhibition of neurotransmitter release by inhaled anesthetics appears to be mediated by inhibition of neurosecretion, rather than by inhibition of transmitter synthesis or storage. The mechanism by which anesthetics act to inhibit neurotransmitter release is not yet defined, but there are several candidate targets. First, Ratnakumari and Hemmings[55] have shown that presynaptic sodium channels are inhibited by halothane. This could reduce depolarization of the presynaptic membrane, attenuating calcium entry and thus the neurosecretory process. There is also evidence that inhaled anesthetics can reduce calcium entry into the presynaptic terminal,[56] perhaps by blocking neuronal voltage-dependent calcium channels.[57] Blockade of voltage-gated calcium channels is responsible for inhaled anesthetic inhibition of secretion in neuroendocrine cells.[58,59] (It should be noted that clinical concentrations of inhaled agents have modest effects on neuronal voltage-activated calcium currents. However, modest inhibition of calcium entry may profoundly inhibit transmitter release because neurosecretion has a steep dependence on intracellular calcium.) Finally, the proteins involved in neurotransmitter vesicle release (syntaxin, synaptobrevin, SNAP-25) have been identified as a major locus for isoflurane action in lower organisms.[60] Regardless of the precise molecular target, the halogenated alkane and ether anesthetics do have substantial effects on neurotransmitter release, and this may be an important mechanism underlying some of components of anesthesia. There is no evidence that N_2O or Xe affects neurotransmitter release, but this may be because of a paucity of investigation.

Other Molecular Targets

Other members of the ligand-gated ion channel family are expressed in the central nervous system and are potential targets of inhaled anesthetic action. Neuronal nicotinic receptors are expressed on presynaptic terminals in the brain and in sympathetic ganglia, and they are inhibited by clinical concentrations of halogenated alkane and ether anesthetics.[61,62] Studies examining various combinations of neuronal nicotinic receptor subunits show that in receptors composed of various combinations of $\alpha2$, $\alpha4$, $\beta2$, and $\beta4$ subunits, acetylcholine-elicited currents are inhibited by subanesthetic concentrations of halothane[63] and isoflurane.[64] The extreme sensitivity of the neuronal nicotinic receptors to inhaled anesthetics makes it unlikely that they are the site of action for anesthetic-induced unconsciousness or loss of response to noxious stimulation. It is plausible that neuronal nicotinic receptors are contributors to anesthetic-induced analgesia or amnesia, both of which occur at concentrations substantially below MAC. The actions of cyclopropane and Xe on neuronal nicotinic receptors are not known, but cyclopropane has recently been shown to block currents mediated by neuronal nicotinic receptors.[48]

Serotonin-3 (5-HT_3) receptors are another member of the superfamily of ligand-gated receptor channels. Clinical concentrations of volatile anesthetics potentiate currents activated by 5-hydroxytryptamine in intact cells[65] and in cloned receptors expressed in oocytes.[66] The potential contribution of 5-HT_3 receptors to the components of general anesthesia is not known; 5-HT_3 receptors may contribute to some unpleasant anesthetic side effects such as nausea and vomiting.

The actions of inhaled anesthetics on ion channels could be mediated by direct anesthetic actions on the channel proteins or indirectly by anesthetic modulation of second messenger systems or regulatory proteins. Phosphorylation is the most important known mechanism for regulation of ion channel function and therefore a plausible target for anesthetic action. In principle, an anesthetic could affect the phosphorylation state of an ion channel either by acting on a protein kinase or a protein phosphatase. Although there is not a substantial body of data concerning the effects of anesthetics on protein kinases and phosphatases, the effects of inhaled anesthetics on protein kinase C (PKC) have been studied. Slater and colleagues[67] showed that several anesthetics inhibit purified brain PKC and that they act through an effect on the regulatory (lipid-binding) subunit. Subsequent studies have shown that halothane has two distinct actions on brain PKC: stimulation of PKC activity and potentiation of activation-induced PKC translocation and down-regulation.[68] Although inhaled anesthetic modulation of PKC may be important in some actions of the drug, it does not appear to be responsible for actions on the $GABA_A$ receptor, because halothane affects $GABA_A$ receptors on excised membrane patches in the absence of ATP and with a time course inconsistent with phosphorylation.[69]

Biochemical Basis of Inhaled Anesthetic Action

For most of the twentieth century it was thought that all anesthetics act by a common mechanism based on physical rather than structural properties of the anesthetic molecule; this idea is called the Unitary Theory of Anesthesia. This theory was based on the Meyer-Overton correlation[70,71] and subsequent refinements,[72] showing that the anesthetic potency of a gas correlates with its solubility in relatively nonpolar solvents. It was widely assumed that inhaled anesthetics dissolved in lipid bilayers (the nonpolar solvent) and acted by perturbing the biophysical properties of biologic membranes. The discovery that different inhaled anesthetics probably act through different mechanisms (e.g., N_2O vs. isoflurane) challenged the Unitary Theory. The finding that certain halogenated alkanes and ethers were incorrectly predicted to be anesthetics by the Meyer-Overton correlation (referred to as nonimmobilizers) suggested that structural and physical properties of a molecule were responsible for determining anesthetic activity.[2] This was confirmed by the finding that enantiomers of isoflurane differed in their potency as anesthetics in animals.[1,73] Enantiomers are "mirror image" molecules that have identical physical properties but different shape. Collectively, the data with nonimmobilizers and enantiomers indicate that inhaled anesthetics probably act by binding to specific sites and have focused attention on potential protein binding sites.

The plausibility that inhaled anesthetics act by binding to specific sites on proteins was established in studies examining isolated model proteins. For example, it was shown that inhaled anesthetics could modulate the function of firefly luciferase in a manner consistent with the Meyer-Overton correlation and that was apparently competitive with respect to substrate binding.[74,75] Subsequent x-ray crystallographic studies provided a high-resolution image of the inhaled anesthetic binding site on firefly luciferase.[76] Similarly, inhaled anesthetics were shown to compete with fatty acids for binding sites on bovine serum albumin.[77] Again, x-ray crystallographic studies provided a high-resolution definition of the precise location and shape of these binding sites.[78]

It has proven more difficult to demonstrate and to characterize binding sites for inhaled anesthetics on membrane protein targets such as the $GABA_A$ receptor. Enantioselective effects of inhaled agents on ion channel function have provided one line of evidence for the existence of specific binding sites on membrane proteins. As discussed earlier, the enantiomers of isoflurane differ by about 40% in their anesthetic potency (R^+ isomer more potent than S^- isomer), as determined using the loss of righting reflex endpoint in rodents.[73,79] Isoflurane shows similar enantioselectivity in its actions on $GABA_A$ receptor–mediated currents[41] and background potassium currents.[61] This contrasts with the actions of isoflurane enantiomers on other ion channels where either no enantioselectivity or opposite ($S > R$) enantioselectivity is observed.[80,81] These results support the existence of specific inhaled anesthetic binding sites on $GABA_A$ receptors and background potassium channels. The similar enantiose-

lectivity observed at the level of behavior (loss of righting reflex) and ion channel physiology is consistent with these sites contributing to isoflurane-induced obtundation.

Molecular biologic approaches including chimeric strategies and site-directed mutagenesis studies have also provided evidence for specific binding sites for inhaled anesthetics on membrane proteins. Initial studies were performed looking at anesthetic effects on chimeric receptors constructed with various portions of the glycine receptor α_1 subunit (function enhanced by inhaled anesthetics) and the $GABA_C$ receptor ρ_1 subunit (function inhibited by inhaled anesthetics). These studies identified a region of the glycine receptor, including portions of transmembrane-spanning regions two and three (TM2, TM3), that was both necessary and sufficient for enhancement of receptor function.[82] Based on these results, site-directed mutagenesis studies were performed that identified two specific amino acid residues in TM2 and TM3 that were critical to inhaled anesthetic potentiation of receptor function (Fig. 23–4D). Specific mutations of these two residues eliminated potentiation by the halogenated ethers—isoflurane and enflurane—in both $GABA_A$ and glycine receptors[82]; these mutations did not, however, affect potentiation by the halogenated alkanes—halothane and chloroform. Subsequent studies have shown that mutations in transmembrane-spanning region 1 (TM1) of $GABA_A$ and glycine receptors can eliminate potentiation by the halogenated alkanes.[83] Recent site-directed mutagenesis studies have identified a specific amino acid residue in TM1 of the $GABA_A$ receptor that is critical for halothane, but not isoflurane potentiation.[84]

The amino acid residues identified as being critical to inhaled anesthetic action could represent residues lining an anesthetic binding pocket(s) or they could be important in transducing the effect of inhaled anesthetic action at a distant site. Currently, two approaches have been taken to address this important question. One approach has been to determine whether the volume of the amino acid side chain at the identified residues differentially alters the actions of anesthetics of different molecular volume. In both $GABA_A$ and glycine receptors, it appears that there is a strong inverse relationship between the molecular volume of amino acid side chains substituted in the TM2 and TM3 sites and the molecular volume of inhaled anesthetics and n-alkanols that retain their ability to potentiate receptor function.[85–88] These data suggest the existence of a cavity of finite size that may be filled either by an anesthetic molecule or by the side chains of amino acids in specific locations in TM2 and TM3. A recent study has shown that when a large amino acid (tryptophan) is placed in the critical residue in TM1, TM2, or TM3 of the $GABA_A$ receptor, sensitivity to both halothane and isoflurane is absent. Based on these results, it is postulated that residues in TM1-3 contribute to a binding cavity with a volume of 250 to 370 $Å^3$ that can accommodate both halogenated alkanes and ethers. Modeling studies further suggest that portions of TM4 may also contribute to the walls of the inhaled anesthetic binding pocket. The postulated alignment of critical residues in TM1-4 that form the binding pocket are illustrated in Figure 23–5.

More direct proof for a binding site for inhaled anesthetic on $GABA_A$ and glycine receptors is found in a study in which the amino acid residue in TM2 shown to be critical for isoflurane effect was mutated to a cysteine. These mutant

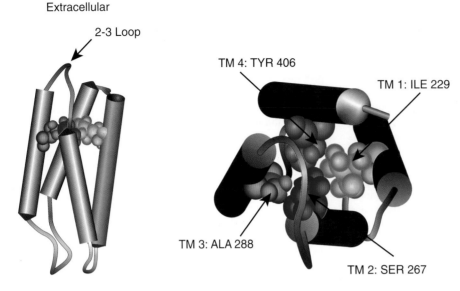

Extracellular

2-3 Loop

TM 4: TYR 406

TM 1: ILE 229

TM 3: ALA 288

TM 2: SER 267

Intracellular

Figure 23–5. A model of the putative site of inhaled anesthetic action on the glycine α1 receptor. Figure shows the amino acid side chains thought to contribute to the anesthetic binding cavity on the glycine and γ-aminobutyric acid type A (GABA$_A$) receptors. The *cylinders* represent the transmembrane-spanning segments (TM1-4) and the colored structures are the amino acid side chains that have been identified as critical to inhaled anesthetic action. *Left,* View in the plane of the membrane; *Right,* view from the extracellular surface. (Courtesy of Dr. James Trudell, Stanford University, Stanford, Ca.)

receptors were then reacted with propanethiol, an anesthetic that contains a sulfhydryl reacting group (i.e., a group that would form a covalent bond with an exposed cysteine). Propanethiol produced irreversible enhancement of the receptors and prevented any further potentiation by halogenated ether anesthetics, indicating that the anesthetic formed a covalent bond with the critical cysteine in TM2.[89] In summary, the weight of current evidence suggests that inhaled anesthetics produce their actions on GABA$_A$ and glycine receptors by binding to a cavity formed by TM1-3 near the extracellular side of the membrane.

Linking Molecular Targets of Inhaled Anesthetics to Components of Anesthesia in the Intact Organism

With the identification of several molecular targets for inhaled anesthetics, the final challenge is determining which of these targets contributes to which of the component behaviors of anesthesia. The most tenable approach to studying the relationship between anesthetic effects observed in vitro and whole animal anesthesia is to alter the structure of putative anesthetic targets and determine how this affects whole animal anesthetic sensitivity. Genetic techniques provide the most reliable and versatile methods for changing the structure of putative anesthetic targets. One useful genetic approach is to generate animals in which suspected inhaled anesthetic targets have been either eliminated (knockouts) or altered so that the target no longer responds to anesthetics (knockins). The knockout approach has been used to advantage to demonstrate that the α$_{2B}$ adrenergic receptor is required for the analgesic effects of N$_2$O.[16,17] This indicates that this receptor is in the neuronal pathway through which N$_2$O produces analgesia but not necessarily that N$_2$O binds to this receptor.

The knockout approach has been less fruitful in studying the actions of the halogenated inhaled agents. Mice lacking

the α$_6$ or δ subunits of the GABA$_A$ receptor have normal sensitivity to the inhaled anesthetics[90,91]; mice lacking the β3 subunit are slightly resistant to enflurane and halothane using the MAC endpoint and have normal sensitivity using the loss-of-righting reflex endpoint.[92] The small effect of these knockouts may be caused by the redundancy of GABA$_A$ receptor subunits and the ease with which one subunit can developmentally replace another. This problem can be circumvented by doing knockin experiments. Studies are in progress to create mice in which the α$_1$ subunit of the GABA$_A$ receptor has been replaced with an α$_1$ subunit that is insensitive to isoflurane (TM2, TM3 mutants). The behavioral effects of inhaled anesthetics on these knockin animals will be an important test of the contribution of GABA$_A$ receptors to the various components of anesthesia.

A second approach to matching molecular targets with behavioral actions is referred to as "forward genetics." This refers to a process of screening animals (either various populations or specifically mutagenized animals) for abnormal behavioral responses to anesthetics. Identification of the mutagenized genes contributing to altered anesthetic response provides a set of molecular targets that are not biased by preconceived notions. This kind of screen is generally performed in lower organisms such as *Caenorhabditis elegans* (a worm) or *Drosophila melanogaster* (the fruit fly) that have fully sequenced genomes and a rapid reproductive cycle. The unclear matching of behavioral anesthetic endpoints in simple organisms to the behavioral endpoints used in higher animals and humans complicates these studies. One set of studies in *C. elegans* has shown that mutations in the proteins involved in synaptic vesicle release (syntaxin, SNAP-25, and synaptobrevin) can produce dramatic changes in inhaled anesthetic sensitivity.[60] This suggests a presynaptic mechanism for inhaled anesthetics. Other studies in *C. elegans* (using a different behavioral endpoint) have identified two proteins, a stomatin analogue[93] and a mitochondrial protein involved in the respiratory chain,[94] as potential targets of inhaled anesthetic action. The novel anesthetic targets discovered in lower organisms need to be studied in higher organisms to delineate their potential role in the various components of anesthesia.

cific anatomic locations in the central nervous system by direct binding of inhaled anesthetic agents to specific molecular targets. The inhaled anesthetics are a heterogeneous group and do not all interact with the same molecular targets. Furthermore, it appears likely that a given inhaled anesthetic may produce its various behavioral effects through interactions with distinct molecular targets.

Summary

Current evidence indicates that inhaled anesthetics produce several behavioral effects, each of which is mediated in spe-

CLINICAL PHARMACOLOGY

Properties of the Ideal Inhaled Anesthetic

Inhaled anesthetics have been used for more than 150 years to render patients insensible to the pain of surgical procedures. With the exception of N_2O, inhaled anesthetics introduced before the 1950s have been abandoned from clinical practice because of unfavorable side effects to the patient, or unfavorable physical properties of the anesthetics, or both (Table 23–1). Although the modern inhaled anesthetics developed during the past few decades are much improved compared with their predecessors, none of the inhaled anesthetics in current clinical use fulfills the requirements of the ideal inhaled anesthetic (Table 23–2). Thus the clinician's decision to administer a particular inhaled anesthetic

(usually in combination with other anesthetics or anesthetic adjuvants) represents the clinician's assessment of benefits versus side effects of that agent for a particular patient undergoing a specific operation.

The current discussion centers on the inhaled anesthetics that are now most commonly used in North America: the methylethylethers isoflurane and desflurane, the methylisopropyl ether sevoflurane, and the gas N_2O (see Fig. 23–1 for chemical structures). Halothane, now in limited clinical use, will also be referred to as a representative alkane anesthetic because extensive clinical information is available for this compound. In addition, Xe will be discussed because of its unique (inert) chemical nature and its increased administration in the clinical setting.[95]

TABLE 23–1.

Some Inhaled Anesthetics That Have Been Abandoned from Clinical Use

Anesthetic	Decade Introduced	Unfavorable Properties
Diethylether ($CH_3CH_2OCH_2CH_3$)	1840s	Enhanced airway secretions; flammable
Chloroform ($CHCl_3$)	1840s	Hepatotoxic; nephrotoxic; dysrhythmias; carcinogen
Cyclopropane (C_3H_6)	1920s, 1930s	Explosive with oxygen and nitrous oxide
Trichloroethylene ($CHCl=CCl_2$)	1930s	Dysrhythmias; may be broken down by soda lime to eventually form phosgene (CCl_2O) (i.e., "war gas")
Fluroxene ($CF_3CH_2OCH=CH_2$)	1950s	Strong emetic properties; flammable
Methoxyflurane ($CH_3OCF_2CHCl_2$)	1950s, 1960s	Nephrotoxic; slow induction and recovery of anesthesia

TABLE 23–2.

Ideal Characteristics of Inhaled Anesthetics

Ideal Characteristics	Comments
1. Be pleasant to inhale, permitting a smooth and rapid induction of anesthesia.	Induction of anesthesia with desflurane at >6% atm can cause airway irritation.
2. Be potent to allow the concomitant administration of high concentrations of oxygen.	Use of nitrous oxide or xenon limits the concentration of oxygen.
3. Be able to produce a rapid emergence and flexibility in adjusting the depth of anesthesia.	The less soluble the anesthetic, the faster the induction of and emergence from anesthesia.
4. Be easy to administer and to measure its concentration.	Vaporizers are needed to administer volatile agents.
5. Be easily and inexpensively prepared in a pure form.	Xenon costs about $10 per liter.
6. Be stable outside the body (e.g., nonflammable, nonreactive with soda lime, environmentally safe) and inside the body (resist metabolism).	Nitrous oxide will support combustion. Sevoflurane may react with soda lime to form compound A. Only xenon is not metabolized inside the body.
7. Specifically act at central nervous system sites involved in the production of unconsciousness.	All inhaled anesthetics may occasionally have stimulant activity.
8. Be devoid of cardiovascular and respiratory side effects and be nontoxic to organs.	In general, side effects will increase with increasing concentrations of inhaled anesthetics.
9. Provide prolonged postoperative pain relief after return to conscious state.	None of the currently available inhaled anesthetics has this property.

Pharmacokinetics

Inhaled anesthetics cannot be directly applied to their site(s) of action in the central nervous system. Instead, these anesthetics are delivered into the lungs through a mask or endotracheal tube, taken up by blood passing through the lungs, and are transported through blood to diffuse into the central nervous system. The amount of time required for an inhaled anesthetic to reach the brain depends on a number of factors (Table 23–3). The most important parameter is the relationship between the inspired (F_I) and alveolar (F_A) anesthetic partial pressures. The alveolar (end tidal) partial pressure of anesthetic controls the partial pressure of anesthetic in all body tissues. With the administration of an inhaled anesthetic, the increase in alveolar partial pressure represents a balance between the amount of anesthetic delivered to the lungs by ventilation and the amount removed from the lungs by uptake into blood and tissues (e.g., vessel-rich tissues [central nervous system, heart, liver, kidney], muscle, and fat).[96]

The more soluble the anesthetic is in blood and tissues, the greater the anesthetic uptake from lung, the lower the F_A/F_I ratio, and the slower the anesthetic induction. Because blood flow to the brain is high, it takes a relatively short time for the partial pressure in the brain to approach that in the alveoli.[96] By using a high gas flow rate and initially administering a higher inspired anesthetic concentration than is required for the maintenance of anesthesia (i.e., "overpressurization"), the clinician can rapidly (<1 minute) render a patient unconsciousness with any of the modern volatile anesthetics. However, there are dangers associated with overpressurization. For example, patients with low cardiac output may develop unexpectedly high alveolar anesthetic concentrations (see Table 23–3) with induction, resulting in a greater probability of anesthetic-induced side effects, including a further decrease in cardiac output.

Maintenance of anesthesia involves adjusting the inspired anesthetic concentration (F_I) to achieve a given endtidal anesthetic concentration (F_A) that will produce the desired clinical effect. If the inspired anesthetic concentration is set at a given level, the endtidal concentration will increase toward the inspired concentration but will always be less because of anesthetic uptake into blood and tissues. Although near-equilibration of partial pressures in alveoli

TABLE 23–3.

Factors Influencing Speed of Action of Inhaled Anesthetics

Factor	Comments
Inspired (F_I) anesthetic partial pressure	Faster anesthetic induction at greater anesthetic concentrations.
Gas flow rate.	It takes time to replace gas in anesthesia circuit with fresh gas.
Alveolar (F_A) anesthetic partial pressure	The alveolar (endtidal) partial pressure of anesthetic controls the partial pressure of anesthetic in all body tissues.
Anesthetic solubility*	F_A/F_I decreases with increasing anesthetic solubility in blood. Slow onset of anesthesia with very soluble anesthetics.
Ventilation	Increased ventilation accelerates the rate of increase of F_A/F_I.
Cardiac output	Decreased cardiac output accelerates the rate of increase of F_A/F_I.

At 37° C, blood/gas partition coefficients (in parentheses) of inhaled anesthetics are halothane (2.5) > isoflurane (1.4) > sevoflurane (0.65) > nitrous oxide (0.47) > desflurane (0.45) > xenon (0.12).
*A larger blood/gas partition coefficient results in greater anesthetic uptake from lung into blood and therefore a lower F_A/F_I ratio.

and vessel-rich tissues may occur in minutes, equilibration may take many hours to days for muscle and fat.

Recovery from anesthesia (with inspired anesthetic concentration = 0) is primarily determined by the alveolar partial pressure of anesthetic and can be influenced by factors listed in Table 23–3. During recovery, the alveolar partial pressure is a balance between elimination of anesthetic from the lung through ventilation and the delivery of anesthetic to the lung from body tissues. A highly soluble agent (e.g., halothane) is more effective than a poorly soluble one (e.g., desflurane) in replacing anesthetic into alveoli because a greater reserve exists in the blood for the more soluble compound. Thus recovery from anesthesia tends to be slower with the more soluble agents. Similarly, an increase in cardiac output delivers more anesthetic to alveoli, thereby increasing alveolar anesthetic concentration and prolonging recovery.

Duration of anesthesia also influences the rate of recovery; the longer the anesthetic duration the more the rate of recovery depends on the solubility of the anesthetic. This is because for short operations muscle and fat (tissues that receive low blood flow compared with brain) take up relatively little anesthetic, have a far lower anesthetic partial pressure than found in alveoli, and thus contribute little to the transfer of anesthetic back to the lungs. For long surgeries (e.g., several hours), more anesthetic is deposited in muscle and fat, and these reservoirs can then supply more anesthetic to blood returning to the lungs and can prolong time to recovery.[97] Healthy volunteers anesthetized with desflurane or sevoflurane for 2 hours require ~11 to 18 minutes to respond to command after discontinuation of anesthesia, whereas those anesthetized for 8 hours require ~14 to 28 minutes to respond.[98]

Clinical Measurements of Anesthetic Potency

A simple definition of anesthesia is the state in which a patient is insensible to the trauma of surgery. However, a more precise definition of anesthesia and the quantitation of its effect remain a matter of debate. One approach is to consider anesthesia as that state that ensures amnesia and absence of movement to noxious stimulation, and that analgesia, muscle relaxation, and blunting of the stress response are desirable supplements to the state of anesthesia.[99]

MAC is the minimum alveolar concentration of inhaled anesthetic (in the absence of all other drugs) at a pressure of 1 atm that produces immobility in 50% of patients in response to a surgical incision.[100] MAC is an equilibrium measurement; that is, quantitation of MAC involves maintaining a constant alveolar concentration for sufficient time (typically > 15 minutes) to allow near equilibration between alveolar gas, arterial blood, and brain before application of the surgical stimulus. MAC is a useful index of clinical anesthetic potency for several reasons: (1) it can be equally applied to all anesthetics (i.e., does not result from anesthetic side effects that vary from agent to agent); (2) it can be measured with relative ease by sampling end tidal gases that after equilibration represent the amount (partial pressure) of anesthetic at the site of action (central nervous system); and (3) the endpoint of lack of movement is an important element of clinical anesthesia. MAC also has the advantage of being relatively constant, with standard deviations of less than 20% of its mean value typically associated with its measurement.

During normal operating room conditions, anesthesia can be achieved with volatile agents and with Xe (barely), but

TABLE 23–4.

Quantitation of Depth of Anesthesia in Humans

Anesthetic	MAC (% atm)	MAC with 60% N_2O (% atm)	MAC-Awake (% atm)	MAC-Intubation (% atm)	MAC-BAR (% atm)
Nitrous oxide	104	NA	66	>120	ND
Xenon	71	ND	31	ND	ND
Desflurane	7.25	4.0	2.60	ND	9.42
Sevoflurane	1.85	0.66	0.67	4.52	4.15
Isoflurane	1.15	0.50	0.37	1.76	1.50
Halothane	0.74	0.29	0.38	1.12	1.07

Values are those of young adults and are expressed as percent of one atmosphere. Standard deviations are ~20% of these mean values. MAC is the minimum alveolar concentration of inhaled anesthetic at a pressure of 1 atmosphere that produces immobility in 50% of patients in response to a surgical incision. MAC-awake is the minimum alveolar concentration of anesthetic that abolishes response to verbal command in 50% of patients. MAC-intubation is the minimum alveolar concentrations of agent required to inhibit movement and coughing response to tracheal intubation in 50% of patients. MAC-BAR is the minimum alveolar concentration of anesthetic needed to block the autonomic response to skin incision in 50% of patients.
NA, not applicable; ND, not determined.

not with N_2O while coadministering adequate amounts of oxygen (i.e., MAC of N_2O determined in a pressure chamber is 1.04 atm) (Table 23–4). However, it is common clinical practice to add N_2O to gas mixtures of a volatile agent and oxygen, which decreases the requirement for volatile anesthetics. In most cases, the addition of N_2O is additive (i.e., ~0.6 MAC N_2O decreases MAC of the volatile anesthetic by about 60%) (see Table 23–4; Fig. 23–6), although exceptions may exist.[101,102]

The concept of MAC has been expanded by the use of other clinical endpoints. MAC-awake is the MAC of anesthetic that abolishes response to verbal command in 50% of patients, appears to correspond to the anesthetic concentration that abolishes learning or memory,[103] and is less than the anesthetic concentration required to prevent movement in response to skin incision (see Table 23–4). In contrast, MAC-intubation[104,105] and MAC BAR[104,106] (the MACs of agent required to inhibit movement and coughing response to tracheal intubation, and to block the autonomic response to skin incision, respectively) are greater than the anesthetic concentrations required to prevent movement to skin incision (see Table 23–4).

An important characteristic of inhaled anesthetics is the steep nature of their concentration-response curve (see Fig. 23–6). Thus at concentrations 20% lower than MAC almost all patients will move in response to surgical stimulation, and at concentrations 20% greater than MAC, less than 5% of patients will move with surgical stimulation. Such steep concentration-response curves are found for all inhaled agents (see Fig. 23–6).

Physiologic Factors and MAC

MAC for a given inhaled anesthetic is maximal in infants at about 6 months of age, after which MAC decreases with increasing age at a rate of ~6% decrease per decade for all inhaled anesthetics.[107] MAC-awake also decreases with increasing age.[108]

Although the influence of aging on MAC can be measured with relative ease, the influence of other physiologic parameters is more difficult to quantitate in patients. Therefore, clinical impressions may be supported by studies in animals. A decrease in body temperature from 37° C to 27° C decreases the MAC of volatile agents by about 50% and is related to increasing anesthetic solubility at lower temperatures.[109] MAC may decrease slightly (<20%) during the prolonged administration of anesthesia and the performance of surgery.[110] Inhaled anesthetic requirement decreases by about 25% with pregnancy and in the immediate postpartum period.[111] Patient sex, and moderate to severe degrees of hypocarbia, hypercarbia, metabolic acidosis, metabolic alkalosis, hypoxia, hyperoxia, hypotension, hypertension, anemia, and thyroid function have little or no influence on MAC. Extreme alterations in physiologic parameters (e.g., mean arterial pressure < 50 mm Hg, PaO_2 < 38 mm Hg, $PaCO_2$ > 90 mm Hg) may decrease MAC.[96,100]

Modulation of the nervous system may also alter anesthetic requirement. In patients, reduced halothane requirements occur after electrical stimulation of periaqueductal gray matter[112] or the application of transcutaneous electrical nerve stimulation.[113] Halothane MAC in children with

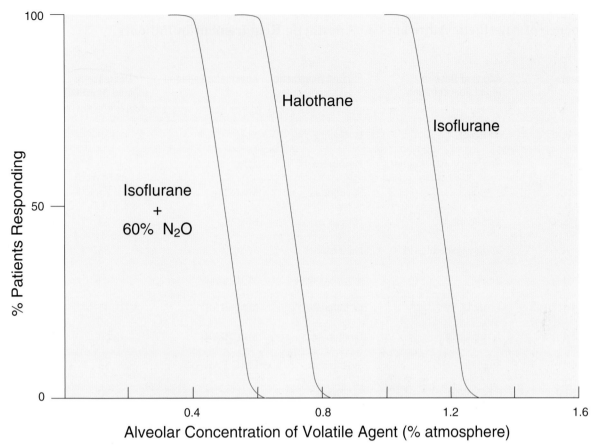

Figure 23–6. Representative dose-response curves for isoflurane, halothane, and isoflurane in the presence of 60% N₂O. The midpoint of the dose-response curve is defined as the minimum alveolar concentration (MAC) of anesthetic that produces immobility in 50% of patients in response to a surgical incision. Note that the anesthetic requirement for isoflurane is greatly decreased by N₂O. Also note the steep nature of the curves, indicating that a patient responding to surgical stimuli may be converted to a nonresponder by a small increase in alveolar anesthetic concentration.

cerebral palsy is ~25% lower than in healthy children.[114] Although it is a common clinical impression that patients with chronic alcoholism are resistant to inhaled agents, only a single abstract[115] that finds a ~30% increase in halothane MAC for these patients provides support for this belief.

Anesthetic Adjuvants and MAC

Many anesthetic adjuvants (e.g., narcotics, benzodiazepines, local anesthetics, α_2 agonists) decrease requirement for inhaled anesthetics. The influence of each of these drug classes on inhaled anesthetic requirements for blunting various clinical endpoints is presented in Table 23–5. These anesthetic adjuvants are thought to have a "ceiling effect," where further increases in adjuvant dose have lesser effects on inhaled anesthetic requirement and even extremely high doses of these adjuvants do not eliminate the requirement for inhaled anesthetics. Although it was previously thought that muscle relaxants decreased MAC, evidence now indicates that atracurium, vecuronium, and pancuronium have no effect on anesthetic requirement.[116]

Side Effects on Organs and Systems

All of the inhaled agents currently available produce side effects. Although some side effects may be favorable (e.g., enhancement of muscle relaxation, deliberate decreasing of blood pressure), many are unfavorable (Fig. 23–7). The inhaled anesthetic and its concentration are chosen to minimize untoward effects.

Cardiovascular System

Hemodynamics

Volatile anesthetics decrease mean arterial blood pressure in a concentration-related fashion. At 1 MAC, the blood pressure is typically 20% lower than baseline values in healthy individuals, but the magnitude of this decrease depends on the patient population and degree of surgical stimulation,[117,118] and severe decreases in blood pressure may occur in patients with cardiovascular disease. The decrease in

TABLE 23–5.

Influence of Anesthetic Adjuvants on Anesthetic Requirement in Patients

Adjuvant	Adjuvant Dose or Blood Concentration	Inhaled Anesthetic	Anesthetic Endpoint	Decrease in Inhaled Anesthetic Requirement (%)	Reference
Fentanyl	0.5 ng/mL	Isoflurane	MAC	50	179
Fentanyl	3 µg/kg IV = 0.78 ng/mL	Desflurane	MAC	59	180
Fentanyl	3 ng/mL	Sevoflurane	MAC	61	181
Fentanyl	3.26 ng/mL	Nitrous oxide	MAC	33	182
Fentanyl	2 µg/kg epidural (T9)	Halothane	MAC	58	183
Fentanyl	3 ng/mL	Sevoflurane	MAC-awake	24	184
Fentanyl	1.5 µg/kg IV	Isoflurane	MAC-BAR	45	106
Fentanyl	1.5 µg/kg IV	Desflurane	MAC-BAR	60	106
Fentanyl	3 ng/mL	Sevoflurane	MAC-BAR	83	181
Sufentanil	0.145 ng/mL	Isoflurane	MAC	50	185
Alfentanil	28.8 ng/mL	Isoflurane	MAC	50	179
Alfentanil	50 ng/mL	Isoflurane	MAC	25	186
Alfentanil	101 ng/mL	Nitrous oxide	MAC	36	187
Remifentanil	1.37 ng/mL	Isoflurane	MAC	50	188
Remifentanil	32 ng/mL	Isoflurane	MAC	91	188
Morphine	0.75 mg intrathecal	Halothane	MAC	43	189
Morphine	4 mg epidural	Halothane	MAC	28	190
Buprenorphine	4 µg/kg IV	Halothane	MAC	35	191
Buprenorphine	4 µg/kg epidural	Halothane	MAC	32	191
Midazolam	0.4 mg/kg IV = 539 ng/mL	Halothane	MAC	70	192
Diazepam	0.5 mg/kg IV	Halothane	MAC	43	100
Lidocaine	3.2 µg/mL	Nitrous oxide	MAC	33	177
Clonidine	4.5 µg/kg PO	Sevoflurane	MAC	35	193
Clonidine	4.5 µg/kg PO	Sevoflurane	MAC-awake	47	193
Dexmedetomidine	0.6 ng/mL	Isoflurane	MAC	47	194
Ethanol	100 mg%	Halothane	MAC	32	195

Note that the adjuvant-induced decreases in inhaled anesthetic requirements reported in this table may depend on the patient population examined and the time between administration of anesthetic adjuvant and measurement of inhaled anesthetic potency.

IV, intravenous; MAC, minimum alveolar concentration; MAC-awake, minimum alveolar concentration of anesthetic that abolishes response to verbal command; MAC-BAR, minimum alveolar concentration of anesthetic needed to block the autonomic response to skin incision; PO, per os (by mouth).

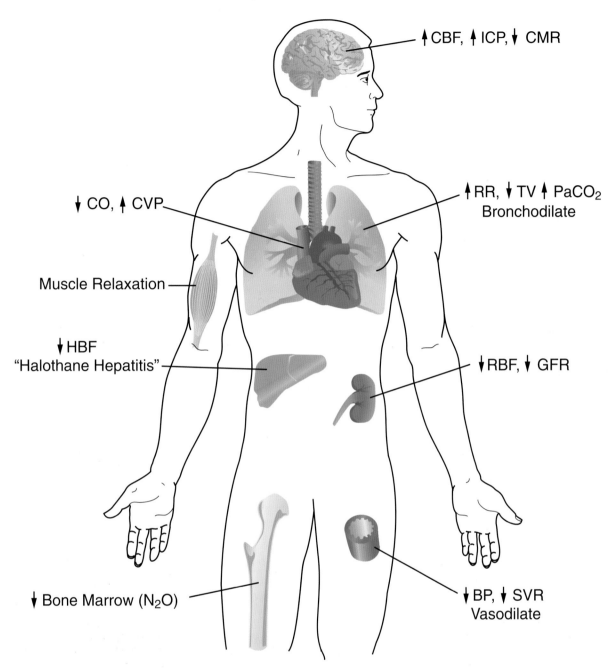

Figure 23–7. Typical side effects of inhaled anesthetics. The magnitude of the side effect depends on the particular inhaled agent and its concentration. BP, blood pressure; CBF, cerebral blood flow; CVP, central venous pressure; GFR, glomerular filtration rate; HBF, hepatic blood flow; ICP, intracranial pressure; N_2O, nitrous oxide; $PaCO_2$, arterial partial pressure of CO_2; RBF, renal blood flow; RR, respiratory rate; SVR, systemic vascular resistance; TV, tidal volume.

blood pressure may be primarily associated with a decrease in cardiac output (e.g., halothane), a decrease in systemic vascular resistance (e.g., isoflurane, desflurane), or an increase in central venous pressure. Desflurane is associated with a transient cardiovascular stimulation (lasting several minutes) when end-tidal concentrations are rapidly increased.[119] The baroreceptor reflex is diminished by the volatile agents, whereas N_2O decreases baroreflex-mediated tachycardia but augments sympathetic nerve activity directed to blood vessels that supply skeletal muscles.[120] The N_2O-enhanced sympathetic outflow may in part be respon-

sible for the lesser circulatory depression of a N_2O/volatile agent mixture compared with equal MAC levels of volatile agents alone. When administered as the sole anesthetic, hyperbaric N_2O results in tachycardia and hypertension.[121]

Coronary Circulation

Concern has been raised that volatile anesthetics (especially isoflurane) might cause ischemia by vasodilating coronary arteries and thereby redistribute intramyocardial coronary blood flow away from areas of myocardium that depend on collateral circulation (coronary steal). However, this concern may be more theoretical than real because patients with "steal prone" coronary anatomy have the same incidence of myocardial ischemia when anesthetized with an isoflurane-, enflurane-, halothane-, or sufentanil-based technique.[122]

Cardiac Dysrhythmias

Inhaled anesthetics alter electrical activity in the heart; their effects include a slowing of sinoatrial discharge and a decrease in the action potential duration of ventricular muscle fibers.[123] N_2O increases the incidence of isorhythmic atrioventricular dissociation in response to epinephrine administration.[124] Production of ventricular extrasystoles in response to epinephrine tends to be greatest with halothane compared with other volatile agents, is greater in adults than children, and is enhanced in the presence of hypercarbia.[125]

Respiratory System

Ventilatory Control

Inhaled anesthetics cause dose-dependent respiratory depression, as manifest by an increase in $PaCO_2$ during spontaneous breathing and depression of the ventilatory response to CO_2.[126] The increase in respiratory rate with anesthesia does not compensate for the reduction in tidal volume, therefore $PaCO_2$ increases. Surgical stimulation counteracts the anesthetic-induced respiratory depression. At anesthetic concentrations of 1 MAC, respiratory depression is greatest with enflurane and desflurane and least with N_2O and halothane. With hypoxia, the usual increase in ventilation may be extremely sensitive to volatile anesthetics, with concentrations as low as 0.1 MAC blunting the response.[127] With normoxia, apnea occurs at anesthetic concentrations of about 2 MAC. The ventilatory response is unaffected by N_2O—that is, substitution of N_2O for an equivalent MAC fraction of volatile agent results in the same degree of respiratory depression as the volatile agent alone.[126]

Hypoxic Pulmonary Vasoconstriction

Inhaled anesthetics may worsen oxygenation in patients with atelectasis. This is because the normal physiologic adaptation of diverting blood away from hypoxic areas of lung (hypoxic pulmonary vasoconstriction) may be blunted by inhaled anesthetic-induced pulmonary artery vasodilation. Although this phenomenon exists, it is usually (but not always) of little clinical consequence.[128]

Airway Resistance

The increase in airway resistance with the loss of lung volume during anesthesia may be counterbalanced by a decrease in airway resistance caused by bronchodilation by volatile agents. The mechanism of bronchodilation by inhaled anesthetics is through complex neural pathways, and in part involves an anesthetic-induced reduction in acetylcholine release from nerve terminals with a resultant decrease in airway muscle contraction. At equal MAC levels, halothane, isoflurane, and sevoflurane cause approximately the same decrease in respiratory resistance, whereas desflurane may slightly increase respiratory resistance.[129]

Of the inhaled agents, desflurane is most pungent[130] and about one half of patients find the smell of desflurane disagreeable.[131] Desflurane is not recommended for the induction of anesthesia through mask in infants or children because of the high incidence of laryngospasm and coughing.

Central Nervous System

Mental Function and Awareness

Changes in mental function by inhaled anesthetics are manifest by loss of response to verbal command at concentrations of MAC-awake and lack of response to noxious stimuli at greater concentrations (see Table 23–4). Even more subtle effects on mental function (e.g., learning) may occur at lower anesthetic concentrations (0.1–0.2 MAC).[132] Of particular clinical importance is the finding that inhaled anesthetics may not be equally effective in preventing awareness. For example, 0.4% atm isoflurane (about one-third MAC) prevents recall and responses to commands in healthy volunteers, whereas 60% N_2O (more than one-half MAC) may not.[132] Surgical stimulation has an unknown effect on (but probably increases) inhaled anesthetic requirement to prevent awareness. N_2O may slightly antagonize the hypnotic properties of volatile agents.[102]

Excitatory Activity

In general, electroencephalographic activity (which represents an integration of cortical postsynaptic potentials) is increasingly depressed with increasing inhaled anesthetic concentrations. However, transient neurologic abnormalities, including hyperreflexia, a positive Babinski reflex, and spasticity, may occur during induction or emergence from anesthesia with inhaled anesthetics.[133] Epileptiform activity may even appear at relatively high anesthetic concentrations (~2 MAC), is well known to occur with enflurane during conditions of hypocapnia, and may occur during anesthesia with sevoflurane.[134]

Intracranial Pressure

Inhaled anesthetics, including N_2O and Xe^{135} increase intracranial pressure. This increase may be direct, by vasodilation resulting in an increase in cerebral blood flow (CBF) and cerebral blood volume, or indirect, by depressing ventilation and increasing $PaCO_2$. A high intracranial pressure may have detrimental effects by reducing cerebral perfusion pressure and causing cerebral ischemia, or by causing brain shift and herniation in patients with brain tumors. The differential effects of inhaled agents on CBF may in part be explained by their differential effects on cerebral metabolic rate and production/reabsorption of cerebrospinal fluid. The increase in CBF can usually, but not always, be ameliorated by hyperventilation before anesthetic administration.[136,137]

Hepatic Function

After halothane administration, mild hepatic reactions occur commonly (incidence of ~20%) and are less frequent with other inhaled anesthetics.[138] Such mild reactions are manifest only by abnormal laboratory values (e.g., increases in serum transaminase and glutathione-S-transferase concentrations) and do not result in clinical evidence of liver disease. Abnormalities in liver function may relate to an anesthetic-induced decrease in hepatic blood flow and decreased oxygen and glucose supply or to breakdown products of the parent anesthetics (see later discussion on metabolism).

Renal Function

Inhaled anesthetics tend to decrease glomerular filtration rate and renal blood flow. For example, administration of an isoflurane/N_2O/O_2 anesthetic to patients undergoing oral/maxillofacial surgery to maintain a mean arterial pressure of 60 mm Hg decreases glomerular filtration rate by about 20%.[139] Transient, but not sustained, abnormalities in renal function in healthy individuals are found after prolonged exposures to inhaled anesthetics.[140,141] A potential cause of renal compromise is the production of fluoride ion that occurs with anesthetic metabolism, or the production of reactive breakdown products on exposure of parent anesthetic compounds to soda lime in the anesthesia circuit, or both (see later).

Muscular Systems

Muscle Relaxation

Volatile anesthetics have muscle relaxant properties by themselves and also potentiate the action of depolarizing and nondepolarizing neuromuscular blocking drugs[142] (see Chapter 33). Uterine smooth muscle is relaxed by volatile anesthetics to approximately the same extent at equal MAC values.[143] Although the potential exists for increased uterine bleeding with the use of volatile agents for cesarean section, this does not appear to be a problem in practice, and the administration of volatile anesthetic to supplement N_2O will decrease the likelihood of maternal awareness of perioperative events.

In contrast to the volatile anesthetics, N_2O tends to increase skeletal muscle activity. When used as the sole anesthetic during hyperbaric conditions, N_2O produces muscle rigidity, jerky limb movements, and even opisthotonus.[121] Xe appears to have minimal influence on neuromuscular block.[144]

Malignant Hyperthermia

Malignant hyperthermia identifies a rare syndrome during general anesthesia that is associated with a rapidly increasing temperature and a high mortality rate if not quickly recognized and treated. Its incidence is approximately 1 in 250,000 anesthetics. Although usually associated with the combined administration of halothane and succinylcholine, any of the volatile anesthetics may be triggering agents, and volatile anesthetics should be avoided in patients susceptible to malignant hyperthermia.

Gastrointestinal System

Many factors contribute to postoperative nausea and vomiting, with the incidence of postoperative emesis ranging from less than 1% to greater than 50% depending on the patient population, type of surgery, and medications administered.[145] Emesis may occur after the administration of inhaled anesthetics in oxygen, and the use of N_2O increases the probability of postoperative nausea and vomiting.[146]

Unique Properties of Nitrous Oxide

Expansion of Closed Gas Spaces

Any closed gas space in the body that contains air (i.e., nitrogen) will increase in size, pressure, or both when N_2O is administered. This is because N_2O is carried to the closed air space and diffuses from a region of high concentration outside to a region of low concentration inside the space. Nitrogen is transferred from inside to outside the space much slower than N_2O enters because nitrogen is much less soluble in blood and tissues (blood/gas partition coefficients at 37° C of 0.47 for N_2O and 0.015 for nitrogen). The increase in volume, pressure, or both of the air space increases with N_2O concentration and duration of exposure.

Untoward outcomes may arise from expansion of air spaces by N_2O and the use of N_2O is contraindicated in these circumstances. The most rapid N_2O-induced increase in closed air space volume occurs with a pneumothorax. Expansion of air emboli in blood vessels by N_2O is of concern, especially air emboli in coronary vessels and in the brain. However, N_2O may be safely used in neurosurgical patients provided that it is immediately discontinued on detection of an air embolus.[147]

N_2O will slowly expand a closed air space in bowel obstruction. Even in patients without bowel obstruction, N_2O may delay return of normal bowel function after surgery if air is present in the bowel at the start of surgery.[148] If air in the bowel is not initially present, the use of N_2O during routine intestinal surgery causes a clinically unnoticeable (but statistically significant) increase in circumference of the ileum.[149] The expansion of gas spaces in bowel by N_2O may contribute to the enhanced postoperative nausea and vomiting often seen after N_2O administration.[146]

A potential for injury also exists when N_2O increases middle ear pressure, expands intraocular gases used to treat retinal detachment, or increases pressures in air-inflated endotracheal tube cuffs to levels that cause tracheal damage.[150]

Inactivation of Methionine Synthase

N_2O is unique among the inhaled anesthetics in its ability to oxidize vitamin B_{12} and inactivate the enzyme methionine synthase, an enzyme that controls interrelations between vitamin B_{12} and folic acid metabolism. Patients given 50% N_2O for 2 hours have more than half of their hepatic methionine synthase inactivated. In almost all cases, exposure to N_2O during surgery and inactivation of methionine synthase are without clinical consequences.[150] However, severe disturbances in vitamin B_{12}/folate metabolism and marked hematologic and neurologic abnormalities may occur after N_2O exposure in individuals who abuse N_2O, in those who are critically ill, and on rare occasions in patients who have a pre-existing subclinical deficiency in vitamin B_{12}, folate, or both.[150] By disrupting vitamin B_{12} and folic acid metabolism, N_2O also increases homocysteine concentrations, and N_2O-induced increases in plasma homocysteine have been associated with increases in myocardial ischemia in patients undergoing carotid endarterectomy.[151]

Degradation of Inhaled Anesthetics

Metabolism

Toxicity of inhaled agents is linked with anesthetic metabolism. Volatile anesthetics are metabolized in the liver by cytochrome P450 proteins (see Chapter 4). Halothane is metabolized the most (~20% of amount taken up) and desflurane the least (~0.02%).[152] Individuals who receive compounds that induce production of cytochrome P450s (e.g., ethanol, isoniazid, phenobarbital) will metabolize anesthetics to a greater extent.

Severe hepatic necrosis after halothane anesthesia ("halothane hepatitis") is a rare event (incidence of 1:35,000 in adults to 1:120,000 in children).[138] Clinical features of halothane hepatitis include malaise, delayed pyrexia, jaundice, eosinophilia, and markedly abnormal liver function tests. Risk factors are multiple exposures to halothane, middle age, obesity, female sex, genetic predisposition, and medications that enhance cytochrome P450 production. For a diagnosis of halothane hepatitis, other possible causes of hepatic necrosis (e.g., viral) need to be excluded. The mechanism of injury probably involves the generation of antibodies against an antigen that is produced by reaction of a trifluoroacetyl [CF_3CO-] moiety (formed after oxidation of halothane) with liver proteins. Such antibodies are found in some (but not all) patients with halothane hepatitis. Oral administration of disulfiram (an inhibitor of cytochrome P450 2E1) before surgery inhibits oxidation of halothane and has been speculated as a method to provide prophylaxis against halothane hepatitis.[153]

Because a reactive trifluoroacetyl moiety can also be formed after oxidative metabolism of isoflurane and desflurane, a possible cross-sensitivity may occur between anesthetics. This possibility is extremely remote,[152] but hepatotoxicity associated with antibodies to trifluoroacetylated proteins has been reported after isoflurane[154] or desflurane[155] anesthesia in patients exposed previously to halothane.

Methoxyflurane was abandoned from clinical use because its prolonged administration led to increasing degrees of nephrotoxicity (e.g., polyuria, hypernatremia, decrease in creatinine clearance). This methoxyflurane-induced nephrotoxicity was associated with serum fluoride ion concentrations greater than $50\,\mu M$. Of the currently used inhaled anesthetics, sevoflurane metabolism results in the highest serum fluoride ion levels and prolonged administration of sevoflurane may result in serum fluoride ion concentrations greater than $100\,\mu M$.[156] However, clinical signs of nephrotoxicity rarely occur in patients who receive sevoflurane for prolonged periods, possibly because the relatively low blood/gas partition coefficient of sevoflurane (0.65 vs. 15 for methoxyflurane) facilitates its elimination from the body on recovery from anesthesia and fluoride ion concentration in serum remains above $50\,\mu M$ for only relatively short time periods after sevoflurane.[157] Another hypothesis is that selective renal metabolism by methoxyflurane but not sevoflurane may underlie the nephrotoxicity of methoxyflurane.[158]

Interaction with Carbon Dioxide Absorbents

Compound A

Economic and environmental concerns demand a limited gas flow rate of inhaled anesthetics, and a carbon dioxide absorbent is a necessary component of an anesthesia circuit to limit side effects related to high inspired CO_2 concentrations. Carbon dioxide absorbents degrade sevoflurane ($CFH_2OCH(CF_3)_2$) to CFH_2-O-C(=CF_2)(CF_3), a vinyl ether known as compound A. Factors that increase compound A concentration in the anesthesia circuit include an increased sevoflurane concentration, increased amounts of carbon dioxide reacting with absorbents, a decreased fresh gas flow rate, increasing temperature, decreasing water content of the absorbent, and increasing concentrations of potassium or sodium hydroxides in carbon dioxide absorbents.[159,160] Inspired concentrations of Compound A may reach greater than 50 ppm.[156] Because compound A is known to be nephrotoxic in rats, concern has been raised about the potential for compound A toxicity in patients anesthetized with sevoflurane. However, as noted earlier, transient biochemical abnormalities found after prolonged sevoflurane anesthesia are not associated with clinical signs of sustained nephrotoxicity.[140,141,156,157] Nevertheless, it remains possible that Compound A contributes to the development of renal failure that is rarely observed after administration of sevoflurane. The use of a carbon dioxide absorbent that does not contain potassium or sodium hydroxides minimally degrades sevoflurane to Compound A and should decrease or eliminate concerns regarding Compound A toxicity from sevoflurane.[160,161]

Carbon Monoxide

There are case reports of intraoperative carbon monoxide poisoning,[162] typically occurring during the first case on a Monday morning when an idle anesthesia machine was used with unchanged carbon dioxide absorbent with oxygen flowing for more than 1 day. In vitro studies demonstrate that desflurane and isoflurane (but not sevoflurane or halothane) may react with carbon dioxide absorbent and produce carbon monoxide.[163] Carbon monoxide production increases with increasing dryness of the absorbent, increasing temperature, increasing concentrations of desflurane or isoflurane,[163] and increasing concentrations of potassium hydroxide in the absorbent.[164] The use of a carbon dioxide absorbent that does not contain potassium or sodium hydroxides prevents the degradation of desflurane or isoflurane to carbon monoxide.[161]

Trace Anesthetic Concentrations

Because of concern that subanesthetic levels of inhaled agents may alter the performance or health of medical personnel, recommendations have been made to minimize pollution in anesthetizing areas.[165] These recommendations include scavenging of waste anesthetic gases and education and work practice to minimize exposure to waste anesthetic gases. In the United States, environmental levels of inhaled anesthetics considered acceptable are less than 2.0 ppm volatile anesthetic when used alone or less than 0.5 ppm volatile anesthetic when used with N_2O.[165] The recommended maximum environmental level of N_2O when used alone (<25 ppm 8-hour time-weighted average) is much less than the concentration of N_2O (~1000 ppm or 0.1%) needed to produce a detectable inactivation of methionine synthase with chronic exposure.[150] Trace levels of anesthetics found in scavenged operating rooms have no detrimental effect on the mood or cognitive functions of anesthetists. Although it remains possible that chronic exposure to trace anesthetic levels have an adverse effect on health, no clear evidence currently exists of harmful effects.

Indications Other Than Surgery

Although inhaled anesthetics are primarily administered in the operating room for surgical procedures, they may also be used at other hospital locations to provide immobility and alleviate discomfort for either invasive (e.g., endoscopy, angiography) or noninvasive (e.g., magnetic resonance imaging) procedures. On occasions, inhaled anesthetics have been used for prolonged sedation (e.g., 0.1–0.6% isoflurane) in the intensive care unit,[166] and to treat refractory cases of seizures,[167] asthma,[168] and arterial and intracranial hypertension.[169] Administration of general anesthesia using a combination of intravenous and inhaled agents has been used to perform rapid opioid detoxification.[170] An earlier claim that isoflurane anesthesia has antidepressant activity has not been substantiated.[171]

Practical Aspects of Anesthetic Administration

There are few absolute contraindications to the administration of inhaled anesthetics. Volatile agents should not be given to patients with known or suspected susceptibility to malignant hyperthermia. In patients who are severely hypotensive (e.g., caused by trauma or sepsis), the administration of even low concentrations of volatile anesthetics may cause death. In patients with "difficult airways" or who are at risk for aspiration of gastric contents into the lungs, unconsciousness should not be produced with inhaled anesthetics (or any other anesthetic or anesthetic adjuvants) without having a well-defined plan and backup plans for airway control, provision of adequate oxygenation, and prevention of aspiration.

The known side effects of individual inhaled anesthetics provide a "common sense guide" on which anesthetics to avoid in certain patient subpopulations. For example, it is unwise to administer halothane (and probably isoflurane or desflurane) to patients with a history of "halothane hepatitis." Inhaled induction of anesthesia with desflurane should not be performed in adults with reactive airway disease or in infants or children. There is no need to give a 10-hour sevoflurane anesthetic at low flow to patients with impaired renal function. N_2O should be avoided in patients with impaired oxygenation, pneumothorax, bowel obstruction, or vitamin B_{12}/folate deficiency.

For most cases, the advantages versus disadvantages of each inhaled anesthetic are more subtle than the situations described earlier, and the clinician's decision to (or not to) administer a particular agent is often based on personal preference. The choice of an anesthetic is usually less important than the vigilance of the anesthetist and the care with which the anesthetic is administered. Consider, for example, the issue of whether N_2O should be administered to the patient undergoing a laparoscopic cholecystectomy. Anesthesiologist A is aware of publications[172,173] demonstrating that N_2O has no clinically apparent deleterious effects during laparoscopic cholecystectomy (as assessed by a "blinded" surgeon evaluating operating conditions and no increased incidence of postoperative nausea and vomiting and no delay in postoperative recovery) and decides to administer N_2O. Anesthesiologist A also prefers to administer N_2O because it is less expensive than other anesthetic alternatives and because N_2O is quickly eliminated at the end of the operation, allowing for a fast "wake-up." Anesthesiologist B is also aware of the studies[172,173] showing no harmful effects of N_2O use during laparoscopic cholecystectomy, but decides not to administer N_2O. Anesthesiologist B knows that the use of N_2O will cause some bowel expansion,[149] that N_2O will support combustion, that there is a small risk for an explosion with N_2O use during laparoscopy,[174] and that the use of the N_2O flowmeter promotes tantrums in the surgeon involved in the case. Instead, Anesthesiologist B decides to administer a relatively higher concentration of volatile agent that will have the beneficial effect of lessening the need for muscle relaxants.[142] Both anesthesiologists may alter their anesthetic management depending on intraoperative changes and the medical condition of the patient. If oxygen saturation decreases, Anesthesiologist A will discontinue N_2O until the cause of impaired oxygenation has been evaluated and corrected. If the patient has known or suspected coronary artery disease, Anesthesiologist B may avoid the use of desflurane or provide additional medications to prevent the tachycardia that may be seen with administration of desflurane.[119] The "best" technique remains a matter of opinion.

Inhaled Versus Intravenous Anesthetics

Both inhaled and intravenous (Chapter 24) anesthetics can produce the desired clinical endpoints (i.e., amnesia and absence of movement to noxious stimulation) required for surgery. Thus rather than be concerned about choosing which of the inhaled anesthetics to use, one might ask why inhaled anesthetics are needed at all? Why not just administer intravenous agents? The answer is that there is no ideal intravenous anesthetic (Chapter 24), just as there is no ideal inhaled anesthetic (see Table 23–2). The clinical challenge is to select a combination of inhaled and intravenous agents at concentrations and doses that produce the appropriate (and easily reversible) anesthetic endpoint while minimizing side effects. Induction of anesthesia in adults with intravenous anesthetics is usually more rapid and involves less coughing and excitatory phenomena than induction with inhaled agents. After control of the airway (e.g., endotracheal intubation, insertion, or laryngeal mask), anesthesia is often maintained with an inhaled anesthetic that can be rapidly eliminated from the body through exhalation at the end of the operation. In infants or children, administration by a skilled clinician of an inhaled anesthetic through mask that is not irritating to the airway (e.g., halothane or sevoflurane with N_2O) can be provided to an anesthetic depth where the insertion of an intravenous line is tolerated. Again, the choice of an inhaled versus intravenous anesthetic is often less important than the vigilance of the anesthetist and the care with which the anesthetic is administered.

Combinations of Drugs and Physiologic Factors

The sole administration of inhaled anesthetics is a rare occurrence in current anesthetic practice, and drugs administered in the perioperative period to treat anxiety or pain or to control hemodynamics may influence inhaled anesthetic requirement (see Table 23–5). For example, consider the 75 year-old patient undergoing a vascular operation who receives 2 mg midazolam intravenously in the preoperative area to treat anxiety, and 250 µg fentanyl intravenously and propofol in the operating room with induction of anesthesia to blunt hemodynamic response to laryngoscopy, and "spraying" of the vocal cords with 4 mL 4% lidocaine (160 mg) to minimize irritation of the endotracheal tube. After tracheal intubation, body temperature monitored from an esophageal stethoscope reads 35° C. Midazolam, fentanyl, lidocaine (see Table 23–5), and propofol (Chapter 24) will all significantly decrease the requirement for inhaled anesthetics, with their effects diminishing with time depend-ing on the pharmacokinetics of these agents. Moreover, there will be a relative decrease in inhaled anesthetic requirement because of the patient's age and presence of mild hypothermia, and blood pressure often decreases shortly after induction of anesthesia in patients with vascular disease while the unstimulated patient is being prepared before surgical incision. Thus little or no inhaled anesthetic (N_2O will probably cause less of a decrease in blood pressure than the volatile agents) may be required during this time period, and vasopressors may be needed to support the blood pressure. If the patient has received muscle relaxants and is paralyzed and unable to move in response to verbal command or noxious stimuli, awareness may be an issue in this setting.

Dosage and Administration

As the name implies, inhaled anesthetics are almost always administered in a gaseous or vaporized form by an inhaled route (e.g., through face or laryngeal mask, endotracheal tube, tracheostomy site). An exception is the delivery of volatile agent into the oxygenator of a cardiopulmonary bypass circuit. Intravenous injection of the liquid form of volatile anesthetics has resulted in severe phlebitis, pulmonary edema, or both.[175]

How Inhaled Anesthetics Are Supplied

N_2O is usually stored in cylinders as a liquid under pressure at room temperature. At room temperature (21° C), the saturated vapor pressure (pressure exerted by the vapor in equilibrium with its liquid form) of N_2O is 735 pounds per square inch gauge (~50 kPa). Large H cylinders (43.5 L capacity) typically supply the hospital's "piped" N_2O system, and E cylinders (4.7 L capacity) are attached to individual anesthesia machines. An unused N_2O E cylinder contains ~85% liquid and can supply greater than 1500 L N_2O in gaseous form. Toxic N_2O contaminants (e.g., nitrogen oxides) are possible but extremely rare with current manufacturing standards.[150]

The volatile anesthetics are provided in liquid form in amber-colored bottles to minimize reaction with light. Halothane contains 0.01% thymol as a stabilizer; isoflurane, sevoflurane, and desflurane do not contain additives.

Anesthesia Systems

Although in 1847 John Snow was quite skillful in providing anesthesia by dripping liquid ether into a chamber attached to the patient's face mask, modern practice requires an anesthesia machine for safe and accurate delivery of inhaled anesthetics. Attached monitors and alarms allow quantitation of anesthetic, O_2 and CO_2 concentrations, and detection of physiologic side effects produced by inhaled agents. Anesthesia machines down-regulate oxygen and N_2O cylinder pressures with specific flowmeters controlling the flow of each gas (flow depends on the viscosity and density of the gas). Oxygen and N_2O combine and flow through a common manifold. The oxygen and N_2O gas mixture may be directed to a vaporizer to pick up a precise amount of volatile agent before exiting the machine at the common gas outlet.

Vaporizers

Concentrations of halothane, isoflurane, and sevoflurane are controlled with temperature-compensated, variable-bypass vaporizers. Variable bypass means that the concentration setting on the vaporizer control dial regulates the amount of gas flow going through the bypass and vaporizing chambers. Gas going to the vaporizing chamber flows over liquid anesthetic, becomes saturated with vapor, and mixes with gas passing through the bypass chamber at the vaporizer outlet to produce the desired concentration of volatile anesthetic. At room temperature (20° C), the saturated vapor pressures of halothane, isoflurane, and sevoflurane are 241, 240, and 160 mm Hg, respectively. These vaporizers are temperature-compensated because the saturated vapor pressures are highly dependent on temperature and evaporation of anesthetic from liquid to gas form would otherwise lead to a cooling of the remaining liquid anesthetic.

Desflurane requires a different type of vaporizer than the other volatile agents because it has a high saturated vapor pressure (669 mm Hg at 20° C) and boils at 22.8° C. The desflurane vaporizer is electrically heated to 39° C (it feels warm to the touch) and contains a reservoir of desflurane vapor maintained at ~2 atm pressure. Electronic regulation of differential pressures between the fresh gas circuit and the vapor circuit allows for the desired concentration of desflurane at a given setting on the concentration dial. Although anesthetic-specific filling systems minimize the chance of misfilling other vaporizers with desflurane, the misfilling of a halothane or isoflurane vaporizer with desflurane can produce a 10-fold anesthetic overdose and result in the administration of a hypoxic mixture.[176]

Anesthesia Circuits

The circle system (named because its components are arranged in a circular manner) is the most commonly used anesthesia circuit. A Y-piece, with one end connected to the patient's airway (e.g., face mask or endotracheal tube), has tubing at its other two connections that lead to unidirectional inspiratory and expiratory valves. Fresh gas flow enters the circuit from the common gas outlet of the anesthesia machine. Other circle system components include a canister with CO_2 absorbent and a means of inflating and deflating the patient's lungs (i.e., reservoir bag, mechanical ventilator, or both, with appropriate pressure alarms and safety valves). This circle system prevents rebreathing of CO_2 but allows partial rebreathing (and conservation) of oxygen and inhaled anesthetics. Complete rebreathing of exhaled gases (except CO_2) occurs when the system is "closed" and the volume of inflow gas exactly matches the volumes of O_2 consumed, the CO_2 absorbed, and the anesthetics taken up by the body.

Safe and Recommended Concentrations of Inhaled Anesthetics

As recently as 1977,[177] healthy individuals were administered 100% N_2O for short time periods (~90 seconds) during induction of anesthesia. Currently, this practice is considered unsafe and the clinician will rarely administer an inspired gas mixture that contains less than 25% oxygen.

In healthy individuals who have received no other medications, steady-state alveolar concentrations of inhaled anesthetics needed to produce a given clinical endpoint can be estimated from the MAC values in Table 23–4. Medications provided in the perioperative period lower MAC (see Table 23–5). Although the MAC values listed in these tables mean that only 50% of individuals will have the desired response, the steep nature of the concentration-response curve of inhaled anesthetics (see Fig. 23–6) means that almost all patients will have the desired clinical result with modest increases in concentrations greater than MAC. It must be emphasized that it is the alveolar (end-tidal) anesthetic concentration, and not the concentration dialed to on the vaporizer, which controls the partial pressure of inhaled anesthetic at its central nervous system sites of action.

A rapid inhaled induction of anesthesia can be achieved by having the patient take a large (vital capacity) breath of 4% halothane or 8% sevoflurane (both with 66% N_2O in oxygen) and "hold" the breath for as long as possible. This "single breath" induction method produces loss of eyelash reflex in ~60 to 90 seconds.[178] Following loss of consciousness, the inspired halothane concentration is decreased to prevent anesthetic overdose, because these induction concentrations of halothane and sevoflurane would cause cardiovascular collapse if maintained for a prolonged period. "Single breath" inductions are more difficult to perform with isoflurane or desflurane because of the airway irritation of these agents.

The administration of inhaled anesthetics must be individualized to the patient's response. Administration of a volatile anesthetic at a concentration of 0.4 MAC to a critically ill patient may be lethal, whereas this same 0.4 MAC concentration of volatile anesthetic given to a healthy patient will produce inadequate anesthesia and may even result in awareness of the surgical incision. The clinician behind the patient is more important than the particular type of inhaled anesthetic administered to the patient.

References

1. Lysko GS, Robinson JL, Casto R, et al: The stereospecific effects of isoflurane isomers in vivo. Eur J Pharmacol 263:25, 1994.
2. Koblin DD, Chortkoff BS, Laster MJ, et al: Polyhalogneated and perfluorinated compounds that disobey the Meyer-Overton hypothesis. Anesth Analg 79:1043, 1994.
3. Newberg LA, Milde JJ, Michenfelder JD: The cerebral metabolic effects of isoflurane at and above concentrations that suppress cortical electrical activity. Anesthesiology 59:23, 1983.
4. de Jong RH, Nace RA: Nerve impulse conduction and cutaneous receptor responses during general anesthesia. Anesthesiology 28:851, 1967.
5. Campbell JN, Raja SN, Meyer RA: Halothane sensitizes cutaneous nociceptors in monkeys. J Neurophysiol 52:762, 1984.

6. MacIver MB, Roth SH: Inhalational anaesthetics exhibit pathway-specific and differential actions on hippocampal synaptic responses in vitro. Br J Anaesth 60:680, 1988.

7. Richards CD, White AN: The actions of volatile anaesthetics on synaptic transmission in the dentate gyrus. J Physiol (Lond) 252:241, 1975.

8. Rampil IJ: Anesthetic potency is not altered after hypothermic spinal cord transection in rats. Anesthesiology 80:606, 1994.

9. Rampil IJ, Mason P, Singh H: Anesthetic potency (MAC) is independent of forebrain structures in the rat. Anesthesiology 78:707, 1993.

10. Antognini JF, Schwartz K: Exaggerated anesthetic requirements in the preferentially anesthetized brain. Anesthesiology 79:1244, 1993.

11. Borges M, Antognini JF: Does the brain influence somatic responses to noxious stimuli during isoflurane anesthesia? Anesthesiology 81:1511, 1994.

12. King BS, Rampil IJ: Anesthetic depression of spinal motor neurons may contribute to lack of movement in response to noxious stimuli. Anesthesiology 81:1484, 1994.

13. Antognini JF, Carstens E, Buzin V: Isoflurane depresses motoneuron excitability by a direct spinal action: An F-wave study. Anesth Analg 88:681, 1999.

14. Fang F, Guo TZ, Davies MF, et al: Opiate receptors in the periaqueductal gray mediate analgesic effect of nitrous oxide in rats. Eur J Pharmacol 336:137, 1997.

15. Guo TZ, Poree L, Golden W, et al: Antinociceptive response to nitrous oxide is mediated by supraspinal opiate and spinal alpha2 adrenergic receptors in the rat. Anesthesiology 85:846, 1996.

16. Sawamura S, Kingery WS, Davies MF, et al: Antinociceptive action of nitrous oxide is mediated by stimulation of noradrenergic neurons in the brainstem and activation of [alpha]2B adrenoceptors. J Neurosci 20:9242, 2000.

17. Zhang C, Davies MF, Guo TZ, et al: The analgesic action of nitrous oxide is dependent on the release of norepinephrine in the dorsal horn of the spinal cord. Anesthesiology 91:1401, 1999.

18. Kendig JJ, MacIver MB, Roth SH: Anesthetic actions in the hippocampal formation. Ann NY Acad Sci 625:37, 1991.

19. Ries CR, Puil E: Mechanism of anesthesia revealed by shunting actions of isoflurane on thalamocortical neurons. J Neurophysiol 81:1795, 1999.

20. Madison DV, Nicoll RA: General anesthetics hyperpolarize neurons in the vertebrate central nervous system. Science 217:1055, 1982.

21. MacIver MB, Kendig JJ: Anesthetic effects on resting membrane potential are voltage-dependent and agent-specific. Anesthesiology 74:83, 1991.

22. Franks NP, Lieb WR: Mechanisms of general anesthesia. Environ Health Perspect 87:199, 1990.

23. Franks NP, Lieb WR: Volatile general anaesthetics activate a novel neuronal K^+ current. Nature 333:662, 1988.

24. Ries CR, Puil E: Ionic mechanism of isoflurane's actions on thalamocortical neurons. J Neurophysiol 81:1802, 1999.

25. Gray AT, Winegar BD, Leonoudakis DJ, et al: TOK1 is a volatile anesthetic stimulated K^+ channel. Anesthesiology 88:1076, 1998.

26. Patel AJ, Honore E, Lesage F, et al: Inhalational anesthetics activate two-pore-domain background K^+ channels. Nat Neurosci 2:422, 1999.

27. Larrabee MG, Posternak JM: Selective action of anesthetics on synapses and axons in mammalian sympathetic ganglia. J Neurophysiol 15:91, 1952.

28. Haydon DA, Urban BW: The effects of some inhalation anesthetics on the sodium current of the squid giant axon. J Physiol 341:429, 1983.

29. Nicoll RA: The effects of anaesthetics on synaptic excitation and inhibition in the olfactory bulb. J Physiol (Lond) 223:803, 1972.

30. Kullman DM, Martin RL, Redman SJ: Reduction by general anaesthetics of group Ia excitatory postsynaptic potentials and currents in the cat spinal cord. J Physiol (Lond) 412:277, 1989.

31. Richards CD, Russel WJ, Smaje JC: The action of ether and methoxyflurane on synaptic transmission in isolated preparations of the mammalian cortex. J Physiol (Lond) 248:121, 1975.

32. Yoshimura M, Higashi H, Fujita S, et al: Selective depression of hippocampal inhibitory postsynaptic potentials and spontaneous firing by volatile anesthetics. Brain 340:363, 1985.

33. Fujiwara M, Higashi H, Nishi S, et al: Changes in spontaneous firing patterns of rat hippocampal neurones induced by volatile anaesthetics. J Physiol (Lond) 402:155, 1988.

34. Mui P, Puil E: Isoflurane-induced impairment of synaptic transmission in hippocampal neurons. Exp Brain Res 75:354, 1989.

35. Tanelian DL, Kosek P, Mody I, et al: The role of the $GABA_A$ receptor/chloride channel complex in anesthesia. Anesthesiology 78:757, 1993.

36. Franks NP, Lieb WR: Molecular and cellular mechanisms of general anesthesia. Nature 367:607, 1994.

37. Banks MI, Pearce RA: Dual actions of volatile anesthetics on $GABA_A$ IPSCs: Dissociation of blocking and prolonging effects. Anesthesiology 90:120, 1999.

38. Wakamori M, Ikemoto Y, Akaike N: Effects of two volatile anesthetics and a volatile convulsant on the excitatory and inhibitory amino acid responses in dissociated central nervous system neurons of the rat. J Neurophysiol 66:2014, 1991.

39. Jones MV, Brooks PA, Harrison NL: Enhancements of gamma-aminobutyric acid-activated Cl^- currents in cultured rat hippocampal neurones by three volatile anesthetics. J Physiol 449:279, 1992.

40. Yeh JZ, Quandt FN, Tanguy J, et al: General anesthetic action on gamma-aminobutyric acid-activated channels. Ann NY Acad Sci 625:155, 1991.

41. Hall AC, Lieb WR, Franks NP: Stereoselective and non-stereoselective actions of isoflurane on the $GABA_A$ receptor. Br J Pharmacol 112:906, 1994.

42. Mascia MP, Machu TK, Harris RA: Enhancement of homomeric glycine receptor function by long-chain alcohols and anaesthetics. Br J Pharmacol 119:1331, 1996.

43. Downie DL, Hall AC, Lieb WR, et al: Effects of inhalational general anaesthetics on native glycine receptors in rat medullary neurons and recombinant glycine receptors in Xenopus oocytes. Br J Pharmacol 118:493, 1996.

44. Mennerick S, Jevtovic-Todorovic V, Todorovic SM, et al: Effect of nitrous oxide on excitatory and inhibitory synaptic transmission in hippocampal cultures. J Neurosci 18:9716, 1998.

45. Jevtovic-Todorovic V, Todorovic SM, Mennerick S, et al: Nitrous oxide (laughing gas) is an NMDA antagonist, neuroprotectant and neurotoxin. Nat Med 4:460, 1998.

46. Franks NP, Dickinson R, de Sousa SL, et al: How does xenon produce anaesthesia? Nature 396:324, 1998.

47. deSousa SLM, Dickinson R, Lieb WR, et al: Contrasting synaptic actions of the inhalational general anesthetics isoflurane and xenon. Anesthesiology 92:1055, 2000.

48. Raines DE, Claycomb RJ, Scheller M, et al: Nonhalogenated alkane anesthetics fail to potentiate agonist actions on two ligand-gated ion channels. Anesthesiology 95:470, 2001.

49. Perouansky M, Kirson E, Yaari Y: Halothane blocks synaptic excitation of inhibitory interneurons. Anesthesiology 85:1431, 1996.

50. Lin LH, Chen LTL, Harris RA: Enflurane inhibits NMDA, AMPA, and kainate-induced currents in xenopus oocytes expressing mouse and human brain messenger RNA. FASEB J 7:479, 1993.

51. Dildy-Mayfield JE, Eger EI, Harris RA: Anesthetics produce subunit-selective actions on glutamate receptors. J Pharmacol Exp Ther 276:1058, 1996.

52. Perouansky M, Baranov D, Salman M, et al: Effects of halothane on glutamate receptor-mediated excitatory postsynaptic currents: A patch-clamp study in adult mouse hippocampal slices. Anesthesiology 83:109, 1995.

53. MacIver M, Bruce M, Mikulec AA, et al: Volatile anesthetics depress glutamate transmission via presynaptic actions. Anesthesiology 85:823, 1996.

54. Schlame M, Hemmings HC Jr: Inhibition by volatile anesthetics of endogenous glutamate release from synaptosomes by a presynaptic. Anesthesiology 82:1406, 1995.

55. Ratnakumari L, Hemmings HCJ: Inhibition of presynaptic sodium channels by halothane. Anesthesiology 88:1043, 1998.

56. Bleakman D, Jones MV, Harrison NL: The effects of four general anesthetics on intracellular calcium in cultured hippocampal neurons. Neuropharmacology 34:541, 1995.

57. Study RE: Isoflurane inhibits multiple voltage-gated calcium currents in hippocampal pyramidal neurons. Anesthesiology 81:104, 1994.

58. Pocock G, Richards CD: The action of volatile anaesthetics on stimulus-secretion coupling in bovine adrenal chromaffin cells. Br J Pharmacol 95:209, 1988.

59. Herrington J, Stern RC, Evers AS, et al: Halothane inhibits two components of calcium current in clonal (GH_3) pituitary cells. J Neurosci 11:2226, 1991.

60. van Swinderen B, Saifee O, Shebester L, et al: A neomorphic syntaxin mutation blocks volatile-anesthetic action in *Caenorhabditis elegans*. Proc Natl Acad Sci USA 96:2479, 1999.

61. Franks NP, Lieb WR: Stereospecific effects of inhalational general anesthetic optical isomers on nerve ion channels. Science 254:427, 1991.

62. Charlesworth P, Richards CD: Anaesthetic modulation of nicotinic ion channel kinetics in bovine chromaffin cells. Br J Pharmacol 114:909, 1995.

63. Violet JM, Downie DL, Nakisa RC, et al: Differential sensitivities of mammalian neuronal and muscle nicotinic acetylcholine receptors to general anesthetics. Anesthesiology 86:866, 1997.

64. Flood P, Ramirez-Latorre J, Role L: alpha4beta2 neuronal nicotinic acetylcholine receptors in the central nervous system are inhibited by isoflurane and propofol, but alpha7-type nicotinic acetylcholine receptors are unaffected. Anesthesiology 86:859, 1997.

65. Jenkins A, Franks NP, Lieb WR: Actions of general anaesthetics on 5-HT3 receptors in N1E-115 neuroblastoma cells. Br J Pharmacol 117:1507, 1996.

66. Machu TK, Harris RA: Alcohols and anesthetics enhance the function of 5-hydroxytryptamine-3 receptors expressed in Xenopus laevis oocytes. J Pharmacol Exp Ther 271:898, 1994.

67. Slater S, Cox KJA, Lombardi JV, et al: Inhibition of protein kinase C by alcohols and anesthetics. Nature 364:82, 1993.

68. Hemmings HCJ, Adamo AI: Effect of halothane on conventional protein kinase C translocation and down-regulation in rat cerebrocortical synaptosomes. Br J Anaesth 78:189, 1997.

69. Li X, Czajkowski C, Pearce RA: Rapid and direct modulation of GABA$_A$ receptors by halothane. Anesthesiology 92:1366, 2000.

70. Overton CE: Studies of Narcosis, 1st ed. London, Chapman and Hall, 1891.

71. Meyer H: Theorie der alkoholnarkose. Arch Exp Pathol Pharmakol 42:109, 1899.

72. Franks NP, Lieb WR: Where do general anaesthetics act? Nature 274:339, 1978.

73. Dickinson R, White I, Lieb WR, et al: Stereoselective loss of righting reflex in rates by isoflurane. Anesthesiology 93:837, 2000.

74. Franks NP, Lieb WR: Do general anaesthetics act by competitive binding to specific receptors. Nature 310:599, 1984.

75. Franks NP, Lieb WR: Mapping of general anaesthetic target sites provides a molecular basis for cutoff effects. Nature 316:149, 1985.

76. Franks NP, Jenkins A, Conti E, et al: Structural basis for the inhibition of firefly luciferase by a general anaesthetic. Biophys J 75:2205, 1998.

77. Dubois BW, Evers AS: An ^{19}F-NMR spin-spin relaxation (T$_2$) method for characterizing volatile anesthetic binding to proteins. Analysis of isoflurane binding to serum albumin. Biochemistry 31:7069, 1992.

78. Bhattacharya AA, Curry S, Franks NP: Binding of the general anesthetics propofol and halothane to human serum albumin. High resolution crystal structures. J Biol Chem 275:38731, 2000.

79. Harris B, Moody E, Skolnick P: Isoflurane anesthesia is stereoselective. Eur J Pharmacol 217:215, 1992.

80. Moody EJ, Harris B, Hoehner P, et al: Inhibition of [3H]isradipine binding to L-type calcium channels by the optical isomers of isoflurane. Anesthesiology 81:124, 1994.

81. Graf BM, Boban M, Stowe DF, et al: Lack of stereospecific effects of isoflurane and desflurane isomers in isolated guinea pig hearts. Anesthesiology 81:129, 1994.

82. Mihic SJ, Ye Q, Wick MJ, et al: Sites of alcohol and volatile anaesthetic action on GABA$_A$ and glycine receptors. Nature 389:385, 1997.

83. Greenblatt EP, Meng X: Divergence of volatile anesthetic effects in inhibitory neurotransmitter receptors. Anesthesiology 94:1026, 2001.

84. Jenkins A, Greenblatt EP, Faulkner JH, et al: Evidence for a common binding cavity for three general anesthetics within the GABA$_A$ receptor. J Neurosci 21:RC136, 2001.

85. Wick MJ, Mihic SJ, Ueno S, et al: Mutations of gamma-aminobutyric acid and glycine receptors change alcohol cutoff: Evidence for an alcohol receptor? Proc Natl Acad Sci USA 95:6504, 1998.

86. Yamakura T, Mihic SJ, Harris RA: Amino acid volume and hydropathy of a transmembrane site determine glycine and anesthetic sensitivity of glycine receptors. J Biol Chem 274:23006, 1999.

87. Ye Q, Koltchine VV, Mihic SJ, et al: Enhancement of glycine receptor function by ethanol is inversely correlated with molecular volume at position alpha267. J Biol Chem 273:3314, 1998.

88. Koltchine VV, Finn SE, Jenkins A, et al: Agonist gating and isoflurane potentiation in the human gamma-aminobutyric acid type A receptor determined by the volume of a second transmembrane domain residue. Mol Pharmacol 56:1087, 1999.

89. Mascia MP, Trudell JR, Harris RA: Specific binding sites for alcohols and anesthetics on ligand-gated ion channels. Proc Natl Acad Sci USA 97:9305, 2000.

90. Homanics GE, Ferguson C, Quinlan JJ, et al: Gene knockout of the alpha6 subunit of the gamma-aminobutyric acid type A receptor: Lack of effect on responses to ethanol, pentobarbital, and general anesthetics. Mol Pharmacol 51:588, 1997.

91. Mihalek RM, Banerjee PK, Korpi ER, et al: Attenuated sensitivity to neuroactive steroids in gamma-aminobutyrate type A receptor delta subunit knockout mice. Proc Natl Acad Sci USA 96:12905, 1999.

92. Quinlan JJ, Homanics GE, Firestone LL: Anesthesia sensitivity in mice that lack the beta3 subunit of the gamma-aminobutyric acid type A receptor. Anesthesiology 88:775, 1998.

93. Rajaram S, Sedensky MM, Morgan PG: Unc-1: A stomatin homologue controls sensitivity to volatile anesthetics in *Caenorhabditis elegans*. Proc Natl Acad Sci USA 95:8761, 1998.

94. Kayser EB, Morgan PG, Sedensky MM: GAS-1: A mitochondrial protein controls sensitivity to volatile anesthetics in the nematode *Caenorhabditis elegans*. Anesthesiology 90:545, 1999.

95. Lynch C, Baum J, Tenbrinck R: Xenon anesthesia. Anesthesiology 92:865, 2000.

96. Eger EI II: Anesthetic Uptake and Action. Baltimore, Williams & Wilkins, 1974.

97. Carpenter RL, Eger EI II, Johnson BH, et al: Does the duration of anesthetic administration affect the pharmacokinetics or metabolism of inhaled anesthetics in humans? Anesth Analg 66:1, 1987.

98. Eger EI II, Gong D, Koblin DD, et al: The effect of anesthetic duration on kinetic and recovery characteristics of desflurane versus sevoflurane, and on the kinetic characteristics of compound A, in volunteers. Anesth Analg 86:414, 1998.

99. Kissin I: A concept for assessing interactions of general anesthetics. Anesth Analg 85:204, 1997.

100. Quasha AL, Eger EI II, Tinker JH: Determination and applications of MAC. Anesthesiology 53:315, 1980.

101. Fisher DM, Zwass MS: MAC of desflurane in 60% nitrous oxide in infants and children. Anesthesiology 76:354, 1992.

102. Katoh T, Ikeda K, Bito H: Does nitrous oxide antagonize sevoflurane-induced hypnosis? Br J Anaesth 79:465, 1997.

103. Chortkoff BS, Eger EI II, Crankshaw DP, et al: Concentrations of desflurane and propofol that suppress response to command in humans. Anesth Analg 81:737, 1995.

104. Zbinden AM, Maggiorini M, Petersen-Felix S, et al: Anesthetic depth defined using multiple noxious stimuli during isoflurane/oxygen anesthesia. Anesthesiology 80:253, 1994.

105. Kimura T, Watanabe S, Asakura N, et al: Determination of end-tidal sevoflurane concentration for tracheal intubation and minimum alveolar anesthetic concentration in adults. Anesth Analg 79:378, 1994.

106. Daniel M, Weiskopf RB, Noorani M, et al: Fentanyl augments the blockade of the sympathetic response to incision (MAC-BAR) produced by desflurane and isoflurane. Anesthesiology 88:43, 1998.

107. Mapleson WW: Effect of age on MAC in humans. Br J Anaesth 76:179, 1996.

108. Katoh T, Bito H, Sato S: Influence of age on hypnotic requirement, bispectral index, and 95% spectral edge frequency associated with sedation induced by sevoflurane. Anesthesiology 92:55, 2000.

109. Franks NP, Lieb WR: Temperature dependence of the potency of volatile general anesthetics. Anesthesiology 84:716, 1996.

110. Petersen-Felix S, Zbinden AM, Fischer M, et al: Isoflurane minimum alveolar concentration decreases during anesthesia and surgery. Anesthesiology 79:959, 1993.

111. Zhou HH, Norman P, DeLima LGR, et al: The minimum alveolar concentration of isoflurane in patients undergoing bilateral tubal ligation in the postpartum period. Anesthesiology 82:1364, 1995.

112. Roizen MF, Newfield P, Eger EI II, et al: Reduced anesthetic requirement after electrical stimulation of periaqueductal gray matter. Anesthesiology 62:120, 1985.

113. Bourke DL, Smith BAC, Erickson J, et al: TENS reduces halothane requirements during hand surgery. Anesthesiology 61:679, 1984.

114. Frei FJ, Haemmerle MH, Brunner R, et al: Minimum alveolar concentration for halothane in children with cerebral palsy and severe mental retardation. Anaesthesia 52:1056, 1997.

115. Barber RE: Anesthetic requirement in alcoholic patients. American Society of Anesthesiologists Annual Meeting Abstracts, 1978, p 623.

116. Fahey MR, Sessler DI, Cannon JE, et al: Atracurium, vecuronium, and pancuronium do not alter the minimum alveolar concentration of halothane in humans. Anesthesiology 71:53, 1990.

117. Weiskopf RB, Cahalan MK, Eger EI II, et al: Cardiovascular actions of desflurane in normocarbic volunteers. Anesth Analg 73:143, 1991.

118. Frink EJ, Malan TP, Atlas M, et al: Clinical comparison of sevoflurane and isoflurane in healthy patients. Anesth Analg 74:241, 1992.

119. Muzi M, Ebert TJ, Hope WG, et al: Site(s) mediating sympathetic activation with desflurane. Anesthesiology 785:737, 1996.

120. Ebert TJ: Differential effects of nitrous oxide on baroreflex control of heart rate and peripheral sympathetic nerve activity in humans. Anesthesiology 72:16, 1990.

121. Russell GB, Snider MT, Richard RB, et al: Hyperbaric nitrous oxide as a sole anesthetic agent in humans. Anesth Analg 70:289, 1990.

122. Slogoff S, Keats AS, Dear WE, et al: Steal-prone coronary anatomy and myocardial ischemia associated with four primary anesthetic agents in humans. Anesth Analg 72:22, 1991.

123. Atlee JL III, Bosnjak ZJ: Mechanisms for cardiac dysrhythmias during anesthesia. Anesthesiology 72:47, 1990.

124. Lampe GL, Donegan JH, Rupp SM, et al: Nitrous oxide and epinephrine-induced arrhythmias. Anesth Analg 71:602, 1990.

125. Rolf N, Coté CJ: Persistent cardiac arrhythmias in pediatric patients: Effects of age, expired carbon dioxide values, depth of anesthesia, and airway management. Anesth Analg 73:720, 1991.

126. Lockhart SH, Rampil IJ, Yasuda N, et al: Depression of ventilation by desflurane in humans. Anesthesiology 74:484, 1991.

127. Knill RL: Interpreting low-dose anesthetic effects on the ventilatory response to hypoxaemia: Facts, findings, and fanciful formulations. Anesthesiology 81:1087, 1994.

128. Benumof JL, Augustine SD, Gibbons JA: Halothane and isoflurane only slightly impair arterial oxygenation during one lung ventilation in patients undergoing thoracotomy. Anesthesiology 67:910, 1987.

129. Goff MJ, Arain SR, Ficke DJ, et al: Absence of bronchodilation during desflurane anesthesia. Anesthesiology 93:404, 2000.

130. TerRiet MF, DeSouza GJA, Jacobs JS, et al: Which is most pungent: Isoflurane, sevoflurane, or desflurane? Br J Anaesth 85:305, 2000.

131. Rampil IJ, Lockhart SH, Zwass MS, et al: Clinical characteristics of desflurane in surgical patients: Minimum alveolar concentration. Anesthesiology 74:429, 1991.

132. Ghoneim MM, Block RI: Learning and memory during general anesthesia. An update. Anesthesiology 87:387, 1997.

133. McCulloch PR, Milne B: Neurologic phenomena during emergence from enflurane or isoflurane anaesthesia. Can J Anaesth 37:739, 1990.

134. Kaisti KK, Jaaskelainen SK, Rinne JO, et al: Epileptiform discharges during 2 MAC sevoflurane in two healthy volunteers. Anesthesiology 91:1952, 1999.

135. Plougmann J, Astrup J, Pedersen J, et al: Effect of stable xenon inhalation on intracranial pressure during measurement of cerebral blood flow in head injury. J Neurosurg 81:822, 1994.

136. Moss E: Volatile anaesthetic agents in neurosurgery. Br J Anaesth 63:4, 1989.

137. Muzzi DA, Losasso TJ, Dietz NM, et al: The effect of desflurane and isoflurane on cerebrospinal fluid pressure in humans with supratentorial mass lesions. Anesthesiology 76:720, 1992.

138. Elliott RH, Strunin L: Hepatotoxicity of volatile anaesthetics. Br J Anaesth 70:339, 1993.

139. Lessard MR, Trepanier CA: Renal function and hemodynamics during prolonged isoflurane-induced hypotension in humans. Anesthesiology 74:860, 1991.

140. Obata R, Bito H, Ohmura M, et al: The effects of prolonged low-flow sevoflurane anesthesia on renal and hepatic function. Anesth Analg 91:1262, 2000.

141. Mazze RI, Callan CM, Galvez ST, et al: The effects of sevoflurane on serum creatinine and blood urea nitrogen concentrations: A retrospective, twenty-two-center, comparative evaluation of renal function in adult surgical patients. Anesth Analg 90:683, 2000.

142. Caldwell JE, Laster MJ, Magorian T, et al: The neuromuscular effects of desflurane, alone and combined with pancuronium or succinylcholine in humans. Anesthesiology 74:412, 1991.

143. Munson ES, Embro WJ: Enflurane, isoflurane, and halothane and isolated uterine muscle. Anesthesiology 46:11, 1977.

144. Nakata Y, Goto T, Morita S: Vecuronium-induced neuromuscular block during xenon or sevoflurane anaesthesia in humans. Br J Anaesth 80:238, 1998.

145. Wachta MF, White PF: Postoperative nausea and vomiting. Anesthesiology 77:162, 1992.

146. Divatia JV, Vaidya JS, Badwe RA, et al: Omission of nitrous oxide during anesthesia reduces the incidence of postoperative nausea and vomiting. A meta-analysis. Anesthesiology 85:1055, 1996.

147. Losasso TJ, Muzzi DA, Dietz NM, et al: Fifty percent nitrous oxide does not increase the risk of venous air embolism in neurosurgical patients operated upon in the sitting position. Anesthesiology 77:21, 1992.

148. Scheinin B, Lindgren L, Scheinin TM: Preoperative nitrous oxide delays bowel function after colonic surgery. Br J Anaesth 64:154, 1990.

149. Boulanger A, Hardy JF: Intestinal distention during elective abdominal surgery: Should nitrous oxide be banished? Can J Anaesth 34:346, 1987.

150. Koblin DD: Toxicity of nitrous oxide (N_2O). In Rice SA, Fish KJ (eds): Anesthetic Toxicity. New York, Raven Press, 1994, pp 135–155.

151. Badner NH, Beattie WS, Freeman D, et al: Nitrous oxide-induced increased homocysteine concentrations are associated with increased postoperative myocardial ischemia in patients undergoing carotid endarterectomy. Anesth Analg 91:1073, 2000.

152. Koblin DD: Characteristics and implications of desflurane metabolism and toxicity. Anesth Analg 75:S10, 1992.

153. Kharasch ED, Hankins D, Mautz D, et al: Identification of the enzyme responsible for oxidative halothane metabolism: Implications for prevention of halothane hepatitis. Lancet 347:1367, 1996.

154. Gunaratnam NT, Benson J, Gandolfi AJ, et al: Suspected isoflurane hepatitis in an obese patient with a history of halothane hepatitis. Anesthesiology 83:1361, 1995.

155. Martin JL, Plevak DJ, Flannery KD, et al: Hepatotoxicity after desflurane anesthesia. Anesthesiology 83:1125, 1995.

156. Eger EI II, Koblin DD, Bowland T, et al: Nephrotoxicity of sevoflurane versus desflurane anesthesia in volunteers. Anesth Analg 84:160, 1997.

157. Kobayashi Y, Ochiai R, Takeda J, et al: Serum and urinary inorganic fluoride concentrations after prolonged inhalation of sevoflurane in humans. Anesth Analg 74:753, 1992.

158. Kharasch ED, Thummel KE: Identification of cytochrome P450 2E1 as the predominant enzyme catalyzing human liver microsomal defluorination of sevoflurane, isoflurane, and methoxyflurane. Anesthesiology 79:795, 1993.

159. Bito H, Ikeuchi Y, Ikeda K: Effects of water content of soda lime on compound A concentration in the anesthesia circuit in sevoflurane anesthesia. Anesthesiology 88:66, 1998.

160. Higuchi H, Adachi Y, Arimura S, et al: Compound A concentrations during low-flow sevoflurane anesthesia correlate directly with the concentration of monovalent bases in carbon dioxide absorbents. Anesth Analg 91:434, 2000.

161. Murray JM, Renfrew CW, Bedi A: Amsorb: A new carbon dioxide absorbent for use in anesthetic breathing systems. Anesthesiology 91:1342, 1999.

162. Woehlck HJ: Severe intraoperative CO poisoning. Should apathy prevail? Anesthesiology 90:353, 1999.

163. Fang ZX, Eger EI II, Laster MJ, et al: Carbon monoxide production from degradation of desflurane, enflurane, isoflurane, halothane, and sevoflurane by soda lime and baralyme. Anesth Analg 80:1187, 1995.

164. Baxter PJ, Garton K, Kharasch ED: Mechanistic aspects of carbon monoxide formation from volatile anesthetics. Anesthesiology 89:929, 1998.

165. American Society of Anesthesiologists: Waste anesthetic gases. Information for management in anesthetizing areas and the postanesthesia care unit (PACU). Task Force on Trace Anesthetic Gases, 1999.

166. Kong KL, Willatts SM, Prys-Roberts C: Isoflurane compared with midazolam for sedation in the intensive care unit. BMJ 298:1277, 1989.

167. Kofke WA, Young RSK, Davis P, et al: Isoflurane for refractory status epilepticus: A clinical series. Anesthesiology 71:653, 1989.

168. Parnass SM, Feld JM, Chamberlin WH, et al: Status asthmaticus treated with isoflurane and enflurane. Anesth Analg 66:193, 1987.

169. Miller LR, Drummond JC, Lamond RG: Refractory arterial and intracranial hypertension in the intensive care unit: Successful treatment with isoflurane. Anesthesiology 74:946, 1991.

170. Gold CG, Cullen DJ, Gonzales S, et al: Rapid opioid detoxification during general anesthesia. Anesthesiology 91:1639, 1999.

171. Greenberg LB, Gage J, Vitkun S, et al: Isoflurane anesthesia therapy: A replacement for ECT in depressive disorders? Convuls Ther 3:269, 1987.

172. Taylor E, Feinstein R, White PF, et al: Anesthesia for laparoscopic cholycystectomy. Is nitrous oxide contraindicated? Anesthesiology 76:541, 1992.

173. Jensen AG, Kullman E, Anderberg B, et al: Peroperative nitrous oxide does not influence recovery after laparoscopic cholycystectomy. Acta Anaesthesiol Scand 37:683, 1993.

174. Neuman GG, Sidebotham G, Negoianu E, et al: Laparoscopy explosion hazards with nitrous oxide. Anesthesiology 78:875, 1993.

175. Dwyer R, Coppel DL: Intravenous injection of liquid halothane. Anesth Analg 69:250, 1989.

176. Andrews JJ, Johnston RV, Kramer GC: Consequences of misfilling contemporary vaporizers with desflurane. Can J Anaesth 40:71, 1993.

177. Himes RS, DiFazio CA, Burney RG: Effects of lidocaine on the anesthetic requirements for nitrous oxide and halothane. Anesthesiology 47:437, 1977.

178. Hall JE, Oldham TA, Stewart JIM, et al: Comparison between halothane and sevoflurane for adult vital capacity induction. Br J Anaesth 79:285, 1997.

179. Westmoreland CL, Sebel PS, Gropper A: Fentanyl or alfentanil decreases the minimum alveolar anesthetic concentration of isoflurane in surgical patients. Anesth Analg 78:23, 1994.

180. Sebel PS, Glass PSA, Fletcher JE, et al: Reduction of the MAC of desflurane with fentanyl. Anesthesiology 76:52, 1992.

181. Katoh T, Kobayashi S, Suzuki A, et al: The effect of fentanyl on sevoflurane requirements for somatic and sympathetic responses to surgical incision. Anesthesiology 90:398, 1999.

182. Glass PSA, Doherty M, Jacobs JR, et al: Plasma concentration of fentanyl, with 70% nitrous oxide, to prevent movement at skin incision. Anesthesiology 78:842, 1993.

183. Inagaki Y, Mashimo T, Yoshiya I: Segmental analgesic effect and reduction of halothane MAC from epidural fentanyl in humans. Anesth Analg 74:856, 1992.

184. Katoh T, Ikeda K: The effects of fentanyl on sevoflurane requirements for loss of consciousness and skin incision. Anesthesiology 88:18, 1998.

185. Brunner MD, Braithwaite P, Jhaveri R, et al: MAC reduction of isoflurane by sufentanil. Br J Anaesth 72:42, 1994.

186. Johansen JW, Schneider G, Windsor AM, et al: Esmolol potentiates reduction of minimum alveolar isoflurane concentration by alfentanil. Anesth Analg 87:671, 1998.

187. Vuyk J, Lim T, Engbers FHM, et al: Pharmacodynamics of alfentanil as a supplement to propofol or nitrous oxide for lower abdominal surgery in female patients. Anesthesiology 78:1036, 1993.

188. Lang E, Kapila A, Shlugman D, et al: Reduction of isoflurane minimum alveolar concentration by remifentanil. Anesthesiology 85:721, 1996.

189. Drasner K, Bernards CM, Ozanne GM: Intrathecal morphine reduces the isoflurane minimum alveolar concentrations of halothane in humans. Anesthesiology 69:310, 1988.

190. Schwieger IM, Klopfenstein CE, Forster A: Epidural morphine reduces halothane MAC in humans. Can J Anaesth 39:911, 1992.

191. Inagaki Y, Kuzukawa A: Effects of epidural and intravenous buprenorphine on halothane minimum alveolar concentration and hemodynamic responses. Anesth Analg 84:100, 1997.

192. Inagaki Y, Sumikawa K, Yoshiya I: Anesthetic interaction between midazolam and halothane in humans. Anesth Analg 76:613, 1993.

193. Inomata S, Yaguchi Y, Toyooka H: The effects of clonidine premedication on sevoflurane requirements and anesthetic induction time. Anesth Analg 89:204, 1999.

194. Aantaa R, Jaakola ML, Kallio A, et al: Reduction of the minimum alveolar concentrations of isoflurane by dexmedetomidine. Anesthesiology 86:1055, 1997.

195. Slee TA, Cullen BF, Unadkat J, et al: The effect of ethanol on MAC of halothane in humans. Anesthesiology 75:A332, 1991.

Intravenous Anesthetics

Neil L. Harrison, PhD • John W. Sear, MA, PhD

BARBITURATES, ETOMIDATE, PROPOFOL, KETAMINE, AND STEROIDS

Despite more than a century of research, the molecular mechanisms of action of general anesthetics in the central nervous system (CNS) have remained elusive, although ligand-gated ion channels have emerged as promising molecular targets to mediate the CNS effects of many general anesthetics. γ-Aminobutyric acid type A (GABA$_A$) and N-methyl-D-aspartate (NMDA) receptors are promising general anesthetic targets, because of their ubiquitous distribution and essential physiologic roles in the CNS. However, given the uncertainty concerning the exact anatomy of the synapses that are disrupted to produce the constellation of behavioral effects seen during general anesthesia, receptors with more limited distribution may con-

ceivably play major roles as molecular mediators of specific components of the general anesthetic state.

It was recognized decades ago that intravenous anesthetics may act on specific targets; in recent years this has in turn led to the study of their effects on the ligand-gated ion channels.

This chapter first considers general issues concerning intravenous anesthetic action, then reviews the clinical pharmacology and mechanisms of action of several important classes of intravenous anesthetic agents in turn, before ending by considering allergic reactions to these agents as a group.

MECHANISMS OF ACTION

There have been a number of excellent reviews during the last decade summarizing work on the molecular and cellular actions of general anesthetics.[1-3] What are the pharmacologic criteria that can help define proteins as plausible molecular targets for general anesthetics?

Pharmacologic Criteria for a Reasonable Intravenous Anesthetic Target Site

Before considering the actions of specific intravenous agents on ligand-gated ion channels, it is worthwhile to define specific criteria that a target molecule (receptor protein or otherwise) must fulfill to qualify as a candidate in mediating the behavioral actions of the intravenous anesthetics.[1,2]

1. The anesthetic must alter the function of the receptor at behaviorally relevant concentrations.
2. The receptor must be expressed in the appropriate anatomic locations to mediate the specific behavioral effects of the anesthetic.
3. If an anesthetic molecule shows stereoselective effects in vivo, these should be mirrored by the in vitro actions at the receptor.
4. Within a homologous series of anesthetics (e.g., the barbiturates or the phenols), the potency of a compound at the receptor should correlate with in vivo anesthetic potency.

What Is the "Clinically Relevant Concentration" for an Intravenous General Anesthetic?

The issue of clinically relevant concentrations for the intravenous anesthetics in humans and other mammals is complicated by pharmacokinetic aspects (absorption/redistribution/metabolism/elimination) of these drugs (see "Clinical Pharmacology of Hypnotic Drugs" for a detailed discussion). One consequence of this is difficulty in ascertaining steady-state drug concentrations in the brain. In some cases (e.g., for propofol and the barbiturates), detailed studies have addressed these issues, and reasonable estimates of free anesthetic concentrations in brain have been obtained (reviewed by Franks and Lieb[1]). In other cases (e.g., ketamine and the steroid anesthetic alphaxalone), only total anesthetic concentrations in blood are known,[4,5] thus invariably overestimating brain concentrations and therefore underestimating the potency of this class of anesthetics, often by as much as one to two orders of magnitude (refer to Franks and Lieb[1] and to an extensive tabulation of anesthetic concentrations recently published elsewhere[6]).

Anatomic Location

This is a more difficult issue to discuss because there is considerable debate about precisely which synaptic circuits are responsible for the various reflexes and complex behaviors that are perturbed by general anesthetics. The immobility produced by general anesthetics, perhaps not surprisingly, appears to involve the depression of monosynaptic and polysynaptic spinal reflex pathways. Immobilization can be demonstrated to occur completely independently of drug actions in the brain during certain defined experimental circumstances.[7-9] What is less clear is whether supraspinal targets can influence these reflex pathways during more normal conditions of anesthetic application.

Stereoselectivity

Stereoselectivity represents one of the most powerful tests for the relevance of a putative intravenous anesthetic target.[1] A number of intravenous anesthetic molecules possess a chiral carbon atom, and some pairs of stereoisomers or enantiomers exert different anesthetic potencies in vivo. The clinical formulation of these anesthetics is usually based on the racemic mixture, because of the difficulty of separating enantiomers in large quantities—an exception is etomidate, which is prepared by a chiral synthesis. Production of pure enantiomers perhaps would improve the clinical profile for other general anesthetics, although cost considerations probably preclude such a development.

Intravenous anesthetic stereoselectivity posed a severe challenge to traditional "lipid theories" of anesthetic action and was pivotal in building the arguments that led to the abandonment of these ideas.[10] For example, stereoselectivity supports the plausibility of the GABA$_A$ receptor as a target in mediating the actions of etomidate,[11] because in vivo potency and activity at the GABA$_A$ receptor display identical trends. Despite the rewards of studying general anesthetic stereoisomers, exemplified by the etomidate work outlined earlier,[11] the stereoselectivity approach has been underused, mainly because of the limited supply and expense of purified stereoisomers.[12] Furthermore, only limited anesthetic endpoints (mainly immobility or loss of righting reflex) have been assessed for the anesthetic stereoisomers. It would be interesting to know whether the additional neurobiologic actions of anesthetics (e.g., amnesia, analgesia) display similar patterns of stereoselectivity.

Homologous Series

The so-called "Meyer-Overton correlation" (MOC), which led to the adoption of the traditional dogma concerning lipid mechanisms, arose from the fundamental observation that the in vivo potency of general anesthetics increases in parallel with increasing hydrophobicity of the anesthetic molecules. This trend holds to some degree for anesthetic molecules with oil/water partition coefficients varying over numerous orders of magnitude; but it is especially striking within homologous series of anesthetic compounds. However, the correlation breaks down when hydrophobic nonanesthetic homologs are included. A major problem for traditional theories arose with the discovery of hydrophobic compounds that disobey the MOC. These so-called "non-immobilizers" have provided some additional clues as to which receptor targets might underlie the behavioral actions of general anesthetics.

The MOC was traditionally interpreted to suggest non-specific mechanisms of action for general anesthetics within membrane lipid compartments; however, a modern (and equally valid) interpretation of the MOC is that anesthetics bind to partially hydrophobic domains of receptor proteins.[1,10] General anesthetic actions at a plausible receptor target usually exhibit similar trends, with the more hydrophobic members of a series being more potent at the target than the more hydrophilic analogs.

Experimental Approaches to Studying General Anesthetic Actions

General anesthetic actions at ligand-gated ion channels have been studied using a variety of methodologies, including protein chemistry, radioligand binding, ion flux studies, and electrophysiology. One of the main foci have been electro-physiologic studies because these generally provide superior time resolution and also offer the possibility of analyzing isolated cells or even single ion channels. The general anesthetics have properties that limit the use of other experimental techniques. For example, specific binding of radiolabeled general anesthetics to ligand-gated ion channels has proven exceedingly difficult to demonstrate, because of the low affinity of the interactions and the high degree of nonspecific binding to neuronal membranes. Allosteric effects of general anesthetics have been monitored using radioligand binding of drugs to other sites on the ligand-gated ion channels. In addition, limited progress has been made in developing intravenous anesthetic congeners useful for photoaffinity labeling or other covalent modification of receptors. These limitations contrast starkly with the studies of other classes of agents at ligand-gated ion channels. For instance, the high-affinity benzodiazepine binding site on the GABA_A receptor has been mapped out in some detail, because of its the ability to perform both specific radioligand binding and photoaffinity labeling, which powerfully complement the extensive literature on electrophysiologic actions of benzodiazepines at GABA_A receptors.

Another exciting tool in the quest to establish the in vivo significance of a putative anesthetic target is the use of targeted gene manipulations in mice.[13] A variety of manipulations are possible, including introducing a gene not normally present (transgenic mice), removing an endogenous gene ("knockout mice"), or replacing an endogenous gene with an altered copy ("knockin mice"). Gene targeting in mice has already been very valuable for elucidating the mechanism of action for some drugs. Knockout of the GABA_A γ_2 receptor subunit gene resulted in mice that were insensitive to the sedative/hypnotic actions of benzodiazepines such as diazepam[14]; whereas another gene targeting experiment in mice involved the replacement of the α_{2A} adrenoreceptor with a dysfunctional receptor mutant. These "knockin" mice failed to show analgesic and sedative responses to α_{2a} adrenoreceptor agonists such as dexmedetomidine (DMD) and clonidine.[15]

Ligand-gated ion channels are certainly not the only possible molecular targets for general anesthetics. Other neuronal proteins such as voltage-gated ion channels and G protein–coupled receptors may also play a role in the overall spectrum of behavioral actions of some of the general anesthetics. Detailed studies of general anesthetic actions on G protein–coupled receptors are scarce, and it can be difficult to distinguish effects on the receptor per se versus general anesthetic perturbations of second messengers or effector molecules such as protein kinases and phospholipases. However, most research confirms that the voltage-gated ion channels are, in general, relatively insensitive to clinically relevant concentrations of general anesthetics.[1]

The ligand-gated ion channels include the GABA_A, glycine, serotonin-3 (5-HT_3), and nicotinic acetylcholine (nACh) receptors, along with the α-amino-3-hydroxy-5-methylisoxazole-4-propionic acid (AMPA)-, kainate-, and NMDA-sensitive subtypes of iontotropic glutamate receptors (GABA, glutamate, 5-HT, and ACh also act on "slow" neurotransmitter receptors, e.g., GABA_B, muscarinic ACh, and metabotropic glutamate receptors, which are coupled to second messenger systems). GABA_A, glycine, 5-HT_3, and nicotinic ACh receptors form part of an evolutionarily related ligand-gated ion channel gene superfamily. Ionotropic glutamate receptors were previously thought to be part of this superfamily but are now considered to belong to a distinct ion channel class.

General Principles for Anesthetics Acting on γ-Aminobutyric Acid Type A and Glycine Receptors

GABA_A and glycine receptors are chloride-selective ion channels. These are generally considered to be inhibitory neurotransmitter receptors, because in most cells, opening of chloride channels results in membrane hyperpolarization or stabilization of the membrane potential away from the threshold for firing action potentials. GABA and glycine are the primary fast inhibitory neurotransmitters in the CNS, with glycine abundant in the spinal cord and brain stem, and GABA predominant in higher brain regions.

GABA_A and glycine receptors, like the other members of the ligand-gated ion channel superfamily to which they belong, appear to have the basic subunit topology, with a large N-terminal extracellular domain, four putative membrane-spanning regions (TM1–TM4), a heterogeneous intracellular loop between TM3 and TM4, and a short extra-cellular C-terminal domain. Residues within the extracellular N-terminal domain form the agonist binding domains, whereas amino acid residues within TM2 line the ion channel pore. Native receptors are composed of pentameric arrangements of individual receptor subunits.

Subunit heterogeneity creates extensive diversity among the inhibitory ligand-gated ion channels, and multiple subunits have been cloned for $GABA_A$ receptors and glycine (α1-4 and β) receptors. $GABA_A$ receptors in vivo predominantly consist of α, β, and γ subunits with a proposed stoichiometry of $2\alpha:2\beta:1\gamma$. The existence of six α subunit isoforms enables considerable anatomic and functional diversity of $GABA_A$ receptors. In particular, the α subunit isoform may influence agonist potency, agonist efficacy, regulation by benzodiazepines, and channel kinetics. The most common neuronal subunit combination is α_1, β_2, γ_1. $GABA_A$ receptors are blocked competitively by bicuculline and noncompetitively by picrotoxinin and Zn^{2+}.

A number of studies now suggest that the key residues of import for anesthetic sensitivity reside within the second transmembrane domain, which is thought to form part of the ion channel pore. The amino acid Asp265 in TM2 of β_3 subunits confer anesthetic activity for etomidate but not for pentobarbital, propofol, or the anesthetic steroids.[16] Other important residues exist within the TM1 and TM3 domains, especially the Try328 residue in TM3 and Gly219 in TM1. Currently, it is not known whether these other sites are part of the binding pocket, or whether ligand/residue interaction influences channel gating.

The strychnine-sensitive glycine receptors in vivo consist of both α homomers and $\alpha\beta$ heteromeric receptors, with a switch from homomeric α_2 to heteromeric $\alpha_1\beta$ receptors occurring during development. The best described physiologic role for glycine receptors is in Renshaw cell-mediated inhibition of motor neurons in the spinal cord; however, glycine receptors are also widely expressed in the brain stem, where they participate in processing of auditory information, and throughout higher regions of the neuraxis, where their functions remain to be elucidated.

Action of Intravenous Anesthetics at γ-Aminobutyric Acid Type A Receptors

General anesthetics act as *positive or negative allosteric modulators* of agonist actions at ligand-gated ion channels. Among the ligand-gated ion channels, there is no known case in which the anesthetic competes for the same binding site as the endogenous neurotransmitter. The most extensively examined ligand-gated ion channel target for general anesthetics has been the $GABA_A$ receptor. Virtually every general anesthetic tested enhances the function of the $GABA_A$ receptor at clinically relevant concentrations.[1,17] The exceptions are ketamine, xenon, possibly nitrous oxide, and cyclopropane.

General anesthetic enhancement of $GABA_A$ receptor function is evident in single cell electrophysiologic experiments as potentiation of a submaximal GABA response or, at the synaptic level, as prolongation of inhibitory postsynaptic potentials or currents. Potentiation of submaximal GABA-induced currents remains the most popular paradigm for electrophysiologic experiments, because it is easily reproducible and can be used to study native $GABA_A$ recep-

tors in dissociated neurons or recombinant receptors expressed in mammalian cell lines or Xenopus oocytes. Some anesthetics, particularly the intravenous agents, open the $GABA_A$ receptor chloride channel in the absence of agonist. This "direct activation" by general anesthetics involves a binding site completely distinct from that for classical $GABA_A$ receptor agonists such as GABA and muscimol. Although direct activation usually occurs at supra-anesthetic concentrations, direct activation effects do sometimes occur at lower concentrations for some anesthetics (e.g., propofol) suggesting possible clinical relevance. Direct activation by anesthetics has been observed in other ligand-gated ion channels (e.g., for the anesthetic isoflurane at the strychnine-sensitive glycine receptor[18]), but it is most pronounced at the $GABA_A$ receptor.

Experimental Approaches to Studying General Anesthetic Actions

General anesthetic actions at ligand-gated ion channels have been studied using a variety of methodologies, including protein chemistry, radioligand binding, ion flux studies, and electrophysiology. This chapter focuses mainly on electrophysiologic studies because these generally provide superior time resolution and offer the possibility of analyzing isolated cells or even single ion channels. Potentiation of submaximal GABA-induced currents remains the most popular paradigm for electrophysiologic experiments, because it is easily reproducible and can be used to study native $GABA_A$ receptors in dissociated neurons or recombinant receptors expressed in mammalian cell lines or Xenopus oocytes.[1,19,20]

Mechanism of Action of Intravenous Anesthetic Agents on Receptors and Ion Channels

Barbiturates

Barbiturates act on several targets within the CNS at concentrations less than or equal to their clinically active concentrations. These include, but are not limited to, $GABA_A$ receptors, AMPA and kainate subtypes of glutamate receptors, adenosine receptors, and neuronal nicotinic acetylcholine (n-nACh) receptors. NMDA receptors and glycine receptors appear to be very insensitive to barbiturates. What is less clear is to what extent the various potential targets are relevant to their clinical effects. Here the potency and stereoselectivity criteria referred to earlier come into play. Stereoselectivity for producing immobility has been documented for the barbiturates.[21] The optical isomers of pentobarbital display the same order of potency for modulatory actions at the $GABA_A$ receptor as for their in vivo anesthetic actions,[1] and the isomers of etomidate show almost identical degrees of stereoselectivity at $GABA_A$ receptors and for producing loss of righting reflex in tadpoles.[11] Conversely, the potency data for the barbiturate isomers acting at the n-nACh receptors are in the opposite direction to their in vivo potency ratio. These data illustrate the use of the stereoselectivity criterion discussed earlier, and indicate that although it is unlikely for n-nACh receptors to be involved in barbiturate, GABA$_A$ receptors are indeed potentially relevant targets.

The actions of barbiturates at GABA$_A$ receptors are twofold: to enhance the actions of GABA at its receptor and to activate the receptor directly in the absence of GABA. The mechanism involved appears to be a modification of the gating of the ion channel associated with the GABA$_A$ receptor. A variety of biophysical studies have shown that long-lived open states of the GABA$_A$ receptor ion channel are stabilized in the presence of barbiturates such as pentobarbital.

At the molecular level, a residue within TM2 of the β_1 subunit of the GABA$_A$ receptor has been identified that is reported to be necessary for GABA potentiation by pentobarbital.[22] Because this is a conserved residue in this subfamily, this residue does not explain the pharmacologic differences between GABA$_A$ and glycine receptors (which are strikingly insensitive to barbiturates). GABA potentiation by barbiturates is not abolished by specific mutations in receptors that abolish potentiation by volatile anesthetics, n-alcohols, propofol, or trichloroethanol. Currently, the binding site for barbiturates on this receptor remains uncertain.

Etomidate

In contrast to the barbiturates, etomidate appears to be relatively selective as a modulator of the GABA$_A$ receptor. The GABA$_A$ receptor fulfills all of the above criteria for a plausible target underlying the anesthetic actions of these compounds. Etomidate does not modulate other ligand-gated ion channels at clinically relevant concentrations. Stereoselectivity supports the plausibility of the GABA$_A$ receptor as a target in mediating the actions of etomidate.[11] As indicated earlier, amino acid residues within the β subunit of the GABA$_A$ receptor have been identified that are essential for potentiation of GABA$_A$ receptor function by etomidate[23] consistent with previous studies suggesting that the β subunit of the receptor may contain a minimal binding site for this anesthetic.

Ketamine

Compared with the other intravenous anesthetic agents discussed earlier, the "dissociative anesthetic" ketamine has a very different in vivo and in vitro profile of action. Ketamine and related arylcycloalkylamines such as phencyclidine produce an atypical behavioural state characterized by a state of sedation, immobility, amnesia, marked analgesia, and a feeling of dissociation from the environment, without true unconsciousness. These compounds can also produce intense hallucinations, especially in adults, and this limits the clinical usefulness of the compounds (see "Clinical Pharmacology of Hypnotic Drugs").

In contrast to many of the agents discussed in this chapter, ketamine has only weak actions at the GABA$_A$ receptor according to most studies; these effects have been reported to occur at ketamine concentrations that are considerably greater than those reported during clinical use.[24]

Ketamine appears instead to produce its actions by inhibition of NMDA subtype of the glutamate receptors.[25] Ketamine also has potent inhibitory actions at nACh receptors. Ketamine shows stereospecificity of action, and the in vivo selectivity of ketamine stereoisomers is paralleled by the inhibitory action of the isomers at the NMDA receptor.

Propofol

As with etomidate, the known neuropharmacologic profile of propofol suggests it to be a relatively selective modulator of the GABA$_A$ receptor. Propofol does not appear to modulate other ligand-gated ion channels at clinically relevant concentrations with the exception of very weak actions at the strychnine-sensitive glycine receptor.[26] A specific amino acid residue, Met 286, within the $\beta2/3$ subunit of the GABA$_A$ receptor has been identified as essential for potentiation of GABA$_A$ receptor function by propofol,[27] consistent with previous studies suggesting that the β subunit of the GABA$_A$ receptor was likely to contain binding sites for these compounds. It is not known, however, whether propofol interacts directly with this Met residue or whether this plays a role in allosteric transitions within the receptor initiated by the binding of propofol elsewhere on the receptor molecule.

Other studies by Flood and colleagues have shown that propofol (in accord with findings for isoflurane) also inhibits nACh receptors.[28] Two types of nACh receptors ($\alpha_4\beta_2$ and α_7) were examined in vitro after expression in Xenopus oocytes. The IC$_{50}$ concentration for propofol was 19 μM for the $\alpha_4\beta_2$ receptors (about three times the effective clinical concentration), whereas the α_7 receptors were unaffected. The exact role that these nicotinic receptors play in the production of general anesthesia remains uncertain.

Further important observations on the site of anesthetic agent action have been provided by a series of in vivo studies by Jurd and colleagues.[29] Using site-directed mutagenesis and knockin gene targeting in mice at the N265M region of the β_3 GABA$_A$ subunit, they have shown that changes to this amino acid residue lead to a dramatic reduction in sensitivity to propofol and etomidate, as well as a reduction in the duration of anesthetic effect. In contrast, no difference in drug sensitivity was seen with alphaxalone when applied to the same system. The authors also observed that the N265M mice had a decreased sensitivity to the immobilizing effects of enflurane and halothane, but no effect on the duration of loss of the righting reflex.

These findings provide evidence supporting the hypothesis that the mechanisms of anesthesia are likely to be agent specific, and that different sites may be involved in the mediation of different components of general.

Steroids

Many steroid anesthetics such as alphaxalone are also relatively selective for the GABA$_A$ receptor, although certain steroids have potent actions on other ligand-gated ion channels. For the steroid anesthetics, structure/activity studies comparing in vivo and in vitro potencies support a role for GABA$_A$ receptors in the actions of these compounds.[30] For example, the nonanesthetic structural isomer betaxalone does not modulate the GABA$_A$ receptor.[31]

Alphaxalone exerts direct GABA-mimetic effects on $\alpha_2\beta_2\gamma_2$ receptors.[32] The N265M residue has already been defined as being key in the modulatory actions of some hypnotic agents. Mutation at N265M has no effect on the direct action of alphaxalone, but the M286W mutation significantly increases the direct, but not the modulatory, effects of alphaxalone. These data demonstrate that the structural requirements for modulation and direct action differ for the different classes of intravenous agents.

Although the GABA$_A$ ligand-gated channels are the most likely site of action of the intravenous agents, there are effects on other channels (as summarized in Table 24–1).

Physicochemical Models for Mechanism of Action of Intravenous Anesthetic Agents

This chapter has focused on the effects of intravenous anesthetic agents on ion channels. However, there have been studies reviewing the physicochemical properties that confer anesthetic properties on a molecule.

The lipid solubility relationship (MOC) seen for the volatile agents does not hold true for all intravenous agents. Based on the EC$_{50}$ free drug concentrations associated with lack of response to the surgical incision, the benchmark model (based on octanol-water partition coefficients [hydrophobic correlation]) explains only 65% of the vari-ance in the observed activities of the compounds; it also fails to predict the potency order for the enantiomers of ketamine and has a predictive power of only 41.8%.[34]

Using the technique of computer modelling to delineate the structure/activity relationships of intravenous anesthetic agents, a model based on combined shape and electrostatic potential similarities to two conformers of eltanolone (the most potent anesthetic agent) explains 82% of the variance in the observed activities of the hypnotic agents. This model had a predictive power of 75.5%; and correctly ordered the potency for the enantiomers of the chiral agent ketamine. When the relationship between the spatial distribution of these properties and associated in vivo potency is performed using comparative molecular field analysis (CoMFA), 93.7% of the observed variance in 14 compounds can be predicted[35]; it also showed good internal predictability (q^2 = 0.763) and was a good predictor of the activity of the five test set compounds (r^2 = 80.0%). The CoMFA models show areas where electrostatic and steric interactions are either favored or disfavored. This mapping of the spatial arrangements facilitates the derivation of a preliminary pharmacophore for the intravenous anesthetic agents.

Using a similar technique, Krasowski and colleagues[36] also derived a 4D-QSAR model for three aspects of biologic activity: namely, loss of righting reflex in tadpoles, enhanced agonist activity at GABA$_A$ receptors, and direct (agonist independent) activation at the GABA$_A$ receptor. The three resulting QSAR models were almost identical; there are key ligand/receptor interaction sites including an intermolecular hydrogen bonding involving the proton of the ligand-OH

TABLE 24–1.

Effects of Intravenous Anesthetics on Ligand-Gated Ion Channels

Receptor Type	Barbiturates	Propofol	Steroids	Etomidate	Ketamine
Glycine	+/0	+	+/0	+/0	0
GABA$_A$	+++	+++	++/+++	+++	0
nACh	––	0	0	0	–
5-HT$_3$	0	0	0	0	0
AMPA	–/0	0	0	0	0
Kainate	0/–	+/0	0	0	0
NMDA	0	0	0	0	––

Symbols indicate the extent of potentiation or inhibition seen at clinically relevant concentrations: (+) or (–): 20–50%; (++) or (––): 50–100%; (+++) or (–––): >100%.

Clinically relevant anesthetic concentrations have been assumed to be: pentobarbital, 50 μM; thiopental, 25 μM; methohexital, 25 μM; propofol, 1 μM; alphaxalone, 5 μM; 3α-OH, 5α-pregnan-20-one, 0.3 μM; etomidate, 5 μM; ketamine, 10 μM.

5-HT$_3$, serotonin-3; AMPA, α-amino-3-hydroxy-5-methylisoxazole-4-propionic acid; GABA$_A$, _-aminobutyric acid type A; nACh, nicotinic acetylcholine; NMDA, *N*-methyl-D-aspartate.

Source: Adapted from Yamakura T, Bertaccini E, Trudell JR, Harris RA: Anesthetics and ion channels: Molecular models and sites of action. Annu Rev Pharmacol Toxicol 41:23–51, 2001.

group and a hydrophobic pocket of binding involving the six-substituent and also the two-substituent. Because there was a striking similarity between the models of the sites responsible for and those mediating effects of the training set of propofol analogs on the GABA$_A$ receptor, this provides further confirmation that the latter receptor is likely to be a main site of propofol's action.

Thus in many respects, these studies provide information on the nature of the "key" in the lock and key relationship among a ligand (here an intravenous anesthetic agent), a putative anesthetic receptor, and its effector system.

Clinical Pharmacology of Hypnotic Drugs

Barbiturates are the archetypal induction agents; thiopental was introduced into practice in 1934 by Lundy and Tovell,[37] and then by Pratt and colleagues.[38] The subsequent introduction of other compounds has been principally led by the desire to overcome some of the perceived disadvantages of the barbiturates.

Barbiturates

These compounds are formed through the "interaction" of malonic acid and urea to form the barbiturate ring structure. There are four main groups of barbiturates:

1. Oxybarbiturates with hydrogen at N_1 and oxygen at C_2 (these have a delayed onset and prolonged duration of action)
2. Thiobarbiturates with hydrogen at N_1 and sulfur at C_2 (e.g., thiopental, thiamylal)
3. Methylbarbiturates with a methyl group at N_1 and oxygen at C_2 (e.g., methohexital)
4. Methylthiobarbiturates—although these are very potent, they show marked excitatory effects and are not used clinically.

Thiopental

Thiopental is presented as a pale yellow powder with added 6% anhydrous sodium carbonate in an ampoule containing an inert atmosphere of nitrogen. Although it is poorly soluble in water, it dissolves in the alkaline solution of the sodium carbonate, in which a 2.5% solution has a pH of 10.5. There is no added preservative, but the alkaline solution is bacteriostatic. The alkaline thiopental is less soluble at the pH of blood, and this results in microcrystal formation.

The rapid onset of hypnosis after an intravenous dose of thiopental is caused by its uptake across the blood–brain barrier (as a result of its high lipid solubility and low degree of ionization at physiologic pH). Barbiturates are almost insoluble in aqueous, but possess weak acidic properties through their "ketoenol tautomerism."

As an induction agent, thiopental has a number of drawbacks; e.g., it is highly alkaline in solution and therefore extremely irritant if injected extravascularly or intra-arterially. It also has a low therapeutic index (median lethal dose [LD$_{50}$]/mean effective dose [ED$_{50}$]:$\approx$4). The kinetics of thiopental and the other intravenous agents are shown in Table 24–2. Recovery to awakening occurs within 15 to 20 minutes after a 3 to 5 mg/kg single bolus dose. However, at the time of awakening, only 18% of the injected dose will have undergone metabolism, compared with about 38% of a dose of methohexital and nearly 70% of propofol. Comparing the pharmacokinetics of the different intravenous induction agents shows that they all have similar distribu-

TABLE 24–2.

Disposition Parameters for Intravenous Hypnotic Agents Used for Induction of Anesthesia

Hypnotic Agent	$T_{(1/2)}\alpha$ (min)	$T_{(1/2)}\beta$ (min)	$T_{(1/2)}\gamma$ (hr)	Cl (mL/min/kg)	% AUCγ
Thiopental	2–7	42–59	5.1–11.5	2.2–3.5	0.72
Methohexital	6	2–58	1.62–3.9	8.2–12.0	0.66
Etomidate	1–3	12–29	2.9–5.5	11.6–25	0.64
Propofol	1–4	5–69	1.62–63.0	23.2–32.9	0.29
Ketamine	1–3	8–18	2.2–3.0	14.0–19.1	0.68

% AUCγ, area under the curve during the terminal elimination phase as a % of the total area under the concentration-time curve (0 to infinity); Cl, systemic clearance; $T_{(1/2)}\alpha$, β, and γ, three half-lives for data described by a three-compartment model.

tion half-lives but vary greatly in their clearance rates and the fraction of drug eliminated during the terminal elimination phase (AUCgamma) (see Table 24–2).

To review the influence of different factors on drug elimination one can reflect on population kinetic/dynamic studies. For thiopental, this has been performed by Stanski and Maitre,[39] who found that although age influenced the kinetics of thiopental, it had no effect on brain responsiveness or pharmacodynamics when the spectral edge was used as a measure of drug effect. Hence the induction dose requirements for thiopental vary with patient age and weight, and most importantly, cardiac output. The blood/brain equilibration rate constant is $0.58\,min^{-1}$; the effect compartment concentration associated with the subject dropping a loaded syringe is about $17\,\mu g/mL$, and the duration of effect of the dose (320 mg) is about 4 minutes.

The nonhypnotic effects of thiopental (and most other induction agents) include dose-related cardiorespiratory depression and an increased sensitivity to somatic pain. The side effect profiles of thiopental differ from other hypnotic agents and are summarized in Table 24–3.

Initial recovery from thiopental is through the decline in the blood (and brain) concentrations, mainly caused by redistribution. Following bolus doses and after short or low-dose infusion regimens, thiopental is eliminated by first-order kinetics and the patient promptly awakens. However, at rates in excess of $300\,\mu g/kg$ per minute, thiopental concentrations increase nonlinearly because peripheral tissue stores become saturated. In addition to the change in kinetics, high doses lead to significant blood levels of the active metabolite, pentobarbital. Metabolism is 10% to 15% per hour, with the sulfur replaced by oxygen to give pentobarbital, and the side chains at the C_5 position being oxidized. The renal excretion of thiopental is very low (about 0.3%).

Thiopental may also be used for maintenance of anesthesia at rates of 150 to $300\,\mu g/kg$ per minute in combination with either nitrous oxide or an opioid (the resulting thiopental concentrations being between 15 and $25\,\mu g/mL$). In the absence of supplements, thiopental concentrations needed to abolish response to squeezing the trapezius muscle (roughly equivalent with the initial surgical incision) are about 40 to $50\,\mu g/mL$.

Advantages of thiopental infusions include minimal cardiovascular depression and cerebral protection during ischemic episodes. Although pentobarbital concentrations between 25 and $35\,\mu g/mL$ are effective in reducing intracranial pressure (ICP) in patients with head injuries, the concentration of thiopental needed to achieve electroencephalogram (EEG) burst suppression is about $73\,\mu g/mL$ (with a range of $42–90\,\mu g/mL$).[40]

Thiamylal

This is also a thiobarbiturate with clinical properties similar to thiopental. It is formulated as a racemic mixture; the

TABLE 24–3.

Comparison of Some Nonanesthetic Side Effects of the Intravenous Hypnotic Agents

Side Effects	Thiopental	Methohexital	Propofol	Etomidate	Ketamine
At induction:					
Change in blood pressure (%)	−8	−8	−17	−2	+28
Change in heart rate (%)	+14	+15	+7	+8	+33
Induction pain (%)	0	30–50	10–30	40–60	0
Induction movement (%)	0	5	5–10	30	Very little
Induction hiccups (%)	0	30	5	20	Very little
Induction apnea (%)	6	20	40	20	Rare
Recovery restlessness (%)	10	5	5	35	Common
Recovery nausea (%)	7–10	7–10	5	20	Common
Recovery vomiting (%)	7–10	5	5	20	Common

potency of the S enantiomer being twice that of the R form. In keeping with other barbiturates, there are some kinetic differences between the enantiomers, but these are thought to have little clinical relevance.[41–44]

The plasma protein binding of the R^+ and S isomer is 82.5% and 88.3%, respectively. The elimination half-life of the R^+ enantiomer is 20.2 hours, the apparent volume of distribution is 3.66 L/kg, and clearance is 0.27 L/kg per hour; the corresponding values for the S compound are 24.1 hours, 2.60 L/kg, and 0.15 L/kg per hour, respectively.[43] The barbiturate in vitro shows greater metabolism by cytochrome P450 (CYP) C29 compared with CYP 2E1 and CYP 3A4, with the metabolism of the R enantiomer being greater than S form.[45]

Dosage and administration: Thiamylal is formulated as for thiopental, and the induction dose of thiamylal is 5 mg/kg.

Methohexital

The barbiturate methohexital has currently been withdrawn in the United Kingdom because of production difficulties, and its future seems uncertain.

Methohexital is used as a 1% solution. Its structure contains two asymmetric carbon atoms, and the barbiturate therefore exists as four enantiomers. The β-1 enantiomer is the most potent, being four to five times more active than the α-1 enantiomer. Because the β pair causes excessive motor activity, the drug is formulated as the α-dL pair. Methohexital has a more appropriate kinetic profile for both induction and maintenance of intravenous anesthesia (elimination half-life of 420–460 minutes, clearance of 700–800 mL/min) when compared with thiopental. Its main metabolite, 4-OH methohexital, has no pharmacologic activity.

In healthy volunteers, venous concentrations of 3 to 4 μg/mL result in sleep and 10 to 12 μg/mL concentrations result in EEG burst suppression. Based on dose-response studies, the ED_{50} infusion rate as a supplement to 67% nitrous oxide is 50 to 65 μg/kg per minute (plasma concentrations 2–5 μg/mL); infusion rates of 100 μg/kg per minute are required in the absence of nitrous oxide.

Methohexital infusions depress both blood pressure and cardiac output, as well as reducing baroreflex sensitivity with a resetting of the response to allow a more rapid heart rate at lower arterial pressures than when awake. Side effects include excitatory movements, pain on injection, and predisposition to convulsions. Epileptiform activity has been recorded by EEG, but clinical fitting is rare. It also causes pain if injected into arteries, but unlike thiopental this does not normally lead to thrombosis.

The combination methohexital/nitrous oxide in opioid premedicated patients may result in significant respiratory depression, but there are no untoward effects of methohexital on liver, renal, or adrenal function. The actions of methohexital are additive with those of other CNS depressants (including ethanol and antihistamines), and administration of the drug should be avoided in patients receiving coumarin-like anticoagulants (because of the possibility of drug/drug binding interaction).

Adverse Effects of Barbiturates

The barbiturates have a number of absolute contraindications to their use, including porphyria. Although not all types of porphyria are adversely affected by thiopental, any suspicion of the disease should be a contraindication to the barbiturates. Known susceptible types of porphyria include acute intermittent porphyria, variegate porphyria, and hereditary coproporphyria. Other contraindications include proven allergy to thiopental or other barbiturates and all patients with airway or potential airway obstruction. In addition, methohexital should be avoided in individuals with a history of epilepsy (because there is a risk it might elicit psychomotor seizures).

In marked hypovolemia including blood loss, cardiovascular collapse, severe uremia, in patients with a history of severe asthma, and in all patients with severe cardiac disease (e.g., ischemic heart disease, malignant or untreated severe hypertension), barbiturates should either be avoided or administered in reduced dosage.

Etomidate

Etomidate (D-ethyl-1(α-methyl-benzyl)imidazole-5carboxylate) is a carboxylated imidazole that is unstable in water and is therefore currently solubilized in either 33% propylene glycol or as an emulsion. The drug has a pH of 8.1 and pKa of 4.2. It is a base with about 99% of the drug is unionized in the blood. Plasma protein binding is about 75% (mainly to albumin). Metabolism occurs in the liver and plasma by esterase hydrolysis; about 2% is excreted in the urine and is unchanged. It is one of the first drugs to be marketed as the single enantiomer of a racemic mixture (the approximate potency ratio of the enantiomers being R:S 1:10).[46] The induction dose for etomidate is 0.3 mg/kg.

Etomidate has many ideal properties (cardiostability; reduction of cerebral blood flow, cerebral metabolic rate, and ICP; no release of histamine and low rate of allergic reactions [see later]; transient and minimal respiratory depression; and no inhibition of the hypoxic pulmonary vasoconstrictor reflex), and it offers advantages during induction of anesthesia in patients with poor cardiac reserve and hypovolemia.

Adverse Effects of Etomidate

Etomidate use is associated with a high incidence of nausea and vomiting, pain on injection and thrombophlebitis (up to 30% by the third postoperative day), especially if administered into the small veins of the hand, excitatory movements, and myoclonia. These excitatory movements and myoclonia can be reduced in both incidence and severity using a pretreatment regimen of a 0.03 mg/kg etomidate dose.[47] Recent studies suggest that the cause of the thrombophlebitis may be the propylene solvent. Recovery may be more uncomfortable after etomidate than for some other drugs because of the increased restlessness, nausea, and vomiting. The action of etomidate is potentiated by the coadministration of other sedative and centrally acting drugs. There are reports of etomidate causing convulsions in unpremedicated patients.[48]

Etomidate causes dose-related reversible inhibition of adrenal steroidogenesis by interaction with the mitochondrial CYP (affecting 11β-, 17α-, and 18-hydroxylases, and 20,22 lyase). This is seen after an induction dose, where the peak time to suppression of the normal plasma cortisol response to surgical stress occurs after about 4 hours after initial exposure[49]; however, the effect is probably not clinically significant unless etomidate is administered by infusion for prolonged periods of time.

Recently, an emulsion formulation of etomidate has been introduced into Europe, including Great Britain. This formulation shows no change in the drug's dynamic properties, but does show decreased incidences of pain on injection, myoclonus, and local thrombophlebitis.[50,51] An additional advantage of an emulsion formulation is its lower osmolality and higher pH (400 mosmol/kg and pH 7.6 compared with 4965 mosmol/kg and pH 5.1 for the propylene glycol formation), which causes less red cell hemolysis.[52] Studies of healthy volunteers comparing the two formulations show the emulsion to be associated with both a decreased incidence of pain on injection and fewer venous sequelae.[53]

A second reformulation of etomidate has used 2-hydroxypropyl-β-cyclodextrin as the solvent[54]; and again, there was a lower incidence of myoclonia and pain (17% vs. 92%; and 8% vs. 58%), thrombophlebitis (0% vs. 42%), and no hemolysis. There were no alterations in the kinetics or dynamics of etomidate.

Although it is widely believed that use of etomidate is associated with an increased incidence of postoperative nausea and vomiting, this was not supported by a recent comparison in which etomidate-lipuro and propofol were used for induction of anesthesia to supplement isoflurane/fentanyl in air in patients undergoing orthopedic procedures.[55] There were no differences in rates of nausea, vomiting, or the intensity of any nausea during the early postoperative period to 24 hours. However, the rates of vomiting after etomidate were greater (26.8% vs. 10%).

Contraindications to Etomidate

As with barbiturates, use of etomidate is contraindicated in patients with acute porphyria, in patients with evidence of or suggestion of depressed adrenocortical activity, and in patients with a known sensitivity to etomidate (although the latter is rare). Because of its effect on steroidogenesis, etomidate is no longer licensed in many countries for administration by continuous infusion.

Propofol (2,6 di-isopropyl phenol)

This sterically hindered alkyl phenol was first studied in 1977 when formulated in Cremophor EL (DASF, Mount Olive, NJ.). However, after reports of adverse allergic reactions, it has been reformulated as an aqueous emulsion containing soya bean oil and egg phosphatide. Propofol has a neutral pH (7.4) and a pKa of 11.0, making it 99.7% non-ionized and highly lipid soluble.

Kinetics

Propofol has a long elimination half-life (up to 45 or more hours), an apparent volume of distribution greater than 1000 to 3940 L, and a systemic clearance between 1.0 and 1.8 L/min. Plasma protein binding is greater than 96%. The population kinetics of propofol have recently been examined using data from 7 studies containing 270 patients and healthy volunteers by Schuttler and Ihmsen.[56] Weight was found to be a significant covariate for elimination clearance, the two intercompartmental clearances of the three-compartment model, and the volumes of the central and two peripheral compartments. For the average 70-kg adult, the best estimates given by the model are 1.44, 2.25, and 0.92 L/min, and 9.3, 44.2, and 266 L, respectively. In older patients (>60 years), elimination clearance decreases linearly, and the central volume compartment also decreases with age. Venous data show decreased elimination clearance compared with arterial values; and bolus dose data were characterized by increases in the volumes of the central and shallow peripheral compartments and rapid distribution clearance, as well as decreased slow distribution clearance.

Because of wide variability in the therapeutic drug concentration window (related to age and type of surgery) and intersubject kinetics, propofol dosing is best titrated to effect. This is easily achieved because it has a short blood/brain equilibration time (k_{eo}) of 0.24 min^{-1}. Drug dosing can be by bolus dosing, continuous infusion, or more recently by target-controlled infusions based on a population/kinetic model. It requires drug concentrations of 4 to 6 μg/mL when propofol supplements either nitrous oxide or an opioid infusion, with recovery occurring at drug concentrations of about 1.0 μg/mL.

Propofol is rapidly metabolized mainly in the liver to inactive metabolites (the glucuronide and corresponding quinol glucuronides and sulphates). Other minor metabolites detected in the urine by gas chromatography-mass spectroscopy include 2-(omega-propanol)-6-isopropylphenol and 2-(omega-propanol)-6-isopropyl-1,4-quinol. It is not known whether any of these have anesthetic potencies. However, as total body clearance is greater than liver blood flow, there is assumed to be extrahepatic metabolism.

Propofol is initially hydroxylated by CYP; the key isoform is CYP P450 2B6, which shows wide individual variability found in human liver microsomes.[57] Other isoforms with a high activity for propofol hydroxylation include CYP 2C9.[58]

Evidence for a role of the lung in the disposition and metabolism of propofol in humans has been provided by two recent studies in surgical patients.[59,60] Although He and colleagues[59] found that pulmonary transit time of propofol was significantly longer than that of indocyanine green (22.4 compared with 2.7 seconds), there were no significant differences in the area under the curve (0–60 minutes) for propofol between the pulmonary and radial arterial curves, indicating that any propofol undergoing pulmonary uptake during the first pass is released back to the circulation by "back-diffusion." There was no pulmonary propofol metabolism. These data contrast with those of Dawidowicz and colleagues[60] who found greater propofol concentrations in pulmonary artery compared with radial artery and the formation of the metabolite 2,6-di-isopropyl-1,4 quinol.

Pharmacodynamics

Propofol has a therapeutic index similar to thiopental (3.4 vs. 3.91); but recovery to consciousness in both animals and humans is faster after propofol than thiopental. The difference in recovery becomes more exaggerated when repeated bolus doses or infusions are administered.

Induction of anesthesia with propofol is smooth and is associated with a low incidence of excitatory side effects. Occasional epileptiform fits have been reported during recovery (see later). Closing of the eyes is delayed after propofol compared with thiopental, and this may lead to a relative overdosing with the drug; the better endpoint for induction is loss of verbal contact.

Although a range of 1.5 to 2.5 mg/kg is recommended as the induction dose, the dose of propofol is variable and depends on many factors including the initial volume of distribution and cardiac output. Recent studies by Kazama and colleagues,[61] using stepwise multiple linear regression modelling, determined four factors that were independently associated with the size of the induction dose (age, lean body mass, central blood volume, and liver blood flow). When the dynamics of propofol are related to age, there are three functions that correlate linearly: blood/brain equilibration rate constant and time to peak effect, the steepness of the concentration/response relationships for EEG activation and depression, and the effect site concentration associated with 50% of peak EEG activation.[62]

The henodynanic effects of induction doses of propofol are similar to those of the thiobarbiturates, but there are also accompanying decreases in systemic vascular resistance. The combination of the drug's vagotonic effect and the decrease in vascular resistance produces significant decreases in blood pressure when used in the hypovolemic patient or the patient receiving other vagotonic drugs (e.g., opioids).[63] Another difference between propofol and barbiturates is that the normal baroreflex increase in heart rate for a decreased blood pressure is not seen for propofol. Propofol causes a resetting of the baroreflex, such that slower heart rates are seen for a given arterial blood when compared with awake values.[64]

Propofol infusions decrease clearance of flow-dependent and capacity-limited drugs by dose-related reductions in liver blood flow and decreases in the hepatic extraction ratio.[65,66] This may be relevant during anenthesia, where coadministered drugs during propofol infusions may show reductions in their total body clearance because of changes in effective liver blood flow or the hepatic extraction ratio. However, simulation studies by Schnider and colleagues[67] suggest that these changes may not be seen using propofol infusion rates in the clinical range, because they found the kinetics of propofol to be linear with regard to infusion rate at those concentrations.

The ventilatory effects of propofol are similar to those of other hypnotic agents—induction doses cause significant decreases in tidal and minute volumes, coupled with episodes of apnea greater than 30 seconds; comparative studies show the duration of apnea after propofol to be greater than those following either eltanolone or thiopental.[68] All induction agents decreased the ribcage and abdominal components of ventilation to a similar amount. When given by continuous infusion, propofol causes a 50% reduction in the ventilatory response to carbon dioxide, as well as in the acute ventilatory response to isocapnic hypoxia.[69,70]

Propofol/Drug Interactions

There is evidence that propofol at clinical concentrations inhibits drug metabolism.[71–73] In vitro studies by Baker and colleagues[72] and Chen and coworkers[73] have demonstrated inhibition of hydroxylation and dealkylation reactions at propofol concentrations between 25 and 1000 µM. The magnitude of inhibition varied from 30% to 71% with the greatest effect on reactions mediated through isocytochrome P450 2B1. The wide range of isozymes that are inhibited (1A1 and 2A1, as well as 2B1) suggests there may indeed be a kinetic basis for many drug/drug interactions. Further studies by Chen and colleagues[74] show that propofol at clinical concentrations inhibits renal mono-oxygenase (as assessed using aniline and benzo(α)pyrene) and defluorinase activities in hamster renal microsomes. There are also in vivo data indicating interactions with propofol leading to a reduced drug clearance. Mertens and colleagues[75] examined for effects of steady-state propofol concentrations on alfentanil disposition. They measured a decreased elimination clearance of 15%, a rapid distribution clearance of 68%, a slow distribution clearance of 51%, and lag time accounting for venous sampling by 62%. Because mean arterial pressure and systemic vascular resistance are also significantly lower, scaling to mean pressure improved the model; hence it appears that the henodynanic interaction induced by propofol may have an important influence on alfentanil kinetics.[75]

In clinical studies, combinations of two hypnotics administered to achieve loss of response to verbal command have been shown to be synergistic rather than directly additive.[76] This principle has been further used in the technique of coinduction. There is also increasing evidence that opioids and hypnotic drugs are synergistic. Billiard and colleagues[77] examined the propofol/fentanyl interaction at induction of anesthesia. They found that 3 mg/kg propofol produced no greater henodynanic response than a dose of 2 mg/kg, and the addition of 2 µg/kg fentanyl blunted the responses to intubation. To achieve optimum efficacy from such combinations, drug concentrations at the effector site (or biophase) need to peak at the same time. The combination of hypnotic/opioid/benzodiazepine results in significant reductions in dose requirements of all three, but no more synergism than can be expected from the various combinations of pairs of the drugs.[78]

The interaction between α_2 agonists and hypnotic agents has been studied by two groups. Peden and colleagues[79] have clearly demonstrated that a 3 ng/kg per minute dose of dexmedetomidine (DMD) (producing a median DMD concentration of 0.20 ng/mL) reduced the ED_{50} infusion rate and EC_{50} concentration for loss of consciousness from 5.79 to 3.45 mg/kg per hour and from 2.3 to 1.69 µg/mL, respectively; but without any significant shift in the position of the dose-response curve. However, this study was originally designed with a higher infusion rate of DMD; but during the pilot phase there were a number of significant side effects (two cases of sinus arrest and one case of severe postural hypotension persisting for 24 hours after anesthesia). Sinus arrest has also been observed in other studies in both patients and healthy volunteers. It is therefore appropriate to pretreat patients (especially those younger than 40 years) with an anticholinergic agent. At the final DMD dose rate used in the study (3 ng/kg per minute), the ic responses to intubation and surgical incision were blunted, and the blood pressure and heart rate remained stable during surgery and into the recovery period. In a separate study, Dutta and colleagues[80] found that the EC_{50} concentration for loss of motor response to electrical stimulation was 6.63 µg/mL in the absence of DMD. When DMD was infused to a concentration of 0.66 ng/mL, the associated EC_{50} propofol concentration was 3.89 µg/mL. Similar reductions were seen for the EC_{50} values for the subject's ability to retain hold of a syringe.

Nonhypnotic Effects of Propofol

As well as being an anesthetic agent, propofol has a number of other important nonhypnotic effects.

Mood-Altering Effects

Subhypnotic doses of propofol administered by a PCA system (10 mg with a 1–5-minute lockout) have been shown to exert sedative and anxiolytic effects in anxious patients presenting for ambulatory surgery.[81,82]

Antiemetic Effects

Although several authors have suggested an antiemetic effect of propofol (in both hypnotic and subhypnotic doses), the site of this action of the drug remains uncertain.[83] It is probable that propofol does not act as an antidopaminergic agent. Propofol is also effective in the prevention of nausea and emesis after cisplatin chemotherapy.[83]

Antipruritic Effects

Subhypnotic doses of propofol (10–20 mg intravenously) are equally effective to naloxone in relieving pruritus caused by both epidural and spinally administered opioids[84,85] and in the treatment of pruritus caused by cholestasis.[86]

Effects on the Central Nervous System

CEREBRAL BLOOD FLOW AND INTRACRANIAL PRESSURE

In vitro studies demonstrate a direct vasodilating effect of propofol caused by calcium channel blockade; however, in vivo studies show infusions of propofol to decrease cerebral blood flow and ICP also decrease both ICP and the cerebral metabolic rate. Propofol does not affect cerebrovascular autoregulation to carbon dioxide,[87] although the slope of the curve is decreased.

CEREBRAL PROTECTION

Evidence for a protective effect in humans and animals is controversial; although high doses of propofol have been used to afford protection during cerebral aneurysm surgery in patients requiring cardiopulmonary bypass and deep hypothermic arrest, as well as in patients undergoing non-pulsatile cardiopulmonary bypass for cardiac surgery.[88,89]

ELECTROENCEPHALOGRAM EFFECTS

Low infusion rates of propofol cause increased β activity and loss of consciousness causes increased theta activity, whereas burst suppression occurs at blood concentrations greater than 6 µg/mL.[90] At these EEG suppression levels, propofol causes significant reductions in cerebral blood flow, oxygen delivery, and metabolic rate; although cerebral autoregulation remains unaltered. These changes are in contrast to the volatile agents.

NEUROEXCITATORY EVENTS AND EPILEPSY

There are many cases of opisthotonos, hyperreflexia and hypertonus, involuntary movements, choreoathetosis, and seizure-like activity associated with propofol.[91] However, the agent has variable effect on the EEG in patients with epilepsy (some show increased spike activity, others show decreased EEG activity). Data from the Committee on Safety of Medicines (CSM) indicate an incidence of convulsions in association with propofol of about 1 in 47,000, with many cases seen as the drug concentration in the body is decreasing, and delayed reactions occurring in about a third of cases.

CARDIORESPIRATORY SYSTEM

The effects of bolus doses and infusions of propofol on the cardiac and respiratory systems are similar to those of the other three groups of drugs in this section (barbiturates, etomidate, and steroids) but excluding ketamine. Rare cardiac events after propofol administration include severe bradycardia, sinus arrest, heart block, and asystole in association with the coadministration of other vagotonic drugs. Induction doses of propofol (2–3 mg/kg) also depress pharyngeal reflexes and allow satisfactory jaw tone for both insertion of the laryngeal mask and endotracheal intubation.[92]

HEPATIC AND RENAL SYSTEMS

Bolus doses of propofol do not alter renal or portal venous blood flows[93]; although dose-related changes in liver blood flow have been reported in dogs during graded infusions.[65] Infusions of propofol in humans cause no significant changes of liver blood flow or liver function tests.[94,95]

Adverse Properties of Propofol

Adverse properties of propofol include pain on injection (especially when given into small veins and to children), hypotension and bradycardia (which are exaggerated in the presence of other vagotonic drugs such as opioids and hypovolemia), apnea in up to 40% patients after induction, and reports of epileptiform movements and true convulsions. The incidence of pain on injection is reduced by the intravenous administration of 1% lidocaine or fentanyl preanesthetic, or by mixing 20 mg lidocaine with an ampoule of propofol; although the latter can destabilize the soya bean emulsion.

A systematic review of techniques aimed at preventing pain on injection with propofol showed intravenous administration of 40 mg lidocaine with a tourniquet 30 to 120 seconds before the hypnotic to be the best option with a number needed to treat of 1.6.[96]

Attempts at decreasing the pain (which varies in incidence between 30% and 70%) include pretreatment with lidocaine, aseptically mixing with lidocaine immediately before dosing, or pretreatment with fentanyl or alfentanil. More recently it has been shown that addition of long chain triglyceride (LCT) to propofol (as Diprivan; AstraZeneca, Wilmington, Del.) will reduce the incidence of severe pain from about 70% to 0%.[97] The mechanism behind this result is thought to be a decrease in propofol concentration in the aqueous phase secondary to the increase in the fat content. However, this change in aqueous drug concentration does not seem to influence the kinetics or dynamics of propofol.[98] In a double-blind comparison, Rau and colleagues[99] found less pain with the LCT/medium chain triglyceride (MCT) emulsion compared with the Intralipid (Kabivitrum, Cal.) emulsion, but there are no other kinetic or dynamic differences between propofol formulations.[100] Attempts to use 2-hydroxypropyl β-cyclodextrin to reformulate propofol were unsuccessful because the drug has caused severe bradycardia and hypotension when administered to rats.[101]

During the past decade, the side effect profile of propofol has become complex. Currently, there are several case reports of allergic reactions to the drug and reports of convulsions after drug administration, although propofol also has anticonvulsant properties.[63]

The aqueous emulsion does not contain any preservative and is therefore a good bacterial medium. In 1996, Bennett and colleagues[102] examined the etiologic factors of multiple outbreaks of postoperative infection. The cause was not surgical, but rather was the repeated use of propofol during nonsterile conditions during the preparation and filling of syringes and the multiuse of single dose drug vials. In a separate study, Sosis and colleagues[103] demonstrated that propofol will support bacterial growth of Corpus albicans when inoculated on to Agar plates. Once propofol is drawn up in the syringe from the ampoule, it should be used immediately for a single patient and the remainder in the syringe should be discarded. Opened ampoules must not stand at room temperature. Once dispensed, a propofol syringe should be used within a few hours. Consequently, a different formulation of propofol containing EDTA has been introduced in the United States in an attempt to decrease bacterial growth.

Recently, there has been a report of profound metabolic acidosis when the bisulphite formulation of propofol was infused over 48 hours in an adult patient after neurosurgery. The peak serum lactate concentration reached 15 mM and was associated with cardiovascular collapse and death.[104] This situation was similar to the one reported after use of the hypnotic for sedation in children.[105] The exact cause of death remains uncertain. As a result of this and other cases, propofol is no longer licensed for sedation in patients younger than 17 years.

There are two absolute contraindications to the use of propofol: in patients with a known hypersensitivity to propofol or related compounds and in patients with disorders of fat metabolism.

Ketamine (2-o-chlorophenyl-2-methylaminocyclohexanone HCl)

Ketamine is a phencyclidine derivative formulated as a racemic mixture. The two stereoisomers R⁻ and S⁺ have different anesthetic potencies (1:3–4) but similar kinetics. Ketamine is soluble in aqueous solutions and can be used as 1%, 5%, and 10% solutions. The pH of the solutions is 3.5 to 5.5, and the pKa 7.5. Ketamine is highly lipid soluble with 12% to 35% plasma protein binding and 44% nonionized at physiologic pH.

Kinetics

There are few kinetic studies or concentration/effect data for continuous infusions of ketamine; the hypnotic and analgesic thresholds are 1.5 to 2.5 µg/mL and 200 ng/mL, respectively. As sole agent, infusion rates of 60 to 80 µg/kg per minute provide clinical anesthesia. Disposition kinetics indicate an elimination half-life of 80 to 180 minutes, clearance of 980 to 1500 mL/min, and apparent volume of distribution (V_{ss}) 130 to 220 L.

Recovery from ketamine anesthesia is by both distribution and metabolism by demethylation and hydroxylation by hepatic CYP. The metabolic fate of ketamine is complex, but one metabolite (norketamine; Metabolite I) is pharmacologically active, with a potency of about 30% that of the parent drug and a longer elimination half-life. The main excretory metabolites are ketamine and metabolite I and II glucuronides; hence efficacy may be enhanced in patients with renal impairment. Most of the ketamine is excreted in the urine as the glucuronides; only 2.5% is unchanged.

Ketamine has advantages over propofol and etomidate in being water soluble (and hence not requiring a lipid solvent) and also in producing profound analgesia at subanesthetic doses. However, although lacking the cardiorespiratory depressive properties of other intravenous agents, its usefulness has been limited by the high incidence of disturbing emergence reactions (in up to 30% of patients). Compared with other induction agents, ketamine increases the pulse rate, blood pressure, and intracranial pressure (ICP). Salivation is increased but this can be attenuated by administration of antimuscarinic agents such as atropine or glycopyrrolate.

It also causes postoperative dreaming and hallucinations. These may be attenuated by benzodiazepine or α_2 agonist premedication, although these classes of drugs prolong the elimination half-life and increase the duration of effect.

Assessment of the Hypnotic Properties of the Enantiomers of Ketamine

Separation of the enantiomers of ketamine has allowed clinicians to examine their relative potencies, side effects, and other pharmacologic effects. The usefulness of ketamine has been limited by a high incidence of disturbing emergence reactions (thought to be caused by the high affinity of the R⁻ enantiomer for the sigma opioid receptor) in up to 30% of patients. Previous studies have shown that these side effects can be reduced in both incidence and severity by the cotreatment of patients with other supplementary drugs (e.g., midazolam and propofol). The separation of the hypnotically active S⁺ enantiomer has been achieved, and this is now available in mainland Europe.

In vivo, S⁺ ketamine is about two times more potent in terms of anesthesia and is associated with faster recovery compared with the racemic mixture, and four times compared with the R⁻ isomer. An initial study of the S⁺ isomer in healthy volunteers by White and colleagues[106] demonstrated that the doses of ketamine of 6 minutes in duration were 275 mg for the racemate, 140 mg for S⁺ ketamine, and 429 mg for R⁻ ketamine with recovery being more rapid after the individual enantiomers. This relates closely to subsequent studies showing inhibition of the metabolism of S⁺ ketamine by the R⁻ isomer.[107] Ketamine concentrations at time of regaining consciousness and orientation were consistent with an S:R potency ratio of 4:1, whereas the ratio for impairment of psychomotor function was between 3:1 and 5:1. At equipotent doses, S⁺ ketamine produces longer hypnosis than the R⁻ isomer with the racemate being intermediate. However, cardiovascular stimulation and psychotomimetic effects are seen with both stereoisomers.

Crossover studies in healthy volunteers have shown that the dynamics of the racemate and S⁺ ketamine are comparable with regard to hemodynamic and metabolic responses.[108,109] However, there was improved recovery with the latter formulation. S⁺ ketamine is also accompanied by decreased locomotor activity, but equipotent analgesia.

In studies of the effects of racemic ketamine and the S⁺ isomer on the EEG spectrum, both increased fast β activity (21–30 Hz) with an accompanying reduction in delta power.[110] Using the IC_{50} (drug concentration of ketamine necessary to achieve a 50% depression of the maximal EEG median frequency reduction) as the index of potency, the S⁺ ketamine concentration was 0.8 μg/mL compared with 1.8 and 2.0 μg/mL for the R⁻ and the racemic preparations.[111]

On the basis of an assumed equipotency ratio of S⁺ ketamine-to-racemate of 1:2, Geisslinger and colleagues[112] compared the kinetics and dynamics of the enantiomers of ketamine in 50 surgical patients. There were no significant kinetic differences between S⁺ ketamine alone and the enantiomer present in the racemic mixture. However, the R⁻ enantiomer showed a lower clearance and smaller apparent volumes of distribution compared with the S⁺ enantiomer when administered as one component of the racemate, but there were no differences in the clearance rates of the S⁺ and R⁻ isomers when given as the racemate. The concentration/effect relationship for S⁺ ketamine therefore lies to the left of that for the racemate and has a steeper curve.

Clinical Evaluation of S⁺ Ketamine

When used as part of the anesthetic technique in surgical patients, ketamine causes considerable side effects. The incidence of emergence reactions is about 37% after the R⁻ enantiomer, 15% after the racemate, and 5% after the S⁺ isomer with comparable incidences of dreaming with all three treatment groups.[113] Another feature of ketamine is the significant increase in blood cortisol, catecholamines, and glucose concentrations[114]; similar increases occur with the S⁺ enantiomer in surgical patients when used for elective lower limb orthopedic surgery, although the increases in circulating plasma epinephrine concentrations were greater after use of the racemic mixture.[115] There are no apparent differences between the enantiomers and racemate in their hemodynamic effects. However, recovery is faster with the S⁺ isomer.

One other important aspect of ketamine's pharmacologic profile is its ability to regulate intracellular calcium levels and inducible nitric oxide synthase activity after hypoxic insults (i.e., its role as a neuroprotectant). There are data from cell culture experiments that the S⁺ enantiomer has a greater protective potential than the racemate, and that its use was accompanied by a greater reoutgrowth of axonal neurites and an increased expression of growth-associated proteins.[116,117] R⁻ ketamine was ineffective as a neuroprotectant.

Adverse Effects of Ketamine

Use of ketamine or S⁺ ketamine is contraindicated in patients with increased ICP or intraocular pressure, and in patients with severe cardiac diseases such as arterial hypertension, ischemic, or valvular heart disease. There is also a relative contraindication to its use in patients with psychotic disorders.

Steroid Anesthetic Agents

The hypnotic properties of steroid molecules were first recognized in 1927 by Cashin and Moravek[118] who induced in cats using a colloidal suspension of cholesterol. There was no apparent relationship between hypnotic (anesthetic) and hormonal properties of steroids, and the most potent anesthetic steroid, pregnane-3,20-dione (pregnanedione), was virtually devoid of endocrinologic activity. The steroids as a group of compounds have been shown to all have greater therapeutic indices than thiopental, but equally important side effects.

Althesin

Althesin is a mixture of alphaxalone and alphadolone acetate, which is solubilized in Cremophor EL because of the two chemicals hydrophobicity. Both steroids possess anesthetic activity, but the potency of the alphaxalone was approximately twice that of the alphadolone acetate, which was present solely to increase the solubility of the alphaxalone in its solvent. The drug continues to be used in veterinary practice, but was withdrawn from clinical use in 1984.

Sear and Sanders[119] studied the pharmacokinetics of Althesin steroids in humans and showed the disposition of alphaxalone to have an elimination half-life of about 30 minutes, a systemic clearance for alphaxalone of about 20 mL/kg per minute, and apparent volume of distribution at steady-state of 0.79 L/kg. The kinetics of alphadolone acetate in man do not differ from those of alphaxalone. The protein binding of alphaxalone and alphadolone was mainly to albumin, but also to β lipoproteins. Recent studies by Visser and colleagues[120] indicate the binding of alphaxalone to be about 97%.

Using gas chromatography-mass spectroscopy, both parent steroids and the metabolite 20α-hydroxy alphaxalone are detectable in blood after single doses and continuous infusions of Althesin.[121] Plasma concentrations of 20α-hydroxy alphaxalone remained low indicating a probable high clearance. Most of the alphaxalone (90–95%) is eliminated in the glucuronide fraction of the urine, mainly as the 20α-reduced alphaxalone glucuronide. Further quantitative studies in humans by Desmet and colleagues[122] confirm that the total urinary excretion of alphaxalone (both free drug and glucuronide conjugates) was less than 1%, which supports a significant role for systemic metabolism in drug elimination.

The clinical effects of bolus doses of Althesin was similar to that of thiopental apart from the more rapid recovery. Althesin also had important effects on cerebral hemodynamics, cerebral metabolism, and ICP with induction doses causing reductions in ICP proportional to the initial ICP. Althesin also caused decreases in cerebrospinal fluid pressure. When given by infusion (300 μg/kg per hour), Althesin decreased both cerebral blood flow and cerebral metabolic rate compared with the awake state in a manner similar to the barbiturates. Althesin also reduced brain blood flow homogenously to all cortical areas.

In humans, Althesin caused only minimal effects on blood pressure, respiration, and temperature homeostasis, suggesting its central depressive effect might be different from that seen with other intravenous agents. Althesin had no significant effects on either renal or hepatic function, but it was not considered safe when administered to patients with acute porphyria (both acute intermittent [Swedish] and variegate [South African] types). It was, however, an important agent for the management of patients who were susceptible to malignant hyperpyrexia.

Recovery

After either single dose administration or incremental dosing to supplement nitrous oxide anesthesia for short surgical procedures, immediate recovery after Althesin was more rapid than after thiopental was and comparable with methohexital. In the few comparative studies existing between Althesin and propofol (formulated as the emulsion), the cardiovascular effects of the two drugs when used for induction of anesthesia were similar, although recovery was faster after propofol.[123]

The main side effects after induction were a dose-related incidence of hiccups, coughing, laryngospasm, and involuntary muscle movements. Advantages included low incidences of postoperative nausea and vomiting and venous sequelae.

Pharmacology of Infusions of Althesin

The high clearance of the Althesin steroids, and their relatively short duration of action, made the drug appropriate for use by continuous infusion. Rates of infusion varied between authors and with the different supplements (e.g., opioids or extradural blockade or nitrous oxide) but ranged between 15 and 30 μg/kg per minute alphaxalone. Side effects (muscle twitching, hiccoughs, salivation) were minimal. There was remarkable cardiovascular stability even at eight times the maintenance rate when given to patients receiving 67% nitrous oxide and controlled ventilation. In the spontaneously breathing patient, rates up to four times the maintenance rate were associated with only small increases in the arterial CO_2 tension.

Adverse Reactions to Althesin

The major adverse side effects of Althesin were the occurrence of allergic reactions with an incidence between 1/1000 and 1/18,000. The immunology of adverse reactions to Althesin probably has many etiologic factors; reactions on first exposure being due either to a direct nonimmunologic effect on mast cells to cause histamine and other autocoids to be released or by alternative pathway complement activation. Reactions to repeat exposure to Althesin resulted from classical complement pathway activation, indicating an antigen/antibody interaction. This latter group of reactions generally had a more severe symptomatology.[124] IgE antibodies were not detected in affected individuals (indeed IgE does not bind to complement), but Moneret-Vautrin and colleagues[125] found anti-Cremophor EL IgG antibodies. In another in vitro study, Tachon and colleagues[126] showed that Althesin (formulated in Cremophor EL), but not the individual steroids, was allergenic. There was also laboratory evidence of subclinical complement activation after both bolus doses and infusions of Althesin.[127]

Whether these reactions to the Cremophor-formulated drugs such as Althesin was caused by the pharmacologically active components with the Cremophor acting as an adjuvant or to the Cremophor itself is a matter of conjecture.

Minaxolone Citrate

Because of the problems with dissolving the steroid molecules, there has been a search for water-soluble steroids.

Figdor and colleagues[128] found that amino esters of 21-hydroxypregnanedione were water-soluble and had general anesthetic properties, whereas Hewett and coworkers[129] investigated derivatives of androstane or pregnane with amino radicals attached at C_2, C_6, or C_{16} and found that the most potent in causing loss of righting reflex was a C_2 morpholino-steroid (3α-hydroxy, 2β-morpholino, 5α-pregnan-20-one: SAV 1710). It had a low therapeutic index of 4.69, a long threshold time to onset of anesthesia, and a long duration of effect. Minaxolone citrate (one of the 11α- or 11β-dialkylaminoacyloxy or dialkylamino steroids) formed water-soluble salts that showed anesthetic activity in mice. It had a high therapeutic index (>5) and was two to three times as potent as Althesin and eight times as potent as thiopental.

The main adverse features of minaxolone were the high incidence of excitatory side effects during induction, increased muscle tone intraoperatively, and involuntary movements during recovery; the latter was often prolonged. Minaxolone was withdrawn from clinical studies because of these adverse features and concern regarding toxicologic results from large doses given to rats.

5β-Pregnanolone (Eltanolone)

Eltanolone is a 5β pregnane steroid with anesthetic properties and a high therapeutic index (>40). Like Althesin, it is water insoluble and is therefore formulated as an emulsion.

The respective potencies of eltanolone to etomidate and propofol were compared because the concentrations needed to achieve hypnosis (0.46, 0.32, and 2.3 µg/mL). Of greater importance was the prolonged blood/brain equilibration time of 6 to 8 minutes compared with values of 1.5 and 3 minutes, respectively, for thiopental and propofol,[130] therefore making eltanolone difficult to administer by titration of dose to effect. A consequence was overdosing when given by incremental doses or continuous infusions, which led to prolonged immediate recovery.

Eltanolone was withdrawn from clinical trials because of its side effects profile (skin rashes and urticaria, especially in children, and four cases of convulsions), as well as the absence of clinical advantages over existing drugs.

ORG 21465

ORG 21465 and ORG 20599 were water-soluble 2-substituted aminosteroids. ORG 21465 (base: ORG 21256) was evaluated in both animals and humans. The steroid had a high therapeutic index in mice (13.8) compared with propofol or thiopental (4–5). In the monkey, ORG 21465 produced rapid-onset hypnosis, but duration of sleep and recovery were longer when the steroid was compared with propofol. As with other steroids investigated in humans, there was a high incidence (70%) of excitatory side effects, but no accompanying EEG spike activity. Although the steroid caused no cardiovascular and respiratory depression, it is not being evaluated further in humans.

Allergic Reactions to Hypnotic Agents

Although the majority of allergic reactions to intravenous agents originate from use of neuromuscular blocking drugs, there are large numbers caused by hypnotic agents. The overall incidence to intravenous agents is between 1/5000 and 1/20,000; for the barbiturates, the incidence is 1/23,000 to 1/30,000 with possible cross-sensitivity between methohexital and the thiobarbiturate. In contrast, the incidence of reactions to etomidate (about 1/45,0000) and ketamine (two cases) is low (Table 24–4).

TABLE 24–4.

Incidence of Adverse Hypersensitivity Reactions to Intravenous Hypnotic Agents

Hypnotic Agent	Incidence
Thiopental	1/14,000–1/20,000
Methohexital	1/1600–1/7000
Propofol (as Cremophor formulation; BASF, Mount Olive, Nj.)	1 in 1131
Etomidate	10+ cases (estimate 1/50,000–1/450,000)
Propofol as emulsion	(estimate 1/80,000–1/100,000)
For comparison:	
Althesin (in Cremophor)	1/400–1/11,000
Propanidid (in Micellophor)	1/500–1/17,000
Neuromuscular blocking drugs	1/5000
Penicillin	1/2500–1/10,000
Dextrans	1/3000
Gelatins	1/900
Hydroxyethyl starch	1/1200

Thiopental and Other Barbiturates

The quoted incidences of adverse reactions to thiopental and methohexital are about 1/14000 and 1/7000, respectively. There have been more than 250 published cases of anaphylactic or anaphylactoid reactions to thiopental. Cutaneous and cardiovascular manifestations predominate (65% and 56%, respectively) with respiratory side effects (laryngospasm or difficulty in ventilating the patient) in about 35% of cases. There are also recorded cases of death after administration of thiopental. Many affected patients give a history of atopy, allergy, or a previous general anesthetic (presumably one of the barbiturates).

Laboratory testing after a suspected reaction usually shows a significant immediate decrease in the plasma levels of IgE with no significant change in the concentration of complement proteins C_3 and C_4. In rarer cases, there is both IgE and complement involvement; complement activation probably occurs secondary to the hypotension. There are currently well-documented cases in which specific IgE antibodies to thiopental have been detected by id. testing.[131,132]

Clarke[133] reported the 15 cases of suspected hypersensitivity to methohexital and the 2 cases associated with thiamylal. The incidence is undoubtedly low and there have been no reported deaths. Most patients showed periorbital and facial edema with no history of allergy. One reaction presented with cutaneous signs of flushing and periorbital edema accompanied by severe hypotension. Clinical signs and laboratory tests indicate an anaphylactic response caused by a type I hypersensitivity reaction due to a possible cross-sensitivity between the two barbiturates.

Data from the CSM (UK) show a total of 84 allergic reactions to thiopental over the past 37 years; the majority are anaphylactic.

Etomidate

The incidence of reactions to etomidate is low. There are five reports between 1978 and 1982 of possible adverse reactions to the drug.[134] Each reaction involved widespread cutaneous flushing or urticaria and the postoperative occurrence of vomiting. None of the patients showed complement activation. An additional two cases reported to Watkins in 1982[134] also exhibited anaphylactoid responses, with signs of cyanosis, marked hypotension, and, in one case, edema. Whether these are caused by etomidate is difficult to decide because the drug was administered concurrently with suxamethonium or alcuronium. Nevertheless, complement C_3 activation was shown in one of the cases.

Further reactions described by Krumholz and colleagues[135] and Sold and Rothhammer[136] report generalized erythema, urticaria, tachycardia and hypotension, and positive skin tests supporting anaphylactoid reactions. Fazackerley and colleagues[137] reported the first case of severe bronchospasm (leading to hypoxic cardiac arrest) and urticaria after induction of anesthesia with etomidate. Complement was not activated, but the patient had an increased

plasma IgE level, which was consistent with atopy. Unlike many of the other reports, a direct release of histamine or other immune mediators by the intravenous hypnotic agent seems the most likely explanation. There have been eight allergic reactions reported to the CSM since 1979.

Ketamine

There are only two reported allergic reactions to ketamine[138,139]; one involving IgE, the other probably having a nonimmune basis.

Di-isopropyl Phenol

The incidence of reactions to propofol appears to be increasing. At least 5 cases of hypersensitivity were reported among the 1131 patients receiving the agent during clinical trials with a formulation made up in Cremophor EL. Reformulation of propofol as an emulsion has currently resulted in 89 cases reported to the CSM (UK). These have been categorized as "allergic, anaphylactoid, or anaphylactic," with one associated death.[63,140] Other side effects occurring with a high incidence (and which may be related to histamine or other mediator release) include pain on injection, erythematous rashes, bronchospasm, flushing, and hypotension. When all of these hypersensitivity reactions are taken together, the overall incidence for propofol is probably between 1/80,000 and 1/100,000 administrations.

Practical Aspects of Drug Administration

Thiopental

This drug is administered for four specific indications:

1. Induction of anesthesia
2. Maintenance of anesthesia by either intermittent administration, or by infusion in combination with analgesics as needed
3. As an anticonvulsant
4. For sedation of and control of ICP in the patient with head injury

Dosage and administration: Thiopental is supplied as a yellow powder with added 6% anhydrous sodium carbonate in vials containing an inert atmosphere of nitrogen and is formulated as a 2.5% solution. The recommended induction dose is 100 to 150 mg over 10 to 15 seconds, followed by additional increments after 30 to 60 seconds; or a single dose up to 4 mg/kg. In children, doses of 2 to 7 mg/kg may be needed.

For the maintenance of thiopental infusions at rates between 150 and 300 μg/kg per minute can be used to supplement either nitrous oxide or as part of a totally intravenous technique with opiates such as morphine, fentanyl, sufentanil, or remifentanil. However, use of the thiobarbiturate for maintenance of may be accompanied by prolonged recovery times.

For the management of convulsions or treatment of increased ICP, doses of 1.5 to 3 mg/kg may be administered, repeated as necessary, and followed by either 25 to 50 mg boluses or an infusion of the barbiturate titrated against the occurrence of further fits or ICP (3–10 mg/kg per hour). Dosing adjustments may be needed in the critically ill patient with either liver or renal failure.

Similar dosing strategies should be adopted with thiamylal.

Methohexital

Like thiopental, methohexital can be used for both induction of anesthesia and by continuous infusion for maintenance of anesthesia.

Methohexital is supplied in vials containing 100 or 500 mg, which is made up as a 1% solution. The usual induction dose is 2.0 to 2.5 mg/kg. Infusions of methohexital up to 100 μg/kg per minute can be used to maintain anesthesia with either 67% nitrous oxide or opioid supplementation.

Etomidate

Etomidate can be used for induction of especially in patients with cardiovascular disease, as well as induction of anesthesia in patients with known drug hypersensitivity or atopy. Because of its effects on adrenal steroidogenesis, the drug is no longer recommended for maintenance of anesthesia by repeat dosing or continuous infusion. Single bolus doses of etomidate (5–20 mg) may be used in the intensive care unit for control of acute increases in ICP.

Etomidate is formulated as a 2 mg/mL solution in 10 mL ampoules made up in propylene glycol or LCT/MCT (Etomidate-Lipuro). The recommended induction dose is 0.3 mg/kg, but is reduced in the elderly to 0.15 to 0.2 mg/kg. In children younger than 15 years, doses up to 0.39 mg/kg may be needed.

Ketamine

There are a number of indications for use of ketamine including:

- induction of anesthesia
- maintenance of anesthesia
- sedation by use as a continuous infusion,
- analgesia (intraoperatively or after surgery) by use as a continuous infusion, or
- the drug may also be given for all of the above by the intramuscular route.

Ketamine is supplied in 10, 50, and 100 mg/mL strengths. The recommended induction dose is 1 to 4.5 mg/kg (usually a dose of 2 mg/kg provides surgical anesthesia for 5–10 minutes). Maintenance of anesthesia can be achieved using a 1 mg/mL solution at a rate of 10 to 45 μg/kg per minute. Anesthesia may also be achieved with intramuscular ketamine in a dose of range 6.5 to 13.0 mg/kg (a dose of 10 mg/kg providing 12 to 25 minutes for diagnostic procedures and manipulations).

S-ketamine is supplied in 5 and 25 mg/mL strengths as 5- and 20-mL vials for the 5 mg/mL and 2- and 10-mL vials for the 25 mg/mL strength. Induction doses of 0.5 to 1.0 mg/kg intravenously and 2 to 4 mg/kg intramuscularly are recommended. The recommended induction dose is 0.5 to 1.0 mg/kg intravenously or 2 to 4 mg/kg intramuscularly. Maintenance can be achieved by repeated boluses of 50% of the induction dose or infusion of 0.5 to 3.0 mg/kg per hour. For analgesia, doses of 0.1 to 0.25 mg/kg intravenously followed by an infusion of 0.2 to 1.0 mg/kg per hour are recommended.

Propofol

Propofol can be used both in the operating room and in the intensive care unit. In the former, propofol is administered intravenously for both induction of anesthesia and maintenance of by intermittent bolus dosing or continuous infusion. In some countries, the use of target controlled infusions of propofol to maintain anesthesia is only licensed for use in adults. Propofol is also widely used for sedation by continuous infusion both as supplement to regional anesthetic techniques for endoscopic procedures and in the intensive care unit. There are reports of the drug being administered by patient control (that is, the patient themselves titrate the amount of hypnotic they receive to produce sedation).

Propofol is formulated as 1% or 2% solutions in oil emulsion (20 and 50 mL) and as a 50-mL vial for use in target-controlled infusion anesthesia and a 1% solution in LCT/MCT. The recommended induction dose is 1.5 to 2.5 mg/kg given at 20 to 40 mg per 10 seconds. The dose should be reduced in the patient older than 55 years. The drug may also be used for induction of anesthesia in children older than 1 month. Maintenance of anesthesia can be achieved using 25 to 50 mg bolus doses or an infusion of 4 to 12 mg/kg per hour (for children older than 3 years, rates of 9–15 mg/kg per hour may be needed). The use of target-controlled infusions for induction and maintenance of is approved only for adults.

In the intensive care unit, initial doses of propofol of about 0.3 to 2 mg/kg followed by 25 to 50 mg boluses may be used to institute sedation for controlled ventilation. In the agitated patient, doses of up to 10 mg/kg per hour may be needed. The average maximum dose per day should not exceed 15 mg/kg per hour, and the use of propofol for intensive therapy unit sedation is not currently recommended in patients younger than 17 years. However, clinical trials in this area are ongoing.

Future Directions in Intravenous Anesthetic Pharmacology

Recent advances in molecular biology and gene targeting have provided tremendous opportunities for understanding the actions of intravenous anesthetics on these receptors. The availability of cDNA encoding receptor subunits, combined with expression systems and methods for the rapid introduction of mutations, has allowed rapid advances toward the culmination of mechanism research—defining molecular sites of anesthetic action in the brain.

There are tantalizing suggestions for the existence of an anesthetic binding site within GABA receptor subunits, but the low affinity of anesthetic binding makes it difficult to prove rigorously that the drug is indeed binding at the site of the mutation. Despite the obstacles, it is likely that the site(s) of anesthetic action on GABA$_A$ receptors will be defined to the satisfaction of many within a few years. These advances in molecular analysis will allow researchers to address the bigger question of which aspects of anesthetic action are caused by enhancement of GABAergic function. This will be accomplished for the GABA$_A$ receptor by constructing mice with mutations in genes encoding specific subunits. Targeted gene manipulations in mice will provide hypothesis-driven tests of the in vivo roles of GABA$_A$ receptors and other ligand-gated ion channels in mediating the diverse behavioral actions of intravenous anesthetics.

Researchers recently have created "global knockout mice" for various subunits of the ligand-gated ion channels. Although these knockout mice may provide initial clues as to the nature of anesthetic targets, experiments on such mice have been difficult to analyze (and interpret) in terms of anesthetic sensitivity, because they often exhibit abnormal behavior, lethality, or gross alterations in neural development.[141] These problems with knockout mice may be circumvented by "conditional" gene knockouts in which the gene of interest is disrupted only in limited brain regions or specified developmental time periods[142] and by knockin mice. Knockin mice experiments potentially provide an elegant bridge between in vitro experiments and whole animal behavior. Ideally, the mutated receptor subunit would differ from its wild-type counterpart only in terms of general anesthetic modulation (i.e., agonist response, voltage-dependence, and kinetics of the receptor would be relatively normal). A complication to gene targeting experiments is the presence of multiple subunit isoforms for the GABA$_A$ receptor subunits; if some or all of these isoforms play a role in general, then targeting of multiple genes may be required to obtain a clear alteration in anesthetic sensitivity.

Currently, there is ample evidence that clinical concentrations of several intravenous general anesthetics enhance the function of GABA$_A$ receptors or inhibit the function of NMDA receptors. We are already on the verge of a molecular understanding of the sites of action of these drugs on GABA$_A$ receptors. However, there is still little information, or at least agreement, about the consequence of intravenous agent actions at GABA$_A$ receptors. This problem reflects our basic ignorance of how the human brain works. We have some concept of how alteration in receptor function perturbs synaptic transmission, but little idea how these changes are translated into alterations in behavior. We can be optimistic that construction of mice with mutant receptors that differ in regulation by anesthetics will indeed help to address the fundamental question of how modulation of specific receptors influences specific anesthetic-sensitive behaviors, including recall, the awareness of pain, and movement. The relative complexity of human neuroanatomy and behavior represents an additional barrier to understanding, yet it is clear that our knowledge of intravenous anesthetic action has advanced more in the last decade than in the entire previous century, and this provides for an optimistic outlook for future developments in anesthetic pharmacology and drug development.

Acknowledgments

Funding to N.L.H. has been generously provided by NIH grants GM 61925, GM45129, GM56850 and by the C.V. Starr Foundation of New York City.

References

1. Franks NP, Lieb WR: Molecular and cellular mechanisms of general anaesthesia. Nature 367:607–614, 1994.
2. Harrison NL, Flood P: Molecular mechanisms of general anesthetic action. Sci Med 5:18–27, 1998.
3. Pearce RA: Effects of volatile anesthetics on GABA$_A$ receptors: Electrophysiological studies. In Moody EJ, Skolnick P (eds): Molecular Bases of Anesthesia. Boca Raton, Fl: CRC Press, 2000.
4. Cohen ML, Chan SL, Way WL, Trevor AJ: Distribution in the brain and metabolism of ketamine in the rat after intravenous administration. Anesthesiology 39:370–376, 1973.
5. Sear JW, Prys-Roberts C: Plasma concentrations of alphaxalone during continuous infusion of Althesin. Br J Anaesth 51:861–865, 1979.
6. Krasowski MD, Harrison NL: General anaesthetic actions on ligand-gated ion channels. Cell Mol Life Sci 55:1278–1303, 1999.
7. Antognini JF, Schwartz K: Exaggerated anesthetic requirements in the preferentially anesthetized brain. Anesthesiology 79:1244–1249, 1993.
8. Rampil IJ, Mason P, Singh H: Anesthetic potency (MAC) is independent of forebrain structures in the rat. Anesthesiology 78:707–712, 1993.
9. Collins JG, Kendig JJ, Mason P: Anesthetic actions within the spinal cord: Contributions to the state of general anesthesia. Trends Neurosci 18:549–553, 1995.
10. Franks NP, Lieb WR: Do general anaesthetics act by competitive binding to specific receptors? Nature 310:599–601, 1984.
11. Tomlin SL, Jenkins A, Lieb WR, Franks NP: Stereoselective effects of etomidate optical isomers on gamma-aminobutyric acid type A receptors and animals. Anesthesiology 88:708–717, 1998.
12. Moody EJ, Harris BD, Skolnick P: The potential for safer anaesthesia using stereoselective anaesthetics. Trends Pharmacol Sci 15:387–391, 1994.
13. Homanics GE, Quinlan JJ, Mihalek RM, Firestone LL: Alcohol and anesthetic mechanisms in genetically engineered mice. Front Biosci 3:D548–D558, 1998.
14. Gunther U, Benson J, Benke D, et al: Benzodiazepine-insensitive mice generated by targeted disruption of the g2 subunit of g-aminobutyric acid type A receptors. Proc Natl Acad Sci USA 92:7749–7753, 1995.
15. Lakhlani PP, MacMillan LB, Guo TZ, et al: Substitution of a mutant α_{2A} adrenergic receptor via "hit and run" gene targeting reveals the role of this subtype in sedative, analgesic, and anesthetic-sparing responses in vivo. Proc Natl Acad Sci USA 94:9950–9955, 1997.

16. Belelli D, Lambert JJ, Peters JA, et al: The interaction of the general anesthetic etomidate with the g-aminobutyric acid type A receptor is influenced by a single amino acid. Proc Natl Acad Sci USA 94:11031–11036, 1997.

17. Zimmerman SA, Jones MV, Harrison NL: Potentiation of g-aminobutyric acid$_A$ receptor Cl$^-$ current correlates with in vivo anesthetic potency. J Pharmacol Exp Ther 270:987–991, 1994.

18. Downie DL, Hall AC, Lieb WR, Franks NP: Effects of inhalational general anaesthetics in native glycine receptors in medullary neurones and recombinant glycine receptors in Xenopus oocytes. Br J Pharmacol 118:493–502, 1996.

19. Tanelian DL, Kosek P, Mody I, MacIver MB: The role of GABA$_A$ receptor/chloride channel complex in anesthesia. Anesthesiology 78:757–776, 1993.

20. Harris RA, Mihic SJ, Dildy-Mayfield JA, Machu TK: Actions of anesthetics on ligand-gated ion channels: Role of receptor subunit composition. FASEB J 9:1454–1462, 1995.

21. Andrews PR, Mark LC: Structural specificity of barbiturates and related drugs. Anesthesiology 57:314–320, 1982.

22. Birnir B, Tierney ML, Dalziel JE, et al: A structural determinant of desensitization and allosteric regulation by pentobarbital of the GABA$_A$ receptor. J Membrane Biol 155:157–166, 1997.

23. Belelli D, Lambert JJ, Peters JA, et al: The interaction of the general anesthetic etomidate with the g-aminobutyric acid type A receptor is influenced by a single amino acid. Proc Natl Acad Sci USA 94:11031–11036, 1997.

24. Flood P, Krasowski MD: Intravenous anesthetics differentially modulate ligand-gated ion channels. Anesthesiology 92:18–25, 2000.

25. Orser BA, Pennefather PS, MacDonald JF: Multiple mechanisms of ketamine blockade on N-methyl-D-aspartate receptors. Anesthesiology 86:903–917, 1997.

26. Pistis M. Belelli D, Peters JA, Lambert JJ: The interaction of general anaesthetics with recombinant GABA$_A$ and glycine receptors expressed in Xenopus laevis oocytes: A comparative study. Br J Pharmacol 122:1707–1719, 1997.

27. Krasowski MD, O'Shea SM, Rick CEM, et al: α subunit isoform influences GABA$_A$ receptor modulation by propofol. Neuropharmacology 36:941–949, 1998.

28. Flood P, Ramirez-Latorre J, Role L: Alpha4 beta2 neuronal acetylchoine receptors in the central nervous system are inhibited by isoflurane and propofol but alpha7-type nicotinic acetylcholine receptors are unaffected. Anesthesiology 86:859–865, 1997.

29. Jurd R, Arras M, Lambert S, et al: General anesthetic actions in vivo strongly attenuated by a point mutation in the GABA$_A$ receptor. FASEB J 17:250–252, 2003.

30. Harrison NL, Vicini S, Barker JL: A steroid anesthetic prolongs inhibitory postsynaptic currents in cultured rat hippocampal neurons. J Neurosci 7:604–609, 1987.

31. Harrison NL, Simmonds MA: Modulation of the GABA receptor complex by a steroid anaesthetic. Brain Res 323:287–292, 1984.

32. Siegwart R, Jurd R, Rudolph U: Molecular determinants for the action of general anesthetics at recombinant $\alpha_2\beta_3g_2$ g-aminobutyric acid$_A$ receptors. J Neurochem 80:140–148, 2002.

33. Yamakura T, Bertaccini E, Trudell JR, Harris RA: Anesthetics and ion channels: Molecular models and sites of action. Annu Rev Pharmacol Toxicol 41:23–51, 2001.

34. Sewell JC, Sear JW: Can molecular similarity-activity models for iv. general anaesthetics help explain their mechanism of action? Br J Anaesth 88:166–174, 2002.

35. Sewell JC, Sear JW: Derivation of preliminary three-dimensional pharmacophoric maps for chemically diverse intravenous general anaesthetics. Br J Anaesth 92: 2004.

36. Krasowski MD, Hong X, Hopfinger AJ, Harrison NL: 4D-QSAR analysis of a set of propofol analogues: Mapping binding sites for an anesthetic phenol on the GABA(A) receptor. J Med Chem 45:3210–3221, 2002.

37. Lundy JS, Tovell RM: Some of the newer local and general anesthetic agents. Methods of their administration. Northwest Medicine (Seattle) 33:308–311, 1934.

38. Pratt TW, Tatum AL, Hathaway HR, Waters RM: Sodium ethyl(1-methylbutyl) thiobarbiturate: Preliminary experimental and clinical study. Am J Surg 31:464, 1936.

39. Stanski DR, Maitre PO: Population pharmacokinetics and pharmacodynamics of thiopental: The effect of age revisited. Anesthesiology 72:412–422, 1990.

40. Cordata DJ, Herkes GK, Mather LE, et al: Prolonged thiopentone infusion for neurosurgical emergencies: Usefulness of therapeutic drug monitoring. Anaesth Intensive Care 29:339–348, 2001.

41. Cordato DJ, Gross AS, Herkes GK, Mather LE: Pharmacokinetics of thiopentone enantiomers following intravenous injection or prolonged infusion of *rac*-thiopentone. Br J Clin Pharmacol 43:355–362, 1997.

42. Nguyen KT, Stephens DP, McLeish MJ, et al: Pharmacokinetics of thiopental and pentobarbital enantiomers after intravenous administration of racemic thiopental. Anesth Analg 83:552–558, 1996.

43. Sueyasu M, Ikeda T, Taniyama T, et al: Pharmacokinetics of thiamylal enantiomers in humans. Int J Clin Pharmacol Ther 35:128–132, 1997.

44. Cook CE, Seltzman TB, Tallent CR, et al: Pharmacokinetics of pentobarbital enantiomers as determined by enantioselective radioimmunoassay after administration of racemate to humans and rabbits. J Pharmacol Exp Ther 241:779–785, 1987.

45. Sueyasu M, Fujito K, Shuto H, et al: Protein binding and the metabolism of thiamylal enantiomers in vitro. Anesth Analg 91:736–740, 2000.

46. Tomlin SL, Jenkins A, Lieb WR, et al: Stereoselective effects of etomidate optical isomers on gamma-aminobutyric acid type A receptors and animals. Anesthesiology 88:708–717, 1998.

47. Doenicke A, Roizen MF, Kugler J, et al: Reducing myoclonus after etomidate. Anesthesiology 90:113–119, 1999.

48. Modica PA, Tempelhoff R, White PF: Pro and anticonvulsant effects of anesthetics (Part II). Anesth Analg 70:433–444, 1990.

49. Preziosi P, Vacca M: Adrenocortical suppression and other endocrine effects of etomidate. Life Sci 42:477–489, 1988.

50. Vanacker B, Wiebalck A, Van Aken H, et al: Induktionsqualitat und nebennierenrindenfunktion: Ein klinischer vergleich von Etomidat-lipuro und hypnomidate. Der Anaesthesist 42:81–89, 1993.

51. Kulka PJ, Bremer F, Schuttler J: Narkoseeinleitung mit etomidat in lipidemulsion. Der Anaesthesist 42:205–209, 1993.

52. Nebauer AE, Doenicke A, Hoernecke R, et al: Does etomidate cause haemolysis? Br J Anaesth 69:58–60, 1992.

53. Doenicke AW, Roizen MF, Hoernecke R, et al: Solvent for etomidate may cause pain and adverse effects. Br J Anaesth 83:464–466, 1999.

54. Doenicke A, Roizen MF, Nebauer AE, et al: Comparison of two formulations of etomidate, 2-hydroxypropyl-β-cyclodextrin (HPCD) and propylene glycol. Anesth Analg 79:933–939, 1994.

55. St Pierre M, Dunkel M, Rutherford A, Hering W: Does etomidate increase postoperative nausea? A double-blind controlled comparison of etomidate in lipid emulsion with propofol for balanced anaesthesia. Eur J Anaesthesiol 17:634–641, 2000.

56. Schuttler J, Ihmsen H: Population pharmacokinetics of propofol: A multicenter study. Anesthesiology 92:727–738, 2000.

57. Court MH, Duan SX, Hesse LM, et al: Cytochrome P-450 2B6 is responsible for interindividual variability of propofol hydroxylation by human liver microsomes. Anesthesiology 94:110–119, 2001.

58. Oda Y, Hamaoka N, Hiroi T, et al: Involvement of human liver cytochrome P4502B6 in the metabolism of propofol. Br J Clin Pharmacol 51:281–285, 2001.

59. He YL, Ueyama H, Tashiro C, et al: Pulmonary disposition of propofol in surgical patients. Anesthesiology 93:986–991, 2000.

60. Dawidowicz Al, Fornal E, Mardarowicz M, Fijalkowska A: The role of human lungs in the biotransformation of propofol. Anesthesiology 93:992–997, 2000.

61. Kazama T, Ikeda K, Morita K, et al: Relation between initial blood distribution volume and propofol induction dose requirement. Anesthesiology 94:205–210, 2001.

62. Schnider TW, Minto CF, Shafer SL, et al: The influence of age on propofol pharmacodynamics. Anesthesiology 90:1502–1516, 1999.

63. Bryson HM, Fulton BR, Faulds D: Propofol: An update of its use in anaesthesia and conscious sedation. Drugs 50:513–559, 1995.

64. Cullen PM, Turtle M, Prys-Roberts C, et al: Effect of propofol on baroreflex activity in humans. Anesth Analg 66:1115–1120, 1987.

65. Sear JW, Diedericks J, Foex P: Continuous infusions of propofol administered to dogs: Effects on ICG and propofol disposition. Br J Anaesth 72:451–455, 1994.

66. Coetzee JF, Glen JB, Wium CA, Boshoff L: Pharmacokinetic model selection for target controlled infusions of propofol. Assessment of three parameter sets. Anesthesiology 82:1328–1345, 1995.

67. Schnider TW, Minto CF, Gambus PL, et al: The influence of method of administration and covariates on the pharmacokinetics of propofol in adult volunteers. Anesthesiology 88:1170–1182, 1998.

68. Spens HJ, Drummond GB: Ventilatory effects of eltanolone during

induction of anaesthesia: Comparison with propofol and thiopentone. Br J Anaesth 77:194–199, 1996.

69. Nagyova B, Dorrington KL, Gill EW, et al: Comparison of the effects of sub-hypnotic concentrations of propofol and halothane on the acute ventilatory response to hypoxia. Br J Anaesth 75:713–718, 1995.

70. Nieuwenhuijs D, Sarton E, Teppema L, et al: Propofol for monitored care: Implications on hypoxic control of cardiorespiratory responses. Anesthesiology 92:46–54, 2000.

71. Janicki PK, James MFM, Erskine WAR: Propofol inhibits enzymatic degradation of alfentanil and sufentanil by isolated liver microsomes in vitro. Br J Anaesth 68:311–312, 1992.

72. Baker MT, Chadam MV, Ronnenberg WC Jr: Inhibitory effects of propofol on cytochrome P450 activity in rat hepatic microsomes. Anesth Analg 76:817–821, 1993.

73. Chen TL, Ueng TH, Chen SH, et al: Human cytochrome P450 mono-oxygenase system is suppressed by propofol. Br J Anaesth 74:558–562, 1995.

74. Chen TL, Chen TG, Tai YT, et al: Propofol inhibits renal cytochrome P450 activity and enflurane defluorination in vitro in hamsters. Can J Anaesth 47:680–686, 2000.

75. Mertens MJ, Vuyk J, Olofsen E, et al: Propofol alters the pharmacokinetics of alfentanil in healthy male volunteers. Anesthesiology 94:949–957, 2001.

76. Short TG. Pharmacodynamic interactions of anaesthetics. Curr Opin Anaesth 8:292–297, 1995.

77. Billard V, Moulla F, Bourgain JL, et al: ic response to induction and intubation. Propofol/fentanyl interaction. Anesthesiology 81:1384–1394, 1994.

78. Vinik HR, Bradley EL, Kissin I: Triple anesthetic combination: propofol-midazolam-alfentanil. Anesth Analg 78:354–358, 1994.

79. Peden CJ, Cloote AH, Stafford N, Prys-Roberts C: The effect of intravenous dexmedetomidine premedication on the dose requirement of propofol to induce loss of consciousness in patients receiving alfentanil. Anaesthesia 56:408–413, 2001.

80. Dutta S, Karol MD, Cohen T, et al: Effect of dexmedetomidine on propofol requirements in healthy subjects. J Pharm Sci 90:172–181, 2001.

81. Ure RW, Dwyer SJ, Blogg CE, White AP: Patient-controlled anxiolysis with propofol (ARS abstract). Br J Anaesth 67:657–658, 1991.

82. Rudkin GE, Osborne GA, Curtis NJ: Intra-operative patient-controlled sedation. Anaesthesia 46:90–92, 1991.

83. Borgeat A, Wilder-Smith O, Forni M, Suter PM: Adjuvant propofol enables better control of nausea and emesis secondary to chemotherapy for breast cancer. Can J Anaesth 41:1117–1119, 1994.

84. Borgeat A, Wilder-Smith OHG, Salah M, et al: Subhypnotic doses of propofol relieve pruritus induced by epidural and intrathecal morphine. Anesthesiology 76:510–512, 1992.

85. Salah M, Borgeat A, Wilder-Smith OH, et al: Epidural morphine-induced pruritus: Propofol versus naloxone. Anesth Analg 78:1110–1113, 1994.

86. Borgeat A, Mentha G, Savoiz D, et al: Prurit associe a une hepatopathie: Propofol, une nouvelle approche therapeutique? Schweiz Med Wochenschr 124:649–650, 1994.

87. Fox J, Gelb AW, Enns J, et al: The responsiveness of cerebral blood flow to changes in arterial carbon dioxide is maintained during propofol-nitrous oxide in humans. Anesthesiology 77:453–456, 1992.

88. Stone JG, Young WL, Marans ZS, et al: Consequences of electroencephalographic suppressive doses of propofol in conjunction with deep hypothermic circulatory arrest. Anesthesiology 85:497–501, 1996.

89. Newman MF, Murkin JM, Roach G, et al: Cerebral physiologic effects of burst suppression doses of propofol during non-pulsatile cardiopulmonary bypass. Anesth Analg 81:452–457, 1995.

90. Illievich UM, Petricek W, Schramm W, et al: Electroencephalographic burst suppression by propofol infusion in humans: ic consequences. Anesth Analg 77:155–160, 1993.

91. Sear JW. Intravenous anaesthetics. Balliere's Clinical Anaesthesiology 3:217–242, 1989.

92. McKeating K, Bali IM, Dundee JW: The effects of thiopentone and propofol on upper airway integrity. Anaesthesia 43:638–640, 1988.

93. Wouters PF, Van de Velde M, Marcus MAE, et al: ic changes during induction of with eltanolone and propofol in dogs. Anesth Analg 81:125–131, 1995.

94. Sear JW, Prys-Roberts C, Dye A: Hepatic function after anaesthesia for major vascular reconstructive surgery: A comparison of four anaesthetic techniques. Br J Anaesth 55:603–609, 1983.

95. Murray JM, Trinick TR: Hepatic function and indocyanine green clearance during and after prolonged anaesthesia with propofol. Br J Anaesth 69:643–644, 1992.

96. Picard P, Tramer MR: Prevention of pain on injection with propofol: A quantitative sytematic review. Anesth Analg 90:963–969, 2000.

97. Doenicke AW, Roizen MF, Rau J, et al: Reducing pain during propofol injection: the role of the solvent. Anesth Analg 82:472–476, 1996.

98. Doenicke A, Roizen MF, Rau J, et al: Pharmacokinetics and pharmacodynamics of propofol in a new solvent. Anesth Analg 85:1399–1404, 1997.

99. Rau J, Roizen MF, Doenicke AW, et al: Propofol in an emulsion of long- and medium-chain triglycerides: The effect on pain. Anesth Analg 93:382–384, 2001.

100. Knibbe CAJ, Aarts LPHJ, Kuks PFM, et al: Pharmacokinetics and pharmacodynamics of propofol 6% SAZN versus propofol 1% SAZN and Diprivan 10 for short-term sedation following coronary artery bypass surgery. Eur J Clin Pharmacol 56:89–95, 2000.

101. Bielen SJ, Lysko GS, Gough WB: The effect of a cyclodextrin vehicle on the cardiovascular profile of propofol in rats. Anesth Analg 82:920–924, 1996.

102. Bennett SN, McNeil MM, Bland LA, et al: Postoperative infections traced to contamination of an intravenous anesthetic propofol. N Engl J Med 333:147–154, 1995.

103. Sosis MB, Braverman B, Villaflor E: Propofol, but not thiopental, supports the growth of Candida albicans. Anesth Analg 81:132–134, 1995.

104. Badr AE, Mychaskiw G, Eichhorn JH: Metabolic acidosis associated with a new formulation of propofol. Anesthesiology 94:536–538, 2001.

105. Matrin PH, Murthy BV, Petros AJ: Metabolic, biochemical and haemodynamic effects of infusion of propofol for long term sedation of children undergoing intensive care. Br J Anaesth 79:276–279, 1997.

106. White PF, Schuttler J, Shafer A, et al: Comparative pharmacology of the ketamine isomers. Br J Anaesth 57:197–203, 1985.

107. Kharasch ED, Labroo R: Metabolism of ketamine stereoisomers by human liver microsomes. Anesthesiology 77:1201–1207, 1992.

108. Adams HA, Thiel A, Jung A, et al: Untersuchumgen mit S+ ketamin an probanden. Endokrine- und kreislaufreaktionen, aufwachverhalten und traumerlebnisse. Der Anaesthesist 41:588–596, 1992.

109. Albrecht S, Hering W, Schuttler J, Schwilden H: Neue intravenose anasthetika. Der Anaesthesist 45:1129–1141, 1996.

110. Hering W, Geisslinger G, Kamp DH, et al: Changes in the EEG power spectrum after midazolam anaesthesia combined with racemic or S+ ketamine. Acta Anaesthesiolog Scand 38:719–723, 1994.

111. Schuttler J, Stanski DR, White PF, et al: Pharmacodynamic modeling of the EEG effects of ketamine and its enantiomers in man. J Pharmacokinet Biopharm 15:241–253, 1987.

112. Geisslinger G, Hering W, Thomann P, et al: Pharmacokinetics and dynamics of ketamine enantiomers in surgical patients using a stereospecific analytical method. Br J Anaesth 70:666–671, 1993.

113. White PF, Ham J, Way WL, Trevor AJ: Pharmacology of ketamine isomers in surgical patients. Anesthesiology 52:231–239, 1980.

114. Doenicke A, Angster R, Maker M, et al: Die wirkung von S+ ketamin auf katecholamine und cortisol im serum. Der Anaesthesist 41:597–603, 1992.

115. Adams HA, Bauer R, Gebhardt B, et al: TIVA mit S+ ketamin in der orthopadischen alterschirugie. Der Anaesthesist 43:92–100, 1994.

116. Pfenninger E, Himmelseher S: Neuroprotektion durch ketamin auf zellularer ebene. Der Anaesthesist 46(suppl 1):s47–s54, 1997.

117. Himmelseher S, Pfenninger E, Georgieff M: The effects of ketamine isomers on neuronal injury and regneration in rat hippocampal neurons. Anesth Analg 83:505–512, 1996.

118. Cashin MF, Moravek V: The physiological action of cholesterol. Am J Physiol 82:294–298, 1927.

119. Sear JW, Sanders RS: Intra-patient comparison of the kinetics of alphaxalone and alphadolone in man. Eur J Anaesthesiol 1:113–121, 1984.

120. Visser SAG, Smulders CJGM, Reijers BPR, et al: Mechanism-based pharmacokinetic-pharmacodynamic modeling of concentration-dependent hysteresis and biphasic electroencephalogram effects of alphaxalone in rats. J Pharmacol Exp Ther 302:1158–1167, 2002.

121. Holly JMP, Trafford DJH, Sear JW, Makin HLJ: The in vivo metabolism of Althesin (alphaxalone + alphadolone acetate) in man. J Pharm Pharmacol 33:427–433, 1981.

122. Desmet G, Nemitz B, Biotieux JL, et al: Dosage de l'alphaxalone dans

le serum et les urines par chromatographie gaz-liquide. Ann Biol Clin (Paris) 37:83–88, 1979.

123. Uppington J, Kay NH, Sear JW: Propofol (Diprivan) as a supplement to nitrous oxide-oxygen for the maintenance of anaesthesia. Postgrad Med J 61(suppl 3):80–83, 1985.

124. Radford SG, Lockyer JA, Simpson PJ: Immunological aspects of adverse reactions to Althesin. Br J Anaesth 54:859–863, 1982.

125. Moneret-Vautrin DA, Laxenaire MC, Viry-Babel F: Anaphylaxis caused by anti-Cremophor EL IgG STS antibodies in a case of reaction to Althesin. Br J Anaesth 55:469–471, 1983.

126. Tachon P, Descotes J, Laschi-Loquerie A, et al: Assessment of the allergenic potential of Althesin and its constituents. Br J Anaesth 55:715–717, 1983.

127. Simpson PJ, Radford SG, Lockyer JA, Sear JW: Some predisposing factors to hypersensitivity reactions following first exposure to Althesin. Anaesthesia 40:420–423, 1985.

128. Figdor SK, Kodet MJ, Bloom BM, et al: Central activity and structure in a series of water soluble steroids. J Pharmacol Exp Ther 119:299–307, 1957.

129. Hewitt CL, Savage DS, Lewis JS, et al: Anticonvulsant and interneuronal blocking activity in some synthetic amino-steroids. J Pharm Pharmacol 16:765–767, 1964.

130. Hering WJ, Ihmsen H, Langer H, et al: Pharmacokinetic-pharmacodynamic modeling of the new steroid hypnotic eltanolone in healthy volunteers. Anesthesiology 85:1290–1299, 1996.

131. Fisher MM, Ross JD, Harle DA, Baldo B: Anaphylaxis to thiopentone: An unusual outbreak in a single hospital. Anaesth Intensive Care 17:361–365, 1989.

132. Moneret-Vautrin DA, Widmer S, Gueant J-L, et al: Simultaneous ana-phylaxis to thiopentone and a neuromuscular blocker: A study of two cases. Br J Anaesth 64:743–745, 1990.

133. Clarke RSJ: Adverse effects of intravenously administered drugs used in anaesthetic practice. Drugs 22:26–41, 1981.

134. Watkins JA: Etomidate: An "immunologically safe" anaesthetic agent. Anaesthesia 38(suppl):34–38, 1983.

135. Krumholz W, Muller H, Gerlach H, et al: Ein fall von anaphylaktoider reaktion nach gabe von etomidat. Der Anaesthesist 33:161–162, 1984.

136. Sold M, Rothhammer A: Lebensbedrohliche anaphylaktoide reaktion nach etomidat. Der Anaesthesist 34:208–210, 1985.

137. Fazackerley EJ, Martin AJ, Tolhurst-Cleaver CL, Watkins J: Anaphylactoid reaction following the use of etomidate. Anaesthesia 43:953–954, 1988.

138. Mathieu A, Goudsouzian N, Snider MT: Reaction to ketamine: Anaphylactoid or anaphylactic. Br J Anaesth 47:624, 1975.

139. Laxenaire MC, Moneret-Vautrin D, Vervloet D: The French experience of anaphylactoid reactions. Int Anesthesiol Clin 23:145–160, 1985.

140. Ducart AR, Watremez C, Louagie YA, et al: Propofol-induced anaphylactoid reaction during for cardiac surgery. J Cardiothoracic Vasc Anesth 14:200–201, 2000.

141. Homanics GE, DeLorey TM, Firestone LL, et al: Mice devoid of g-aminobutyric acid type A receptor β_3 subunit have epilepsy, cleft palate, and hypersensitive behavior. Proc Natl Acad Sci USA 94:4143–4148, 1997.

142. Homanics GE, Quinlan JJ, Mihalek RM, Firestone LL: Alcohol and anesthetic mechanisms in genetically engineered mice. Front Biosci 3:D548-D558, 1998.

25

Sedatives, Anxiolytics, and Amnestics

Uwe Rudolph, MD • Florence Crestani, PhD • Hanns Möhler, PhD • Juliana Barr, MD • Timothy M. DeLorey, PhD • Jelveh Lameh, PhD • M. Frances Davies, PhD

The inhibitory tone for information processing in the central nervous system (CNS) can be enhanced pharmacologically to various degrees. This is exploited therapeutically in the treatment of mental disorders such as generalized anxiety states, panic attacks, post-traumatic stress disorders, and anxious depression, as well as in the treatment of epilepsy, muscle tension, and sleep disorders. In its most extreme case, the reduction of CNS activity is associated with a loss of consciousness as induced by anesthetic agents. Many of the agents used for these conditions act by enhancing the fast neuronal inhibition mediated by the neurotransmitter γ-aminobutyric acid (GABA).

The GABA type A (GABA$_A$) receptor is the target for the action of anxiolytics, sedatives, and amnestic agents such as the benzodiazepines, sedative barbiturates (see Chapter 24), neurosteroids (see Chapter 24), and general anesthetics (see Chapter 23). An anxiolytic activity can also be mediated through the serotonin (5-HT) system as shown by the clinical use of the 5-HT$_{1A}$ receptor ligand buspirone and of selective serotonin reuptake inhibitors (SSRIs). However, the 5-HT system mediates an adaptive process because the onset of the anxiolytic drug action is not immediate but occurs as a response with a delay of up to 2 weeks.

The modulation of GABA$_A$ receptor function by ligands of the benzodiazepine site remains a powerful means to induce anxiolytic activity and sedation. These ligands include the classical benzodiazepines as well as chemically different agents such as zolpidem. The pharmacology of GABA$_A$ receptor subtypes is being further dissected by genetically engineered reagents. These studies have revealed that the α$_1$-subunit mediates sedation, whereas receptors containing the α$_2$-subunit mediate anxiolytic activity.[1,2]

The insights into the subtype-specificity of benzodiazepine actions obtained by analyzing point-mutated mice provide a blueprint for the development of novel drugs with a better clinical profile than the benzodiazepines currently in clinical use. If a sedative action is to be avoided, a ligand should fail to interact with the α$_1$ receptor or should display no or only a minimal intrinsic activity at this receptor. The novel ligand L 838417 represents a major step forward in this direction providing hope for a nonsedative anxiolytic agent.[3] In the future, an even more specific profiling of ligands toward GABA$_A$ receptors containing the α$_2$ subunit may lead to even more selective anxiolytic drugs.

In addition, the 5-HT system can indirectly mediate anxiolytic activity as shown mainly by the use of SSRIs in the treatment of anxiety disorders. Surprisingly, 5-HT receptor subtypes had no major impact as anxiolytic drug targets apart from buspirone acting on 5-HT$_{1A}$ receptors.

MECHANISMS OF DRUG ACTION

GABA is the major inhibitory neurotransmitter in the CNS operating in local feedback and feed-forward circuits. Generated in presynaptic nerve endings from glutamate by the action of the enzyme glutamic acid decarboxylase, GABA undergoes vesicular release on the arrival of an action potential (Fig. 25–1). Two types of receptors serve as targets for the neurotransmitter, the ionotropic GABA$_A$ receptor and the metabotropic, G protein–coupled GABA$_B$ receptor, the latter mediating a comparatively slow response. Most GABA$_A$ receptors possess binding sites for various modulators (Fig. 25–2). These include benzodiazepines, barbiturates, neuro-

steroids, loreclezole, γ-butyrolactones, ethanol, zinc, volatile anesthetics (e.g., enflurane and isoflurane), and intravenous (IV) anesthetics (e.g., etomidate and propofol).[4–7]

The GABA$_A$ receptors do not represent a single uniform signal transduction system. Based on the presence of 7 subunit families comprising at least 18 subunits in the CNS (α_{1-6}, β_{1-3}, γ_{1-3}, δ, ε, θ, ρ_{1-3}) the GABA$_A$ receptors display an extraordinary structural heterogeneity. Most GABA$_A$ receptors subtypes *in vivo* are believed to be composed of α-, β-, and γ-subunits. The role of the δ, ε, and θ subunits, which have a limited expression pattern in brain, remains to be

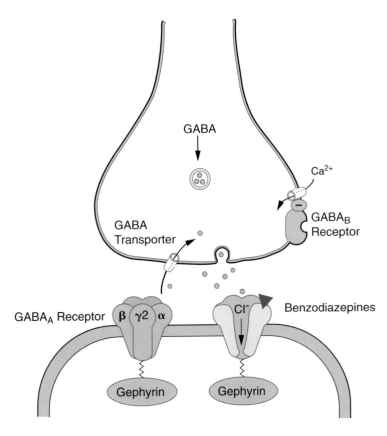

Figure 25–1. GABAergic synapse. Scheme of the GABAergic synapse, depicting the major elements of signal transduction. GABA$_A$ receptors in the brain are pentameric ligand-gated ion channels assembled from various types of subunits. On the cytoplasmic side they are indirectly linked to the anchoring protein gephyrin. GABA, γ-aminobutyric acid.

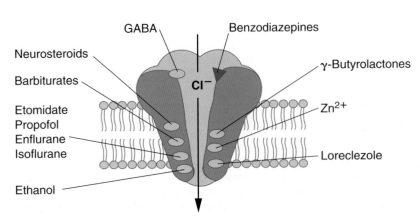

Figure 25–2. Model of a γ-aminobutyric acid type A (GABA$_A$) receptor complex and its binding sites. In addition to the binding sites for the physiologic neurotransmitter GABA, GABA$_A$ receptors have modulatory binding sites for benzodiazepines, barbiturates, neurosteroids, γ-butyrolactones, Zn^{2+}, loreclezole, and ethanol and also for general anesthetics such as etomidate, propofol, isoflurane, and enflurane. The positioning and size of the binding sites is arbitrary.

determined, but it is possible that they may substitute for the γ-subunit in αβγ combinations. The physiologic significance of the structural diversity of $GABA_A$ receptors lies in the provision of receptors that differ in their channel kinetics, affinity for GABA, rate of desensitization, and subcellular positioning (see reviews[4,5,8–11]). Thus in addition to the mechanisms outlined earlier, the receptor properties shape the response to a benzodiazepine drug in a region- or neuron-specific manner (Table 25–1).

Receptors containing the α_1-, α_2-, α_3-, or α_5-subunits in combination with any β-subunit and the γ_2-subunit are most prevalent in the brain and sensitive to modulation by benzodiazepines (see Table 25–1). They are differentially distributed in the mammalian brain.[12] The α_1-containing $GABA_A$ receptors are the most abundant receptor subtype, making up about 60% of all $GABA_A$ receptors in the brain. They are highly abundant in cerebral and cerebellar cortices, mainly in interneurons, as well as in thalamus and pallidum. The α_2-containing $GABA_A$ receptors are found mainly in hippocampus, amygdala, accumbens, and striatum. The α_3-containing $GABA_A$ receptors are unique for noradrenergic and serotonergic neurons of the brain stem, basal forebrain cholinergic neurons, and the reticular nucleus of the thalamus. The α_5-containing $GABA_A$ receptors are mainly found in the hippocampus and are differentiated from receptors containing the α_1-, α_2-, and α_3-subunits by a virtual lack of affinity for zolpidem (see Table 25–1).

$GABA_A$ receptors that do not respond to classical benzodiazepine drugs are of low abundance and are largely characterized by α_4- and α_6-subunits. Receptors containing the α_6-subunit are restricted to the granule cell layer of the cerebellum. In the retina, homomeric ρ-subunit–containing receptors are likewise insensitive to benzodiazepines and have also been termed $GABA_C$ receptors.[5,13]

$GABA_A$ receptors are clustered in GABAergic synapses but also occur ubiquitously in extrasynaptic sites particularly in cerebellum, thalamus, and cerebral cortex.[14] Receptors containing the δ-subunit in the cerebellum are exclusively found in extrasynaptic sites[15] mediating tonic inhibition of neuronal activity.[16] Synaptic receptors can be differentially targeted to specific synapses. For instance, the receptors containing the α_2 subunit in hippocampal pyramidal cells are concentrated in synapses on the axon initial segment.[17,18] In addition, synaptic and extrasynaptic receptors can differ in their desensitization kinetics, in line with their distinct functional roles. Extrasynaptic receptors containing the δ-subunit display a high affinity for GABA and low desensitization; thus these are ideal for tonic inhibition.[19]

The benzodiazepines do not activate the $GABA_A$ receptors by themselves. Benzodiazepines rather modulate the response to GABA by enhancing the affinity of the receptor for GABA. In many synapses, not all $GABA_A$ receptors are occupied by GABA when the neurotransmitter is released into the synaptic cleft. In the presence of a benzodiazepine drug, more receptors can be recruited for activation by the neurotransmitter GABA and the peak current amplitude is enhanced (Fig. 25–3). Other synapses operate in such a way that all $GABA_A$ receptors are occupied by GABA when the neurotransmitter is released into the synaptic cleft and no further recruitment of receptors is possible. In this case, benzodiazepine drugs do not directly enhance the amplitude of

the receptor response. Thus benzodiazepines have a built-in ceiling effect that prevents them from exceeding the physiologic maximum of GABA inhibition. The low toxicity of the benzodiazepine drugs and their corresponding clinical safety is attributed to this built-in limitation of their effect on GABAergic neurotransmission. However, irrespective of

TABLE 25–1.

$GABA_A$ Receptor Subtypes

Subunit Composition	Pharmacologic Characteristics
$\alpha_1\beta_2\gamma_2$	Major subtype (60% of all $GABA_A$ receptors). Mediates the sedative, amnestic, and to a large extent the anticonvulsant action of benzodiazepine site agonists. High affinity for classical benzodiazepines, zolpidem, and the antagonist flumazenil.
$\alpha_2\beta_3\gamma_2$	Minor subtype (15–20%). Mediates anxiolytic action of benzodiazepine site agonists. High affinity for classical benzodiazepine agonists and the antagonist flumazenil. Intermediate affinity for zolpidem.
$\alpha_3\beta_n\gamma_2$	Minor subtype (10–15%). High affinity for classical benzodiazepine agonists and the antagonist flumazenil. Intermediate affinity for zolpidem
$\alpha_4\beta_n\gamma/\alpha_4\beta_n\delta$	Less than 5% of all receptors. Insensitive to classical benzodiazepine agonists and zolpidem.
$\alpha_5\beta_{(1/3)}\gamma_2$	Less than 5% of all receptors. High affinity for classical benzodiazepine agonists and the antagonist flumazenil. Very low affinity for zolpidem.
$\alpha_6\beta_{2,3}\gamma_2$	Less than 5% of all receptors. Insensitive to classical benzodiazepine agonists and zolpidem.
$\alpha_6\beta_n\delta$	Minor population. Lacks benzodiazepine site.
ρ	Homomeric receptors. Insensitive to bicuculline, barbiturates, baclofen, and all benzodiazepine site ligands. Also termed *GABA_C receptor* (for nomenclature see Löw and colleagues[2] and Sigel and Buhr[25]).

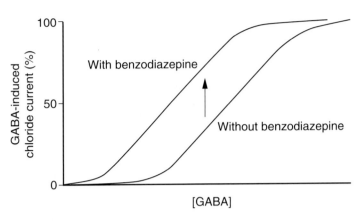

Figure 25–3. Benzodiazepine-induced potentiation of γ-aminobutyric acid (GABA) action. The GABA dose-response curve is shifted to the left in the presence of a benzodiazepine drug such as diazepam. The chloride current, which is induced at a given submaximal concentration of GABA, is increased. Benzodiazepines are effective only in the presence of GABA (use-dependence). The maximal inhibition by GABA (100%) cannot be further increased by benzodiazepine drugs. This activity-dependent and self-limiting modulation of the GABA_A receptor is the basis for the therapeutic actions of benzodiazepines.

the degree of synaptic receptor occupancy by GABA, the decay of the GABA response is prolonged in the presence of a benzodiazepine drug. This effect slightly enhances the GABA response even in those synapses that display a maximal receptor occupancy by GABA.[20,21] These principles of the synaptic action of the benzodiazepine drugs extend to ligands of the benzodiazepine site that are chemically unrelated to benzodiazepines such as zolpidem, zaleplon, or zopiclone (see "Non-benzodiazepine Ligands").

Tranquilizing actions are usually achieved at low doses of benzodiazepine drugs. The neuronal networks that mediate the anxiolytic activity are therefore considered to be those with a high receptor reserve. At higher drug doses, additional neuronal networks with a lower receptor reserve

are thought to be invoked, because the affinity of the drug was the same for all GABA_A receptors. This view provided a rational basis for the dose-dependent spectrum of benzodiazepine effects. The concept of differential receptor reserve was validated in animal experiments.[22,23] Partial agonists acting at the benzodiazepine site were therefore expected to provide a better separation between the desired anxiolytic effect and the unwanted side effects compared with the classical full agonistic drugs. A preferential anxiolytic activity of partial agonists was proven in animal models.[24] However, the partial agonists bretazenil and abecarnil largely failed to substantiate their promise in clinical trials.

PRECLINICAL PHARMACOLOGY

Ligands for the Benzodiazepine Binding Site on γ-Aminobutyric Acid Type A Receptors

The benzodiazepine binding site is thought to be located at the interface between α- and γ-subunits of the GABA_A receptors.[25] Wieland and collaborators[26] identified the histidine residue 101 in the extracellular N-terminal region of the α_1-subunit of the GABA_A receptor as being essential for diazepam (Valium) binding.[27] When this histidine residue in the α_1-subunit was replaced by an arginine, the point-mutated, α_1-containing, GABA_A receptor was no longer able to bind diazepam. This molecular switch was confirmed to be operative in all benzodiazepine-sensitive GABA_A receptors—that is, also those containing the α_2-, α_3-, and α_5-subunits as tested in recombinant systems.[28] In point-mutated mice, the mutated receptor subunits were expressed at normal levels and with a regional and subcellular distribution indistinguishable from that of wild type control mice, as shown by Western blotting, immunohistochemistry, and immunofluorescence. The diazepam insensitivity of the mutated GABA_A receptor subtypes was confirmed in ligand

binding studies, which showed that the affinity for diazepam was reduced at least 300-fold. Importantly, the physiologic functions of the GABA_A receptors appeared to be unchanged in the mutant mouse lines.

Benzodiazepines

Benzodiazepine is a chemical term that has become the hallmark of an entire class of drugs. Since their first introduction in the late 1950s, the benzodiazepine drugs have been widely used in the treatment of sleep disorders, generalized anxiety disorders, panic attacks, status epilepticus, and muscle tension. All actions of the benzodiazepine drugs including their side effects such as anterograde amnesia and ethanol potentiation are generated by their interaction with GABA_A receptors. This is demonstrated by the ability of the benzodiazepine antagonist flumazenil (Anexate; Roche Product Limited, Isando, South Africa) to alleviate all of these actions.[29] The benzodiazepine binding site was discovered by [3H]-diazepam binding to brain membranes and originally termed benzodiazepine receptor.[30,31] When a benzodiazepine was covalently crosslinked, its target protein was identified, which was to become the first known component of the $GABA_A$ receptor,[32] later termed *α-subunit*.[33]

Classical benzodiazepine drugs such as diazepam, clonazepam, or alprazolam were found to interact with comparable affinity with most $GABA_A$ receptors in the brain with only a small population of $GABA_A$ receptors being benzodiazepine-insensitive. It was therefore somewhat surprising that the modulation of a single, ubiquitously distributed receptor system would result in such a diversity of therapeutic drug actions. However, the sophisticated mode of action of benzodiazepines is only currently becoming fully appreciated.

Sedation, Anterograde Amnesia, and Anticonvulsant Activity

The sedative action of diazepam is mediated by the $GABA_A$ receptors containing the $α_1$-subunit.[1,3] This conclusion is based on the finding that the diazepam-induced impairment of the horizontal motor activity, monitored in a familiar environment, was absent in $α_1$ dysfunctional mice, even at a high dose (30 mg/kg).[1] Furthermore, the sedative action of diazepam was not impaired in $α_2$ or $α_3$ dysfunctional mice.[2]

The anterograde amnesia induced by diazepam was likewise absent in $α_1$ dysfunctional mice, as tested in a passive-avoidance paradigm. The specificity of this effect was confirmed by the finding that the muscarinic antagonist, scopolamine, retained its amnesic action in $α_1$ dysfunctional (H101R) mice. Thus the anterograde amnesic action of diazepam is mediated by $GABA_A$ receptors containing the $α_1$ subunit.[1]

The anticonvulsant activity of diazepam was determined in the pentylenetetrazole convulsion test. Doses of diazepam that were able to protect all wild type mice from tonic seizures were only partially effective in $α_1$-deficient mice, with about half of the animals being protected from tonic seizures.[1] The anticonvulsant activity of diazepam in the pentylenetetrazole convulsion test did not differ among the $α_2$- and $α_3$-deficient mice and their wild type control subjects.[2]

Anxiolytic Activity

It had been speculated that the anxiolytic action of benzodiazepines would be caused by inhibition of noradrenergic neurons in the locus ceruleus and its interaction with serotonergic neurons. The major neurons in the reticular-activating system (i.e., noradrenergic, dopaminergic, and serotonergic neurons of the brain stem) and in the basal forebrain (cholinergic neurons) are exceptional in that they express $GABA_A$ receptors that are characterized by the $α_3$-subunit. However, the anxiolytic activity of diazepam was unimpaired in several tests of anxiety in the $α_3$-deficient mice compared with wild type mice.[2]

Brain areas involved in the processing of fear include the thalamus, cerebral cortex, hippocampus, and amygdala.[34] Neurons that express $GABA_A$ receptors containing the $α_2$-subunit, about 15% of all $GABA_A$ receptors in the brain,[35] are found in limbic areas (e.g., hippocampus, amygdala,

cortex, and striatum). When $α_2$-deficient mice were tested, the anxiolytic activity of diazepam was absent in the light/dark choice test and the elevated plus maze test,[2] indicating that the neurons expressing $GABA_A$ receptors containing the $α_2$-subunit specifically mediate the anxiolytic action of diazepam (Table 25–2). Interestingly, the output synapses of cholecystokinin/vasoactive intestinal polypeptide–containing basket cells on soma and proximal dendrites are also rich in $α_2$-subunit–containing synaptic receptors; furthermore, the cholecystokinin/vasoactive intestinal polypeptide–containing basket cells express presynaptic type 1 cannabinoid receptors.[36] Both cannabinoid agonists and cholecystokinin type B receptor antagonists are known to have anxiolytic actions.[37–39]

Myorelaxant Activity

Diazepam (10 mg/kg) induced significant myorelaxation in wild type mice as tested in the horizontal wire test; however, the same dose of diazepam had no myorelaxant effect when tested in $α_2$-deficient mice, indicating that the myorelaxant action of diazepam is largely mediated by $GABA_A$ receptors containing the $α_2$-subunit.[40] At a dose of 30 mg/kg diazepam, however, diazepam displayed some residual myorelaxant activity in $α_2$-deficient mice, causing a minority of mice to fall from the horizontal wire.[40] This indicates that at high doses of diazepam other $GABA_A$ receptor, subtypes are

TABLE 25–2.

Dissection of the Benzodiazepine Pharmacology

	$α_1$	$α_2$	$α_3$
Sedation	+	−	−
Anterograde amnesia	+	ND	ND
Anticonvulsion	+	−	−
Anxiolysis	−	+	−
Myorelaxation	−	+	(+)

The functional roles of γ-aminobutyric acid type A receptor subtypes mediating particular actions of diazepam are indicated. The analysis is based on the pharmacology of mice that carry a histidine to arginine point mutation in the respective α-subunit [$α_1$(H101R), $α_2$(H101R), or $α_3$(H126R)]. (−) Indicates that the response is not mediated by the respective receptor in wild-type mice. This is based on the finding that the response is indistinguishable from wild-type in the respective point-mutated mice. (+) Indicates that the response is mediated by the respective receptor in wild-type mice. This is based on the finding that the response is missing in the respective point-mutated mouse line. See text for details on the behavioral tests used.
ND, not determined.

involved in the mediation of the myorelaxant action of diazepam. The agonist at the $GABA_B$ receptor, baclofen, induced myorelaxation in both wild type and α_2-deficient mice,[40] demonstrating the specificity of the interruption. In α_3-deficient mice, diazepam produced a similar impairment of the grasping reflex as wild type mice at doses up to 10 mg/kg diazepam.[40] At 30 mg/kg, however, a significantly smaller percentage of mice (62%) displayed an impaired grasping reflex compared with wild type mice (100%).[40] Taken together, these data demonstrate that the myorelaxant activity of diazepam is primarily mediated by $GABA_A$ receptors containing the α_2-subunit but at greater concentrations and also by $GABA_A$ receptors containing the α_3 subunit (see Table 25–2). This finding is consistent with the presence of α_2- and α_3-subunits in the spinal cord.[41]

Hypnotic Activity

Because the sedative activity of diazepam is clearly mediated by $GABA_A$ receptors containing the α_1-subunit, it was expected that the hypnotic activity as analyzed by electroencephalogram (EEG) measurements would also be mediated by $GABA_A$ receptors containing the α_1-subunit. After all, sedative/hypnotic drugs display a sedative activity at lower doses and a hypnotic activity at higher doses. Surprisingly, the α_1-deficient mice, which are resistant to the sedative effect of diazepam, expressed a similar reduction in initial rapid eye movement (REM) sleep as observed in wild type mice; furthermore, the increase in power density greater than 21 Hz in non-REM sleep and waking and the suppression of slow-wave activity (0.75–4 Hz) in non-REM sleep were present in both genotypes and even more pronounced in the α_1-deficient mice. The number of brief awakenings per hour of sleep was decreased, and thus sleep continuity enhanced only in α_1-deficient mice.[42] These data suggest that the sedative and hypnotic action of diazepam are likely to be mediated by different receptor subtypes and are thus qualitatively different phenomena mediated by distinct neuronal circuits. These results also raise the intriguing question whether the hypnotic activity of zolpidem (see discussion of zolpidem, zaleplon, and zopoclone in "Nonbenzodiazepine Ligands of the Benzodiazepine Site") is indeed caused by its preferential affinity for $GABA_A$ receptors containing the α_1-subunit or rather is caused by its intermediate affinity for $GABA_A$ receptors containing the α_2- and α_3-subunits.

Non-Benzodiazepine Ligands of the Benzodiazepine Site

Ligands of the benzodiazepine site of $GABA_A$ receptors comprise not only drugs that contain the benzodiazepine ring structure but also ligands with different chemical structures, such as zolpidem, zaleplon, and zopiclone. The imidazopyridine zolpidem is widely used as hypnotic. It differs from the classical benzodiazepine drugs in that it interacts preferentially with $GABA_A$ receptor containing the α_1 subunit. When tested at recombinant receptors, zolpidem displays a high potency at $GABA_A$ receptors containing the α_1-subunit and medium potency at $GABA_A$ receptors containing the α_2- and α_3-subunits but fails to interact with $GABA_A$ receptors containing the α_5-subunit. Thus it was postulated that its sedative/hypnotic effect[43] would be mediated by the $GABA_A$ receptors containing the α_1-subunit. However, the similarly α_1-selective imidazopyridine alpidem has been characterized as a selective anxiolytic.[44,45] An alternative explanation for the preferential sedative/hypnotic effect of zolpidem was the extraordinary strong GABA shift—an increase in the affinity of zolpidem by a factor of 3 in the presence of 100 μM GABA in vitro. In α_1-deficient mice, the sedative effect of zolpidem was absent, indicating that the sedative action is exclusively mediated by $GABA_A$ receptors containing the α_1-subunit.[46] Similarly, the activity of zolpidem against pentylenetetrazole-induced tonic convulsions is also completely mediated by $GABA_A$ receptors containing the α_1-subunit.[46] Although these results clearly point to α_1 receptors as mediators of the sedative and anticonvulsant activity of zolpidem, it is not clear whether this also holds for the hypnotic action as assessed by changes in the EEG spectrum.

Zaleplon (CL284,846) is a pyrazolopyrimidine hypnotic developed for the treatment of insomnia.[47,48] At recombinant receptors, zaleplon binds preferentially to $GABA_A$ receptors containing the α_1-subunit and to receptors containing the γ_3-subunit but binds 8- to 20-fold less to $GABA_A$ receptors containing the α_2- or α_5-subunits.[49] Thus zaleplon is largely a ligand with preference for $GABA_A$ receptors containing the α_1-subunit. The contribution to the hypnotic action of its interaction with $GABA_A$ receptors containing the γ_3-subunit is unclear because these receptors represent only a small population in the brain.

Unlike zolpidem and zaleplon, the cyclopyrrolone zopiclone does not display preferential affinity to specific $GABA_A$ receptor subtypes.[50] It is used as a hypnotic and also displays sedative, anticonvulsant, and muscle relaxant actions.

Drugs Acting at the Serotonin System

Azaperone

Azaperones (e.g., buspirone) have a high affinity at $5\text{-}HT_{1A}$ receptors and a low affinity at $5\text{-}HT_2$ receptors. At somatodendritic $5\text{-}HT_{1A}$ receptors, they act as partial agonists, leading to decreased firing of dorsal raphe serotonin neurons and decreased synthesis and release of serotonin.[51,52] Buspirone can be used to treat generalized anxiety disorder with an onset of its anxiolytic effect after several days. It is therefore assumed that adaptations to the long-term antiserotonergic actions of azaperone form the basis of their anxiolytic action. Unlike currently used benzodiazepines, buspirone has no sedative side effects. It can be used, for example, in patients with anxiety of moderate intensity but not in those with severe anxiety with panic attacks.[53,54]

Selective Serotonin Reuptake Inhibitors

SSRIs (e.g., fluoxetine) inhibit the neuronal reuptake of serotonin. Although they are used primarily as antidepressants, they are also effective in the treatment of panic disorder, obsessive/compulsive disorder, social phobia, and potentially post-traumatic stress disorder.[55]

CLINICAL PHARMACOLOGY OF THE BENZODIAZEPINES

Benzodiazepines have sedative, amnestic, anxiolytic, and muscle relaxant properties that make them effective perioperative sedative agents. They are also used for the treatment of seizures and symptoms associated with alcohol withdrawal. Midazolam, lorazepam (Ativan), and diazepam are the most commonly used benzodiazepines for perioperative sedation. Patients may receive either single intramuscular (IM) or IV bolus injections for short-term sedation during a surgical procedure or repeated IV boluses or continuous infusions for postoperative sedation in the intensive care unit (ICU). The observed differences in the onset, duration, and offset of effects with midazolam (Versed; Hoffman-LaRoche, Nutley, N. J.), lorazepam, and diazepam are explained by differences in their (1) receptor binding affinities (which determines potency), (2) lipid solubilities (which determines the speed with which each drug crosses the blood–brain barrier and the degree to which it redistributes into peripheral tissues), and (3) pharmacokinetics (which determines the uptake, distribution, and elimination of each drug).

Physicochemical Properties

Midazolam, lorazepam, and diazepam are available in parenteral form and are therefore the primary benzodiazepines used in anesthetic practice. Clinically, their observed differences relate to differences in their pharmacokinetic and pharmacodynamic properties. All benzodiazepines have a high lipid/water distribution coefficients in the nonionized form. The lipophilicity of these agents can vary more than 50-fold. They are highly bound to plasma proteins, particularly albumin, as a function of their lipophilicity.[56] Approximately 94% to 97% of midazolam is bound to plasma proteins, whereas 85% of lorazepam and 99% of diazepam is bound to plasma proteins. Patients with hypoalbuminemia (e.g., caused by cirrhosis or chronic renal failure) have a greater unbound fraction of benzodiazepines, which may increase their sensitivity to these agents. All benzodiazepines are essentially completely absorbed with oral administration. After IV administration, they are rapidly taken up into the brain and other highly perfused organs, with the benzodiazepine concentration in the cerebrospinal fluid (CSF) approximating the concentration of the free drug in the plasma.

Midazolam is a crystalline compound with the chemical formula 8-chloro-6-(2-fluorophenyl)-1-methyl-4H-imidazol[1,5-a][1,4]benzodiazepine. Midazolam itself is insoluble in water; however, its hydrochloride salt is soluble in aqueous solutions. In the acidic environment used to solubilize midazolam, it exists in an equilibrium between closed and open ring forms; however, at the physiologic pH, midazolam reverts to being in the closed ring form, which is lipophilic and the pharmacologically active form.[69] The chemical formula for lorazepam is 7-chloro-5(2-chlorophenyl)-1,3-dihydro-3-hydroxy-2H-1,4-benzodiazepin-2-one. Lorazepam is a nearly white powder, which is extremely insoluble in water. The chemical formula for diazepam is 7-chloro-1,3-dihydro-1-methyl-5-phenyl-2H-1,4-benzodiazepin-2-one. Diazepam is a colorless crystalline compound that is also insoluble in water.

Metabolism

Midazolam is rapidly metabolized by the liver through oxidative hydroxylation to active (1- and 4-hydroxymidazolam) and inactive metabolites.[58,59] The hepatic clearance of midazolam is reduced in the presence of drugs that inhibit the cytochrome P450 enzyme system, such as cimetidine, erythromycin, calcium channel blockers, and antifungal agents. The principal active metabolite of midazolam, 1-hydroxymidazolam, is conjugated in the liver to 1-hydroxymidazolam glucuronide, which is subsequently cleared by the kidneys.[60–63] This glucuronide metabolite of midazolam has substantial pharmacologic activity.[64] In patients with renal failure who receive repeated IV boluses or continuous infusions of midazolam over several days, plasma levels of the 1-hydroxymidazolam glucuronide may become significantly elevated and may have synergistic sedative effects with the parent compound.[65,66]

Lorazepam is extensively conjugated to the inactive 3-O-phenolic glucuronide in the liver, undergoes enterohepatic recirculation, and is excreted mainly by the kidneys.[67]

Diazepam is hepatically metabolized through oxidative N-demethylation to two active metabolites: desmethyldiazepam and oxazepam.[68] The active metabolites of diazepam are further metabolized through hepatic glucuronidation to inactive metabolites that are then excreted by the kidneys. The principal active diazepam metabolite, desmethyldiazepam, is only slightly less potent than diazepam and is metabolized much more slowly, with an elimination half-life that is 2 to 3 times that of diazepam.[69] Desmethyldiazepam may accumulate to a significant degree with chronic administration of diazepam, thereby prolonging the sedative effect of the parent compound.[70] In contrast, oxazepam does not accumulate with chronic administration of diazepam.

Pharmacokinetics

The clinical pharmacology of midazolam, lorazepam, and diazepam differ significantly during varying clinical circumstances including duration of drug administration, total dose of drug administered, and patient characteristics such as age, weight, and liver disease.

Midazolam

The pharmacokinetics of short-term midazolam infusion regimens are best described by a two-compartment model with an estimated elimination half-life of 1.5 to 3.5 hours.[64,71] The elimination half-life of midazolam is increased in elderly patients because of decreases in metabolic clearance and in obese patients because of increases in the total volume of distribution.[71] In patients with severe liver disease, the volume of distribution for midazolam is increased, whereas the metabolic clearance is decreased, resulting in a prolonged elimination half-life.[72] Opioids may also decrease the metabolic clearance of midazolam.[73]

The pharmacokinetics of long-term continuous IV infusions of midazolam for sedation of ICU patients differ significantly from the pharmacokinetics of single IV bolus injections of midazolam. Both two- and three-compartment pharmacokinetic models have been derived for midazolam infusions in ICU patients.[65,74,75] ICU patients receiving continuous infusions of midazolam have both a slower metabolic clearance and a larger volume of distribution at steady-state, resulting in a much longer elimination half-life for midazolam.[65,74,75] In addition, the pharmacokinetics of long-term midazolam infusions in ICU patients are more dependent on patient characteristics such as age, height, weight, and body surface area.[65,74] Previous estimates of the elimination half-life for midazolam in these patients range from 1.5 to 50 hours.[74,76–80] With long-term administration, peripheral tissues become relatively saturated with midazolam, and midazolam clearance from the circulation becomes less dependent on redistribution into peripheral tissues and more dependent on hepatic metabolism. During these circumstances, midazolam plasma levels decrease much more slowly after discontinuation of the infusion and the apparent elimination half-life of midazolam (i.e., the context-sensitive half-life) is increased.[81] Table 25–3 compares the estimated pharmacokinetic parameters of midazolam after a single IV bolus injection in a healthy individual with those estimated for an ICU patient receiving a continuous IV infusion of midazolam for postoperative sedation.[65,71]

Lorazepam

The pharmacokinetics of lorazepam are best described by a two-compartment model.[57,65] Because the metabolism of lorazepam is somewhat independent of hepatic microsomal enzymes, lorazepam clearance is not altered significantly with age, liver disease, or by drugs such as cimetidine.[82] The volume of distribution and the elimination half-life of lorazepam are increased in obese patients. Compared with midazolam, lorazepam has a much slower metabolic clearance. This may be explained by that the hepatic glucuronidation of lorazepam occurs much more slowly than the oxidative hydroxylation of midazolam by the liver.[83,84] As a result, the elimination half-life of lorazepam is twice that of midazolam. The estimated volume of distribution of lorazepam increases with long-term administration, which increases the estimated elimination half-life of lorazepam during these circumstances by about 30%.[57,65] Table 25–4 compares the estimated pharmacokinetic parameters of lorazepam after a single IV bolus injection in a healthy individual with those estimated for a typical ICU patient receiving a continuous IV infusion of lorazepam for postoperative sedation.[57,65]

TABLE 25–3.

Midazolam Pharmacokinetic Parameters*

Model Parameters	Short-Term Sedation[†]	Long-Term Sedation[‡]
Volumes (L):		
Central (V_1)	29.6	28.2
Peripheral (V_2)	99.4	131
Steady-state (V_{ss})	129	159.2
Clearances (L • min^{-1}):		
Metabolic (Cl_1)	0.34	0.25
Peripheral (Cl_2)	0.99	0.6
Fractional coefficients:		
A	0.845	0.896
B	0.155	0.104
Exponents (min^{-1}):		
α	0.053	0.033
β	0.002	0.001
Rate constants (min^{-1}):		
k_{10}	0.011	0.009
k_{12}	0.034	0.021
k_{21}	0.01	0.005
Half-lives (min):		
$t_{(1/2)}\alpha$	13.1	20.71
$t_{(1/2)}\beta$	319.8	572.3

*Typical values derived from population pharmacokinetic models (65-year-old man, weight = 70 kg, height = 180 cm).

[†]Model derived from healthy volunteers receiving a single intravenous bolus (≤5 mg) of midazolam.

Source: Modified from Depoortere H, Zivkovic B, Lloyd KG, et al: Zolpidem, a novel nonbenzodiazepine hypnotic. I. Neuropharmacological and behavioral effect. J Pharmacol Exp Ther 237:649–658, 1986.

[‡]Model derived from intensive care unit patients receiving midazolam infusions for up to 72 hours (age- and weight-adjusted).

Source: Modified from Mohler H, Okada T: Benzodiazepine receptor: Demonstration in the central nervous system. Science 198:849–851, 1977.

Diazepam

Most studies of diazepam pharmacokinetics have been performed using noncompartmental analysis techniques, which yield single estimates of the total volume of distribution at steady-state, the clearance, and the elimination half-life of diazepam.[85,86] The pharmacokinetics of diazepam are complicated by the fact that diazepam undergoes enterohepatic circulation and that the accumulation of its principal metabolite, desmethyldiazepam, impairs the hepatic clearance

TABLE 25–4.

Lorazepam Pharmacokinetic Parameters*

Model Parameters	Short-term Sedation[†]	Long-term Sedation[‡]
Volumes (L):		
Central (V_1)	32.2	40.8
Peripheral (V_2)	41.3	102
Steady-state (V_{ss})	73.5	142.8
Clearances (L·min^{-1}):		
Metabolic (Cl_1)	0.07	0.11
Peripheral (Cl_2)	3.01	1.86
Fractional coefficients:		
A	0.570	0.731
B	0.430	0.269
Exponents (min^{-1}):		
α	0.166	0.066
β	0.001	0.001
Rate constants (min^{-1}):		
k_{10}	0.002	0.003
k_{12}	0.093	0.046
k_{21}	0.072	0.018
Half-lives (min):		
$t_{1/2}\alpha$	4.1	10.6
$t_{1/2}\beta$	736.0	952.5

*Typical values derived from population pharmacokinetic models (65-year-old man, weight = 70 kg, height = 180 cm).
[†]Model derived from healthy volunteers receiving a single intravenous bolus (2–4 mg) of lorazepam.
Source: Modified from Barnard ED, Skonick P, Olsen RW, et al: International Union of Pharmacology. XV. Subtypes of gamma-aminobutyric acid$_A$ receptors: Classification on the basis of subunit structure and receptor function. Pharmacol Rev 2:291–313, 1998.
[‡]Model derived from intensive care unit patients receiving lorazepam infusions for up to 72 hours.
Source: Modified from Mohler H, Okada T: Benzodiazepine receptor: Demonstration in the central nervous system. Science 198:849–851, 1977.

TABLE 25–5.

Diazepam Pharmacokinetic Parameters

Model Parameters	Values
Volumes (L):	
Central (V_1)	3.43
Rapid redistribution (V_2)	8.47
Slow redistribution (V_3)	87.51
Steady-state (V_{ss})	99.41
Clearances: (L·min^{-1})	
Metabolic (Cl_1)	0.03
Rapid peripheral (Cl_2)	1.10
Slow peripheral (Cl_3)	0.34
Fractional coefficients:	
A	0.793
B	0.176
C	0.031
Exponents (min^{-1}):	
α	0.532
β	0.029
γ	0.000
Rate constants (min^{-1})	
k_{10}	0.008
k_{12}	0.322
k_{13}	0.098
k_{21}	0.130
k_{31}	0.004
Half-lives (min):	
$t_{1/2}\alpha$	1.3
$t_{1/2}\beta$	24.0
$t_{1/2}\gamma$	2713.1

Typical values derived from a population pharmacokinetic model for diazepam in healthy adults receiving a single (30 mg) intravenous dose of diazepam.
Source: Möhler H, Fritschy JM, Rudolph U: A new benzodiazepine pharmacology. J Pharmacol Exp Ther 300:2–8, 2001.

of diazepam itself.[87,88] The few studies that have used multicompartmental analysis techniques to describe the pharmacokinetics of diazepam have been limited to healthy individuals receiving single IV doses of diazepam.[70,81,88] Currently, there have been no studies conducted to determine the pharmacokinetics of diazepam administered either as repeated IV boluses or as continuous infusions to critically ill patients for long-term sedation. Table 25–5 summarizes the estimated pharmacokinetic parameters of diazepam in a healthy adult receiving a single IV dose of diazepam.

From single-dose diazepam studies, the estimated volume of distribution for diazepam is between that of midazolam and lorazepam. However, the metabolic clearance of diazepam is much slower resulting in a long elimination half-life for diazepam with estimates ranging from 20 to 50 hours.[85] The elimination half-life of diazepam is further increased in elderly patients and in obese patients because of an increased volume of distribution.[70,87] Hepatic clearance of diazepam is not affected by age. Patients with cirrhosis typically demonstrate a fivefold increase in the elimination half-life of diazepam because of the combined effects of reduced metabolic clearance and an increased volume of distribution for diazepam.[87] Cimetidine reduces the hepatic clearance of both diazepam and desmethyldiazepam, which prolongs the elimination half-life of both the parent compound and its active metabolite.[89]

Pharmacodynamics

Midazolam

As a sedative, midazolam is twice as potent as diazepam, but only 1/3 to 1/2 as potent as lorazepam. As with other benzodiazepines, the amnestic effects of midazolam are more potent than its sedative effects. As a result, patients who are conscious after receiving midazolam may still be amnestic for events and relevant conversations for several hours. Midazolam potency is significantly increased in elderly patients.[65,90] The water solubility of midazolam is pH-dependent, with midazolam going into solution at a pH of 3. However, at physiologic pH (7.4), midazolam is highly lipid-soluble, enabling it to quickly cross the blood–brain barrier.[57] The equilibration half-life between midazolam blood levels and the EEG effects of midazolam is approximately 1 to 2 minutes.[64,91] The onset of effect after a single IV bolus injection of a typical sedative dose of midazolam (e.g., 1–2 mg) occurs within 30 seconds to 1 minute, with a time-to-peak effect of 3 to 5 minutes and a duration of sedation ranging from 15 to 80 minutes.[64,92] Midazolam may also be used for the induction of general anesthesia. A typical IV induction dose of midazolam (e.g., 0.2–0.35 mg/kg in adults) administered over 20 to 30 seconds will induce general anesthesia in about 110 seconds.[93] This is about twice as long as the induction time associated with thiopental administration. The onset of unconsciousness with midazolam induction is hastened in patients who have been premedicated with small amounts of opioid (e.g., 50–100 µg IV fentanyl or 1–2 mg IV morphine) administered within 3 to 5 minutes of administering the midazolam. Emergence from general anesthesia after induction with midazolam is up to 2.5 times longer than emergence after induction with thiopental, although discharge times from the recovery room are similar for both agents.[94,95]

With short-term administration of midazolam, emergence from sedation is relatively rapid because of redistribution of midazolam into peripheral tissues and its rapid metabolic clearance. With long-term administration in critically ill patients, midazolam accumulation in peripheral tissues together with a decreased hepatic clearance in these patients results in prolonged elevation of midazolam plasma levels after discontinuation of the infusion leading to delayed emergence from sedation.[65,74,96–98] Emergence time is also a function of the midazolam plasma concentration at the time that the infusion is discontinued. Patients maintained at deeper levels of sedation take longer to awaken than patients who are more lightly sedated for comparable periods. Figure 25–4 compares the predicted emergence times from midazolam in a typical patient following a single IV bolus with a continuous infusion of midazolam titrated to maintain either light or deep levels of sedation for 3 days. The predicted emergence time from a single 4 mg IV bolus injec-

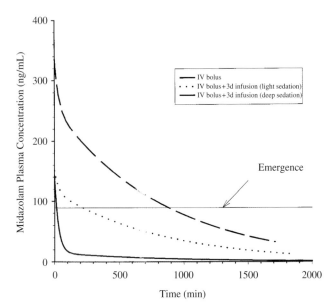

Midazolam Sedation Recovery Profiles

Figure 25–4. Sedation emergence times after a single (4 mg) intravenous (IV) bolus of midazolam compared with emergence from light and deep sedation midazolam regimens lasting 3 days: (1) light sedation (*initial bolus:* 4 mg; *infusion regimen:* 6 mg/hr × 3 hours, then 3 mg/hr × 12 hours, then 2.25 mg/hr thereafter); (2) deep sedation (*initial bolus:* 9.5 mg; *infusion regimen:* 12 mg/hr × 3 hours, then 8 mg/hr × 6 hours, then 5 mg/hr thereafter). Patient is a 65-year-old man (weight = 70 kg, height = 180 cm).

tion of midazolam is 20 minutes versus 4.5 hours after a 3-day infusion adjusted to maintain a light level of sedation and 15.5 hours after a 3-day infusion adjusted to maintain a deep level of sedation. The coadministration of analgesic doses of opioids significantly reduces midazolam requirements in these patients and leads to a more rapid emergence from sedation following discontinuation of the midazolam infusion.[65] If the midazolam and opioid infusions are discontinued simultaneously, emergence time is shortened by approximately 20%.[65] The emergence time from midazolam increases significantly with age, obesity, and in patients with severe liver disease because of increases in the elimination half-life of midazolam in these patients. The amnestic effects of midazolam after long-term sedation may last up to 24 hours beyond the sedative effects of midazolam.[65]

Lorazepam

Lorazepam as a sedative is 2 to 3 times more potent than midazolam and 5 to 6 times more potent than diazepam. Although the sedative potency of lorazepam is twice that of midazolam, the amnestic potency of lorazepam to midazolam is 4:1.[65] Like midazolam, lorazepam potency is increased in elderly patients.[65] Lorazepam has a slower onset of action than midazolam or diazepam because of its lower lipid solubility and its slower entry into the CSF.[99] After a single IV bolus injection of a sedative dose of lorazepam (e.g., 1–4 mg), the onset of effect occurs within of 1 to 2 minutes, with a time-to-peak effect of 20 to 30 minutes, and a duration of sedative effects ranging from 6 to 10 hours.[99] Emergence time is increased in obese patients because of the larger volume of distribution and the longer elimination half-life. The coadministration of analgesic doses of opioids significantly reduces lorazepam requirements and shortens the emergence time by 20% following discontinuation of the lorazepam infusion, assuming that the opioid infusion is discontinued simultaneously.[65] The slow onset and long duration of effect limits the usefulness of IV lorazepam either for induction of anesthesia or for conscious sedation during regional anesthesia or invasive procedures.

Lorazepam is often used as an economic alternative to midazolam for long-term sedation of ICU patients.[92] The slower onset and offset of sedation with lorazepam, together with its greater potency compared with midazolam, significantly increases the risk for oversedation and delayed emergence from sedation with lorazepam in ICU patients.[65] As with midazolam infusions, emergence time from a continuous infusion of lorazepam is a function of the duration of the infusion and the lorazepam plasma concentration at the time that the infusion is discontinued. Figure 25–5 compares the predicted emergence times from lorazepam after a single IV bolus with a continuous infusion of lorazepam titrated to maintain either light or deep levels of sedation for 3 days. The predicted emergence time from a single 3-mg IV bolus injection of lorazepam is 55 minutes, including the 30-minute equilibration time between the plasma and the CSF.

The emergence times from 3 days of light sedation with lorazepam is 13 hours versus 32 hours after 3 days of deep sedation with lorazepam.[65] As with midazolam, the coadministration of analgesic doses of opioids significantly reduces lorazepam requirements in these patients and shortens emergence time by about 20% once both drugs are discontinued.[65] The amnestic effects of lorazepam also last longer than with midazolam; patients receiving lorazepam infusions may be amnestic for up to several days even after the sedative effects of lorazepam have resolved.[65] In general, the time to emergence from the sedative and amnestic effects of lorazepam infusions is much longer than with midazolam infusions, particularly with deep sedation. These differences have clinically significant implications for the recovery of ICU patients who are intubated and mechanically ventilated, because delays in emergence lead to delays in weaning and extubation of these patients.[65] This may more than offset any cost savings realized from substituting lorazepam for midazolam for sedation of ICU patients.

Diazepam

Diazepam is only half as potent as midazolam, and one sixth as potent as lorazepam. As with the other benzodiazepines, the amnestic potency of diazepam is greater than its sedative potency, resulting in a longer duration of amnesia than sedation. Diazepam potency is also increased in elderly patients. The lipid solubility of diazepam is similar to that of midazolam in vivo. As a result, the onset of sedation with diazepam is quite rapid. Following a single 10 mg IV dose of diazepam, the onset of sedation occurs within 60 seconds, with a peak effect occurring within 3 to 4 minutes, and a duration of sedation ranging from 1 to 6 hours.[99–101] Diazepam may also be used for the induction of general anesthesia, although its long duration of action limits its use in this regard. A typical induction dose of diazepam (0.5 mg/kg given over 5 to 15 seconds) induces unconsciousness in approximately 40 seconds, but its duration of effect may last for several hours.[102]

Diazepam is sometimes administered for sedation of ICU patients as an economic alternative to either midazolam or lorazepam. Although there are no pharmacologic studies of diazepam in ICU patients, the pharmacokinetics of diazepam make drug accumulation with delayed emergence from sedation likely in these patients. Figure 25–6 compares the predicted emergence times after a single 10-mg IV bolus of diazepam with repeated dosing of 10 mg intravenously every 6 hours for 3 days versus a 10-mg IV bolus followed by an intermittent dosing regimen of 5 mg intravenously every 6 hours for 3 days. With a single IV bolus of diazepam, the emergence time is 10 minutes versus 31 minutes after a 3-day regimen of 5 mg intravenously every 6 hours versus 24 hours following a 10 mg intravenously every 6 hours regimen administered for 3 days. The rapid emergence time following single bolus injections is caused by the rapid redistribution of diazepam into peripheral tissues. With repeated bolus dosing of diazepam over several days, peripheral tissues become progressively saturated with diazepam and its duration of effect becomes more a function of its metabolic clearance and its long elimination half-life. Furthermore, the actual emergence times are probably

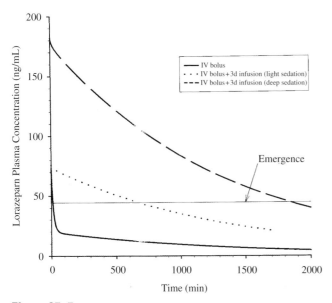

Lorazepam Sedation Recovery Profiles

Figure 25–5. Sedation emergence times after a single (3 mg) intravenous (IV) bolus of lorazepam compared with emergence from light and deep sedation lorazepam regimens lasting 3 days: (1) light sedation (*initial bolus:* 3 mg; *infusion regimen:* 2.5 mg/hr × 3 hours, then 0.75 mg/hr × 12 hours, then 0.5 mg/hr thereafter); (2) deep sedation (*initial bolus:* 7 mg; *infusion regimen:* 5 mg/hr × 3 hours, then 2 mg/hr × 6 hours, then 1.2 mg/hr thereafter). Patient is a 65 year-old-man (weight = 70 kg, height = 180 cm).

Diazepam Midazolam Sedation Recovery Profiles

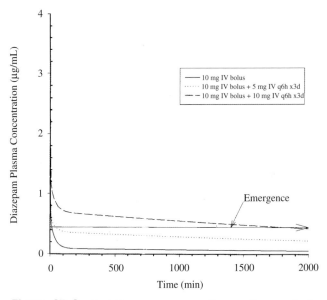

Figure 25–6. Sedation emergence times after a single (10 mg) intravenous (IV) bolus of diazepam compared with repeated dosing of high and low dose diazepam (10 mg intravenously every 6 hours vs. 10 mg IV bolus, then 5 mg intravenously every 6 hours) over 3 days. Patient is a 65 year-old-man (weight = 70 kg, height = 180 cm).

much longer in ICU patients receiving diazepam over several days than those predicted in Figure 25–6, because the volume of distribution and the elimination half-life of diazepam in these patients is likely to be even greater than those estimated in healthy individuals receiving individual doses of diazepam. The sedative effect of diazepam is further prolonged in ICU patients because of the accumulation of desmethyldiazepam, its long-acting metabolite. Desmethyldiazepam may also reduce the hepatic clearance of diazepam in these patients, further prolonging the elimination half-life and duration of effect of diazepam itself. Finally, the administration of cimetidine or other H_2-blockers in ICU patients may also prolong the effect of diazepam.

Adverse Effects

The most significant side effect of benzodiazepine administration is respiratory depression caused by a decrease in hypoxic drive.[103] The respiratory depressant effects of midazolam are greater than lorazepam and diazepam at equipotent doses.[104] The respiratory depressant effects of benzodiazepines are amplified in the presence of opioids and other sedatives and in patients with chronic obstructive pulmonary disease.

During certain circumstances, benzodiazepines may also cause significant cardiovascular depression primarily caused by systemic vasodilatation.[105] In addition, diazepam also causes myocardial depression. In healthy patients receiving small doses of benzodiazepines, the cardiovascular depres-

sion associated with benzodiazepine administration is minimal. Patients who are hemodynamically unstable or who are otherwise debilitated may develop clinically significant hypotension with parenteral benzodiazepine administration.[102] In addition, the administration of even small doses of benzodiazepines in conjunction with opioids, propofol, or thiopental can also result in significant hypotension caused by the synergistic effect of these agents.[106–109]

The efficacy of benzodiazepines may be reduced in patients who take oral benzodiazepines on a chronic basis, and it may be necessary to adjust the dose to achieve the desired pharmacologic effect. These patients are also at risk for having a withdrawal seizure if given the benzodiazepine antagonist flumazenil.[110]

Drug Interactions

Benzodiazepines have synergistic sedative effects with other CNS depressants including inhalational and IV anesthetics, opiates, and α_2 agonists. Benzodiazepines reduce anesthetic requirements for both inhalation anesthetics,[111] and intravenous anesthetics (*e.g.*, propofol[112,113] and thiopental[114]) Benzodiazepine interaction with opiates is not straightforward. There is a synergistic interaction of midazolam and fentanyl for the induction of anesthesia,[115] and midazolam potentiates the respiratory depressant effects of alfentanil.[116] However, the analgesic action of opiates is reduced in the presence of benzodiazepines.[117] Further evidence that benzodiazepines inhibit the analgesia effects of opioids is that flumazenil, a benzodiazepine antagonist, enhances the postoperative analgesic effects of morphine, reduces morphine requirements, and decreases the sedative, emetic, and cardiopulmonary depressant effects of morphine in patients who have received benzodiazepine after surgery.[116,118,119] Preclinical studies of α_2 agonists, such as dexmedetomidine, have shown synergistic sedative effects while reversing the cardiovascular depressant effects of benzodiazepines.[120]

Dosage and Administration Guidelines

Midazolam, lorazepam, and diazepam may be administered for preoperative sedation, induction, and maintenance of general anesthesia, conscious sedation for invasive procedures, or for postoperative sedation of ICU patients. The dose-response relationship of these drugs varies considerably among patients and during different clinical circumstances. It is therefore important to carefully titrate these drugs to the desired level of sedation in patients to prevent inadequate or excessive sedation and unwanted side effects. Benzodiazepine dosing must be decreased in the presence of other drugs with sedative and cardiopulmonary depressant effects such as opioids, other sedative/hypnotics, antipsychotics, and general anesthetics. Patients receiving benzodiazepines for postoperative sedation may have increasing dose requirements over the first 24 to 36 hours as the patient emerges from the residual sedative effects of general anesthesia and surgery.[65] Thereafter, as drug accumulation occurs, the dose requirements for benzodiazepines to maintain constant levels of sedation may decrease. Administering opioid infusions to ICU patients for analgesia in conjunction with benzodiazepines reduces the amount of benzodiazepine required to achieve adequate sedation and hastens the emergence from sedation in these patients when both drugs are discontinued simultaneously. Integration of the pharmacokinetics and pharmacodynamics for each agent allows us to predict patterns of sedation and to develop dosing guidelines for each agent during different clinical circumstances.

Midazolam

Midazolam is commercially available in both 1 and 5 mg/mL concentrations, packaged either in 1-mL vials (5 mg/mL

only), in 2-, 5-, or 10-mL vials (both 1 and 5 mg/mL concentrations), or in 2 mL Tel-E-Ject disposable syringes (5 mg/mL only; Hoffman-LaRoche). All midazolam solutions are compounded with 0.8% sodium chloride, 0.01% edetate disodium, and 1% benzyl alcohol with the pH adjusted to 3 with hydrochloric acid and sodium hydroxide.

Table 25–6 summarizes the parenteral dosing regimens for midazolam during a variety of clinical circumstances. Midazolam doses should be decreased by 25% to 50% in elderly patients, in patients with severe liver disease or other high-risk surgical patients, and in patients receiving concomitant opioids or other sedative medications. Obese patients may require greater initial doses of midazolam to achieve adequate sedation, but they may exhibit delayed emergence from sedation. Individual midazolam doses may be given either intravenously or intramuscularly. Because of the interpatient variability in absorption and the dose-response relationship for midazolam, the use of IM mid-

TABLE 25–6.

Dosing Guidelines for Parenteral Administration of Benzodiazepines in Adults

Indication	Midazolam[a]	Lorazepam[b]	Diazepam[c]
Preoperative medication:[d]	0.5–5 mg[e]	0.5–2 mg[f]	2–10 mg
Conscious sedation:			
Initial dose	0.5–5 mg IV[e]	NA	NA
Maintenance dose	0.25–2 mg IV q 15–80 min[g]	NA	NA
Induction of anesthesia	0.2–0.35 mg/kg IV[h]	0.1 mg/kg IV[i]	0.3–0.5 mg/kg IV[j]
ICU sedation:			
Loading dose	0.5–4 mg IV[k]	3–6 mg IV	2–10 mg IV q6h[l]
Maintenance dose[m]	1–7 mg/h IV infusion[n]	0.5–2 mg/h IV infusion[o]	2–10 mg IV q6h[l]

[a]In elderly or debilitated patients, in patients with liver disease, and in the presence of opioids or other sedatives, midazolam doses should be reduced by 25% to 50%.

[b]In elderly and debilitated patients and in patients receiving opioids or other sedatives, reduce lorazepam doses by 20% to 50% and carefully titrate to the desired level of sedation.

[c]In elderly or debilitated patients, in patients with liver disease, and in the presence of opioids or other sedatives, diazepam doses should be reduced by 25% to 50%.

[d]Single preoperative benzodiazepine dose may be given either intramuscularly or IV; intramuscular doses should only be given to healthy patients younger than 60 years old.

[e]Administer intravenously midazolam boluses in 0.5- to 1-mg increments every 5 minutes, titrating to desired level of sedation; single intramuscular doses should be given 30 to 60 minutes before surgery.

[f]Must administer intravenous lorazepam 20 to 30 minutes before surgery.

[g]Repeat boluses for maintenance sedation with midazolam = 25% of initial dose; titrate to desired effect.

[h]Reduce midazolam induction dose by 25% if opioid or other sedative premed is given.

[i]The slow onset and long duration of effect with lorazepam make it a poor induction agent.

[j]Diazepam induction should not be used in patients requiring rapid emergence from anesthesia.

[k]Administer midazolam loading dose over 5 minutes; may repeat loading dose after 15 minutes if necessary.

[l]No studies of long-term dosing of diazepam in ICU patients. Titrate to minimum dose is required.

[m]Benzodiazepine dosing requirements generally decrease over time because of drug accumulation. Titrate all dosing regimens daily to maintain the desired level of sedation, with daily suspensions of sedative infusions to minimize risk for oversedation.

[n]Higher midazolam infusion rates required in some patients. Lower doses with opioid administration.

[o]Titrate lorazepam infusion to lowest possible infusion rate within 24 hours to prevent oversedation.

ICU, intensive care unit; IV, intravenously.

azolam should be reserved for healthy patients without IV access who receive a single IM dose of midazolam for preoperative sedation. IM midazolam must be administered 30 to 60 minutes in advance of the desired time-to-peak effect, whereas IV midazolam boluses for preoperative sedation can be administered 3 to 5 minutes before the start of a procedure. IV doses of midazolam for induction of anesthesia should be administered over 20 to 30 seconds with a peak effect occurring within 2 minutes. Patients undergoing general anesthesia who are premedicated with opioids or other sedatives should have their midazolam induction dose reduced by 25%. Subsequent doses of midazolam (approximately 25% of the induction dose) may be given intraoperatively in response to signs of lightening anesthesia. Because of the interpatient variability in the dose-response relationship for midazolam, IV midazolam boluses given for conscious sedation during procedures should be administered in divided doses and carefully titrated to the desired level of sedation for each patient, waiting at least 5 minutes between each dose.

With long-term midazolam administration for sedation of patients in the ICU, the emergence time from midazolam may last hours or even days with deep sedation. Midazolam infusions should be titrated frequently during the first 24 to 48 hours after surgery because midazolam requirements increase initially with the resolving effects of anesthesia then decrease with drug accumulation over time. Patients who are initially awake in the ICU before initiation of midazolam infusion should receive an IV loading dose of midazolam to achieve therapeutic levels of midazolam more quickly. The loading dose of midazolam should be administered in divided doses to prevent hemodynamic instability in these patients. Patients should be maintained at a level of sedation with midazolam that allows them to respond to simple commands without agitation if possible. The use of a sedation scoring system to monitor depth of sedation can help to optimize the dosing of midazolam infusions in ICU patients. In addition, midazolam infusions should be suspended each day to prevent oversedation and to minimize drug accumulation, and then they should be resumed at the lowest possible infusion rate to maintain the desired level of sedation. Such sedative holidays have been shown to significantly reduce the emergence time from sedation after discontinuation of sedative infusions. The concurrent use of opioid infusions for analgesia in ICU patients also significantly reduces their midazolam requirements and hastens their emergence from midazolam sedation when the opioid and midazolam infusions are discontinued simultaneously. ICU patients with a creatinine clearance less than 50 mL/min who receive continuous infusions of midazolam over several days may accumulate significant amounts of 1-hydroxymidazolam glucuronide, the active metabolite of midazolam, resulting in deeper levels of sedation and an even greater prolonged emergence from sedation. Alternative sedative regimens may be indicated in these patients.

Lorazepam

Lorazepam is supplied in Tubex Blunt Pointe Sterile Cartridge Units and Sterile Cartridge-Needle Units (Wyeth-Ayerst, Madison, N. J.) for use with various injection systems (2 and 4 mg/mL concentrations in 0.5- and 1-mL cartridges), and in glass vials (2 and 4 mg/mL concentrations in 1- and 10-mL vials). Because of its water insolubility, each milliliter of lorazepam is dissolved in 0.18 mL polyethylene glycol 400 in propylene glycol with 2% benzyl alcohol as a preservative.

Lorazepam dosing must take into account the slower onset and longer duration of action with lorazepam compared with midazolam. In addition, lorazepam is more potent than midazolam; therefore patients generally require much smaller doses of lorazepam than midazolam. The potency of lorazepam is increased in elderly patients; for every 10 years of patient age over 60 years, lorazepam potency increases by about 18% therefore doses should be reduced accordingly in these patients. Lorazepam doses should also be decreased in debilitated patients and in the presence of opioids or other preoperative sedatives to avoid cardiorespiratory depression. Obese patients may require greater initial doses of lorazepam to achieve adequate sedation, but may exhibit delayed emergence from sedation compared with nonobese patients.

Table 25–6 summarizes the parenteral dosing regimens for lorazepam for various clinical indications. Lorazepam may be administered either intramuscularly or intravenously. When administered intravenously, lorazepam can cause venous irritation and thrombophlebitis and should be diluted with an equal volume of compatible diluent. Continuous infusions of lorazepam should be administered through central venous catheter. Because of its longer onset of effect, IM lorazepam must be administered at least 2 hours before surgery. In addition, 17% of patients experience significant pain and burning sensations with IM injections of lorazepam. For these reasons, oral administration of lorazepam may be preferable for preoperative sedation of patients. Lorazepam should not be used as a preoperative sedative in cases in which rapid emergence from anesthesia at the end of the procedure is desired. Because of its slow onset of action and its long duration of effect, lorazepam is a poor choice for the induction or maintenance of anesthesia or for use in conscious sedation.

Continuous infusions of IV lorazepam or intermittent bolus injections may be used for sedation of patients in the ICU who are intubated and mechanically ventilated. Because of its slower onset of action and its prolonged effect, lorazepam may be more difficult to titrate to a desired level of sedation compared with midazolam. As with midazolam, lorazepam infusions should be preceded by IV loading doses in awake patients to initially achieve the desired level of sedation, and then the lorazepam infusion should be frequently titrated over the first 24 hours to maintain optimal levels of sedation. Patients emerging from anesthesia will require less lorazepam for the first 24 hours after surgery than awake patients. Patients may still experience prolonged emergence times from sedation with lorazepam leading to significant delays of up to several days in weaning these patients from mechanical ventilation and extubation. Strategies to minimize emergence time after discontinuation of lorazepam infusions in ICU patients include: (1) using sedation scoring systems to target the desired level of sedation with lorazepam; (2) maintaining the lightest possible level of sedation with lorazepam, ideally where the patient is still able to follow commands without being agitated; (3) using opioids together with lorazepam to minimize the amount of lorazepam required; (4) using lorazepam holidays with daily suspension of lorazepam infusions to prevent oversedation; and (5) swapping lorazepam for a shorter acting sedative, such a propofol, 48 to 72 hours in advance of discontinuing sedation to allow for the lorazepam to wash out and to hasten emergence. The delays in patient care resulting from the longer emergence time from lorazepam sedation may offset the lower cost of lorazepam compared with midazolam.

Diazepam

Diazepam is supplied in 2-mL vials, 10-mL ampules, or 2-mL Tel-E-Ject disposable syringes (5 mg/mL each). Diazepam is dissolved in 40% propylene glycol, 10% ethyl alcohol, 5% sodium benzoate and benzoic acid as buffers, and 1.5% benzyl alcohol as a preservative. Diazepam may be given either intramuscularly or intravenously. Because the benzyl alcohol additive can cause venous irritation and thrombophlebitis, IV diazepam should be administered through a central venous catheter. Only small amounts of diazepam (≤5 mg) should be administered very slowly through peripheral IV (no more than 5 mg/min) avoiding small peripheral veins.

Diazepam doses should be reduced in elderly or debilitated patients (especially in patients with cirrhosis) because of an increased sensitivity and longer elimination half-life for diazepam in these patients leading to oversedation and delayed emergence. Diazepam doses should also be reduced in patients receiving opioids, other sedatives, or H_2 blockers. Obese patients require greater initial doses of diazepam but may experience prolonged sedation with diazepam.

Table 25–6 summarizes the parenteral dosing regimens for diazepam for various clinical indications. As a preoperative sedative, IV diazepam may be administered within 3 to 5 minutes of the start of the procedure versus 15 to 30 minutes before for IM dosing. Although the rapid onset of IV diazepam makes it a good induction agent, the larger doses required for induction of anesthesia necessitate administering diazepam only through a central venous catheter. In addition, diazepam should not be used for induction of anesthesia in which rapid emergence from anesthesia and extubation are anticipated at the end of the procedure. Diazepam dosing in ICU patients should be carefully titrated to the desired level of sedation, adjusting the dose and dosing interval over time as diazepam and desmethyldiazepam accumulation occurs. Emergence from sedation with diazepam in these patients may be hastened by switching from diazepam to a shorter-acting sedative, such as propofol, several days in advance of discontinuing sedation altogether. Diazepam should not be used for sedation of ICU patients with end-stage liver disease because these patients may experience prolonged sedation caused by the decreased clearance of both diazepam and desmethyldiazepam.

Reversal Agent: Flumazenil

Flumazenil is a benzodiazepine antagonist. Chemically, flumazenil is ethyl 8-fluoro-5,6-dihydo-5-methyl-6-oxo-4H-imidazo[1,5-a](1,4)benzodiazepine-3-carboxylate. Flumazenil is metabolized by hydroxylation through hepatic microsomal enzymes to inactive metabolites with a half-life of about 1 hour. Flumazenil (Romazicon; Hoffman-LaRoche) is supplied in both 5- and 10-mL vials (0.1 mg/mL). Each milliliter of flumazenil is dissolved with 1.8 mg methylparaben, 0.2 mg propylparaben, 0.9% sodium chloride, 0.01% edetate disodium, and 0.01% acetic acid with the pH adjusted to 4 with hydrochloric acid.

Flumazenil is used clinically as a rescue agent to reverse the cardiopulmonary depressant effects or the excessive sedative effects of benzodiazepines. The onset of flumazenil is quite rapid. After a single IV bolus injection of flumazenil, the onset of effect is 1 to 2 minutes, with a peak effect occurring in 2 to 10 minutes and duration of effect that lasts between 45 to 90 minutes, depending on benzodiazepine plasma concentrations at the time of flumazenil administration. Flumazenil is administered in 0.2- to 1.0-mg IV boluses titrated to the patient's response; up to 3 mg per hour may be administered. After an initial response, patients may become resedated once the effects of flumazenil have subsided. In this case, a flumazenil infusion may be continued (0.5–1.0 mg/kg/min) until the benzodiazepine effects have resolved. A lack of response by a patient to a total dose of 5 mg flumazenil strongly suggests that a benzodiazepine is not the cause of excessive sedation or cardiorespiratory depression. In addition, the use of flumazenil to reverse benzodiazepine-induced sedation should be avoided in patients currently using benzodiazepines to control seizure activity as it may precipitate an acute withdrawal seizure.[110]

References

1. Rudolph U, Crestani F, Benke D, et al: Benzodiazepine actions mediated by specific γ-aminobutyric acid_A receptor subtypes. Nature 401:796–800, 1999.
2. Löw K, Crestani F, Keist R, et al: Molecular and neuronal substrate for the selective attenuation of anxiety. Science 290:131–134, 2000.
3. McKernan RM, Rosahl TW, Reynolds DS, et al: Sedative but not anxiolytic properties of benzodiazepines are mediated by the GABA_A receptor α_1 subtype. Nat Neurosci 3:587–592, 2000.
4. Sieghart W: Structure and pharmacology of γ-aminobutyric acid_A receptor subtypes. Pharmacol Rev 47:181–234, 1995.
5. Barnard EA, Skolnick P, Olsen RW, et al: International Union of Pharmacology. XV. Subtypes of gamma-aminobutyric acid_A receptors: Classification on the basis of subunit structure and receptor function. Pharmacol Rev 2:291–313, 1998.
6. Krasowski MD, Harrison NL: General anaesthetic actions on ligand-gated ion channels. Cell Mol Life Sci 55:1278–1303, 1999.
7. Antkowiak B: How do general anesthetics work? Naturwissenschaften 88:201–213, 2001.
8. Olsen RW, Homanics GE: Function of GABA_A receptors: Insights from mutant and knockout mice. In Martin DL, Olsen RW (eds): GABA and the Nervous System, Philadelphia, Lippincott Williams & Wilkins, 2000, pp 81–96.
9. Möhler H: Pharmacology and pathophysiology of GABA_A-receptor subtypes. In Möhler H (ed): Pharmacology of GABA and Glycine

Neurotransmission, Handbook of Experimental Pharmacology, vol 150, New York, Springer, 2001, pp 101–116.

10. Möhler H, Crestani F, Rudolph U: GABA$_A$-receptor subtypes: A new pharmacology. Curr Opin Pharmacol 1:22–25, 2001.

11. Rudolph U, Crestani U, Möhler H: GABA$_A$ receptor subtypes: Dissecting their pharmacological functions. Trends Phamacol Sci 22:188–194, 2001.

12. Fritschy JM, Möhler H: GABA$_A$-receptor heterogeneity in the adult rat brain: Differential regional and cellular distribution of seven major subunits. J Comp Neurol 359:154–194, 1995.

13. Bormann J: The 'ABC' of GABA receptors. Trends Pharmacol Sci 21:16–19, 2000.

14. Möhler H, Fritschy JM, Rudolph U: A new benzodiazepine pharmacology. J Pharmacol Exp Ther 300:2–8, 2001.

15. Nusser Z, Sieghart W, Somogyi P: Segregation of different GABA$_A$ receptors to synaptic and extrasynaptic membranes of cerebellar granule cells. J Neurosci 18:1693–1703, 1998.

16. Brickley SG, Revilla V, Cull-Candy SG, et al: Adaptive regulation of neuronal excitability by a voltage independent potassium conductance. Nature 409:88–92, 2001.

17. Nusser Z, Sieghart W, Benke D, et al: Differential synaptic localization of two major γ-aminobutyric acid type A receptor α subunits on hippocampal pyramidal cells. Proc Natl Acad Sci USA 93:11939–11944, 1996.

18. Fritschy JM, Weinmann O, Wenzel A, et al: Synapse-specific localization of NMDA and GABA$_A$ receptor subunits revealed by antigen-retrieval immunohistochemistry. J Comp Neurol 390:194–210, 1998.

19. Mody I, Nusser Z: Differential activation of synaptic and extrasynaptic GABA$_A$ receptors. Eur J Neurosci 12(Suppl 11):398, 2000.

20. Mody I, De Koninck Y, Otis TS, et al: Bridging the cleft at GABA synapses in the brain. Trends Neurosci 17:517–525, 1994.

21. Hajos N, Nusser Z, Rancz EA, et al: Cell type- and synapse-specific variability in synaptic GABA$_A$ receptor occupancy. Eur J Neurosci 12:810–818, 2000.

22. Facklam M, Schoch P, Haefely W: Relationship between benzodiazepine receptor occupancy and potentiation of GABA-stimulated chloride flux in vitro of four ligands of differing intrinsic efficacies. J Pharmacol Exp Ther 261:1106–1112, 1992.

23. Facklam M, Schoch P, Bonetti EP, et al: Relationship between benzodiazepine receptor occupancy and functional effects in vivo of four ligands of differing intrinsic efficacies. J Pharmacol Exp Ther 261:1113–1121, 1992.

24. Haefely W, Martin JR, Schoch P: Novel anxiolytics that act as partial agonists at benzodiazepine receptors. Trends Pharmacol Sci 11:452–456, 1990.

25. Sigel E, Buhr A: The benzodiazepine binding site of GABA$_A$ receptors. Trends Pharmacol Sci 18:425–429, 1997.

26. Wieland HA, Lüddens H, Seeburg PH: A single histidine in GABA$_A$ receptors is essential for benzodiazepine agonist binding. J Biol Chem 267:1426–1429, 1992.

27. Kleingoor C, Wieland HA, Korpi ER, et al: Current potentiation by diazepam but not GABA sensitivity is determined by a single histidine residue. Neuroreport 4:187–190, 1993.

28. Benson JA, Löw K, Keist R, et al: Pharmacology of recombinant γ-aminobutyric acid$_A$ receptors rendered diazepam-insensitive by point-mutated α-subunits. FEBS Lett 431:400–404, 1998.

29. Hunkeler W, Mohler H, Pieri L, et al: Selective antagonists of benzodiazepines. Nature 290:514–516, 1981.

30. Mohler H, Okada T: Benzodiazepine receptor: Demonstration in the central nervous system. Science 198:849–851, 1977.

31. Braestrup C, Albrechtsen R, Squires RF: High densities of benzodiazepine receptors in human cortical areas. Nature 269:702–704, 1977.

32. Mohler H, Battersby MK, Richards JG: Benzodiazepine receptor protein identified and visualized in brain tissue by a photoaffinity label. Proc Natl Acad Sci USA 77:1666–1670, 1980.

33. Schofield PR, Darlison MG, Fujita N, et al: Sequence and functional expression of the GABA$_A$ receptor shows a ligand-gated receptor super-family. Nature 328:221–227, 1987.

34. Armony JL, Le Doux JE: How danger is encoded: Toward a sytems, cellular and computational understanding of cognitive-emotional interactions in fear. In Gazzaniga MS (ed): The New Cognitive Neuroscience. Cambridge, MIT Press, 2000, pp 1067–1080.

35. Marksitzer R, Benke D, Fritschy JM, et al: GABA$_A$-receptors: Drug binding profile and distribution of receptors containing the α2-subunit in situ. J Recept Res 13:467–477, 1993.

36. Katona I, Sperlagh B, Sik A, et al: Presynaptically located CB1 cannabinoid receptors regulate GABA release from axon terminals of specific hippocampal interneurons. J Neurosci 19:4544–4558, 1999.

37. Navarro M, Hernandez E, Munoz RM, et al: Acute administration of the CB1 cannabinoid receptor antagonist SR 141716A induces anxiety-like responses in the rat. Neuroreport 8:491–496, 1997.

38. Singh L, Lewis AS, Field MJ, et al: Evidence for an involvement of the brain cholecystokinin B receptor in anxiety. Proc Natl Acad Sci USA 88:1130–1133, 1991.

39. Dauge V, Lena I: CCK in anxiety and cognitive processes. Neurosci Biobehav Rev 22:815–825, 1998.

40. Crestani F, Löw K, Keist R, et al: Molecular targets for the myorelaxant action of diazepam. Mol Pharmacol 59:442–445, 2001.

41. Bohlhalter S, Weinmann O, Möhler H, et al: Laminar compartmentalization of GABA$_A$-receptor subtypes in the spinal cord: An immunohistochemical study. J Neurosci 16:283–297, 1996.

42. Tobler I, Kopp C, Deboer T, et al: Diazepam-induced changes in sleep: Role of the α1 GABA$_A$ receptor subtype. Proc Natl Acad Sci USA 98:6464–6498, 2001.

43. Depoortere H, Zivkovic B, Lloyd KG, et al: Zolpidem, a novel non-benzodiazepine hypnotic. I. Pharmacological and behavioural effects. J Pharmacol Exp Ther 237:649–658, 1986.

44. Zivkovic B, Morel E, Joly D, et al: Pharmacological and behavioural profile of alpidem as an anxiolytic. Pharmacopsychiatry 23:108–113, 1990.

45. Morselli PL: Anxiolytic therapy in the elderly. Experiences with alpidem. In Bartholini G, Garreau M, Morselli PL, Zivkovic B (eds): Imidazopyridines in Anxiety Disorders: A Novel Experimental and Therapeutic Approach. New York, Raven Press, 1993, pp 215–225.

46. Crestani F, Martin JR, Möhler H, et al: Mechanism of action of the hypnotic zolpidem in vivo. Br J Pharmacol 131:1251–1254, 2000.

47. Allen D, Curran HV, Lader M: The effects of single doses of CL284,846, lorazepam, and placebo on psychomotor and memory function in normal male volunteers. Eur J Clin Pharmacol 45:313–320, 1993.

48. Sanger DJ, Morel E, Perrault G: Comparison of the pharmacological profiles of the hypnotic drugs, zaleplon and zolpidem. Eur J Pharmacol 313:35–42, 1996.

49. Dämgen K, Lüddens H: Zaleplon displays a selectivity to recombinant GABA$_A$ receptors different from zolpidem, zopiclone and benzodiazepines. Neurosci Res Commun 25:139–148, 1999.

50. Doble A: New insights into the mechanism of action of hypnotics. J Psychopharmacol 13:S11–S20, 1999.

51. Tunnicliff G: Molecular basis of buspiron's anxiolytic action. Pharmacol Toxicol 69:149–156, 1991.

52. Eison AS, Eison MS: Serotonergic mechanisms in anxiety. Prog Neuropsychopharmacol Biol Psychiatry 18:47–62, 1994.

53. Baldessarini RJ: Drugs and the treatment of psychiatric disorders. Psychosis and anxiety. In Hardman JG, Limbird LE, Molinoff PB, et al (eds): Goodman's and Gilman's. The Pharmacological Basis of Therapeutics, 9th ed. New York, McGraw-Hill, 1996, pp 399–430.

54. Pecknold JC: A risk-benefit assessment of buspirone in the treatment of anxiety disorders. Drug Safety 16:118–132, 1997.

55. Allgulander C: Documented effects of SSRI preparations in anxiety [Swedish]. Lakartidningen 95:2464–2467, 1998.

56. Moschitto LJ, Greenblatt DJ: Concentration-independent plasma protein binding of benzodiazepines. J Pharm Pharmacol 35:179, 1983.

57. Greenblatt DJ, Shader RI, Franke K, et al: Pharmacokinetics and bioavailability of intravenous, intramuscular, and oral lorazepam in humans. J Pharm Sci 68:57, 1979.

58. Thummel KE, Shen DD, Podoll TD, et al: Use of midazolam as a human cytochrome P450 3A probe: I. In vitro-in vivo correlations in liver transplant patients. J Pharmacol Exp Ther 271:549, 1994.

59. Ardent RM, Greenblatt DJ, Garland WA: Quantitation by gas chromatography of the 1- and 4-hydroxy metabolites of midazolam in the human plasma. Pharmacology 29:158, 1984.

60. Jochemsen R, Rijin PA, Hazelzet TGM, et al: Assay of midazolam and brotizolam in plasma by gas chromatography and radioreceptor technique. Pharmaceutisch Weekblad Scientific Edition 5:308, 1983.

61. Heinzmann P, Eckert M, Zeigler WH: Pharmacokinetics and bioavailibility of midazolam in man. Br J Clin Pharmacol 165:43S, 1983.

62. Taylor KM, Paton DM, Boas RA: Radioreceptor assay of the pharmacokinetics of midazolam and chlordiazepoxide. Clin Exp Pharmacol Physiol 10:693, 1983.

63. Vree TB, Baars AM, Booij LHD, et al: Simultaneous determination and pharmacokinetics of midazolam and its hydroxymetabolites in plasma and urine of man and dog by means of high performance liquid chromatography. Arzneimittel-Forschung 31:2215, 1981.

64. Mandema JW, Tuk B, van Stevenick AL, et al: Pharmacokinetic-pharmacodynamic modeling of the central nervous system effects of midazolam and its main metabolite alpha-hydroxymidazolam in healthy volunteers. Clin Pharmacol Ther 51:715, 1992.

65. Barr J, Zomorodi K, Bertaccini E, et al: A double-blind, randomized comparison of IV lorazepam vs. midazolam for sedation of ICU patients via a pharmacologic model. Anesthesiology 95:286–298, 2001.

66. Bauer TM, Ritz R, Haberthur C, et al: Prolonged sedation due to accumulation of conjugated metabolites of midazolam. Lancet 346: 145, 1995.

67. Greenblatt DJ, Schillings RT, Kyriakopoulos AA, et al: Clinical pharmacokinetics of lorazepam. I. Absorption and disposition of oral ^{14}C-lorazepam. Clin Pharmacol Ther 20:329, 1976.

68. Schwartz MA, Koechlin BA, Postma E, et al: Metabolism of diazepam in rat, dog, and man. J Pharmacol Exp Ther 149:423, 1965.

69. van der Klejin E, van Rossum JM, Muskens ET, et al: Pharmacokinetics of diazepam in dogs, mice and humans. Acta Pharmacol Toxicol (Copenhagen) 29:109, 1971.

70. Herman RJ, Wilkinson GR: Disposition of diazepam in young and elderly subjects after acute and chronic dosing. Br J Clin Pharmacol 42:147, 1996.

71. Greenblatt DJ, Abernethy DR, Locniskar A, et al: Effect of age, gender, and obesity on midazolam kinetics. Anesthesiology 61:27, 1984.

72. MacGilchrist AJ, Birnie GG, Cook A, et al: Pharmacokinetics and pharmacodynamics of intravenous midazolam in patients with severe alcoholic cirrhosis. Gut 27:190, 1986.

73. Hase I, Oda Y, Tanaka K, et al: I.V. fentanyl decreases the clearance of midazolam. Br J Anaesth 79:740, 1997.

74. Zomorodi K, Donner A, Somma J, et al: Population pharmacokinetics of midazolam administered by target controlled infusion for sedation following coronary artery bypass grafting. Anesthesiology 89:1418, 1998.

75. Maitre PO, Funk B, Crevoisier C, et al: Pharmacokinetics of midazolam in patients recovering from cardiac surgery. Eur J Clin Pharmacol 37:161, 1989.

76. Dirksen MS, Vree TB, Driessen JJ: Clinical pharmacokinetics of long-term infusion of midazolam in critically ill patients—preliminary results. Anaesth Intensive Care 15:440, 1987.

77. Malacrida R, Fritz ME, Suter PM, et al: Pharmacokinetics of midazolam administered by continuous intravenous infusion to intensive care patients. Crit Care Med 20:1123, 1992.

78. Oldenhof H, de Jong M, Steenhoek A, et al: Clinical pharmacokinetics of midazolam in intensive care patients, a wide interpatient variability? Clin Pharmacol Ther 43:263, 1988.

79. Shafer A, Doze VA, White PF: Pharmacokinetic variability of midazolam infusions in critically ill patients. Crit Care Med 18:1039, 1990.

80. Behne M, Asskali F, Steuer A, et al: Continuous midazolam infusion for sedation of respirator patients. Anaesthesist 36:228, 1987.

81. Hung OR, Dyck JB, Varvel J, et al: Comparative absorption kinetics of intramuscular midazolam and diazepam. Can J Anaesth 43:450, 1996.

82. Kraus JW, Desmond PV, Marshall JP, et al: Effects of aging and liver disease on disposition of lorazepam. Clin Pharmacol Ther 24:411, 1978.

83. Ameer B, Greenblatt DJ: Lorazepam: A review of its clinical pharmacological properties and therapeutic uses. Drugs 21:162, 1981.

84. Reves JG, Fragen RJ, Vinik HR, et al: Midazolam: Pharmacology and uses. Anesthesiology 62:310, 1985.

85. Ochs HR, Greenblatt DJ, Kaschell HJ, et al: Diazepam kinetics in patients with renal insufficiency or hyperthyroidism. Br J Clin Pharmacol 12:829, 1981.

86. Mould DR, DeFeo TM, Reele S, et al: Simultaneous modeling of the pharmacokinetics and pharmacodynamics of midazolam and diazepam. Clin Pharmacol Ther 58:35, 1995.

87. Klotz U, Avant GR, Hoyumpa A, et al: The effects of age and liver disease on the disposition and elimination of diazepam in adult man. J Clin Invest 55:347, 1975.

88. Klotz U, Reimann I: Clearance of diazepam can be impaired by its major metabolite desmethyldiazepam. Eur J Clin Pharmacol 21:161, 1981.

89. Greenblatt DJ, Abernethy DR, Morse DS, et al: Clinical importance of the interaction of diazepam and cimetidine. N Engl J Med 310: 1639, 1984.

90. Greenblatt DJ, Sellers EM, Shader RI: Drug therapy: Drug disposition in old age. N Engl J Med 306:1081, 1982.

91. Breimer LT, Burm AG, Danhof M, et al: Pharmacokinetic-pharmacodynamic modelling of the interaction between flumazenil and midazolam in volunteers by aperiodic EEG analysis. Clin Pharmacokinet 20:497, 1991.

92. Shapiro BA, Warren J, Egol AB, et al: Practice parameters for intravenous analgesia and sedation for adult patients in the intensive care unit: An executive summary. Society of Critical Care Medicine, Crit Care Med 23:1596, 1995.

93. Sarnquist FH, Mathers WD, Brock-Utne J, et al: A bioassay for a water-soluble benzodiazepine against sodium thiopental. Anesthesiology 52:149, 1980.

94. Jensen S, Schou-Olesen A, Huttel MS: Use of midazolam as an induction agent: Comparison with thiopentone. Br J Anaesth 54:605, 1982.

95. Crawford ME, Carl P, Andersen RS, et al: Comparison between midazolam and thiopentone-based balanced anaesthesia for day-case surgery. Br J Anaesth 56:165, 1984.

96. Somma J, Donner A, Zomorodi K, et al: Population pharmacodynamics of midazolam administered by target controlled infusion in SICU patients after CABG surgery. Anesthesiology 89:1430, 1998.

97. Byatt CM, Lewis LD, Dawling S, et al: Accumulation of midazolam after repeated dosage in patients receiving mechanical ventilation in an intensive care unit. Br Med J (Clin Res Ed) 289:799, 1984.

98. Byrne AJ, Yeoman PM, Mace P: Accumulation of midazolam in patients receiving mechanical ventilation. BMJ 289:1309, 1984.

99. Greenblatt DJ, Ehrenberg BL, Gunderman J, et al: Kinetic and dynamic study of intravenous lorazepam: Comparison with intravenous diazepam. J Pharmacol Exp Ther 250:134, 1989.

100. Cole SG, Brozinsky S, Isenberg JI: Midazolam, a new more potent benzodiazepine, compared with diazepam: A randomized, double-blind study of preendoscopic sedatives. Gastrointest Endosc 29:219, 1983.

101. Greenblatt DJ, Ehrenberg BL, Gunderman J, et al: Pharmacokinetic and electroencephalographic study of intravenous diazepam, midazolam, and placebo. Clin Pharmacol Ther 45:356, 1989.

102. Samuelson PN, Reves JG, Kouchoukos NT, et al: Hemodynamic responses to anesthetic induction with midazolam or diazepam in patients with ischemic heart disease. Anesth Analg 60:802, 1981.

103. Mora CT, Torjman M, White PF: Effects of diazepam and flumazenil on sedation and hypoxic ventilatory response. Anesth Analg 68:473, 1989.

104. Gross JB, Zebrowski ME, Carel WD, et al: Time course of ventilatory depression after thiopental and midazolam in normal subjects and in patients with chronic obstructive pulmonary disease. Anesthesiology 58:540, 1983.

105. van der Bijl P, Roelofse JA, Joubert JJ, et al: Comparison of various physiologic and psychomotor parameters in patients sedated with intravenous lorazepam, diazepam, or midazolam during oral surgery. J Oral Maxillofac Surg 49:672, 1991.

106. Heikkila H, Jalonen J, Arola M, et al: Midazolam as adjunct to high-dose fentanyl anaesthesia for coronary artery bypass grafting operation. Acta Anaesthesiol Scand 28:683, 1984.

107. Windsor JP, Sherry K, Feneck RO, et al: Sufentanil and nitrous oxide anaesthesia for cardiac surgery. Br J Anaesth 61:662, 1988.

108. Ruff R, Reves JG: Hemodynamic effects of a lorazepam-fentanyl anesthetic induction for coronary artery bypass surgery. J Cardiothorac Anesth 4:314, 1990.

109. Benson KT, Tomlinson DL, Goto H, et al: Cardiovascular effects of lorazepam during sufentanil anesthesia. Anesth Analg 67:996, 1988.

110. Spivey WH: Flumazenil and seizures: Analysis of 43 cases. Clin Ther 14:292, 1992.

111. Melvin MA, Johnson BH, Quasha AL, et al: Induction of anesthesia with midazolam decreases halothane MAC in humans. Anesthesiology 57:238, 1982.

112. Short TG, Chui PT: Propofol and midazolam act synergistically in combination. Br J Anaesth 67:539, 1991.

113. McClune S, McKay AC, Wright PM, et al: Synergistic interaction between midazolam and propofol. Br J Anaesth 69:240, 1992.

114. Tverskoy M, Fleyshman G, Bradley EL Jr, et al: Midazolam-thiopental anesthetic interaction in patients. Anesth Analg 67:342, 1988.

115. Ben-Shlomo I, abd-el-Khalim H, Ezry J, et al: Midazolam acts synergistically with fentanyl for induction of anaesthesia. Br J Anaesth 64:45, 1990.

116. Gross JB, Blouin RT, Zandsberg S, et al: Effect of flumazenil on ventilatory drive during sedation with midazolam and alfentanil. Anesthesiology 85:713, 1996.

117. Daghero AM, Bradley EL Jr, Kissin I: Midazolam antagonizes the analgesic effect of morphine in rats. Anesth Analg 66:944, 1987.

118. Weinbroum AA, Weisenberg M, Rudick V, et al: Flumazenil potentiation of postoperative morphine analgesia. Clin J Pain 16:193, 2000.

119. Gear RW, Miaskowski C, Heller PH, et al: Benzodiazepine mediated antagonism of opioid analgesia. Pain 71:25, 1997.

120. Bol CJ, Vogelaar JP, Tang JP, et al: Quantification of pharmacodynamic interactions between dexmedetomidine and midazolam in the rat. J Pharmacol Exp Ther 294:347, 2000.

26

Analgesics

Peter Isakson, PhD • Richard Hubbard, MD

NONSTEROIDAL ANTI-INFLAMMATORY DRUGS

Nonsteroidal anti-inflammatory drugs (NSAIDs) represent a diverse class of agents with analgesic, anti-inflammatory, and anti-pyretic activity. NSAIDs are used extensively to manage pain and inflammation associated with surgical procedures, inflammatory diseases such as osteoarthritis (OA) and rheumatoid arthritis (RA), and more moderate pain associated with migraine, dysmenorrhea, myalgia, and dental pain. NSAIDs have been used in one form or another for centuries. Extracts and preparations from plants such as

the willow tree *Salix alba* have been used for hundreds of years for relief from pain and fever. These plants contain derivatives of salicylic acid, which were characterized as their active components in the eighteenth century and were chemically synthesized for the first time in 1860. Commercial production of salicylates began by 1874, and reports of salicylate (5–6 g/day) being able to "cure" rheumatic disorders were first published in 1876.

The mechanism of action of NSAIDs was described in **435**

1971[1] and is characterized by the inhibition of the enzyme cyclo-oxygenase (COX, also known as prostaglandin endoperoxide synthase) resulting in the inhibition of prostaglandin (PG) production. In the late 1980s and early 1990s, a second isoform of COX, COX-2, was identified, cloned, and sequenced. The two isoforms of COX (COX-1 and COX-2) are distinct with respect to genetic structure, transcriptional regulation, and tissue expression patterns. COX-2 is induced by cytokines in inflammatory cells such as macrophages and monocytes, in tissue at localized sites of injury, and in the spinal cord in response to tissue damage.[2-5] In contrast, COX-1 is constitutively expressed at low levels in many tissues and is responsible for maintaining homeostatic pathways,[6] for example, in platelets. COX-2 may be important in certain physiologic processes, particularly in female reproduction.[7,8]

Conventional NSAIDs are nonspecific inhibitors of both isoforms of COX. COX-2 is the therapeutic target for conventional NSAIDs, its inhibition accounting for the analgesic and anti-inflammatory activity of these drugs. However, the inhibition of COX-1 by conventional NSAIDs leads to the disruption of several homeostatic mechanisms, including maintenance of platelet function and protection of the gastric mucosa. It is widely accepted that the inhibition of COX-1 is responsible for many of the adverse side effects associated with conventional NSAIDs. In recent years, the development of inhibitors that demonstrate high specificity for COX-2 at therapeutic doses without concomitant inhibition of COX-1 has provided an alternative to conventional NSAIDs in managing pain. The COX-1 sparing nature of this new class of agents accounts for their improved gastrointestinal (GI) and platelet safety profile compared with conventional NSAIDs.[9-13] The improved long-term upper gastrointestinal series safety profile of the COX-2–specific inhibitors celecoxib and rofecoxib relative to conventional NSAIDs has been demonstrated in two large-scale trials, each involving more than 8000 patients with arthritis.[11,12] In the Celecoxib Long-Term Arthritis Safety study, patients with OA and RA receiving a supratherapeutic dosage of celecoxib (400 mg twice daily) had a significantly lower incidence of symptomatic ulcers and ulcer complications compared with patients receiving standard therapeutic doses of the conventional NSAIDs ibuprofen (800 mg three times daily) or diclofenac (75 mg twice daily).[11] Similarly, patients with RA receiving rofecoxib (50 mg daily) in the VIOXX (Merck & Co., Whitehouse Station, N.J.) GI Outcomes Research study had a significantly lower risk for clinically important upper GI events than those receiving naproxen (500 mg twice daily).[12]

In 1998, approximately 41.5 million inpatient surgical procedures were performed in the United States.[14] The benefit of effective pain management after these procedures is crucial to providing the best patient comfort and satisfaction possible. Effective pain management after surgery not only improves patient recovery and care but also provides fiscal benefits, resulting from earlier patient mobilization and reduction in length of hospital stay. This chapter examines the mechanism of action of NSAIDs and COX-2–specific inhibitors, including the role that they play in the reduction of inflammation and in the perception of pain, and reviews some of the pharmacokinetic properties and clinical uses of these agents.

Mechanism of Action of Nonsteroidal Anti-inflammatory Drugs

Perception of Pain

Understanding the role that COX and PGs play in the pain pathway is critical to the understanding of the mechanism of action of conventional NSAIDs and COX-2–specific inhibitors. Pain perception involves the process of nociception, whereby extremes of temperature, painful mechanical stimuli, and noxious chemical stimuli are detected by the distal ends of primary afferent (nociceptive) neurons.[15,16] The neural axons of these primary afferent neurons also have central branches terminating in the dorsal horn of the spinal cord, and the cell bodies of these neurons are located in the dorsal root ganglia.[15] The details of transmission of nociceptive signals from peripheral nociceptors to the spinal cord and higher centers are reviewed in detail in Chapters 11 through 13.

Role of Cyclo-oxygenase and Prostaglandins in Inflammation and Sensitization

Prostaglandins (PGs) are produced during inflammation by the action of COX. They increase the sensitivity of nociceptors and nociceptive neurons to other pain-producing stimuli, such as bradykinin, histamine, and serotonin, and to mechanical, chemical, and thermal stimuli (peripheral sensitization) (Fig. 26–1). For example, pretreatment of sensory neurons in culture with prostaglandin E_2 (PGE_2) potentiates bradykinin-mediated release of substance P.[17] Substance P enhances synaptic transmission in the dorsal horn and is at least partly involved in the production of inflammatory hyperalgesia.[18]

In the early stages of peripheral sensitization, PG release leads to post-translational protein modifications in the peripheral terminals of nociceptors and in dorsal horn neurons.[15-17,19] This sensitization alters transduction sensitivity by nociceptive neurons.[16,19-21] These early changes are followed by transcription-dependent changes in the dorsal root ganglion of primary afferent neurons and in the dorsal horn.[20,21] These translational and transcriptional changes within the cell potentiate nociception and lead to "phenotypic switching" of sensory neurons—i.e., biochemical changes that alter the physiologic responses of low-threshold Aβ neuron inputs, to such an extent that normal stimuli such as touch elicit a painful response.[22,23] In simple terms, the production of excessive PGs in the periphery leads to modifications in gene expression in the central nervous system (CNS) that result in hyperalgesia and allodynia (central sensitization) (see Fig. 26–1).

Prostaglandin Signal Transduction Pathway

COX oxygenates arachidonate to form the endoperoxide derivative PGG_2.[24] A wide variety of stimuli, including

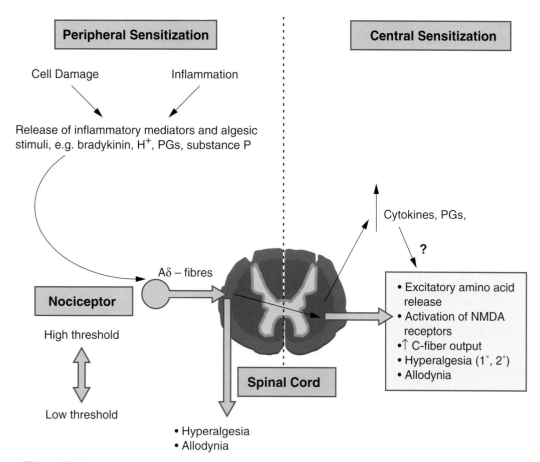

Figure 26–1. Peripheral and central sensitization to inflammatory pain. Cell damage and inflammatory stimuli in the periphery induce the release of mediators of inflammation and pain, which transmit signals through nociceptors and Aδ neurons to the central nervous system (CNS) leading to hyperalgesia and allodynia (peripheral sensitization). Peripheral sensitization, tissue injury, and inflammatory signals such as inflammatory cytokines act directly on the CNS to induce transcriptional and post-translational changes in the CNS (e.g., COX-2 up-regulation) that increase pain sensitivity to mechanical, thermal, chemical, and inflammatory stimuli (central sensitization). NMDA, *N*-methyl-D-aspartate; PGs, prostaglandins.

cytokines, hormones, allergens, neuropeptides, mechanical and oxidative stress, and tissue damage activate phospholipases (PLAs) through G proteins and intracellular kinases.[25–30] Certain of these PLAs (primarily PLA$_2$) specifically release arachidonate from the SN-2 position of membrane phospholipids.[30] Free arachidonate is then available for oxidation by COX to the endoperoxide PGG$_2$, which is converted by the COX enzyme to PGH$_2$, the unstable precursor of all PGs and thromboxane (Tx).[24] The biologically active PGs and Tx are formed in a highly tissue-specific manner by PGE$_2$, PGD, and PGF isomerases, and by prostacyclin (PGI$_2$) and TxA$_2$ synthase (Fig. 26–2).[24]

Depending on the cell type and tissue, one or all of these may be produced in response to a stimulus. For example, most platelet-derived endoperoxide is converted to TxA$_2$,[31] whereas in most vascular tissues PGI$_2$ predominates,[32] and mast cells produce mainly PGD$_2$.[33] The monocyte/macrophage lineage can produce the entire spectrum of endoperoxide metabolites, but in inflamed tissue PGE$_2$ is typically found in abundance.[34] Recent discoveries have

shown that this enhanced production of PGE$_2$ is caused by a PGE isomerase whose expression parallels COX-2 in many respects—e.g., synthesis of both enzymes is induced by inflammatory stimuli and down-regulated by glucocorticoids.[35] Each of the PGs interacts with specific G protein–coupled receptors. Single receptor types have been identified for PGF$_{2\alpha}$, PGI$_2$, and TxA$_2$ (referred to as FP, IP, and TP, respectively); two subtypes of the PGD$_2$ (DP) receptor are known and four distinct PGE$_2$ (EP) receptors have been identified.[36] In general, there is scant sequence similarity between the major receptor classes and little cross-reactivity of PGs on heterologous receptor types. Future development of specific receptor antagonists and isomerase/synthase inhibitors will allow further elucidation of the functional role of each PG and receptor subtype.

There are two distinct isoforms of COX (COX-1 and COX-2) associated with PG production. COX-1 and COX-2 are encoded by two genes that are differentially expressed in a variety of tissues.[36–41] COX-1 is constitutively expressed in many tissues, including lung, liver, spleen, kidney, and

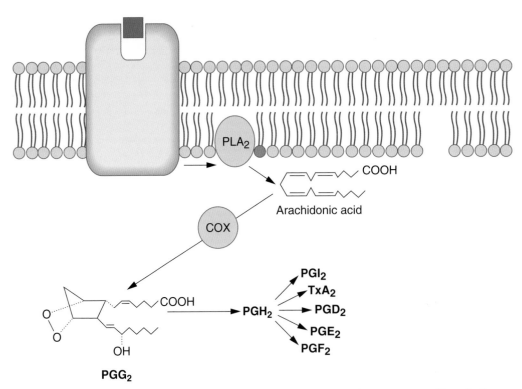

Figure 26–2. Cyclo-oxygenase (COX)–mediated prostaglandin (PG) production. Phospholipase A_2 (PLA$_2$) converts membrane phospholipids to arachidonate in response to cytokines and other extracellular stimuli, binding to membrane receptors. Arachidonate is further metabolized by COX to prostaglandin G_2 (PGG$_2$), the precursor for a variety of other prostaglandins including PGI$_2$, thromboxane A$_2$ (TxA$_2$), PGD$_2$, PGE$_2$, and PGF$_2\alpha$.

stomach.[6] In particular, COX-1 is expressed in platelets and in the gastric mucosa (see Fig. 26–3). Nonspecific inhibition of COX-1 in these tissues by conventional NSAIDs results in reduced platelet aggregation, prolonged bleeding, damage to gastric mucosa, and GI tract erosion and ulceration.[42–45] COX-2, the therapeutic target for conventional NSAIDs and COX-2–specific inhibitors,[6,46,47] is induced in inflamed tissues in response to mitogenic stimuli and inflammatory cytokines such as interleukin-1 (IL-1) and tumor necrosis factor-α.[2–4] COX-2 is also expressed in the spinal cord and the brain[5,48–50] (Fig. 26–3) and may be involved in pain responses at greater levels in the CNS.

The relative roles of the individual PGs in pain and inflammation is still uncertain, partly because of the paucity of specific pharmacologic antagonists of their receptors noted earlier. An alternate approach to the use of antagonists is the injection of PGs into tissue. Such studies have shown that PGE$_2$ causes some of the cardinal signs of inflammation, including swelling and sensitization to hyperalgesia, and PGI$_2$ can elicit similar effects. These studies are hampered by the nonphysiologic nature of the delivery method, rapid clearance from the site (as opposed to continuous production in situ during inflammation), and the lability of PGI$_2$ and especially TxA$_2$. A study using an antibody to PGE$_2$ showed that neutralizing this mediator was as effective as COX inhibition in reducing edema and hyperalgesia,[51] suggesting that PGE$_2$ was an essential mediator of pain and inflammation in this rat model. Because antibodies do not readily cross the blood–brain barrier, these experiments

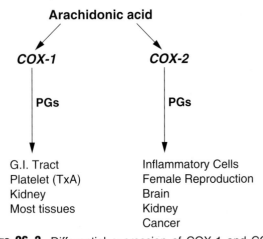

Figure 26–3. Differential expression of COX-1 and COX-2 isoenzymes in different tissues. COX-1 is constitutively expressed in most tissues including platelets and in epithelial cells of the gastric mucosa and intestine. In contrast, COX-2 is induced in response to inflammatory stimuli, including inflammatory cytokines such as interleukin-1β (IL-1β) and tumor necrosis factor alpha (TNF-α), in inflammatory cells, in sites of inflammation and tissue damage, in the synovium of joints, in endothelial cells, and in the central nervous system. NSAIDs are nonselective inhibitors of both isoforms of COX, whereas COX-2–specific inhibitors do not inhibit COX-1 at therapeutic doses. GI, gastrointestinal; PGs, prostaglandins; Tx, thromboxane.

also point to a peripheral site of action of PGE_2; however, they do not eliminate an important role for central PGs in higher pain pathways. The role of COX-2 and the production of PGs in inflammation and pain after surgery and in inflammatory diseases such as arthritis have also been demonstrated in a number of animal models and among surgical patients and those with chronic inflammatory disease.

Peripheral Cyclo-oxygenase-2 Expression in Response to Tissue Damage

A number of animal models have been developed to study physiologic processes governing inflammation and pain and to assess the effects of pharmacologic manipulation of the mediators of inflammation. These experimental models have demonstrated that PGs are produced at the site of inflammation and that inhibition of their production by NSAIDs reduces swelling and pain. Over the past decade, a wealth of data has accumulated indicating that COX-2 mRNA and protein is abundantly expressed after an inflammatory stimulus or tissue damage, and is responsible for the concomitant production of PGE_2.[6,46] A correlation between tissue damage, inflammation, and COX-2 expression has also been shown in animal surgical models. For example, COX-2 mRNA and protein levels were increased in rat hepatocytes 3 hours after a partial hepatectomy, whereas COX-1 and PLA_2 levels were unchanged.[52]

Increased production of PGs at localized sites of injury has also been demonstrated in many human surgical models. Increased PG production, particularly of PGE_2, has been demonstrated in tissue surrounding surgical sites in patients who have undergone oral surgery and after major surgical procedures.[53-55] Increases in PG production have also been shown in other surgical models, including coronary artery bypass grafts and abdominal aortic aneurysmectomy.[56-58] In all of these studies, patients who were administered NSAIDs before or after surgery showed reduced PG levels in localized surgical sites. In addition, increased levels of COX-2, but not COX-1, have been demonstrated in synovial tissue and cartilage from patients with inflammatory disease such as RA and OA.[59-61]

Induction of Cyclo-oxygenase-2 in the Central Nervous System

In addition to peripheral COX production in damaged tissue, studies in several animal models have demonstrated COX-2 expression and activity and concomitant PG production in the CNS in response to tissue and nerve damage. Allodynia, artificially induced in rats by the ligation of the left lumbar L5 and L6 spinal nerves, was associated with increased expression of COX-2 protein in the dorsal spinal cord and thalamus.[62] Low basal levels of COX-2 are detectable in rat dorsal horn neurons and substantial up-regulation of COX-2 mRNA and protein occurs in response to injection of carrageenan or Freund's complete adjuvant.[48,49,63] This induction of COX-2 in the spinal cord is associated with marked hyperalgesia and a substantial increase of PGE_2 in cerebrospinal fluid (CSF).[63] Freund's complete adjuvant also leads to massive up-regulation of IL-1β at the injection site and in the CSF and increased expression of type I IL-1β receptors.[63] IL-1β given systemically is a potent hyperalgesic agent.[64] Therefore it is likely that the proinflammatory cytokine IL-1β is responsible for increased levels of COX-2, and thus increased levels of PGE_2, in the spinal cord, with concomitant pain hypersensitivity.[63] No increase in COX-1 expression has been detected after similar nerve injury, suggesting that increased COX-2 activity is primarily responsible for increased prostanoid signaling in the CNS.[62]

It appears, therefore, that the involvement of COX-2 in the perception of pain is twofold. Localized production of COX-2 at sites of tissue damage in response to inflammatory stimuli, whether at surgical sites or in inflamed joints in patients with arthritis, sensitizes primary afferent neurons and leads to the transmission of pain stimuli to the dorsal horn. In addition, COX-2 and PG levels in spinal neurons are increased in response to both peripheral inflammatory stimuli and the direct action of inflammatory cytokines such as IL-1β on dorsal horn neurons. This central sensitization is responsible for the perception of pain associated with inflammatory disease and with tissue damage sustained during surgery.

Mechanism of Action of Conventional Nonsteroidal Anti-inflammatory Drugs and Cyclo-oxygenase-2–Specific Inhibitors on Cyclo-oxygenase-1 and Cyclo-oxygenase-2 Inhibition

Conventional NSAIDs are nonselective inhibitors of both COX-1 and COX-2. The anti-inflammatory activity of NSAIDs is mediated by inhibition of COX-2.[47] Individual NSAIDs function by binding to and blocking the active site of COX, although their inhibition kinetics vary considerably. X-ray crystallography studies have advanced our understanding of the inhibitory mechanism of conventional NSAIDs and the selectivity of COX-2–specific inhibitors.[65,66] The crystal structure of COX-1 reveals that the substrate-binding site of the enzyme is located within the catalytic domain in a pocket surrounded by three α-helices at the mouth of the channel, with charged amino acid residues at each turn in the helices.[65,66] Conventional NSAIDs bind to a charged arginine residue (Arg-120) near the active site of the enzyme, thereby blocking substrate access to amino acid residues such as tyrosine-385 that are essential for catalysis.[67,68]

Single amino acid differences in the active sites of COX-1 and COX-2 account for the selectivity of COX-2–specific inhibitors, the most critical of which seems to be the substitution of the valine residue (Val-509) in COX-2 for isoleucine in COX-1.[69] In the COX-2 isoform, the valine residue, with its smaller side chain, makes a side pocket adjacent to the active site accessible to COX-2–specific inhibitors.[70,71] In contrast, the COX-1 substrate channel is much narrower, because of the presence of the larger isoleucine residue, and therefore is unable to accommodate the COX-2–specific inhibitors with their bulky side chains (Fig. 26–4).

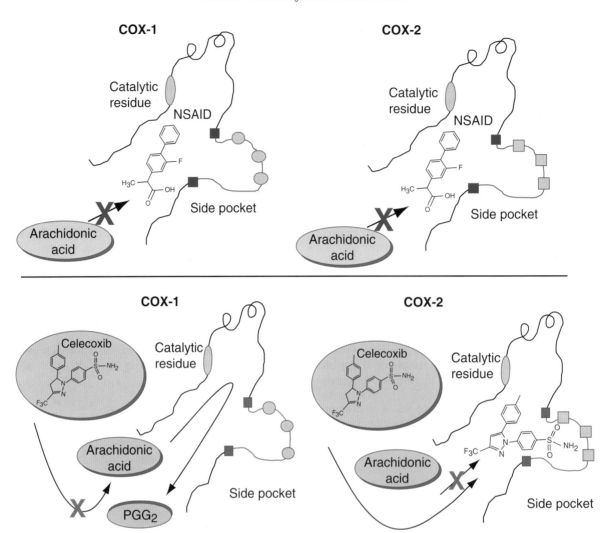

Figure 26–4. Cyclo-oxygenase-1 (COX-1) and COX-2 inhibition: mechanism of action. Conventional nonsteroidal anti-inflammatory drugs (NSAIDs) inhibit COX-1 and COX-2 by binding to the active site in the catalytic domain of the protein. COX-2–specific inhibitors such as celecoxib are characterized by a bulky side chain, which prohibits binding of the inhibitor in the narrow catalytic pocket of COX-1. A single amino acid change in the catalytic pocket of COX-2 exposes a side pocket that is able to accommodate the bulky side chain of COX-2–specific inhibitors.

Preclinical Pharmacology

Enzyme Kinetics of Conventional Nonsteroidal Anti-inflammatory Drugs and Cyclo-oxygenase-2–Specific Inhibitors

Conventional NSAIDs can be subdivided into four groups depending on their inhibition kinetics. The first group comprises competitive, reversible inhibitors (e.g., ibuprofen) that display the same inhibition kinetics for both COX-1 and COX-2.[69] The second group consists of time-dependent inhibitors (e.g., indomethacin) that exhibit increased in vitro inhibition of the enzyme as the preincubation time of the inhibitor with the enzyme is increased.[69,72] Inhibitors that function in this manner are thought to induce a conforma-

tional change in the enzyme active site, rendering it unable to catalyze substrate conversion. The third group of conventional NSAIDs comprises those with mixed kinetics that produce initial time-dependent inhibition but do not reach a zero endpoint—i.e., they never completely disable the enzyme[69] and are often slow, weakly binding inhibitors. This group includes many commonly used conventional NSAIDs, such as naproxen. The final group, which consists solely of aspirin, forms a covalent bond within the active site, thereby irreversibly inhibiting the enzyme. Thus acetylation of serine residues in the active site of COX-1 and COX-2 (Ser-530 and Ser-516, respectively) by aspirin causes irreversible inhibition of both enzymes. It is not clear whether these different modes of inhibition have any clinical consequences, although the slow reversibility of time-dependent inhibitors (off rate of hours) may prolong the pharmacodynamic effects of these drugs. A notable exception is aspirin, in which covalent modification of an active site serine found in both COX-1 and COX-2 permanently inactivates the enzyme.

Early inhibitor binding studies with the COX-2–specific inhibitor DuP-697[76] demonstrated a difference in the inhibition kinetics of the two COX isoforms that account for COX-2 selectivity.[76] Like most COX-2–specific inhibitors, DuP-697 binds COX-1 weakly and displays modest competitive inhibition of the enzyme. In contrast, DuP-697 displays time-dependent, noncompetitive, inhibition kinetics with COX-2, resulting in a tightly bound inhibitor/enzyme complex that is only slowly reversible.[77] The COX-2–specific inhibitors, celecoxib, valdecoxib and rofecoxib, all derive their selectivity for COX-2 through this mechanism—i.e., weak competitive inhibition of COX-1 but tight binding, which is time-dependent and slowly reversible, to COX-2.

Quantitation of the in vitro potency and selectivity (half-maximal inhibition, IC_{50}) of conventional NSAIDs and COX-2–specific inhibitors can vary widely depending on the type of assay used. The in vitro potency of NSAIDs such as ibuprofen, aspirin, and indomethacin can be affected by differences in the source of the enzyme used—i.e., purified enzyme, crude broken cell preparations, or intact cell preparations, and especially by the enzyme assay conditions. Also, different methods of quantitation of COX activity—e.g., enzyme-linked immunosorbent assay of PGE_2, NNN "N"-tetramethyl-p-phenylenediamine oxidation, and oxygen uptake—can give widely varying IC_{50} values for individual NSAIDs and COX-2–specific inhibitors.[69,78] Therefore, although in vitro data provide a valuable guide to the relative potency of both conventional NSAIDs and COX-2–specific inhibitors, it is not possible to predict clinical efficacy or specificity based solely on these types of study. In particular, it is difficult to make a direct comparison between the inhibition of COX-1 and COX-2 by a single agent when the inhibitor displays different enzyme kinetics for each isoform.[69]

In Vivo Models for Cyclo-oxygenase Inhibition

As noted earlier, animal models have been extensively used to analyze the processes of inflammation and hyperalgesia.[6,46,79–81] These models have also been used to evaluate the efficacy of NSAIDs in managing inflammation and pain. Intramuscular (IM), intravenous (IV), and oral administration of aspirin, indomethacin, diclofenac, naproxen, ibuprofen, piroxicam, and ketorolac reduce inflammation and pain, assessed by the extent of footpad swelling and the rate of withdrawal on application of mechanical or thermal stimuli, in animals with experimental inflammation.[81–85] Notably, direct application of small quantities of NSAIDs to the spinal cord is as effective in reducing inflammatory hyperalgesia as conventional doses delivered systemically. This suggests that there may be a CNS component to the action of COX inhibitors including the NSAIDs.[81] This is further supported by the observation that PG levels are markedly increased in the CSF after peripheral inflammation.[48,49,86] CSF PG levels were reduced in this model by a COX-2 inhibitor but were not affected by a COX-1–specific agent.[83]

Clinical Pharmacology

Conventional Nonsteroidal Anti-inflammatory Drugs: Pharmacokinetic Parameters

NSAIDs are a heterogeneous class of compounds, often chemically unrelated, which share a similar therapeutic and side effect profile.[87,88] The pharmacokinetic properties of some of the most commonly used NSAIDs are described in Table 26–1. The rates of absorption of NSAIDs are affected by a number of factors.[88,89] Consumption of NSAIDs with food often delays their absorption because of the reduction in the rate of gastric emptying. The formulation of NSAIDs affects absorption, and for most compounds soluble preparations are more rapidly absorbed.[88] However, recently developed enteric-coated tablets and sustained release preparations have demonstrated improved bioavailability.[89,90] Absorption, peak plasma concentration, and metabolism of NSAIDs can also be significantly affected by GI pH, patient age, concomitant administration of other drugs, and the disease state of the patient.[88–95] Elimination of conventional NSAIDs is largely dependent on hepatic biotransformation and renal excretion.[88–95] Therefore patients with hepatic and renal disease often demonstrate greater and more prolonged peak plasma concentrations because rates of metabolism and elimination of the drugs are often reduced.[88]

Absorption

In general, conventional NSAIDs are rapidly and well absorbed from the GI tract. Orally administered aspirin is rapidly absorbed by passive diffusion of unionized lipophilic molecules, but it also undergoes a high degree of presystemic hydrolysis to form salicylate before absorption.[89] The remainder is hydrolyzed to salicylate after absorption (half-life [$t_{1/2}$] 15–20 minutes) by nonspecific esterases found in many body tissues.[96] Commercially available suppositories and soluble or enteric-coated tablet preparations of diclofenac are reported to be almost totally absorbed in the GI tract.[97,98] However, other reports suggest that diclofenac undergoes presystemic elimination with ~60% of the initial dose detected in the systemic circulation unchanged.[99]

Oral doses of ibuprofen are rapidly and almost completely absorbed (>80%) in the GI tract.[88,91] Ibuprofen exists as two enantiomers: R-(−)-ibuprofen and S-(+)-ibuprofen. The majority of the anti-inflammatory and analgesic effects of ibuprofen have been attributed to the S-enantiomer. The R-enantiomer undergoes unidirectional metabolic inversion to form the S-enantiomer.[91] It has been suggested that the rate of bioinversion of ibuprofen is affected by the rate of absorption. The longer ibuprofen remains in the GI tract the more likely presystemic inversion is to take place, thereby increasing the S:R enantiomer ratio.[100] Conversely, a significant correlation between the S:R ratio and time-to-peak plasma concentration (T_{max}) has been observed, with a greater S:R area under the time-concentration curve (AUC)

TABLE 26–1.

Pharmacokinetic Parameters of Commonly Used Conventional NSAIDs and COX-2–Specific Inhibitors

NSAID/COX-2–Specific Inhibitors	C_{max} (Peak Plasma Concentration)	T_{max}	$t_{1/2}$	Clearance (L/hr or L/hr/kg)	Excretion
Aspirin Soluble Tablet	150–300 µg/mL	25 min, 4–6hr	0.25hr	39 L/hr	Excreted as salicylic acid or as glycine, glucuronidate conjugates
Diclofenac 50 mg Soluble Tablet	0.7–1.2 µg/mL, 0.5–1.5 µg/mL	10–40 min, 1.5–2hr	1–1.5hr	15.6 L/hr	90% excreted within 96hr
Ibuprofen Solution 300 mg, Tablet 200–400 mg	37.9 mg/mL, 20–30 mg/mL	1.39hr, ~3hr	2–2.5hr	~0.04–0.1 L/hr/kg	70–90% excreted within 24 hr
Ketorolac 10 mg IV, IM, Oral (tablet)	2.39 µg/mL, 0.6–1.44 µg/mL, 0.7–0.9 µg/mL	5 min, 20–60 min, 1 hr	~5 hours	~0.01 L/hr/kg, ~0.01 L/hr/kg, ~0.3 L/hr/kg	91% excreted within 2 days (75% as glucuronidate conjugate; ~12% as *para*-hydroxylated form)
Naproxen 250–500 mg	20–80 µg/mL		12–15hr	0.3 L/hr	~80% of daily does excreted as glucuronidate conjugates
Acetaminophen 0.5–2 g		20–90 min	1.9–2.5 hr	~20–30 L/hr	85–95% excreted within 24 hr
Celecoxib 100–200 mg	0.6–0.7 µg/mL	2–4hr	11.2–15.6 hr	~20–40 L/hr	<2% recovered unchanged in urine
Rofecoxib 25–50 mg	207 µg/mL	2–3hr	~17hr	~7 L/hr	<1% recovered unchanged in urine
Parecoxib sodium IV 10–20 mg Parecoxib, Valdecoxib	2–4 µg/mL, 0.1–0.4 µg/mL	2–3 min, 1 hr	15–40 min, 5–8hr	~30–35 L/hr, ~6.5–7.5 L/hr	~95% excreted 5–8hr
Parecoxib sodium IM 10–20 mg Parecoxib, Valdecoxib	0.4–1 µg/mL, 0.13–0.27 µg/mL	~15 min, ~2.5 hr	~0.5 hr, 5.5–10hr	~35–38 L/hr, ~6–8 L/hr	~95% excreted 5–8hr

COX-2, cyclo-oxygenase; IM, intramuscularly; IV, intravenously; NSAIDs, nonsteroidal anti-inflammatory drugs.

ratio in individuals with a longer T_{max}, suggesting that the absorption rate is dependent on enantiomer inversion.[101] Detection of S-(+)-ibuprofen after IV administration of R-(−)-ibuprofen also suggests systemic enantiomer inversion. Oral, IM, and subcutaneous doses of ketorolac are rapidly absorbed, reaching C_{max} in 30 to 60 minutes.[72,73,94,95] The relative bioavailability after oral, IM, and IV administration is 80% to 100%.[102] Oral naproxen is rapidly and almost completely absorbed whether it is administered in suspension, capsule, or tablet form.[92] Naproxen suppositories are also readily absorbed with 94.6% bioavailability compared with tablets.[92]

Although acetaminophen is not classified as an NSAID because it is not an anti-inflammatory, it is frequently used to treat similar conditions (i.e., acute and chronic pain). Acetaminophen displays analgesic and antipyretic actions similar to aspirin and should therefore be considered in any discussion of conventional NSAIDs.[103] Oral acetaminophen is rapidly absorbed from the GI tract with C_{max} reached 20 to 90 minutes after ingestion. Its systemic bioavailability is dose-dependent and ranges from 70% to 90%, being reduced by first pass metabolism. Similar to NSAIDs, the absorption of acetaminophen is heavily dependent on factors such as the rate of gastric emptying, pH, and formulation.[103]

Distribution

All conventional NSAIDs are highly bound to plasma proteins, particularly albumin, limiting their distribution to extracellular spaces. As a result, volumes of distribution are often very low (<0.2 L/kg).[88] At therapeutic concentrations, a high proportion of NSAIDs such as salicylate (80–90%),[89] diclofenac (99%),[90,93] ibuprofen (99%),[91] ketorolac (99%),[94,95] and naproxen (99.6%)[92] are bound to plasma protein. NSAIDs are generally distributed throughout most body tissues, including synovial fluid and CSF. Total concentrations are generally lower in the synovium and CSF than in plasma, and T_{max} is longer; but lower protein concentrations in these fluids generally lead to lower concentrations of protein-bound NSAIDs, and elimination time is longer.[88] However, unlike NSAIDs, acetaminophen does not bind to plasma proteins at therapeutic doses, although approximately 15% to 20% of the drug is bound at concentrations associated with an overdose.[103] Therefore acetaminophen is distributed throughout most tissues, and its elimination is very rapid.

Metabolism and Excretion

There is a high degree of variability in the processes of metabolism and excretion of NSAIDs (see discussion later and outline in Table 25–1). Aspirin is rapidly hydrolyzed by nonspecific esterases into salicylate (within 15–20 minutes after absorption). Salicylate is excreted by renal elimination or by metabolism to salicyluric acid, salicyl phenolic glucuronide, salicyl acetyl glucuronide, and gentisic acid, which are subsequently excreted in urine.[88,89] The plasma $t_{1/2}$ of salicylate after low-dose aspirin is 2 to 3 hours, compared with 15 to 30 hours for high doses. Thus high salicylate concentrations, such as those used for anti-inflammatory

therapy, can be maintained by administration of aspirin every 8 to 12 hours.

Diclofenac is eliminated largely by metabolism to glucuronide, hydroxy, and sulphate conjugates, followed by excretion in the urine and bile.[93] Less than 1% is excreted in an unchanged form, and elimination is rapid, with 90% of the clearance occurring within 3 to 4 hours of administration. Ibuprofen is primarily eliminated by biotransformation and is metabolized to adenylate, glucuronidate, hydroxyl, or carboxyl derivatives; approximately 60% of the excreted drug is in the form of hydroxyl or carboxyl conjugates and less than 1% is recovered in the urine as unchanged ibuprofen.[91] Ketorolac is primarily metabolized by glucuronidation (~75%) and by *para*-hydroxylation (~12%). Approximately 91% of ketorolac or its metabolites is excreted in the urine within 2 days of administration.[94,95] Glucuronidation is also the main elimination pathway for naproxen; ~60% is recovered from the urine as naproxen glucuronidate. Naproxen is metabolized by dealkylation by cytochrome P450 (CYP) oxidase to an *o*-demethylated metabolite, followed by acyl glucuronidation. Less than 10% is excreted unchanged in the urine. Approximately 80% of each daily dose is excreted in conjugated form in the urine within 24 hours of administration.[92]

Acetaminophen is extensively metabolized to sulphate and glucuronidate derivatives in the liver, with only 2% to 5% being excreted unchanged. A minor fraction is converted in the liver and is oxidized by CYP to a highly reactive alkylating metabolite, which is rapidly deactivated by conjugation with reduced glutathione. Large doses of acetaminophen cause hepatic necrosis due to depleted glutathione and covalent binding of excess reactive metabolite to liver cell constituents. Between 85% and 95% of acetaminophen or its metabolites is excreted in the urine within 24 hours of administration in healthy subjects.[103]

Cyclo-oxygenase-2–Specific Inhibitors: Pharmacokinetic Parameters

The oral COX-2 inhibitors, including celecoxib, rofecoxib, and valdecoxib, differ from earlier NSAIDs in that they are all highly lipophilic, neutral, nonacidic molecules with very limited solubility in aqueous media. All three have been shown to have specificity for COX-2 versus COX-1 in vitro and in vivo and to spare COX-1 in humans at therapeutic doses. Parecoxib sodium is a water-soluble prodrug of valdecoxib that is rapidly converted to the active moiety (valdecoxib) in vivo, and thus is suitable for parenteral IV and IM administration.

Absorption

Oral celecoxib is well absorbed with C_{max} reached 2 to 4 hours after a single dose of 100 to 200 mg.[104,105] Rofecoxib is rapidly absorbed in the GI tract with peak plasma concentrations occurring 2 to 3 hours after oral administration.[106] Valdecoxib is currently the only COX-2–specific inhibitor with a parenteral formulation in development. IV parecoxib sodium, the inactive prodrug of valdecoxib, rapidly reaches C_{max} within 30 minutes after injection over a dose range of 1 to 100 mg. Plasma concentrations of parecoxib sodium are short-lived, because the drug is rapidly hydrolyzed to valdecoxib with peak valdecoxib plasma concentrations being reached approximately 1 hour after injection of parecoxib sodium.[107,108] Like conventional NSAIDs, the absorption of COX-2–specific inhibitors is affected by a number of factors—for example, administration of celecoxib with high fat meals extends T_{max} by 1 to 2 hours. Similarly, coadministration with aluminum- or magnesium-containing antacids results in ~37% decrease in C_{max} for celecoxib.[104]

Distribution

Celecoxib, like conventional NSAIDs, is highly protein-bound in plasma (~97%), primarily to albumin. Approximately 87% of rofecoxib is bound to plasma protein.

Metabolism and Excretion

Celecoxib is converted by hepatic biotransformation to hydroxy, carboxylic acid, and glucuronidate derivatives. Oxidative metabolism by the CYP 2C9 isoenzyme is the primary metabolic pathway, resulting in oxidation of the methyl moiety to a carboxyl group followed by glucuronidation of this carboxyl metabolite to form the major metabolite, SC-62807. A minor metabolite SC-60613 is also formed by partial oxidation of the methyl moiety to form a hydroxyl group. Only 2% of celecoxib is excreted in the urine unchanged.[104] None of the metabolites has appreciable activity on COX-1 or COX-2.

Rofecoxib is metabolized by an uncharacterized cytosolic reductase to *cis*-dihydro and *trans*-dihydro derivatives, most likely in the liver; these metabolites can undergo further hepatic biotransformation to carboxylic acid and glucuronidate derivatives. Most of a single daily dose is excreted in the urine within 17 hours of administration, and less than 1% of excreted drug is unchanged.[106]

After parenteral administration, peak plasma concentrations of parecoxib are short-lived (15–40 minutes) as parecoxib sodium is rapidly converted in vivo to its active metabolite, valdecoxib. Valdecoxib is in turn metabolized by hydroxylation to SC-66905, a derivative that is also a COX-2–specific inhibitor. The circulating concentrations of the parent compound are 7- to 20-fold greater than those of SC-66905. Valdecoxib and its hydroxylated active metabolite undergo extensive hepatic metabolism by CYP, as well as glucuronidation in some species.[108]

Drug/Drug Interactions of Conventional Nonsteroidal Anti-inflammatory Drugs and Cyclooxygenase-2–Specific Inhibitors

Nonsteroidal anti-inflammatory agents are used routinely to manage pain and inflammation and many formulations are available in nonprescription form. Therefore the likelihood of coadministration with other drugs is high and may have implications for the absorption, pharmacokinetics, and elimination of either compound.[88]

Conventional NSAIDs are associated with increased bleeding risks, including prolonged postoperative bleeding and upper GI bleeding, because of their inhibition of COX-1.[42] It is, therefore, important when prescribing these drugs to consider the potential for increased bleeding risks associated with the coadministration of NSAIDs with anticoagulant agents (e.g., the coumarin derivative warfarin). Pyrazole NSAIDs, like phenylbutazone, have been shown to be particularly hazardous when coadministered with warfarin; and aspirin, at the high doses used for the treatment of severe pain (>3 g/day), can cause increased bleeding when coadministered with warfarin.[109–111] COX-2–specific inhibitors, however, do not appear to have any significant interactions with anticoagulant agents.[104,106] The steady-state concentration of warfarin is not altered by coadministration with celecoxib, and prothrombin times are not significantly affected.[104,105] Rofecoxib has shown clinically insignificant interactions with warfarin, although coadministration of the two drugs results in an 8% increase in prothrombin time in healthy subjects.[106] Coadministration of the COX-2–specific inhibitor parecoxib sodium with aspirin, administered at doses recommended for cardiovascular prophylaxis, does not appear to cause any clinically significant changes in the effects of aspirin on platelet aggregation or bleeding times.[112] Currently, there are no published data on the interaction of valdecoxib with anticoagulants.

NSAIDs are frequently administered with opioid agents to enhance their analgesic potential, particularly in the treatment of postoperative pain. There is no strong evidence suggesting that the absorption, pharmacokinetics, or clearance of conventional NSAIDs or COX-2–specific inhibitors are adversely affected by opioids.[109,111]

Antacids, mucoprotective agents, and absorbent antidiarrheal agents can delay the absorption of NSAIDs, which is dependent on the relative doses, the timing of dosing, formulation of the medications, and the gastric contents.[113] High doses of aluminum-magnesium hydroxide can increase urinary pH and enhance excretion of salicylates, although it has no effect on the pharmacokinetics of other NSAIDs (e.g., ibuprofen or ketorolac).[88]

Mucosal protective agents such as sulglicotide and PG analogs are frequently coadministered with conventional NSAIDs to limit gastroduodenal ulceration.[109] However, they have been shown to reduce C_{max} and T_{max} of certain conventional NSAIDs, including naproxen and ketoprofen, although not diclofenac.[109] Other more lipophilic NSAIDs can be coadministered with β-cyclodextrins, which increase their absorption and may provide gastrocytoprotective effects. The mucosal protective agent misoprostol, a PG analog, can be administered with NSAIDs to reduce gastroduodenal ulceration without altering their bioavailability.[88]

Effect of Disease on Pharmacokinetics

The effects of disease state on the pharmacokinetics of conventional NSAIDs and COX-2–specific inhibitors are also important considerations for prescribing these drugs. Because most of these agents are metabolized through hepatic biotransformation and substantial proportions of each drug are eliminated through renal excretion, there are particular concerns for patients with hepatic and renal disorders.[88–95] Many patients with RA have some degree of renal function impairment making them susceptible to NSAID-induced renal failure. Also, patients with RA may have diminished serum albumin concentrations, thus alterations in free NSAID concentration may occur.

Renal dysfunction is expected to lead to changes in volume of distribution caused by decreased plasma protein binding of NSAIDs and accumulation of biotransformation products in the kidneys.[88] Unbound salicylate is increased in patients with renal failure; however, there is no concomitant change in other pharmacokinetic properties.[89] Total body clearance and volume of distribution of naproxen is significantly increased among patients with renal failure.[92] In patients with similar disorders, the elimination kinetics of diclofenac and ibuprofen are delayed mainly because of accumulation of diclofenac conjugates and primary metabolites.[90,91,93]

Celecoxib and rofecoxib display 47% and 69% decrease in AUC, respectively, in patients with moderate renal insufficiency.[104] Plasma clearance of ketorolac is reduced, the AUC is greater, and $t_{(1/2)}$ is prolonged in patients with renal impairment compared with healthy individuals.[94] Acetaminophen plasma concentrations and half-life are similar in healthy subjects and patients with chronic renal disease. However, there is an accumulation of its sulphate and glucuronidate conjugates in plasma up to four times greater than in healthy subjects.[103]

Free plasma salicylate concentrations are increased among patients with liver disease because of decreased plasma protein binding and clearance of salicylate.[88,89] AUC, C_{max}, and clearance values for ketorolac among patients with alcoholic cirrhosis were similar to healthy individuals, although T_{max} and $t_{(1/2)}$ were increased after IM and oral administration, respectively.[94,95] Patients with mild or moderate hepatic insufficiency demonstrated 22% and 63% decreases in clearance of celecoxib, respectively.[104] There are no published studies on the pharmacokinetics of rofecoxib, valdecoxib, or parecoxib sodium in patients with hepatic disease. Patients with liver disease who have abnormally low albumin concentrations and increased prothrombin time ratios display grossly abnormal elimination kinetics for acetaminophen because of the correlation between plasma half-life and clearance of the drug, serum albumin, and prothrombin time ratio.

Practical Aspects of Drug Administration

Conventional NSAIDs are used extensively in the management of pain associated with surgery. The predominant use of these agents in managing acute postoperative pain is as part of balanced multimodal analgesia in combination with opioids after major surgical procedures.[113–119] However, other studies have shown that they can be used as an alternative to opiates for more minor surgical procedures.[120–128] Diclofenac, naproxen, ibuprofen, and ketorolac are effective in reducing pain and opioid consumption in a multitude of surgical pain models including laparoscopic procedures, and dental, orthopedic, abdominal, and thoracic surgery.[120–123,125,127,128] Although some clinical trials show a lack of effective pain relief and opioid sparing effects with diclofenac after invasive surgical models associated with severe pain,[115,124,126] in general, the literature overwhelmingly supports the efficacy of NSAIDs in managing postoperative pain.

Conventional NSAIDs in the Management of Postsurgical Pain

NSAIDs have been used for the management of acute postoperative pain for the last 15 years, either alone for the treatment of mild to moderate pain or in combination with other analgesics as part of a multimodal therapeutic strategy. The use of NSAIDs in multimodal therapy is usually associated with major invasive surgical procedures such as abdominal, thoracic, and orthopedic surgery (e.g., joint arthroplasty).

Conventional NSAIDs, administered as an alternative to opioids, are effective in managing mild to moderate pain associated with less invasive surgical procedures, including maxillofacial surgery, minor orthopedic surgery, and some laparoscopic procedures. There is a high degree of variability between different NSAIDs in terms of their efficacy in managing postoperative pain. Thus ketorolac, which is generally considered to be one of the more powerful NSAIDs, is a more effective analgesic in surgical models than many other agents. As the efficacy of NSAIDs is not confined to reducing peripheral inflammation but also involves antinociceptive effects in the CNS, those agents that are able to cross the blood–brain barrier may be particularly effective in managing acute pain.

Conventional NSAIDs are also routinely used as an alternative to opioids in ambulatory surgical procedures because of the drawbacks of opioids in these patients. The strong sedative effects of opioids and their adverse effect profile, particularly increased nausea and vomiting, generally results in a slower time to patient recovery.

In clinical trials, naproxen sodium reduced postoperative pain intensity levels and pain relief scores after laparoscopic tubal ligation and exploratory laparoscopic surgery, reducing the requirement for other analgesics and shortening the length of each patient's hospital stay.[128,129] Preoperative administration of naproxen in daycare surgery patients also provided improved postoperative analgesia in the first few hours after surgery compared with postoperative administration.[121] Similarly, administration of ibuprofen after diagnostic laparoscopy reduced postoperative pain relief scores.[127] In this study, ibuprofen demonstrated analgesic efficacy that was equivalent to the opioid fentanyl, with a longer duration of action. Patients receiving ibuprofen also experienced a lower incidence of postoperative nausea, probably as a result of their reduced requirement for other postoperative analgesics.

Reported data on the postoperative analgesic efficacy of diclofenac are conflicting. Diclofenac effectively reduced postoperative pain after diagnostic laparoscopic procedures, although it did not significantly affect the rate of mobilization of patients and was considerably less effective in more invasive procedures such as laparoscopic tubal ligation or sterilization.[124–126] However, other studies report reduced pain scores in patients treated with diclofenac undergoing laparoscopic tubal ligation and major orthopedic surgery.[120,130] Diclofenac has also provided effective pain relief and has reduced the requirement for opiate rescue analgesics after maxillofacial surgery.[131] In addition, in a head-to-head comparison with ketorolac, diclofenac demonstrated equivalent efficacy to ketorolac in managing acute pain associated with the removal of impacted third molars.[132] In this study, both diclofenac and ketorolac produced improved pain scores, a rapid onset of analgesia, and a significantly longer time to requirement for rescue medication compared with placebo. Diclofenac and ketorolac are also reported to be equally effective in managing pain and reducing opioid use after thorascopic surgery.[133]

Ketorolac is considered to be one of the stronger NSAIDs and is often indicated for the management of acute pain that traditionally requires opioid analgesia. Ketorolac effectively reduces postoperative pain and the requirement for postoperative opioid analgesics in patients undergoing laparoscopic sterilization and cholecystectomy. In single dose trials, ketorolac was as effective as morphine or pethidine in treating acute pain and provided longer lasting analgesia.[134] In addition, in both major and minor surgical procedures, single doses of ketorolac (10–30 mg) IV or IM have been shown to be as effective as opiates such as IV morphine (20–100 mg) or pethidine (10–20 mg) in treating pain associated with surgery.[135] Ketorolac provided excellent analgesic efficacy that was equivalent to morphine after radical retropubic prostatectomy and allowed for earlier recovery and concomitant lower overall hospital costs.[117] Ketorolac is currently the only NSAID available in the United States as a parenteral formulation. The availability of both oral and parenteral formulations combined with its powerful analgesic efficacy means that it is often used in multimodal therapeutic strategies to reduce opioid requirements in surgical patients.

Acetaminophen alone has been shown to be ineffective in alleviating postoperative pain after dental surgery[136] and cesarean section.[137] However, acetaminophen (1000 mg) combined with oxycodone (10 mg; Tylox, Ortho-McNeil Pharmaceuticals, Springhouse, Pa.) is a strong analgesic in the treatment of acute postoperative pain,[136,137] as demonstrated in significant reductions in pain intensity levels and improved pain relief scores after dental surgery and cesarean section compared with placebo, acetaminophen, or oxycodone alone.

Although conventional NSAIDs are effective analgesics after minor surgical procedures, more invasive surgical techniques require more powerful analgesic combinations. The use of NSAIDs in combination with opioids has proved effective in reducing postoperative opioid requirements while maintaining effective analgesia. The reduction of opioid consumption has obvious benefits in reducing specific opioid-related side effects. However, although NSAIDs are opioid-sparing, they too are associated with a range of adverse effects that often make them less than ideal for administration to surgical patients.

Nonsteroidal Anti-inflammatory Drugs as Part of Multimodal Therapy

Opioids are extensively used for managing pain associated with surgery and are highly effective analgesics particularly during rest. They are less effective during mobilization after surgery and have strong sedative effects that limit their use in outpatient surgery. Opioids also produce a host of other adverse effects including impaired respiratory function with reduced sensitivity to hypoxemia and hypercapnia, reduced expiratory force and respiratory depression, marked sedative effects contributing to alveolar hypoventilation, sleep disturbances, nausea and vomiting, ileus, and urinary retention.[138–140] A multimodal approach to postoperative pain management has been recommended in surgical patients to reduce the use of opioid analgesics and therefore reduce opioid-related side effects. This opioid-sparing effect of NSAIDs is clinically relevant because it may reduce sedation,[141] improve respiratory function,[142] improve GI motility allowing earlier oral nutrition,[143] and reduce urinary retention.[144] In addition to improving patient comfort, multimodal therapy has a large pharmacoeconomic impact. Patients who receive opioids in combination with nonopioid analgesics require less direct nursing care, fewer doses of supplemental analgesia, meet recovery measures sooner, and have shorter hospital stays, resulting in a reduction of overall hospitalization costs.[117,128,129,143]

The opioid-sparing effects of the NSAIDs ketorolac, naproxen, and diclofenac in major surgical procedures are well documented. Coadministration of ketorolac (10–30 mg IV or IM) with morphine significantly improved pain control compared with morphine alone and allowed 25% to 50% less morphine use in the first 24 hours after several surgical procedures, including laparoscopy,[145,146] abdominal surgery,[113,118,119,143,147,148] orthopedic surgery,[149–151] and thoracic surgery.[116] The clinical importance of the opioid-sparing effects of ketorolac is not confined to improved pain relief. The incidence of opioid-related adverse effects is also reduced. Patients experienced earlier recovery of bowel function,[117] and, as a result, the length of hospital stay was significantly shortened and patient mobilization was more rapid. In one study, patients receiving ketorolac self-administered 40% less morphine compared with placebo patients, and consequently experienced a lower incidence of cardiorespiratory depression.[148] Furthermore, coadministration of ketorolac with morphine has been demonstrated to reduce myocardial ischemia in patients undergoing total hip or knee arthroplasty.[149] The withdrawal rate was also lower in thoracotomy patients who received ketorolac in combination with patient-controlled morphine than in those who received morphine alone.[116] There are also clear pharmacoeconomic benefits of including ketorolac in multimodal analgesic strategies; e.g., earlier patient mobilization and oral feeding, more rapid recovery of bowel function, and generally greater patient satisfaction are observed leading to overall reduction in hospital costs for individual patients.[117,152]

Diclofenac and naproxen have also been shown to have significant opioid-sparing effects in abdominal,[129,153–158] thoracic,[133,159] and orthopedic surgery,[130,160] reducing consumption of opiates such as morphine and fentanyl by up to 40% and improving analgesia compared with opioid treatment alone. However, data reporting the effectiveness of diclofenac as an opioid-sparing agent are conflicting. Although many studies have reported its effectiveness, other studies have demonstrated that diclofenac did not provide opioid-sparing effects after procedures such as cholecystectomy, major orthopedic surgery, or in the management of cancer pain.[114,115,161]

The optimal timing for multimodal analgesia is also controversial. It has been shown that preoperative and intraoperative administration of NSAIDs improves pain relief and reduces the requirement for additional postoperative analgesia.[162,163] Patients undergoing hip arthroplasty or abdominal hysterectomy experienced decreased pain during the recovery period and reduced morphine requirements when ketorolac (60 mg IV) was administered before the incision compared with administration of the same dose at closure of the incision.[162,163] In contrast, other studies that examined the benefits of preoperative versus postoperative administration of multimodal analgesia in thoracotomy patients demonstrated no, or only modest, benefits with respect to reduction in postoperative pain levels. However, the increased bleeding risks associated with conventional NSAIDs often prohibit their administration before and during surgery, therefore denying patients the advantage of pre-emptive analgesia.

Adverse Effects of Conventional Nonsteroidal Anti-inflammatory Drugs Versus Cyclo-oxygenase-2–Specific Inhibitors

Although NSAIDs are effective in managing the acute pain associated with surgery and inflammatory disorders and these agents are used routinely in daily clinical practice, they have an extensive side effect profile that contraindicates their use in many patients. COX-1 is constitutively expressed in platelets, the gastric mucosa, and renal tissue and is thought to be responsible for maintaining homeostasis in these tissues. The nonselective inhibition of both isoforms of COX by conventional NSAIDs interferes with normal GI and platelet function and leads to clinically important adverse events.[42]

As noted earlier, COX-1 catalyzes formation of PGH_2 from arachidonate released from the cell membranes of platelets, where it is subsequently metabolized to TxA_2, a potent stimulus of platelet aggregation. The inhibition of COX-1 in platelets by conventional NSAIDs results in the modulation of platelet function leading to prolonged bleeding. For surgical patients, the increased risk for bleeding associated with conventional NSAIDs is probably the most pertinent side effect.[43,164,165]

Studies have shown that most conventional NSAIDs are associated with reduced platelet aggregation in response to arachidonate and collagen, and there is a subsequent increase in bleeding times. Although NSAIDs are used routinely in the treatment of postoperative pain, many clinicians are reluctant to use these drugs in the perioperative period, even during minor surgical procedures like oral surgery. Preoperative and intraoperative administration of NSAIDs are considered to pose a greater risk in terms of increased wound site bleeding, particularly in orthopedic and abdominal surgery that already have a high risk for bleeding (see "Benefits of Administration of Injectable Versus Oral Compounds in Managing Surgical Pain"). This antiplatelet function of conventional NSAIDs contraindicates their use in many patients, particularly the elderly and those already being prescribed anticoagulants such as warfarin. Other studies have shown that patients who routinely take NSAIDs, including aspirin, ibuprofen, and naproxen, reported significantly more perioperative bleeding complications, including GI tract bleeding and hypotension.[164] In addition, such complications were considerably more frequent with NSAIDs with longer half lives (>6 hours).[164] Therefore it is recommended that patients who are routinely prescribed conventional NSAIDs for the management of chronic pain associated with inflammatory disorders or prophylactic aspirin should stop taking the NSAIDs before surgery to allow time for their elimination.

In addition to increased bleeding risks during surgery, conventional NSAIDs present a greater risk for GI side effects, ranging from mild irritation and intolerability to life-threatening complications. Conventional NSAIDs are associated with low GI tolerability leading to symptoms such as nausea, dyspepsia, abdominal pain, diarrhea, and constipation.[166,167] These side effects can be apparent even with short-term use of NSAIDs. More clinically important GI complications include gastroduodenal and intestinal ulceration that can lead to potentially life-threatening upper GI bleeding and GI perforation.[44,45,165] The dangers of GI perforation and bleeding are compounded by the inhibition of platelet function observed with conventional NSAIDs, leading to bleeding episodes that dramatically increase patient mortality rates. NSAIDs such as naproxen, diclofenac, ibuprofen, and piroxicam lead to gastroduodenal ulcer rates ranging from 15% to 40%, and GI complications among patients with arthritis are common, with an estimated 16,800 deaths per year in the United States caused by conventional NSAID-related gastroduodenal injury.[168] Although GI complications are more often associated with long-term prescription of NSAIDs in conditions such as RA and OA, GI erosion and ulceration can also occur with short-term use of conventional NSAIDs. Ketorolac in particular demonstrates a high incidence of GI tract ulceration after a few days of use, and it is recommended that it be prescribed for no more than 5 days (see "Benefits of Administration of Injectable Versus Oral Compounds in Managing Surgical Pain").

Conventional NSAIDs are also associated with renal side effects. PGs are involved in the control of renin release, regulation of vascular tone, and control of tubular function. Therefore one of the drawbacks of conventional NSAID therapy is its adverse effect on renal function. These NSAIDs are most frequently associated with a transient imbalance of electrolyte and water levels that is generally mild in most patients. However, patients with renal disease, elderly patients, and patients with cardiovascular problems are at risk for more serious renal complications including acute ischemic renal failure, interstitial nephritis, and renal papillary necrosis. An increased rate of acute renal failure has been observed in patients treated with ketorolac for more than 5 days.[169]

In recent years, the development of COX-2–specific inhibitors, such as celecoxib and rofecoxib, has allowed effective management of pain and inflammation associated with OA and RA, while eliminating many of the side effects caused by conventional NSAIDs.[11,13] COX-2–specific inhibitors provide analgesic and anti-inflammatory activity equivalent to conventional NSAIDs with improved safety due to their COX-1–sparing effects.[9,11,13] COX-1 is the only COX isoform expressed in platelets, therefore COX-2–specific inhibitors display a significantly reduced bleeding risk compared with nonspecific COX inhibitors.[112,170–174] The improved platelet safety of COX-2–specific inhibitors makes them valuable agents for the management of pain associated with surgical procedures. COX-2–specific inhibitors can be safely administered for the management of postoperative pain, and because they do not present a risk for increased bleeding, they are suitable analgesics for preoperative and intraoperative administration.

Cyclo-oxygenase-2–Specific Inhibitors in the Treatment of Postsurgical Pain

There is limited published information on the effectiveness of the new COX-2–specific inhibitors in managing postoperative pain. However, both celecoxib and rofecoxib have been shown to be as effective as the conventional NSAIDs naproxen, ibuprofen, and diclofenac in reducing pain after oral[175–180] and spinal fusion surgery.[181] Not only were these first generation COX-2 inhibitors effective in reducing pain and inflammation after surgery, but they also reduced the requirement for postoperative opiates in many patients.[182] More recently, numerous clinical trials have shown that valdecoxib, a novel COX-2–specific inhibitor, and parecoxib sodium, the injectable prodrug of valdecoxib, are effective in treating postoperative pain.[183–188] Valdecoxib and parecoxib sodium effectively reduce postoperative pain associated with a range of surgical procedures, including oral,[183,185] orthopedic,[186–188] and abdominal surgery.[189,190] Valdecoxib and parecoxib sodium demonstrate opioid-sparing effects when administered perioperatively in patients who were undergoing orthopedic surgery.[191,192] In addition, the same trials demonstrated improved pain intensity levels and pain relief in postoperative patients, despite the reduction in morphine use.[191,192]

Benefits of Administration of Injectable Versus Oral Compounds in Managing Surgical Pain

A substantial number of surgical patients cannot tolerate postoperative oral medication, and some procedures, including oral and maxillofacial surgery, prohibit the preoperative administration of oral medication. Therefore there is a need for injectable analgesic agents that can be administered to surgical patients. Ketorolac (Toradol, Roche Pharmaceuti-

cals, Nutley, N.J.) was approved by the Food and Drug Administration (FDA) in 1989 for the short-term management of pain and was the first (and is currently the only) injectable conventional NSAID available in the United States. Its early indications were for the management of postoperative pain, either alone or as part of multimodal therapy. The efficacy of ketorolac in treating postoperative pain has been highlighted earlier. The relatively short T_{max} of ketorolac compared with oral analgesics results in rapid onset of analgesia. In addition, some clinical trial data have shown that the requirements for additional postoperative analgesics are fewer with IV compared with oral ketorolac administration, and continuous IV infusion leads to lower postoperative morphine use compared with intermittent administration of ketorolac.[113]

Ketorolac has obvious benefits as an injectable NSAID that has strong analgesic effects. Despite this, serious side effects, characteristic of conventional NSAIDs, are associated with the drug. Between 1990 and 1993, ketorolac was prescribed to 16 million people in the United States and was implicated in 97 deaths, half of which were caused by GI bleeding and perforation. The side effects of ketorolac range from GI irritation to serious ulceration and include low GI tolerability (nausea, dyspepsia, GI pain and fullness, diarrhea, vomiting, constipation, and so on),[193] in addition to serious GI bleeding, perforation, and gastroduodenal ulceration.[44,45,94,95] Gastric and duodenal ulcers are most common, but there have also been incidences of colonic ulcers indicating that the ulcerogenic effects of ketorolac may be mediated systemically.[194] In addition to increased risk for GI bleeding, a number of studies have demonstrated clinically significant increases in bleeding at the wound site during surgical procedures.[195,196] Increases in bleeding episodes in pediatric surgery (tonsillectomy) in response to ketorolac compared with codeine and morphine have also been reported.[195,196,198] The risk for these effects is increased if ketorolac is used in higher doses (>105 mg/day), in elderly patients, and is administered for more than 5 days.[165] These findings negate any benefit of the drug for preoperative and intraoperative analgesia, particularly in procedures such as orthopedic surgery in which the risk for bleeding is already high.

Parecoxib sodium is currently the only parenteral COX-2–specific inhibitor in development in the United States. Clinical trials have shown that, like ketorolac, parecoxib sodium is effective in managing postoperative pain associated with a variety of surgical procedures, including oral and orthopedic surgery and abdominal hysterectomy. Parecoxib sodium also demonstrates strong opioid-sparing effects, with patients requiring up to 40% less morphine than patients receiving placebo.[192] In addition, preoperative administration of parecoxib sodium demonstrates greater efficacy in managing pain associated with surgery.[184,185] The improved platelet safety profile of parecoxib sodium and the consequent reduction in bleeding times compared with conventional NSAIDs means that its preoperative administration presents far fewer risks for increased bleeding during surgery than conventional NSAIDs.[112,173,174] Thus the availability of an injectable COX-2–specific inhibitor will provide greater flexibility when prescribing preoperative and postoperative analgesia to manage surgical pain and inflammation.

Dosing and Administration

Conventional Nonsteroidal Anti-inflammatory Drugs

It has been difficult to establish relationships between plasma concentrations of NSAIDs and the clinical efficacy of these drugs in managing acute pain and inflammatory disorders. Moreover, the response to different NSAIDs is highly variable between different patients; thus a patient who responds well to diclofenac may not necessarily respond in a similar manner to naproxen or ibuprofen. However, some correlations have been drawn between analgesic efficacy and drug plasma concentrations (correlations are outlined later in this chapter).

In contrast to opioids, the analgesic effects of NSAIDs reach a plateau, although they may be dose-dependent at lower concentrations. Therefore NSAIDs by themselves may not adequately control severe pain. However, they have a valuable role as adjuvant analgesics in balanced multi-modal therapy, particularly in surgical patients experiencing severe acute pain. The recommended dosing levels for some of the most commonly used NSAIDs are outlined in Table 26–2. Some of the clinical considerations of dosing and administration of NSAIDs are discussed later in this chapter.

Aspirin is used for analgesic, anti-inflammatory, and antipyretic indications. The optimal plasma therapeutic range of aspirin for analgesia and anti-inflammatory activity in patients with chronic inflammatory disorders is 15 to 30 mg/100 mL, requiring daily doses in excess of 3 g.[89] As this optimal plasma concentration is only slightly less than toxic levels, care should be taken in the clinical use of salicylates. Recommended doses for cardiovascular prophylaxis vary. Significant reduction of platelet aggregation has been demonstrated after administration of a 650-mg dose of aspirin.[199] Aspirin is also used to reduce temperature, for relief of headache, and for relief of muscle and joint pain associated with minor febrile conditions such as colds or influenza. Aspirin is available as plain, uncoated, buffered tablets, dispersible tablets, enteric-coated tablets, and modified release tablets, or as suppositories. Oral aspirin should be taken with food to reduce gastric irritation.[89]

The usual recommended initial dose for diclofenac is 75 to 150 mg daily (25–50 mg three times daily) for the relief of pain and inflammation in patients with RA and OA, ankylosing spondylitis, gout, and after surgery. Linear pharmacokinetics are observed within this dose range.[90,93]

Ibuprofen is recommended for the management of mild to moderate pain in dysmenorrhea, migraine, postoperative procedures, ankylosing spondylitis, OA and RA, including juvenile RA, and other musculoskeletal and joint disorders.[91] Its anti-inflammatory properties may be weaker than some other conventional NSAIDs. The usual recommended analgesic daily dose of ibuprofen is 200 to 400 mg every 4 to 6 hours. In inflammatory conditions, the recommended dosage is 400 to 800 mg three to four times daily, up to a maximum daily dosage of 3200 mg/day in patients with RA.[91] Ibuprofen has a wide therapeutic range between 10 and 50 mg/L and is toxic at greater than 100 mg/L. The $t_{1/2}$ of ibuprofen is short, resulting in the need for frequent administration to maintain peak plasma concentrations within the therapeutic range.[91] A positive correlation has been shown between total ibuprofen concentration and analgesic effect in patients with mild to moderate pain following third molar extraction.[200]

Ketorolac is used as an oral analgesic, anti-inflammatory, and antipyretic agent, and as an IM or IV injection for short-term management of pain.[94] Ketorolac is indicated for the management of acute pain that traditionally requires opioid analgesia over short-term periods. Ketorolac is generally used for the treatment of postoperative acute pain, but is on occasion recommended for other painful conditions such as acute back pain.[113,116,132–135] The serious GI and platelet adverse effects of ketorolac are such that long-term use or use in children are not recommended.[165] The side effects of ketorolac have also resulted in a high degree of variability in dosing recommendations in different countries, and in some cases the removal of the drug's license (e.g., in France and Germany). The maximum recommended IM dose is 60 mg. In the United States and the United Kingdom, 10 to 30 mg ketorolac may be administered intravenously or intramuscularly as a single dose or every 4 to 6 hours.[94] Total dosage should not exceed 90 mg/day in the United Kingdom or 120 mg/day in the United States for parenteral administration, and 40 mg/day for oral therapy.[94] Parenteral ketorolac should not be administered for more than 5 days in the United States or 2 days in the United Kingdom, and patients should be switched to oral therapy as soon as possible.[94] A lower 15-mg loading dose, up to 60 mg/day, is generally prescribed for patients older than 65 years, and exceeding this dosage in this population is not recommended. This is also the recommended daily dosage in patients with renal impairment and should not be exceeded.[94]

Naproxen is used in musculoskeletal and joint disorders such as ankylosing spondylitis, OA, and RA, and to manage mild to moderate pain in conditions such as dysmenorrhea, migraine, and acute gout.[92] The recommended initial dosage for naproxen is 250 to 375 mg twice daily, and the maintenance dosage in inflammatory conditions is 375 to 750 mg in 2 separate doses. A linear relationship has been suggested between the dose and AUC for dosages up to 500 mg twice daily. However, other studies have suggested dose-dependent kinetics occurring between 250 and 500 mg.[92]

Acetaminophen has analgesic and antipyretic activity and is given orally or as a rectal suppository. For long-term therapy, the daily dosage should not exceed 2.6 g.[103]

Conventional NSAIDs share many contraindications in patients with a history of bleeding complications, GI disease, and NSAID hypersensitivity. They should also be used with caution in elderly patients, children, and patients with congestive heart failure, hepatic impairment, and hypertension. Concomitant use of NSAIDs with other NSAIDs, probenecid, pentoxifylline, or lithium should be avoided, and they should be administered with caution in patients on anticoagulant therapy (including warfarin and heparin).

Cyclo-oxygenase-2–Specific Inhibitors

The availability of COX-2–specific inhibitors that provide analgesic and anti-inflammatory efficacy that is equivalent

TABLE 26-2.

Dosing Guidelines for Commonly Used Conventional NSAIDs and COX-2–Specific Inhibitors

NSAID/COX-2–Specific Inhibitors	Route of Administration	Acute Pain (Postoperative Analgesia)	Acute Pain (Dysmenorrhea/Myalgia/Dental Pain, etc.)	Inflammatory Disorders (RA/OA/Ankylosing Spondulitis/Gout, etc.)	Juvenile RA
Aspirin	Oral	N/A	0.3–0.9 g every 4–6hr, up to 4 g/day	4–8 g/day	N/A
Diclofenac	Oral suppository	75–150 mg/day		75–100 mg/day 100 mg/day	1–3 mg/kg body weight
Ibuprofen	Oral	N/A	1.2–1.8 g/day	1.2–1.8 g/day	20 mg/kg body weight
Ketorolac	IV or IM	30–60 mg loading dose plus 15–30 mg every 6 hr (15 mg prescribed for patients >65 yr)	N/A	N/A	N/A
Naproxen	Oral		500 mg loading dose, followed by 250 mg every 6–8 hr	500–1000 mg/day (daily or twice daily)	10 mg/kg body weight
Acetaminophen	Oral	N/A	0.5–1 g every 4–6hr up to max 4 g/day	0.5–1 g every 4–6hr (for long-term therapy should not exceed 2.4 g/day	N/A
Celecoxib	Oral	50–400 mg/day	N/A	200 mg daily or 100 mg twice daily	N/A
Rofecoxib	Oral	50 mg loading dose (up to 75 mg/day)	50 mg loading dose (up to 75 mg/day)	12.5–25 mg/day	N/A
Parecoxib sodium	IV or IM	20–40 mg loading dose (up to 80 mg/day)	N/A	N/A	N/A
Valdecoxib	Oral	20–40 mg loading dose (up to 80 mg/day)	20–40 mg/day (with optional second dose if required)	10–20 mg/day	N/A

COX-2, cyclo-oxygenase-2; IM, intramuscularly; IV, intravenously; N/A, not applicable; OA, osteoarthritis; RA, rheumatoid arthritis.

to most NSAIDs, while providing an improved platelet and GI safety profile, has broadened the physician's analgesic armentarium.

Celecoxib was the first COX-2–specific inhibitor to be approved by the U.S. FDA (in 1998) and is recommended for the treatment of pain and inflammation associated with OA and RA.[104] For patients with OA, an initial dosage of 200 mg daily, administered as a single dose or as 100 mg twice daily, is recommended. In patients with RA, a therapeutic dosage of 100 to 200 mg twice daily is recommended.[104]

The recommended dosing of rofecoxib for acute pain, including pain associated with surgery, is a loading dose of 50 mg followed by a further 25 mg daily.[106] A single daily dose of 12.5 or 25 mg daily is recommended for patients with OA. Rofecoxib (50 mg) demonstrates similar analgesic efficacy to naproxen sodium and ibuprofen for treatment of postoperative dental pain.[175,177] A loading dose of 50 mg followed by a further 25 mg daily is recommended for the treatment of menstrual pain associated with primary dysmenorrhea and is equivalent to 550 mg naproxen.[201] In inflammatory disorders, the recommended daily dosage of rofecoxib is 5 to 50 mg once daily for treatment of OA of the hip or knee. Rofecoxib has similar clinical efficacy to diclofenac and ibuprofen in alleviating chronic pain and inflammation associated with OA.[202]

A once daily dose of valdecoxib 40 mg is recommended for the management of pain, including the treatment of menstrual pain associated with primary dysmenorrhea. Valdecoxib may be administered before surgery for relief of postoperative pain; 40 mg administered 1 hour before the surgical procedure, and an additional 40 mg to be taken after surgery on the first day of treatment if required.[183,184,191] The recommended dosage for the treatment of the signs and symptoms of OA and RA is 10 mg once daily, although some patients may receive additional benefit from a 20-mg once daily dosage.[203,204] Parecoxib sodium is currently the only parenteral form of a COX-2–specific inhibitor in development. Pending approval by the FDA, a once daily dose of 40 mg parecoxib sodium is recommended for the management of pain. Parecoxib sodium may be administered before surgery for relief of postoperative pain, 40 mg administered 1 hour before the surgical procedure, and an additional 40 mg to be taken after surgery on the first day of treatment if required.[185,186,205] Dosing can be increased to 40 mg twice a day if required.[185,186,205]

References

1. Vane JR: Inhibition of prostaglandin synthesis as a mechanism of action for aspirin-like drugs. Nat New Biol 231:232, 1971.
2. Huang Z, Massey J: Differential regulation of cyclooxygenase-2 (COX-2) mRNA stability by interleukin-1 beta (IL-1 beta) and tumor necrosis factor-alpha (TNF-alpha) in human in vitro differentiated macrophages. Biochem Pharmacol 59:187, 2000.
3. Porreca E, Reale M, Febbo CD, et al: Down-regulation of cyclooxygenase-2 (COX-2) by interleukin-receptor antagonist in human monocytes. Immunology 89:424, 1996.
4. Kang RY, Freire-Moar, Sigal E, et al: Expression of cyclooxygenase-2 in human and an animal model of rheumatoid arthritis. Br J Rheumatol 35:711, 1996.
5. Vanegas H, Schaible HG: Prostaglandins and cyclooxygenases in the spinal cord. Prog Neurobiol 64:327, 2001.
6. Seibert K, Zhang Y, Leahy K, et al: Pharmacological and biochemical demonstration of the role of cyclooxygenase 2 in inflammation and pain. Proc Natl Acad Sci USA 91:12013, 1994.
7. Matsumoto H, Ma W, Smalley W, et al: Diversification of cyclooxygenase-2-derived prostaglandins in ovulation and implantation. Biol Reprod 64:1557, 2001.
8. Pall M, Frieden B, Brännström M: Induction of delayed follicular rupture in the human by the selective COX-2 inhibitor rofecoxib: A randomized double-blind study. Hum Reprod 16:1323, 2001.
9. Bensen WG, Zhao SZ, Burke TA, et al: Upper gastrointestinal tolerability of celecoxib, a COX-2 specific inhibitor, compared to naproxen and placebo. J Rheumatol 27:1876, 2000.
10. Simon LS, Lanza FL, Lipsky PE, et al: Preliminary study of the safety and efficacy of SC-58635, a novel cyclooxygenase 2 inhibitor: Efficacy and safety in two placebo-controlled trials in osteoarthritis and rheumatoid arthritis, and studies of gastrointestinal and platelet effects. Arthritis Rheum 41:1591, 1998.
11. Silverstein FE, Faich G, Goldstein JL, et al: Gastrointestinal toxicity with celecoxib vs. nonsteroidal anti-inflammatory drugs for osteoarthritis and rheumatoid arthritis: The CLASS study: A randomized controlled trial. Celecoxib Long-term Arthritis Safety Study. JAMA 284:1247, 2000.
12. Bombardier C, Laine L, Reicin AS: Risk factors for clinically important upper GI events: The Vigor Study. European League against Rheumatism Annual Congress, June 13–16, 2001, Prague, Czech Republic.
13. Watson DJ, Harper SE, Zhao PL, et al: Gastrointestinal tolerability of the selective cyclooxygenase-2 (COX-2) inhibitor rofecoxib compared with nonselective COX-1 and COX-2 inhibitors in osteoarthritis. Arch Intern Med 160:2998, 2000.
14. National Center for Health Statistics on line: Available at www.cdc.gov/nchs/fastats/insurg.htm/
15. Doubell TP, Mannion RJ, Woolf CJ: The dorsal horn: State-dependent sensory processing, plasticity and the generation of pain. In Wall PD, Melzack R (eds): Textbook of Pain. Hong Kong, Churchill Livingstone, 1999.
16. Woolf CJ, Salter MW: Neuronal plasticity: Increasing the gain in pain. Science 288:1765, 2000.
17. Vasko MR, Campbell WB, Waite KJ: Prostaglandin E2 enhances bradykinin-stimulated release of neuropeptides from rat sensory neurons in culture. J Neurosci 14:4987, 1994.
18. Okano K, Kuraishi Y, Satoh M: Involvement of spinal substance P and excitatory amino acids in inflammatory hyperalgesia in rats. Jpn J Pharmacol 76:15, 1998.
19. Woolf CJ, Mannion RJ: Neuropathic pain: Aetiology, symptoms, mechanisms, and management. Lancet 353:1959, 1999.
20. Woolf CJ, Costigan M: Transcriptional and posttranslational plasticity and the generation of inflammatory pain. Proc Natl Acad Sci USA 96:7723, 1999.
21. Ji R-R, Woolf CJ: Neuronal plasticity and signal transduction in nociceptive neurons: Implications for the initiation and maintenance of pathological pain. Neurobiol Dis 8:1, 2001.
22. Mannion RJ, Costigan M, Decosterd I, et al: Neurotrophins: Peripherally and centrally acting modulators of tactile stimulus-induced inflammatory pain hypersensitivity. Proc Natl Acad Sci USA 96:9385, 1999.
23. Neumann S, Doubell TP, Leslie T, et al: Inflammatory pain hypersensitivity mediated by phenotypic switch in myelinated primary sensory neurons. Nature 384:360, 1996.
24. O'Banion MK: Cyclooxygenase-2: Molecular biology, pharmacology, and neurobiology. Crit Rev Neurobiol 13:45, 1999.
25. Dorsam G, Taher MM, Valerie KC, et al: Diphenyleneiodium blocks inflammatory cytokine-induced up-regulation of group IIA phospholipase A(2) in rat mesangial cells. J Pharmacol Exp Ther 292:271, 2000.
26. Han HJ, Park SH, Koh HJ, et al: Mechanism of regulation of Na+ transport by angiotensin II in primary renal cells. Kidney Int 57:2457, 2000.
27. Sun G, Stacey MA, Schmidt M, et al: Interactions of mite allergens der p3 and der p9 with protease-activated receptor-2 expressed by lung epithelial cells. J Immunol 167:1014, 2001.
28. Poulin B, Rich N, Mitev Y, et al: Differential involvement of calcium channels and protein kinase-C activity in GnRH-induced

phospholipase-C, -A2 and -D activation in a gonadotrope cell line (alpha T3-1). Mol Cell Endocrinol 122:33, 1996.

29. Rawlinson SC, Wheeler-Jones CP, Lanyon LE: Arachidonic acid for loading induced prostacyclin and prostaglandin E(2)-release from osteoblasts and osteocytes is derived from the activity of different forms of phospholipase A(2). Bone 27:241, 2000.

30. Triggiani M, Granata F, Oriente A, et al: Secretory phospholipases A2 induce beta-glucuronidase release and IL-6 production from human lung macrophages. J Immunol 164:4908, 2000.

31. Kuehl FA, Egan RW: Prostaglandins, arachidonic acid, and inflammation. Science 210:978, 1980.

32. Dominguez Z, Merhi-Soussi F, MacOvschi O, et al: Endothelial cell prostacyclin synthesis induced by lymphocytes is independent of the membrane fatty acid composition of both cell types and of E-selectin, VCAM-1 or ICAM-1-mediated adhesion. Br J Haematol 113:521, 2001.

33. Hart PH: Regulation of the inflammatory response in asthma by mast cell products. Immunol Cell Biol 79:149, 2001.

34. Hahn G, Stuhlmüller B, Hain N, et al: Modulation of monocyte activation in patients with rheumatoid arthritis by leukapheresis therapy. J Clin Invest 91:862, 1993.

35. Goppelt-Struebe M, Wolter D, Resch K: Glucocorticoids inhibit prostaglandin synthesis not only at the level of phospholipase A2 but also at the level of cyclooxygenase/PGE isomerase. Br J Pharmacol 94:1287, 1989.

36. Breyer R, Bagdassarian C, Myers S, et al: Prostanoid receptors: Subtypes and signaling. Annu Rev Pharmacol Toxicol 41:661, 2001.

37. Kujubu DA, Fletcher BS, Varnum BC, et al: TIS10, a phorbol ester tumor promoter-inducible mRNA from Swiss 3T3 cells, encodes a novel prostaglandin synthase/cyclooxygenase homologue. J Biol Chem 266:12866, 1991.

38. Merlie JP, Fagan D, Mudd J, et al: Isolation and characterization of the complementary DNA for sheep seminal vesicle prostaglandin endoperoxide synthase (cyclooxygenase). J Biol Chem 263:3550, 1988.

39. O'Banion MK, Sadowski HB, Winn V, et al: A serum- and glucocorticoid-regulated 4-kilobase mRNA encodes a cyclooxygenase-related protein. J Biol Chem 266:23261, 1991.

40. Raz A, Wyche A, Needleman P: Temporal and pharmacological division of fibroblast cyclooxygenase expression into transcriptional and translational phases. Proc Natl Acad Sci USA 86:1657, 1989.

41. Xie WL, Chipman JG, Robertson DL, et al: Expression of a mitogen-responsive gene encoding prostaglandin synthase is regulated by mRNA splicing. Proc Natl Acad Sci USA 88:2692, 1991.

42. Borda IT, Koff R: NSAIDs: A profile of adverse effects. Philadelphia, Hanley and Belfus, 1995.

43. Born BVR, Cross MJ: The aggregation of blood platelets. J Physiol 168:178, 1963.

44. Gabriel SE, Jaakkimainen L, Bombardier C: Risk for serious gastrointestinal complications related to use of nonsteroidal anti-inflammatory drugs. A meta-analysis. Ann Intern Med 115:787, 1991.

45. Garcia Rodriguez LA, Jick H: Risk of upper gastrointestinal bleeding and perforation associated with individual non-steroidal anti-inflammatory drugs. Lancet 343:769, 1994.

46. Masferrer JL, Zweifel BS, Manning PT, et al: Selective inhibition of inducible cyclooxygenase 2 in vivo is antiinflammatory and nonulcerogenic. Proc Natl Acad Sci USA 91:3228, 1994.

47. Laneuville O, Breuer DK, Dewitt DL, et al: Differential inhibition of human prostaglandin endoperoxide H synthases-1 and -2 by nonsteroidal anti-inflammatory drugs. J Pharmacol Exp Ther 271:927, 1994.

48. Hay C, de Belleroche J: Carrageenan-induced hyperalgesia is associated with increased cyclooxygenase-2 expression in spinal cord. Neuroreport 8:1249, 1997.

49. Hay CH, Trevethick MA, Wheeldon A, et al: The potential role of spinal cord cyclooxygenase-2 in the development of Freund's complete adjuvant-induced changes in hyperalgesia and allodynia. Neuroscience 78:843, 1997.

50. Yamagata K, Andreasson KI, Kaufmann WE, et al: Expression of a mitogen-inducible cyclooxygenase in brain neurons: Regulation by synaptic activity and glucocorticoids. Neuron 11:371, 1993.

51. Zhang Y, Shaffer A, Portanova J, et al: Inhibition of cyclooxygenase-2 rapidly reverses inflammatory hyperalgesia and prostaglandin E2 production. J Pharmacol Exp Ther 283:1069, 1997.

52. Watanabe A, Nakashima S, Adachi T, et al: Changes in the expression of lipid-mediated signal-transducing enzymes in the rat liver after partial hepatectomy. Surg Today 30:622, 2000.

53. O'Brien TP, Roszkowski MT, Wolff LF, et al: Effect of a non-steroidal anti-inflammatory drug on tissue levels of immunoreactive prostaglandin E2, immunoreactive leukotriene, and pain after periodontal surgery. J Periodontol 67:1307, 1996.

54. Power I, Cumming AD, Pugh GC: Effect of diclofenac on renal function and prostacyclin generation after surgery. Br J Anaesth 69:451, 1992.

55. Roszkowski MT, Swift JQ, Hargreaves KM: Effect of NSAID administration on tissue levels of immunoreactive prostaglandin E2, leukotriene B4, and (S)-flurbiprofen following extraction of impacted third molars. Pain 73:339, 1997.

56. Huval WV, Lelcuk S, Allen PD, et al: Determinants of cardiovascular stability during abdominal aortic aneurysmectomy (AAA). Ann Surg 199:216, 1984.

57. Lewin J, Swedenborg J, Egberg N, et al: Effect of acetyl salicylic acid on increased production of thromboxane after aortic graft surgery. Eur J Vasc Surg 3:213, 1989.

58. Subramanian VA, Hernandez Y, Tack-Goldman K, et al: Prostacyclin production by internal mammary artery as a factor in coronary artery bypass grafts. Surgery 100:376, 1986.

59. Amin AR, Attur M, Patel RN, et al: Superinduction of cyclooxygenase-2 activity in human osteoarthritis-affected cartilage. Influence of nitric oxide. J Clin Invest 99:1231, 1997.

60. Sano H, Hla T, Maier JA, et al: In vivo cyclooxygenase expression in synovial tissues of patients with rheumatoid arthritis and rats with adjuvant and streptococcal cell wall arthritis. J Clin Invest 89:97, 1992.

61. Siigle I, Klein T, Backman JT, et al: Expression of cyclooxygenase-1 and cyclooxygenase-2 in human synovial tissue: Differential elevation of cyclooxygenase in inflammatory joint disease. Arthritis Rheum 41:122, 1998.

62. Zhao Z, Chen SR, Eisenach JC, et al: Spinal cyclooxygenase-2 is involved in development of allodynia after nerve injury in rats. Neuroscience 97:743, 2000.

63. Samad TA, Moore KA, Sapirstein A, et al: Interleukin-1 beta-mediated induction of COX-2 in the CNS contributes to inflammatory pain hypersensitivity. Nature 410:471, 2001.

64. Ferreira SH, Lorenzetti BB, Bristow AF, et al: Interleukin-1 beta as a potent hyperalgesic agent antagonized by a tripeptide analogue. Nature 334:698, 1988.

65. Garavito RM: The three dimensional structure of cyclooxygenases. In Vane JR, Botting J, Botting RS (eds): Improved nonsteroidal anti-inflammatory drugs: COX-2 enzyme inhibitors. Dordrecht, Kluwer Academic Publishers, 1996.

66. Picot D, Loll PJ, Garavito RM: The X-ray crystal structure of the membrane protein prostaglandin H2 synthase. Nature 367:243, 1994.

67. Loll PJ, Picot D, Ekabo O, et al: Synthesis and use of iodinated nonsteroidal anti-inflammatory drug analogs as crystallographic probes of the prostaglandin H2 synthase cyclooxygenase active site. Biochemistry 35:7330, 1996.

68. Mancini JA, Riendeau D, Falgueyret JP, et al: Arginine 120 of prostaglandin G/H synthase-1 is required for the inhibition by nonsteroidal anti-inflammatory drugs containing a carboxylic acid moiety. J Biol Chem 270:29372, 1995.

69. Gierse JK, Koboldt CM, Walker MC, et al: Kinetic basis for selective inhibition of cyclo-oxygenases. Biochem J 339:607, 1999.

70. Kurumbail RG, Stevens AM, Gierse JK, et al: Structural basis for selective inhibition of cyclooxygenase-2 by anti-inflammatory agents. Nature 384:644, 1996.

71. Luong C, Miller A, Barnett J, et al: Flexibility of the NSAID binding site in the structure of human cyclooxygenase-2. Nat Struct Biol 3:927, 1996.

72. Rome LH, Lands WE: Structural requirements for time-dependent inhibition of prostaglandin biosynthesis by anti-inflammatory drugs. Proc Natl Acad Sci USA 72:4863, 1975.

73. Loll PJ, Picot D, Garavito RM: The structural basis of aspirin activity inferred from the crystal structure of inactivated prostaglandin H2 synthase. Nat Struct Biol 2:637, 1995.

74. Lecomte M, Laneuville O, Ji C, et al: Acetylation of human prostaglandin endoperoxide synthase-2 (cyclooxygenase-2) by aspirin. J Biol Chem 269:13207, 1994.

75. Wennogle LP, Liang H, Quintavalla JC, et al: Comparison of recombinant cyclooxygenase-2 to native isoforms: Aspirin labeling of the active site. FEBS Lett 371:315, 1995.

76. Gans KR, Galbraith W, Roman RJ, et al: Anti-inflammatory and safety profile of DuP 697, a novel orally effective prostaglandin synthesis inhibitor. J Pharmacol Exp Ther 254:180, 1990.

77. Copeland RA, Williams JM, Giannaras J, et al: Mechanism of selective inhibition of the inducible isoform of prostaglandin G/H synthase. Proc Natl Acad Sci USA 91:11202, 1994.

78. Mitchell JA, Akarasereenont P, Thiemermann C, et al: Selectivity of nonsteroidal anti-inflammatory drugs as inhibitors of constitutive and inducible cyclooxygenase. Proc Natl Acad Sci USA 90:11693, 1993.

79. Winter CA, Risely EA, Nuss GW: Carrageenan-induced edema in hind paw of the rat as an assay for anti-inflammatory drugs. Proc Soc Exp Biol Med 111:544, 1962.

80. Hargreaves KM, Dubner R, Brown F, et al: A new and sensitive method for measuring thermal nociception in cutaneous hyperalgesia. Pain 32:77, 1988.

81. Ferreira SH, Lorenzetti BB, Correa FM: Central and peripheral antialgesic action of aspirin-like drugs. Eur J Pharmacol 53:39, 1978.

82. Clarke GD, MacPherson IS, Petrone G, et al: Antinociceptive effects of nonsteroidal anti-inflammatory drugs in a rat model of unilateral hindpaw inflammation. Eur J Pharmacol 257:103, 1994.

83. Dirig DM, Isakson PC, Yaksh TL: Effect of COX-1 and COX-2 inhibition on induction and maintenance of carrageenan-evoked thermal hyperalgesia in rats. J Pharmacol Exp Ther 285:1031, 1998.

84. Jett MF, Ramesha CS, Brown CD, et al: Characterization of the analgesic and anti-inflammatory activities of ketorolac and its enantiomers in the rat. J Pharmacol Exp Ther 288:1288, 1999.

85. Tonussi CR, Ferreira SH: Mechanism of diclofenac analgesia: Direct blockade of inflammatory sensitization. Eur J Pharmacol 14:173, 1994.

86. Dirig DM, Yaksh TL: In vitro prostanoid release from spinal cord following peripheral inflammation: Effects of substance P, NMDA and capsaicin. Br J Pharmacol 126:13330, 1999.

87. Fenner H: Differentiating among nonsteroidal anti-inflammatory drugs by pharmacokinetic and pharmacodynamic profiles. Semin Arthritis Rheum 26:28, 1997.

88. Verbeeck RK, Blackburn JL, Loewen GR: Clinical pharmacokinetics of non-steroidal anti-inflammatory drugs. Clin Pharmacokinet 8:297, 1983.

89. Needs CJ, Brooks PM: Clinical pharmacokinetics of the salicylates. Clin Pharmacokinet 10:164, 1985.

90. Brodgen RN, Heel RC, Pakes GE, et al: Diclofenac sodium: A review of its pharmacological properties and therapeutic use in rheumatic diseases and pain of varying origin. Drugs 20:24, 1980.

91. Davies NM: Clinical pharmacokinetics of ibuprofen. The first 30 years. Clin Pharmacokinet 34:101, 1998.

92. Davies NM, Anderson KE: Clinical pharmacokinetics of naproxen. Clin Pharmacokinet 32:268, 1997.

93. Davies NM, Anderson KE: Clinical pharmacokinetics of diclofenac. Therapeutic insights and pitfalls. Clin Pharmacokinet 33:184, 1997.

94. Gillis JC, Brogden RN: Ketorolac. A reappraisal of its pharmacodynamic and pharmacokinetic properties and therapeutic use in pain management. Drugs 53:139, 1997.

95. Litvak KM, McEvoy GK: Ketorolac, an injectable nonnarcotic analgesic. Clin Pharm 9:921, 1990.

96. Rowland M, Riegleman S, Harris P, et al: Absorption kinetics of aspirin in man following oral administration of an aqueous solution. J Pharmaceut Sci 61:379, 1972.

97. Kendal M, Thornhill D, Willis J: Factors affecting the pharmacokinetics of diclofenac sodium. Rheumatol Rehabil (Suppl 2):38, 1979.

98. Riess W, Stierlin H, Degen P, et al: Pharmacokinetics and metabolism of the anti-inflammatory agent Voltaren. Scand J Rheumatol Suppl 22:17, 1978.

99. Willis J, Kendal M, Flinn R, et al: The pharmacokinetics of diclofenac sodium following intravenous and oral administration. Eur J Clin Pharmacol 16:405, 1979.

100. Jamali F, Singh N, Pasutto F: Pharmacokinetics of ibuprofen enantiomers in man following oral administration of tablets with different absorption rates. Pharm Res 5:40, 1988.

101. Cox S, Brown M, Squires D: Comparative human study of ibuprofen enantiomer plasma concentrations produced by two commercially available ibuprofen tablets. Biopharm Drug Disp 9:539, 1988.

102. Brocks D, Jamali F: Clinical pharmacokinetics of ketorolac tromethamine. Clin Pharmacokinet 23:415, 1992.

103. Forrest JA, Clements JA, Prescott LF: Clinical pharmacokinetics of paracetamol. Clin Pharmacokinet 7:93, 1982.

104. Davies NM, McLachlan AJ, Day RO, et al: Clinical pharmacokinetics and pharmacodynamics of celecoxib: A selective cyclo-oxygenase-2 inhibitor. Clin Pharmacokinet 38:225, 2000.

105. Karim A, Tolbert D, Piergies A, et al: Celecoxib does not significantly alter the pharmacokinetics or hypoprothrombinemic effect of warfarin in healthy subjects. J Clin Pharmacol 40:655, 2000.

106. Scott LJ, Lamb HM: Rofecoxib. Drugs 58:499, 1999.

107. Karim A, Laurent A, Kuss M, et al: Single dose tolerability and pharmacokinetics of parecoxib sodium, a COX-2 specific inhibitor, following intramuscular administration. American Society of Anesthesiology Annual Congress, October 14–18, 2000, San Francisco, Calif.

108. Karim A, Laurent A, Kuss ME, et al: Single dose tolerability and pharmacokinetics of parecoxib sodium, a COX-2 specific inhibitor following intravenous administration. American Society of Anesthesiology Annual Congress, October 14–18, 2000, San Fransisco, Calif.

109. Brouwers JR, de Smet PA: Pharmacokinetic-pharmacodynamic drug interactions with nonsteroidal anti-inflammatory drugs. Clin Pharmacokinet 27:462, 1994.

110. Chan TY: Adverse interactions between warfarin and nonsteroidal anti-inflammatory drugs: Mechanisms, clinical significance, and avoidance. Ann Pharmacother 29:1274, 1995.

111. Harder S, Thurmann P: Clinically important drug interactions with anticoagulants. An update. Clin Pharmacokinet 30:416, 1996.

112. Noveck RJ, Kuss M, Qian J, et al: Parecoxib sodium, an injectable COX-2 specific inhibitor, does not affect aspirin-mediated platelet function. American Society of Regional Anesthesia Annual Congress, May 2001, Vancouver, Canada.

113. Burns JW, Aitken HA, Bullingham RE, et al: Double-blind comparison of the morphine sparing effect of continuous and intermittent i.m. administration of ketorolac. Br J Anaesth 67:235, 1991.

114. Bjorkman R, Ullman A, Hedner J: Morphine-sparing effect of diclofenac in cancer pain. Eur J Clin Pharmacol 44:1, 1993.

115. Colquhoun AD, Fell D: Failure of rectal diclofenac to augment opioid analgesia after cholecystectomy. Anaesthesia 44:57, 1989.

116. Power I, Bowler GM, Pugh GC, et al: Ketorolac as a component of balance analgesia after thoracotomy. Br J Anaesth 72:224, 1994.

117. See WA, Fuller JR, Toner ML: An outcome study of patient-controlled morphine analgesia, with or without ketorolac, following radical retropubic prostatectomy. J Urol 154:1429, 1995.

118. Sevarino FB, Sinatra RS, Paige D, et al: Intravenous ketorolac as an adjunct to patient-controlled analgesia (PCA) for management of postgynecologic surgical pain. J Clin Anesth 6:23, 1994.

119. Sevarino FB, Sinatra RS, Paige D, et al: The efficacy of intramuscular ketorolac in combination with intravenous PCA morphine for postoperative pain. J Clin Anesth 4:285, 1992.

120. Buggy DJ, Wall C, Carton EG: Preoperative or postoperative diclofenac for laparoscopic tubal ligation. Br J Anaesth 73:767, 1994.

121. Bunemann L, Thorshauge H, Herlevsen P, et al: Analgesia for outpatient surgery: Placebo versus naproxen sodium (a nonsteroidal anti-inflammatory drug) given before or after surgery. Eur J Anaesthesiol 11:461, 1994.

122. Ding Y, Fredman B, White PF: Use of ketorolac and fentanyl during outpatient gynecologic surgery. Anesth Analg 77:205, 1993.

123. Ding Y, White PF: Comparative effects of ketorolac, dezocine and fentanyl as adjuvants during outpatient anesthesia. Anesth Analg 75:566, 1992.

124. Edwards ND, Barclay K, Catling SJ, et al: Day case laparoscopy: A survey of postoperative pain and an assessment of the value of diclofenac. Anaesthesia 46:1077, 1991.

125. Hovorka J, Kallela H, Korttila K: Effect of intravenous diclofenac on pain and recovery profile after day-case laparoscopy. Eur J Anaesthesiol 10:105, 1993.

126. Grace D, Milligan KR, Loughran PG, et al: Diclofenac sodium versus fentanyl for analgesia in laparoscopic sterilization. Acta Anaesthesiol Scand 38:342, 1994.

127. Rosenblum M, Weller RS, Conrad PL, et al: Ibuprofen provides longer lasting analgesia than fentanyl after laproscopic surgery. Anesth Analg 73:255, 1991.

128. van EE R, Hemrika DJ, van der Linden CT: Pain relief following day-case diagnostic hysteroscopy-laparoscopy for infertility: A double-blind randomized trial with preoperative naproxen versus placebo. Obstet Gynecol 82:951, 1993.

129. Comfort VK, Code WE, Rooney ME, et al: Naproxen premedication reduces post-operative tubal ligation pain. Can J Anaesth 39:349, 1992.

130. Claeys M, Camu F, Maes V: Prophylactic diclofenac infusions in major orthopedic surgery: Effects on analgesia and acute phase proteins. Acta Anaesthesiol Scand 36:270, 1992.

131. Niemi L, Tuominen M, Pitkanen M, et al: Comparison of parenteral diclofenac and ketoprofen for postoperative pain relief after maxillo-facial surgery. Acta Anaesthesiol Scand 39:96, 1995.

132. Walton GM, Rood JP, Snowdon AT, et al: Ketorolac and diclofenac for postoperative pain relief following oral surgery. Br J Oral Maxillofacial Surg 31:158, 1993.

133. Perttunen K, Nilsson E, Kalso E: I.V. diclofenac and ketorolac for pain after thorascopic surgery. Br J Anaesth 82:221, 1999.

134. DiPalma JR: Ketorolac: An injectable NSAID. Am Fam Physician 43:207, 1991.

135. Buckley MM, Brogden RN: Ketorolac. A review of its pharmacody-namic and pharmacokinetic properties, and therapeutic potential. Drugs 39:86, 1990.

136. Cooper SA, Precheur H, Rauch D, et al: Evaluation of oxycodone and acetaminophen in treatment of postoperative dental pain. Oral Surg Oral Med Oral Pathol 50:496, 1980.

137. Sunshine A, Olson NZ, Zighelboim I, et al: Ketoprofen, aceta-minophen plus oxycodone, and acetaminophen in the relief of postoperative pain. Clin Pharmacol Ther 54:546, 1993.

138. Hamilton GR, Baskett TF: In the arms of Morpheus, the development of morphine for postoperative pain relief. Can J Anaesth 47:367, 2000.

139. Kehlet H, Rung GW, Callesen T: Postoperative opioid analgesia: Time for a reconsideration? J Clin Anesth 8:441, 1996.

140. Mulroy MF: Monitoring opioids. Reg Anesth 21:89, 1996.

141. Wong HY, Carpenter RL, Kopacz DJ, et al: A randomized, double-blind evaluation of ketorolac tromethamine for postoperative analge-sia in ambulatory surgery patients. Anesthesiology 78:6, 1993.

142. Krimmer H, Bruch HP, Hoffman G, et al: Comparison of the respira-tory effects of ketorolac and morphine in postoperative analgesia. Curr Ther Res 55:1293, 1994.

143. Parker RK, Holtmann B, Smith I, et al: Use of ketorolac after lower abdominal surgery. Effect on analgesic requirement and surgical outcome. Anesthesiology 80:6, 1994.

144. Stahlgren LR, Trierweiler M, Tommeraasen M, et al: Comparison of ketorolac and meperidine in patients with post-operative pain—impact on health care utilization. Clin Ther 15:571, 1993.

145. Liu J, Ding Y, White PF, et al: Effects of ketorolac on postoperative analgesia and ventilatory function after laparoscopic cholecystec-tomy. Anesth Analg 76:1061, 1993.

146. Shapiro MH, Duffy BL: Intramuscular ketorolac for postoperative analgesia following laparoscopic sterilization. Anaesth Intensive Care 22:22, 1994.

147. Blackburn A, Stevens JD, Wheatley RG, et al: Balanced analgesia with intravenous ketorolac and patient-controlled morphine follow-ing lower abdominal surgery. J Clin Anesth 7:103, 1995.

148. Kenny GN, McArdle CS, Aitken HA: Parenteral ketorolac: Opiate-sparing effect and lack of cardiorespiratory depression in the perioperative patient. Pharmacotherapy 10:127S, 1990.

149. Beattie W, Warriner C, Etches R, et al: The addition of continuous intravenous infusion of ketorolac to a patient-controlled analgesic morphine regime reduced postoperative myocardial ischemia in patients undergoing elective total hip or knee arthroplasty. Anesth Analg 84:715, 1997.

150. Fogarty DJ, O'Hanlon JJ, Milligan KR: Intramuscular ketorolac fol-lowing total hip replacement with spinal anaesthesia and intrathecal morphine. Acta Anaesthesiol Scand 39:191, 1995.

151. Fragen RJ, Stulberg SD, Wixson R, et al: Effect of ketorolac tromethamine on bleeding and on requirements for analgesia after total knee arthroplasty. J Bone Joint Surg Am 77:998, 1995.

152. Moiniche S, Bulow S, Hesselfeldt P, et al: Convalescence and hospi-tal stay after colonic surgery with balanced analgesia, early oral feeding and enforced mobilization. Eur J Surg 1661:283, 1995.

153. Cardoso MM, Carvalho JC, Amaro AR, et al: Small doses of intrathe-cal morphine combined with systemic diclofenac for postoperative pain control after cesarean delivery. Anesth Analg 86:538, 1998.

154. Moffat AC, Kenny GN, Prentice JW: Postoperative nefopam and diclofenac. Evaluation of their morphine-sparing effect after upper abdominal surgery. Anaesthesia 45:302, 1990.

155. Olofsson CI, Legeby MH, Nygards EB, et al: Diclofenac in the treat-ment of pain after caesarean delivery. An opioid-saving strategy. Eur J Obstet Gynecol Reprod Biol 88:143, 2000.

156. Rockemann MG, Seeling W, Bischof C, et al: Prophylactic use of epidural mepivacaine/morphine, systemic diclofenac and matamizole reduces postoperative morphine consumption after major abdominal surgery. Anesthesiology 84:1027, 1996.

157. Sun HL, Wu CC, Lin MS, et al: Effects of epidural morphine and intramuscular diclofenac sodium in postcesarean analgesia: A dose-range study. Anesth Analg 76:284, 1993.

158. Sun HL, Wu CC, Lin MS, et al: Combination of low-dose epidural morphine and intramuscular diclofenac sodium in postcesarean analgesia. Anesth Analg 75:64, 1992.

159. Rhodes M, Conacher I, Morritt G, et al: Nonsteroidal anti-inflammatory drugs for posthoracotomy pain. A prospective con-trolled trial after lateral thoracotomy. J Thorac Cardiovasc Surg 103:17, 1992.

160. Laitinen J, Nuutinen LS, Puranen J, et al: Effect of a non-steroidal anti-inflammatory drug, diclofenac, on haemostasis in patients undergoing total hip replacement. Acta Anaesthesiol Scand 36:486, 1992.

161. Fredman B, Zohar E, Tarabykin A, et al: Continuous intravenous diclofenac does not induce opioid-sparing or improve analgesia in geriatric patients undergoing major orthopedic surgery. J Clin Anesth 12:531, 2000.

162. Fletcher D, Zetlaoui P, Monin S, et al: Influence of timing on the analgesic effect of intravenous ketorolac after orthopedic surgery. Pain 61:291, 1995.

163. Parke TJ, Lowson SM, Uncles DR: Pre-emptive versus post-surgical administration of ketorolac for hysterectomy. Eur J Anaesthesiol 12:549, 1995.

164. Connelly CS, Panush RS: Should nonsteroidal anti-inflammatory drugs be stopped before elective surgery. Arch Intern Med 151:1963, 1991.

165. Strom BL, Berlin JA, Kinman JL, et al: Parenteral ketorolac and risk of gastrointestinal and operative site bleeding. A postmarketing surveillance study. JAMA 275:376, 1996.

166. Singh G, Rosen Ramey D: NSAID induced gastrointestinal compli-cations: The ARAMIS perspective- 1997. Arthritis, rheumatism, and aging medical information system. J Rheumatol Suppl 51:8, 1998.

167. Singh G, Ramey DR, Morfeld D, et al: Gastrointestinal tract compli-cations of nonsteroidal anti-inflammatory drug treatment in rheuma-toid arthritis. A prospective observational cohort study. Arch Intern Med 156:1530, 1996.

168. Fries JF: The assessment of disability: From first to future principles. Br J Rheumatol 22:48, 1983.

169. Feldman H, Kinman J, Berlin J, et al: Parenteral ketorolac: The risk of acute renal failure. Ann Intern Med 126:193, 1997.

170. Leese P, Recker D, Kuss M: The novel COX-2 specific inhibitor, valdecoxib, does not affect platelet function in healthy adults. Euro-pean League Against Rheumatism Annual Congress, June 13–16, 2001, Prague, Czech Republic.

171. Leese P, Recker D, Kuss M: A double-blind, placebo-controlled study to evaluate the effects of valdecoxib, a novel COX-2 specific inhibitor, on platelet function in the elderly, European League Against Rheumatism Annual Congress, Prague, Czech Republic, 13–16 June, 2001.

172. Leese PT, Hubbard RC, Karim A, et al: Effects of celecoxib, a novel cyclooxygenase-2 inhibitor, on platelet function in healthy adults: A randomized, controlled trial. J Clin Pharmacol 40:124, 2000.

173. Noveck RJ, Kuss M, Qian J, et al: Parecoxib sodium, an injectable COX-2 specific inhibitor, does not affect heparin-regulated blood coagulation parameters. American Society of Regional Anesthesia Annual Congress, May 2001, Vancouver, Canada.

174. Noveck RJ, Laurent A, Kuss M, et al: The COX-2 specific inhibitor, parecoxib sodium, does not impair platelet function in healthy elderly and nonelderly subjects: Two randomized, controlled trials [in press].

175. Brown J, Morrison BW, Christensen S: MK-966 50 mg versus ibuprofen 400 mg in post-surgical dental pain [abstract PI-4]. Clin Pharmacol Ther 65:118, 1999.

176. Brugger AM, Richardson ET, Kotey P: Comparison of celecoxib, hydrocodone/acetaminophen and placebo for relief of postsurgical pain. American Pain Society Annual Congress, Oct 21, 1999.

177. Fricke J, Morrison BW, Fite S: MK-966 versus naproxen sodium 550 mg in post-surgical dental pain [abstract No. PI-7]. Clin Pharmacol Ther 65:119, 1999.

178. Hubbard RC, Mehlisch DR, Jasper DR: SC-58635, a highly selective inhibitor of COX-2, is an effective analgesic in an acute post-surgical pain model [abstract]. J Invest Med 44:293A, 1996.

179. Malmstrom K, Daniels S, Kotey P, et al: Comparison of rofecoxib and

celecoxib, two cyclooxygenase-2 inhibitors, in postoperative dental pain: A randomized, placebo- and active-comparator-controlled clinical trial. Clin Ther 21:1653, 1999.

180. Mehlisch DR, Hubbard RC, Isakson PC: Analgesic efficacy and plasma levels of a highly selective inhibitor of COX-2 (SC-58635) in patients with post-surgical dental pain [abstract PIII-2]. Clin Pharmacol Ther 61:195, 1997.

181. Reuben SS, Connelly NR: Postoperative analgesic effects of celecoxib or rofecoxib after spinal fusion surgery. Anesth Analg 91:1221, 2000.

182. Reuben SS, Connelly NR, Lurie S, et al: Dose-response of ketorolac as an adjunct to patient-controlled analgesia morphine in patients after spinal fusion surgery. Anesth Analg 87:98, 1998.

183. Daniels SE, Talwalker S, Hubbard RC, et al: Pre-operative valdecoxib, a COX-2 specific inhibitor, provides effective and long lasting pain relief following oral surgery. American Society of Anesthesiology Annual Congress, October 13–17, 2001, New Orleans, La.

184. Desjardins PJ, Talwalker S, Hubbard RC, et al: Pre-operative administration of valdecoxib, a potent COX-2 specific inhibitor, provides effective post-operative analgesia. American Society of Anesthesiology Annual Congress, October 13–17, 2001, New Orleans, La.

185. Desjardins PJ, Grossman E, Kuss M, et al: The COX-2 specific inhibitor, parecoxib sodium, has analgesic efficacy when administered preoperatively. Anesth Analg [in press].

186. Rasmussen GL, Steckner K, Hogue C, et al: Intravenous parecoxib sodium for acute pain after postorthopedic knee surgery. Am J Orthopedics [in press].

187. Teeny S, Grossman E, Kuss M, et al: Pre-operative administration of parecoxib sodium effectively reduces post-operative pain in bunionectomy patients. American Society of Anesthesiology Annual Congress, October 13–17, 2001, New Orleans, La.

188. Torri S, Kuss M, Talwalker S, et al: The injectable COX-2 specific inhibitor parecoxib sodium, is effective in treating post-operative pain in total hip arthroplasty patients. American Society of Anesthesiology Annual Congress, October 13–17, 2001, New Orleans, La.

189. Bikhazi GB, Bajwa ZH, Snabes MC, et al: Parecoxib sodium effectively treats post-laparotomy pain. American Society of Reproductive Medicine Annual Congress, 2001, Orlando, Fla.

190. Wender RH, Desai PM, Snabes MC, et al: Parecoxib sodium demonstrates opioid sparing effects in post-laparotomy surgical patients. American Society of Reproductive Medicine Annual Congress, 2001, Orlando, Fla.

191. Camu F, Beecher T, Talwalker S, et al: The COX-2 specific inhibitor, valdecoxib is opioid-sparing and provides effective analgesia in primary hip arthroplasty patients. American Society of Anesthesiology Annual Congress, October 13–17, 2001, New Orleans, La.

192. Camu F, Kuss M, Talwalker S, et al: The COX-2 specific inhibitor parecoxib sodium is an effective, opioid-sparing agent in patients undergoing knee replacement surgery. American Society Anesthesiology Annual Congress, October 13–17, 2001, New Orleans, La.

193. Syntex Laboratories I. Ketorolac Prescribing Information.

194. Buchman AL, Schwartz MR: Colonic ulceration associated with the systemic use of non-steroidal anti-inflammatory medication. J Clin Gastroenterol 22:224, 1996.

195. Gallagher JE, Blauth J, Fornadley JA: Perioperative ketorolac tromethamine and postoperative hemorrhage in cases of tonsillectomy and adenoidectomy. Laryngoscope 105:606, 1995.

196. Judkins JH, Dray TG, Hubbell RN: Intraoperative ketorolac and post-tonsillectomy bleeding. Arch Otolaryngol Head Neck Surg 122:937, 1996.

197. Gunter JB, Varughese AM, Harrington JF, et al: Recovery and complications after tonsillectomy in children: A comparison of ketorolac and morphine. Anesth Analg 81:1136, 1995.

198. Rusy LM, Houck CS, Sullivan LJ: A double-blind evaluation of ketorolac tromethamine versus acetaminophen in pediatric tonsillectomy: Analgesia and bleeding. Anesth Analg 80:226, 1995.

199. Ross-Lee L, Elms M, Cham B, et al: Plasma levels of aspirin following effervescent and enteric-coated tablets, and their effect on platelet function. Clin Pharm 23:545, 1982.

200. Laska E, Sunshine A, Marrero I: The correlation between blood levels of ibuprofen and analgesic response. Clin Pharm Ther 40:1, 1986.

201. Morrison BW, Daniels SE, Kotey P, et al: Rofecoxib, a specific cyclooxygenase-2 inhibitor, in primary dysmenorrhea: A randomized controlled trial. Obstet Gynecol 94:504, 1999.

202. Day R, Morrison B, Luza A, et al: A randomized trial of the efficacy and tolerability of the COX-2 inhibitor rofecoxib vs. ibuprofen in patients with osteoarthritis. Rofecoxib/Ibuprofen Comparator Study Group. Arch Intern Med 160:1781, 2000.

203. Fiechtner J, Sikes D, Recker D: A double-blind, placebo-controlled dose ranging study to evaluate the efficacy of valdecoxib, a novel COX-2 specific inhibitor, in treating the signs and symptoms of osteoarthritis of the knee. European League against Rheumatism Annual Congress, May 13–16, 2001, Prague, Czech Republic.

204. Kivitz AJ, Eisen G, Zhao WW, et al: The COX-2 specific inhibitor valdecoxib is as effective as naproxen in treating symptomatic osteoarthritis of the knee and demonstrates reduced gastrointestinal ulceration. J Family Prac [submitted].

205. Daniels S, Grossman E, Kuss M, et al: A double-blind, randomized comparison of intramuscularly and intravenously administered parecoxib sodium versus ketorolac and placebo in a post-oral surgery pain model. Clin Therap [in press].

27

Analgesics

Christoph Stein, MD • Carl E. Rosow, MD

RECEPTOR LIGANDS AND OPIATE NARCOTICS

History

Ancient writings and archeologic data indicate that the Sumerians, who inhabited what is today Iraq, cultivated poppies and isolated opium from their seed capsules at the end of the third millennium BC.[1] At first, opium may have been used as a euphoriant in religious rituals, but by the second century BC it was used medicinally. As early as the eighth century AD, Arab traders brought opium to India and China, and between the 10th and 13th centuries, opium reached all parts of Europe.[1]

With the drug came addiction. Starting in the 16th century, manuscripts describe drug abuse in Turkey, Egypt, Germany, England, and China. In 1806, Sertürner isolated the active ingredient in opium, naming it morphine after the god of dreams. After the invention of the hypodermic syringe and hollow needle in the 1850s, morphine began to be used for surgical procedures, for postoperative and chronic pain, and as an adjunct to general anesthetics. Because morphine had just as much potential for abuse as opium, much effort was expended in developing a safer, more efficacious, nonaddicting opiate. In 1898, heroin was synthesized and pronounced free from the liability of abuse. This was the first of many such claims for new opiates, however, no such substances currently have been introduced into clinical practice.

The first two opiates that differed structurally from morphine were discovered in 1939 (meperidine) and 1946 (methadone). In 1942, nalorphine, the first opiate antagonist, was produced.[1] Nalorphine, however, not only countered the actions of morphine but also produced limited analgesia– i.e., it acted as a mixed agonist/antagonist. Its discovery led to the development of naloxone, a relatively pure antagonist.

Terminology

Opiates are drugs derived from opium and include morphine, codeine, and a wide variety of related alkaloids. The term *opioid* is broader and includes all agonists and antagonists that have alkaloid structures, as well as naturally occurring and synthetic peptides that bind to opioid receptors. The term *narcotic* originally referred to any drug that induced sleep but then became associated with the strong opiate analgesics. It is now used for a wide variety of opioid and nonopioid abused substances and is no longer useful in a pharmacologic context.

MECHANISMS OF DRUG ACTION

Classification of Opioid Receptors

By the mid-1960s it became evident that the effects of opiate agonists, antagonists, and mixed agonist/antagonists could be explained by postulating actions on multiple opiate receptors. In 1973, Pert and Snyder,[2] Simon and colleagues,[3] and Terenius[4] almost simultaneously demonstrated stereospecific opiate binding sites in the central nervous system (CNS). Subsequently, extensive pharmacologic research led to the discrimination of three major classes of opioid receptors: designated μ, δ, and κ. (Early studies had also described σ- and ϵ-receptors, but these are no longer considered opioid receptors.) During certain experimental conditions, the activation of all three classes of opioid receptors results in pain relief.[5]

Advances in molecular biology have led to the cloning and characterization of three cloned deoxyribonucleic acids (cDNA) encoding the μ-, δ-, and κ-opioid receptors, respectively.[6–9] The availability of these clones from rodents then allowed the cloning of the human homologues and the identification of their respective genes.[10,11] Comparing DNA sequences among a number of species displays 96% to 98% homologies, indicating that the opioid receptor gene family has been conserved during vertebrate evolution.[10] Another opioid receptor-related cDNA with high sequence homology to the three cloned opioid receptors was isolated but did not encode an opioid binding site. Thus it remained an "opioid receptor-like 1" orphan receptor with hitherto controversial functions.[12]

The availability of a host of synthetic opioid ligands and their use in biologic assays has indicated a possible heterogeneity within each opioid receptor class. Thus the existence of receptor subtypes μ_1, μ_2, δ_1, δ_2, κ_{1a}, κ_{1b}, κ_2, and κ_3 has been proposed.[5] However, only one receptor gene has been cloned for each class. Therefore the issue of subtype diversity remains a matter of debate. Several mechanisms are conceivable for creating this diversity, including currently uncloned opioid receptor genes, alternative splicing from the known genes, post-translational modifications, ligand-induced changes in receptor conformation, association with distinct sets of G proteins, receptor oligomers, or cellular compartmentalization.[10,13,14]

Genes

The organization of the opioid receptor genes has been studied in mice and humans. The three opioid receptor genes share a similar pattern of exons (coding sequences leading to mature messenger ribonucleic acid [mRNA]) and introns (noncoding intervening sequences that are spliced out of mRNA before translation). The coding regions are distributed over three exons, and their splice sites are found at homologous positions after the first and fourth transmembrane (TM) regions. This suggests that the three opioid receptor genes evolved from a single ancestral gene. The μ-opioid receptor gene differs from the δ- and κ-receptor genes at the level of exon 3, which terminates before the stop codon such that the 12 C-terminal amino acids are encoded by a fourth exon. Transcription initiation sites and promoter regions have been identified for all three opioid receptor genes, and alternative splicing mechanisms have been demonstrated for all three receptor mRNA.[10] Messenger RNA isoforms with distinct C-terminal sequences have been described for the μ-opioid receptor. The receptor protein of one isoform (MOR-1B) shows desensitization properties different from those of the classically described μ-opioid receptor, which may be of interest with regard to mechanisms by which tolerance develops.[14] Currently, the search for alternative transcripts has provided unusual mRNA isoforms but no evidence for altered binding properties or subtypes of receptor proteins.[10]

Transgenic Studies on Receptors

In addition to classic pharmacologic methodology, genetic approaches now make it possible to assess the contribution of each receptor to opioid actions in vivo. Synthetic antisense oligodeoxynucleotides hybridize to complementary sequences in the target gene or its mRNA, thereby leading to reduced transcription, translation, and protein levels. Antisense studies have confirmed the contribution of μ- and δ-receptors in opioid-induced analgesia. Furthermore, an antisense oligonucleotide against a coding region in TM 2 that is conserved (identical) between the three receptors indeed diminished the antinociceptive actions of μ-, δ-, and κ-receptor agonists.[10]

The availability of techniques to remove ("knockout") genes on the chromosomes now permits unprecedented selectivity in the removal of responses mediated by the respective encoded protein. Although this approach circumvents some of the shortcomings of conventional pharmacology (e.g., limited duration of action and variable selectivity of agonists, antagonists, or antibodies), it is itself limited by compensatory developmental changes during embryogenesis and adolescence and variable genetic backgrounds.[15] Nevertheless, knockout studies have shown that the removal of any single opioid receptor does not result in major changes in basal pain thresholds or other behaviors. Such studies have confirmed that all three classes of opioid receptors mediate analgesia induced by their respective agonists, and that there is only one gene encoding for each receptor.[11,16] Even though conventional pharmacology has suggested that morphine might also activate κ- and δ-receptors, μ-receptor knockout animals show a complete loss of analgesic, reinforcing, respiratory, and gastrointestinal effects of morphine.[17] This result is corroborated by the finding that morphine analgesia is unchanged in δ- and κ-receptor knockout animals, thus establishing the μ-receptor as a mandatory target for morphine. In addition, synergistic interactions between μ- and δ-receptors have been confirmed.[11,14]

Structural Characteristics

Opioid receptors belong to the family of G protein–coupled receptors that have the typical structure of seven putative TM regions. Sequence comparisons among the receptor family shows high similarity in several protein regions such as TM 2, 3, 5, 6, and 7; the three intracellular loops; and a short region of the C-terminal tail proximal to the membrane. In contrast, little or no homology is found in the extracellular N-terminal, in the intracellular C-terminal, and in the extracellular loops. These structural features are important for ligand recognition. The seven TM bundle forms a binding pocket, which is highly similar across receptor types. The extracellular domains, which differ among opioid receptor types, play a role in discriminating μ-, δ-, and κ-receptor ligands.[10] Intracellular regions are implicated in receptor signaling and regulation. The third intracellular loop and the juxtamembranous part of the C-terminus participate in the coupling to G proteins. The strong sequence homology in these regions suggests that the three opioid receptors interact with similar G proteins.

Signal Transduction

Three signaling pathways have been well characterized: all three opioid receptor classes couple to G proteins (mainly G_i/G_o) and subsequently inhibit adenylyl cyclase, decrease the conductance of voltage-gated Ca^{++} channels, or open inwardly rectifying K^+ channels. Any of these effects ultimately results in decreased neuronal activity. More recently,

opioid receptors were also found to modulate the phosphoinositide-signaling cascade,[18] the mitogen-activated protein kinase cascade, and phospholipase C.[14] The prevention of Ca^{++} influx results in the suppression of pronociceptive neurotransmitter release in many neuronal systems. A prominent example is the inhibition of substance P release from primary afferent sensory neurons in the spinal cord and from their peripheral terminals.[19] This is a plausible mechanism for opioid-induced spinal analgesia, although its importance has recently been questioned.[20] At the postsynaptic membrane, opioid receptors produce hyperpolarization by activating K^+ channels, thereby preventing excitation or propagation of action potentials. Apart from Ca^{++} and K^+ channels, opioid receptors may regulate the functions of other ion channels. For example, excitatory postsynaptic currents evoked by *N*-methyl-D-aspartate (NMDA) receptors or tetrodotoxin-resistant Na^+ channels in primary sensory neurons are inhibited by μ-receptor agonists.[14,21]

Desensitization, Internalization, Down-Regulation, and Drug Tolerance

The prolonged activation of opioid receptors leads to the expression of compensating mechanisms in many neurons or neuronal systems. These adaptations can take the form of a reduced sensitivity of the receptor through which the agonist acts (homologous desensitization), a reduced sensitivity of receptors with similar functions coexpressed in the same neuron (heterologous desensitization), or a change in the effector systems in the same or functionally related neurons, or both. The initiating step of receptor desensitization involves phosphorylation by G protein–coupled receptor kinases at the carboxyl tail of the receptor.[14] Thereafter, binding of regulatory proteins (e.g., arrestin, dynamine) leads to a removal of receptors from the cell membrane without reduction in the total number of receptors (internalization) and to clustering in clathrin-coated pits. Internalized receptors are either recycled to the cell surface after dephosphorylation or degraded in lysosomes (down-regulation, i.e., reduction in the total number of receptors expressed by the cell).

These and other mechanisms (e.g., reduced receptor synthesis, altered drug metabolism) may partially explain the apparent loss of effectiveness of agonists (tolerance) with prolonged activation of receptors.[14,22] In vivo animal experiments have shown that development of tolerance can be counteracted by use of NMDA antagonists.[22] In the clinical situation, however, tolerance is not observed ubiquitously and is often caused by increasing nociceptive stimulation with progressing disease.[22] Similarly, animal models of pathologic conditions (e.g., persistent inflammatory pain) have also shown a diminished development of tolerance to opioid analgesia.[21] These findings indicate a potential for plastic changes in the opioid system and highlight the importance of studying animal models of persistent pain. Because clinical pain is frequently associated with inflammatory tissue injury (e.g., postoperative pain, arthritis, neurogenic inflammation), such models will mirror the clinical situation more closely than traditional models of acute thermal stimuli (e.g., as used in the hot plate and tail-flick tests).

PRECLINICAL PHARMACOLOGY

Endogenous Ligands

Soon after the discovery of opiate receptors, brain extracts were found to contain a factor that inhibits release of acetylcholine from nerves in the guinea pig ileum in a naloxone-reversible fashion.[23] Also, electrical stimulation of specific brain regions in the rat was found to elicit a profound analgesia that was reversible by naloxone.[24] These findings implied the existence of endogenous opioid factors. These factors were subsequently identified as two structurally related pentapeptides: Tyr-Gly-Gly-Phe-Met and Tyr-Gly-Gly-Phe-Leu.[23] These peptides were named methionine-enkephalin (Met-enkephalin) and leucine-enkephalin (Leu-enkephalin).

More than 20 peptides have since been identified from the brain, the pituitary gland, the adrenal glands, immune cells, and other tissues.[1,25–27] The amino-terminal of all opioid peptides contains the Tyr-Gly-Gly-Phe-[Met/Leu] sequence, later known as the opioid motif, followed by various carboxy-terminal extensions. The resulting peptides have 5 to 31 amino acids in total. Two interesting peptides are β-endorphin, an extremely potent opioid analgesic with long-lasting effects,[28,29] and dynorphin A.[30]

The three precursors of these peptides were cloned between 1979 and 1982. The first was pro-opiomelanocortin (POMC), the common precursor for β-endorphin and corticotropin.[31] The observation that a given precursor can give rise to multiple active peptides held true for the other two opioid precursors. Proenkephalin encodes multiple copies of Met-enkephalin and one copy of Leu-enkephalin.[32] Prodynorphin encodes the opioid peptides dynorphin A, dynorphin B, and α-neoendorphin.[33–35] Biologically active opioid peptides are later cleaved into inactive fragments by peptidases. Accordingly, peptidase inhibitors were found to elicit or potentiate antinociceptive effects by increasing the extracellular levels of endogenous opioids.[36]

Ligand/Receptor Relationships

The existence of three families of opioid peptides and three cloned receptors might suggest a one-to-one correspondence between the peptides and receptors. However, such a pattern does not exist. Although proenkephalin products are generally associated with δ-receptors, and prodynorphin derivatives are generally associated with κ-receptors, a fair amount of "cross-talk" is evident. High-affinity interactions are possible among each of the peptide families and each of the three receptors, with the exception of POMC peptides and κ-receptors, which do not have a high affinity for each other.[35]

The relatively low affinity of the μ-receptor for all currently known endogenous ligands had long been the subject of intense investigations. These studies led to the recent discovery of novel peptides called endormorphins.[37] Endomorphin-1 (Tyr-Pro-Trp-Phe) and endomorphin-2 (Tyr-Pro-Phe-Phe) are tetrapeptides that do not contain the pan-opioid motif but nevertheless bind to the μ-receptor with unprecedented affinity and selectivity. Both endomorphins have been detected in various regions of the CNS and peripheral nervous system relevant to pain processing, as well as in immune cells.[38] A precursor has not yet been identified.

Studies on the opioid receptor-like 1 orphan receptor led to the discovery of its endogenous ligand—a 17-amino acid peptide termed orphanin FQ/nociceptin with a sequence similar to that of dynorphin A but with negligible affinity for opioid receptors. Although the exact nature of the functions of this peptide is controversial, an interplay with the endogenous opioid system seems likely.[39,40]

Transgenic Studies on Ligands

Similar to the genetic ablation of opioid receptors, knockout animals have been produced for the three known precursors of opioid peptides.[17] Mice lacking β-endorphin exhibit normal analgesia in response to morphine, indicating the presence of functional and unaltered μ-receptors. Whereas basal sensitivity to acute pain does not change, these animals do not produce the opioid-mediated analgesia that would normally occur in response to cold water swim, an environmental stressor commonly used to study endogenous systems that inhibit pain. However, these mice exhibit a greater nonopioid component of stress-induced analgesia, suggesting a compensatory up-regulation of alternative central pain control mechanisms.[17] Mice lacking proenkephalin exhibit normal stress-induced analgesia but a lower basal pain threshold (hyperalgesia) to heat stimuli.[17] Studies in prodynorphin knockout mice suggest that the maintenance of neuropathic pain may depend on an increase in spinal dynorphin expression.[41]

With all the caveats in mind,[15] this limited number of knockout studies suggests that β-endorphin is necessary for stress-induced analgesia, that enkephalins are involved in setting the basal sensitivity to acute painful stimuli, and that dynorphin may have pronociceptive properties in chronic neuropathic pain. Similar adverse effects of dynorphin have been confirmed in a number of functional and morphologic studies.[42]

Exogenous Agonists and Antagonists

Ligands may either drive (agonists), not affect (neutral antagonists), or inhibit (inverse agonists) G protein coupling. Opioid agonists are distinguished by their ability to induce a subsequent response (e.g., inhibition of adenylyl cyclase or analgesia) of a given magnitude. Partial agonists must occupy a greater fraction of the available pool of functional receptors than full agonists to induce a response of equivalent magnitude.[22] Mixed agonists/antagonists (e.g., buprenorphine, butorphanol, nalbuphine, pentazocine) may act as agonists at low doses and as antagonists (at the same or a different receptor) at greater doses. Such compounds typically exhibit ceiling effects for analgesia, and they may precipitate an acute withdrawal syndrome when administered to subjects physically dependent on pure μ-agonists.

The three opioid receptor types have been studied extensively by means of highly selective agonists (DAMGO, DPDPE, and U-69,593 for μ-, δ-, and κ-receptors, respectively) and antagonists (CTOP, naltrindole, and norbinaltorphimine for μ-, δ-, and κ-receptors, respectively). These ligands made it possible to define binding characteristics, anatomic distribution, and function of each receptor. All three receptors mediate analgesic effects. In addition, μ- and δ-receptors mediate respiratory depression, sedation, reward and euphoria, and constipation. κ-Receptors mediate dysphoric, aversive, and diuretic effects. The most commonly used agents in the clinical setting (morphine and fentanyl and its derivatives) are μ-receptor agonists, and naloxone is a nonselective antagonist at all three receptors.

Sites of Analgesic Opioid Action

Until the late 1980s, opioids were believed to be prototypic of centrally active analgesics. Currently, it is clear that opioid receptors and opioid peptides are located not only in the CNS but also in the peripheral nervous system. Such areas include primary afferent neurons, dorsal root ganglia, spinal cord, brain stem, midbrain, and cortex.[19,43] In addition, opioid peptides and receptors are expressed by neuroendocrine (pituitary, adrenal), immune, and ectodermal tissues.[26,27]

Supraspinal Sites

Studies using intracerebroventricular or regional microinjections of opioid ligands, stress-induced analgesia, and electrical stimulation or ablation of various brain regions have identified the periaqueductal gray (PAG), the locus ceruleus, and the rostral ventral medulla (RVM) as major areas containing opioid peptides and receptors. The stimulation of midbrain areas leads to activation of descending monoaminergic pathways in the dorsolateral funiculus and to a net inhibitory effect on nociceptive processing in the spine.[44] In the PAG, opioid agonists can presynaptically inhibit release of γ-aminobutyric acid (GABA), thereby disinhibiting descending nociceptive controls.[45] Both μ- and δ-receptors play major roles in the PAG and RVM. The endogenous ligands in the PAG are presumed to be derived from intrinsic enkephalinergic interneurons and from β-endorphin–containing projections arising from the arcuate nucleus. Other supraspinal sites supporting opioid analgesia include the ventral tegmental area, globus pallidus, hypothalamus, and insular cortex. In addition, the amygdala has reciprocal connections with the PAG and contains high levels of all three opioid receptors.

Persistent inflammatory pain can lead to an increase in the levels of Met- and Leu-enkephalin in the RVM and PAG. Some investigators believe that these peptides may interact in a synergistic or additive manner when opioid agonists are microinjected into the RVM and may thus contribute to the enhanced efficacy of such exogenous agents in inflammatory pain.[46]

Spinal Sites

All three types of opioid receptors are present in the dorsal horn of the spinal cord. Morphologic, electrophysiologic, and functional studies all indicate that opioid receptors are located on intrinsic spinal cord neurons and on terminals of primary afferents originating in the dorsal root ganglion.[47] Opioid agonists (μ-, δ-, and κ-receptors) applied directly to the cord produce profound analgesia.[48] Presynaptically, μ- and δ-receptor agonists can inhibit Ca^{++} influx and the subsequent release of glutamate and neuropeptides (e.g., substance P, calcitonin gene-related peptide) from primary afferent terminals. Postsynaptically, opioids (particularly μ-receptor agonists) hyperpolarize ascending projection neurons by increasing conductance of K^+. The dorsal horn is rich in enkephalinergic and dynorphinergic neurons. These neurons include terminals of primary afferents, spinal interneurons, and projection neurons. Primary afferent neurons also contain endomorphins. Noxious stimuli can release these opioids (particularly enkephalins), which some researchers believe act on primary afferent autoreceptors or postsynaptically, or both.[47,49] Persistent inflammatory pain is associated with increased levels of proenkephalin- and prodynorphin-derived peptides in the dorsal horn. It appears that enkephalins act to suppress noxious input through μ- and κ-receptors, but the nature of the role of dynorphin and κ-receptors is controversial.[47] Several studies indicate pronociceptive and excitotoxic effects of spinal dynorphin.[42]

Peripheral Sites

In the late 1980s, reports appeared regarding the existence of opioid receptors outside the CNS and the generation of analgesia by these kinds of peripheral receptors.[19] Such analgesic effects are particularly prominent in peripheral inflamed tissue and have been demonstrated in animals and humans.[25,49,50] All three opioid receptors are expressed in primary afferent neurons, and expression increases during the development of inflammation.[21] Endogenous ligands (mainly β-endorphin and Met-enkephalin), mRNA-encoding POMC, and proenkephalin are present within the lymphocytes, monocytes, and granulocytes of inflamed tissue.[25,26,51] Environmental stimuli (stress) and releasing agents (corticotropin-releasing factor, cytokines) can liberate these opioid peptides to elicit local analgesia, whereas suppression of the immune system abolishes these effects.[52] Selectins have recently been identified as important adhesion molecules governing the homing of these opioid cells to injured tissue.[53] (Fig. 27–1.)

The activation of opioid receptors on primary afferent neurons inhibits voltage-activated calcium channels through G proteins (G_i/G_o) and decreases the release of proinflammatory neuropeptides (substance P) into peripheral tissues.[19,21] These mechanisms not only generate analgesia but also potent anti-inflammatory effects (particularly with μ- and κ-receptor agonists). It appears that relatively little analgesic tolerance develops after repeated administration of peripheral opioid agonists in inflamed tissue.[21] Human studies have amply demonstrated effective analgesia after the peripheral (e.g., intraarticular, topical) administration of morphine and other μ-receptor agonists to acutely inflamed tissue (e.g., knee joint, cornea, and surgical and dental wounds).[50,54] Clinical studies are now moving into the field of chronic arthritic pain, with particular attention directed toward the possible anti-inflammatory effects of peripheral opioids.[21,50] Two novel peripherally selective κ-opioid peptides have recently undergone preliminary testing.[55]

Clinical Opioid Pharmacology

Opioids Tested in Humans

The remainder of this chapter focuses on morphine-like agonists that are relatively selective for μ-receptors, because such agents constitute most of the clinically useful opioids. Although many attempts have been made to create selective κ- and δ-receptor agonists for clinical use, other than the

agonist-antagonist opioids, only a few compounds have been tested in humans.

- The highly selective *κ-receptor agonists* of the arylacetamide series were a disappointment because they produced unacceptable dysphoria, an effect that some theorize is inherent in the κ-receptor mechanism.[56] Several of the available agonist/antagonist opioids (e.g., nalbuphine, butorphanol) have significant effects at more than one receptor—they are strong agonists at κ-receptors and antagonists or partial agonists at μ-receptors. Despite their κ-receptor activity, these drugs do not produce much dysphoria, and they have proven clinically useful.
- A few opioid *peptides with δ- or μ-receptor activity, or both* have been tried in humans.[57,58] None has shown any marked advantages as analgesics. Most opioid peptides are significantly limited by a lack of oral bioavailability, poor CNS penetration, and a variety of side effects.
- Various *nonpeptide δ-receptor agonists* have undergone preclinical screening, but only one has reached phase I clinical testing.[59] This compound is δ-

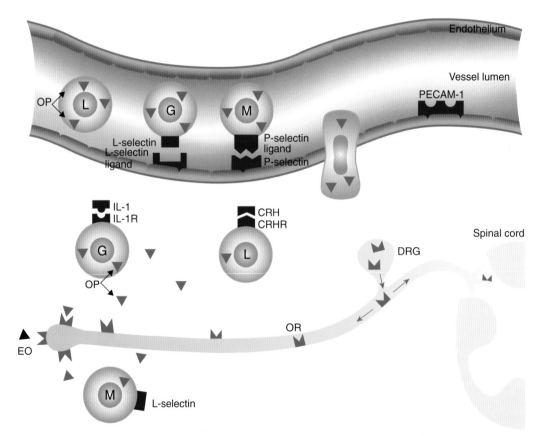

Figure 27–1. Migration of opioid-producing cells and opioid secretion within inflamed tissue. P-selectin and platelet-endothelial cell adhesion molecule-1 (PECAM-1) are upregulated on vascular endothelium. L-selectin is coexpressed by immune cells producing opioid peptides (OP). L- and P-selectin mediate rolling of opioid-containing cells along the vessel wall. PECAM-1 (among other molecules) mediates their diapedesis. Adhesion molecules interact with their respective ligands. In response to stress or releasing agents (corticotropin-releasing hormone [CRH], interleukin-1b [IL-1]), the cells secrete OP. CRH and IL-1 elicit OP release by activating CRH receptors (CRHR) and IL-1 receptors (IL-1R), respectively. OP or exogenous opioids (EO) bind to opioid receptors on primary afferent neurons leading to analgesia. Afterwards immune cells, depleted of the opioids, migrate to regional lymph nodes.

receptor–selective but retains some μ- and κ-receptor activity, and initial data show that it is active against experimental pain.

The μ-receptor agonists come from many different chemical classes, and they vary widely in potency and physicochemical properties. Given the common receptor mechanism, it is not surprising that all of them produce a broadly similar set of effects (Table 27–1). All of these compounds have sufficient intrinsic activity to produce profound analgesia and respiratory depression. The few pharmacodynamic differences between them are usually caused by nonopioid mechanisms (such as histamine release) or the presence of active metabolites. The opioids have marked differences in onset, duration, and physicochemical properties, therefore the clinical choice of a particular opioid is often based on pharmacokinetic considerations (route of administration, desired onset or duration).

Clinical Opioid Analgesia

Opioids are the most broadly effective analgesics available, possibly a reflection of their supraspinal, spinal, and peripheral sites of action. Opioids are traditionally said to be most effective for visceral or burning pain, less effective for sharp pain (e.g., on incision), and least effective for neuropathic pain.[60] The opioid effect is selective for nociception, because touch, pressure, and other sensory modalities are generally unaffected. After systemic administration, forebrain mechanisms play a prominent role in the production of clinical

effects, and a common clinical manifestation of opioid analgesia is a change in the effective response to pain. Patients given systemic opioids will typically report that pain is still present, but that the intensity is reduced and the pain discomfort is also less. The mental clouding and dissociation from pain are often accompanied by mood elevation.[61] This effect may explain the relatively high patient acceptance of opioids, but it may also contribute to their potential for abuse. Spinal mechanisms become proportionately more important when the opioids are given by neuraxial injection.

Opioids produce a dose- and concentration-dependent reduction in the intensity of acute pain. Many textbooks have lists of equianalgesic doses for various opioids, usually based on data from postoperative pain models. Information on relative potency is useful, but it must be emphasized that for many patients the "usual" doses can produce inadequate or excessive opioid effect. For example, one study shows that an initial 100-mg intramuscular dose of meperidine was adequate for only 20% of adults with postsurgical pain.[62] Austin and colleagues[63] demonstrated that the intensity of self-rated postsurgical pain decreases with increasing plasma concentrations of meperidine (Fig. 27–2). Their data show two important characteristics of opioid analgesia: (1) for each patient, the pain scores decrease dramatically over a small range of concentrations of meperidine; and (2) the threshold concentration varies fourfold to fivefold among patients. The large interindividual variation in opioid requirement has been almost a universal finding in pain studies and makes it clear why opioids need to be titrated for optimal effect.

These considerations apply equally well to the use of opioids for intraoperative pain. Because it is not possible to use subjective reports of pain during general anesthesia, opioids are commonly titrated to surrogate endpoints, such as blood pressure, heart rate, and movement. Ausems and colleagues[64] showed that alfentanil produces a concentration-dependent suppression of autonomic responses and movement during surgery. The data from this study were quite similar to those described for postoperative pain—i.e.,

TABLE 27–1.

Effects of Short- and Long-Term Administration of Opioids

Administration of Opioids	Effects
Short-term:	Analgesia
	Respiratory depression
	Sedation
	Euphoria
	Vasodilatation
	Bradycardia
	Cough suppression
	Miosis
	Nausea and vomiting
	Skeletal muscle hypertonus
	Constipation
	Urinary retention
	Biliary spasm
Long-term:	Tolerance to the effects of the opioid
	Physical dependence

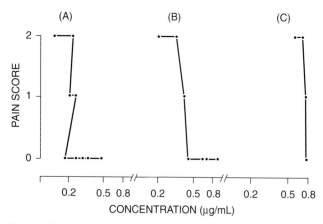

Figure 27–2. For three postoperative patients (*A, B,* and *C*), intensity of self-rated postsurgical pain (*0* = no pain, *1* = moderate pain, and *2* = severe pain) decreased with increasing plasma concentrations of meperidine. (From Austin KL, Stapleton JV, Mather LE: Relationship between blood meperidine concentrations and analgesic response: A preliminary report. Anesthesiology 53:460, 1980.)

the slope of the concentration-response curves for each patient was steep, and the threshold concentrations for analgesia were highly variable.

Numerous factors contribute to interindividual variability in opioid requirement for analgesia, making it difficult to isolate the effect of any one variable on clinical pain relief.

- The location and intensity of the pain stimulus is obviously important. For example, postoperative thoracotomy pain requires more opioid than pain of hernia repair; intraoperative responses to laryngoscopy are harder to blunt than those to skin incision.
- As with other subjective responses, a huge variety of psychological factors may come into play. For example, previous positive or negative experiences with anal-gesics can influence subsequent responses. It follows logically that a crossover study comparing analgesic and placebo should always be randomized for the order of treatment.
- Therapeutic drug interactions are tremendously important in clinical analgesia. Treatment with other analgesics (nonsteroidal anti-inflammatory drugs, α_2-agonists) and certain sedative/hypnotics (e.g., hydroxyzine) can reliably potentiate opioid analgesia and are frequently used for this purpose. Other CNS depressants (benzodiazepines, alcohol, barbiturates) do not have as clear an effect on analgesia but can increase toxicity.
- Age affects opioid requirement. On average, the elderly are more sensitive to opioids, although some older patients may require surprisingly high doses for adequate analgesia.[65] The age effect is partly because of pharmacokinetic changes (decreased clearance, decreased volumes of distribution). Pharmacokinetic and pharmacodynamic studies on fentanyl and remifentanil have also demonstrated an increase in pharmacodynamic sensitivity (i.e., a decrease in dose requirement) with age.[66,67] Sensitive or not, many elderly patients are underdosed and receive inadequate relief of pain. A recent large study of morphine for postoperative pain suggests that it may be appropriate to give adults of all ages similar incremental doses of morphine.[68]
- Certain pathophysiologic conditions, such as hypothyroidism or pre-existing CNS disease, can increase sensitivity. Although no studies demonstrate increased opioid sensitivity in patients with asthma or mild chronic obstructive pulmonary disease, opioids should be used with care, because decreased cough or deep breathing can lead to inspissation of secretions and bronchospasm.
- Hepatic and renal dysfunction can lead to accumulation of parent drug or active metabolites, but CNS sensitivity does not appear to be greatly altered. One pharmacokinetic and pharmacodynamic study demonstrated that patients with severe hepatic disease have only a slight increase in sensitivity to the ventilatory depressant effects of remifentanil.[69] Also, a similar study showed that patients with severe renal failure (who were not uremic) had no change in sensitivity to the ventilatory effects of remifentanil when compared with healthy control subjects.[70]
- Preliminary data suggest that sex can influence the response to opioids. There are complex sex-related differences in the ventilatory responses to a given concentration of morphine.[71] The clinical relevance of these differences for pain treatment currently has not been established.

- Genetic differences in drug disposition may also influence opioid requirement. For example, the analgesic effect of codeine is almost entirely caused by its conversion to morphine by O-demethylation. This reaction is catalyzed by CYP2D6, a cytochrome P450 enzyme that shows important genetic polymorphisms. About 10% of whites[72] and most Chinese[73] are "poor metabolizers" who may have an inadequate analgesic effect from codeine. One study found that Colombian Indians are more sensitive than white or Latino patients to the respiratory depressant effects of morphine.[74] Notably, they also have less capacity to form morphine glucuronides.

Opioid Pharmacokinetics

Absorption

Almost all opioids are rapidly absorbed after oral administration, although many undergo substantial first-pass metabolism. Much effort has been directed at *delaying* absorption with sustained-release opioid preparations, because adequate duration of analgesia is a bigger clinical problem than slow onset. Sometimes, almost no absorption is desirable; loperamide and diphenoxylate are potent opioids used in the treatment of diarrhea because they are poorly absorbed and produce minimal CNS effects. Actually, loperamide is absorbed but is rapidly pumped out of the CNS by the P-glycoprotein efflux pump.[75] This property is a potentially important source of drug interaction; loperamide can produce respiratory depression in healthy volunteers given quinidine, a known inhibitor of P-glycoprotein.[75]

The opioids vary tremendously in their lipid solubility (Table 27–2), which largely determines the efficiency of

TABLE 27–2.

Physicochemical Properties of Opioid Agonists

Drug	pK_a*	% Ionized Drug at pH 7.4	Partition Coefficient†
Morphine	7.9/9.4	76	1.4
Meperidine	8.5	93	38.8
Fentanyl	8.4	9.1	860
Sufentanil	8.0	80	1778
Alfentanil	6.5	11	130
Remifentanil	7.1	33	17.9

*Acid base ionization constant.
†The n-octanol/water partition coefficient (corrected for the percentage of drug un-ionized at pH 7.4) is a measure of lipid solubility.

absorption from peripheral sites. For example, after sublingual administration, the bioavailability of morphine is only 12%, whereas highly lipid-soluble drugs such as fentanyl and buprenorphine are 60% to 70% absorbed.[76] Lipophilic opioids are now commercially available in buccal, intranasal, and transdermal preparations. By using a special nebulizer apparatus, it is possible to administer morphine by inhalation and achieve almost 60% bioavailability.[77]

Distribution

All opioids are distributed rapidly and extensively throughout the body. After a bolus intravenous injection, the rapid increase and decrease in plasma concentrations look quite similar for morphine and fentanyl. The difference in onset and duration of effect for these two drugs is a function of the rate at which concentrations in the blood equilibrate with those in the brain. For a lipophilic opioid such as fentanyl, the concentration in the CNS closely follows the concentration in plasma—increasing, then decreasing rapidly as the drug is redistributed from highly perfused tissues into muscle and fat.[78] In this respect, fentanyl is similar to thiopental or propofol—i.e., its short duration of action is caused by the rapidity of physical translocation out of the CNS. The slow onset and offset of morphine are because it enters and exits the CNS slowly.[79] The concentrations of morphine in the brain and cerebrospinal fluid (CSF) lag far behind the concentration in the plasma.

Distribution after neuraxial administration of opioids deserves special mention. When an opioid is administered intrathecally or epidurally, the onset of spinal effect depends on the rate at which drug penetrates the spinal cord to reach opioid receptors in the dorsal horn. Because little metabolism of opioids occurs in the CNS, the effects are terminated by redistribution of opioid into blood vessels. A lipophilic opioid moves quickly from CSF into the substance of the cord, producing the rapid onset of a highly segmental block. Redistribution and offset of effect are also rapid. In contrast, the slow entry of morphine into the cord accounts for its slow onset and the substantial concentrations of morphine that remain in the CSF for a period of time. Once in the dorsal horn, morphine redistributes slowly.

These properties help explain the clinical behavior of epidurally and intrathecally administered morphine, specifically:

- Morphine has an extraordinarily long duration of effect when given neuraxially. High concentrations in the CSF and slow clearance of the drug tend to maintain the analgesic effect.
- CSF circulates slowly, taking 6 or more hours to move a water-soluble compound from lumbar cistern to brain. As a result, the pool of morphine in the CSF can move rostrally, and the effect of the opioid can spread from the point of injection. Rostral spread can be desirable or undesirable. In rare instances, high concentrations of morphine have reached the brain stem and caused respiratory depression 6 to 10 hours after injection. More commonly, clinicians use rostral spread to advantage. For example, when administering morphine, the clinician can often use just a lumbar epidural catheter to provide analgesia for the thorax.

Metabolism and Excretion

All opioids undergo extensive hepatic metabolism to polar metabolites that are excreted by the kidney. The notable exception is remifentanil, which is rapidly hydrolyzed by nonspecific esterases in peripheral tissues and plasma. In general, morphine and its close congeners undergo mainly synthetic biotransformation to glucuronides, whereas meperidine and the fentanyl derivatives undergo oxidative metabolism by cytochrome P450 enzymes. Both morphine and fentanyl have high hepatic extraction ratios (0.7 and 0.6, respectively); this means that the clearance of these drugs is sensitive to factors that alter liver blood flow. (The clearance of morphine can be dramatically increased if a patient has congestive heart failure.) Conversely, clearance is relatively unaffected by inducers or inhibitors of liver enzymes.

Much has been written about the influence of the active metabolites of morphine and meperidine. Although the major metabolite of morphine is 3-glucuronide, approximately 15% forms morphine 6-glucuronide (M6G), a compound that has substantial opioid activity in animals. It is not clear from clinical studies whether M6G contributes significantly to the opioid effect of a single dose of morphine.[80,81] Conversely, it is likely that this highly polar metabolite enters the CNS slowly and accumulates over time.[82] Thus M6G may account for an increasing part of the overall opioid effect with chronic dosing.[83,84] Morphine toxicity has been reported in patients with renal failure, and inability to clear M6G may be playing a role.

Meperidine is mainly cleared by *N*-demethylation to normeperidine. This compound is an analgesic in animals and a convulsant in animals and humans. Patients with renal insufficiency who are given repeated doses of meperidine may accumulate toxic concentrations of normeperidine and may have seizures.[85]

Sedation and Hypnosis

Opioids produce sedation, and sleep often accompanies relief of pain. Given alone, opioids do not generally produce hypnosis. Even with very high doses of fentanyl or its analogues, the hypnotic effect may be brief and unreliable.[86,87] Notably, alfentanil, given at 3 µg/kg (a dose that is probably subanalgesic), can double the hypnotic potency of midazolam.[88] Similar interactions of opioids have been demonstrated with propofol[89] and barbiturates. The κ-receptor agonist butorphanol produces a strong sedative effect at doses less than those used for analgesia, and butorphanol has been used clinically for this purpose.[90]

Central Nervous System Toxicity

Occasionally, opioids produce agitation and dysphoria, and some opioids are proconvulsant. Fortunately, the convulsant effects of most opioids occur at concentrations greater than those needed for analgesia. In patients with head injury, opioids can increase intracranial pressure by causing hypercarbia. Some opioids can produce a modest direct cerebral vasodilation, but this is easily overcome when ventilation is controlled.[91] The pupillary effects can also mask changing neurologic signs.

Respiratory Depression

Opioids produce a dose-dependent depression of the ventilatory response to hypercapnia and hypoxia through actions on μ_2-receptors in respiratory centers of the medulla.[92] These effects may be detectable well before changes in respiratory rate and depth become clinically apparent. Because none of the available opioids is selective for μ_2-receptors, analgesic doses will always produce some effect on ventilatory drive. With increasing doses of opioid, ventilatory rate slows, tidal volume increases, and then eventually decreases. Sufficiently high doses can produce apnea, and a small number of patients still die each year from opioid-induced ventilatory depression. The potential for such disasters is greatest in heavily medicated patients who are unstimulated and unmonitored. The classic study of Forrest and Bellville[93] shows that the occurrence of natural sleep greatly increases the ventilatory depressant effects of morphine. Fentanyl, alfentanil, and sufentanil have all been reported to produce "recurrent" ventilatory depression—i.e., dangerous postoperative depression of breathing in patients who previously seemed to be breathing well.[94] It seems likely that these episodes were actually caused by variations in the level of postoperative stimulation.

Because the analgesic and ventilatory effects of opioids occur by similar receptor mechanisms, the following statements are possible. (1) Equianalgesic doses of all opioid agonists will produce about the same effect on ventilation. In this regard, no drug is any more dangerous or any more safe than morphine. (2) Reversal of ventilatory depression with an opioid antagonist such as naloxone almost always involves some reversal of analgesia. (3) A patient who is tolerant to an opioid and requires increased doses for pain relief will also be tolerant to the ventilatory effects of the opioid.

Cough Suppression

Opioids depress cough by effects on medullary cough centers that are distinct from the effects of the opioids on ventilation. The structure/activity requirements for the antitussive effects are not the same as those for typical μ-receptor effects. The greatest activity occurs with drugs such as codeine and heroine—morphine congeners that have bulky substitutions at the 3 position. The stereospecificity of the response is also different—i.e., cough suppression is produced by dextrorotatory isomers of opioids (e.g., dextromethorphan) that do not have analgesic activity.

Nausea and Vomiting

Opioids stimulate nausea and vomiting by a direct effect on the chemoreceptor trigger zone in the area postrema.[95] This effect is increased by labyrinthine input, therefore patients who are moving are much more likely to experience nausea than those who are lying quietly. Some patients always vomit after morphine, whereas some never do. Many tolerate one opioid but not another; the basis for these differences is not known. There is no clear dose/response relationship for this effect. Wang[96] showed in animals that high doses of opioids can actually have antiemetic effects by depressing the vomiting center proper. The relevance of this finding to clinical practice is uncertain.

Constriction of the Pupils

The miotic effect of opioids occurs through a direct action on the autonomic (Edinger-Westphal) nucleus of the oculomotor nerve; the result is an increase in parasympathetic tone. Although this effect can be detected after extremely small doses of fentanyl or alfentanil, the minimum effective concentration for alfentanil-induced miosis is close to that for analgesia.[97] Relatively little tolerance to this effect develops, therefore patients taking very high doses of opioids for pain will continue to have constricted pupils. Pupillary responses have been useful for simultaneous pharmacokinetic/pharmacodynamic modeling of opioids.[97]

Skeletal Muscle Rigidity

This phenomenon, often incorrectly called *truncal* or *chest wall* rigidity, is actually a generalized hypertonus of striated muscle throughout the body.[98] The condition is usually seen when potent opioids are administered rapidly and is most commonly produced by fentanyl and its congeners. The mechanism appears to be an inhibition of striatal γ-aminobutyric acid release and an increase in dopamine production.[99] In rats, selective antagonism at the nucleus raphe magnus can completely prevent the increase in tone.[100] Opioid-induced rigidity usually occurs during induction of anesthesia (and rarely during emergence) and can make a patient extremely difficult to ventilate. The problem does not seem to be loss of chest wall compliance, but rather hypertonus of the pharyngeal and laryngeal musculature, leading to narrowing of the laryngeal inlet.[101] The presence of a tracheostomy prevents much of the difficulty in ventilating. When rigidity is recognized, it can be treated quickly with a muscle relaxant or reversed with naloxone, depending on the circumstances.

Cardiovascular Effects

Normal analgesic doses of opioids may cause bradycardia and vasodilation. In a healthy individual, the most common effect is mild orthostatic hypotension that responds to administration of fluids and recumbency. More significant bradycardia and vasodilation are seen at greater doses and when opioids are combined with other anesthetic drugs.

Bradycardia is produced by a direct stimulant effect on the central vagal nuclei.[102] It may be reversed or prevented by atropine, pancuronium, or other vagolytic drugs. Meperidine, which is weakly atropinic, does not usually cause bradycardia. The increase in vagal tone can prolong atrioventricular conduction. Also, in animals, meperidine has had a direct depressant effect on the sinoatrial node.[103]

Preload and afterload are decreased by opioid-induced depression of vasomotor centers in the medulla and a consequent decrease in central sympathetic tone. The effects of morphine on skeletal muscle vascular resistance are mediated neurally and most likely occur during conditions of high sympathetic tone.[104] Venodilation may lead to significant pooling of blood, especially in the splanchnic vasculature.[105] In humans and animals, opioid-induced venodilation seems to occur later and last longer than the effect on arterioles.[106]

The cardiovascular effects that are *not* produced by opioids are equally significant for the practice of anesthesia. At clinically relevant concentrations, opioids do not produce significant myocardial depression, and they do not predispose the heart to arrhythmias. Opioids do not block high- or low-pressure baroreceptor reflexes,[107] and they preserve the cardiovascular responses to circulating catecholamines.[108] For these reasons, opioid-based anesthesia is often a good choice for a critically ill patient with diminished cardiovascular reserve.

Histamine Release

Although patients who have experienced hives and itching after administration of an opioid frequently report that they are allergic to the drug, true allergy to opioids is in fact extremely rare. As with many other low-molecular weight basic drugs, morphine, codeine, and meperidine can cause displacement of histamine from tissue mast cells. This is a nonimmunologic response that most often manifests as local itching, redness, or hives near the site of intravenous injection. Fentanyl and its congeners do not release histamine.

If sufficient histamine is liberated, it may cause a transient decrease in systemic vascular resistance, hypotension, and tachycardia.[109] These effects usually occur when very large doses of opioids are given rapidly. The cardiovascular effects may be prevented by pretreatment with H_1- and H_2-receptor antagonists, such as chlorpheniramine and cimetidine.[110]

Opioid-related itching also may be produced by other mechanisms. Opioids frequently cause itching and warmth over the neck and face, especially over the malar area. Epidural opioids can produce troublesome generalized itching.[111] These dysesthesias appear to be opioid-specific effects. They are produced by opioids such as fentanyl, which do not release histamine, and can be reversed by naloxone.

Smooth Muscle Spasm

Opioid receptors are found throughout the enteric nervous system in the plexus of the bowel, in the sacral plexus, along the biliary tree, in the ureters, and in the bladder. Opioids stimulate tonic contraction of smooth muscle at all of these sites, while reducing normal propulsive activity. These effects can be a source of significant morbidity:

- Inhibition of normal intestinal secretions and peristalsis can lead to increased water absorption and *constipation*. Very little tolerance develops to this effect, therefore patients taking opioids chronically can experience severe constipation. This is a common problem for patients with cancer.
- *Delay of gastric emptying* may not only decrease the absorption of some drugs but also increase the likelihood that a surgical patient will have a "full stomach" despite restriction of food and liquids before surgery.
- Opioid-induced *postoperative ileus* is common and may be an important factor in delaying hospital discharge of surgical patients. Both central and peripheral mechanisms play a part in this gastrointestinal effect.[112] Several clinical studies have shown that poorly absorbed quaternary opioid antagonists such as methylnaltrexone[113] and ADL8-2698[114] can reverse or prevent the peripheral component of opioid-induced ileus and constipation. Because these antagonists are permanently charged, they do not enter the CNS and therefore do not reverse opioid analgesia.
- Stimulation of smooth muscle along the gallbladder and cystic duct and contraction of the sphincter of Oddi may produce an *increase in intrabiliary pressure* that can lead to biliary colic and false-positive cholangiograms. The increase in pressure can be completely reversed by naloxone and partially reversed by atropine or nitroglycerin. Reversal appears to be much less likely with κ-receptor–type opioid agonists/antagonists.[115]
- Opioids can cause *urinary retention* by decreasing bladder detrusor tone and increasing tone in the urinary sphincter. Opioids also cause decreased awareness of bladder distention and inhibition of the reflex urge to void. This complication is more common in male patients and is more likely to occur when opioids are given by epidural or intrathecal injection.

Effects of Chronic Use of Opioids

Drug Tolerance

Because tolerance to the effects of repeatedly administered opioids can be profound, it is sometimes a barrier to the use of these drugs in chronic painful conditions. In humans and animals, two types of tolerance, acute and chronic, seem to exist.[116] Acute tolerance (i.e., tachyphylaxis) can be demonstrated within hours, after a single high dose or a rapid infusion. Acute tolerance occurs in fairly restricted circumstances, and the clinical relevance remains to be proved. Chronic tolerance takes more time to develop (although morphine-pelleted rats and mice can become highly tolerant in a day or two), and it can last even longer. The earliest clinical manifestation of tolerance is a decrease in the duration of effect after a bolus dose; a decrease in the intensity of effect usually follows. With tolerance to one μ-receptor agonist, there is simultaneous cross-tolerance to other μ-receptor agonists. This cross-tolerance is often incomplete. Tolerance develops most rapidly to opioid-induced depressant effects, such as analgesia and respiratory depression, and very slowly to opioid-induced stimulant effects, such as constipation or miosis.

The mechanisms of tolerance to opioids are unknown. The speed of the changes in acute tolerance suggests rapid cellular autoregulatory responses, whereas chronic tolerance appears to be a much more permanent alteration in cellular structure and function. As stated earlier, receptor phosphorylation, G protein uncoupling, and receptor internalization (removal of receptors from the cell membrane) may all play a role. Recent research suggests that opioid tolerance also involves the activation of NMDA receptors and the production of nitric oxide. As a result, recent experiments have tried to modulate tolerance to opioids by administering NMDA antagonists (dizocilpine, dextromethorphan) or nitric oxide synthase inhibitors.[117,118]

Physical Dependence

After sufficient doses have been administered, all opioids induce a state of physical dependence. Discontinuation of the drug causes a stereotypical withdrawal syndrome that includes restlessness, mydriasis, gooseflesh, runny nose, diarrhea, shaking chills, and drug-seeking behavior. The rate of onset of these symptoms depends on the speed of opioid elimination. Administration of an opioid antagonist can cause an immediate "precipitated" withdrawal that can sometimes be quite violent. Withdrawal symptoms can be terminated rapidly by intravenous administration of a small dose of morphine.

When a patient with known physical dependence is to be detoxified, he or she is commonly switched to administration of methadone, and the dosage is reduced slowly. The result is a mild, although protracted, withdrawal syndrome. When a person dependent on heroin or methadone seeks medical treatment on an emergency basis, he or she is generally not an appropriate candidate for detoxification.

It seems likely that most patients administered opioids chronically have some clinically imperceptible level of physical dependence. In most instances, withdrawal may take place without the patient or physician being aware of its occurrence. Physical dependence must be distinguished from psychological dependence or addiction, which includes compulsive drug-seeking behavior. The data of Porter and Jick[119] suggest that drug addiction resulting from appropriate medical treatment is an unusual event.

Use of Opioids for Chronic Pain

The use of opioids for chronic pain is controversial. Few would deny opioids to the patient with terminal cancer, but what about the patient without cancer (or the cancer patient with substantial time remaining)? Despite that many patients have received opioids chronically without apparent problems,[120] it is not really known how well such opioids work. Recently, much attention has been given to the finding that neuropathic pain and centrally mediated pain are less responsive to opioids than other types of pain. Some preclinical data even suggest that chronic neuropathic pain may be worsened by use of opioids.[121] Unfortunately, a large percentage of chronic pain (both cancer and noncancer) falls into the neuropathic category.

The efficacy of opioids for low back pain and neuropathic pain has been supported (sometimes enthusiastically) by an accumulation of case reports and uncontrolled open studies.[122] Few controlled studies investigating the efficacy and side effects of opioids in these clinical settings are available.[123-126] Currently, the maximum duration of opioid treatment investigated in a double-blind, placebo-controlled study is 9 weeks.[123] All other studies have lasted a maximum of 4 weeks. These trials found a reduction in subjective pain scores, but only one study examined psychosocial features, quality of life, drug dependence, or functional status in detail.[123] No significant differences in any of the functional status parameters were detected, and there was a lack of overall patient preference for the opioid. The authors concluded that morphine may confer analgesic benefit with a low risk for addiction, but that it is unlikely to yield psychological or functional improvement.[123] Adverse opioid-induced side effects were reported in all of these investigations and led to large numbers (up to 60%) of patients withdrawing from the study.

Thus there is a lack of prospective, controlled studies examining the long-term (at least several months) administration of opioids. Future studies need to demonstrate positive outcomes, not only in subjective pain reports, but also in terms of reduced depression, functional improvement, rates of patient re-employment, and decreased use of the health care system.

References

1. Brownstein MJ: A brief history of opiates, opioid peptides, and opioid receptors. Proc Natl Acad Sci USA 90:5391, 1993.
2. Pert CB, Snyder SH: Opiate receptor: Demonstration in nervous tissue. Science 179:1011, 1973.
3. Simon EJ, Hiller JM, Edelman I: Stereospecific binding of the potent narcotic analgesic (3H) Etorphine to rat-brain homogenate. Proc Natl Acad Sci USA 70:1947, 1973.
4. Terenius L: Characteristics of the "receptor" for narcotic analgesics in synaptic plasma membrane fraction from rat brain. Acta Pharmacol Toxicol (Copenh) 33:377, 1973.
5. Pasternak GW: Pharmacological mechanisms of opioid analgesics. Clin Neuropharmacol 16:1, 1993.
6. Kieffer BL, Befort K, Gaveriaux-Ruff C, et al: The delta-opioid receptor: Isolation of a cDNA by expression cloning and pharmacological characterization. Proc Natl Acad Sci USA 89:12048, 1992.

7. Evans CJ, Keith DE, Morrison H, et al: Cloning of delta opioid receptor by functional expression. Science 258:1952, 1992.
8. Yasuda K, Raynor K, Kong H, et al: Cloning and functional comparison of kappa and delta opioid receptors from mouse brain. Proc Natl Acad Sci USA 90:6736, 1993.
9. Chen Y, Mestek A, Liu J, et al: Molecular cloning and functional expression of a mu-opioid receptor from rat brain. Mol Pharmacol 44:8, 1993.
10. Gaveriaux-Ruff C, Kieffer B: Opioid receptors: Gene structure and function. In Stein C (ed): Opioids in Pain Control: Basic and Clinical Aspects. Cambridge, Cambridge University Press, 1999.
11. Kieffer BL: Opioids: First lessons from knockout mice. Trends Pharmacol Sci 20:19, 1999.
12. Kieffer BL: Recent advances in molecular recognition and signal transduction of active peptides: Receptors for opioid peptides. Cell Mol Neurobiol 15:615, 1995.
13. Jordan BA, Devi LA: G-protein-coupled receptor heterodimerization modulates receptor function. Nature 399:697, 1999.
14. Law PY, Wong YH, Loh HH: Molecular mechanisms and regulation of opioid receptor signaling. Annu Rev Pharmacol Toxicol 40:389, 2000.
15. Mogil JS, Yu L, Basbaum AI: Pain genes? Natural variation and transgenic mutants. Annu Rev Neurosci 23:777, 2000.
16. Simonin F, Slowe S, Becker JA, et al: Analysis of [3H]bremazocine binding in single and combinatorial opioid receptor knockout mice. Eur J Pharmacol 414:189, 2001.
17. Clarke S, Kitchen I: Opioid analgesia: New information from gene knockout studies. Curr Opin Anaesth 12:609, 1999.
18. Narita M, Mizoguchi H, Narita M, et al: Involvement of spinal protein kinase C gamma in the attenuation of opioid mu-receptor-mediated G-protein activation after chronic intrathecal administration of [D-Ala2,N-MePhe4,Gly-Ol(5)]enkephalin. J Neurosci 21:3715, 2001.
19. Stein C: The control of pain in peripheral tissue by opioids. N Engl J Med 332:1685, 1995.
20. Trafton JA, Abbadie C, Marchand S, et al: Spinal opioid analgesia: How critical is the regulation of substance P signaling? J Neurosci 19:9642, 1999.
21. Stein C, Machelska H, Schäfer M: Peripheral analgesic and antiinflammatory effects of opioids. Z Rheumatol 60:416, 2001.
22. Cox BM: Mechanisms of tolerance. In Stein C (ed): Opioids in pain control: Basic and clinical aspects. Cambridge, UK, Cambridge University Press, 1999.
23. Hughes J, Smith TW, Kosterlitz HW, et al: Identification of two related pentapeptides from the brain with potent opiate agonist activity. Nature 258:577, 1975.
24. Akil H, Mayer DJ, Liebeskind JC: Antagonism of stimulation-produced analgesia by naloxone, a narcotic antagonist. Science 191:961, 1976.
25. Stein C, Schäfer M, Cabot PJ, et al: Peripheral opioid analgesia. Pain Reviews 4:171, 1997.
26. Slominski A, Wortsman J, Luger T, et al: Corticotropin releasing hormone and pro-opiomelanocortin involvement in the cutaneous response to stress. Physiol Rev 80:979, 2000.
27. Machelska H, Stein C: Immune mechanisms of pain and analgesia. Georgetown, TX, Landes Bioscience, 2001.
28. Li CH, Chung D: Isolation and structure of an untriakontapeptide with opiate activity from camel pituitary glands. Proc Natl Acad Sci USA 73:1145, 1976.
29. Loh HH, Tseng LF, Wei E, et al: Beta-endorphin is a potent analgesic agent. Proc Natl Acad Sci USA 73:2895, 1976.
30. Goldstein A, Tachibana S, Lowney LI, et al: Dynorphin-(1-13), an extraordinarily potent opioid peptide. Proc Natl Acad Sci USA 76:6666, 1979.
31. Nakanishi S, Inoue A, Kita T, et al: Nucleotide sequence of cloned cDNA for bovine corticotropin-beta-lipotropin precursor. Nature 278:423, 1979.
32. Comb M, Seeburg PH, Adelman J, et al: Primary structure of the human Met- and Leu-enkephalin precursor and its mRNA. Nature 295:663, 1982.
33. Kakidani H, Furutani Y, Takahashi H, et al: Cloning and sequence analysis of cDNA for porcine beta-neo-endorphin/dynorphin precursor. Nature 298:245, 1982.
34. Höllt V: Opioid peptide processing and receptor selectivity. Annu Rev Pharmacol Toxicol 26:59, 1986.
35. Akil H, Owens C, Gutstein H, et al: Endogenous opioids: Overview and current issues. Drug Alcohol Depend 51:127, 1998.
36. Roques BP, Noble F, Fournie-Zaluski MC: Endogenous opioid peptides and analgesia. In Stein C (ed): Opioids in Pain Control: Basic and Clinical Aspects. Cambridge, UK, Cambridge University Press, 1999.
37. Zadina JE, Hackler L, Ge LJ, et al: A potent and selective endogenous agonist for the mu-opiate receptor. Nature 386:499, 1997.
38. Horvath G: Endomorphin-1 and endomorphin-2: Pharmacology of the selective endogenous mu-opioid receptor agonists. Pharmacol Ther 88:437, 2000.
39. Grisel JE, Mogil JS: Effects of supraspinal orphanin FQ/nociceptin. Peptides 21:1037, 2000.
40. Reinscheid RK, Nothacker H, Civelli O: The orphanin FQ/nociceptin gene: Structure, tissue distribution of expression and functional implications obtained from knockout mice. Peptides 21:901, 2000.
41. Wang Z, Gardell LR, Ossipov MH, et al: Pronociceptive actions of dynorphin maintain chronic neuropathic pain. J Neurosci 21:1779, 2001.
42. Caudle RM, Mannes AJ: Dynorphin: Friend or foe? Pain 87:235, 2000.
43. Millan MJ: Multiple opioid systems and chronic pain. In Herz A (ed): Opioids II, Berlin, Heidelberg, Springer-Verlag, 1993.
44. Heinricher MM, Morgan MM: Supraspinal mechanisms of opioid analgesia. In Stein C (ed): Opioids in Pain Control: Basic and Clinical Aspects. Cambridge, UK, Cambridge University Press, 1999.
45. Christie MJ, Connor M, Vaughan CW, et al: Cellular actions of opioids and other analgesics: Implications for synergism in pain relief. Clin Exp Pharmacol Physiol 27:520, 2000.
46. Hurley RW, Hammond DL: Contribution of endogenous enkephalins to the enhanced analgesic effects of suprasinal mu opioid receptor agonists after inflammatory injury. J Neurosci 21:2536, 2001.
47. Cesselin F, Benoliel JJ, Bourgoin S, et al: Spinal mechanisms of opioid analgesia. In Stein C, (ed): Opioids in Pain Control: Basic and Clinical Aspects. Cambridge, UK, Cambridge University Press, 1999.
48. Yaksh TL: Pharmacology and mechanisms of opioid analgesic activity. Acta Anaesthesiol Scand 41:94, 1997.
49. Trafton JA, Abbadie C, Marek K, et al: Postsynaptic signaling via the [mu]-opioid receptor: Responses of dorsal horn neurons to exogenous opioids and noxious stimulation. J Neurosci 20:8578, 2000.
50. Schäfer M: Peripheral opioid analgesia: From experimental to clinical studies. Curr Opin Anaesth 12:603, 1999.
51. Rittner HL, Brack A, Machelska H, et al: Opioid peptide-expressing leukocytes: Identification, recruitment, and simultaneously increasing inhibition of inflammatory pain. Anesthesiology 95:500, 2001.
52. Cabot PJ, Carter L, Gaiddon C, et al: Immune cell-derived β-endorphin: Production, release and control of inflammatory pain in rats. J Clin Invest 100:142, 1997.
53. Machelska H, Cabot PJ, Mousa SA, et al: Pain control in inflammation governed by selectins. Nat Med 4:1425, 1998.
54. Gupta A, Bodin L, Holmstrom B, et al: A systematic review of the peripheral analgesic effects of intraarticular morphine. Anesth Analg 93:761, 2001.
55. Binder W, Machelska H, Mousa S, et al: Analgesic and antiinflammatory effects of two novel kappa-opioid peptides. Anesthesiology 94:1034, 2001.
56. Pfeiffer A, Brantl V, Herz A, et al: Psychotomimesis mediated by κ opiate receptors. Science 233:774, 1986.
57. Coombs DW, Saunders RL, Lachance D, et al: Intrathecal morphine tolerance: Use of intrathecal clonidine, DADLE, and intraventricular morphine. Anesthesiology 62:358, 1985.
58. Bloomfield SS, Barden TP, Mitchell J: Metkephamid and meperidine analgesia after episiotomy. Clin Pharmacol Ther 34:240, 1983.
59. Glass PSA, Chavis II, Ginsberg B, et al: Analgesic and cardiorespiratory effects of the first mixed mu/delta/kappa opioid agonist DP13290. Anesthesiology 91(3A Suppl):A985, 1999.
60. McQuay HJ: Pharmacological treatment of neuralgic and neuropathic pain. Cancer Surv 7:141, 1988.
61. Kaiko RF, Wallenstein SL, Rogers AG, et al: Intramuscular meptazinol and morphine in postoperative pain. Clin Pharmacol Ther 37:589, 1985.
62. Austin KL, Stapleton JV, Mather LE: Multiple intramuscular injections: A major source of variability in analgesic response to meperidine. Pain 8:47, 1980.

63. Austin KL, Stapleton JV, Mather LE: Relationship between blood meperidine concentrations and analgesic response: A preliminary report. Anesthesiology 53:460, 1980.

64. Ausems ME, Hug CC, Stanski DR, et al: Plasma concentrations of alfentanil required to supplement nitrous oxide anesthesia for general surgery. Anesthesiology 65:362, 1986.

65. Rooke GA, Reves JG, Rosow CE: Anesthesiology and geriatric medicine: mutual needs and opportunities. Anesthesiology 96:2, 2002.

66. Scott JC, Stanski DR: Decreased fentanyl and alfentanil dose requirements with age. A simultaneous pharmacokinetic and pharmacodynamic evaluation. J Pharmacol Exp Ther 240:159, 1987.

67. Minto CF, Schnider TW, Egan TD, et al: Influence of age and gender on the pharmacokinetics and pharmacodynamics of remifentanil. I. Model development. Anesthesiology 86:10, 1997.

68. Aubrun F, Moncel S, Langeron O, et al: Postoperative titration of intravenous morphine in the elderly patient. Anesthesiology 96:17, 2002.

69. Dershwitz M, Hoke JF, Rosow CE, et al: Pharmacokinetics and pharmacodynamics of remifentanil in volunteer subjects with severe liver disease. Anesthesiology 84:812, 1996.

70. Hoke JF, Shlugman D, Dershwitz M, et al: Pharmacokinetics and pharmacodynamics of remifentanil in persons with renal failure compared with healthy volunteers. Anesthesiology 87:533, 1997.

71. Dahan A, Sarton E, Teppema L, et al: Sex-related differences in the influence of morphine on ventilatory control in humans. Anesthesiology 88:903, 1998.

72. Eichelbaum M, Evert B: Influence of pharmacogenetics on drug disposition and response. Clin Exp Pharmacol Physiol 23:983, 1996.

73. Caraco Y, Sheller J, Wood AJ: Impact of ethnic origin and quinidine coadministration on codeine's disposition and pharmacokinetic effects. J Pharmacol Exp Ther 290:413, 1999.

74. Cepeda MS, Farrar JT, Roa JH, et al: Ethnicity influences morphine pharmacokinetics and pharmacodynamics. Clin Pharmacol Ther 70:351, 2001.

75. Sadeque AJM, Wandel C, He H, et al: Increased drug delivery to the brain by P-glycoprotein inhibition. Clin Pharmacol Ther 68:231, 2000.

76. Weinberg DS, Inturrisi CE, Reidenberg B, et al: Sublingual absorption of selected opioid analgesics. Clin Pharmacol Ther 44:335, 1988.

77. Dershwitz M, Walsh JL, Morishige RJ, et al: Pharmacokinetics and pharmacodynamics of inhaled versus intravenous morphine in healthy volunteers. Anesthesiology 93:619, 2000.

78. Hug CC, Murphy MR: Fentanyl disposition in cerebrospinal fluid and plasma and its relationship to ventilatory depression in the dog. Anesthesiology 50:342, 1979.

79. Herz A, Teschemacher JH: Activities and sites of antinociceptive action of morphine like analgesics. In Harper NJ, Simmonds AB (eds): Advances in Drug Research, New York, Academic Press, 1971.

80. Osborne RJ, Joel SP, Trew D, et al: The analgesic activity of morphine-6-glucuronide. Lancet 1:828, 1988.

81. Lötsch J, Kobal G, Stockmann A, et al: Lack of analgesic activity of morphine 6-glucuronide after short-term intravenous administration in healthy volunteers. Anesthesiology 87:1348, 1997.

82. Portenoy RK, Khan E, Layman M, et al: Chronic morphine therapy for cancer pain: Plasma and cerebrospinal fluid morphine and morphine-6-glucuronide concentrations. Neurology 41:1457, 1991.

83. Lötsch J, Weiss M, Ahne G, et al: Pharmacokinetic modeling of M6G formation after oral administration of morphine in healthy volunteers. Anesthesiology 90:1026, 1999.

84. Portenoy RK, Thaler HT, Inturrisi CE, et al: The metabolite morphine-6-glucuronide contributes to the analgesia produced by morphine infusion in patients with pain and normal renal function. Clin Pharmacol Ther 51:422, 1992.

85. Kaiko RF, Foley KM, Grabinski PY, et al: Central nervous system excitatory effects of meperidine in cancer patients. Ann Neurol 13:180, 1983.

86. Bailey PL, Wilbrink J, Zwanikken P, et al: Anesthetic induction with fentanyl. Anesth Analg 64:48, 1985.

87. Silbert BS, Rosow CE, Keegan CR, et al: The effect of diazepam on induction of anesthesia with alfentanil. Anesth Analg 65:71, 1986.

88. Kissin I, Vinik HR, Castillo R, et al: Alfentanil potentiates midazolam-induced unconsciousness in subanalgesic doses. Anesth Analg 71:65, 1990.

89. Short TG, Plummer JL, Chui PT: Hypnotic and anaesthetic interactions between midazolam, propofol and alfentanil. Br J Anaesth 69:162, 1992.

90. Dershwitz M, Rosow CE, DiBiase PM, et al: Comparison of the sedative effects of butorphanol and midazolam. Anesthesiology 74:717, 1991.

91. Shupak RC, Harp JR: Comparison between high-dose sufentanil-oxygen and high-dose fentanyl-oxygen for neuroanesthesia. Br J Anaesth 57:375, 1985.

92. Weil JV, McCullough RE, Kline JS, et al: Diminished ventilatory response to hypoxia and hypercapnia after morphine in normal man. N Engl J Med 292:1103, 1975.

93. Forrest WH, Bellville JW: The effect of sleep plus morphine on the respiratory response to carbon dioxide. Anesthesiology 25:137, 1964.

94. Becker LD, Paulson BA, Miller RD, et al: Biphasic respiratory depression after fentanyl-droperidol or fentanyl alone used to supplement nitrous oxide anesthesia. Anesthesiology 44:291, 1976.

95. Wang SC, Glaviano VV: Locus of emetic action of morphine and hydergine in dogs. J Pharmacol Exp Ther 111:329, 1954.

96. Wang SC: Emetic and antiemetic drugs. In Root WS, Hoffman FG (eds): Physiological Pharmacology II (part B). New York, Academic Press, 1963.

97. He Y-L, Walsh JL, Denman WT, et al: Pharmacodynamic modeling of the miotic effects of alfentanil in humans measured with infrared pupillometry. Anesthesiology 95:A55, 2001. Available at www.asa-abstracts.com/

98. Benthuysen JL, Smith NT, Sanford TJ, et al: Physiology of alfentanil-induced rigidity. Anesthesiology 64:440, 1986.

99. Costall B, Fortune DH, Naylor RJ: Involvement of mesolimbic and extrapyramidal nuclei in the motor depressant action of narcotic drugs. J Pharm Pharmacol 30:566, 1978.

100. Weinger MB, Smith NT, Blasco TA, et al: Brain sites mediating opiate-induced muscle rigidity in the rat: Methylnaloxonium mapping study. Brain Res 544:181, 1991.

101. Arandia HY, Patil VU: Glottic closure following large dose of fentanyl. Anesthesiology 66:574, 1987.

102. Laubie M, Schmitt H, Vincent M: Vagal bradycardia produced by microinjections of morphine-like drugs into the nucleus ambiguus in anaesthetized dogs. Eur J Pharmacol 59:287, 1979.

103. Urthaler F, Isobe JH, James T: Direct and vagally mediated chronotropic effects of morphine studied by selective perfusion of the sinus node of awake dogs. Chest 68:222, 1975.

104. Lowenstein E, Whiting DA, Bittar CA, et al: Local and neurally mediated effects of morphine on skeletal muscle vascular resistance. J Pharmacol Exp Ther 180:359, 1972.

105. Green JF, Jackman AP, Krohm KA: Mechanism of morphine-induced shifts in blood volume between extracorporeal reservoir and the systemic circulation of the dog under conditions of constant blood flow and vena caval pressures. Circ Res 2:479, 1978.

106. Hsu HO, Hickey RF, Forbes AR: Morphine decreases peripheral vascular resistance and increases capacitance in man. Anesthesiology 50:98, 1979.

107. Ebert TJ, Kortly KJ: Fentanyl-diazepam anesthesia with or without nitrous oxide does not attenuate cardiopulmonary baroreflex-mediated vasoconstrictor responses to controlled hypovolemia in humans. Anesth Analg 67:548, 1988.

108. Ward JW, McGrath RL, Weil JV: Effects of morphine on the peripheral vascular response to sympathetic stimulation. Am J Cardiol 29:656, 1972.

109. Rosow CE, Moss J, Philbin DM, et al: Histamine release during morphine and fentanyl anesthesia. Anesthesiology 56:93, 1982.

110. Philbin DM, Moss J, Rosow CE, et al: Histamine release with intravenous narcotics: protective effects of H1 and H2 receptor antagonists. Klin Wochenschr 60:1056, 1982.

111. Ballentyne JC, Loach AB, Carr DB: Itching after epidural and spinal opiates. Pain 33:149, 1988.

112. Steward JJ, Weisbrodt NW, Burks TF: Central and peripheral actions of morphine on intestinal transit. J Pharmacol Exp Ther 205:547, 1978.

113. Yuan CS, Foss JF, Osinski J, et al: The safety and efficacy of oral methylnaltrexone in preventing morphine-induced delay in oral-cecal transit time. Clin Pharmacol Ther 61:467, 1997.

114. Taguchi A, Sharma N, Saleem RM, et al: Selective postoperative inhibition of gastrointestinal opioid receptors. N Engl J Med 345:935, 2001.

115. Radnay PA, Duncalf D, Novakovic M, et al: Common bile duct pressure changes after fentanyl, morphine, meperidine, butorphanol, and naloxone. Anesth Analg 63:441, 1984.

116. Rosow CE: Acute and chronic tolerance: Relevance for clinical practice. In Problems of Drug Dependence. Research monograph 76, National Institute on Drug Abuse. U.S. Government Printing Office, Washington, DC, 1987, pp 29–34.

117. Trujillo KA, Akil H: Inhibition of morphine tolerance and dependence by the NMDA receptor antagonist MK-801. Science 251:85, 1991.

118. Elliott K, Minami N, Kolesnikov YA, et al: The NMDA receptor antagonists, LY274614 and MK-801, and the nitric oxide synthase inhibitor, NG-nitro-L-arginine, attenuate analgesic tolerance to the mu-opioid morphine but not to kappa opioids. Pain 56:69, 1994.

119. Porter J, Jick H: Addiction rare in patients treated with narcotics. N Engl J Med 302:123, 1980.

120. Portenoy RK: Chronic opioid therapy in nonmalignant pain. J Pain Symptom Manage 5(1 Suppl):S46, 1990.

121. Mao J, Price DD, Mayer DJ: Mechanisms of hyperalgesia and morphine tolerance: A current view of other possible interactions. Pain 62:259, 1995.

122. Stein C: What is wrong with opioids in chronic pain? Curr Opin Anaesth 13:557, 2000.

123. Moulin DE, Iezzi A, Amireh R, et al: Randomized trial of oral morphine for chronic non-cancer pain. Lancet 347:143, 1996.

124. Watson CP, Babul N: Efficacy of oxycodone in neuropathic pain: A randomized trial in postherpetic neuralgia. Neurology 50:1837, 1998.

125. Caldwell JR, Hale ME, Boyd RE, et al: Treatment of osteoarthritis pain with controlled release oxycodone or fixed combination oxycodone plus acetaminophen added to nonsteroidal antiinflammatory drugs: A double blind, randomized, multicenter, placebo controlled trial. J Rheumatol 26:862, 1999.

126. Peloso PM, Bellamy N, Bensen W, et al: Double blind randomized placebo control trial of controlled release codeine in the treatment of osteoarthritis of the hip or knee. J Rheumatol 27:764, 2000.

28

Analgesics

Mervyn Maze, MB, ChB • Francis Bonnet, MD

RECEPTOR LIGANDS—α_2 ADRENERGIC RECEPTOR AGONISTS

History and Background

Clonidine, the prototypical α_2 adrenergic receptor agonist ("α_2 agonist"), was developed as a nasal decongestant in the early 1970s. Soon its potent sympatholytic effect on the cardiovascular system was noted, and clonidine was then used as an antihypertensive. However, because sedation also occurred, clonidine became only a second- or third-line antihypertensive. A decade after its first clinical use, anesthesiologists realized that the sedative properties, which were

considered undesirable by cardiologists, could be used to clinical advantage. Thereafter, α_2 agonists have been used as both a premedication and supplementation to general anesthesia in humans.

Xylazine, a weak and relatively nonselective α agonist, had already been used for these purposes in veterinary anesthesia. In the early 1990s, the racemic compound medetomidine was introduced as a more selective α_2 agonist for veterinary anesthesia. Subsequently, its active enantiomer dexmedetomidine was developed for use as a perioperative sedative and analgesic for humans.

MECHANISM OF ACTION

Receptor Subtypes

α_2 Agonists exert their properties by activating α_2 adrenergic receptors, of which there are three subtypes. Initially, Bylund and colleagues[1] classified these subtypes according to their susceptibility to activation or inactivation by a series of agonists and antagonists. The nomenclature "A," "B," and "C" was used, although there was confusion about a species homologue of "A" that was initially referred to as "D." Subsequently, it was suggested that there are four rather than three subtypes. However, with the advent of cloning, Kobilka and colleagues[2] confirmed that there are only three subtypes. Further confusion reigned when molecular biologists adopted a nomenclature based on the chromosome on which the genetic sequence resided. Thus α_{2A} was referred to as C_{10}, α_{2B} was referred to as C_2, and α_{2C} was referred to as C_4. Fortunately, pharmacologists and molecular biologists have fully reconciled, and the receptor subtypes currently are conventionally referred to as α_{2A}, α_{2B}, and α_{2C}.

Structure of α_2 Adrenoceptors

Figure 28–1 shows the secondary structure of the α_2 adrenergic receptor (adrenoceptor). As with other G protein–coupled receptors, α_2 adrenoceptors course back and forth across the plasma membrane in a serpiginous manner. The orientation of the transmembrane domains was shown to be identical to that of the transmembrane protein bacteriorhodopsin.[3] Because high-fidelity structural information exists for bacteriorhodopsin, this protein was used as a template to deduce the structure of the α_2 adrenoceptors. With the advent of x-ray crystallographic resolution of bovine rhodopsin, however, bovine rhodopsin replaced bacteriorhodopsin as the homologous model.[4] The binding site for the agonist remains uncertain, although it is thought to involve three contact points, with amino acid residues on at least two separate transmembrane domains. Further understanding of these sites will allow the creation of agonists that are selective for the receptor subtypes.[5]

Responses Mediated by the α_2 Adrenoceptor Subtypes

Figure 28–2 shows the physiologic functions mediated by α_2 adrenoceptors. Each of the receptor subtypes is distributed ubiquitously throughout the body, including the central nervous system. Thus it is not possible to ascribe a particular response based on the location of the individual receptor subtype. The α_{2A} adrenoceptor has been positively identified as mediating sedation and hypnosis, analgesia, and sympatholysis,[6] whereas the α_{2B} adrenoceptor mediates vasoconstriction[7] and probably the antishivering action[5] and the endogenous analgesic mechanism.[8] The α_{2C} adrenoceptor has been linked to learning and to the startle response.[9]

Transmembrane Signal Transduction

Each of the receptor subtypes is capable of inhibiting adenyl cyclase through the α_i subunit of the G protein. The resulting decrease in the accumulation of cyclic adenosine monophosphate (cAMP) will limit stimulation of cAMP-dependent protein kinase, and hence phosphorylation of target regulatory proteins. Although such inhibition of adenylyl cyclase may be a cellular response of α_2 agonists,[10] it may not necessarily be causally related to the observed response. There is evidence of direct coupling, through the appropriate subunit, to ligand-gated ion channels. Several species of these channels currently have been linked to activation of the α_2 adrenoceptor including the N-type Ca^{++} channel (inhibition),[11] the P/Q-type Ca^{++} channel (inhibition),[12] the I_A K^+ channel (activation),[13] the calcium-activated potassium channel (activation),[14] and the Na^+/H^+ antiporter (activation).[15] The α_{2B} adrenoceptor subtype appears to be positively coupled to the L-type Ca^{++} channel[16] and, in keeping with its vasoconstrictive action, appears more like an "excitatory" subtype rather than an "inhibitory" subtype.

Modulation of Responses Mediated by α_2 Adrenoceptors

The development of tolerance is a widespread biologic process in which responsiveness to a drug decreases with continuing exposure to the drug. For example, in rats, the anesthetic properties of dexmedetomidine wane after continuous administration of the drug.[17] Likewise, in humans, the sedative effects of clonidine decrease over time.[18] The induction of tolerance involves both *N*-methyl-D-aspartate–type glutamate receptors and nitric oxide synthetase,[19] whereas the expression of tolerance involves the L-type Ca^{++} channel.[20]

Preclinical Pharmacology

Analgesia

Experimental models have confirmed the analgesic action of α_2 agonists. Clonidine and dexmedetomidine increase the latency of tail withdrawal during the hot-plate or tail-flick

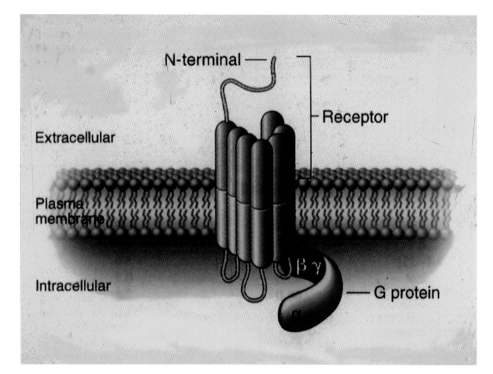

Figure 28–1. Secondary structure of the α_{2A} adrenergic receptor. The receptor weaves its way back and forth through the membrane seven times with a extracellular amino terminus and an intracellular carboxy terminus. The transmembrane domains are arranged in an anticlockwise manner when viewed from the extracellular surface.

test in a dose-related manner.[21] This increase can be prevented by administration of the specific antagonist of α_2 adrenoceptors, yohimbine. Because of its greater selectivity, dexmedetomidine may be more effective than clonidine.[22] After injection of irritating substances such as capsaicin or formalin, α_2 adrenergic agonists inhibit not only the immediate response (paw flinching) but also the secondary response, which is thought to be similar to the hyperalgesia and allodynia of neuropathic pain.[23] Moreover, clonidine impairs the perception of visceral pain[24] and increases the threshold of vocalization during inflation of colonic balloons in rats.[25] Numerous studies show that α_2 adrenergic agonists reduce or prevent allodynia after nerve lesioning models of neuropathic pain.[26] Although the precise site of action is not known, neuraxially administered clonidine may induce release of nitric oxide, thereby providing a possible explanation for the analgesic effect of clonidine.[27] Some authors believe a peripheral site is possible for the analgesic mechanism.[26]

At the level of the spinal cord, α_2 adrenergic agonists produce analgesia through stimulation of specific receptors in the dorsal horn. Exposure to chronic pain increases the number of these receptors in areas of the spinal cord dorsal horn associated with nociception.[30] The endogenous neurotransmitter norepinephrine is released through activation of descending inhibitory pathways originating from the periaqueductal gray, the locus ceruleus (LC), and the dorsal raphe nucleus.[31,32] Norepinephrine depresses the activity of wide-dynamic-range neurons in the superficial dorsal horn, evoked by stimulation of Aδ and C peripheral nociceptive fibers,[33] an effect that is prevented or reversed by yohimbine.

In animal behavioral studies, α_2 adrenergic agonists interact pharmacodynamically with both opioid and cholinergic agonists (or cholinesterase inhibitors such as neostigmine).[28]

After spinal administration, isobolographic analysis reveals that the interaction is synergistic, whereas after oral or parenteral administration, the interaction may be only additive.[29]

Neuraxially administered clonidine and related substances mimic the effect of norepinephrine on widedynamic-range neurons[34] in a dose-related fashion. Subthreshold doses of clonidine can inhibit wide-dynamic-range activity in the presence of nonantinociceptive doses of opioid or cholinergic agonists.[35] Clonidine stimulates intermediate, spontaneously active neurons located in the deeper layers of the dorsal horn of the spinal cord[34]; these neurons are believed to release acetylcholine, enkephalins, or both, and in this way inhibit the activity of wide-dynamic-range neurons. In fact, acute pain is associated with an increase in norepinephrine and acetylcholine levels in the cerebrospinal fluid (CSF).[36] Moreover, spinal clonidine increases the CSF concentrations of acetylcholine and nitric oxide.[28] α_2 Adrenergic agonists are also reported to act presynaptically to inhibit the release of calcitonin generelated peptide and substance P from primary afferent neurons.[37]

Which antinociceptive mechanisms, if any, are involved supraspinally remains controversial. For example, earlier studies reported that supraspinal administration of α_2 adrenergic agonists in dogs did not produce antinociception,[21] whereas localized administration of clonidine into the periaqueductal gray region (a potent site for the production of opioid receptor–mediated analgesia) did produce antinociception.[38] Furthermore, administration of α_2 agonists into other areas of the brain stem also produces antinociception.[39] Guo and colleagues[39] suggest that the LC tonically inhibits the activity of A5 and A7 neurons (two nuclei within the brainstem) and that discrete application of α_2 adrenergic agonists inhibits firing of the LC. This releases the tonic

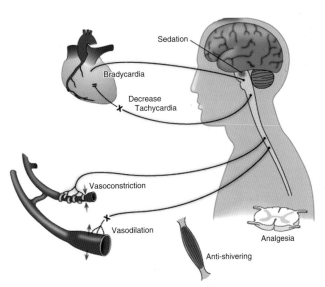

Figure 28–2. Functions mediated by α_2 adrenoceptors. The site for the sedative action is in the locus ceruleus of the brain stem, whereas the principal site for the analgesic action is probably in the spinal cord, although there are data supporting both a peripheral and a supraspinal site of action. In the heart, α_2 agonists decrease tachycardia (through block of the cardioaccelerator nerve) and produce bradycardia (through a vagomimetic action). In the peripheral vasculature, there are both a vasodilatory action (through sympatholysis) and vasoconstriction (by a direct action on the α_2 adrenoceptors on the smooth muscle cells).

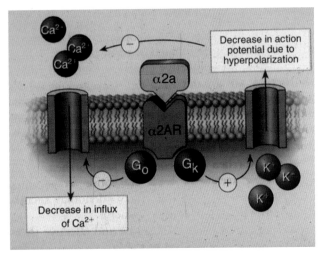

Figure 28–3. Molecular mechanism for hypnotic effect in the locus ceruleus. When a selective α_2 adrenoceptor agonist binds to an α_{2A} adrenoceptor in the locus ceruleus (LC), transmembrane signaling is activated through an inwardly rectifying potassium channel allowing for a K^+ efflux and by inhibition of voltage-gated Ca^{2+} channels. The resulting hyperpolarization decreases the firing rate in LC projections.

inhibition of A5 and A7, resulting in activation of a descending noradrenergic pathway.[39]

Clonidine can also produce its analgesic action through nonspinal mechanisms. Intra-articularly administered clonidine has a local analgesic effect that may be mediated by release of enkephalins at nerve endings[40]; such a mechanism is not related to plasma absorption of the drug or to stimulation of receptors in the spinal cord.[41]

Sedation

Sedation results from inactivation of the LC,[42] a relay station in the brain stem that has long been implicated in the sleep/wake cycle in rodents. Within the LC, it is the α_{2A} adrenoceptor subtype that transduces the response[6] that is coupled, by means of pertussis toxin-sensitive G proteins,[43] to effector mechanisms involved in hyperpolarization of the LC neurons (see Fig. 28–3).[44]

Recently, Nelson and colleagues[45] demonstrated that the mechanism for the sedative state produced by α_2 agonists converges on the pathway transducing natural sleep in rats. Dexmedetomidine induced a pattern of c-Fos (an immediate early gene product) expression that was qualitatively similar to that occurring during normal sleep—i.e., a decrease in the LC, an increase in the ventrolateral preoptic nucleus, and a decrease in the tuberomamillary nucleus.[45] These investigators confirmed that this endogenous sleep pathway is causally involved in dexmedetomidine-induced hypnosis by demonstrating that the hypnotic response was attenuated in rats with ventrolateral preoptic lesions (Fig. 28–4).[45]

The sedative effect of α_2 adrenergic agonists is antagonized by α_1 adrenergic agonists,[46] explaining why agents that have a relatively low α_2/α_1, such as clonidine, do not produce complete anesthesia.

The effect of α_2 adrenergic agonists on the LC has been suggested as an explanation for the anesthetic-sparing effect of α_2 adrenergic agonists and as a site for the prevention or treatment of drug withdrawal syndrome after administration of opiates or cocaine.[47]

Hemodynamic Effects

The most notable hemodynamic effects of α_2 adrenergic agents are hypotension and bradycardia,[48] which may be mediated by central and peripheral mechanisms. Because α_2 adrenergic agents have no direct effect on the contractile properties of the isolated myocardium,[49] the hemodynamic properties of these agents are produced by mechanisms other than cardiac contractility.

α_2 Adrenergic agonists depress both spontaneous and evoked sympathetic activity[50] through a decrease in the firing rate of the adrenergic cardiovascular neurons located in the vasomotor center of the brain stem.[51] Activation of α_2 adrenergic receptors in neurons of the nucleus tractus solitarius enhances the inhibitory action of this nucleus on the sympathetic neurons of the medulla.[51]

When considering the effects of α_2 adrenergic agonists on the baroreflex, it is necessary to distinguish the tonic elements from the phasic elements of the reflex. Administration of clonidine produces a shift in the set point of the baroreflex. Therefore, for a given level of arterial pressure, heart rate is lower because of a decrease in tonic

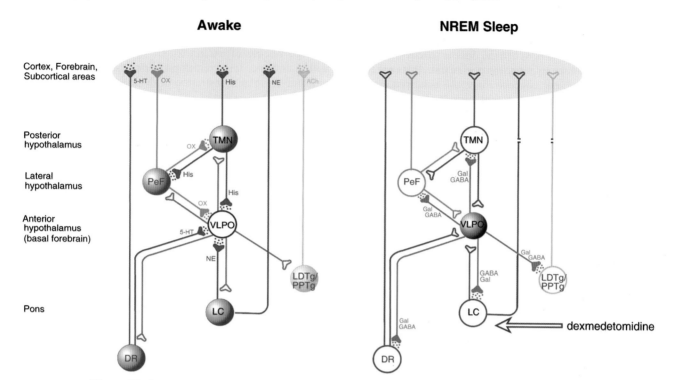

Figure 28–4. Neural substrates for sedative effect. During the hypnotic response induced by α_2 adrenoceptor agonist, a qualitatively similar pattern of neural activation is seen in rats as that observed during normal sleep; there is a decrease in the locus ceruleus (LC) and tuberomamillary nucleus (TMN) and an increase in the ventrolateral preoptic nucleus (VLPO). These changes are attenuated by a selective α_2 adrenenoceptor antagonist and are not seen in mice lacking functional α_{2A} adrenoceptors (which do not show a hypnotic response to α_2 adrenoceptor agonists). There is a hierarchical sequence of changes in which inhibition of the LC disinhibits the VLPO to release g-aminobutyric acid (GABA) and galanin at the projections that terminate at the TMN. These inhibitory neurotransmitters inhibit firing of the TMN projections to the cortical and subcortical regions. ACh, acetylcholine 5-HT, serotonin; His, histamine; LDTg, laterodorsal tegmental nucleus; NE, norepinephrine; NREM, non–rapid eye movement; OX, orexin PPTg, pedunculopontine tegmental nucleus.

activity.[52] Conversely, changes in arterial pressure from the set point cause a phasic response, the amplitude of which may be even greater in the presence of α_2 adrenergic agonists.[53]

Many of the studies examining the hemodynamic effects of α_2 adrenergic agonists have used agents that have an imidazoline structure. Therefore it is possible that some of the hemodynamic properties that are observed may be produced by the imidazoline I_1 receptors in the rostral ventrolateral medulla.[54] This may in part explain why hypotension produced by α_2 adrenergic agonists with an imidazoline structure cannot be completely reversed by yohimbine, the nonimidazoline α_2 adrenergic antagonist. In contrast, idazoxan, which preferentially blocks imidazoline-preferring sites in the brainstem, blocks the hypotensive action completely. A cooperative relationship between α_2 adrenergic and imidazoline receptors in the brainstem should also be considered as a possible mechanism for the hypotension and bradycardia that follow use of α_2 agonists having an imidazole ring in their structure.[55]

In ewes, Eisenach and Tong[56] showed that although intrathecal clonidine interferes with the initial regulatory mechanisms that maintain arterial pressure during hemorrhage, the level of arterial pressure at the end of blood withdrawal was unaffected. Furthermore, arterial blood gas measurements were unaffected by clonidine. α_2 Adrenergic agonists inhibit presynaptic sympathetic neuronal activity in the lateral horn of the thoracic spinal cord, an effect that is reversed by local administration of the cholinesterase inhibitor neostigmine.[56]

Ganglionic transmission is also depressed by several mechanisms, including through a presynaptic auto feedback mechanism that reduces the release of acetylcholine.[57] Consequently, intrathecal administration of α_2 adrenergic agonists produces a more marked hypotension than epidural or parenteral administration of the same drug at the same dose.[58]

Hypotension induced by α_2 adrenergic agonists can be reversed by standard vasoactive agents. There appears to be an enhanced pressor response to ephedrine,[59] phenylephrine, and dobutamine, but not to norepinephrine.[60] The response to dopamine (which partly depends on the release of norepinephrine) and to atropine are somewhat attenuated.[60]

Besides central effects, α_2 adrenergic agents produce peripheral vasoconstriction through stimulation of α_2 adrenergic receptors in the peripheral vasculature.[61] After rapid intravenous bolus administration of clonidine, the vasoconstrictive effect of the drug is believed to be responsible for a transient hypertension. When the dose is slowly increased in a stepwise manner, hypotension occurs initially but is then reversed when greater concentrations are achieved, as the peripheral vasoconstrictive action overcomes the sympatholytic effect.[62] At therapeutic doses of α_2 adrenergic agonists given by oral, intravenous, or epidural routes of administration, sympatholysis predominates.[63]

The effects of α_2 adrenergic agonists on ischemic myocardium and coronary artery circulation are complex. α_2 Adrenergic agonists have a direct vasoconstrictive effect on the coronary arteries that is partly opposed by nitric oxide, which is indirectly released by α_2 adrenergic agonists.[64] The overall impact on myocardial oxygen balance is an aggregate of the effects produced by a reduction in myocardial oxygen demand and by a decrease in coronary perfusion pressure (as a consequence of hypotension). On balance, myocardial energetics is usually improved; however, in some patients, hypotension may produce myocardial ischemia.[65] In experimental studies, α_2 adrenergic agonists have produced anti-ischemic effects,[66,67] also partly related to the attenuation of sympathetically mediated coronary vasoconstriction.[68] Consequently, in patients with myocardial ischemia, α_2 adrenergic agonists have an antianginal effect[69] and improve exercise tolerance.[70]

Abrupt discontinuation of α_2 adrenergic agonists after chronic administration may induce a drug withdrawal syndrome, including rebound hypertension possibly leading to myocardial ischemia. Such a syndrome has been noted even after a relatively brief administration of drugs such as clonidine.[71]

Cerebral Circulation

Activation of α_2 adrenergic receptors in the cerebral vessels produces vasoconstriction[72] and reduces cerebral blood flow without influencing the metabolic rate for oxygen, indicating an uncoupling of flow and metabolic activity.[73] Reactivity of cerebral blood flow to carbon dioxide is either preserved or modestly attenuated by dexmedetomidine[74] and clonidine.[75] Despite this, both agents improve neurologic outcome and histopathologic lesions after cerebral ischemia in animals when the agents are administered either before or even after the start of cerebral injury.[76] Although the precise mechanism for this neuroprotective effect is unknown, some

investigators note a correlation with circulating levels of norepinephrine.[77] Others suggest a decrease in ischemia-induced release of excitotoxins.[78] In animals anesthetized with halothane, intracranial pressure does not change significantly with administration of dexmedetomidine.[79]

Respiratory Effects

α_2 Adrenergic agonists are known to induce hypoxemia in ungulates such as sheep.[80,81] This effect is reversed by α_2 adrenergic antagonists, such as idazoxan, and is independent of changes in respiratory pattern. Hypoxemia is believed to result from activation of platelet aggregation, which is responsible for microemboli,[82] and from respiratory shunting. α_2 Agonist–induced hypoxemia is an effect that is specific for ungulates and has never been documented in humans.

Gastrointestinal Effects

α_2 Adrenergic agents reduce gastrointestinal motility because of a central and peripheral action.[83] Gastric emptying is not delayed by administration of α_2 adrenergic agents, but transit time is prolonged.[84] Concurrent administration of opioids and α_2 adrenergic agonists produces a supra-additive inhibition of gastrointestinal transit.[84] α_2 Adrenergic agents have no deleterious effect on splanchnic perfusion and do not induce mucosal ischemia in laboratory animals during surgery.[85] Moreover, in laboratory animals, clonidine also prevents stress-induced gastric ulcer.[86]

Endocrine Effects

α_2 Adrenergic agonists blunt the neuroendocrine stress response to surgery, with regard to cortisol, β-endorphins, arginine vasopressin,[87,88] epinephrine, and norepinephrine. Growth hormone is released by α_2 adrenergic agonists. These effects may alter postoperative metabolism; for example, protein catabolism is attenuated in patients administered clonidine.[89] Like most imidazoline compounds (e.g., etomidate), dexmedetomidine (at concentrations that are 100 to 1,000 times greater than those used clinically) blocks steroidogenesis in vitro.[90]

CLINICAL PHARMACOLOGY

Pharmacokinetics

α_2 Adrenergic agonists can be divided into three main chemical classes: phenylethylates (e.g., methyldopa, guanabenz), imidazolines (e.g., clonidine, dexmedetomidine, mivazerol, azepexole), and oxaloazepines.

Clonidine, the prototypical α_2 adrenergic agonist, has a 200-fold greater selectivity for α_2 adrenoceptors than for α_1

adrenoceptors. Clonidine is moderately lipid-soluble and is absorbed almost completely after oral administration; the peak effect occurs at 60 to 90 minutes, and the peak plasma concentration occurs at 1 to 3 hours.[91] After epidural administration, the peak plasma concentration occurs earlier from 15 to 20 minutes.[92] Clonidine has a large volume of distribution (approximately 2 L/kg) and a relatively long terminal elimination half-life of 12 to 24 hours.[91] In healthy volunteers, the analgesic and hemodynamic effects of clonidine were out of phase with the plasma concentrations[62] because of a lag in penetration of the drug into the effect site. Rather, the analgesic effect of clonidine is more closely related to its concentration in the CSF, the minimal CSF concentration producing analgesia being 76 ng/mL.[62] In patients, the morphine-sparing effect of clonidine, estimated from patient-controlled administration, is also closely related to its concentration in the CSF.[93] Placental transfer of clonidine has been demonstrated after oral and epidural administration.[94] Concentrations in breast milk are approximately twice those in maternal plasma, whereas concentrations in the plasma of neonates are about half those in their mothers.[95]

Dexmedetomidine, the dextroisomer of medetomidine, is also an imidazoline compound. It has an eight times greater affinity for α_2 adrenoceptors than does clonidine. The pharmacokinetics of dexmedetomidine were derived using a variety of intravenous infusion regimens; the distribution half-life of the drug is approximately 6 minutes, and the terminal elimination half-life is 2 hours. Both of these half-lives are considerably shorter than those of clonidine. The steady-state volume of distribution of dexmedetomidine is 1.33 L/kg.[96] Dexmedetomidine is highly bound (±94%) to albumin and α_1 glycoprotein and undergoes extensive biotransformation in the liver; the resulting methyl and glucuronide conjugates are excreted by the kidneys. Dexmedetomidine has a weak inhibiting effect on cytochrome P450 enzyme systems in vitro.[97] An in vitro study concluded that dexmedetomidine may impair the metabolism of alfentanil,[98] which could result in greater plasma concentrations of alfentanil. Therefore, it is possible that part of the interaction between dexmedetomidine and anesthetic agents may be related to changes in pharmacokinetics.[99]

Pharmacodynamics

Analgesia

Eisenach and colleagues[62] confirmed that the spinal cord is a site for the analgesic action of clonidine. Lumbar epidural injection of the drug attenuated cold-induced pain in the foot but not the hand.[62] Furthermore, the analgesic effectiveness of clonidine appears to be better after spinal or epidural administration than after intravenous administration.[100,101]

Sedation

Sedation and changes on electroencephalogram may occur after epidural administration of clonidine, suggesting rostral spread of the drug.[102] In "equivalently sedated" states, produced by dexmedetomidine or midazolam, there are distinctive differences in the blood oxygen level-dependent functional magnetic resonance responses. Whereas there are few changes compared with placebo in the dexmedetomidine-sedated state, there are several brain regions that differ in the midazolam-sedated state from their placebo state (Fig. 28–5).[103] These data support the sugges-

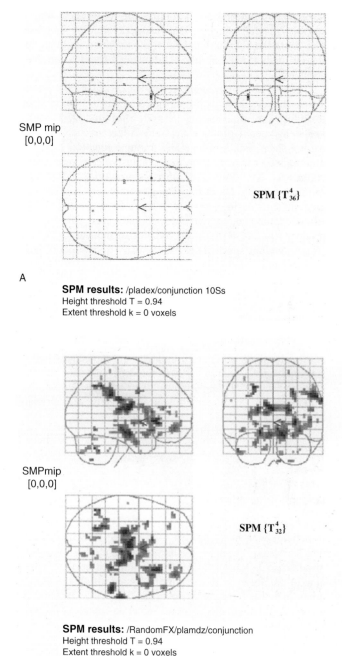

SPM results: /pladex/conjunction 10Ss
Height threshold T = 0.94
Extent threshold k = 0 voxels

SMPmip
[0,0,0]

SPM {T_{32}^4}

SPM results: /RandomFX/plamdz/conjunction
Height threshold T = 0.94
Extent threshold k = 0 voxels

Figure 28–5. Functional magnetic resonance imaging at equisedative states produced by dexmedetomidine and midazolam in healthy volunteers. Statistical Parametric Mapping (SPM) projections of areas of brain, shown in sagittal, coronal, and transverse views, illustrating statistical change in activity when dexmedetomidine (*A*) and midazolam (*B*) are compared with a placebo state ($P < 0.001$). The images represent a transparent "glass brain" and not a two-dimensional "slice."

tion by Nelson and colleagues[45,104] that α_2 agonists converge on the endogenous substrates for natural sleep to produce their sedative action. Subjects deeply sedated by α_2 agonists can immediately rouse themselves to almost full consciousness when required to participate in clinical testing.[105] Recent research suggests that dexmedetomidine increases activity in the pulvinar nucleus of the thalamus and that this region mediates the ability of arousing stimuli to produce attention.[103]

The potential implications of using sedative/hypnotic agents that act through similar mechanisms as natural sleep to induce loss of consciousness are profound. A hypnotic agent that could produce the same reparative changes as natural sleep (i.e., hormone and immune function changes) might speed recovery time in an intensive care setting and counteract the effects of sleep deprivation, a common problem for patients in the intensive care unit and for surgical patients during recovery. It has been suggested that α_2 adrenoceptor agonist sedatives activate sleep pathways to produce more restorative sleep than that induced by downstream modulation of the same pathway by γ-aminobutyric acid mimetic agents.[104]

Cardiovascular System

Although all α_2 adrenergic agonists produce hypotension and bradycardia, there may be some differences in the clinical importance of their effects. Even though comparative studies of the hemodynamic effects of the α_2 agonists are lacking, mivazerol appears to induce less change than other clinically available compounds (e.g., clonidine and dexmedetomidine).[106–108]

Cerebral Circulation

In patients with head injuries, clonidine and dexmedetomidine decrease plasma catecholamines and do not affect intracranial pressure.[109–111] However, administration of clonidine in the presence of intracranial hypertension can sometimes increase intracranial pressure transiently.[112] This, in theory, could aggravate cerebral ischemia because of a possible decrease in perfusion pressure.[112]

Shivering

α_2 Adrenergic agonists alter thermoregulatory control and decrease the threshold for vasoconstriction and shivering during hypothermia.[113] Conversely, during hyperthermia, the threshold for sweating increases only slightly.[113] Clonidine inhibits active shivering and the related increase in oxygen consumption.[114] In patients undergoing elective ear, nose, or pharyngeal surgery under general anesthesia (induction with propofol, vecuronium, and fentanyl; maintenance with isoflurane in 70% nitrous oxide), the high incidence of postoperative shivering (40%) could be completely eliminated by administration of clonidine (1.5 µg/kg) before emergence from anesthesia.[115] The antishivering effects probably result from central thermoregulatory inhibition rather than peripheral action on thermogenic muscular activity.

Respiratory Effects

Although α_2 adrenergic agonists have no significant effect on respiratory rate or tidal volume during resting ventilation, ventilatory drive is modestly attenuated in both healthy volunteers[116] and patients.[117,118] This reduction in ventilatory drive can produce an obstructive upper airway ventilatory pattern.[119] In American Society of Anesthesiologists (ASA) physical status I patients, the epidural administration of 300 µg clonidine modestly decreases the slope of the ventilatory response to carbon dioxide.[118] The ventilatory response to hypoxia is also mildly depressed.[120] Nevertheless, compared with opiates, clonidine has little depressive effect on ventilation.[121] Moreover, it does not potentiate the respiratory depressant effects of opiates.[122] However, the simultaneous intravenous administration of clonidine and fentanyl may lead to accumulation of fentanyl, which, if the dose of fentanyl is not significantly reduced, may increase the risk for respiratory depression.[123]

Practical Aspects of Drug Administration

Most of the clinical applications of α_2 adrenergic agonists in anesthesia and intensive care involve clonidine, which has been used in Europe in this setting for more than 15 years. More recently, dexmedetomidine has been introduced for sedation in the postoperative intensive care setting. Also, multiple clinical studies have examined the clinical efficacy of dexmedetomidine in other perioperative settings—e.g., as a premedication, in the prevention of perioperative myocardial ischemia, and for postoperative analgesia.

Premedication

α_2 Adrenergic agonists may be used as premedication to provide sedation and relieve anxiety. These effects extend into the intraoperative period and make it possible to significantly reduce the dose of concomitantly administered anesthetics. Clonidine and dexmedetomidine decrease anxiety[124] and can induce amnesia.[125] However, the dose of clonidine must be adapted to the age of the patient, so that elderly patients do not become deeply sedated and hypotensive on induction of anesthesia.[126] Young ASA I or II patients may receive a dose of 2 to 4 µg/kg, whereas 1 to 2 µg/kg is more appropriate for elderly patients.[126] In children, clonidine premedication is well accepted and improves tolerance of the facemask for induction of anesthesia.[127]

Although sedation with α_2 agonists is associated with a statistically significant depression in ventilatory drive, this effect is no greater than the respiratory depression or upper airway obstruction associated with natural sleep. Premedication with α_2 agonists has two important effects on the gastrointestinal system: xerostomia and decreased gastrointestinal transit. Although dry mouth occasionally can be distressing for the patient, it is often a desirable circumstance if the airway is to be instrumented. Also, the decrease in gastrointestinal transit does not appear to significantly delay gastric emptying of liquids.[128]

Premedication with α_2 adrenergic agonists allows a significant reduction in anesthetic requirement for induction of anesthesia, regardless of the agent used. α_2 Adrenergic agonists reduce the minimum alveolar concentrations (MACs) of coadministered volatile anesthetic agents necessary to produce anesthesia (their MAC values),[129] as well as the dose of intravenous hypnotic needed for induction of anesthesia and orotracheal intubation,[130] whether hemodynamic or nonhemodynamic clinical signs are used as an endpoint.[131] The use of α_2 adrenergic agonists as premedication blunts sympathetic activation and the resulting hypertension and tachycardia consequent to orotracheal intubation.[130] These agonists can also blunt the sympathetic activation related to administration of anesthetic agents such as ketamine or desflurane.[132] In clinical studies in which the double-blind study design resulted in patients receiving a "full" dose of anesthetic agents when premedicated with clonidine or dexmedetomidine, elderly patients became particularly susceptible to hypotension and bradycardia.[133] In clinical practice, these side effects can be mitigated by appropriately decreasing the dose of coadministered hypnotic anesthetic agent. Nevertheless, bradycardia may still occur in relatively young, unstimulated ASA I or II patients administered dexmedetomidine.[134]

Intraoperative administration of α_2 adrenergic agonists decreases requirements for analgesic agents after surgery and prevents tachycardia and hypertension on emergence from anesthesia.[135] One potential adverse effect of the use of α_2 adrenergic agonists is prolongation of anesthesia and delayed emergence from anesthesia; however, recovery from anesthesia is only delayed when rigidly adhering to anesthetic protocols, which precludes reduction of the amount of hypnotic agent given to the patients.[136]

Although the occurrence of hypotension and bradycardia may prevent the more cautious practitioner from using α_2 agonists in all patients, there are some clinical conditions in which their use outweighs concerns about decreases in blood pressure and heart rate.

- In *drug addicts and alcoholics*, sympathetic hyperactivity is well controlled by α_2 adrenergic agonists.[68] When administered as premedication and continued after surgery, α_2 adrenergic agonists may reduce the risk for drug withdrawal syndrome.
- Because patients who have *chronic cancer* or *noncancer pain* are often given large doses of opioids, their opioid requirements are considerably increased in the perioperative period. These requirements may be significantly reduced by the use of α_2 adrenergic agonists as premedication.
- *Patients with hypertension* are particularly vulnerable to marked swings in blood pressure perioperatively. Use of α_2 adrenergic agonists as premedication provides a useful way of reducing this hyper-reactivity.[137] As with other antihypertensive medications, α_2 adrenergic agonists must not be discontinued before surgery because of the risk for a hypertensive crisis and myocardial ischemia and infarction. Several studies have demonstrated that cloni-

dine premedication reduces the number of hypertensive episodes,[138] albeit with more frequent hypotensive or bradycardic episodes.[65,139] In summary, if one were to customize an "ideal" range of arterial blood pressures for surgery, patients administered α_2 adrenergic agonists would be found to spend more time within that ideal range than patients given a placebo.

- *Hypotension* is required to perform certain types of surgery (e.g., ear or orthopedic surgery). Premedication with clonidine is an easy way to induce mild to moderate hypotension without using excessive amounts of anesthetic agents.[140]
- During *ophthalmic surgery*, premedication with clonidine or dexmedetomidine has the advantage of decreasing intraocular pressure and is the preferred premedicant in patients with increased intraocular pressure.[126]
- In patients anesthetized with *ketamine*, premedication with an α_2 adrenergic agonist may prevent postanesthetic delirium.[141]

Anesthetic-Sparing Effects

Because of their sedative properties, α_2 adrenergic agents have a significant anesthetic-sparing effect. The effect results from the action of the agents at α_2 adrenergic receptors and is unrelated to their imidazoline structure.[142] The anesthetic-sparing effect is best documented during induction of anesthesia,[143] but may also occur during maintenance of anesthesia.[138]

Premedication with a 3-μg/kg dose of clonidine reduces the propofol and thiopental requirements for induction of anesthesia by 30% to 35%.[144] The same dose of clonidine decreases the minimum end-tidal concentration of isoflurane required for induction of burst suppression on electroencephalogram from 1.4% to 0.9%.[145] Within a dose range of 0.5 to 5 μg/kg, the anesthetic-sparing effect of clonidine is dose-dependent.[143,144] In children administered 2 or 4 μg/kg clonidine, the MAC of sevoflurane required for endotracheal intubation decreased from 2.9% to 2.5% and 1.9% (35% decrease), respectively; the MAC of sevoflurane required for skin incision decreased from 2.3% to 1.8% and 1.3%, respectively.[146]

The MAC of isoflurane is decreased by dexmedetomidine in a dose-dependent fashion.[129] Unlike clonidine, for which the effect "plateaus" between 25% and 40% (depending on the anesthetic agent), dexmedetomidine may reduce anesthetic requirements by up to 90%.[133] Moreover, dexmedetomidine acts synergistically with opioids (fentanyl) to further reduce the MAC of volatile agents.[147]

The anesthetic-sparing effect is also documented on awakening from anesthesia. The MAC-awake of isoflurane (the endtidal concentration of isoflurane corresponding to opening of the eyes on verbal command) is reduced from 0.28% to 0.22% by clonidine administered before surgery.[148]

Even though α_2 adrenergic agonists produce flaccidity and prevent opioid-induced muscle rigidity, these compounds have no clinically significant effect on the neuromuscular blocking action of muscle relaxants.[149,150]

Sedation

Clonidine and dexmedetomidine both produce dose-dependent sedation.[126] Patients appear to be calm and relaxed and to breathe spontaneously while being easily roused.[105,125] Dexmedetomidine (0.2 to 0.7 mg • kg^{-1} • h^{-1}) has been studied as a sedative agent after major surgical procedures. It was found to effectively reduce the amount of propofol or midazolam necessary to sedate intensive care patients. Dexmedetomidine sedation offers the advantage of being maintained after extubation in spontaneously breathing patients without producing respiratory depression.[151] Qualitatively, dexmedetomidine induces a sedative response that exhibits properties similar to natural sleep, unlike other sedative/hypnotic agents such as midazolam and propofol. Both clonidine and dexmedetomidine can be given to patients in the intensive care unit to prevent drug withdrawal syndrome after long-term sedation with benzodiazepines and opioids or to facilitate invasive endoscopic and radiologic procedures.

Hemodynamic Stability

α_2 Adrenergic agonists have been advocated to prevent hemodynamic instability ("Alpine anesthesia") during surgery[152] based on that increases in plasma catecholamines in response to nociceptive and surgical stimulations are blunted.[130] If one considers plasma catecholamine levels to be reflective of sympathetic activity, α_2 adrenergic agonists attenuate sympathetic activity during surgery and on emergence from anesthesia.[153]

Administration of α_2 adrenergic agonists before anesthesia reduces myocardial energy requirements and improves myocardial oxygen balance.[154] Functionally, this translates to improved myocardial energetics. For example, clonidine has been shown to improve recovery from myocardial stunning.[155] During anesthesia, cardiac output is more increased after clonidine or dexmedetomidine administration than after placebo; after pretreatment with dexmedetomidine, cardiac output is better maintained during isoflurane anesthesia than during desflurane anesthesia.[156] Conversely, dexmedetomidine does not significantly affect the hemodynamic response to induction of anesthesia with propofol and etomidate[157] and does not potentiate the cardiovascular depressant effects of alfentanil.[158] In addition, α_2 adrenergic agonists prevent hypertension and tachycardia both during intubation of the trachea and during surgical stimulation.[159] Clonidine premedication has also been shown to protect against the development of cardiac arrhythmias (apart from bradycardia) and myocardial ischemia in at-risk patients undergoing microlaryngoscopy and rigid bronchoscopy.[160] Prevention of tachycardia and hypertension also has been documented during recovery from anesthesia.[107,137,161]

In patients with hypertension, clonidine preserves baroreflex function after surgery, thereby stabilizing the circulation and controlling hemodynamic changes.[137] Therefore, if α_2 agonists are used during cardiac or vascular surgery, the improved hemodynamic control may prevent myocardial ischemia[107,162,163] and reduce cardiac morbidity and mortality rates.[164] A further improvement in cardiovascular performance may be attributed to a decrease in the incidence of shivering and a reduction of oxygen consumption.[114,132]

Improvement of Local Anesthetic Blocks

Intrathecal Administration

The effect of intrathecal clonidine on the kinetics of coadministered drugs is controversial; no effect,[165] improved effect,[166] and poorer absorption[167] have all been reported. Compared with epinephrine, epidural clonidine probably causes less vasoconstriction and decreases plasma absorption to a lesser extent. Any decrease in cardiac output (and hence a decrease in hepatic blood flow) induced by clonidine could have the effect of decreasing the clearance of lidocaine and increasing plasma concentrations of the drug. Offsetting the possible lidocaine toxicity is that clonidine increases the plasma concentration at which bupivacaine causes its toxicity.[168] Parenthetically, a premedication dose of clonidine does not preclude the use of an epinephrine-containing solution to test for intravascular injection during epidural administration.[169]

The combined administration of clonidine with a local anesthetic improves the quality and duration of the block[170] but may cause more hypotension. Consequently, when used in combination with local anesthetics, the maximum dose of intrathecal clonidine should not exceed 1 µg/kg. In laboratory animals and humans, clonidine enhances the sensory and motor block.[171] The use of clonidine as an adjunct to intrathecal local anesthesia for orthopedic surgery appears to convey benefit compared with morphine, because use of clonidine obviates the need for a urinary catheter.[172] Also, when cesarean section is performed under spinal anesthesia, long-lasting postoperative analgesia is provided by the addition of clonidine.[173]

Epidural Administration

Epidural administration of clonidine (1–4 µg/kg) improves the quality of the block, prolongs postoperative analgesia,[174] and prevents shivering during labor.[175] Unlike intrathecal administration, the addition of clonidine to the epidural space is not associated with more hypotension.[176] Similar to effects when opiate narcotics are used with 2-chloroprocaine, clonidine appears to antagonize the analgesic block provided by that local anesthetic.[177]

Caudal Administration

When clonidine (0.75–3 µg/kg) is added to caudal local anesthetic solutions, the duration of anesthesia and analgesia increases twofold to threefold.[178] Furthermore, in pediatric patients, hemodynamic parameters play a diminished role, possibly because this age group is less dependent on sympathetic tone for control of blood pressure.[178]

Peripheral Nerve Blocks

Clonidine is commonly used as an adjuvant to local anesthetics in brachial plexus blocks because it significantly prolongs (up to 24 hours) the duration of the anesthesia and analgesia of these blocks in the postoperative period.[179] This effect appears to originate from the site of administration (possibly through a decrease in the plasma absorption of coadministered local anesthetics), as parenteral administration of the same dose of clonidine does not prolong the duration of the block.[180] The effect of clonidine is dose-related.[179] After brachial plexus block with mepivacaine, the minimum effective doses that significantly prolong analgesia and anesthesia are 0.1 and 0.5 μg/kg, respectively.[181] Also, at these relatively low doses, the risk for hemodynamic alterations is minimized. In the absence of local anesthetic, 150 μg clonidine does not produce postoperative analgesia when administered into the brachial plexus sheath.[182]

Clonidine is also used for several other peripheral blocks, including Bier block, in which a 1- to 2-μg/kg dose of clonidine significantly improves the quality of intravenous regional anesthesia with lidocaine, and especially tolerance to tourniquet-induced pain.[100,183] Clonidine has also been particularly beneficial in retrobulbar blocks with local anesthetic agents—not only is the block prolonged, but also intraocular pressure and ocular akinesia are decreased.[184] In addition, clonidine, which by itself produces local analgesia when administered intra-articularly, improves analgesia produced by intra-articular administration of bupivacaine after knee arthroscopy.[185]

Postoperative Analgesia

Clonidine and dexmedetomidine both have been studied as postoperative analgesics. Whereas dexmedetomidine can only be given intravenously for this purpose, clonidine can be administered intravenously, transdermally, orally, epidurally, spinally, intra-articularly, and perineurally.

Epidural analgesia has long been the preferred technique after surgery because of the previous demonstration of spinal α$_2$ adrenoceptors and because of the opportunity for continuous administration through a catheter. When using clonidine as the sole agent after surgery, bolus administration of the drug by the epidural route provides analgesia for some [186,187] but not all surgeries.[188] Compared with morphine, clonidine has a lower efficacy and shorter duration.[189] Pain relief is improved when clonidine is administered by continuous infusion. However, with clonidine alone, doses as high as 100 to 150 μg/hr are required for complete pain relief.[191] At these doses, hypotension, bradycardia, and sedation do occur but are well tolerated.[190] Nevertheless, one can anticipate that some postoperative patients may be adversely affected, and the occurrence of these side effects is the reason epidural clonidine has not been universally adopted.[191]

Conversely, urinary retention, a frequent problem with epidural opioids, occurs much less frequently with epidural clonidine. Therefore, the use of epidural clonidine for postoperative analgesia is recommended, especially in combination with other analgesic drugs (e.g., opioids) in which

analgesia is enhanced[192]; and, as a consequence of the lowered required, fewer side effects are experienced. Although the interaction between opioids and α$_2$ agonists is known to be synergistic in animals, this characteristic currently has not been demonstrated in humans.[29]

Spinal clonidine can be used in lieu of spinal opioids for postoperative analgesia.[173] The duration of analgesia after intrathecal clonidine is dose-dependent,[173] but pain relief may not be as effective as that produced by intrathecal morphine. However, significantly fewer adverse effects occur with clonidine (although sedation may occur[193]) than with morphine.[172] Coadministration of an opioid and clonidine prolongs the analgesic effect when doses up to 75 μg of clonidine are used.[194] Recently, the combination of spinal neostigmine and clonidine was shown to prolong the duration of postoperative analgesia.[195]

Analgesia and opioid-sparing effects can also be demonstrated when clonidine is administered by non-neuraxial routes.[138] Again, lower blood pressures and heart rates are notable after parenteral administration of α$_2$ agonists for postoperative analgesia.[196]

Intra-articular analgesia is a technique that has gained in popularity in recent years, especially for arthroscopic procedures. Intra-articular clonidine produces analgesia by means of a local, but currently unknown, mechanism of action.[185] Because plasma absorption is slow, minimal systemic effects occur after intra-articular administration. Intra-articular clonidine produces a degree of analgesia similar to that of intra-articular morphine, and the combination of the two moderately increases the duration of analgesia and moderately decreases the pain score.[185]

Analgesia for Labor

In the parturient, epidural doses of clonidine from 30 to 150 μg prolong the analgesic effect of epidural bupivacaine. In addition, 150 μg clonidine prolongs bupivacaine analgesia significantly more than 100 μg fentanyl; moreover, the combination of 75 μg clonidine and 50 μg fentanyl more than doubles the duration of analgesia produced by bupivacaine alone.[197] Although a combination of 120 μg epidural clonidine and 50 μg epidural fentanyl produces less effective analgesia than 25 mg epidural bupivacaine, the combination induces less motor impairment.[198] Although epidural clonidine has the advantage of inhibiting shivering in parturients, its disadvantages include greater incidences of sedation, hypotension, and bradycardia.[175] Epidural clonidine also decreases the heart rate of the fetus in animals[81] and humans,[199] although no deleterious effect has been reported in newborns. Because clonidine crosses the placenta,[200,201] the dose of epidural clonidine should be limited to 1 μg/kg in parturients.

Intrathecal clonidine (50 to 200 μg) produces satisfactory analgesia during the first stage of labor.[202] Although intervention with ephedrine is more often required at the highest dose of clonidine, no adverse effect has been documented in neonates. Intrathecal clonidine also produces long-lasting analgesia after cesarean section and is devoid of the side effects associated with intrathecal morphine, including urinary retention, pruritus, and nausea.[172]

Chronic Pain

Neuropathic Pain

Epidural clonidine has been used successfully for deafferentation pain after spinal cord injury.[203] Spasticity, associated with incomplete paraplegia following spinal cord lesion, impairs the ability to walk and produces pain that can be treated with intrathecal clonidine.[204] Epidural clonidine is also useful for the management of pain in some patients with chronic arachnoiditis.[205] Chronic pain states of different origins have been successfully treated with a combination of epidural lidocaine and clonidine,[206] but the side effects, particularly at initiation of treatment, can prove troublesome.[207] Clonidine may also be applied transdermally and produces an analgesic effect in some patients with painful neuropathy, especially in those who describe sharp and shooting pains.[208]

Sympathetically Maintained Pain

In patients with intractable sympathetically maintained pain (pain dependent on efferent sympathetic activity), a continuous epidural infusion of clonidine has been reported to relieve pain, even though the associated trophic changes are unaffected.[209] Some investigators have reported a benefit from intrathecal clonidine that lasts as long as 18 months.[210] The application of a transdermal clonidine patch produces a local effect in patients with sympathetically maintained pain, alleviating hyperalgesia and allodynia. This suggests a peripheral analgesic effect of the drug that could be mediated by a depression in peripheral release of norepinephrine.[211] Repeated blocks with intravenous clonidine may be an alternative to guanethidine, reserpine, bretylium, or steroids in some patients with sympathetically maintained pain.[212]

Cancer Pain

In patients with intractable cancer pain, epidural clonidine (100–900 μg) produces a dose-dependent analgesia lasting up to 8 hours.[213] Treatment with a continuous epidural infusion of clonidine at the rate of 30 μg/hr alleviates cancer pain over a 2-week period, during which time the initial sedative and xerostomic effects have dissipated.[214] Patients most likely to benefit are those who have not been treated previously with opioids in which the addition of clonidine restores analgesic responsiveness for opiate analgesia. Clonidine is thus a "second-line" drug in the treatment of cancer pain, for which it can be used to decrease the amount of opioids administered or as an alternative when tolerance to opioids is developing.[215]

Prevention of Drug Withdrawal Syndrome

α_2 Adrenergic agonists prevent the occurrence of drug withdrawal syndrome in patients with addiction, whatever the cause of addiction. After interruption of morphine treatment in animals, α_2 adrenergic agonists inhibit neural firing in the LC[216,217] and prevent hyperalgesia and symptoms related to opiate withdrawal.[218,219] In the intensive care unit, continuous intravenous administration of clonidine is used to prevent or treat alcohol withdrawal symptoms in patients at risk for addiction.[220]

Prevention and Treatment of Shivering

Postoperative shivering is easily treated by intravenous administration of boluses of clonidine; for this purpose, clonidine is as effective or more effective than other agents.[114] For most patients, a dose of 0.5 to 1 μg/kg eliminates shivering within a few minutes. Clonidine can also prevent shivering and the related increase in oxygen consumption.[221]

Conclusions

α_2 Adrenergic agonists provide a useful and efficient solution to a number of problems encountered in the perioperative setting. As such, they deserve to be more widely used and are a useful addition to the anesthesiologist's armamentarium.

References

1. Bylund DB, Eikenberg DC, Hieble JP, et al: International union of pharmacology nomenclature of adrenoceptors. Pharmacol Rev 46:121, 1994.
2. Kobilka BK, Matsui H, Kobilka TS, et al: Cloning, sequencing, and expression of the gene coding for the human platelet alpha 2-adrenergic receptor. Science 30:650, 1987.
3. Mizobe T, Maze M, Lam V, et al: Arrangement of transmembrane domains in adrenergic receptors. Similarity to bacteriorhodopsin. J Biol Chem 271:2387, 1996.
4. Palczewski K, Kumasaka T, Hori T, et al: Crystal structure of rhodopsin: A G protein-coupled receptor. Science 289:739, 2000.
5. Takada K, Clark DJ, Davies MF, et al: Meperidine exerts agonist activity at the alpha 2b-adrenoceptor subtype. Anesthesiology 96:1420, 2002.
6. Lakhlani PP, MacMillan LB, Guo TZ, et al: Substitution of a mutant alpha2a-adrenergic receptor via "hit and run" gene targeting reveals the role of this subtype in sedative, analgesic, and anesthetic-sparing responses in vivo. Proc Natl Acad Sci USA 94:9950, 1997.
7. Link RE, Desai K, Hein L, et al: Cardiovascular regulation in mice lacking alpha 2-adrenergic receptor subtypes B and C. Science 273:803, 1996.
8. Sawamura S, Kingery WS, Davies MF, et al: Antinoceptive action of nitrous oxide is mediated by stimulation of noradrenergic neurons in the brainstem and activation of (alpha) 2B adrenoceptors. J Neurosci 20:9242, 2000.
9. Lahdesmaki J, Sallinen J, MacDonald E, et al: Behavioral and neurochemical characterization of alpha(2A)-adrenergic receptor knockout mice. Neuroscience 113:289, 2002.
10. Andrade R, Aghajanian GK: Opiate- and a_2-adrenoceptor-induced hyperpolarization of locus ceruleus neurons in brain slices: Reversal

by cyclic adenosine 3′:5′-monophosphate analogues. J Neurosci 5:2359, 1985.

11. Adamson P, Xiang JZ, Mantzourides T, et al: Presynaptic alpha 2-adrenoceptor and kappa-opiate receptor occupancy promotes closure of neuronal (N-type) calcium channels. Eur J Pharmacol 174:63, 1989.

12. Ishibashi H, Akaike N: Norepinephrine modulates high voltage-activated calcium channels in freshly dissociated rat nucleus tractus solitarii neurons. Neuroscience 68:1139, 1995.

13. North RA, Williams JT, Surprenant A, et al: M and d opioid receptors belong to a family of receptors that are coupled to potassium channels. Proc Natl Acad Sci USA 84:5487, 1987.

14. Ryan JS, Tao QP, Kelly ME: Adrenergic regulation of calcium-activated potassium current in cultured rabbit pigmented ciliary epithelial cells. J Physiol 511(Pt 1):145, 1998.

15. Isom LL, Cragoe EJ Jr, Limbird LE: Alpha 2-adrenergic receptors accelerate Na+/H+ exchange in neuroblastoma X glioma cells. J Biol Chem 262:6750, 1987.

16. Soini SL, Duzic E, Lanier SM, et al: Dual modulation of calcium channel current via recombinant alpha2-adrenoceptors in pheochromocytoma (PC-12) cells. Pflugers Arch 435:280, 1998.

17. Reid K, Hayashi Y, Guo T-Z, et al: Chronic administration of an alpha 2 adrenergic agonist desensitizes rats to the anesthetic effects of dexmedetomidine. Pharmacol Biochem Behav 47:171, 1994.

18. Ferder L, Inserra F, Medina F: Safety aspects of long-term antihypertensive therapy (10 years) with clonidine. J Cardiovasc Pharmacol 10(Suppl 12):S104, 1987.

19. Davies MF, Reid K, Guo TZ, et al: Sedative but not analgesic alpha2 agonist tolerance is blocked by NMDA receptor and nitric oxide synthase inhibitors. Anesthesiology 95:184, 2001.

20. Reid K, Guo T-Z, Davies MF, et al: Nifedipine, a L-type calcium channel blocker, restores the hypnotic response in rats made tolerant to the alpha-2-adrenergic agonist dexmedetomidine. J Pharmacol Exp Ther 283:993, 1997.

21. Sabbe MB, Penning JP, Ozaki GT, et al: Spinal and systemic action of the alpha 2 receptor agonist dexmedetomidine in dogs. Anesthesiology 80:1057, 1994.

22. Takano Y, Yaksh TL: Relative efficacy of spinal alpha-2 agonists, dexmedetomidine, clonidine and ST-91, determined in vivo by using N-ethoxycarbonyl-2-ethoxy-1,2-dihydroquinoline, an irreversible antagonist. J Pharmacol Exp Ther 258:438, 1992.

23. Malmberg AB, Yaksh TL: Pharmacology of the spinal action of ketorolac, morphine, ST-91, U50488H, and L-PIA on the formalin test and the isobolographic analysis of the NSAID interaction. Anesthesiology 79:270, 1993.

24. Harada Y, Nishioka K, Kitahata LM, et al: Visceral antinociceptive effects of spinal clonidine combined with morphine, (D-Pen², D-Pen⁵) enkephalin, or U50,488H. Anesthesiology 83:344, 1995.

25. Iwasaki H, Collins JG, Saito Y, et al: Low dose clonidine enhances pregnancy-induced analgesia to visceral but not somatic stimuli in rats. Anesth Analg 72:325, 1991.

26. Poree LR, Guo TZ, Kingery WS, et al: The analgesic potency of dexmedetomidine is enhanced after nerve injury: A possible role for peripheral a2-adrenoceptors. Anesth Analg 87:941, 1998.

27. Pan HL, Eisenach JC: Role of spinal NO in antiallodynic effect of intrathecal clonidine in neuropathic rats. Anesthesiology 89:1518, 1998.

28. Detweiler DJ, Eisenach JC, Tong C, et al: A cholinergic interaction in alpha2 adrenoceptor-mediated antinociception in sheep. J Pharmacol Exp Ther 265:536, 1993.

29. Eisenach JC, D'Angelo R, Taylor C, et al: An isobolographic study of epidural clonidine and fentanyl after cesarean section. Anesth Analg 79:285, 1994.

30. Brandt SA, Livingston A: Receptor changes in the spinal cord of sheep associated with exposure to chronic pain. Pain 42:323, 1990.

31. Jones SL, Gebhart GF: Characterization of coerulospinal inhibition of the nociceptive tail-flick reflex in the rat: Mediation by spinal a2-adrenoceptors. Brain Res 364:315, 1986.

32. Tjolsen A, Lund A, Hole K: The role of descending noradrenergic systems in regulation of nociception: The effects of intrathecally administered a adrenoceptor antagonists and clonidine. Pain 43:113, 1990.

33. Fleetwood-Walker SM, Mitchell R, Hope PJ, et al: An alpha 2 receptor mediates the selective inhibition by noradrenaline of nociceptive

responses of identified dorsal horn neurones. Brain Res 334:243, 1985.

34. Millar J, O'Brien FE, Williams GV, et al: The effect of iontophoretic clonidine on neurones in the rat superficial dorsal horn. Pain 53:137, 1993.

35. Sullivan AF, Dashwood MR, Dickensen AH: a2-adrenoceptor modulation of nociception in rat spinal cord: Location, effects and interactions with morphine. Eur J Pharmacol 138:169, 1987.

36. Eisenach JC, Detweiler DJ, Tong C, et al: Cerebrospinal fluid norepinephrine and acetylcholine concentrations during acute pain. Anesth Analg 82:621, 1996.

37. Takano Y, Yaksh TL: Release of calcitonin gene-related peptide (CGRP), substance P (SP), and vasoactive intestinal polypeptide (VIP) from rat spinal cord: Modulation by alpha 2 agonists. Peptides 14:371, 1993.

38. Ossipov MH, Gebhart GF: Absence of antinociceptive effect of alpha-2-agonists microinjected in the periaqueductal gray of the rat. Brain Res 289:349, 1983.

39. Guo TZ, Jiang JY, Buttermann AE, et al: Dexmedetomidine injection in the locus ceruleus produces antinociception. Anesthesiology 84:873, 1996.

40. Nakamura M, Ferreira SH: Peripheral analgesic action of clonidine: Mediation by enkephalin-like substances. Eur J Pharmacol 146:223, 1988.

41. Buerkle H, Schäpsmeier M, Bantel C, et al: Thermal and mechanical antinociceptive action of spinal vs peripherally administered clonidine in the rat inflamed knee joint. Br J Anaesth 83:436, 1999.

42. Correa-Sales C, Rabin BC, Maze M: A hypnotic response to dexmedetomidine, an a-2 agonist, is mediated in the locus coeruleus in rats. Anesthesiology 76:948, 1992.

43. Doze VA, Chen BX, Tinklenberg JA, et al: Pertussis toxin and 4-amidopyridine differential affect the hypnotic-anesthetic action of dexmedetomidine and pentobarbital. Anesthesiology 73:304, 1990.

44. Nacif-Coelho C, Correa-Sales C, Lenoir Chang L, et al: Perturbation of ion channel conductance alters the hypnotic response to the a2-adrenergic agonist dexmedetomidine in the locus coeruleus of the rat. Anesthesiology 81:1527, 1994.

45. Nelson LE, Lu J, Guo T, et al: The alpha2-adrenoceptor agonist dexmedetomidine converges on an endogenous sleep-promoting pathway to exert its sedative effects. Anesthesiology 98:428, 2003.

46. Guo TZ, Tinklenberg BS, Oliker R, et al: Central a1-adrenoreceptor stimulation functionally antagonizes the hypnotic response to dexmedetomidine and a2-adrenoreceptor agonist. Anesthesiology 75:252, 1991.

47. Pertovaara A, Hämäläinen MM: Spinal potentiation and supraspinal additivity in the antinociceptive interaction between systemically administered alpha 2-adrenoceptor agonist and cocaine in the rat. Anesth Analg 79:261, 1994.

48. Kallio A, Scheinin M, Koulu M, et al: Effects of dexmedetomidine, a selective a2-adrenoreceptor agonist, on hemodynamic control mechanisms. Clin Pharmacol Ther 46:33, 1989.

49. Housmans PR: Effects of dexmedetomidine on contractility, relaxation, and intracellular calcium transients of isolated ventricular myocardium. Anesthesiology 73:919, 1990.

50. Wang C, Knowles PM, Chakrabarti MK, et al: Clonidine has comparable effects on spontaneous sympathetic activity and afferent Ad- and C-fiber-mediated somatosympathetic reflexes in dogs. Anesthesiology 81:710, 1994.

51. Bruandet N, Rentero N, Debeer L, et al: Catecholamine activation in the vasomotor center on emergence from anesthesia: The effects of a2 agonists. Anesth Analg 86:240, 1998.

52. Saunier CF, Akaoka H, de la Chapelle B, et al: Activation of brain noradrenergic neurons during recovery from halothane anesthesia. Persistence of phasic activation after clonidine. Anesthesiology 79:1072, 1993.

53. Muzi M, Goff DR, Kampine JP, et al: Clonidine reduces sympathetic activation but maintains baroreflex responses in normotensive humans. Anesthesiology 77:864, 1992.

54. Tibiriça E, Feldman J, Mermet C, et al: An imidazoline specific mechanism for the hypotensive effect of clonidine: A study with yohimbine and idazoxan. J Pharmacol Exp Ther 256:606, 1990.

55. Bruban V, Estato V, Schann S, et al: Evidence for synergy between alpha(2)-adrenergic and nonadrenergic mechanisms in central blood pressure regulation. Circulation 105:1116, 2002.

56. Eisenach JC, Tong C: Site of hemodynamic effects of intrathecal a2-adrenergic agonists. Anesthesiology 74:766, 1991.

57. McCallum JB, Boban N, Hogan Q, et al: The mechanism of a2-adrenergic inhibition of sympathetic ganglionic transmission. Anesth Analg 87:503, 1998.

58. Castro MI, Eisenach JC: Pharmacokinetics and dynamics of intravenous, intrathecal and epidural clonidine in sheep. Anesthesiology 71:418, 1989.

59. Nishikawa T, Kimura T, Taguchi N, et al: Oral clonidine preanesthetic medication augments the pressor responses to intravenous ephedrine in awake or anesthetized patients. Anesthesiology 74:705, 1991.

60. Ohata H, Iida H, Watanabe Y, et al: Hemodynamic responses induced by dopamine and dobutamine in anesthetized patients premedicated with clonidine. Anesth Analg 89:843, 1999.

61. Talke PO, Caldwell JE, Richardson CA, et al: The effects of clonidine on human digital vasculature. Anesth Analg 91:793, 2000.

62. Eisenach J, Detweiler D, Hood D: Hemodynamic and analgesic actions of epidurally administered clonidine. Anesthesiology 78:277, 1993.

63. Kirnö K, Lundin S, Elam M: Epidural clonidine depresses sympathetic nerve activity in humans by a supraspinal mechanism. Anesthesiology 78:1021, 1993.

64. Coughlan MG, Lee JG, Bosnjak ZJ, et al: Direct coronary and cerebral vascular responses to dexmedetomidine: Significance of endogenous nitric oxide synthesis. Anesthesiology 77:998, 1992.

65. Engelman E, Lipszyc M, Gilbart E, et al: Effects of clonidine on anesthetic drug requirements and hemodynamic response during aortic surgery. Anesthesiology 71:178, 1989.

66. Roekaerts PM, Prinzen FW, Willigers HM, et al: The effects of a2-adrenergic stimulation with mivazerol on myocardial blood flow and function during coronary artery stenosis in anesthetized dogs. Anesth Analg 82:702, 1996.

67. Kono M, Morita S, Hayashi T, et al: The effects of intravenous clonidine on regional myocardial function in a canine model of regional myocardial ischemia. Anesth Analg 78:1047, 1994.

68. Kersten J, Pagel PS, Hettrick A, et al: Dexmedetomidine partially attenuates the sympathetically mediated systemic and coronary hemodynamic effects of cocaine. Anesth Analg 80:114, 1995.

69. Thomas MG, Quiroz AC, Rice JC, et al: Antianginal effects of clonidine. J Cardiovasc Pharmacol 8:S69, 1986.

70. Wright RA, Decroly P, Karkevitch T, et al: Exercise tolerance in angina is improved by mivazerol: An alpha 2-adrenoreceptor agonist. Cardiovasc Drugs Ther 7:929, 1993.

71. Weber MA: Discontinuation syndrome following cesation of treatment with clonidine and other antihypertensive agents. J Cardiovasc Pharmacol 1:S73, 1980.

72. Ishiyama T, Dohi S, Iida H, et al: Mechanisms of dexmedetomidine-induced cerebrovascular effects in canine in vivo experiments. Anesth Analg 81:1208, 1995.

73. Zornow MH, Fleischer JE, Scheller MS, et al: Dexmedetomidine, an a2-adrenergic agonist, decreases cerebral blood flow in the isoflurane-anesthetized dog. Anesth Analg 70:624, 1990.

74. Takenada M, Iida H, Iida M, et al: Intrathecal dexmedetomidine attentiuates hypercapnic but not hypoxic cerebral vasodilation in anesthetized rabbits. Anesthesiology 92:1376, 2000.

75. Lee HW, Caldwell JE, Dodson B, et al: The effect of clonidine on cerebral blood flow velocity, carbon dioxide cerebral vasoreactivity, and response to increased arterial pressure in human volunteers. Anesthesiology 87:553, 1997.

76. Maier C, Steinberg GK, Sun GH, et al: Neuroprotection by the alpha-2 adrenoreceptor agonist dexmedetomidine in a focal model of cerebral ischemia. Anesthesiology 79:306, 1993.

77. Hoffman WE, Kochs E, Werner C, et al: Dexmedetomidine improves neurologic outcome from incomplete ischemia in the rat. Anesthesiology 75:328, 1991.

78. Matsumoto M, Zornow MH, Rabin BC, et al: The alpha-2 adrenergic agonist, dexmedetomidine, selectively attenuates ischemia-induced increases in striatal norepinephrine concentrations. Brain Res 627:325, 1993.

79. Zornow MH, Scheller MS, Sheehan PB, et al: Intracranial pressure effects of dexmedetomidine in rabbits. Anesth Analg 75:232, 1992.

80. Eisenach JC: Intravenous clonidine produces hypoxemia by a peripheral alpha-2 adrenergic mechanism. J Pharmacol Exp Ther 244:247, 1988.

81. Eisenach JC, Dewan DM: Intrathecal clonidine in obstetrics: Sheep studies. Anesthesiology 72:663, 1990.

82. Rosenfeld BA, Faraday N, Campbell D, et al: Perioperative platelet reactivity and the effects of clonidine. Anesthesiology 79:255, 1993.

83. Jiang QI, Sheldon RJ, Porreca F: Sites of clonidine action to inhibit gut propulsion in mice: Demonstration of a central component. Gastroenterology 95:1265, 1988.

84. Asai T, Mapleson WW, Power I: Interactive effect of morphine and dexmedetomidine on gastric emptying and gastrointestinal transit in the rat. Br J Anaesth 80:63, 1998.

85. Lawrence CJ, Prinzen FW, de Lange S: The effect of dexmedetomidine on nutrient organ blood flow. Anesth Analg 83:1160, 1996.

86. Yelken B, Dorman T, Erkasap S, et al: Clonidine pretreatment inhibits stress-induced gastric ulcer in rats. Anesth Analg 89:159, 1999.

87. Aho M, Lehtinen AM, Laatikainen T, et al: Effects of intramuscular clonidine on hemodynamic and plasma beta-endorphin responses to gynecologic laparoscopy. Anesthesiology 72:797, 1990.

88. Aho M, Scheinin M, Lehtinen AM, et al: Intramuscular administered dexmedetomidine attenuates hemodynamic and stress hormone responses to gynecologic laparoscopy. Anesth Analg 75:932, 1992.

89. Mertes N, Goeters C, Kuhmann M, et al: Postoperative a2-adrenergic stimulation attenuates protein catabolism. Anesth Analg 82:258, 1996.

90. Maze M, Virtanen R, Daunt D, et al: Effects of dexmedetomidine, a novel imidazole sedative-anesthetic agent, on adrenal steroidogenesis: In vivo and in vitro studies. Anesth Analg 73:204, 1991.

91. Arndts D, Doevendans J, Kirsten R, et al: New aspects of the pharmacokinetics and pharmacodynamics of clonidine in man. Eur J Clin Pharmacol 24:21, 1983.

92. Bonnet F, Boico O, Rostaing S, et al: Clonidine-induced analgesia in postoperative patients: epidural versus intramuscular administration. Anesthesiology 72:423, 1990.

93. Mendez R, Eisenach JC, Kashtan K: Epidural clonidine analgesia after cesarean section. Anesthesiology 73:848, 1990.

94. Cigarini I, Kaba A, Bonnet F, et al: Epidural clonidine combined with bupivacaine for analgesia in labor: Effect on mother and neonate. Reg Anesth 20:113, 1995.

95. Hartikainen-Sorri AL, Heikkinen JE, Koivisto M: Pharmacokinetics of clonidine during pregnancy and nursing. Obstet Gynecol 69:598, 1987.

96. Khan ZP, Munday IT, Jones RM, et al: Effects of dexmedetomidine on isoflurane requirements in healthy volunteers. 1: Pharmacodynamic and pharmacokinetic interactions. Br J Anaesth 83:372, 1999.

97. Rodrigues AD, Roberts EM: The in vitro interaction of dexmedetomidine with human liver microsomal cytochrome P450D6 (CYP2D6). Drug Metab Dispos 65:128, 1997.

98. Kharash ED, Hill HF, Eddy AC: Influence of dexmedetomidine on human liver microsomal alfentanil metabolism. Anesthesiology 75:520, 1991.

99. Bührer M, Mappes A, Lauber R, et al: Dexmedetomidine decreases thiopental dose requirement and alters distribution pharmacokinetics. Anesthesiology 80:1216, 1994.

100. Bernard JM, Kick O, Bonnet F: Comparison of intravenous and epidural clonidine for postoperative patient-controlled analgesia. Anesth Analg 81:706, 1995.

101. Eisenach JC, Hood DD, Curry R: Intrathecal, but not intravenous, clonidine reduces experimental thermal or capsaicin-induced pain and hyperalgesia in normal volunteers. Anesth Analg 87:591, 1998.

102. De Kock M, Martin N, Scholtes JL: Central effects of epidural and intravenous clonidine in patients anesthetized with enflurane/nitrous oxide. An electroencephalographic analysis. Anesthesiology 77:457, 1992.

103. Coull JT, Jones MEP, Egan TD, et al: Attentional effects of noradrenaline vary with arousal level: Selective activation of thalamic pulvinar in humans. Neuropsychopharmacology [in press].

104. Nelson LE, Guo TZ, Lu J et al: The sedative component of anesthesia is mediated by GABA(A) receptors in an endogenous sleep pathway. Nat Neurosci 5:979, 2002.

105. Hall JE, Uhrich TD, Barney JA, et al: Sedative, amnestic, and analgesic properties of small-dose dexmedetomidine infusions. Anesth Analg 90:699, 2000.

106. Richer C, Gobert J, Noyer M et al: Peripheral alpha 2-adrenoceptor-mediated sympathoinhibitory effects of mivazerol. Fundam Clin Pharmacol 10:529, 1996.

107. McSPI-EUROPE Research Group: Perioperative sympatholysis. Beneficial effects of the alpha 2-adrenoreceptor agonist mivazerol on hemodynamic stability and myocardial ischemia. Anesthesiology 86:346, 1997.

108. Zhang X, Wülfert E, Hanin I: Mivazerol, a new a2-adrenergic agonist, blunts cardiovascular effects following surgical stress in pentobarbital-anesthetized rats. Acta Anaesthesiol Scand 41:694, 1997.

109. Payen D, Quintin L, Plaisance P, et al: Head injury: Clonidine decreases plasma catecholamines. Crit Care Med 18:392, 1990.

110. Asgeirsson B, Grände PO, Nordström CH, et al: Effects of hypotensive treatment with a₂-agonist and b₁-antagonist on cerebral haemodynamics in severely head injured patients. Acta Anaesthesiol Scand 39:347, 1995.

111. Talke P, Tong C, Lee HW, et al: Effect of dexmedetomidine on lumbar cerebrospinal fluid pressure in humans. Anesth Analg 85:358, 1997.

112. Ter Minassian A, Beydon L, Decq P, et al: Changes in cerebral hemodynamics after a single dose of clonidine in head injured patients. Anesth Analg 84:127, 1997.

113. Talke P, Tayefeh F, Sessler DI, et al: Dexmedetomidine does not alter the sweating threshold, but comparably and linearly decreases the vasoconstriction thresholds. Anesthesiology 87:835, 1997.

114. Joris J, Banache M, Bonnet F, et al: Clonidine and ketanserin both are effective treatment for postanesthetic shivering. Anesthesiology 79:532, 1993.

115. Horn EP, Standl T, Sessler DI, et al: Physostigmine prevents postanesthetic shivering as does meperidine or clonidine. Anesthesiology 88:108, 1998.

116. Belleville JP, Wards DS, Bloor DC, et al: Effects of intravenous dexmedetomidine in humans. Sedation, ventilation, and metabolic rate. Anesthesiology 77:1125, 1992.

117. Narchi P, Benhamou D, Hamza J, et al: Ventilatory effects of epidural clonidine during the first 3 hours after cesarean section. Acta Anaesthesiol Scand 36:791, 1992.

118. Penon C, Ecoffey C, Cohen SE: Ventilatory response to carbon dioxide after epidural clonidine injection. Anesth Analg 72:761, 1991.

119. Benhamou D, Veillette Y, Narchi P, et al: Ventilatory effects of premedication with clonidine. Anesth Analg 73:799, 1991.

120. Foo IT, Warren PM, Drummond GB: Influence of oral clonidine on the ventilatory response to acute and sustained isocapnic hypoxia in human males. Br J Anaesth 76:214, 1996.

121. Bailey PL, Speng RJ, Johnson GK, et al: Respiratory effects of clonidine alone and combined with morphine in humans. Anesthesiology 74:43, 1991.

122. Jarvis DA, Duncan S, Segan IS, et al: Ventilatory effects of clonidine alone, and the presence of alfentanil, in human volunteers. Anesthesiology 76:899, 1992.

123. Bernard JM, Lagarde D, Souron R: Balanced postoperative analgesia: Effect of intravenous clonidine on blood gases and pharmacokinetics of intravenous fentanyl. Anesth Analg 79:1126, 1994.

124. Scheinin H, Jaakola M-L, Sjövall S, et al: Intramuscular dexmedetomidine as premedication for general anesthesia. Anesthesiology 78:1065, 1993.

125. Hall JE, Uhrich TD, Ebert TJ: Sedative, analgesic and cognitive effects of clonidine infusions in humans. Br J Anaesth 86:5, 2001.

126. Filos KS, Patroni O, Goudas LC, et al: A dose-response study of orally administered clonidine as premedication in the elderly: Evaluating hemodynamic safety. Anesth Analg 77:1185, 1993.

127. Mikawa K, Maekawa N, Nishina K, et al: Efficacy of oral clonidine premedication in children. Anesthesiology 79:926, 1993.

128. Asai T, McBeth C, Tewart JIM, et al: Effect of clonidine on gastric emptying of liquids. Br J Anaesth 78:28, 1997.

129. Aantaa R, Jaakola ML, Kallio A, et al: Reduction of the minimum alveolar concentration of isoflurane by dexmedetomidine. Anesthesiology 86:1055, 1997.

130. Ghignone M, Noe C, Calvillo O, et al: Anesthesia for ophthalmic surgery in the elderly: The effects of clonidine on intraocular pressure, perioperative hemodynamics, and anesthetic requirements. Anesthesiology 68:707, 1988.

131. Ghignone M, Quintin L, Duke PC, et al: Effects of clonidine on narcotic requirements and hemodynamic response during induction of fentanyl anesthesia and endotracheal intubation. Anesthesiology 64:36, 1986.

132. Taittonen MT, Kirvelä OA, Aantaa R, et al: The effect of clonidine or midazolam premedication on perioperative responses during ketamine anesthesia. Anesth Analg 87:161, 1998.

133. Erkola O, Korttrila K, Aho M, et al: Comparison of intramuscular dexmedetomidine and midazolam premedication for elective abdominal hysterectomy. Anesth Analg 79:646, 1994.

134. Aantaa R, Kanto J, Scheinin M: Intramuscular dexmedetomidine, a novel alpha 2-adrenoreceptor agonist, as premedication for minor gynaecological surgery. Acta Anaesthesiol Scand 35:283, 1991.

135. Bernard JM, Bourreli B, Hommeril JL, et al: Effects of oral clonidine premedication and postoperative IV infusion on haemodynamic and adrenergic responses during recovery from anaesthesia. Acta Anaesthesiol Scand 35:54, 1991.

136. Aantaa R, Jaakola ML, Kallio A, et al: A comparison of dexmedetomidine, an alpha 2-adrenoreceptor agonist and midazolam as i.m. premedication for minor gynaecological surgery. Br J Anaesth 67:402, 1991.

137. Quintin L, Bouilloc X, Butin E, et al: Clonidine for major vascular surgery in hypertensive patients: A double-blind, controlled, randomized study. Anesth Analg 83:687, 1996.

138. Segal IS, Jarvis DJ, Duncan SR, et al: Clinical efficacy of oral-transdermal clonidine combination during the perioperative period. Anesthesiology 74:220, 1991.

139. Pluskwa F, Bonnet F, Saada M, et al: Effect of clonidine on changes in blood pressure during carotid artery surgery. J Cardiothor Anesth 5:431, 1991.

140. Woodcock TE, Millard RK, Dixon J, et al: Clonidine premedication for isoflurane-induced hypotension. Br J Anaesth 60:388, 1988.

141. Levanen J, Mäkelä ML, Scheinin H: Dexmedetomidine premedication attenuates ketamine-induced cardiostimulatory effects and postanesthetic delirium. Anesthesiology 82:1117, 1995.

142. Kagawa K, Mammoto T, Hayashi Y, et al: The effect of imidazoline receptors and a2-adrenoreceptors on the anesthetic requirement (MAC) for halothane in rats. Anesthesiology 87:963, 1997.

143. Carabine UA, Wright PMC, Moore J: Preanaesthetic medication with clonidine: A dose-response study. Br J Anaesth 67:79, 1991.

144. Marinangeli F, Cocco C, Ciccozzi A, et al: Haemodynamic effects of intravenous clonidine on propofol or thiopental induction. Acta Anaesthesiol Scand 44:150, 2000.

145. Entholzner EK, Mielke LL, Hargasser SR, et al: Intravenous clonidine decreases minimum end-tidal isoflurane for induction of electroencephalographic burst suppression. Anesth Analg 85:193, 1997.

146. Inomata S, Kihara S, Yaguchi Y, et al: Reduction in standard MAC and MAC for intubation after clonidine premedication in children. Br J Anaesth 85:700, 2000.

147. Salmenperä MT, Szlam F, Hug CC: Anesthetic and hemodynamic interactions of dexmedetomidine and fentanyl in dogs. Anesthesiology 80:837, 1994.

148. Goyagi T, Tanaka M, Nishikawa T: Oral clonidine premedication reduces the awakening concentration of isoflurane. Anesth Analg 86:410, 1998.

149. Weinger MB, Segal IS, Maze M: Dexmedetomidine, acting through central alpha-2 adrenoreceptors, prevents opiate-induced muscle rigidity in the rat. Anesthesiology 71:242, 1989.

150. Talke PO, Caldwell JE, Richardson CA, et al: The effects of dexmedetomidine on neuromuscular blockade in human volunteers. Anesth Analg 88:633, 1999.

151. Venn RM, Bradshaw CJ, Spencer R, et al: Preliminary UK experience of dexmedetomidine, a novel agent for postoperative sedation in the intensive care unit. Anaesthesia 54:1136, 1999.

152. Longnecker DE: Alpine anesthesia: Can pretreatment with clonidine decrease the peaks and valleys? Anesthesiology 67:1, 1987.

153. Kulka PJ, Tryba M, Zenz M: Dose-response effects of intravenous clonidine on stress response during induction of anesthesia in coronary artery bypass graft patients. Anesth Analg 80:263, 1995.

154. Lawrence CJ, Prinzen FW, de Lange S: The effect of dexmedetomidine on the balance of myocardial energy requirement and oxygen supply and demand. Anesth Analg 82:544, 1996.

155. Meissner A, Weber T, Van Aken H, et al: Clonidine improves recovery from myocardial stunning in conscious chronically instrumented dogs. Anesth Analg 87:1009, 1998.

156. Kersten J, Pagel PS, Tessmer JP, et al: Dexmedetomidine alters the hemodynamic effects of desflurane and isoflurane in chronically instrumented dogs. Anesthesiology 79:1022, 1993.

157. Proctor LY, Schmeling WT, Warltier DC: Premedication with oral clonidine alters hemodynamic action of intravenous anesthetic agents in chronically instrumented dogs. Anesthesiology 77:554, 1992.

158. Furst SR, Weinger MB: Dexmedetomidine, a selective a2-agonist, does not potentiate the cardiorespiratory depression of alfentanil in the rat. Anesthesiology 72:882, 1990.

159. Ellis JE, Drijvers G, Pedlow S, et al: Premedication with oral and transdermal clonidine provides safe and efficacious postoperative sympatholysis. Anesth Analg 79:1133, 1994.

160. Matot I, Sichel JY, Yofe V, et al: The effect of clonidine premedication on hemodynamic responses to microlaryngoscopy and rigid bronchoscopy. Anesth Analg 91:828, 2000.

161. Jalonen J, Hynynen M, Kuitunen A, et al: Dexmedetomidine as an anesthetic adjunct in coronary artery bypass grafting. Anesthesiology 86:331, 1997.

162. Talke P, Li J, Jain U, et al: The study of perioperative ischemia research group. Effects of perioperative dexmedetomidine infusion in patients undergoing vascular surgery. Anesthesiology 82:620, 1995.

163. Dorman BH, Zucker JR, Verrier ED, et al: Clonidine improves perioperative myocardial ischemia, reduces anesthetic requirements, and alters hemodynamic parameters in patients undergoing coronary artery bypass surgery. J Cardiothor Anesth 78:386, 1993.

164. Oliver MF, Goldman L, Julian DG, et al: Effect of mivazerol on perioperative cardiac complications during non-cardiac surgery in patients with coronary artery disease: The European Mivazerol Trial (EMIT). Anesthesiology 91:951, 1999.

165. Boico O, Bonnet F, Mazoit X: Effect of epinephrine and clonidine on pharmacokinetics of spinal bupivacaine. Acta Anaesthesiol Scand 36:684, 1992.

166. Nishikawa T, Dohi S: Clinical evaluation of clonidine added to lidocaine solution for epidural anesthesia. Anesthesiology 73:853, 1990.

167. Mazoit JX, Benhamou D, Veillette Y, et al: Clonidine and or adrenaline decrease lignocaine plasma peak concentration after epidural injection. Br J Clin Pharmacol 42:242, 1996.

168. De Kock M, Le Polain B, Henin D, et al: Clonidine pretreatment reduces the systemic toxicity of intravenous bupivacaine in rats. Anesthesiology 79:282, 1993.

169. Ohata H, Iida H, Wanatabe Y, et al: The optimal test dose of epinephrine for epidural injection with lidocaine solution in awake patients premedicated with oral clonidine. Anesth Analg 86:1010, 1998.

170. Bonnet F, Diallo A, Saada M, et al: Prevention of tourniquet pain by spinal isobaric bupivacaine with clonidine. Br J Anaesth 63:93, 1989.

171. Bonnet F, Brun-Buisson V, Boico O, et al: Dose-related prolongation of hyperbaric tetracaine spinal anesthesia by clonidine in humans. Anesth Analg 68:619, 1989.

172. Gentili M, Bonnet F: Spinal clonidine produces less urinary retention than spinal morphine. Br J Anaesth 76:872, 1996.

173. Filos KS, Goudas LC, Patroni O, et al: Intrathecal clonidine as a sole analgesic for pain relief after cesarean section. Anesthesiology 77:267, 1992.

174. Mogensen T, Eliasen K, Ejlersen E, et al: Epidural clonidine enhances postoperative analgesia from combined low-dose epidural bupivacaine and morphine regimen. Anesth Analg 75:607, 1992.

175. Capogna G, Celleno D: IV clonidine for post-extradural shivering in parturients: A preliminary study. Br J Anaesth 71:294, 1993.

176. Klimscha W, Chiari A, Krafft P, et al: Hemodynamic and analgesic effects of clonidine added repetitively to continuous epidural and spinal blocks. Anesth Analg 80:322, 1995.

177. Huntoon M, Eisenach JC, Boese P: Epidural clonidine after cesarean section. Appropriate dose and effect of prior local anesthetic. Anesthesiology 76:187, 1992.

178. Lee JJ, Rubin AP: Comparison of a bupivacaine-clonidine mixture with plain bupivacaine for caudal analgesia in children. Br J Anaesth 72:258, 1994.

179. Bernard JM, Macaire P: Dose-range effects of clonidine added to lidocaine for brachial plexus block. Anesthesiology 87:277, 1997.

180. Gaumann D, Forster A, Griessen M, et al: Comparison between clonidine and epinephrine admixture to lidocaine in brachial plexus block. Anesth Analg 75:69, 1992.

181. Singelyn FJ, Gouverneur JM, Robert A: A minimum dose of clonidine added to mepivacaine prolongs the duration of anesthesia and analgesia after axillary brachial plexus block. Anesth Analg 83:1046, 1996.

182. Sia S, Lepri A: Clonidine administered as an axillary block does not affect postoperative pain when given as the sole analgesic. Anesth Analg 88:1109, 1999.

183. Lurie SD, Reuben SS, Gibson CS, et al: Effect of clonidine on upper extremity tourniquet pain in healthy volunteers. Reg Anesth Pain Med 25:502, 2000.

184. Mjahed K, Harrar N, Hamdani M, et al: Lidocaine-clonidine retrobulbar block for cataract surgery in the elderly. Reg Anesth 21:569, 1996.

185. Joshi W, Scott SR, Kilaru PR, et al: Postoperative analgesia for outpatient arthroscopic knee surgery with intraarticular clonidine and/or morphine. Anesth Analg 90:1102, 2000.

186. Kalia PK, Madan R, Batra RK, et al: Clinical study on epidural clonidine for postoperative analgesia. Indian J Med Res 83:550, 1986.

187. Bonnet F, Boico O, Rostaing S, et al: Postoperative analgesia with extradural clonidine. Br J Anaesth 63:465, 1989.

188. Gordh T: Epidural clonidine for treatment of postoperative pain after thoracotomy. A double blind placebo controlled study. Acta Anaesthesiol Scand 32:702, 1988.

189. Rockemann MG, Seeling W, Brinkmann A, et al: Analgesic and hemodynamic effects of epidural clonidine/morphine and morphine after pancreatic surgery. A double-blind study. Anesth Analg 80:869, 1995.

190. De Kock M, Famenne F, Deckers G, et al: Epidural clonidine or sufentanil for intraoperative and postoperative analgesia. Anesth Analg 81:1154, 1995.

191. Rockemann MG, Seeling W, Duschek S, et al: Epidural bolus clonidine/morphine versus epidural patient-controlled bupivacaine/sufentanil: Quality of postoperative analgesia and cost-identification analysis. Anesth Analg 85:864, 1997.

192. Rostaing S, Bonnet F, Levron JC, et al: Effect of epidural clonidine on analgesia and pharmacokinetics of epidural fentanyl in postoperative patients. Anesthesiology 75:420, 1991.

193. Filos KS, Goudas LC, Patroni O, et al: Hemodynamic and analgesic profile after intrathecal clonidine in humans. A dose-response study. Anesthesiology 81:591, 1994.

194. Grace D, Bunting H, Milligan KR, et al: Postoperative analgesia after co-administration of clonidine and morphine by the intrathecal route in patients undergoing hip replacement. Anesth Analg 80:86, 1995.

195. Pan PM, Huang CT, Wei TT, et al: Enhancement of analgesic effect of intrathecal neostigmine and clonidine on bupivacaine spinal anesthesia. Reg Anesth Pain Med 23:49, 1998.

196. Aho MS, Olli A, Scheinin H, et al: Effect of intravenously administered dexmedetomidine on pain after laparoscopic tubal ligation. Anesth Analg 73:112, 1991.

197. Celleno P, Capogna G, Costantino P: Comparison of fentanyl with clonidine as adjuvants for epidural analgesia with 0.125% bupivacaine in the first stage of labor. Int J Obstet Anesth 4:426, 1995.

198. Buggy DJ, MacDowell C: Extradural analgesia with clonidine and fentanyl compared with 0.25% bupivacaine in the first stage of labour. Br J Anaesth 76:319, 1996.

199. Chassard D, Mathon L, Dailler F, et al: Extradural clonidine combined with sufentanil and 0.625% bupivacaine for analgesia in labour. Br J Anaesth 77:458, 1996.

200. Boutroy MJ, Gisonna CR, Legagneur M: Clonidine: Placental transfer and neonatal adaptation. Early Hum Dev 17:275, 1988.

201. Ala-Kokko TI, Pienimäki P, Lampela E, et al: Transfer of clonidine and dexmedetomidine across the isolated perfused placenta. Acta Anaesthesiol Scand 41:313, 1997.

202. Chiari A, Lorber C, Eisenach JC, et al: Analgesic and hemodynamic effects of intrathecal clonidine as the sole analgesic agent during first stage of labor: A dose-response study. Anesthesiology 91:388, 1999.

203. Glynn CJ, Jamous MA, Teddy PJ, et al: Role of spinal noradrenergic system in transmission of pain in patients with spinal cord injury. Lancet 2:1249, 1986.

204. Rémy-Néris O, Barbeau H, Daniel O, et al: Effects of intrathecal clonidine injection on spinal reflexes and human locomotion in incomplete paraplegic subjects. Exp Brain Res 129:433, 1999.

205. Glynn C, Dawson D, Sanders R: A double-blind comparison between epidural morphine and epidural clonidine, in patients with chronic non-cancer pain. Pain 34:123, 1988.

206. Glynn C, O'Sullivan K: A double-blind randomized comparison of the effects of epidural clonidine, lignocaine and the combination of clonidine and lignocaine in patients with chronic pain. Pain 64:337, 1995.

207. Carroll D, Jadad A, King V, et al: Single-dose, randomized, double-blind, double-dummy cross-over comparison of extradural and IV clonidine in chronic pain. Br J Anaesth 71:665, 1993.

208. Byas-Smith MG, Max MB, Muir J, et al: Transdermal clonidine compared to placebo in painful diabetic neuropathy using a two-stage "enriched enrollment" design. Pain 60:267, 1995.

209. Rauck RL, Eisenach JC, Jackson K, et al: Epidural clonidine for refractory reflex sympathetic dystrophy. Anesthesiology 79:1163, 1993.

210. Kabeer AA, Hardy PAJ: Long-term use of subarachnoid clonidine for analgesia in refractory reflex sympathetic dystrophy. Reg Anesth 21:249, 1996.

211. Davis KD, Treede RD, Raja SN, et al: Topical application of clonidine relieves hyperalgesia in patients with sympathetically maintained pain. Pain 47:309, 1991.

212. Reuben SS, Steinberg RB, Madabhushi L, et al: Intravenous regional clonidine in the management of sympathetically maintained pain. Anesthesiology 89:527, 1998.

213. Eisenach J, Rauck RLR, Buzzanell C, et al: Epidural clonidine analgesia for intractable cancer pain: Phase I. Anesthesiology 71:647, 1989.

214. Eisenach JC, DuPen S, Dubois M, et al: Epidural clonidine analgesia for intractable cancer pain. The Epidural Clonidine Study Group. Pain 61:391, 1995.

215. Coombs DW, Saunders RL, Lachance D, et al: Intrathecal morphine tolerance: Use of intrathecal clonidine, DADLE, and intraventricular morphine. Anesthesiology 62:358, 1985.

216. Marwaha J, Kehne JH, Commissaris RL, et al: Spinal clonidine inhibits neural firing in locus coeruleus. Brain Res 276:379, 1983.

217. Aghajanian GK: Tolerance of locus coeruleus neurons to morphine and suppression of withdrawal response by clonidine. Nature 275:186, 1978.

218. Milne B, Cervenko FW, Jhamandas K, et al: Intrathecal clonidine: Analgesia and effect on opiate withdrawal in the rat. Anesthesiology 62:34, 1985.

219. Fielding S, Wilker J, Hynes M, et al: A comparison of clonidine with morphine for antinociceptive and antiwithdrawal actions. J Pharmacol Exp Ther 207:899, 1978.

220. Spies CD, Dubisz N, Neumann T, et al: Therapy of alcohol withdrawal syndrome in intensive care unit patients following trauma. Results of a prospective, randomized trial. Crit Care Med 24:414, 1996.

221. Delaunay L, Bonnet F, Duvaldestin P: Clonidine decreases postoperative oxygen consumption in patients recovering from general anaesthesia. Br J Anaesth 67:397, 1991.

29

Analgesics

Andrew S.C. Rice, MD • Ken Mackie, MD

CANNABINOIDS

Although herbal cannabis has enjoyed a reputation as a therapeutic agent in many cultures for thousands of years, its use in Western medicine died out in the 1930s when fears regarding its abuse potential were aroused. However, in the last 30 years there have been considerable advances in the understanding of the scientific basis of cannabinoid therapeutics, which has led to a resurgence of interest in potential medicinal applications. Not least amongst these discoveries was the identification of a system of cannabinoid receptors and ligands that constitute the "endocannabinoid system"; the physiologic role is being actively investigated. These scientific advances have been paralleled by a sometimes vociferous public lobby seeking to promote the legal use of herbal cannabis, with the boundaries between "recreational" and therapeutic uses often being obfuscated.

Although there are data attesting to therapeutic effects of cannabinoids in many important areas of medicine, such as relief of spasticity and tremor in multiple sclerosis,[1] nausea and vomiting,[2] and bronchospasm,[3] this chapter discusses potential analgesic applications only. This subject has been the topic of several recent comprehensive reviews that contain detailed information beyond the scope of this chapter.[4-7]

Historical Aspects

Cannabis sativa has been a valuable source of hemp fiber for many thousands of years, and abuse of its psychoactive constituents has also been evident in many cultures for a considerable time. One of the first references to the therapeutic use of cannabis is in the Chinese pharmacopoeia *Pen ts'ao,* published in 2800 BC, and analgesia was among the first recommended uses. Indian writings in the *Athera Veda,* which were based on an oral tradition dating to about 2000 BC, also refer to the therapeutic effects of cannabis.[8] There is archaeologic evidence from Israel that cannabis was used therapeutically during obstructed childbirth, possibly as an analgesic.[9] In Greek and Roman histories, both the Herbal of Dioscorides and the subsequent writings of Galen refer to the therapeutic effects of cannabis. Cannabis was introduced into Western medicine much later; although Culpepper's medieval herbal does mention cannabis, it was the Indian Army physician William O'Shaughnessy who, in 1842, was credited with introducing cannabis for medicinal use to the West after his observations in India. He recommended a tincture for a wide range of uses, including analgesia, and it has been suggested that Queen Victoria was prescribed it for relief of dysmenorrhea. The medicinal use of cannabis faded with the advent of superior medications and it was removed from the U.S. pharmacopoeia in 1942, but continued to be included in the British pharmacopoeia until 1976 when it was reclassified as a schedule 1 drug (of no therapeutic benefit). In the 1990s, considerable public pressure has forced the re-evaluation of cannabinoids as useful therapeutics, and a number of influential bodies have considered this issue.[10-13]

The last 30 years have seen considerable advances in the understanding of cannabinoids, which include the identification of the psychoactive constituents of *C. sativa,* the receptors at which they act, and the corresponding endogenous ligands, and the synthesis of synthetic cannabinoids, which is discussed in this chapter.

Endocannabinoid System

Receptors

For many years, the mechanism of action of Δ^9 tetrahydrocannabinol (THC) was enigmatic. Because it is a very lipophilic molecule, the dominant belief was that it acted by perturbing membranes, much in the same way as general anesthetics were thought to act. The first hints of a receptor-mediated action of cannabinoids can be found in careful studies performed in the 1970s showing that cannabinoids exhibited enantiomeric selectivity,[14] a property not predicted by a lipid perturbing mechanism of action. In the 1980s, Allyn Howlett and colleagues demonstrated conclusively the existence of cannabinoid receptors and identified them as members of the G protein–coupled receptor superfamily.[15,16]

The simultaneous development of high-affinity cannabinoid ligands (the nonclassical cannabinoids and aminoalkylindoles) and their radiolabeling permitted the anatomic distribution of cannabinoid receptor binding to be determined. Interestingly, these studies show that cannabinoid binding was greatest in brain regions implicated in the behavioral effects of cannabinoids. Conversely, regions not involved in the physiologic effects of cannabinoids (for example, brain stem respiratory nuclei) had very low levels of cannabinoid binding.[17] An interesting feature of these studies is that cannabinoid receptors are often expressed at very high levels in the brain; for example, in the striatum, their density is ~2-fold greater than that of dopamine receptors.[18] Importantly, these studies and later immunocytochemical studies demonstrate that cannabinoid receptors are especially enriched in axons and particularly axon terminals.[19,20]

Identification of a cannabinoid receptor was quickly followed by the serendipitous cloning of a cannabinoid receptor cDNA (designated CB_1) by Lisa Matsuda working in Tom Bonner's laboratory.[21] The mRNA for this receptor was widely expressed in the brain, expressed in low levels in the periphery, and its regional distribution closely matched that found in binding studies.[22] Evidence from two CB_1 knockout mice suggests most, if not all, of the behavioral effects of cannabinoids observed at doses relevant for human ingestion are mediated by CB_1 receptors.[23,24] A few years later, a second cannabinoid receptor (designated CB_2) was cloned from a macrophage cell line.[25] There is little evidence that CB_2 receptors are expressed in neurons, but they are expressed in a number of immune cells. Their role, if any, in mediating the purported immunomodulatory properties of cannabis remains obscure. However, strong evidence suggests that CB_2 receptors may have a role in analgesia, particularly during inflammation.[7,26]

CB_1 receptors belong to the Gi/o class of G protein–coupled receptors. Work from Howlett and colleagues demonstrates that CB_1 receptor activation led to the inhibition of adenylyl cyclase.[15] This action will affect neuronal function in a variety of ways—for example, by slowing inactivation of rapidly inactivating potassium channels[27]—and may contribute to inhibition of neurotransmission. Subsequent work found that CB_1 receptors, independent of their actions on adenylyl cyclase, inhibited N and P/Q type calcium channels, activated inwardly rectifying potassium channels, and stimulated mitogen-activated protein kinase.[28–31] Other less well-studied actions also attributed to CB_1 receptor activation include: stimulation of ceramide synthesis,[32] activation of JNK,[33] and activation of neuronal nitric oxide synthase.[34] Undoubtedly other effectors modulated by cannabinoid receptors remain to be identified.

Studies using knockout mice and cannabinoid receptor antagonists have identified that other receptors, including G protein–coupled receptors, might be targets of cannabimimetic drugs, particularly endocannabinoids (see later).[35] Although it is unlikely that these receptors are involved in mediating the psychoactive effects of cannabis preparations, they may play a role in the physiologic actions of endogenous cannabinoids in processes such as analgesia.[36]

Endocannabinoids

The existence of cannabinoid receptors suggests the existence of endogenous ligand(s).[37] Currently, three distinct endogenous ligands for CB_1 receptors have been identified; two of these have been well characterized. Undoubtedly, more remain to be identified and characterized. The first to be discovered was arachidonyl ethanolamide, designated anandamide (AEA).[38] AEA appears to be formed by its cleavage from a lipid precursor existing in the membrane.[39] After its generation, it diffuses to its site of action where it binds to and activates CB_1 receptors. Its actions are terminated by a combination of cellular uptake[40] and hydrolysis.[41] Interestingly, AEA has a lower intrinsic efficacy than the synthetic cannabinoids often used in animal studies[42] and a lower intrinsic efficacy compared with the other well-described endocannabinoid, arachidonyl glycerol (2-AG).[43] Further complicating the use of AEA in experimental models is its rapid hydrolysis after systemic administration. Indeed, few studies have convincingly demonstrated CB_1-mediated central nervous system (CNS) effects after its systemic administration. A recent exception is a report using the fatty acid amide hydrolase (FAAH) (see later) knockout mouse. This mouse, which degrades AEA at a very slow rate, shows clear CB_1 effects when AEA is administered systemically. AEA has also been shown to interact with cell surface proteins in addition to CB_1 receptors, such as vanilloid receptors type-1 (VR1) and the TASK-1 potassium channel.[44,45] While these interactions occur at concentrations one or two orders of magnitude greater than AEA's affinity for CB_1 receptors, they should be considered when evaluating studies using pharmacologic concentrations of AEA and may be important during pathophysiologic states in which cell death releases membrane lipids, including endocannabinoid precursors.

The second endogenous cannabinoid to be identified was 2-AG.[46] Like AEA, this endocannabinoid exists as a precursor in the membrane where it is released after activation of specific phospholipases.[46] Although less well studied, 2-AG action appears to be terminated by some of the same mechanisms as AEA action. In particular, 2-AG appears to be a substrate for the AEA membrane transporter and the fatty acid aminohydrolase. Although there are structural similarities between AEA and 2-AG, factors controlling their release have distinguishing features and in vivo studies have demonstrated the release of one or the other in different brain regions.[47,48]

The third endogenous cannabinoid to be identified was 2-arachidonyl glyceryl ether. This compound is the *ether* of arachidonic acid and glycerol, again at the 2 position. 2-Arachidonyl glyceryl ether has been given the trivial name of noladin ether. This compound has been isolated from brain and has been shown in a limited series of assays to possess the properties expected of an endogenous cannabinoid.[49] There have been preliminary reports of additional endocannabinoids, such as the *ester* of arachidonic acid and ethanolamine. Undoubtedly, there are a number of endogenous compounds that qualify as "endocannabinoids." A major research challenge will be to identify additional compounds and to determine the relative biologic role of these various endocannabinoids in physiologic and pathophysiologic states.

Palmitoylethanolamide (PEA) is a fatty acid amide that is structurally similar to AEA and has many cannabinomimetic effects. However, it does not bind to known cannabinoid receptors, although its analgesic effects are sensitive to the CB_2 receptor antagonist SR144528, suggesting that it acts at CB_2-like receptors or enhances the effects of endocannabinoids at these receptors.[36,50–52]

Although the physiologic role of endocannabinoids is largely unknown, three important articles recently have been published that indicate that endocannabinoids are released from postsynaptic neurons in response to depolarization. These endocannabinoids act as a general short-range ($<20\mu m$) interneuronal retrograde modulator of neurotransmitter release by binding to and activating presynaptic CB_1 receptors.[53–55] That this occurs at both GABAergic (essentially inhibitory) and glutamatergic (essentially excitatory) synapses suggests that it is a ubiquitous mode of action of endocannabinoids. In the context of regulating pain transmission, it is likely that endocannabinoids have a similar role in the dorsal horn of the spinal cord. In this way, endocannabinoids will be released during intense activation of dorsal horn neurons and may inhibit neurotransmitter release from adjacent CB_1 receptor–expressing primary afferents and interneurons (Fig. 29–1).

Biosynthesis of Endocannabinoids

The biosynthesis of endocannabinoids[37] differs from that of more classical neurotransmitters such as glutamate and acetylcholine. Rather than being synthesized ahead of time and stored in synaptic vesicles, much evidence suggests that endocannabinoid precursors exist in the lipid bilayer. Endocannabinoids then are released either after activation of specific enzymes in a regulated fashion or after cell death and unregulated activation of these enzymes with the destruction of the plasma membrane. Both of these routes of synthesis

have direct implications for the role of endocannabinoids after tissue damage and the initiation of pain responses.

It is likely that the precursor to AEA is the lipid N-arachidonyl phosphatidylethanolamine (NAPE) (Fig. 29–2*A*). NAPE is found at quite low levels in the brain and other tissues compared with other lipids. Interestingly, NAPE levels are raised by increases in intracellular calcium or cyclic adenosine monophosphate, suggesting a means for modulating AEA production.[56] Hydrolysis of the bond between the phosphate and ethanolamine in NAPE by a phospholipase D will liberate AEA and phosphatidic acid.

The synthetic pathway for 2-AG is distinct from that for AEA and is regulated differently. This may explain why in certain experimental models elevation of one rather than the other endocannabinoid is seen. The current hypothesis for the formation of 2-AG shares commonality with the synthetic pathway for inositol 1,4,5-triphosphate and 1,2 diacylglycerol, which is important in the release of intracellular calcium and activation of protein kinase C, respectively (Fig. 29–2*B*). In this scheme, a phospholipase C cleaves inositol 1,4,5-triphosphate from a phospholipid containing an arachidonic acid moiety in the 2 position, leaving diacylglycerol. Diacylglycerol is then cleaved by a sn-1(3) diacylglycerol lipase, yielding 2-AG and a fatty acid.[57]

Inactivation of Endocannabinoids[37]

Endocannabinoids are inactivated by defined pathways in a two-step process. Manipulation of these pathways may prove to be therapeutically beneficial. The first step is the uptake of 2-AG or AEA through a carrier.[40] Transport likely occurs by facilitated diffusion. Once inside the cell, both endocannabinoids can be hydrolyzed by a rather nonspecific enzyme, FAAH.[58,59] Although its substrate specificity is broad, knockout of FAAH greatly increases tissue AEA levels and strongly potentiates the effects of exogenously administered AEA, suggesting that this enzyme degrades most AEA. A second, less well-characterized acid hydrolase can also degrade AEA.[60] In addition to catabolism by FAAH, 2-AG is also degraded by a monoacylglycerol lipase. Because inhibition of endocannabinoid degradation strongly diminishes uptake,[61] it is unlikely that cells accumulate much intact endocannabinoid. PEA is also metabolized by FAAH and is transported by a similar, but not identical, transporter as that for AEA.[62,63]

Fowler and colleagues[65–67] have demonstrated that certain nonsteroidal anti-inflammatory drugs (NSAIDs), at mildly acidic pH and at clinically relevant concentrations (i.e., that can be reached in tissues), inhibit AEA degradation by FAAH. This raises the tantalizing hypothesis that the CNS-mediated analgesia actions of certain NSAIDs may be attributable to inhibition of endocannabinoid breakdown (Fig. 29–3).

Plant-Derived and Synthetic Cannabinoids

Herbal cannabis contains a complex and variable mixture of psychoactive cannabinoids and it is difficult to envisage how

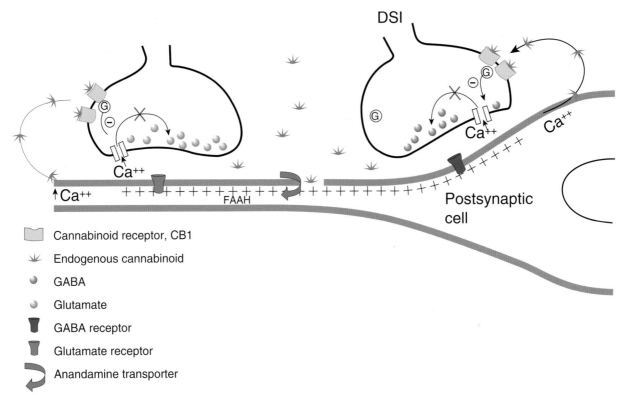

Figure 29–1. Endocannabinoids act as short-range retrograde modulators of neurotransmitter release. In response to ligand binding, endocannabinoids are rapidly synthesized and released from postsynaptic neurons, a process that is Ca^{++}-dependent. They then diffuse retrogradely across the synaptic cleft to bind to presynaptic CB_1 receptors. Activation of CB_1, through a number of mechanisms, then modulates both glutamate and γ-aminobutyric acid (GABA) release at their respective synapses. Endocannabinoids are then inactivated by re-uptake from the synaptic cleft by a transporter molecule into postsynaptic neurons where they are hydrolyzed by fatty acid amide hydrolase (FAAH). Endocannabinoids probably act as interneuronal retrograde at short distances less than 20 μm. Depolarisation induced suppression of inhibition (DSI). (Modified from Wilson RI, Nicoll RA: Endogenous cannabinoids mediate retrograde signaling at hippocampal synapses. Nature 410:588–592, 2001; Kreitzer AC, Regehr WG: Retrograde inhibition of presynaptic calcium influx by endogenous cannabinoids at excitatory synapses onto purkinje cells. Neuron 29:717–727, 2001; and Ohno-Shosaku T, Maejima T, Kano M: Endogenous cannabinoids mediate retrograd signals from depolarized postsynaptic terminals. Neuron 29:729–738, 2001.)

the type of simple horticulturally derived preparations, commonly used for "recreational" purposes, could be approved as 21st century therapeutics. Δ^9THC, along with cannabidiol and cannabinol, are the major psychoactive ingredients of herbal cannabis[68]; and oral preparations of THC (Marinol; Unimed Pharmaceuticals, Marietta, Ga.) and synthetic THC in sesame oil (dronabinol) have been granted regulatory approval in the United States for chemotherapy-induced nausea and vomiting and acquired immune deficiency syndrome–related anorexia. There is extensive literature on the pharmacology of THC and one particular feature of plant-derived cannabinoids is their high lipid solubility, which dictates that limited gastrointestinal absorption and bioavailability are significant barriers to their development as therapeutics.[69] For this reason, cannabis is traditionally smoked for "recreational" purposes, providing the most predictable and titratable route for administration; however, it is difficult to make a case for inhalation of cannabis smoke as a route for therapeutic development, given the potential health risks. Pulmonary delivery of cannabinoid aerosols are being

investigated as an alternative. Oral and rectal administration of THC and other plant-derived cannabinoids tends to be unpredictable and of limited bioavailability, but the rectal route does appear to have some advantage over the oral, at least for the THC prodrug THC hemisuccinate.[70] The lipid solubility of these compounds predicates that they are rapidly sequestered into fatty tissue and the elimination half-life is considerable, extending from days to weeks. THC is a substrate for the P450 mixed function oxidases, is biotransformed in the liver, and its metabolites are excreted in feces and urine as glucuronide conjugates.

A number of synthetic cannabinoids have been developed, predominately for experimental use, which can be classified as follows (for a comprehensive review see Barth[71] and Pertwee[72]).

- *Classical cannabinoids:* These are predominately substances that are structurally related to THC based on its dibenzopyran ring and are the only class of synthetic cannabinoids that have so far been granted regulatory approval. For example, in the United Kingdom, a synthetic derivative of THC has been approved for the treatment of chemotherapy-induced nausea and vomiting.[13] Mechoulam and his colleagues[73] have synthesized a number of classical cannabinoids, for example, HU210 and HU243. Some classical cannabinoids have been described that have some selectivity for CB_2 over CB_1, for example, L759,633, L759,656, and 1-deoxy-HU210 (JWH-051).[74,75] Although some water-soluble cannabinoids have been synthesized, an important recent advance was the pharmacologic characterization of a novel potent water-soluble THC analogue (O-1057). This compound is an agonist at both CB receptors and possesses cannabinomimetic properties including antinociception.[76]

■ *Nonclassical cannabinoids:* This term refers to bicyclic or tricyclic THC analogues that lack a pyran ring, for example, CP 55,940 and levonantradol. Radiolabeled CP 55,940 has been widely used in radioligand binding studies,[77] whereas levonantradol was administered to humans in early analgesic clinical trials but was associated with unacceptable side effects.[78] Levonantradol derivatives have been described that possess a degree of CB_2 selectivity,[71] and HU308 is a CB_2 receptor agonist,

devoid of CB_1-mediated effects, which has analgesic properties.[79]

■ *Aminoalkyindoles:* These compounds were serendipitously discovered during the search for novel NSAIDs. The best example is WIN 55,212-2, which has high affinity for both CB_1 and CB_2 receptors, with a modest selectivity for CB_2, and has cannabinomimetic properties.[71,72] A number of CB_2-selective ligands are based on the structure of WIN 55,212-2, including indomethacin morpholinylamide.[80] Further developments on this theme have included the synthesis of CB_2-selective agonists, for example, JWH-015, L-768,242, and L-759,787.[71]

■ *Endocannabinoid analogues[71]:* In an effort to prolong the duration of action of endocannabinoids, their molecular structure has been manipulated, for example, methanandamide and fluoroanandamide, both of which display some selectivity for CB_1 over CB_2. There have also been reports of PEA being investigated in clinical trials[81] and of the synthesis of PEA analogues.[82] The CB receptor antagonists developed by Sanofi have proven useful in dissecting CB-mediated effects. This is an important issue given the lack of $CB_{1/2}$ selectively of most available ligands and the early theories of nonreceptor-mediated

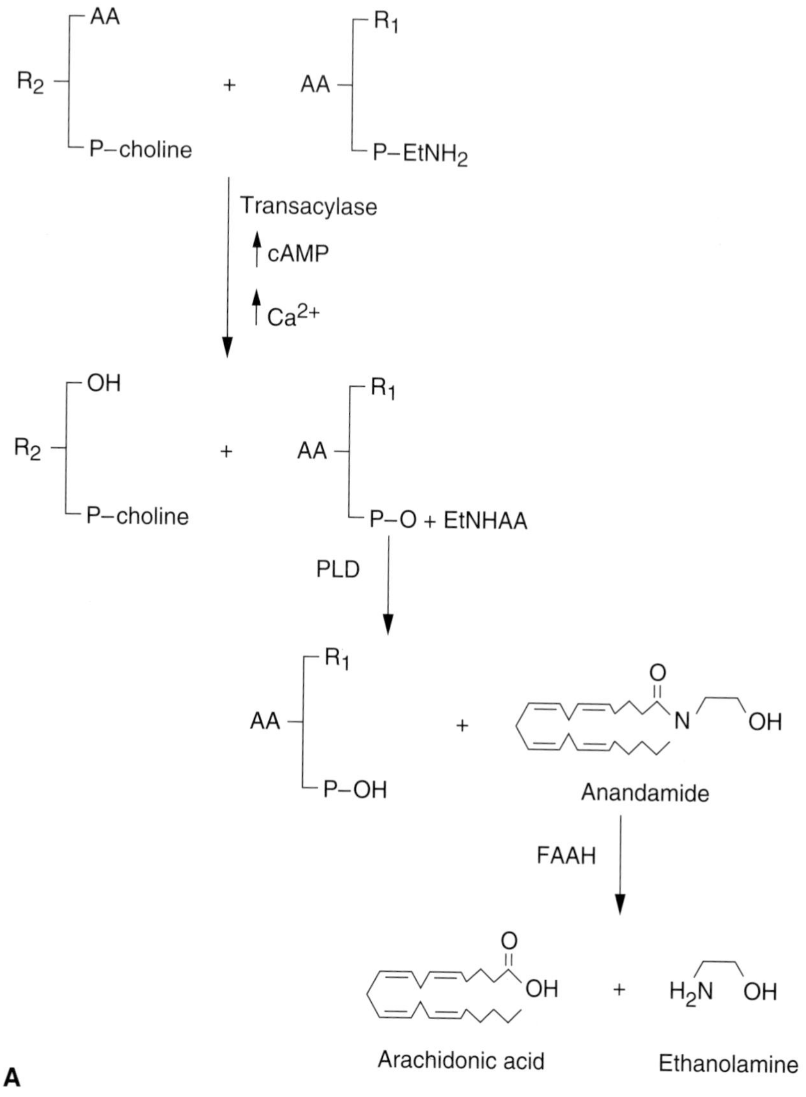

Figure 29–2. Metabolic pathways for the synthesis and degradation of the endogenous cannabinoids, anandamide, and 2-arachidonyl glycerol. *A*, Anandamide. The precursors to anandamide are the N-arachidonyl phosphatidylethanolamine (NAPE) lipids. NAPE is likely formed by a transacylation reaction between arachidonic acid (AA)–containing and phosphatidyl ethanolamine–containing lipids. NAPE levels are increased by raised cyclic adenosine monophosphate (cAMP) or intracellular calcium. Anandamide is formed by the action of a phospholipases D (PLD) on NAPE. Most anandamide appears to be degraded by fatty acid amino hydrolase (FAAH). R_1 and R_2 refer to alkyl chains of futty acid. *B*, 2-Arachidonyl glycerol (2-AG). A phospholipase C (PLC) cleaves inositol triphosphate (PI) from a phospholipid containing an AA moiety in the 2 position, leaving diacylglycerol. The diacylglycerol is then cleaved by *sn-1* diacylglycerol lipase, yielding 2-AG and a free fatty acid. Alternate pathways involving phospholipase A2 or starting with other lipids also participate. Most 2-AG is degraded by a monoacylglycerol lipase (MAG lipase); in addition, 2-AG may be degraded by FAAH and cyclooxygenase 2 (COX-2). EtNH, ethanolamine.

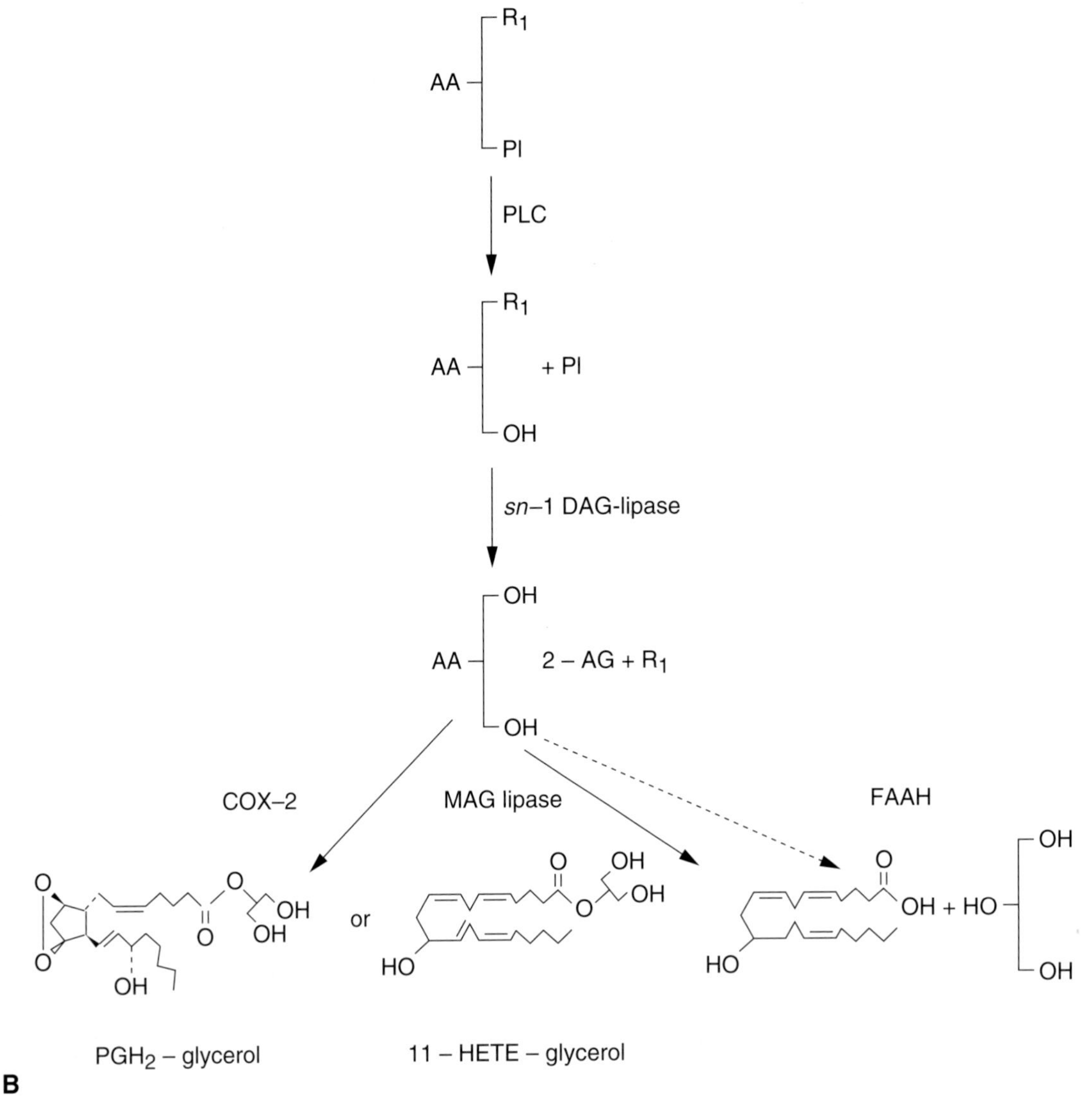

B

Figure 29–2.—*cont'd*

effects of cannabinoids. SR141716A[83,84] and SR144528[85] are competitive CB$_1$ and CB$_2$ receptor antagonists, respectively, although there is strong evidence that these compounds actually behave as inverse agonists and are capable of exerting biologic effects by suppressing constitutive activity in CB receptors.[86,87] Apart from its usefulness as a pharmacologic tool to dissect CB$_1$ receptor–mediated actions of cannabinoids, SR141716A is currently undergoing clinical trials for a variety of psychiatric disorders[71] and has also been used as a radioligand for imaging studies in primates.[88] Other CB$_1$ receptor antagonists have also been reported (e.g., LY-320135[89]).

Bioavailability, Kinetics, Metabolism, and Excretion of Plant-Derived Cannabinoids

The pharmacokinetics of plant-derived cannabinoids are complex with several issues that need to be considered.

These include the THC content of the preparation, the route of administration, the chronicity of use, and other cannabinoid compounds that may be present. Depending on the cultivar, parts of the plant included in cannabis joint, and processing, a cannabis cigarette may contain anywhere from 0.5% to 5% THC (up to 20% for hashish). It has been calculated that, at best, only 50% of the THC is absorbed when smoked. The actual value is strongly dependent on the smoking pattern. When smoked, plasma THC levels peak quickly, with maximal levels of approximately 500 nM within 5 to 10 minutes.[90] However, peak psychoactive effects lag peak plasma levels by 5 to 15 minutes. Plasma levels of Δ^9THC also decline quickly, decreased to less than 50 nM within 30 minutes of consumption of an entire joint.[90] Presumably, this reflects rapid redistribution to body lipids. However, elimination of THC metabolites is slow, with many metabolites detectable for days after consumption of a single joint.[91] When THC is taken orally, almost all of the compound is absorbed, but metabolism is significant as it passes through enterocytes and then the liver, resulting in a bioavailability of about 5%.[92] Onset of psychoactive effects

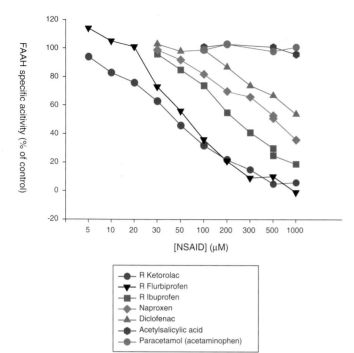

Figure 29–3. The effect of various nonsteroidal anti-inflammatory drugs (NSAIDs) on rat brain fatty acid amide hydrolase (FAAH) activity measured using anandamide as substrate. Ketorolac, flurbiprofen, and ibuprofen are particularly effective inhibitors at biologically relevant concentrations. (From Fowler CJ, Jonsson K, Tiger G: Fatty acid amid hydrolase: Biochemistry, pharmacology, and therapeutic possibilities for an enzyme hydrolysing anandamide, 2-arachidonylglycerol, palmitoylethanolamide, and oleamide. Biochem Pharm 62:517–526, 2001).

is considerably slower after oral administration compared with inhalation, occurring between 30 and 60 minutes after ingestion and peaking after 2 to 3 hours.

Cannabinoid metabolism and excretion occurs by several routes.[93] Δ^9THC is the primary psychoactive cannabinoid in cannabis preparations. Although minute quantities of Δ^8THC are also present, the pharmacology of this compound is similar to the more abundant Δ^9THC. Δ^9THC is extensively metabolized to more than 80 distinct compounds. Initial metabolism is by hydroxylation to 11-OH-Δ^9THC. This compound is approximately threefold more potent than Δ^9THC. This metabolite likely contributes to psychoactive effects when cannabis preparations are ingested because peak levels of 11-OH-Δ^9THC are greater after ingestion.[94] Subsequent metabolism is 8,11 dihydroxy THC, which is inactive. The majority of ingested THC is excreted through bile to feces as an array of metabolic products. The primary urinary metabolite is 11-*nor*-9-carboxy THC, which is also inactive. Another major constituent of cannabis preparations, cannabidiol, inhibits cytochrome P450 (CYPA1) thus impeding metabolism of THC (and many other drugs).[95] It remains controversial whether inhibition of cytochrome P450 contributes to a prolonged duration of effect in chronic cannabis users.

Analgesic Effects of Cannabinoids

As is the case for opioids, potential analgesic sites of action for cannabinoids have been identified at brain,[19,96] spinal cord, and peripheral levels. The evidence for brain-mediated analgesic effects of cannabinoids is most convincing, with good evidence suggesting that neurones in the rostroventral medulla and periaqueductal gray are involved.[70,97–99] However, in terms of developing therapeutics, the goal is to identify cannabinoids, or routes of administration, where analgesic effects can be achieved at doses not associated with troublesome psychotropic events. For this purpose, the spinal cord and periphery would appear to present better targets than the brain; therefore this chapter focuses on these aspects of cannabinoid-induced analgesia.

Spinal Mechanisms of Analgesia

CB_1 receptors have been identified in the spinal cord using autoradiography[100–103] and immunohistochemistry[19,104–106] in both rodents and primates. Detailed immunocytochemical mapping and colocalization studies using an antibody directed against the C-terminal of the CB_1 receptor has recently been published.[106] These studies reveal the presence of intense CB_1-like immunoreactivity in the superficial dorsal horn, dorsolateral funiculus, and lamina X; all areas intimately associated with the processing of nociceptive information. In the superficial dorsal horn, immunoreactivity was observed as a double band corresponding with lamina I and II_{inner}, where double-labeling studies suggest that the greatest colocalization was with markers for the central terminals of the nerve growth factor (NGF)-dependent peptidergic class of primary afferent nociceptor, at least at a laminal rather than cellular level. Although agreement exists regarding the general pattern of CB_1 expression in the spinal cord at a supracellular level, there is some uncertainty as to their exact cellular location. Current evidence suggests that there may be two distinct subpopulations of CB_1 (or CB_1-like) receptors—one on spinal interneurons and one on the central terminals of primary afferent neurones. Supporting the existence of the interneuronal expression is that CB_1 immunoreactivity is essentially unaffected by dorsal rhizotomy or rostral hemisection of the spinal cord, which, when taken together with colocalization of CB_1 for markers of spinal interneurons, suggests that some spinal CB_1 expression is on spinal interneurons.[106] This is supported by that there is minimal change in CB radioligand binding after destruction of primary afferent nociceptors by neonatal capsaicin therapy.[107] However, radioligand binding in cervical spinal cord harvested from animals subjected to more extensive rhizotomy suggests that about 50% of spinal CB_1 expression is on primary afferent neurons, but postsynaptic changes in response to such an extensive rhizotomy may have complicated this picture.[108] However, it is also clear that primary afferent neurons also express CB_1, as the gene encoding the CB_1 receptor has been identified in dorsal root ganglion cells[109] where CB_1 mRNA is also found[102] and CB radioligand binding sites are axonally transported in peripheral neurons.[77] This is further supported by a immunocytochemical study of cultured dorsal root ganglion cells with an antibody directed against the N-terminal of CB_1, CB_1-like immunoreactivity with a very high degree of colocalization with VR1-like immunoreactive small diameter cells of nociceptive phenotype[110]; however, studies using a different antibody on dorsal root ganglion tissue sections suggest a smaller percentage of small-diameter cells express CB_1 and that large-diameter cell bodies also express CB_1.[111]

Electrophysiologic studies arrive at similar conclusions with evidence of CB_1 expression on both interneurons inhibiting the release of γ-aminobutyric acid and glycine[112] and primary afferent neurons inhibiting glutamate release.[113] Further evidence of cannabinoid-evoked attenuation of neurotransmitter release from the central terminals of primary afferent nociceptors was provided by the observation that AEA prevented capsaicin and K^+-evoked release of the calcitonin gene–related peptide from primary afferent nociceptors.[114,115] Other electrophysiologic data support the concept of spinal antinociceptive effects of CBs. Noxious thermal and mechanical-evoked activity in spinal wide-dynamic-range neurons is attenuated by systemically and intrathecally administered WIN 55,212-2.[101,116,117] Systemic administration of this compound also reduced the augmented activity ("wind-up") in dorsal horn neurons evoked by a sustained noxious input.[118] Evidence of tonic modulation of spinal nociceptive systems by cannabinoids was suggested by augmentation of neuronal responses to a noxious stimulus in the presence of the CB_1 receptor antagonist SR141716A[119]; however, it is possible that these observations were a result of the inverse agonist properties of this compound as opposed to blocking the effects of endocannabinoids at this receptor.[86,87]

A compelling case for spinally mediated effects of cannabinoids is supported by the finding that systemically administered THC retains its antinociceptive properties after spinal transection.[120] Studies of spinal intrathecal administration of cannabinoids in animal models of pain adds further weight to this argument. Biodisposition studies reveal that intrathecally administered cannabinoids tend to remain at the site of action and are not rapidly redistributed to the brain.[4] Spinal intrathecal administration of the water soluble cannabinoid O-1057 has been reported to be associated with antinociception[76] and systemic administration of THC accompanied by intrathecal administration of an α_2 noradrenergic antagonists suggested that the antinociceptive effects of cannabinoids are mediated, at least partly, by an adrenergic mechanism.[121] There is also evidence that endocannabinoids regulate the effects of glutamate (*N*-methyl-D-aspartate)-mediated central sensitization.[122] Hargreaves and colleagues[100] have demonstrated that intrathecal administration of AEA blocked the thermal hyperalgesia associated with carrageenan injection to the skin of the hind paw at doses that did not alter sensory thresholds to noxious heat in the absence of inflammation. Similarly, intrathecal administration of Win 55,212-2 reversed the mechanical allodynia and prevented the appearance of Fos-like immunoreactivity in spinal neurons, which follows subcutaneous injection of complete Freund's adjuvant into the hindpaw.[123] The precise function of Fos protein in the spinal cord is unknown, but

the appearance of this product of the early/immediate gene *c-fos* is widely held to be a marker of persistent activation of spinal nociceptive systems.[124] Prevention of the appearance of Fos immunoreactivity in the dorsal horn after vesical inflammation,[125] or subcutaneous formalin injection[126] by systemic administration of Win 55,212-2, AEA, or PEA has been demonstrated. Spinal intrathecal administration of Win 55,212-2 has also been shown to reverse the mechanical hyperalgesia that is associated with the partial sciatic nerve ligation model of neuropathic pain.[127]

Peripheral Mechanisms of Analgesia

There is an increasing body of evidence supporting the hypothesis of a peripheral analgesic action of cannabinoids, particularly during inflammation. This presents an obvious target for the development of cannabinoid-based analgesics that are largely devoid of centrally mediated psychotropic effects. The primary line of evidence comes from studies that have demonstrated analgesic effects of locally delivered cannabinoids at doses that were not systemically effective. For example, locally administered AEA (0.01 ng) attenuated carrageenan-induced thermal hyperalgesia and cutaneous edema, the effect of AEA was sensitive to the CB_1 receptor antagonist SR141716A, but CB_2 effects were not investigated.[115] Calcitonin gene–related peptide release studies suggest that one mechanism for this effect may be that cannabinoids prevent neuropeptide release from primary afferent neurones, which not only locally contributes to primary hyperalgesia[6,7,114,128] but also centrally through release of neuropeptides from the central terminals of primary afferent nociceptors.[115] In the formalin model of cutaneous inflammatory hyperalgesia, Piomelli and colleagues have shown that local administration of Win 55,212-2, HU210, and methanandamide attenuated both phases of the behavioral response to subcutaneous formalin injection, through a CB_1 but not CB_2 or opioid receptor–mediated mechanism.[52] AEA was similarly active, although only for the first phase of the behavioral response, probably reflecting its rapid degradation. PEA also reduced both phases of the response, but by a CB_2-like not CB_1-mediated mechanism. Peripheral analgesia effects of cannabinoids have also been reported in neuropathic pain models.[127] Further circumstantial support for a peripheral analgesic effect of cannabinoids in neuropathy was provided by a preliminary report indicating that systemically administered PEA is effective at reducing mechanical hyperalgesia in a model of neuropathic pain, but the mechanism of this effect was not elucidated.[129]

The mechanisms of these peripheral analgesic actions are not completely understood, but they appear to be related to the well-known anti-inflammatory effects of cannabinoids.[6,7,128] Certainly there is evidence that both CB_2 and CB_1 receptors are present locally and the mechanisms for synthesizing, releasing, and inactivating endocannabinoids are present during inflammation, as discussed earlier. The pivotal role of the neurotrophin NGF in inflammatory hyperalgesia is well established, and the endocannabinoid apparatus is strategically placed to physiologically modulate these effects. Such an interaction could provide an explanation for the mechanism of the antihyperalgesic effects of cannabinoids during inflammation.[7,128] To discuss this hypothesis, the evidence supporting a key role for NGF in inflammatory hyperalgesia must be briefly examined.

Direct sensitization of primary afferent nociceptors through the high-affinity NGF receptor (tyrosine kinase A [trkA]), which is selectively expressed on primary afferent nociceptors, is probably the major event underlying NGF-evoked hyperalgesia. After ligand binding, the NGF/trkA complex is rapidly internalized and transported to the dorsal root ganglia, where it exerts profound effects on cellular process, particularly on the synthesis of peptide neurotransmitters, receptors, and ion channels.[130] NGF also regulates the spinal expression of another neurotrophin, brain-derived neurotrophic factor, which modulates *N*-methyl-D-aspartate receptor–induced central sensitization.[131] However, many of the features of NGF-induced hyperalgesia are observed before axonal transport of the NGF/trkA complex has occurred, therefore other locally mediated events, such as receptor phosphorylation, may be responsible for the initial phase of NGF-induced hyperalgesia. NGF appears to up-regulate the binding sites for, and responsiveness of nociceptors to, several molecules of known importance in inflammatory hyperalgesia, including the potent algogen bradykinin,[132] $Na_v1.8$-type sodium channels,[133] and the noxious heat-gated VR1, which participates in mediating the effects of protons and capsaicin.[134] Not only is direct interaction with sensory neurons important to the NGF-evoked component of inflammatory hyperalgesia, but the role of immune cells must also be considered.[135] Mast cells appear to be particularly important in this regard, because they effectively amplify the NGF signal by degranulating in response to NGF activation of mast cell-expressed trkA receptors and releasing other prohyperalgesic mediators (e.g., serotonin), which, in turn, sensitize sensory neurons.[128,136–138] In addition, in a positive feedback process, mast cells synthesize and release further NGF during degranulation, thus further amplifying the biologic signal.[136,139] The hyperalgesic response to NGF is attenuated in animals prophylactically treated with a mast cell degranulating compound.[135]

The evidence for CB_1 expression in primary afferent nociceptors has been already discussed in detail, but notably, the gene encoding the CB_1 receptor has been identified in dorsal root ganglion cells that are NGF-dependent[109] and there is evidence suggesting that endocannabinoids suppress expression of trk receptors, at least in vitro.[140] Also, CB_1 receptor expression colocalizes in the same regions of the spinal dorsal horn as the central terminals of the NGF-dependent peptidergic class of primary afferent neurons.[106]

Further support for the hypothesis of local cannabinoid modulation of the NGF-driven aspects of inflammatory hyperalgesia is provided by examining the role of mast cell CB_2 receptors.[141] Both CB_2 and trkA have been identified on mast cells[128,141] and, as discussed earlier, mast cells amplify the NGF signal during inflammation. What are the biologic controls on this process? Certainly, there is mounting evidence that the PEA attenuates this amplification of NGF effects by participating in the process dubbed "autacoid local inflammation antagonism."[141] PEA accumulates in inflamed tissue, prevents mast cell degranulation, and suppresses inflammatory hyperalgesia and edema, although the

exact role of CB_2 receptors in this process in unclear and is discussed elsewhere in this chapter.[141,142]

Attenuation of other proinflammatory hyperalgesia processes by endocannabinoids probably contributes to the local analgesic effects of cannabinoids during inflammation; for example, we have shown that cutaneous NGF-induced thermal hyperalgesia and the associated neutrophil accumulation are diminished by endocannabinoids.[36,143] Also, the CB_2-mediated cannabinoid attenuation of nitric oxide from macrophages when stimulated by lipopolysaccharide has been demonstrated.[144] The effects of Win 55,212-2 in these cells was shown to be antagonized by SR144528, suggesting CB_2-mediated effects, whereas that of PEA was not. Cannabinoids also have profound effects on cytokine production, although the direction of such effects is variable and is not always mediated by cannabinoid receptors.[145]

Endogenous Analgesic Tone

Several reports have suggested the presence of a physiologic analgesic tone exerted by the endocannabinoid system. This hypothesis is predominately based on studies in which SR141716A was administered to experimental animals and signs of increased pain-related behavior were observed. For example, when SR141716A was administered to rodents, thermal nociceptive thresholds were reduced,[122,146] and the behavioral signs related to formalin injection were prolonged and enhanced.[26,148] Intrathecal injection of SR141716A increased the number of Fos-like–immunoreactive neurons in the spinal cord of both healthy and inflamed rats.[123] Similar findings have been reported for the chronic constriction injury model of painful neuropathy,[148] and Chapman showed that SR141716A, but not SR144528, selectively facilitated nociceptive responses of dorsal horn neurons in the rat.[119] These observations are further supported by the observation that thermal nociceptive thresholds were elevated after intrathecal injection of anti-CB_1 oligonucleotide.[122] Arguing against the hypothesis of endogenous tone, it should be noted that these findings for SR141716A have not been replicated by others who examined the response to administration of this antagonist in the formalin or arthritis models of persistent inflammation nor in the spinal nerve ligation model of neuropathic pain.[149–151] Also in the original characterization study, SR141716A failed to evoke any changes in murine behavioral models of nociception (e.g., tail-flick latency).[84] It is also possible that the observations related to SR141716A administration, which have been used to support the hypothesis of endogenous tone, are attributable to its inverse agonist properties (see earlier) rather than blocking of any endogenous tone. Furthermore, the levels of endocannabinoids present in formalin-treated tissue do not differ significantly from control-treated tissue, suggesting that they are insufficient to activate CB receptors.[151] Finally, two studies using "knockout" mice in which the gene encoding the cannabinoid CB_1 receptor was disrupted did not confirm results of studies in which SR141716A was used to "block" the putative endogenous tone, although of course the obfuscating effect of developmental compensation for the lack of the *CB1* gene by other systems in these mice cannot be excluded.[23,24] The attractive hypothesis of an endogenous cannabinoid analgesic tone thus remains unproven.

Interactions with Other Systems

Opioid

Although it is clear that the endocannabinoid and opioids systems are biologically distinct, it does appear that there is a degree of interaction at a functional level. Although naloxone generally does not antagonize the antinociceptive effect of THC, antagonists at certain opioid receptors subtypes (e.g., kappa) do block the analgesic effects of THC.[4] Furthermore, certain cannabinoids (e.g., THC, CP55,940) provoke dynorphin and enkephalin release.[152] Recent data from experiments using CB_1 knockout mice indicate that although the endocannabinoid system does not participate in the analgesic response to exogenously administered opioids, it is necessary for activation of stress-induced opioid analgesia.[153] However, detailed review of this complex area is outside the scope of this chapter but is available elsewhere.[4,152,154]

Noradrenaline and Serotonin

Noradrenaline is a neurotransmitter in the descending control of nociception,[155] and the antinociceptive effects of cannabinoids are reduced by perturbation of noradrenergic neurotransmission.[4] This appears to be an α_2 effect, because the α_2 antagonist yohimbine blocks the antinociceptive effects of THC at a spinal level, whereas the serotonergic and α_1 adrenergic systems do not seem to influence cannabinoid-induced analgesia.[121]

Studies in Models of Human Disease

There is ample evidence of cannabinoid-induced antinociceptive activity in animal models in which a physiologic response to an ephemeral noxious stimulus (e.g., the tail-flick test) was examined.[4] However, these models are rather poor reflections of the clinical state, when the excitability of a dynamic nervous system is considerably altered by the consequences of tissue inflammation or peripheral nerve injury.[151,155,156] To obtain a better prediction of clinical usefulness, it is necessary to examine the analgesic effect of cannabinoids in animal models that encompass a significant persistent inflammatory or peripheral nerve injury component. These are discussed in this chapter under three main headings: persistent somatic inflammation, persistent visceral inflammation, and peripheral nerve injury (neuropathic pain).

Persistent Somatic Inflammation

The behavioral response to a dilute formalin injection into the skin of the rodent hind paw is a widely used model of

persistent cutaneous inflammatory pain.[157-159] After injection, a characteristic biphasic behavioral response is observed: the first phase lasts about 15 minutes and is thought to represent the acute response to the injection of a noxious chemical. This is followed, after a short quiescent phase, by a second response that lasts about 50 minutes and represents sensitization of primary afferent and spinal components of the nociceptive "pathway." AEA and PEA have been shown to dose-dependently attenuate the second phase of this response in the rat.[142] Endocannabinoid tissue concentrations are not increased in this model, indicating an absence of a local endocannabinoid effect,[151] but formalin injection is associated with release of AEA in the periaqueductal gray matter of the brain.[48] These findings of analgesic activity in the formalin test have been confirmed for Win 55,212-2, methanandamide and HU 210, and a CB_1-mediated effect was identified.[26] In the latter study, the effects of AEA were restricted to the first phase of the behavioral response, probably reflecting its limited duration of action. PEA attenuated both phases of the response and its effects were blocked by SR144528 rather than SR141716A, indicating a CB_2-like mediated response. Others have shown that the CB_2 agonist HU 308 reduces the second phase of the formalin test by an SR144528-sensitive mechanism[79] and that formalin behavior and the associated increase in the number of dorsal horn cells staining immunopositive for Fos protein are attenuated by WIN 55,212-2.[126]

After carrageenan injection to the skin, there is a reduction in the limb withdrawal threshold to noxious thermal stimulus, indicating the development of a thermal hyperalgesia.[160] Locally administered AEA attenuates this effect, through a CB_1-mediated mechanism, although CB_2-mediated effects were not assessed. Similar effects have been described for the hyperalgesia that is associated with capsaicin injection.[161] The mechanical hyperalgesia and spinal Fos expression related to cutaneous injection of complete Freund's adjuvant is similarly attenuated by intrathecal administration of Win 55,212-2.[123] There is also evidence that AEA attenuates NGF-induced hyperalgesia in the skin.[36,162]

Persistent Visceral Inflammation

Visceral and somatic pain differ significantly in their clinical and pathophysiologic aspects, which predicates that each requires study using appropriate models.[163] The effects of cannabinoids in persistent visceral pain have been studied in a model of cystitis that shares features of a more persistent condition, interstitial cystitis.[125,128,143,164,165] In this model, inflammation is accompanied by:

1. An increase in excitability of the spinal reflexes that control micturition (viscero-visceral hyper-reflexia)[166]
2. Sensitization of primary afferent neurons[167,168]
3. Dorsal horn neuronal sensitization[168]
4. Referred hyperalgesia[169,170]
5. An increase in the number of dorsal horn neurons displaying Fos-like immunoreactivity[171-173]

Cannabinoids (AEA, PEA, and Win 55,212-2) attenuate the viscero-visceral hyper-reflexia, spinal Fos expression, and referred hyperalgesia associated with cystitis at doses that do not interfere with normal micturition[165,174] (Farquhar-Smith WP, Jaggar SI, Rice ASC, unpublished data). We have also shown that NGF is crucial to the development of inflammatory hyperalgesia in this model,[7,128,169,175,176] and the evidence of endocannabinoid involvement in the modulation of the NGF-driven components of inflammatory hyperalgesia has already been discussed. Both AEA and PEA dose-dependently prevent the viscero-visceral hyper-reflexia associated with NGF treatment of the urinary bladder.[177] The effects of AEA are reversed by SR141716A and partially by SR144528 implying that its effects may be mediated by both CB_1 and CB_2 receptors. The antihyperalgesic effect of PEA is only antagonized by SR144528, further supporting a CB_2-like effect of PEA. In support of this, we have also obtained preliminary evidence that the appearance of Fos protein in the spinal dorsal horn after NGF treatment of bladder is prevented by cannabinoids.[125]

Neuropathic Pain

The chronic pain that occasionally follows peripheral nerve injury differs fundamentally from inflammatory pain and is an area of considerable unmet therapeutic need.[150] Although controversial, it is generally accepted that opioid analgesics are less effective when used to treat neuropathic compared with inflammatory pain. One explanation is that after peripheral nerve injury there is a depletion of opioid receptor expression in the spinal dorsal horn.[107,178,179] Destruction of primary sensory afferent input to the dorsal horn, by dorsal rhizotomy[106] or neonatal capsaicin therapy,[107] is not associated with such a depletion of CB_1 receptor–like immunoreactivity or binding, thus giving cannabinoids a potential therapeutic advantage over cannabinoids in neuropathic pain.

The effectiveness of cannabinoids has been examined in several animal models of neuropathic pain: Win 55,212-2 attenuated the thermal hyperalgesia and the mechanical and cold allodynia, which developed 8 days after chronic constriction injury of the rat sciatic nerve.[148] Antagonism of the effects of Win 55,212-2 by SR141716A confirmed CB_1-mediated effects, but CB_2 effects were not excluded. However, there is a significant inflammatory component to most of the neuropathic pain models in common use (particularly in the chronic constriction injury model) and the anti-inflammatory effects of cannabinoids may have obfuscated any true antineuropathy effects.[180–182] Therefore, we have investigated Win 55,212-2 in the spinal nerve ligation model, which may be associated with a lesser inflammatory component.[183] Systemic administration of Win 55,212-2 dose-dependently reversed the thermal hyperalgesia and the mechanical and cold allodynia by a CB_1, but not CB_2-mediated, effect. Similar results have been described for the partial sciatic nerve ligation model for Win 55,212-2, CP55,940, and HU210.[127] The effect of Win 55,212-2 was antagonized by a CB_1 receptor antagonist, but the possibility of CB_2-mediated effects were not examined. The effectiveness of Win 55,212-2 after intrathecal and peripheral administration (in doses not systemically active) were also reported in that article, suggesting that a potential peripheral site of action may be exploited to divorce the psychotropic

effects of cannabinoids from their analgesic effects. However, the extent to which the inherent inflammation involved in this model obfuscates this finding is currently unclear. A preliminary report has shown that PEA reduces the mechanical hyperalgesia in the chronic sciatic nerve constriction model, and although the role of cannabinoid receptors in this effect were not investigated, it does lend some weight to the arguments supporting a possible peripheral CB_2-like analgesic effect of PEA in neuropathic pain[129]; these findings are supported by clinical trial data (see later).

Clinical Evidence of Analgesia

In contrast to the strong preclinical data, the clinical evidence supporting cannabinoid-induced analgesia is of insufficient quality to support or refute the basic scientific data.[10–13,184] The anecdotal nature, low quality, or limited power of those studies that have been reported predicates that they would not be acceptable as evidence of benefit by today's standards.[12,13] No reports of studies examining cannabinoids in modern human volunteer models of pain, as opposed to acute nociception, have been located. However, the effect of intravenous THC on nociceptive thresholds in dental patients has been reported and no significant effect has been noted, although the methodology makes it difficult to draw conclusions from this study.[185]

Most of those small clinical trials that have been reported examined the efficacy of drugs such as THC or levonantradol and indicated that analgesia was only possible at doses that were associated with unacceptable CNS-mediated side effects. For example, in a small trial of intramuscular levonantradol in postoperative pain, levonantradol (1.5–3 mg) was superior to placebo, but a dose response could not be demonstrated and the drug was associated with an unacceptable side effect profile.[78] Study of the analgesic effects of oral THC in a small number of patients with cancer pain revealed that 20 mg THC was equianalgesic to 120 mg codeine, but was associated with unacceptable side effects.[186,187] Both codeine and THC were associated with analgesia superior to that afforded by placebo. A systematic review of the limited clinical data has been reported, but the manner in which the outcomes were reported in the constituent studies dictated that this could only be interpreted in a *qualitative* fashion.[188] However, it was concluded that the cannabinoids that had been examined in these studies possessed an insufficiently broad therapeutic index to be useful as analgesics, at least for acute pain management. Therefore, clinical availability of cannabinoids with a favorable side effect profile is required before this issue can be examined further. One candidate for such a role is PEA. An unconfirmed report of a large clinical trial undertaken in patients with sciatica compared the effectiveness of 300 or 600 mg/day oral PEA with placebo is interesting, but the lack of formal publication precludes assessment of the trial's quality.[81] PEA was more effective at reducing pain intensity scores than placebo and there was evidence of a dose/response relationship. This suggests that peripherally acting cannabinoid-type analgesic are effective analgesic for neuropathic pain and may provide a method of divorcing psychotropic effects from analgesia, although, as discussed earlier, the contribution of cannabinoid receptors to PEA-induced analgesia is unclear.

Well-designed clinical trails are therefore required, but are currently premature until a suitable cannabinoid, with a satisfactory therapeutic window for analgesia (especially as far as psychotropic side effect are concerned) that is of proven bioavailability when administered by a practical route, is available for human study. PEA fulfills some of these criteria, but the extent to which its actions are mediated by cannabinoid receptors is unclear. Furthermore, such trials should be performed in an area of therapeutic need (e.g., neuropathic pain) or where the anti-inflammatory or antiemetic effects of cannabinoids may confer an additional benefit over existing therapies.[184]

Conclusion

There is a wealth of strong laboratory evidence supporting the concept of cannabinoid-induced analgesia, but the corresponding clinical evidence to support this hypothesis is not currently available. Before gathering such clinical evidence can be attempted, two major issues must be resolved: first, the development of cannabinoids with predictable bioavailability suitable for practical human administration; and second, the development of cannabinoid analgesics with a suitable therapeutic ratio, with brain-mediated side effects being a particular problem. One way of addressing this latter issue may be to target sites of action remote from the brain (e.g., spinal cord or periphery) or by enhancing the activity of endocannabinoids by inhibiting their degradation in areas of nerve injury where they are selectively elevated.

Acknowledgment

Some sections of this chapter have been previously published in review form.

References

1. Baker D, Pryce G, Croxford JL, et al: Cannabinoids control spasticity and tremor in a multiple sclerosis model. Nature 404:84–87, 2000.
2. Tramer M, Carroll D, Campbell F, et al: Cannabinoids for control of chemotherapy induced nausea and vomiting: Quantitative systematic review. BMJ 323:16–20, 2001.
3. Calignano A, Katona I, Desarnaud F, et al: Bidirectional control of airway responsiveness by endogenous cannabinoids. Nature 408:96–101, 2000.
4. Martin BR, Lichtman AH: Cannabinoid transmission and pain perception. Neurobiol Dis 5:447–461, 1998.
5. Pertwee RG: Cannabinoids and pain. Prog Neurobiol 63:569–611, 2001.
6. Rice ASC: Cannabinoids and pain. Curr Opin Invest Drugs 2:399–414, 2001.
7. Rice ASC: Mechanisms of inflammatory pain: Role of neurotrophins and cannabinoids. In Soulsby L, Morton D: Pain: Nature and Management in Man and Animals. London, Royal Society of Medicine Press, 35–45, 2001.
8. Iversen L: The Science of Marijuana. Oxford, Oxford University Press, 2000.
9. Zias J, Stark H, Sellgman J, et al: Early medical use of cannabis. Nature 363:215, 1993.
10. American Medical Association. Medical Marijuana, 1997.
11. Select Committee on Science and Technology & House of Lords: Cannabis. The scientific and medical evidence. 1998.
12. Lachmann PJ, Edwards JG, Pertwee RG, et al: The Use of Cannabis and Its Derivatives for Medical and Recreational Purposes. London, The Royal Society/The Academy of Medical Sciences, 1998, p 8.
13. Ashton CH: Therapeutic Uses of Cannabis. Harwood, Amsterdam, British Medical Association, 1997.
14. Roth SH: Stereospecific presynaptic inhibitory effect of delta9-tetrahydrocannabinol on cholinergic transmission in the myenteric plexus of the guinea pig. Can J Physiol Pharmacol 56:968–975, 1978.
15. Howlett AC, Fleming RM: Cannabinoid inhibition of adenylate cyclase. Pharmacology of the response in neuroblastoma cell membranes. Mol Pharmacol 26:532–538, 1984.
16. Devane WA, Dysarz FA 3rd, Johnson MR, et al: Determination and characterization of a cannabinoid receptor in rat brain. Mol Pharmacol 34:605–613, 1988.
17. Herkenham M, Lynn AB, Little MD, et al: Cannabinoid receptor localization in brain. Proc Natl Acad Sci USA 87:1932–1936, 1990.
18. Herkenham M, Lynn AB, de Costa BR, Richfield EK: Neuronal localization of cannabinoid receptors in the basal ganglia of the rat. Brain Res 547:267–274, 1991.
19. Tsou K, Brown S, Mackie K, et al: Immunohistochemical distribution of cannabinoid CB1 receptors in the rat central nervous system. Neuroscience 83:393–411, 1998.
20. Katona I, Sperlagh B, Sik A, et al: Presynaptically located CB1 cannabinoid receptors regulate GABA release from axon terminals of specific hippocampal interneurons. J Neurosci 19:4544–4559, 1999.
21. Matsuda LA, Lolait SJ, Brownstein MJ, et al: Structure of a cannabinoid receptor and functional expression of the cloned cDNA. Nature 346:561–564, 1990.
22. Matsuda LA, Bonner TI, Lolait SJ: Localization of cannabinoid receptor mRNA in rat brain. J Comp Neurol 327:535–550, 1993.
23. Ledent C, Valverde O, Cossu G, et al: Unresponsiveness to cannabinoids and reduced addictive effects of opiates in CB1 receptor knock-out mice. Science 283:401–404, 1999.
24. Zimmer A, Zimmer AM, Hohmann AG, et al: Increased mortality, hypoactivity, and hypoalgesia in cannabinoid CB1 receptor knockout mice. Proc Natl Acad Sci USA 96:5780–5785, 1999.
25. Munro S, Thomas KL, Abu-Shaar M: Molecular characterization of a peripheral receptor for cannabinoids. Nature 365:61–65, 1993.
26. Calignano A, La Rana G, Giuffrida A, Piomelli D: Control of pain initiation by endogenous cannabinoids. Nature 394:277–281, 1998.
27. Mu J, Zhuang SY, Hampson RE, Deadwyler SA: Protein kinase-dependent phosphorylation and cannabinoid receptor modulation of potassium A current (IA) in cultured rat hippocampal neurons. Pflugers Arch 439:541–546, 2000.
28. Bouaboula M, Poinot-Chazel C, Bourrie B, et al: Activation of mitogen-activated protein kinases by stimulation of the central cannabinoid receptor CB1. Biochem J 312:637–641, 1995.
29. Mackie K, Hille B: Cannabinoids inhibit N-type calcium channels in neuroblastoma-glioma cells. Proc Natl Acad Sci USA 89:3825–3829, 1992.
30. Mackie K, Lai Y, Westenbroek R, Mitchell R: Cannabinoids activate an inwardly rectifying potassium conductance and inhibit Q-type calcium currents in AtT20 cells transfected with rat brain cannabinoid receptor. J Neurosci 15:6552–6561, 1995.
31. Twitchell W, Brown S, Mackie K: Cannabinoids inhibit N- and P/Q-type calcium channels in cultured rat hippocampal neurons. J Neurophysiol 78:43–50, 1997.
32. Guzman M, Galve-Roperh I, Sanchez C: Ceramide: A new second messenger of cannabinoid action. Trends Pharmacol Sci 22:19–22, 2001.
33. Rueda D, Galve-Roperh I, Haro A, Guzman M: The CB(1) cannabinoid receptor is coupled to the activation of c-Jun N-terminal kinase. Mol Pharmacol 58:814–820, 2000.
34. Azad SC, Marsicano G, Eberlein I, et al: Differential role of the nitric oxide pathway on delta(9)-THC-induced central nervous system effects in the mouse. Eur J Neurosci 13:561–568, 2001.
35. Breivogel CS, Griffin G, Di Marzo V, Martin BR: Evidence for a new G-protein coupled cannabinoid receptor in mouse brain. Mol Pharmacol 60:155–163, 2001.

36. Farquhar-Smith WP, Rice ASC: Palmitoylethanolamide (PEA) attenuates NGF-induced hyperalgesia by reducing neutrophil accumulation via cannabinoid CB2-like receptors. Soc Neurosci Abstr (in press).

37. Di Marzo V, Deutsch DG: Biochemistry of the endogenous ligands of cannabinoid receptors. Neurobiol Dis 5:386–404, 1998.

38. Devane WA, et al: Isolation and structure of a brain constituent that binds to the cannabinoid receptor. Science 258:1946–1949, 1992.

39. Di Marzo V, Fontana A, Cadas H, et al: kL Formation and inactivation of endogenous cannabinoid anandamide in central neurons. Nature 372:686–691, 1994.

40. Beltramo M, Stella N, Calignano A, et al: Functional role of high-affinity anandamide transport, as revealed by selective inhibition. Science 277:1094–1097, 1997.

41. Deutsch DG, Chin SA: Enzymatic synthesis and degradation of anandamide, a cannabinoid receptor agonist. Biochem Pharmacol 46:791–796, 1993.

42. Mackie K, Devane WA, Hille B: Anandamide, an endogenous cannabinoid, inhibits calcium currents as a partial agonist in N18 neuroblastoma cells. Mol Pharmacol 44:498–503, 1993.

43. Gonsiorek W, Lunn C, Fan X, et al: Endocannabinoid 2-arachidonyl glycerol is a full agonist through human type 2 cannabinoid receptor: Antagonism by anandamide. Mol Pharmacol 57:1045–1050, 2000.

44. De Petrocellis L, Bisogno T, Davis JB, et al: Overlap between the ligand recognition properties of the anandamide transporter and the VR1 vanilloid receptor: Inhibitors of anandamide uptake with negligible capsaicin-like activity. FEBS Lett 483:52–56, 2000.

45. Maingret F, Patel AJ, Lazdunski M, Honore E: The endocannabinoid anandamide is a direct and selective blocker of the background K(+) channel TASK-1. Embo J 20:47–54, 2001.

46. Stella N, Schweitzer P, Piomelli D: A second endogenous cannabinoid that modulates long-term potentiation. Nature 388:773–778, 1997.

47. Giuffrida et al: 1999.

48. Walker JM, Huang SM, Strangman NM, et al: Pain modulation by release of the endogenous cannabinoid anandamide. Proc Natl Acad Sci USA 96:12198–12203, 1999.

49. Hanus L, Abu-Lafi S, Fride E, et al: 2-arachidonyl glyceryl ether, an endogenous agonist of the cannabinoid CB1 receptor. Proc Natl Acad Sci USA 98:3662–3665, 2001.

50. Lambert DM, Vandevoorde S, Govaerts SJ, et al: Anticonvulsant activity of palmitoylethanolamide, a putative endocannabinoid, in mice. Epilepsia 42:321–327, 2001.

51. Lambert DM, Vandevoorde S, Jonsson K, Fowler CJ: The palmitoylethanolamide family: A new class of anti-inflammatory agent? Curr Med Chem 45:1748–1756, 2002.

52. Calignano A, La Rana G, Piomelli D: Antinocieptive activity of the endogenous fatty acid amide, palmitoylethanolamide. Eur J Pharmacol 419:191–198, 2001.

53. Kreitzer AC, Regehr WG: Retrograde inhibition of presynaptic calcium influx by endogenous cannabinoids at excitatory synapses onto purkinje cells. Neuron 29:717–727, 2001.

54. Maejima T, Ohno-Shosaku T, Kano M: Endogenous cannabinoid as a retrograde messenger from depolarized postsynaptic neurons to presynaptic terminals. Neurosci Res 40:205–210, 2001.

55. Wilson RI, Nicoll RA: Endogenous cannabinoids mediate retrograde signaling at hippocampal synapses. Nature 410:588–592, 2001.

56. Cadas H, Gaillet S, Beltramo M, et al: Biosynthesis of an endogenous cannabinoid precursor in neurons and its control by calcium and cAMP. J Neurosci 16:3934–3942, 1996.

57. Hillard CJ: Biochemistry and pharmacology of the endocannabinoids arachidonylethanolamide and 2-arachidonylglycerol. Prostaglandins Other Lipid Mediat 61:3–18, 2000.

58. Cravatt BF, Giang DK, Mayfield SP, et al: Molecular characterization of an enzyme that degrades neuromodulatory fatty-acid amides. Nature 384:83–87, 1996.

59. Ueda N, Puffenbarger RA, Yamamoto S, Deutsch DG: The fatty acid amide hydrolase (FAAH). Chem Phys Lipids 108:107–121, 2000.

60. Ueda N, Yamanaka K, Terasawa Y, Yamamoto S: An acid amidase hydrolyzing anandamide as an endogenous ligand for cannabinoid receptors. FEBS Lett 454:267–270, 1999.

61. Deutsch DG, Glaser ST, Howell JM, et al: The cellular uptake of anandamide is coupled to its breakdown by fatty-acid amide hydrolase. J Biol Chem 276:6967–6973, 2001.

62. Tiger G, Stenstrom A, Fowler CJ: Pharmacological properties of rat brain fatty acid amidohydrolase in different subcellular fractions using palmitoylethanolamide as substrate. Biochem Pharmacol 59:647–653, 2000.

63. Jacobsson SOP, Fowler CJ: Characterization of palmitoylethanolamide transport in mouse neuro-2a neuroblastoma cells and rat RBL-2H3 basophilic leukaemia cells: Comparison with anandamide. Br J Pharmacol 132:1743–1754, 2001.

64. Holt S, Nilsson J, Omier R, et al: Effects of pH on the inhibition of fatty acid amidohydrolase by ibuprofen. Br J Pharmacol 133:513–520, 2001.

65. Fowler CJ: Ibuprofen inhibits rat brain deamidation of anandamide at pharmacologically relevant concentrations. Mode of inhibition and structure-activity relationship. J Pharmacol Exp Ther 283:729–734, 1997.

66. Fowler CJ, Janson U, Johnson RM, et al: Inhibition of anandamide hydrolysis by the enantiomers of ibuprofen, ketorolac and flurbiprofen. Arch Biochem Biophys 362:191–196, 1999.

67. Fowler CJ, Stenstrom A, Tiger G: Ibuprofen inhibits the metabolism of the endogenous cannabimimetic agent anandamide. Pharmacol Toxicol 80:103–107, 1997.

68. Gaoni Y, Mechoulam R: Isolation, structure and partial synthesis of an active constituent of hashish. J Am Chem Soc 86:1646–1647, 1964.

69. Harvey DJ: Absorption, distribution, and biotransformation of the cannabinoids. In Nahas GG, Sutin KM, Harvey DJ, Agurell S (eds): Marihuana and Medicine. Totowa, N.J., Humana Press, 1999. pp 91–103.

70. Walker LA, Harland EC, Best AM, ElSohly MA: Delta^9 THC hemisuccinate in suppository form as an alternative to oral and smoked THC. In Nahas GG, Sutin KM, Harvey DJ, Agurell S (eds): Totowa, N.J., Human Press, 1999, pp 123–135.

71. Barth F: Cannabinoid receptor agonists and antagonists. Exp Opin Ther Patents 8:301–313, 1998.

72. Pertwee RG: Pharmacology of cannabinoid CB1 and CB2 receptors. Pharmacol Ther 74:129–180, 1997.

73. Mechoulam et al:

74. Ross RA, Brockie HC, Stevenson LA, et al: Agonist-inverse agonist characterization at CB1 and CB2 cannabinoid receptors of L759633, L759656, and AM630. Br J Pharmacol 126:665–672, 1999.

75. Huffman JW: The search for selective ligands for the CB2 receptor. Curr Pharm Des 6:1323–1337, 2000.

76. Pertwee RG, Gibson TM, Stevenson LA, et al: O-1057, a potent water-soluble cannabinoid receptor agonist with antinociceptive properties. Br J Pharmacol 129:1577–1584, 2000.

77. Hohmann AG, Herkenham M: Cannabinoid receptors undergo axonal flow in sensory nerves. Neuroscience 92:1171–1175, 1999.

78. Jain AK, Ryan JR, McMahon FG, Smith G: Evaluation of intramuscular levonantradol and placebo in acute postoperative pain. J Clin Pharmacol 21:320S-326S, 1981.

79. Hanus L, Breuer A, Tchilibon S, et al: HU 308: A specific agonist for CB(2), a peripheral cannabinoid receptor. Proc Natl Acad Sci USA 96:14228–14233, 1999.

80. Gallant M, Dufresne C, Gareau Y, et al: New class of potent ligands for the human peripheral cannabinoid receptor. Bioorg Med Chem Lett 6:2263–2268, 1996.

81. Jack DB: Aliamides: A new approach to the treatment of inflammation. Drugs News Perspect 9:93–98, 1996.

82. Lambert DM, DiPaolo FG, Sonveaux P, et al: Analogues and homologues of N-palmitoylethanolamide, a putative endogenous CB(2) cannabinoid, as potential ligands for the cannabinoid receptors. Biochim Biophys Acta 1440:266–274, 1999.

83. Compton DR, Aceto MD, Lowe J, Martin BR: In vivo characterization of a specific cannabinoid receptor antagonist (SR141716A): Inhibition of delta 9-tetrahydrocannabinol-induced responses and apparent agonist activity. J Pharmacol Exp Ther 277:586–594, 1996.

84. Rinaldi Carmona M, Barth F, Heaulme M, et al: Biochemical and pharmacological characterization of SR141716A, the first potent and selective brain cannabinoid receptor antagonist. Life Sci 56:1941–1947, 1995.

85. Rinaldi Carmona M, Barth F, et al: SR 144528, the first potent and selective antagonist of the CB2 cannabinoid receptor. J Pharmacol Exp Ther 284:644–650, 1998.

86. Bouaboula M, Desnoyer N, Carayon P, et al: Gi protein modulation induced by a selective inverse agonist for the peripheral cannabinoid receptor CB2: Implication for intracellular signalization cross-regulation. Mol Pharmacol 55:473–480, 1999.

87. Landsman RS, Burkey TH, Consroe P, et al: SR141716A is an inverse agonist at the human cannabinoid CB1 receptor. Eur J Pharmacol 334:R1–2, 1997.

88. Gatley SJ, Lan R, Volkow ND, et al: Imaging the brain marijuana receptor: Development of a radioligand that binds to cannabinoid CB1 receptors in vivo. J Neurochem 70:417–423, 1998.

89. Felder CC, et al: LY320135, a novel cannabinoid CB1 receptor antagonist, unmasks coupling of the CB1 receptor to stimulation of cAMP accumulation. J Pharmacol Exp Ther 284:291–297, 1998.

90. Huestis MA, Sampson AH, Holicky BJ, et al: Characterization of the absorption phase of marijuana smoking. Clin Pharmacol Ther 52:31–41, 1992.

91. Huestis MA, Mitchell JM, Cone EJ: Urinary excretion profiles of 11-nor-9-carboxy-delta 9-tetrahydrocannabinol in humans after single smoked doses of marijuana. J Anal Toxicol 20:441–452, 1996.

92. Ohlsson A, Lindgren JE, Wahlen A, et al: Plasma delta-9-tetrahydrocannabinol concentrations and clinical effects after oral and intravenous administration and smoking. Clin Pharmacol Ther 28:409–416, 1980.

93. Yamamoto I, Watanabe K, Narimatsu S, Yoshimura H: Recent advances in the metabolism of cannabinoids. Int J Biochem Cell Biol 27:741–746, 1995.

94. Wall ME, Sadler BM, Brine D, et al: Metabolism, disposition, and kinetics of delta-9-tetrahydrocannabinol in men and women. Clin Pharmacol Ther 34:352–363, 1983.

95. Bornheim LM, Everhart ET, Li J, Correia MA: Characterization of cannabidiol-mediated cytochrome P450 inactivation. Biochem Pharmacol 45:1323–1331, 1993.

96. Egertova M, Elphick MR: Localization of cannabinoid receptors in the rat brain using antibodies to the intracellular C-terminal of CB1. J Comp Neurol 422:159–171, 2000.

97. Lichtman AH, Cook SA, Martin BR: Investigation of brain sites mediating cannabinoid-induced antinociception in rats: Evidence supporting periaqueductal gray involvement. J Pharmacol Exp Ther 276:585–593, 1996.

98. Martin WJ, Hohmann AG, Walker JM: Suppression of noxious stimulus-evoked activity in the ventral posterolateral nucleus of the thalamus by a cannabinoid agonist: Correlation between electrophysiological and antinociceptive effects. J Neurosci 16:6601–6611, 1996.

99. Meng ID, Manning BH, Martin WJ, Fields HL: An analgesic circuit activated by cannabinoids. Nature 395:381–383, 1998.

100. Richardson JD, Aanonsen L, Hargreaves KM: Antihyperalgesic effects of spinal cannabinoids. Eur J Pharmacol 345:145–153, 1998.

101. Hohmann AG, Tsou K, Walker JM: Cannabinoid suppression of noxious heat-evoked activity in wide dynamic range neurons in the lumbar dorsal horn of the rat. J Neurophysiol 81:575–583, 1999.

102. Hohmann AG, Herkenham M: Localization of central cannabinoid CB1 receptor messenger RNA in neuronal subpopulations of rat dorsal root ganglia: A double-label in situ hybridization study. Neuroscience 90:923–931, 1999.

103. Herkenham M, Lynn AB, Johnson MR et al: Characterization and localization of cannabinoid receptors in rat brain: A quantitative in vitro autoradiographic study. J Neurosci 11:563–583, 1991.

104. Sanudo-Pena MC, Strangman NM, Mackie K, et al: CB1 receptor localization in rat spinal cord and roots, dorsal root ganglion and peripheral nerve. Zhongguo Yao Li Xue Bao 20:1115–1120, 1999.

105. Ong WY, Mackie K: A light and electron microscopic study of the CB1 cannabinoid receptor in the primate spinal cord. J Neurocytol 28:39–45, 1999.

106. Farquhar-Smith WP, Egertova M, Bradbury EJ, et al: Cannabinoid CB1 receptor expression in rat spinal cord. Mol Cell Neurosci 15:510–521, 2000.

107. Hohmann AG, Herkenham M: Regulation of cannabinoid and mu opioid receptors in rat lumbar spinal cord following neonatal capsaicin treatment. Neurosci Lett 252:13–16, 1998.

108. Hohmann AG, Briley EM, Herkenham M: Pre- and postsynaptic distribution of cannabinoid and mu opioid receptors in rat spinal cord. Brain Res 822:17–25, 1999.

109. Friedel RH, Schnurch H, Stubbusch J, Barde Y: Identification of genes differentially expressed by nerve growth factor and neurotrophin-3 dependent sensory neurons. Proc Natl Acad Sci USA 94:12670–12675, 1997.

110. Ahluwalia J, Urban L, Capogna M, et al: Cannabinoid 1 receptors are expressed in nociceptive primary sensory neurones. Neuroscience 100:685–688, 2000.

111. Bridges D, Rice ASC, Egertova M, et al: The cannabinoid CB1 receptor is localised predominantly on N52 within the rat dorsal root ganglion. Soc Neurosci Abstr (in press).

112. Jennings EA, Vaughan CW, Christie MJ: Effects of cannabinoids on neurons in the superficial medullary dorsal horn of the rat. Soc Neurosci Abstr 26:812.13, 2000.

113. Morisset V, Urban L: Cannabinoid-induced presynaptic inhibition of glutamatinergic EPSCs in substantia gelatinosa neurons of the rat spinal cord. J Neurophysiol 86:40–48, 2001.

114. Millns PJ, Chapman V, Kendall DA: Cannabinoid inhibition of the capsaicin-induced calcium response in rat dorsal root ganglion neurones. Br J Pharmacol 132:969–971, 2001.

115. Richardson JD, Kilo S, Hargreaves KM: Cannabinoids reduce hyperalgesia and inflammation via interaction with peripheral CB1 receptors. Pain 75:111–119, 1998.

116. Hohmann AG, Tsou K, Walker JM: Cannabinoid modulation of wide dynamic range neurons in the lumbar dorsal horn of the rat by spinally administered WIN 55,212. Neurosci Lett 257:119–122, 1998.

117. Hohmann AG, Martin WJ, Tsou K, Walker JM: Inhibition of noxious stimulus-evoked activity of spinal cord dorsal horn neurons by the cannabinoid WIN 55,212-2. Life Sci 56:2111–2118, 1995.

118. Strangman NM, Walker JM: Cannabinoid WIN 55,212-2 inhibits the activity-dependent facilitation of spinal nociceptive responses. J Neurophysiol 82:472–477, 1999.

119. Chapman V: The cannabinoid CB1 receptor antagonist, SR141716A, selectively facilitates nociceptive responses of dorsal horn neurones in the rat. Br J Pharmacol 127:1765–1767, 1999.

120. Smith PB, Martin BR: Spinal mechanisms of delta 9-tetrahydrocannabinol-induced analgesia. Brain Res 578:8–12, 1992.

121. Lichtman AH, Martin BR: Cannabinoid-induced antinociception is mediated by a spinal alpha 2-noradrenergic mechanism. Brain Res 559:309–314, 1991.

122. Richardson JD, Aanonsen L, Hargreaves KM: Hypoactivity of the spinal cannabinoid system results in NMDA-dependent hyperalgesia. J Neurosci 18:451–457, 1998.

123. Martin WJ, Loo CM, Basbaum AI: Spinal cannabinoids are anti-allodynic in rats with persistent inflammation. Pain 82:199–205, 1999.

124. Chapman V, Besson JM: Pharmacological studies of nociceptive systems using the C-Fos immunohistochemical technique: An indicator of noxiously activated spinal neurones. In Dickenson AH, Besson JM: The Pharmacology of Pain. Berlin, Springer, 1997, pp 235–280.

125. Farquhar-Smith WP, Rice ASC: Expression of spinal Fos after nerve growth factor-induced inflammation of the rat urinary bladder is attenuated by cannabinoids. Paper presented at the European Winter Conference on Brain Research, 2001 (abstract).

126. Tsou K, Lowitz KA, Hohmann AG, et al: Suppression of noxious stimulus-evoked expression of FOS protein-like immunoreactivity in rat spinal cord by a selective cannabinoid agonist. Neuroscience 70:791–798, 1996.

127. Fox A, Kesingland A, Gentry C, et al: The role of central and peripheral cannabinoid1 receptors in the antihyperalgesic activity of cannabinoids in a model of neuropathic pain. Pain 92:91–100, 2001.

128. Rice ASC: Local neuro-immune interactions in visceral hyperalgesia: Bradykinin, neurotrophins and cannabinoids. In Bountra C, Schmidt W, Munglani R (eds): Pain: Current Understanding, Emerging Therapies and Novel Approaches to Drug Discovery. New York, Marcel Dekker, 2000.

129. Mazzari S, Canella R, Leon A: N-(2-hydroxyethyl)hexadecamide reduces mechanical hyperalgesia following sciatic nerve constriction injury. Soc Neurosci Abstr 21:263.15, 1995.

130. McMahon SB, Bennett DLH: Trophic factors and pain. In Wall PD, Melzack R (eds): Textbook of Pain, 4th ed. Edinburgh, Churchill Livingstone, 1999, pp 105–128.

131. Thompson SWN, Bennett DLH, Kerr BJ, et al: Brain-derived neurotrophic factor is an endogenous modulator of nociceptive responses in the spinal cord. Proc Natl Acad Sci USA 96:7714–7718, 1999.

132. Petersen M, Segond von Banchet G, Heppelmann B, Koltzenburg M: Nerve growth factor regulates the expression of bradykinin binding sites on adult sensory neurons via the neurotrophin receptor p75. Neuroscience 83:161–168, 1998.

133. Fjell J, Cummins TR, Fried K, et al: In vivo NGF deprivation reduces SNS expression and TTX-R sodium currents in IB4-negative DRG neurons. J Neurophysiol 81:803–810, 1999.

134. Bevan S, Winter J: Nerve growth factor (NGF) differentially regulates the chemosensitivity of adult rat cultured sensory neurons. J Neurosci 15:4918–4926, 1995.

135. Woolf CJ, Ma QP, Allchorne A, Poole S: Peripheral cell types contributing to the hyperalgesic action of nerve growth factor in inflammation. J Neurosci 16:2716–2723, 1996.

136. Nilsson G, Forsberg Nilsson K, Xiang Z, et al: Human mast cells express functional trkA and are a source of nerve growth factor. Eur J Immunol 27:2295–2301, 1997.

137. Tal M, Liberman R: Local injection of nerve growth factor (NGF) triggers degranulation of mast cells in rat paw. Neurosci Lett 221:129–132, 1997.

138. Horigome K, Pryor JC, Bullock ED, Johnson EM Jr: Mediator release from mast cells by nerve growth factor. Neurotrophin specificity and receptor mediation. J Biol Chem 268:14881–14887, 1993.

139. Leon A, Buriani A, Dal Toso R, et al: Mast cells synthesize, store, and release nerve growth factor. Proc Natl Acad Sci USA 91:3739–3743, 1994.

140. Melck D, De Petrocellis L, Orlando P, et al: Suppression of nerve growth factor Trk receptors and prolactin receptors by endocannabinoids leads to inhibition of human breast and prostate cancer cell proliferation. Endocrinology 141:118–126, 2000.

141. Levi-Montalcini R, Skaper SD, Dal Toso R, et al: Nerve growth factor: From neurotrophin to neurokine. Trends Neurosci 19:514–520, 1996.

142. Jaggar SI, Hasnie FS, Sellaturay S, Rice ASC: The anti-hyperalgesic actions of the cannabinoid anandamide and the putative CB2 agonist palmitoylethanolamide investigated in models of visceral and somatic inflammatory pain. Pain 76:189–199, 1998.

143. Farquhar-Smith WP, Rice ASC: The effects of endocannabinoids on peripheral NGF-induced neutrophil accumulation in rat skin. Paper presented at the 2001 Symposium on the Cannabinoids, International Cannabinoid Research Society, 2001, p 76.

144. Ross RA, Brockie HC, Pertwee RG: Inhibition of nitric oxide production in RAW264.7 macrophages by cannabinoids and palmitoylethanolamide. Eur J Pharmacol 401:121–130, 2000.

145. Klein TW, Lane B, Newton CA, Friedman H: The cannabinoid system and cytokine network. Proc Soc Exp Biol Med 225:1–8, 2000.

146. Richardson JD, Aanonsen L, Hargreaves KM: SR141716a, a cannabinoid receptor antagonist, produces hyperalgesia in untreated mice. Eur J Pharmacol 319:R3–4, 1997.

147. Strangman NM, Patrick SL, Hohmann AG, et al: Evidence for a role of endogenous cannabinoids in the modulation of acute and tonic pain sensitivity. Brain Res 813:323–328, 1998.

148. Herzberg U, Eliav E, Bennett GJ, Kopin IJ: The analgesic effects of R(+)-WIN55,212-2 mesylate, a high affinity cannabinoid agonist, in a rat model of neuropathic pain. Neurosci Lett 221:157–160, 1997.

149. Smith FL, Fujimore K, Lowe J, Welch SP: Characterisation of delta9 Tetrahydrocannabinol and anandamide antinociception in nonarthritic and arthritic rats. Pharmacol Biochem Behav 60:183–191, 1998.

150. Bridges D, Thompson SWN, Rice ASC: Mechanisms of neuropathic pain. Br J Anaesth 87:12–26, 2001.

151. Beaulieu P, Bisogno T, Punwar S, et al: Role of the endogenous cannabinoid system in the formalin test of persistent pain in the rat. Eur J Pharmacol 396:85–92, 2000.

152. Welch SP, Eads M: Synergistic interactions of endogenous opioids and cannabinoid systems. Brain Res 848:183–190, 1999.

153. Valverde O, Ledent C, Beslot F, et al: Reduction of stress-induced analgesia but not of exogenous opioid effects in mice lacking CB1 receptors. Eur J Neurosci 12:533–539, 2000.

154. Manzanares J, Corchero J, Romero J, et al: Pharmacological and biochemical interactions between opioids and cannabinoids. Trends Pharmacol Sci 20:287–294, 1999.

155. Rice ASC, Justins DM: Pain mechanisms and pathways. Curr Anaesth Crit Care 10:98–104, 1999.

156. Rice ASC: Recent developments in the pathophysiology of acute pain. Acute Pain 1:27–36, 1998.

157. Tjolsen A, Berge OG, Hunskaar S, et al: The formalin test: An evaluation of the method [see comments]. Pain 51:5–17, 1992.

158. Watson GS, Sufka KJ, Coderre TJ: Optimal scoring strategies and weights for the formalin test in rats. Pain 70:53–58, 1997.

159. Dubuisson D, Dennis SG: The formalin test: A quantitative study of the analgesic effects of morphine, meperidine, and brain stem stimulation in rats and cats. Pain 4:161–174, 1977.

160. Hargreaves KM, Dubner R, Brown F, et al: A new and sensitive method for measuring thermal nociception in cutaneous hyperalgesia. Pain 32:77–88, 1988.

161. Li J, Daughters RS, Bullis C, et al: The cannabinoid receptor agonist WIN 55,212-2 blocks the development of hyperalgesia produced by capsaicin in rats. Pain 81:25–34, 1999.

162. Farquhar-Smith WP, Rice ASC: Anandamide attenuates a nerve growth factor-induced hyperalgesia via cannabinoid CB$_1$ receptors. J Physiol (Lond) 2000, p 528.

163. McMahon SB: Are there fundamental differences in the peripheral mechanisms of visceral and somatic pain? Behav Brain Sci 20:381–391, 1997.

164. Farquhar-Smith WP, Rice ASC: Administration of endocannabinoids prevents a referred hyperalgesia associated with inflammation of the urinary bladder. Anesthesiology 94:507–513, 2001.

165. Jaggar SI, Sellaturay S, Rice ASC: The endogenous cannabinoid anandamide, but not the CB2 ligand palmitoylethanolamide, prevents the viscero-visceral hyper-reflexia associated with inflammation of the rat urinary bladder. Neurosci Lett 253:123–126, 1998.

166. McMahon SB, Abel C: A model for the study of visceral pain states: Chronic inflammation of the chronic decerebrate rat urinary bladder by irritant chemicals. Pain 28:109–127, 1987.

167. McMahon SB, Koltzenburg M: Changes in the afferent innervation of the inflamed urinary bladder. In Mayer EA, Raybould H: Basic and Clinical Aspects of Chronic Abdominal Pain. Amsterdam, Elsevier, 1993, pp 155–172.

168. McMahon SB: Neuronal and behavioural consequences of chemical inflammation of rat urinary bladder. Agents Actions 25:231–233, 1988.

169. Jaggar SI, Scott HCF, Rice ASC: Inflammation of the rat urinary bladder is associated with a referred thermal hyperalgesia which is nerve growth factor dependant. Br J Anaesth 83:442–448, 1999.

170. Scott HCF, Jaggar SI, Rice ASC: Mechanical hyperalgesia is referred to the hind limb following inflammation of the urinary bladder in the rat. J Physiol (Lond) 18:507, 1998.

171. Dmitrieva N, Iqbal R, Shelton D, McMahon SB: c-fos induction in a rat model of cystitis: Role of NGF. Soc Neurosci Abstr 22:301.6, 1996.

172. Cruz F, Avelino A, Lima D, Coimbra A: Activation of the c-fos proto-oncogene in the spinal cord following noxious stimulation of the urinary bladder. Somatosens Mot Res 11:319–325, 1994.

173. Birder LA, de Groat WC: Increased c-fos expression in spinal neurons after irritation of the lower urinary tract in the rat. J Neuroscience 12:4878–4883, 1992.

174. Rice ASC, Farquhar-Smith WP: Endocannabinoids prevent the referred viscero-somatic hyperalgesia associated with inflammation of the rat urinary bladder. Paper presented at the 2000 Symposium on the Cannabinoids, International Cannabinoid Research Society, 2000, p 84.

175. Dmitrieva N, McMahon SB: Sensitisation of visceral afferents by nerve growth factor in the adult rat. Pain 66:87–97, 1996.

176. Dmitrieva N, Shelton D, Rice ASC, McMahon SB: The role of nerve growth factor in a model of visceral inflammation. Neuroscience 78:449–459, 1997.

177. Farquhar-Smith WP, Jaggar SI, Rice ASC: Cannabinoids attenuate NGF-induced viscero-visceral hyper-reflexia via both CB$_1$ and CB$_2$ receptors. Soc Neurosci Abstr 25:373.2, 1999.

178. Besse D, Lombard MC, Besson JM: Time-related decreases in mu and delta opioid receptors in the superficial dorsal horn of the rat spinal cord following a large unilateral dorsal rhizotomy. Brain Res 578:115–127, 1992.

179. Besse D, Lombard MC, Perrot S, Besson JM: Regulation of opioid binding sites in the superficial dorsal horn of the rat spinal cord following loose ligation of the sciatic nerve: Comparison with sciatic nerve section and lumbar dorsal rhizotomy. Neuroscience 50:921–933, 1992.

180. Cui J, Holmin S, Mathiesen T, et al: Possible role of inflammatory mediators in tactile hypersensitivity in rat models of mononeuropathy. Pain 88:239–248, 2000.

181. Clatworthy AL, Illich PA, Castro GA, Walters ET: Role of peri-axonal inflammation in the development of thermal hyperalgesia and guarding behavior in a rat model of neuropathic pain. Neurosci Lett 184:5–8, 1995.

182. Okamato K, Martin DP, Schmelzer JD, et al: Pro- and anti-inflammatory cytokine messenger RNA changes in chronic constriction injury model. Soc Neurosci Abstr 25:578.1, 1999.

183. Bridges D, Ahmad KS, Rice ASC: The synthetic cannabinoid WIN 55,212-2 attenuates hyperalgesia and allodynia in a rat model of neuropathic pain. Br J Pharmacol 133:586–594, 2001.

184. Kalso E: Cannabinoids for pain and nausea. BMJ 323:2–4, 2001.

185. Raft D, Gregg J, Ghia J, Harris L: Effects of intravenous tetrahydrocannabinol on experimental and surgical pain. Psychological correlates of the analgesic response. Clin Pharmacol Ther 21:26–33, 1977.

186. Noyes R, Brunk SF, Baram DA, Canter A: The analgesic properties of delta-9-THC and codeine. Clin Pharmacol Ther 18:84–89, 1975.

187. Noyes R Jr, Brunk SF, Baram DA, Canter A: Analgesic effect of delta-9-tetrahydrocannabinol. J Clin Pharmacol 15:139–143, 1975.

188. Campbell F, Tramer M, Carroll D, et al: Are cannabinoids an effective and safe option in the management of pain? A qualitative systematic review. BMJ 323:13–16, 2001.

189. Barinaga, M. How cannabinoids work in the brain. Science 291:2530, 2001.

190. Christie MJ, Vaughan CW: Cannabinoids act backwards. Nature 410:527–530, 2001.

191. Elphick MR, Egertova M: The neurobiology and evolution of cannabinoid signaling. Philos Trans R Soc Lond B Biol Sci 356:381–408, 2001.

192. Montgomery JM, Madison DW: The grass roots of synapse suppression. Neuron 29:567–570, 2001.

30

Analgesics

Francis V. Salinas, MD • Spencer L. Liu, MD • Andreas M. Scholz, PD, MD

ION CHANNEL LIGANDS/SODIUM CHANNEL BLOCKERS/LOCAL ANESTHETICS

Despite widespread use of local anesthetics for more than a century, the molecular mechanisms by which they alter specific peripheral nervous system functions have remained unclear. This chapter presents evidence implicating the Na^+ channel protein as a target for specific, clinically important LA effects in mammalian neurons. The elucidation of the primary and secondary structure of the Na^+ channel protein has provided key insights into this target for mechanism of LA action.[1] Na^+ channels are not the only targets of local anesthetics at clinically relevant concentrations. K^+ and Ca^{2+} channels are also affected, which might elucidate some side effects of local anesthetics; therefore they also will be described in this chapter. Recent findings indicate that local anesthetics also act on intracellular mechanisms, which may explain the toxicity associated with local anesthetics.

MECHANISMS OF ACTION

Historical View

Interestingly, cocaine was first used as a local anesthetic by Carl Koller and Sigmund Freud. They noticed a numbing effect on the tongue after swallowing cocaine, and Koller, an intern in the ophthalmology department in Vienna who was intent on finding a drug to anesthetize the cornea, knew that Freud had relieved pain with cocaine.[2] In fact, they demonstrated on themselves—taking pins and trying in front of a mirror to touch their cornea—that within minutes they could not feel anything. They reported in the same year that they had enucleated painlessly a dog's eye. Leonard Corning, a neurologist in New York City, had already tried in 1885 to inject cocaine solution (2%) between the spinous process in a young dog, which resulted in insensibility within 5 minutes[3]; this was later transferred to patients, with the drug presumably acting in the epidural space. The lumbar puncture later introduced by Quincke allowed spinal anesthesia.[4] Cocaine was widely used despite its disadvantages of high toxicity, short duration of anesthesia, impossibility of sterilizing the solution, and its high cost (not to mention addiction). Alfred Einhorn synthesized procaine by degrading cocaine and commented that: "The anesthetic capability of cocaine is therefore a function of its acid group called by Paul Ehrlich the 'anesthesiophoric' group—the most potent being the benzoyl group."[5] From this structural starting point the majority of clinically used local anesthetics (see "Clinical Pharmacology") consist of the benzene ring linked through an amide or ester to an amine group, and their names still end in "caine."

Peripheral Nerve and Local Anesthetics

Differential and Use-dependent Block by Local Anesthetics

At that time the basic mechanism of nerve blockade was relatively unknown, but it was noticed soon afterward that a selective block of specific nerve fiber groups occurred termed *differential nerve block*. This differential block was revealed as a block of sensory information; Bier provided evidence for the progression of the block to involve attenuation of sharp pain, cold, warmth and contact or touch, then finally motor fibers (Bier, 1899). A quantitative neurophysiologic technique was used by Gasser and Erlanger in 1929.[6] Based on their classification of nerve fiber size and conduction velocity (from Aα-fastest to C-fibers-slowest), they compared the ability of these fibers to generate a compound action potential in response to pressure when exposed to cocaine-containing solutions. They suspected that diameter might be the main parameter accounting for differential nerve block. They observed with cocaine that small fibers

(slowly conducting) tended to be blocked before large fibers, but in all cases, a varying proportion of large fibers were blocked well before the compound action potential for small fibers had disappeared. That is why they concluded: "Such a simple mechanism as has just been described should cause the fibers to be blocked systematically on a size basis; and since this does not rigidly hold the problem can be considered to be only partly solved. Some other as yet undetermined factor must be operating."[6] Within the C fibers, the Na$^+$ current could be decreased to 20% before conduction was blocked, resulting in a safety factor of fivefold.

Later experiments with compound action potentials of peripheral nerves from various species revealed that some C fibers are affected when A fibers start to be blocked. However, the half-maximal concentration necessary to block the C fiber compound action potential was two to four times greater than for A fibers depending on the type of local anesthetic used.[7–9] It seemed that local anesthetics with an ester structure have an inherently more potent action than the amide.

C Fibers and Nociceptors

Later experiments especially in humans[10–12] showed that C fibers themselves could be further categorized based on their diverse physiologic and electrical responses; thus a large subgroup responds to mechanical, chemical, and noxious stimuli and are termed *polymodal receptors,* whereas others do not respond except after sensitization (e.g., with capsaicin) and are called *silent nociceptors.*[13,14] This variability within the same fiber type raises another possible mechanism for differential local anesthetic effects, i.e. different populations of ion channels. Recent findings supporting this idea show that in small fibers, besides classical Na$^+$ channels sensitive to tetrodotoxin (TTX), there are also TTX-resistant Na$^+$ channels and Ca^{2+} channels present with different susceptibility to block by local anesthetics.[15,16]

Mechanisms of Block

QX 314 is a quaternary derivative of local anesthetics with a permanent positive charge. It is not in clinical use but has shown interesting features which have helped in understanding the mechanisms whereby the Na$^+$ channel is blocked by LA. This drug blocks only when applied to the internal side.[17] Nearly all local anesthetics are amine compounds, which are charged at a pH of below 6 (except benzocaine); the uncharged form is more lipid-soluble.[18] Biophysical calculations of the electric field[19] reveal that the distance of the binding site from the outer face of the membrane is about 0.6 of the total membrane thickness. From these calculations emerged the notion that the "receptor" is within the pore and that drugs must pass through the lipid membrane to act through their charged form at the channel.

Nearly full-sized Na$^+$ currents could be elicited during the *first* depolarizing impulse even in the presence of the local anesthetic (or of internal QX 314), but *subsequent* impulses elicited progressively smaller currents.[20] This phenomenon was interpreted to be produced by cumulative binding through the open channels. This accumulation of inhibition has been called *use-dependent block* or phasic block.[21,22] The overall theory was called the *guarded receptor hypothesis*,[23] and it proposed that the receptor is protected in the pore and needs the channel to be open to be accessible. The impact of use-dependent block can be seen at greater firing frequencies in nerve fibers in which lower concentrations of local anesthetics are required for block than those required for block single compound action potentials (Fig. 30–1).[9]

Function and Structure of Na$^+$ Channels

Structure of the Na$^+$ Channel

Isolation and purification of the protein that forms the Na$^+$ channel uncovered a single polypeptide of relative molecular mass ~260,000,[24] which is called the *α-subunit*.[1,25] The functional amino acid sequence encoded by the corresponding cDNA results in a ~1950 amino acid chain that crosses the cell membrane several times. The channel consists of four domains (D I to D IV, see Fig. 30–1A),[26] each containing six transmembrane helices: S1 to S6 segments. The link between the S5 and S6 segments in each domain is of particular interest because these "pore loops" form the outer pore and contain the amino acid sequence of aspartic acid,

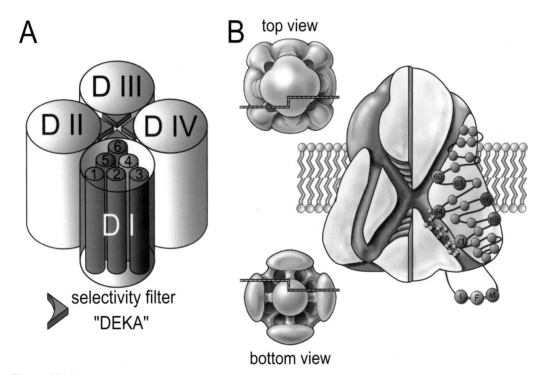

Figure 30–1. *A*, Schematic diagram of the structure of a α-subunit of a Na$^+$ channel. Each of the four domains (D I–D IV) consists of six segments that span the membrane. Part of the "pore" loops, the amino acid link between S5 and S6 segments, is specially highlighted because the four amino acids "DEKA" form in the outer pore mouth the selectivity filter (see "Function and Structure of Na$^+$ channels"). *B*, Sketch of the three-dimensional view of a Na$^+$ channel with cross section. From cryoelectron microscopic and single particle analysis data, a three-dimensional model of the Na$^+$ channel was derived[95]; *top* and *bottom* views show the cross section of the large sketch. *Left*, The cross section is through the S4 segment (the function of the cavity marked in red is currently unclear). *Right*, The cross section is through the S6 segment overlaid with the amino acid sequence of rat brain Na$^+$ channel (Na$_v$ 1.2). Those residues that are important for the affinity of local anesthetics are colored and numbered (60 for amino acid 1760, and so on). (*B*, Adapted from Ragsdale DS, McPhee JC, Scheuer T, et al: Molecular determinants of state-dependent block of Na$^+$ channels by local anesthetics. Science 265:1724, 1994; Catterall WA: Structural biology—A 3D view of sodium channels. Nature 409:988, 2001.)

glutamic acid, lysine, and alanine [DEKA] in each link, which represent the selectivity filter allowing primarily Na$^+$ ions to pass (see Fig. 30–1A). The region of the outer pore mouth is also involved in the binding of toxins like TTX, batrachotoxin, and conotoxins.[27–29] Although batrachotoxin is localized at the *outer* pore mouth, it in particular seems to influence the binding of local anesthetics at the *inner* pore regions.[30–32]

An intracellular link between D III and D IV underlies "fast" inactivation (see Fig. 30–1B). Aside from the pore-forming α-subunit (of which 9 of the 11 genes are known to be expressed), three auxiliary subunits (β1–3) influence the activation and inactivation parameters of an expressed α-subunit or the level of channel protein expression.[33–36] Another type of inactivation, the slow "C-type,"[37] appears to involve the pore loops mentioned earlier.

Molecular Functions of the Na$^+$ Channel

In its simplest form, the channel functions in three steps. First, the channel is closed at potentials less than −70 mV. The pore in the channel is occluded so that no Na$^+$ ion can pass from one side to the other. From experiments with K$^+$ channels, it appears that the outer pore interacts directly with the S4 voltage sensor.[38,39] The segments in the K$^+$ channel were found to twist and move inward causing the closing of

the outer pore. The structure/function motifs in the K$^+$ channel parallel those in the Na$^+$ channel, suggesting that similar gating mechanisms may be operating.

The opening of the channel is initiated by a depolarization so that the transmembrane potential becomes more positive than the threshold potential (usually greater than −40 mV). Now the channel opens within a millisecond and allows Na$^+$ ion to pass through the pore causing an inward current that continues a self-driven depolarization. This underlies the upstroke of the action potential of most excitable cells (see Chapter 8). During channel opening, the S4 segment twists back because of changes in potential difference and intrinsic charge, which allow the outer pore mouth to expand, thus resulting in a 20-degree twist of the α helix.[34]

After activation (during prolonged depolarization), the channel enters into the inactivated state (Fig. 30–2). After depolarization, the macroscopic Na$^+$ current reaches a peak and the current decreases in time, often monoexponentially, even if the membrane potential is clamped positive. Together with the outward currents through voltage-gated K$^+$ channels, the self-decreasing inward current provides the conditions for repolarization after an action potential. Previously it was thought that the inactivated state existed as a nonconducting mode even though gating currents were measured.[40] Currently, it is known that the inactivation gate is positioned on the inner side of the channel protein, like

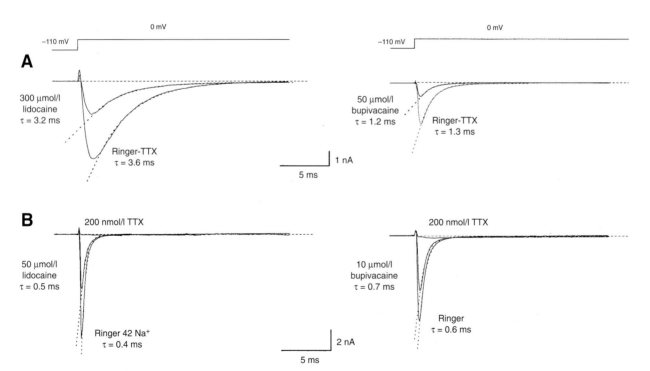

Figure 30–2. Tetrodotoxin (TTX)-sensitive and TTX-resistant Na$^+$ currents in rat dorsal root ganglia neurons blocked by lidocaine and bupivacaine, respectively. *A*, Fits to the decaying parts of TTX-resistant Na$^+$ currents *(dotted lines)* showed a time constant of 3.6 milliseconds in Ringer-TTX solution and 3.2 milliseconds in the presence of 300 µmol/L lidocaine. *B*, The TTX-sensitive Na$^+$ currents decayed faster with a time constant of 0.4 millisecond in Ringer solution and 0.5 millisecond in the presence of 50 µmol/L lidocaine. Less than 2% of the current remained in the presence of 200 nmol/L TTX. AP, action potential. (Adapted from Scholz A, Kuboyama N, Hempelmann G, et al: Complex blockade of TTX-resistant Na$^+$ currents by lidocaine and bupivacaine reduce firing frequency in DRG neurons. J Neurophysiol 79:1746, 1998.)

a ball on a chain, and a sequence of three amino acids (isoleucine, methionine, phenylalanine; IMF) has been identified as the "occluder" providing "fast" inactivation. The IMF sequence is on the linker between domain D III and D IV facing the cytoplasmic side of the membrane (see Fig. 30–1*B*).[34] Thus "fast" inactivation may function like a "lid" plugging the pore by binding to sites situated on or near the inner vestibule. The role of the IMF sequence in binding of local anesthetics is not fully understood but it seems that this "lid" retains open channel blockers inside the pore during use-dependent blockade.[34,41] This situation would mean that the Na$^+$ ions could no longer pass through the pore even though the pore is open at the outer mouth. For two reasons the fast inactivated state is interesting in anesthesia; first, this state seems to play an important role in high-affinity binding (as discussed later) and, secondly the movement of S4 segment in gating (important for activation and closing as described earlier) directly influences fast inactivation.[42]

Na$^+$ Channelopathies

Na$^+$ channel mutations causing multiple inherited diseases of hyperexcitability in humans were first described in skeletal muscle Na$^+$ channel. The familial periodic paralysis syndromes, hyperkalemic periodic paralysis[43,44] and paramyotonia congenita,[45,46] were found to be due to mutations in either the inactivation gate, in regions thought to serve as the inactivation gate receptor, or in the S4 segment. Each of these impairs inactivation and voltage dependence, resulting in hyperactive Na$^+$ channels. Interestingly, mutations in the heart Na$^+$ channel in the region of the linker D III to D IV and in the S4 segment have been found to underlie some diseases like long QT syndrome.[41] Mutations of only a few amino acids are necessary to disturb fast inactivation, resulting in a slowly diminishing or persistent Na$^+$ current with sustained depolarization. Although the remaining current is miniscule (0.5–2% from peak values), it facilitates arrhythmic activity that has been confirmed by quantitative modeling.[47] No mutations have been found in Na$^+$ channels on neurons that cause an inherited disease to date, but a mutation in the β_1-subunit might be connected with inherited febrile seizures with indirect effects on Na$^+$ channel function.[48] Currently, it is not well understood whether these mutants might have different susceptibility to local anesthetics. These Na$^+$ "channelopathies" are targets for the development of therapeutic drugs.

Molecular Determinants of Local Anesthetic Action on Na$^+$ Channels

Experiments on the rat brain Na$^+$ channel IIa (Na$_v$ 1.2) revealed that exchanging the amino acid phenylalanine (F) at position 1764 with alanine (A) made the channel virtually insensitive to use-dependent block. Measurements of the IC$_{50}$ for the wild type Na$^+$ channel inactivated with depolarizing prepulses were described by a 1:1 binding relation with 300-fold smaller values compared with tonic blockade. In contrast, in the F1764A mutation, in which the IC$_{50}$ values for tonic inhibition were threefold greater than wild type Na$^+$

channels, the IC$_{50}$ values in inactivated Na$^+$ channels were only six times smaller than for tonic blockade. The mutant Y1771A rat exhibited less use-dependent block and reduced drug binding at depolarized potentials, but the effect was smaller than for F1764A rats.[42] These results led to a model for the "receptor" site of local anesthetics in the pore of the Na$^+$ channel. The residues F1764A and Y1771A described earlier are hydrophobic aromatic residues separated by two turns on the same face of the protein helix of the pore-forming S6 segment (see Fig. 30–1*B*). These amino acids are about 11 Å apart, and most effective local anesthetics are about 10 to 15 Å in length. The local anesthetics have positively charged moieties at either end, which could interact through hydrophobic or π electrons with these amino acid residues.[49,50] The substitution with alanine changed the size and the chemical properties with minimal effect on the protein's secondary structure[51] in these mutants. These substitutions revealed an affinity in open and inactivated channels of one or two orders of magnitude smaller than in wild-type channels. These residues are well positioned to modulate the extracellular access route of local anesthetics and are probably the main determinants of drug binding for the open channel. This idea is supported by experiments with the permanently charged local anesthetic QX314, which showed a use-dependent block of more than 50% in the wild-type Na$^+$ channel, but produced virtually no use-dependent block in the F1764A mutant expressed in oocytes. In these types of experiments, the only possible access route to this site is the open channel; recovery times comparable to those in the wild type indicate that the escape pathway of the local anesthetic is not altered.

Another mutation oriented toward the pore, I1760A (see Fig. 30–1*B*), did not alter the local anesthetic affinity of either the open or the inactivated state of the Na$^+$ channel. Notably, the rate of drug dissociation from the mutant channel was found to be eight times faster than for wild type channels. Because I1760A mutation is close to the extracellular side of S6 segment at the channel mouth, and isoleucine is a bulky residue, it seems likely that the drugs could escape more easily from the mutated channel. Indeed, QX314, usually ineffective when applied externally, rapidly blocked this mutant; thus the mutation created a pathway for the extracellular drug to enter, supporting the idea that faster recovery from drug bound states is due to easier escape of the drug from the channel.[42]

The emerging picture suggests two binding sites in the pore of brain Na$^+$ channel (position 1764 and 1771), whose hydrophobic parts interact with the corresponding regions of the local anesthetic molecule. The residue oriented more toward the mouth of the pore (1760) guards the fast escape of the drug molecule to the extracellular side and protects the channel from extracellular drugs.

D III, the neighbor domain of D IV, also appears important in binding of local anesthetics.[32,52] Both groups demonstrated by point mutations in the S6 segment in this domain a reduction in affinity of local anesthetics in neuronal and muscle Na$^+$ channels. This indicates that at least some drug molecules bind primarily at the S6 segment in D IV, but the molecule also binds on the other side of the channel pore at the S6 segment of D III.

In one respect the local anesthetic benzocaine is remarkable: it is the sole clinically used drug that is not charged (because of its low pKa; see "Clinical Pharmacology"). Up to now it has been suggested that benzocaine shares the same binding site as other local anesthetics,[53] at least in the neuronal and muscle Na$^+$ channel. However, the low affinity of benzocaine in comparison to other local anesthetics (IC$_{50}$ ~800 μM) and the lack of use-dependent block[53,54] do not suggest a high-affinity binding site for local anesthetics which are charged.

The small differences in potency and toxicity of enantiomers that were found in clinical studies seems to have a counterpart on the molecular level. A stereoselectivity of about 1.5 was found for Na$^+$ channels from skeletal muscle and human heart cells (Na$_v$ 1.5).[55] It was demonstrated that the binding residues 1760 and 1765 (the corresponding position in Na$_v$ 1.2 is 1764 and 1771) contribute to the weak stereoselectivity, especially in the human heart channel.

Other Ion Channels as Targets

Tetrodotoxin-Resistant Na$^+$ Channels

The description of the molecular mechanism described earlier is derived mainly from those Na$^+$ channels that are sensitive in the nanomolar range to tetrodotoxin (TTX), apart from the cardiac channel (which is less sensitive but not insensitive). The typical TTX-resistant Na$^+$ channels, referred to originally as SNS/PN3 and SNS2/NaN but now as Na$_v$ 1.8 and Na$_v$ 1.9 in the new nomenclature,[56] are primarily found in neurons of dorsal root ganglia (DRG).[57-60] Apart from their different sensitivity to TTX, their current kinetics were described as slower compared with the "fast" TTX-sensitive Na$^+$ currents, and their threshold for activation and half-maximal inactivation was found at more depolarized potentials (see Fig. 30–2). Their distribution is predominantly in the small- to medium-diameter sized neurons which are part of the Aδ and C-fibers; this reflects their function in pair conduction. Indeed, null mutant mice lacking the SNS/PN3 Na$^+$ channel reveal partial analgesia.[61] The question whether this TTX-resistant Na$^+$ current is sensitive to local anesthetics had already been raised in previous studies. Indeed, the blocking mechanisms found were similar to those in TTX-sensitive Na$^+$ currents, but the main difference was the two to six times lower affinity of local anesthetics to TTX-resistant Na$^+$ channels depending on the type of local anesthetic (see Fig. 30–2).[62-64] Other than the presence of TTX-resistant Na$^+$ channels in the soma of DRG neurons, electrophysiologic and immunohistochemical evidence demonstrates their presence in the peripheral nerve[15,16,65] on nociceptor nerve terminals.[66,67] The latter work in particular clearly shows that in experiments with sensory nerve, 50% of small Aδ and 85% of the C fibers were unaffected by 1 μM TTX! This indicates that TTX-resistant Na$^+$ channels are important elements of transduction in the smallest terminals.

In one study it was demonstrated that TTX-resistant action potentials in small sensory neurons, which are involved in the generation and conduction of pain-related impulses, were suppressed by lidocaine and bupivacaine in a concentration-dependent manner at clinically relevant concentrations (Fig. 30–3).[68] These concentrations were about three to four times greater than the concentrations required to block TTX-sensitive Na$^+$ currents in the same type of neurons. A marked ability of bupivacaine and lidocaine to reduce the number of TTX-sensitive action potentials during repetitive firing at concentrations that are lower by a factor of 10 to 20 than those required to reduce the amplitude of the TTX-sensitive action potentials was also shown (see Fig. 30–3). This observation may be relevant to their analgesic properties, especially on the basis that strength of pain sensation is encoded by frequency. However, it emphasizes that concentrations of a drug measured for half-maximal blockade of ion currents do not necessarily reflect the relevant concentration that may be required for blockade of a function of a cell.

Potassium Channels

Interestingly, not only voltage-dependent Na$^+$ channels are blocked by local anesthetics, but also voltage-dependent K$^+$ channels.[69,70] This is of interest because voltage-dependent K$^+$ channels have been investigated in DRG and dorsal horn neurons, and one could speculate that the channels present on the nerve fibers might be the same. The major difference compared with Na$^+$ currents is the lower affinity; depending on current type, it is a 4- to 10-fold lower affinity for bupivacaine and 10- to 80-fold lower affinity for lidocaine.[69,71] However, block of K$^+$ channels might be an additional explanation for broadening the action potential in the presence of local anesthetics, because the repolarization phase of an action potential is caused by the activation of voltage-gated K$^+$ currents as well as the decreasing Na$^+$ current because of its inactivation.

Not only voltage-gated K$^+$ currents, but also a voltage-independent K$^+$ channel, were found to be blocked by local anesthetics in sensory neurons.[72] This *flicker* K$^+$ channel (termed because of its flickering openings in high K$^+$ solutions) was found mainly in thin myelinated fibers of frog sciatic nerves and was highly sensitive to local anesthetics, requiring only 0.21 μM bupivacaine for half-maximal blockade. This is the most sensitive ion channel in this preparation even though this flicker channel currently has not been described in mammalian fibers.

In addition to these K$^+$ channels, the ATP-sensitive K$^+$ channel in heart muscle cells was found to be sensitive to lidocaine and bupivacaine.[73,74] This blockade of K$^+$ channels raises the possibility of explaining side effects and toxic effects of local anesthetics in organs other than the peripheral nervous system, especially if K$^+$ channel subtypes are differentially sensitive.

Calcium Channels

Because of the close structural similarity between voltage-dependent Ca^{2+} channels and Na$^+$ channels, it is not surprising that Ca^{2+} currents, especially in DRG, were found to be blocked by local anesthetics.[75-77] A dose-response curve for tetracaine in high voltage-activated Ca^{2+} currents (L-, N-, Q- and P-type) revealed an apparent dissociation constant of 80 μM. When specific blockers were used for L- and N-type

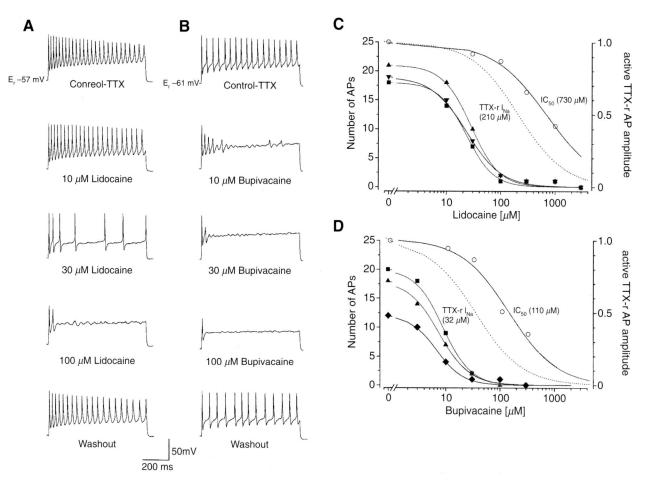

Figure 30–3. Reduction of firing frequency of tetrodotoxin-resistant (TTX-r) action potentials (APs) by lidocaine and bupivacaine in the slice preparation of rat dorsal root ganglia. *A,* Trains of TTX-r action potentials blocked by increasing concentrations of lidocaine. Oscillations can be observed after the action potential at 100 μM lidocaine. Note that the remaining single action potential at the beginning of the current injection is only slightly diminished. *B,* Reduction of firing frequency and number of TTX-resistant action potentials by bupivacaine in another neuron. The oscillation after the AP are mainly at 10 and 30 μM bupivacaine. Seven hundred fifty milliseconds current stimuli of 400 pA. *C,* Lidocaine concentration/effect curve for the number of TTX-r APs and blockade of active amplitudes of TTX-r APs. A Michaelis-Menten equation was fitted to the data revealing IC$_{50}$ values of 24, 27, and 23 μM for 300 *(squares),* 400 *(triangles)* and 500 pA *(inverted triangles)* current stimuli, respectively, from a single neuron. Blockade of active amplitudes of TTX-r APs from the same neuron *(open circles,* right ordinate) revealed an IC$_{50}$ of 730 μM lidocaine. For comparison, the reduction of TTX-r Na$^+$ current *(dotted line;* from Butterworth and Strichartz[97]) is given with IC$_{50}$ of 210 μM lidocaine. *D,* Bupivacaine concentration/effect curve for the number of TTX-r action potentials and blockade of active amplitudes of TTX-r action potentials. IC$_{50}$ values of 7, 9, and 7 μM bupivacaine for 200 *(diamonds),* 300 *(squares),* and 400 pA *(triangles)* stimuli, respectively. IC$_{50}$ of reduction of active TTX-r AP amplitudes *(open circles,* same neuron) was 110 μM bupivacaine. IC$_{50}$ of reduction of TTX-r Na$^+$ current *(dotted line)* was 32 μM bupivacaine. (Adapted from Scholz A, Vogel W: Tetrodotoxin-resistant action potentials in dorsal root ganglion neuron are block by local anesthetics. Pain 89:47, 2000.)

Ca^{2+} channels, it was found that the L-type was more sensitive to local anesthetics than either the N-type Ca^{2+} channel or low voltage-activated Ca^{2+} current (T-type). Local anesthetics other than tetracaine also depressed high voltage-activated Ca^{2+} currents but were of different potency; the rank sequence was dibucaine > tetracaine > bupivacaine >> procaine = lidocaine. Ca^{2+} channels are extremely important in synaptic transmission and in muscle cells, coupling electric excitability with mechanical function. In the peripheral nerve in humans, not only the central end of the fibers in the

dorsal horn contains Ca^{2+} channels but also some thin (mainly C) fibers.[15] This might suggest that in some axons Ca^{2+} channels are sufficient to propagate action potentials in the absence of TTX-sensitive Na$^+$ channels. Although the half maximal blockade occurred at greater concentrations compared with Na$^+$ channels (~5–15 times), their blockade might contribute to interrupting the transmission at concentrations required for spinal anesthesia. What effect this has on the synaptic transmission in the dorsal horn which is triggered by Ca^{2+} channels remains to be investigated. This raises the question whether their effects on Ca^{2+} channels underlie the side effects or toxic effects of local anesthetics in the nervous system as well as in other organs.

Other than these unwanted effects, some similarities of local anesthetics with Ca^{2+} channel blockers (e.g., verapamil) were described that showed a use-dependence like local anesthetics.[78]

Other Targets of Local Anesthetics

Signalling Through G Protein-Coupled Receptors

Although local anesthetics are considered primarily ion channel blockers, studies suggest these may act on additional intracellular sites of action involved in the signal transduction of G protein-coupled receptors.[79] From a series of experiments involving recombinant G protein-coupled receptors (LPA, M1, trypsin, and angiotensin [1A]), and antisense oligonucloetides in an oocyte preparation, it was deduced that the most likely site of action of local anesthetics on the signaling process was at the level of the α_q subunit of the G proteins. Additionally the same group has suggested that local anesthetics produce antagonism of the M3 muscarinic acetylcholine receptor subtype; this cannot be in the same manner as has been demonstrated for the M1 receptor which possesses residues in the extracellular amino terminus which are lacking in the M3 subtype.[80]

There is additional evidence that G-protein-gated inwardly rectifing K^+ channels are blocked by local anesthetics.[81] In addition, in sensory neurons it was shown that bupivacaine, via the IP_3 signalling cascade, mobilized intracellular calcium ions.[82] Taken together these pathways might explain why local anesthetics exhibit side effects in other organs and justify future work to elucidate whether they act in the same way on signal transduction through the endogenous G protein-coupled receptors present in the brain or heart.

Neuropathic and Inflammatory Pain

There is growing evidence that TTX-resistant Na^+ channels play an important role in various types of chronic pain states and hyperalgesia.[83–85] One major outcome in recent studies is that depending on the kind of lesion to the peripheral nerve (cut, crush, ligation, or inflammation), different types of Na^+ channels are down-regulated or up-regulated.[86] This might even result in spontaneous activity whether coming from the neuroma of the nerve or the dorsal root ganglion itself.[87] This was explained by an up-regulation of TTX-sensitive Na^+ channels, because low doses of systemically applied lidocaine blocked this spontaneous activity while only minimally affecting normal sensory receptors.[88]

Pain hypersensitivity was found to be a consequence of early post-translational changes, both in the peripheral terminals of the nociceptor and in dorsal horn neurons, as well as later transcription-dependent changes in effector genes, again in primary sensory and dorsal horn neurons, termed the "wind-up" phenomenon.[89,90] This inflammatory neuroplasticity is the consequence of a combination of activity-dependent changes in the neurons and specific signal molecules initiating particular signal-transduction pathways. It could be demonstrated that the systemic administration of local anesthetics that increase the inactivation of sodium channels can produce a selective central block of certain types of afferent-evoked activity in the spinal cord. The local anesthetics used at these concentrations produced evidence of a block in the conduction of action potentials in Aβ, Aδ, or C fibers.[91]

In a recent study, the sensitivity of the "late" TTX-sensitive Na^+ current generated by large-diameter DRG neurons (>50 μm), as well as of the transient TTX-sensitive Na^+ current in these neurons, was determined.[92] The late Na^+ current was found to be more sensitive to lidocaine and benzocaine than the transient Na^+ current. The late Na^+ current was suggested to be involved in ectopic impulse generation in these neurons, because of its low threshold for activation, and the authors therefore suggest that block of late Na^+ current by systemic local anesthetic may play a part in preventing ectopic impulse generation in sensory neurons.

However, in situations in which other depolarizing currents excite pain fibers above the threshold (ligand-gated or mechanically gated channels, e.g., vanilloid receptor type-1 or dorsal root acid-sensing ion channel) low concentrations of local anesthetics might be expected to have little effect on impulse generation and the associated pain would be refractory.

Neurotoxicity

Evidence from both clinical studies and animal models suggests that the local anesthetic, lidocaine, is neurotoxic. However, the mechanism of lidocaine-induced toxicity is unknown. The hypothesis that toxicity results from a direct action of lidocaine on sensory neurons has been tested in vitro with histologic, electrophysiologic, and fluorometrical experiments on isolated dorsal root ganglion neurons from the adult rat.[93] It was observed that lidocaine induced neuronal death after a 4-minute exposure of DRG neurons to lidocaine concentrations as small as 30 mM. Consistent with an excitotoxic mechanism of neurotoxicity, lidocaine depolarized DRG neurons at concentrations that induced cell death (EC_{50} of 14 mM). This depolarization occurred even though voltage-gated Na^+ currents and action potentials were blocked effectively at much lower concentrations. At concentrations similar to those that induced neurotoxicity and depolarization, lidocaine also induced an increase in the concentration of intracellular Ca^{2+} ions (EC_{50} of 21 mM) through Ca^{2+} influx through the plasma membrane and release of Ca^{2+} from intracellular stores. Finally, lidocaine-induced neurotoxicity was attenuated significantly when lidocaine was applied in the presence of nominally Ca^{2+}-free bath solution to DRG neurons preloaded with BAPTA. These results indicate that lidocaine is neurotoxic to sensory neurons, that toxicity results from a direct action on sensory neurons, and that a lidocaine-induced increase in intracellular Ca^{2+} is a mechanism of lidocaine-induced neuronal toxicity. This may be a convincing path to explain neurotoxicity, and it can be assumed that other local anesthetic act similarly only at different concentrations.[82]

Perspectives for Local Anesthetics

Early hypotheses based on nonspecific interactions of lipid-soluble anesthetics with membrane bilayers have largely given way to the current idea that membrane-associated proteins, particularly ion channels, are specifically modulated by local anesthetics. Indeed, Na^+ channels have been identified as major targets with two different blocking mechanisms.

The use-dependent (phasic) block by local anesthetics seems to be the mechanism that underlies the high sensitivity of Na^+ channels. A recent investigation focused on the goal of testing a substance that produces pronounced use-dependence—a benzomorphan derivative (BIII 890) with phasic blockade ~2000 more potent than its tonic blockade.[31] Even though it was designed to protect the brain after permanent focal cerebral ischemia, its highly use-dependent Na^+ channel block makes it a possible candidate as a local anesthetic and treatment for neuropathic pain.[94]

A selective action on pain might be expected from a drug that targets TTX-resistant Na^+ channels (e.g., Na_v 1.8 and Na_v 1.9), whose expression is confined to Aδ and C fibers transmitting pain.[35,59,65] Unfortunately, no drug currently exhibits this selective property of blocking neuronal TTX-resistant Na^+ channels; however, this remains an attractive goal.

CLINICAL PHARMACOLOGY

Chemical Properties and Relationship to Activity and Potency

The clinically useful local anesthetics consist of a lipophilic, substituted benzene ring linked to a hydrophilic amine group (tertiary or quaternary depending on pKa and pH) through an intermediate chain consisting of either an ester or amide linkage (Fig. 30–4). The type of linkage separates the local anesthetics into two chemically distinct classes. Aminoamides are metabolized in the liver by microsomal enzymes, and plasma cholinesterase enzymes hydrolyze aminoesters. The clinical activity of local anesthetics is dependent on several important chemical properties.

Clinically useful local anesthetics are weak bases that exist in equilibrium between the lipid-soluble, neutral form or as the charged, hydrophilic form. The pKa, or dissociation constant, is the pH at which the two different forms are present in equivalent amounts. The combination of environmental pH and pKa of a local anesthetic determines how much of the compound exists in each form (Table 30–1). The primary site of action of local anesthetics appears to exist on the intracellular side of the sodium channel, and the charged form appears to be the predominantly active form.[97] Penetration by the lipid-soluble form across lipid membranes appears to be the primary mechanism to gain access to the local anesthetic binding site, although some access by the charged form can be gained through the aqueous sodium channel pore (Fig. 30–5).[98] The percentage of local anesthetic found in the neutral lipophilic form at the normal tissue pH of 7.4 is inversely proportional to the pKa of a specific agent. Thus a local anesthetic with a lower pKa will have a relatively more rapid onset of action.

Lipid solubility is another important determinant of clinical activity. Although increasing lipid solubility may hasten penetration of neural membranes, it may also result in increased sequestration of the lipid-soluble form within myelin and other lipid-soluble compartments. Thus the net effect of increasing lipid solubility usually slows the rate of onset of action.[99] In addition, duration of action is increased as absorption of local anesthetic molecules into myelin and surrounding neural compartments creates a depot for slow release of local anesthetics.[99] Finally, increased lipid solubility parallels intrinsic local anesthetic potency.[100] This observation may be explained by a correlation between lipid solubility and both sodium channel receptor affinity and the ability to alter sodium channel conformation by direct effects on lipid cell membranes.

Degree of protein binding also determines activity of local anesthetics, because only the unbound form is free for pharmacologic activity. Increasing protein binding is associated with increased duration of action. Studies suggest that dissociation of local anesthetic molecules from the sodium channel receptor occurs in a matter of seconds regardless of degree of protein binding of the local anesthetic.[101] Thus prolongation in duration of action associated with increased degree of protein binding must include other extracellular or membranous proteins.

Enantiomers of local anesthetics appear to have potentially different effects on pharmacodynamics, pharmacokinetics, and systemic toxicity.[102,103] All currently available local anesthetics are racemic mixtures (50:50 mixture) with the exception of lidocaine (achiral), ropivacaine (S-enantiomer), and levobupivacaine (S-enantiomer).[102,104] R-enantiomers appear to have greater in vitro potency for conduction blockade of both neural and cardiac sodium channels and may thus have greater therapeutic efficacy and potential systemic toxicity.[105] In contrast to their R-enantiomers, both ropivacaine and levobupivacaine possess inherent vasoconstrictor activity, which may explain their

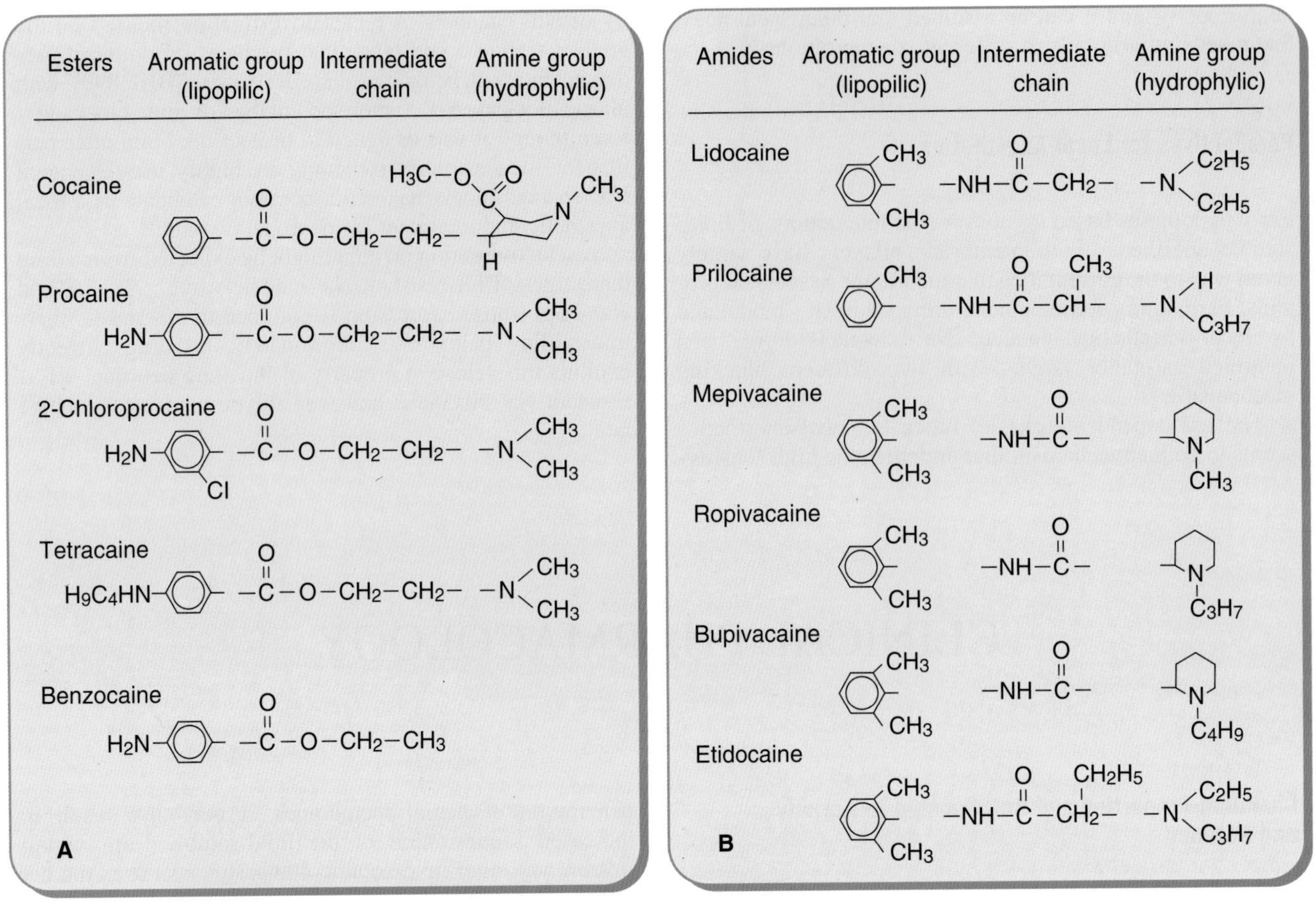

A

Esters	Aromatic group (lipopilic)	Intermediate chain	Amine group (hydrophylic)

Cocaine

Procaine

2-Chloroprocaine

Tetracaine

Benzocaine

B

Amides	Aromatic group (lipopilic)	Intermediate chain	Amine group (hydrophylic)

Lidocaine

Prilocaine

Mepivacaine

Ropivacaine

Bupivacaine

Etidocaine

Figure 30–4. Local anesthetic structures. Clinically useful local anesthetics consist of an aromatic benzene ring linked to a hydrophilic amine group through an intermediate chain consisting of either an ester *(A)* or amide *(B)* linkage. Benzocaine, an agent used primarily for topical anesthesia, is the only clinically useful local anesthetic lacking a tertiary amine group. Local anesthetics connected through an ester linkage are metabolized by plasma cholinesterases; local anesthetics connected through an amide linkage are metabolized in the liver by microsomal enzymes. (Adapted from Butterworth J: Mechanisms of local anesthetic action. In Miller RA, Schwinn DA (eds): Atlas of Anesthesia, vol 2, Scientific Principles of Anesthesia, Philadelphia, Churchill-Livingstone, p 162, 1998.)

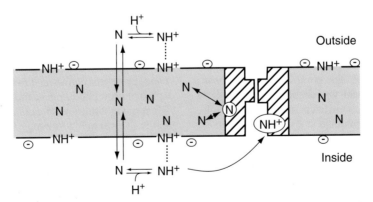

Figure 30–5. Diagram of bilayer lipid membrane of conductive tissue with sodium channel *(crosshatching)* spanning the membrane. Clinically useful local anesthetics exist in equilibrium between the lipid-soluble neutral (N) base and the charged (NH^+) hydrophilic form. The neutral base (N) preferentially partitions into the lipophilic membrane interior and easily passes into the membrane. The charged hydrophilic form (NH^+) binds to the sodium channel at the negatively charged membrane surface. The neutral form can cause membrane expansion and closure of the sodium channel. The charged form directly inhibits the sodium channel by binding with a local anesthetic receptor. (Adapted from Strichartz GR: Neural physiology and local anesthetic action. In Cousins MJ, Bridenbaugh PO (eds): Neural Blockade in Clinical Anesthesia and Management of Pain, Philadelphia, Lippincott-Raven, p 42, 1998.)

TABLE 30–1.

Physicochemical Properties of Clinically Used Local Anesthetics

Local Anesthetic	pKa	% Ionized (at pH 7.4)	Partition Coefficient (lipid solubility)	% Protein Binding
Amides				
Bupivacaine	8.1	83	3420	95
Levobupivacaine	8.1	83	3420	>97%
Etidocaine	7.7	66	7317	94
Lidocaine	7.9	76	366	64
Mepivacaine	7.6	61	130	77
Prilocaine	7.9	76	129	55
Ropivacaine	8.1	83	775	94
Esters				
Chloroprocaine	8.7	95	810	N/A
Procaine	8.9	97	100	6
Tetracaine	8.5	93	5822	94

N/A, not available.

Source: Liu SS: Local anesthetics and analgesia. In Ashburn MA, Rice LJ (eds): The Management of Pain. New York, Churchill Livingstone, 1997, pp 141–170.

longer duration of sensory blockade.[106] A complete analysis of clinical effects from the potential differences in pharmacology between enantiomers has not been determined, nor have optimal mixtures of enantiomers been determined. Future production and commercial release of specific local anesthetic enantiomers may allow for precise selection of not only type of local anesthetic but also exact racemic mixtures for specific applications.

Relative in vitro potencies of the clinically used local anesthetics have been identified and vary depending on individual nerve fibers and frequency of stimulation (Table 30–2). However, clinical use of local anesthetics is more complex than the bathing of nerve fibers in solutions, and in vivo potencies often do not correlate with in vitro determinants.[107] Local factors affecting diffusion and spread of anesthetic will have great impact on clinical effects and will vary with different applications (e.g., peripheral nerve block versus spinal injection). Furthermore, clinical use may not require absolute suppression of the compound action potential, but rather a disruption of information coding in the pattern of discharges. Few rigorous studies have been performed to evaluate relative clinical potencies of local anesthetics; commonly accepted values are listed in Table 30–3.

Mixtures of Local Anesthetics

The practice of combining different local anesthetic agents has been adopted in an attempt to provide a single local anesthetic solution with both a short latency and a long duration of action. The value of such combinations is unclear, because previous studies have reported inconsistent results on both the onset and duration of action, which may vary with type of local anesthetic mixtures, ratio of local anesthetic mixtures, and type of neural block.[108] These disparate findings may reflect the complexity of potential interactions of mixtures of local anesthetics, and current evidence has not shown any clinically significant advantages regarding the practice of combining local anesthetics. Conversely, systemic toxicity appears to be additive, and caution should be used to limit total doses of local anesthetic mixtures.[109]

Tachyphylaxis to Local Anesthetics

Tachyphylaxis to local anesthetics is a clinical phenomenon whereby repeated injection of the same dose of a local anesthetic agent leads to decreasing efficacy.[110] Tachyphylaxis has been described after different regional anesthetic techniques and for different local anesthetics agents.[110] An important clinical feature of tachyphylaxis is its dependence on the dosing interval. If dosing intervals are short enough that pain does not occur, then tachyphylaxis does not occur. Conversely, a longer period of patient discomfort before redosing hastens development of tachyphylaxis.[110] The lack of an underlying mechanism coupled with the clinical observation of the importance of pain for the development of tachyphylaxis led to a hypothesis of a central, spinal mechanism of tachyphylaxis through spinal cord sensitization. A recent series of studies lend support to this hypothesis.[111,112] Tachyphylaxis did not develop in rats receiving repeated sciatic nerve blocks in the absence of sufficient noxious stimulation. However, exposure to increasingly noxious degrees of thermal hyperalgesia hastened development of

TABLE 30–2.

Relative Potency of Local Anesthetics for Block of Different Nerve Fibers

Local Anesthetic	Nerve Fiber					
	Tonic Block			Use-Dependent Block		
	A	B	C	A	B	C
Bupivacaine	12.3	8.4	5.9	16	21.3	24.7
Levobupivacaine	16.4	11.2	7.8	24	32	37
Etidocaine	22.9	20	14.5	35.5	26.7	21.3
Lidocaine	3	2.3	0.8	3.4	4.8	3.4
Mepivacaine	1.7	1.3	0.7	2	2.9	2
Procaine	1	0.7	0.3	1.1	1.1	0.5
Ropivacaine	9.4	6.4	3.5	10.7	15.2	9.7

Source: Wildsmith JA, Brown DT, Paul D, Johnson S: Structure-activity relationships in differential nerve block at high and low frequency stimulation. Br J Anaesth 63:444, 1989; Lee-Son MB, Wang GK, Concus A, et al: Stereoselective inhibition of neuronal sodium channels by local anesthetics. Anesthesiology 77:324–335, 1992.

tachyphylaxis. Conversely, pretreatment of rats with an N-methyl-D-aspartate antagonist that prevents spinal cord sensitization prevented development of tachyphylaxis.[111] Nitric oxide appears to act as a second messenger in N-methyl-D-aspartate pathways, and the administration of a nitric oxide synthase inhibitor also prevented development of tachyphylaxis in a dose-dependent manner in the same model.[112] The clinical relevance of these findings needs to be explored, but the development of a plausible mechanism for local anesthetic tachyphylaxis may lead to useful clinical interventions for its prevention.

Additives to Increase Local Anesthetic Activity

Epinephrine

Reported benefits of epinephrine include prolongation of local anesthetic block,[113] increased intensity of both sensory and motor block,[114] and decreased systemic absorption of local anesthetic.[115] The mechanism whereby epinephrine augments local anesthetic actions remains uncertain. It is commonly theorized that epinephrine-mediated vasoconstriction plays an important role,[116] because most local anesthetics, with the exception of ropivacaine,[117] possess intrinsic vasodilator properties.[118] Local vasoconstriction would theoretically slow clearance from the injection site, thus allowing a greater mass of drugs available for blocking

activity while decreasing the amount available for systemic absorption. This pharmacokinetic mechanism is supported by the fact that peak plasma concentrations of local anesthetics are decreased,[119] whereas tissue levels of local anesthetics are increased when epinephrine is used as an additive for neural blockade.[120] Further analgesic effects from epinephrine may also occur through interaction with α_2 adrenergic receptors in the brain and spinal cord,[121] especially because local anesthetics increase the vascular uptake of epinephrine.[122] Although most reports support adding epinephrine, reported effectiveness depends on the amount of epinephrine added, local anesthetic used, and type of regional block (Table 30–4). It is unfortunate that few data are available concerning the optimal amount of epinephrine as an additive. The most commonly used dose is 5 µg/mL (1:200,000 concentration), but doses as low as 1 to 2 µg/mL may be sufficient. The smallest dose should be used, because epinephrine combined with local anesthetics may have toxic affects on tissue,[123] the cardiovascular (CV) system,[124] peripheral nerves, and the spinal cord.[125]

Alkalinization of Local Anesthetic Solutions

Alkalinization has been shown to shorten the onset of neural blockade, enhance the depth of sensory and motor blockade,[127] and increase the spread of epidural blockade.[128] The pH of commercial preparations of local anesthetics ranges from 3.9 to 6.47 and is especially acidic if prepackaged with

TABLE 30–3.

Relative Potency of Local Anesthetics for Different Clinical Applications

Local Anesthetic	Peripheral Nerve	Spinal	Epidural
Lidocaine	1	1	1
Prilocaine	0.8	N/A	1
Mepivacaine	2.6	1	1
Bupivacaine	3.6	9.6	4
Etidocaine	0.7	6.7	2
Ropivacaine	3.6	4.8	4
Levobupivacaine	3.6	9.6	4
Chloroprocaine	N/A	N/A	0.5

N/A, not available.

Source: Hassan HG: On the relative potency of amino-amide local anesthetics in vivo. Acta Anaesth Scand 38:505, 1994; Langerman L: Duration of spinal anesthesia is determined by the partition coefficient of local anesthetic. Br J Anaesth 72:456, 1994; Langerman L: The partition coefficient as a predictor of local anesthetic potency for spinal anesthesia: Evaluation of five local anesthetics in a mouse model. Anesth Analg 79:490, 1994; Smith C: Pharmacology of local anesthetic agents. Br J Hosp Med 52:455, 1994; Morrison LM: Efficacy of kinetics of extradural ropivacaine: Comparison with bupivacaine. Br J Anaesth 72:164, 1994; Wahedi W: [The equipstency of ropivacaine, bupivacaine and etidocaine]. Reg Anaesth 13:66, 1990; Nolte H: Local anesthetic efficacy of ropivacaine (LEA 103) in ulnar nerve block. Reg Anesth 15:118, 1990; Pateromichelakis S, Prokopiar AA: Local anesthesia office. Discrepancies between in vitro and in vivo studies. Acta Anaesthesiol Scand 32:672, 1988; and Vainionpaa VA: A clinical and pharmacokinetic comparison of ropivacaine and bupivacaine in axillary plexus block. Anesth Analg 81:534, 1995.

epinephrine.[129] As the pKa of commonly used local anesthetics ranges from 7.6 to 8.9 (see Table 29–1), less than 3% of the commercially prepared local anesthetic solution exists as the lipid-soluble, neutral form. The rationale for alkalinization is to increase the percent of local anesthetic existing as the lipid-soluble, neutral form available to diffuse across the neural membrane. Alkalinization is especially effective with local anesthetics prepackaged with epinephrine secondary to the increased acidity of the solution that allows increased shelf-life of the epinephrine. Typically, adding 1 mL sodium bicarbonate per 10 mL lidocaine will hasten the onset of epidural and peripheral nerve blockade by 3 to 5 minutes.

Opioids

Opioids have multiple central neuraxial and peripheral mechanisms of analgesic action (see Chapter 26). Spinal administration of opioids provides analgesia primarily by attenuating C fiber nociception[130] and is independent of supraspinal mechanisms.[131] Coadministration of opioids with most local anesthetics epidurally[132] and intrathecally[133] results in synergistic analgesia.[134] An exception to this analgesic synergy is 2-chloroprocaine (2-CP), which appears to decrease the effectiveness of epidural opioids when used for epidural anesthesia.[135] The mechanism for this action is unclear but does not appear to involve direct antagonization of opioid receptors.[136] Overall, clinical studies support central neuraxial coadministration of opioids with local anesthetics in humans for prolongation and intensification of analgesia and anesthesia[137]; however, the optimal mixtures have yet to be determined.[138] The recent discovery of peripheral opioid receptors offers yet another avenue in which the coadministration of local anesthetics and opioids may be useful.[139] The most promising clinical results have been from intra-articular and infiltration administration of local anesthetic/opioid combinations for postoperative analgesia,[140] whereas combining local anesthetics and opioids for nerve blocks appears to be ineffective.[141]

α_2 Adrenergic Agonists

α_2 Adrenergic agonists can be a useful adjuvant to local anesthetics. α_2 Agonists, such as clonidine, produce analgesia through supraspinal and spinal adrenergic receptors.[142] Clonidine also has direct inhibitory effects on peripheral nerve conduction (A and C nerve fibers).[143] Thus addition of clonidine may have multiple routes of action depending on type of application. Preliminary evidence suggests that coadministration of α_2 agonists and local anesthetic results in central neuraxial and peripheral nerve analgesic synergy,[144] whereas systemic (supraspinal) effects are additive.[145] Overall, clinical trials indicate that clonidine enhances intrathecal and epidural anesthesia,[142] peripheral nerve blocks,[146] and intravenous regional anesthesia (IVRA)[147] without evidence for neurotoxicity.[126] Dexmedetomidine is a potent α_2 adrenergic agonist with eight times greater affinity for the α_2 receptor than clonidine[148,149] that has been approved in the United States for use as a sedative in the intensive care unit setting. Studies with human volunteers have demonstrated that dexmedetomidine not only has sedative properties, but also has analgesic properties that merit further clinical research to determine its place as an adjunct to local anesthetics.[150]

Pharmacokinetics of Local Anesthetics

Clinical effects of neural blockade from local anesthetics are primarily dependent on local factors (as discussed in "Clinical Pharmacology"). However, systemic toxicity is primarily dependent on blood levels of local anesthetics. Resultant blood levels after administration of local anesthetics for

TABLE 30–4.

Effects of Addition of Epinephrine to Local Anesthetics

	Increase Duration	Decrease Blood Levels (%)	Dose/Concentration of Epinephrine
Nerve block			
Bupivacaine	++	10–20	1 : 200,000
Lidocaine	++	20–30	1 : 200,000
Mepivacaine	++	20–30	1 : 200,000
Ropivacaine	−−	0	1 : 200,000
Epidural			
Bupivacaine	++	10–20	1 : 300,000–1 : 200,000
Levobupivacaine*	−−	0	1 : 200,000–1 : 400,000
Chloroprocaine	++		1 : 200,000
Lidocaine	++	20–30	1 : 600,000–1 : 200,000
Mepivacaine	++	20–30	1 : 200,000
Ropivacaine	−−	0	1 : 200,000
Spinal			
Bupivacaine	++		0.2 mg
Lidocaine	++		0.2 mg
Tetracaine	++		0.2 mg

*Data from Kopacz DJ: Anesth Analg 92:S334, 2001.
(++), Overall supported; (−−) overall not supported.
Source: Liu SS: Local anesthetics and analgesia. In Ashburn MA, Rice LJ (eds): The Management of Pain. New York: Churchill Livingstone, 1997, 141–170.

neural blockade are determined by the rate of absorption from the site of injection, the rate of tissue distribution, and the rate of elimination of the specific local anesthetic agent.

Systemic Absorption

In general, local anesthetics with decreased systemic absorption will have a greater margin of safety in clinical use. The site of injection, dose of local anesthetic, physicochemical properties of local anesthetic agent, and addition of epinephrine determine the rate and extent of systemic absorption.

The relative amounts of fat and vasculature surrounding the site of local anesthetic injection will interact with the physicochemical properties of the local anesthetic to affect rate of systemic uptake. In general, areas with greater vascularity will have more rapid and complete uptake compared with those with more fat, regardless of type of local anesthetic. Thus rates of absorption generally decrease in the following order: interpleural > intercostal > caudal > epidural > brachial plexus > sciatic/femoral > subcutaneous tissue (Table 30–5).[151]

The greater the total dose of local anesthetic injected, the greater the systemic absorption and peak blood levels (Cmax). Within the clinical range of doses used for local anesthetics, this relationship is nearly linear and is relatively

unaffected by anesthetic concentration[152] and speed of injection.[151]

Physicochemical properties of local anesthetics will affect systemic absorption. In general, the more potent agents with greater lipid solubility and protein binding will result in lower systemic absorption and Cmax. Increased binding to neural and non-neural tissue probably explains this observation.

Effects of epinephrine have been previously discussed. In brief, epinephrine can counteract the inherent vasodilating characteristics of most local anesthetics. The reduction in Cmax with epinephrine is most effective for the less lipid-soluble, less potent, shorter acting agents (see Table 30–5), because increased tissue binding rather than local blood flow may be a greater determinant of absorption for the long-acting agents.

Distribution

After systemic absorption, local anesthetics are rapidly distributed throughout all body tissues, but the relative concentration in different tissues depends on organ perfusion, partition coefficient, and plasma protein binding. The end organs of main concern for toxicity are the cardiovascular system (CVS) and central nervous system (CNS), because they are considered members of the "vessel rich group" and will have local anesthetic rapidly distributed to them.

TABLE 30–5.

Typical Cmax after Regional Anesthetics with Commonly Used Local Anesthetics

Local Anesthetic	Technique	Dose (mg)	Cmax (µg/mL)	Tmax (min)	Toxic Plasma Concentration (µg/mL)
Bupivacaine	Brachial plexus	150	1.00	20	3
	Celiac plexus	100	1.50	17	
	Epidural	150	1.26	20	
	Intercostal	140	0.90	30	
	Lumbar sympathetic	52.5	0.49	24	
	Sciatic/Femoral	400	1.89	15	
Lidocaine	Brachial plexus	400	4.00	25	5
	Epidural	400	4.27	20	
	Intercostal	400	6.80	15	
Mepivacaine	Brachial plexus	500	3.68	24	5
	Epidural	500	4.95	16	
	Intercostal	500	8.06	9	
	Sciatic/Femoral	500	3.59	31	
Ropivacaine	Brachial plexus	190	1.30	53	4
	Epidural	150	1.07	40	
	Intercostal	140	1.10	21	
Levobupivacaine*	Brachial plexus	2 mg/kg	0.96	43	
	Epidural	150	1.02	24	

Cmax, peak plasma levels; Tmax, time until Cmax.
*Data from Foster RH, Markham A: Levobupivacaine: A review of its pharmacology and use as a local anesthetic. Drugs 59:551, 2000.
Source: Liu SS: Local anesthetics and analgesia. In Ashburn MA, Rice LJ (eds): The Management of Pain. New York, Churchill Livingstone, 1997, pp 141–170; and Berrisford RG, Sabanathan S, Mearns AJ, et al: Plasma concentrations of bupivacaine and its enantiomers during continuous extrapleural intercostal nerve block. Br J Anaesth 70:201–204, 1993.

Despite the high blood perfusion, regional blood and tissue levels of local anesthetics within these organs will not initially correlate with systemic blood levels due to hysteresis.[153] Because regional and not systemic pharmacokinetics govern subsequent pharmacodynamic effects, systemic blood levels may not correlate with effects of local anesthetics on end organs.[154] Regional pharmacokinetics of local anesthetics for the heart and brain have not been fully delineated, thus the volume of distribution at steady state (VD_{ss}) is often used to describe local anesthetic distribution (Table 30–6). However, VD_{ss} describes the extent of total body distribution and may be inaccurate for specific organ systems.

Elimination

Clearance of aminoesters is primarily dependent on hydrolysis of the ester bond by plasma cholinesterases. The rate of enzymatic degradation varies, with chloroprocaine being the most rapid, tetracaine being the slowest, and procaine being intermediate. Aminoamide clearance is dependent on enzymatic degradation primarily in the liver by the mixed-function oxidase system.[155] Thus hepatic extraction, hepatic perfusion, hepatic metabolism, and protein binding determine the rate of clearance of aminoamides (see Table 30–6). In general, local anesthetics with greater rates of clearance will have a greater margin of safety.

Clinical Pharmacokinetics

The primary benefit of systemic pharmacokinetics is in prediction of Cmax after administration of local anesthetics, with the goal of avoiding administration of toxic doses (see Tables 30–5 through 30–7). Both physical and pathophysiologic characteristics will affect an individual's pharmacokinetics, making pharmacokinetics difficult to predict. There is some evidence for increased systemic levels of local anesthetics in the very young and in the elderly caused by decreased clearance and increased absorption.[156] The correlation of resultant systemic blood levels between dose of

TABLE 30–6.

Pharmacokinetic Parameters of Clinically Used Local Anesthetics

Local Anesthetic	VD_{ss} (L/kg)	CL (L/kg/hr)	$T_{1/2}$ (hr)
Bupivacaine	1.02	0.41	3.5
Levobupivacaine	0.78	0.32	2.6
Chloroprocaine	0.50	2.96	0.11
Etidocaine	1.9	1.05	2.6
Lidocaine	1.3	0.85	1.6
Mepivacaine	1.2	0.67	1.9
Prilocaine	2.73	2.03	1.6
Procaine	0.93	5.62	0.14
Ropivacaine	0.84	0.63	1.9

Source: Denson DD: Physiology and pharmacology of local anesthetics. In: Sinatra RS, Hord AH, Ginsberg B, Preble LM (eds): Acute Pain. Mechanisms and Management. St. Louis, Mosby Year Book, 1992, pp 124; and Burm AG, van der Meer AD, van Kleef JW, et al: Pharmacokinetics of the enantiomers of bupivacaine following intravenous administration of the racemate. Br J Clin Pharmacol 38:125–129, 1994.

TABLE 30–7.

Relative Potency for Systemic Central Nervous System Toxicity by Local Anesthetics and Ratio of Dosage Needed for Cardiovascular System: Central Nervous System System (CVS:CNS) Toxicity

Agent	Relative Potency for CNS Toxicity	CVS:CNS
Bupivacaine	4	2.0
Levobupivacaine	2.9	2.0
Chloroprocaine	0.3	3.7
Etidocaine	2.0	4.4
Lidocaine	1.0	7.1
Mepivacaine	1.4	7.1
Prilocaine	1.2	3.1
Procaine	0.3	3.7
Ropivacaine	2.9	2.2
Tetracaine	2.0	

Source: Liu SS: Local anesthetics and analgesia. In Ashburn MA, Rice LJ (eds): The Management of Pain. New York, Churchill Livingstone, 1997, pp 141–170.

local anesthetic and patient weight is often inconsistent.[157] Effects of gender on clinical pharmacokinetics of local anesthetics have not been well defined, although pregnancy may decrease clearance.[156] Pathophysiologic states such as low cardiac output and hepatic disease will alter expected pharmacokinetic parameters (Table 30–8), and lower doses of local anesthetics should be used in these clinical conditions. As expected, renal disease has little effect on pharmacokinetic parameters of local anesthetics (see Table 30–8). Although commonly accepted maximum dosages are listed in Table 30–9, all of these factors should be considered in clinical use of local anesthetics to minimize potential systemic toxicity.

Toxicity of Local Anesthetics

Systemic Toxicity of Local Anesthetics

Central Nervous System Toxicity

Local anesthetics readily cross the blood-brain barrier and produce a dose-dependent pattern of CNS symptoms. Signs of generalized CNS toxicity caused by local anesthetics are dependent on the plasma concentration of the particular drug (Table 30–10). Low plasma concentrations produce CNS depression, whereas higher plasma concentrations result in progressive CNS excitation that may lead to seizures.[158] As the plasma concentration of local anesthetics progressively increases, both inhibitory and facilitatory neurons are blocked leading to generalized CNS depression. The incidence of seizures varies after different regional anesthetic techniques, as would be expected because of differences in the likelihood of unintentional intravascular injection or systemic absorption (Table 30–11).[159]

The potential for systemic CNS toxicity approximately parallels the intrinsic anesthetic potency of the various local anesthetic agents (see Tables 29–3 and 29–7). In addition, decreased local anesthetic protein binding and clearance will increase potential CNS toxicity. A more rapid rate of intravenous administration of local anesthetic will also affect signs of CNS toxicity, because the accelerated rate of increase in plasma concentration will decrease the plasma concentration needed to induce seizures.[160] External factors

TABLE 30–8.

Clinical Profile of Local Anesthetics

Local Anesthetic	Concentration (%)	Clinical Use	Onset	Duration (hr)	Recommended Maximum Single Dose (mg)
Amides					
Bupivacaine	0.25	Infiltration	Fast	2–8	175/225 + epinephrine
	0.25–0.5	Peripheral nerve block	Slow	4–12	175/225 + epinephrine
	0.5–0.75	Epidural anesthesia	Moderate	2–5	175/225 + epinephrine
	0.03–0.25	Epidural analgesia		N/A	
	0.5–0.75	Spinal anesthesia	Fast	1–4	20
Etidocaine	0.5	Infiltration	Fast	2–8	300/400 + epinephrine
	0.5–1	Peripheral nerve block	Fast	3–12	300/400 + epinephrine
	1–1.5	Epidural anesthesia	Fast	2–4	300/400 + epinephrine
Lidocaine	0.5–1	Infiltration	Fast	1–4	300/500 + epinephrine
	0.25–0.5	IV regional anesthesia	Fast	0.5–1	300
	1–1.5	Peripheral nerve block	Fast	1–3	300/500 + epinephrine
	1.5–2	Epidural anesthesia	Fast	1–2	300/500 + epinephrine
	1.5–5	Spinal anesthesia	Fast	0.5–1	100
	4	Topical	Fast	0.5–1	300
Mepivacaine	0.5–1	Infiltration	Fast	1–4	400/500 + epinephrine
	1–1.5	Peripheral nerve block	Fast	2–4	400/500 + epinephrine
	1.5–2	Epidural anesthesia	Fast	1–3	400/500 + epinephrine
	2–4	Spinal anesthesia	Fast	1–2	100
Prilocaine	0.5–1	Infiltration	Fast	1–2	600
	0.25–0.5	IV regional anesthesia	Fast	0.5–1	600
	1.5–2	Peripheral nerve block	Fast	1.5–3	600
	2–3	Epidural	Fast	1–3	600
Ropivacaine	0.2–0.5	Infiltration	Fast	2–6	200
	0.5–1	Peripheral nerve block	Slow	5–8	250
	0.5–1	Epidural anesthesia	Moderate	2–6	200
	0.05–0.2	Epidural analgesia	N/A	N/A	N/A
Levobupivacaine	0.25	Infiltration	Fast	2–8	150
	0.25–0.5	Peripheral nerve block	Slow	14–17	150
	0.5–0.75	Epidural anesthesia	Moderate	5–9	150
	0.125–0.25	Epidural analgesia	N/A	N/A	N/A
	0.5–0.75	Spinal anesthesia	Fast	1–6	20
Mixture Lidocaine + prilocaine	2.5/2.5	Skin topical	Slow	3–5	20 gm
Esters					
Benzocaine	up to 20%	Topical	Fast	0.5–1	200
Chloroprocaine	1	Infiltration	Fast	0.5–1	800/1000 + epinephrine
	2	Peripheral nerve block	Fast	0.5–1	800/1000 + epinephrine
	2–3	Epidural anesthesia	Fast	0.5–1	800/1000 + epinephrine
Cocaine	4–10	Topical	Fast	0.5–1	150
Procaine	10	Spinal anesthesia	Fast	0.5–1	1000
Tetracaine	2	Topical	Fast	0.5–1	20
	0.5	Spinal anesthesia	Fast	2–6	20

Source: Covino BG, Wildsmith JAW: Clinical pharmacology of local anesthetic agents. In Cousins MJ, Bridenbaugh PO (eds): Neural Blockade in Clinical Anesthesia and Management of Pain. Philadelphia, Lippincott-Raven, 1988 pp 97–128 and Foster RH, Markham A: Levobupivacaine: A review of its pharmacology and use as a local anesthetic. Drugs 59:551, 2000.

TABLE 30–9.

Effects of Cardiac, Hepatic, and Renal Disease on Lidocaine Pharmacokinetics

	VD$_{ss}$ (L/kg)	CL (mL/kg/min)	T$_{1/2}$ (hr)
Normal	1.32	10.0	1.8
Cardiac failure	0.88	6.3	1.9
Hepatic disease	2.31	6.0	4.9
Renal disease	1.2	13.7	1.3

CL, total body clearance; T$_{1/2}$, terminal elimination half life; VD$_{ss}$, volume of distribution at steady state.
Source: Thomson PD: Ann Intern Med 78:499, 1973.

can increase potential for CNS toxicity, such as acidosis and increased PCO_2, perhaps through increased cerebral perfusion or decreased protein binding of local anesthetic.[158] There are also external factors that can decrease the potential for generalized CNS toxicity. For example, seizure thresholds of local anesthetics are increased by administration of barbiturates and benzodiazepines.[161]

Cardiovascular Toxicity of Local Anesthetics

In general, significantly larger doses of local anesthetics are required to produce CV toxicity than CNS toxicity. Similar to CNS toxicity, potential for CV toxicity parallels the anesthetic potency of the agent (see Tables 29–3 and 29–7). The more potent, more lipid-soluble agents (bupivacaine, etidocaine, ropivacaine) appear to have an inherently greater cardiotoxicity than the less potent agents.[102] In addition, the

TABLE 30–10.

Dose-Dependent Systemic Effects of Lidocaine

Plasma Concentration (µg/mL)	Effect
1–5	Analgesia
5–10	Lightheadedness Numbness of tongue Tinnitus Muscular twitching
10–15	Seizures Unconsciousness
15–25	Coma Respiratory arrest
>25	Cardiovascular depression

more potent agents also appear to have a different sequence of CV toxicity compared with the less potent agents. For example, increasing doses of lidocaine lead to hypotension, bradycardia, and hypoxia, whereas bupivacaine often results in sudden CV collapse caused by ventricular dysrhythmias that are resistant to resuscitation.[162]

The more potent local anesthetics appear to possess greater potential for direct cardiac electrophysiologic toxicity. A previous study examining lidocaine, bupivacaine, and ropivacaine in rats has demonstrated equivalent peak effects on myocardial contractility but much greater effects on electrophysiology (prolongation of QRS) from bupivacaine

TABLE 30–11.

Incidence of Seizures after Regional Anesthesia in the United States and Europe

Anesthesia	Procedures (n)	Seizures (n)	Incidence of Seizures (incidence/10,000)
Peripheral nerve blocks*	28,810	31	11/10,000
Epidural*	45,578	15	3/10,000
Intravenous regional	11,229	3	3/10,000

*Increased incidence of seizures with bupivacaine vs. lidocaine.
Source: Auroy Y, Narchi P, Messiah A, et al: Serious complications related to regional anesthesia: Results of a prospective survey in France. Anesthesiology 87:479–486, 1997; and Brown DL, Ransom DM, Hall JA, et al: Regional anesthesia and local anesthetic-induced systemic toxicity: Seizure frequency and accompanying cardiovascular changes. Anesth Analg 81:321–328, 1995.

and ropivacaine than lidocaine.[163] Although all local anesthetics block the cardiac conduction system through a dose-dependent block of sodium channels, two features of bupivacaine's sodium channel blocking abilities may enhance its cardiotoxicity. First, bupivacaine exhibits a much stronger binding affinity to resting and inactivated sodium channels than lidocaine.[164] Second, local anesthetics bind to sodium channels during systole and dissociate during diastole. Bupivacaine dissociates from sodium channels during cardiac diastole much more slowly than lidocaine. Indeed, bupivacaine dissociates so slowly that the duration of diastole at physiologic heart rates (60–180 bpm) does not allow enough time for complete recovery of sodium channels and bupivacaine conduction block accumulates (Fig. 30–6). In contrast, lidocaine fully dissociates from sodium channels during diastole and little accumulation of conduction block occurs.[182] Thus enhanced electrophysiologic effects of more potent local anesthetics on the cardiac conduction system may explain their increased potential to produce sudden CV collapse through cardiac dysrhythmias.

Increased potency for direct myocardial depression from the more potent local anesthetics is another contributing factor to increased cardiotoxicity. However, potency of myocardial depression roughly parallels anesthetic potency,[163] thus appropriate use of bupivacaine, levobupivacaine, etidocaine, and ropivacaine will not lead to excessive myocardial depression. Indeed, blood concentrations of bupivacaine and ropivacaine that typically occur from systemic absorption after regional blocks do not result in significant myocardial depression in animals or humans.[102]

CNS-mediated mechanisms may be involved in the increased cardiotoxicity of bupivacaine. The nucleus tractus solitarii in the medulla is an important region for autonomic control of the CVS.[165] Neural activities within the nucleus tractus solitarii of rats are markedly diminished by intravenous doses of bupivacaine immediately before the development of hypotension.[165] Furthermore, direct intracerebral injection of bupivacaine can elicit sudden dysrhythmias and CV collapse.[166]

Peripheral effects of bupivacaine on the autonomic and vasomotor systems may also augment its CV toxicity. Bupivacaine possesses potent peripheral inhibitory effects on sympathetic reflexes[167] and also has potent direct vasodilating properties that may exacerbate CV collapse.[118] The multitude of different cardiac and neural mechanisms of cardiotoxicity may in part explain the reported difficulties of resuscitation after CV collapse from bupivacaine. Once CV collapse occurs, maintenance of respiration and myocardial perfusion are vital, because hypercapnia, hypoxia, acidosis, hypothermia, hyperkalemia, hyponatremia, and myocardial ischemia will all sensitize the heart to bupivacaine cardiotoxicity.[168]

Neurotoxicity of Local Anesthetics

In addition to systemic toxicity, local anesthetics can cause injury to the central and peripheral nervous system from direct exposure. Mechanisms for local anesthetic neurotoxicity remain speculative, but previous studies have demonstrated local anesthetic-induced injury to Schwann cells, inhibition of fast axonal transport, disruption of the blood-nerve barrier, and decreased neural blood flow with associated ischemia.[169] Local anesthetics can cause concentration-dependent nerve fiber damage in peripheral nerves when used in high enough concentrations; however, studies have demonstrated that local anesthetics in clinically used concentrations are safe for peripheral nerves.[170] The spinal cord and the nerve root,[171] in contrast, are more prone to injury. Spinal cord or nerve root toxicity may present as neurohistopathologic, physiologic, or behavioral/clinical

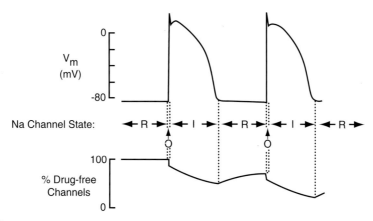

Figure 30–6. Diagram illustrating the relationship between cardiac action potential (*top*), sodium channel state (*middle*), and sodium channel block by bupivacaine (*bottom*). Sodium channels are predominantly in the resting (R) form during diastole, open (O) transiently during the upstroke of the action potential, and are in the inactive (I) form during the plateau of the action potential. Block of sodium channels by bupivacaine accumulates during the action potential (systole) with recovery occurring during diastole. Recovery of sodium channels occurs by dissociation of bupivacaine and is time-dependent. Recovery during each diastolic interval is incomplete and results in accumulation of sodium channel block with successive heartbeats. (Adapted from Clarkson CW, Hondeghem LM: Mechanisms for bupivacaine depression of cardiac conduction: Fast block of sodium channels during the action potential with slow recovery from block during diastole. Anesthesiology 62:396, 1985.)

changes such as pain, motor and sensory deficits, and bowel and bladder dysfunction.

In 1985, Ready et al.[172] evaluated the neurotoxic effects of single intrathecal injections of clinically relevant concentrations of tetracaine, lidocaine, bupivacaine, or chloroprocaine in rabbits, after which spinal cord histopathology remained normal and persistent behavioral deficits were not seen. However, histopathologic changes and neurologic deficits did occur with greater concentrations of tetracaine (1%) and lidocaine (8%). Desheathed peripheral nerve models, designed to mimic unprotected nerve roots in the cauda equina, have been used to further assess electrophysiologic neurotoxicity of local anesthetics.[173] Five percent lidocaine and 0.5% tetracaine caused irreversible conduction block in these models, whereas 1.5% lidocaine, 0.75% bupivacaine, and 0.06% tetracaine did not. Electrophysiologic toxicity of lidocaine in isolated nerve preparations represented by incomplete recovery of neuromuscular function occurs at 40 mM (approximately 1%) with irreversible ablation of the compound action potential seen at 80 mM (approximately 2%). In addition, lidocaine and tetracaine have been shown to cause axonal degeneration in a dose-dependent fashion. Although such studies do not reflect in vivo conditions, they suggest that lidocaine and tetracaine may be especially neurotoxic in a concentration-dependent fashion, and that neurotoxicity could theoretically occur with clinically used solutions.

Neurohistopathologic data in humans after intrathecal exposure to local anesthetics are not available. Electrophysiologic parameters such as somatosensory-evoked potentials, monosynaptic H-reflex,[174] and cutaneous current perception thresholds[175] have been used to evaluate recovery after spinal anesthesia. These measurements have shown complete return to baseline activity after 5% lidocaine spinal anesthesia in small study populations. Recent epidemiologic studies report a 0% to 0.7% incidence of postoperative neurologic injury in patients undergoing spinal anesthesia.[126] Thus despite findings that all local anesthetics have the potential for neurotoxicity in laboratory and animal models, spinally administered local anesthetics currently have not notably manifested their neurotoxic potential in human studies.

Transient Neurologic Symptoms After Spinal Anesthesia

Prospective, randomized, controlled studies reveal up to a 40% incidence of pain radiating from the lower back to the buttocks or lower extremities after lidocaine spinal anesthesia.[176] These symptoms have been labeled as transient neurologic symptoms (TNS) and also have been reported with other local anesthetics, but it is clear that the incidence of TNS is greater after lidocaine spinal anesthesia (Table 30–12). Clinical studies have identified the use of lidocaine,

TABLE 30–12.

Incidences of Transient Neurologic Symptoms (TNS) after Spinal Anesthesia

Agent	Preparation	Position	Approximate TNS Incidence
Lidocaine	Hyperbaric 2–5%	Lithotomy	30–40%
	Hyperbaric 0.5–5%	Knee arthroscopy	20–30%
	Hyperbaric 5%	Supine/unspecified	5–10%
	Hyperbaric 5%	Supine/cesarean section	0–3%
	Hyperbaric 5%[†]	Supine/postpartum tubal ligation	3%
Bupivacaine	Isobaric/hyperbaric	Lithotomy/others	Rare
Tetracaine	Hyperbaric	General use	Rare
	Hyperbaric + phenylephrine	Lower extremity/perineal	12%
Procaine	Hyperbaric 5%	Knee arthroscopy	6%
	Isobaric 5%	Supine/other	1%
Mepivacaine	Hyperbaric 4%	Lithotomy/other	30–40%
	Isobaric 1.5%	Knee arthroscopy	Rare
Ropivacaine	Hyperbaric 0.25%	Supine volunteers	Rare

Source: Hodgson PS, Neal JM, Pollock JE, et al: The neurotoxicity of drugs given intrathecally (spinal). Anesth Analg 88:797–809, 1999;
*Aouad MT, Siddik SS, Jalbout MI, et al: Does pregnancy protect against intrathecal lidocaine-induced transient neurologic symptoms? Anesth Analg 92:401, 2001; and
[†]Philip J, Sharma SK, Gottumukkala VNR, et al: Transient neurologic symptoms after spinal anesthesia with lidocaine in obstetric patients. Anesth Analg 92:405, 2001.

lithotomy position, ambulatory surgical status, arthroscopic knee surgery, and obesity as factors that place patients at increased risk for development of TNS.[177] The lowest incidence of TNS in patients receiving spinal lidocaine has been found in obstetric patients undergoing cesarean section (see Table 30–12).[178]

Patients typically manifest symptoms of TNS within 12 to 24 hours after surgery and recover within 1 week. Current treatment modalities include traditional classes of medications: opioids, nonsteroidal anti-inflammatory drugs, and muscle relaxants.[179] Nonpharmacologic modalities include symptomatic treatment with warm heat and positioning as well as trigger-point injections. Currently, there are no reported cases of TNS with abnormal neurologic examinations or motor weakness. When a patient has symptoms of back and leg pain after spinal anesthesia, other potentially serious causes (hematoma, abscess, cauda equina syndrome) must be eliminated before symptomatic treatment is inititated.[180]

Contemporary reports of cauda equina syndrome after single-shot or continuous lidocaine spinal anesthesia and the potential concentration-dependent neurotoxicity of lidocaine have led several authors to label TNS as a manifestation of subclinical neurotoxicity.[181] As discussed earlier, laboratory work in both intrathecal and desheathed peripheral nerve models has proven that the concentration of lidocaine is a critical factor in neurotoxicity. As concentrations of lidocaine less than 40 mM (approximately 1.0%) are not neurotoxic to desheathed peripheral nerve, such dilute concentrations of spinal lidocaine should not cause TNS if the syndrome is due to subclinical concentration-dependent neurotoxicity. However, the dilution of lidocaine to 0.5% does not decrease the incidence of TNS.[176] The high incidence of TNS observed with lidocaine concentrations less than 1% despite further dilution in cerebrospinal fluid would appear to lessen the plausibility of a concentration-dependent neurotoxic etiologic factor. Electrophysiologic studies of nerve conduction velocity, electromyography, and somatosensory-evoked potentials in human volunteers both before and after episodes of TNS show no changes, even in the posterior nerve roots, which are particularly susceptible to local anesthetic toxicity.[182] Other potential causes for TNS include patient positioning, early mobilization, needle trauma, neural ischemia secondary to sciatic stretching, maldistribution of local anesthetics secondary to pooling caused by small-gauge pencil point needles, muscle spasm, myofascial trigger points, or irritation of DRG.[176,179] Clearly, the cause of TNS remains undetermined and further studies are needed to elucidate the underlying mechanism.

In summary, all local anesthetics have the potential to be neurotoxic, particularly in concentrations and doses greater than those used clinically. In neurohistopathologic, electrophysiologic, behavioral, and in vitro models, lidocaine and tetracaine appear to have greater potential for neurotoxicity than bupivacaine at clinically relevant concentrations. Nonetheless, large-scale surveys of the complications of spinal anesthesia attest to the relative safety of spinal local anesthetics.

Clinical Use of Local Anesthetics

Amino Ester Agents

Procaine

Procaine is a chemical derivative of para-aminobenzoic acid with a high pKa and poor lipid solubility. It is a relatively weak local anesthetic with a slow onset and a short duration of action of 30 to 60 minutes. Its rapid hydrolysis by plasma cholinesterases limits the potential for systemic toxicity. Procaine can be used for infiltration anesthesia in 0.25% to 1.0% concentrations, but most commonly it is used for spinal anesthesia with 50 to 200 mg of the 10% solution. The use of procaine for topical anesthesia is not recommended, and it has limited use for epidural anesthesia, peripheral nerve blockade, or intravenous regional anesthesia (IVRA).

Chloroprocaine

2-CP is a derivative of procaine with a rapid onset of action and an even more rapid metabolism than procaine. The short plasma half-life of 2-CP (<30 seconds) limits its potential for systemic toxicity. It can be used in 1% concentrations to produce rapid analgesia or anesthesia for infiltration. At 2% to 3% concentrations, rapid onset of anesthesia for epidural and peripheral nerve blockade is achieved, with the total dose primarily determining the degree of blockade.[183] 2-CP has been most commonly used for epidural anesthesia for cesarean section because of its rapid onset and low potential for systemic toxicity in both the parturient and fetus. In addition, the predictable short duration of action of 2-CP facilitates a rapid recovery and discharge in the ambulatory surgery setting.[184] Intravenous 2-CP has been effective for rapid, short-term inhibition of sympathetic responses to laryngoscopy and intubation.[185] Older preparations of 2-CP contained sodium metabisulfite as a preservative, which had been linked to severe neurologic injury in the event of an accidental subarachnoid injection of doses intended for epidural anesthesia. Subsequently, 2-CP was reformulated with ethylenediaminetetraacetic acid as the preservative, but in doses larger than 40 mL; the chelating action of ethylenediaminetetraacetic acid has been implicated as the cause of severe paravertebral muscle spasm that occurs after resolution of epidural blockade.[186] To minimize this potential problem, the use of 2-CP should be limited to doses less than 25 mL with the newer preservative-free formulation.

Tetracaine

Tetracaine is the butylaminobenzoic acid derivative of procaine. It is a potent, long-acting local anesthetic that produces dense sensory and motor blockade. It remains a popular choice for spinal anesthesia, with a relatively fast onset of 3 to 5 minutes, and duration of 2 to 3 hours, which can be extended to 4 to 6 hours with the addition of epinephrine. It is available in a 0.5% to 1.0% solution or in lyophilized crystalline form. The crystalline form can be reconstituted either with 10% dextrose for a hyperbaric solution, with sterile water for a hypobaric solution, or with cerebrospinal fluid for an isobaric solution. Tetracaine has the slowest rate of hydrolysis of the clinically used ester agents, but its half-life is shorter than any of the amide agents. It has excellent topical anesthetic properties, and remains the agent of choice for topical ophthalmologic anesthesia. The use of tetracaine for epidural anesthesia, peripheral nerve blockade, or IVRA is limited as the larger doses required increase the potential for systemic toxicity.

Cocaine

Cocaine has the unique property of combining local anesthetic activity with intense vasoconstriction. It is most commonly used as a 4% to 10% solution before instrumentation of the nasopharyngeal mucosa or otolaryngologic surgical procedures. Its low therapeutic index and potential for illicit abuse limits its use to only for topical anesthesia.

Benzocaine

Benzocaine is unique among clinically useful local anesthetics because it is a secondary amine and a weak acid (pKa 3.5). Benzocaine is found only in its uncharged form at physiologic pH, making it ideally suited for topical anesthesia of mucous membranes before endoscopy, bronchoscopy, or fiberoptic intubation of the trachea. It is most commonly available as a 20% solution, with an extremely rapid onset and duration of action of 30 to 60 minutes. Doses greater than 200 to 300 mg can result in methemoglobinemia potentially leading to cyanosis and a decrease in oxygen-carrying capacity,[187] with neonates at greater risk because of the more readily oxidized fetal hemoglobin. In the event of symptomatic methemoglobinemia, 1% methylene blue, in a 1 to 2 mg/kg dose over 20 minutes, should be administered.

Amino Amide Agents

Lidocaine

Lidocaine was the first aminoamide local anesthetic introduced into clinical practice, and remains the most widely used agent because of its potency, short latency, and intermediate duration of action. Lidocaine's versatility is demonstrated by clinical application for almost any regional anesthetic application. At concentrations of 0.5% to 1.0%, lidocaine provides anesthesia of rapid onset with a duration of 60 to 120 minutes. It is excellent for topical anesthesia when used in 4% concentration. Tumescent anesthesia, whereby large volumes of dilute lidocaine in combination with epinephrine are injected into subcutaneous tissue, is most often used by plastic surgeons for liposuction procedures. Despite the use of large doses (up to 55 mg/kg), there

have been few reports of systemic toxicity, although plasma concentrations may peak more than 10 to 12 hours after completion of surgery.[188] Lidocaine is the most commonly used local anesthetic for IVRA. Fifty milliliters of the 0.5% concentration provides 45 to 60 minutes of anesthesia for upper extremity surgery. Lidocaine remains a popular choice for spinal anesthesia or epidural anesthesia providing dense sensory anesthesia and complete motor block for surgery of the trunk and lower extremities, although controversy regarding lidocaine neurotoxicity has tempered its popularity for spinal anesthesia.

Intravenous or laryngotracheal administration of lidocaine has been used with variable success to blunt hemodynamic responses to tracheal intubation and extubation.[189] Intravenous lidocaine can be effective for decreasing airway sensitivity by depressing airway reflexes and decreasing calcium influx in airway smooth muscle. Doses of 2 to 2.5 mg/kg are required to consistently blunt hemodynamic and airway responses to tracheal instrumentation.[190] Intravenous lidocaine is also effective for attenuating increases in intraocular, intracranial, and intra-abdominal pressure during airway instrumentation and may be beneficial in selected clinical situations (e.g., open eye injury or increased intracranial pressure).[191]

Intravenous lidocaine has well-recognized antidysrhythmic properties and acts by inhibiting phase 3 repolarization and suppressing ventricular ectopy.[192] It is administered as an intravenous bolus dose of 100 to 200 mg followed by continuous infusion of 1 to 4 mg/min with minimal potential for systemic toxicity.

Finally, intravenous lidocaine (1–5 mg/kg) is an effective systemic analgesic and has been used to treat both acute postoperative pain[193] and chronic neuropathic pain.[194] The mechanism of analgesia remains unclear,[195] but does not involve typical block of impulse conduction in peripheral nerves. Both peripheral inhibition of spontaneous ectopic discharges in injured nerve fibers and DRG, as well as central inhibition of activity of hippocampal and thalamic neurons,[196] probably contribute to systemic analgesic effects of lidocaine. The ability of lidocaine to provide systemic analgesic effects at peripheral and central sites may in part explain the ability of a single neural block to provide long-lasting analgesia from neuropathic pain.[195] In addition, oral congeners of lidocaine such as mexiletine have been used successfully to treat chronic pain conditions such as peripheral neuropathies[197] and central spinal cord pain.[198]

Prilocaine

The clinical profile of prilocaine is similar to that of lidocaine except that it causes significantly less vasodilation and thus can be used without epinephrine. The most popular clinical application of prilocaine is for topical anesthesia when used within eutectic mixture of LA cream (25 mg/mL prilocaine and 25 mg/mL lidocaine). The application of eutectic mixture of LA cream to intact skin for 60 to 90 minutes underneath an occlusive dressing provides cutaneous anesthesia for painful superficial procedures such as vascular cannulation[199] or spinal puncture.[200] Because of its extremely rapid metabolism, prilocaine is considered the least toxic of the amide agents.[201] However, the metabolite of prilocaine (o-toluidine) is associated with dose-related formation of methemoglobin, which has limited its widespread clinical use.

Mepivacaine

Mepivacaine is similar to lidocaine with regard to clinical applicability to regional anesthesia. It is a potent local anesthetic, with a short latency and intermediate duration of action that is slightly longer than lidocaine.[202] In can be used for topical or infiltration anesthesia, but is seldom used because of the widespread popularity of lidocaine. There has been a renewed interest in mepivacaine for spinal anesthesia because of the current concerns of lidocaine neurotoxicity. The anesthetic and recovery profile of plain 1.5% to 2.0% isobaric mepivacaine makes it a suitable alternative to lidocaine for ambulatory spinal anesthesia, with a lower or similar reported incidence of TNS (0–33%) than has been reported for lidocaine.[203] The use of mepivacaine for epidural anesthesia in 1.5% to 2.0% solutions provides a profound depth of surgical anesthesia obtained within 10 to 15 minutes, with a slightly longer time (70–90 minutes) to two-segment regression than lidocaine.[204] The use of 1.0% to 1.5% mepivacaine for peripheral nerve blockade will provide anesthesia for 2 to 4 hours. The systemic toxicity profile of mepivacaine is similar to lidocaine, with the exception of use for surgical obstetric anesthesia. The fetus poorly metabolizes mepivacaine, and the doses required for surgical anesthesia can lead to accumulation of high levels of mepivacaine in the fetal circulation resulting in poor fetal muscle tone.[205]

Bupivacaine

Bupivacaine was the first long-acting amide agent to gain widespread use. The physiochemical properties of bupivacaine confer a relatively slow onset time with the exception of infiltration and spinal anesthesia. The main disadvantage of bupivacaine is its potential for significant systemic toxicity.

Bupivacaine in concentrations of 0.25% provides extended duration anesthesia and analgesia after infiltration in surgical wounds. The intraperitoneal administration of bupivacaine has been found to decrease postoperative pain and nausea after gynecologic laparoscopic procedures,[206] but has been less effective after laparoscopic cholecystectomy.[207]

Bupivacaine is commonly used for spinal anesthesia with relatively fast onset within 5 minutes and a dose-dependent duration of sensory and motor block persisting for 1 to 4 hours. It can be administered as either a hyperbaric solution (0.75% with 8.25% glucose) or an isobaric solution (0.5%), with the isobaric solution generally exhibiting less hypotension because of its slower onset and lower overall peak block height. The synergistic combination of very low doses of spinal bupivacaine administered with fentanyl provides reliable lower extremity surgical anesthesia, providing shorter discharge times in the ambulatory setting,[208] as well as less need for hemodynamic support than higher doses of plain bupivacaine.[209]

The unique property of sensory and motor dissociation with bupivacaine makes it ideal for continuous epidural labor analgesia and postoperative epidural analgesia. The degree of motor block begins to decrease significantly below 0.25%. At concentrations of 0.1% or less, epidural bupivacaine provides sensory analgesia with minimal motor block, allowing the capability of ambulation with assistance. Concentrations of 0.5% to 0.75% provide complete sensory anesthesia with variable degrees of motor block. The 0.75% solution is no longer recommended for surgical obstetric anesthesia because of the selective cardiotoxicity of bupivacaine.

The use of bupivacaine for peripheral nerve block is ideal when the goal is to provide long-lasting sensory anesthesia. The average duration of sensory anesthesia is from 4 to 12 hours, occasionally lasting up to 24 hours. The concern for cardiac toxicity has limited its use for IVRA.

Etidocaine

Etidocaine is a potent, highly lipophilic local anesthetic with relatively rapid onset of action, but a duration of action similar to bupivacaine. It can be use for infiltration, epidural anesthesia, and peripheral nerve blockade. Etidocaine is the only local anesthetic agent that is selectively more potent for motor blockade than sensory anesthesia, thus making it particularly useful when a profound depth of muscle relaxation is required for a surgical procedure. However, in clinically used doses, limited sensory anesthesia can accompany profound motor block, thus limiting its widespread use. Etidocaine has the same electrophysiologic effects as bupivacaine and the potential for significant CV toxicity.

New Local Anesthetics with Decreased Systemic Toxicity

In 1979, Albright[210] published an editorial drawing attention to the potential for sudden CV collapse with the accidental intravascular administration of potent, highly lipophilic local anesthetics bupivacaine and etidocaine. Heightened awareness of potential CV toxicity led to the withdrawal of U.S. Food and Drug Administration approval of high concentrations of bupivacaine (0.75%) for obstetric use. Subsequently, changes in clinical practice, such as the use of a test dose, intermittent aspiration, and incremental dosing[211] indicate that the current clinical use of potent local anesthetics is safe, with an incidence of CNS toxicity with epidural anesthesia of approximately 3/10,000 and an incidence of 11/10,000 with peripheral nerve blockade[159] (see Table 30–11). Interestingly, there continues to be a greater incidence of accidental intravascular injection of local anesthetics during peripheral nerve blockade, perhaps because of differences in clinical practice or less clinical awareness. This observation is consistent with Albright's original editorial,[210] because three out of the six cases reported were observed during attempted brachial plexus blockade. Unfortunately, accidental intravenous injection of local anesthetics can occur even in experienced hands and despite the current practice of safety checks. Based on the findings that the cardiotoxicity observed with racemic bupivacaine is more pronounced with the R-enantiomer, the S-enantiomer preparations of ropivacaine and levobupivacaine have been introduced into clinical practice to provide long-acting agents with a greater safety margin than racemic bupivacaine.

Ropivacaine was released for widespread clinical use in 1996. Ropivacaine has a three-carbon substitution (isopropyl) on the tertiary amine and is structurally similar to mepivacaine (methyl substitution) and bupivacaine (butyl substitution). The lower lipid solubility of ropivacaine may explain the in vitro and clinical observations that, at lower concentrations, ropivacaine causes less motor block than bupivacaine.[212]

Animal studies and human volunteer studies have confirmed that ropivacaine is approximately 30% to 40% less cardiotoxic than bupivacaine (Table 30–13; Fig. 30–7).[213,214] In both animal and human studies, ropivacaine has been found to cause less prolongation of QRS duration, less depression of myocardial contractility,[215] and less depression of myocardial mitochondrial activity than equivalent doses of bupivacaine.[216] In addition, the symptoms and severity of CNS toxicity of bupivacaine were greater than ropivacaine.[217] Currently, clinical experience has shown that serious systemic cardiac toxicity with ropivacaine is extremely rare, with only one case report occurring during a sciatic nerve block and the patient fully recovered.[218]

Overall, ropivacaine appears clinically equivalent to racemic bupivacaine. Clinical data have shown that epidural 0.1% to 0.25% ropivacaine provides labor analgesia with similar efficacy to bupivacaine.[219] Epidural anesthesia with 0.5% ropivacaine is as efficacious as 0.5% bupivacaine for cesarean section,[220] lower limb orthopedic surgeries,[221] and urologic surgery[222] without significant differences in onset, duration, or regression of sensory block, and intensity and duration of motor block. Limited experience with spinal administration of ropivacaine indicates that it provides a pattern of sensory and motor blockade similar to equivalent doses of spinal bupivacaine.[223] Recent studies with ropiva-

caine for brachial plexus[224] and peripheral nerve blockade demonstrate similar clinical outcomes to comparable doses and concentrations of racemic bupivacaine. Ropivacaine has the unique property of vasoconstriction and may provide either an advantage or disadvantage when used for local infiltration, depending on the surgical site.

Levobupivacaine is the S^- enantiomer of racemic bupivacaine. Clinical evidence confirms that levobupivacaine has similar potency to bupivacaine.[225] However, levobupivacaine also appears to have approximately 30% to 40% less systemic toxicity on a mg:mg basis in human volunteer studies,[226] which is likely because of reduced affinity for brain and myocardial tissue compared with the racemic preparation of bupivacaine. Animal studies have demonstrated that levobupivacaine has less cardiotoxicity than either racemic bupivacaine (Table 30–14; see Fig. 30–7) or the R^+ enantiomer dexbupivacaine.[214] Levobupivacaine was shown to produce both less of a negative inotropic effect and less prolongation of the QT_C interval than bupivacaine.[226] Animal studies suggest that the uptake of levobupivacaine by the CNS is slower than for dexbupivacaine and may explain the decreased CNS toxicity observed in human volunteer studies.[226] Clinical studies have established that levobupivacaine has a clinical profile that is similar to equivalent doses of racemic bupivacaine when used for epidural[227] and brachial plexus anesthesia,[228] although there was a trend toward a longer duration of sensory block with levobupivacaine. Levobupivacaine in concentrations of 0.125% to 0.25% has been shown to provide equianalgesic potency to bupivacaine for epidural labor analgesia.[229]

Extended Duration Local Anesthetics

There is potential clinical application for extended duration of local anesthetic action. Use of extended duration local anesthetic formulations could be used for infiltration and peripheral nerve or plexus blockade and could significantly

TABLE 30–13.

Animal Studies Evaluating Relative Cardiotoxicity of Lidocaine, Ropivacaine, and Bupivacaine

Species	Measurement	Lidocaine	Ropivacaine	Bupivacaine
Dog	Ventricular fibrillation (%)	0	33	83
	Resuscitate (%)	75	100	66
Sheep	Ventricular fibrillation (%)	—	40	75
Pig	Myocardial depression (%)	13	38	50
	Death (%)	0	0	25

Source: Carpenter RL: Am J Anesthesiol 24:4, 1997.

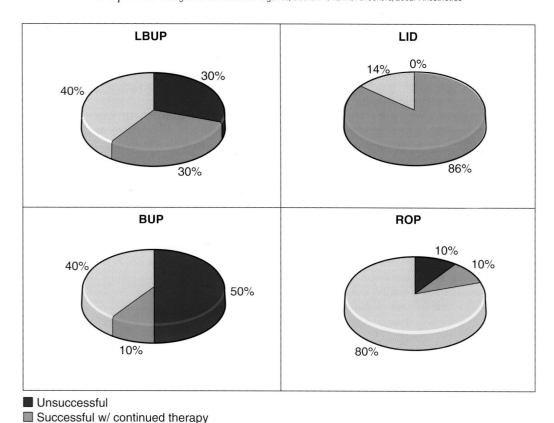

■ Unsuccessful
■ Successful w/ continued therapy
□ Successful

Figure 30–7. Pie diagram representing resuscitative outcomes for each group of anesthetized dogs after incremental overdosage with levobupivacaine (LBUP), bupivacaine (BUP), lidocaine (LID), and ropivacaine (ROP). (Adapted from Groban L, Deal DD, Vernon JC, et al: Cardiac resuscitation after incremental overdosage with lidocaine, bupivacaine, levobupivacaine, and ropivacaine in anesthetized dogs. Anesth Analg 92:37, 2001.)

TABLE 30–14.

Animal Studies Evaluating Relative Cardiotoxicity of Bupivacaine and Levobupivacaine

Species	Measurement	Bupivacaine	Levobupivacaine
Pig*	Minimum lethal dose injected into LAD (mg)	5	8
Sheep[†]	Ventricular arrhythmias (%)	45	28
	Death (%)	14	0
Dogs[‡]	Cumulative dose to cardiovascular collapse (mg/kg)	21.7	27.3
	Successful resuscitation (%)	50	70

LAD, left anterior descending Coronary artery.

Source: *Morrison SG, Dominguez JJ, Frascarolo P, et al: Reg Anesth Pain Med 23:S50, 1998; [†]Huang YF, Pryor ME, Mather LE, et al: Cardiovascular and central nervous system effects of intravenous levobupivacaine and bupivacaine in sheep. Anesth Analg 86:797, 1998; and [‡]Groban L, Deal DD, Vernon JC, et al: Cardiac resuscitation after incremental overdosage with lidocaine, bupivacaine, levobupivacaine, and ropivacaine in anesthetized dogs. Anesth Analg 92:37, 2001.

decrease the need for postoperative systemic analgesics. In addition, intra-articular injections of extended duration formulations could treat chronic arthritic pain, whereas central neuraxial administration would probably be limited to treatment of chronic or cancer pain syndromes because of the possibility of associated motor block. Current technology for extending duration of action typically involves extended delivery of commercially available local anesthetics rather than development of new local anesthetics. Delivery systems include encapsulation of local anesthetic in liposomes (Fig. 30–8), microspheres, or polymers with slow degradation and release.[230] Animal studies using controlled release microspheres containing a combination of bupivacaine and dexamethasone provided peripheral nerve block analgesia from 2 days to greater than 2 weeks.[231] In addition to extended clinical duration, these delivery systems also appear to decrease potential for both CNS and CV toxicity caused by slow release of local anesthetic and altered tissue uptake.[232] The potential for extended local analgesic activity of these delivery systems merits further clinical research.

Local Anesthetics with Combined Mechanisms of Action

An increased understanding of mechanisms of pain has led to the realization that multiple neurotransmitters are involved in the spinal cord and peripheral nervous system, and these neurotransmitters may play a role in central sensitization of the CNS responses to pain. Local anesthetics are somewhat effective for prevention of pain and central sensitization when administered centrally or peripherally.[233] However, targeted modulation of multiple receptors involved in mechanisms of pain and central sensitization could produce multimodal analgesia, with added efficacy and decreased side effects, in contrast to local anesthetics alone. Molecules that have local anesthetic activity in combination with analgesic activities through other mechanisms (opioid receptors, alpha adrenergic receptors, and so on) could potentially provide this multimodal analgesia by either central neuraxial or peripheral delivery. Sameridine is a mixed local anesthetic and opioid agonist compound that is undergoing clinical trials as a spinal agent,[234] and other mixed function compounds may soon be tested.

Calcium Channel Ligands

Neuronal-type, voltage-dependent, calcium channels are located on presynaptic nerve terminals where they allow calcium influx required for depolarization-induced neurotransmitter release. Administration of voltage-dependent, calcium channel antagonists results in hyperpolarization of cell membranes, resistance to electrical stimulation from nociceptive afferents, and intense analgesia. Ziconotide is a

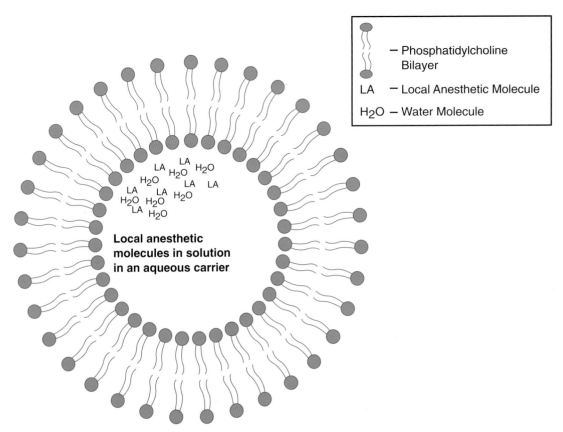

— Phosphatidylcholine Bilayer

LA — Local Anesthetic Molecule

H_2O — Water Molecule

Local anesthetic molecules in solution in an aqueous carrier

Figure 30–8. Schematic structure of a liposome. (Adapted from Kuzma PJ, Kline MD, Calkins MD, et al: Progress in the development of ultra-long-acting local anesthetics. Reg Anesth 22:543, 1997.)

new synthetic conopeptide that specifically blocks neuronal-type, voltage-dependent, calcium channels.[235] Ziconotide has been shown to be effective in various animal models of acute, chronic, and neuropathic pain.[236] Currently human studies indicate that a constant spinal infusion of ziconotide may have a potential role in the management of chronic neuropathic pain.[237] In addition, spinal infusion of ziconotide has also been shown to have opioid-sparing activity in patients with acute postoperative pain.[238] Future studies are needed to investigate the clinical application of this potentially useful class of antinociceptive agents.

References

1. Noda M, Ikeda T, Suzuki H, et al: Expression of functional sodium channels from cloned cDNA. Nature 322:826, 1986.
2. Freud S: Über Coca. Zentralbl Ges Ther 2:289, 1884.
3. Corning JL: Spinal anaesthesia and local medication of the cord. NY Med J 42:183, 1885.
4. Quincke H: Die Lumbalpunktion des Hydrozephalus. Berl Klin Wochenschr 28:929, 1891.
5. Einhorn A: On the chemistry of local anesthetics. MMW 46:1218, 1899.
6. Gasser HS, Erlanger J: Role of fibre size in the establishment of nerve block by pressure or cocaine. Am J Physiol 88:581, 1929.
7. Gissen AJ, Covino BG, Gregus J: Differential sensitivities of mammalian nerve fibers to local anesthetic agents. Anesthesiology 53:467, 1980.
8. Wildsmith JA, Gissen AJ, Takman B, et al: Differential nerve blockade: Esters v. amides and the influence of pKa. Br J Anaesth 59:379, 1987.
9. Raymond SA, Gissen AJ: Mechanisms of differential nerve block. In Strichartz GR (ed): Local Anesthetics. Berlin, Heidelberg, Springer-Verlag, 1987, pp 95–165.
10. Ochoa JL, Torebjork HE: Paraesthesiae from ectopic impulse generation in human sensory nerves. Brain 103:835, 1980.
11. Weidner C, Schmelz M, Schmidt R, et al: Functional attributes discriminating mechano-insensitive and mechano-responsive C nociceptors in human skin. J Neurosci 19:10184, 1999.
12. Schmelz M, Schmidt R, Bickel A, et al: Specific C-receptors for itch in human skin. J Neurosci 17:8003, 1997.
13. Wall PD, Melzack R: Textbook of Pain, 4th ed. New York, Churchill Livingstone, 1999.
14. Belmonte C, Cervero F: Neurobiology of Nociceptors, 1st ed. Oxford, Oxford University Press, 1996.
15. Quasthoff S, Grosskreutz J, Schroder JM, et al: Calcium potentials and tetrodotoxin-resistant sodium potentials in unmyelinated C fibres of biopsied human sural nerve. Neuroscience 69:955, 1995.
16. Kobayashi JI, Ohta M, Terada Y: Tetrodotoxin resistant na+ spikes of c fibers have at least two subtypes in the isolated bullfrog sciatic nerve. Neurosci Lett 221:9, 1996.
17. Frazier DT, Narahashi T, Yamada M: The site of action and active form of local anesthetics. II. Experiments with quaternary compounds. J Pharmacol Exp Ther 171:45, 1970.
18. Hille B: Ionic Channels of Excitable Membranes, 2nd ed. Sunderland, Mass., Sinauer Associates, 1992.
19. Woodhull AM: Ionic blockage of sodium channels in nerve. J Gen Physiol 61:687, 1973.
20. Strichartz GR: The inhibition of sodium currents in myelinated nerve by quaternary derivatives of lidocaine. J Gen Physiol 62:37, 1973.
21. Courtney KR: Mechanism of frequency-dependent inhibition of sodium currents in frog myelinated nerve by the lidocaine derivative GEA. J Pharmacol Exp Ther 195:225, 1975.
22. Ulbricht W: Kinetics of drug action and equilibrium results at the node of Ranvier. Physiol Rev 61:785, 1981.
23. Starmer CF, Grant AO, Strauss HC: Mechanisms of use-dependent block of sodium channels in excitable membranes by local anesthetics. Biophys J 46:15, 1984.
24. Agnew WS, Levinson SR, Brabson JS, et al: Purification of the tetrodotoxin-binding component associated with the voltage-sensitive sodium channel from electrophorus electricus electroplax membranes. Proc Natl Acad Sci USA 75:2606, 1978.
25. Noda M: Structure and function of sodium channels. Ann NY Acad Sci 20:20–37, 1993.
26. Vassilev PM, Scheuer T, Catterall WA: Identification of an intracellular peptide segment involved in sodium channel inactivation. Science 241:1658, 1988.
27. Terlau H, Heinemann SH, Stuhmer W, et al: Mapping the site of block by tetrodotoxin and saxitoxin of sodium channel II. FEBS Lett 293:93, 1991.
28. Shon KJ, Olivera BM, Watkins M, et al: mu-Conotoxin PIIIA, a new peptide for discriminating among tetrodotoxin-sensitive Na channel subtypes. J Neurosci 18:4473, 1998.
29. Wang SY, Wang GK: Batrachotoxin-resistant Na+ channels derived from point mutations in transmembrane segment D4-S6. Biophys J 76:3141, 1999.
30. Wang SY, Barile M, Wang GK: Disparate role of Na+ channel D2-S6 residues in batrachotoxin and local anesthetic action. Mol Pharmacol 59:1100, 2001.
31. Carter AJ, Grauert M, Pschorn U, et al: Potent blockade of sodium channels and protection of brain tissue from ischemia by BIII890CL. Proc Natl Acad Sci USA 97:4944, 2000.
32. Wang SY, Nau C, Wang GK: Residues in Na+ channel D3-S6 segment modulate both batrachotoxin and local anesthetic affinities. Biophys J 79:1379, 2000.
33. Isom LL, De Jongh KS, Patton DE, et al: Primary structure and functional expression of the beta 1 subunit of the rat brain sodium channel. Science 256:839, 1992.
34. Catterall WA: From ionic currents to molecular mechanisms: The structure and function of voltage-gated sodium channels. Neuron 26:13, 2000.
35. Baker MD, Wood JN: Involvement of Na+ channels in pain pathways. Trends Pharmacol Sci 22:27, 2001.
36. Malhotra JD, Kazen-Gillespie K, Hortsch M, et al: Sodium channel beta subunits mediate homophilic cell adhesion and recruit ankyrin to points of cell-cell contact. J Biol Chem 275:11383, 2000.
37. Benitah JP, Chen Z, Balser JR, et al: Molecular dynamics of the sodium channel pore vary with gating: Interactions between P-segment motions and inactivation. J Neurosci 19:1577, 1999.
38. Loots E, Isacoff EY: Molecular coupling of S4 to a K+ channel's slow inactivation gate. J Gen Physiol 116:623, 2000.
39. Perozo E, Cortes DM, Cuello LG: Structural rearrangements underlying K+-channel activation gating. Science 285:73, 1999.
40. Armstrong CM: Voltage-dependent ion channels and their gating. Physiol Rev 72:S5, 1992.
41. Balser JR: The cardiac sodium channel: Gating function and molecular pharmacology. J Mol Cell Cardiol 33:599, 2001.
42. Ragsdale DS, McPhee JC, Scheuer T, et al: Molecular determinants of state-dependent block of Na+ channels by local anesthetics. Science 265:1724, 1994.
43. Ptacek LJ, George AL Jr, Griggs RC, et al: Identification of a mutation in the gene causing hyperkalemic periodic paralysis. Cell 67:1021, 1991.
44. Rojas CV, Wang JZ, Schwartz LS, et al: A Met-to-Val mutation in the skeletal muscle Na+ channel alpha-subunit in hyperkalemic periodic paralysis. Nature 354:387, 1991.
45. McClatchey AI, McKenna-Yasek D, Cros D, et al: Novel mutations in families with unusual and variable disorders of the skeletal muscle sodium channel. Nat Genet 2:148, 1992.
46. Ptacek LJ, George AL Jr, Barchi RL, et al: Mutations in an S4 segment of the adult skeletal muscle sodium channel cause paramyotonia congenita. Neuron 8:891, 1992.
47. Clancy CE, Rudy Y: Linking a genetic defect to its cellular phenotype in a cardiac arrhythmia. Nature 400:566, 1999.
48. Wallace RH, Wang DW, Singh R, et al: Febrile seizures and generalized epilepsy associated with a mutation in the Na+-channel beta1 subunit gene SCN1B. Nat Genet 19:366, 1998.
49. Bokesch PM, Post C, Strichartz G: Structure-activity relationship of lidocaine homologs producing tonic and frequency-dependent impulse blockade in nerve. J Pharmacol Exp Ther 237:773, 1986.
50. Heginbotham L, Abramson T, MacKinnon R: A functional connection between the pores of distantly related ion channels as revealed by mutant K+ channels. Science 258:1152, 1992.
51. Richardson JS: The anatomy and taxonomy of protein structure. Adv Protein Chem 34:167, 1981.

52. Yarov-Yarovoy V, Brown J, Sharp EM, et al: Molecular determinants of voltage-dependent gating and binding of pore-blocking drugs in transmembrane segment IIIS6 of the Na⁺ channel alpha subunit. J Biol Chem 276:20, 2001.

53. Schmidtmayer J, Ulbricht W: Interaction of lidocaine and benzocaine in blocking sodium channels. Pflügers Arch 387:47, 1980.

54. Wang GK, Quan C, Wang S: A common local anesthetic receptor for benzocaine and etidocaine in voltage-gated mu1 Na+ channels. Pflugers Arch 435:293, 1998.

55. Nau C, Wang SY, Strichartz GR, et al: Block of human heart hH1 sodium channels by the enantiomers of bupivacaine. Anesthesiology 93:1022, 2000.

56. Goldin AL, Barchi RL, Caldwell JH, et al: Nomenclature of voltage-gated sodium channels. Neuron 28:365, 2000.

57. Akopian AN, Souslova V, England S, et al: The tetrodotoxin-resistant sodium channel SNS has a specialized function in pain pathways. Nat Neurosci 2:541, 1999.

58. Tate S, Benn S, Hick C, et al: Two sodium channels contribute to the TTX-R sodium current in primary sensory neurons. Nat Neurosci 1:653, 1998.

59. Scholz A, Appel N, Vogel W: Two types of TTX-resistant and one TTX-sensitive Na⁺ channel in rat dorsal root ganglion neurons and their blockade by halothane. Eur J Neurosci 10:2547, 1998.

60. Rush AM, Brau ME, Elliott AA, et al: Electrophysiological properties of sodium current subtypes in small cells from adult rat dorsal root ganglia. J Physiol 511:771, 1998.

61. Cummins TR, DibHajj SD, Black JA, et al: A novel persistent tetrodotoxin-resistant sodium current in SNS-null and wild-type small primary sensory neurons. J Neurosci 19:1, 1999.

62. Roy ML, Narahashi T: Differential properties of tetrodotoxin-sensitive and tetrodotoxin-resistant sodium channels in rat dorsal root ganglion neurons. J Neurosci 12:2104, 1992.

63. Scholz A, Kuboyama N, Hempelmann G, et al: Complex blockade of TTX-resistant Na⁺ currents by lidocaine and bupivacaine reduce firing frequency in DRG neurons. J Neurophysiol 79:1746, 1998.

64. Brau ME, Elliott JR: Local anaesthetic effects on tetrodotoxin-resistant Na+ currents in rat dorsal root ganglion neurones. Eur J Anaesthesiol 15:80, 1998.

65. Fjell J, Hjelmstrom P, Hormuzdiar W, et al: Localization of the tetrodotoxin-resistant sodium channel NaN in nociceptors. Neuroreport 11:199, 2000.

66. Brock JA, McLachlan EM, Belmonte C: Tetrodotoxin-resistant impulses in single nociceptor nerve terminals in guinea-pig cornea. J Physiol 512:211, 1998.

67. Strassman AM, Raymond SA: Electrophysiological evidence for tetrodotoxin-resistant sodium channels in slowly conducting dural sensory fibers. J Neurophysiol 81:413, 1999.

68. Scholz A, Vogel W: Tetrodotoxin-resistant action potentials in dorsal root ganglion neurons are blocked by local anesthetics. Pain 89:47, 2000.

69. Komai H, McDowell TS: Local anesthetic inhibition of voltage-activated potassium currents in rat dorsal root ganglion neurons. Anesthesiology 94:1089–1095, 2001.

70. Olschewski A, Hempelmann G, Vogel W, et al: Blockade of Na+ and K+ currents by local anesthetics in the dorsal horn neurons of the spinal cord. Anesthesiology 88:172, 1998.

71. Brau ME, Vogel W, Hempelmann G: Fundamental properties of local anesthetics: Half-maximal blocking concentrations for tonic block of Na+ and K+ channels in peripheral nerve. Anesth Analg 87:885, 1998.

72. Brau ME, Nau C, Hempelmann G, et al: Local anesthetics potently block a potential insensitive potassium channel in myelinated nerve. J Gen Physiol 105:485, 1995.

73. Olschewski A, Olschewski H, Brau ME, et al: Effect of bupivacaine on ATP-dependent potassium channels in rat cardiomyocytes. Br J Anaesth 82:435, 1999.

74. Olschewski A, Brau ME, Olschewski H, et al: ATP-dependent potassium channel in rat cardiomyocytes is blocked by lidocaine. Possible impact on the antiarrhythmic action of lidocaine. Circulation 93:656, 1996.

75. Xiong ZL, Strichartz GR: Inhibition by local anesthetics of Ca2+ channels in rat anterior pituitary cells. Eur J Pharmacol 363:81, 1998.

76. Sugiyama K, Muteki T: Local anesthetics depress the calcium current of rat sensory neurons in culture. Anesthesiology 80:1369, 1994.

77. Scholz A, Kuboyama N, Bischoff U, et al: Local anesthetics and ketamine are inhibiting Ca2+ channels in rat DRG neurones. Pflügers Arch 426, 1994.

78. Sperelakis N: Electrophysiology of calcium antagonists. J Mol Cell Cardiol 19(suppl 2):19, 1987.

79. Hollmann MW, Wieczorek KS, Berger A, et al: Local anesthetic inhibition of G protein-coupled receptor signaling by interference with Galpha(q) protein function. Mol Pharmacol 59:294, 2001.

80. Hollmann MW, Ritter CH, Henle P, et al: Inhibition of m3 muscarinic acetylcholine receptors by local anaesthetics. Br J Pharmacol 133:207, 2001.

81. Slesinger PA: Ion selectivity filter regulates local anesthetic inhibition of G-protein-gated inwardly rectifying K+ channels. Biophys J 80:707, 2001.

82. Kuboyama N, Nakao S, Moriya Y, et al: Bupivacaine-included Ca²⁺ release on intracellular Ca²⁺ stores in rat DRG neurones. Jpn J Pharmacol 73:O-103, 1997.

83. Gold MS, Reichling DB, Shuster MJ, et al: Hyperalgesic agents increase a tetrodotoxin-resistant Na+ current in nociceptors. Proc Natl Acad Sci USA 93:1108, 1996.

84. Dib-Hajj SD, Tyrrell L, Black JA, et al: NaN, a novel voltage-gated Na channel, is expressed preferentially in peripheral sensory neurons and down-regulated after axotomy. Proc Natl Acad Sci USA 95:8963, 1998.

85. Novakovic SD, Tzoumaka E, McGivern JG, et al: Distribution of the tetrodotoxin-resistant sodium channel PN3 in rat sensory neurons in normal and neuropathic conditions. J Neurosci 18:2174, 1998.

86. Okuse K, Chaplan SR, McMahon SB, et al: Regulation of expression of the sensory neuron-specific sodium channel SNS in inflammatory and neuropathic pain. Mol Cell Neurosci 10:196, 1997.

87. Wall PD, Devor M: Sensory afferent impulses originate from dorsal root ganglia as well as from the periphery in normal and nerve injured rats. Pain 17:321, 1983.

88. Devor M, Wall PD, Catalan N: Systemic lidocaine silences ectopic neuroma and DRG discharge without blocking nerve conduction. Pain 48:261, 1992.

89. Woolf CJ: Evidence for a central component of post-injury pain hypersensitivity. Nature 306:686, 1983.

90. Woolf CJ, Costigan M: Transcriptional and posttranslational plasticity and the generation of inflammatory pain. Proc Natl Acad Sci USA 96:7723, 1999.

91. Woolf CJ, Wiesenfeld-Hallin Z: The systemic administration of local anaesthetics produces a selective depression of C-afferent fibre evoked activity in the spinal cord. Pain 23:361, 1985.

92. Baker MD: Selective block of late Na⁺ current by local anaesthetics in rat large sensory neurones. Br J Pharmacol 129:1617, 2000.

93. Gold MS, Reichling DB, Hampl KF, et al: Lidocaine toxicity in primary afferent neurons from the rat. J Pharmacol Exp Ther 285:413, 1998.

94. Krause U, Weiser T, Carter AJ, et al: Potent, use-dependent blockade of TTX-resistant Na⁺ channels in dorsal root ganglion neurones by BIII 890 CL. Eur J Neurosci 12:S387, 2000.

95. Sato C, Ueno Y, Asai K, et al: The voltage-sensitive sodium channel is a bell-shaped molecule with several cavities. Nature 409:1047, 2001.

96. Scholz A, Kuboyama N, Hempelmann G, et al: Complex blockade of TTX-resistant Na⁺ currents by lidocaine and bupivacaine reduce firing frequency in DRG neurons. J Neurophysiol 79:1746, 1998.

97. Butterworth JF, Strichartz GR: Molecular mechanisms of local anesthetics: A review. Anesthesiology 72:711, 1990.

98. Frazier DY, Narahashi T, Yamada M: The site of action and active form of local anesthetic. II. Experiments with quaternary compounds. J Pharmacol Exp Ther 171:45, 1970.

99. Gissen AJ, Covino BG, Gregus J: Differential sensitivity of fast and slow fibers in mammalian nerve. Anesth Analg 61:561, 1982.

100. Brau ME, Vogel W, Hempelmann G: Fundamental properties of local anesthetic: Half-maximal blocking concentrations for tonic block of Na⁺ and K⁺ channels in peripheral nerve. Anesth Analg 87:885, 1998.

101. Ulbricht W: Kinetics of drug action and equilibrium results at the node of Ranvier. Physiol Rev 61:785, 1981.

102. McClellan KJ, Spencer CM: Levobupivacaine. Drugs 56:355;discussion 363, 1998.

103. McClure JH: Ropivacaine. Br J Anesthesia 76:300, 1996.

104. Burns AG, van der Meer AD, van Kleef JW, et al: Pharmacokinetics of the enantiomers of bupivacaine following intravenous administration of the racemate. Br J Clin Pharmacol 38:125, 1994.

105. Lee-Son MB, Wang GK, Concus A, et al: Stereoselective inhibition of neuronal sodium channels by local anesthetics. Anesthesiology 77:324, 1992.

106. Reynolds F: Ropivacaine. Anaesthesia 46:339, 1991.
107. Pateromichelakis S, Prokopiou AA: Local anaesthesia efficacy: Discrepancy between in vitro and in vivo studies. Acta Anaesthesiol Scand 32:672, 1988.
108. Hassan HG, Youssef H, Renck H: Duration of experimental nerve block by combinations of local anesthetic agents. Acta Anaesthesiol Scand 37:70, 1993.
109. Spiegel DA, Dexter F, Warner DS: Central nervous system toxicity of local anesthetic mixtures in the rat. Anesth Analg 75:922, 1992.
110. Bromage PR, Pettigrew RT, Crowell DE: Tachyphylaxis in epidural anesthesia: I. Augmentation and decay of local anesthetics. J Clin Pharmacol 9:30, 1969.
111. Lee K-C, Wilder RT, Smith RL, et al: Thermal hyperalgesia accelerates and MK-801 prevents the development of tachyphylaxis to rat sciatic nerve blockade. Anesthesiology 81:1284, 1994.
112. Wilder RT, Sholas MG, Berde CB: NG-nitro-L-arginine methyl ester (L-NAME) prevents tachyphylaxis to local anesthetics in a dose-dependent manner. Anesth Analg 83:1251, 1996.
113. Kito K, Kata H, Shibata M, et al: The effects of varied doses of epinephrine on duration of lidocaine spinal anesthesia in the thoracic and lumbosacral dermatomes. Anesth Analg 86:1018, 1998.
114. Chiu AA, Liu S, Carpenter RL: Effects of epinephrine on lidocaine spinal anesthesia: A crossover study. Anesth Analg 80:735, 1995.
115. Niemi G, Breivik H: Adrenaline markedly improves thoracic epidural analgesia produced by a low-dose infusion of bupivacaine, fentanyl, and adrenaline after major surgery. Acta Anaesthesiol Scand 42:897, 1998.
116. Liu S, Carpenter RL, Chiu AA: Epinephrine prolongs duration of subcutaneous infiltration of local anesthetics in a dose related manner: Correlation with magnitude of vasoconstriction. Reg Anesth 20:378, 1995.
117. Cederholm I, Evers H, Lofstrom JB: Skin blood flow after intradermal injection of ropivacaine in various concentrations with and without epinephrine evaluated by laser Doppler flowmetry. Reg Anesth 17:322, 1992.
118. Lofstrom JB: 1991 Labat Lecture. The effect of local anesthetics on the peripheral vasculature. Reg Anesth 17:1, 1992.
119. Scott D, Jebson P, Braid D, et al: Factors affecting plasma levels of lignocaine and prilocaine. Br J Anaesth 44:1040, 1972.
120. Bernards CM, Kopacz DJ: Effect of epinephrine on lidocaine clearance in vivo: A microdialysis study in humans. Anesthesiology 91:962, 1999.
121. Curatolo M, Peterson-Felix S, Arendt-Nielsen L, et al: Epidural epinephrine and clonidine. Segmental analgesia and effects on different pain modalities. Anesthesiology 87:785, 1997.
122. Ueda W, Hirakawa M, Mori: Acceleration of epinephrine absorption by lidocaine. Anesthesiology 63:717, 1985.
123. Magee C, Rodeheaver GT, Edgerton MT, et al: Studies of the mechanisms by which epinephrine damages tissue defenses. J Surg Res 23:126, 1977.
124. Hall JA, Ferro A: Myocardial ischemia and ventricular arrhythmias precipitated by physiological concentrations of adrenaline in patients with coronary artery disease. Br Heart J 67:419, 1992.
125. Rowlingson JC: Toxicity of local anesthetics additives. Reg Anesth 18:453, 1993.
126. Hodgson PS, Neal JM, Pollock JE: The neurotoxicity of drugs given intrathecally (spinal). Anesth Analg 88:797, 1999.
127. Curatolo M, Petersen-Felix S, Arendt-Nielsen L, et al: Adding sodium bicarbonate to lidocaine enhances the depth of epidural blockade. Anesth Analg 86:341, 1998.
128. Capogna G, Celleno D, Laudano D, et al: Alkalinization of local anesthetics. Which block, which local anesthetic? Reg Anesth 20:369, 1995.
129. Ikuta PT, Raza SM, Durrani Z: pH adjustment schedule for the amide local anesthetics. Reg Anesth 14:229, 1989.
130. Wang C, Chakrabarti MK, Galletly DC, et al: Relative effects of intrathecal administration of fentanyl and midazolam on A delta and C fibre reflexes. Neuropharmacology 31:439, 1992.
131. Niv D, Nemirovsky A, Rudick V: Antinociception induced by simultaneous intrathecal and intraperitoneal administration of low doses of morphine. Anesth Analg 80:886, 1995.
132. Kaneko M, Saito Y, Kirihara Y, et al: Synergistic antinociception after epidural coadministration of morphine and lidocaine in rats. Anesthesiology 80:137, 1994.
133. Saito Y, Kaneko M, Kirihara Y, et al: Interaction of intrathecally infused morphine and lidocaine in rats (part I): Synergistic antinociceptive effects. Anesthesiology 89:1455, 1998.
134. Solomon RE, Gebhart GF: Synergistic antinociceptive interactions among drugs administered to the spinal cord. Anesth Analg 78:1164, 1994.
135. Karambelkar DJ, Ramanathan S: 2-Chloroprocaine antagonism of epidural morphine analgesia. Acta Anaesth Scand 41:774, 1997.
136. Coda B, Bausch S, Haas M, et al: The hypothesis that antagonism of fentanyl analgesia by 2-chloroprocaine is mediated by direct action on opioid receptors. Reg Anesth 22:43, 1997.
137. Curatolo M, Petersen-Felix S, Scaramozzino P, et al: Epidural fentanyl, adrenaline and clonidine as adjuvants to local anaesthetics for surgical analgesia: Meta-analyses of analgesia and side effects. Acta Anaesth Scand 42:910, 1998.
138. Curatolo M, Schnider TW, Petersen-Felix SW, et al: A direct search procedure to optimize combinations of epidural bupivacaine, fentanyl, and clonidine for postoperative analgesia. Anesthesiology 92:325, 2000.
139. Stein C, Yassouridis A: Peripheral morphine analgesia [editorial]. Pain 71:119, 1997.
140. Allen GC, St Amand MA, et al: Postarthroscopy analgesia with intraarticular bupivacaine/morphine. Anesthesiology 79:475, 1993.
141. Picard PR, Tramer MR, Mcquay HJ, et al: Analgesic efficacy of peripheral opioids (all except intra-articular): A qualitative systematic review of randomized controlled trials. Pain 72:309, 1997.
142. Eisenach JC, De Kock M, Klimscha W: alpha₂-adrenergic agonists for regional anesthesia. A clinical review of clonidine (1984–1995). Anesthesiology 85:655, 1996.
143. Butterworth JF, Strichartz GR: The alpha2-adrenergic agonists clonidine and guanfacine produce tonic and phasic block of conduction in rat sciatic nerve fibers. Anesth Analg 76:295, 1993.
144. Gaumann DM, Brunet PC, Jirounek P: Clonidine enhances the effects of lidocaine on C fiber action potential. Anesth Analg 74:719, 1992.
145. Pertovaara A, Hamalainen MM: Spinal potentiation and supraspinal additivity in the antinociceptive interaction between systemically administered alpha 2-adrenoreceptor agonist and cocaine in the rat. Anesth Analg 79:261, 1994.
146. Bernard JM, Macaire P: Dose-range effects of clonidine added to lidocaine for brachial plexus block. Anesthesiology 87:277, 1997.
147. Reuben SS, Steinberg RB, Klatt JL, et al: Intravenous regional anesthesia using lidocaine and clonidine. Anesthesiology 91:654, 1999.
148. Bhana N, Goa KL, McClellan: Dexmedetomidine. Drugs 59:263, 2000.
149. Kamibayashi T, Maze M: Clinical uses of alpha₂-adrenergic agonists. Anesthesiology 93:1345, 2000.
150. Hall JE, Uhrich TD, Barney JA, et al: Sedative, amnestic, and analgesic properties of small-dose dexmedetomidine infusions. Anesth Analg 90:699, 2000.
151. Tucker GT, Moore DC, Bridenbaugh PO: Systemic absorption of mepivacaine in commonly used regional block procedures. Anesthesiology 37:277, 1972.
152. Morrison LM, Emanuelsson BM, McClure JH: Efficacy and kinetics of extradural ropivacaine: Comparison with bupivacaine. Br J Anaesth 72:164, 1994.
153. Huang YF, Upton RN, Runciman WB: I.V. bolus administration of subconvulsive doses of lignocaine to conscious sheep: Myocardial pharmacokinetics. Br J Anaesth 70:326, 1993.
154. Huang YF, Upton RN, Runciman WB: I.V. bolus administration of subconvulsive doses of lidocaine to conscious sheep: Relationships between myocardial pharmacokinetics and pharmacodymanics. Br J Anaesth 70:556, 1993.
155. Rutten AJ, Mather LE, Nancarrow C: Cardiovascular effects and regional clearances of intravenous ropivacaine in sheep. Anesth Analg 70:577, 1990.
156. Tucker GT, Mather LE: Properties, absorption, and disposition of local anesthetic agents. In Cousins MJ, Bridenbaugh PO (eds): Neural Blockade in Clinical Anesthesia and Management of Pain, 3rd ed. Philadelphia, Lippincott-Raven, 1998, pp 55–96.
157. Braid DP, Scott DB: Dosage of lignocaine in epidural block in relation to toxicity. Br J Anaesth 38:596, 1966.
158. McCaughey W: Adverse effects of local anaesthetics. Drug Safety 7:178, 1992.
159. Auroy Y, Narchi P, Messiah A, et al: Serious complications related to regional anesthesia: Results of a prospective survey in France [see comments]. Anesthesiology 87:479, 1997.
160. Shibata M, Shingu K, Murakawa M: Tetraphasic actions of local anes-

thetics on central nervous system electrical activity in cats. Reg Anesth 19:255, 1994.

161. Bernards CM, Carpenter RL, Rupp SM: Effects of midazolam and diazepam premedication on central nervous system and cardiovascular toxicity of bupivacaine. Anesthesiology 70:318, 1989.

162. Groban L, Deal DD, Vernon JC, et al: Cardiac resuscitation after incremental overdosage with lidocaine, bupivacaine, levobupivacaine, and ropivacaine, in anesthetized dogs. Anesth Analg 92:38, 2001.

163. Reiz S, Haggmark S, Johansson G, et al: Cardiotoxicity of ropivacaine: A new amide local anaesthetic agent. Acta Anaesthesiol Scand 33:93, 1989.

164. Guo XT, Castle NA, Chernoff DM, et al: Comparative inhibition of voltage-gated cation channels by local anesthetics. Ann NY Acad Sci 625:181, 1991.

165. Denson DD, Behbehani MM, Gregg RV: Effects of an intravenously administered arrhythmogenic dose of bupivacaine at the nucleus tractus solitarius in the conscious rat. Reg Anesth 15:76, 1990.

166. Bernards CM, Artruu AA: Hexamethonium and midazolam terminate dysrhythmias and hypertension caused by intracerebroventricular bupivacaine in rabbits. Anesthesiology 74:89, 1991.

167. Szocik JF, Gardner CA, Webb RC: Inhibitory effects of bupivacaine and lidocaine on adrenergic neuroeffector junctions in rat-tail artery. Anesthesiology 78:911, 1993.

168. Freysz M, Timour Q, Bertrix L, et al: Bupivacaine hastens the ischemia-induced decrease of the electrical ventricular fibrillation threshold. Anesth Analg 80:657, 1995.

169. Kalichman MW: Physiologic mechanisms by which local anesthetics may cause injury to nerve and spinal cord. Reg Anesth 18:448, 1993.

170. Selander D: Neurotoxicity of local anesthetics: Animal data. Reg Anesth 18:461, 1993.

171. Takenami T, Yagishita S, Asato F, et al: Neurotoxicity of intrathecally administered tetracaine commences at the posterior roots near entry into the spinal cord. Reg Anesth Pain Med 25:372, 2000.

172. Ready LB, Plumer MH, Haschke RH, et al: Neurotoxicity of intrathecal local anesthetics in rabbits. Anesthesiology 63:364, 1985.

173. Lambert L, Lambert D, Strichartz G: Irreversible conduction block in isolated nerve by high concentrations of local anesthetics. Anesthesiology 80:1082, 1994.

174. Chabal C, Jacobson L, Little J: Effects of intrathecal fentanyl and lidocaine on somatosensory-evoked potentials, the H-reflex, and clinical responses. Anesth Analg 67:509, 1988.

175. Liu S, Kopacz D, Carpenter R: Quantitative assessment of differential sensory nerve block after lidocaine spinal anesthesia. Anesthesiology 82:60, 1995.

176. Pollock JE, Liu SS, Neal JM, et al: Dilution of lidocaine does not decrease the incidence of transient neurologic symptoms. Anesthesiology 90:445, 1999.

177. Freedman J, Li D, Jaskela M: Risk factors for transient neurologic symptoms after spinal anesthesia. Anesthesiology 89:633, 1998.

178. Aouad MT, Siddik SS, Jalbout MI, et al: Does pregnancy protect against intrathecal lidocaine-induced transient neurologic symptoms? Anesth Analg 92:401, 2001.

179. Pollock JE: Management of the patient who develops transient neurologic symptoms after spinal anesthesia with lidocaine. Tech Reg Anesth Pain Management 4:155, 2000.

180. Horlocker TT, Wedel DJ: Neurologic complications of spinal and epidural anesthesia. Reg Anesth Pain Med 25:83, 2000.

181. Drasner K: Lidocaine spinal anesthesia: A vanishing therapeutic index? Anesthesiology 87:469, 1997.

182. Pollock JE, Burkhead D, Neal J: Spinal nerve function in five volunteers experiencing transient neurologic symptoms after lidocaine subarachnoid anesthesia. Anesth Analg 90:658, 2000.

183. Liu SS, Ware PD, Rajendran S: Effects of concentration and volume of 2-chloroprocaine on epidural anesthesia in volunteers. Anesthesiology 86:1288, 1997.

184. Mulroy MF, Larkin KL, Hodgson PS, et al: A comparison of spinal, epidural, and general anesthesia for outpatient knee arthroscopy. Anesth Analg 91:860, 2000.

185. Durrani M, Barwise JA, Johnson RF, et al: Intravenous chloroprocaine attenuates hemodynamic changes associated with direct laryngoscopy and tracheal intubation. Anesth Analg 90:1208, 2000.

186. Stevens RA, Urmey WF, Urquhart BL, et al: Back pain after epidural anesthesia with chloroprocaine. Anesthesiology 78:492, 1993.

187. Grauer SE, Giraud GD: Toxic methemoglobinemia after topical anes-

thesia for transesophageal echocardiography. J Am Soc Echocardiogr 9:874, 1996.

188. Choi RH, Birkness JK, Popitz-Bergez FA, et al: Safety of tumescent liposuction in 15,336 patients: National survey results. Dermatol Surg 21:459, 1995.

189. Kindler CH, Schumacher PG, Schneider MC, et al: Effects of intravenous lidocaine and/or esmolol on hemodynamic responses to laryngoscopy and intubation: A double-blind, controlled clinical trial. J Clinical Anesth 8:491, 1996.

190. Helfman SM, Gold MI, DeLisser EA, et al: Which drug prevents tachycardia and hypertension associated with tracheal intubation: Lidocaine, fentanyl, or esmolol? [see comments]. Anesth Analgesia 72:482, 1991.

191. Nakayama M, Fujita S, Kanaya N, et al: Effect of intravenous lidocaine on intraabdominal pressure response to airway stimulation. Anesth Analg 78:1149, 1994.

192. Chamberlain DA: Antiarrhythmic drugs in resuscitation. Heart 80:408, 1998.

193. Cassuto J, Wallin G, Hogstrom S, et al: Inhibition of postoperative pain by continuous low-dose intravenous infusion of lidocaine. Anesth Analg 64:971, 1985.

194. Mao J, Chen LL: Systemic lidocaine for neuropathic pain relief. Pain 87:7, 2000.

195. Chaplan SR, Bach FW, Shafer SL, et al: Prolonged alleviation of tactile allodynia by intravenous lidocaine in neuropathic rats. Anesthesiology 83:775, 1995.

196. Schwarz SK, Puil E: Analgesic and sedative concentrations of lignocaine shunt tonic and burst firing in thalamocortical neurones. Br J Pharmacol 124:1633, 1998.

197. Jarvis B, Coukell AJ: Mexiletine: A review of its therapeutic use in painful diabetic neuropathy. Drugs 56:691, 1998.

198. Kemper CA, Kent G, Burton S, et al: Mexiletine for HIV-infected patients with painful peripheral neuropathy: A double-blind, placebo-controlled, crossover treatment trial. J Acquir Immune Defic Syndr Hum Retrovirol 19:367, 1998.

199. Joly LM, Spaulding C, Monchi M, et al: Topical lidocaine-prilocaine cream (EMLA) versus local infiltration for radial artery cannulation. Anesth Analg 87:403, 1998.

200. Koscielniak-Nielsen Z, Hesselbjerg L, Brushoj J, et al: EMLA patch for spinal puncture. A comparison of EMLA patch with lignocaine infiltration and placebo patch. Anaesthesia 53:1218, 1998.

201. Arthur GR, Scott DH, Boyes RN, et al: Pharmacokinetic and clinical pharmacological studies with mepivacaine and prilocaine. Br J Anaesth 51:481, 1979.

202. Salazar F, Bogdanovich A, Adalia R, et al: Transient neurologic symptoms after spinal anesthesia using isobaric 2% mepivacaine and isobaric 2% lidocaine. Acta Anaesth Scand 45:240, 2001.

203. Pawlowski J, Sukhani R, Pappas AL, et al: The anesthetic and recovery profile of two doses (60 and 80 mg) of plain mepivacaine for ambulatory spinal anesthesia. Anesth Analg 91:580, 2000.

204. Terai T, Yukioka H, Fujimori M: A double-blind comparison of lidocaine and mepivacaine during epidural anaesthesia. Acta Anaesth Scand 37:607, 1993.

205. Meffin P, Long GJ, Thomas J: Clearance and metabolism of mepivacaine in the human neonate. Clin Pharm Exp Ther 14:218, 1972.

206. Goldstein A, Grimault P, Henique A, et al: Preventing postoperative pain by local anesthetic instillation after laparoscopic gynecologic surgery: A placebo controlled comparison of bupivacaine and ropivacaine. Anesth Analg 91:403, 2000.

207. Joris J, Thiry E, Paris P, et al: Pain after laparoscopic cholecystectomy: Characteristics and effects of intraperitoneal bupivacaine. Anesth Analg 81:379, 1995.

208. Ben-David B, Solomon E, Levin H, et al: Intrathecal fentanyl with small-dose dilute bupivacaine: Better anesthesia without prolonging recovery. Anesth Analg 85:560, 1997.

209. Ben-David B, Frankel R, Arzumonov T, et al: Minidose bupivacaine-fentanyl spinal anesthesia for surgical repair of hip fracture in the aged. Anesthesiology 92:6, 2000.

210. Albright GA: Cardiac arrest following regional anesthesia with etidocaine or bupivacaine. Anesthesiology 51:285, 1979.

211. Mulroy MF, Norris MC, Liu SS: Safety steps for epidural injection of local anesthetics: Review of the literature and recommendations. Anesth Analg 85:1346, 1997.

212. Bader AM, Datta S, Flanagan H, Covino BG: Comparison of bupivacaine and ropivacaine-induced conduction blockade in the isolated rabbit vagus nerve. Anesth Analg 68:724, 1989.

213. Carpenter RL. Local anesthetic toxicity: The case for ropivacaine. Am J Anesthesiol 24:4, 1997.

214. Groban L, Deal DD, Vernon JC, et al: Cardiac resuscitation after incremental overdosage with lidocaine, bupivacaine, levobupivacaine, and ropivacaine in anesthetized dogs. Anesth Analg 92:37, 2001.

215. Scott B, Lee AL, Fagen D, et al: Acute toxicity of ropivacaine compared with that of bupivacaine. Anesth Analg 69:563, 1989.

216. Sztark F, Malgat M, Dabadie P, et al: Comparison of the effects of bupivacaine and ropivacaine on heart cell mitochondrial bioenergetics. Anesthesiology 88:1340, 1998.

217. Knudsen K, Beckman Suurkula M, Blomberg S, et al: Central and cardiovascular effects of i.v. infusions of ropivacaine and placebo in volunteers. Br J Anaesth 78:507, 1997.

218. Reutsch YA, Fattinger KE, Borgeat A: Ropivacaine-induced convulsions and severe cardiac dysrhythmia after sciatic block. Anesthesiology 90:1784, 1999.

219. Campbell DC, Zwack RM, Crone L, et al: Ambulatory labor epidural analgesia: Bupivacaine versus ropivacaine. Anesth Analg 90:1384, 2000.

220. Griffin RP, Reynolds F: Extradural anaesthesia for cesarean section: A double-blind comparison of 0.5% ropivacaine with 0.5% bupivacaine. Br J Anaesth 74:512, 1995.

221. Gautier PhE, De Kock M, Van Steenberge A, et al: Intrathecal ropivacaine for ambulatory surgery: A comparison between intrathecal bupivacaine and intrathecal ropivacaine for knee arthoscopy. Aneshthesiology 91:1239, 1999.

222. Kerkamp HEM, Axelsson KH, Edstrom HH, et al: An open study comparison of 0.5%, 0.75%, and 1.0% ropivacaine, with epinephrine in epidural anesthesia in patients undergoing urologic surgery. Reg Anesth 15:53, 1990.

223. Levin A, Datta S, Camann WR: Intrathecal ropivacaine for labor analgesia: A comparison with bupivacaine. Anesth Analg 87:624, 1998.

224. McGlade DP, Kalpokas MV, Mooney PH, et al: A comparison of 0.5% ropivacaine and 0.5% bupivacaine for axillary brachial plexus anesthesia. Anesth Intens Care 26:515, 1998.

225. Beardsley H, Gristwood R, Watson N, et al: The local anesthetic activity of levobupivacaine does not differ from racemic bupivacaine (Marcain): First clinical evidence. Expert Opin Invest Drug 6:1883, 1997.

226. Beardsley H, Gristwood R, Baker H, et al: A comparison of cardiovascular and effects of levobupivacaine and rac-bupivacaine following intravenous administration to healthy volunteers. Br J Clin Pharmacol 46:245, 1998.

227. Kopacz DJ, Allen HW, Thompson GE: A comparison of epidural levobupivacaine 0.75% with racemic bupivacaine for lower abdominal surgery. Anesth Analg 90:642, 2000.

228. Cox CR, Checketts MR, Mackenzie N, et al: Comparison of S⁻ bupivacaine with racemic (R,S) bupivacaine in supraclavicular brachial plexus block. Br J Anaesth 80:594, 1998.

229. Burke D, Henderson DJ, Simpson AM, et al: Comparison of 0.25% S⁻ bupivacaine with 0.25% RS bupivacaine for epidural analgesia in labor. Br J Anaesth 83:750, 1999.

230. Kuzma PJ, Kline MD, Calkins MD, et al: Progress in the development of ultra-long-acting local anesthetics. Reg Anesth 22:543, 1997.

231. C, Benzinger D, Gao F, et al: Prolonged intercostal nerve blockade in sheep using controlled release of bupivacaine and dexamethasone from polymer microspheres. Anesthesiology 89:969, 1998.

232. Boogaerts J, Declercq A, Lafont N, et al: Toxicity of bupivacaine encapsulated into liposomes and injected intravenously: Comparison with plain solutions. Anesth Analg 76:553, 1993.

233. Curatolo M, Petersen-Felix S, Arendt-Nielsen L, et al: Spinal anaesthesia inhibits central temporal summation. Br J Anaesth 78:88, 1997.

234. Mulroy MF, Greengrass R, Ganapathy S, et al: Sameridine is safe and effective for spinal anesthesia: A comparative dose-ranging study with lidocaine for inguinal hernia repair. Anesth Analg 88:815, 1999.

235. Chaplan SR: Neuropathic pain: Role of voltage-dependent calcium channels. Reg Anesth Pain Med 25:283, 2000.

236. Wang YX, Pettus M, Gao D, et al: Effects of intrathecal ziconotide, a selective neuronal N-type calcium channel blocker, on mechanical allodynia and heat hyperalgesia in a rat model of postoperative pain. Pain 84:151, 2000.

237. Brose WG, Gutlove DP, Luther RR, et al: Use of intrathecal SNX-111, a novel N-type, voltage-sensitive, calcium channel blocker, in the management of intractable brachial plexus avulsion pain. Pain 13:256, 1997.

238. Atanassoff PG, Hartmnnsgruber MWB, Thrasher J, et al: Ziconotide, a new N-type calcium channel blocker, administered intrathecally for acute postoperative pain. Reg Anesth Pain Med 25:274, 2000.

31

Anticonvulsant Drugs

Dean A. Cowie, MB • Adrian W. Gelb, MB

Definitions and Classification of Seizure Disorders

Anticonvulsant drugs are used to treat a wide variety of seizures. Table 31–1 provides definitions for commonly used terms regarding seizure disorders. These disorders have been classified by the International League Against Epilepsy, using a system based on clinical seizure types and changes on the electroencephalogram (EEG) (Table 31–2).[1–4]

Initiation and Propagation of Seizures

Approximately 65% of seizure disorders are idiopathic.[5] One large study identified the most frequent known causes of epilepsy as cerebrovascular disease (11%), congenital abnormalities (8%), trauma (6%), neoplasms (4%), degenerative neurologic diseases (4%), and infections of the central nervous system (3%).[5] Table 31–3 lists some of the factors that can precipitate seizures.

Despite a wealth of information from experimental models of epilepsy,[6] our understanding of the generation and propagation of seizures remains incomplete.[7] Certain general points can be made. The pathophysiology of epilepsy is complex, and no single mechanism accounts for all the types of seizures.[8–10] This is not surprising, given the wide variety of clinical forms of seizures. Although seizure activity may originate in apparently healthy areas of the brain,[11] when a focus is detectable, it tends to arise in areas where cells have the greatest functional plasticity, i.e., areas concerned with learning and memory.[9,12] For normal functioning to occur, the cortex must be kept in a state of fine balance between excitation and inhibition. An increase in activity sufficient to cause a clinical seizure may result from an increase in excitatory influences or a decrease in inhibitory influences. Conceptually, changes may occur at three levels: within the neuron, between neurons, and among groups of neurons.[9]

The rapidly inactivating sodium channel is responsible for the brief, rapid depolarization of the normal action potential. A slowly inactivating sodium current has been identified in many neurons and, when activated by excitatory postsynaptic potentials, may contribute to the long-lasting depolarization required to initiate hyperexcitability.[9] Several calcium currents have been described, of which the low-threshold T-type current has been intensely studied in relation to thalamocortical rhythms and generalized seizures. The T current is normally inactivated during the resting phase. Removal of the inactivation (deinactivation) occurs during membrane hyperpolarization, and additional depolarization (by excitatory synaptic transmission) then opens the T channels and causes calcium influx and depolarization.[13] This low-threshold calcium current is thought to contribute to the thalamic spike/wave activity seen in some forms of seizure. High-threshold calcium currents, such as the N, P, Q, and L types, require greater depolarization for activation and may play a role in presynaptic or postsynaptic neuronal plasticity. Several potassium channels exist, the

539

TABLE 31–1.

Definitions of Frequently Used Terms

Seizure	A transient change in behavior caused by the disordered, synchronous, and rhythmic firing of populations of central nervous system neurons.[11,101]
Epilepsy	A family of disorders characterized by recurrent, spontaneous seizures.[32,102] The term implies that there is no specific provocation for the seizure.[31]
Nonepileptic seizure	A seizure that arises in the normal brain as a result of a provocative stimulus, such as electric shock, chemicals, drugs, or altered physiology.[31]
Partial seizure	A seizure that begins focally at a cortical site. It may be a *simple partial seizure* with preservation of consciousness or a *complex partial seizure* in which the conscious state is impaired[101]; it is also called *focal or local seizures.*[103]
Generalized seizure	A seizure with widespread involvement of both cerebral hemispheres from the onset.[101]
Epileptic syndrome	A specific epilepsy disease, diagnosed by the presence of a cluster of symptoms and including factors such as seizure type, cause, and age of onset.[4]
Status epilepticus	A seizure that lasts for more than 30 minutes and is associated with loss of consciousness.

primary function of which is to repolarize the cell after an action potential.[14,15] Compromise of the function of these channels may cause uncontrolled depolarization.

The concentration and distribution of ions around the cell membrane may affect excitability. For example, extracellular hyperkalemia, as occurs with prolonged or repeated ictal episodes, impairs the normal outward potassium current and reduces the effectiveness of potassium as a regulator of cell excitability.[16,17] Experimental evidence shows that the morphology of a neuron can affect its electrical behavior. Synapses close to the cell body have a greater effect than those on distal processes, suggesting that shorter cells may be excitable for a given degree of input.[9] It is possible that chronic excitability, as occurs with long-lasting epilepsy, may lead to similar changes in cortical neurons, including shortening and widening of the dendritic spinal stalks.[18] It has been shown that hypersynchrony can occur in cortical structures even in the absence of chemical transmission.[19] This may occur by the transmission of current through gap junctions and along the extracellular space (ephaptic interactions) or by an increase in glutamate and potassium ions in the extracellular environment.

The excitability of neurons is greatly affected by interaction among cells. The primary excitatory transmitter in the brain is glutamate. Generation of an excitatory postsynaptic potential occurs mainly by the binding of glutamate to ligand-gated sodium and potassium channels that are of the non-NMDA (*N*-methyl-D-aspartate) type.[20] The depolarization that results from activation of these currents is relatively short-lived. A second group of receptors, the NMDA receptors, are normally inactive because of the presence of magnesium inside the cation channel.[21] Recurrent or prolonged depolarization liberates the channel from the magnesium

blockade, allowing the influx of calcium through the NMDA channel.[22] An increase in intracellular calcium results in chronic potentiation of the excitable tissue and also contributes to the cell damage seen with seizure discharge.[23,24] Reorganization of the neuronal circuitry occurs with repeated seizure discharges.[25,26] This reorganization may involve selective death of inhibitory interneurons or a reduction in their function and is probably mediated by activation of NMDA receptors.[7]

γ-Aminobutyric acid (GABA) is the primary inhibitory transmitter in the brain. It acts by binding to the $GABA_A$ receptor, which activates a ligand-gated chloride channel to produce an inhibitory postsynaptic potential, usually around −70 mV; that is, it inhibits postsynaptic cell firing. Epileptic activity can be generated experimentally by blocking GABA receptors,[27] and a 20% reduction in GABA activity is sufficient to allow spread of synchronized cortical activity.[28] In certain situations, $GABA_A$ activation may favor depolarization.[29] For example, depolarizing $GABA_A$ action is observed in neurons that have a relatively hyperpolarized resting potential, such as immature cells, or in neurons subjected to repeated exposure to GABA.[9] Potential mechanisms include a change in the chloride gradient across the cell membrane and altered conductance of bicarbonate ions.[30]

Focal Seizures

The mechanisms by which hyperexcitability and hypersynchronization events occur has been studied extensively in models of epilepsy. The most frequently studied models

TABLE 31–2.

Classification of Epileptic Seizures[2]

I. **Partial seizures**
   A. Simple partial seizures
      - Motor
      - Sensory
      - Autonomic–visceral
      - Psychic
   B. Complex partial seizures
      - Simple partial seizures followed by an impairment of consciousness
      - With impairment of consciousness at onset
   C. Partial seizures evolving to secondarily generalized seizures
      1. Generalization of a simple partial seizure
      2. Generalization of a complex partial seizure
      3. Generalization of a complex partial seizure which evolved from a simple partial seizure

II. **Generalized seizures**
   A. Absence seizures
      1. Typical absence
      2. Atypical absence
   B. Myoclonic seizures
   C. Clonic seizures
   D. Tonic seizures
   E. Tonic-clonic seizures
   F. Atonic seizures

III. **Unclassified epileptic seizures**

TABLE 31–3.

Factors That May Precipitate Seizures

Physiologic derangement	Heavy metals
■ Hypoxia	■ Mercury
■ Hypocapnia	■ Lead
■ Hypoglycemia	■ Aluminum
■ Hypomagnesemia	■ Lithium
■ Hypocalcemia	
■ Uremia	
■ Hepatic failure	

Lifestyle and hormonal factors	Drug withdrawal
■ Sleep deprivation	■ Alcohol
■ Psychological or physical stress	■ Barbiturates
■ Menstrual cycle changes	■ Benzodiazepines
■ Cocaine	■ Anticonvulsants
■ Amphetamine and related substances	
■ Phensyclidine	

Psychiatric disorders	Prescription drugs
■ Conversion disorder	■ Penicillin
■ Hyperventilation/Panic attacks	■ Isoniazid
■ Depression	■ Gancyclovir
	■ Tricyclic antidepressants
	■ Lithium
	■ Cyclosporin

have been those of focal seizures, for which the region of the brain primarily involved can be identified. The EEG characteristically shows a spike discharge between seizures (Fig. 31–1).[8,31] These interictal spike discharges occur in the region of the brain responsible for the seizure discharge[31] but may be a reflection rather than a cause of focal seizures. The interictal spike discharges themselves do not appear to affect cerebral function.[32]

Focal seizures usually produce a characteristic series of events.[8] The first is a depolarizing shift in which thousands of neurons in the focus undergo an unusually large and prolonged depolarization. This event is an exaggerated expression of the normal excitatory influences on the cell and is caused by inward sodium and calcium currents influenced by the excitatory neurotransmitters, particularly glutamate. The depolarizing shift is followed by a large, prolonged hyperpolarization mediated by GABA and, in some cells, potassium.[7] These cells undergo cycles of excitation and inhibition. With repeated cycles, the hyperpolarization becomes gradually smaller[27] and is eventually replaced by a large depolarization on top of which are smaller depolarizing waves. Finally, the neurons remain depolarized long enough to cause repetitive firing that spreads to neighboring

cells. Repeated stimulation of normal areas of the brain tends to favor further excitation by reducing function in inhibitory interneurons[33] and increasing extracellular potassium and presynaptic calcium levels. Thus transition to a seizure is likely. Epileptic activity may be spatially limited by inhibitory influences or may spread to involve the entire cortex. Such activity will present as a secondarily generalized focal seizure.

Primarily Generalized Seizures

The mechanisms involved in the initiation of primarily generalized seizures are less well understood. It has not been possible to identify a localized abnormality in the brain. Typically, during an absence seizure, the EEG contains bilateral synchronous spike and wave discharges (Fig. 31–2).[32] These discharges are generated in the corticothalamic tracts[31] and are similar to slow-wave activity normally seen in this region during sleep.[7] The rhythmicity of these 3- to 4-Hz waves may be caused by T-type calcium currents alternating with hyperpolarization in thalamic neurons.[13,34]

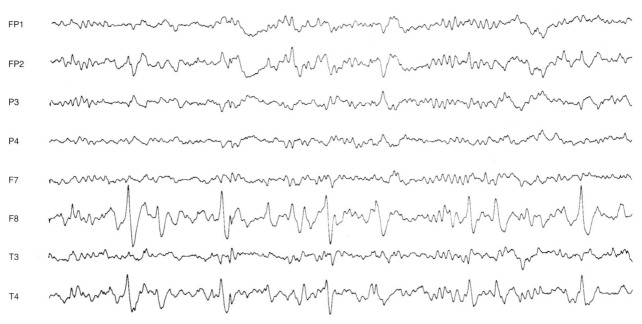

Figure 31–1. Frequent right temporal (F8, T4) spikes on a common average reference sleep recording.

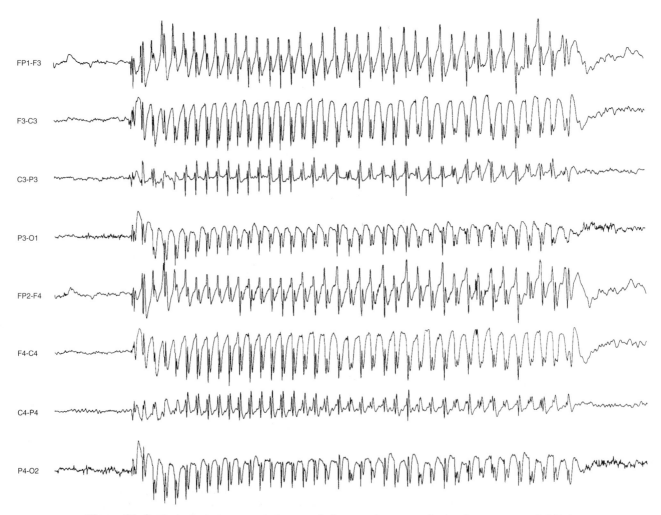

Figure 31–2. Typical electroencephalogram during an absence seizure shows sequential 3- to 4-Hz bilaterally synchronous spike and wave discharges. Note the sudden onset and offset and the normal background activity before and after.

During a generalized tonic-clonic seizure, the EEG has a less ordered appearance, with bilateral onset (Fig. 31–3). For comparison, a normal EEG is shown in Figure 31–4.

In summary, the mechanisms underlying the propensity for epilepsy and the initiation of a seizure are not completely understood. Just as there are different forms of epilepsy, so too are there various mechanisms by which seizures may occur. More is known about the mechanisms underlying focal seizures than primarily generalized seizures, because the neurons involved in the interictal spike or seizure focus can be studied. The occurrence of seizures increases the likelihood of additional seizures. An understanding of the cellular and metabolic mechanisms of seizure formation promotes an understanding of the mechanisms of anticonvulsant drug action.

Anticonvulsant Drugs

Antiepileptic drugs are a diverse group of compounds that have become significantly more numerous in recent years. (Figures 31–5 and 31–6 show the molecular structure of some of the drugs introduced before and after 1980, respectively.) Antiepileptic drugs are usually classified according to their principal mechanism of action (Table 31–4), although they may also be grouped according to the conditions for which they are used clinically (Table 31–5). An appreciation of the pharmacokinetic properties of antiepileptic agents is important for good perioperative care (Table 31–6). Anesthetic drugs have a variety of effects on the EEG in healthy subjects and in patients with epilepsy. The proconvulsant and anticonvulsant effects of these agents and other drugs used by anesthesia practitioners have been reviewed extensively.[35–37]

TABLE 31–4.

Classification of Available Antiepileptic Medications According to the Primary Mechanism of Action

A. Reduction of the slowly-inactivating sodium current
   Phenytoin
   Carbamazepine
   Oxcarbazepine
   Lamotrigine

B. Enhanced concentration or activity of γ-aminobutyric acid
   Barbiturates
   Benzodiazepines
   Tiagabine
   Vigabatrin
   Gabapentin

C. Reduction of the T-type calcium current
   Ethosuximide

D. Multiple actions
   Valproic acid
   Felbamate
   Topiramate
   Zonisamide

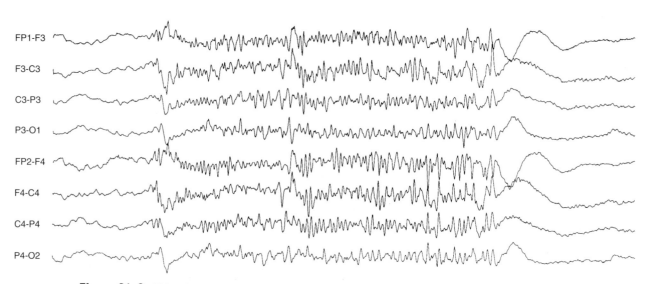

FP1-F3

F3-C3

C3-P3

P3-O1

FP2-F4

F4-C4

C4-P4

P4-O2

Figure 31–3. This electroencephalogram shows an epileptic recruiting rhythm in a drowsy or lightly sleeping patient. Note the sudden onset and offset of high-voltage, diffuse, rhythmic, occasionally sharply contoured waves. Such potentials may occur at the onset of a generalized tonic-clonic (grand mal) seizure, in patients with tonic seizures, and in some patients with absence (petit mal) attacks.

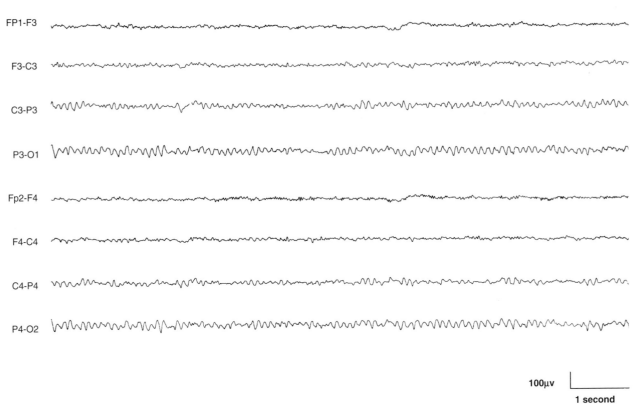

FP1-F3

F3-C3

C3-P3

P3-O1

Fp2-F4

F4-C4

C4-P4

P4-O2

100μv

1 second

Figure 31-4. This normal awake electroencephalogram in a healthy 16-year-old patient shows bilaterally synchronous and symmetrical 9-Hz alpha activity occurring principally in the fourth and eighth channels.

Phenytoin

Phenytoin is an hydantoin drug that was developed in 1938 by Merritt and Putnam[38] as the result of a systematic search for drugs that were structurally similar to barbiturates but caused little or no sedation.

Mechanism of Action

At therapeutic concentrations of 10 to 20 μg/mL, phenytoin prevents the sustained repetitive firing that normally results from extended depolarization in the epileptogenic focus.[39] The central mechanism is voltage-dependent blockade of fast sodium conductance.[40] Phenytoin prolongs the inactivated and blocked state of the channel.[41,42] The use-dependent nature of the blockade means that neurons with fewer depolarizations will be less affected, a property that reduces the adverse effects of this agent, as normal brain activity is less affected. This characteristic also explains why phenytoin is not an effective local anesthetic despite being a sodium channel blocker.

Adverse Reactions

At the time of its introduction, phenytoin set a new standard as a safe and reliable agent. Nevertheless, numerous adverse reactions are known to occur with prolonged use or high doses. Toxic neurologic effects, which tend to occur with plasma levels greater than 20 μg/mL, include nystagmus, ataxia, and incoordination. The therapeutic index for motor impairment is 6.9.[40] Adverse systemic effects include hirsutism, gingival hyperplasia (20%), and a coarsening of the features, an effect that may limit its use in children and young adults. Phenytoin can inhibit the secretion of insulin, leading to impaired glucose tolerance. Other adverse endocrine effects include hypocalcemia and osteomalacia. Adverse gastrointestinal side effects include anorexia, nausea, and vomiting. Prolonged use has been associated with mild peripheral neuropathy (30%), which is usually not a significant problem.[31] As many as 5% of patients administered phenytoin have rashes, including benign morbilliform rash and the more serious Stevens-Johnson syndrome. Although rare, serious hematologic abnormalities, such as aplastic anemia, and hypersensitivity reactions have been reported.

Acute administration of high doses of phenytoin has caused reduced consciousness, cardiac arrhythmias, and profound hypotension.[43] Reactions are more likely to occur when the agent is infused at rates greater than 50 mg/min.[31]

Drug Interactions

Phenytoin causes a variety of drug interactions because of its tendency to induce metabolic pathways in the liver and its high degree of binding to plasma proteins. Coadministration with phenobarbital reduces the absorption of pheny-

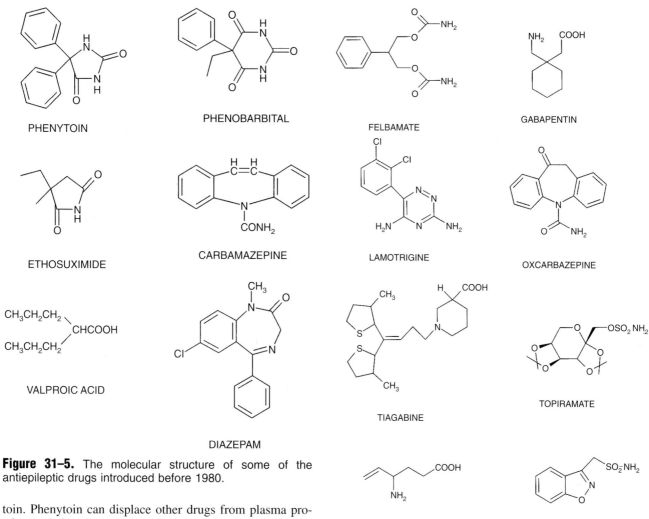

Figure 31–5. The molecular structure of some of the antiepileptic drugs introduced before 1980.

Figure 31–6. The molecular structure of some of the antiepileptic drugs introduced during or after 1980.

toin. Phenytoin can displace other drugs from plasma proteins and thus increase the free plasma concentration of those drugs. Such drugs include valproic acid, phenylbutazone, salicylates, and tolbutamide.

Phenytoin competes with other drugs at the cytochrome P450 level, and some of these agents reduce the metabolism of phenytoin and increase its plasma concentration. Chloramphenicol, disulfiram, isoniazid, cimetidine, sulfonamides, valproic acid, phenylbutazone, and theophylline can all have this effect. Conversely, the metabolism of phenytoin is greater when agents such as carbamazepine, phenobarbital, and alcohol are also used.

By inducing hepatic enzymes, phenytoin reduces the plasma concentration of corticosteroids, oral contraceptives, theophylline, and benzodiazepines. Phenytoin can also reduce folate levels and hence predispose a fetus to abnormalities. The mechanism is unknown but appears to relate to a reduction in folate liver stores rather than inhibition of gastrointestinal uptake.[44] An unproved drug interaction is the induction of halothane metabolism, which might increase the incidence of halothane hepatitis in individuals administered phenytoin.

Clinical Use

Phenytoin is a widely used first-line antiepileptic drug that is as effective as carbamazepine and valproic acid for treat-

ment of generalized (tonic-clonic) and complex partial seizures.[40] However, it is not effective for myoclonic seizures and can increase the incidence and duration of absence seizures.

Phenobarbital

Phenobarbital is the oldest antiepileptic drug in current clinical use. Before its introduction in 1912, seizures could only be managed with sedative/hypnotic agents such as the bromides. Phenobarbital was the first agent to demonstrate that anticonvulsant effects could be achieved without marked sedation.

Mechanism of Action

Used at therapeutic concentrations (10–40 µg/mL), this barbiturate primarily enhances the effect of GABA at the

TABLE 31–5.

Effective Anticonvulsants for Various Forms of Epilepsy

Seizure Type	Anticonvulsants	
	First-line	Additional/ Alternative
Focal seizures		
All types	Carbamazepine	Gabapentin
	Phenytoin	Lamotrigine
	Valproic acid	Oxcarbazepine
		Tiagabine
		Topiramate
		Vigabatrin
		(Felbamate)*
Generalized seizures		
Tonic-clonic	Valproic acid	Topiramate
	Carbamazepine	Oxcarbazepine
	Phenytoin	Zonisamide
		Phenobarbital
Absence	Ethosuximide	Lamotrigine
	Valproic acid	Topiramate
		Zonisamide
		Clonazepam
Myoclonic	Valproic acid	Clonazepam
		Primidone
		Zonisamide
Atonic	Valproic acid	Clonazepam
		(Felbamate)*

*Because of the risk for life-threatening toxic reactions, felbamate is reserved for patients with intractable seizures.

GABA$_A$ receptor on postsynaptic neurons. It does this by binding to one or more subunits on the GABA$_A$ receptor and increasing the affinity of the receptor for GABA.[45] As a result, the mean duration of opening of the chloride channel increases.[10]

Phenobarbital has other actions as well.[40] It can reduce release of the excitatory neurotransmitter glutamate by inhibiting presynaptic N-type calcium conductance. At high concentrations, phenobarbital also affects other voltage-gated ionophores. By decreasing the conductance of sodium and increasing the conductance of potassium, the neuronal membrane reverts to a hyperpolarized state.

Adverse Reactions

Sedation often follows initiation of phenobarbital.[31] Fortunately, tolerance to the sedative effects is greater than tolerance to the anticonvulsant effects.[40] Other central nervous system reactions include ataxia, confusion, diplopia, dizzi-

ness, and depression. Phenobarbital can adversely affect learning, memory, and behavior, with irritability and hyperactivity being common problems in children.[40] Older patients may experience confusion or agitation.

The adverse systemic effects of phenobarbital are numerous. A scarlatiniform or morbilliform rash,[46] most common in patients with asthma,[10] develops in as many as 2% of patients administered the drug. When the drug is given to pregnant women, the neonate can suffer a bleeding diathesis caused by a reduction in prothrombin levels. Uncommon reactions include megaloblastic anemia, an increase in antidiuretic hormone levels, renal impairment, and mild hypothermia. Phenobarbital can induce porphyria and should be avoided in patients with disorders of heme metabolism.

Drug Interactions

Because of its effects on the hepatic cytochrome P450 system, phenobarbital undergoes many of the same drug interactions as phenytoin. In addition, concurrent administration of valproic acid can increase plasma levels of phenobarbital. In addition to reducing metabolism of the barbiturate, valproic acid can also reduce renal excretion of the unchanged drug.[46]

Clinical Use

Phenobarbital effectively reduces the occurrence of generalized, partial, and myoclonic seizures. However, the somnolence that almost always occurs with phenobarbital, in addition to behavioral disturbances in children, has made the drug less popular than it had been previously.

Ethosuximide

Before 1960, the available treatments for absence seizures were limited to the toxic oxazolidinediones.[31] The succinimide anticonvulsants resulted from a screening program for antiabsence drugs that were safer. Ethosuximide is the agent in this group that is used clinically.

Mechanism of Action

Ethosuximide does not have the same mechanism of action as barbiturates and hydantoins, and it was not until 1989 that its mechanism of action was elucidated.[47] Ethosuximide reduces the voltage-dependent, T-type, calcium current that is involved in the generation of thalamic spike and wave discharges in absence seizures.

Adverse Reactions

Ethosuximide is relatively nontoxic and sedation is unusual.[40] Neurologic effects can include ataxia, lethargy, headache, euphoria, dizziness, and hiccups. Rarely,

TABLE 31–6.

Pharmacokinetic Properties of Antiepileptic Drugs

Anticonvulsant	F (%)	T_{max} (hr)	PPB (%)	V_d (1/kg)	Hepatic Enzyme Induction	Elimination	Clearance (mL/min)	$T_{1/2}$(hr)
Carbamazepine	80	4–8	75	1.4	Moderate	Oxidation, glucuronide	60–90	10–20
Clonazepam	80	2	85	3.2	—	Hepatic	80–120	20–40
Diazepam	90	1–4	95	1.1	—	Desmethyl'n	30	20–35 (60–90)*
Ethosuximide		3	0	0.7	Low	Oxidation	15	60
Felbamate	80	2–6	25	0.8	High	Oxidation	35	16–22
Gabapentin	60	2–3	0	0.98	—	Renal	100–300	6–7
Lamotrigine	90	1–3	55	1.2	Low	Glucuronide conjugation	30–60	15–30
Lorazepam	80	2–5	80	1.2	—	Hepatic		14
Oxcarbazepine*	90	1–2	40		Low	Renal		8–10
Phenobarbital	98	4–6	50	0.5	High	Oxidation	4	96
Phenytoin	98	3–12	90	0.6	High	Oxidation		24–60
Primidone	90	3	20	0.6	Moderate	Oxidation	20–55	56
Tiagabine	98	1–2	95	1.2	—	Oxidation	120–200	5–8
Topiramate	80	2–4	10	0.7	—	Renal, oxidation	27–50	8–15
Valproic acid	99	2	90	0.2	Low	Oxidation, glucuronide	8	14
Vigabatrin	70	1–2	0	0.8	—	Renal	100–140	5–8
Zonisamide	60	2–5	50	1.5	Low	Glucuronide, acetylation, oxidation	17–24	50–70

F, oral bioavailability; T_{max}, time to maximum concentration; V_d, volume of distribution; $T_{1/2}$, elimination half-life.
*Values given refer to principal metabolite.

photophobia and a parkinsonian disorder occur.[31] Uncommon systemic effects are blood dyscrasias, including bone marrow suppression, and gastrointestinal irritation. Connective tissue disorders such as systemic lupus erythematosus and Stevens-Johnson syndrome also can occur.

Drug Interactions

No clinically important drug interactions for ethosuximide have been reported.

Clinical Use

Ethosuximide has been, and probably remains, the agent of choice for use in absence seizures. Most patients experience more than 50% fewer seizures when prescribed the drug.[48]

Carbamazepine

Carbamazepine is an anticonvulsant that is structurally similar to the tricyclic antidepressants. Its clinical use in the treatment of trigeminal neuralgia symptoms began in the 1960s. Carbamazepine was first used as an antiseizure agent in the United States in 1974.

Mechanism of Action

Carbamazepine is an iminostilbene compound that blocks voltage- and frequency-dependent fast sodium currents. The sodium channels are kept in the inactivated state, which inhibits the spread of synchronized depolarization that is associated with the onset of seizures.

Adverse Reactions

Oral carbamazepine is relatively nontoxic. The therapeutic index for neurologic side effects is 8.1.[40] Negative side effects include diplopia, ataxia, vertigo, and sedation. Tolerance to the sedative effects occurs with continued use. Gastrointestinal irritation can be a negative side effect. An increase in hepatic enzymes and mild leukopenia occur in 5% to 10% of patients administered carbamazepine. More serious blood dyscrasias, such as aplastic anemia, are rare.[10] Acute intoxication may lead to respiratory depression, unconsciousness, and seizures. Carbamazepine can also increase the frequency of absence seizures in susceptible patients, even at therapeutic plasma concentrations of 4 to 12 μg/mL.

Drug Interactions

Carbamazepine can induce hepatic enzyme function to hasten the metabolism of numerous compounds, including itself. Hence the half-life tends to decrease with regular use. Other affected agents include phenytoin and primidone, whose plasma levels may decrease as a result. Carba-

mazepine can also reduce the plasma concentration of valproic acid and haloperidol. Careful monitoring of patients previously stabilized who are taking any of these medications is advised when introducing carbamazepine. Erythromycin, isoniazid, cimetidine, and propoxyphene are among the drugs that can inhibit the hepatic metabolism of carbamazepine, which leads to an increase in the drug's plasma level and the possibility of toxic effects.

Clinical Use

Carbamazepine effectively reduces the frequency of complex partial seizures and primarily generalized seizures by 83% and 55%, respectively.[49] Previously, its high degree of safety made carbamazepine a popular choice for those forms of epilepsy; however, its relatively short half-life necessitates dosing three times a day. Currently, the drug is administered less frequently because of newer agents.

Valproic Acid

This structurally simple yet clinically diverse agent was first synthesized in 1882. Its anticonvulsant activity was discovered by accident in the 1960s, when used on experiments as a solvent carrier for other agents being tested as antiepileptic drugs.[31]

Mechanism of Action

Valproic acid is a branched-chain carboxylic acid. At least three important mechanisms have been identified, and the therapeutic effects of the drug most likely result from a combination of the mechanisms.[40] First, valproic acid produces a voltage-dependent blockade of sodium currents. It delays the recovery of the channel from its inactive state. A second action is inhibition of the low-threshold (T-type) calcium currents in certain neurons.[50] Finally, valproic acid increases the concentration of GABA by inhibiting the GABA transaminase metabolic pathway[42] and by inducing the synthesis of glutamic acid decarboxylase.[31]

Adverse Reactions

Despite its low therapeutic index of 1.6 for neurologic complications in animal studies, valproic acid is generally well tolerated.[40] As with other agents, ataxia, sedation, and tremor have been reported. Adverse systemic reactions include rashes, alopecia, and appetite stimulation. Adverse gastrointestinal effects include gastric irritation, acute pancreatitis, and increase of liver enzymes. Fulminant hepatitis occurs in approximately 1/10,000 treated individuals, with most cases occurring in patients younger than 2 years who have been administered multiple antiseizure medications. Other anticonvulsants, particularly phenytoin and phenobarbital, can induce the transformation of valproic acid to toxic metabolites. Neutropenia, thrombocytopenia, and abnormalities of platelet function are among the adverse hematologic reactions that have occurred.

Drug Interactions

Because valproic acid has high plasma protein binding, it can displace phenytoin from these sites, increasing the free concentration of that drug. In addition, valproic acid prolongs the duration of action of barbiturates, benzodiazepines, and narcotics. Used with clonazepam, valproic acid has been associated on rare occasion with increased frequency of absence seizures. Plasma levels of the drug are decreased by coadministration of agents that induce hepatic metabolism, including carbamazepine, phenobarbital, and phenytoin.

Clinical Use

The multiple mechanisms by which valproic acid inhibits seizure activity are reflected in its broad clinical profile. It has been used to treat both focal and primarily generalized seizures, including absence, atypical absence, and myoclonic seizures. Comparative studies have shown that valproic acid has a lower efficacy than carbamazepine or phenytoin in the treatment of secondarily generalized partial seizures.[40]

Diazepam

Benzodiazepines have sedative, hypnotic, and amnestic effects. Diazepam was the first benzodiazepine to be used clinically. It was introduced into clinical practice in 1968, 7 years after it was first synthesized.[51] Many of the features of diazepam that are discussed in this section of the chapter also apply to other benzodiazepines used in the management of seizure disorders.

Mechanism of Action

Benzodiazepines have a structure characterized by attachment of a benzene ring to a diazepine moiety. The primary action is to bind to the $GABA_A$ receptor and enhance the effect of GABA.[45] A specific benzodiazepine binding site exists on the $GABA_A$ receptor,[52] and the site may involve more than one of the receptor subunits.[53] Occupation of this site increases the receptor's affinity for GABA[10] and the frequency of opening of the ligand-gated chloride channel.[45]

Adverse Reactions

Chronic diazepam ingestion causes tolerance, dependence, and physical and psychological addiction, along with anxiety and insomnia on withdrawal. These effects have prevented diazepam as an ongoing treatment for epilepsy.

In the acute treatment of seizures, diazepam is safe and effective. It has a wide range of therapeutic indices for neurologic reactions.[10] For example, the median effective dose for prevention of seizures in the pentylenetetrazol model of epilepsy is 0.3 mg/kg, compared with a median toxic dose of 57 mg/kg for motor incoordination.[40] Toxic concentrations can lead to hypotonia, dysarthria, drowsiness, dys-

equilibrium, or dizziness. Behavioral disturbances may occur in children. Cardiovascular and respiratory depression occur with high-dose intravenous administration. A more common problem is venous thrombosis or phlebitis at the site of injection of the propylene glycol-containing preparation, and pain on injection of either preparation.

Drug Interactions

Benzodiazepines are free from clinically important drug interactions. Administration with other anticonvulsant agents increases the incidence of cardiovascular and respiratory depression.

Clinical Use

Diazepam has been a mainstay in the treatment of status epilepticus. Administered intravenously or rectally, high brain levels can be achieved rapidly. In one comparative study, diazepam was effective in terminating 79% of episodes of status epilepticus.[54] However, because effectiveness is limited to 1 hour, initiation of a longer term therapy with a second agent, such as phenytoin, is recommended. Diazepam is also effective in terminating focal status epilepticus in 70% of cases. Administered rectally, it is the preferred agent for management of febrile convulsions.[55]

Chronic use of diazepam for prophylaxis of seizure disorders is not recommended. Oral dosing produces unstable blood levels, and tolerance develops with time. Monitoring of plasma levels is not useful, because one plasma level can be toxic in one person but subtherapeutic in another.

Felbamate

Felbamate was the first of the new anticonvulsants introduced in the last 20 years. Initially popular, felbamate has since been associated with serious adverse events.

Mechanism of Action

Felbamate has the structure of a dicarbamate and, in vitro, reduces sustained repetitive firing in spinal neurons,[56] suggesting activity at the slowly recovering sodium channels. Additional activity has been shown at calcium channels, where this agent reduces non–T-type calcium currents.[57] The underlying mechanism is binding of felbamate to a glycine regulatory site, causing inhibition of the glycine-enhanced calcium current at the NMDA-induced calcium channels.[58]

Adverse Reactions

The toxicity of felbamate has been a concern. On the positive side, the neurologic reactions described are usually minor. Felbamate causes relatively little central nervous system depression. Somnolence or insomnia may occur, especially in children. Gastric symptoms occur frequently, with many patients experiencing a 3% to 5% weight loss during the first 3 months of therapy.[58] Weight loss can be accompanied by nausea, vomiting, and anorexia.

In 1994, just 18 months after the introduction of felbamate, the U.S. Food and Drug Administration (FDA) issued a warning in response to several case reports of serious hematologic and hepatic reactions with felbamate. Aplastic anemia has been positively associated, predominantly in females, with use of felbamate. It occurs at the annual rate of 127/1,000,000[59] compared with an incidence of 2/1,000,000 in the general population. The mortality rate associated with this complication is as great as 40%. Identified risk factors include a history of cytopenia, autoimmune diseases, and previous allergy to antiepileptic drugs. Hepatotoxicity and acute liver failure also occur at an increased rate, the overall incidence being approximately 1/20,000. Although these two effects have caused additional concern, the incidence is not greater than with valproic acid therapy. Routine laboratory testing has not been effective in preventing serious reactions.[58]

Drug Interactions

Because felbamate is metabolized by the hepatic cytochrome P450 system, its metabolism is affected by concurrent administration of drugs that alter the function of that system. In particular, the plasma level of felbamate is reduced by phenytoin or carbamazepine use. Conversely, because felbamate is a potent inhibitor of enzyme function, it can reduce the metabolism of phenytoin, phenobarbital, and valproic acid. Felbamate also increases the plasma levels of carbamazepine epoxide and, to a lesser extent, lamotrigine and vigabatrin. The efficacy of the oral contraceptive pill is reduced because of the effect of felbamate on steroid metabolism.

Clinical Use

Because of the risk for life-threatening toxic reactions, felbamate is not used as a first-line drug but is reserved for patients with intractable epilepsy. After the FDA warning, the number of patients taking felbamate decreased by almost 90%.[58] However, felbamate use is currently increasing, because the drug is particularly effective in certain clinical situations. Felbamate is used mainly for poorly controlled partial and secondarily generalized seizures.[6] It also effectively reduces the frequency of seizures in Lennox-Gastaut syndrome and myoclonic and atonic forms of epilepsy.[58,60]

Gabapentin

Gabapentin was developed to produce an agent that could cross the blood–brain barrier and increase the concentration of GABA or have an effect at the GABA receptor. Structurally, gabapentin resembles the inhibitory neurotransmitter GABA, but the inclusion of a carbon ring greatly enhances its lipid solubility.

Mechanism of Action

Gabapentin acts through a unique but poorly understood mechanism that does not involve direct interaction with the $GABA_A$ receptor. Gabapentin also does not inhibit the reuptake of GABA.[10] At concentrations greater than those used clinically, this drug is a weak inhibitor of the metabolic enzyme GABA transaminase.[41] The most likely mechanism of action is an increase in synthesis of GABA, although the pathways involved are not clearly understood.[61]

Adverse Reactions

The most common adverse reactions associated with gabapentin have been dizziness, somnolence, headache, ataxia, and fatigue.[61] Nausea and vomiting occur infrequently. Generally, gabapentin is well tolerated, and serious reactions have not been reported. The incidence of adverse events is not related to the rate at which gabapentin is introduced.[62]

Drug Interactions

With no plasma protein binding and no metabolism or effect on the metabolic pathways of other drugs, gabapentin is almost totally free of drug interactions. Gastric absorption may be reduced by administration of antacid medications that contain hydroxides of aluminum or magnesium.[63] The renal clearance of gabapentin can be reduced by administration of cimetidine.[64]

Clinical Use

Gabapentin is a safe and effective anticonvulsant with proven clinical efficacy as either monotherapy or as an additive agent for partial seizures in children or adults.[61] In controlled trials of its efficacy as an add-on agent, the odds ratio for a 50% reduction in seizure frequency is 2.3.[65] Because of its short half-life, administration several times per day is required. A relationship between plasma concentration and efficacy has not been established.

Lamotrigine

Lamotrigine was introduced into clinical practice in 1994.

Mechanism of Action

Lamotrigine is a phenyltriazine that acts on voltage-sensitive sodium channels, inhibiting the slowly inactivating sodium current.[66] Lamotrigine also has some activity at the P-type and N-type calcium channels.[57,67]

Adverse Reactions

Lamotrigine is generally well tolerated. Neurologic reactions include headache, asthenia, dizziness, and somnolence. The most frequent reason for discontinuation is rash, usually a benign macropapular or erythematous rash, suggesting a delayed hypersensitivity reaction. On occasion, more serious reactions occur, including the Stevens-Johnson syndrome or toxic epidermal necrolysis. The incidence of serious skin reactions appears to be greater if a patient is also taking valproic acid.[66] A few cases of disseminated intravascular coagulation have occurred.[31] Gastrointestinal complaints are infrequent, and blood dyscrasias have not been reported.

Drug Interactions

The clearance of lamotrigine is increased by the concurrent administration of agents that induce the hepatic microsomal cytochrome P450 system, including phenytoin and barbiturates. Valproic acid has the opposite effect, increasing the half-life of lamotrigine to about 60 hours.[68]

Clinical Use

Lamotrigine is used as adjunct therapy for the control of partial and secondarily generalized seizures.[69] The odds ratio for a 50% response is 2.2.[65] Recently, lamotrigine has been shown to be effective in the treatment of absence seizures, with one third of patients obtaining a 50% or greater reduction in seizure frequency.[66] Lamotrigine may be useful as monotherapy and in the treatment of Lennox-Gastaut syndrome.

Oxcarbazepine

Oxcarbazepine was developed to provide the clinical efficacy of carbamazepine with fewer toxic side effects. Oxcarbazepine does not form carbamazepine oxide, which increases its safety.

Mechanism of Action

Oxcarbazepine is a keto analog of carbamazepine. After administration, it is quickly reduced to its active metabolite 10-hydroxycarbazepine, the 10-monohydroxy derivative (MHD). Because the actions and kinetic profile of oxcarbazepine can be attributed to MHD, oxcarbazepine can be regarded as a prodrug.[70] It blocks sustained firing of voltage- and frequency-dependent sodium currents in a manner similar to carbamazepine.

Adverse Reactions

Oxcarbazepine is a relatively safe drug that has greater tolerability than carbamazepine. Possible adverse neurologic side effects include sedation, headache, dizziness, vertigo, ataxia, and diplopia. The therapeutic index for motor ataxia is about 10.[71] Nausea and rash are infrequent. Oxcarbazepine has a mild antidiuretic effect, accounting for the mild and reversible hyponatremia that occurs in some individuals. Although some alteration in hepatic enzyme or sex hormone levels may occur, these changes are usually not clinically apparent. Hypersensitivity reactions can occur. Cross-sensitivity occurs in 25% of patients administered oxcarbazepine who are allergic to carbamazepine.

Drug Interactions

Oxcarbazepine and MHD do not induce hepatic microsomal enzymes, and their metabolism is not altered by drugs that do. When polytherapy is instituted with oxcarbazepine, the plasma level of phenytoin or valproic acid may increase because of removal of another agent that does induce hepatic enzymes.[72] Oxcarbazepine and MHD do not displace other agents from plasma protein binding sites. MHD can reduce the effectiveness of oral contraceptives.[73]

Clinical Use

Compared with carbamazepine, oxcarbazepine offers equivalent seizure reduction but with fewer adverse events. Oxcarbazepine can be used to treat complex partial and primarily generalized seizure disorders. Its use is not established for absence or myoclonic seizures, for the Lennox-Gastaut syndrome, or in pregnancy.

Tiagabine

The anticonvulsant effects of nipecotic acid have been useful experimentally for decades. However, because of its insolubility in lipids, nipecotic acid does not cross the blood–brain barrier and must be administered directly into the ventricles of the brain. Tiagabine is a modification of nipecotic acid that can be administered systemically.

Mechanism of Action

Structurally, tiagabine is a nipecotic acid moiety connected to a lipophilic anchor with an aliphatic chain. Tiagabine is a potent inhibitor of GABA reuptake.[39] It acts primarily on the most important of the four known GABA transporters: GAT-1.[74]

Adverse Reactions

Possible adverse neurologic reactions include dizziness, asthenia, poor concentration, aphasia, and tremor. Depression is more frequent with tiagabine than with placebo,[65] possibly because of the ability of tiagabine to increase resting concentrations of GABA. Depression also occurs with vigabatrin, an antiepileptic drug that inhibits the breakdown of GABA. Gastrointestinal effects, such as abdominal pain, have been reported with tiagabine.

Drug Interactions

Despite being 98% bound to plasma proteins, tiagabine has no clinically important effects on the protein binding of other agents, because the amount of tiagabine administered (2- to 20-mg tablets) is quite small.[63] Although tiagabine has no effect on hepatic enzymes, its own half-life is reduced by administration of agents that stimulate hepatic metabolism.

Clinical Use

Tiagabine is indicated as adjunctive therapy for complex partial seizures, having an odds ratio of 3.0 for a 50% reduction in seizure frequency compared with placebo.[65,75–77] Efficacy has been demonstrated against simple partial and secondarily generalized seizures.[78] Preliminary investigations suggest that tiagabine may be useful for status epilepticus[79] and as a neuroprotective agent.[80] Its efficacy in monotherapy has not been established.

Topiramate

Topiramate is a new broad-spectrum antiepileptic drug that has a favorable pharmacokinetic profile and low toxicity.

Mechanism of Action

Topiramate is a monosaccharide that is produced by sulfamate substitution from the R-enantiomer of fructose. Topiramate reduces the voltage-dependent sodium current.[39] It also enhances GABA-mediated inhibition of the postsynaptic potential. This action does not occur at the same site at which barbiturates and benzodiazepines produce their effects but rather seems to involve a novel interaction at the $GABA_A$ receptor.[81] Topiramate also antagonizes the action of glutamate at the AMPA (alpha-amino-3-hydroxy-5-methylisoxazole-4-propionic acid) subtype receptor.[82,83] Finally, topiramate is a weak inhibitor of carbonic anhydrase. This characteristic may be important because the presence of high intracellular concentrations of bicarbonate can cause cell depolarization when GABA (normally inhibitory) activates the anionic channel.[41]

Adverse Reactions

Although topiramate usually does not produce adverse effects,[82] dizziness, ataxia, altered concentration, confusion, fatigue, and somnolence have been reported. These side effects may be more common if the drug is rapidly titrated to higher doses. The therapeutic index for motor impairment is 12.[40] Nephrolithiasis occurs in 1.5% of patients administered topiramate, presumably because of the drug's action on carbonic anhydrase.

Drug Interactions

Enzyme-inducing drugs reduce the plasma concentration of topiramate, therefore it may be necessary to adjust the dose when phenytoin or carbamazepine is started or discontinued.[84] By contrast, topiramate has no effect on the pharmacokinetics of other drugs, because it does not affect hepatic enzyme systems and undergoes little plasma protein binding.[85] Serum digoxin levels may decrease by 10% to 15% in the presence of topiramate.[63]

Clinical Use

Topiramate has a broad clinical profile. It reduces the frequency of partial, generalized tonic-clonic and absence seizures. As an add-on therapy, the odds ratio for 50% response is 4.3.[65] Topiramate has the additional advantage of daily or twice daily dosing. New applications might include the Lennox-Gastaut and West epilepsies and as a monotherapy for partial seizures.[86–88]

Vigabatrin

Vigabatrin has been used clinically in Europe and Australia for two decades. However, its safety is still being reviewed, and currently it has not been approved for use in the United States.

Mechanism of Action

Vigabatrin (γ-vinyl GABA) is a structural analog of the inhibitory neurotransmitter GABA. It was the first anticonvulsant to be designed with a specific mechanism of action in mind. Vigabatrin causes inhibition of GABA transaminase (GABA-T), the enzyme that biotransforms GABA. The inhibition is irreversible, with GABA-T activity increasing to only 60% of baseline 5 days after administration.[89] In addition to its primary action, chronic vigabatrin administration can reduce glutamate levels in the brain, probably through inhibition of glutamate synthetase activity.[41]

Adverse Reactions

Adverse neurologic side effects such as headache, dizziness, and anxiety have been reported. Drowsiness occurs in as many as 40% of patients, particularly after the start of therapy.[89] Depression or psychosis occurs three times more frequently with vigabatrin than with placebo. After several months of vigabatrin therapy, 10% of patients experience a characteristic visual field defect: peripheral vision decreases, with sparing of the nasal segment. Gastrointestinal reactions include irritation and mild weight gain. One case of overdose had encephalopathy.[89]

The adverse event that led to discontinuation of clinical trials in the United States in 1983 was intramyelinic edema, reversible microvacuolation in the outer laminar myelin sheaths. This condition was observed at autopsy in rats and dogs administered vigabatrin.[40] The importance of these findings was unclear, because the animals did not appear to be neurologically impaired. Also, no clinical or autopsy findings suggest that this condition occurs in humans.[89]

Drug Interactions

The plasma concentration of phenytoin decreases 15% to 20% in patients treated concurrently with vigabatrin.[90] The mechanism is not known, because there is no basis for enzyme induction or protein binding displacement. No other interactions are known to occur.

Clinical Use

The countries that have a long clinical experience with vigabatrin use it primarily as add-on therapy for poorly controlled partial seizures. For that purpose, vigabatrin reduces the frequency of seizures by at least 50% in about half of the subjects;[91] the odds ratio is 3.7 compared with placebo.[65] Vigabatrin has no efficacy against generalized seizures, including absence, myoclonus, and Lennox-Gastaut syndrome. The drug has been used successfully to treat infantile spasms, for which it has an efficacy equivalent to corticosteroids but with less toxicity.[92-94]

Zonisamide

Zonisamide is a recently approved broad-spectrum anticonvulsant.

Mechanism of Action

In cultured spinal cord neurons, zonisamide reduces the voltage-dependent calcium current in the same manner as phenytoin and carbamazepine.[95] Zonisamide also provides activity against the voltage-dependent T-type calcium currents, an effect that would account for the efficacy of the drug in models of absence seizures.[96,97] An additional effect is enhancement of the GABA-mediated postsynaptic inhibition of cell firing.

Adverse Reactions

Possible adverse neurologic effects include somnolence, ataxia, anorexia, confusion, altered thinking, fatigue, and dizziness. Behavioral disorders may affect children, and manic episodes in adults have been reported.[98] Acute overdose causes a depressed conscious state.

Nephrolithiasis is a problem in 3% of patients administered zonisamide.[98] Most renal calculi have been small and have not required surgical treatment.

Drug Interactions

The use of zonisamide does not result in drug interactions because of displacement of other drugs from plasma protein binding sites. Administration has little effect on the metabolism of other agents, although the metabolism of carbamazepine to its epoxide may be enhanced.[98] Conversely, pretreatment with phenobarbital or carbamazepine reduces the half-life and plasma level of zonisamide, because of induction of hepatic clearance mechanisms.[63]

Clinical Use

Zonisamide is an anticonvulsant with low toxicity and a broad spectrum of clinical activity. It is useful as an adjunctive agent in the management of partial and secondarily generalized seizures. Zonisamide also has activity against tonic-clonic, absence, and myoclonic seizures, as well as the Lennox-Gastaut syndrome and infantile spasms.[98] In studies of add-on antiepileptic drugs, the overall odds ratio for a 50% reduction in seizure frequency was 2.5 with zonisamide.[65] The use of the drug as monotherapy currently is not supported by clinical studies.

Anesthesia and Anticonvulsant Drugs

Patients taking anticonvulsant drugs have an increased requirement for nondepolarizing muscle relaxants, opioids, sedatives, and anesthetic agents such as thiopental, propofol, and midazolam.[99,100] For fentanyl, the increased requirement seems to relate to the number of anticonvulsant drugs being administered.[99] The exact causes for the increased requirements are unknown. Possibilities include enzyme induction by hepatic microsomes, resulting in enhanced drug clearance; changes in protein binding; changes in the number or dynamics of receptors; and interactions with endogenous neurotransmitters.

Although gastrointestinal symptoms are commonly associated with anticonvulsants, increased postoperative nausea and vomiting have not been demonstrated. Bleeding from the gums may occasionally complicate endotracheal intubation in patients who have gingival hyperplasia from chronic ingestion of phenytoin. Hematologic complications from anticonvulsant drugs rarely affect intraoperative management significantly.

Acknowledgments
The authors thank Dr. Warren Blume for providing the electroencephalograms used in this chapter, Drs. Stan Leung and Ian Herrick for editorial assistance, and Ms. Jeanette Mikulic for assistance in the preparation of the manuscript.

References

1. Gastaut H: Clinical and electroencephalographical classification of epileptic seizures. Epilepsia 11:102, 1970.
2. Proposal for revised clinical and electroencephalographic classification of epileptic seizures. From the Commission on Classification and

Terminology of the International League Against Epilepsy. Epilepsia 22:489, 1981.

3. Proposal for classification of epilepsies and epileptic syndromes. Commission on Classification and Terminology of the International League Against Epilepsy. Epilepsia 26:268, 1985.

4. Proposal for revised classification of epilepsies and epileptic syndromes. Commission on Classification and Terminology of the International League Against Epilepsy. Epilepsia 30:389, 1989.

5. Hauser WA, Annegers JF, Kurland LT: Incidence of epilepsy and unprovoked seizures in Rochester, Minnesota: 1935–1984. Epilepsia 34:453, 1993.

6. McNamara JO: Development of new pharmacological agents for epilepsy: Lessons from the kindling model. Epilepsia 30(suppl 1):S13;discussion S64, 1989.

7. Lowenstein DH: Seizures and epilepsy. In Fauci AS, Braunwald E, Isselbacher KJ, et al (eds): Harrison's Principles of Internal Medicine, 14th ed. New York, McGraw-Hill, 1998.

8. Dichter MA, Ayala GF: Cellular mechanisms of epilepsy: A status report. Science 237:157, 1987.

9. Schwartzkroin P: Basic mechanisms of epileptogeneis. In Wyllie E (ed): The treatment of Epilepsy: Principles and Practice. Philadelphia, Lea & Febiger, 1993.

10. Carvey PM: Antiepileptic drugs. In Drug Action in the Central Nervous System. New York, Oxford University Press, 1998.

11. Schwartzkroin PA: Cellular electrophysiology of human epilepsy. Epilepsy Res 17:185, 1994.

12. Dichter MA: Emerging insights into mechanisms of epilepsy: Implications for new antiepileptic drug development. Epilepsia 35(suppl 4):S51, 1994.

13. McCormick DA, Pape HC: Properties of a hyperpolarization-activated cation current and its role in rhythmic oscillation in thalamic relay neurones. J Physiol 431:291, 1990.

14. Crill WE, Schwindt PC: Role of persistent inward and outward membrane currents in epileptiform bursting in mammalian neurons. Adv Neurol 44:225, 1986.

15. Storm JF: Action potential repolarization and a fast afterhyperpolarization in rat hippocampal pyramidal cells. J Physiol 385:733, 1987.

16. Haglund MM, Schwarzkroin PA: Role of Na-K pump potassium regulation and IPSPs in seizures and spreading depression in immature rabbit hippocampal slices. J Neurophysiol 63:225, 1990.

17. Fisher RS, Pedley TA, Moody WJ Jr, et al: The role of extracellular potassium in hippocampal epilepsy. Arch Neurol 33:76, 1976.

18. Fifkova E: A possible mechanism of morphometric changes in dendritic spines induced by stimulation. Cell Mol Neurobiol 5:47, 1985.

19. Jefferys JG, Haas HL: Synchronized bursting of CA1 hippocampal pyramidal cells in the absence of synaptic transmission. Nature 300:448, 1982.

20. Collingridge GL, Kehl SJ, McLennan H: Excitatory amino acids in synaptic transmission in the Schaffer collateral-commissural pathway of the rat hippocampus. J Physiol 334:33, 1983.

21. Nowak L, Bregestovski P, Ascher P, et al: Magnesium gates glutamate-activated channels in mouse central neurones. Nature 307:462, 1984.

22. Dingledine R: N-methyl aspartate activates voltage-dependent calcium conductance in rat hippocampal pyramidal cells. J Physiol 343:385, 1983.

23. Choi DW, Rothman SM: The role of glutamate neurotoxicity in hypoxic-ischemic neuronal death. Annu Rev Neurosci 13:171, 1990.

24. Tanaka K, Graham SH, Simon RP: The role of excitatory neurotransmitters in seizure-induced neuronal injury in rats. Brain Res 737:59, 1996.

25. Goddard GV, McIntyre DC, Leech CK: A permanent change in brain function resulting from daily electrical stimulation. Exp Neurol 25:295, 1969.

26. Sutula T, Cascino G, Cavazos J, et al: Mossy fiber synaptic reorganization in the epileptic human temporal lobe. Ann Neurol 26:321, 1989.

27. Dichter M, Spencer WA: Penicillin-induced interictal discharges from the cat hippocampus. I. Characteristics and topographical features. J Neurophysiol 32:649, 1969.

28. Chagnac-Amitai Y, Conners BW: Horizontal spread of synchronized activity in neocortex and its control by GABA-mediated inhibition. J Neurophysiol 61:747, 1989.

29. Manuel NA, Davies CH: Pharmacological modulation of GABA(A) receptor-mediated postsynaptic potentials in the CA1 region of the rat hippocampus. Br J Pharmacol 125:1529, 1998.

30. Staley KJ, Soldo BL, Proctor WR: Ionic mechanisms of neuronal excitation by inhibitory GABAA receptors. Science 269:977, 1995.

31. McNamara JO: Drugs effective in the therapy of the epilepsies. In Hardman JG, Limbird LE (eds): Goodman & Gilman's Pharmacological Basis of Therapeutics, 9th ed, New York, McGraw-Hill, 1996.

32. Dichter MA: Basic mechanisms of epilepsy: Targets for therapeutic intervention. Epilepsia 38(suppl 9):S2, 1997.

33. Deisz RA, Prince DA: Frequency-dependent depression of inhibition in guinea-pig neocortex in vitro by GABAB receptor feed-back on GABA release. J Physiol 412:513, 1989.

34. Coulter DA, Huguenard JR, Prince DA: Calcium currents in rat thalamocortical relay neurones: Kinetic properties of the transient, low-threshold current. J Physiol 414:587, 1989.

35. Modica PA, Tempelhoff R, White PF: Pro- and anticonvulsant effects of anesthetics (part I). Anesth Analg 70:303, 1990.

36. Modica PA, Tempelhoff R, White PF: Pro- and anticonvulsant effects of anesthetics (part II). Anesth Analg 70:433, 1990.

37. Herrick IA: Seizure activity and anesthetic agents and adjuvants. In Albin MS (ed): Textbook of Neuroanesthesia with Neurosurgical and Neuroscience Perspectives. New York, McGraw-Hill, 1997.

38. Merritt HH, Putnam TJ: A new series of anti-convulsant drugs tested by experiments on animals. Arch Neurol Psychiatry 39:1003, 1938.

39. White HS: Comparative anticonvulsant and mechanistic profile of the established and newer antiepileptic drugs. Epilepsia 40(suppl 5):S2, 1999.

40. Rogawski MA, Porter RJ: Antiepileptic drugs: Pharmacological mechanisms and clinical efficacy with consideration of promising developmental stage compounds. Pharmacol Rev 42:223, 1990.

41. Meldrum BS: Update on the mechanism of action of antiepileptic drugs. Epilepsia 37(suppl 6):S4, 1996.

42. Ferrendelli JA, Mathews GC: Neuropharmacology of antiepileptic medications: Mechanisms of action. In Wyllie E (ed): The Treatment of Epilepsy: Principles and Practice. Philadelphia, Lea & Febiger, 1993.

43. Berry JM, Kowalski A, Fletcher SA: Sudden asystole during craniotomy: Unrecognized phenytoin toxicity. J Neurosurg Anesthesiol 11:42, 1999.

44. Carl GF, Hudson FZ, McGuire BS Jr: Phenytoin-induced depletion of folate in rats originates in liver and involves a mechanism that does not discriminate folate form. J Nutr 127:2231, 1997.

45. Twyman RE, Rogers CJ, Macdonald RL: Differential regulation of gamma-aminobutyric acid receptor channels by diazepam and phenobarbital. Ann Neurol 25:213, 1989.

46. Julien RM: Antiepileptic agents. In Smith NT, Corbascio AN (eds): Drug Interactions in Anesthesia. Philadelphia, Lea & Febiger, 1986.

47. Coulter DA, Huguenard JR, Prince DA: Characterization of ethosuximide reduction of low-threshold calcium current in thalamic neurons. Ann Neurol 25:582, 1989.

48. Browne TR, Dreifuss FE, Dyken PR, et al: Ethosuximide in the treatment of absence (peptit mal) seizures. Neurology 25:515, 1975.

49. Rodin EA, Rim CS, Rennick PM: The effects of carbamazepine on patients with psychomotor epilepsy: Results of a double-blind study. Epilepsia 15:547, 1974.

50. Kelly KM, Gross RA, Macdonald RL: Valproic acid selectively reduces the low-threshold (T) calcium current in rat nodose neurons. Neurosci Lett 116:233, 1990.

51. Sternbach LH, Reeder E: Quinzalones and 1,4-benzodiazepines. IV. Transformations of 7-chloro-2-methylamino-5-phenyl-3H-1,4-benzodiazepine-4-oxide. J Org Chem 26:4936, 1961.

52. Squires RF, Brastrup C: Benzodiazepine receptors in rat brain. Nature 266:732, 1977.

53. Pritchett DB, Sontheimer H, Shivers BD, et al: Importance of a novel GABAA receptor subunit for benzodiazepine pharmacology. Nature 338:582, 1989.

54. Leppik IE, Derivan AT, Homan RW, et al: Double-blind study of lorazepam and diazepam in status epilepticus. JAMA 249:1452, 1983.

55. Henriksen O: An overview of benzodiazepines in seizure management. Epilepsia 39(suppl 2):S2, 1998.

56. Pisani A, Stefani A, Siniscalchi A, et al: Electrophysiological actions of felbamate on rat striatal neurones. Br J Pharmacol 116:2053, 1995.

57. Stefani A, Spadoni F, Bernardi G: Voltage-activated calcium channels: Targets of antiepileptic drug therapy? Epilepsia 38:959, 1997.

58. Pellock JM: Felbamate. Epilepsia 40(suppl 5):S57, 1999.
59. Kaufman DW, Kelly JP, Anderson T, et al: Evaluation of case reports of aplastic anemia among patients treated with felbamate. Epilepsia 38:1265, 1997.
60. Efficacy of felbamate in childhood epileptic encephalopathy (Lennox-Gastaut syndrome). The Felbamate Study Group in Lennox-Gastaut Syndrome. N Engl J Med 328:29, 1993.
61. Morris GL: Gabapentin. Epilepsia 40(suppl 5):S63, 1999.
62. Morris GL 3rd: Efficacy and tolerability of gabapentin in clinical practice. Clin Ther 17:891, 1995.
63. Perucca E: The clinical pharmacokinetics of the new antiepileptic drugs. Epilepsia 40(suppl 9):S7, 1999.
64. Goa KL, Sorkin EM: Gabapentin. A review of its pharmacological properties and clinical potential in epilepsy. Drugs 46:409, 1993.
65. Chadwick DW, Marson T, Kadir Z: Clinical administration of new antiepileptic drugs: An overview of safety and efficacy. Epilepsia 37(suppl 6):S17, 1996.
66. Matsuo F: Lamotrigine. Epilepsia 40(suppl 5):S30, 1999.
67. Stefani A, Spadoni F, Siniscalchi A, et al: Lamotrigine inhibits Ca2+ currents in cortical neurons: Functional implications. Eur J Pharmacol 307:113, 1996.
68. Binnie CD, van Emde Boas W, Kasteleijn-Nolste-Trenite DG, et al: Acute effects of lamotrigine (BW430C) in persons with epilepsy. Epilepsia 27:248, 1986.
69. Matsuo F, Bergen D, Faught E, et al: Placebo-controlled study of the efficacy and safety of lamotrigine in patients with partial seizures. U.S. Lamotrigine Protocol 0.5 Clinical Trial Group. Neurology 43:2284, 1993.
70. Jensen PK, Gram L, Schmutz M: Oxcarbazepine. Epilepsy Res Suppl 3:135, 1991.
71. Tecoma ES: Oxcarbazepine. Epilepsia 40(suppl 5):S37, 1999.
72. Houtkooper MA, Lammertsma A, Meyer JW, et al: Oxcarbazepine (GP 47.680): A possible alternative to carbamazepine? Epilepsia 28:693, 1987.
73. Klosterskov Jensen P, Saano V, Haring P, et al: Possible interaction between oxcarbazepine and an oral contraceptive. Epilepsia 33:1149, 1992.
74. Meldrum BS, Chapman AG: Basic mechanisms of gabitril (tiagabine) and future potential developments. Epilepsia 40(suppl 9):S2, 1999.
75. Richens A, Chadwick DW, Duncan JS, et al: Adjunctive treatment of partial seizures with tiagabine: A placebo-controlled trial. Epilepsy Res 21:37, 1995.
76. Uthman BM, Rowan AJ, Ahmann PA, et al: Tiagabine for complex partial seizures: A randomized, add-on, dose-response trial. Arch Neurol 55:56, 1998.
77. Kalviainen R, Brodie MJ, Duncan J, et al: A double-blind, placebo-controlled trial of tiagabine given three-times daily as add-on therapy for refractory partial seizures. Northern European Tiagabine Study Group. Epilepsy Res 30:31, 1998.
78. Ben-Menachem E: International experience with tiagabine add-on therapy. Epilepsia 36(suppl 6):S14, 1995.
79. Halonen T, Nissinen J, Jansen JA, et al: Tiagabine prevents seizures, neuronal damage and memory impairment in experimental status epilepticus. Eur J Pharmacol 299:69, 1996.
80. Inglefield JR, Perry JM, Schwartz RD: Postischemic inhibition of GABA reuptake by tiagabine slows neuronal death in the gerbil hippocampus. Hippocampus 5:460, 1995.
81. White HS, Brown SD, Woodhead JH, et al: Topiramate enhances GABA-mediated chloride flux and GABA-evoked chloride currents in murine brain neurons and increases seizure threshold. Epilepsy Res 28:167, 1997.
82. Shorvon SD: Safety of topiramate: Adverse events and relationships to dosing. Epilepsia 37(suppl 2):S18, 1996.
83. Gibbs JW 3rd, Sombati S, DeLorenzo RJ, et al: Cellular actions of topiramate: Blockade of kainate-evoked inward currents in cultured hippocampal neurons. Epilepsia 41(suppl 1):S10, 2000.
84. Perucca E: Pharmacokinetic profile of topiramate in comparison with other new antiepileptic drugs. Epilepsia 37(suppl 2):S8, 1996.
85. Bourgeois BF: Drug interaction profile of topiramate. Epilepsia 37(suppl 2):S14, 1996.
86. Glauser TA: Topiramate. Epilepsia 40(suppl 5):S71, 1999.
87. Glauser TA: Topiramate use in pediatric patients. Can J Neurol Sci 25:S8, 1998.
88. Sachdeo RC, Reife RA, Lim P, et al: Topiramate monotherapy for partial onset seizures. Epilepsia 38:294, 1997.
89. French JA: Vigabatrin. Epilepsia 40(suppl 5):S11, 1999.
90. Rimmer EM, Richens A: Interaction between vigabatrin and phenytoin. Br J Clin Pharmacol 27(suppl 1):27S, 1989.
91. Ben-Menachem E: Expanding antiepileptic drug options: Clinical efficacy of new therapeutic agents. Epilepsia 37(suppl 2):S4, 1996.
92. Aicardi J, Mumford JP, Dumas C, et al: Vigabatrin as initial therapy for infantile spasms: A European retrospective survey. Sabril IS Investigator and Peer Review Groups. Epilepsia 37:638, 1996.
93. Chiron C, Dulac O, Beaumont D, et al: Therapeutic trial of vigabatrin in refractory infantile spasms. J Child Neurol Suppl 2:S52, 1991.
94. Chiron C, Dumas C, Jambaque I, et al: Randomized trial comparing vigabatrin and hydrocortisone in infantile spasms due to tuberous sclerosis. Epilepsy Res 26:389, 1997.
95. Schauf CL: Zonisamide enhances slow sodium inactivation in Myxicola. Brain Res 413:185, 1987.
96. Suzuki S, Kawakami K, Nishimura S, et al: Zonisamide blocks T-type calcium channel in cultured neurons of rat cerebral cortex. Epilepsy Res 12:21, 1992.
97. Kito M, Maehara M, Watanabe K: Mechanisms of T-type calcium channel blockade by zonisamide. Seizure 5:115, 1996.
98. Leppik IE: Zonisamide. Epilepsia 40(suppl 5):S23, 1999.
99. Tempelhoff R, Modica PA, Spitznagel EL Jr: Anticonvulsant therapy increases fentanyl requirements during anaesthesia for craniotomy. Can J Anaesth 37:327, 1990.
100. Tempelhoff R, Modica PA, Jellish WS, et al: Resistance to atracurium-induced neuromuscular blockade in patients with intractable seizure disorders treated with anticonvulsants. Anesth Analg 71:665, 1990.
101. McNamara JO: Cellular and molecular basis of epilepsy. J Neurosci 14:3413, 1994.
102. Noebels JL: Targeting epilepsy genes. Neuron 16:241, 1996.
103. Dreifuss FE: Classification of the epileptic seizures. In Engel J Jr, Pedley TA (eds): Epilepsy: A Comprehensive Textbook. Philadelphia, Lippincott-Raven, 1998.

32

Neuroprotective Agents

Vesna Jevtovic-Todorovic, MD, PhD • John W. Olney, MD

Protecting the central nervous system (CNS) against injury, either acute injury (e.g., stroke, trauma, status epilepticus) or chronic neurodegeneration (e.g., amyotrophic lateral sclerosis [ALS], Parkinson, Huntington, or Alzheimer diseases [AD]), is an issue of enormous societal importance. The costs to society associated with brain injury and neurodegeneration are huge, and the money currently being spent by the pharmaceutical industry in attempts to develop neuroprotective drugs is of corresponding magnitude.

For many years, both acute CNS injury and chronic neurodegeneration were considered hopelessly untreatable conditions. A major impetus giving new hope was the discovery that glutamate (Glu), the predominant excitatory transmitter in the mammalian CNS, has neurotoxic (excitotoxic) properties[1,2] that play a major role in triggering neuronal cell death in a wide variety of acute CNS injury conditions, including stroke, head and spinal cord trauma, hypoglycemia, and status epilepticus (see reviews[3-7]). Identifying a molecule (Glu) as the culprit and a process (hyperactivation of Glu excitatory receptors) as the mechanism responsible for triggering the cascade of events leading to neuronal cell death provided tangible therapeutic targets for drug development by the pharmaceutical industry.

The first major drug development efforts were focused on drugs that block Glu receptors, especially the N-methyl-D-aspartate (NMDA) receptor. This development had special significance for the field of anesthesiology, because simultaneous with the identification of NMDA receptor blockade as a therapeutic objective was the discovery that drugs known for several decades as dissociative anesthetics (phencyclidine [PCP] and ketamine)[8] owe their anesthetic properties to a powerful blocking action at the NMDA Glu receptor. Reinforcing the significance for anesthesiology was the more recent discovery that nitrous oxide, a general anesthetic used in human medicine and dentistry for more than a century, and xenon have NMDA antagonist properties.[9,10] Thus when the neuroprotective properties of NMDA antagonists became known, the pharmaceutical industry already had examples of drugs that have the desired mechanism of action, and the challenge was to develop analogs that would provide optimal neuroprotection with minimal side effects.

Two decades of research aimed at bringing Glu antagonist drugs to the clinical setting has been disappointing—not a single new agent with this mode of action has been approved for use in humans. Although the reasons are complex, in essence, all Glu antagonists were found to be effective neuroprotectants in preclinical animal studies, but those antagonists tested in human clinical trials were ineffective at the doses used. The most important limiting factors were that blockade of NMDA receptors was found consistently to trigger psychotic reactions[11,12] similar to those that PCP and ketamine are known to cause,[13-15] and it was discovered in animal studies that NMDA antagonists predictably induce pathomorphologic changes in cerebrocortical neurons at doses in the range of those considered necessary for neuroprotection.[16-18] Several different classes of drugs[19,20] have been shown to prevent the neurotoxic side effects of NMDA antagonists, including γ-aminobutyric acid (GABA) mimetic agents,[9,17,21,22] which have been used in anesthesia for many years to attenuate the psychotomimetic effects of ketamine.[14,23,24] However, the strategy of administering NMDA antagonists together with adjunctive drugs that enhance their safety has been uniformly rejected by the pharmaceutical industry because of the costs inherent in developing drug combinations. Efforts to develop NMDA antagonists that have negligible adverse side effects are ongoing, but exceptionally promising candidates currently have not materialized.

Other recent efforts to develop neuroprotective therapies have been directed toward blockade of non-NMDA Glu receptors, presynaptic inhibition of Glu release, manipulation of intracellular processes that participate in excitotoxic cascades, and modulation of inflammatory responses. Drugs in one or more of these categories have recently been approved or are in the process of being approved. For many years, up to the current time, there have been waxing and waning efforts to protect the brain against injurious processes by administering drugs that increase GABAergic inhibition, many of which drugs are anesthetic agents. New insights pertaining to the advantages and disadvantages of using this strategy in the adult versus the developing CNS are discussed in this chapter.

An additional major thrust of the pharmaceutical industry has evolved in relation to the recent groundswell of interest in apoptosis as a mechanism of cell death that putatively may play a role in acute CNS injury and in chronic neurodegeneration. It has been proposed that, whereas excitotoxic neurodegeneration tends to transpire to end-stage necrosis within a few hours, apoptotic neurodegeneration may evolve more slowly or occur on a delayed time schedule, thereby providing a wider window for therapeutic intervention. Moreover, because the pathophysiology of apoptotic cell death is different from the pathophysiology of excitotoxic cell death, entirely new and different pharmacologic approaches can be developed for the management of apoptotic cell death. Currently, considerable money and effort have been invested in the development of a new drug armamentarium, but it remains uncertain whether apoptotic mechanisms are really operative in either acute or chronic diseases of the adult nervous system.

Recent evidence pertaining to the developing CNS supports the conclusion that apoptosis plays an important role in ischemic[25] and trauma-induced[26–28] neurodegeneration during the synaptogenesis stage of development. Moreover, in the course of studying developmental models of cell death, it was discovered that certain neuroprotective drugs— namely NMDA antagonists—trigger widespread apoptotic neurodegeneration in the developing brain.[29] It was demonstrated that both competitive and noncompetitive NMDA antagonists, if administered to immature rats during the period of synaptogenesis, also known as the brain growth spurt period, cause developing neurons to commit suicide (die by apoptosis).[29] Following up on this discovery, it was learned that other classes of drugs that suppress neuronal activity (GABA mimetic agents and sodium channel blockers), if administered during the brain growth spurt period, trigger widespread apoptotic neurodegeneration throughout the developing brain.[30–32] Because the brain growth spurt period in humans extends from the sixth month of gestation to several years after birth[33] and because GABA mimetic and NMDA antagonist drugs are widely used in pediatric and obstetric anesthesia, and GABA mimetic and sodium channel blocking drugs are widely used as sedatives and anticonvulsants in pediatric and obstetric neurology, these recent results from animal studies are reviewed and discussed in this chapter in terms of their potential relevance in a human medical context.

Because there are striking differences in the way the mature and immature CNS respond to anesthetic drugs that are of interest in a neuroprotection context, the effects of such drugs on the adult and developing CNS are discussed separately.

Neuroprotection in Adult Central Nervous System

The pathophysiology of nervous system injury and nerve cell death is complex and remains poorly understood, despite significant advances in recent years. Before addressing mechanisms of drug action, information pertaining to mechanisms of nervous system dysfunction, injury, and nerve cell death are reviewed.

Mechanisms of Nervous System Dysfunction, Injury, and Nerve Cell Death

Glutamate Excitotoxicity

A large body of evidence, reviewed by many authors,[3–7,34] implicates excessive ("excitotoxic") activation of Glu receptors as the triggering mechanism that initiates the pathologic chain of events leading to nerve cell death in all of the major forms of acute CNS injury, including hypoxia/ischemia (stroke), status epilepticus, hypoglycemia, and trauma. However, many auxiliary mechanisms come into play at one stage or another in what is commonly referred to as the *excitotoxic cascade* that ensues after the triggering event. Because of the desirability of interrupting the excitotoxic cascade as early as possible, a major emphasis of neuroprotection research has been preventing Glu receptors from being hyperstimulated, but significant attention has also been given to methods of interrupting the excitotoxic cascade at later stages.

In addition to being the most prevalent excitatory neurotransmitter in the CNS, Glu plays an important role in CNS metabolism and is the sole precursor molecule for the synthesis of GABA, which is the most prevalent inhibitory transmitter in the CNS. Accordingly, Glu is found in very high concentration throughout the CNS, some of it being stored in metabolic and some in synaptic compartments. Release of Glu from presynaptic axon terminals is triggered by an action potential, and its action at postsynaptic receptors on dendritic or somal membranes results in excitation (depolarization) of these membranes. During physiologic conditions, the excitatory action of Glu is terminated by energy-dependent transporter systems that remove Glu from the synaptic cleft and transport it back into the presynaptic terminal, into astroglial processes, or into both.

A great variety of receptor interactions involving Glu are possible in that there exists in the CNS a large variety of Glu receptor subtypes. The Glu receptor family is composed of two major categories: inotropic and metabotropic. The inotropic category is further divided into three subcategories based on receptor binding affinities of specific synthetic ligands: NMDA receptors, amino-3-hydroxy-5-methyl-4-isoxazole propionic acid (AMPA receptors), and kainic acid (KA receptors). Because pharmacologic probes for studying AMPA and KA receptors have shown a great deal of cross-reactivity, making it difficult to separately characterize these receptors, they are commonly referred to as AMPA/KA (also as non-NMDA) receptors. Many receptor subunits or splice variants have been identified within each subcategory of inotropic receptor, and these join together in various combinations to yield heteromeric assemblies that serve as the functional synaptic receptors. There are many receptor subtypes within the metabotropic receptor category and these have been assigned to three separate groups based on their selective sensitivity to specific agonist molecules. Signal transduction is affected at metabotropic receptors by direct activation of intracellular second messenger systems and at inotropic receptors by opening of a receptor-linked ion channel with consequent sodium/calcium influx and potassium efflux.

Excitotoxic cascades entail disruptions at several levels of organization—network, cellular, and molecular. At a network level, because many CNS neurons use Glu as transmitter and also receive Glu synaptic inputs, hyperactivation of Glu receptors on one set of neurons entails injury of these neurons, but also excessive release of Glu from these neurons onto a second set of neurons, which causes both injury of the second set and excessive firing onto a third set, and so forth. In ischemia and hypoglycemia, energy deficiency causes dysfunction of presynaptic release mechanisms leading to excessive Glu release while disabling energy-dependent Glu uptake mechanisms, thereby causing excessive accumulation of Glu at its various excitatory receptors.[35] During energy-deficient conditions, there is also evidence that Glu transporter systems become deranged and begin acting in reverse to facilitate movement of Glu out of rather than into the cell.[36] In this case, the Glu leaking out of the cell may come from metabolic and synaptic compartments. In other acute injury syndromes (e.g., status epilepticus), energy deficiency also plays a role, in that persistent excessive excitatory activity depletes energy reserves. Head trauma, by mechanisms that are poorly understood, entails sudden release of Glu from metabolic and synaptic pools. The excitotoxic action of Glu on millions of neurons causes them to accumulate edema fluid and massively swell. In fact, at the site of excitotoxic injury there is also massive swelling of astroglia, possibly because astroglia take up large amounts of potassium released from neurons, and this is accompanied by influx of osmolar equivalents of water. Brain swelling results in intracranial hypertension, which, by itself, can cause considerable morbidity and mortality.

At a cellular and molecular level, Mg^{++} normally performs a voltage-dependent blockade of the NMDA Glu receptor ion channel, which has a high conductance for calcium. During physiologic circumstances, this Mg^{++} block serves a protective function preventing excessive calcium from entering the cell. However, it is an integral feature of the excitotoxic cascade that at least partial membrane depolarization will occur because of hyperactivation of non-NMDA Glu receptors. This causes the Mg^{++} blocking mechanism to fail, thereby allowing persistent sodium and

calcium entry through NMDA receptors, even if concentrations of Glu at the NMDA receptor are not excessive. It is hypothesized that overload of intracellular free calcium plays a critical role by promoting intracellular enzyme activation (e.g., lipases, proteases, endonucleases), resulting in massive production of free oxygen radicals, synthesis of nitric oxide and related toxic reaction products, and culminating in degradation of cellular structure and ultimately cell death.[3,37–39] It is believed that mitochondria normally exert a strong protective effect by buffering calcium, but this protective mechanism fails when calcium concentrations exceed a certain threshold level. Many studies, especially those using cell culture preparations in which NMDA receptors are the primary mediators of excitotoxicity, have demonstrated a close relationship between excessive calcium influx and cell injury.[40] However, uncontrolled build-up of intracellular calcium ions is probably not an absolute requirement for cell death, in that hyperactivation of KA or AMPA receptors, most of which do not have a high conductance for calcium, triggers a fulminating excitotoxic cell death reaction in the adult in vivo brain.[34] Moreover, in some in vitro systems, excitotoxic cell death is triggered more readily when extracellular concentrations of calcium are deficient than when they are excessive.[41]

It has been reported that inflammatory mechanisms activated in late stages of the excitotoxic cascade contribute to the final infarct size in cerebral ischemia.[42] Glu excitotoxicity associated with cerebral ischemia typically causes extreme cytotoxic edema, which is believed to allow leakage of cellular constituents (e.g., chemokines and cytokines) that evoke a strong inflammatory response,[5,43–45] including local accumulation of leukocytes, which can cause secondary injury by several mechanisms, such as vasospasm and capillary occlusion,[5,46] free oxygen radical formation,[47] increased vascular permeability,[48] and increased release of IL-8.[49]

There is also evidence that a Glu excitotoxic mechanism may play a role in chronic neurodegenerative diseases, for example, ALS. Rothstein and colleagues[50–52] have developed considerable evidence suggesting that dysfunction of Glu transporter mechanisms resulting in abnormally high concentrations of Glu at AMPA/KA receptors may be responsible for motor neuron degeneration in sporadic ALS. Using organotypic cultures containing motor neurons and specific Glu transport inhibitors to cause slow degeneration of these neurons, it was demonstrated that such degeneration could be prevented by drugs that block AMPA/KA receptors, by agents that block presynaptic release, or by synthesis of Glu. In the mid 1990s, human clinical trials[53,54] showed that riluzole, a drug that blocks release of Glu, significantly prolonged survival of patients with ALS. Consequently, riluzole was approved by the U.S. Food and Drug Administration for the treatment of ALS and currently remains the first and only drug ever shown to favorably alter the clinical course of ALS.

N-*methyl*-D-*aspartate Receptor Blockade and Cerebrocortical Neurotoxicity*

In the course of testing NMDA antagonist drugs for their ability to protect against ischemic- and seizure-mediated neurodegeneration, it was discovered[16,17] that various drugs that block NMDA Glu receptors, including the commonly used general anesthetic, ketamine, have acute neurotoxic effects on cerebrocortical neurons when administered subcutaneously to adult rats. Extensive studies during the past decade have traced the mechanism of this neurotoxic action to a polysynaptic network disturbance in which blockade of NMDA receptors disinhibits excitatory pathways, both glutamatergic and cholinergic, leaving these pathways in a state of hyperactivity that results in excitotoxic overstimulation and injury of cerebrocortical neurons. Thus what begins as a potentially neuroprotective blocking action at NMDA receptors on certain types of neurons in specific brain regions, culminates in an excitotoxic hyperactivation and injury of certain other neurons in other specific brain regions. Paradoxically, this signifies that in the adult rat brain, either hyperactivation or hypoactivation of NMDA Glu receptors can result in excitotoxic neuronal injury. A more detailed description of this neurotoxic phenomenon is discussed in this section of the chapter.

It was demonstrated[16] that administration of a single low dose of any of several NMDA antagonist drugs to adult rats caused pathomorphologic changes confined to specific neurons in the posterior cingulate/retrosplenial cortex (PC/RSC). These changes were initially described as reversible, and consisted of conspicuous swelling of endoplasmic reticulum and mitochondria, which gave the affected cell a striking vacuolated appearance. The vacuoles became evident within 2 to 4 hours after a single low dose of the NMDA antagonist drug, and they gradually disappeared at approximately 12 to 16 hours after treatment. It was subsequently found[17] that the powerful NMDA antagonists, MK801 or PCP, at greater doses or repeated administration of low doses over several days caused irreversible neurodegeneration of neurons in a widely disseminated pattern involving several corticolimbic brain regions in addition to the PC/RSC.[55-58] These findings signify that severity of this pathologic reaction and its reversibility depend on how long the NMDA receptor blockade is maintained.

Recognition that NMDA antagonist drugs can cause neurotoxic side effects led serendipitously to a new discovery of considerable interest to the field of anesthesiology. Because ketamine was among the agents that caused an acute vacuole reaction in the adult rat brain, various other anesthetic drugs were screened to rule out the possibility that they might also have this property. A dose-response study performed on nitrous oxide revealed that at concentrations moderately greater than those used in human anesthesia, this agent triggered a robust vacuole reaction in the PC/RSC of the adult rat brain. Additional studies were then performed[9] that revealed that nitrous oxide has many of the properties that well-known NMDA antagonists, such as MK801, PCP, and ketamine, have. It was found that nitrous oxide protects neurons in the rat hypothalamus against excitotoxic degeneration induced by NMDA and, like other NMDA antagonists, nitrous oxide dose-dependently blocked inward currents elicited by NMDA in cultured hippocampal neurons, while having no significant effect on GABA-induced chloride currents.[9,10] After this discovery, another inhalational agent with anesthetic properties, xenon, was

shown to block NMDA receptor-mediated ion currents and to have negligible effects on GABA_A transmission.[59]

Although both ketamine and nitrous oxide have been shown to cause the reversible vacuole reaction in PC/RSC neurons that other NMDA antagonists cause, it remains to be clarified if or during what circumstances they might have irreversible neurotoxic effects. However, recent findings indicate that nitrous oxide and ketamine, when administered to adult rats in combination at low doses, augment each other's reversible neurotoxic effect by an apparently synergistic mechanism.[60] Surprisingly, xenon does not share the neurotoxic property of other NMDA antagonist-type anesthetics and may in fact *protect* against ketamine-induced toxicity.[61]

Many classes of pharmacologic agents protect against the excitotoxic effects of NMDA antagonist drugs, including agents that block transmission through muscarinic cholinergic or AMPA/KA Glu receptors, agents that block release of Glu at AMPA/KA receptors, and agents that promote transmission through GABA_A, 5-HT_{2A}, or α_2 adrenergic receptors (see reviews for more details[19,20]). Based on these and related observations, a circuit diagram (Fig. 32–1) has been

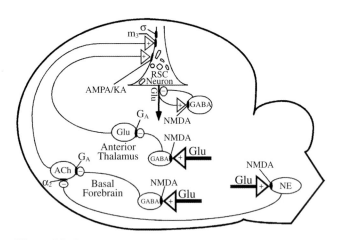

Figure 32–1. Proposed circuitry to explain how hypofunction of the *N*-methyl-D-aspartate (NMDA) receptor system can induce dysfunction and injury of neurons in the posterior cingulate/retrosplenial (PC/RS) cortex by a disinhibition principle. Glutamate (Glu) acting at NMDA receptors on γ-aminobutyric acid (GABA) and norepinephrine (NE) neurons maintains tonic inhibition over two excitatory inputs (+) to the PC/RS neuron. Both excitatory inputs are subject to disinhibition when NMDA receptors are blocked. In addition, the PC/RS neuron uses Glu as transmitter and gives off a recurrent collateral that terminates at an NMDA receptor on a GABAergic neuron; through this collateral circuit, the PC/RS neuron regulates its own firing. An NMDA antagonist would abolish inhibition in this collateral circuit, thereby removing inhibitory restraint over firing of the PC/RS neuron at the same time that the PC/RS neuron is being hyperstimulated through two disinhibited excitatory pathways. In addition to the components of the circuit illustrated here, there is evidence for involvement of serotonergic neurons acting through a 5-HT_{2a} receptor, but the point in the circuitry where this interaction occurs remains to be clarified. (-), inhibitory input; ACh, acetylcholine; α_2, α_2 subtype of adrenergic receptor; G_A, GABA_A subtype of GABA receptor; m_3, m_3 subtype of muscarinic cholinergic receptor.

devised that can explain, on the basis of a disinhibition mechanism, how NMDA antagonist drugs can cause reversible injury of cerebrocortical neurons. To understand this mechanism, it is first necessary to recognize that Glu, in addition to its more straightforward excitatory actions, is a major regulator of inhibitory tone. Glu regulates inhibitory tone by tonically stimulating NMDA receptors on inhibitory neurons. Thus as is depicted in Figure 32–1, Glu, acting at NMDA receptors on GABA and norepinephrine neurons, maintains tonic inhibition over two major excitatory inputs to PC/RS cortical neurons. One excitatory input is cholinergic and innervates a muscarinic receptor; the other input is glutamatergic and innervates an AMPA/KA receptor. When the NMDA receptors are blocked, Glu ceases driving the inhibitory neurons, and this leaves both of the excitatory pathways disinhibited and hyperactive, a condition that leads to excessive (excitotoxic) stimulation and injury of PC/RS neurons. Consistent with this disinhibition hypothesis, GABAergic agents that restore GABA tone (e.g., barbiturates, benzodiazepines, inhalational anesthetics, propofol),[17,21,22] antimuscarinic agents (e.g., scopolamine, atropine)[17] that block muscarinic receptors, and α_2 adrenergic agonists (clonidine, lofedipine, guanabenz)[62] that prevent excessive release of acetylcholine activity also suppress the neurotoxic effect of NMDA antagonists. In addition, agents that block AMPA/KA receptors or suppress the release of Glu directed at these receptors prevent the neurotoxic reaction.[20] Collectively, these and related findings signify that for the neurotoxic reaction to occur, it requires simultaneous hyperactivation of both cholinergic muscarinic and Glu AMPA/KA receptors on any given neuron.

Major components of the circuitry proposed in Figure 32–1 have been confirmed in microdialysis studies. This research[63] demonstrates that systemic administration of MK801 or ketamine to adult rats causes a sustained three-fold increase in the release of acetylcholine in the PC/RSC, and this increased acetylcholine release was abolished if the GABA$_A$ agonist, pentobarbital, was coadministered with MK801.[64] Consistent with these findings is evidence that in the adult rat cerebral cortex, release of acetylcholine is significantly increased by the NMDA antagonist anesthetic, nitrous oxide,[65] and is decreased by the GABA mimetic anesthetics, isoflurane and sevoflurane.[66] Microdialysis studies also show that MK801-induced acetylcholine release is significantly suppressed if the α-2 adrenergic agonist, clonidine, is coadministered with MK-801.[63,67] Other studies demonstrate that systemically administered NMDA antagonists trigger release of Glu in the cerebral cortex and that microinjection of nanomole amounts of a cholinergic agonist (carbachol) plus KA into the PC/RSC reproduces the type of PC/RSC vacuole reaction that systemic NMDA antagonists cause. These and other findings corroborating the circuitry and receptor mechanisms that mediate the neurotoxic reaction induced in the PC/RSC by NMDA antagonist drugs have been reviewed recently.[20]

The cerebrocortical neurotoxic action of NMDA antagonist drugs is an age-dependent phenomenon to which adult animals are highly sensitive and pre-adult animals are insensitive. Experiments[68] focusing on the reversible vacuole reaction induced in cerebrocortical neurons 4 hours after administration of the powerful NMDA antagonists, MK801 or PCP, revealed that very high doses of these agents do not induce a vacuole reaction in immature rats younger than 45 days. At this age, the reaction is mild, and with increasing age it gradually increases in severity but does not reach peak severity until full adulthood at 120 days of age.

N-*methyl-D-aspartate Receptor Blockade and Psychosis*

It has been recognized for many years that the dissociative anesthetics PCP and ketamine have psychotomimetic properties. Shortly after PCP was introduced into clinical medicine as a general anesthetic, it was withdrawn because of its prominent and sometimes prolonged psychotomimetic actions. Because the psychotomimetic reactions associated with ketamine anesthesia, referred to as *emergence* reactions, were less pronounced and less prolonged, and because it was found that they can be attenuated by coadministration of benzodiazepines[14,24] or barbiturates,[23,24] this adverse side effect of ketamine has been regarded for many years as undesirable but manageable. The clinical observation that adults are more susceptible than children to ketamine-induced emergence reactions has resulted in a tendency for ketamine to be used more frequently in pediatric than adult anesthetic practice.

Although the mechanisms underlying the psychotomimetic actions of PCP and ketamine are not fully understood, pieces of the puzzle are beginning to fall in place. A major step toward understanding this type of side effect came with the discovery that PCP and ketamine are NMDA antagonists and that other NMDA antagonist drugs also produce psychotomimetic side effects. For example, all NMDA antagonists classified as either competitive or noncompetitive (Fig. 32–2) that have been administered to humans for anesthestic purposes,[24] for neuroprotection against stroke,[11,12] or to alleviate neuropathic pain[69] produce psychotic symptoms when administered in a clinically relevant dose range with the possible exception of xenon. This signifies that effective blockade of the NMDA receptor channel complex, regardless of whether this is achieved by an action at the PCP recognition site or the NMDA/Glu recognition site (see Fig. 32–2), results in production of psychotic symptoms.

The observation that PCP produces a schizophrenia-like psychosis and that ketamine has similar but less pronounced properties, prompted contemporary researchers to undertake studies in which ketamine is administered to human volunteers at doses substantially lower than an anesthetizing dose for the purpose of producing mild schizophrenia-like symptoms and studying methods of preventing such symptoms. Although this line of research is relatively new, interesting observations have been made. For example, it has been found that cognitive or psychotic disturbances, or both, induced by ketamine can be prevented by coadministration of the Glu release inhibitor, lamotrigine,[70] or the α_2 adrenergic agonist, guanabenz.[70] Consistent with the latter finding, it was recently reported that coadministration of clonidine (α_2 adrenergic agonist) with ketamine in a human anesthesia setting reduced the incidence of psychotomimetic side effects.[72] Also relevant is evidence from veterinary literature that administration of ketamine to certain animal

NMDA RECEPTOR
ION CHANNEL COMPLEX

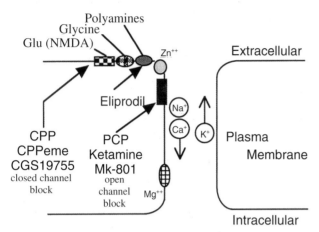

Figure 32–2. Associated with the *N*-methyl-D-aspartate (NMDA) receptor complex are multiple recognition sites through which receptor channel function is modulated. Currently, it is recognized that NMDA receptor hypofunction (NRHypo) results in psychosis in humans and cerebrocortical injury in rats regardless of whether the NRHypo condition is induced by agents acting at the phencyclidine (PCP) site to perform an open channel block (PCP, ketamine, MK-801) or by agents acting at the NMDA-specific glutamate (Glu) site to perform a closed channel block (CPP, CPPeme, CGS 19755).

species, especially dogs, triggers an agitated excitement reaction (possible psychosis equivalent syndrome) that can be prevented by coadministration of xylazine, an α_2 adrenergic agonist. Similarly, in recent behavioral studies, it was found that motor hyperactivity induced by MK-801 in adult rats is prevented by coadministration of clonidine.[73]

It is instructive to compare the above findings with those pertaining to methods of preventing the cerebrocortical neurotoxic side effects of NMDA antagonists in adult rats. In rats, administration of any GABA mimetic agent (benzodiazepines, barbiturates, halothane, isoflurane, propofol)[9,17,21,22,60] prevents the neurotoxic side effects of NMDA antagonists, just as GABA mimetic agents are well known to suppress the psychotomimetic side effects of ketamine.[14,23] In rats, administration of any α_2 adrenergic agonist[62] or lamotrigine[74] prevents the neurotoxic side effects of NMDA antagonists, just as α_2 adrenergic agonists or lamotrigine suppress the psychomimetic side effects of ketamine. Based on extensive evidence (see review[20]), the neurotoxic side effects in the rat studies are interpreted as the result of a disinhibition phenomenon that can be aborted if inhibition is restored by administration of a GABA mimetic agent or if excessive release of ACh or Glu in the cerebral cortex is prevented by administration of an α_2 adrenergic agonist or a Glu release inhibitor, respectively. These parallels suggest that a similar disinhibition mechanism involving excessive cerebrocortical release of ACh and Glu may underlie the neurotoxic and psychotomimetic effects of NMDA antagonists in animals and humans, respectively.

Apoptosis

Many authors have reported data during the past decade that they have interpreted as evidence that an apoptotic mechanism may mediate nerve cell death in both acute and chronic adult neurologic disorders. In addition, it has been claimed that an excitotoxic stimulus can trigger apoptosis; this has been interpreted as the sequence of events that occur in the penumbral region surrounding the central core of infarcted brain tissue in cerebral ischemia.[75,76] Currently, however, there is no compelling evidence that an excitotoxic stimulus can trigger apoptosis or that neurons die from an apoptotic mechanism in adult neurologic disorders. A major problem is that methods used (primarily DNA fragmentation analysis) for diagnosing apoptosis have not been validated for that purpose. In fact, the methods being used have been shown by many authors to yield false-positive results, because they are nonspecific procedures that mark a DNA fragmentation phenomenon that occurs in both apoptotic and nonapoptotic cell death.[26,77–81] In contrast to the uncertain status of evidence pertaining to apoptosis in the adult CNS, there is strong evidence that apoptotic neurodegeneration does occur in the developing CNS and may contribute to developmental neuropathologic conditions that occur in humans.

Mechanisms of Neuroprotective Drug Action

Interrupting the Glutamate Excitotoxic Cascade

Many approaches have been taken to prevent the excitotoxic cascade or to arrest it in its early stages. These approaches are discussed in order of their potential promise for interrupting the excitotoxic cascade in as timely a manner as possible.

Postsynaptic Excitatory Receptor Blockade

N-METHYL-D-ASPARTATE RECEPTOR BLOCKADE

The most studied and reportedly the most widely and densely distributed of the Glu receptor subtypes is the NMDA receptor (see Fig. 32–2). Several features of the NMDA receptor distinguish it from other subtypes of Glu receptor. This receptor is linked to a cation channel that has a much greater Ca^{++} conductance than ion channels associated with other Glu receptor subtypes, and the NMDA ion channel is subject to a voltage-dependent Mg^{++} blockade, which prevents current flow through the channel at physiologic membrane potential. The NMDA receptor is functionally coupled to a strychnine-insensitive glycine receptor and a polyamine receptor where glycine and polyamines, respectively, act to facilitate opening of the NMDA ion channel. There is evidence that Zn^{++}, acting at a site near the mouth of the NMDA ion channel, serves as an inhibitory modulator of channel function, and there is a site within the ion channel where PCP and its analogs such as MK801 and ketamine act to perform an open channel block.

Several different classes of drugs have been developed as postsynaptic NMDA receptor antagonists. Terminology used in referring to these classes is as follows: *competitive NMDA antagonists* refer agents that compete with Glu for binding at the NMDA recognition site; *noncompetitive antagonists* refer to agents that perform an open channel block at the PCP recognition site (they are noncompetitive with respect to binding to the NMDA recognition site, but, of course, are competitive with respect to binding to the PCP site); *glycine site antagonists* refer to agents that inhibit the action of glycine at the glycine recognition site; and *polyamine site antagonists* refers to agents that exert a blocking action at the polyamine recognition site.

COMPETITIVE AND NONCOMPETITIVE N-METHYL-D-ASPARTATE ANTAGONISTS

Initially, the primary focus of attention was on noncompetitive NMDA antagonists, especially MK801 (dizocilpine), which is the most powerful NMDA antagonist currently known. MK801 and various other noncompetitive NMDA antagonists were shown to be quite effective in preventing NMDA or various NMDA agonists from triggering excitotoxic degeneration, and then were shown to prevent neurodegeneration in various in vivo animal models for studying ischemia, hypoglycemia, head and spinal cord trauma, and status epilepticus. MK801 was entered into clinical trials for neuroprotection against stroke in the same year that it was reported that MK801 and various other NMDA antagonists trigger pathomorphologic changes in cerebrocortical neurons in the adult rat brain.[16] Shortly thereafter, clinical trials were halted, and with little explanation MK801 was retired from drug development. The next NMDA antagonist in clinical trials for neuroprotection in stroke was a competitive NMDA antagonist, CGS 19775 (Selfotel). Like MK801, Selfotel showed a promising neuroprotection profile in animal studies, but in human clinical trials, the greatest doses tested were suboptimal for adequate neuroprotection and produced agitation and psychotic reactions. It was then tested for efficacy in reducing morbidity in unconscious patients with head injury. Although preliminary reports suggested it might be beneficial for this indication,[82] Selfotel was withdrawn shortly thereafter from drug development. During the past decade, numerous other competitive and noncompetitive NMDA antagonists were developed and then abandoned, usually at some point near the beginning of clinical trials. In view of the numerous agents available for preventing the adverse side effects of NMDA antagonist drugs, the question arises why the pharmaceutical industry has shown no interest in seeking regulatory approval for coadministering such agents with an NMDA antagonist. The answer is that the costs are deemed prohibitive for performing a safety evaluation on three drugs (drug A, drug B, drug A + B) compared with costs for developing a single drug.

GLYCINE SITE ANTAGONISTS

The existence of an allosteric site on the NMDA receptor where glycine acts as an essential coagonist to assist Glu in NMDA channel activation[83,84] is well established. Several major pharmaceutical companies, after unsuccessful attempts to develop competitive or noncompetitive NMDA antagonists for stroke therapy, began intensively developing glycine site antagonists with the belief that these agents might confer neuroprotection with fewer side effects. Although in theory it would seem that any agent that is effective in blocking NMDA receptor channel function will also be effective in producing psychotomimetic or neurotoxic side effects, the preclinical information that has been reported suggests that these agents provide effective protection against hypoxic/ischemic neurodegeneration at doses that are free from untoward side effects. However, these representations have been heard now for more than 10 years and no glycine site antagonist has emerged as a successful neuroprotection candidate. For example, gavestinel (GV 150526), a glycine site antagonist described as highly effective in protecting against focal cerebral ischemia in rats,[85,86] has now been subjected to international clinical trials that, for reasons that remain unclear, failed to show neuroprotection against stroke in humans.[87]

POLYAMINE SITE ANTAGONISTS

The polyamine site within the NMDA receptor complex has also been represented as a promising target for neuroprotective therapy. Polyamine site antagonists, such as Ifenprodil (Regis Technologies, Morton Grove, Ill.) and Eliprodil (Syntholabe Recherche), have been described as effective neuroprotective agents in acute brain injury models and reportedly do not trigger abnormal metabolic activation patterns in the brain[88] or cause pathomorphologic changes in rat cerebrocortical neurons.[89] Theoretically, it is possible that these agents may be able to block NMDA receptors without causing cerebrocortical neurotoxic side effects, because, in addition to their action at the polyamine NMDA receptor site, they have strong binding affinity for sigma receptors, and sigma receptor ligands protect against the neurotoxic side effects of NMDA antagonist drugs. However, Eliprodil, the more favorable agent because it is orally bioavailable and penetrates biologic barriers better than Ifenprodil, was entered into clinical stroke trials and these trials were prematurely terminated for reasons that remain unclear.[87]

AMPA/KAINIC ACID RECEPTOR BLOCKADE

In early research, after it was learned that Glu plays a major role in acute CNS injury syndromes, attention was focused almost exclusively on NMDA receptors. But in the early 1990s, it was reported that NBQX, a newly developed competitive antagonist of non-NMDA (AMPA/KA) receptors, was neuroprotective in a global ischemia model[90] and in focal ischemia.[91] However, because of poor solubility and nephrotoxicity, quinoxalinedione molecules such as NBQX were withdrawn from drug development. Other quinoxalinedione analogs that are more soluble and reportedly have comparable neuroprotective properties have been developed (e.g., YM872[92,93]), as well as a class of 2,3-benzodiazepine noncompetitive AMPA-selective antagonists, but none of these agents have been entered into clinical trials. Another distinct class of agents that target AMPA/KA receptors is the decahydroisoquinolines.[94] Various molecules in this series have shown varying degrees of selectivity for AMPA or KA receptor subtypes and have been reported to have good blood–brain barrier penetrability and to provide excellent neuroprotection in several acute brain injury models. However, none of these classes of agents has reached the clinical trial stage, therefore essentially nothing is currently known about either the safety or efficacy of AMPA/KA receptor antagonists as neuroprotectants in human medicine. Notably, however, topiramate, a drug recently approved by the U.S. Food and Drug Administration as an anticonvulsant that blocks seizure activity by an unknown mechanism, has been shown in vitro to exert electrophysiologic blocking activity at KA receptors.

Combined Blockade of N-*methyl-D-aspartate and AMPA/Kainic Acid Receptors*

It is well established that excessive activation of Glu receptors is responsible for triggering nerve cell death in acute brain injury conditions, and that hyperactivation of either NMDA or AMPA/KA receptors can trigger excitotoxic neurodegeneration in the adult CNS.[34] It is also reasonably clear that during hypoxic/ischemic conditions, excessive release of Glu and impaired reuptake of Glu cause Glu to accumulate at both NMDA and AMPA/KA receptors. It is logical, therefore, to conclude that for optimal protection against ischemic neurodegeneration in the adult CNS, it may be necessary to prevent Glu from hyperactivating NMDA and AMPA/KA receptors. This principle has been largely ignored by the pharmaceutical industry because of an industry-wide bias favoring the development of drugs that act selectively at only one receptor or another, and an even stronger bias against developing therapeutic strategies that use drug combinations. In addition, this principle has been largely overlooked by academic researchers who for hypoxia/ischemia research have tended to use in vitro cerebrocortical cell culture models featuring immature neurons dissociated from the fetal mammalian brain. An important difference between the immature and mature mammalian brain is that in the adult brain both NMDA and AMPA/KA receptors are sensitive mediators of excitotoxic neurodegeneration, whereas in the immature brain NMDA receptors are exquisitely sensitive to excitotoxic stimulation and AMPA/KA receptors are relatively insensitive.[95] Also relevant is that NMDA receptors have a high conductance for calcium, whereas most AMPA/KA receptors do not. There has been a strong tendency to extrapolate from the *in vitro* immature model to the *in vivo* mature CNS and assume that because simulated ischemic neurodegeneration in the immature model is mediated almost exclusively by NMDA receptor stimulation, which entails excessive calcium entry into the cell, targeting NMDA receptors and calcium overload is the preferred strategy for protecting the adult CNS against ischemic neurodegeneration.

Using an in vivo adult rat dye-photothrombosis model of retinal ischemia,[96] it has been shown that it requires simultaneous blockade of both NMDA and AMPA/KA receptors to achieve complete protection against ischemic neurodegeneration, whereas pretreatment with NMDA or AMPA/KA antagonists individually provided only partial and

relatively weak protection.[97] These findings signify that the anti-excitotoxic treatment approach pursued as the preferred strategy by the pharmaceutical industry for the last 15 years, which features an emphasis on selective blockade of NMDA receptors or prevention of calcium overload, may be a misguided strategy that has left essentially untested the central hypothesis that effective protection against ischemic neurodegeneration can be achieved by preventing excessive stimulation of Glu receptors (all inotropic Glu receptors). No drugs that effectively block NMDA and AMPA/KA receptors have been entered into clinical trials, and there has been no interest in developing such drugs.

Presynaptic Modulation of Glutamate Release

Na+ Channel Blockers

It has been shown in several recent studies that a sustained increase in intracellular Na^+ can contribute to the excitotoxic effect of Glu by two major mechanisms: impairment of Na^+-dependent Glu re-uptake[98] and an increase in Na^+-dependent Glu release from presynaptic Glu axon terminals.[99] For example, it has been demonstrated in vitro that veratridine, an alkaloid that induces a persistent activation of Na^+ channels and persistent increase in intracellular Na^+ concentration, kills cultured hippocampal, cortical, or cerebellar neurons,[100–102] and that Na^+ channel blockers protect against this cell killing effect.[103–106]

Another important mechanism by which excess Na^+ influx can contribute to neuronal damage during energy-deficient conditions is by overstimulation of Na/K-TPase, thereby increasing energy demand on cells that already are subject to impaired adenosine triphosphate production.[107] In addition, the Na^+/Ca^{2+} exchanger of the plasma membrane works in reverse when intracellular Na^+ increases excessively, forcing Ca^{2+} into cells in exchange for Na^+ and causing build-up of intracellular calcium.[108]

A wide range of drugs able to inhibit voltage-dependent Na^+ channels are reportedly neuroprotective in various models of neuronal injury. Among these are phenytoin, carbamazepine, lidoflazine, the benzothiazole derivatives, riluzole and lubeluzole,[109] and the lubefolate-antagonist derivatives, lamotrigine and BW619C89.[110] It has been argued that the efficacy of these agents for treatment of ischemia may be due more to an anti-excitotoxic effect of sodium channel blockade than to inhibition of Glu release, because some (lubeluzole and BW619C89) provide neuroprotection even 6 hours after ischemia, whereas increased Glu release is evident for less than 1 hour after ischemia.

From a practical standpoint, perhaps the most important observation about Na^+ channel blockers is that several of these agents (phenytoin, carbamazepine, riluzole, lamotrigine) are already being marketed, which signifies that they are considered safe for human pharmaceutical use. However, three are being marketed as anticonvulsants, one (riluzole) for treatment of ALS, and none for neuroprotection against hypoxia/ischemia or head trauma. Another potentially important observation is that lubeluzole underwent extensive clinical trials as a neuroprotectant against stroke; in the first two trials, it was reported to provide effective treatment, but was ineffective in a more recent trial.[87] This is important because many other classes of agents that have been entered into clinical trials for stroke were deemed less promising (often because of adverse side effects) and therefore were eliminated in earlier stages.

Opioid Receptor Antagonists

Although the mechanism by which endogenous opioids contribute to the pathogenesis of neuronal damage is not fully understood, there are several studies that indicate that the opiate antagonists naloxone and nalmefene provided protection in animal models of spinal cord injury.[111–113] It is thought that the beneficial effects of the opiate antagonists are mediated by an interaction between the dynorphin opioid system (kappa receptors) and NMDA Glu system.[114] Nalmefene is currently being used in clinical trials, the results of which have not been reported.

Adenosine Agonists

Adenosine and its agonists are known to decrease calcium-mediated Glu release and to increase potassium conductance through A_1 receptors, thereby causing postsynaptic membrane hyperpolarization.[82] Adenosinergic agents have been shown by intracerebroventricular administration to protect against ischemic neurodegeneration, but agents in this class have not been entered into human clinical trials.

Metabotropic Glutamate Receptors

Metabotropic Glu receptors (mGluRs) represent a large family of Glu-activated receptors that are coupled to second messenger systems. These receptors are involved in fine modulation of fast synaptic responses elicited by inotropic Glu receptors.[115] They are very diverse and widely distributed in the CNS and therefore are potentially attractive therapeutic targets. Taxonomy of the mGluR family is confusing because these receptors were initially divided into eight cloned receptor subtypes numbered mGluR 1 through 8, then rearranged into three groups numbered mGluR I through III, based on preferential interaction with specific agonist molecules. Thus original subtypes 1 and 5 belong to group I, original subtypes 2 and 3 belong to Group II, and original subtypes 4, 6, 7, and 8 belong to group III. Group I mGluRs are coupled to phospholipase C and the production of the second messengers inositol 1,4,5-triphosphate and 1,2,-diacylglycerol, which release intracellular Ca^{++} and activate protein kinase C. Group II and III mGluRs are negatively coupled to (and inhibit) forskolin-sensitive, cyclic adenosine monophosphate production and voltage-dependent Ca^{++} channels.

The most prominent physiologic effect that currently has been attributed to mGluRs is an action at presynaptic autoreceptors, resulting in reduction in Glu transmission through inotropic Glu receptors. A growing body of evidence suggests that activation of mGluRs, primarily groups II and III, can be neuroprotective. Most of this evidence pertains to protection against excitotoxic neurodegeneration in vitro,[116–118] although neuroprotection in vivo against focal ischemia has been reported.[119] Activation of group I mGluRs during ischemia may significantly contribute to the excitotoxic cascade by increasing the release of Ca^{++} from intracellular stores.[120] Therefore a successful mGluR-based strategy for neuroprotection will probably require manipulating some components of the mGluR transmitter system in one direction, whereas manipulating other components in another direction. Currently, it appears that the complexities of the metabotropic Glu transmitter system are considerable, and obstacles remain in developing successful strategies. No agents in this class have been entered into neuroprotection clinical trials.

Manipulation of Intracellular Targets

Intracellular Calcium

Calcium ions (Ca^{++}) are important intracellular messengers that mediate many important cellular functions such as membrane excitability, synaptic activity, cell growth, viability, and differentiation. Therefore it is not surprising that disruption of intracellular Ca^{++} homeostasis has been suspected of playing a major role in many forms of cellular injury, or that controlling intracellular Ca^{++} overload has been considered an important target of neuroprotection therapy. Currently, the majority of research has been focused on inhibiting Ca^{++} channels (calcium channel blockers) and on blocking calcium-activated enzyme reactions that are harmful when excessive.

Although there are at least four major types of voltage-gated Ca^{++} channels (L, P, N, and T), only the N and P types are believed to be involved in Glu-mediated excitotoxicity. It is thought that calcium channel blockers may be neuroprotective by a dual mechanism: (1) prevention of Ca^{++} influx into the cell, and (2) vasodilatation, which increases blood flow and tissue perfusion. Preclinical neuroprotection studies with various Ca^{++} channel blockers yielded inconsistent results, suggesting that the protective effects of these agents may be demonstrable only in certain species or certain injury models. Nimodipine was identified in early studies as the most promising Ca^{++} channel blocker and became the lead molecule for development of this class of drugs. Nimodipine primarily blocks L-type Ca^{++} channels, resulting in vasodilatation that may be beneficial in preventing vasospasm, especially after subarachnoid hemorrhage.[35] Unfortunately, extensive neuroprotection clinical trials with nimodipine yielded negative results, with hypotensive side effects being a significant problem, therefore nimodipine was withdrawn from drug development.

Ca^{++} homeostasis research is currently focusing attention on membrane permeability transition (MPT), a concept that refers to the phenomenon whereby mitochondria, when overloaded with Ca^{++}, develop a large, nonspecific pore that not only spills accumulated calcium into the cytosol, but also damages the normal functioning of the inner mitochondrial membrane, leading to decreased adenosine triphosphate production and energy deficiency.[121] MPT is postulated to be the final step in determining neuronal fate in acute CNS injury conditions. The most studied agent that can suppress MPT is the immunosuppressive agent cyclosporine.[122] This action is distinct from its immunosuppressive action. Cyclosporine was demonstrated to preserve axonal mitochondrial integrity, to limit calcium-induced axonal damage in a rat model of traumatic CNS injury,[123] and to limit lipid peroxidation in spinal cord injury.[122] Ca^{++} homeostasis research is also currently focusing attention on ways of inhibiting calcium-activated proteolysis, which is viewed as a promising therapeutic target in traumatic brain injury.[124] Suppression of MPT and inhibition of calcium-activated proteases are both lines of research that are in early stages of development.

Reactive Oxygen Species

That oxidative stress may contribute to cell death in various disease conditions is a concept that has been around for a long time. In recent years, the concept has become incorporated into the excitotoxic cascade hypothesis, the assumption being that reactive oxygen species generated as byproducts of the cascade join in to add their own kind of insult to the injury that is already taking place. Scavengers of reactive oxygen species (e.g., superoxide dismutase, catalase, and glutathione) are naturally present in the CNS, and in the case of acute brain injury, it is postulated that the generation of oxidative free radicals exceeds the scavenger capacity of these endogenous molecules. However, two agents that are considered free radical scavengers, Citicoline (Indevus Pharmaceuticals, Lexington, Mass.) and tirilazad, have been thoroughly tested in stroke neuroprotection human clinical trials with negative results.[87]

It is postulated that reactive oxygen species also play a role in chronic neurodegenerative diseases, such as AD and ALS. The putative link to AD is based on evidence that the free radical scavenger vitamin E may delay the progression of cognitive deterioration in AD.[126] In a familial form of ALS, there is evidence for a genetic anomaly affecting the superoxide dismutase gene. In addition, there is recent evidence that riluzole, the only drug that has been approved for treatment of ALS (based on evidence that it prolongs survival), directly inhibits the activity of protein kinase C, an enzyme that is thought to mediate oxidative stress. This suggests that in addition to an anti-excitotoxic action of riluzole, it may counteract oxidative stress more directly by inhibition of protein kinase C. If this finding is corroborated it would suggest that direct inhibition of protein kinase C may be a good strategy to pursue for protection against neuronal degeneration in ALS.

There is evidence from animal studies that corticosteroids, based on their ability to inhibit free radical-induced lipid peroxidation, may be beneficial in management of brain or spinal cord injury. Based on a National Acute Spinal Cord Injury Study[126] reporting favorable outcome of human spinal cord injury achieved by high-dose methylprednisolone therapy, this agent has been used extensively in the United States in recent years for treatment of nonpenetrating acute spinal cord injury. However, it remains controversial whether high-dose methylprednisolone therapy is truly beneficial,[127] and questions have been raised regarding whether it might be associated with increased morbidity, mortality, or both.[128] In a recent study[129] on spinal cord injury in adult rats, a comparison was made between methylprednisolone, riluzole, or both of these agents combined, and the only treatment that promoted tissue sparing at the lesion epicenter or that provided significantly improved behavioral recovery was the combined therapy.

Nitric Oxide

Nitric oxide is a gas that in recent years has been described as a novel neurotransmitter that is synthesized in the brain by the calcium-activated enzyme nitric oxide synthase. As is clear from a recent review by Lipton,[130] the biochemical behaviors of nitric oxide and related molecules (referred to as nitric oxide-related species) are exceedingly complex, in that the nitric oxide molecule can exist in several different redox states, and depending on which state is present, it can have either a neuroprotective or neurodestructive effect in the brain. In acute brain injury conditions, it is thought that intracellular accumulation of calcium results in excessive calcium-activated synthesis of nitric oxide, which combines with superoxide to form peroxynitrite, a powerful oxidative free radical that can damage proteins, lipids, and DNA. Therefore the thrust of neuroprotection drug development has been on inhibiting the synthesis of nitric oxide. The only agent characterized as an inhibitor of nitric oxide synthase that also has been evaluated in human clinical trials for neuroprotective properties is lubeluzole. Although two early clinical trials pertaining to lubeluzole use in stroke were promising, a third trial provided completely negative results and was terminated prematurely. Lubeluzole is considered a Na^{++} channel blocker and an inhibitor of nitric oxide synthase, therefore it is not clear which mechanism was on trial, but the negative results diminish hopes that either mechanism, or both operating jointly, can prevent ischemic neurodegeneration in the human clinical setting.

Modulation of Inflammatory Response

It is believed that after acute CNS injury there is a secondary wave of injury that is mediated by inflammatory mechanisms. Even if methods for preventing the initial CNS injury are not available, it would be beneficial to prevent, or at least diminish, any additional injury that might ensue. Accordingly, significant research attention has been focused on suppressing the inflammatory process that inevitably occurs in the late stages of acute CNS injury. Because leukocyte interaction with the endothelium at the site of tissue injury appears to play an important role in secondary tissue injury, there has been a major effort to develop therapeutic strategies aimed at controlling this interaction. In preclinical animal studies, it was shown that the use of antibodies to neutralize leukocyte adhesion molecules that are present at the surface of leukocytes resulted in the reduction of infarct volume in an ischemia/reperfusion model.[131,132] However, an antibody product (Enlimomab; Boehringer Ingelheim, Ridgefield, Conn.) based on this principle was evaluated in human clinical trials with negative results.

Enhancing Inhibitory Neurotransmission

In the absence of any other effective method for the clinical management of acute brain injury conditions, such as stroke, cardiac arrest or head trauma, a method referred to as *barbiturate coma* was sometimes relied on in past decades before much was known about either the Glu or GABA transmitter systems. This approach entailed keeping the patient in a comatose state throughout the acute period after the adverse event and was based largely on the assumption that it was beneficial, during conditions of profound cerebral energy deficiency or increased intracranial pressure, to reduce metabolic activity in the brain to a bare minimum and suppress abnormal increases in intracranial pressure. The assumption that barbiturates may be beneficial during such circumstances was supported by evidence from human studies that barbiturates decrease cerebral oxygen consumption[133] and decrease intracranial pressure after head injury.[134] In the late 1970s, favorable results were reported by Safar and colleagues[135-137] pertaining to an uncontrolled feasibility study to evaluate the efficacy of barbiturate coma for preventing brain damage in patients sustaining prolonged anoxia or ischemia from various causes. Because of these favorable results, in the mid-1980s, a controlled multicenter randomized study was conducted in which thiopental loading was commenced 10 to 50 minutes after restoration of spontaneous circulation in patients with cardiac arrest. It was found in this study that thiopental loading, although showing a trend toward improved outcome in patients with cardiac arrest lasting longer than 5 minutes, did not confer an overall statistically significant benefit. These negative results caused the barbiturate coma approach to be abandoned as a treatment for acute brain injury conditions. Notably, in the studies reported by Safar and colleagues,[135-137] some of the most dramatic cases of recovery after prolonged cerebral ischemic episodes were obtained by use of the thiobarbiturate, thiamylal. However, it was a different thiobarbiturate, thiopental, that provided negative results in the multicenter clinical trials. This is of particular interest because it has been shown that some barbiturates, in addition to their GABA mimetic properties, have blocking activity at both NMDA and AMPA/KA Glu receptors.[138] In fact, when numerous barbiturates were tested, thiamylal proved to have the most potent Glu receptor blocking activity and was three times more potent than thiopental in this regard.

Neuroprotective Agents in the Developing Central Nervous System

Mechanisms of Nervous System Injury and Nerve Cell Death

Excitotoxic Neurodegeneration

In the immature CNS, like the mature CNS, nerve cell death in all acute injury syndromes (e.g., hypoxia/ischemia, CNS trauma, status epilepticus) is triggered by excessive activation of Glu receptors. However, a major difference between the adult and developing CNS is that in the adult CNS both NMDA and non-NMDA Glu receptors participate in the neurotoxic process, whereas during important stages of development (e.g., migration and synaptogenesis) it appears that NMDA receptors play the primary role and non-NMDA receptors make little if any contribution.[139-141]

Apoptotic Neurodegeneration

It has been demonstrated that both excitotoxic and apoptotic neurodegeneration (confirmed ultrastructurally) occur in the in vivo developing brain during hypoxic/ischemic or head trauma conditions.[27,142,143] Recent experiments[25,26] aimed at clarifying how the excitotoxic and apoptotic cell death mechanisms relate to one another revealed the following: both hypoxia/ischemia and head trauma in the developing CNS produce an acute wave of excitotoxic cell death that is followed, after a delay interval, by a secondary wave of apoptotic cell death. The delayed apoptotic response affects different neuronal populations than those affected by the initial excitotoxic response and, at least in those cases that lend themselves to analysis, the neurons that die from a delayed apoptotic mechanism are neurons that would be expected to send synaptic projections to, or receive synaptic projections from, the neurons deleted in the initial wave of excitotoxic degeneration. Thus it appears that the delayed wave of apoptotic neurodegeneration does not occur as a direct effect of ischemia, but rather as a secondary consequence of the primary excitotoxic event. This interpretation is consistent with other evidence that during synaptogenesis, the natural response of a neuron that has lost either its synaptic targets or synaptic inputs is to commit suicide.[144]

In recent years, it has become increasingly evident that neurons with NMDA receptors are exceedingly sensitive to Glu stimulation during the synaptogenesis period; and of particular importance is the observation that during this critical period either *overstimulation* or *understimulation* of these receptors can trigger neuronal cell death. Equally important is the observation that whereas overstimulation leads to excitotoxic neurodegeneration,[141] understimulation leads to apoptotic neurodegeneration.[29]

Neuroprotection Against Excitotoxic Neurodegeneration in Hypoxia/Ischemia and Head Trauma

If ischemia or head trauma triggers excitotoxic neurodegeneration by excessive activation of NMDA Glu receptors, a rational strategy for neuroprotection would be to prevent such activation by blocking NMDA receptors. In fact, it has been shown in the infant rat brain that this does confer protection against the acute wave of excitotoxic neurodegeneration in both ischemia[141] and head trauma.[143] If apoptotic neurodegeneration occurs in ischemia or head trauma as a secondary consequence of the initial excitotoxic neuronal

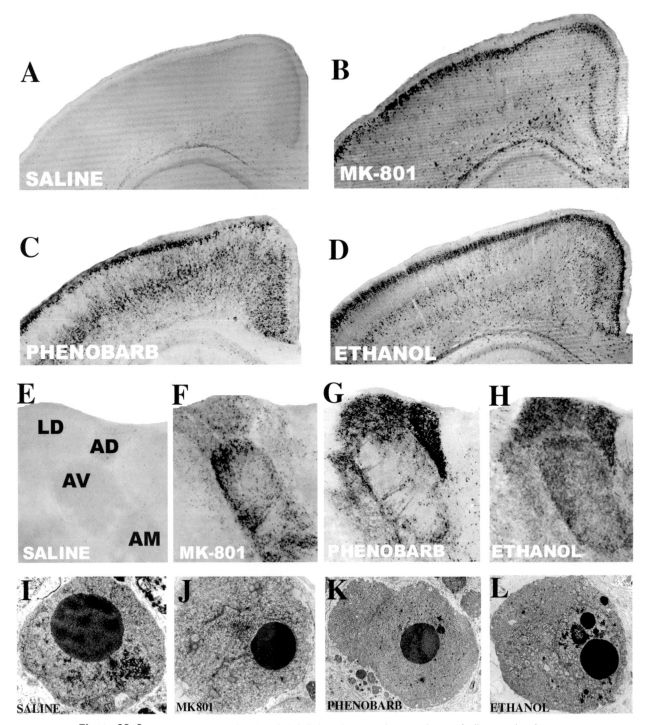

Figure 32–3. *A-D,* Low magnification (x25) light microscopic overviews of silver-stained transverse sections from the parietal and cingulate cortex of 8-day-old rats treated 24 hours previously with saline, MK-801 (NMDA antagonist), phenobarbital (GABA mimetic), or ethanol. Degenerating neurons (*small dark dots*) are abundantly present in several brain regions following MK-801, phenobarbital, or ethanol but are only sparsely present after saline treatment. Note that MK-801 and phenobarbital both affect neurons superficial to the cortical surface, whereas the middle cortical layers are affected very prominently by phenobarbital and are relatively spared by MK-801. The ethanol pattern resembles a combination of the MK-801 and phenobarbital patterns. *E-H,* Light micrographs (x55) depicting the anterior thalamus at the level of the laterodorsal (LD), anterodorsal (AD), anteroventral (AV), and anteromedial (AM) nuclei. Note that MK-801 affects the LD, AV, and AM nuclei but not the AD nucleus, and phenobarbital affects the LD and AD very prominently but almost entirely spares the AV and AM nuclei. The ethanol pattern includes all four nuclei, which is expected if it acts by a combined action involving blockade of

Figure 32–3.—*cont'd* N-methyl-D-aspartate (NMDA) receptors plus activation of γ-aminobutyric acid type A (GABA$_A$) receptors. *I-L*, Electron micrographs (x1800) illustrating that apoptotic neurodegeneration induced by MK801 *(J)*, phenobarbital *(K)*, or ethanol *(L)* has the same ultrastructural appearance as physiological cell death *(I)*, an apoptotic phenomenon that occurs spontaneously to a limited degree in the normal (saline) developing brain. As described recently,[26,145] in both spontaneous and induced apoptosis, the earliest signs are the formation of spherical chromatin masses and flocculent densities in the nucleus, whereas the nuclear envelope remains intact and cytoplasmic organelles are relatively unaltered; this is followed in the middle and late stages by fragmentation of the nuclear envelope, intermixing of nucleoplasmic and cytoplasmic contents, and progressive condensation of the entire cell. All four examples shown here have a similar appearance because they are all in the middle stage of apoptotic neurodegeneration.

loss, preventing the excitotoxic event might be expected to provide protection against the secondary apoptotic event as well. However, experiments designed to test this hypothesis have provided results contrary to this expectation.

Neurotoxic Consequences of Blocking N-methyl-D-aspartate Receptors During Synaptogenesis

It has been shown in an infant rat model of concussive head trauma that the concussive force induces an acute excitotoxic lesion at the impact site, which is followed several hours later by apoptotic neurodegeneration at numerous distant sites in the brain. The number of neurons dying from an apoptotic mechanism at numerous distant sites was substantially larger than the number dying from an excitotoxic mechanism at the local impact site. Blockade of NMDA receptors by any of several NMDA antagonist drugs was found to protect against the acute excitotoxic lesion, but resulted in a substantial augmentation of the delayed apoptotic neurodegeneration.[27] This finding has the important clinical implication that using an NMDA antagonist to treat head trauma in the developing brain may prevent excitotoxic degeneration of a small number of neurons at the expense of destroying a much larger number by apoptosis. It also raised the important question whether blockade of NMDA receptors during synaptogenesis might augment the natural process referred to as *physiologic cell death*, whereby neurons that are unsuccessful in making their synaptic connections commit suicide. If blockade of NMDA receptors in the normal developing brain can trigger apoptosis, independent of head trauma, this would explain why treatment of head trauma with NMDA antagonist drugs would augment apoptotic neurodegeneration while preventing excitotoxic degeneration. Experiments undertaken to test this hypothesis revealed that NMDA antagonist drugs trigger a robust apoptotic neurodegenerative response in the normal developing brain, independent of head trauma (Fig. 32–3).[29,145]

Neurotoxic Consequences of Stimulating γ-Aminobutyric Acid Type A Receptors or Blocking Sodium Channels During Synaptogenesis

The results discussed earlier raise the question whether the observed neurotoxic effect was specific for NMDA receptors or may also be triggered by drugs that interfere with other transmitter receptor systems in the developing brain. Experiments addressing this issue revealed that two other classes of drugs can trigger apoptosis during the synaptogenesis period, namely those that enhance GABA$_A$ inhibitory transmission (see Fig. 32–3)[30] and those that inhibit action potentials by blocking sodium channels.[31,32]

Susceptibility of Immature Animals, During Synaptogenesis, to Apoptotic Neurodegeneration Induced by N-methyl-D-aspartate Antagonist or γ-Aminobutyric Acid Mimetic Drugs

As described earlier, a series of recent studies have documented that several classes of drugs, namely those that block NMDA receptors, those that block sodium channels and those that hyperactivate GABA$_A$ receptors, trigger widespread apoptotic neurodegeneration in the developing rat brain. Because most agents used in general anesthesia, including obstetrical and pediatric anesthesia, have either NMDA or GABA mimetic properties, these findings are necessarily of interest to anesthesiologists. Because the findings are recent, it is too early to draw any conclusions regarding human risk.

References

1. Olney JW: Brain lesions, obesity and other disturbances in mice treated with monosodium glutamate. Science 164:719, 1969.
2. Olney JW, Ho OL, Rhee V: Cytotoxic effects of acidic and sulphur-containing amino acids on the infant mouse central nervous system. Exp Brain Res 14:61, 1971.
3. Rothman SM, Olney JW: Glutamate and the pathophysiology of hypoxic-ischemic brain damage. Ann Neurol 19:105, 1986.
4. Meldrum, Garthwaite J: Excitatory amino acid neurotoxicity and neurodegenerative disease. Trends Pharmacol Sci 11:379, 1990.
5. Siesjo BK: Pathophysiology and treatment of focal cerebral ischemia. Part II. Mechanisms of damage and treatment. J Neurosurg 77:337, 1992.
6. Choi DW: Excitotoxic cell death. J Neurobiol 23:1261, 1992.
7. Lipton SA, Rosenberg PA: Excitatory amino acids as a final common pathway for neurologic disorders. N Engl J Med 330:613, 1994.
8. Lodge D, Anis NA: Effects of phencyclidine on excitatory amino acid activation of spinal interneurons in the cat. Eur J Pharmacol 77:203, 1982.
9. Jevtovic-Todorovic V, Todorovic, SM, Mennerick S, et al: Nitrous oxide (laughing gas) is an NMDA antagonist, neuroprotectant and neurotoxin. Nat Med 4:460, 1998.
10. Mennerick S, Jevtovic-Todorovic V, Todorovic SM, et al: Effect of nitrous oxide on excitatory and inhibitory synaptic transmission in hippocampal cultures. J Neurosci 18:9716, 1998.
11. Herrling PL: D-CPPene (SDZ EAA 494), A competitive NMDA antagonist: Results from animal models and first results in humans. Neuropsychopharmacology 10(suppl 3, part 1):591S, 1994.
12. Grotta J: Why do all drugs work in animals but none in stroke patients? 2: Neuroprotective therapy. J Intern Med 237:89, 1995.

13. Luby ED, Gottlieb JS, Cohen BD, et al: Model psychosis and schizophrenia. Am J Psych 119:61, 1962.

14. Reich DL, Silvay G: Ketamine: An update on the first twenty years of clinical experience. Can J Anaesth 36:186, 1989.

15. Krystal JH, Karper LP, Seibyl JP, et al: Dose-related effects of the NMDA antagonist, Ketamine, in healthy humans. Schizophrenia Res 9:240, 1993.

16. Olney JW, Labruyere J, Price MT: Pathological changes induced in cerebrocortical neurons by phencyclidine and related drugs. Science 244:1360, 1989.

17. Olney JW, Labruyere J, Wang G, et al: NMDA antagonist neurotoxicity: Mechanism and protection. Science 254:1515, 1991.

18. Hargreaves RJ, Rigby M, Smith D, et al: Competitive as well as uncompetitive NMDA receptor antagonists affect cortical neuronal morphology and cerebral glucose metabolism. Neurochem Res 18:1263, 1993.

19. Olney J, Farber NB: NMDA antagonists as neurotherapeutic drugs, psychotogens, neurotoxins and research tools for studying schizophrenia. Neuropsychopharmacology 13:335, 1995.

20. Farber NB, Kim SH, Dikranian K, et al: Receptor mechanisms and circuitry underlying NMDA antagonist neurotoxicity. Mol Psychiatry 7:32, 2002.

21. Ishimaru M, Fukamauchi F, Olney JW: Halothane prevents MK-801 neurotoxicity in the rat cingulate cortex. Neurosci Lett 193:1, 1995.

22. Jevtovic-Todorovic V, Kirby CO, Olney JW: Isoflurane and propofol block neurotoxicity caused by MK-801 in the rat posterior cingulate/retrosplenial cortex. J Cereb Blood Flow Metab 17:168, 1997.

23. Magbagbeola JAO, Thomas NA: Effect of thiopentone on emergence reactions to ketamine anaesthesia. Can Anaesth Soc J 21:321, 1974.

24. White PF, Way WL, Trevor AJ: Ketamine-its pharmacology and therapeutic uses. Anesthesiology 56:119, 1982.

25. Olney JW, Price MT, Labruyere J, Tenkova T: Perinatal hypoxia/ischemia kills neurons directly by excitotoxic necrosis and indirectly by deafferentation apoptosis. Soc Neurosci Abst 26:1880, 2000.

26. Ishimaru MJ, Ikonomidou C, Tenkova TI, et al: Distinguishing excitotoxic from apoptotic neurodegeneration in the developing rat brain. J Comp Neurol 408:461, 1999.

27. Pohl D, Bittigau P, Ishimaru MJ, et al: *N*-methyl-D-aspartate antagonists and apoptotic cell death triggered by head trauma in developing rat brain. Proc Natl Acad Sci USA 96:2508, 1999.

28. Bittigau P, Sifringer M, Pohl D, et al: Apoptotic neurodegeneration following trauma is markedly enhanced in the immature brain. Ann Neurol 45:724, 1999.

29. Ikonomidou C, Bosch F, Miksa M, et al: Blockade of NMDA receptors and apoptotic neurodegeneration in the developing brain. Science 283:70, 1999.

30. Ikonomidou C, Bittigau P, Ishimaru MJ, et al: Ethanol-induced apoptotic neurodegeneration and fetal alcohol syndrome. Science 287:1056, 2000.

31. Ikonomidou C, Genz K, Engelbrechten Sv, et al: Antiepileptic drugs which block sodium channels cause neuronal apoptosis in the developing rat brain. Soc Neurosci Abst 26:323, 2000.

32. Dikranian K, Tenkova T, Bittigau P, et al: Histological characterization of apoptotic neurodegeneration induced in the developing rat brain by drugs that block sodium channels. Soc Neurosci Abst 26:323, 2000.

33. Dobbing J, Sands J: The brain growth spurt in various mammalian species. Early Hum Dev 3:79, 1979.

34. Olney JW: Neurotoxicity of excitatory amino acids. In McGeer E, Olney JW, McGeer P (eds): Kainic Acid as a Tool in Neurobiology. New York, Raven Press, 1978.

35. Verma A: Opportunities for neuroprotection in traumatic brain injury. J Head Trauma Rehabil 15:1149, 2000.

36. Billups B, Rossi D, Oshima T, et al: Physiological and pathological operation of glutamate transporters. Prog Brain Res 116:45, 1998.

37. MacDermott AB, Mayer ML, Westbrook GL: NMDA-receptor activation increases cytoplasmic calcium concentration in cultured spinal cord neurons. Nature 321:519, 1986.

38. Rothman SM: Excitotoxins: Possible mechanisms of action. Ann NY Acad Sci 648:132, 1992.

39. Obrenovitch TP, Urenjak J: Altered glutamatergic transmission in neurological disorders: From high extracellular glutamate to excessive synaptic efficacy. Prog Neurobiol 51:39, 1997.

40. Choi DW: Glutamate neurotoxicity in cortical cell cultures is calcium dependent. Neurosci Lett 58:293, 1985.

41. Price MT, Olney JW, Samson L, et al: Calcium influx accompanies but does not cause excitotoxin-induced neuronal necrosis in retina. Brain Res Bull 14:369, 1985.

42. DeGraba TJ: The role of inflammation after acute stroke: Utility of pursuing anti-adhesion molecule therapy. Neurology 51:S62, 1998.

43. Horikawa Y, Naruse S, Hirakawa K, et al: In vivo studies of energy metabolism in experimental cerebral ischemia using topical magnetic resonance: Changes in ^{31}P-nuclear magnetic resonance spectra compared with electroencephalograms and regional cerebral blood flow. J Cereb Blood Flow Metab 5:235, 1985.

44. Pantoni L, Sart C, Domenico I: Cytokines and cell adhesion molecules in cerebral ischemia. Arterioscler Thromb Vasc Biol 18:503, 1998.

45. Nicotera P, Lipton S: Excitotoxins in neuronal apoptosis and necrosis. J Cereb Blood Flow Metab 19:583, 1999.

46. Akopov S, Sercombe R, Seylaz J: Cerebrovascular reactivity: Role of endothelium/platelet/leukocyte interaction. Cerebrovasc Brain Metab Rev 8:11, 1996.

47. Murota S, Fujita H, Wakabayashi Y, Morita I: Cell adhesion molecule mediates endothelial cell injury caused by activated neutrophils. Keio J Med 45:207, 1996.

48. Bjork J, Hedqvist P, Arfors KE: Increase in vascular permeability induced by leukotriene B4 and the role of polymorphonuclear leukocytes. Inflammation 6:189, 1982.

49. Baggiolini M, Loetscher P, Moser B: Interleukin-8 and the chemokine family. Int J Immunopharmacology 17:103, 1995.

50. Rothstein JD, Van Kammen M, Levey AI, et al: Selective loss of glial glutamate transporter GLT-1 in amyotrophic lateral sclerosis. Ann Neurol 38:73, 1995.

51. Rothstein JD: Therapeutic horizons for amyotrophic lateral sclerosis. Curr Opin Neurobiol 6:679, 1996.

52. Rothstein JD: Excitotoxicity hypothesis. Neurology 47(4 suppl 2):S19-25;discussion S26, 1996.

53. Bensimon G, Lacomblez L, Meininger V: A controlled trial of riluzole in amyotrophic lateral sclerosis. ALS/Riluzole Study Group. N Engl J Med 330:585, 1994.

54. Mitsumoto H: Riluzole—what is its impact in our treatment and understanding of amyotrophic lateral sclerosis? Ann Pharmacother 31:779, 1997.

55. Fix AS, Horn JW, Wightman KA, et al: Neuronal vacuolization and necrosis induced by the non-competitive N-methyl-D-aspartate (NMDA) antagonist MK (+)801 (Dizocilipine Maleate): A light and electron microscopic evaluation of the rat retrosplenial cortex. Exp Neurol 123:204, 1993.

56. Ellison G: The *N*-methyl-D-aspartate antagonists phencyclidine, ketamine and dizocilipine as both behavioral and anatomical models of the dementia. Brain Res Rev 20:250, 1995.

57. Wozniak DF, Dikranian K, Ishimaru MJ, et al: Disseminated corticolimbic neuronal degeneration induced in rat brain by MK-801: Potential relevance to Alzheimer's disease. Neurobiol Dis 5:305, 1998.

58. Corso TD, Sesma MA, Tenkova TI, et al: Multifocal brain damage induced by phencyclidine is augmented by pilocarpine. Brain Res 752:1, 1997.

59. Franks NP, Dickinson R, de Sousa SLM, et al: How does xenon produce anaesthesia? Nature 396:324, 1998.

60. Jevtovic-Todorovic V, Benshoff N, Olney JW: Ketamine potentiates cerebrocortical damage induced by the common anaesthetic agent nitrous oxide in adult rats. Br J Pharmacol 130:1692, 2000.

61. Nagata A, Nakao Si S, Nishizawa N, et al: Xenon inhibits but N$_2$O enhances ketamine-induced c-Fos expression in the rat posterior cingulate and retrosplenial cortices. Anesth Analg 92:362, 2001.

62. Farber NB, Foster J, Duhan NL, Olney JW: A2 adrenergic agonists prevent MK-801 neurotoxicity. Neuropsychopharmacology 12:347, 1995.

63. Kim SH, Price MT, Olney JW, Farber NB: Excessive cerebrocortical release of acetylcholine induced by NMDA antagonists is reduced by GABAergic and alpha2-adrenergic agonists. Mol Psychiatry 4:344, 1999.

64. Kim SH, Farber NB, Price MT, Olney JW: Clonidine suppresses MK-801-induced acetylcholine release in rat posterior cingulate cortex: In vivo microdialysis study. Soc Neurosci Abst 23:2308, 1997.

65. Shichino T, Murakawa M, Adachi T, et al: Effects of inhalational anaesthetics on the release of acetylcholine in the rat cerebral cortex in vivo. Br J Anaesth 80:365, 1998.

66. Bertorelli R, Hallstrom A, Hurd YL, et al: Anaesthesia effects on in vivo acetylcholine transmission: Comparison of radioenzymatic and HPLC assays. Eur J Pharmacol 175:79, 1990.

67. Kim SH, Olney JW, Farber NB: Clonidine prevents NMDA antagonist neurotoxicity by activating α_2 adrenergic receptors in the diagonal band. Soc Neurosci Abst 24, 1998.

68. Farber NB, Wozniak DF, Price MT, et al: Age-specific neurotoxicity in the rat associated with NMDA receptor blockade: potential relevance to schizophrenia? Biol Psychiatry 38:788, 1995.

69. Backonja M, Arndt G, Gombar KA, et al: Response of chronic neuropathic pain syndromes to ketamine: A preliminary study. Pain 56:51, 1994.

70. Anand A, Charney DS, Berman RM, et al: Reduction in ketamine effects in humans by lamotrigine. Soc Neurosci Abstr 27:310, 1997.

71. Newcomer JW, Farber NB, Selke G, et al: Guanabenz effects on NMDA antagonist-induced mental symptoms in humans. Soc Neurosci Abst 24:525, 1998.

72. Handa F, Tanaka M, Nishikawa T, Toyooka H: Effects of oral clonidine premedication on side-effects of intravenous ketamine anesthesia: a randomized double-blind placebo contolled study. J Clin Anesth 12:19, 2000.

73. Jevtovic-Todorovic V, Wozniak DF, Nardi A, et al: Clonidine potentiates the neuropathic pain relieving action of MK-801 while preventing its neurotoxic and hyperactivity side effects. Brain Res 781:202, 1998.

74. Jevtovic-Todorovic V, Olney JW, Farber NB: Lamotrigine prevents NMDA antagonist neurotoxicity. Soc Neurosci Abst 24:745, 1998.

75. Linnik MD, Zobrist RH, Hatfield MD: Evidence supporting a role for programmed cell death in focal cerebral ischemia in rats. Stroke 24:2002, 1993.

76. MacManus MP, Hill I, Huang ZG, et al: DNA damage consistent with apoptosis in transient focal ischaemic neocortex. Neuroreport 5:493, 1994.

77. Collins RJ, Harmon BB, Gobé GC, Kerr JFR: Internucleosomal DNA cleavage should not be the sole criterion for identifying apoptosis. Int J Radiat Biol 61:451, 1992.

78. van Lookeren Campagne M, Lucassen PJ, Vermeulen JP, Balazs R: NMDA and kainate induce internucleosomal DNA cleavage associated with both apoptotic and necrotic cell death in the neonatal rat brain. Eur J Neurosci 7:1627, 1995.

79. Charriaut-Marlangue C, Ben-Ari Y: A cautionary note on the use of the TUNEL stain to determine apoptosis. Neuroreport 7:61, 1995.

80. Grasl-Kraupp B, Ruttkay-Nedecky B, Koudelka H, et al: In situ detection of fragmented DNA (TUNEL assay) fails to discriminate among apoptosis, necrosis, and autolytic cell death: A cautionary note. Hepatology 21:1465, 1995.

81. Gwag BJ, Koh JY, DeMaro JA, et al: Slowly triggered excitotoxicity occurs by necrosis in cortical cultures. Neuroscience 77:393, 1997.

82. Muir KW, Lees KR: Clinical experience with excitatory amino acid antagonist drugs. Stroke 26:503, 1995.

83. Johnson JW, Ascher P: Glycine potentiates the NMDA response in cultured mouse brain neurons. Nature 325:529, 1987.

84. Kemp JA, Leeson PD: The glycine site on NMDA receptor-five years on. Trends Pharmacol Sci 14:20, 1993.

85. Di Fabio R, Cugola A, Donati D, et al: Identification and pharmacological characterization of GV 150526, a novel glycine antagonist as a potent neuroprotective agent. Drugs Future 23:62, 1998.

86. Bordi F, Pietra C, Ziviani L, Reggiani A: The glycine antagonist GV 150526 protects somatosensory evoked potentials and reduces the infarct area in the MCAO model of focal ischemia in the rat. Exp Neurol 145:425, 1997.

87. DeGraba TJ, Pettigrew LC: Why do neuroprotective drugs work in animals but not humans? Neurol Clin 18:475, 2000.

88. Cudennec A, Duverger D, Benavides J, et al: Effect of eliprodil, an NMDA receptor antagonist acting at the polyamine modulatory site, on local cerebral glucose use in the rat in the rat brain. Brain Res 664:41, 1994.

89. Duval D, Roome N, Gauffeny C, et al: SL 82.0715, an NMDA antagonist acting at the polyamine site, does not induce neurotoxic effects on rat cortical neurons. Neurosci Lett 137:193, 1992.

90. Sheardown MJ, Nielsen EO, Hansen AJ, et al: 2,3-Dihydroxy-6-nitro-7-sulfamoyl-benzo(F)quinoxaline: A neuroprotectant for cerebral ischemia. Science 247:571, 1990.

91. Gill R, Nordholm L, Lodge D: The neuroprotective actions of 2,3-dihydroxy-6-nitro-7-sulfamoyl-benzo(F)quinoxaline (NBQX) in a rat focal ischaemia model. Brain Res 580(1-2):35, 1992.

92. Kawasaki-Yatsugi S, Yatsugi S, Takahashi M, et al: A novel AMPA receptor antagonist, YM872, reduces infarct size after middle cerebral artery occlusion in rats. Brain Res 793(1-2):39, 1998.

93. Shimizu-Sasamata M, Kano T, Rogowska J, et al: YM872, a highly water-soluble AMPA receptor antagonist, preserves the hemodynamic penumbra and reduces brain injury after permanent focal ischemia in rats. Stroke 29:2141, 1998.

94. O'Neill MJ, Bogaert L, Hicks CA, et al: LY377770, a novel iGlu5 kainate receptor antagonist with neuroprotective effects in global and focal cerebral ischaemia. Neuropharmacology 39:157, 2000.

95. Campochiaro P, Coyle JT: Ontogenetic development of kainate neurotoxicity: Correlates with glutamatergic innervation. Proc Natl Acad Sci USA 75:2025, 1978.

96. Mosinger JL, Olney JW: Photothrombosis-induced ischemic neuronal degeneration in the rat retina. Exp Neurol 105:110, 1989.

97. Mosinger JL, Price MT, Bai HY, et al: Blockade of both NMDA and non-NMDA receptors is required for optimal protection against ischemic neuronal degeneration in the in vivo adult mammalian retina. Exp Neurol 113:10, 1991.

98. Nicholls DG: Release of glutamate, aspartate and gamma-aminobutyric acid from isolated nerve terminals. J Neurochem 52:331, 1989.

99. Sitges M, Nekrassov V: Vinpocetine selectively inhibits neurotransmitter release triggered by sodium channel activation. Neurochem Res 24:1585, 1999.

100. Lysko PG, Webb CL, Yue TL, et al: Neuroprotective effects of tetrodotoxin as Na^+ channel modulator and glutamate release inhibitor in cultured rat cerebellar neurons and in gerbil global brain ischemia. Stroke 25:2476, 1994.

101. Catterall WA: Neurotoxins that act on voltage-sensitive sodium channels in excitable membranes. Annu Rev Pharmacol Toxicol 20:15, 1980.

102. Deri Z, Adam-Vizi V: Detection of intracellular free Na^+ concentration of synaptosomes by a fluorescent indicator, $Na^{(+)}$-binding benzofuran isophthalate: The effect of veratridine, ouabain, and alpha-latrotoxin. J Neurochem 61:818, 1993.

103. Rothman S: Synaptic release of excitatory amino acid neurotransmitter mediates anoxic neuronal death. J Neurosci 4:1884, 1984.

104. Carter AJ: The importance of voltage-dependent sodium channels in cerebral ischaemia. Amino Acids 14:159, 1998.

105. Narahashi T, Huang CS, Song JH, Yeh JZ: Ion channels as targets for neuroprotective agents. Ann NY Acad Sci 825:380, 1997.

106. Obrenovitch TP: Neuroprotective strategies: Voltage-gated Na+-channel down-modulation verses presynaptic glutamate release inhibition. Rev Neurosci 9:203, 1998.

107. Bonoczk P, Gulyas B, Adam-Vizi V, et al: Role of sodium channel inhibition in neuroprotection: Effect of vinpocetine. Br Res Bull 53:245, 2000.

108. Stys PK, Waxman SG, Ransom BR: Ionic mechanism of anoxic injury in mammalian CNS white matter: Role of Na^+ channels and $Na^{(+)}$-Ca^{2+} exchanger. J Neurosci 12:430, 1992.

109. Urenjak J, Obrenovitch TP: Pharmacological modulation of voltage-gated Na^+ channels: A rational and effective strategy against ischemic brain damage. Pharmacol Rev 48:21, 1999.

110. Kawaguchi K, Henshall DC, Simon RP: Parallel dose-response studies of the voltage-dependent Na^+ channel antagonist BW619C89, and the voltage-dependent Ca^{2+} channel antagonist nimodipine, in rat transient focal cerebral ischaemia. Eur J Pharmacol 364(2-3):99, 1999.

111. Yum SW, Faden AI: Comparison of the neuroprotective effects of the NMDA antagonist MK-801 and the opiate-receptor antagonist nalmefene in experimental SCI. Arch Neurol 47:277, 1990.

112. Robertson C, Foltz R, Grossman R, et al: Protection against experimental ischemic spinal cord injury. J Neurosurg 64:633, 1986.

113. Faden AI, Jacobs TP, Smith MT, et al: Naloxone in experimental spinal cord ischemia: Dose-response studies. Eur J Pharmacol 103:115, 1984.

114. Faden AI: Opioid and nonopioid mechanisms may contribute to dynorphin's pathophysiological actions in spinal cord injury. Ann Neurol 27:67, 1990.

115. Conn PJ, Pin JP: Pharmacology and functions of metabotropic glutamate receptors. Ann Rev Pharmacol Toxicol 37:205, 1997.

116. Pizzi M, Fallacara C, Arrighi V, et al: Attenuation of excitatory amino acid toxicity of metabotropic glutamate receptor agonists and aniracetam in primary cultures of cerebellar granule cells. J Neurochem 61:683, 1993.

117. Bruno V, Battaglia G, Copani A, et al: Activation of class II or III metabotropic glutamate receptors protects cultured cortical neurons against excitotoxic degeneration. Eur J Neurosci 7:1906, 1995.

118. Siliprandi R, Lipartiti M, Fadda E, et al: Activation of glutamate metabotropic receptor protects retina against N-methyl-D-aspartate toxicity. Eur J Pharmacol 219:173, 1992.

119. Chiamulera C, Albertini P, Valerio E, Reggiani A: Activation of metabotropic receptors has a neuroprotective effect in a rodent model of focal ischaemia. Eur J Pharmacol 216:335, 1992.

120. Kristian T, Gido G, Kuroda S, et al: Calcium metabolism of focal and penumbral tissues in rats subjected to transient middle cerebral artery occlusion. Exp Brain Res 120:503, 1998.

121. Murphy AN, Fiskum G, Beal MF: Mitochondria in neurodegeneration: Bioenergetic function in cell life and death. J Cereb Blood Flow Metab 19:231, 1999.

122. Diaz-Ruiz A, Rios C, Duarte I, et al: Cyclosporine A inhibits lipid peroxidation after spinal cord injury in rats. Neurosci Lett 266:61, 1999.

123. Okonkwo DO, Buki A, Siman R, Povlishock JT: Cyclosporin A limits calcium-induced axonal damage following traumatic brain injury. Neuroreport 10:353, 1999.

124. Kampfl A, Posmantur RM, Zhao X, et al: Mechanism of calpain proteolysis following traumatic brain injury: Implications for pathology and therapy: A review and update. J Neurotrauma 14:121, 1997.

125. Sano M, Ernesto C, Thomas RG, et al: A controlled trial of selegiline, alpha-tocopherol, or both as treatment for Alzheimer's disease. The Alzheimer's Disease Cooperative Study. N Engl J Med 336:1216, 1997.

126. Bracken MB: Methylprednisolone in the management of acute spinal cord injuries. Med J Aust 153:368, 1990.

127. Qian T, Campagnolo D, Kirshblum: High-dose methylprednisolone may do more harm for spinal cord injury. Med Hypotheses 55:452, 2000.

128. Hurlbert RJ: Methylprednisolone for acute spinal cord injury: An inappropriate standard of care. J Neurosurg 93(1 suppl):1, 2000.

129. Mu X, Azbill RD, Springer JE: Riluzole and methylprednisolone combined treatment improves functional recovery in traumatic spinal cord injury. J Neurotrauma 17:773, 2000.

130. Lipton SA: Neuronal protection and destruction by NO. Cell Death Differ 6:943, 1999.

131. Clark WM, Lauten JD, Lessov N, et al: The influence of antiadhesion therapies on leukocyte subset accumulation in central nervous system ischemia in rats. J Mol Neurosci 6:43, 1995.

132. Clark WM, Madden KP, Rothlein R, Zivin JA: Reduction of central nervous system ischemic injury by monoclonal antibody to intercellular adhesion molecule. J Neurosurg 75:623, 1991.

133. Shapiro HM: Barbiturates in brain ischaemia. Br J Anaesth 57:82, 1985.

134. Eisenberg HM, Frankowski RF, Contant CF, et al: High-dose barbiturate control of elevated intracranial pressure in patients with severe head injury. J Neurosurg 69:15, 1988.

135. Safar P: Brain resuscitation in metabolic-toxic infectious encephalopathy. Crit Care Med 6:68, 1978.

136. Safar P, Bleyaert A, Nemoto EM, et al: Resuscitation after global brain ischemia-anoxia. Crit Care Med 6:215, 1978.

137. Safar P, Nemoto E: Brain resuscitation. Acta Anaesthesiol Scand Suppl 70:60, 1978.

138. Olney JW. Endogenous excitotoxins and neuropathological disorders. In Lodge D (ed): Excitatory Amino Acids in Health and Disease. West Sussex, England, John Wiley & Sons, 1988, p 337.

139. MacDonald JF, Schneiderman JH, Miljkovic Z: Excitatory amino acids and regenerative activity in cultured neurons. Adv Exp Med Biol 203:425, 1986.

140. Komuro, Rakic P: Modulation of neuronal migration by NMDA receptors. Science 260:95, 1993.

141. Ikonomidou C, Mosinger JL, Salles KS, et al: Sensitivity of the developing rat brain to hypobaric/ischemic damage parallels sensitivity to N-methyl-D-aspártate neurotoxicity. J Neurosci 9:2809, 1989.

142. Ikonomidou C, Price MT, Mosinger JL, et al: Hypobaric-ischemic conditions produce glutamate-like cytopathology in infant rat brain. J Neurosci 9:1693, 1989.

143. Ikonomidou C, Qin Y, Labruyere J, et al: Prevention of trauma-induced neurodegeneration in infant rat brain. Pediatr Res 39:1020, 1996.

144. Stefanis L, Burke RE: Transneuronal degeneration in substantia nigra pars reticulata following striatal excitotoxic injury: Time-course, distribution and morphology of cell death. Neuroscience 74:997, 1996.

145. Dikranian K, Ishimaru MJ, Tenkova T, et al: Apoptosis in the in vivo mammalian forebrain. Neurobiol Dis 8:359, 2001.

33

Neuromuscular Blocking Agents and Reversal Drugs

Heidrun Fink, MD • Manfred Blobner, MD • J. A. Jeevendra Martyn, MD

The French physiologist Claude Bernard (1811–1878) discovered that the arrow poison curare extracted from the plant *Chondodendron tomentosum* induces paralysis without interrupting nerve conductivity, making the muscle still susceptible for contraction by direct stimulation.[1,2] This finding was a milestone in the discovery of the interface between muscle and nerve, the neuromuscular junction. Currently, muscle relaxants are used in the anesthetized patient to temporarily paralyze the muscles to facilitate endotracheal intubation or to improve the operative conditions. Muscle relaxants are also an integral part of a balanced anesthesia. Less commonly, muscle relaxants are used in the critically ill patient in the intensive care unit (ICU) to facilitate mechanical ventilation, decrease oxygen consumption, and attenuate increases in intracranial or intrathoracic pressures resulting from suctioning or coughing.

Neuromuscular Transmission

The physiologic and biochemical basis of neuromuscular transmission is discussed in detail in Chapter 10. This chapter highlights several specific aspects of neuromuscular transmission that are germane to the pharmacology of neuromuscular blockade.

Presynaptic Physiology and Pharmacology

The presynaptic release of acetylcholine is triggered by the influx of calcium through voltage-dependent calcium channels. Different drugs can inhibit the calcium influx into the nerve terminal and the consequent release of acetylcholine. These drugs can therefore impair neuromuscular transmission and potentiate the effect of muscle relaxants. Magnesium (e.g., during prophylaxis against pre-eclampsia) can competitively inhibit calcium influx into the nerve terminals, whereas calcium channel antagonists and aminoglycoside antibiotics can also block the channel. As a corollary, toxic effects of magnesium, calcium channel antagonists, and aminoglycosides could be partially reversed by exogenous calcium.

Notably, there are acetylcholine receptors located on the presynaptic terminal. They are similar to the acetylcholine receptors on the postsynaptic membrane, but differ in one subunit (α_3 rather than α_1, see later). The function of these presynaptic acetylcholine receptors is to facilitate the liberation of acetylcholine to the neuromuscular junction using a positive feedback mechanism. This mechanism prevents a premature fade of transmitter release with increasing impulse rate of the motor nerve. Nondepolarizing neuromuscular blocking drugs not only bind to the postsynaptic receptor, but can also block presynaptic acetylcholine receptors. In the presence of neuromuscular blocking drugs, therefore, during high-frequency nerve action potentials, the facilitated acetylcholine release can be impaired because of the block of the positive feedback. Clinically this is described as "fade" during repetitive nerve stimulation at a frequency of 2 Hz or greater.

Postsynaptic Physiology and Pharmacology

In the healthy innervated muscle, the acetylcholine receptors (also termed *mature* acetylcholine receptors) are highly localized to the neuromuscular endplate region. However, when there is deprivation of neural influence or activity, as in the fetus or after denervation, the muscle expresses acetylcholine receptors where the ϵ-subunit has been replaced by a γ-subunit.[7] These "immature" or "fetal" receptors are no longer localized to the endplate region but are inserted throughout the muscle membrane into the junctional and extrajunctional area. This "ϵ to γ switch" of the acetylcholine receptor subunit has some important physiologic and metabolic consequences for the receptor itself. The mature acetylcholine receptor is metabolically more stable, with a half-life approximating 2 weeks, whereas immature acetylcholine receptors have a metabolic half-life of about 24 hours. Immature receptors have a smaller single channel conductance but a 2- to 10-fold longer mean channel open time. In addition, the sensitivity and affinity to ligands are different. Agonists, such as acetylcholine, and also succinylcholine depolarize immature receptors more easily; one tenth to one hundredth of normal doses of these agonists can affect depolarization.[8,9]

Margin of Safety of Neurotransmission

Approximately 10% of the total number of acetylcholine receptors at the endplate must be opened for the flow of ions to increase the endplate potential to a threshold at which a muscle action potential is initiated. The muscle action potential then runs across the muscle membrane resulting in the activation and contraction of muscle fibers. The action potential signal is usually carried out by more molecules of transmitter than are needed, and these evoke an action potential response that is greater than needed. At the same time, only a small fraction of the available vesicles and receptors are used to send each action potential signal. Consequently, neuromuscular transmission is said to have a substantial margin of safety or a system that has substantial reserve capacity.[6] Reinforcing the idea of margin of safety, in practice, approximately 75% of the acetylcholine receptors can be occupied by an antagonist (neuromuscular blocker) before any effect (fade) can be seen during the administration of neuromuscular blockers. At least 95% receptor occupancy is necessary for complete suppression of twitch (Fig. 33–1). The percent receptor occupancy, and not the absolute number blocked, varies with dose, and therefore concentrations reached at the neuromuscular junction vary. In other words, if the receptor number is increased in the perijunctional area and if antagonists occupy the same percentage of receptors, the absolute number of receptors remaining unblocked is still high. In these instances, a given concentration or dose of muscle relaxant will produce a smaller effect on twitch height, provided that other factors such as acetylcholine release are unaltered. Clinically, this can be described as a resistance to antagonists (muscle relaxants).

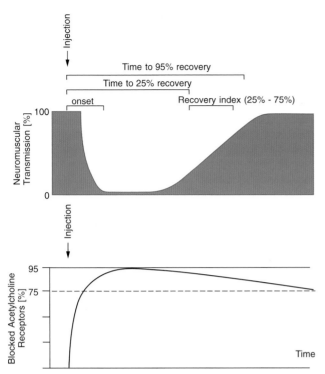

Figure 33–1. Definitions of neuromuscular parameters (see text for explanation).

Mechanisms of Action of Muscle Relaxants

Clinically, muscle paralysis by muscle relaxants is primarily achieved by blocking the function of the postsynaptic acetylcholine receptor. Aside from the competitive block of the acetylcholine receptor produced by nondepolarizing neuromuscular blocking drugs and the noncompetitive block by depolarizing muscle relaxants (Fig. 33–2), numerous other anesthetic and nonanesthetic drugs, often used during anesthesia, influence neuromuscular transmission at the receptor level.

Competitive Block

Nondepolarizing neuromuscular blocking drugs, just like acetylcholine, bind to the α-subunit of the acetylcholine receptor. They do not, however, possess any intrinsic agonist activity, meaning that they do not cause a conformational change of the receptor from the closed to open state. One molecule of nondepolarizing muscle relaxant is sufficient to occupy the receptor and to prevent the opening of the ion channel and consequent ion flow. Therefore, acetylcholine and the nondepolarizing muscle relaxant compete for the same binding site at the receptor; hence the term *competitive* block. The probability of binding is solely dependent on the concentration of each ligand present at the neuromuscular junction and their affinity for the receptor. As soon as the neuromuscular blocking drug diffuses out of the junction, the probability for acetylcholine to bind to the receptor increases and the muscle blocking effect of the drug diminishes.

Noncompetitive Block

The neuromuscular block (paralysis) produced by depolarizing neuromuscular blocking drugs, typified by succinylcholine, is noncompetitive. Succinylcholine, which is structurally two molecules of acetylcholine bound together, is a partial agonist of the acetylcholine receptor, and depolarizes (opens) the ion channel. This opening requires the binding of only one molecule of succinylcholine to the α-subunit. The other α-subunit of the receptor can be occupied by either acetylcholine or succinylcholine. Succinylcholine cannot be hydrolyzed by acetylcholinesterase; it can therefore detach from the receptor and repeatedly bind to other acetylcholine receptors until it is cleared from the junctional area into the plasma where it is hydrolyzed by plasma (pseudo-) cholinesterase. Because succinylcholine is an agonist of the acetylcholine receptor, binding induces muscle fasciculation (uncoordinated minicontraction), which occurs only during the initial phase, followed by a relaxation period. Because the endplate membrane is continuously depolarized by the presence of succinylcholine, the voltage-gated sodium channels in the perijunctional

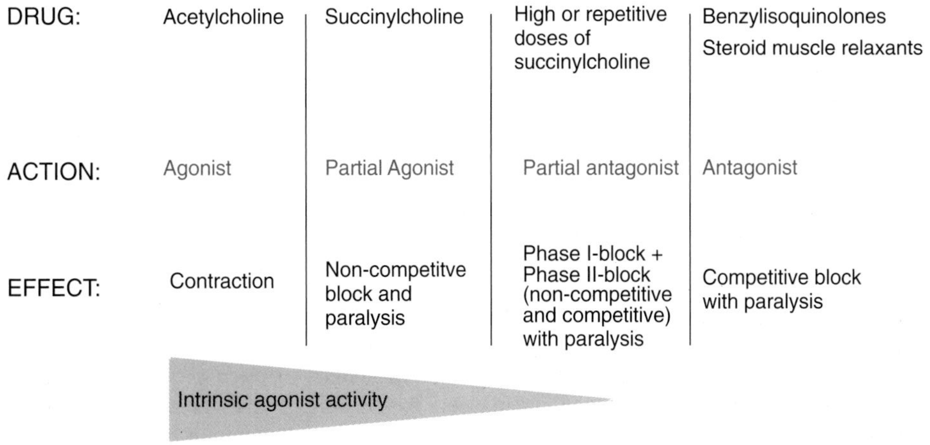

DRUG:	Acetylcholine	Succinylcholine	High or repetitive doses of succinylcholine	Benzylisoquinolones Steroid muscle relaxants
ACTION:	Agonist	Partial Agonist	Partial antagonist	Antagonist
EFFECT:	Contraction	Non-competitve block and paralysis	Phase I-block + Phase II-block (non-competitive and competitive) with paralysis	Competitive block with paralysis

Intrinsic agonist activity

Figure 33–2. Agonistic and antagonistic interactions at the nicotinic acetylcholine receptor.

region, which initiate the muscle action potential, are not activated after the initial depolarization. The musculature relaxes after the initial fasciculation, although the cell membrane beyond the perijunctional area is repolarized. Therefore, muscle contraction can be elicited by direct electrical stimulation of the muscle.

Phase II Block

A phase II block is a complex phenomenon seen not only after high single or cumulative doses of a depolarizing muscle relaxant, but also after normal doses of succinylcholine during lack or functional inefficiency of pseudocholinesterase (the metabolizing enzyme of succinylcholine). In the latter situation, the initial phase I (depolarization) block is converted into a phase II (nondepolarizing) block[11]; the decreased metabolism of succinylcholine produces a relative overdose causing an increased concentration in the synaptic cleft. The exact mechanism underlying a phase II block remains unclear. It is probably caused by an electrical imbalance at the junctional membrane caused by the repeated opening of the channels by succinylcholine. The junction is depolarized by the initial action of succinylcholine; the muscle membrane potential then, however, recovers to normal resting potential even though the junction is still exposed to the drug. Clinically, a phase II block is characterized by a tetanic or train-of-four (TOF) fade. Acetylcholinesterase inhibitors usually reverse a phase II block, but they can also enhance the block.

Desensitization Block

The acetylcholine receptor can exist in a number of conformational states. The desensitized state is one in which acetylcholine can bind to the receptor but cannot activate (open) the channel. The desensitized state is probably a physiologic response of the acetylcholine receptor designed to prevent an excessive muscle response to extreme neural stimulation.[12] An increase in desensitized receptors can be induced by an unphysiologically high concentration of agonist—e.g., high acetylcholine levels caused by inhibition of acetylcholinesterase enzyme, or high doses of succinylcholine concentrations after repetitive administration or decreased metabolism. Nicotine itself can also cause a desensitization of the receptor. The exact mechanism that induces a desensitization block is not fully understood. However, it is believed that it might be caused by a certain acetylcholine receptor subtype, containing $\alpha_8\beta_2$-subunits instead of $\alpha_1\beta_1$-subunits. This receptor subtype is especially stimulated at high concentrations of agonist, at which the ion channel opens with a high selectivity for calcium ions. Calcium influx activates protein kinase C, which in turn phosphorylates the "normal" $[(\alpha_1)_2\beta_1\delta\epsilon]$ acetylcholine receptor and thereby desensitizes it.[13]

Apart from high levels of agonists or cholinesterase inhibitors, desensitization can also be caused by certain inhalation anesthetics, barbiturates, alcohols, local anesthetics (including cocaine), phenothiazines, verapamil, and polymyxin B. A decrease in the margin of safety or an increase in the ability of nondepolarizing muscle relaxants to block neurotransmission, a concomitant feature of desensitization block, is independent of the classical effect based on competitive inhibition of acetylcholine. These effects are mediated by allosteric inhibition of receptors by binding of the drug to sites other than acetylcholine binding sites. The presence of desensitized receptors means that fewer functional receptor channels than usual are available to induce a transmembrane current. Therefore the production of desensitized receptors decreases the efficacy or margin of safety of neuromuscular transmission. This increases the susceptibility to antagonists, i.e., nondepolarizing neuromuscular blocking drugs. If many receptors are desensitized, insufficient nondesensitized normal receptors are left to depolarize the motor endplate, and effective neuromuscular transmission will not occur.

Channel Block

A noncompetitive method to block the physiologic opening and closing of the acetylcholine receptor channel and thus depolarization is through direct channel block. This happens if molecules binding to the acetylcholine receptor change its conformation in such a way that any further binding of acetylcholine to the α-subunit is prevented. However, because the site of action is not at the acetylcholine recognition site, it is not a competitive antagonism with acetylcholine and therefore cannot be reversed by acetylcholinesterase inhibitors. Depending on the conformation of the acetylcholine receptor, time of the block, and size of the blocking molecule, the result can be either an open channel block, a closed channel block, or a flickering between both states. Some drug-induced alterations in neuromuscular function are thought to be caused by closed channel block. Drugs that produce closed channel block include antibiotics, cocaine, quinidine, piperocaine, tricyclic antidepressants, naltrexone, naloxone, and histrionicotoxin. Open channel block is usually produced by positively charged (cationic) molecules. They enter the open channel then physically clog the pore and prevent ion flow. This mechanism may also play a role in the channel depolarization and paralysis during phase I block.[14,15] Pancuronium, gallamine, and succinylcholine are typical open channel blockers. *d*-Tubocurarine has a biphasic action: at low doses it is a pure competitive antagonist, at larger doses it enters the channel and causes open channel blockade.

Acetylcholine receptors are especially susceptible to channel block if a profound (deep) paralysis by nondepolarizing neuromuscular block is antagonized by acetylcholinesterase inhibitors. The increased number of acetylcholine molecules displace and replace the muscle relaxant molecules from binding to the α-subunit causing the channel to open. The muscle relaxant molecules, which are still present in a high concentration, can then enter the open channel and block the receptor for a longer duration than the original block produced by binding at the α-subunit.

In addition, the acetylcholinesterase inhibitors themselves can cause channel block.

Acetylcholinesterase

Acetylcholinesterase hydrolyses acetylcholine within 1 msec after its release from the presynaptic nerve terminal to acetic acid and choline. The enzyme is synthesized underneath the postsynaptic endplate membrane and, although it is secreted into the synaptic cleft, it remains attached to the basement membrane through thin stalks of collagen.

Acetylcholinesterase Inhibition

Specific inhibition of acetylcholinesterase prevents the metabolism of acetylcholine and increases its concentration in the synaptic cleft. In a clinical setting, this is used to advantage to reverse the effect of nondepolarizing neuromuscular blocking drugs. During a competitive block of neuromuscular transmission by muscle relaxants, an increase in acetylcholine concentration decreases the probability of the muscle relaxant binding to the receptor and neuromuscular transmission is thus restored. Because acetylcholinesterases are nonspecific, they inhibit all esterases including those at parasympathetic nerve endings. Increased parasympathetic activity, caused by increased levels of acetylcholine from acetylcholinesterase inhibition, leads to increased salivary secretions and slowing of the heart. These can be prevented by simultaneous use of parasympatholytic drugs (atropine, glycopyrrolate). An irreversible inhibition of the acetylcholinesterase can be caused by pesticides (e.g., E605, malathion) or nerve gases (e.g., Sarin). These toxic chemicals have both muscular and central nervous system effects; they have received increased attention recently because of the potential for chemical warfare.

Chemical Structure and Specific Properties of Muscle Relaxants

In 1935, H. King identified the chemical structure of the Indian arrow poison curare, isolated from the *C. tomentosum*.[16] In 1942, Griffith and Johnson used *d*-tubocurarine for the first time in humans during ether anesthesia.[17] Nine years later, succinylcholine was introduced into clinical practice, although it had been synthesized for the first time in 1906.[18] Bovet realized that succinylcholine and *d*-tubocurarine had different mechanisms of action at the neuromuscular junction, which led to the classification of depolarizing and nondepolarizing muscle relaxants.[19] Pancuronium, a compound derived from the Central African plant *Malouetia bequaertiana,* was introduced into clinical practice in 1967 as the second nondepolarizing muscle relaxant.[20]

Structure/Activity Relationship of Muscle Relaxants

Analogous to acetylcholine, all muscle relaxants have at least one quaternary amine group, which is involved in binding to the α-subunit of the nicotinic acetylcholine receptor. Succinylcholine consists of two acetylcholine molecules joined together, forming diacetylcholine (Fig. 33–3). Succinylcholine retains the depolarizing capacity of acetylcholine but is not susceptible to hydrolysis by acetylcholinesterase. Degradation is only achieved by the pseudocholinesterase after diffusion from the synaptic cleft into the plasma. The delayed degradation of succinylcholine (compared with acetylcholine) results in a sustained high concentration of the drug within the synaptic cleft.

Most nondepolarizing neuromuscular blocking drugs contain two amine groups. Some, but not all, of these compounds have two quaternary amines. *d*-Tubocurarine, vecuronium, and rocuronium are monoquaternary at a physiologic pH. The second amine group is protonated and is therefore present in an uncharged state as a tertiary amine (Fig. 33–4). The bisquaternary structure of the steroid muscle relaxants favors the block of postganglionic muscarinic acetylcholine receptors, and these drugs therefore have a vagolytic effect. This effect is much weaker in monoquaternary substances (e.g., vecuronium, rocuronium). Stereochemical aspects of a compound also have a role in structure/activity relationships. Muscle relaxants of the benzylisoquinoline type, including *d*-tubocurarine, mivacurium, and atracurium, tend to have histaminergic side effects. Some stereoisomers of atracurium have histaminergic properties as opposed to several other isomers (e.g., cisatracurium, Fig. 33–5), which have no histaminergic side effects in clinical doses.

The binding affinity of a neuromuscular blocker for the nicotinic acetylcholine receptor is an important determinant for the onset time of muscle relaxation.[21] This principle was used when developing rocuronium from vecuronium (see Fig. 33–4). Muscle relaxants with a lower affinity need to be administered in greater doses to achieve complete neuromuscular block. The high initial bolus dose required for this low-affinity drug, however, is associated with a greater

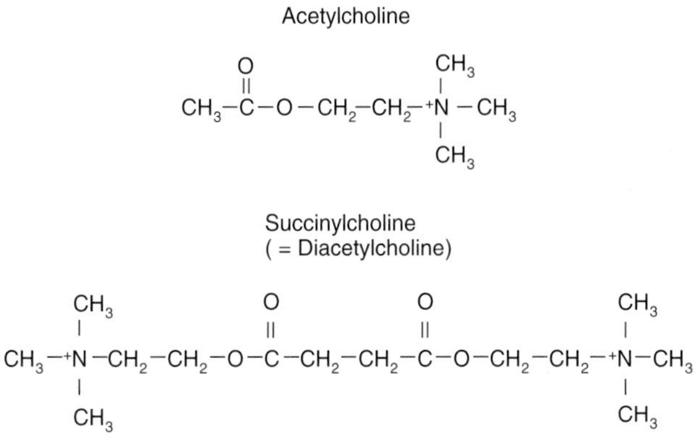

Figure 33–3. Chemical structure of acetylcholine and succinylcholine

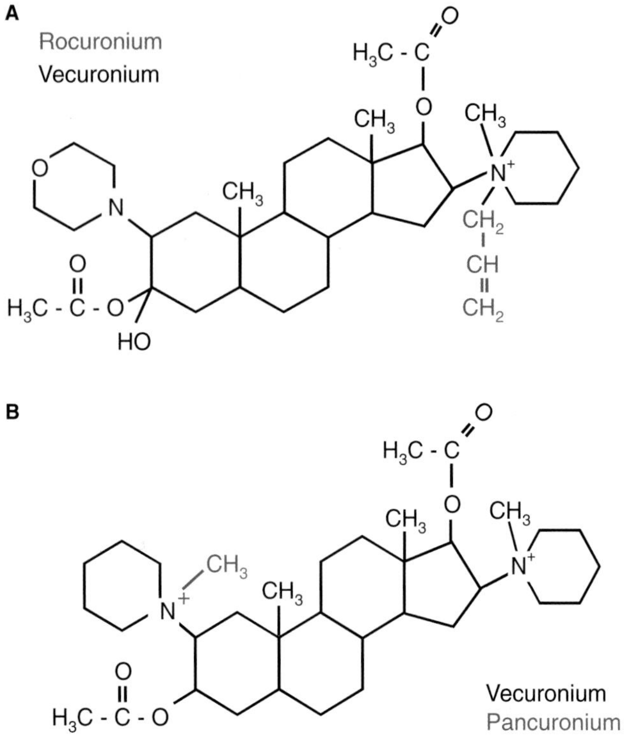

A

B

Figure 33–4. *A,* Chemical structure of the steroidal muscle relaxants, vecuronium and rocuronium. The longer aliphatic tail at the quaternary amine reduces the affinity toward the acetylcholine receptor. The hydroxyl tail at position 3 (A-Ring) ensures an adequate molecular stability of rocuronium during storage. *B,* Chemical structure of the steroidal muscle relaxants, vecuronium and pancuronium. The bisquaternary structure of pancuronium blocks the postganglionic muscarinic acetylcholine receptors (vagolysis) as opposed to the monoquaternary, vecuronium.

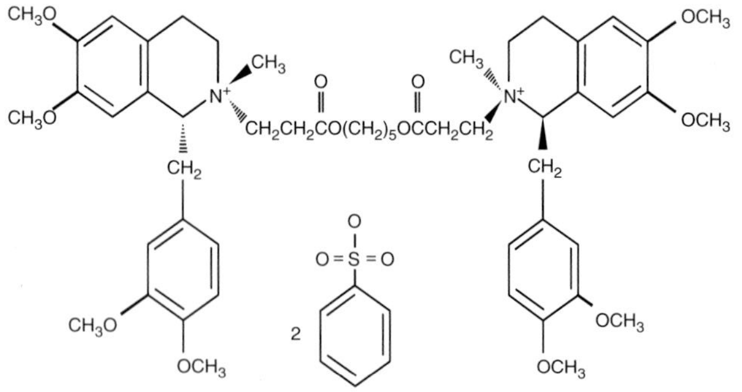

Figure 33–5. Chemical structure of cis-atracurium. Cis-atracurium is 1 of the 16 possible isomers of atracurium. The R-cis,R′-cis-conformation is approximately five times more potent than the racemate and induces almost no histamine release.

concentration gradient between the central compartment and the neuromuscular junction, and this results in the rapid diffusion to the acetylcholine receptor and faster onset of paralysis. Therefore less potent muscle relaxants, in equipotent doses, have a relatively shorter onset time.[22]

Intrinsic Activity of Relaxants at the Neuromuscular Nicotinic Acetylcholine Receptor

Molecules binding to the nicotinic acetylcholine receptor, depending on their intrinsic activity, are either agonists, partial agonists, or antagonists (see Fig. 33–2). The classic agonist of the acetylcholine receptor is acetylcholine: after binding of two acetylcholine molecules (one to each of the α-subunits), the receptor-associated ion channel opens. Succinylcholine acts as a partial agonist: it opens the ion channel after binding to the receptor; however, it elicits only an initial depolarization with subsequent muscle contraction. If high concentrations of succinylcholine induce a phase II block, the antagonistic or primarily the blocking action become more obvious. For practical purposes, nondepolarizing muscle relaxants display no intrinsic agonist activity (i.e., they are antagonists or competitive blockers of the acetylcholine receptor).

Relaxant Effects on Acetylcholine Receptors of the Central and Autonomic Nervous System

Nicotinic acetylcholine receptors are not only located at the neuromuscular junction, but can also be found in the central nervous system and in autonomic ganglia. These receptors are termed *nicotinic* because nicotine can elicit a response in all of these sites. Although these nicotinic receptors differ in their subunit composition, they all contain α-subunits with acetylcholine binding capacity. The acetylcholine receptors located in the brain contain other α-subunits (α_1 to α_9) or β-subunits (β_1 to β_4).[10] Therefore it is obvious that all muscle relaxants that bind to the acetylcholine receptors of the neuromuscular junction can also potentially interact with the receptors located in the central and autonomic nervous system. Aside from the clinically apparent effects of individual compounds on the receptors of the autonomic nervous system, a central effect, especially after prolonged use and disrupted blood–brain barrier, is possible. Intrathecal administration of muscle relaxants to animals induces seizures.[23] Individual case reports of accidental intrathecal injection have confirmed this.[24] Atracurium and its main metabolite, laudanosine, present agonistic and antagonistic actions at central nicotinic acetylcholine receptors, yet the clinical implications of these findings still remain undetermined. However, most muscle relaxants in current clinical use have high specificity for the α_1-subunit, which is almost exclusively located within the acetylcholine receptors at the neuromuscular junction.

Ganglia of the autonomic nervous system transduce either sympathetic or parasympathetic signals. In both ganglia, acetylcholine is the neurotransmitter. Succinylcholine stimulates the sympathetic and the parasympathetic ganglia, as well as the postsynaptic parasympathetic muscarinic receptors. Thus it is not unusual to see increased salivary secretions and bradycardia even in adults, especially with repetitive doses of succinylcholine. Nondepolarizing neuromuscular blocking drugs have no effect on autonomic ganglia (Table 33–1). High doses of *d*-tubocurarine, however, can result in ganglionic blockade giving rise to hypotension and pupillary dilatation.

TABLE 33–1.

Effect of Muscle Relaxants on the Autonomic Nervous System and Histamine Release

Muscle Relaxant	Ganglion Blockade*	Vagolysis*	Histamine Liberation†
Steroids			
Pancuronium	>100	3	None
Rocuronium	Ø	3	None
Vecuronium	>100	20	None
Rapacuronium‡	>250	3–5	~5‡
Benzylisoquinolines			
Mivacurium	>100	>50	~3
Atracurium	40	16	~2.5
Cisatracurium	>50	>50	None
Others			
Alcuronium	~3	~4	None

Data are expressed as the ratio of $ED_{50}SE/ED_{95}NMB$ where $ED_{50}SE$ is the dose at which there is a 50% probability of a specific side effect, and $ED_{95}NMB$ is the effective dose for 95% twitch depression of a muscle relaxant. The greater the ratio $ED_{50}SE/ED_{95}NMB$, the safer the drug. Values less than 3 can be considered as low. The ratio does not provide information about the magnitude of the side effect.
*Determined in cats.
†Estimated from the clinical signs of histamine liberation.
‡Withdrawn from the market because of severe bronchopulmonary side effects.

The actions of succinylcholine on the autonomic nervous system are not limited to stimulation of the nicotinic acetylcholine receptor on sympathetic and parasympathetic ganglia. It also stimulates postganglionic parasympathetic muscarinic receptors throughout the body, which transmit signals to the sinus node of the heart, carotid and aortic bodies, and visceral organs and modulate the sympathetic activity through cross-connections to the sympathetic nervous system. Because of their helical structure and seven transmembrane domains, the muscarinic receptors have a greater similarity to adrenergic receptors than to the nicotinic acetylcholine receptor, and like the adrenergic receptors, they belong to the class of G protein–coupled receptors. When succinylcholine is administered, whether the sympathetic or parasympathetic action in the autonomic nervous system dominates is dependent on the pre-existing dynamic equilibrium. Children, for example, often have an elevated vagal tone and therefore are prone to react with bradycardia or arrhythmia to administration of succinylcholine. To prevent this, prophylactic block of the muscarinic receptors with atropine can be attempted. Bradycardia also may be seen in adults with repeated dosing of succinylcholine.

Pancuronium is the only currently used nondepolarizing muscle relaxant that blocks muscarinic receptors in clinically relevant doses. For rocuronium to display such an effect, twice the clinically applicable dose must be administered. In a clinical setting, the cardiac vagolytic effect of pancuronium is evidenced as tachycardia after its injection (see Table 33–1).

Histamine Release and Anaphylaxis by Relaxants

Histamine release from mast cells can be induced either by an antigen/antibody reaction as a result of a true anaphylaxis (IgE), by activation of the complement system (IgG or IgM), or by direct action of molecules on the surface of mast cells. Two types of mast cells are differentiated: mucosal (in the bronchial system and gastrointestinal tract) and serosal (vascular endothelium, skin, connective tissue).[25]

Direct Effects on Mast Cells

In comparison with tertiary amines (e.g., morphine), the quaternary ammonium structure of muscle relaxants presents a weak histaminergic effect on mast cells. In clinical doses, succinylcholine and benzylisoquinolines (atracurium, mivacurium) can directly liberate histamine from serosal mast cells. Clinical symptoms are erythema, blistering, tachycardia, and in rare cases hypotension. In contrast, the pharmacologically selective and more potent cis-atracurium isoform (cis-atracurium) has no direct histaminergic effects,[26] nor do any of the commonly used steroid muscle relaxants (pancuronium, vecuronium, rocuronium). Rapacuronium, which recently has been taken off the market, is the first steroid muscle relaxant thought to have a histaminergic side effect, acting more on mucosal rather than serosal mast cells.[27,28] These side effects (e.g., bronchospasm) recurred even in the absence of increased plasma levels of histamine.[27] The direct effect on the surface of mast cells is subject to tachyphylaxis, meaning that slower, graduated, or repetitive administration of the drug decreases the histaminergic side effect. Prophylactic administration of histamine (H_1 and H_2) receptor blockers can suppress the clinical side effects of histamine release.[29]

Anaphylactic Reactions

Anaphylactic reactions toward muscle relaxants are rare and are probably not related to other drug allergies, atopic disposition, or sensitivity toward direct mast cell activation by individual substances. Anaphylactic reactions have also been observed at the first contact with a drug, and often crossover allergies are present. Female patients have a greater propensity to anaphylactic reactions with muscle relaxants (male : female = 2.5 : 1). A causal relationship with cosmetics and cleaning chemicals, which often also have quaternary ammonium structures, is speculated. Relative to the frequency by which they are used, the incidence of anaphylactic reactions after succinylcholine are approximately three times greater than after administration of nondepolarizing neuromuscular blocking drugs. The anaphylactic potential (with the exception of rapacuronium, which led to its withdrawal from the market) of individual neuromuscular blocking drugs does not differ among each other (see Table 33–1).[30]

Preclinical Pharmacology and Pharmacologic Variables of Neuromuscular Block

The neuromuscular blocking action of muscle relaxants is characterized by a decreased muscular response to the stimulation of a motor nerve. The onset, maximal effect, and duration of block after administration of a muscle relaxant depends on the individual muscle group and its blood supply. To determine clinical (pharmacologic) response to a muscle relaxant, the twitch depression of a skeletal muscle (e.g., adductor pollicis muscle) in response to its nerve stimulation is measured after single or incremental doses of the muscle relaxant. A twitch of 100% is the response in absence of any neuromuscular block, 0% is complete paralysis. Although there is substantial variability between patients in terms of response to muscle relaxants, the compounds are characterized by determining the following pharmacologic variables as endpoints in large groups of patients (see Fig. 33–1):

1. *Potency:* The potency of a muscle relaxant is described by its "effective dose" (ED): ED_{95} and ED_{50} are the doses of muscle relaxant necessary to suppress the twitch response by 95% (5% twitch height) or 50% (50% twitch height) of baseline (100%) twitch height, respectively.

2. *Onset:* Onset describes the interval between injection of the muscle relaxant and development of maximal neuromuscular block.

3. *Clinical duration of action (dur25/dur95):* The clinical duration of action is the interval between injection of the muscle relaxant and recovery of the twitch to 25% or 95% of baseline twitch height (i.e., 75% and 5% twitch suppression), respectively. If the surgical conditions require continued relaxation, reinjection of the muscle relaxant becomes necessary at or before 25% recovery.

4. *Recovery index:* The recovery index describes the offset speed of the effect of a muscle relaxant and is defined as the time taken for recovery from 25% to 75% twitch height.

5. *Total duration of action:* The total duration of action is best described by the interval between injection of the muscle relaxant and a recovery of the TOF ratio to ≥0.7. Recent studies, however, advocate a TOF ratio of ≥0.9 as the parameter for complete neuromuscular recovery.[31]

Pharmacokinetics (Absorption and Distribution)

Muscle relaxants are usually administered intravenously to ensure a rapid onset, fast distribution, and predictable elimination. The desired effect after subcutaneous or intramuscular application (as in the Amazon Indian's arrow poisoning) can only be achieved with high doses of muscle relaxants. Furthermore, the pharmacodynamics of intramuscular nondepolarizing relaxants are unpredictable. Therefore an intramuscular administration of a muscle relaxant can be justified only in few instances—e.g., laryngospasm in the absence of intravenous access.[32] Muscle relaxants are not absorbed through the gastrointestinal tract so that prey killed with curare could be eaten without risking muscle paralysis. Succinylcholine, in contrast, is absorbed effectively and rapidly through the intramuscular route and therefore can be used to treat laryngospasm in the absence of any contraindication to its use.

Pharmacokinetic Models and Parameters

Pharmacokinetics attempts to describe mathematically the relationship between time and plasma concentration of a drug and its metabolites. The parameters for muscle relaxants are mostly calculated using a two-compartment model. After injection, the muscle relaxant is immediately distributed in the first, "central" compartment, before it is redistributed to the second "peripheral" compartment (Fig. 33–6). Metabolism and elimination of the drug begin almost instantaneously. Parameters that are used to describe muscle relaxant pharmacokinetics are the initial total volume of distribution (V_1), volume of distribution (V_d) at steady-state, plasma clearance (Cl), and elimination half-life ($t^1/_2\beta$). The term *context-sensitive half-life* describes the pharmacokinetics after repeated or continuous administration. In

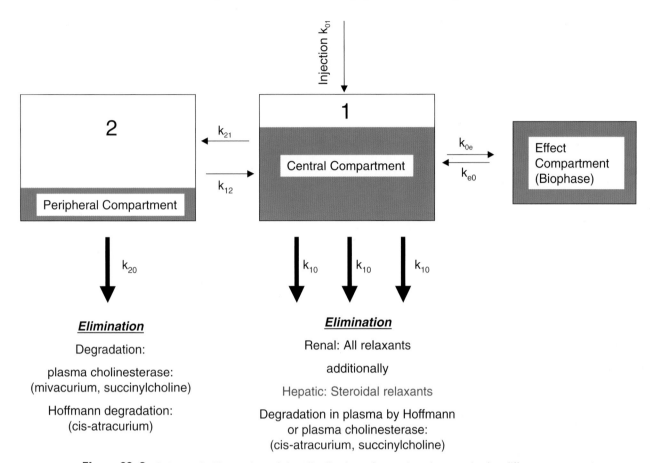

Figure 33–6. Schematic illustration of the distribution of muscle relaxants in the different compartments. The propagated model can be used to mathematically determine pharmacokinetic parameters. k_{x-y} describes the distribution constants between the different compartments.

pharmacokinetic/pharmacodynamic (PK/PD) models, the term *biophase* describes the compartment of action—i.e., in the case of muscle relaxants, the neuromuscular junction.

Factors Influencing Pharmacokinetics of Relaxants

Volume of distribution: All muscle relaxants have a positively charged quaternary ammonium group, which remains ionized independent of the pH value. The positive charge makes it almost impossible for muscle relaxants to bind to lipids. Therefore the V_d of muscle relaxants is the extracellular space and consists of 0.2 to 0.5 L/kg. If muscle relaxants are administered repetitively or continuously over a prolonged period (>24 hours), distribution into less perfused tissue, such as connective tissue, occurs resulting in a V_d that can then increase up to 10-fold.[33]

Plasma protein binding: After injection, muscle relaxants bind to plasma proteins, particularly to albumin and γ-globulins. The published values as to the percentage of protein binding of individual muscle relaxants are inconsistent and highly dependent on the method of determination.

Pharmacologic potency: The pharmacologic potency of a muscle relaxant is described by its affinity toward the acetylcholine receptor. For many relaxants, a reciprocal

relationship between pharmacologic potency and onset time could be shown. If a low-affinity drug requires a high dose of muscle relaxant (e.g., ED_{95}) to achieve a defined twitch depression, the concentration gradient between central compartment and biophase is high resulting in faster delivery of the drug to the receptor. In contrast, for drugs with high affinity toward the acetylcholine receptor, the dose administered would be smaller (lower ED_{95}) and the gradient for transfer of drug lower; therefore a slower onset will result.[21,22] Even though all muscle relaxants do not show these characteristics,[22] pharmaceutical research has oriented according to this postulate when developing and synthesizing new muscle relaxants such as rocuronium and rapacuronium.

Speed of injection: Fast injection of muscle relaxant generates a high concentration gradient between central compartment and the biophase (i.e., neuromuscular junction), and therefore expedites onset time. However, in the case of benzylisoquinolines, especially atracurium and mivacurium, histaminergic side effects can be associated with rapid injection.[34]

Perfusion: Intravenously applied muscle relaxants must be transported through the bloodstream to their effect compartment. If cardiac output is reduced, onset of neuromuscular block is delayed.[35] Differences in regional blood flow result in different onset times in the individual muscle groups (diaphragm < laryngeal muscles < orbicular ocular muscle < adductor pollicis muscle).[36]

Obesity: At normal doses, the positive charge of muscle relaxants prevents its absorption into fat tissue. Therefore, the body weight-related volume of distribution (V_d/kg) and clearance in obese patients is markedly reduced compared with patients who are not obese. The elimination half-life, however, remains almost unaltered.[37]

Age: V_d for muscle relaxants is larger in children compared with adults. Therefore, a greater dose of muscle relaxant must be injected into children to achieve a given concentration of relaxant. The neuromuscular junction is also more sensitive in children,[38] thus the higher dose can result in prolonged duration of action. With aminosteroidal derivatives, the greater V_d of the drug can result in a prolonged duration of action and prolonged elimination.[39] Because of the higher heart rate and cardiac index in children, onset time of neuromuscular block is faster compared with adults. Despite the widening of the neuromuscular junction and decrease of acetylcholine receptors with aging,[40,41] the sensitivity toward neuromuscular blocking drugs remains unaltered.[40,42,43] However, distribution and elimination kinetics are often delayed in the elderly. This is largely the consequence of impaired organ function of, for example, heart, liver, and kidneys. Of the currently used drugs, it is primarily the organ-dependent metabolism and elimination of aminosteroidal muscle relaxants that are affected by age (Table 33–2).

Pregnancy: During pregnancy, the pharmacokinetics and pharmacodynamics of muscle relaxants remain almost unaltered. However, an increased potency and duration of action must be considered with the use of nondepolarizing muscle relaxants when magnesium is used as treatment for premature contractions or pre-eclampsia. The ionized state of muscle relaxants minimizes the passage of drug through the blood–placenta barrier. Only after extended use—for example, during prolonged mechanical ventilation with relaxants in an ICU setting—can sufficient levels of muscle relaxant reach the fetus to affect muscle function.[44]

Temperature: Duration of action of muscle relaxants is prolonged during hypothermia because of reduced hepatic and renal function and clearance.[45] With atracurium and cis-atracurium, it is also caused by slowed Hoffman elimination.[46] The differentiation between pharmacodynamic and pharmacokinetic causes of prolonged neuromuscular block during hypothermia is difficult. A possible exception is mivacurium, which is degraded by temperature-independent plasma cholinesterase.[47]

Elimination and Metabolism of Relaxants

The neuromuscular effect of a single dose of muscle relaxant is primarily terminated by redistribution from the neuromuscular junction and the central compartment into the peripheral compartment. After repeated injection or continuous infusion, however, the redistribution capacity might be saturated and the muscle relaxants and their active metabolites can be distributed back into the central compartment. In this case, neuromuscular recovery is determined primarily by elimination of the drug.

Renal Elimination

All muscle relaxants can be eliminated through the kidney, although this route may not be the primary pathway. At physiologic pH, muscle relaxants are ionized as quaternary

TABLE 33–2.

Pharmacokinetic Parameters at Different Ages

	Plasma Clearance (mL/kg/min)			Volume of Distribution (mL/kg)			Elimination Half-Life (min)		
	Children	Adults	Elderly	Children	Adults	Elderly	Children	Adults	Elderly
Atracurium	5.1–9.1	5.0–6.2	5.4–6.5	113–210	100–140	150–190	14–20	17–23	22–23
Cis-atracurium		4.1–6.5			110–180			19–25	
Mivacurium		40–120	54		120–410	290		1–3	2
Vecuronium	2.8–5.9	4.2–6.3	2.6–3.7	130–360	210–280	180–440	28–123	50–90	58–125
Rocuronium	11.4–13.5	2.2–3.5	3.4	220–300	140–220	620	38–56	70–106	137
Pancuronium	1.7	1.0–2.0	0.8–1.2	200	100–280	220–320	103	115–155	151–204

amines. Patients with healthy renal function can eliminate muscle relaxants at a rate of approximately 1 to 2 mL/kg per minute, which is equivalent to the normal glomerular filtration rate. Reabsorption from the tubules does not take place. Decreased renal function therefore naturally prolongs the elimination half-life of muscle relaxants such as pancuronium, alcuronium, doxacurium, and pipecuronium that are primarily renally excreted (Table 33–3).

Metabolism: Ester Hydrolysis

Succinylcholine and mivacurium are the only neuromuscular blocking drugs inactivated through enzymatic cleavage by plasma cholinesterase. This takes place as long as the molecules are in the extracellular space or diffuse back into it from the synaptic cleft.

Atypical plasma cholinesterases: The incidence of individuals with heterozygous atypical plasma cholinesterases is 1:480. The duration of action of succinylcholine and mivacurium in these cases is prolonged only minimally.

Homozygous carriers of the atypical plasma cholinesterase (incidence: 1:3200), however, can present with a prolonged neuromuscular blockade for hours. Numerous genotypes of plasma cholinesterase, in heterozygous or homozygous form, can be differentiated: E_1^u (usual = normal form), E_1^a (atypical form = dibucaine-resistant), E_1^f (fluoride-resistant), E_1^s (silent form = no enzyme activity at all). The "dibucaine test," introduced in 1957 by Kalow and Genest, uses the local anesthetic dibucaine to inhibit plasma cholinesterase in vitro.[48] Normal isoforms of plasma cholinesterases are more easily inhibited than the atypical isoforms. The percentage of inhibition of the plasma cholinesterase is referred to as *dibucaine-number.* Normal plasma cholinesterases will be inhibited about 70% by dibucaine; abnormal cholinesterases are less inhibited (Table 33–4).

Acquired cholinesterase deficiency: Different drugs can inhibit the activity of the plasma cholinesterase, and thereby decrease the metabolism of succinylcholine and mivacurium. This is most obvious with the cholinesterase inhibitors, neostigmine and pyridostigmine. Pancuronium has a considerable capacity to inhibit cholinesterase, as does the antiemetic metoclopramide and different antiasthmatic

TABLE 33–3.

Metabolism and Elimination of Muscle Relaxants

Muscle Relaxant	Metabolism	Renal Elimination	Biliary Elimination
Succinylcholine	98–99% (plasma cholinesterase)	<2% High elimination in presence of plasma cholinesterase deficiency	—
Mivacurium	95–99% (plasma cholinesterase)	<5% (metabolites) High elimination in presence of plasma cholinesterase deficiency	—
Atracurium	70–90% (Hoffmann elimination and esterases)	10–30% (laudanosine)	(laudanosine)
Cis-atracurium	70–90% (Hoffmann elimination and esterases)	10–30% (laudanosine)	(laudanosine)
Alcuronium	—	80–90%	10–20%
Vecuronium	30–40% (hepatic)	~40% (metabolites)	10–20% (metabolites)
Pancuronium	10–20% (hepatic)	60–80%	~10%
Rocuronium	Minimal (hepatic)	30–40%	~60%

TABLE 33–4.

Dibucaine Number, Atypical Plasma Cholinesterase, and Neuromuscular Recovery after Succinylcholine or Mivacurium

Dibucaine Number	Plasma Cholinesterase	Neuromuscular Recovery	Incidence
>70%	Normal	Normal	
35–65%	Heterozygous atypical	Minimal increase	1:480
<30%	Homozygous atypical	Prolonged by hours	1:3200

drugs. If the plasma cholinesterase activity is reduced to values approximately 500 IU/L (e.g., during liver failure or burn injury), the neuromuscular block induced by succinylcholine or mivacurium can be prolonged up to 2.5 times.[48a] Patients with renal insufficiency or pregnant women may also have reduced plasma cholinesterase activity.

Metabolism: Nonenzymatic Decay (Hoffmann Elimination)

Atracurium and its isomer cis-atracurium are inactivated by spontaneous degradation by the so-called *Hoffmann elimination*. They are degraded into the inactive metabolites, laudanosine and monacrylate, which are inactive at the neuromuscular junction. Hoffmann elimination takes place in the central and peripheral compartment and in the synaptic cleft. In addition, atracurium is degraded through ester hydrolysis into a quaternary acid and quaternary alcohol. It is, however, still a subject of discussion if cis-atracurium also displays this additional pathway.[49]

Metabolism: Hepatic Elimination

Steroidal relaxants, rocuronium, pancuronium, and vecuronium, are eliminated through the kidneys and the liver. Hepatic elimination of the drugs and their metabolites can be important during renal failure, but this pathway is still slightly slower than the dissipation of action caused by redistribution of the drug after a single dose. Therefore, the duration of action of each repetitive injection increases, or the dose of muscle relaxant required to establish a defined neuromuscular block decreases, because the distribution volume of the drug is small. This accumulation during repetitive dosing, however, in no way compares with the accumulation of parent drug and metabolites during liver or kidney failure. In contrast to the benzylisoquinolines, the deacetylation by the liver of steroidal muscle relaxants in position 3 and 17 leads to metabolites, which themselves have a neuromuscular blocking effect and are slowly eliminated. This is of clinical relevance if these muscle relaxants are used over a long time, as accumulation of the metabolites can potentiate the paralysis and delay neuromuscular recovery (e.g., in the ICU).

Clinical Pharmacology of Depolarizing Relaxant, Succinylcholine

Succinylcholine is the only depolarizing muscle relaxant currently in clinical use.[18] In 1951, succinylcholine was introduced into clinical practice in Sweden by Thesleff[50] and in Austria by Mayrhofer[51] before it gained international recognition based on research by Foldes.[52] The molecular size is smaller than that of nondepolarizing muscle relaxants. Both nitrogen atoms are quaternary, i.e., positively charged and therefore polar, water-soluble, and almost fat-insoluble. The pH of a 2% solution is about 2 to 3. The commercially available solutions also contain stabilizers and buffers (benzylalcohol, benzoate, and sodium chloride), which might account for some of the side effects (Table 33–5). The absolute and relative contraindications for use of succinylcholine are based on these side effects (Table 33–6). In current clinical practice, succinylcholine is almost exclusively used for rapid-sequence intubation in patients with increased risk for aspiration of stomach contents, or it is used to counteract laryngospasm.

After intravenous injection, most of the succinylcholine is immediately metabolized by the plasma cholinesterase to succinylmonocholine and choline, even before it reaches the synaptic cleft. Thus only a small fraction reaches the neuromuscular junction and displays its depolarizing effect within 20 to 40 seconds. Clinically, this can be visible within the first minute after injection as muscle fasciculations, followed by complete muscle relaxation. The ED$_{95}$ for succinylcholine is about 0.35 to 0.5 mg/kg body weight. In clinical practice, to ensure fast and complete paralysis, a dose of $2 \times$ ED$_{95}$ (0.8–1.0 mg/kg) is given. Neuromuscular recovery begins after succinylcholine diffuses out of the neuromuscular junction into the extracellular space, where it is enzymatically metabolized. Despite the development of newer nondepolarizing neuromuscular blocking drugs with faster onset times (rocuronium, rapacuronium), or shorter

TABLE 33-5.

Adverse Effects of Succinylcholine

Stimulation of muscarinic acetylcholine receptors of the cardiac sinus node
Bradycardia
AV-node dysrhythmia
Ventricular arrhythmia

Depolarization of the endplate
Increased intracranial pressure
Increased intraocular pressure
Increased intragastric pressure
Release of intracellular potassium
Myalgia
Masseter spasm
Trigger for malignant hyperthermia

Allergic Reactions

TABLE 33-6.

Contraindications to Succinylcholine

Neuromuscular diseases

Denervation (after 2 days)

Immobilization (after 3 days)

Burns (after 2 days)

Disposition to malignant hyperthermia

Allergy to succinylcholine

Homozygous for atypical plasma cholinesterase

Sepsis/infection

Basal serum K^+ level $\geq 5.5\,mEq/L$

fraction of the acetylcholine receptors without any evidence of weakness or fade, is administered before giving the succinylcholine.[53] Some patients, however, may show signs of muscle weakness (e.g., diplopia) with the precurarizing dose. Precurarization is not advised in patients with existing muscle weakness (e.g., myasthenia gravis).

Side Effects of Succinylcholine on Autonomic Ganglia and Muscarinic Receptors

The effects of succinylcholine on the cardiovascular system are diverse, because it binds to all types of cholinergic receptors in the autonomic nervous system (see Table 33–5). Complete suppression of the sinus node, idioventricular rhythm, and ventricular arrhythmias can all occur as a result of a stimulation of the vagal muscarinic receptors, especially after the second and subsequent injections. This is often seen if a high vagal tone is present, which is common in pediatric patients or after vagal stimulation induced by the laryngoscopy blade. Stimulation of other parasympathetically innervated structures (dilation of cervix, stimulation of carotid body or eye balls) can potentiate the bradycardia. Succinylcholine-induced high levels of catecholamines and serum potassium can potentiate the dysrhythmias. By premedicating with atropine, bradyarrhythmias can be prevented; however, ventricular arrhythmias are not attenuated by atropine pretreatment. In addition, a preceding injection of a small dose of succinylcholine ("self-taming")[54] or the injection of lidocaine[55] or opioids[56] cannot attenuate these unwanted cardiovascular effects, but it may attenuate the side effects related to fasciculations.

Effects of Succinylcholine at the Neuromuscular Junction

Succinylcholine induces fasciculation (uncoordinated contraction) of all skeletal muscles, causing a variety of unwanted side effects (see Table 33–5). Although a causative relationship has not yet been established, the increases in intragastric, intracranial, and intraocular pressures and myalgia have generally been attributed to the fasciculations. The relationship between fasciculations and side effects is controversial, because of the observation that a precurarizing dose can weaken the intensity of the fasciculations but does not reduce the side effects in toto. It is especially difficult to explain the reason behind increased intracranial pressure. It has been suggested that the increase in cerebral perfusion due to an increase in afferent excitation, in the context of the generalized muscle fasciculations, causes the increase in intracranial pressure. Prior hyperventilation can attenuate the increase in intracranial pressure. Other studies do not confirm the increase in intracranial pressure.[57]

Succinylcholine leads to a temporary small increase in serum potassium levels in healthy patients. Pathologic states, which lead to a quantitative increase, or qualitative changes of the acetylcholine receptor, or both, are often associated with larger succinylcholine-induced increases of serum potassium. During certain circumstances, the

duration of action (mivacurium), succinylcholine remains the only muscle relaxant that combines both properties: short onset time (<1 minute) and short duration of action (5–10 minutes). To prevent some of the unwanted side effects of succinylcholine related to general muscle fasciculations, the concept of precurarization was introduced: a small dose of nondepolarizing neuromuscular blocking drug (e.g., 0.05 mg vecuronium in an adult), which occupies a hyperkalemia can reach life-threatening levels (see Table 33–6). If a patient has pre-existing hyperkalemia, succinylcholine is contraindicated. It is difficult, however, to provide an exact number above which succinylcholine should not be used; a number that is usually referred to is 5.5 mEq/L.[58] The serum potassium level does not reflect the potential for increased potassium release from the muscle after succinylcholine injection. This dilemma will hopefully become moot as techniques for rapid intubation with fast-onset nondepolarizing neuromuscular blocking drugs are established. There seems no contraindication to succinylcholine in normokalemic patients with renal insufficiency, especially in the absence of uremic neuropathy.[58] Finally, other than volatile anesthetics, succinylcholine is the strongest inducer of malignant hyperthermia.

Histamine Release and Allergic Reactions Following Succinylcholine

Although rare, succinylcholine is the most common inducer of anaphylactoid reactions among the relaxants. Should severe cardiopulmonary side effects occur after injection of succinylcholine, after exclusion of a hyperkalemic response, one must consider an allergic reaction and treat the patient accordingly. Postoperative allergy testing should be performed.

Clinical Pharmacology of Nondepolarizing Neuromuscular Blocking Drugs

Nondepolarizing neuromuscular blocking drugs can be classified according to their clinical duration of action (short, intermediate, and long acting) or their chemical structure (benzylisoquinolines, aminosteroidal, and others; Table 33–7). In this review, the nondepolarizing muscle relaxants have been classified according to their chemical structure. The following section discusses the pharmacodynamic effects.

Standard Intubation

One of the main reasons for using muscle relaxants in the context of general anesthesia is to facilitate an atraumatic or rapid tracheal intubation. If the muscles of the oral cavity, larynx, diaphragm, and abdomen are completely relaxed, that goal is achieved. In clinical practice, little emphasis is placed on neuromuscular monitoring when determining the optimal time point of intubation. Most anesthesiologists judge the time point when adequate depth of anesthesia and muscle relaxation is achieved by their clinical assessment. Normally, a 1 to 3 × ED_{95} dose of a muscle relaxant is

TABLE 33–7.

Classification of Nondepolarizing Muscle Relaxants

Muscle Relaxant	ED_{95} (mg/kg)	Year of Clinical Introduction	Chemical Classification	Duration of Action
Rapacuronium	1–1.2	2000 (USA)	Aminosteroid	Short
Rocuronium	0.3	1992	Aminosteroid	Intermediate
Vecuronium	0.05–0.06	1980	Aminosteroid	Intermediate
Pancuronium	0.06–0.07	1960	Aminosteroid	Long
Mivacurium	0.08	1997	Benzylisoquinoline	Short
Atracurium	0.25	1980	Benzylisoquinoline	Intermediate
Cis-atracurium	0.05	1995	Benzylisoquinoline	Intermediate
d-Tubocurarine	0.5	1942	Dibenzyl-tetrahydro-isoquinoline	Long
Alcuronium	0.2–0.25	1964	Strychnine-derivate	Long

Muscle relaxants can be classified according to their potency (ED_{95}), duration of action, chemical structure, or chronologically, depending on the relevance to discussion.

injected, and an intubation attempt is started after the standard onset time (Table 33–8). Aside from muscle relaxation, the depth of anesthesia determines the ease of intubation.

Rapid Sequence Induction with Nondepolarizers

When there is substantial risk for aspiration of gastric contents, the goal of anesthesia induction is to secure the airway as rapidly as possible, usually within 60 to 90 seconds after loss of the protective airway reflexes. Currently, succinylcholine is the only muscle relaxant with the pharmacologic characteristics to enable this. If contraindications to succinylcholine are present (see Table 33–6), alternative techniques or a nondepolarizing muscle relaxant can be used (Table 33–9).

"Priming": Two successive injections of a nondepolarizing muscle relaxant can increase the onset of muscle paralysis. Thus a small subparalytic ("priming") dose is injected about 3 minutes before the full intubating dose (see Table 33–9). By doing so, it is possible to achieve onset times in the range of 1 minute.

Increased intubating dose: By increasing the dose of nondepolarizing muscle relaxant, the onset time for paralysis can be decreased. However, by increasing the dose, the likelihood of cardiovascular side effects is increased and the time to complete neuromuscular recovery is prolonged (see Table 33–9). The limitations of currently available nondepolarizing muscle relaxants for use in rapid sequence induction are: (1) their relatively long onset time for paralysis; the time to intubation is longer than with succinylcholine unless large doses of nondepolarizing agent are given; and (2) their prolonged duration of action, particularly when given in high doses to speed onset of paralysis; this can pose problems related to surgery of shorter duration and can produce a crisis when difficult intubating conditions result in a "cannot intubate, cannot ventilate" scenario. For these reasons, many anesthesiologists prefer not to use nondepolarizing muscle relaxants for rapid sequence induction.

Neuromuscular Recovery from Nondepolarizers

Clinical recovery from neuromuscular block is usually described by the "recovery index." The index determined in one muscle (e.g., the adductor pollicis muscle) can be used to compare recovery index in another muscle (e.g., diaphragm) within the same subject to compare the sensitivity of different muscles groups to a drug. The recovery index in the same muscle among individuals, however, is mainly used for studying the effect of variables, such as age, drugs, diseases, and so on.

Residual neuromuscular block is a common sequela of muscle relaxant use. Approximately 30% of all patients who receive a muscle relaxant have residual paralysis at the time they leave the operating room.[59–61] This can be a serious unrecognized and relevant clinical problem with a potential for severe cardiorespiratory complications. Older patients are more likely to be affected. Clinical consequences of this include hypoventilation,[62–64] atelectasis, aspiration of gastric

TABLE 33–8.

Onset and Duration of Action after $2 \times ED_{95}$ Dose

	Onset (min)	Dur$_{25}$ (min)	Duration of Action Until TOF $\geq$ 0.9 (min)	Recovery Index (min)
Rapacuronium	1–1.5	15–20	25–50	5–15
Rocuronium	1.5–2.5	35–50	55–80	10–15
Vecuronium	2–3	30–40	50–80	10–20
Pancuronium	3.5–6	70–120	130–220	30–50
Mivacurium	2.5–4.5	15–20	25–40	5–9
Atracurium	2–3	35–50	55–80	10–15
Cis-atracurium	3–6	40–55	60–90	10–15
Alcuronium	3.5–6	80–120	170–240	45–60

Refer to Figure 33–2 for definitions of onset, Dur$_{25}$, train-of-four (TOF) $\geq$ 0.9, and recovery index.

TABLE 33–9.

Muscle Relaxants Used for Rapid Sequence Induction

Muscle Relaxant	"Priming"-Dose (mg/kg)	Intubation Dose (mg/kg)	Complete Recovery (min)
Succinylcholine	None	0.8–1.0	5–10
Succinylcholine	Precurarization	1.5–2.0	5–10
Rocuronium	None	0.6–1.0	60–120
Vecuronium	0.01	0.15–0.4	90–180
Mivacurium	0.02	0.25	25–40
Atracurium	0.05	0.7–0.8	60–90
Cis-atracurium	0.01	0.2–0.4	75–120

Primary goal of a rapid sequence induction is to achieve intubation within the shortest possible time after loss of protective airway reflexes.

content,[65,66] lung infiltrates, pneumonia, and even death.[67] This emphasizes the utmost importance of monitoring neuromuscular block and its residual effects to evaluate the need for prolonged intubation or reversal of the neuromuscular block.

Clinical Pharmacology of Reversal Drugs

The pharmacologic reversal of residual neuromuscular block produced by nondepolarizing neuromuscular blocking drugs is achieved by inhibition of acetylcholinesterase. Inhibition of acetylcholinesterase will lead to increased concentrations of acetylcholine in the synaptic cleft. Because nondepolarizing neuromuscular blocking drugs act through a competitive mechanism, the increase in acetylcholine concentration increases the chance for an acetylcholine molecule to bind to a vacant acetylcholine receptor. Therefore, the likelihood of sufficient acetylcholine receptors to be occupied by acetylcholine and the likelihood for the nerve action potential to be transferred to a muscle membrane potential increases. In addition, the fraction of relaxant not bound to the acetylcholine receptor also increases with a concentration gradient of relaxant decreased away from the neuromuscular junction. The commonly used acetylcholinesterase inhibitors are pyridostigmine (0.25 mg/kg), neostigmine (0.03–0.06 mg/kg), and edrophonium (0.5–1.0 mg/kg). The deeper (more profound) the residual neuromuscular block, the longer the recovery interval for the muscle relaxant action to be reversed, and the greater the dose of reversal drug required. Cholinesterase inhibitors not only inhibit the junctional acetylcholinesterase at the

neuromuscular junction, but also the plasma cholinesterase. Despite this, mivacurium-induced neuromuscular block recovers faster after reversal drugs than after no antagonism.

If a residual neuromuscular blockade is caused by a presynaptic mechanism (e.g., magnesium overdose), calcium can enhance the synthesis and liberation of acetylcholine and therefore act as a reversal drug. A new and thus far clinically untested method of reversing residual neuromuscular block is the concept of direct binding of the relaxant drug by an antibody (e.g., fab fraction) or by chemical interaction. A latter compound currently being investigated in clinical trials is ORG25969, a γ-cyclodextrin derivative with a high affinity for steroid structures. The cyclodextrin forms inactive complexes with steroidal muscle relaxants, with the highest affinity for rocuronium. These complexes are then removed through the kidney. Although the preliminary results seem promising, the full extent of possible side effects remains to be determined.

Pharmacokinetics of Anticholinesterases

Cholinesterase inhibitors are ionized water-soluble molecules, which are eliminated through the kidneys. Renal insufficiency therefore leads to protracted clearance (Table 33–10). Pyridostigmine has a slightly longer duration of action than neostigmine. Any aberrations in the acid-base balance (both acidosis or alkalosis) or the electrolyte status not only prolongs the duration of action of muscle relaxants but also inhibits the action of cholinesterase inhibitors.[55,68] Pancuronium and alcuronium have longer half-lives than pyridostigmine, neostigmine, and edrophonium. Therefore there is a potential for a successfully antagonized

TABLE 33–10.

Pharmacokinetics of Cholinesterase-Inhibitors during Kidney Failure

Cholinesterase Inhibitor	Plasma Clearance (mL/kg/min)		Volume of Distribution (mL/kg)		Elimination Half-time (min)	
	Normal	Kidney Failure	Normal	Kidney Failure	Normal	Kidney Failure
Neostigmine	9.1	4.8–7.8	700	1600	77	181
Pyridostigmine	8.6	2.1–3.1	1100	1200	113	379
Edrophonium	9.5	3.9	1100	1100	110	304

neuromuscular paralysis to re-occur ("recurarization"). This can be prevented by additional subcutaneous injection of half of the dose of the cholinesterase inhibitor.

Side Effects of Anticholinesterases

Inhibition of acetylcholinesterase not only increases the concentration of acetylcholine at the neuromuscular junction but also at all other synapses that use acetylcholine as transmitter. These include the muscarinic receptors of the parasympathetic nervous system, the nicotinic receptors of the autonomic ganglia, and the smooth muscles, especially of the respiratory and gastrointestinal tract. The increase in acetylcholine levels at these parasympathetic sites leads to predictable unwanted side effects (Table 33–11), which can be attenuated with atropine (10–35 µg/kg) or glycopyrrolate (5–20 µg/kg). The dose of parasympatholytic used depends on the dose of cholinesterase inhibitor used. The contraindications and dose restrictions of atropine and glycopyrrolate should be kept in mind.

Factors Confounding the Clinical Pharmacology of Relaxants

Renal Insufficiency and Muscle Relaxants

If renal function is impaired or completely absent, there is reduced clearance (prolonged renal elimination) of both relaxants and cholinesterase inhibitors. However, because the neuromuscular effect of a single injection of a muscle relaxant is mainly terminated by redistribution, reduced renal elimination rate does not usually cause prolonged recovery times after a single dose. After repetitive injections or continuous infusion, however, the decreased renal clearance of relaxants prolongs the neuromuscular effect of muscle relaxants eliminated primarily by the renal route.

TABLE 33–11.

Adverse Effects of Cholinesterase Inhibitors (Pyridostigmine, Edrophonium and Neostigmine)

Cardiovascular system
Bradycardia
Hypotension (Vasodilatation)

Respiratory system
Bronchoconstriction, Bronchorrhea

Central nervous system
Increased postoperative nausea and vomiting

Gastrointestinal system
Hypersalivation, lacrimation
Increased bowel motility

Thus despite the decreased elimination of cholinesterase inhibitors in renal dysfunction, the potential for recurarization exists.

The elimination pathways of cis-atracurium, mivacurium, and rocuronium make their terminal elimination mainly independent of renal function. However, even these primarily kidney-independent pathways are often impaired by concomitant diseases (Table 33–12). The activity of pseudocholinesterase is reduced in renal failure, probably related to its loss through dialysis filter membranes and its reduced synthesis from uremic hepatopathy. This leads to a prolonged effect of succinylcholine[69] and mivacurium.[70] In addition, altered fluid balance during dialysis changes the V_d of the muscle relaxants, making it difficult to predict their neuromuscular blocking effect. Changes in acid base balance and electrolyte status can also influence the clinical response to muscle relaxants.

TABLE 33–12.

Pharmacokinetic Parameters in Normal, and Hepatic or Renal Failure

	Plasma Clearance (mL/kg/min)			Volume of Distribution (mL/kg)			Elimination Half-life (min)		
	Normal	Kidney Failure	Liver Failure	Normal	Kidney Failure	Liver Failure	Normal	Kidney Failure	Liver Failure
Atracurium	6.8	5.5–7.0	6.5–8.0	172	140–220	200–280	21	18–25	20–25
Cis-atracurium	4.3–5.3	3.8	6.6	195	161	161	22–30	25–34	24
Mivacurium	1.8	1.8	0.9	112	112	124	1–3	—	—
Vecuronium	3.0–5.3	2.5–4.5	2.4–4.3	200–510	240–470	210–250	50–110	80–150	49–98
Rocuronium	2.9	3	3	175	260	320	87	97	97
Pancuronium	1.8	0–0.9	1.1–1.5	274	210–260	310–430	132	240–1050	208–270

Hepatic Diseases and Muscle Relaxants

Liver failure is often associated with secondary hyperaldosteronism, which results in fluid retention and an increase in the V_d of muscle relaxants. Consequently, greater than normal doses must be administered to achieve a given level of paralysis. The higher dose, once administered, may stay in the central compartment for a longer time because of poor elimination by the liver. Therefore, patients with hepatobiliary diseases often have a prolonged duration of action of muscle relaxants. After a single dose, however, the elimination (clearance) times are relatively unimportant because redistribution within the compartments is the major factor determining duration of action. However, after repetitive or continuous administration, vecuronium, rocuronium, and pancuronium accumulation occurs, because their elimination is partly dependent on hepatic function. Plasma-cholinesterase activity is also decreased in liver dysfunction because of decreased synthesis; the ester hydrolysis of mivacurium is proportionately reduced.[71] The elimination times for atracurium and cis-atracurium are independent of hepatic function. Because cis-atracurium is prescribed in lower doses due to its higher potency, a relatively smaller amount of laudanosine is produced. The plasma protein deficiency associated with liver failure hardly increases the free fraction of muscle relaxant since the overall plasma protein binding of relaxants is relatively low.

Neuromuscular Diseases and Muscle Relaxants

The integrity and function of presynaptic structures is important for development, function, and maintenance of the neuromuscular endplate.[72] Any neuromuscular disease that influences nerve conduction or electrical activity of the muscle membrane therefore influences neuromuscular architecture and receptor function. These changes in turn can affect the response to a relaxant (Fig. 33–7).

Increased Expression of the Acetylcholine Receptor

When innervation and electrical conductivity are established between muscle and nerve, the mature receptors are localized to the neuromuscular junction. Deprivation of the neural influences to the muscle leads to an up-regulation of acetylcholine receptors, as well as a spread of the receptors away from the neuromuscular junction into the perijunctional and extrajunctional areas. During this time, receptors containing a γ-subunit, rather than an ε-subunit, termed *fetal*

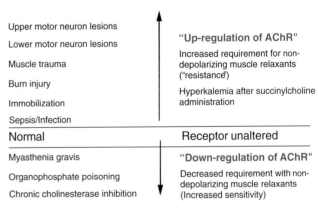

Figure 33–7. Diseases with altered acetylcholine receptor (AChR) expression.

or *immature* receptors, are re-expressed (see section 2.3.). The ligand sensitivity and affinity of these immature receptors are altered. Agonists such as succinylcholine depolarize immature receptors more easily and can lead to altered and exaggerated cation fluxes. Clinically, this means that less succinylcholine is needed to open the receptor channels. Because potassium is transported from intracellular to extracellular fluid during channel opening, the up-regulated acetylcholine receptors can efflux dangerously high levels of potassium into the bloodstream. Conversely, the increased number of acetylcholine receptors in the perijunctional area results in increased margin of safety for neuromuscular block in terms of response to muscle relaxants and leads to a resistance to nondepolarizing neuromuscular blocking drugs. Examples of diseases that induce an up-regulation of acetylcholine receptors are denervation, immobilization, burns, and possibly sepsis, as well as chronic neuromuscular blockade (see Fig. 33–7).[73]

Lower and Upper Motor Neuron Lesion

The potential for succinylcholine-induced hyperkalemia after lower motor neuron lesion has been well established.[74] An increase in sensitivity to succinylcholine is already present 3 to 4 days after denervation and reaches a critical level after 7 to 8 days. Because the reason for this agonist hypersensitivity is up-regulated acetylcholine receptors, patients also display a resistance to nondepolarizing neuromuscular blocking drugs. The shorter the nerve segment distal to the lesion, the earlier the receptors are up-regulated.[75] However, even a polyneuropathy, in the absence of a complete transection of the nerve, can cause a high potassium response to succinylcholine.[76,77] Lesions such as strokes, cerebral hemorrhage,[78] head trauma,[79] multiple sclerosis,[80] syringomyelia, and paraplegia or quadriplegia[81] also result in up-regulated acetylcholine receptors, with the potential of hypersensitivity toward succinylcholine and resistance toward nondepolarizing neuromuscular blocking drugs. Upper motor neuron lesions can lead to unilateral or bilateral changes, whereas lower motor neuron injury causes changes only in the distribution of the affected nerve. The exact time period over which the receptors remain up-regulated remains unclear. There have been reports of increased succinylcholine sensitivity present several years after the nerve injury.[78] The risk for hyperkalemia after upper or lower motor neuron injury is probably absent once resistance to nondepolarizing muscle relaxants disappears, but no studies have defined this period. Because it is difficult to predict how a patient with neurologic symptoms will react to muscle relaxants, succinylcholine should be avoided and neuromuscular function should be monitored when using nondepolarizing muscle relaxants.

Immobilization

The physiologic state of immobilization contrasts with denervation syndromes in that there is no direct damage to cord or nerve roots, and the muscle fibers remain innervated. However, immobilization (from isolated limbs with plaster cast to total body immobilization in an ICU setting) also induces an up-regulation of acetylcholine receptors.[82,83] The peak effect on acetylcholine receptor regulation occurs at 14 days after onset of immobilization, but the duration of this change is unclear in humans.[83]

Burn Injury

Burn injury induces an up-regulation of acetylcholine receptors in the musculature underneath the burn site, but not at distant muscles.[84] The iatrogenically induced immobilization in bed may, however, cause receptor changes even in distant muscles. There is no evidence that the burn injury per se leads to a direct chemical or physical denervation, because the mRNA for all (α, β, δ, γ, and ϵ) subunits are *not* increased, as in denervation. To what extent circulating mediators or the inhibition of cell signaling pathways is involved in the up-regulation remains to be investigated. Burn of a single limb (8–9% body surface area) is sufficient to cause lethal hyperkalemia after succinylcholine.[85] The prolonged administration of muscle relaxants to facilitate mechanical ventilation can accentuate the up-regulation.[86] Because it takes some time to initiate the up-regulation, it is safe to use succinylcholine for up to 48 hours after acute burn injury. Any use beyond this time point, however, should be avoided.[87]

Infection and Systemic Inflammation

The effect of systemic inflammation and infectious diseases on acetylcholine receptor remains controversial. There have been reports of hyperkalemia after succinylcholine administration in septic patients.[88,89] However, it is difficult in critically ill patients receiving intensive care treatment to isolate the factor of infection/inflammation per se from concomitant factors such as immobilization, long-term administration of muscle relaxants, or steroid treatment. Other than an increase in acetylcholine receptors, the resistance toward nondepolarizing muscle relaxants can also be explained by increased binding to acute phase reactant proteins, namely α_1-acid glycoprotein, which is increased in inflammatory processes and can bind to nondepolarizing muscle relaxants. In rodents, inflammation alone has not been shown to increase acetylcholine receptors, but does cause increased protein binding of the relaxant.[90] A completely new pathophysiology behind acetylcholine receptor regulation was recently reported. In rats, after induction of a chronic abdominal infection, autoantibodies to the acetylcholine receptor could be detected, which lead to a decrease in receptor number, creating a myasthenia gravis-like clinical picture.[91] The clinical significance of this is unclear.

Decreased Number of Acetylcholine Receptors

Myasthenia Gravis

Myasthenia gravis is an autoimmune disease, with the clinical picture of increasing muscle weakness and fatigue. Antibodies against the acetylcholine receptor are present in approximately 80% of the patients ("antibody-positive"). Some of the "antibody-negative" patients have antibodies against a receptor tyrosine kinase, Muscle-Specific Kinase, important for the clustering and maturation of the receptors at the neuromuscular junction.[92] It is therefore likely that antibody-negative patients may have antibodies against other proteins related to the neuromuscular junction. The autoantibodies to the acetylcholine receptor in myasthenics leads to a decrease in receptor number. Interestingly, the level of antibody correlates poorly with the clinical status. Symptoms of myasthenic patients generally start with ptosis and diplopia, and proceed to bulbar paralysis. In the later stages of the disease, dysarthria, dysphagia, and weakness of extremities and of respiratory muscles occur.[93,94] Therapeutic approach to myasthenia, aside from thymectomy (to remove the origin of the autoantibodies), is the administration of cholinesterase inhibitors (mostly pyridostigmine). Because of the down-regulation of acetylcholine receptors, patients with myasthenia are sensitive to nondepolarizing muscle relaxants. If muscle relaxants are used during clinical anesthesia, neuromuscular function monitoring throughout the duration of anesthesia is advisable. The reduced number of acetylcholine receptors, however, also means that succinylcholine cannot depolarize the endplate effectively. This also results in a greater dose requirement for succinylcholine. For rapid sequence induction, it is advisable to increase the dose of succinylcholine to 1.5 to 2 mg/kg. Greater doses, however, may cause a nondepolarizing block (see "Phase II Block" and "Desensitization Block"). The continuation of the treatment of myasthenics with cholinesterase inhibitors, during the perioperative period, can cause delayed hydrolysis of succinylcholine and a prolongation of the neuromuscular block.[95]

Lambert-Eaton Myasthenic Syndrome

Lambert-Eaton myasthenic syndrome is a paraneoplastic disease associated with small-cell carcinoma of various tissue (usually lung) origin. It is an autoimmune disorder caused by the presence of antibodies directed against the PQ-type, voltage-gated calcium channels,[96] possibly because of a cross-reaction with the calcium channels on the carcinomatous cells.[94] It is therefore caused by a prejunctional mechanism resulting in a decreased quantal release of acetylcholine. The acetylcholine receptor number on the postsynaptic membrane remains normal. Clinically, patients with Lambert-Eaton syndrome display an increased sensitivity to both nondepolarizing and depolarizing muscle relaxants.[97] Again, monitoring neuromuscular function during use of muscle relaxants will provide continuous assessment. In contrast to myasthenia gravis, repetitive stimulation (e.g., TOF) results in enhancement, and not fade, of twitch.

Interaction of Relaxants with Other Drugs

Although some drugs have neuromuscular effects, because of the high margin of safety of neuromuscular transmission,

the effects can often be seen only as a potentiation of muscle relaxant effect. The neuromuscular effect of these "nonmuscle relaxant" drugs are dose-dependent and the onset is much slower than the muscle relaxants themselves. The neuromuscular effect of nonmuscle relaxants, however, can outlast the primary effects of the relaxant drug. Clinically relevant interactions between these drugs and muscle relaxants can be classified into three main areas: pharmacokinetic, junctional, and muscular effects.

Pharmacokinetic Interaction of Relaxants with Other Drugs

Hemodynamic effects of drugs coadministered with relaxants can affect the onset time of muscle relaxants. This can play a major role in a rapid sequence induction. If these drugs decrease the cardiac output or decrease muscle perfusion, onset time of muscle paralysis will be slowed. Steroidal muscle relaxants are eliminated or metabolized by the liver to a greater (e.g., rocuronium) or lesser (e.g., pancuronium) extent (see Table 33–2). Drugs that inhibit the cytochrome P450 enzyme system (e.g., cimetidine) or reduce liver perfusion delay hepatic elimination and prolong the effect of muscle relaxants when high doses are administered.[98] Conversely, drugs that induce the cytochrome P450 system (e.g., antiepileptic drugs), increase the rate of elimination of hepatic metabolized drugs. Thus the requirement for drugs such as vecuronium and rocuronium is increased, but not for drugs such as mivacurium, which is metabolized independent of the liver.[99–102]

Relaxant and Nonrelaxant Interaction at the Neuromuscular Junction

Neuromuscular transmission can be influenced by drugs, which have actions on the nerve terminal or receptor. Presynaptically, three mechanisms have been identified, all of which decrease the release of acetylcholine. First, cyclic adenosine monophosphate and adenosine triphosphate are necessary to synthesize acetylcholine. Furosemide is a drug, which inhibits the synthesis of the former, thereby also decreasing presynaptic acetylcholine synthesis. Second, volatile anesthetics block presynaptic acetylcholine receptors, which decreases the availability of acetylcholine at the presynaptic membrane during repetitive stimulation. Finally, volatile anesthetics, magnesium,[103,104] calcium antagonists, and aminoglycoside antibiotics[105] reduce acetylcholine release by blocking presynaptic calcium channels. Postsynaptically, numerous drugs block the α-subunit of the acetylcholine receptor in a dose-dependent fashion. These include: inhalational anesthetics,[106] aminoglycoside antibiotics,[107] quinidine,[108] tricyclic antidepressants,[109] ketamine,[110] midazolam,[111] and barbiturates.[112] Aside from binding to the α-subunit, these drugs often also block the channel itself, or desensitize the acetylcholine receptor by allosteric mechanisms (see "Phase II Block," "Desensitization Block," and "Channel Block"). Which of these mechanisms has the greatest effect on neuromuscular transmission and potentiate muscle relaxants is difficult to determine.

Muscular Effects of Other Drugs

Dantrolene inhibits calcium release and its re-uptake into the sarcoplasmatic reticulum and is used for treatment of malignant hyperthermia. It can potentiate the effects of nondepolarizing muscle relaxants at a muscular level without having any effect on neuromuscular transmission.[113] The effects of dantrolene cannot be monitored electromyographically but only using mechanomyography.

Practical Aspects of Drug Administration

Few surgical procedures absolutely require continuous neuromuscular paralysis. In many cases, it is not necessary to continue paralysis after intubation. Operations in the abdomen usually require relaxation. If the depth of anesthesia is not sufficient and cannot be achieved because of other factors (e.g., hemodynamic instability), the patient might move or cough. If this must be avoided, one can either give repetitive doses of muscle relaxant or start an infusion with close monitoring of neuromuscular function. The infusion rate is determined by the clearance of the drug during steady-state and the V_d (see Table 33–3), both of which can vary greatly from patient to patient (see Table 33–12). The most commonly used muscle relaxants for infusion are mivacurium or cis-atracurium, because they do not accumulate, and their off-set indices stay the same even after repetitive injection or continuous infusion (Table 33–13).[114,115]

TABLE 33–13.

Infusion Rates for a Continuous Neuromuscular Block and Clinical Recovery after Continuous Infusion

	IR_{90}-IR_{95} (µg/kg/min)	Recovery Time Until T1/T4 > 0.9 (min)
Mivacurium	3–15	10–20*
Atracurium	4–12	30–70*
Cis-atracurium	0.4–4	30–70*
Rocuronium	3–12	30–90†

IR_{90}, Infusion rate for a 90% neuromuscular block; IR_{95}, infusion rate for a 95% neuromuscular block; recovery until T1/T4 > 0.9 (min), time from end of infusion until complete neuromuscular recovery.

*Independent of infusion time.

†Recovery after infusion of up to 2 hours is significantly increased compared with single-shot injection.

Differential Diagnosis and Therapy of Residual Neuromuscular Block

Before reversal of residual neuromuscular block, the presence or absence of paralysis should be evaluated. The TOF ratio is the common method of assessment of muscle weakness, and a ratio of ≥0.9 is usually recommended for full recovery from paralysis.[31,64,65] If a nondepolarizing neuromuscular blocking drug was used, the muscle weakness might be caused by delayed elimination of or increased sensitivity to the drug. After the use of reversal drugs (anticholinesterases), patients should be closely monitored in the recovery room, because the half-life of the reversal drug might be shorter than that of the muscle relaxant, thus recurarization can occur.

If succinylcholine or mivacurium was used, the underlying cause could be a plasma cholinesterase deficiency or atypical plasma cholinesterases. In both cases, antagonism with cholinesterase inhibitors will not be of much benefit. Patients should be mechanically ventilated until spontaneous recovery occurs, after renal elimination of the drug. This may take as long as 4 to 6 hours. The activity of the plasma cholinesterase should be determined. If the activity of the plasma cholinesterase is reduced because of a genetic factor, the patient should be advised about this so that the same complication can be avoided in future anesthetic procedures.

Use of Muscle Relaxants During Rapid Sequence Induction

In patients with increased risk for aspiration of gastric contents, one of the goals during induction of anesthesia is to secure the airway as quickly as possible. As stated earlier, succinylcholine is the only drug currently available to achieve this. However, succinylcholine has clinically relevant side effects (see Table 33–5). Myalgias are treated either with analgesics or by reducing muscle fasciculations. To what extent opioids are beneficial for succinylcholine-induced myalgia remains to be answered.[56] It is most common in clinical practice to treat myalgias after the fact with nonsteroidal anti-inflammatory drugs. Prophylactic administration of nonsteroidal anti-inflammatory drugs can also be beneficial. Both options, however, should be carefully reviewed in terms of bleeding complications.[116] Prevention of muscle fasciculations not only reduces the incidence of myalgias but also attenuates increases in intraocular[117] and intragastric[55] pressures. The clinically most applied method to reduce fasciculations is by "precurarization," which implies the administration of a small dose of nondepolarizing muscle relaxant (e.g., 0.05 mg vecuronium) preceding the administration of succinylcholine. Preadministration of small doses of succinylcholine ("self-taming"),[54] lidocaine (100 mg),[55] or opioids[56] are alternative strategies. In one study, 37.5% of precurarized patients showed paralytic symptoms such as diplopia, heavy eyelids, difficulty with speech, and swallowing. In some patients, other signs of respiratory insufficiency were noted.[118] This suggests that precurarization has its own problems and side effects.

The efficacy of precurarization in terms of reducing fasciculations is undisputed. The basis for this effect is the antagonism of the depolarizing effect of succinylcholine by the blocking effect of nondepolarizing muscle relaxant at the presynaptic and postsynaptic acetylcholine receptors. However, because the antagonism also affects the actual mechanism of action of succinylcholine, precurarization leads to prolonged onset time, shorter duration of action, and reduced maximal neuromuscular block.[119] To overcome these effects, an increased dose of succinylcholine by approximately 25% to 75% is recommended (1.05–2.0 mg/kg).[120] Our experience, however, indicates that an increase in succinylcholine dose also increases the probability for muscle fasciculations. A higher dose of succinylcholine after precurarization and a normal dose without precurarization may show no difference in terms of incidence of muscle fasciculations.

Succinylcholine can induce bradycardia, especially in children. This side effect is prevented by premedication with atropine, which at the same time can cause tachycardia. This tachycardia can confound the assessment of depth of anesthesia and fluid status. It remains to be demonstrated if a reduction of succinylcholine dose used for intubation can reduce bradycardias as effectively as premedication with atropine. Precurarization with nondepolarizing muscle relaxants does not affect muscarinic receptors and therefore does not prevent the cardiac effects of succinylcholine.

Since the introduction of short- and medium-acting nondepolarizing muscle relaxants, the indications for use of succinylcholine in patients not at risk for aspiration of stomach contents is decreasing. For patients in which rapid sequence induction is indicated, the goal of administering muscle relaxants is to achieve fast and complete muscle paralysis, ideal for rapid intubation. This goal, however, is not evidence based—i.e., there is no controlled study showing the benefit of rapid sequence induction itself or the specific impact of succinylcholine use on patient outcome. Conversely, generations of anesthetists believe that rapid sequence induction is a useful tool for anesthesiologists and that succinylcholine is the neuromuscular blocking drug that is best in this context.[121] All other pharmacologic attempts to either reduce the side effects of succinylcholine or to replace succinylcholine with other drugs have their own unwanted effects that can be more dangerous than the potential side effects of succinnylcholine.[122]

Sustained Neuromuscular Block in the Critically Ill Patient

Continuous administration of neuromuscular blocking drugs in the ICU is primarily performed to facilitate mechanical ventilation or to manage patients with head trauma. The cause of prolonged muscle weakness in patients in the ICU has always been uncertain and is multifactorial. Extended use of muscle relaxants, however, definitely plays a role in the muscle weakness. It is well known that prolonged disruption of neuromuscular transmission can cause profound changes at the neuromuscular junction resulting in aberrant

responses to future use of both depolarizing and nondepolarizing muscle relaxants. Therefore, the American College of Critical Care Medicine has published clinical practice guidelines for the sustained neuromuscular block in the adult critically ill patient[123] (see later).

Before initiating neuromuscular block, patients should be medicated with sedative and analgesic drugs to provide adequate sedation and analgesia. Only after all other means have been tried without success should neuromuscular blocking drugs be added to the armamentarium. Indications for muscle relaxant therapy could include facilitation of mechanical ventilation, prevention of increased intracranial pressure during coughing and suctioning, treatment of muscle spasms (e.g., tetanus), and decrease of oxygen consumption. Patients receiving neuromuscular blocking drugs should be monitored with a nerve stimulator, with the goal of adjusting the dose to achieve at least one twitch during TOF pattern of stimulation. Regular discontinuation of the administered neuromuscular blocking drugs until forced to restart them, based on the patient's condition, might be beneficial to the patient in terms of decreasing the incidence of neuromuscular complications during prolonged use.

Pancuronium or vecuronium are popular choices for relaxants in the ICU because they are inexpensive. However, for patients in whom vagolysis is contraindicated (i.e., those with cardiovascular disease), neuromuscular blocking drugs other than pancuronium should be used. The steroidal relaxants have also been implicated to have more profound effects on the muscle, potentiating the effect of endogenous and exogenous steroids. This hypothesis has not been proved convincingly. For patients receiving neuromuscular blocking drugs and corticosteroids, every effort should be made to discontinue neuromuscular blocking drugs as soon as possible. Because of their unique metabolism (Hoffmann degradation) cis-atracurium is recommended for patients with significant hepatic or renal disease. If tachyphylaxis to one neuromuscular blocking drug develops, a different neuromuscular blocking drug could be tried, although cross-tolerance does exist. In general, all patients receiving neuromuscular blocking drugs should have prophylactic eye care, physical therapy, and prophylaxis for deep vein thrombosis.[123]

References

1. Bernard C: Lecon sur les effets de substances toxiques et medicamenteuses. Paris, Bailliere, 1851, pp 164–190.
2. Bernard C: Etudes Etudes physiologiques sur quelques poisons americains. Rev Deux Mondes 53:164–190, 1864.
3. Catterall WA: Structure and regulation of voltage-gated Ca2+ channels. Annu Rev Cell Dev Biol 16:521–555, 2000.
4. Calakos N, Scheller RH: Synaptic vesicle biogenesis, docking, and fusion: A molecular description. Physiol Rev 76:1–29, 1996.
5. Rash JE, Walrond JP, Morita M: Structural and functional correlates of synaptic transmission in the vertebrate neuromuscular junction. J Electron Microsc Tech 10:153–185, 1988.
6. Paton WD, Waud DR: The margin of safety of neuromuscular transmission. J Physiol (Lond) 191:59–90, 1967.
7. Gu Y, Hall ZW: Immunological evidence for a change in subunits of the acetylcholine receptor in developing and denervated rat muscle. Neuron 1:117–125, 1988.

8. Fambrough DM: Control of acetylcholine receptors in skeletal muscle. Physiol Rev 59:165–227, 1979.

9. Maclagan J, Vrbova G: A study of the increased sensitivity of denervated and re-innervated muscle to depolarizing drugs. J Physiol (Lond) 182:131–143, 1966.

10. Leonard S, Bertrand D: Neuronal nicotinic receptors: From structure to function. Nicotine Tob Res 3:203–223, 2001.

11. Lingle CJ, Steinbach JH: Neuromuscular blocking agents. Int Anaesthesiol Clin 26:288–301, 1988.

12. Martyn JAJ, Standaert FG, Miller RD: In Miller RD (ed): Neuromuscular Physiology and Pharmacology, Anesthesia, 5th ed. New York, Churchill Livingstone, 1999, pp 735–751.

13. Prince RJ, Sine SM: The ligand binding domains of the nicotinic acetylcholine receptor. In Barrantes FJ (ed): The Nicotinic Acetylcholine Receptor: Current Views and Future Trends. Berlin, Springer-Verlag, 1988, pp 32–59.

14. Adams PR, Sakmann B: Decamethonium both opens and blocks endplate channels. Proc Natl Acad Sci USA 75:2994–2998, 1978.

15. Marshall CG, Ogden DC, Colquhoun D: The actions of suxamethonium (succinyldicholine) as an agonist and channel blocker at the nicotinic receptor of frog muscle. J Physiol 428:155–174, 1990.

16. King H: Curare alkaloids. Part I. Tubocurarine. Journal of the Chemical Society London 57:1381–1389, 1935.

17. Griffith HR, Johnson GE: The use of curare in general anesthesia. Anesthesiology 3:418–420, 1942.

18. Hunt R, Taveau RdM: On physiological action of certain choline derivates and new methods for detecing choline. Br Med II 1906, p 1788.

19. Bovet D: Some aspects of the relationship between chemical structure and curare-like activity. Ann NY Acad Sci 54:407–410, 1951.

20. Baird WL, Reid AM: The neuromuscular blocking properties of a new steroid compound, pancuronium bromide. A pilot study in man. Br J Anaesth 39:775–780, 1967.

21. Bowmann WC, Rodger IW, Houston J, et al: Structure: action relationships among some desacetoxy analogues of pancuronium and vecuronium in the anesthetized cat. Anesthesiology 69:57–62, 1988.

22. Kopman AF, Klewicka MM, Kopman DJ, Neuman GG: Molar potency is predictive of the speed of onset of neuromuscular block for agents of intermediate, short, and ultrashort duration. Anesthesiology 90:425–431, 1999.

23. Szenohradszky J, Trevor AJ, Bickler P, et al: Central nervous system effects of intrathecal muscle relaxants in rats. Anesth Analg 76:1304–1309, 1993.

24. Cardone C, Szenohradszky J, Spencer Y, Bickler P: Activation of brain acetylcholine receptors by neuromuscular blocking drugs. Anesthesiology 80:1155–1161, 1994.

25. Lowman MA, Rees PH, Benyon RC, Church MK: Human mast cell heterogeneity: Histamine release from mast cells dispersed from skin, lung, adenoids, tonsils, and colon in response to IgE-dependent and nonimmunologic stimuli. J Allergy Clin Immunol 81:590–597, 1988.

26. Lien CA, Belmont MR, Abalos A, et al: The cardiovascular effects and histamine-releasing properties of 51W89 in patients receiving nitrous oxide/opioid/barbiturate anesthesia. Anesthesiology 82:1131–1138, 1995.

27. Levy JH, Pitts M, Thanopoulos A, et al: The effects of rapacuronium on histamine release and hemodynamics in adult patients undergoing general anesthesia. Anesth Analg 89:290–295, 1999.

28. Blobner M, Mirakhur RK, Wierda JM, et al: Rapacuronium 2.0 or 2.5 mg kg-1 for rapid-sequence induction: Comparison with succinylcholine 1.0 mg kg-1. Br J Anaesth 85:724–731, 2000.

29. Scott RP, Savarese JJ, Basta SJ, et al: Atracurium: Clinical strategies for preventing histamine release and attenuating the haemodynamic response. Br J Anaesth 57:550–553, 1985.

30. Laxenaire MC: [Epidemiology of anesthetic anaphylactoid reactions. Fourth multicenter survey (July 1994-December 1996)]. Ann Fr Anesth Reanim 18:796–809, 1999.

31. Eriksson LI: Residual neuromuscular blockade. Incidence and relevance. Anaesthesist 1:S18–19, 2000.

32. Berry FA Jr: Intramuscular rocuronium in infants and children—is there a need? Anesthesiology 85:229–230, 1996.

33. Waser PG, Wiederkehr H, Sin-Ren AC, Kaiser-Schonenberger E: Distribution and kinetics of 14C-vecuronium in rats and mice. Br J Anaesth 59:1044–1051, 1987.

34. Savarese JJ, Ali HH, Basta SJ, et al: The clinical neuromuscular pharmacology of mivacurium chloride (BW B1090U): A short-acting nondepolarizing ester neuromuscular blocking drug. Anesthesiology 68:723–732, 1988.

35. Iwasaki H, Igarashi M, Yamauchi M, Namiki A: The effect of cardiac output on the onset of neuromuscular block by vecuronium. Anaesthesia 50:361–362, 1995.

36. Donati F, Meistelman C, Plaud B: Vecuronium neuromuscular blockade at the diaphragm, the orbicularis oculi, and adductor pollicis muscles. Anesthesiology 73:870–875, 1990.

37. Parker CJ, Hunter JM: Relationship between volume of distribution of atracurium and body weight. Br J Anaesth 70:443–445, 1993.

38. Goudsouzian NG, Martyn JJ, Liu LM, Ali HH: The dose response effect of long-acting nondepolarizing neuromuscular blocking agents in children. Can Anaesth Soc J 31:246–250, 1984.

39. Fisher DM, Miller RD: Neuromuscular effects of vecuronium (ORG NC45) in infants and children during N_2O, halothane anesthesia. Anesthesiology 58:519–523, 1983.

40. Courtney J, Steinbach JH: Age changes in neuromuscular junction morphology and acetylcholine receptor distribution on rat skeletal muscle fibres. J Physiol 320:435–447, 1981.

41. Sanes JR, Lichtman JW: Induction, assembly, maturation and maintenance of a postsynaptic apparatus. Nat Rev Neurosci 2:791–805, 2001.

42. Matteo RS, Backus WW, McDaniel DD, et al: Pharmacokinetics and pharmacodynamics of d-tubocurarine and metocurine in the elderly. Anesth Analg 64:23–29, 1985.

43. Yang HS, Goudsouzian NG, Cheng M, Martyn JA: The influence of the age of the rat on the neuromuscular response to mivacurium in vitro. Paediatr Anaesth 6:367–672, 1996.

44. Guay J, Grenier Y, Varin F: Clinical pharmacokinetics of neuromuscular relaxants in pregnancy. Clin Pharmacokinet 34:483, 1998.

45. Smeulers NJ, Wierda JM, van den Broek L, et al: Hypothermic cardiopulmonary bypass influences the concentration-response relationship and the biodisposition of rocuronium. Eur J Anaesthesiol Suppl 11:91–94, 1995.

46. Leslie K, Sessler DI, Bjorksten AR, Moayeri A: Mild hypothermia alters propofol pharmacokinetics and increases the duration of action of atracurium. Anesth Analg 80:1007–1014, 1995.

47. Rump AF, Schierholz J, Biederbick W, et al: Pseudocholinesterase-activity reduction during cardiopulmonary bypass: The role of dilutional processes and pharmacological agents. Gen Pharmacol 32:65–69, 1999.

48. Kalow W, Genest K: A method for the detection of atypical forms of human serum cholinesterase. Determination of dibucaine numbers. Can J Biochem Physiol 35:339–346, 1957.

48a. Martyn JAJ, Chang Y, Goudsouzian NG, Patel SS: Pharmacodynamics of mivacurium chloride in 13- to 18-year-old adolescents with thermal injury. Br J Anaesth 89:580–585, 2002.

49. Welch RM, Brown A, Ravitch J, Dahl R: The in vitro degradation of cisatracurium, the R, cis-R′-isomer of atracurium, in human and rat plasma. Clin Pharmacol Ther 58:132–142, 1995.

50. Thesleff S: Farmakologiska och kliniska forsok med L.T.I. (O,O-succinylcholine jodid). Nord Med 46:1045, 1951.

51. Mayrhofer OMH: Kurz wirkende Muskelerschlaffungsmittel. Selbstversuche und klinische Erprobung am narkotisierten Menschen. Wien Klin Wochenschr 63:885–889, 1951.

52. Foldes FF, Rendell-Baker L, Birch J: Causes and prevention of prolonged apnea with succinylcholine. Anesth Analg 25:609, 1956.

53. Mayrhofer O: Die Wirksamkeit von d-Tubocurarin zur Verhütung der Muskelschmerzen nach Succinylcholin. Der Anaesthesist 8:313–315, 1959.

54. Wald-Oboussier G, Lohmann C, Viell B, Doehn M: ["Self-taming": An alternative to the prevention of succinylcholine-induced pain]. Anaesthesist 36:426–430, 1987.

55. Miller RD, Way WL: Inhibition of succinylcholine-induced increased intragastric pressure by nondepolarizing muscle relaxants and lidocaine. Anesthesiology 34:185–188, 1971.

56. Polarz H, Bohrer H, Fleischer F, et al: Effects of thiopentone/suxamethonium on intraocular pressure after pretreatment with alfentanil. Eur J Clin Pharmacol 43:311–313, 1992.

57. Kovarik WD, Mayberg TS, Lam AM, et al: Succinylcholine does not change intracranial pressure, cerebral blood flow velocity, or the electroencephalogram in patients with neurologic injury. Anesth Analg 73:469–473, 1994.

58. Schow AJ, Lubarsky DA, Olson RP, Gan TJ: Can succinylcholine be used safely in hyperkalemic patients? Anesth Analg 95:119–122, 2002.

59. Baillard C, Gehan G, Reboul-Marty J, et al: Residual curarization in the recovery room after vecuronium. Br J Anaesth 84:394–395, 2000.

60. Hayes AH, Mirakhur RK, Breslin DS, et al: Postoperative residual block after intermediate-acting neuromuscular blocking drugs. Anaesthesia 56:312–318, 2001.

61. Viby-Mogensen J, Chraemer Jorgensen B, Ording H: Residual curarization in the recovery room. Anesthesiology 50:539–541, 1979.

62. Eriksson LI: The effects of residual neuromuscular blockade and volatile anesthetics on the control of ventilation. Anesth Analg 89:243–251, 1999.

63. Eriksson LI: Reduced hypoxic chemosensitivity in partially paralysed man. A new property of muscle relaxants? Acta Anaesthesiol Scand 40:520–523, 1996.

64. Eriksson LI, Sato M, Severinghaus JW: Effect of a vecuronium-induced partial neuromuscular block on hypoxic ventilatory response. Anesthesiology 78:693–699, 1993.

65. Eriksson LI, Sundman E, Olsson R, et al: Functional assessment of the pharynx at rest and during swallowing in partially paralyzed humans: Simultaneous videomanometry and mechanomyography of awake human volunteers. Anesthesiology 87:1035–1043, 1997.

66. Sundman E, Witt H, Olsson R, et al: The incidence and mechanisms of pharyngeal and upper esophageal dysfunction in partially paralyzed humans: Pharyngeal videoradiography and simultaneous manometry after atracurium. Anesthesiology 92:977–984, 2000.

67. Berg H: Is residual neuromuscular block following pancuronium a risk factor for postoperative pulmonary complications? Acta Anaesthesiol Scand Suppl 110:156–158, 1997.

68. Miller RD, Van Nyhuis LS, Eger EI 2nd, Way WL: The effect of acid-base balance on neostigmine antagonism of d-tubocurarine-induced neuromuscular blockade. Anesthesiology 42:377–383, 1975.

69. Ryan DW: Preoperative serum cholinesterase concentration in chronic renal failure. Clinical experience of suxamethonium in 81 patients undergoing renal transplant. Br J Anaesth 49:945–949, 1977.

70. Cook DR, Freeman JA, Lai AA, et al: Pharmacokinetics of Mivacurium in normal patients and in those with hepatic or renal failure. Br J Anaesth 69:580–585, 1992.

71. Martyn JA, Goudsouzian NG, Chang Y, et al: Neuromuscular effects of mivacurium in 2- to 12-yr-old children with burn injury. Anesthesiology 92:31–37, 2000.

72. Mathiesen I, Rimer M, Ashtari O, et al: Regulation of the size and distribution of agrin-induced postsynaptic-like apparatus in adult skeletal muscle by electrical muscle activity. Mol Cell Neurosci 13:207–217, 1999.

73. Martyn JAJ, White DA, Gronert GA, et al: Up-and-down regulation of sceletal muscle acetylcholine receptors. Anesthesiology 76:822–843, 1992.

74. John DA, Tobey RE, Homer LD, Rice CL: Onset of succinylcholine-induced hyperkalemia following denervation. Anesthesiology 45:294–299, 1976.

75. McArdle JJ: Molecular aspects of the trophic influence of nerve on muscle. Prog Neurobiol 21:135–198, 1983.

76. Fergusson RJ, Wright DJ, Willey RF, et al: Suxamethonium is dangerous in polyneuropathy. Br Med J (Clin Res Ed) 282:298–299, 1981.

77. Hogue CW Jr, Itani MS, Martyn JA: Resistance to d-tubocurarine in lower motor neuron injury is related to increased acetylcholine receptors at the neuromuscular junction. Anesthesiology 73:703–709, 1990.

78. Cooperman LH: Succinylcholine-induced hyperkalemia in neuromuscular disease. JAMA 213:1867–1871, 1970.

79. Frankville DD, Drummond JC: Hyperkalemia after succinylcholine administration in a patient with closed head injury without paresis. Anesthesiology 67:264–266, 1987.

80. Brett RS, Schmidt JH, Gage JS, et al: Measurement of acetylcholine receptor concentration in skeletal muscle from a patient with multiple sclerosis and resistance to atracurium. Anesthesiology 66:837–839, 1987.

81. Tobey RE: Paraplegia, succinylcholine and cardiac arrest. Anesthesiology 32:359–364, 1970.

82. Ibebunjo C, Martyn JA: Fiber atrophy, but not changes in acetylcholine receptor expression, contributes to the muscle dysfunction after immobilization. Crit Care Med 27:275–285, 1999.

83. Ibebunjo C, Nosek MT, Itani MS, Martyn JA: Mechanisms for the paradoxical resistance to d-tubocurarine during immobilization-induced muscle atrophy. J Pharmacol Exp Ther 283:443–451, 1997.

84. Ward JM, Martyn JA: Burn injury-induced nicotinic acetylcholine receptor changes on muscle membrane. Muscle Nerve 16:348–354, 1993.

85. Viby Mogensen J, Hanel HK, Hansen E, Graae J: Serum cholinesterase activity in burned patients. II: Anaesthesia, suxamethonium and hyperkalaemia. Acta Anaesthesiol Scand 19:169–179, 1975.

86. Kim C, Hirose M, Martyn JA: d-Tubocurarine accentuates the burn-induced upregulation of nicotinic acetylcholine receptors at the muscle membrane. Anesthesiology 83:309–315, 1995.

87. Martyn JA: Succinylcholine hyperkalemia after burns. Anesthesiology 91:321–322, 1999.

88. Khan TZ, Khan RM: Changes in serum potassium following succinylcholine in patients with infections. Anesth Analg 62:327–331, 1983.

89. Kohlschütter B, Baur H, Roth F: Suxamethonium-induced hyperkalaemia in patients with severe intra-abdominal infections. Br J Anaesth 48:557–562, 1976.

90. Fink H, Blobner M, Martyn JAJ: Up-regulation of AChRs during chronic pancuronium is caused by a post-transcriptional mechanism due to disuse. Anesthesiology (in press).

91. Tsukagoshi H, Morita T, Takahashi K, et al: Cecal ligation and puncture peritonitis model shows decreased nicotinic acetylcholine receptor numbers in rat muscle: Immunopathologic mechanisms? [see comments]. Anesthesiology 91:448–460, 1999.

92. Hoch W, McConville J, Helms S, et al: Auto-antibodies to the receptor tyrosine kinase MuSK in patients with myasthenia gravis without acetylcholine receptor antibodies. Nat Med 7:365–368, 2001.

93. Grob D, Arsura EL, Brunner NG, Namba T: The course of myasthenia gravis and therapies affecting outcome. Ann NY Acad Sci 505:472–499, 1987.

94. Boonyapisit K, Kaminski HJ, Ruff RL: Disorders of neuromuscular junction ion channels. Am J Med 106:97–113, 1999.

95. Baraka A: Suxamethonium block in the myasthenic patient. Correlation with plasma cholinesterase. Anaesthesia 47:217–219, 1992.

96. Vincent A, Drachman DB: Myasthenia gravis. Adv Neurol 88:159–188, 2002.

97. Engel AG: Myasthenia gravis and myasthenic syndromes. Ann Neurol 16:519–534, 1984.

98. McCarthy G, Mirakhur RK, Elliott P, Wright J: Effect of H2-receptor antagonist pretreatment on vecuronium- and atracurium-induced neuromuscular block. Br J Anaesth 66:713–715, 1991.

99. Hatta V, Saxena A, Kaul HL: Phenytoin reduces suxamethonium-induced myalgia. Anaesthesia 47:664–667, 1992.

100. Kim CS, Arnold FJ, Itani MS, Martyn JA: Decreased sensitivity to metocurine during long-term phenytoin therapy may be attributable to protein binding and acetylcholine receptor changes. Anesthesiology 77:500–506, 1992.

101. Soriano SG, Kaus SJ, Sullivan LJ, Martyn JA: Onset and duration of action of rocuronium in children receiving chronic anticonvulsant therapy. Paediatr Anaesth 10:133–136, 2000.

102. Soriano SG, Sullivan LJ, Venkatakrishnan K, et al: Pharmacokinetics and pharmacodynamics of vecuronium in children receiving phenytoin or carbamazepine for chronic anticonvulsant therapy. Br J Anaesth 86:223–229, 2001.

103. Fuchs-Buder T, Wilder Smith OH, Borgeat A, Tassonyi E: Interaction of magnesium sulphate with vecuronium-induced neuromuscular block. Br J Anaesth 74:405–409, 1995.

104. Ghoneim MM, Long JP: The interaction between magnesium and other neuromuscular blocking agents. Anesthesiology 32:23–27, 1970.

105. Fiekers JF: Sites and mechanisms of antibiotic-induced neuromuscular block: A pharmacological analysis using quantal content, voltage clamped end-plate currents and single channel analysis. Acta Physiol Pharmacol Ther Latinoam 49:242–250, 1999.

106. Scheller M, Bufler J, Schneck H, et al: Isoflurane and sevoflurane interact with the nicotinic acetylcholine receptor channels in micromolar concentrations. Anesthesiology 86:118–127, 1997.

107. Liu M, Kato M, Hashimoto Y: Neuromuscular blocking effects of the aminoglycoside antibiotics arbekacin, astromicin, isepamicin and netilmicin on the diaphragm and limb muscles in the rabbit. Pharmacology 63:142–146, 2001.

108. Shorten GD, Crawford MW, St Louis P: The neuromuscular effects of mivacurium chloride during propofol anesthesia in children. Anesth Analg 82:1170–1175, 1996.

109. Fryer JD, Lukas RJ: Antidepressants noncompetitively inhibit nicotinic acetylcholine receptor function. J Neurochem 72:1117–1124, 1999.
110. Scheller M, Bufler J, Hertle I, et al: Ketamine blocks currents through mammalian nicotinic acetylcholine receptor channels by interaction with both the open and the closed state. Anesth Analg 83:830–836, 1996.
111. Hertle I, Scheller M, Bufler J, et al: Interaction of midazolam with the nicotinic acetylcholine receptor of mouse myotubes. Anesth Analg 85:174–181, 1997.
112. Krampfl K, Schlesinger F, Dengler R, et al: Pentobarbital has curare-like effects on adult-type nicotinic acetylcholine receptor channel currents. Anesth Analg 90:970–974, 2000.
113. Driessen JJ, Wuis EW, Gielen MJ: Prolonged vecuronium neuromuscular blockade in a patient receiving orally administered dantrolene. Anesthesiology 62:523–524, 1985.
114. Ali HH, Savarese JJ, Embree PB, et al: Clinical pharmacology of mivacurium chloride (BW B1090U) infusion: Comparison with vecuronium and atracurium. Br J Anaesth 61:541–546, 1988.
115. Brandom BW, Woelfel SK, Ryan Cook D, et al: Comparison of mivacurium and suxamethonium administered by bolus and infusion. Br J Anaesth 62:488–493, 1989.
116. McLoughlin C, Nesbitt GA, Howe JP: Suxamethonium induced myalgia and the effect of pre-operative administration of oral aspirin. A comparison with a standard treatment and an untreated group. Anaesthesia 43:565–567, 1988.
117. Meyers EF, Krupin T, Johnson M, Zink H: Failure of nondepolarizing neuromuscular blockers to inhibit succinylcholine-induced increased intraocular pressure, a controlled study. Anesthesiology 48:149–151, 1978.
118. Engbaek J, Viby Mogensen J: Precurarization: A hazard to the patient? Acta Anaesthesiol Scand 28:61–62, 1984.
119. Walts LF, Dillon JB: Clinical studies of the interaction between d-tubocurarine and succinylcholine. Anesthesiology 31:39–44, 1969.
120. Erkola O, Salmenpera A, Kuoppamaki R: Five non-depolarizing muscle relaxants in precurarization. Acta Anaesthesiol Scand 27:427–432, 1983.
121. Goulden MR, Hunter JM: Rapacuronium (Org 9487): Do we have a replacement for succinylcholine? Br J Anaesth 82:489–492, 1999.
122. Goudsouzian NG: Rapacuronium and bronchospasm. Anesthesiology 94:727–728, 2001.
123. Murray MJ, Cowen J, DeBlock H, et al: Clinical practice guidelines for sustained neuromuscular blockade in the adult critically ill patient. Crit Care Med 30:142–156, 2002.

34

Sympathomimetic, Sympatholytic Drugs, Parasympathomimetic, and Parasympatholytic Drugs

Imre Rédai, MD • Berend Mets, MD

Sympathomimetic Drugs

Sympathomimetics are agents that produce effects similar to those produced by impulses conveyed by adrenergic postganglionic fibers of the sympathetic nervous system. Because these agents resemble epinephrine (adrenaline) in physiologic action, they are also called adrenergics.

Stimulation of postganglionic sympathetic nerve terminals, with a few exceptions, liberates norepinephrine, the main neurotransmitter at the sympathetic nerve terminal. Stimulation of the adrenal medulla releases epinephrine and norepinephrine into the systemic circulation. Dopamine, the third naturally occurring sympathomimetic amine, serves as a neurotransmitter in multiple systems.

Background and History

Therapeutic use of a sympathomimetic agent was first described in China around 3000 BC.[1] The plant Ma-huang was used as a diaphoretic, a circulatory stimulant, an antipyretic, and a sedative for cough. Ephedrine, the main alkaloid of Ma-huang, was isolated in 1886.[2] In 1895,

adrenal extracts were described,[3] and, in 1910, the phenylethanolamines were first analyzed.[4]

Mechanisms of Drug Action

The adrenergic receptors, which play a central role in many physiologic processes, belong to the family of G protein–coupled receptors and are subjects of intensive research.[5] Sympathomimetics produce their effects by either direct stimulation of α and β adrenergic receptors or indirectly by displacement of norepinephrine from vesicular or extravesicular binding sites in the presynaptic adrenergic nerve terminal (see Chapter 13). The displaced norepinephrine then stimulates α and β adrenergic receptors at the neuroeffector junction. Pretreatment with reserpine depletes presynaptic norepinephrine stores, allowing separation of direct and indirect sympathomimetic effects.[6] Many drugs—"mixed-acting sympathomimetics"—have both direct and indirect actions.[7]

The sympathomimetic amines are derivatives of β-phenylethanolamine (Fig. 34–1). This versatile molecule allows substitutions on the benzene ring (O-dihydroxybenzene is known as catechol, thus the name catecholamines), on the two carbons of the ethyl side chain, resulting in enan-

599

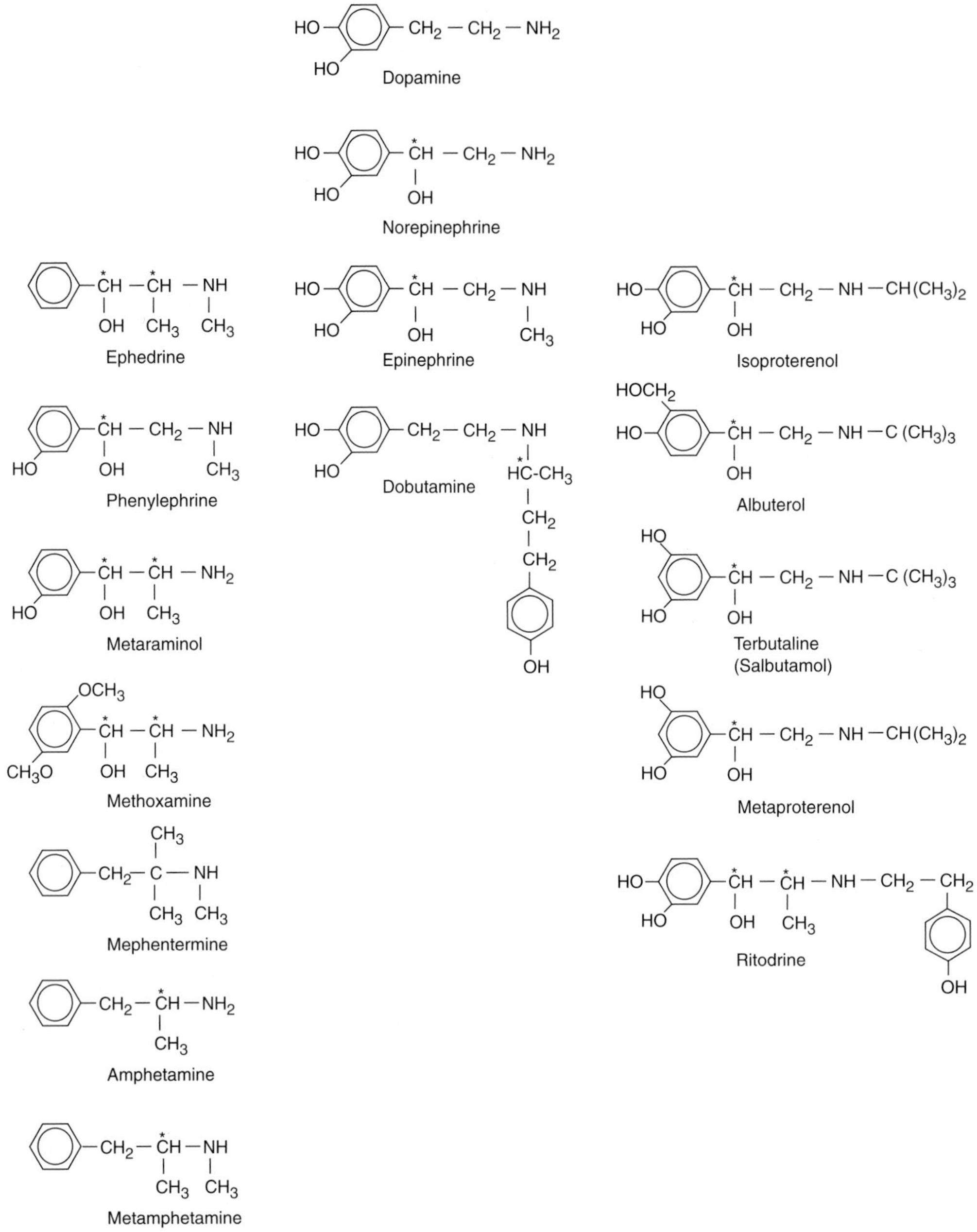

Part III Pharmacologic Basis of Clinical Practice

Dopamine

Norepinephrine

Ephedrine Epinephrine Isoproterenol

Phenylephrine Dobutamine Albuterol

Metaraminol Terbutaline (Salbutamol)

Methoxamine Metaproterenol

Mephentermine Ritodrine

Amphetamine

Metamphetamine

Figure 34–1. Structural formulas of phenylethanolamine sympathomimetics. *Left,* Agents with predominantly α receptor agonist activity. *Right,* β Receptor agonists. *Middle,* Agents representing both receptor groups. *Asterisk* signals asymmetric carbons and existence of enantiomers.

tiomers, and on the amine terminal. The subtle differences in structure produce not only marked differences in receptor binding and activation and metabolism of the drug but also effects on uptake mechanisms and the ratio of central to peripheral action.[8] The two-carbon distance between the benzene ring and the amine group ensures maximal sympathomimetic activity.[9]

The understanding of interactions between drugs and receptors at the molecular level elucidates the significance of the subtle differences between the ligands. Computer-simulated docking arrangements to the β_2 receptor of epinephrine, ritodrine (a β_2-selective agonist), and propranolol (a β_2 antagonist) are illustrated in Figure 34–2.[10] The amine

terminal of the agonist or antagonist forms a link with an aspartic carboxylate group (113 on the β_2 receptor) in the third transmembrane helix of the β adrenergic receptor, and the result of this interaction affects coupling to, and activation of, adenylyl cyclase by the receptor.[11] Except for phenylephrine, alkyl substitution on the amino group results in increased potency on the β_2 receptor. However, β_2 selectivity requires further substitutions on the phenylethanolamine base.

Hydrophobic substitutions on the aromatic ring and an increase in the distance between the amine group and the aromatic ring result in antagonist ligands.[12] A pouch is formed between the second and seventh transmembrane domains: in

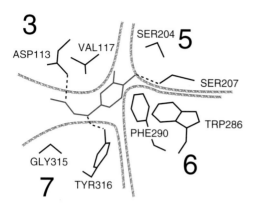

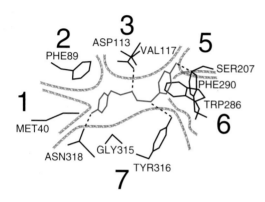

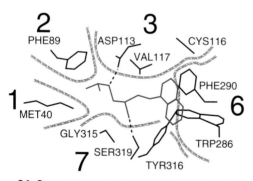

Figure 34–2. Ligand binding to the β_2 receptor. Computer-simulated models of docking of epinephrine *(top)*, the β_2 agonist ritodrine *(middle)*, and the nonselective β antagonist propranolol *(bottom)*. The simulation presents a cross-section of the receptor—the ligand binding site is located toward the center portion. The ligands are displayed in blue. The corresponding numbers indicate the relative positions of the seven transmembrane helices. The 4th helix does not participate in the binding interaction. The amino groups of all three ligands proximate with aspartate$_{113}$ (ASP113) of the third transmembrane helix. Only the two agonist are linked with hydrogen bonds to the serine residues of the fifth helix. This interaction plays a central role in receptor activation. The tyrosine residue overhanging the binding pocket also forms links only with the agonists. Complex van der Waals interactions between hydrophobic amino acid residues and propranolol allow easy docking to the binding site. (Modified from Kontoyianni M, DeWeese C, Penzotti, JE, et al: Three-dimensional models for agonist and antagonist complexes with B$_2$ adrenergic receptor. J Med Chem 39:4406, 1996.)

β_1 receptors, a threonine is located at the base of this pocket, whereas in β_2 receptors, a tyrosine residue overhangs the binding pocket.[13] Hydroxyl groups in the third and fifth position and large alkyl or aryl groups on the amino terminal contribute to β_2 receptor selectivity; the latter groups interact with the tyrosine residue in the seventh transmembrane domain.[14] Maximal α- and β-agonist activities depend on the presence of hydroxyl groups on positions 3 and 4 on the aromatic ring. Hydroxyl residues of serine 204 and 207 of the fifth transmembrane helix on the β receptor are believed to form hydrogen bonds with the catecholic hydroxyl groups[15] (see Fig. 34–2, *top* and *middle*). These amino acid residues not only serve as docking sites but also play an important role in regulating equilibrium dynamics between the receptor's active and inactive forms.[16] Loss of one or both hydroxyls results in dramatic reduction or complete loss of direct agonist activity. Noncatecholamine sympathomimetics, which are agents that are missing one or both hydroxyl groups on the aromatic ring, elicit their effect by stimulating release of norepinephrine from sympathetic nerve terminals[6] (see below: indirect-acting sympathominetics). Furthermore, loss of aromatic hydroxyl groups increases the lipophilic characteristics of the compounds, allowing better penetration of the blood–brain barrier and enhancing central effects. These drugs are also resistant to metabolism by catechol *O*-methyltransferase (COMT), which improves bioavailability and prolongs the duration of action.

Substitution at the α-carbon prevents oxidation of the compound by monoamine oxidases (MAOs), resulting in longer half-life and prolonged presence at the effector nerve terminals. This later effect may cause prolonged presynaptic effects with sustained release of norepinephrine. One example is ephedrine (see Fig. 34–1), an indirect-acting sympathomimetic.

Substitution on the β-carbon increases potency on α and β receptors, but also reduces lipophilicity and lessens central nervous system (CNS) effects. For example, β-hydroxylation of methamphetamine produces ephedrine (see Fig. 34–1), an agent with reduced central potency but increased peripheral potency. β-Hydroxylation is necessary for storage in vesicles at the adrenergic presynaptic terminal. α- and β-carbon substitutions result in stereoisomers. In general, α-carbon *d*-substitutions and β-carbon *l*-substitutions confer greater potency—*l*-epinephrine is 12 times more potent than *d*-epinephrine.[17] Coupling with an asparagine residue in the sixth transmembrane domain is responsible for the stereoselectivity of β-hydroxyl ligand binding.[18]

Clinical Pharmacology

Depending on the relative potency at the different subtypes of α and β receptors, the route of administration, and the degree of lipid solubility and biotransformation, a myriad of pharmacologic effects can be achieved by carefully selecting the drug to be used. In the next part of this chapter, the physiologic effects and clinical applications of the commonly used α- and β-agonists are reviewed, starting from pure agonists and ending with agents that have multiple effects.

α_1 Adrenergic Receptor Agonists

Phenylephrine

The physiologic effects of phenylephrine were first described in 1933.[19] The drug was first used in anesthetic practice to sustain blood pressure during spinal anesthesia.[20]

Phenylephrine (see Fig. 34–1) is administered intravenously to counteract hypotension and to increase coronary and cerebral perfusion pressure. This drug is an almost pure α_1-selective agonist—only very high doses produce an effect on β receptors. Nevertheless, phenylephrine is only a partial agonist of the α_1 receptor. Because it increases vascular resistance in the skin, muscles, and renal and mesenteric vascular beds, systolic and diastolic blood pressures increase. Little direct effect accrues to the coronary and cerebral circulation or to intracranial blood volume. Heart rate slows secondary to vagally mediated reflex bradycardia. Phenylephrine is probably a pulmonary arterial vasoconstrictor in man,[21] although the increases in diastolic and mean pulmonary artery blood pressures are more likely caused by translocation of the circulating blood volume from the systemic to the pulmonary capillary and venous pools. Compared with ephedrine, phenylephrine is inferior in maintaining placental blood flow during cesarean delivery under spinal anesthesia.[22] Table 34–1 shows the recommended parenteral doses for phenylephrine and other α_1 receptor agonists.

Topical phenylephrine is popular as a nasal decongestant or mydriatic. It is available in 0.25%, 0.5%, or 1% solutions for nasal decongestion and as 2.5% or 10% eye drops. However, when large doses are instilled to constrict nasal mucosa before ear, nose, and throat surgery, or to control bleeding after adenoidectomy, severe systemic effects (pulmonary edema, cardiac arrest) may occur; fatalities have been described in even American Society of Anesthesiologist's physical status I patients.[23] Inadequate management by the anesthesiologist, including deepening of inhalational anesthesia and administration of intravenous beta-blocking drugs, contributed to the adverse outcome; on the contrary, no intervention to reduce severe hypertension produced a good outcome.[23] An advisory committee for the New York State Department of Health recommended that the initial dose of phenylephrine should not exceed 0.5 mg (four drops of the 0.25% solution) in adults or 20 µg/kg in children. Mild-to-moderate hypertension should be observed, and severe hypertension should be treated with either α_1 adrenergic antagonists, such as phentolamine or tolazoline, or direct-acting vasodilating drugs, such as hydralazine.[23] Excessive doses of phenylephrine for patients undergoing cataract surgery under general anesthesia has caused severe hypertension soon after surgery, necessitating administration of vasodilating drugs (I.R., personal observation). This effect was eliminated by reducing the concentration of the solution and by judicious administration of the drug.

Methoxamine

The pharmacologic properties of methoxamine were first described in 1948,[24] and, in 1950, methoxamine was used to maintain blood pressure during spinal anesthesia.[25]

Although methoxamine (see Fig. 34–1) has similar pharmacologic properties but longer duration of action then phenylephrine, large doses of methoxamine have an inhibitory effect on β receptors and may produce bradycardia.[26] In the elderly and in those with a history of myocardial ischemia, a slow intravenous infusion of methoxamine may be superior to ephedrine in maintaining blood pressure during spinal anesthesia, because the potential for atrial tachyarrhythmias is less with methoxamine while coronary perfusion is maintained. Methoxamine has a prolonged duration of action when compared with other α_1 receptor agonists, and rebound hypertension may occur more frequently after recovery from spinal anesthesia.[25]

Midodrine is an orally absorbed α_1-agonist used to treat autonomic failure and dialysis-related hypotension.[27] Its

TABLE 34–1.

Recommended Parenteral Doses of α_1 Receptor Agonist Drugs

Drug	IV Bolus	Infusion (rate adjusted to effect)	IM/SC
Phenylephrine	40–200 µg (maximum 500 µg)	40–180 µg/min	2–5 mg IM or SC
Methoxamine	3–5 mg (1 mg/min)	0.1–0.3 mg/min	10–15 mg IM
Metaraminol	0.5–5 mg	5 µg/kg/min	2–10 mg IM or SC
Mephentermine	15–30 mg	—	30–45 mg IM
Ephedrine	5–25 mg	0.5–5 mg/min	10–50 mg IM or SC

IM, Intramuscularly; SC, subcutaneously.

active metabolite desglymidodrine differs from methoxamine only by lacking a methyl group.

Metaraminol, Mephentermine, and the Topical α₁ Receptor Agonists

Metaraminol (see Fig. 34–1) was first used in anesthetic practice in 1954.[28] It not only directly stimulates α_1 receptors but also has a significant indirect effect on adrenergic terminals—the *l*-isomer is responsible for the presynaptic effects.[29] The positive inotropic effect of metaraminol on the myocardium and the peripheral release of norepinephrine and its cotransmitters may lead to profound peripheral vasoparalysis if phenylephrine has not produced adequate vascular resistance.

Mephentermine (see Fig. 34–1) is also a combined direct- and indirect-acting agonist that produces a variable heart rate response, depending on the balance between indirect sympathetic stimulation and baroreflex-mediated inhibition of the heart.

Topically active imidazoline derivatives (naphazoline, oxymetazoline, xylometazoline, and tetrahydrozoline) (Fig. 34–3) are used for the vasoconstriction of the conjunctiva and nasal mucosa. Their systemic absorption is much less

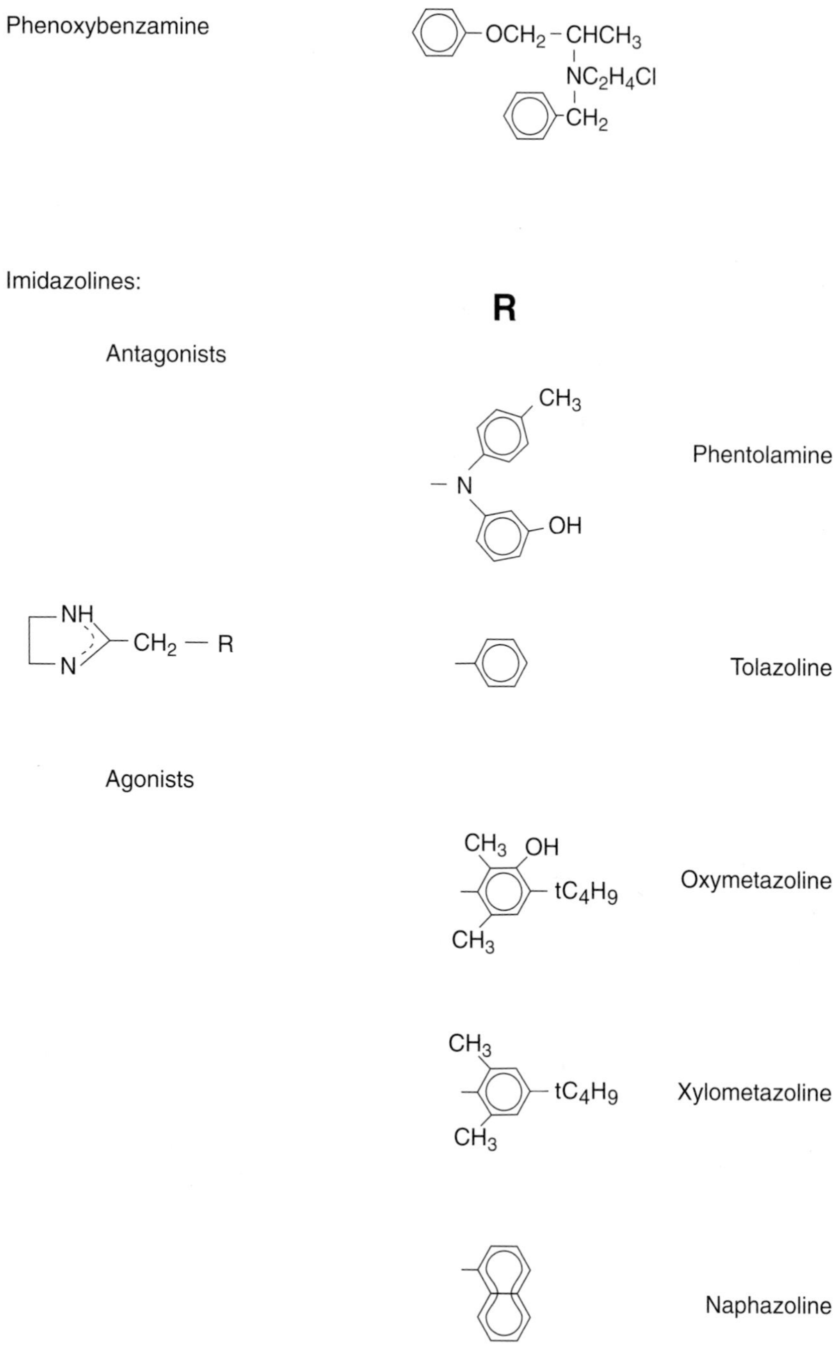

Figure 34–3. Structural formulas of phenoxybenzamine and the imidazoline derivative α receptor agonists and antagonists.

than that of phenylephrine, and they are regarded as safer than phenylephrine for nasal vasoconstriction.[30]

α_2 Adrenergic Receptor Agonists

Clonidine

The clinical pharmacology of clonidine is discussed in Chapter 28.

Guanidine Derivatives and α-Methyldopa

Guanfacine and guanabenz are guanidine derivative antihypertensive drugs that are structurally and functionally similar to clonidine. Guanabenz is metabolized extensively and may be safer in patients with renal failure but more problematic in those with cirrhosis.[31] Side effects of the guanidine derivatives are similar but milder than those for clonidine, and withdrawal symptoms occur less frequently.[32]

α-Methyldopa is a precursor drug and is converted to α-methylnorepinephrine, its active form in the sympathetic nerve terminals. α-Methylnorepinephrine exerts its antihypertensive effect by central α_2 receptor stimulation.[33] In addition, α-methylnorepinephrine inhibits dopa decarboxylase and being resistant to breakdown by MAO replaces norepinephrine in the storage vesicles leading to the depletion of presynaptic norepinephrine stores. Rebound hypertension is unusual after discontinuation of the drug. In addition to the side effects associated with the other members of this group, acquired hemolytic anemia and liver dysfunction may occur in patients taking α-methyldopa, and the drug is contraindicated in patients with cirrhosis or active liver disease. A positive direct Coombs' test (formation of antibodies against red blood cells) that was associated with α-methyldopa therapy has been noted in 10% to 20% of patients. Because a positive test result may delay or interfere with the cross-matching of blood for transfusion, the blood bank should be notified about the possibility as soon as possible. The pharmacokinetic characteristics and recommended dosing of the guanidine derivatives and α-methyldopa are presented in Table 34–2.

β Adrenergic Receptor Agonists

Stimulation of β adrenergic receptors increases heart rate, the force of myocardial contractility, and therefore cardiac output. Myocardial relaxation and diastolic filling time also increase. Stimulation of β_2 receptors results in peripheral arteriolar dilatation in muscular, splanchnic, and renal vasculature. This leads to a reduction in vascular resistance and a decrease in diastolic blood pressure, whereas the increase or decrease of systolic blood pressure is a function of the change in cardiac output. Stimulation of β_2 receptors, abundant in bronchial and enteric smooth muscle, leads to bronchodilation and slowing of peristalsis; it also inhibits activation of T cells[34] and release of cytokines from airway smooth muscle cells.[35] Increased glycogenolysis in the liver is partially counterbalanced by activation of pancreatic islet cells by β receptors. Lipolysis is mediated by activation of β_3 receptors.[36] The commonly observed skeletal muscle tremor with β-agonist therapy is mediated by β_2 receptors.[37]

Isoproterenol (Isoprenaline)

Isoproterenol (see Fig. 34–1), the isopropyl derivative of norepinephrine, was the first synthetic β receptor agonist in clinical use.

Isoproterenol is nonselective in its β receptor effects and has low affinity for α receptors. Its chronotropic and dromotropic effects are caused by stimulation of β_1 and β_2 receptors,[38] whereas the inotropic effect is mediated predominantly by β_1 receptors.[39]

Isoproterenol is rapidly absorbed if applied to mucous membranes but undergoes extensive metabolism by liver COMT if administered enterally. Although isoproterenol is a poor substrate of MAO, and its neuronal uptake is less than

TABLE 34–2.

Pharmacokinetic Characteristics and Recommended Dosing of Some Common α_2 Adrenergic Receptor Agonist Drugs

Drug	Bioavailability	Protein Binding	Metabolism	Excretion	Half-life	Recommended Dose
Guanfacine	~80%	70%	55%, liver	Renal	14 hr	1–2 mg daily
Guanabenz	20–30%	10%	~100%, liver	Gastrointestinal, renal	3–4 hr	8–32 mg daily
α-Methyldopa	8–62%	83%	Liver	Renal	1.5–2 hr	1–2 g daily; max 4 g*

*In children, the recommended starting daily dose is 10 mg/kg with a maximum of 65 mg/kg or 3 g, whichever is less.

that of norepinephrine, its duration of action is brief when administered parenterally. Hence isoproterenol is administered as a continuous infusion. Current clinical indications include bradycardia caused by heart block and treatment of torsades de pointes ventricular tachycardia. The use of isoproterenol as an inotrope has declined since the emergence of dobutamine and phosphodiesterase inhibitors.[40] As a bronchodilator, isoproterenol has largely been replaced by the β_2-selective drugs. Palpitations, headache, anxiety and restlessness, tremor, and skin flushes are common side effects of isoproterenol.

β_2 Adrenergic Receptor Agonists

Agonists that are selective for the β_2 adrenergic receptors were developed to reduce the cardiovascular side effects of nonselective β receptor agonists in the treatment of bronchial asthma. Changing the catechol ring (3,4-dihydroxybenzene) to a resorcinol ring (3,5-dihydroxybenzene) improved bioavailability, because these molecules are not methylated by COMT. Further substitutions on the amino group resulted in increased β receptor activity and reduced α receptor activity. This chemical change also increased the duration of action caused by decreased metabolism by MAOs.[41] However, all currently used β_2-selective agonists are only relatively selective; thus they also stimulate the β_1 receptor at greater concentrations. Further reduction in systemic side effects is achieved by aerosolized administration of these drugs, as the drug reaches therapeutic concentrations in the bronchi with minimal activation of cardiac and peripheral β receptors.[42] However, the use of an inhalational β_2 receptor agonist still increases the risk for arrhythmias (predominantly atrial fibrillation), necessitating hospital admission for patients with congestive heart failure.[43] (See Chapter 39 regarding use of β_2-selective agonists for bronchial asthma and chronic obstructive airway disease.)

Use of inhaled albuterol (see Fig. 34–1) has been described in hyperkalemic familial periodic paralysis; two to four metered doses of albuterol halted the progress of both hyperkalemia and paralysis.[44] Similar emergency treatment for hyperkalemia was successful for patients in renal failure.[45] Therefore, not surprisingly, continuous infusion of β-agonists may lead to hypokalemia.

Ritodrine

The β_2-selective agonist ritodrine (see Fig. 34–1) is used as a uterine relaxant to arrest premature labor.[46] Ritodrine is usually started intravenously and is continued as an oral drug if uterine contractions have stopped. Oral bioavailability is about 30%. Ritodrine is metabolized in the liver to form inactive conjugates, and about half the drug is excreted unchanged in the urine. Although ritodrine therapy reduces the incidence of delivery within 48 hours of the start of treatment, this immediate effect has not led to a decrease in the overall rate of preterm delivery or to a reduction in neonatal morbidity or mortality.[47] Pulmonary edema with normal pulmonary capillary wedge pressures has been attributed to ritodrine therapy.[48]

α and β Adrenergic Receptor Agonists

Norepinephrine (Noradrenaline), Epinephrine (Adrenaline), Dopamine, and Dobutamine

These agents are discussed in detail in Chapter 37.

Indirect-Acting Sympathomimetics

Ephedrine

Although the physiologic effects of ephedrine were described in 1887,[49] it was not until the 1920s that the drug was introduced into Western medicine[1] and clinical anesthesia. Ephedrine (see Fig. 34–1) is a mixed-acting sympathomimetic—it has both direct and indirect stimulating effects on α and β adrenergic receptors. Intravenous administration causes rapid increases in heart rate, cardiac output, and blood pressure that last 10 to 15 minutes; repeat doses have a decreasing effect (tachyphylaxis[50]). Intramuscular injection has a slower rate of onset (5–10 minutes) but a longer duration of effect (35–45 minutes). Ephedrine has a half-life of 3 to 6 hours and is eliminated largely unchanged in the urine.

Ephedrine has a stimulatory effect on the CNS, relaxes bronchial smooth muscle, and increases trigone and sphincter muscle tone in the urinary bladder. Uterine and placental artery blood flow is not adversely affected when ephedrine is used to sustain blood pressure during spinal anesthesia for cesarean section,[22] and umbilical artery vascular resistance remains unchanged.[51,52]

Although ephedrine is effective in maintaining or restoring blood pressure during spinal anesthesia when administered intravenously,[53] preemptive intramuscular administration of the drug is not a reliable preventive measure.[54]

Amphetamine and Other Central Nervous System Stimulants

Amphetamine and methamphetamine are powerful stimulants of the CNS. They cause the release, and inhibit the reuptake, of stimulatory neurotransmitters in the cortex, the motor nuclei, and the reticular activating system. These two drugs have mild analgesic effects and may stimulate respiration obtunded by centrally acting drugs. This class of drugs also possesses peripheral indirect sympathomimetic activity, leading to an acute increase in blood pressure and secondary bradycardia; large doses may cause arrhythmias.[55] Chronic use may lead to a decrease in blood pressure, because *d*-amphetamine and *d*-methamphetamine are metabolized to a false neurotransmitter.[56] Although amphetamine and methamphetamine are sometimes used to suppress appetite,[57] their effect is not sustained, and tolerance and dependence often occur.[58] Even though the therapeutic use of amphetamine and methamphetamine has declined, their respective methylenedioxy derivatives "Ice" and "Ecstasy" remain popular illicit recreational drugs.[59]

Acute intoxication with amphetamine or its synthetic congeners is characterized by increasing restlessness, agitation, and irritability that progress to confusion, aggressive behavior, delirium, and paranoid delusions. Differentiation from acute schizophrenia may be difficult. Headache, shivering, palpitation and tachycardia, hypertension, and flushed or pale skin are followed by central chest pain, cardiac arrhythmias, and hypotension. Dry mouth, a metallic taste, nausea, vomiting, and abdominal cramps are the leading gastrointestinal symptoms. In fatal poisoning, convulsions, coma, and circulatory collapse are the terminal events. Gross hyperpyrexia, rhabdomyolysis, disseminated intravascular coagulopathy, and hepatorenal failure leading to death are most common with "Ecstasy" but has also been attributed to amphetamine overdose.

Treatment of acute intoxication consists of acidification of urine to enhance elimination, administration of sedatives, and control of cardiovascular side effects. Dantrolene is indicated in the event of hyperpyrexia.[60]

Methylphenidate is a structural relative of amphetamine. It has milder CNS-stimulating activity and less effect on motor function. Methylphenidate is used to treat narcolepsy and attention-deficit hyperactivity disorder. Side effects of insomnia, anorexia, weight loss, suppression of growth, and abdominal pain have been described in children. Overdose causes symptoms similar to those of overdose with amphetamine; again, treatment is supportive.

Ergot Alkaloids

Known as St. Anthony's fire in the Middle Ages, the poisoning caused by contamination of wheat or rye with the fungus *Claviceps purpurea* was characterized by mental disturbance and severe, painful peripheral vasoconstriction often leading to gangrene of the extremities.

The ergot alkaloids stimulate contraction of a variety of smooth muscles, both directly and indirectly by adrenergic and serotoninergic receptors. Contraction of vascular smooth muscle leads to coronary, cerebral, and peripheral vasoconstriction. Reflex bradycardia is commonly associated with the increase in blood pressure.

When taken orally, the alkaloids are slowly absorbed from the gut, and bioavailability is approximately 10%. The drugs are eliminated mainly in metabolized form in the bile. A number of ergot alkaloids have been isolated: ergotamine is used to treat migraine headaches, and ergonovine (also called ergometrine) is used to enhance postpartum uterine contractions.

Intravenous administration of the ergot alkaloids can produce sudden severe hypertension and should be avoided. The oral dose of ergotamine for acute migraine is 2 mg, followed by 1-mg dosages every half hour to a maximum of 6 mg. The intramuscular dosage is 0.5 mg, repeated every half hour to a maximum of 3 mg. Intramuscular administration of ergonovine, 0.2 mg, is used to enhance postpartum uterine contractions; this dosage may be continued up to a week postpartum as an oral preparation. Contraindications to ergot alkaloids include peripheral and coronary artery disease, thyrotoxicosis, and porphyria.[61]

Sympatholytic Drugs

Sympatholytics (also known as antiadrenergics) are drugs or agents that oppose the effects of impulses conveyed by adrenergic postganglionic fibers of the sympathetic nervous system.

Mechanisms of Drug Action

Sympatholytics may produce their effects in three ways: they can block α adrenergic receptors, the main result being dilation of peripheral blood vessels; they can selectively block β adrenergic receptors, the principal pharmacologic target being the heart and vascular smooth muscle; or they can block nicotinic transmission in the sympathetic ganglia. This chapter reviews the first two mechanisms.

Clinical Pharmacology

α Adrenergic Receptor Antagonists ("Alpha-Blockers")

Phenoxybenzamine

Phenoxybenzamine (see Fig. 34–3) is a haloalkylamine compound and an irreversible noncompetitive blocker of α adrenergic receptors. It forms a covalent link with the receptor, and recovery of receptor function requires synthesis of new receptor molecules. This sympatholytic binds to and inactivates not only α_1 and α_2 receptors, but also proteins responsible for neuronal and non-neuronal uptake of norepinephrine.

The reduction in peripheral vascular resistance is accompanied by reflex sympathetic stimulation of cardiac β_1 receptors and an increase in cardiac output. Phenoxybenzamine blocks sympathetic presynaptic inhibitory α_2 receptors in the heart and decreases elimination of myocardial norepinephrine secondary to inhibition of uptake mechanisms; these effects also contribute to the observed increase in cardiac output. Orthostatic hypotension is a characteristic of phenoxybenzamine, because baroreceptor mechanisms cannot be activated when the patient is erect.[62] Furthermore, unopposed vascular β_2 receptor stimulation may decrease vascular resistance even more.

Phenoxybenzamine is administered orally to induce hypotension. Although half-life is approximately 18 to 24 hours, duration of action depends on the cellular turnover rate of the alkylated α receptors.

Phenoxybenzamine remains the preferred drug for management of pheochromocytoma.[63] The unique noncompetitive nature of its α receptor blockade prevents receptor activation by sudden catecholamine surges during surgical manipulation of the tumor. The recommended daily dose is 1 to 2 mg/kg. Phenoxybenzamine is also used to alleviate urinary retention caused by neurogenic bladder or benign prostatic hypertrophy.[64] The recommended dose for relief of obstruction in neurogenic bladder is 0.3 to 0.5 mg/kg per day in children and 10 to 20 mg per day in adults.

Imidazoline Receptor Drugs: Phentolamine and Tolazoline

Phentolamine and tolazoline (see Fig. 34–3) are competitive nonselective α receptor antagonists. Although these drugs have cardiovascular effects similar to those of phenoxybenzamine, α blockade is short-lived and the effects are reversible with α receptor agonists. Phentolamine is discussed in Chapter 39.

Tolazoline is used to treat persistent pulmonary hypertension of the newborn.[65] Major side effects are hypotension with reflex tachycardia, arrhythmias, and pulmonary and gastrointestinal hemorrhages. Unfortunately, improved oxygenation in these newborns did not result in an improved survival rate. Since the introduction of inhaled nitric oxide, the use of tolazoline in the treatment of pulmonary hypertension has declined.[66] Tolazoline has a plasma half-life of 3 to 13 hours. It is excreted mainly unchanged by the kidney. The recommended dose for the treatment of persistent pulmonary hypertension of the newborn is 0.5 to 2 mg/kg per hour following a 0.5- to 2-mg/kg loading dose administered over 10 minutes. Using a 0.5-mg load and 0.5-mg/kg per hour infusion rate appears to prevent accumulation of the drug.

Piperazinyl Quinazoles

Prazosin and other piperazinyl quinazoles are discussed in Chapter 39.

β Adrenergic Receptor Antagonists ("Beta-Blockers")

The first synthetic β adrenergic receptor-blocking compounds appeared in the late 1950s.[67] In these compounds, the two-carbon distance between the amino terminal and the aryl group of phenylethanolamine was extended by substituting either an amino-oxypropanol or a hydroxyaminoethyl backbone. This substitution abolishes sympathomimetic activity whereas still allowing docking of the molecule to the β receptor (see Fig. 34–2). Since then, numerous side-chain modifications have produced a large family of structurally related compounds (Fig. 34–4). Desirable pharmacodynamic characteristics include enhanced selectivity to β_1 receptors, partial agonist activity on β_2 receptors (known as intrinsic sympathomimetic activity), or the addition of α_1 receptor antagonism or quinidine-like membrane stabilizing activity. Desirable pharmacokinetic characteristics include prolonged half-life, which allows single daily dosing, and reduced lipophilicity, which limits CNS penetration and hence CNS side effects. The introduction of esterase-dependent metabolism for rapid elimination has resulted in the development of an ultra-short–acting antagonist: esmolol.

The cardiovascular system is the primary target of β adrenergic antagonist drugs. These drugs block the effect of adrenergic stimulation, thereby reducing heart rate and cardiac output, which is dependent on tonic stimulation of β receptors. These effects are more pronounced in patients with greater sympathetic tone, such as younger patients and those with congestive heart failure. β Receptor antagonists attenuate exercise- or stress-induced increases in heart rate and cardiac output, whereas stroke volume is relatively well preserved.[68] Blockade of β receptors reduces the pacemaker rate of the sinus node, suppresses the rate of depolarization in ectopic pacemaker foci, and increases the refractory period in the atrioventricular node.

Although acute postsynaptic β_2 receptor blockade increases peripheral vascular resistance, in patients with hypertension, long-term administration of β receptor antagonists produces vasodilatation and a reduction in diastolic blood pressure.[69] Blockade of presynaptic stimulatory β_2 receptors reduces release of norepinephrine and contributes to the hypotensive effect of β receptor antagonists.[70] This suppression of adrenergic reactivity was found to be beneficial in patients with severe hypertension undergoing aortic surgery.[71]

Nonselective β receptor antagonists inhibit β_2 receptor-dependent bronchodilation and increase airway obstruction in patients with asthma and chronic obstructive bronchopulmonary disease; even β_1-selective antagonists may exacerbate obstructive airway disease. Celiprolol, a drug with intrinsic β_2-agonist activity, increases rather than decreases forced expiratory volume (FEV_1) in patients with asthma.[72]

Glucose mobilization is inhibited by β receptor antagonists; this effect may be particularly pernicious in patients with diabetes, in whom the ensuing hypoglycemia may remain concealed because of the suppression of signs of sympathetic response.[73] Hypoglycemia-induced perspiration, mediated by cholinergic mechanisms, may remain the only warning sign in these patients. Nonselective beta-blockers adversely affect lipid metabolism and lipoprotein levels.[74]

Propranolol,[75] metoprolol,[76] timolol, nadolol, and atenolol[77] (see Fig. 34–4) are used to prevent migraine headache; and pindolol was found to accelerate the antidepressant response to selective serotonin uptake inhibitors by blocking the serotoninergic 5-HT_{1A} receptors.[78] Nebivolol, a new β_1-selective antagonist, also enhances vascular nitric oxide production and hence vasodilation.[79] Carvedilol (see Fig. 34–4), a nonselective β receptor antagonist with α receptor-blocking activity, was shown to inhibit HERG (human *ether-a-go-go*–related gene) potassium channels (a class III antiarrhythmic effect)[80]; this effect may be responsible for the prevention of cardiac arrhythmias and sudden death.[81]

Although β receptor antagonists may cause neonatal bradycardia and retarded intrauterine growth, chronic therapy with atenolol or labetalol for pregnancy-associated hypertension has not resulted in significant fetal morbidity.[82]

Tables 34–3 and 34–4 provide the characteristics and recommended doses for commonly used β receptor antagonists (see also Chapters 35 and 38).

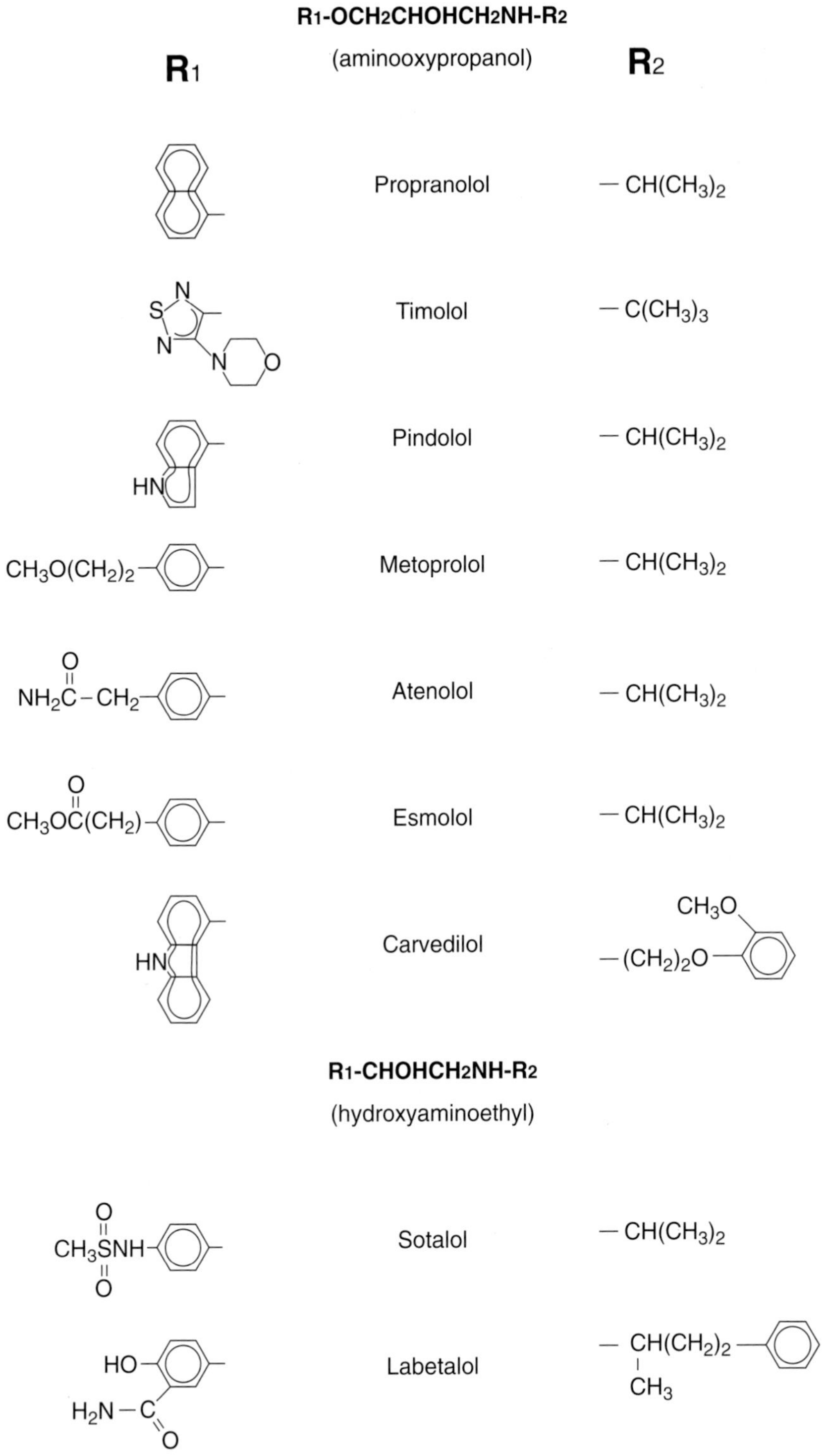

R₁-OCH₂CHOHCH₂NH-R₂

R_1-OCH₂CHOHCH₂NH-R_2

R₁ (aminooxypropanol) **R₂**

R_1		R_2
(naphthalene)	Propranolol	— CH(CH₃)₂
(thiadiazole–morpholine)	Timolol	— C(CH₃)₃
(indole)	Pindolol	— CH(CH₃)₂
CH₃O(CH₂)₂— (benzene)	Metoprolol	— CH(CH₃)₂
NH₂C(O)–CH₂—(benzene)	Atenolol	— CH(CH₃)₂
CH₃OC(O)(CH₂)—(benzene)	Esmolol	— CH(CH₃)₂
(carbazole)	Carvedilol	—(CH₂)₂O—(CH₃O-benzene)

R₁-CHOHCH₂NH-R₂

(hydroxyaminoethyl)

CH₃SNH—(benzene)	Sotalol	— CH(CH₃)₂
HO—(benzene), H₂N—C(O)	Labetalol	— CH(CH₂)₂—(benzene), CH₃

Figure 34–4. The β receptor antagonists. The variety of side chains linking to common backbones determines the diversity of drug characteristics.

Parasympathomimetic Drugs

Parasympathomimetics are drugs or agents that produce effects similar to those produced by stimulation of the parasympathetic nerves. These agents preferentially stimulate postsynaptic effector muscarinic receptors. Their actions are cholinergic—resembling those of acetylcholine.

Background and History

Muscarinic receptors are present not only on postsynaptic visceral effectors in the periphery, but also in the brain and ganglionic cells, on blood vessels, and in numerous presynaptic sites, where they modulate a variety of centrally mediated functions such as locomotion, learning and memory, antinociception, regulation of circadian rhythm,

TABLE 34–3.

Pharmacokinetic Characteristics of Some Commonly Used β Adrenergic Antagonists

Antagonist	Absorption	First-pass Metabolism	Blood Level Variability	Protein Binding	Metabolism	Excretion	Half-life
Propranolol	~100%	~75%	High	90%	~Full, liver	Renal	3–5 hr
Pindolol	~100%	10–15%	Mild	40%	50%, liver	Renal	3–4 hr
Oxprenolol	~70–90%	20–65%	High	80–90%	~95%, liver	Renal	1.5–4 hr
Nadolol	~37%	Minimal	Minimal	30%	Minimal	Renal	20–24 hr
Timolol	~100%	~50%	Moderate	80%	~80%, liver	Renal	3–5 hr
Labetalol	~100%	~70%	High	50%	~Full, liver	Renal, biliary	6–8 hr PO, 5.5 hr IV
Sotalol	~100%	~10%	Mild	Minimal	Minimal	Renal	7–15 hr
Metoprolol	~100%	~60%	High	5–10%	~90%	Renal	3–4 hr
Atenolol	~50%	<10%	Minimal	~3%	~10%	Renal	5–8 hr
Acebutolol	~100%	~60%	Mild	26%	~Full, liver	Renal, biliary	3–4 h*
Esmolol	IV only	NA	Minimal	50%	Erythrocyte esterase	Renal	8 min
Carvedilol	~100%	60–75%	Moderate	98%	Liver	Biliary	6–10 hr
Celiprolol	30–70%	Minimal	Mild	30%	Minimal	Renal	4–6 hr

*Diacetolol, the active metabolite of Acebutolol has a half-life of 8 to 12 hours.
IV, Intravenously; NA, not available; PO, per os (by mouth).

generation of epileptic seizures, and thermoregulation.[84] Acetylcholine is the endogenous neurotransmitter for all cholinergic receptors, both muscarinic and nicotinic. Whereas the exogenous parasympathomimetics are relatively selective for the muscarinic receptor, some cross-reactivity also may result in activation or inhibition of nicotinic receptors.

Muscarine, pilocarpine, and arecoline are three parasympathomimetic alkaloids derived from plants. Muscarine (Fig. 34–5), an alkaloid found in some mushroom species, was shown to produce the same effect on the heart as did stimulation of the vagus nerve.[85] Pilocarpine was isolated from the leaves of the shrub pilocarpus. A South American herbal product, Jaborandi, contains about 0.5% pilocarpine.[86] Arecoline is found in betel nuts *(Areca catechu)*. Betel nut is the fourth most widely used recreational drug

(after nicotine, alcohol, and caffeine) and is used in masticatory mixtures by millions of people living between the east coast of Africa and the western Pacific.[87]

Mechanisms of Drug Action

Five distinct muscarinic receptors have been identified[88] and their genes have been cloned.[89] These G protein–coupled receptors are characterized by seven highly conserved membrane-spanning domains. The receptors are divided into two subgroups, depending on their signal transduction. The M_1, M_3, and M_5 receptors activate G_q/G_{11} proteins, leading to phospholipase C stimulation and calcium mobilization. The M_2 and M_4 receptors activate pertussis toxin-sensitive

TABLE 34–4.

Pharmacodynamic Characteristics and Recommended Dosage of Some Commonly Used β Adrenergic Antagonists

Antagonist	Receptor	Other Effects	Oral Dose (daily)	Intravenous Dose
Propranolol	β_1, β_2	Mem stab, 5-HT$_{1C}$ 5-HT$_2$	40–320 mg	0.5–1 mg to maximum 3 mg
Pindolol	β_1, β_2	ISA, 5-HT$_{1A}$	15–45 mg	0.1–0.4 mg slowly
Oxprenolol	β_1, β_2	ISA	120–480 mg	1–2 mg slowly, maximum 5 mg
Nadolol	β_1, β_2	None	80–240 mg (maximum 320 mg)	
Timolol	β_1, β_2	None	15–45 mg (maximum 60 mg)	*
Labetalol	$\alpha_1, \beta_1, \beta_2$[†]	ISA	400–1200 mg	5–20 mg IV every 5–10 minutes to maximum 300 mg; infusion start at 2 mg/min
Sotalol	β_1, β_2[‡]	Class III antiarrhythmic	160–320 mg (maximum 640 mg)	20–120 mg over 10 min or 1.5 mg/kg followed by 0.2–0.5 mg/kg/hr (maximum 640 mg daily)
Metoprolol	β_1	None	100–400 mg	5 mg every 2 minutes to 15 mg total
Atenolol	β_1	None	50–100 mg	2.5 mg over 2.5 min every 5 min to 10 mg or 0.15 mg/kg over 20 min
Acebutolol	β_1	ISA	200–800 mg	
Esmolol	$\beta\beta_1$	None	NA	50–100 mg bolus, 0.05–0.3 mg/kg/min infusion
Carvedilol	$\alpha_1, \beta_1, \beta_2$[§]	Mem stab, antioxidant	12.5–50 mg	
Celiprolol	β_1	Partial β_2 agonist	200–600 mg	

5-HT$_{1A}$, 5HT$_{1A}$ receptor antagonism; 5-HT$_{1C}$, 5-HT$_2$, 5-HT$_{1C}$, 5-HT$_2$ receptor antagonism[83]; ISA, intrinsic sympathomimetic activity (partial agonist at the β$_2$ receptor); IV, intravenously; mem stab, membrane stabilizing effect; NA, not available.
*Used as ophthalmic preparation 0.25 to 0.5 mg/mL for treatment of glaucoma.
[†]Four stereoisomers: R,R responsible for most of β activity (antagonism and ISA), S,R and S,S responsible for α$_1$ antagonism, R,S is inactive; β to α activity is 7:1 when given IV, 5:1 when given orally.
[‡]The *l*-stereoisomer is responsible for the β antagonist activity; both stereoisomers possess class III antiarrhythmic activity.
[§]S(-) stereoisomer is responsible for the β antagonist activity, the stereoisomers are equipotent in α$_1$ antagonist activity; β to α potency is 10:1.
[¶]4'-hydroxyphenol metabolite is 13 times more potent β receptor antagonist than the parent drug; two of the hydroxy-carbazole metabolites are 30 to 80 times more potent antioxidants than the parent drug.

G$_i$/G$_o$ proteins, which mediate inhibition of adenylyl cyclase, activation of inwardly rectifying potassium currents, and inhibition of voltage-sensitive calcium channels.[90] The structural core of the muscarinic receptor is the third transmembrane helix. Helix 1 is relatively exposed, whereas the rest of the transmembrane helices are arranged in a bundle around the central third helix. In the inactive state, this arrangement is tight on the cytoplasmic surface but has an open ligand binding surface at the outer leaflet of the phospholipid bilayer. The binding of the agonist results in rearrangement of the intracellular portion, exposing the G protein binding site.[91] The ligand binding site involves the formation of a cleft between the transmembrane domains, by multiple amino acid residues. Residue of aspartate 105

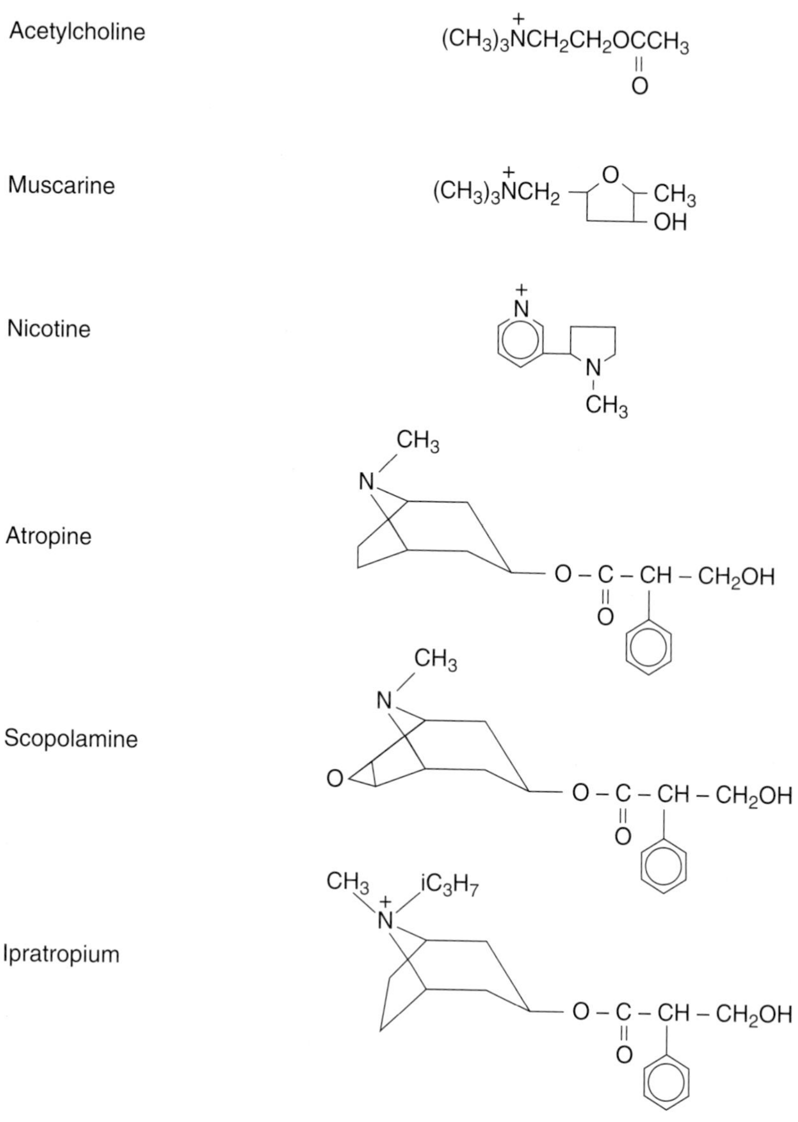

Figure 34–5. Acetylcholine, cholinergic agonists and muscarinic antagonists.

within the third transmembrane helix was identified as the likely binding site for the cationic nitrogen of acetylcholine.[92,93] Whereas the amino acid sequence of the muscarinic receptors is highly conserved across the subtypes, this does not apply to the third intracellular loop, which is responsible for G protein binding.[94]

Clinical Pharmacology

Acetylcholine

The pharmacologic effect of acetylcholine (see Fig. 34–5) results from stimulation of muscarinic and nicotinic receptors in combination with further regulatory and adaptive reflexes. The result is a complex response. In isolated preparations, acetylcholine produces negative chronotropy, dromotropy, and inotropy and vasodilation; however, in the intact animal, intravenous injection of a small dose of acetylcholine generally produces a decrease in blood pressure with concomitant reflex tachycardia. If the effect of stimulation of muscarinic receptors is blocked with atropine, administration of acetylcholine may increase blood pressure. This is the result of the release of catecholamines secondary to stimulation of nicotinic receptors in the sympathetic ganglia and the adrenal gland.[95] Dilatation of vascular beds by choline esters is mediated predominantly by M_3 muscarinic receptors located on the luminal surface of endothelial cells.[96] Stimulation of these receptors is followed by release of nitric oxide and vasodilatation. However, direct stimulation of vascular smooth muscle cells by choline esters results in pertussis toxin-sensitive vasoconstriction that suggests involvement of M_2, or M_4, or both receptors.[97]

Cardiac M_2 muscarinic receptors densely populate specialized cardiac conductive tissue such as the sinoatrial and atrioventricular nodes and the Purkinje fibers but are sparse in the ventricular myocardium.[98] In the sinoatrial node, cholinergic stimulation causes the opening of inwardly rectifying potassium channels by activated G protein α-[99] or βγ-subunits.[100] Acetylcholine has an additional strong inhibitory action on the hyperpolarization-activated i_f

current, a nonspecific cation current normally carried by Na^+ and K^+ ions.[101] This leads to a decrease in the rate of spontaneous diastolic depolarization, resulting in slowing of heart rate. In the atrioventricular node and in the Purkinje fibers, cholinergic stimulation increases the refractory period and slows impulse conduction. If cholinergic stimulation is overwhelming, complete heart block may occur. However, cholinergic stimulation can be clinically beneficial by reducing the ventricular rate in atrial fibrillation.

In atrial muscle, acetylcholine shortens the duration of the action potential and the effective refractory period.[102] Stimulation of muscarinic receptors affects ventricular function indirectly by inhibiting the effects of adrenergic, cyclic adenosine monophosphate–dependent activation.[103] Indeed, muscarinic receptor–mediated negative inotropic effect on the ventricles is only observed when the force of myocardial contraction is increased by stimulation of β adrenergic receptors.[104,105] In addition, activation of presynaptic M_1 receptors on adrenergic sympathetic fibers inhibits release of norepinephrine and contributes to reduced myocardial response to catecholamines. The density of muscarinic receptors in the myocardium decreases with age[106] but does not change in chronic heart failure.[107]

Stimulation of muscarinic receptors reduces heart rate and myocardial oxygen consumption,[108] and chronic hypoxia increases the density of M_2 receptors in the ventricles.[109] M_2 receptor agonists may become clinically useful in the treatment of acute myocardial ischemia,[110] based on their ability to reduce myocardial oxygen consumption and catecholamine-induced arrhythmias through a mechanism mediated by the inhibitory G_i protein.

M_3 receptors were found to predominate on both the sphincter muscle of iris of the eye, which regulates the amount of light reaching the retina, and the ciliary body, which continually adjusts the focal characteristics of the lens.[111]

Bronchoconstriction may occur secondary to cholinergic stimulation.[112] Both M_2 and M_3 receptors were identified in bronchial smooth muscle[113]; bronchial M_3 receptors mediate muscarinic agonist-induced bronchoconstriction,[114] whereas M_2 receptors functionally antagonize β receptor–mediated bronchodilation through inhibition of adenylyl cyclase activity.[115] M_3 receptor–dependent activation of protein kinase C causes uncoupling of β receptors from adenylyl cyclase,[116] whereas dysfunctional parasympathetic prejunctional M_2 receptors do not inhibit acetylcholine release, an effect that contributes to exaggerated cholinergic bronchoconstriction.[117] Tone, peristaltic activity, and the amplitude of contractions within the gastrointestinal tract increase with cholinergic stimulation.[118] Postganglionic cholinergic efferent fibers make direct contact with enteral smooth muscle cells, and muscarinic receptors are present in the longitudinal and circumflex muscles in the entire length of the gut.[119] When unopposed, this may result in intestinal cramps, belching, nausea and vomiting, and involuntary defecation. Muscarinic M_2 and M_3 receptors were identified in the stomach, ileum, and cecum; the M_3 receptor appears to mediate contraction,[120,121] whereas M_2 receptors modulate cyclic adenosine monophosphate–driven relaxation.[122] In the colon, parasympathetic stimulation causes sodium and fluid absorption and mucus secretion.[123]

In the genitourinary tract, acetylcholine increases ureteral peristalsis, contracts the detrusor muscle, and relaxes the trigone and external sphincter. Parasympathetic stimulation results in increased secretion of tears, saliva, and sweat, as well as tracheobronchial and digestive mucus.[124]

Synthetic Choline Esters

Rapid hydrolysis of acetylcholine at the neuroeffector junction and in the plasma by cholinesterases precludes systemic use of acetylcholine for therapeutic purposes. However, an 1:100 intraocular preparation is available to rapidly induce miosis during ophthalmic surgery.

Muscarinic receptors can be activated by agonists that are resistant to cholinesterases, or by blocking the degradation of susceptible agonists by cholinesterase inhibitors.[125]

Cholinesterase-resistant choline esters were initially synthesized in the 1930s. Methacholine (acetyl-β-methylcholine) is resistant to hydrolysis by plasma cholinesterases and is only slowly hydrolyzed by acetylcholinesterase. Methacholine acts predominantly on the muscarinic receptors but retains mild agonist properties for nicotinic receptors. The methacholine inhalation challenge test is used in the investigation of cholinergic involvement in patients with reactive airway disease.[126]

Both bethanechol and carbachol are carbamoyl ester derivatives of acetylcholine. They are resistant to hydrolysis, both by acetylcholinesterase and plasma cholinesterases. Bethanechol acts predominantly on muscarinic receptors, whereas carbachol has significant effect on nicotinic receptors, particularly in the autonomic ganglia.[127] Bethanechol and carbachol stimulate the urinary tract and the gastrointestinal tract rather selectively, and bethanechol is used in the treatment of neurogenic bladder paralysis after spinal cord injury. Bethanechol also increases lower esophageal sphincter tone and esophageal and gastric motility.[128] However, its popularity in the treatment of gastroesophageal reflux has faded with the emergence of more specific prokinetic drugs, such as metoclopramide and cisapride (see Chapter 44). The usual oral dose of bethanechol is 10 to 50 mg two to four times a day, and the subcutaneous dose is 2.5 to 5 mg.

Bethanechol and carbachol should only be administered orally or subcutaneously, because the usual oral doses decrease diastolic blood pressure only slightly. When administered intravenously or intramuscularly, bethanechol and carbachol lose their relative selectivity, and the incidence and severity of side effects increase. Muscarinic side effects are readily reversed by intravenous administration of atropine, but severe cardiovascular or bronchial side effects may need immediate treatment with epinephrine.

Cholinomimetic Alkaloids

Muscarine (see Fig. 34–5) causes diaphoresis, salivation, abdominal cramps, nausea, and severe vomiting commonly accompanied by visual disturbances, hypotension, and bradycardia. Bronchospasm may be induced in susceptible individuals. Symptoms usually occur within 15 to

30 minutes of ingestion, and victims recover within 24 hours. In severe muscarine poisoning, death is usually caused by respiratory failure. The antidote is atropine; severe cases may need supportive ventilation. The lethal dose of muscarine in humans is 0.2 g.

Whereas muscarine acts predominantly on muscarinic receptors, pilocarpine and arecoline affect both muscarinic and nicotinic receptors. Pilocarpine, the only parasympathomimetic alkaloid currently in clinical use, is used to treat glaucoma and xerostomia. When instilled in the eye, pilocarpine causes miosis lasting several hours. A transient increase in intraocular pressure is followed by the main therapeutic effect: a prolonged (up to 8 hours) decrease in intraocular pressure. The usual solutions for treatment of open-angle glaucoma are 0.5% to 4%, but solutions to 10% are also available. Oral doses of 5 to 10 mg four times a day are used to treat xerostomia associated with Sjögren syndrome[129] and radiation therapy[130] involving the salivary glands. The most common side effect is diaphoresis, which is usually well tolerated. However, severe symptomatic atrioventricular block induced by pilocarpine eye drops has occurred in an elderly man.[131]

Arecoline is a chemical found in the nut of the betel palm tree. Arecoline crosses the blood–brain barrier rapidly and elicits a variety of central and parasympathetic effects.[132] Although arecoline has a plasma half-life of only 1 to 9 minutes, if the betel quid (a wad of the mixture used for chewing) is held in the mouth, first-pass metabolism of the drug is not a factor, and the alkaloid stays in the blood for extended periods of time. Severe and occasionally fatal cardiac dysrhythmias,[133] myocardial infarction,[134] acute severe asthma,[135] and extrapyramidal symptoms[136] have been attributed to ingestion of betel nut.

Parasympatholytic Drugs

Parasympatholytics are drugs that oppose the effects of the parasympathetic nervous system through anticholinergic action—that is, they prevent acetylcholine from acting as a neurotransmitter at muscarinic receptors.

Muscarinic receptor antagonists competitively block the binding of acetylcholine to the muscarinic receptor and have little or no effect on the binding of acetylcholine to the nicotinic receptor.

Background and History

Several plants contain parasympatholytic alkaloids. Scopolamine (hyoscine) is found in the common Eurasian weed henbane *(Hyoscyamus niger)*.[137] In the Middle Ages, henbane extract was used to enhance the inebriating qualities of beer (the word "pilsner" is related to the German word for henbane). Medieval "witches" consumed and rubbed their skin with belladonna and henbane to produce flushed skin, vivid hallucinations of flying in the air, and wild dancing.

Atropine is an alkaloid found in several plants, the two most common being deadly nightshade and jimsonweed.[137] Deadly nightshade *(Atropa belladonna)* was named after Atropa, who, according to Greek mythology, cuts the thread of life.[138] The name belladonna ("pretty woman") comes from the ancient custom of treating the face with nightshade to produce a flushed complexion and dilated pupils. Deadly nightshade is a perennial plant found widely in Euro-Asia and the Middle East. Its poisonous qualities were long exploited: the emperor Claudius was among its victims. Also, legend has it that barrels of beer laced with belladonna sap saved Scotland from the invading Danes. Medicinal use of belladonna extracts dates back to Galen (129–210 AD), who recommended it for nonhealing ulcers. The use of henbane and nightshade for sedation and anesthesia was described by Avicenna (980–1037 AD).[139]

Jimsonweed or thorn apple *(Datura stramonium,* "thorny fruit") is a decorative but extremely poisonous plant. Originally from Asia, jimsonweed was spread all over the world by gypsies. In India, smoke from burned jimsonweed was long used to treat asthma. The plant was first used for Western medicinal purposes—to treat psychosis and epilepsy—in 1762. Accidental henbane and jimsonweed poisoning still occurs, mainly in children and adolescents experimenting with these plants for their hallucinogenic effect.[140] Plants contain up to 0.5% alkaloid in their leaves, roots, and fruit.[141] Prompt recognition of poisoning is important, although in most cases (the exception being children) the outcome is not fatal.

Atropine, scopolamine, and their synthetic quaternary ammonium derivatives are esters of an aromatic acid containing an asymmetrical carbon atom (tropic acid or mandelic acid) and an organic base (tropine, scopine, or an *N*-methylated derivative of tropine) closely similar in structure. Only the *l*-isomers have a pharmacologic effect, and the intact ester link and the hydroxyl group on the acid portion are essential for the antimuscarinic action.

Mechanisms of Drug Action

The structural similarity of the intramolecular arrangement around the cationic quaternary nitrogen in acetylcholine and the organic base of the antagonists is the basis for the competitive antagonism on the muscarinic receptor. The antagonists are believed to compete with acetylcholine to form a link with the residue of aspartate 105 of the third transmembrane helix. Binding of acetylcholine to the muscarinic receptor results in coupling of the receptor with a G protein. The resulting complex remains stable after the dissociation of acetylcholine after the binding of guanosine triphosphate. In one study, atropine was able to cause dissociation of the receptor/G protein complex even after the agonist was removed.[142] Atropine also abolished the basal level of G protein activation in the absence of acetylcholine.[143] Conformational change after antagonist binding to the receptor may explain these findings. Scopolamine has been shown to close inwardly rectifying acetylcholine-sensitive potassium channels, which were open at rest.[144] These findings suggest a negative intrinsic activity of atropine and scopolamine.[90]

Clinical Pharmacology

Atropine and scopolamine are nonselective inhibitors at the muscarinic receptor (see Fig. 34–5). Both are readily absorbed from the gastrointestinal tract and mucous membrane surfaces. Because scopolamine is poorly absorbed from the skin, the transdermal preparation is applied to the postauricular area to enhance absorption. When instilled intratracheally, atropine is readily absorbed.[145] Although atropine is stable when stored in glass syringes, it is adsorbed to plastic; in plastic syringes, atropine content decreases by 52% over 4 days.[146] Pharmacokinetic characteristics of atropine and scopolamine are summarized in Table 34–5.

Atropine

When atropine is administered intravenously, a transient reduction in heart rate occurs before the onset of tachycardia.[147] This paradoxic effect was once thought to be caused by a central vagal stimulating activity of atropine.[148] However, the effect is present with antimuscarinic drugs that do not penetrate the blood–brain barrier.[149] The phenomenon probably results from blockade of presynaptic inhibitory M_1 autoreceptors on vagus nerve terminals, which usually provide negative feedback on further acetylcholine release. This inhibition leads to an increase in acetylcholine release, which initially overcomes the muscarinic blockade on sinoatrial M_2 receptors.[150] Although atropine does increase resting heart rate, the maximal heart rate achieved during exercise does not change. Atropine is also less effective in increasing resting heart rate at the two extremes of age—in infants, the resting tone is predominantly sympathetic; and, in the elderly, the density of muscarinic receptors is lower.[106]

Atropine shortens the functional refractory period of the atrioventricular node, which may accelerate the ventricular rate in patients with atrial flutter or fibrillation. In complete heart block, the idioventricular rate may accelerate after atropine, although this response is unpredictable. Atropine has no effect on the denervated, acutely transplanted heart, although parasympathetic reinnervation occurs in the long term after orthotopic heart transplantation.[151] Intravenous atropine is used to counteract the cardiodecelerator effect of vagus stimulation and to prevent the parasympathomimetic effects of cholinesterase inhibitors and succinylcholine. Atropine has little, if any, effect on resting vascular tone, although larger doses produce cutaneous vasodilatation. Vasodilatation may be a compensatory response to the loss of the ability to perspire that occurs with even small doses of atropine, or a presynaptic effect on sympathetic nerves supplying the blush to areas of the body. Atropine markedly decreases baroreflex sensitivity and suppresses parasympathetic control mechanisms. Return to baseline functions takes 3 hours in healthy adults after a single 20-µg/kg intravenous dose.[152]

Atropine does not readily penetrate the blood–brain barrier and, in the usual clinical doses of 0.5 to 1 mg, has negligible effect on the CNS. Larger (5- to 10-mg) doses cause restlessness, hallucinations, and delirium. Massive intoxication leads to CNS depression and coma followed by circulatory collapse, paralysis, and respiratory failure. Elderly patients may be more vulnerable to the CNS effects of atropine than children or young adults.[153]

Topical application of atropine on the conjunctiva causes mydriasis and cycloplegia. Near vision becomes blurred, and the loss of accommodation and pupillary reflexes may not fully recover for 7 to 12 days. These unpleasant side effects can be reversed by topical parasympathomimetics or cholinesterase inhibitors. Synthetic muscarinic antagonists such as cyclopentolate and tropicamide have a much shorter duration of action and are the preferred drugs to elicit brief mydriasis and cycloplegia.

Large doses of atropine instilled in the eye and absorbed from the nasal mucosa or by swallowing may produce significant systemic effects. Delirium and psychosis have been reported for adults who used atropine eye drops.[154] Systemic administration of atropine rarely causes ocular effects and only mildly increases intraocular pressure. Nevertheless, in patients with narrow-angle glaucoma, sphincter constriction may lead to a sudden, dangerous increase in intraocular pressure.[155] For patients who have the more common open-angle glaucoma, parenteral use of atropine and scopolamine is regarded as safe.

Because of the suppression of evaporative heat loss, infants and small children who have febrile disease may develop life-threatening hyperthermia if given atropine.

Bronchial tone and secretions are partially regulated by M_3 receptors. Blockade of these receptors decreases bronchial tone[156] and thickens bronchial secretions. Although anticholinergics are most effective in alleviating

TABLE 34–5.

Pharmacokinetic Characteristics of Atropine and Scopolamine

	Bioavailability	Protein Binding	Half-life	Metabolism	Excretion
Atropine	10–25%	50%	2–4 hr (terminal: 12.5 hr)	50–75%, liver	Renal
Scopolamine	11–48%	Variable	1.5–4.5 hr	~100%, liver	Renal

bronchoconstriction from cholinergic stimulation, they also partially antagonize the effects of inflammatory mediators, suggesting a role for local or central parasympathetic reflexes in the pathophysiology of asthma and allergic airway disease. In addition, atropine has an inhibitory effect on mucociliary clearance[157] and helps suppress excessive bronchial secretions induced by ether or ketamine anesthesia. Administration of atropine produces dry mouth and difficulty in swallowing.

Atropine reduces gastric secretion of acid, mucin, and proteolytic enzymes. It also delays gastric and intestinal emptying and reduces lower esophageal sphincter tone[158,159]; this effect is not abolished by metoclopramide.[158] Because acetylcholine is only one of the mediators of gastrointestinal tone and function, use of anticholinergic agents only partially reduces gut motility and secretion. Atropine has little or no effect on the biliary sphincter mechanism and does not relieve biliary colic.

Atropine has no significant effect on the uterus. Also, even though atropine does readily cross the placenta, clinically relevant doses have no harmful effect on the fetus.[160,161]

The clinical dose of atropine is 0.5 to 1 mg (20 µg/kg) intravenously or intramuscularly, 1 to 2 mg (20–40 µg/kg) orally, or 2 mg (50 µg/kg) intratracheally. In the past, atropine has been routinely used as a premedicant or before induction of general anesthesia. This practice has diminished both in adults[162] and children[163] because anesthetic agents and skills have improved.

Scopolamine

Parenteral scopolamine is more likely than atropine to produce bradycardia, either as the only response or after an initial tachycardia.[164] Scopolamine readily penetrates the blood–brain barrier and, in the usual clinical doses of 0.3 to 0.6 mg, causes drowsiness, fatigue, amnesia, and occasionally euphoria,[165] making it a popular premedication before surgery. However, restlessness, hallucinations, and delirium may occur in the elderly or in the presence of pain, even with the usual clinical doses. These adverse effects are avoidable by combining scopolamine with a benzodiazepine or an opiate.

Although scopolamine is used to prevent and treat motion sickness, it is less effective in preventing and treating perioperative nausea and vomiting.[166] Delirium and psychosis have been reported for even transdermal use of the drug for motion sickness in children[167] and the elderly.[168]

Ocular and bronchopulmonary effects of scopolamine are similar to those of atropine. The drying effect on mucous membranes is better tolerated because of the associated sedation. Like atropine, scopolamine readily crosses the placenta.[169]

Adverse Effects of Atropine or Scopolamine Overdose

Accidental overdose or ingestion of plant alkaloids is the common cause of atropine or scopolamine poisoning. The diagnosis is suggested by dilated pupils, dry mucous membranes, difficulty in swallowing, dry and flushed skin, and the absence of sweating in a patient who is warm or hot. Usually, tachycardia, blurred vision, and headache also occur. Larger doses lead to ataxia, restlessness, delirium, and coma.

The diagnosis may be confirmed by administering 1 mg physostigmine intramuscularly. If salivation, intestinal hypermotility, and sweating do not occur, anticholinergic poisoning is likely. If the poison has been ingested, gastric lavage and administration of charcoal should be initiated without delay to limit intestinal absorption of the drug. Treatment consists of slow intravenous administration of physostigmine (up to 4 mg in adults and 0.5 mg in small children), which usually rapidly reverses delirium and coma. The patient should be observed continuously, because physostigmine is metabolized more rapidly than atropine, and a second dose may be needed in 1 or 2 hours. If physostigmine is not available, benzodiazepines may be used to achieve sedation and control seizures. Children may need active cooling by means of alcohol sponges or immersion in cold water. Severe cases may require artificial ventilation.

Many drugs used in anesthesia and intensive care may cause blockade of central cholinergic transmission—the central anticholinergic syndrome.[170] The syndrome has the clinical characteristics of central atropine poisoning. The peripheral signs of anticholinergic overdose, such as mydriasis, are often absent immediately after general anesthesia. Although restlessness, agitation, and hallucinations may occur, motionlessness and depression rather than agitation are more often the presenting clinical features perioperatively. The central anticholinergic syndrome is often mistaken for delayed recovery from anesthesia. Respiratory drive may be suppressed. Differentiation of the syndrome from other causes of perioperative confusion is possible with slow intravenous administration of physostigmine, 0.04 mg/kg. Treatment of the syndrome also consists of administration of physostigmine, which may need to be repeated every 1 to 2 hours.

Glycopyrrolate (Glycopyrronium Bromide)

Glycopyrrolate is a potent quaternary antagonist of muscarinic receptors. The commercially available drug is a mixture of the four stereoisomers. Although the mixture was reported to be highly selective for M_1 receptors,[171] the individual stereoisomers and the corresponding tertiary amines do not show selectivity to the individual muscarinic receptor subtypes.[172]

Cardiovascular responses to glycopyrrolate are similar to those for atropine. Bradycardia may occur at lower doses, but tachycardia is usually less prominent and shorter in duration.[173] Impairment of autonomic and baroreceptor reflex is about half the duration of that with atropine.[152] Its antisialagogue effect is more pronounced and lasts up to 8 hours,[174] which is two to five times longer than that of atropine.[175,176] Although glycopyrrolate reduces gastric volume and acidity, the clinical usefulness of this effect is offset by the relaxing effect of the drug on the lower esophageal sphincter.

Glycopyrrolate is poorly absorbed from the gut. When given parenterally, its elimination half-life is 0.8 to 1.2 hours. Glycopyrrolate is eliminated by the kidneys, mainly in the unchanged form, and its effects are markedly prolonged in renal failure.[177] Transplacental transfer of glycopyrrolate is negligible.[178]

Other Anticholinergic Agents

Several synthetic tertiary amine muscarinic receptor antagonists are in clinical use. Table 34–6 shows the pharmacokinetic characteristics and recommended dosing for these agents.

Benztropine (a synthetic compound containing the tropine base of atropine and the benzohydryl portion of diphenhydramine) and trihexyphenidyl are used in the treatment of parkinsonism. These two drugs are also useful in treating extrapyramidal side effects of antidopaminergic drugs such as metoclopramide and some antipsychotic drugs. Hyoscine butylbromide is used to relieve symptoms of acute renal or biliary colic and to reduce spasm during esophagogastroduodenoscopy. Oxybutynin is recommended as the main therapy for detrusor instability or urge incontinence.[179] Propantheline is indicated as adjunctive therapy for peptic ulcer disease, gastritis, and irritable bowel syndrome. Dryness of the mouth and pupillary side effects are more common with oxybutynin. Tolterodine[180] and vamicamide[181] may have fewer side effects because of tissue selectivity[182] or accumulation in the urinary bladder.[183] However, initial optimism was not confirmed in additional clinical trials.[184]

Intensive research is being done to identify receptor subtype–specific muscarinic antagonists for gastrointestinal use. Numerous compounds were synthesized and used in laboratory research. The M_1 receptor-selective pirenzepine is used clinically in several countries to treat peptic ulcers. Dry mouth and blurred vision are common side effects. Darifenacin is an M_3 antagonist that has preferential inhibitory action on muscarinic receptors in the gut and bladder.[185]

Alkylation of the nitrogen atom on the base of the belladonna alkaloids results in quaternary ammonium compounds. This alkylation results in poor absorption from the gut and mucous membranes, prolonged duration of action compared with that of the parent drug, increased activity on the nicotinic acetylcholine receptors, inability to cross the blood–brain barrier, and an increased potency in the gastrointestinal tract. The *N*-isopropyl derivative of atropine, ipratropium bromide (see Fig. 34–5), is used as an inhaled bronchodilator in patients with chronic obstructive airway disease. Because ipratropium is poorly absorbed from mucous membranes of the mouth or the tracheobronchial tree, systemic side effects are minimal. However, ipratropium is minimally effective against leukotriene-induced bronchoconstriction and thus has reduced effectiveness in bronchial asthma. Tiotropium bromide, an antagonist with a preferential slow dissociation rate from M_3 receptors,[186] and revatropate, a selective M_1 and M_3 antagonist,[185] may be the first steps toward selective muscarinic antagonists in the treatment of reactive airway disease.

TABLE 34–6.

Pharmacokinetic Characteristics and Recommended Doses of Some Parasympatholytic Drugs

Drugs	Bioavailability	Half-life	Metabolism	Elimination	Usual Dose
Benztropine	NA	NA	NA	NA	1–2 mg IV or IM,* 0.5–6 mg PO daily
Trihexyphenidyl	Well absorbed	NA	NA	NA	1–2 mg starting dose up to 20 mg daily
Hyoscine butylbromide	(parenteral)	5 hr	50%, liver	Renal	20 mg slow IV or IM
Oxybutynin	21%	2–2.5 hr	Liver: metabolite active	Renal	10–15 mg daily (5 mg in elderly)
Propantheline	50%	1.3–2 hr	95%, hydrolysis	Renal	75–120 mg daily
Tolterodine	17%[†]	2–3 hr[#]	99%, liver	Renal	2–4 mg daily
Vamicamide	Well absorbed	5.5 hr	20% liver	Renal	12–36 mg daily
Pirenzepine	25%	10 hr	Minimal	Renal	150 mg daily

*For acute dystonic reaction.
[†]In poor metabolizers (CYP2D6 deficiency), bioavailability is 65% and half-life is 10 hours.

References

1. Chen KK, Schmidt GF: The action of ephedrine, the active principle of the Chinese drug Ma Huang. J Pharmacol Exp Ther 24:339, 1924.
2. Nagai T: Ephedrin. Pharm Zeit 32:700, 1887.
3. Oliver G, Schäfer EA: The physiologic action of extract of the suprarenal capsules. J Physiol 18:230, 1895.
4. Barger G, Dale HH: Chemical structure and sympathomimetic action of amines. J Physiol 41:19, 1910.
5. Kobilka B: Adrenergic receptors as models for G protein-coupled receptors. Annu Rev Neurosci 15:87, 1992.
6. Burn JH, Rand MJ: The action of sympathomimetic amines in animals treated with reserpine. J Physiol 144:314, 1958.
7. Hoffman BB, Lefkowitz RJ: Catecholamines, sympathomimetic drugs, and adrenergic receptor antagonists. In Hardman JG, Gilman AG, Limbird LE (eds): Goodman and Gilman's The Pharmacological Basis of Therapeutics, 9th ed. New York, McGraw-Hill, 1996.
8. Patil PN, Miller DD, Trendelenburg U: Molecular geometry and adrenergic drug activity. Pharmacol Rev 26:323, 1975.
9. Bilezikian JP, Dornfeld Am, Gammon DE: Structure-binding-activity analysis of β-adrenergic amines: I. Binding to the β-receptor and activation of adenylyl cyclase. Biochem Pharmacol 27:1445, 1978.
10. Kontoyianni M, DeWeese C, Penzotti JE, et al: Three-dimensional models for agonist and antagonist complexes with β2 adrenergic receptor. J Med Chem 39:4406, 1996.
11. Strader CD, Sigal IS, Candelore MR, et al: Conserved aspartic acid residues 79 and 113 of the β-adrenergic receptor have different roles in receptor function. J Biol Chem 263:10267, 1998.
12. Bilezikian JP, Dornfeld Am, Gammon DE: Structure-binding-activity analysis of β-adrenergic amines: II. Binding to the β-receptor and inhibition of adenylyl cyclase. Biochem Pharmacol 27:1455, 1978.
13. Isogaya M, Sugimoto Y, Tanimura R, et al: Binding pockets of the β1- and β2-adrenergic receptors for subtype-specific agonists. Mol Pharmacol 56:875, 1999.
14. Kurose H, Isogaya M, Kikkawa H, et al: Domains of β1 and β2 adrenergic receptors to bind subtype selective agonists. Life Sci 62:1513, 1998.
15. Strader CD, Candelore MR, Hill WS, et al: Identification of two serine residues involved in agonist activation of the β-adrenergic receptor. J Biol Chem 264:13572, 1989.
16. Ambrosio C, Molinari P, Cotecchia S, et al: Catechol-binding serines of β2-ardrenergic receptors control the equilibrium between active and inactive receptor states. Mol Pharmacol 57:198, 2000.
17. Cushny AR: Biological relations of optically isomeric substances. Baltimore, Md, Williams and Wilkins, 1926.
18. Wieland K, Zuurmond HM, Krasel C, et al: Involvement of Asn-293 in stereospecific agonist recognition and in activation of the β2-adrenergic receptor. Proc Natl Acad Sci USA 93:9276, 1996.
19. Tainter ML, Stockton AB: Comparative actions of sympathomimetic compounds: The circulatory and local actions of the optical isomers of meta-synephrine and possible therapeutic applications. Am J Med Sci 185:832, 1933.
20. Lorhan PH, Oliverio RM: A study of the use of neosynephrine hydrochloride in spinal anesthesia in place of ephedrine for the sustaining of blood pressure. Curr Res Anesth Analg 17:44, 1938.
21. Rich S, Gubin S, Hart K: The effects of phenylephrine on right ventricular performance in patients with pulmonary hypertension. Chest 98:1102, 1990.
22. Alahuhta S, Räsänen J, Jouppila P, et al: Ephedrine and phenylephrine for avoiding maternal hypotension due to spinal anaesthesia for Caesarean section. Int J Obstet Anesth 1:129, 1992.
23. Groudine SB, Hollinger I, Jones J, et al: New York State Guidelines on the topical use of phenylephrine in the operating room. Anesthesiology 92:859, 2000.
24. Hjort AM, Randall LO, de Beer EJ: Pharmacology of compounds related to β-2,5-dimethoxy phenethyl amine; ethyl, isopropyl and propyl derivations. J Pharmacol Exp Ther 92:283, 1948.
25. King BD, Dripps RD: Use of methoxamine for maintenance of the circulation during spinal anesthesia. Surg Gynec Obstet 90:659, 1950.
26. Poe MF: Use of methoxamine hydrochloride as a pressor agent during spinal analgesia. Anesthesiology 13:89, 1952.
27. Cruz DN: Midodrine: A selective α-adrenergic agonist for orthosta-

tic hypotension and dialysis hypotension. Expert Opin Pharmacother 1:835, 2000.
28. Poe MF: The use of Aramine® as a pressor agent during spinal anesthesia. Anesthesiology 15:547, 1954.
29. Albertson NF, McKay FC, Lape HE, et al: The optical isomers of metaraminol. Synthesis and biological activity. J Med Chem 13:132, 1970.
30. Riegle EV, Gunter JB, Lusk RP, et al: Comparison of vasoconstrictors for functional endoscopic sinus surgery in children. Laryngoscope 102:820, 1992.
31. Lasseter KC, Shapse D, Pascucci VL, et al: Pharmacokinetics of guanabenz in patients with impaired liver function. J Cardiovasc Pharmacol 6:S766, 1984.
32. Sorkin EM, Heel RC: Guanfacine. A review of its pharmacodynamic and pharmacokinetic properties and therapeutic efficacy in the treatment of hypertension. Drugs 31:301, 1986.
33. Van Zwieten PA, Thoolen MJ, Timmermans PB: The hypotensive activity and the side effects of methyldopa, clonidine and guanfacine. Hypertension 6(SII):28, 1984.
34. Paegelow I, Werner H: Influence of adrenergic agonists and antagonists on lymphokine secretion in vitro. Int J Immunopharmacol 9:761, 1987.
35. Halsworth CH, Lee TH, Hirst SJ: β2-adrenoceptor agonists inhibit release of eosinophil-activating cytokines from human airway smooth muscle cells. Br J Pharmacol 132:729, 2001.
36. Arch JRS, Ainsworth AT, Cawthorne MA, et al: Atypical β-adrenoceptor on brown adipocytes as a target for anti-obesity drugs. Nature 309:163, 1984.
37. Larsson S, Svedmyr N: Tremor caused by sympathomimetics is mediated by β2-adrenoceptors. Scand J Respir Dis 58:5, 1977.
38. McDewitt DG: In vivo studies on the function of cardiac β-adrenoceptors in man. Eur Heart J 10(suppl B):22, 1989.
39. Brodde OE, Michel MC: Adrenergic and muscarinic receptors in the human heart. Pharmacol Rev 51:651, 1999.
40. Loeb HS, Khan M, Sandye A, et al: Acute hemodynamic effects of dobutamine and isoproterenol in patients with low output cardiac failure. Circ Shock 3:55, 1976.
41. Nelson HS: Beta adrenergic agonists. Chest 82(S):33, 1982.
42. Newhouse MT, Dolovich MB: Control of asthma by aerosols. N Eng J Med 315:870, 1986.
43. Bouvy ML, Heerdink ER, De Bruin ML, et al: Use of sympathomimetic drugs leads to increased risk of hospitalization for arrhythmias in patients with congestive heart failure. Arch Intern Med 160:2477, 2000.
44. Wang P, Clausen T: Treatment of attacks of hyperkalemic familial periodic paralysis by inhalation of salbutamol. Lancet I:221, 1976.
45. Brown MJ: Hypokalemia from beta2-receptor stimulation by circulating epinephrine. Am J Cardiol 56:3D, 1985.
46. Barden TP, Peter JB, Merkatz IR: Ritodrine hydrochloride: A betamimetic agent for use in preterm labor. I. Pharmacology, clinical history, administration, side effects, and safety. Obstet Gynecol 56:1, 1980.
47. Moutquin JM, Milner RA, Mohide PT, et al: Treatment of preterm labor with the beta-adrenergic agonist ritodrine. N Engl J Med 327:308, 1992.
48. Wheeler AS, Patel KF, Spain J: Pulmonary edema during beta-2-tocolytic therapy. Anesth Analg 60:695, 1981.
49. Miura K: Vorläufige Mittheilung über ephedrine, ein neues mydriaticum. Berl Klin Wochens 24:707, 1887.
50. Patil PN, Tye A, LaPidus JB: A pharmacological study of the ephedrine isomers. J Pharmacol Exp Ther 148:158, 1965.
51. Lindblad A, Bernow J, Vernersson E, et al: Effect of extradural anaesthesia on human foetal blood flow in utero. Br J Anaesth 59:1265, 1987.
52. Räsänen J, Alahuhta S, Kangas-Saarela T et al: The effects of ephedrine and etilephrine on uterine and fetal blood flow and on fetal myocardial function during spinal anesthesia for caesarian section. Int J Obstet Anaesth 1:3, 1991.
53. Ferguson LK, North JP: Observations on experimental spinal anaesthesia. Surg Gynecol Obstet 54:62, 1932.
54. Dripps RD, van Deming M: An evaluation of certain drugs used to maintain blood pressure during spinal anesthesia. Comparison of ephedrine, paredrine, pitressin-ephedrine and methedrine in 2500 cases. Surg Gynecol Obstet 83:312, 1946.
55. Moore KE: Toxicity and catecholamine releasing actions of d- and

l-amphetamine in isolated and aggregated mice. J Pharmacol Exp Ther 142:6, 1963.

56. Vidrio H, Parra J, Padro EG: Characterization of the antihypertensive effects of *d*-amphetamine. Fed Proc 29:150, 1970.

57. Silverstone T: Appetite suppressants. A review. Drugs 43:820, 1992.

58. Bray GA: Use and abuse of appetite-suppressant drugs in the treatment of obesity. Ann Intern Med 119:707, 1993.

59. Hall AP: "Ecstasy" and the anaesthetist. Br J Anaesth 79:697, 1997.

60. Singarajah MH, Lavies NG: An overdose of ecstasy. A role for dantrolene. Anaesthesia 47:686, 1992.

61. Saxena VK, De Deyn PP: Ergotamine: Its use in the treatment of migraine and its complications. Acta Neurol (Napoli) 14:140, 1992.

62. Carruthers SG: Adverse effects of α 1-adrenergic blocking drugs. Drug Saf 11:12, 1994.

63. Kinney MA, Warner ME, vanHeerden JA, et al: Perianesthetic risks and outcomes of pheochromocytoma and paraganglioma resection. Anesth Analg 91:1118, 2000.

64. Caine M, Perlberg S, Meretyk S: A placebo-controlled double-blind study of the effect of phenoxybenzamine in benign prostatic obstruction. Br J Urol 50:551, 1978.

65. Stevenson DK, Kasting DS, Darnall RA, et al: Refractory hypoxemia associated with neonatal pulmonary disease: The use and limitations of tolazoline. J Pediatr 95:595, 1979.

66. Weinberger B, Weiss K, Heck DE, et al: Pharmacologic therapy of persistent pulmonary hypertension of the newborn. Pharmacol Ther 89:67, 2001.

67. Black JW, Stephenson JS: Pharmacology of a new adrenergic beta-receptor blocking compound. Lancet 2:311, 1962.

68. Van Baak MA: Beta-adrenoceptor blockade and exercise: An update. Sports Med 5:209, 1988.

69. Man in't Veld AJ, Van den Meiracker AH, Schalekamp MA: Do beta-blockers really increase peripheral vascular resistance? Review of the literature and new observations under basal conditions. Am J Hypertens 1:91, 1988.

70. Mitchell HC, Pettinger WA: Dose-response of clonidine on plasma catecholamines in the hypernoradrenergic state associated with vasodilator β-blocker therapy. J Cardiovasc Pharmacol 3:647, 1981.

71. Prys-Roberts C: Interactions of anaesthesia and high pre-operative doses of β-receptor antagonists. Acta Anaesthesiol Scand 76(S):47, 1982.

72. Matthys H, Doshan HD, Rühle KH et al: The bronchosparing effects of celiprolol, a new beta-1 alpha-2-receptor antagonist on pulmonary function of propranolol sensitive asthmatics. J Clin Pharmacol 25:354, 1985.

73. Van Zwieten PA: The role of adrenoceptors in circulatory and metabolic regulation. Am Heart J 116:1384, 1988.

74. Rabkin SW: Mechanism of action of adrenergic receptor blockers on lipids during antihypertensive drug treatment. J Clin Pharmacol 33:286, 1993.

75. Nadelmann JW, Phil M, Stevens J, et al: Propranolol in the prophylaxis of migraine. Headache 26:175, 1986.

76. Ljung O: Treatment of migraine with metoprolol. N Engl J Med 303:156, 1980.

77. Becker WJ: Evidence based migraine prophylactic therapy. Can J Neurol Sci 26:S27, 1999.

78. Blier P, Bergeron R, de Montigny C: Selective activation of postsynaptic 5-HT1A receptors induces rapid antidepressant response. Neuropsychopharmacology 16:333, 1997.

79. Broeders MAW, Doevendans PA, Bekkers BCAM, et al: Nebivolol: A third-generation β-blocker that augments vascular nitric oxide release. Endothelial β2-adrenergic receptor-mediated nitric oxide production. Circulation 102:677, 2000.

80. Karle CA, Kreye VAW, Thomas D, et al: Antiarrhythmic drug carvedilol inhibits HERG potassium channels. Cardiovasc Res 49:361, 2001.

81. Packer M, Bristow MR, Cohn JN et al: The effect of carvedilol on morbidity and mortality in patients with chronic heart failure. US Carvedilol Heart Failure Group. N Engl J Med 334:1349, 1996.

82. Magee LA, Elran E, Bull SB, et al: Risks and benefits of β-receptor blockers for pregnancy hypertension: Overview of randomized trials. Eur J Obstet Gynecol Reprod Biol 88:15, 2000.

83. Nishio H, Nagakura Y, Segawa T: Interactions or careolol and other beta-adrenoceptor blocking agents with serotonin receptor subtypes. Arch Int Pharmacodyn Ther 302:96, 1989.

84. Gainetdinov RR, Caron MG: Delineating muscarinic receptor functions. Proc Natl Acad Sci USA 96:12222, 1999.

85. Schmiedeberg O, Koppe R: Das Muscarin. Das giftige Alkaloid des Fliegenpilzes. Leipzig, 1869.

86. Grieve M: Jaborandi. In A modern herbal on-line at http://www.botanical.com/botanical/mgmh/j/jabora01.html, 2000.

87. Marshall M: An overview of drugs in Oceania. In Lindström L (ed): Drugs in Western Pacific Societies: Relations of Substance. ASAO Monograph No II. Lanham, Md, University Press of America, 1987.

88. DörjeF, Levey AI, Brann MR: Immunological detection of muscarinic receptor subtype proteins (m1-m5) in rabbit peripheral tissues. Mol Pharmacol 40:459, 1991.

89. Hulme EC, Birdsall NJM, Buckley NJ: Muscarinic receptor subtypes. Annu Rev Pharmacol Toxicol 30:633, 1990.

90. Caulfield MP: Muscarinic receptors—characterization, coupling and function. Pharmacol Ther 58:319, 1993.

91. Hulme EC, Curtis CAM, Page KM, et al: Agonist activation of muscarinic acetylcholine receptors. Cell Signal 5:687, 1993.

92. Curtis CA, Wheatley M, Bansal S, et al: Propylbenzylcholine mustard labels an acidic residue in transmembrane helix 3 of the muscarinic receptor. J Biol Chem 264:489, 1989.

93. Wess J: Molecular basis of muscarinic acetylcholine receptor function. Trends Pharmacol Sci 14:308, 1993.

94. Felder CC: Muscarinic acetylcholine receptors: Transduction through multiple effectors. FASEB J 9:619, 1995.

95. Brown JH, Taylor P: Muscarinic receptor agonists and antagonists. In Hardman JG, Gilman AG, Limbird LE (eds): Goodman and Gilman's The Pharmacological Basis of Therapeutics, 9th ed. New York, McGraw-Hill, 1996.

96. Eglen RM, Whiting RL: Heterogeneity of vascular muscarinic receptors. J Auton Pharmacol 19:233, 1990.

97. Hohlfeld J, Liebau S, Forstermann U: Pertussis toxin inhibits contractions but not endothelim-dependent relaxations of rabbit pulmonary artery in response to acetylcholine and other agonists. J Pharmacol Exp Ther 252:260, 1990.

98. Deighton NM, Motomura S, Borquez D, et al: Muscarinic cholinoceptors in the human heart: demonstration, subclassification and distribution. Naunyn-Schmiedebergs Arch Pharmacol 341:14, 1990.

99. Yatani A, Codina J, Brown AM, et al: Direct activation of mammalian atrial muscarinic potassium channels by GTP regulatory protein Gk. Science 235:207, 1987.

100. Yamada M, Inanobe A, Kurachi Y: G protein regulation of potassium ion channels. Pharmacol Rev 50:723, 1998.

101. Difrancesco D, Tromba C: Acetylcholine inhibits activation of the cardiac pacemaker current, if. Pflüger Arch 410:139, 1987.

102. Giles W, Noble SJ: Changes in the membrane currents in bullfrog atrium produced by acetylcholine. J Physiol 261:103, 1976.

103. Levy MN: Sympathetic-parasympathetic interactions in the heart. Circ Res 29:437, 1971.

104. Loffelholz K, Pappano A: The parasympathetic neuroeffector junction of the heart. Pharmacol Rev 37:1, 1985.

105. Von Scheidt, W, Böhm M, Stäblein A, et al: Antiadrenergic effect of *m*-cholinoceptor stimulation on human ventricular contraction in vivo. Am J Physiol 263:H1927, 1992.

106. Brodde OE, Konschak U, Becker K, et al: Cardiac muscarinic receptors decrease with age. In vitro and in vivo studies. J Clin Invest 101:471, 1998.

107. Giessler C, Dhein S, Pönicke K, et al: Muscarinic receptors in the failing human heart. Eur J Pharmacol 375:197, 1999.

108. Nuutinen EM, Wilson DF, Erecinska M: The effect of cholinergic agonists on coronary flow rate and oxygen consumption in isolated perfused rat heart. J Mol Cell Cardiol 17:31, 1985.

109. Favret F, Richalet JP, Henderson KK, et al: Myocardial adrenergic and cholinergic receptor function in hypoxia: Correlation with O2 transport in exercise. Am J Physiol Regul Integr Comp Physiol 280:R730, 2001.

110. Rauch B, Niroomand F: Specific M2-receptor activation: An alternative to treatment with β-receptor blockers? Eur Heart J 12(suppl F):76, 1991.

111. Woldemussie E, Feldmann BJ, Chen J: Characterization of muscarinic receptors in cultured human iris sphincter and ciliary smooth muscle cells. Exp Eye Res 56:385, 1993.

112. Richardson JB. Nerve supply to the lung. Am Rev Resp Dis 119:785, 1979.

113. Mak JCW, Barnes PJ: Autoradiographic visualization of muscarinic receptor subtypes in human and guinea-pig lung. Am J Resp Dis 141:1559, 1990.

114. Meurs H, Timmermans A, Van Amsterdam RMG, et al: Muscarinic

receptors in human airway smooth muscle are coupled to phospho-inositide metabolism. Eur J Pharmacol 164:369, 1989.

115. Gunst SJ, Stropp JQ, Flavahan NA: Muscarinic receptor reserve and β-adrenergic sensitivity in tracheal smooth muscle. J Appl Physiol 67:1294, 1989.

116. Zaagsma J, Roffel AF, Meurs H: Muscarinic control of airway function. Life Sci 60:1061, 1997.

117. Barnes PJ, Haddad EB, Rousell J: Regulation of muscarinic M₂ receptors. Life Sci 60:1015, 1997.

118. Goyal RK: Identification, localization and classification of muscarinic receptor subtypes in the gut. Life Sci 43:2209, 1988.

119. Buckley N, Burnstock G: Autoradiographic localization of muscarinic receptors in guinea pig intestine: Distribution of low and high affinity sites. Brain Res 295:15, 1984.

120. Eglen RM, Harris GC: Selective inactivation of muscarinic M₂ and M₃ receptors in guinea-pig ileum and atria in vitro. Br J Pharmacol 109:946, 1993.

121. Kerr PM, Hillier K, Wallis RM, et al: Characterization of muscarinic receptors mediating contractions of circular and longitudinal muscle of human colon. Br J Pharmacol 115:1518, 1995.

122. Ehlert FJ, Thomas EA: Functional role of M₂ muscarinic receptors in the guinea-pig ileum. Life Sci 56:965, 1995.

123. Venglarik CJ, Dawson DC: Cholinergic regulation of Na absorption by turtle colon: Role of basolateral K conductance. Am J Physiol 251:C563–C570, 1986.

124. Hirschowitz BI, Keeling D, Lewin M, et al: Pharmacological aspects of acid secretion. Dig Dis Sci 40:3S, 1995.

125. Cushny AR: The action of atropine, pilocarpine and physostigmine. J Physiol 41:233, 1910.

126. Maclagan J, Barnes PJ: Muscarinic pharmacology of the airways. Trends Pharmacol Sci 5:88, 1989.

127. Brown DA, Ftaherazi S, Garthwaite J, et al: Muscarinic receptors in rat sympathetic ganglia. Br J Pharmacol 70:577, 1980.

128. Humphries TJ: Effects of long-term medical treatment with cimetidine and bethanechol in patients with esophagitis and Barrett's esophagus. J Clin Gastroenterol 9:28, 1987.

129. Nusair S, Rubinow A: The use of oral pilocarpine in xerostomia and Sjögren's syndrome. Semin Arthritis Rheum 28:360, 1999.

130. Horiot JC, Lipinski F, Schraub S, et al: Post-radiation severe xerostomia relieved by pilocarpine: A prospective French cooperative study. Radiother Oncol 55:233, 2000.

131. Littmann L, Kempler P, Rohla M, et al: Severe symptomatic atrioventricular block induced by pilocarpine eye drops. Arch Intern Med 147:586, 1987.

132. Asthana S, Greig NH, Holloway HW, et al: Clinical pharmacokinetics of arecholine in subjects with Alzheimer's disease. Clin Pharmacol Ther 60:276, 1996.

133. Chiang WT, Yang CC, Deng JF, et al: Cardiac arrhythmia and betel nut chewing—is there a casual effect? Vet Hum Toxicol 40:287, 1998.

134. Hung DZ, Deng JF: Acute myocardial infarction temporally related to betel nut chewing. Vet Hum Toxicol 40:25, 1998.

135. Taylor RF, al-Jarad N, John LM, et al: Betel-nut chewing and asthma. Lancet 339(8802):1134, 1992.

136. Deahl M: Betel nut-induced extrapyramidal syndrome: An unusual drug interaction. Mov Disord 4:330, 1989.

137. Iliev I, Varbanova M, Zhekov O, et al: Poisonous plants and animals. On-line at http://library.thinkquest.org/C007974/1plants.htm, 2000.

138. Graves R: The Greek Myths. New York, Penguin, 1993.

139. Aziz E, Nathan B, McKeever J: Anesthetic and analgesic practices in Avicenna's Canon of Medicine. Am J Chinese Med 28:147, 2000.

140. Turgul L: Abuse of henbane by children in Turkey. Bull Narc 37:75, 1985.

141. Adriani J: The chemistry and physics of anesthesia, ed 2, Springfield, CC Thomas, 1962.

142. Matesic DF, Luthin GR: Atropine dissociates complexes of muscarinic acetylcholine receptor and guanine nucleotide-binding protein in heart membranes. FEBS Lett 284:184, 1991.

143. Hilf G, Jakobs KH: Agonist-independent inhibition of G protein activation by muscarinic acetylcholine receptor antagonists in cardiac membranes. Eur J Pharmacol 225:245, 1992.

144. Soejima M, Noma A: Mode of regulation of the Ach-sensitive K-channel by the muscarinic receptor in rabbit atrial cells. Pflüger Arch 409:424, 1984.

145. Hornchen U, Schutter J, Stoeckel H, et al: Comparison of intravenous and endobronchial atropine: A pharmacokinetic and dynamic study in pigs. Eur J Anaesthesiol 6:95, 1989.

146. Lewis B, Jarvi E, Cady P: Atropine and ephedrine adsorption to syringe plastic. AANA J 62:257, 1994.

147. Morton HJV, Thomas ET: Effect of atropine on the heart rate. Lancet ii:1313, 1958.

148. Das G, Talmers FN, Weissler AM: New observations on the effects of atropine on the sinuatrial and atrioventricular nodes. Am J Cardiol 36:281, 1975.

149. Kottmeier CA, Gravenstein JS: The parasympathomimetic activity of atropine and atropine methylbromide. Anesthesiology 29:1125, 1968.

150. Wellstein A, Pitschner HF: Complex dose-response curves of atropine in man explained by different functions of M₁- and M₂-cholinoceptors. Naunyn Schmiedebergs Arch Pharmacol 338:19, 1988.

151. Überführ P, Frey AW, Reichart B: Vagal reinnervation in the long term after orthotopic heart transplantation. J Heart Lung Transplant 19:946, 2000.

152. Parlow JL, van Vlymen JM, Odell MJ: The duration of impairment of autonomic control after anticholinergic drug administration in humans. Anesth Analg 84:155, 1997.

153. Smith DS, Orkin FK, Gardner SM, et al: Prolonged sedation in the elderly after intraoperative atropine administration. Anesthesiology 51:348, 1979.

154. Kounis NG: Letter: Atropine eye-drops delirium. Can Med Assoc J 110:759, 1974.

155. Mendak JS, Minerva P, Wilson TW, et al: Angle closure glaucoma complicating systemic atropine use in the cardiac catheterization laboratory. Cath Cardiovasc Diagn 39:262, 1996.

156. Gal TJ, Suratt PM: Atropine and glycopyrrolate effects on lung mechanics in normal man. Anesth Analg 60:85, 1981.

157. Annis P, Landa J, Lichtiger M: Effects of atropine on velocity of tracheal mucus in anesthetized patients. Anesthesiology 44:74, 1976.

158. Cotton BR, Smith G: Single and combined effects of atropine and metoclopramide on the lower esophageal sphincter pressure. Br J Anaesth 53:869, 1981.

159. Opie JC, Chaye H, Steward DJ: Intravenous atropine rapidly reduces lower esophageal sphincter pressure in infants and children. Anesthesiology 67:989, 1987.

160. Kanto J, Virtanen R, Iisalo E, et al: Placental transfer and pharmacokinetics of atropine after a single maternal intravenous and intramuscular administration. Acta Anaesthesiol Scand 25:85, 1981.

161. Abboud T, Raya J, Sadri S, et al: Fetal and maternal cardiovascular effects of atropine and glycopyrrolate. Anesth Analg 62:426, 1983.

162. Leighton KM, Sanders HD: Anticholinergic premedication. Can Anaesth Soc J 34:259, 1976.

163. Jöhr, M: Is it time to question the routine use of anticholinergic agents in paediatric anaesthesia? Paediatr Anaesth 9:99, 1999.

164. List WF, Gravenstein JS: Effects of atropine and scopolamine on the cardiovascular system in man: II. Secondary bradycardia after scopolamine. Anesthesiology 26:299, 1965.

165. Ostfeld AM, Arguete A: Central nervous system effects of hyoscine in man. J Pharmacol Exp Ther 137:133, 1962.

166. Gibbons PA, Nicolson SC, Betts EK, et al: Scopolamine does not prevent postoperative emesis after pediatric eye surgery. Anesthesiology 61:A435, 1984.

167. Osterholm RK, Camoriano JK: Transdermal scopolamine psychosis. JAMA 247:3081, 1982.

168. Wilkinson JA: Side effects of transdermal scopolamine. J Emerg Med 5:389, 1987.

169. Kanto J, Kentala E, Kaila T, et al: Pharmacokinetics of scopolamine during caesarian section: Relationship between serum concentration and effect. Acta Anaesth Scand 33:482, 1989.

170. Schnesk HJ, Ruphert J: Central anticholinergic syndrome in anaesthesia and intensive care. Acta Anaesthesiol Belg 40:219, 1989.

171. Fuder H, Meincke M: Glycopyrronium blocks differentially responses mediated by muscarinic receptor subtypes. Naunyn Schmiedebergs Arch Pharmacol 347:591, 1993.

172. Czeche S, Elgert M, Noe C, et al: Antimuscarinic properties of the stereoisomers of glycopyrronium bromide. Life Sci 60:1167, 1997.

173. Mirakhur RK: Intravenous administration of glycopyrronium: Effects on cardiac rate and rhythm. Anaesthesia 34:458, 1979.

174. Ali-Melkkilä T, Kaila T, Kanto J, Iisalo E: Pharmacokinetics of i.m. glycopyrronium. Br J Anaesth 64:667, 1990.

175. Wyant GM, Kao E: Glycopyrrolate methobromide. I. Effect on salivary secretions. Can Anaesth Soc J 21:230, 1974.

176. Mirakhur RK, Dundee JW: Glycopyrrolate: Pharmacology and clinical use. Anaesthesia 38:1195, 1983.

177. Ali-Melkkilä T, Kanto J, Iisalo E: Pharmacokinetics and related pharmacodynamics of anticholinergic drugs. Acta Anaesthesiol Scand 37:633, 1993.

178. Ali-Melkkilä T, Kaila T, Kanto J, et al: Pharmacokinetics of glycopyrronium in parturients. Anaesthesia 45:634, 1990.

179. Hieble JP, McCafferty GP, Naselsky DP, et al: Recent progress in the pharmacotherapy of diseases of the urinary tract. Eur J Med Chem 30:269, 1995.

180. Nilvebrant L, Glass G, Jonsson A, et al: The in vitro pharmacological profile of Tolterodine—a new agent for the treatment of urinary urge incontinence. Neurourol Urodyn 13:433, 1994.

181. Yamamoto T, Matsuo M, Yamazaki S, et al: Antimuscarinic properties of vamicamide, a novel compound for the treatment of pollakicuria. Drug Dev Res 34:9, 1995.

182. Gillberg PG, Modiri AR, Sparf B: Tolterodine—a new agent with tissue selectivity for urinary bladder. Neurourol Urodyn 13:435, 1994.

183. Oyasu H, Yamamoto T, Sato N, et al: Urinary bladder selective action of the new antimuscarinic compound vamicamide. Arzneimittelforschung 4:1242, 1994.

184. Withdrawal of NDA for antipollakiuria agent. Fujisawa Pharmaceutical, 1998. On-line at http://www.fujisawa.co.jp/english/ir/release/e981001.shtm/

185. Alabaster VA: Discovery and development of selective M_3 antagonists for clinical use. Life Sci 60:1053, 1997.

186. Haddad EB, Mak JC, Barnes PJ: Characterization of [^{3}H]Ba 679 Br, a slowly dissociating muscarinic antagonist, in human lung: Radioligand binding and autoradiographic mapping. Mol Pharmacol 45:899, 1994.

187. Pharmacokinetic data and recommended dosing of drugs were compiled from the following Internet databases: http://emc.vhn.net/public/; www.medsafe.govt.nz/search.htm; www.rxmed.com; http://www.pflegeintensiv.de/notfallmedis/; www.biam2.org

35

Antiarrhythmic Agents

Marye J. Gleva, MD • Charles W. Hogue, Jr., MD

Cardiac arrhythmias are common perioperatively ranging in frequency from less than 1% for serious ventricular arrhythmias to 40% for atrial fibrillation (AF) after cardiac surgery.[1,2] Antiarrhythmic drugs are compounds whose actions affect the cellular and subcellular mechanisms of arrhythmia initiation and maintenance. The use of antiarrhythmic drugs for treating and preventing cardiac arrhythmias has undergone critical reappraisal over the last several decades partly because of concerns regarding the potential of these drugs to depress left ventricular function and to precipitate arrhythmias (proarrhythmic effects).[3–6] Furthermore, results from randomized clinical trials showing improved survival for patients receiving implantable cardioverter-defibrillator devices compared with antiarrhythmic drugs has revolutionized treatment paradigms for patients with ventricular arrhythmias.[7] Finally, advances in catheter ablation techniques now make these methods the therapy of choice for many supraventricular arrhythmias including atrial flutter and subtypes of paroxysmal AF.[8] As a result, antiarrhythmic drug therapy, beyond the acute arrhythmic episodes, is now primarily used for patients with AF and

atrial flutter not amenable to catheter ablation treatment, for patients who have failed catheter ablation therapy, and for patients with implantable cardioverter-defibrillator devices who are receiving frequent, yet appropriate shocks or cardiac pacing treatments. This chapter reviews the pharmacology of antiarrhythmic drugs and their indications along with the basic principles of acute arrhythmia management.

Mechanism of Drug Action

The cardiac action potential (AP) is the result of multiple inward and outward ion currents with specific ion channels responsible for each of the five phases (Fig. 35–1).[9] The duration of each phase of the AP varies regionally in the heart, and the specialized conduction system exhibits regional differences in ion channel density. This relationship between ion channels and AP phase is fundamental to

A

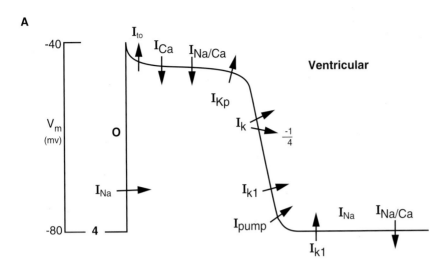

B

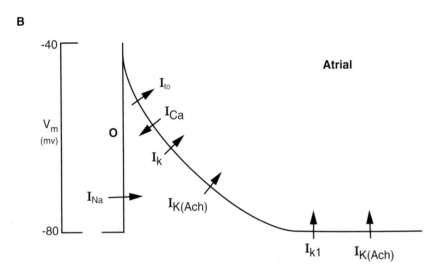

Figure 35–1. Ion channels that comprise the cardiac action potential. *A,* Represents the action potential in ventricular myocardium. *B,* Represents an atrial action potential. I_{Ca}, Ca^+ current; I_K, delayed (outwardly rectifying) K^+ current; I_{K2}, inwardly rectifying K^+ current; $I_{K(Ach)}$, acetylcholine activated K^+ current; I_{Kp}, plateau K^+ current; I_{Na}, Na^+ current; $I_{Na/Ca}$, Na^+Ca^{2+} exchanger; I_{pump}, Na^+K^+ pump current; I_{to}, transient outward current. (Redrawn from Whalley DW, Wendt DJ, Grant AO: Basic concepts in cellular cardiac electrophysiology: Part II: Block of ion channels by antiarrhythmic drugs. Pacing Clin Electrophysiol 18:1565, 1995.)

understanding the cellular, antiarrhythmic, and electrocardiogram (ECG) effects of antiarrhythmic drugs. At the molecular level, antiarrhythmic drugs exert their effect on *ion channels, pumps,* or *receptors.* Ion-specific channels exist for sodium, potassium, calcium, and chloride. Membrane pump targets for antiarrhythmic drug therapy include the Na^+-K^+ ATPase, the Na^+/Ca^{++} exchanger, the Na^+-H^+ exchanger, the Cl-$HCO3$- exchanger, and the Na^+K^+/Cl^- cotransporter. Membrane receptor targets for antiarrhythmic treatments include the β_1 and β_2 adrenergic receptors, muscarinic M_2 receptor, and purinergic A_1 and A_2 receptors. However, much of the current interest in the development of new antiarrhythmic drugs is focused on ion channel or channel subgroup-specific agents.

Ion Channels

Ion channels are large membrane-bound glycoproteins that change configuration or function in response to a stimulus, thus providing a pathway of low electrical resistance across the hydrophobic lipid bilayer of the cell membrane.[10,11] Ion channels exist in different states, specifically the *open, inactivated,* or *closed state.* In the open state, the channel has changed its configuration to allow passive flux of an ion along an electrochemical gradient. An activated channel progresses first to the inactivated state, at which time further ion conductance stops, and then to the closed state (i.e., resting state). Whereas an inactivated channel is unresponsive to a continued or new stimulus, a resting channel can open in response to a subsequent stimulus. The resting ion channel state is more prevalent during diastole. The active state occurs during the upstroke of the AP (see Fig. 35–1), and the inactivated state occurs during the plateau of repolarization.

The net direction of ion flow through a channel is channel-specific and is referred to as *rectification.* An inward rectifying current produces a larger current when the ions are moving into the cell versus out of the cell. Ion channels that carry inward currents include the Na^+ channel (I_{Na}), Ca^{++} channels (I_{Ca-L} and I_{Ca-T}), and the nonselective hyperpolarization Na^+ channel (I_f). Specific channel densities differ in different regions of the myocardium. For example, I_f is more prominent in pacemaker cells, and I_{Ca-T} is more dense in the sinus node complex. The main outward rectifying channels are the K$^+$ channels, I$_{kl}$, I$_k$, with the subsets, I$_{kr}$ and I$_{ks}$, and the transient outward current, I$_{to}$. Newer antiarrhythmic drugs target the I$_{kr}$ and I$_{ks}$ potassium channels.

Two populations of channels exist in the presence of antiarrhythmic drugs: those blocked by the drug and those not blocked. In both the blocked and unblocked states, the three morphologic configurations of resting, active, or inactive are present. Drug association and dissociation time constants can be defined for the progression between the number of channels in each state. These rate constants in turn are affected by factors in the cellular milieu such as hyperkalemia, hypoxia, pH changes, catecholamine release, and depolarization. The net changes in channel blocking and state as a function of time can be described by sets of differential equations.[12,13] Antiarrhythmic drugs can be characterized in vitro based on the rate of block development and rate of recovery during repetitive stimulation. Binding kinetics of drugs to activated or inactivated channels are quantitative, but can be qualitatively described as slow, intermediate, or fast. These kinetic properties determine overall effect on the AP and QRS duration.

Use-dependent block refers to drug effect on an ion channel that is more pronounced at more rapid heart rates, or after longer periods of stimulation, or both. It results when the drug affinity for open or inactivated channels exceeds the drug affinity for resting channels. *Reverse use-dependent* block, usually seen with drugs that prolong repolarization, occurs when a drug exerts a greater effect at slower heart rates. The latter is not ideal insofar as lengthening repolarization may be more desirable during tachycardia.

Specific Ion Channels

The cardiac I$_{Na}$ is a large transmembrane glycoprotein with multiple subunits.[9] Two gates control the flow of Na$^+$ ions through this channel. The m gate controls activation and the h gate controls inactivation. In the resting or closed channel configuration, the activation (m) gate is in the closed position and the inactivation (h) gate is in the open position. With membrane depolarization, the activation m gate joins the h gate in the open position, allowing the passage of Na$^+$ ions into the cell along their electrochemical gradient. Inward ion movement is terminated when the h gate moves to the closed position (inactivated state). The m gate then moves to the closed position (deactivation). When the h gate subsequently moves to the open position, the channel is ready to respond to the next stimulus (recovery from inactivation). Sodium channel blockers slow conduction and decrease the maximum upstroke velocity of phase 0 of the AP (V$_{max}$).

Multiple K$^+$ channels have been identified in human cardiac tissue.[9] The voltage-gated channels include: I$_{kl}$, the inward rectifying channel; I$_{to}$, the transient outward current; and I$_k$, the delayed rectifier channel. I$_k$ has two subunits: the rapid subunit I$_{kr}$ and the slowly rectifying subunit I$_{ks}$. Ligand-gated potassium channels include I$_{kACh}$, I$_{kATP}$, and I$_{kNa}$. The different K$^+$ channels exhibit a diverse structural spectrum. The simplest is minK, a single polypeptide chain with a single crossing point on the cell membrane. Other K$^+$ channels have four subunits and multiple transmembrane helices. Potassium channel block prolongs the refractory period increasing the effective refractory period (ERP) and AP duration, but it does not effect V$_{max}$. They exhibit reverse use-dependence with decreased effectiveness in prolonging the AP at increased heart rates.

There are two extracellular and two intracellular types of Ca^{++} channels identified in human cardiac cells.[9] L- and T-type Ca^{++} channels are voltage-dependent plasma membrane ion channels, whereas the IP$_3$ receptor and the Ca^{++} release channel (ryanodine receptor) are ligand-gated ion channels that control calcium release from the sarcoplasmic reticulum. The L- and T-type Ca^{++} channel are multiple subunit proteins; the α-subunit is the target of antiarrhythmic drugs and shares homology with the voltage-dependent sodium channel.

Preclinical Pharmacology

There have been multiple classification schemes applied to antiarrhythmic drugs. The two most frequently implemented schemes in clinical practice are the Vaughn Williams classification (Table 35–1) and the Sicilian Gambit (Table 35–2).[14,15] The Vaughan Williams classification describes four main drug actions. This classification is based on the predominant effect of the drug seen in healthy tissue. This approach is limited insofar as many of the drugs exert multiple effects and they may have active metabolites with differing mechanisms of action. Furthermore, drug effects are dependent on species, type of cardiac tissue, the presence of pathophysiologic perturbations, and other factors.[16] Moreover, the effects of drugs in the same class often differ. In 1991, the Working Group on Arrhythmias from the European Society of Cardiology proposed the Sicilian Gambit.[15] This organizational construct emphasizes first the identification of the mechanism of the arrhythmia and its vulnerable parameter susceptible to modification, followed by identification of the target likely to affect the vulnerable parameter, and finally, selection of an antiarrhythmic drug that may effect the target.

The effects of each antiarrhythmic drug on the AP and the ERP of cardiac cells are important effects that dictate clinical effect. Drugs that primarily block the inward I$_{Na}$ current attenuate or suppress the upstroke of the AP or V$_{max}$. Potassium channel blockers primarily prolong repolarization, by prolonging the AP duration and the ERP, thus prolonging the QT interval. The net effect of a particular drug on the ECG is a combination of the electrophysiologic, pharmacodynamic, and pharmacokinetic effects. The following section describes drug effect as determined in healthy human tissue.

Sodium Channel Blockers with Intermediate Binding Kinetics (Class Ia Agents)

Sodium channel blockers with intermediate binding kinetics include procainamide, quinidine, and disopyramide.[16–19]

TABLE 35–1.

Vaughan Williams Classification

Class	Major Electrophysiologic Effect	Drugs
Ia	Block Na^+ channels leading to $\downarrow V_{max}$ and prolong AP duration, $\downarrow$ amplitude of AP, $\downarrow$ diastolic depolarization. Intermediate (<5 sec) binding kinetics.	Procainamide, quinidine, disopyramide
Ib	Block Na^+ channels, shortened AP duration, no reduction in V_{max}. Fast onset/offset binding kinetics (<500 msec).	Lidocaine, mexiletine, phenytoin, tocainide
Ic	Block Na^+ channels leading to $\downarrow V_{max}$, slow conduction but minimal prolongation of refractoriness. Slow binding kinetics (10 to 20 sec).	Flecainide, propafenone, moricizine
II	Blockade of β adrenergic receptor.	Propranolol, atenolol, metoprolol, timolol, esmolol, and so on
III	Block K^+ channels, prolong repolarization.	Amiodarone, sotalol, bretylium, azimilide, dofetilide, and ibutilide
IV	Block slow Ca^{++} channel.	Verapamil, diltiazem, nifedipine, and so on

Binding kinetics refer to the rate of onset and offset of Na^+ channel blockade.
AP, Action potential; V_{max}, upstroke velocity of phase 0.

TABLE 35–2.

Summary of the More Important Actions of Drugs on Membrane Ion Channels, Receptors, and Pumps

Drug	Channels					Receptors					Pumps
	Na^+			Ca^{++}	K^+	I_f	α	β	M_2	P	Na^+/K^+ ATPase
	Fast	Medium	Slow								
Lidocaine	I*										
Mexiletine	I*										
Tocainide	*										
Phenytoin	I*				I*						
Moricizine	I†										
Procainamide		A†			‡						
Disopyramide		A†			‡				*		

TABLE 35–2.

Summary of the More Important Actions of Drugs on Membrane Ion Channels, Receptors, and Pumps—*cont'd*

Drug	Channels — Na$^+$ Fast	Medium	Slow	Ca^{++}	K$^+$	Receptors — I$_f$	α	β	M$_2$	P	Pumps — Na$^+$/K$^+$ ATPase
Quinidine		A†			‡		*		*		
Propafenone		A, I†		*	*			‡			
Flecainide			A†		*						
Encainide			A†								
Bepridil	*			†	‡						
Verapamil	*			†				‡			
Diltiazem				‡							
Bretylium					†		§	§			
Sotalol					†			†			
Amiodarone	*			*	†		‡	‡			
Alinidine					‡	†					
Ibutilide		¶			(Ikr)†						
Dofetilide					(Ikr)†						
Azimilide					(Iks, Ikr)†						
Nadolol								†			
Propranolol	*							†			
Atropine									†		
Adenosine										¶	
Digoxin									¶		†

Relative blocking potency: *low; †high; ‡ moderate.
¶Agonist.
§Agonist/Antagonist.
A, Activated state blocker; I, inactivated state.

These drugs prolong AP duration, decrease V_{max}, decrease conduction velocity, and decrease maximum diastolic potential. The depression of V_{max} is more pronounced than the prolongation of the AP duration. They prolong atrial, His Purkinje, and ventricular refractoriness, and thus are effective in the treatment of reentrant arrhythmias and those attributed to abnormal automaticity. These Na^+ channel blocking agents exert little effect on cells in the sinus node. Procainamide, quinidine, and disopyramide shorten the refractory period of the atrioventricular node (AVN) through anticholinergic effects. These effects are more pronounced during hyperkalemia in experimental tissue preparations. Procainamide has less anticholinergic properties than quinidine or disopyramide. Procainamide's major metabolite, *N-acetyl procainamide (NAPA)*, neither suppresses the rate of phase 4 diastolic depolarization of Purkinje fibers nor effects resting membrane potential or V_{max}; it does prolong AP duration through K^+ channel blockade (class III effect).[16]

Unlike procainamide, quinidine blocks the rapid component of the K^+ channel, I_{kr}. Quinidine has both use-dependent and reverse use-dependent effects. At slow heart rates, the K^+ channel is more occupied than the Na^+ channel and prolongation of the AP occurs, resulting in reverse use-dependence. At fast heart rates, blockage of the Na^+ channel predominates consistent with use-dependent block.

Disopyramide is a racemic mixture of two stereoisomers. The S^+ isomer exhibits the electrophysiologic properties of increasing the ventricular AP duration and the QTc. The QTc prolongation is generally less than that seen with quinidine. The R^- isomer shortens the AP duration and has no effect on the QT. Disopyramide's effects on I_k, I_{Ca}, and I_{kl} account for prolongation of AP duration. Disopyramide, like quinidine, has anticholinergic effects and blocks the cardiac M_2 receptor. It has about one-thousandth the potency of atropine.

Sodium Channel Blockers with Rapid Binding Kinetics (Class Ib Agents)

This group of antiarrhythmic agents includes lidocaine, tocainide, mexiletine, and phenytoin.[16,20–23] These agents exhibit rapid association and dissociation from the Na^+ channel and preferentially block inactivated channels. These drugs slow the upstroke and prolong the duration of the AP in Purkinje fibers. They exhibit little effect on refractory periods in the sinus node, atrium, or AVN. No vagolytic effects have been described.

Lidocaine suppresses abnormal automaticity in depolarized ventricular myocardium and Purkinje tissue. Modest suppression of early and delayed after depolarizations occurs with lidocaine. Mexiletine blocks inactivated Na^+ channels more readily than activated channels. In diseased myocardium, mexiletine administration slows conduction at the level of the AVN and His-Purkinje system. Phenytoin preferentially blocks inactivated Na^+ channels and also blocks inactivated T-type Ca^{++} channels in ventricular myocytes. Suppression of delayed after depolarizations also has been described. Tocainide is a mixture of two stereoisomers; the R^- isomer is electrically active. Tocainide shortens the AP duration in Purkinje fibers and ventricular

myocytes. There is no effect on refractory periods in the atrium, ventricle, or specialized conduction system.

Sodium Channel Blockers with Slow Binding Kinetics (Class Ic Agents)

Flecainide, encainide, propafenone, and moricizine are potent Na^+ channel blockers with slow kinetics.[23–25] Flecainide is a potent depressant of V_{max}. It was developed as a fluorinated analogue of procainamide, and it demonstrates tonic block of I_{Ca} and Na^+ channel block. This combined effect is responsible for the minimal net effect on repolarization. Block of I_k in ventricular muscle has also been described. In Purkinje tissue, both the AP duration and ERP are shortened. In ventricular tissue, the AP duration and ERP are prolonged. The AH, HV, PR, and QRS intervals are all prolonged.

Propafenone blocks primarily active and inactivated Na^+ channels. As with flecainide, I_k, I_{kl}, and I_{to} are also blocked; the latter two at supratherapeutic concentrations. Propafenone demonstrates mild block of the L-type Ca^{++} channel. AH, HV, PR, QRS, and QT intervals are all prolonged. The ERP of the atrium, AVN, and ventricle are all prolonged. Propafenone is a weak β adrenergic receptor blocker.

Moricizine has multiple effects on the Na^+ channel. Its predominate action is to block the I_{Na} and for that reason is grouped with the Class I agents in the Vaughan Williams scheme. Moricizine exhibits use-dependent properties. It slows retrograde AV nodal and His Purkinje conduction and has minimal effect on atrial, ventricular, and antegrade AVN refractoriness.

β-Adrenergic Receptor Blockers (Class II Agents)

Beta-blockers exhibit antiadrenergic effects and membrane stabilizing effects.[16,26,27] The former effect results from competitive inhibition of catecholamine binding to the β receptor by the levo-stereoisomer of the various compounds. The antiadrenergic effects decrease phase 4 depolarization and spontaneous firing and automaticity of pacemaker cells, especially those in the AVN. As with other antiarrhythmic drugs, sinus node automaticity is depressed in pre-existing sinus node dysfunction. Beta-blockers prevent β-agonist enhancement of L-type Ca^{++} currents. Membrane stabilization results from decreased Na^+ current depressing V_{max} of the AP. The membrane stabilizing effects have no clinical significance because this occurs only at concentrations 10 times greater than necessary for β-blockade.

Class III Potassium Channel Blockers

This group of antiarrhythmic drugs includes K^+ channel–specific agents and those that affect multiple channels. The K^+ channel–specific agents include azimilide, sotalol, dofetilide, and ibutilide.[28–32] These agents prolong the ERP and increase AP duration; as such, they prolong the QT interval without other ECG effects. The pure K^+ channel blockers exhibit reverse use-dependence; the degree of block of the K^+ channel is more pronounced at slow heart rates, and there is less block at more rapid heart rates. Sotalol blocks I_{kr}, and nonspecifically blocks β_1 and β_2 receptors. Ibutilide blocks I_{kr} and the slow inward Na^+ channel. Dofetilide specifically targets I_{kr}. Azimilide blocks both I_{kr} and I_{ks}.

Class III Agents That Block Multiple Channels

Bretylium and amiodarone are two agents in Vaughn Williams Class III that exert their electrophysiologic effect on multiple channels.[16,33,34] Bretylium has adrenergic and antiadrenergic action, and a direct effect on K^+ channels that prolongs the AP duration and the ERP.

The electrophysiologic effects of amiodarone are protean. It blocks inactivated Na^+ channels in a use-dependent fashion, blocks α and β adrenergic receptors, increases AP duration and ERP, and blocks inactivated Ca^{++} channels.[34] The oral form of the drug prolongs the ERP and AP duration in all cardiac tissue. In animal models, it also suppresses sinus node and AVN automaticity. Amiodarone blocks the slow component of the inward rectifying K^+ channel and does not exhibit reverse use-dependence. The intravenous form of amiodarone is a more potent antiadrenergic compound and Ca^{++} channel blocker than the oral agent. There is no use-dependent block of Na^+ channels with intravenous amiodarone. The ECG demonstrates PR prolongation, QRS prolongation, and QT prolongation with chronic oral use.

Calcium Channel Blockers (Class IV Agents)

All currently available Ca^{++} channel antagonists block the α-subunit of the L-type Ca^{++} channel reducing the plateau height of the AP, slightly shortening myocardial AP, and slightly prolonging Purkinje fiber AP.[35] Verapamil and diltiazem depress the slope of diastolic depolarization of phase 0 and decrease maximum diastolic potential and the amplitude of the sinus node and AVN AP. Spontaneous sinus rate is slightly decreased and AV nodal conduction is prolonged. Heart rate may change slightly because of reflex sympathetic stimulation from systemic vasodilation (an effect attenuated with coadministration of a beta-blocker). T-type Ca^{++} channels exist in the sinus node. No currently available agents interact with T-type calcium channels. Verapamil is a racemic mixture and its dextrostereoisomer exerts mild I_{Na} blocking effects.

Other Antiarrhythmic Drugs

Adenosine is an endogenous nucleoside whose action on cardiac ion channels is affected by catecholamine stimulation.[36,37] It directly activates the outward K^+ current present in the sinus node, atrium, and AVN (I_k, I_{Ach}, I_{Ado}), an effect similar to acetylcholine. This results in a negative chronotropic and negative dromotropic response, and it also explains why adenosine can terminate some atrial arrhythmias.[36] Adenosine also decreases the inward Ca^{++} current, the transient inward current, and the hyperpolarization current by stimulating a G protein that inhibits cyclic adenosine monophosphate generation. In the presence of catecholamines, adenosine also inhibits I_{ks}.

Digoxin is a cardiac glycoside that blocks the Na^+/K^+ ATPase and exerts a positive inotropic, negative dromotropic, and negative chronotropic response on the heart (see Chapter 37 for a discussion of inotropic effects). Intracellular Ca^{++} is increased through the slow inward Ca^{++} current. This in turn inhibits the Na^+-Ca^{++} exchange. Digoxin augments vagal tone and increases the ERP of the AVN. As seen with beta-blockers, sinus node automaticity is depressed in underlying sick sinus syndrome. At supratherapeutic levels, digoxin increases delayed afterdepolarizations.

Clinical Pharmacology

Procainamide

Indications

Procainamide is approved for the treatment of life-threatening ventricular arrhythmias. Procainamide is also used for the treatment of supraventricular arrhythmias including the conversion of AF to sinus rhythm.[38,39] Procainamide can depress conduction of accessory pathways and thus is useful in treating AV re-entrant tachycardia and pre-excited AF—two rhythms associated with Wolff-Parkinson-White (WPW) syndrome. Procainamide slows the conduction of atrial impulses through the accessory pathway. Patients with complete heart block should not be given procainamide because ventricular pacemakers can be suppressed leading to asystole. Procainamide should be avoided for patients with second-degree AV block.

Pharmacokinetics

The volume of distribution of procainamide is approximately 2 L/kg, 20% of the drug is bound to serum proteins, and the elimination half-life is 3 to 5 hours. Fifty percent to 60% of the elimination occurs through the kidneys and 10% to 30% through hepatic metabolism.[16] Active renal tubular excretion of procainamide occurs using a base-secreting pathway also used for elimination of cimetidine, ranitidine, flecainide, triamterene, and other drugs. Procainamide undergoes acetylation in the liver to NAPA. The rate of acetylation varies widely. "Fast acetylators" have up to 33% of procainamide converted to NAPA compared with up to 21% in "slow acetylators."[16] NAPA has an elimination half-life of 7 to 8 hours and is excreted through the kidneys. As with the parent compound, serum concentrations of NAPA need to be monitored and dosage adjusted for older patients, patients with left ventricular dysfunction, those with myocardial infarction, and patients with renal dysfunction.

Adverse Effects

Parenteral administration of procainamide can produce hypotension. Procainamide has negative inotropic effects and may lead to cardiac conduction abnormalities, prolonged QT interval, and polymorphic ventricular tachycardia (VT).[40] Procainamide has anticholinergic properties that can speed the conduction of atrial impulses leading to rapid ventricular response when used in patients with AF. Drugs to slow AV nodal conduction are given before starting procainamide.

Central nervous system, gastrointestinal, hematologic, and skin adverse effects have been related to procainamide. A reversible systemic lupus erythematosus syndrome manifesting as arthralgias, pleural effusion, pericarditis, and pericardial tamponade can occur with procainamide use. Positive antinuclear antibodies with or without the lupus-type syndrome are common in patients receiving chronic procainamide.

Quinidine

Indications

Quinidine is indicated for the conversion of AF to sinus rhythm, or the maintenance of sinus rhythm after cardioversion, or both. Conversion to sinus rhythm with quinidine is reported to occur in 20% of patients but meta-analysis of clinical trials suggests a greater mortality rate for patients receiving quinidine compared with patients in the placebo groups.[16] Quinidine is also indicated for the treatment of life-threatening ventricular arrhythmias. Quinidine may be used for the treatment of supraventricular arrhythmias caused by re-entry including those involving accessory pathways or AV nodal re-entry.

Pharmacokinetics

Quinidine is available in sulfate and gluconate forms with similar bioavailability but different patterns of absorption and peak effect. Quinidine is 80% bound to serum proteins, primarily α_1-acid glycoprotein. α_1-Acid glycoprotein concentrations are increased by stress responses, which could alter drug binding. The volume of distribution is 2 to 3 L/kg but varies with different conditions including poor ventricular function. The clearance of quinidine is 3 to 5 mL/kg per minute and elimination half-life is 6 to 8 hours in adults. Quinidine is metabolized in the liver by cytochrome P450 (CYP) $IIIA_4$ to metabolites with antiarrhythmic properties. One metabolite, 3-hydroxyquinidine, has approximately 50% of the antiarrhythmic effectiveness of the parent compound. Quinidine metabolism is inducible with drugs such as phenytoin, whereas quinidine can inhibit the metabolism

of drugs eliminated through $CYPIID_6$ pathways, although quinidine itself is not metabolized by the latter pathway. Renal clearance through glomerular filtration and tubular secretion is inversely related to urine pH. Twenty percent of quinidine is excreted unchanged when the urine pH is less than 7, but lower percentages occur when the urine is alkaline. Drugs that alkalinize the urine (e.g., carbonic anhydrase inhibitors and sodium bicarbonate) can alter renal excretion. Dosage adjustments are needed for patients with renal and hepatic diseases. Serum quinidine concentrations are increased by amiodarone and cimetidine, but are decreased by nifedipine.

Adverse Effects

By slowing AF/flutter rate, quinidine may reduce the degree of AV block. This leads to increased conduction of atrial impulses to the ventricle and produces an accelerated ventricular rate. The anticholinergic properties of quinidine may also lead to accelerated ventricular responses warranting the prior administration of AV nodal blocking drugs before starting quinidine. Quinidine may cause hypotension because of α adrenergic receptor blockade or direct vascular relaxation effects. Quinidine can slow cardiac conduction producing AV block and sinus nodal dysfunction particularly in patients with sick sinus syndrome. Torsade de pointes occurs in 1% to 3% of patients receiving quinidine.[41]

Gastrointestinal adverse effects such as nausea, vomiting, and diarrhea are common with quinidine therapy. Other adverse effects include tinnitus (cinchonism), reversible hearing loss, diplopia, photophobia, and delirium. Autoimmune reactions, rash, thrombocytopenia, and other central nervous system adverse reactions can occur.

Disopyramide

Indications

Disopyramide is indicated for the treatment of life-threatening ventricular arrhythmias. Disopyramide is also used to treat supraventricular arrhythmias caused by re-entrant mechanisms including those using accessory pathways. It is similar in effectiveness to procainamide for the conversion of AF/flutter to sinus rhythm. Disopyramide should not be used in patients with cardiogenic shock, AV block, or long QT intervals.

Pharmacokinetics

Disopyramide is nearly completely absorbed, and serum protein binding varies between 50% and 65%. In healthy volunteers, the mean elimination half-life of disopyramide is almost 7 hours, but it is 10 hours or longer in patients with cardiac disease. Nearly 50% of disopyramide is excreted unchanged in the urine and 20% as the mono-N-dealkylated metabolite that has about one-tenth the antiarrhythmic effects of the parent compound. The dosage of disopyramide must be adjusted for patients with renal disease. Disopyramide is metabolized in the liver by CYP3A4 enzyme. Interactions can occur with drugs, including clarithromycin and erythromycin, that use this pathway.

Adverse Effects

Disopyramide has strong anticholinergic side effects that can facilitate AV conduction of atrial impulses in AF/flutter. As with procainamide and quinidine, drugs that slow AV conduction should be given before beginning disopyramide for patients with AF/flutter. Negative inotropic properties of disopyramide can exacerbate left ventricular dysfunction. Second- and third-degree AV block can occur. Disopyramide can lead to the development of torsade de pointes. Anticholinergic effects can be prominent with disopyramide and include dry mouth, constipation, urinary retention, and exacerbation of glaucoma.

Lidocaine

Indications

Lidocaine is used for the treatment of life-threatening ventricular arrhythmias, particularly those associated with myocardial ischemia. Lidocaine is not effective for the treatment of supraventricular arrhythmias including AF/flutter. Lidocaine has commonly been used after coronary artery revascularization surgery as prophylaxis for ventricular arrhythmias despite little efficacy data.[42,43] Prophylactic lidocaine treatment after myocardial infarction is associated with greater mortality rates and is no longer recommended.[44]

Pharmacokinetics

Lidocaine undergoes significant first-pass metabolism and thus is not effective after oral administration. Binding of lidocaine to serum protein is inversely related to serum concentrations. At therapeutic concentrations, 60% to 80% is bound to serum proteins, particularly α_1-acid glycoprotein. The elimination half-life of lidocaine is approximately 1 to 2 hours. Lidocaine is extensively metabolized in the liver, and clearance is directly related to hepatic blood flow. Glycinexylidide and monoethylglycinexylidide metabolites possess antiarrhythmic properties that are considerably less potent than the parent compound. Ninety percent of lidocaine is excreted in the urine as metabolites and 10% is excreted unchanged. Hepatic disease but not renal disease may interfere with lidocaine clearance, but renal dysfunction can impair excretion of metabolites.

Adverse Effects

Lidocaine administration is typically well tolerated without hypotension. Cardiac conduction delays in the His-Purkinje system and myocardial depression are seen at toxic concentrations. Proarrhythmic side effects may occur even at therapeutic concentrations. Central nervous system adverse effects such as tinnitus, lightheadedness, blurred vision, confusion, and seizures occur in a dose-related manner at greater concentrations.

Mexiletine

Indications

Mexiletine is structurally related to lidocaine. It is indicated for the treatment of life-threatening ventricular arrhythmias. Mexiletine and tocainide may be useful for treating ventricular arrhythmias for patients with prolonged QT interval.

Pharmacokinetics

Mexiletine is well absorbed from the gastrointestinal tract and does not undergo significant first-pass metabolism. In healthy volunteers, the distribution is 5 to 7 L/kg, the elimination half-life 10 to 12 hours, and 50% to 60% is bound to plasma proteins. Mexiletine is extensively metabolized in the liver, and only 10% of the drug is excreted in the urine unchanged. N-methylmexiletine, a major metabolite, possess 20% of the antiarrhythmic effects of the parent compound. Metabolism is enhanced by phenobarbital, phenytoin, and rifampin but is reduced by cimetidine. The dose of mexiletine requires adjustment for liver disease but not for renal dysfunction. Markedly acidic urine enhances excretion, whereas markedly alkaline urine retards excretion of mexiletine. Metabolism is altered in the CYP206 genotype.[45]

Adverse Effects

Mexiletine administration is not associated with marked hemodynamic changes and only mild depression of myocardial contractility. As with other agents, proarrhythmic adverse effects may occur. Toxic effects can occur at concentrations only slightly greater than therapeutic levels. Cardiovascular side effects of mexiletine are similar to those of lidocaine. Increases in liver enzymes are reported, particularly in patients with congestive heart failure. Central nervous system and gastrointestinal adverse effects can occur including lightheadedness, blurred vision, and confusion. Blood dyscrasias are reported in a small subset of patients.

Tocainide

Indications

Tocainide is an orally active, amide analog of lidocaine that is indicated for the treatment of life-threatening ventricular arrhythmias.

Pharmacokinetics

Tocainide is nearly completely absorbed after oral administration. It is 10% bound to plasma proteins and has an elimination half-life of approximately 15 hours in healthy volunteers. Tocainide undergoes hepatic metabolism, but 40% of the drug is excreted unchanged in the urine.

Adverse Effects

Tocainide administration is usually not associated with marked hemodynamic effects and only mild cardiac contractile depression. Small increases in systemic and pulmonary vascular resistance have been observed experimentally. Gastrointestinal and CNS adverse effects are similar to those observed with lidocaine. Hematologic abnormalities including agranulocytosis have been reported with tocainide use primarily within the first 12 weeks of treatment. Pulmonary fibrosis, pneumonitis, and other pulmonary complications have been associated with tocainide therapy.

Flecainide

Indications

Flecainide is indicated for the treatment of supraventricular tachycardias (SVTs) caused by re-entrant mechanisms (e.g., AV nodal reentry, accessory pathways, AF/flutter) in patients without structural heart disease.[39,46–51] In one study, flecainide was more effective than procainamide in converting AF to sinus rhythm.[39] Flecainide is also indicated for the treatment of life-threatening ventricular arrhythmias for patients without structural heart disease.[52] There is no evidence, however, that such treatment will improve survival. Flecainide should not be used for patients with recent myocardial infarction or for patients with non–life-threatening ventricular arrhythmias. Flecainide is contraindicated for patients with severe forms of heart block unless there is a pacemaker present and for patients with cardiogenic shock. Flecainide should not be used for patients with chronic AF.

Pharmacokinetics

Flecainide is nearly completely absorbed and does not undergo significant first-pass hepatic metabolism. The elimination half-life is variable ranging from 12 to 27 hours. Steady-state plasma levels require 3 to 5 days to be attained, after which there is no additional drug accumulation. Thirty percent of flecainide is excreted unchanged in the urine, and about 40% of the drug is bound to plasma proteins. Major metabolites are meta-o-dealkylated flecainide, which has 20% the antiarrhythmic activity of the parent compound, and meta-o-dealkylated lactam of flecainide, which is inactive. Dosage should be adjusted in patients with renal impairment. Hepatic metabolism includes $CYPIID_6$ pathways. Flecainide will compete with other drugs using this

metabolic pathway increasing slowing elimination. An important drug interaction has been demonstrated between flecainide and propranolol. Coadministration of amiodarone and flecainide can double serum flecainide concentrations. Phenytoin and other drugs that activate CYP enzymes can increase the elimination of flecainide by 30%, whereas cimetidine can increase serum levels by 30% and elimination half-life by 10%.

Adverse Effects

The most serious adverse effects of flecainide are worsening of supraventricular and ventricular arrhythmias. Proarrhythmic adverse effects with flecainide can occur in 5% to 30% of patients depending on the dose, history of left ventricular dysfunction, myocardial infarction, and cardiac arrest. Flecainide has important negative inotropic properties that may worsen ventricular dysfunction, but its use is usually not associated with hemodynamic alterations. Flecainide should not be used in patients with second- and third-degree heart block without the presence of a pacemaker. Sinus arrest may occur in patients with sinus node dysfunction. Pacemaker thresholds can increase during flecainide treatment. Central nervous system and gastrointestinal adverse effects can occur.

Propafenone

Indications

Propafenone is approved for the treatment of paroxysmal AF and SVT for patients without structural heart disease. Propafenone is effective for treating supraventricular arrhythmias caused by re-entrant mechanisms including AV nodal re-entrant and accessory pathways and AF/flutter.[48,51,52] Propafenone is also indicated for the treatment of life-threatening ventricular arrhythmias. Propafenone has been used for treating recent onset AF after cardiac surgery.[53] Similar to flecainide, propafenone can increase the pacing threshold requiring adjustments for patients with permanent pacemakers.[54]

Pharmacokinetics

Propafenone is rapidly absorbed from the gastrointestinal tract and undergoes saturable first-pass metabolism resulting in a dose-dependent bioavailability. There is large interindividual variability in the bioavailability of propafenone. The rate of metabolism is genetically determined. In more than 90% of individuals, the drug is rapidly metabolized and the elimination half-life is 2 to 10 hours. The major metabolites in these individuals are 5-hydroxypropafenone and N-depropylpropafenone. Both have antiarrhythmic potency equal to the parent compound, but they are usually only present in concentrations less than 20% of the parent compound. In 10% of individuals, the 5-hydroxy metabolite is not formed or is slowly formed, leading to slower metabolism with an elimination half-life of 10 to 32 hours. Plasma concentrations between slow and extensive metabolizers vary almost twofold. Propafenone is 97% protein bound, predominately to α_1-acid glycoprotein. Slow metabolizers may have more pronounced beta-blocking effects.

Because of extensive hepatic metabolism, bioavailability of propafenone increases by up to 70% in patients with liver disease, requiring dosage adjustments. Renal elimination of active metabolites warrants caution in propafenone use in patients with renal dysfunction. Small doses of quinidine inhibit the metabolism of propafenone, whereas propafenone increases serum digoxin levels by 35% to 85%. Propafenone interferes with the metabolism of propranolol and metoprolol, resulting in increased concentrations of the two beta-blocking drugs. Warfarin concentrations are also increased during propafenone treatment, resulting in a 25% increase in prothrombin time. Other drug interactions may increase (cimetidine) or decrease (rifampin) propafenone concentrations, whereas propafenone therapy may increase serum concentrations of desipramine, cyclosporin, and theophylline. Calcium channel blocking effects of propafenone may lead to interactions with verapamil, diltiazem, and other calcium channel blocking drugs.

Adverse Effects

Proarrhythmic side effects of propafenone occur in 4% to 5% of patients with pre-existing ventricular arrhythmias and in up to 2% of patients receiving treatment for supraventricular arrhythmias. Propafenone may worsen congestive heart failure and lead to conduction disturbances. Other adverse effects include hematologic suppression, dizziness, blurred vision, taste disturbance, gastrointestinal side effects, and central nervous system abnormalities including confusion.

Moricizine

Indications

Moricizine is indicated for the treatment of documented ventricular arrhythmias viewed as life threatening.

Pharmacokinetics

Moricizine is chemically similar to phenothiazines. The drug undergoes extensive first-pass metabolism resulting in 35% to 40% bioavailability. Peak plasma levels are attained in less than 2 hours, but antiarrhythmic effects have a slow onset and offset. The rate, but not peak effect, is altered when moricizine is taken with food. The efficacy of moricizine is not related to serum concentrations of the parent compound or short-lived metabolites. Moricizine is 95% bound to serum proteins. There is extensive hepatic metabolism resulting in less than 1% of the parent drug excreted in the urine. Metabolism of moricizine results in formation of multiple metabolites, but few attain significant plasma

concentrations. The half-life of moricizine is 1.5 to 3.5 hours.

Adverse Effects

Proarrhythmic side effects are reported in 3% to 15% of patients. Moricizine is tolerated in patients with impaired ventricular function and causes worsening congestive heart failure in only a minority of patients. Small increases in blood pressure and heart rate may be observed. Nausea, headache, tremor, mood changes, dizziness, and vertigo are reported with moricizine use. Cimetidine may have small effects on moricizine plasma concentrations, whereas theophylline concentrations may increase because of moricizine therapy.

Amiodarone

Indications

Amiodarone is approved for the treatment of VT and ventricular fibrillation (VF), especially when the arrhythmia has been refractory to other antiarrhythmic drugs. Furthermore, amiodarone is effective for a wide variety of supraventricular arrhythmias including AF and those caused by AV nodal re-entry and AV re-entry.[55-59] Several trials have suggested that amiodarone is effective for the prevention of AF after cardiac surgery.[60-62] Although these preliminary data show favorable benefit, several important confounding variables, such as preoperative beta-blocker use, were not controlled for in these studies. Moreover, the safety of this therapy has only been demonstrated in small trials.

Pharmacokinetics

Amiodarone is slowly and variably absorbed after oral administration with little first-pass metabolism. The bioavailability is approximately 50%. Peak plasma levels occur 5 to 7 hours after oral administration but the onset of action may be 2 to 3 days to weeks. Amiodarone is widely and variably distributed with accumulation in adipose tissue, skin, and highly perfused organs. The volume of distribution is 60 L/kg. The drug is 96% protein bound and plasma concentrations with doses between 100 and 600 mg/day are nearly dose-related averaging of 0.5 mg/L/100 mg dose. N-desethylamiodarone is a major metabolite with antiarrhythmic effects. This metabolite accumulates with chronic therapy to nearly equal plasma concentrations as the parent compound, but its role for the clinical effects of amiodarone is not clear. Amiodarone is mainly excreted by the liver into bile with some enterohepatic circulation. There is minimal renal excretion of the parent drug or its major metabolite, and dosage does not need to be adjusted for renal dysfunction. Amiodarone undergoes a biphasic elimination with half-lives of 2.5 to 10 days, and 26 to 107 days, respectively. Thus a loading dose is needed to achieve relatively rapid effective plasma and tissue concentrations. The onset of electrophysiologic effects requires at least 2 to 3 days to 1 to 3 weeks, and continued antiarrhythmic effects occur for weeks to months after its discontinuation.

Parenteral amiodarone undergoes rapid distribution; plasma concentrations decrease to 10% of peak levels within 30 to 45 minutes. Metabolism of amiodarone is through CYP3A pathways with large interindividual variability. Concentrations of N-desethylamiodarone can accumulate after several days of infusion.

The clearance of amiodarone is inversely related to age and ranges from 98 to 158 mL/hr per kilogram. The onset of action of intravenous amiodarone is within several hours.

Adverse Effects

Antiadrenergic and Ca^{++} channel blocking effects of amiodarone contribute to peripheral vasodilation, bradycardia, conduction disturbances, negative inotropic effects, and hypotension. Hemodynamic effects are more prevalent with parenteral administration, and their occurrence is dependent on the rate of administration. Congestive heart failure can occur, but this is uncommon with oral treatment. Volatile anesthetics, beta-blockers, diltiazem, and verapamil can potentiate the cardiovascular and negative inotropic effects of amiodarone.[63,64] Early retrospective series have reported increased need for inotropic support and vasoconstrictive medications after cardiopulmonary bypass for patients receiving amiodarone, although many of these patients had pre-existing left ventricular dysfunction.[63-65] Proarrhythmic side effects of amiodarone are reported in less than 1% to 2% of patients.[66]

Pulmonary toxicity is a severe complication of amiodarone that may occur as early as 1 week after initiation of treatment, but it is more common with chronic therapy.[67] Clinical presentation includes cough, fever, dyspnea, hypoxemia, chest radiograph changes, and reduced carbon monoxide diffusion capacity. Pulmonary complications may progress to adult respiratory distress syndrome and pulmonary fibrosis. The mechanism is unknown but it may be secondary to hypersensitivity pneumonitis or phospholipidoses. The mainstay of treatment of amiodarone pulmonary toxicity is discontinuation of the drug. Steroids may also be useful. Pulmonary toxicity occurs in up to 17% of patients treated long-term with 400 mg/day amiodarone. Pulmonary complications were reported to be more frequent in patients receiving amiodarone before surgery involving cardiopulmonary bypass.[64,65] Others reported adult respiratory distress syndrome in a high percentage of patients receiving amiodarone before cardiac surgery.[68] The latter was unrelated to duration of treatment and often occurred after an initial uncomplicated postoperative course.

Both hypothyroidism and hyperthyroidism can occur with chronic amiodarone therapy. Amiodarone is a source of iodine and interferes with the peripheral conversion of thyroxin to triiodothyronine. Amiodarone treatment may also lead to malaise, nausea, and increased liver function tests.[67] Ocular abnormalities including corneal microdeposits and optic neuritis have been reported in patients receiving amiodarone. Pulmonary and gastrointestinal complications are the most frequent causes of drug discontinuation. Peripheral neuropathy and tremor may also occur. Photosensitivity and blue-gray skin discoloration are seen in patients receiving amiodarone. Current recommendations for amiodarone monitoring include yearly ophthalmologic examinations, pulmonary function tests with carbon monoxide diffusing capacity, serum liver function tests, serum thyroid tests, and chest radiographs. Amiodarone inhibits CYP metabolisms resulting in increased serum levels of digoxin, procainamide, quinidine, warfarin, and cyclosporine. Cimetidine can reduce the metabolism of amiodarone, and phenytoin increases its metabolism. Cholestyramine increases the elimination of amiodarone by interfering with its enterohepatic circulation.

Bretylium

Indications

Bretylium is approved for the treatment of life-threatening ventricular arrhythmias that are not responsive to other therapies.

Pharmacokinetics

Bretylium is available only in a parenteral form. Onset of action is rapid, but full effects are not observed for 30 to 120 minutes. Elimination is primarily renal, and dosage adjustment should be made for patients with renal insufficiency. The elimination half-life is 5 to 13 hours.

Adverse Effects

Administration of bretylium may result in a transient increase in blood pressure, tachycardia, and worsening of ventricular arrhythmias caused by catecholamine release. These effects are followed by hypotension resulting from the sympatholytic properties of bretylium, but there are no associated negative inotropic effects from the drug. Nausea and vomiting are reported after parenteral bretylium, and parotid inflammation may occur with longer term therapy.

Sotalol

Indications

Sotalol is indicated for the treatment of sustained VT or VF.[29] Sotalol is also approved for the treatment of atrial tachyarrhythmias including AF after cardiac surgery.[69-71] Sotalol is contraindicated in patients with asthma and cardiac conduction abnormalities including long-QT intervals, and it should be used with caution in patients with left ventricular dysfunction.

Pharmacokinetics

Sotalol is readily absorbed from the gastrointestinal tract with 90% to 100% bioavailability. Peak plasma concentrations occur in 2.5 to 4 hours. Elimination is primarily through the kidneys, and the mean elimination half-life is 12 hours. The dosage must be reduced for patients with renal impairment. The drug does not bind to plasma proteins, is not metabolized, and there is little penetration of the blood–brain barrier. Although the *d*- and *l*-isomers of this racemic mixture have electrophysiologic effects, beta-blocking effects primarily result from *l*-sotalol. These non-selective, beta-blocking effects are maximal at doses between 320 and 640 mg/day but are half-maximal at doses of 80 mg/day.

Adverse Effects

The beta-blocking effects of sotalol result in negative inotropic effects, bradycardia, and prolonged AV conduction.[72] Bronchospasm and other side effects of beta-blockers are possible. Sinus nodal dysfunction is also reported with sotalol. The risk for torsade de pointes is dose-related with reported frequencies of 0.5% and 5.8% for daily doses of 160 mg and more than 640 mg/day, respectively.[73] Torsades de pointes most often occurs within 7 days of initiating the drug or increasing the dose. Sotalol is discontinued in as many as 17% of patients, most often for fatigue, bradycardia, bronchospasm, dyspnea, proarrhythmia, or dizziness. Increased liver enzymes have also been reported.

Ibutilide

Indications

Ibutilide is approved for the conversion of AF or atrial flutter of recent onset to sinus rhythm. In a trial of patients with AF after cardiac surgery, ibutilide was more effective than placebo in converting AF to sinus rhythm (placebo 15%, ibutilide 40% to 57%, *P* < 0.05).[74] Reversion to AF may occur after initial effective treatment especially for patients with long-standing atrial arrhythmias. However, 53% and 72% of patients administered 0.5 and 1.0 mg ibutilide, respectively, remained in sinus rhythm for at least 24 hours. Therapy for maintenance of sinus rhythm is considered based on individual risk for proarrhythmic side effects.

Pharmacokinetics

The pharmacokinetics of ibutilide show marked interindividual variability. Systemic clearance is high and is approximately equal to liver blood flow (~29 mL/min/kg). The volume of distribution is high (~11 L/kg), but there is little binding to plasma proteins. The mean elimination half-life is about 6 hours. In healthy volunteers, 82% of ibutilide is excreted in the urine mostly as a metabolite and 19% was recovered from the feces. There are approximately eight metabolites of ibutilide, but only the ω-hydroxy metabolites posses Class III antiarrhythmic effects. The plasma concentrations of the latter are only 10% of ibutilide.

Adverse Effects

Ibutilide use is typically not associated with hemodynamic alterations. Polymorphic VT with or without lengthening of the QTc interval may occur with ibutilide treatment. Most events occur 40 minutes after the start of therapy but recurrence occurs within 3 hours of the infusion. Ibutilide-related polymorphic VT is reported in up to 8% of patients, but the frequency was 1.8% when used for AF after cardiac surgery.[32,74,75] The manufacturer reports polymorphic VT in 2.9% of patients administered 1 mg ibutilide for conversion of AF after cardiac surgery. Polymorphic VT is more likely for patients with impaired left ventricular function, history of polymorphic VT, long QT intervals, hypokalemia, or hypomagnesemia.

Dofetilide

Indications

Dofetilide is indicated for the conversion of AF or atrial flutter to sinus rhythm and for the maintenance of sinus rhythm (or delay of recurrence) for patients with AF for more than 7 days who have been successfully cardioverted. Dofetilide is not effective for patients with paroxysmal AF. In a small study of patients with AF after cardiac surgery, conversion to sinus rhythm occurred in 36% to 44% of patients administered dofetilide, but this was not significantly different than with placebo (24%).[31] In nonsurgical patients, dofetilide is more effective than placebo for converting AF to sinus rhythm.[76] After 1 year of treatment, dofetilide was more effective in maintaining sinus rhythm than placebo or sotalol.[76]

Pharmacokinetics

Bioavailability is greater than 90% with peak effects occurring within 2 to 3 hours of ingestion. Plasma protein binding is 60% to 70%, and volume of distribution 3 L/kg. The terminal half-life is approximately 10 hours. Eighty percent of dofetilide is excreted unchanged in the urine, whereas 20% is in the form of inactive or minimally active metabolites. Dofetilide is metabolized in the liver by CYP3A4 with low affinity. Renal elimination is through glomerular filtration and tubular secretion. Trimethoprim, cimetidine, prochlorperazine, and megestrol can inhibit renal clearance. Ketoconazole inhibits liver metabolism of dofetilide and increases the plasma concentrations. Dosage adjustments are necessary in accordance with creatinine clearance, but not with mild or moderate hepatic impairment. Verapamil, as well as the drugs listed earlier, is contraindicated in patients taking dofetilide because of the increased risk for proarrhythmia.

Adverse Effects

Dofetilide does not posses negative inotropic effects, and its use does not affect cardiac output or systemic vascular resistance. Torsades de pointes occurs in a dose-related fashion in patients administered dofetilide.[31,77] This occurs in 3.3% of patients with congestive heart failure, compared with 0.9% of patients without left ventricular dysfunction. Proarrhythmia is most likely within 1 to 3 days of initiation of therapy.[77] Dofetilide therapy is initiated in an approved hospital setting with continuous telemetry monitoring. The dosage is determined by the QT interval and creatinine clearance.

β-Adrenergic Receptor Blocking Drugs

Indications

β-Adrenergic receptor blocking drugs are effective for treating arrhythmias related to enhanced adrenergic states (e.g., thyrotoxicosis, pheochromocytoma, perioperative stress). Esmolol and propranolol are specifically approved for the treatment of supraventricular arrhythmias.[16] Beta-blockers are effective for controlling ventricular rate during AF and atrial flutter, and this class of drugs is suggested to be effective for preventing these arrhythmias after cardiac surgery.[78,79] By slowing AV conduction, beta-blockers may slow, terminate, or prevent recurrence of SVT involving the AVN as part of the re-entrant pathway (e.g., AV nodal re-entrant tachycardia and orthodromic tachycardia with WPW syndrome).[16] Notably, slowing AV nodal conduction may accelerate SVT with antegrade conduction associated with the WPW syndrome. Multifocal atrial tachycardia may respond to esmolol or metoprolol[80] but is best treated with amiodarone. Acebutolol and propranolol are approved for the treatment of frequent premature ventricular beats and VT, respectively. Beta-blockers, particularly propranolol, may be effective for controlling torsade de pointes for patients with long QT intervals.[81] Acebutolol, metoprolol, atenolol, propranolol, and timolol are approved for prevention of sudden death after myocardial infarction most likely caused by anti-ischemic, autonomic and possibly direct antiarrhythmic properties of the drugs.[16] Labetalol is thought to be effective for treating ventricular arrhythmias associated with pre-eclampsia.[82]

Pharmacokinetics

Esmolol is a β_1-selective, beta-blocker that is rapidly hydrolyzed by esterases in the cytosol of red blood cells (not plasma esterases) resulting in an elimination half-life of about 9 minutes. Metabolism is not limited by blood flow to the liver, kidney, or other tissues. Steady-state blood levels are achieved in about 5 and 30 minutes with and without a loading dose, respectively. Elimination kinetics are dose-independent. These pharmacokinetic properties allow rapid intravenous titration of esmolol. Approximately 2% of the drug is excreted unchanged in the urine, whereas about 88% is recovered as the acid metabolite of esmolol. The acid metabolite has 1/1500th the potency of the parent compound, and its elimination half-life is 3.7 hours, but this is prolonged for patients with renal dysfunction. Propranolol is a nonselective beta-blocker with bioavailability of 25% to 30% because of substantial first pass metabolism, but there is great interindividual variability. Propranolol readily passes the blood–brain barrier. The drug is primarily metabolized in the liver and one metabolite (4-hydroxypropranolol) has weak beta-blocking effects. The volume of distribution is 4 L/kg and about 90% of the drug is bound to plasma proteins. Reduced hepatic blood flow from low cardiac output decreases hepatic extraction of propranolol. Although the plasma half-life is approximately 4 hours, the pharmacologic effect may persist for a longer duration.

Metoprolol and atenolol are β_1-selective antagonists available in oral and parenteral formulations. Metoprolol has about 40% bioavailability and atenolol about 50% bioavailability. The plasma half-lives are 3 to 4 hours for metoprolol and 5 to 8 hours for atenolol. The liver extensively metabolizes metoprolol with marked interindividual variability. Approximately 10% of the drug is excreted unchanged in the urine. Plasma concentrations of atenolol show markedly less interindividual variability than metoprolol. Atenolol is excreted mostly unchanged in the urine, and it will accumulate in patients with renal dysfunction.

Adverse Effects

Bradycardia, hypotension, myocardial depression, and bronchospasm are the primary adverse effects of beta-blockers. These drugs can precipitate heart failure when administered to patients with impaired left ventricular function, although lower doses of the drugs are well tolerated even in this group of patients for whom chronic beta-blocker therapy decreased mortality rates.[83] Cold extremities and worsening of Raynaud disease can occur. Catecholamines promote glucose mobilization, thus beta-blockers may interfere with recovery from hypoglycemia in patients with diabetes, although the latter effect is less with β_1-selective compounds. Hypotension is more marked for patients receiving catecholamine-depleting drugs such as reserpine. Central nervous system side effects include dizziness, headache, and mental status changes. The predominant gastrointestinal side effects are nausea, vomiting, abdominal cramps, and constipation, whereas other adverse effects such as alopecia and lupus reactions are rare. Up-regulation of β adrenergic receptors occurs with chronic beta-blocker therapy such that abrupt withdrawal may lead to tachycardia that is not tolerated by patients with coronary artery disease. These drugs should not be abruptly discontinued, but rather should be slowly tapered before stopping.

Ca^{++} Channel Blocking Drugs

Indications

Calcium channel blocking drugs of clinical use fall into three broad classifications: phenylalkylamines (e.g., verapamil), benzothiazepines (e.g., diltiazem), and dihydropyridines (e.g., nifedipine). Verapamil and diltiazem are indicated for the termination of supraventricular arrhythmias because of re-entry (e.g., sinus nodal re-entry, AV nodal re-entry, and orthodromic tachycardia with WPW syndrome) if maneuvers enhancing vagal tone or adenosine were not successful. As with beta-blockers, slowing AV nodal conduction may accelerate SVT with antegrade conduction associated with the WPW syndrome. When the diagnosis of wide QRS complex tachycardia is in question, it is prudent to avoid Ca^{++} channel blockers. Verapamil and diltiazem are effective for slowing the ventricular rate during AF or atrial flutter, and rarely they can convert recent onset atrial arrhythmias to sinus rhythm. Verapamil and diltiazem are not generally useful for ventricular arrhythmias, although some efficacy is seen in patients with idiopathic VT.[16]

Pharmacokinetics

Verapamil undergoes considerable first-pass metabolism in the liver (bioavailability 25% to 30%), but it is effective in slowing ventricular rate in 30 minutes. The drug is 90% bound to plasma proteins and its half-life is 4 to 6 hours with nearly 70% of the drug excreted in the kidneys. One metabolite, norverapamil, exerts clinically significant electrophysiologic effects. The bioavailability of diltiazem after oral administration is approximately 40%, and the plasma elimination half-life 3 to 4.5 hours. Diltiazem is 70% to 80% bound to plasma proteins. Other drugs that inhibit hepatic microsomal enzymes may increase blood concentrations of diltiazem. Active metabolites of diltiazem have a much slower elimination (~20 hours). Major metabolites include desacetyldiltiazem and desmethyldiltiazem. Dosage adjustments of verapamil and diltiazem are necessary for patients with hepatic impairment.

Adverse Effects

The major adverse effects from Ca^{++} channel blockers result from vasodilation leading to hypotension, lightheadedness, and nausea. Verapamil and diltiazem also have negative inotropic effects. Bradycardia and transient asystole have been reported with intravenous verapamil when administered to patients with cardiac conduction abnormalities or those also receiving beta-blockers. Verapamil can increase serum digoxin concentrations by 50% to 75% the first week of treatment. Downward adjustments in cyclosporine dose are necessary when coadministered with diltiazem. Coadministration of oral diltiazem and carbamazepine results in increased serum levels of the latter drug. Peripheral edema, constipation, and rashes may occur with use of Ca^{2+} channel blockers.

Adenosine

Indications

Adenosine is approved for the termination of re-entrant SVTs. Adenosine does not convert AF or atrial flutter to sinus rhythm, but may serve as a diagnostic maneuver by facilitating the appearance of flutter waves during transient depression of AV conduction. Adenosine may also terminate adrenergic-sensitive idiopathic VT originating from the right ventricular outflow tract in patients with no structural heart disease.[84,85]

Pharmacokinetics

Adenosine has a half-life of seconds. It is taken up into most cells including the endothelium and is metabolized to inosine by adenosine deaminase. Dipyridamole inhibits adenosine uptake and hence potentiates the effects of adenosine. Caffeine and methylxanthines block the adenosine receptor, requiring larger doses of adenosine for clinical effect.

Adverse Effects

Because of its rapid offset, adverse effects of adenosine are short-lived with the possible exception of patients administered dipyridamole. Transient asystole usually follows bolus administration. Adenosine rarely results in bronchospasm in patients with asthma. Prior cardiac transplantation may also result in hypersensitivity to adenosine.

Practical Aspects of Drug Administration

Proarrhythmia refers to bradyarrhythmias or tachyarrhythmias that directly result from drugs. These complications are caused by the electrophysiologic effects of the drugs such as slowed conduction, prolonged repolarization, possibly early afterdepolarizations, and alterations in re-entrant circuits, especially those resulting from dynamic interactions of existing substrate in the setting of myocardial ischemia or electrolyte disturbances.[4-6,16,40,86-88] Patients particularly prone to proarrhythmic side effects include those with primary or drug-induced prolonged QT intervals, with a history of VT, patients with left ventricular hypertrophy, myocardial ischemia, or impaired left ventricular function.[3,89-92] For the most part, Class Ic antiarrhythmic drugs are avoided for patients with structural heart disease. The use of two or more antiarrhythmic agents is avoided when a first agent was ineffective.

In some situations, treating reversible imbalances may be sufficient for terminating arrhythmias. Examples of reversible imbalances include myocardial ischemia, hypoxemia, hypercarbia, acidosis, anemia, electrolyte abnormalities (e.g., hypokalemia, hypomagnesemia, and so on), thyrotoxicosis, hypothermia, microshock or macroshock from medical equipment and monitors, and direct mechanical irritation to the heart (e.g., central venous or pulmonary artery catheters, mediastinal drainage tubes, and so on). An exhaustive search for such factors should be initiated whenever an arrhythmia develops perioperatively.

Direct electrical cardioversion or defibrillation is used when the patient is hemodynamically unstable or the arrhythmia is associated with evidence of myocardial ischemia or congestive heart failure. Using an evidence-based approach, antiarrhythmic agents for treating hemodynamically unstable VT or VF after failure of electrical interventions are given "acceptable based only on fair evidence of benefit (Class IIb, amiodarone)" or "class indeterminate (lidocaine)" ACLS recommendation.[93] There is no evidence that the use of any drug in these settings is associated with improved survival to hospital discharge or improved longer term outcomes. Treatment options for hemodynamically stable monomorphic VT include parenteral procainamide, amiodarone, beta-blockers, and sotalol where available.[93,94]

Polymorphic VT in the absence of pre-existing QT prolongation and associated with stable hemodynamics is treated similar to monomorphic VT when cardioversion is not desirable.[93] The treatment of polymorphic VT with pre-existing QT interval prolongation (torsades de pointes) should include an exhaustive search for reversible causes of such as electrolyte abnormalities, medications, and ischemia. When hemodynamically stable and when cardioversion is not desirable, torsade de pointes can be treated with overdrive atrial or ventricular pacing along with beta-blockers and magnesium (ACLS class of indeterminate).[93]

The treatment aims for hemodynamically stable AF and atrial flutter include heart rate control, conversion to sinus rhythm, and anticoagulation. Verapamil, diltiazem, or beta-blockers can be used to slow the ventricular response in the absence of ventricular dysfunction.[95–97] Digoxin is useful in the setting of left ventricular dysfunction, but is less efficacious when there is enhanced sympathetic drive as seen in the postoperative state.[96] Drugs that slow AV conduction can actually precipitate fast, potentially life-threatening heart rates for patients with AF who have an accessory pathway (WPW syndrome). In these situations, antiarrhythmic drugs that slow conduction (e.g., procainamide or propafenone) are used.[50] Drugs that are effective for treating AF/flutter are given an ACLS Class IIa (acceptable based on good or very good evidence) or Class IIb rating (e.g., sotalol and disopyramide).[93] The drug choice is dependent on individual risk for proarrhythmia and left ventricular function. Left atrial thrombus is present in 13% to 29% of patients with AF.[98–101] When atrial flutter or fibrillation have been present for more than 48 hours, anticoagulation for 3 weeks is typically recommended before pharmacologic or electrical cardiover-sion, but transesophageal echocardiography can be used to exclude left atrial thrombus.[98]

Paroxysmal SVT usually results from a concealed accessory pathway, dual AV nodal physiology (AVNRT), or an atrial tachycardia. In the setting of stable hemodynamics, adenosine may be given. When it is successful in terminating the arrhythmia, adenosine often results in a brief period of asystole followed by sinus rhythm. Antiarrhythmic agents such as procainamide, amiodarone, sotalol, and flecainide are considered for treating paroxysmal SVT when adenosine or AV nodal blocking agents are unsuccessful and cardioversion is not desirable (Class IIa recommendation).[51,93,102,103]

Dosage and Administration

The doses of most antiarrhythmic drugs are adjusted based on therapeutic plasma concentrations, although the exact plasma levels that achieve therapeutic versus toxic effects may vary. Dosing guidelines for antiarrhythmics are listed in Table 35–3.

Procainamide: Oral forms available include 250-, 375-, and 500-mg capsules; 250-, 500-, and 750-mg extended release tablets; and 500- and 1000-mg extended release formulations. Parenteral procainamide is available in 2- (500 mg/mL) and 10-mL (100 mg/mL) multidose vials. Therapeutic plasma concentrations are 4 to 8 μg/mL for the parent compound, whereas NAPA levels are 10 to 20 μg/mL.

Quinidine: Extended release 300- (sulfate) and 324-mg (gluconate) extended release tablets are available. Oral doses of gluconate are 30% more potent than sulfate. Therapeutic plasma concentrations are 2 to 5 μg/mL.

Disopyramide: Capsules and extended release capsules both containing 100 and 150 mg are available. Therapeutic plasma concentrations are 2 to 5 μg/mL.

Lidocaine: Formulations included 50- and 100-mg syringes, 100-mg 5-mL ampules, and 1- and 2-g vials. Therapeutic plasma concentrations are 1.5 to 5.0 μg/mL.

TABLE 35–3.

Dosing for Vaughan Williams Class I and III Drugs

Drug	Oral Dose	Parenteral Dose
Procainamide	500 mg to 1 gm, then 350 to 1000 mg QID	1 gm IV at 20 mg/min or until arrhythmia stops, hypotension develops, QRS ↑ by 50%
Quinidine	600 mg to 1 gm, then 300 to 600 mg QID	
Disopyramide	300 mg, then 150 to 300 mg QID	
Lidocaine		1 to 1.5 mg/kg repeated to maximum of 300 mg, then 1 to 4 mg/min

TABLE 35–3.

Dosing for Vaughan Williams Class I and III Drugs—*cont'd*

Drug	Oral Dose	Parenteral Dose
Mexiletine	400 to 600 mg, then 50 to 300 mg TID or 450 mg BID	
Tocainide	400 to 600 mg TID or BID, then 400 to 600 mg TID	
Flecainide	50 to 100 mg BID then ↑ by 50 mg/day until 400 mg/day	
Propafenone	150 mg TID ↑ to 300 mg TID over 3 to 4 days to maximum 900 mg/day	
Moricizine	200 to 300 mg TID	
Amiodarone	800 to 1600 mg/day for 1 to 3 weeks, then lowest effective dose usually 200 to 600 mg/day	150 mg IV over 10 min, then 1 mg/min for 6 hr, then 0.5 mg/min for 18 hr. Bolus may be repeated for recurrent arrhythmias.
Bretylium		5 to 10 mg/kg at 1 to 2 mg/kg/min repeated every 15 to 30 min as needed to maximum of 30 mg/kg, then 1 to 4 mg/min
Sotalol	80 mg BID, then ↑ every 2 to 3 days to 80 to 160 mg BID	
Ibutilide		1 mg over 10 min. If <60 kg give 0.01 mg/kg. Repeat after 10 min if needed.
Dofetilide	0.125 to 0.5 mg BID based on creatinine clearance	
Diltiazem		0.25 to 0.35 mg/kg IV over 10 min, then 5 to 15 mg/hr
Verapamil		5 to 10 mg IV over 2 min. May give additional 10 mg after 15 to 30 min.
Esmolol		500 μg/kg/min IV, then ↑ in 50 to 100 μg/kg/min increments every 5 min until desired effect
Propranolol		1 to 3 mg IV at 1 mg/min. Repeat after 2 min then give effective dose every 4 hours
Metoprolol	For MI, after IV loading, 50 mg QID for 48 hr, then 100 mg BID or 25 to 50 mg QID	1 to 5 mg IV
Atenolol	For MI, after IV loading, 50 mg BID, ↑ dose to 100 mg/day; for arrhythmias, 0.3 mg/kg/day	1 to 5 mg IV
Acebutolol	200 mg BID ↑ until desired effect, usually 600 to 1200 mg/day	
Timolol	10 mg BID for MI	

IV, intravenously; MI, myocardial infarction.

Mexiletine: Capsules containing 150, 200, and 250 mg mexiletine are available. The therapeutic plasma concentrations are 0.5 to 2.0 μg/mL.

Tocainide: Tablets containing 400 and 600 mg of tocainide are available. Therapeutic plasma concentrations are 3 to 11 μg/mL.

Flecainide: The drug is available in 50-, 100-, and 150-mg tablets. Therapeutic plasma concentrations are 0.2 to 1.0 μg/mL.

Propafenone: Tablets containing 150, 225, and 300 mg are available. Therapeutic plasma concentrations are less than 1 μg/mL.

Moricizine: Tablets containing 200, 250, and 300 mg are available.

Amiodarone: Tablets containing 200 mg amiodarone are available. Amiodarone for injections contains 50 mg/mL amiodarone, 20.2 mg benzyl alcohol, and 100 mg polysorbate 80. The parenteral drug should be given, when possible, through a central venous catheter using an in-line filter. Infusion lasting more than 2 hours must be administered in glass or polyolefin bottles containing D_5W because amiodarone adsorbs to polyvinylchloride tubing. Amiodarone is incompatible with heparin, sodium bicarbonate, aminophylline, cefamandole nafate, cefazolin sodium, and mezlocillin sodium. Transition from intravenous to oral amiodarone is with 800 to 1600 mg, 600 to 800 mg, and 400 mg, for infusions less than 1 week, 1 to 3 weeks, and greater than 3 weeks, respectively.

Bretylium: Solution containing 50 mg/mL bretylium is available for parenteral use. Dilution of the bolus dose in 50 to 100 mL D_5W is recommended.

Sotalol: Tablets containing 80, 120, 160, and 240 mg are available. Parenteral formulations of sotalol are not available in the United States. The dose is individualized when creatinine clearance is less than 10 ml/min. Sotalol is only partially removed by dialysis, and a rebound in plasma concentrations may follow after dialysis. Plasma concentrations of approximately 2.5 μg/mL are considered therapeutic.

Ibutilide: Ibutilide for injection contains 0.1 mg/mL of the drug in 10-mL, single-dose, clear vials. The drug can be given without dilution or after dilution in 0.9% normal saline or D_5W. The QTc interval should be monitored closely during administration and for 4 hours after infusion or until it has returned to normal. The ECG should be monitored longer for patients for whom ventricular arrhythmias develop during ibutilide treatment.

Dofetilide: The drug is supplied in 0.125-, 0.25-, and 0.5-mg tablets. The dose of dofetilide is individualized, depending on the QTc interval and renal function, and it must be administered in the hospital under continuous ECG monitoring for 3 days by staff trained to administer the drug (or for 12 hours after conversion to sinus rhythm). Dofetilide should not be administered to patients with a QTc interval greater than 440 milliseconds, or 500 milliseconds for those with ventricular conduction abnormalities. The patient's creatinine clearance must be calculated before administering dofetilide. The dose is then adjusted accordingly for creatinine clearance greater than 60 mL/min, 40 to 60 mL/min, and 20 to less than 40 mL/min. Dofetilide is contraindicated for patients with creatinine clearance less than 20 mL/min. The QTc interval should be calculated every 2 to 3 hours after starting therapy and after each subsequent dose for the first 3 days of therapy. The dose is reduced if the QTc increases by 15% from baseline, and the drug is discontinued if the QTc is greater than 500 milliseconds, or 550 milliseconds for patients with pre-existing ventricular conduction abnormalities. Renal function and QTc interval are monitored every 3 months or when otherwise indicated during maintenance therapy.

Diltiazem: Parenteral diltiazem is most often used for antiarrhythmic indications. The drug is supplied in 5- and 10-mL vials containing 5 mg/mL.

Verapamil: Parenteral formulation contains 5 mg/mL.

Esmolol: Esmolol is supplied as ready to use in 10-mL (10 mg/mL) multidose vials and in 10-mL ampules containing 2500 mg of the drug. The latter form must be diluted before use usually in a 250- or 500-mL container of IV solution.

Propranolol: Tablets containing 10, 20, 40, 60, and 80 mg propranolol are available. Extended release tablets contain 80 and 160 mg. The injectable form of propranolol contains 1 mg/mL of the drug in light-resistant ampules. As with other beta-blockers, close monitoring of the ECG and blood pressure is required during parenteral administration of propranolol.

Metoprolol: Metoprolol comes in oral tablets containing 50 and 60 mg of the drug and extended release tablets containing 50, 100, and 200 mg. The parenteral form of the drug contains 1 mg/mL.

Atenolol: Tablets of atenolol come in 25, 50, and 100 mg forms. Atenolol for injection is available as 5 mg in 10-mL solution.

Acebutolol: Tablets containing 200 and 400 mg acebutolol are available.

Timolol: Timolol is available in tablets containing 5, 10, and 20 mg of the drug.

References

1. Smith RC, Leung JM, Keith FM, et al: Ventricular dysrhythmias in patients undergoing coronary artery bypass graft surgery: Incidence, characteristics, and prognostic importance. Am Heart J 123:73, 1992.
2. Creswell LL, Schuessler RB, Rosenbloom M, et al: Hazards of postoperative atrial arrhythmias. Ann Thorac Surg 56:539, 1993.
3. The Cardiac Arrhythmia Suppression Trial (CAST) Investigators: Preliminary report: Effect of encainide and flecainide on mortality in a randomized trial of arrhythmia suppression after myocardial infarction. N Engl J Med 321:406, 1989.
4. Ben-David J, Zipes DP: Torsades de pointes and proarrhythmia. Lancet 341:1578, 1993.
5. Lazzara R: Mechanistic and clinical aspects of acquired long QT syndromes. Ann NY Acad Sci 644:48, 1992.
6. Stanton MS, Prystowsky EN, Fineberg NS, et al: Arrhythmogenic effects of antiarrhythmic drugs: A study of 506 patients treated for ventricular tachycardia or fibrillation. J Am Coll Cardiol 14:209, 1989.
7. Zipes DP: Implantable cardioverter-defibrillator: A Volkswagen or Rolls Royce. Circulation 103:1372, 2001.
8. Morady F: Radio-frequency ablation as treatment for cardiac arrhythmias. N Engl J Med 340:534, 1999.
9. Whalley DW, Wendt DJ, Grant AO: Basic concepts in cellular cardiac electrophysiology: Part I: Ion channels, membrane currents, and the action potential. Pacing Clin Electrophysiol 8:1556, 1995.
10. Whalley DW, Wendt DJ, Grant AO: Basic concepts in cellular cardiac electrophysiology: Part II: Block of ion channels by antiarrhythmic drugs. Pacing Clin Electrophysiol 18:1686, 1995.

11. Grant AO, Whalley DW: Mechanisms of cardiac arrhythmias. In Topol EJ (ed): Textbook of Cardiovascular Medicine. Philadelphia, Lippincott-Raven, 1998.

12. Hondeghem LM: Antiarrhythmic agents: Modulated receptor applications. Circulation 75:514, 1987.

13. Hondeghem LM, Katzung BG: Time- and voltage-dependent interactions of antiarrhythmic drugs with cardiac sodium channels. Biochim Biophys Acta 14:373, 1977.

14. Vaughan Williams EM: A classification of antiarrhythmic actions reassessed after a decade of new drugs. J Clin Pharmacol 24:129, 1984.

15. Task Force of the Working Group on Arrhythmias of the European Society of Cardiology: The Sicilian gambit, a new approach to the classification of antiarrhythmic drugs based on their actions on arrhythmogenic mechanisms. Circulation 84:1831, 1991.

16. Zipes DP: Management of cardiac arrhythmias: Pharmacological, electrical, and surgical techniques. In Braunwald E (ed): Heart Disease. Philadelphia, WB Saunders, 1997.

17. Grace AA, Camm AJ: Drug therapy—quinidine. N Engl J Med 338:35, 1998.

18. Cain ME, Josephson ME: Procainamide. In Gould LA (ed): Drug Treatment of Cardiac Arrhythmias. New York, Futura Publishing, 1982.

19. Koch-Weser J: Drug therapy—disopyramide. N Engl J Med 300:957, 1979.

20. Manolis AS, Deering TF, Cameron J, et al: Mexiletine: Pharmacology and therapeutic use. Clin Cardiol 13:349, 1990.

21. Holmes B, Brogden RC, Heel TM, et al: Tocainide: A Review of Its Pharmacological Properties and Therapeutic Efficacy, Drugs. Auckland, New Zealand, Adis International, 1983.

22. Roden DM, Woosley RL: Drug therapy—tocainide. N Engl J Med 315:41, 1986.

23. Kreeger RW, Hammill SC: New antiarrhythmic drugs: Tocainide, mexiletine, flecainide, encainide, and amiodarone. Mayo Clin Proc 62:1033, 1987.

24. Funck-Brentano C, Kroemer HK, Lee JT, et al: Drug therapy—propafenone. N Engl J Med 322:518, 1990.

25. Fitton A, Buckley MM-T: Moricizine: A Review of Its Pharmacological Properties and Therapeutic Efficacy in Cardiac Arrhythmias, drugs. Auckland, New Zealand, Adis International, 1990.

26. Lefkowitz RJ: β-Adrenergic receptors: Recognition and regulation physiology in medicine. Physiol Med 295:323, 1976.

27. Frishman WH: β-Adrenoceptor antagonists: New drugs and new indications. N Engl J Med 305:500, 1981.

28. Fitton A, Sorkin EM: Sotalol, An Updated Review of its Pharmacological Properties and Therapeutic Use in Cardiac Arrhythmias, Drugs. Auckland, New Zealand, Adis International Limited, 1994.

29. Hohnloser SH, Woosley RL: Sotalol. N Engl J Med 331:31, 1994.

30. Karam R, Marcello S, Brooks RR, et al: Azimilide dihydrochloride, a novel antiarrhythmic agent. Am J Cardiol 81:40, 1998.

31. Frost L, Mortensen PE, Tinglef J, et al: Efficacy and safety of dofetilide, a new class III antiarrhythmic agent, in acute termination of atrial fibrillation or flutter after coronary artery bypass surgery. Int J Cardiol 58:135, 1997.

32. Murray K: Ibutilide. Circulation 97:493, 1998.

33. Koch-Weser J: Drug therapy—bretylium. N Engl J Med 300:473, 1979.

34. Zipes DP, Prystowsky EN, Heger JJ: Amiodarone: Electrophysiologic actions, pharmacokinetics and clinical effects. J Am Coll Cardiol 3:1059, 1984.

35. Abernethy DR, Schwartz JB: Calcium-antagonist drugs. Drug Therapy 341:1447, 1999.

36. DiMarco JP, Sellers TD, Berne RM, et al: Adenosine: Electrophysiologic effects and therapeutic use for terminating paroxysmal supraventricular tachycardia. Circulation 68:1254, 1983.

37. Belardinelli L, Linden J, Berne RM: The cardiac effects of adenosine. Prog Cardiovasc Dis Vol 32:73, 1989.

38. Evardsson N: Comparison of class I and class III action in atrial fibrillation. Eur Heart J 14(suppl H):62, 1993.

39. Madrid AH, Moro C, Marin-Huerta E, et al: Comparison of flecainide and procainamide in conversion of atrial fibrillation. Eur Heart J 14:1127, 1993.

40. Steinberg JS, Sahar BI, Rosenbaum M, et al: Proarrhythmic effects of procainamide and tocainide in a canine infarction model. J Cardiovasc Pharmacol 19:52, 1992.

41. Lazzara R: Antiarrhythmic drugs and torsade de pointes. Eur Heart J 14(suppl H):88, 1993.

42. Johnson RG, Goldberger AL, Thurer RL, et al: Lidocaine prophylaxis in coronary revascularization patients: A randomized, prospective trial. Ann Thorac Surg 55:1180, 1993.

43. King FG, Addetia AM, Peters SD, et al: Prophylactic lidocaine for postoperative coronary artery bypass patients, a double-blind, randomized trial. Can J Anaesth 37:363, 1990.

44. Hine LK, Laird N, Hewitt P, et al: Meta-analytic evidence against prophylactic use of lidocaine in acute myocardial infarction. Arch Intern Med 49:2694, 1989.

45. Buchert E, Woosley RL: Clinical implications of variable antiarrhythmic drug metabolism. Pharmacogenetics 2:2, 1992.

46. Hohnloser SH, Zabel M: Short- and long-term efficacy and safety of flecainide acetate for supraventriuclar arrhythmias. Am J Cardiol 70:3A, 1992.

47. Lau CP, Leung WH, Wong CK: A randomized double-blind crossover study comparing the efficacy and tolerability of flecainide and quinidine in the control of patients with symptomatic paroxysmal atrial fibrillation. Am Heart J 124:645, 1992.

48. Auricchio A: Reversible protective effect of propafenone or flecainide during atrial fibrillation in patients with an accessory atrioventricular connection. Am Heart J 124:932, 1992.

49. Kingma JH, Suttorp MJ: Acute pharmacologic conversion of atrial fibrillation and flutter: The role of flecainide, propafenone and verapamil. Am J Cardiol 70:56A, 1992.

50. O'Nunain S, Garratt CJ, Linker NJ, et al: A comparison of intravenous propafenone and flecaindie in the treatment of tachycardias associated with the Wolff-Parkinson-White syndrome. Pacing Clin Electrophysiol 14:2028, 1991.

51. O'Nunain S, Garrat CJ, Linker NJ, et al: A comparison of intravenous propafenone and flecainide in the treatment of tachycardia associated with the Wolff-Parkinson-White syndrome. Pacing Clin Electrophysiol 14:2028, 1991.

52. Gill JS, Mehta D, Ward DE, et al: Efficacy of flecainide, sotalol and verapamil in the treatment of right ventricular tachycardia in patients without overt cardiac abnormality. Br Heart J 68:392, 1992.

53. Gentili C, Giordano F, Alois A, et al: Efficacy of intravenous propafenone in acute atrial fibrillation complicating open-heart surgery. Am Heart J 123:1225, 1992.

54. Bianconi L, Boccadamo R, Toscano S, et al: Effects of oral propafenone therapy on chronic myocardial pacing threshold. Pacing Clin Electrophysiol 15:148, 1992.

55. Estes NA III: Evolving strategies for the management of atrial fibrillation: The role of amiodarone. JAMA 267:3332, 1992.

56. Gosselink AT, Crijn HJ, VanGelder IC, et al: Low-dose amiodarone for maintenance of sinus rhythm after cardioversion of atrial fibrillation or flutter. JAMA 267:3289, 1992.

57. Roden DM: Current status of class III antiarrhythmic drug therapy. Am J Cardiol 72:62F, 1993.

58. Cochrane AD, Siddins M, Rosenfeldt FL, et al: A comparison of amiodarone and digoxin for treatment of supraventricular arrhythmias after cardiac surgery. Eur J Cardiothorac Surg 8:194, 1994.

59. Holt P, Crick JC, Davies DW, Curry P: Intravenous amiodarone in the acute termination of supraventricular arrhythmias. Int J Cardiol 8:67, 1985.

60. Daoud EG, Strickberger SA, Man KC, et al: Preoperative amiodarone as prophylaxis against atrial fibrillation after heart surgery. N Engl J Med 337:1785, 1997.

61. Guarnieri T, Nolan S, Gottlieb SO, et al: Intravenous amiodarone for the prevention of atrial fibrillation after open heart surgery: The Amiodarone Reduction in Coronary Heart (ARCH) trial. J Am Coll Cardiol 34:343, 1999.

62. Lee SH, Chang CM, Lu MJ, et al: Intravenous amiodarone for prevention of atrial fibrillation after coronary artery bypass grafting. Ann Thorac Surg 70:157, 2000.

63. Liberman BA, Teasdale SJ: Anesthesia and amiodarone. Can Anaesth Soc J 32:629, 1985.

64. Feinberg BI, LaMantia KR, Levy WJ: Amiodarone and general anesthesia: A retrospective analysis. Anesth Analg 65:549, 1986.

65. Schmid JP, Rosengant TK, McIntosh CL, et al: Amiodarone-induced complications after cardiac operation for obstructive hypertrophic cardiomyopathy. Ann Thorac Surg 48:359, 1989.

66. Hohnloser SH, Klingenheben T, Singh BN: Amiodarone-associated proarrhythmic effects: A review with special reference to torsade de pointes tachycardia. Ann Intern Med 121:529, 1994.

67. Weinberg BA, Miles WM, Klein LS, et al: Five-year follow-up of 589 patients treated with amiodarone. Am Heart J 125:109, 1993.

68. Greenspon AJ, Kidwell GA, Hurley W, et al: Amiodarone-related postoperative adult respiratory distress syndrome. Circulation 84(suppl III):III-407, 1991.

69. Nystrom UJ, Edvardsson N, Berggren H, et al: Oral sotalol reduces the incidence of atrial fibrillation after coronary artery bypass surgery. J Thorac Cardiovasc Surg 41:34, 1993.

70. Suttorp MJ, Kingma JH, Peels HO, et al: Effectiveness of sotalol in preventing supraventricular tachyarrhythmias shortly after coronary artery bypass grafting. Am J Cardiol 68:1163, 1991.

71. Campbell TJ, Gavaghan TP, Morgan JJ: Intravenous sotalol for the treatment of atrial fibrillation and flutter after cardiopulmonary bypass. Comparison with disopyramide and digoxin in a randomized trial. Br Heart J 54:86, 1985.

72. Hohnloser SH, Zabel M, Krause T, et al: Short- and long-term antiarrhythmic and hemodynamic effects of d, l-sotalol in patients with symptomatic ventricular arrhythmias. Am Heart J 123:1220, 1992.

73. MacNeil DJ, Davies RO, Beitchman D: Clinical safety profile of sotalol in the treatment of arrhythmias. Am J Cardiol 72:44A, 1993.

74. VanderLugt JT, Mattioni T, Denker S, et al: Efficacy and safety of ibutilide fumarate for the conversion of atrial arrhythmias after cardiac surgery. Circulation 100:369, 1999.

75. Stambler BS, Wood MA, Ellenbogen KA, et al: Efficacy and safety of repeated intravenous doses of ibutilide for rapid conversion of atrial flutter or fibrillation. Ibutilide Repeat Dose Study Investigators. Circulation 94:1613, 1996.

76. Singh S, Zoble RG, Yellen L, et al: Efficacy and safety of oral dofetilide in converting to and maintaining sinus rhythm in patients with chronic atrial fibrillation or atrial flutter: The SAFIRE-D study. Circulation 102:2385, 2000.

77. Torp-Pedersen C, Møller M, Bloch-Thomsen PE, et al: Dofetilide in patients with congestive heart failure and left ventricular dysfunction. N Engl J Med 341:857, 1999.

78. Andrews TC, Reimold SC, Berlin JA, et al: Prevention of supraventricular arrhythmias after coronary artery bypass surgery: A meta-analysis of randomized controlled trials. Circulation 84(suppl I):I-236, 1991.

79. Kowey PR, Taylor JE, Rials SJ, et al: Meta-analysis of the effectiveness of prophylactic drug therapy in preventing supraventricular arrhythmia early after coronary artery bypass grafting. Am J Cardiol 69:963, 1992.

80. Hill GA, Owens SD: Esmolol in the treatment of multifocal atrial tachycardia. Chest 101:1726, 1992.

81. Malfatto G, Beria G, Sala S, et al: Quantitative analysis of T wave abnormalities and their prognostic implications in the idiopathic long QT syndrome. J Am Coll Cardiol 23:296, 1994.

82. Bhorat IE, Naidoo DP, Rout CC, et al: Malignant ventricular arrhythmias in eclampsia: A comparison of labetolol with dihydralazine. Am J Obstet Gynecol 168:1292, 1993.

83. Heidenreich PA, Lee TT, Massie BM: Effect of beta-blockade on mortality in patients with heart failure: A meta-analysis of randomized clinical trials. J Am Coll Cardiol 30:27, 1997.

84. Griffith MJ, Garratt CJ, Rowland E, et al: Effects of intravenous adenosine on verapamil-sensitive idiopathic ventricular tachycardia. Am J Cardiol 1994;73:759.

85. Lerman BB: Response of nonreentrant catecholamine-mediated ventricular tachycardia to endogenous adenosine and acetylcholine. Evi-dence for myocardial receptor-mediated effects. Circulation 87:382, 1993.

86. Roden DM: Early after-depolarizations and torsade de pointes: Implications for the control of cardiac arrhythmias by prolonging repolarization. Eur Heart J 14:H56, 1993.

87. Sicouri S, Antzelevitch C: Drug-induced afterdepolarizations and triggered activity occur in a discreet subpopluation of ventricular muscle cells (M cells) in the canine heart: Quinidine and digitalis. J Cardiovasc Electrophysiol 4:48, 1993.

88. Sager PT, Perlumutter RA, Rosenfeld LE, et al: Antiarrhythmic drug exacerbation of ventricular tachycardia inducibility during electrophysiologic study. Am Heart J 123:926, 1992.

89. Kowey PR, Levine JH, Herre JM, et al: Randomized, double-blind comparison of intravenous amiodarone and bretylium in the treatment of patients with recurrent, hemodynamically destabilizing ventricular tachycardia or fibrillation. Circulation 92:3255, 1995.

90. Kudenchuk PJ, Cobb LA, Copass MK, et al: Amiodarone for resuscitation after out-of-hospital cardiac arrest due to ventricular fibrillation. N Engl J Med 341:871, 1999.

91. Herlitz J, Ekstrome L, Wennerblom B, et al: Lidocaine in out-of-hospital ventricular fibrillation: Does it improve survival? Resuscitation 33:199, 1997.

92. Stiell IG, Wells GA, Hebert PC, et al: Association of drug therapy with survival in cardiac arrest: Limited role of advanced cardiac life support drugs. Acad Emerg Med 2:264, 1995.

93. Guidelines 2000 for cardiopulmonary resuscitation and emergency cardiovascular care. Circulation 102:I-112, 2000.

94. Gorgels AP, van den Dool A, Hofs A, et al: Comparison of procainamide and lidocaine in terminating sustained monomorphic ventricular tachycardia. Am J Cardiol 78:43, 1996.

95. Tommaso C, McDonough T, Parker M, et al: Atrial fibrillation and flutter: Immediate control and conversion with intravenously administered verapamil. Arch Intern Med 143:877, 1983.

96. Tisdale JE, Padhi ID, Goldberg AD, et al: A randomized, double-blind comparison of intravenous diltiazem and digoxin for atrial fibrillation after coronary artery bypass surgery. Am Heart J 135:739, 1998.

97. Schwartz M, Michelson EL, Sawain HS, et al: Esmolol: Safety and efficacy in postoperative cardiothoracic patients with supraventricular tachyarrhythmias. Chest 93:705, 1988.

98. Mugge A, Kuhn H, Daniel WG: The role of transesophageal echocardiography in the detection of left atrial thrombi. Echocardiography 10:405, 1993.

99. Brown J, Sadler DB: Left atrial thrombi in non-rheumatic atrial fibrillation: Assessment of prevalence by transesophageal echocardiography. Int J Card Imaging 9:65, 1993.

100. Stoddard MF, Dawkins PR, Prince CR, et al: Left atrial appendage thrombus is not uncommon in patients with acute atrial fibrillation and a recent embolic event: A transesophageal echocardiographic study. J Am Coll Cardiol 25:452, 1995.

101. Aberg H: Atrial fibrillation. 1. A study of atrial thrombosis and systemic embolism in a necropsy material. Acta Med Scand 185:373, 1969.

102. Chapman MJ, Moran JL, O'Fathartaigh MS, et al: Management of atrial tachyarrhythmias in the critically ill: A comparison of intravenous procainamide and amiodarone. Intensive Care Med 19:48, 1993.

103. Jordaens L, Gorgels A, Stroobandt R, et al: Efficacy and safety of intravenous sotalol for termination of paroxysmal supraventricular tachycardia. Am J Cardiol 68:35, 1991.

36

Agents Used to Treat Myocardial Ischemia

Hugh Dorman, MD, PhD • David Feldman, MD, PhD • Joseph G. Reves, MD

Nitrates
   Mechanism of Action
   Clinical Pharmacology
   Practical Aspects of Drug Administration
β Adrenergic Receptor Antagonists
   Mechanism of Action and Preclinical
      Pharmacology
   Clinical Pharmacology
   Practical Aspects of Drug Administration

Calcium Channel Blockers
   Preclinical Science
   Clinical Pharmacology
   Practical Aspects of Drug Administration
Anticoagulation Drugs
Antiplatelet Drugs
Antithrombin Drugs
Thrombolytic Drugs

This chapter focuses on the pharmacologic treatment and prevention of the acute coronary syndrome (ACS). The American Heart Association and the American College of Cardiology have defined ACS as any constellation of clinical signs or symptoms suggestive of acute myocardial infarction or unstable angina. ACS encompasses both non-Q- and Q-wave myocardial infarctions.[1] The most frequent cause of ACS is atherosclerotic coronary artery disease, which commonly precedes myocardial infarction and death. The cascade of ACS is frequently precipitated by plaque rupture and thrombus formation.[2] This pathology causes a mismatch between myocardial oxygen supply and demand.[3] Other causes of ACS include spasm, fixed coronary obstruction, hypermetabolic states, coronary arterial inflammation, and increased intracardiac filling pressures. Irrespective of the etiologic factors, the signs and symptoms of patient presentation are similar with some well-known caveats (e.g., diabetes, elderly age, and so on). Unstable angina may present with prolonged rest symptoms (>20 minutes), new onset exertional angina, or an acceleration of symptoms in a patient previously diagnosed with coronary artery disease.[4,5] In 1996, the National Center for Health Statistics reported more than 1.4 million hospital admissions for unstable angina or myocardial infarction without ST elevation. With advances in medical therapy, the rate of myocardial infarction in patients with ACS has plummeted to 10%, and mortality rate has decreased to approximately 5%.[6–8]

This chapter describes the most common pharmacologic agents used in the treatment of ACS. For the sake of brevity, controversial issues and several medical therapies are not discussed either because it is beyond the intended purpose of this chapter or because these therapies are included elsewhere in this book. Specifically, therapies that are not discussed in this chapter known to be of therapeutic use in ACS and acute myocardial infarction are: opiates, diuretics, anxiolytics, hepatic hydroxymethyl glutaryl coenzyme reductase inhibitors, mechanical support devices, percutaneous cardiac interventions, and cardiac surgery. All approved antianginal drugs seek to either improve cardiac oxygen balance, optimize cardiac hemodynamics (e.g., decrease heart rate and wall stress), or increase myocardial blood supply.

Nitrates

One of the most widely used groups of antianginal drugs is the organic nitrates, of which nitroglycerin, isosorbide dinitrate, and isosorbide-5-mononitrate are the clinically relevant compounds.

Mechanism of Action

At low doses, nitroglycerin and isosorbide dinitrate act on the vascular smooth muscle of venous capacitance vessels to produce peripheral blood pooling, resulting in a reduction in venous return and a decrease in cardiac wall tension.[9] Consequently, organic nitrates reduce myocardial oxygen demand and are thus useful in the treatment of angina pectoris. At greater doses, these compounds also relax arterial smooth muscle, and this effect may be important in relieving coronary artery spasm.[10] The organic nitrates act by releasing nitric oxide (NO) in an endothelium-independent manner. Several mechanisms appear to underlie the biotransformation of organic nitrates to NO, including enzymatic biotransformation mediated by glutathione-S-transferase,[11] nonenzymatic biotransformation by thiol-containing compounds such as cysteine,[12] and hemoprotein-mediated bioconversion.[13] NO released from organic nitrates activates soluble guanylate cyclase in vascular smooth muscle, stimulating the production of cyclic guanosine monophosphate (cGMP). CGMP activates cGMP-dependent protein kinase, which phosphorylates a number of proteins in the vascular smooth muscle cell, ultimately resulting in phosphorylation of myosin light chain and vascular smooth muscle relaxation. (Further details about the NO-guanylate cyclase pathway in vascular smooth muscle are discussed in Chapter 19.)

Clinical Pharmacology

The nitrates must undergo biotransformation to NO to produce their intended therapeutic effect on vascular tone. The nitrates are rapidly absorbed through mucous membranes, gastrointestinal mucosa, and intact skin. Nitroglycerin is quickly metabolized by hepatic and intravenous mechanisms, with a plasma half-life of 2 to 4 minutes. Whereas nitroglycerin is well absorbed after oral administration, it is largely inactive because of first-pass hepatic metabolism. Isosorbide dinitrate has a half-life of approximately 40 minutes with extensive hepatic metabolism into two active metabolites: isosorbide-2-mononitrate (2-hour half-life) and isosorbide-5-mononitrate (4-hour half-life). Isosorbide-5-mononitrate is also available as a synthetic nitrate that does not undergo hepatic transformation and has 100% bioavailability subsequent to oral administration.

Nitrates exert an antianginal effect through many complex and integrated physiologic mechanisms. Nitroglycerin increases oxygen delivery to myocardium, whereas oxygen demand is decreased. Dilation of venous capacitance vessels, particularly splanchnic and mesenteric vasculature, reduces ventricular preload, which decreases ventricular wall tension, a major determinant of myocardial oxygen consumption.[14,15] Additional modest vasodilatory effects on the arterial vasculature cause reduction in systolic wall stress or afterload, which results in further reductions in oxygen consumption. The nitrates also dilate large epicardial and collateral coronary arteries and prevent episodic coronary artery vasoconstriction, which can improve global and regional blood flow and favorably influence the ratio of subendocardial to epicardial blood flow.[16,17] Dilation of severely obstructed atherosclerotic regions with endothelial dysfunction improves blood flow to stenotic areas of myocardium without altering the caliber of coronary resistance vessels.[14] Thus the nitrates promote blood flow to myocardium, including collateral flow and redistribution of flow to ischemic regions, without precipitating coronary steal.

Nitrates also may improve symptoms of ACS through several indirect mechanisms. The nitrates reduce platelet adherence and aggregation, which should decrease thrombosis within the coronary vasculature.[18] The NO liberated from the nitrates reduces platelet function by modulating intracellular calcium, thereby reducing platelet secretion of aggregatory factors.[18,19] Nitroglycerin is effective in the treatment of acute pulmonary edema associated with myocardial ischemia by decreasing ventricular volume and pressure. Finally, concurrent mitral regurgitation is improved with nitrate administration by decreasing papillary muscle ischemia, allowing more appropriate coaptation of valve leaflets, and promoting forward stroke volume.

There are several, significant adverse effects related to administration of the nitrates. Headaches are frequently observed, and dose reduction may be necessary to resolve symptoms. In the perioperative setting, symptoms may be significantly attenuated with concordant administration of acetaminophen. Exacerbation of hypoxemia by increasing ventilation/perfusion mismatch may become significant in patients with marginal pulmonary function. Skin erythema and inflammation at the site of transdermal nitroglycerin patch application may necessitate varying the application site. The most dangerous side effect of the nitrates involves hypotension from widespread systemic vasodilation, which can precipitate reflex tachycardia and myocardial ischemia in patients with limited myocardial reserve. Syncope, nausea, and postural hypotensive symptoms have also been described as side effects of the nitrates;[19] initial treatment with small doses of nitrates with incremental increases may prevent some of the adverse events. Nitroglycerin-mediated vasodilation can be significantly enhanced and prolonged when administered in the presence of sildenafil (Viagra; a phosphodiesterase type V inhibitor that prevents the breakdown of cGMP). Concurrent use of nitrates and sildenafil within 24 hours has resulted in profound vasodilatation and death and is therefore contraindicated. In addition, high-dose nitrate therapy may produce methemoglobinemia in patients with significant hepatic dysfunction. Fortunately, prolonged infusion of intravenous nitroglycerin at high doses has only rarely been shown to increase methemoglobin levels to clinically significant levels.[20]

A substantial limitation to the use of nitrates involves the development of tolerance, defined as a loss of antianginal and hemodynamic effects with sustained treatment.[21] Tolerance is dose- and duration-dependent, usually manifesting after 24 hours, regardless of formulation. If ischemia occurs during continuous nitrate therapy, responsiveness to the anti-ischemic effects of the nitrate can usually be restored by increasing the dose. Although the mechanism of tolerance is not completely understood, continuous exposure to nitrates appears to cause a change in the vasculature that limits the vasodilatory effects. There are several major theories proposed to explain nitrate tolerance.[22–26] First, there is evidence that a depletion of sulfhydryl groups occurs with prolonged exposure, which limits the production of NO. Second, nitrate exposure can result in a neurohumoral activation and a reflex release of vasoactive compounds such as renin, catecholamines, and endothelin, which could counteract the vasodilatory effects of the nitrates. Third, plasma expansion consistently occurs with nitrate administration, which could blunt the beneficial effects on ventricular preload. A drug-free interval of 14 hours is recommended to reverse nitrate tolerance.[21] However, intermittent nitroglycerin therapy has been shown to result in rebound myocardial ischemia during the drug-free interval. Moreover, a reduction in exercise tolerance during nitroglycerin withdrawal has been demonstrated.[27–29] Finally, a potential drug interaction may occur when intravenous nitroglycerin and heparin are administered together. There is evidence that nitroglycerin may decrease sensitivity to heparin by interfering with the binding of heparin to AT-III.[30,31] Therefore, an increased dose of heparin may be required to achieve a therapeutic endpoint in the presence of nitroglycerin, and excessive heparin-induced anticoagulation may result after withdrawal of nitroglycerin therapy during heparin infusion.

Practical Aspects of Drug Administration

Intravenous nitroglycerin is a first-line drug in the management of ACS. Long-acting oral nitrate formulations are not recommended for the treatment of acute coronary ischemic events, because intravenous administration of nitroglycerin allows for more precise control of hemodynamic profile and symptom relief. There is convincing evidence that intravenous administration of nitroglycerin can improve regional myocardial function and reduce infarct size in patients with ACS, and it might also reduce the left ventricular remodeling that can occur after a transmural infarction.[32,33] Data from randomized clinical trials also indicate that nitrates can reduce mortality in the setting of acute myocardial infarction. Nitroglycerin may be especially useful for 24 to 48 hours after acute myocardial infarction in patients with congestive heart failure, hypertension, or recurrent ischemia. Intravenous nitroglycerin should be initiated at $0.25\,\mu g/kg$ per minute and increased in $0.25\,\mu g/kg$ per minute increments every 3 to 5 minutes until either ischemic signs and symptoms are resolved or hypotension ensues, typically defined as a systolic blood pressure less 90 mm Hg or a mean arterial blood pressure less than 70 mm Hg. Because the autoregulation curve for cerebral perfusion is shifted to the right in patients with chronic hypertension, caution should be observed when blood pressure is reduced more than 30% from baseline in this population. Tolerance frequently develops with continuous intravenous nitroglycerin therapy after 24 hours; incremental increases in dosage may be necessary to continue drug efficacy and symptom control, especially in patients for whom recurrent ischemia develops. Although there is no absolute maximal dose limit, significant hypotension usually occurs at doses greater than 3 to $4\,\mu g/kg$ per minute. Tachycardia may develop in patients at

high doses of intravenous nitroglycerin, especially in hyperadrenergic patients. Combination therapy with a short-acting beta-blocker, such as esmolol, is usually efficacious and well tolerated. Nitroglycerin should be used cautiously in patients with suspected inferioposterior myocardial ischemia because the right ventricle may be involved.[34] Patients with right ventricular infarction are extremely dependent on preload and thus can become acutely hypotensive when vasodilation from nitroglycerin occurs. Invasive monitoring of blood pressure is not mandatory, but it is useful when high doses of nitroglycerin are administered or hypotension develops. Documentation of right and left ventricular filling pressures with a Swan-Ganz catheter is also recommended if there is uncertainty about the adequacy of preload during nitroglycerin administration.

β Adrenergic Receptor Antagonists

Mechanism of Action and Preclinical Pharmacology

The majority of β adrenergic receptor antagonists are competitive antagonists. Considerations used to select the appropriate β adrenergic receptor antagonists include receptor subtype selectivity, bioavailability, half-life, lipid solubility, route of clearance, membrane stabilizing effects, intended indication (e.g., angina, postinfarction, or hypertension), and intrinsic sympathetic activity.

β_1 Receptors account for approximately 75% of all the β receptors in the heart; the β_2 ($\geq 20\%$) and β_3 receptors ($<5\%$) comprise the balance. These receptors are G protein–coupled receptors and are found throughout the myocardium and nodal conduction tissue.[35] The structure and signal transduction pathways of the various β adrenergic receptor subtypes are discussed in detail in Chapter 34. Briefly, agonist (norepinephrine, epinephrine) occupancy of the β adrenergic receptor stimulates the G protein, G_S, which in turn activates adenylate cyclase to produce cyclic adenosine monophosphate (cAMP). cAMP activates protein kinase A, which phosphorylates a variety of protein targets in the myocardium, including L-type voltage-dependent calcium channels, troponin C, and other proteins involved in intracellular calcium homeostasis. The net effect of β adrenergic stimulation of the heart is to produce positive chronotropic, inotropic, and lusitropic effects. (See Chapter 37 for a more detailed discussion of the mechanisms of β adrenergic inotropic and lusitropic effects). Thus the actions of β-adrenergic receptor antagonists is to prevent the positive chronotropic, inotropic, and lusitropic effects of endogenous catecholamines. In pathologic states (prolonged ischemia or heart failure), alterations in β adrenergic receptor function and number can occur. In heart failure and with prolonged ischemic conditions, pathologic changes in β adrenergic function may include a decrease in receptor number or ratio (less β_1, more β_2 and β_3), uncoupling of the receptor from its respective G protein, and an alteration of cell signaling.[36–42] Similarly, changes in β adrenergic receptor number and function can be observed after cardiopulmonary bypass.[43]

Clinical Pharmacology

The first beta-blocker used for the treatment of angina in the United States was propranolol. From the introduction of propranolol and then subsequent release of other beta-blockers, the efficacy of beta adrenergic receptor blockade in attenuating morbidity and mortality rates in the treatment of patients with ACS has been demonstrated in countless clinical trials.[1,44–52] Beta-blockers are efficacious in reducing anginal symptoms in the setting of stable and unstable angina with or without other antianginal drugs.[53] In addition, beta-blockers are efficacious in preventing of ischemic events whether in the setting of silent monitoring, unstable coronary syndrome, chronic management of ischemic heart disease, or in provoked ischemia with exercise (Fig. 36–1). Not surprisingly, the best results are often obtained when beta-blockers are combined with nitrates or other antianginal treatments.[55–58] Although less information is available on the initiation of beta-blockers for acute myocardial ischemia in the intraoperative setting, it has been established that patients with unstable coronary syndrome on beta-blocker therapy should have their medications continued throughout the operative period if clinically tolerated. One representative study supporting this strategy enrolled 444 patients undergoing coronary artery bypass surgery.[59] Patients receiving beta-blockers had less intraoperative ischemia (39% vs. 53%), and this protective ischemic effect was enhanced in patients with tachycardia (defined as heart rate > 109 beats per minute). Presumably, these authors would advocate that beta-blockers should be considered as a first-line therapy by anesthesiologists (*vide infra*) in the treatment and prevention of myocardial ischemia in the perioperative setting. As discussed in Chapter 38, beta-blockers have also been shown to reduce mortality when administered prophylactically to patients undergoing major vascular surgery who are at high risk for ischemia.[60]

The major rationale for the use of beta-blockers in patients with ACS is the attenuation of myocardial oxygen demand through β adrenergic receptor antagonism. β Adrenergic receptor antagonism alters myocardial function by a reduction in heart rate, a decrement in contractility, a decrease in afterload, and an increase in diastolic perfusion.[10,61] The preponderance of evidence also suggests that β adrenergic receptor blockade increases the relative ratio of blood flow in ischemic and borderline zones.[62] Additional mechanisms of β adrenergic receptor blockade altering the cardiovascular milieu include a reduction in renin and angiotensin II, and an alteration of central adrenergic and baroceptor signaling. Further reputed mechanisms may include an increase in prostacyclin synthesis, a decrease in apoptosis, improved myocardial energetics, and a reduction in oxidative stress. Although β receptor antagonists clearly alter long-term mortality, β-adrenergic receptor blockade should be initiated with caution in the perioperative setting to avoid adverse effects such as bronchoconstriction, myocardial depression, and exacerbation of atrioventricular nodal blockade. For this reason, the drugs must be used judiciously in patients with severe obstructive pulmonary disease, bradycardia (<55 beats per minute), heart block, or uncompensated congestive heart failure. With these exceptions, recent studies have shown that high-risk patients do benefit from the use of beta-blockers during the perioperative period.[63–65] If there is a relative contraindication for the use of beta-blockers in a patient with ACS, a trial of intravenous esmolol ($t_{1/2}$ of 7 to 8 minutes) may be attempted with minimal risk to the patient.

Beta-blockers belong to two general classifications based on whether they are selective β_1 antagonists or combined β_1 and β_2 antagonists. The β_1 antagonists are "cardioselective" because they predominantly block the receptors in the heart and have little effect on the β_2 receptors of the bronchial musculature and the arterioles and veins.[44,66] The nonselective beta-blockers are antagonists of both β_1 and β_2 receptors. Table 36–1 lists the beta-blockers according to their receptor subtype selectivity. There are two primary differences between the cardioselective and nonselective drugs: (1) cardioselective drugs are better suited for use in patients with asthma and bronchospastic disease, and (2) cardioselective blockers are theoretically better suited in patients with hypertension (no inhibition of peripheral vessel β_2 receptors that mediate vasodilation). With increasing doses of the cardioselective drugs, there is a decrease in receptor specificity. Conversely, nonselective beta-blockers would be the preferred drug for thyrotoxicosis, pheochromocytoma, or catecholamine storm.

The major difference in pharmacokinetics between beta-blockers is their elimination half-life (Table 36–2). Esmolol has a short elimination half-life (10 minutes), whereas the other drugs have much longer half-lives (hours). Thus if a short-lived response is required, esmolol is clearly the preferred drug. Of course, esmolol must be given by continuous infusion if β-blockade is required for a prolonged period. Because many patients about to have surgery are taking beta-blockers, one should be aware of the half-life of

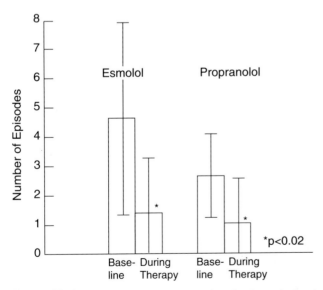

Figure 36–1. Incidents of number of episodes of chest pain ± standard deviation during a 24-hour baseline period compared with the subsequent study period. A significant reduction in chest pain ($p < 0.02$) was seen in both groups. (From Wallis DE, Pope C, Littman WJ, Scanlon PJ: Safety and efficacy of esmolol for unstable angina pectoris. Am J Cardiol 62:1033–1037, 1988.)

TABLE 36–1.

Properties of Beta-Blockers in Clinical Use

	Drug	Selectivity	Partial Agonist Activity	Oral Dose	Intravenous Dose
1	Propranolol	None	No	20–80 mg twice daily	1–10 mg
2	Metoprolol	β_1	No	12.5–100 mg twice daily (total dose usually does not exceed 200 mg/day)	1–15 mg
3	Atenolol	β_1	No	50–200 mg/day	5–10 mg
4	Nadolol	None	No	20–80 mg/day	
5	Timolol	None	No	10 mg twice daily	0.4–1 mg
6	Acebutolol	β_1	Yes	200–600 mg twice daily	12.5–50 mg
7	Betaxolol	β	No	5–20 mg/day	
8	Bisoprolol	β	No	2.5–20 mg/day	
9	Esmolol (intravenous)	β_1	No		50–300 mg/kg/min
10	Labetalol*	None	Yes	100–1200 mg twice daily	20–300 mg 0.5–2 mg/min (titrating up slow push)
11	Pindolol	None	Yes	5–60 mg twice daily	0.4–2.0 mg
12	Carvedilol	None	No	3.125–25 mg twice daily	

*Labetalol is a combined alpha- and beta-blocker.
Data from Drayer D: Lipophilicity, hydrophilicity, and the central nervous system: Side effects of beta blockers. Pharmacotherapy 7:87–91, 1987; McDevitt DG: Comparison of pharmacokinetic properties of beta-adrenoceptor blocking drugs. Eur Heart J 8:9–14, 1987.

TABLE 36–2.

Pharmacokinetic Characteristics of Commonly Used Beta-Blockers

Drug	Trade Name	Relative Potency	Elimination	Elimination Half-life	Therapeutic Level	Protein Binding	Lipid Solubility
Atenolol	Tenormin	1	Renal	6–9 hr	0.2–2 mg/mL	Low	Low
Esmolol	Brevibloc	<0.1	Blood	10 min	—	—	—
Metoprolol	Lopressor	1	Liver	3–4 hr	50–100 mg/mL	Low	Moderate
Propranolol	Inderal	1	Liver	4–6 hr	50–100 mg/mL	High	High
Timolol	Blocadren	6	Renal and liver	4–5 hr	5–10 mg/mL	Low	Low

the beta-blocker administered before surgery. This has clinical implications regarding redosing or conversion to another beta-blocker.

Of the commonly used drugs listed in Table 36–2, only propranolol is highly protein bound. Therefore, the acute response to propranolol may be slightly reduced compared with other beta-blockers. The volume of distribution for all of the beta-blockers is high and generally exceeds the physiologic body space.[44] Thus a drug given intravenously will be rapidly and widely distributed.

Beta-blockers are eliminated by several metabolic pathways. Esmolol is biotransformed in the blood by esterases, propranolol and metoprolol are metabolized by the liver, atenolol is excreted by the kidney, and timolol is eliminated by the kidney and the liver. The metabolism and route of excretion is important when considering patients with renal or hepatic disease. The therapeutic plasma level varies greatly among drugs and between patients (interpatient variability). The reasons given for the marked interpatient variability are: (1) underlying sympathetic tone varies between patients; (2) many beta-blockers have "flat" dose-response curves, therefore changes in plasma level make small differences in response; (3) active metabolites could influence the responses; and (4) genomic β receptor polymorphisms could affect how a given patient responds to a given drug or dose.

The oral and intravenous dose ranges of the beta-blockers are listed in Table 36–1. For initiation of parenteral beta-blockade in patients who are not already receiving beta-blockers, an initial loading dose is required and will probably require a repeat lesser dose within 30 minutes to 2 hours. When administering beta-blockers intravenously, the effect is relatively rapid, and with most drugs the peak onset would be expected within about 10 minutes, possibly longer with the less lipid-soluble drugs, with an onset of about 40 minutes.[53] Esmolol has a more rapid (about 1 minute) onset and a much more rapid offset (about 10 minutes). Titration with repeated dose to the desired heart rate is the most appropriate method of dosing with beta-blockers. An additional consideration in choosing the dose of a beta-blocker is the level of sympathetic tone. With significant endogenous catecholamines, greater doses of beta-blockers are required because these drugs are competitive antagonists at the beta-adrenergic receptor. Overdose of a beta-blocker can be counteracted with either a β-agonist such as dopamine or isoproterenol or with glucagon (which stimulates adenylyl cyclase independent of the β adrenergic receptor). In the setting of acute ischemia, glucagon or dopamine is the preferred agent.

Practical Aspects of Drug Administration

The intent in this section is to discuss the intravenous use of beta-blockers to prevent myocardial infarction by either the prevention of myocardial ischemia or the treatment of it when it occurs. Unfortunately, in contrast to the many outcome studies of the use beta-blockers in patients with ischemic heart disease, there are no large-scale properly powered clinical trials that give evidence for all of the recommendations made in this chapter. As mentioned earlier,

there is evidence that patients presenting for coronary artery bypass graft surgery (and presumably any surgery) with ischemic heart disease have less myocardial ischemia when they are either kept on their beta-blocker regimen or are given beta-blockers during surgery.[59,60] Thus the first recommendation is to *continue beta-blockers during the perioperative period* in all patients taking them for coronary artery disease. If patients cannot be given oral medications during the perioperative period, then one of the longer acting drugs like atenolol (5 mg) or metoprolol (5 mg) should be given intravenously to maintain a heart rate in the desired range. This prophylactic use of beta-blockers should result in less perioperative myocardial ischemia and infarction. The second recommendation is that *patients at high risk for myocardial ischemia presenting for major surgery should be administered beta-blockers before surgery and should continue receiving these agents throughout the perioperative period.*

When myocardial ischemia does occur, as evident from the electrocardiographic display or new onset regional wall motion abnormalities on the echocardiogram, the anesthesiologist must determine what treatment is indicated. If there is no contraindication such as severe bronchospastic disease, shock, or severe ventricular dysfunction, *beta-blockers are indicated to treat the myocardial ischemia*. The anesthesiologist is well advised to select a familiar drug from among a list that includes esmolol (1–1.5 mg/kg bolus followed by infusion of 50–300 μg/kg/min), metoprolol (5 mg), atenolol (5–10 mg), or propranolol (1–10 mg). All drugs should be administered intravenously and titrated to the desired heart rate (50–65 beats per minute) to attenuate ischemia. Often the beta-blocker will be given with nitroglycerin. The advantage of esmolol is that it can be titrated to the desired heart rate with greater ease than the other drugs. The perioperative use of esmolol has been more widely reported than other beta-blockers, probably because of its unique suitability for titration during the many stresses of surgery and the perioperative period.[67,68] When used intraoperatively and then stopped, there is a rapid (15 minute) return to the non-β-blocked condition.[69] Esmolol has been safely and effectively used to treat myocardial ischemia that occurs during surgery, but esmolol has not been definitively shown to prevent myocardial infarction or death.[70,71] When myocardial ischemia is detected, the first action is to increase the depth of anesthesia with inhalation anesthetics. Thereafter, use of nitroglycerin, beta-blockers, and morphine are suggested to decrease ischemic burden and to improve myocardial oxygen consumption.

Calcium Channel Blockers

Preclinical Science

Calcium channel blockers (also referred to as *calcium antagonists*) bind to specific drug receptors on voltage-gated calcium channels in a voltage-dependent manner. Binding of the calcium channel blockers maintains the channels in an inactive state, thus reducing the probability that the channels will open. The resultant attenuation of calcium influx produces a marked reduction in intracellular calcium, and decreases phase II electrical conduction and myocyte contractility.[72,73] Voltage-gated calcium channels have been classified on the basis of their voltage sensitivity, their conductance, and their primary amino acid sequence. The three most thoroughly described channels are the L, N, and T subtypes (others include P/Q and R). All of the commercially available calcium channel blockers are targeted toward the L-type channel, which is the predominant type of channel in heart and vascular smooth muscle.

The L-type calcium channel is a multisubunit protein composed of five subunits: α_1, α_2, β, γ, δ. The α_1-subunit contains the calcium pore, the voltage sensor, and the binding sites for the three major classes of calcium channel blockers. This α_1-subunit can be subdivided into four discrete homologous domains, each composed of six transmembrane segments labeled S1-S6 (see Chapter 3 for a more detailed discussion). The activity of L-type calcium channels is heavily regulated by protein phosphorylation. Protein kinase A is a particularly important regulator of channel activity. Increases in intracellular cAMP activate protein kinase A, which in turn phosphorylates sites in the carboxy terminus of the α_1-subunit; this renders the channel available for activation. Thus agents that increase cAMP, such as the β adrenergic agonists, can enhance the activity of L-type calcium channels and increase inotropy in the heart or vasoconstriction in vascular smooth muscle.

There are three major classes of calcium channel blockers: the dihydropyridines, the phenylalkylamines, and the benzothiazepines. Each class of calcium channel blocker binds to a unique site on the α_1-subunit of the L-type calcium channel and thus diminishes calcium entry into the cells.[74–76] The dihydropyridine (e.g., nifedipine and amlodipine) binding site is on the outer portion of the S5 and S6 segments on domains III and IV of the α_1-subunit.[77] Verapamil (phenylalkylamine) binds to the S6 subunit of the fourth domain of α_1, whereas diltiazem (benzothiazepine) binds to the cytoplasmic bridge on α_1 between domains III and IV (S6).

Clinical Pharmacology

Calcium channel blockers represent a structurally diverse group of compounds that selectively interfere with inward calcium movement through slow (L-type) calcium channels. Calcium flux through the L-type calcium channels is responsible for phase 2 of the cardiac action potential, which is important in excitation/contraction coupling in cardiac and vascular smooth muscle, and depolarization in sinoatrial and atrioventricular nodal tissue.[78–80] Thus blockade of slow calcium channels by calcium antagonists should result in decreased heart rate, a reduction in myocardial contractile function, a decreased rate of conduction through the atrioventricular node, and vascular smooth muscle relaxation.[80] However, the profile of pharmacologic effects (e.g., vascular vs. cardiac) of the various calcium channel blockers differs among the compounds. The various calcium antagonists thus vary in their potential as anti-ischemic agents and their usefulness in ACS.

The clinically relevant calcium channel blockers that have been used for the treatment of ACS in the past include: verapamil, diltiazem, nifedipine, and the long-acting agent, amlodipine. Verapamil can be administered by oral and intravenous routes. Extensive first-pass metabolism by the liver after oral administration results in a bioavailability of only 10% to 20%, such that the oral adult dose (80–120 mg TID or QID) is approximately 10-fold greater than the intravenous dose (0.075–0.15 mg/kg) to achieve a therapeutic plasma concentration of 100 to 300 ng/mL.[81] Metabolism to demethylated metabolites occurs with an elimination half-life of 2 to 6 hours, with significant prolongation to greater than 13 hours in the presence of liver disease.[82] The activity of oral verapamil peaks in 30 to 45 minutes, compared with only 15 minutes after intravenous administration. Although clinical activity after an intravenous bolus begins within 2 to 3 minutes, the duration of action can approach 6 hours. Because verapamil is highly protein bound (90%), the clinical effect can be enhanced by drugs such as lidocaine or diazepam, which increase the pharmacologically active unbound fraction.

Diltiazem can also be administered by either oral or intravenous routes.[79,83] Oral absorption is excellent with an onset of action within 15 minutes and a peak effect within 30 minutes. Elimination half-life is 4 to 6 hours with 60% metabolism by the liver and the remainder by the kidneys.[83] The adult oral dose of diltiazem is 30 to 90 mg, TID or QID, and the intravenous dose is 0.25 to 0.35 mg/kg; an infusion of 0.15 mg/kg per hour can be initiated for prolonged effect. As with verapamil, liver disease may necessitate a reduced dosing regimen.

Nifedipine can only be administered by the oral route.[79,80] Oral administration (10–30 mg TID or QID) has an onset of action within 20 minutes, with a peak effect in 1 to 1.5 hours. Nifedipine is also available in an extended release formulation, which can be administered once daily (30–60 mg); onset of action, however, is approximately 6 hours. Elimination half-life of nifedipine is 3 to 7 hours, with a predominance of hepatic metabolism to inactive metabolites. Like verapamil, protein binding is high (>90%), and thus the unbound active fraction can be significantly altered. Amlodipine is only available for oral administration in the United States. The typical adult dose is 5 to 10 mg daily, with a time-to-peak plasma level of 6 to 12 hours; steady-state plasma drug concentration is achieved after 5 to 7 days.[84] Elimination half-life is 30 to 40 hours, with 90% hepatic conversion to inactive metabolites, and 10% is excreted unchanged in the urine.[85,86] Nicardipine is the only dihydropyridine available for parenteral administration. It is available in 25-mg ampules and must be diluted to 0.1 mg/mL for infusion. The starting rate for infusion is 5.0 mg/hr with a maximum recommended dose of 15 mg/hr. Because nicardipine has a long terminal elimination half-life (14 hours), steady-state infusion rates are not achieved for 1 to 2 days. Nicardipine is metabolized in the liver and is highly protein bound ($\approx$95%).

The calcium channel blockers cause a number of physiologic changes that could impact on the progression and severity of the ACS. Total coronary blood flow increases after treatment with calcium antagonists because of coronary artery dilation.[87–89] The calcium channel blockers also improve collateral coronary flow distal to obstructive lesions, dilate coronary stenotic areas, and improve subendocardial flow relative to subepicardial flow.[90,91] Platelet aggregation is inhibited by calcium antagonists, which appears to be caused by an effect on internal redistribution of calcium.[92] An inhibition of myocardial contractile function and afterload reduction from peripheral arterial vasodilation occurs with the calcium antagonists, contributing to a reduction in myocardial oxygen demand.[79,80,85,86,93] The reduction in contractile function is most apparent with verapamil and may be exaggerated in patients with pre-existing ventricular dysfunction. Diltiazem also possesses a negative inotropic influence; cardiac output and stroke volume, however, may not change in patients with normal contractile function because of the concurrent peripheral vasodilation. Although diltiazem is less likely to enhance congestive heart failure compared with verapamil, caution should be exercised when administering this agent to patients with aortic stenosis, pre-existing left ventricular failure, or patients receiving β_1 adrenergic antagonist therapy. Nifedipine and amlodipine are the most potent arterial dilators with minimal negative inotropic and chronotropic effects. Reflex activation of the sympathetic nervous system after nifedipine administration may, however, cause increases in heart rate and cardiac output with an overall reduction in systemic blood pressure. Finally there are both clinical and animal model studies that suggest that chronic treatment with calcium channel blockers may retard the progression of atherosclerotic disease.[94,95] Verapamil and nifedipine have been demonstrated to slow coronary artery atherosclerosis in humans, whereas diltiazem appears to decrease the formation of coronary disease after heart transplantation.

Use of calcium channel blockers may result in a number of adverse effects and potentially harmful drug interactions. Verapamil and diltiazem have depressant effects on the generation of the action potential at the sinoatrial node and slow antegrade movement of the cardiac impulse through the atrioventricular node.[79,96,97] Thus patients with pre-existing abnormalities in cardiac conduction may experience greater degrees of conduction blockade after the administration of verapamil and diltiazem. There are also reports of various degrees of atrioventricular heart block with concurrent administration of verapamil and a β_1 adrenergic antagonist or digoxin. As previously discussed, calcium antagonists are vasodilators and can depress myocardial contractile function, although amlodipine appears to have minimal effect on contractility. Therefore, it may be prudent to initiate therapy with reduced doses of calcium antagonists in patients with left ventricular dysfunction or hypovolemia. Furthermore, reduction in blood pressure from the administration of volatile anesthetics can be potentiated by concurrent administration of calcium channel blockers.[98] The effects of depolarizing and nondepolarizing neuromuscular blocking drugs are exaggerated by calcium antagonists, and antagonism of a nondepolarizing neuromuscular blockade may be blunted in the presence of calcium channel blockade.[99,100] The mechanism for potentiation of neuromuscular blockade by calcium channel antagonism may involve diminished presynaptic release of acetylcholine, because calcium is essential for the release of acetylcholine at the neuromuscular junction. Edrophonium may be more effective than neostigmine in reversing neuromuscular blockade that has been potenti-

ated by calcium channel blockers.[101] Verapamil and diltiazem have significant local anesthetic activity, as shown by the capacity to block fast sodium channels, and therefore the risk for local anesthetic toxicity may be increased in patients taking these calcium antagonists when a regional block is performed.[102] Cimetidine and ranitidine increase the plasma level of calcium channel blockers, presumably by either alterations in hepatic enzyme activity or hepatic blood flow. Overdose with calcium channel blockers can be partially reversed with intravenous calcium or dopamine.

Practical Aspects of Drug Administration

The use of calcium channel blockers in ACS is controversial. Nifedipine does not appear to have a role in the treatment of patients with coronary disease. Nifedipine does not decrease the incidence of mortality or reinfarction in patients with ACS, irrespective of sex, coronary artery involvement, or comorbid conditions, and it may have a deleterious effect on patient outcomes.[103–109] The pronounced arterial dilation provided by immediate-release nifedipine may be detrimental by causing a decrease in coronary perfusion pressure and reflex activation of the sympathetic nervous system, resulting in worsening myocardial oxygen demand and "steal" from ischemic areas. In contrast, verapamil and diltiazem may have some limited usefulness in the treatment of ACS in certain subpopulations of patients. Both verapamil and diltiazem may be considered with caution after implementation of nitrates, beta-blockers, morphine, and anticoagulation, if clinically indicated. As previously mentioned, patients with refractory tachycardia, contraindication to beta-blockers, or non Q-wave myocardial infarctions with normal liver function may all cautiously be considered for therapy with calcium channel blockers.[110–112]

Intravenous administration of verapamil or diltiazem makes these drugs useful for treatment of acute myocardial ischemia in the perioperative setting.[113–115] The anesthesiologist should remember that calcium channel blockers have not been shown to offer any advantage over beta-blockers in the management of ACS. In fact, studies suggest that administration of verapamil or diltiazem may have a negative impact on mortality rates in patients with ACS and associated left ventricular dysfunction, congestive heart failure, or bradyarrhythmias.[111,113,116–118] Conversely, the longer acting amlodipine is well tolerated and has been shown to provide comparable anti-ischemic effects in patients with ACS as beta-blockers with no increase in mortality rates.[119–124] Moreover, the combination of amlodipine and beta-blockade may be more effective in the treatment of myocardial ischemia than either drug alone. Amlodipine also improves clinical outcome after angioplasty and results in fewer hospitalizations for unstable angina or coronary revascularization.[123,124] However, oral formulation and slow onset limits usefulness in acute coronary episodes. There are no data examining the efficacy of intravenous nicardipine in improving patient outcomes for ACS. There is a single study comparing the efficacy of continuous infusions of nicardipine and nitroglycerin at reducing electrocardiographic evidence of ischemia during coronary artery bypass surgery. This study showed that nicardipine was more effective than either nitroglycerin or no treatment, but the study was modest in size and requires confirmation.[125]

In summary, there is no direct evidence for any beneficial effect of nifedipine in ACS; such therapy may increase the risk for morbidity and mortality. Diltiazem and verapamil may result in beneficial effects in small populations of patients. Because efficacy over beta-blockade has not been demonstrated, these calcium channel blockers should be reserved for treatment failure or intolerance to other drugs discussed in this chapter. They, therefore, appear appropriate only as alternate choices after the initiation of nitrates and beta-blockers when needed for refractory symptom control or in the management of ACS when beta-blockers cannot be used.[1,52] Although amlodipine may be efficacious and well tolerated for chronic management of myocardial ischemia, any role for treatment of ACS in the perioperative setting is limited by the requirement for oral administration and the extremely slow onset of clinical effects.

Anticoagulation Drugs

Patients with ACS may present to the operating room for coronary artery bypass or vascular surgery after treatment with an array of drugs that either interfere with the coagulation process or eliminate pre-existing thrombus in the coronary arteries. Such drugs can result in a number of problems in the perioperative period that complicate patient management. Urgent surgery may not allow adequate time for interventions to minimize adverse effects of these drugs. Therefore the anesthesiologist must understand both the potential adverse effects of drugs that alter coagulation and how to manage them in the perioperative period. The following section is a brief overview that is specifically pertinent to the anesthesiologist in the operating room (see Chapter 53 for a more detailed discussion).

Antiplatelet Drugs

Antiplatelet drugs are widely used in patients with acute myocardial ischemia. The four major subdivisions of antiplatelet drugs are: cyclo-oxygenase inhibitors, adenosine diphosphate (ADP) receptor antagonists, thrombin inhibitors, and platelet glycoprotein receptor (IIb/IIIa or $gp\alpha_{IIb}\beta_3$) inhibitors.

Aspirin is the most widely used antiplatelet drug. Average bleeding time is prolonged because of inhibition of platelet cyclo-oxygenase, thereby inhibiting platelet aggregation. Aspirin permanently acetylates platelets and inhibits thromboxane synthesis and platelet aggregation by ADP and collagen. Hence megakaryocytes must produce new platelets before the full effect of a single dose of aspirin (325 mg) is reversed. It is unusual for aspirin to cause generalized bleeding unless there are other predisposing features for a coagulopathy, such as uremia or other anticoagulant therapy.[126] Hence it is ideal to discontinue aspirin for 7 to 10 days (the

lifetime of a usual platelet) before surgery to minimize adverse platelet effects. In the event of acute perioperative ischemia, aspirin (162–325 mg) should be considered as part of a primary treatment strategy.

Clopidogrel (Plavix; Bristol-Myers Squibb, Princeton, NJ.) inhibits platelet aggregation by irreversible, noncompetitive antagonism of the ADP receptor.[127] Concurrent use of aspirin results in a synergistic inhibition of platelet function.[128] Although clopidogrel has beneficial effects in patients with ACS caused by inhibition of ADP-induced platelet aggregation, the risk for major bleeding, incidence of re-exploration for bleeding, and blood product requirement after coronary artery bypass surgery is increased.[129] These concerns are particularly germane to the anesthesiologist, because cardiologists frequently administer 75 to 300 mg clopidogrel at the time of percutaneous interventions. Because recovery of platelet function after clopidogrel administration requires 3 to 5 days, therapy should be stopped as soon as possible before surgery, but this is often not feasible.[130] The mainstay of treatment for hemorrhage secondary to complications with aspirin or ADP antagonists is platelet transfusion, and this has been recommended for patients with a bleeding diathesis in the perioperative period, even with a normal platelet count.

Three of the most common intravenous platelet IIb/IIIa inhibitors used in patients with ACS include the monoclonal antibody abciximab (ReoPro; Eli Lilly, Indianapolis, Ind.) and the small molecular inhibitors eptifibatide (Integrilin; Millennium Pharmaceuticals, Cambridge, Mass.) and tirofiban (Aggrastat; Merck, Whitehouse Station, NJ.).[131,132] Blockade of glycoprotein IIb/IIIa receptors on platelets does not allow for normal binding of fibrinogen and cross-bridging of platelets, preventing platelet activation, platelet aggregation, and formation of platelet thrombi.[132] Unlike the ADP antagonists and aspirin, the IIb/IIIa inhibitors block the final common pathway between platelet aggregation and coagulation factor activation. This direct receptor antagonism blocks platelet aggregation by excluding fibrinogen, and markedly attenuates thrombus propagation. Although eptifibatide and tirofiban have short circulating half-lives of 2 to 4 hours, the binding of abciximab to platelets has a much longer duration.[133] Increased risk for hemorrhage is present in patients when surgery is performed within 12 hours of discontinuation of abciximab.[134,135] In contrast, patients treated with the shorter acting glycoprotein IIb/IIIa inhibitors (eptifibatide, tirofiban) do not experience increased bleeding with immediate coronary artery bypass surgery. In patients treated with abciximab, platelet transfusions after cardiopulmonary bypass may be helpful in reducing serious hemorrhagic complications. Moreover, a reduction in heparin dosage (150–200 U/kg) may adequately maintain activated clotting time in the therapeutic range (>400 seconds) and reduce the potential for excessive bleeding. The use of a hemoconcentrator during cardiopulmonary bypass may reduce plasma levels of abciximab and allow transfused platelets to remain fully functional.[136] Aprotinin has been shown to be efficacious in reducing bleeding after cardiopulmonary bypass and may prove useful in controlling blood loss in patients presenting for surgery who are taking antiplatelet drugs.[137] Finally, recombinant activated factor VIIa has been reported to reduce blood loss in patients undergoing cardiac surgery and may have a role in improving hemostasis after antiplatelet drug therapy.[138] Although the antiplatelet drugs are not routinely used to treat ACS in the perioperative setting, anesthesiologists should feel comfortable with this class of drugs because they will frequently encounter patients on various kinds of antiplatelet therapy.

Antithrombin Drugs

Patients with ACS may also present to the operating room on antithrombin drugs. Heparin is commonly used preoperatively in patients with unstable angina. Heparin is a mucopolysaccharide polymer, which potentiates the affinity of antithrombin III for thrombin. When the antithrombin III-thrombin complex is formed, it decreases the ability of thrombin to form a functional clot. Unfractionated heparin is very heterogeneous with only 20% of the sugar being biologically active. Chronic heparin treatment can result in heparin resistance, which is usually a consequence of antithrombin-III (AT-III) deficiency or immune-mediated heparin antibodies.[139] Preparations of purified AT-III are available for intravenous use and can improve the anticoagulant activity of heparin and may also result in reduced bleeding after surgery.[140] Fresh-frozen plasma can also be given if commercial preparations of AT-III are not available. Thrombocytopenia can occur with chronic heparin therapy. There are two major forms of heparin-induced thrombocytopenia: type I, which represents a benign, nonimmune reduction in platelet count with limited clinical sequelae; and type II, which is an immune-mediated thrombocytopenia with significant morbidity and paradoxic thromboembolic complications.[141] Diagnosis of type II is by history with laboratory confirmation by the heparin-induced platelet aggregation test or the C-serotonin release assay.[141] Prompt discontinuation of heparin is required. Hirudin (a direct thrombin inhibitor) or danaparoid can be used in patients who require continued anticoagulation or extracorporeal circulation for surgery.[142,143] These drugs, however, have long half-lives and have increased bleeding complications. The reversal of heparin is accomplished by protamine, a basic polypeptide isolated from salmon sperm. A broad spectrum of adverse reactions can occur with protamine, including life-threatening anaphylactic reactions.[144]

An increasing number of patients with acute coronary events are receiving low molecular weight heparin (LMWH) as part of a therapeutic regimen. As with heparin, the anticoagulant action of LMWH is caused by AT-III activation. In fact, many cardiologists are advocating LMWH as the antithrombin drug of choice with ACS. LMWH is produced by depolymerizing unfractionated heparin to yield a uniform heparin molecule of approximately 4000 to 6000kD. The inactivation of thrombin is not as severe, resulting in an increase ratio of factor XA/thrombin inhibition.[145] Other than bleeding, adverse effects of LMWH include increase of liver transaminases and the rare development of heparin-induced thrombocytopenia (significantly lower percentage than with unfractionated heparin).[146] The use of LWMH is gaining popularity because of a long half-life, ease of dosing, and the lack of need for laboratory monitoring.

However, common coagulation tests are not affected by LMWH, and protamine does not effectively reverse its effects, which may complicate subsequent surgery. As opposed to heparin and LMWH, hirudin (and its similar analogs) is a specific, direct, and irreversible inhibitor of thrombin derived from leach saliva. Hirudin does not require AT-III or other cofactors to produce its inhibition. Hirudin therapy can be followed with traditional partial thromboplastin times.

Finally, long-term anticoagulation is often accomplished with warfarin, which inhibits vitamin K epoxide reductase and vitamin K reductase. This impairs vitamin K regeneration and inactivates clotting factors II, VII, IX, and X, prolonging the prothrombin time.[147–149] Patients presenting for surgery taking warfarin with an elevated international normalized ratio greater than 4 are at risk for excessive bleeding. If surgery is not urgent, low-dose oral vitamin K safely and reliably reverses the excessive anticoagulation within 24 hours.[148] For emergent surgery, patients should be treated with vitamin K intravenously (1 mg) or subcutaneously (1–10 mg). Fresh-frozen plasma administration should also be considered in actively bleeding patients.

Thrombolytic Drugs

The thrombolytic agents streptokinase, alteplase, and reteplase are frequently used for patients with ACS because of their well-documented reduction in overall mortality rates and improved success rate for establishing patency of coronary conduits when administered before coronary angioplasty.[150–156] In acute myocardial infarction, thrombolytic drugs are used primarily to cause lysis of fibrin within thrombus in the coronary circulation by activation of the proteolytic enzyme plasminogen. The circulating, unbound activated plasmin can also degrade fibrinogen and factors V and VIII, resulting in various degrees of systemic fibrinolysis. Streptokinase is not fibrin-specific, binding to both bound and unbound plasminogen, creating both clot lysis and a pronounced systemic fibrinolysis.[150] Alteplase and reteplase are more fibrin-specific, resulting in less systemic effects. Although the half-lives of the commonly used thrombolytic agents are relatively short, ranging from 5 minutes (alteplase) to 25 minutes (streptokinase), fibrinogen levels may not normalize for up to 48 hours. The most prominent adverse side effect associated with thrombolytic therapy is hemorrhage, especially in patients undergoing urgent surgery soon after administration. Patients with ACS who are exposed to fibrinolytic therapy and require immediate coronary artery bypass surgery are prime candidates for antifibrinolytic therapy with aprotinin, epsilon-aminocaproic acid, or tranexamic acid. In addition, any fibrinolytic agent should be immediately discontinued. Bleeding during surgery may become severe, necessitating rapid volume administration. Coagulation profiles need to be established early so that fibrinogen, platelets, and fresh-frozen plasma can be immediately available. Thrombolytic agents such as streptokinase, which are derived from bacterial products, are antigenic and can cause anaphylactic shock.[157,158] Hypotension can also occur after administration of thrombolytic agents because of vasodilation from increased plasmin-induced activation of kallikrein and bradykinin. In addition, arrhythmias are not uncommon.

Conclusion

Myocardial ischemia is a common perioperative occurrence. The pharmacologic treatment and prevention of the ACS requires knowledge of the many drugs used in this setting. Many drugs are effective, and usually there is more than one drug that can be used alone or in combination with others. It is important to understand the implications of these drugs in the setting of surgery and anesthesia because there is the potential for interaction with anesthetic drugs and there are some potential untoward effects on such variables as clotting and response to surgical stress. The mechanism of anti-ischemic drugs, the clinical pharmacology, and the various indications and methods of drug delivery have been discussed. This knowledge combined with the material in the other chapters in this book is intended to improve the clinical care of the perioperative patient.

References

1. Braunwald E, et al: ACC/AHA guidelines for the management of patients with unstable angina and non-ST-segment elevation myocardial infarction. A report of the American College of Cardiology/American Heart Association Task Force on Practice Guidelines (Committee on the Management of Patients With Unstable Angina). J Am Coll Cardiol 36:970–1062, 2000.
2. Anderson HV, et al: One-year results of the Thrombolysis in Myocardial Infarction (TIMI) IIIB clinical trial. A randomized comparison of tissue-type plasminogen activator versus placebo and early invasive versus early conservative strategies in unstable angina and non-Q wave myocardial infarction. J Am Coll Cardiol 26:1643–1650, 1995.
3. Robertson R, Friesinger G: Hemodynamics in stable angina pectoris. In Julian D (ed): Angina Pectoris, 1985, pp 25–37.
4. Braunwald E: Unstable angina: An etiologic approach to management. Circulation 98:2219–2222, 1998.
5. Braunwald E: Unstable angina. A classification. Circulation 80:410–414, 1989.
6. Graves EJ: Detailed diagnoses and procedures, national hospital discharge survey, 1990. Vital & Health Statistics—Series 13: Data From the National Health Survey, 1992, pp 1–225.
7. American Heart Association: Heart and Stroke Facts and Statistics. Dallas, Tx, American Heart Association, 1992.
8. Kopecky S: Unstable angina. In Mayo Clinic Cardiology Review. Philadelphia, Lippincott Williams & Wilkins, 2000, pp 159–170.
9. Brady P: Nitrates. In Murphy JG (ed): Mayo Clinic Cardiology Review. Philadelphia, Lippincott Williams & Wilkins, 2000, pp 1227–1230.
10. Opie L: Pharmacologic options for the treatment of ischemic disease. In Smith T (ed): Cardiovascular Therapeutics, Philadelphia, WB Saunders, 1996.
11. Torfgard KE, Ahlner J: Mechanisms of action of nitrates. Cardiovasc Drugs Therapy 8:701–717, 1994.
12. Feldman RL, Pepine CJ, Conti CR: Magnitude of dilatation of large and small coronary arteries of nitroglycerin. Circulation 64:324–333, 1981.
13. Harrison DG, Bates JN: The nitrovasodilators: New ideas about old drugs. Circulation 87:1461–1467, 1993.
14. Brown BG, et al: The mechanisms of nitroglycerin action: Stenosis vasodilatation as a major component of the drug response. Circulation 64:1089–1097, 1981.
15. Goldstein RE, et al: Intraoperative coronary collateral function in patients with coronary occlusive disease. Nitroglycerin responsiveness and angiographic correlations. Circulation 49:298–308, 1974.
16. Gorman MW, Sparks HV Jr: Nitroglycerin causes vasodilatation within ischaemic myocardium. Cardiovasc Res 14:515–521, 1980.
17. Needleman P, Jakschik B, Johnson EM Jr: Sulfhydryl requirement for relaxation of vascular smooth muscle. J Pharmacol Exp Ther 187:324–331, 1973.
18. Loscalzo J: N-Acetylcysteine potentiates inhibition of platelet aggregation by nitroglycerin. J Clin Invest 76:703–708, 1985.
19. Parker JD, Parker JO: Nitrate therapy for stable angina pectoris. N Engl J Med 338:520–531, 1998.
20. Cheitlin MD, et al: ACC/AHA expert consensus document. Use of sildenafil (Viagra) in patients with cardiovascular disease. American College of Cardiology/American Heart Association. J Am Coll Cardiol 33:273–282, 1999.
21. Parker JO, et al: Tolerance to isosorbide dinitrate: Rate of development and reversal. Circulation 68:1074–1080, 1983.
22. Needleman P, Johnson EM Jr: Mechanism of tolerance development to organic nitrates. J Pharmacol Exp Ther 184:709–715, 1973.
23. Munzel T, et al: Evidence for enhanced vascular superoxide anion production in nitrate tolerance. A novel mechanism underlying tolerance and cross-tolerance. J Clin Invest 95:187–194, 1995.
24. Munzel T, et al: Evidence for a role of endothelin 1 and protein kinase C in nitroglycerin tolerance. Proc Natl Acad Sci USA 92:5244–5248, 1995.
25. Dupuis J, et al: Tolerance to intravenous nitroglycerin in patients with congestive heart failure: Role of increased intravascular volume, neurohumoral activation and lack of prevention with N-acetylcysteine. J Am Coll Cardiol 16:923–931, 1990.
26. Parker JD, et al: Effects of diuretic therapy on the development of tolerance during continuous therapy with nitroglycerin. J Am Coll Cardiol 20:616–622, 1992.
27. DeMots H, Glasser SP: Intermittent transdermal nitroglycerin therapy in the treatment of chronic stable angina. J Am Coll Cardiol 13:786–795, 1989.
28. Ferratini M, et al: Intermittent transdermal nitroglycerin monotherapy in stable exercise-induced angina: A comparison with a continuous schedule. Eur Heart J 10:998–1002, 1989.
29. Parker JD, et al: Intermittent transdermal nitroglycerin therapy. Decreased anginal threshold during the nitrate-free interval. Circulation 91:973–978, 1995.
30. Becker RC, et al: Intravenous nitroglycerin-induced heparin resistance: A qualitative antithrombin III abnormality. Am Heart J 119:1254–1261, 1990.
31. Gonzalez ER, et al: Assessment of the drug interaction between intravenous nitroglycerin and heparin. Ann Pharmacother 26:1512–1514, 1992.
32. Jugdutt BI, Warnica JW: Intravenous nitroglycerin therapy to limit myocardial infarct size, expansion, and complications. Effect of timing, dosage, and infarct location. Circulation 78:906–919, 1988.
33. Bussmann WD, et al: Reduction of CK and CK-MB indexes of infarct size by intravenous nitroglycerin. Circulation 63:615–622, 1981.
34. Kinch JW, Ryan TJ: Right ventricular infarction. N Engl J Med 330:1211–1217, 1994.
35. Murphree SS, Saffitz JE: Delineation of the distribution of beta-adrenergic receptor subtypes in canine myocardium. Circ Res 63:117–125, 1988.
36. McLeod AA, et al: Differentiation of hemodynamic, humoral and metabolic responses to beta 1- and beta 2-adrenergic stimulation in man using atenolol and propranolol. Circulation 67:1076–1084, 1983.
37. Inglese J, et al: Structure and mechanism of the G protein-coupled receptor kinases. J Biol Chem 268:23735–23738, 1993.
38. Ping P, et al: Adenylyl cyclase and G protein receptor kinase expression during development of heart failure. Am J Physiol 273:H707–717, 1997.
39. Koch WJ, et al: Cardiac function in mice overexpressing the beta-adrenergic receptor kinase or a beta ARK inhibitor. Science 268:1350–1353, 1995.
40. Neer E, Clapham D: Signal transduction through G-proteins in the cardiac myocyte. 6–11, 1992.
41. Koch WJ, et al: The binding site for the beta gamma subunits of heterotrimeric G proteins on the beta-adrenergic receptor kinase. J Biol Chem 268:8256–8260, 1993.

42. Luttrell L, Leftwitz J: The role of b-amestmis in the termination and transduction of G protein-coupled receptor signals. J Cell Sci 455–465, 2002.

43. Booth JV, et al: Acute depression of beta-adrenergic receptor signaling during cardiopulmonary bypass: Impairment of the adenylyl cyclase moiety. Anesthesiology 89:602–611, 1998.

44. Frishman W: Clinical pharmacology of the new beta-adrenergic blocking drugs. Part 1. Pharmacodynamic and pharmacokinetic properties. Am Heart J 97:663–670, 1979.

45. Frishman WH: Drug therapy: Atenolol and timolol, two new systemic beta-adrenoceptor antagonists. N Eng J Med 306:1456–1462, 1982.

46. Opie LH: Drugs and the heart. Lancet 1:693–698, 1980.

47. Tijssen JG, et al: Nifedipine and metoprolol in suspected unstable angina. Unstable angina pectoris. Eur Heart J 8:3–15, 1987.

48. Yusuf S, et al: Beta blockade during and after myocardial infarction: An overview of the randomized trials. Prog Cardiovasc Dis 27:335–371, 1985.

49. Yusuf S, Wittes J, Friedman L: Overview of results of randomized clinical trials in heart disease. I. Treatments following myocardial infarction. JAMA 260:2088–2093, 1988.

50. Mehta JL: Emerging options in the management of myocardial ischemia. Am J Cardiol 73:18A–27A, 1994.

51. Thadani U: Treatment of stable angina. Curr Opin Cardiol 14:349–358, 1999.

52. Ryan TJ, et al: 1999 update: ACC/AHA guidelines for the management of patients with acute myocardial infarction. A report of the American College of Cardiology/American Heart Association Task Force on Practice Guidelines (Committee on Management of Acute Myocardial Infarction). J Am Coll Cardiol 34:890–911, 1999.

53. Frishman WH, Teicher M: Antianginal drug therapy for silent myocardial ischemia. Med Clin N Am 72:185–196, 1988.

54. Wallis DE, et al: Safety and efficacy of esmolol for unstable angina. Am J Cardiol 62:1033–1037, 1988.

55. Dargie HJ, et al: Nifedipine and propranolol: A beneficial drug interaction. Am J Med 71:676–682, 1981.

56. Gottlieb SO, et al: Effect of the addition of propranolol to therapy with nifedipine for unstable angina pectoris: A randomized, double-blind, placebo-controlled trial. Circulation 73:331–337, 1986.

57. Packer M, et al: Hemodynamic and clinical effects of combined verapamil and propranolol therapy in angina pectoris. Am J Cardiol 50:903–912, 1982.

58. Anonymous: Early treatment of unstable angina in the coronary care unit: A randomized, double blind, placebo controlled comparison of recurrent ischaemia in patients treated with nifedipine or metoprolol or both. Report of The Holland Interuniversity Nifedipine/Metoprolol Trial (HINT) Research Group. Br Heart J 56:400–413, 1986.

59. Slogoff S, Keats AS: Does chronic treatment with calcium entry blocking drugs reduce perioperative myocardial ischemia? Anesthesiology 68:676–680, 1988.

60. Poldermans D, et al: The effect of bisoprolol on perioperative mortality and myocardial infarction in high risk patients undergoing vascular surgery. N Engl J Med 341:1789–1794, 1999.

61. Frishman WH: Multifactorial actions of beta-adrenergic blocking drugs in ischemic heart disease: current concepts. Circulation 67:I11–18, 1983.

62. Becker LC, Fortuin NJ, Pitt B: Effect of ischemia and antianginal drugs on the distribution of radioactive microspheres in the canine left ventricle. Circ Res 28:263–269, 1971.

63. Gottlieb SS, McCarter RJ, Vogel RA: Effect of beta-blockade on mortality among high-risk and low-risk patients after myocardial infarction. N Engl J Med 339:489–497, 1998.

64. Soumerai SB, et al: Adverse outcomes of underuse of beta-blockers in elderly survivors of acute myocardial infarction. JAMA 277:115–121, 1997.

65. Krumholz HM, et al: National use and effectiveness of beta-blockers for the treatment of elderly patients after acute myocardial infarction: National Cooperative Cardiovascular Project. JAMA 280:623–629, 1998.

66. Koch-Weser J: Drug therapy: Metoprolol. N Engl J Med 301:698–703, 1979.

67. Reves JG, Flezzani P: Perioperative use of esmolol. Am J Cardiol 56:57F–62F, 1985.

68. Wolman RL, Fiedler MA: Esmolol and beta-adrenergic blockade. AANA J 59:541–548, 1991.

69. Menkhaus PG, et al: Cardiovascular effects of esmolol in anesthetized humans. Anesth Analg 64:327–334, 1985.

70. Miller DR, Martineau RJ: Bolus administration of esmolol for the treatment of intraoperative myocardial ischaemia. Can J Anaesth 36:593–597, 1989.

71. Harrison L, et al: The role of an ultra short-acting adrenergic blocker (esmolol) in patients undergoing coronary artery bypass surgery. Anesthesiology 66:413–418, 1987.

72. Schwartz A: Molecular and cellular aspects of calcium channel antagonism. Am J Cardiol 70:6F–8F, 1992.

73. Kerins D, Robertson R, Robertson D: Drugs used in the treatment of myocardial ischemia. In Hardman J, Limbird L (eds): Goodman and Gilman's The Pharmacologic Basis of Therapeutics, 10th ed. New York, McGraw-Hill, 2001, pp 843–870.

74. Hulin R, et al: Tissue-specific expression of calcium channels. Trends Cardiovasc 48–53, 1993.

75. Pragnell M, et al: Calcium channel beta-subunit binds to a conserved motif in the I–II cytoplasmic linker of the alpha 1-subunit. Nature 368:67–70, 1994.

76. Taira N: Differences in cardiovascular profile among calcium antagonists. Am J Cardiol 59:24B–29B, 1987.

77. Striessnig J, Murphy BJ, Catterall WA: Dihydropyridine receptor of L-type Ca2+ channels: Identification of binding domains for [3H](+)-PN200-110 and [3H]azidopine within the alpha 1 subunit. Proc Natl Acad Sci USA 88:10769–10773, 1991.

78. Adams RJ, Schwartz A: Comparative mechanisms for contraction of cardiac and skeletal muscle. Chest 78:123–139, 1980.

79. Reves JG, et al: Calcium entry blockers: Uses and implications for anesthesiologists. Anesthesiology 57:504–518, 1982.

80. Reves JG: The relative hemodynamic effects of Ca++ entry blockers. Anesthesiology 61:3–5, 1984.

81. Somogyi A, et al: Pharmacokinetics, bioavailability and ECG response of verapamil in patients with liver cirrhosis. Br J Clin Pharmacol 12:51–60, 1981.

82. Woodcock BG, et al: Verapamil disposition in liver disease and intensive-care patients: Kinetics, clearance, and apparent blood flow relationships. Clin Pharmacol Ther 29:27–34, 1981.

83. Rovei V, et al: Pharmacokinetics and metabolism of diltiazem in man. Acta Cardiol 35:35–45, 1980.

84. Williams DM, Cubeddu LX: Amlodipine pharmacokinetics in healthy volunteers. J Clin Pharmacol 28:990–994, 1988.

85. Faulkner JK, et al: The pharmacokinetics of amlodipine in healthy volunteers after single intravenous and oral doses and after 14 repeated oral doses given once daily. Br J Clin Pharmacol 22:21–25, 1986.

86. van Zwieten PA: Clinical pharmacology of calcium antagonists as antihypertensive and anti-anginal drugs. J Hypertens Suppl 14:S3–9, 1996.

87. Larsson-Backstrom C, Arrhenius E, Sagge K: Comparison of the calcium-antagonistic effects of terodiline, nifedipine and verapamil. Acta Pharmacol Toxicol 57:8–17, 1985.

88. Brown BG, Bolson EL, Dodge HT: Dynamic mechanisms in human coronary stenosis. Circulation 70:917–922, 1984.

89. Sato M, et al: Inhibitory effect of a calcium antagonist (diltiazem) on aortic and coronary contractions in rabbits. J Molecul Cell Cardiol 14:741–744, 1982.

90. Henry PD, et al: Effect of nifedipine on myocardial ischemia: Analysis of collateral flow, pulsatile heat and regional muscle shortening. Am J Cardiol 44:817–824, 1979.

91. da Luz PL, et al: Effect of verapamil on regional coronary and myocardial perfusion during acute coronary occlusion. Am J Cardiol 45:269–275, 1980.

92. Ware JA, et al: Inhibition of human platelet aggregation and cytoplasmic calcium response by calcium antagonists: Studies with aequorin and quin2. Circ Res 59:39–42, 1986.

93. Josephson MA, Hopkins J, Singh BN: Hemodynamic and metabolic effects of diltiazem during coronary sinus pacing with particular reference to left ventricular ejection fraction. Am J Cardiol 55:286–290, 1985.

94. Henry PD: Atherosclerosis, calcium, and calcium antagonists. Circulation 72:456–459, 1985.

95. Lichtlen PR, et al: Retardation of angiographic progression of coronary artery disease by nifedipine. Results of the International Nifedipine Trial on Antiatherosclerotic Therapy (INTACT). INTACT Group Investigators. Lancet 335:1109–1113, 1990.

96. Rowland E, Evans T, Krikler D: Effect of nifedipine on atrioventric-

ular conduction as compared with verapamil. Intracardiac electrophysiological study. Br Heart J 42:124–127, 1979.

97. Sugimoto T, et al: Electrophysiologic effects of diltiazem, a calcium antagonist, in patients with impaired sinus or atrioventricular node function. Angiology 31:700–709, 1980.

98. Kapur PA, Campos JH, Buchea OC: Plasma diltiazem levels, cardiovascular function, and coronary hemodynamics during enflurane anesthesia in the dog. Anesth Analg 65:918–924, 1986.

99. Durant NN, Nguyen N, Katz RL: Potentiation of neuromuscular blockade by verapamil. Anesthesiology 60:298–303, 1984.

100. Lawson NW, Kraynack BJ, Gintautas J: Neuromuscular and electrocardiographic responses to verapamil in dogs. Anesth Analg 62:50–54, 1983.

101. Jones RM, et al: Verapamil potentiation of neuromuscular blockade: Failure of reversal with neostigmine but prompt reversal with edrophonium. Anesth Analg 64:1021–1025, 1985.

102. Rosenblatt R, et al: Verapamil potentiates the toxicity of local anesthetics. Anesth Analg 175–284, 1984.

103. Silvestry FE, Kimmel SE: Calcium-channel blockers in ischemic heart disease. Curr Opin Cardiol 11:434–439, 1996.

104. Muller JE, et al: Nifedipine therapy for patients with threatened and acute myocardial infarction: A randomized, double-blind, placebo-controlled comparison. Circulation 69:740–747, 1984.

105. Wilcox RG, et al: Trial of early nifedipine in acute myocardial infarction: The Trent study. Br Med J (Clin Res Ed) 293:1204–1208, 1986.

106. Anonymous: Secondary prevention reinfarction Israeli nifedipine trial (SPRINT). A randomized intervention trial of nifedipine in patients with acute myocardial infarction. The Israeli Sprint Study Group. Eur Heart J 9:354–364, 1988.

107. Goldbourt U, et al: Early administration of nifedipine in suspected acute myocardial infarction. The Secondary Prevention Reinfarction Israel Nifedipine Trial 2 Study. Arch Intern Med 153:345–353, 1993.

108. Opie LH, Messerli FH: Nifedipine and mortality. Grave defects in the dossier. Circulation 92:1068–1073, 1995.

109. Furberg CD, Psaty BM, Meyer JV: Nifedipine. Dose-related increase in mortality in patients with coronary heart disease. Circulation 92:1326–1331, 1995.

110. Pepine CJ, Faich G, Makuch R: Verapamil use in patients with cardiovascular disease: An overview of randomized trials. Clin Cardiol 21:633–641, 1998.

111. Anonymous: Verapamil in acute myocardial infarction. The Danish Study Group on Verapamil in Myocardial Infarction. Eur Heart J 5:516–528, 1984.

112. Anonymous: Effect of verapamil on mortality and major events after acute myocardial infarction (the Danish Verapamil Infarction Trial II—DAVIT II). Am J Cardiol 66:779–785, 1990.

113. Gheorghiade M: Calcium channel blockers in the management of myocardial infarction patients. Henry Ford Hosp Med J 39:210–216, 1991.

114. Theroux P, et al: Intravenous diltiazem in acute myocardial infarction. Diltiazem as adjunctive therapy to activase (DATA) trial. J Am Coll Cardiol 32:620–628, 1998.

115. Moss AJ, et al: Effects of diltiazem on long-term outcome after acute myocardial infarction in patients with and without a history of systemic hypertension. The Multicenter Diltiazem Postinfarction Trial Research Group. Am J Cardiol 68:429–433, 1991.

116. Hilton TC, Miller DD, Kern MJ: Rational therapy to reduce mortality and reinfarction following myocardial infarction. Am Heart J 122:1740–1750, 1991.

117. Gibson RS, et al: Diltiazem and reinfarction in patients with non-Q-wave myocardial infarction. Results of a double-blind, randomized, multicenter trial. N Engl J Med 315:423–439, 1986.

118. Hansen JF, et al: Cardiac event rates after acute myocardial infarction in patients treated with verapamil and trandolapril versus trandolapril alone. Danish Verapamil Infarction Trial (DAVIT) Study Group. Am J Cardiol 79:738–741, 1997.

119. Estrada JN, et al: Antiischemic properties of amlodipine, a new calcium antagonist, in patients with severe coronary artery disease: A prospective trial. Am Heart J 118:1130–1132, 1989.

120. Opie LH: First line drugs in chronic stable effort angina: The case for newer, longer-acting calcium channel blocking agents. J Am Coll Cardiol 36:1967–1971, 2000.

121. Davies RF, et al: Effect of amlodipine, atenolol and their combination on myocardial ischemia during treadmill exercise and ambulatory

monitoring. Canadian Amlodipine/Atenolol in Silent Ischemia Study (CASIS) Investigators. J Am Coll Cardiol 25:619–625, 1995.

122. Singh S: Long-term double-blind evaluation of amlodipine and nadolol in patients with stable exertional angina pectoris. The Investigators of Study 152. Clin Cardiol 16:54–58, 1993.

123. Pitt B, et al: Effect of amlodipine on the progression of atherosclerosis and the occurrence of clinical events. PREVENT Investigators. Circulation 102:1503–1510, 2000.

124. Jorgensen B, et al: Restenosis and clinical outcome in patients treated with amlodipine after angioplasty: Results from the Coronary Angio-Plasty Amlodipine REStenosis Study (CAPARES). J Am Coll Cardiol 35:592–599, 2000.

125. Apostolidou I, et al: Effects of nicardipine and nitroglycerin on perioperative ischemia in patients undergoing coronary artery bypass surgery. Semin Thorac Cardiovasc Surg 11:77–83, 1999.

126. Tuman KJ, et al: Aspirin does not increase allogeneic blood transfusion in reoperative coronary artery surgery. Anesth Analg 83:1178–1184, 1996.

127. Quinn MJ, Fitzgerald DJ: Ticlopidine and clopidogrel. Circulation 100:1667–1672, 1999.

128. Herbert JM, et al: The antiaggregating and antithrombotic activity of clopidogrel is potentiated by aspirin in several experimental models in the rabbit. Thromb Haemost 80:512–518, 1998.

129. Yende S, Wunderink RG: Effect of clopidogrel on bleeding after coronary artery bypass. Crit Care Med 29:1–11, 2001.

130. Boneu B, Destelle G: Platelet anti-aggregating activity and tolerance of clopidogrel in atherosclerotic patients. Thromb Haemost 76:939–943, 1996.

131. Coller BS: Platelet GPIIb/IIIa antagonists: The first anti-integrin receptor therapeutics. J Clin Invest 100:S57–60, 1997.

132. Lefkovits J, Plow EF, Topol EJ: Platelet glycoprotein IIb/IIIa receptors in cardiovascular medicine. N Engl J Med 332:1553–1559, 1995.

133. Mascelli MA, et al: Pharmacodynamic profile of short-term abciximab treatment demonstrates prolonged platelet inhibition with gradual recovery from GP IIb/IIIa receptor blockade. Circulation 97:1680–1688, 1998.

134. Gammie JS, et al: Abciximab and excessive bleeding in patients undergoing emergency cardiac operations. Ann Thorac Surg 65:465–469, 1998.

135. Aguirre FV, et al: Bleeding complications with the chimeric antibody to platelet glycoprotein IIb/IIIa integrin in patients undergoing percutaneous coronary intervention. EPIC Investigators. Circulation 91:2882–2890, 1995.

136. Silvestry SC, Smith PK: Current status of cardiac surgery in the abciximab-treated patient. Ann Thorac Surg 70:S12–19, 2000.

137. Lemmer JH Jr, et al: Aprotinin for primary coronary artery bypass grafting: A multicenter trial of three dose regimens. Ann Thorac Surg 62:1659–1667; discussion 1667–1668, 1996.

138. Al Douri M, et al: Effect of the administration of recombinant activated factor VII (rFVIIa; NovoSeven) in the management of severe uncontrolled bleeding in patients undergoing heart valve replacement surgery. Blood Coagul Fibrinolysis 11:S121–127, 2000.

139. Despotis GJ, et al: Anticoagulation monitoring during cardiac surgery: A review of current and emerging techniques. Anesthesiology 91:1122–1151, 1999.

140. Levy JH: Pharmacologic preservation of the hemostatic system during cardiac surgery. Ann Thorac Surg 1814–1820, 2001.

141. Shorten GD, Comunale ME: Heparin-induced thrombocytopenia. J Cardiothorac Vasc Anesth 10:521–530, 1996.

142. Greinacher A, Lubenow N: Recombinant hirudin in clinical practice: Focus on lepirudin. Circulation 103:1479–1484, 2001.

143. Gillis S, et al: Danaparoid for cardiopulmonary bypass in patients with previous heparin-induced thrombocytopenia. Br J Haematol 98:657–659, 1997.

144. Levy JH, Zaidan JR, Faraj B: Prospective evaluation of risk of protamine reactions in patients with NPH insulin-dependent diabetes. Anesth Analg 65:739–742, 1986.

145. Cohen M, et al: A comparison of low-molecular–weight heparin with unfractionated heparin for unstable coronary artery disease. Efficacy and Safety of Subcutaneous Enoxaparin in Non-Q-Wave Coronary Events Study Group. N Engl J Med 337:447–452, 1997.

146. Anonymous: Low-molecular–weight heparin during instability in coronary artery disease, Fragmin during Instability in Coronary Artery Disease (FRISC) study group. Lancet 347:561–568, 1996.

147. Abu-Hajir M, Mazzeo AJ: Perioperative use of anticoagulants and

thrombolytics: The pharmacology of antithrombotic and antiplatelet agents. Anesthesiol Clin N Am 17:749–786, 1999.

148. Crowther MA, et al: Low-dose oral vitamin K reliably reverses over-anticoagulation due to warfarin. Thromb Haemost 79:1116–1118, 1998.

149. Fetrow CW, Overlock T, Leff L: Antagonism of warfarin-induced hypoprothrombinemia with use of low-dose subcutaneous vitamin K1. J Clin Pharmacol 37:751–757, 1997.

150. Collins R, et al: Aspirin, heparin, and fibrinolytic therapy in suspected acute myocardial infarction. N Engl J Med 336:847–860, 1997.

151. Anonymous: Trial of abciximab with and without low-dose reteplase for acute myocardial infarction. Strategies for Patency Enhancement in the Emergency Department (SPEED) Group. Circulation 101:2788–2794, 2000.

152. White HD, Van de Werf FJ: Thrombolysis for acute myocardial infarction. Circulation 97:1632–1646, 1998.

153. Anonymous: An international randomized trial comparing four thrombolytic strategies for acute myocardial infarction. The GUSTO investigators. N Engl J Med 329:673–682, 1993.

154. Bizjak ED, Mauro VF: Thrombolytic therapy: A review of its use in acute myocardial infarction. Ann Pharmacother 32:769–784, 1998.

155. Noble S, McTavish D: Reteplase. A review of its pharmacological properties and clinical efficacy in the management of acute myocardial infarction. Drugs 52:589–605, 1996.

156. Zeller FP, Spinler SA: Alteplase: A tissue plasminogen activator for acute myocardial infarction. Drug Intell Clin Pharm 22:6–14, 1988.

157. Gemmill JD, et al: The incidence and mechanism of hypotension following thrombolytic therapy for acute myocardial infarction with streptokinase-containing agents—lack of relationship to pretreatment streptokinase resistance. Eur Heart J 14:819–825, 1993.

158. Woo KS, White HD: Comparative tolerability profiles of thrombolytic agents. A review. Drug Saf 8:19–29, 1993.

159. Drayer D: Lipophilicity, hydrophilicity and the central nervous system: side effects of beta blockers. Pharmacotherapy 7:87–91, 1987.

160. McDevitt DG: Comparison of pharmacokinetic properties of beta-adrenoceptor blocking drugs. Eur Heart J 8:9–14, 1987.

37

Cardiovascular Pharmacology of Positive Inotropic Drugs

Paul S. Pagel, MD, PhD • Judy R. Kersten, MD •
David C. Warltier, MD, PhD

Heart failure occurs when this organ is unable to generate sufficient output to serve cellular metabolic requirements. Heart failure most often occurs as a result of decreases in intrinsic myocardial contractility, but abnormalities in diastolic function may also be responsible in the absence of or preceding significant impairment of systolic performance.[1,2] The heart serves two major functional roles: propelling blood into the high-pressure arterial circulation during systole and collecting blood for subsequent ejection from the low-pressure venous vasculature.[3,4] Thus pathologic conditions that restrict left ventricular (LV) inflow may also produce heart failure independent of pump performance. Reductions in contractile function occur in a variety of disease states including myocardial ischemia, stunning, hibernation, or infarction, pressure or volume overload hypertrophy, and myocyte injury produced by drugs, infectious disease, or infiltrative processes. Diastolic dysfunction may also result from these pathologic conditions or may be produced by forces outside the LV chamber (e.g., pericardial tamponade, constrictive pericarditis, ventricular interaction) that act to impair filling and compliance. Regardless of the underlying cause, heart failure activates a series of compensatory reflexes including sympathetic nervous system stimulation, parasympathetic nervous system withdrawal, stimulation of the renin-angiotensin-aldosterone axis, and increased vasopressin release that serve to increase perfusion pressure and improve cardiac output.[5] Although these compensatory mechanisms may be adequate to maintain cardiovascular homeostasis at rest, cardiac function may subsequently decline, and clinical signs and symptoms of heart failure may ensue during periods of hemodynamic stress. This "cardiac reserve" is diminished by further reductions in contractility or exacerbations in diastolic dysfunction, and cardiac output may eventually become inadequate even during resting conditions. This progressive decline in functional reserve characterizes the well-known stages of the New York Heart Association classification in which patients demonstrate significant cardiac reserve in stage I but suffer end-stage heart failure during resting conditions in stage IV.

Although activation of neural and endocrine reflexes initially maintain overall cardiovascular performance in evolving heart failure, these responses also cause adverse consequences that may eventually lead to disease progression, end-organ hypoperfusion, and death.[5] Activation of the sympathetic nervous system and the renin-angiotensin system preserve or modestly increase arterial pressure by causing arteriolar vasoconstriction. Unfortunately, these actions also produce undesirable increases in LV afterload that further compromise already reduced LV systolic function. Aldosterone release causes retention of sodium (Na^+) and water by the kidney, but resulting increases in plasma volume combine with sympathetic nervous system–mediated reductions in venous capacitance to further exacerbate pre-existing central venous and pulmonary arterial congestion. These increases in LV afterload and preload increase LV end-systolic and end-diastolic volume and wall stress, respectively, and cause detrimental increases in myocardial oxygen consumption. The Frank-Starling mechanism that normally results in enhanced myocardial contractility, cardiac output, and stroke work in response to augmentation of LV preload is exhausted in the failing heart.[6] In fact, further reductions in LV systolic function may occur concomitant with progressive LV dilation. Lastly, increased sympathetic and decreased parasympathetic nervous system activity cause compensatory tachycardia, but this response is an energetically wasteful means of enhancing cardiac output and is especially deleterious in patients with coronary artery disease.

The search for new drugs that enhance contractility in failing myocardium has been remarkably *unsuccessful*.[7] The digitalis glycosides remain the only positive inotropic drugs currently available for the chronic oral treatment of heart failure. Heart failure resulting from LV systolic or diastolic dysfunction appears to be most successfully treated using drugs that optimize LV loading conditions by decreasing preload (e.g., diuretics, nitrates) or afterload (e.g., angiotensin-converting enzyme inhibitors, calcium channel blockers).[8] Low doses of β_1 adrenoceptor antagonists have also been shown to exert beneficial effects in patients with heart failure[9] by reversing down-regulation of the receptor and increasing responsiveness to endogenous catecholamines. The use of these pharmacologic approaches is limited in end-stage heart failure, however, and the lack of an effective, orally-administered positive inotropic drug has led to use of procedures such as optimally-timed sequential atrioventricular (AV) pacing, LV reduction surgery (e.g., Batista procedure), and skeletal muscle augmentation (e.g., cardiomyoplasty), which unfortunately are only beneficial in a small minority of patients. In contrast, a variety of drugs have been used successfully in the intravenous treatment of acute LV failure. Endogenous and synthetic catecholamines, inhibitors of the cardiac isoform of phosphodiesterase, and new drugs such as the myofilament calcium (Ca^{2+}) sensitizers are currently used or will find future use for the treatment of reduced myocardial contractility. This chapter discusses the cardiovascular pharmacology of drugs used for the treatment of acute and chronic heart failure.

Mechanisms of Drug Action: An Overview

Myocardial contractility is determined by several factors that affect the interaction between actin and myosin in the sarcomere.[10] This event is dependent on the concentration of Ca^{2+} in the myoplasm and requires energy in the form of adenosine triphosphate (ATP) to occur. A transient increase in the intracellular Ca^{2+} concentration from less than 10^{-7} to 10^{-5} M causes the cardiac myocyte to contract. Membrane depolarization causes a small amount of Ca^{2+} to enter the myocyte through voltage-regulated Ca^{2+} channels located within the sarcolemma. The total quantity of Ca^{2+} that enters the myocyte depends on the number of open channels and how long these channels remain in the open state. This small increase in intracellular Ca^{2+} concentration causes the release of stored Ca^{2+} from the cisternae of the sarcoplasmic reticulum. This process is known as Ca^{2+}-induced Ca^{2+} release and forms the basis of the "Ca^{2+} transient" measured in the experimental laboratory. Calcium-induced Ca^{2+} release from the sarcoplasmic reticulum is directly related to the quantity of and rate at which Ca^{2+} enters through sarcolemmal Ca^{2+} channels. Calcium binds to the troponin C regulatory protein of the troponin/tropomyosin complex and causes a conformational change that allows the ATP-dependent cycling of crossbridges between actin and myosin. The troponin/tropomyosin complex normally prevents the interaction of these contractile elements and inhibits contraction of the cardiac myocyte. However, the increased intracellular Ca^{2+} concentration observed after sarcolemmal depolarization permits the formation of actin/myosin crossbridges to occur. Thus the degree of tropomyosin disinhibition, the extent of actin/myosin interaction, and the force of contraction at constant load (i.e., inotropic state) are directly related to Ca^{2+} concentration within the myocyte.

Drugs that enhance myocardial contractility either increase the amount of Ca^{2+} for contractile activation through a variety of mechanisms[11] or directly augment the efficacy of this ion at the contractile apparatus[12] (Fig. 37–1). Calcium chloride and Ca^{2+} gluconate directly increase extracellular Ca^{2+} concentration and facilitate a greater influx of Ca^{2+} through sarcolemmal Ca^{2+} channels. This action leads to an increase in intracellular Ca^{2+} concentration and enhanced contractility. However, because most of the Ca^{2+} available for contractile activation is derived from the sarcoplasmic reticulum, exogenously administered Ca^{2+} may not provide a reliable, clinically-evident increase in contractile function. For example, bolus doses of Ca^{2+} do not consistently increase cardiac output in patients after cardiopulmonary bypass,[13,14] most likely because Ca^{2+} also increases LV afterload by arteriolar vasoconstriction, impeding LV ejection. Cardiac glycosides (e.g., digitalis) exert positive inotropic activity by indirectly increasing intracellular Ca^{2+} concentration through reversal of the Na^+-Ca^{2+} exchanger independent of the intracellular second messenger cyclic adenosine monophosphate (cAMP). In contrast, catecholamines (e.g., epinephrine, norepinephrine) and phosphodiesterase inhibitors (e.g., inamrinone, milrinone) increase Ca^{2+} concentration by positively modulating the actions of cAMP. Myofilament Ca^{2+} sensitizers (e.g., pimobendan, levosimendan) increase contractile performance by enhancing the sensitivity of the contractile proteins to Ca^{2+} without specifically affecting the intracellular concentration of this ion.

Rapid extrusion of Ca^{2+} from the myoplasm, and dissociation of Ca^{2+} from troponin C after contraction are required for relaxation of the sarcomere to occur. Delays in this process result in incomplete myocardial relaxation and may be clinically manifested by diastolic dysfunction.[3,4] Thus simultaneous increases in the elimination of Ca^{2+} must also occur during augmentation of contractile state produced by inotropic drugs. Calcium is extruded from the myoplasm by Ca^{2+}-ATPases located within the sarcolemmal membrane and the sarcoplasmic reticulum. The ATP-dependent Ca^{2+} transporter in the sarcoplasmic reticulum is a primary determinant of removal of Ca^{2+} from the cytosol. Calcium is also passively extruded from the myoplasm by the sarcolemmal Na^+-Ca^{2+} transporter. This ion exchanger allows Ca^{2+} to be removed from the cell in exchange for Na^+.

Pharmacology of Positive Inotropic Agents

Digitalis Glycosides

Preclinical Pharmacology

Cardiac glycosides are naturally occurring substances found in a variety of plants including "foxglove" or *Digitalis*

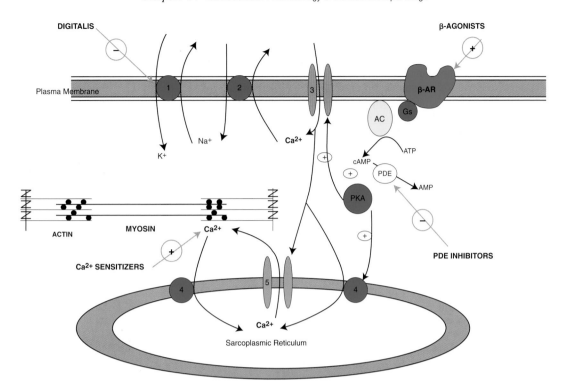

Figure 37–1. Sites of action of positive inotropic agents. Digitalis glycosides indirectly increase intracellular Ca^{2+} by inhibiting the Na^+-K^+ ATPase.[1] This increases intracellular Na^+, thus reducing the activity of the Na^+-Ca^{2+} exchange.[2] β adrenergic agonists also increase intracellular Ca^{2+}. They act by stimulating the production of cyclic adenosine monophosphate (cAMP), which activates protein kinase A (PKA). PKA in turn phosphorylates and activates both voltage-dependent Ca^{2+} channels (VDCC[3]) and the sarcoplasmic reticulum Ca^{2+}-ATPase.[4] The increased activity of VDCC increases "trigger calcium" leading to greater activation of the calcium release channel in sarcoplasmic reticulum.[5] Activation of the Ca^{2+}-ATPase increases Ca^{2+} uptake by sarcoplasmic reticulum, producing a positive lusitropic effect. Phosphodiesterase inhibitors increase cAMP by inhibiting its breakdown, and thus act synergistically with β agonists to increase intracellular Ca^{2+}. Ca^{2+} sensitizers increase the sensitivity of the contractile apparatus to Ca^{2+} without changing intracellular Ca^{2+} concentrations. AC, adenylyl cyclase; ATP, adenosine triphosphate; β-AR, β adrenergic receptor; PDE.

purpurea. The chemical structure of digitalis glycosides contains a hydrophobic steroid nucleus and a hydrophilic unsaturated lactone ring. Digitalis glycosides are the only positive inotropic drugs that are currently available for the chronic oral treatment of heart failure.[15] Digitalis glycosides enhance contractile function, but this positive inotropic effect is relatively minor when compared with the actions produced by other drugs used for the treatment of acute LV dysfunction. The most commonly used cardiac glycosides include digoxin and digitoxin, but a large number of related compounds also have been used clinically.[16] Digitalis glycosides selectively and reversibly inhibit sarcolemmal Sodium-potassium ATPase by binding to the α-subunit on the extracellular surface of the enzyme complex.[17] This digitalis-sarcolemmal Na^+-K^+ ATPase binding is inhibited by increases in extracellular K^+ concentration,[18] and, as a result, digitalis toxicity may be reversed to some degree by the administration of K^+. Conversely, digitalis toxicity is markedly increased in the presence of hypokalemia. Inhibition of sarcolemmal Na^+-K^+ ATPase indirectly increases Ca^{2+} availability during systole, thereby augmenting myocardial contractility. The Na^+-K^+ ATPase enzyme exchanges three intracellular Na^+ ions for two extracellular K^+ ions against concentration gradients in an energy-dependent fashion. This action produces a slight increase in

intracellular Na^+ concentration that, in turn, reduces extrusion of Ca^{2+} from the myoplasm by the sarcolemmal Na^+-Ca^{2+} exchanger.[19] This additional Ca^{2+} is stored by the sarcoplasmic reticulum, providing additional Ca^{2+} for subsequent release during the next contraction. In contrast to other drugs that increase myocardial contractility, tachyphylaxis to the positive inotropic effects of digitalis glycosides does not appear to occur.[20] The mechanism of action of digitalis glycosides is similar to that implicated for the treppe phenomenon observed in cardiac and skeletal muscle. Rapid increases in muscle stimulation or heart rate cause a lag in activity of the Na^+-K^+ ATPase, a transient increase in intracellular Na^+ concentration, and an increase in contractile force mediated by advantageous Na^+-Ca^{2+} exchange.

Clinical Pharmacology

The increase in myocardial contractility produced by digitalis glycosides occurs without change in heart rate and is associated with reductions in LV preload and afterload, LV wall tension, and myocardial oxygen consumption in the failing heart.[21] Heart failure is characterized by a compensatory increase in sympathetic nervous system tone, and digitalis glycosides have been shown to reduce sympathetic activity[22] by enhancing contractility and improving cardiac output. This withdrawal of sympathetic tone is accompanied by reductions in circulating and cardiac norepinephrine concentrations[23,24] and reduces impedance to LV ejection. The decrease in sympathetic nervous system activity observed with digitalis glycosides is also related to the direct actions of these drugs on cardiac baroreceptors[25] and may play an important role in reducing morbidity and mortality rates in patients with chronic congestive heart failure.[26–28] However, dramatic alterations in the electrophysiology of primary pacemaker cells and in the remainder of the cardiac conduction pathway may also occur as a result of digitalis-induced inhibition of the sarcolemmal Na^+-K^+ ATPase because this enzyme is responsible for maintaining the normal resting membrane potential of the myocyte. These direct electrophysiologic effects are further complicated by indirect actions mediated by withdrawal of sympathetic and increases in parasympathetic nervous system activity. Administration of digitalis glycosides frequently leads to the development of a wide variety of arrhythmias including sinus bradycardia or arrest, AV conduction delays, and second- or third-degree heart block. Toxic levels of digitalis glycosides may paradoxically increase sympathetic nervous system tone and may precipitate the formation of malignant ventricular tachyarrhythmias. The digitalis glycosides have a low therapeutic ratio and narrow margin of safety, and mortality rates resulting from arrhythmias have been shown to be directly related to the plasma concentrations of these drugs.[28]

Digitalis glycosides are most often used during the perioperative period for the management of supraventricular tachyarrhythmias associated with a rapid ventricular response, because these drugs prolong conduction time in the AV node. Digitalis glycosides are not commonly used to increase myocardial contractility in patients with acute LV dysfunction because of the availability of far more potent drugs with substantially less toxicity. However, digitalis glycosides continue to play an important role in the treatment of chronic congestive heart failure.

Catecholamines

Preclinical Pharmacology

The cardiovascular effects of both endogenous (e.g., epinephrine, norepinephrine, dopamine) and synthetic (e.g., isoproterenol, dobutamine, dopexamine) catecholamines are mediated by activation of α and β adrenoceptors.[29] These drugs mimic stimulation of the sympathetic nervous system and may be divided into those that act directly on adrenoceptors and those that act indirectly by promoting the release of norepinephrine from sympathetic nerve terminals.[30] Catecholamines enhance myocardial contractility by activation of cardiac β_1 adrenoceptors located on the sarcolemmal surface. The β_1 adrenoceptor is coupled to the enzyme adenylyl cyclase by a stimulatory guanine nucleotide-binding (G_s) protein located in the cell membrane. Adenylyl cyclase converts ATP to cAMP. This second messenger binds to the regulatory subunit of protein kinase A and enhances the activity of this enzyme, resulting in the subsequent phosphorylation of sarcolemmal Ca^{2+} channels,

troponin I, and phospholamban. These actions directly increase Ca^{2+} influx through voltage-dependent Ca^{2+} channels, indirectly stimulate release of Ca^{2+} from the sarcoplasmic reticulum, augment Ca^{2+} binding to the contractile apparatus, and accelerate Ca^{2+} uptake by the sarcoplasmic reticulum. Thus catecholamines exert positive inotropic effects through β_1 adrenoceptor stimulation by increasing the amount of Ca^{2+} available for contractile activation and enhancing the efficacy of Ca^{2+} at the myofilaments. Catecholamines also simultaneously accelerate myocardial relaxation (i.e., lusitropy) and improve diastolic function by augmenting removal of Ca^{2+} from the sarcoplasm after contraction has occurred.[31] In addition to positive inotropic and lusitropic actions, β_1 adrenoceptor stimulation by catecholamines increases heart rate and conduction velocity (e.g., chronotropic and dromotropic effects) and may contribute to the development of supraventricular or ventricular tachyarrhythmias.

Catecholamines are used extensively to enhance myocardial contractility in the setting of acute and chronic LV dysfunction. However, the efficacy of β_1 adrenoceptor agonists in the failing heart may be influenced by the relative density and function of the β_1 adrenoceptor. This receptor is markedly down-regulated and its signal transduction cascade is adversely affected in heart failure.[32,33] There is also strong evidence indicating that cardiopulmonary bypass[34] and intraoperative adrenoceptor stimulation during routine surgery[35] acutely depress β_1 adrenoceptor signaling. Recognition of this phenomenon has led some investigators[36] to advocate the use of β_1-adrenoceptor antagonists during cardiopulmonary bypass to reverse down-regulation of this receptor and enhance the contractile response to exogenously administered catecholamines after bypass.

Catecholamines exert a variety of pharmacologic effects in other circulatory beds, because of the widespread location and heterogenous distribution of α and β adrenoceptor subtypes.[30] The peripheral vascular actions of catecholamines are dependent on the specific drug as a result of differences in chemical structure and selectivity for adrenoceptors. This selectivity may also be highly dose-dependent. For example, low doses of dopamine stimulate dopamine subtype 1 and 2 (DA_1 and DA_2, respectively) receptors to produce arterial vasodilation, whereas progressively greater doses activate β_1 followed by α_1 adrenoceptors, thereby enhancing contractility and causing arterial vasoconstriction, respectively. α_1 Adrenoceptors are located primarily in small arterioles and veins and mediate increases in systemic vascular resistance and decreases in venous capacitance, respectively. Activation of α_1 adrenoceptors located on the sarcolemmal surface of vascular smooth muscle cells increases the activity of phospholipase C through a G protein–mediated mechanism and leads to cleavage of cell membrane phospholipids and the production of inositol 1,4,5-triphosphate.[37] This intracellular second messenger opens receptor-operated Ca^{2+} channels, stimulates Ca^{2+} release from the sarcoplasmic reticulum, and causes activation of Ca^{2+}-dependent protein kinases and phosphorylation of respective substrates. These actions result in an increased intracellular Ca^{2+} concentration and lead to contraction of the vascular smooth muscle cell. In contrast to cutaneous blood vessels that contain primarily α_1 adrenoceptors, skeletal muscle contains β_2 adrenoceptors, whose activation produces arteriolar vasodilation through an adenylyl cyclase–mediated mechanism.

The effects of a catecholamine on arterial pressure are determined by its actions on heart rate, myocardial contractility, arterial resistance (i.e., afterload), and venous tone (i.e., preload). For example, a pure α_1 adrenoceptor agonist produces an increase in systemic vascular resistance and a decrease in venous capacitance, actions that combine to increase arterial pressure. In contrast, a pure β adrenoceptor agonist causes increases in heart rate, stroke volume, and cardiac output, and a decrease in systemic vascular resistance. These effects may result in a modest decline in arterial pressure. In general, catecholamines produce deleterious increases in myocardial oxygen consumption[38] and may cause myocardial ischemia. Use of these drugs to improve LV performance in patients with coronary artery disease or congestive heart failure must be approached with caution. Thus afterload reduction is most commonly used as an initial therapeutic approach to increase cardiac output in the pharmacologic management of acute or chronic heart failure.

Clinical Pharmacology

Epinephrine

Epinephrine is an agonist of α_1, β_1, and β_2 adrenoceptors.[39] Intravenous infusion of epinephrine produces an increase in mean arterial pressure characterized by selectively enhanced systolic pressure with little change in diastolic pressure. Epinephrine exerts positive chronotropic and inotropic actions by stimulation of β_1 adrenoceptors located on the cell membranes of sinoatrial node cells and cardiac myocytes, respectively. Epinephrine also increases the rate of myocardial relaxation and enhances early LV filling, thereby improving diastolic function. These combined effects result in a dramatic increase in cardiac performance. For example, cardiac index increased by 0.1, 0.7, and 1.2 L/min per m² with the administration of epinephrine (0.01, 0.02, and 0.04 µg/kg per minute, respectively) in humans.[40] The initial tachycardia observed with administration of epinephrine may be followed by a subsequent reduction in heart rate resulting from activation of baroreceptor reflexes. Epinephrine (0.01 to 0.03 µg/kg per minute) has been shown to produce similar hemodynamic effects with less pronounced tachycardia than dobutamine (2.5 to 5.0 µg/kg per minute) in patients after coronary artery bypass graft (CABG) surgery.[41] In fact, use of epinephrine as the primary inotropic drug for the management of LV dysfunction after cardiopulmonary bypass has been advocated by some investigators[14,42,43] because of the predictable increase in cardiac performance observed with this catecholamine. Epinephrine has also been shown to increase cardiac index and oxygen delivery without affecting heart rate in patients with sepsis-induced hypotension that is unresponsive to dopamine.[44] However, the use of epinephrine as an inotropic drug in these settings may be limited to some degree by the propensity of this catecholamine to precipitate arrhythmias. Epinephrine causes direct positive dromotropic effects as indicated by an increase in conduction velocity and reduction of the refractory period of the AV node, His bundle, Purkinje

fibers, and ventricular muscle. The increase in AV nodal conduction may produce detrimental increases in ventricular rate in patients with atrial flutter or fibrillation. The automaticity of latent pacemakers also may increase because spontaneous diastolic depolarization is accelerated. These alterations in electrophysiology caused by epinephrine may contribute to the occurrence of benign or malignant ventricular arrhythmias including premature ventricular contractions, ventricular tachycardia, and ventricular fibrillation.[45]

Stimulation of α_1 adrenoceptors by epinephrine constricts arteriolar vascular smooth muscle located in the cutaneous, splanchnic, and renal circulations. Conversely, epinephrine-induced activation of β_2-adrenoceptors in skeletal muscle vascular beds produces vasodilation. Thus the overall effect of epinephrine on blood flow to a specific organ depends on the relative balance of α_1 and β_2 adrenoceptors located in the vasculature. The effects of epinephrine on organ blood flow are also dose-dependent. β_2 Adrenoceptors are sensitive to lower doses of epinephrine and, as a result, peripheral vasodilation and modest reductions in arterial pressure are observed. In contrast, the effects of epinephrine on α_1 adrenoceptors predominate at greater doses. This action produces marked increases in systemic vascular resistance and arterial pressure. The intense vasoconstriction produced by high doses of epinephrine may adversely impede LV ejection by increasing afterload after cardiopulmonary bypass. Thus greater doses of epinephrine may be used in combination with arterial vasodilators such as nitroprusside to optimize contractile performance during these conditions. The venous circulation also contains a relatively high density of α_1 adrenoceptors, and venoconstriction produced by epinephrine enhances venous return. α_1 Adrenoceptors also mediate direct vasoconstriction of the pulmonary vasculature produced by epinephrine and contribute to increases in pulmonary arterial pressures produced by this catecholamine. Both α_1 and β_2 adrenoceptors are located in the coronary circulation, but these receptors do not usually play a major role in determining myocardial perfusion. In contrast, epinephrine-induced increases in myocardial oxygen consumption produced by tachycardia, enhanced LV preload, augmented inotropic state, and increased afterload cause increases in coronary blood flow by metabolic autoregulation.[46] However, during conditions of maximal coronary vasodilation, such as may be observed during myocardial ischemia, direct stimulation of α_1 adrenoceptors by epinephrine may reduce epicardial coronary artery diameter and decrease coronary blood flow.[47]

The hemodynamic effects of epinephrine are affected by prior administration of α or β adrenoceptor antagonists and other vasoactive drugs. For example, the nonselective beta-blocker propranolol abolishes decreases in systemic vascular resistance produced by epinephrine-induced stimulation of β_2 adrenoceptors and contributes to substantially greater peripheral vasoconstriction mediated by unopposed α_1 adrenoceptors. Clearly, the positive inotropic and chronotropic effects of epinephrine are also markedly attenuated in the presence of pre-existing beta-blockade. β adrenoceptor antagonists competitively inhibit these adrenoceptors, and greater doses of epinephrine are required to overcome this competitive blockade. Complete pharmacologic blockade of β_1 and β_2 adrenoceptors may theoretically make the hemodynamic effects of epinephrine essentially indistinguishable from those of the pure α_1 adrenoceptor agonist phenylephrine.

Norepinephrine

Norepinephrine is the endogenous neurotransmitter released from adrenergic nerve terminals during activation of the sympathetic nervous system. Norepinephrine stimulates α_1 and β_1 adrenoceptors, but in contrast to epinephrine, this catecholamine has little effect on β_2 adrenoceptors. These actions produce positive inotropic effects, intense vasoconstriction, increases in arterial pressure, and relative maintenance of cardiac output.[15] In contrast to epinephrine, norepinephrine does not substantially affect heart rate because activation of baroreceptor reflexes resulting from arterial vasoconstriction usually counteracts β_1 adrenoceptor–mediated, direct, positive, chronotropic effects. Norepinephrine causes relatively greater increases in systemic vascular resistance and diastolic arterial pressure than epinephrine. Norepinephrine increases arterial pressure while simultaneously enhancing contractile state and venous return by reductions in venous capacitance, thereby augmenting stroke volume and ejection fraction. In contrast, pure α_1 adrenoceptor agonists such as phenylephrine and methoxamine further compromise cardiac output in failing myocardium and contribute to peripheral hypoperfusion despite an increase in arterial pressure.

The cardiovascular actions of norepinephrine make this catecholamine a useful drug for the treatment of refractory hypotension during severe sepsis. For example, intravenous infusions of norepinephrine (0.03 to 0.90 µg/kg per minute) have been shown to increase arterial pressure, LV stroke work index, cardiac index, and urine output in septic patients with hypotension that was unresponsive to volume administration, dopamine, or dobutamine.[48] The hypertensive actions of norepinephrine may be beneficial for maintenance of coronary artery perfusion pressure in patients with severe coronary artery disease. The efficacy of norepinephrine in the treatment of "low systemic vascular resistance" syndrome that is occasionally observed after cardiopulmonary bypass has also been demonstrated.[49] However, although norepinephrine usually produces coronary vasodilation by indirect metabolic effects, internal mammary, gastroepiploic, or radial artery graft spasm mediated by direct α_1 adrenoceptor activation may occur in patients undergoing CABG surgery as a consequence of administration of this catecholamine. However, norepinephrine may produce ventricular and supraventricular ectopy; its arrhythmogenic potential is considerably less than that of epinephrine. Thus substitution of norepinephrine for epinephrine may be appropriate in the therapeutic management of cardiogenic shock when atrial or ventricular arrhythmias are present.

Norepinephrine-induced stimulation of pulmonary vascular α_1 adrenoceptors and simultaneous increases in venous return may increase pulmonary arterial pressures and contribute to the development of right ventricular (RV) failure. The combined use of norepinephrine administered through the left atrium and the relatively selective pulmonary vasodilator prostaglandin E_1 administered intravenously has been advocated to prevent RV dysfunction in patients with reactive pulmonary vasculature after cardiopulmonary bypass.[39] The use of prostaglandin E_1 has been largely supplanted in recent years in favor of the inhaled highly selective pulmonary vasodilator nitric oxide,[50,51] but lower doses of norepinephrine administered through the left atrium continue to be beneficial in treating RV failure associated with pulmonary hypertension, because metabolism in peripheral tissue limits the plasma concentrations of norepinephrine returning to the pulmonary vasculature. During these conditions, norepinephrine enhances RV coronary perfusion by increasing diastolic arterial pressure while simultaneously increasing RV contractility. These actions lead to reductions in biventricular filling pressures and increase cardiac output in an experimental model of acute RV dysfunction.[52]

Norepinephrine directly reduces hepatic, skeletal muscle, splanchnic, and renal blood flow through α_1 adrenoceptor activation. However, an increase in perfusion pressure produced by norepinephrine during the treatment of profound hypotension may result in enhanced blood flow to these vascular beds. Nevertheless, decreased perfusion of renal and splanchnic beds represents a major limitation of the prolonged use of high doses of norepinephrine. Activation of renal dopamine receptors with low-dose dopamine[53] or the selective DA_1 agonist fenoldopam,[54,55] to counteract the deleterious actions of norepinephrine on renal blood flow, may preserve renal perfusion in patients with hypotension. For example, norepinephrine (between 0.5 and 1.5 µg/kg per minute) and dopamine (approximately 1.5 µg/kg per minute) increased urine output and enhanced renal function compared with dopamine alone in patients with sepsis.[56]

Dopamine

Dopamine is an endogenous catecholamine that is the immediate biochemical precursor of norepinephrine. The pharmacology of dopamine is complex because this agent differentially activates a variety of dopaminergic and adrenergic receptor subtypes.[57] Low doses of dopamine (<3 µg/kg per minute) selectively stimulate DA_1 receptors in and increase blood flow to renal and mesenteric vascular beds. Activation of DA_2 receptors in autonomic nervous system ganglia and adrenergic nerves also reduces norepinephrine release. The combined effects of dopamine on DA_1 and DA_2 receptors may cause a decrease in arterial pressure during administration of lower doses of this catecholamine. Greater doses (3 to 8 µg/kg per minute) of dopamine appear to nonselectively stimulate both α and β adrenoceptors. However, dopamine activates vascular smooth muscle α_1-adrenoceptors almost exclusively and produces arterial and venous vasoconstriction at doses exceeding 10 µg/kg per minute, similar to pure α_1 agonists.

Although pedagogically useful, this traditional dose-response description of dopamine pharmacodynamics may be somewhat simplistic and may not be consistently observed even in healthy individuals.[58,59] In fact, a wide range of clinical responses to dopamine is more typically observed resulting from differences in receptor regulation, the presence of drug interactions, and individual patient variability in pharmacokinetics.[60] Thus although lower doses of dopamine are frequently used for renal protection mediated through DA_1 receptors, these doses may also activate α and β adrenoceptors that obscure the intended dopaminergic effects in some patients. Conversely, high-dose dopamine may continue to stimulate DA_1 receptors despite simultaneous α_1 adrenoceptor–mediated vasoconstriction, as indicated by maintenance of renal perfusion and urine output.[60] The renal vasodilating effects of lower doses of dopamine may be particularly useful in patients with impaired renal function or those at risk for decreases in renal perfusion associated with reduced cardiac output.[61] Dopamine may also preserve renal function during simultaneous administration of other α_1 adrenoceptor agonists that directly reduce renal blood flow.[53,62] The increase in renal blood flow produced by dopamine occurs as a result of direct vasodilation of afferent and indirect vasoconstriction of efferent arterioles, respectively. These renal vascular effects enhance glomerular filtration rate, sodium excretion, and urine output.[63]

Dopamine is commonly used for inotropic support in the perioperative period.[64] This catecholamine produces positive chronotropic, dromotropic, inotropic, and lusitropic effects by stimulation of β_1-adrenoceptors. Concomitant activation of arterial and venous α_1 adrenoceptors by greater doses of dopamine also increases LV preload and afterload. These combined effects enhance contractile performance and increase arterial pressure. However, dopamine may not be the ideal drug of choice for inotropic support in patients with elevated pulmonary arterial or LV filling pressures. For example, atrial and mean arterial pressures were greater in patients receiving dopamine compared with those treated with dobutamine after cardiopulmonary bypass, despite similar levels of cardiac function.[65] Dopamine may also produce more pronounced tachycardia than epinephrine in this clinical setting.[66] Dopamine-induced increases in LV afterload may be reduced or eliminated by simultaneous administration of an arterial vasodilator such as sodium nitroprusside. This combined therapy preserves the positive inotropic actions of dopamine mediated through β_1 adrenoceptors and further enhances cardiac output by reducing impedance to LV ejection.[67] Dopamine increases myocardial oxygen consumption in the normal and failing heart, impairs the functional recovery of stunned myocardium,[68] and exacerbates injury after coronary occlusion in vivo.[69] These data suggest that dopamine may not be the preferred agent to increase contractile function in the presence of a critical coronary artery stenosis.

Dopexamine

Dopexamine is a synthetic catecholamine that exerts activity at dopaminergic and β adrenergic receptors.[70] Dopexamine is structurally related to dopamine but is devoid of α adrenoceptor activity and has a greater affinity (9.8 times) for β_2 than β_1 adrenoceptors.[71] As a result of dopamine and β_2 receptor stimulation, dopexamine acts primarily as a vasodilator. Dopexamine also enhances myocardial contractility by inhibiting presynaptic norepinephrine reuptake.[72] Direct β_1 adrenoceptor activation by dopexamine does not appear to play a substantial role in the positive inotropic actions of this drug. Dopexamine has been shown to increase splanchnic and renal perfusion, reduce systemic vascular

resistance, and enhance cardiac output concomitant with a baroreceptor-mediated increase in heart rate in healthy volunteers[73] and in patients with heart failure.[70] Several studies also indicate that dopexamine (1 to 4 µg/kg per minute) enhances stroke volume and cardiac output and reduces systemic and pulmonary vascular resistances in patients after cardiopulmonary bypass.[74–76] Dopexamine may also improve renal function and reduce the inflammatory response to cardiopulmonary bypass.[77] The use of dopexamine as a positive inotropic drug in patients with severe coronary artery disease may be limited, however, because tachycardia and increases in myocardial oxygen consumption occur at greater doses of the drug. Dopexamine may also play a role in circulatory support during sepsis because this agent preferentially increases splanchnic and renal perfusion by activation of dopaminergic and β_2 adrenergic receptors. Studies conducted in experimental models[78] of and in patients[79] with sepsis suggest that dopexamine increases cardiac output and oxygen delivery concomitant with beneficial redistribution of splanchnic blood flow.

Dobutamine

Dobutamine is a synthetic catecholamine composed of two stereoisomers.[80] The (−) and (+) isomers are both β adrenoceptor agonists, but these isomers exert opposing agonist and antagonist activity on α_1 adrenoceptors, respectively. Dobutamine produces potent β adrenoceptor agonist stimulation with little or no effect on α_1 adrenoceptors at doses less than 5 µg/kg per minute. As a result, dobutamine increases myocardial contractility and causes a modest degree of peripheral vasodilation by stimulation of cardiac β_1 and vascular smooth muscle β_2 adrenoceptors, respectively, at these concentrations. These pharmacodynamic properties of dobutamine account for the reductions in LV preload and afterload and improvements in LV/arterial coupling and mechanical efficiency concomitant with enhanced contractile function observed in patients with LV dysfunction.[81] The salutary actions of dobutamine on LV/arterial matching may also account for the reductions in functional mitral insufficiency that occur with the administration of dobutamine to patients with dilated cardiomyopathy and increased LV filling pressures.[82] The (−) isomer of dobutamine stimulates the α_1 adrenoceptor at greater doses and prevents further vasodilation from occurring. As a result, LV preload, afterload, and arterial pressure are relatively maintained, whereas cardiac output is increased, and less pronounced baroreceptor reflex-mediated tachycardia may be observed.[83] Nevertheless, dobutamine may substantially increase heart rate by direct chronotropic and dromotropic effects mediated by β_1 adrenoceptors in some patients. In fact, doses of dobutamine that enhance cardiac output and stroke volume have been shown to produce significantly greater increases in heart rate than epinephrine in patients after CABG surgery.[41] Dobutamine-induced tachycardia and increases in myocardial contractility produce direct increase of myocardial oxygen consumption and may cause ischemia in patients with coronary artery disease. This observation forms the basis for the use of dobutamine stress-echocardiography as a diagnostic tool for the detection of functional coronary artery stenoses, because easily detected abnormalities in regional wall motion occur during these conditions.[84] Conversely, dobutamine may indirectly reduce heart rate in patients with severe heart failure if increases in cardiac output and oxygen delivery[85] result in a simultaneous reduction of sympathetic nervous system tone that is known to be chronically increased during these conditions. Dobutamine may also indirectly decrease myocardial oxygen consumption by reducing LV end-systolic and end-diastolic wall stress in the failing heart.[86]

The β_2 adrenoceptor–stimulating actions of dobutamine also cause modest reductions in pulmonary arterial pressure and vascular resistance. As a result, dobutamine is often used to increase cardiac output in the presence of increased pulmonary vascular resistance after cardiopulmonary bypass. In contrast, dopamine-induced, α_1 adrenoceptor–mediated vasoconstriction of pulmonary vascular smooth muscle increases pulmonary arterial pressure and results in greater LV filling pressures concomitant with augmented pulmonary venous return. Thus dobutamine may have distinct advantages compared with dopamine in patients with heart failure and increased pulmonary arterial and LV filling pressures.[87] However, pulmonary vasodilation produced by dobutamine may worsen ventilation/perfusion mismatch and increase pulmonary shunting. In contrast to dopamine and dopexamine, dobutamine does not exert activity at dopaminergic receptors or selectively alter renal perfusion.[88] Nevertheless, dobutamine may indirectly enhance renal function in heart failure by augmenting cardiac output and improving renal perfusion.

Isoproterenol

Isoproterenol is a nonselective agonist of β adrenoceptors.[30] This synthetic catecholamine has a low affinity for, and consequently, does not exert activity at α adrenoceptors. Isoproterenol increases heart rate and reduces systemic vascular resistance by β_2 adrenoceptor–mediated arteriolar vasodilation in skeletal muscle, and to a lesser degree, renal and splanchnic vascular beds. As a result of this reduction in LV afterload, decreases in diastolic and mean arterial pressures along with relative maintenance of systolic arterial pressure are typically observed during the administration of isoproterenol. Tachycardia produced by isoproterenol results from direct stimulation of β_1 adrenoceptors in the sinoatrial node and AV conduction system combined with activation of baroreceptor reflexes in response to decreases in arterial pressure. Isoproterenol produces dose-dependent positive inotropic effects, but clinical increases in cardiac output may be limited to some degree because tachycardia interferes with LV filling dynamics, and dilatation of venous capacitance vessels occurs that further reduces LV preload. For example, isoproterenol did not significantly enhance cardiac output in patients after CABG or valve replacement surgery, in contrast to dobutamine.[89] The hemodynamic effects of isoproterenol contribute to dose-related increases in myocardial oxygen consumption concomitant with reductions in coronary perfusion pressure and diastolic filling time. As a result, myocardial ischemia or subendocardial

necrosis may occur even in a healthy coronary circulation. Thus the use of isoproterenol may be especially detrimental in patients with severe coronary artery disease.

Isoproterenol is frequently used to provide sustained increases in heart rate during symptomatic bradyarrhythmias or AV conduction block before the insertion of a temporary or permanent pacemaker. However, isoproterenol increases automaticity and may precipitate supraventricular and ventricular tachyarrhythmias. Isoproterenol is also commonly used after cardiac transplantation to increase heart rate and myocardial contractility in the denervated transplanted heart.[90] Finally, isoproterenol decreases pulmonary vascular resistance and may be useful in the management of RV dysfunction resulting from pulmonary hypertension, valvular or congenital heart disease,[91] or after cardiac transplantation.

Ephedrine and Metaraminol

Ephedrine is a sympathomimetic drug that exerts direct and indirect actions on adrenoceptors. This drug produces arterial and venous vasoconstriction and enhances myocardial contractility primarily by releasing norepinephrine from adrenergic nerve terminals and indirectly stimulating α_1 and β_1 adrenoceptors.[30] Ephedrine is transported into the presynaptic terminals of adrenergic nerves and displaces norepinephrine from binding sites within and outside of the synaptic vesicles. The displaced norepinephrine is subsequently released from the presynaptic nerve terminal and stimulates postsynaptic adrenergic receptors. Although the indirect effects are the predominant pharmacologic consequences of ephedrine, this drug also produces direct activation of β_2 adrenoceptors that tend to limit the increases in arterial pressure observed with its administration.[92] Ephedrine is frequently administered in bolus doses to treat hypotension in the presence of bradycardia. Ephedrine causes dose-related increases in heart rate, cardiac output, and systemic vascular resistance, hemodynamic effects that are similar to those produced by epinephrine. Unlike epinephrine, however, tachyphylaxis to the hemodynamic effects of ephedrine may rapidly occur because repetitive administration of the drug acutely depletes presynaptic norepinephrine stores. Other drugs that deplete norepinephrine from or inhibit the uptake of ephedrine into adrenergic nerves (e.g., reserpine or cocaine, respectively) will markedly reduce the cardiovascular action of this indirect-acting sympathomimetic. Metaraminol has a similar mechanism but more prolonged duration of action than ephedrine.

Phosphodiesterase Inhibitors

Preclinical Pharmacology

Phosphodiesterases are a group of structurally related enzymes that are responsible for a wide range of physiologic actions. The tissue distribution and subcellular isoforms of these enzymes have been intensively studied, and at least seven different subtypes that hydrolyze the second messengers cAMP or cyclic guanosine monophosphate (cGMP) have been identified. The phosphodiesterase inhibitors augment the intracellular actions of cAMP and cGMP by preventing their degradation.[80] Clinically used phosphodiesterase inhibitors may demonstrate some degree of selectivity for a particular isoenzyme, but this selectivity is dose-dependent. Human cardiac and vascular smooth muscle contain the type III phosphodiesterase isoenzyme bound to the sarcoplasmic reticulum[93] that facilitates the cleavage of cAMP to AMP. Unlike aminophylline and caffeine that attenuate that activity of most phosphodiesterase isoforms, selective inhibition of cardiac phosphodiesterase III by bypiridines (e.g., milrinone and inamrinone) or imidazoline (e.g., enoximone and piroximone) produces a series of alterations in intracellular Ca^{2+} regulation that enhance myocardial contractility independent of catecholamine release or β adrenoceptor activation. Increases in cAMP concentration produced by these drugs augment the activity of protein kinase A and lead to the phosphorylation of the voltage-dependent Ca^{2+} channel[94] and the sarcoplasmic reticulum regulatory protein phospholamban.[95] The normal inhibition of sarcoplasmic reticular Ca^{2+}-ATPases produced by phospholamban is attenuated by this cAMP-mediated phosphorylation,[95,96] leading to enhanced diastolic Ca^{2+} storage in and increased systolic Ca^{2+} release from this organelle.[97] Thus cardiac phosphodiesterase III inhibitors not only exert positive inotropic actions by increasing the amount of Ca^{2+} available for contractile activation but also facilitate diastolic relaxation by enhancing Ca^{2+} removal from the myoplasm. This latter positive lusitropic effect may contribute to improvements in diastolic function observed after administration of these drugs to patients with heart failure.[98]

Clinical Pharmacology

Phosphodiesterase III inhibitors cause dose-dependent arterial and venous vasodilation by increasing cAMP concentration and indirectly activating cGMP-dependent protein kinase[99] in vascular smooth muscle. In fact, the propensity of phosphodiesterase III inhibitors to enhance contractile function and simultaneously act as potent vasodilators led to use of the term *inodilator* to describe their cardiovascular effects. All phosphodiesterase III inhibitors, including isoproterenol, produce more pronounced vasodilation than β adrenoceptor agonists.[100] Reductions in systemic and pulmonary vascular resistances enhance LV and RV ejection, respectively. The reduction in LV afterload contributes to the increases in cardiac output, LV/arterial coupling, and mechanical efficiency observed with these drugs in vivo.[101] The relative importance of the positive inotropic effects versus the LV afterload-reducing properties of phosphodiesterase III inhibitors in augmenting cardiac output has been intensely debated,[102] but it is likely that both actions contribute substantially to improvements in overall cardiovascular performance. The declines in pulmonary vascular resistance[103] produced by phosphodiesterase III inhibitors may be especially beneficial in patients with pulmonary hypertension who are undergoing cardiac surgery[104,105] or heart transplantation.[106] However, the pulmonary vasodilat-

ing properties of phosphodiesterase III inhibitors may increase intrapulmonary shunt fraction and cause arterial hypoxemia.[107] Phosphodiesterase III inhibition also causes dilation of venous capacitance vessels, leading to reductions in LV and RV preload (e.g., pulmonary capillary occlusion and central venous pressures, respectively). The decreases in preload and afterload produced by phosphodiesterase III inhibitors may contribute to reductions in myocardial oxygen consumption observed with these drugs in patients with heart failure, despite simultaneous positive inotropic and chronotropic effects.[108] Mean arterial pressure is preserved or modestly reduced during administration of phosphodiesterase III inhibitors as long as LV preload is adequately maintained, because increases in cardiac output compensate for simultaneous declines in systemic vascular resistance.[109]

Phosphodiesterase III inhibitors produce less tachycardia than catecholamines, but these drugs are arrhythmogenic because they increase intracellular cAMP and Ca^{2+} concentration.[110,111] The tachycardia caused by phosphodiesterase III inhibitors may be eliminated by concomitant administration of a selective β_1 adrenoceptor antagonist without adversely affecting the positive inotropic response.[112] Phosphodiesterase III inhibitors block platelet aggregation,[113] suppress neointimal hyperplasia associated with endothelial injury,[114] and attenuate inflammatory cytokine formation after cardiopulmonary bypass.[115] Phosphodiesterase III inhibitors also dilate native epicardial coronary arteries and arterial bypass conduits[116,117] and may produce anti-ischemic effects in patients with chronic stable angina.[118] These data suggest that phosphodiesterase III inhibitors may exert further beneficial actions in addition to their favorable effects on LV systolic and diastolic function in patients with coronary artery disease or heart failure. Notably, the relative pharmacologic efficacy of phosphodiesterase III inhibitors may be reduced to some degree in the failing heart,[119,120] but not to the extent observed with β adrenoceptor agonists. This observation has been attributed to up-regulation of inhibitory G proteins in heart failure[121] and not direct structural or functional alterations in the phosphodiesterase III isoenzyme itself.[93] Nevertheless, phosphodiesterase III inhibitors remain effective positive inotropic drugs in heart failure, in contrast to the markedly attenuated actions of β adrenoceptor agonists on contractile function in this setting.[108]

Phosphodiesterase III inhibitors are orally absorbed, and several large-scale, placebo-controlled, clinical trials[122-124] have been conducted to evaluate the efficacy of these drugs in the treatment of chronic New York Heart Association class IV heart failure. These drugs were shown to enhance cardiac performance in this patient population, but the long-term results of these studies were discouraging because significant increases in mortality rates were observed. The increase in mortality rates that occurred in these investigations was attributed to an increase in malignant ventricular arrhythmias and sudden death.[122] Nevertheless, interest in phosphodiesterase III inhibitors for use in chronic heart failure has been rekindled in recent years by the use of lower doses that do not produce substantial hemodynamic effects[125] with or without simultaneous administration of β adrenoceptor antagonists[126] to counteract adverse electrophysiologic side effects. Despite their apparently limited applicability in the setting of chronic heart failure, phosphodiesterase III inhibitors remain a mainstay in the treatment of acute LV dysfunction.

Milrinone

Milrinone is a bypiridine phosphodiesterase III inhibitor that has been used extensively during and after cardiac surgery. Milrinone is approximately 15 to 20 times more potent than the closely related bypiridine, inamrinone.[127] In contrast to inamrinone, milrinone does not cause thrombocytopenia after prolonged use in cardiac surgical patients.[128] Intravenous milrinone enhances LV function and produces arterial and venous vasodilation in patients emerging from cardiopulmonary bypass.[129,130] Milrinone also improves the probability of successful weaning of high-risk patients from cardiopulmonary bypass.[104] The pharmacokinetics and pharmacodynamics of milrinone have been extensively studied, and a 50 μg/kg loading dose was shown to be optimal compared with either 25 or 75 μg/kg doses for patients separating from cardiopulmonary bypass.[131] This 50 μg/kg loading dose may be used in combination with[132] or without[133] a 0.5 μg/kg per minute infusion to increase cardiac output and oxygen delivery. A similar pharmacokinetic profile may be used to improve oxygen delivery in patients in the intensive care unit.[134]

Inamrinone

Inamrinone was the first clinically used bypiridine phosphodiesterase III inhibitor. Inamrinone produces cardiovascular effects that are almost identical to milrinone.[130] Inamrinone increases cardiac output, reduces LV and RV filling pressures, and causes systemic and pulmonary vasodilation while heart rate and mean arterial pressure are relatively maintained in patients with severe congestive heart failure.[135] Inamrinone and dobutamine were shown to cause similar improvements in LV performance in patients with reduced cardiac output after CABG surgery.[136] Inamrinone and epinephrine were also equally efficacious in cardiac surgical patients with poor preoperative LV function.[137] Unlike milrinone, inamrinone rapidly produces clinically significant thrombocytopenia,[138] and its use for the treatment of acute and chronic LV failure has essentially been abandoned.

Enoximone

Enoximone is a highly selective, imidazoline-derivative, phosphodiesterase III inhibitor that is used in Europe and is currently being investigated in clinical trials in the United States. The cardiovascular actions of intravenous enoximone are similar to those produced by milrinone and inamrinone.[139] Recent evidence indicates that oral enoximone administered in doses that do not cause hemodynamic effects may increase functional capacity in patients with severe congestive heart failure.[125] These data suggest that enoximone may play a role in the treatment of chronic

heart failure, but further study is needed to support this hypothesis.

Myofilament Calcium Sensitizers

Preclinical Pharmacology

A new class of positive inotropic drugs, the myofilament Ca^{2+} sensitizers, has been the subject of considerable experimental and clinical investigation in recent years. These drugs, including pimobendan, sulmazole, MCI-154, and levosimendan, may represent an important therapeutic approach in the pharmacologic management of heart failure.[12,140] Unlike catecholamines, phosphodiesterase III inhibitors, and digitalis glycosides, myofilament Ca^{2+} sensitizers improve contractile function independent of increases in intracellular cAMP or Ca^{2+} concentration. Instead, myofilament Ca^{2+} sensitizers enhance the response of the myofilament regulatory proteins or contractile elements to Ca^{2+} without specifically altering the availability of this ion. As a result, interaction between actin and myosin filaments is prolonged, and a positive inotropic effect is observed. Desensitization of the myofilaments to activator Ca^{2+} is known to occur during myocardial hypoxia, ischemia, and stunning,[141] and myofilament Ca^{2+} sensitizers may be particularly useful drugs during these pathologic conditions.[142] Because of their mechanism of action, myofilament Ca^{2+} sensitizers have the potential to adversely inhibit diastolic dissociation of Ca^{2+} from the contractile apparatus, delay relaxation of the cardiac myocyte, and produce diastolic dysfunction. However, the majority of drugs in this class are potent inhibitors of cardiac phosphodiesterase III, an action that accelerates LV isovolumic relaxation and enhances early LV filling during myofilament Ca^{2+} sensitization. The phosphodiesterase III-inhibiting properties of the majority of myofilament Ca^{2+} sensitizers also produce arterial and venous vasodilation and further enhance inotropic state. The myofilament Ca^{2+} sensitizing characteristics of these drugs have been demonstrated convincingly in vitro,[143] but the relative contribution of this Ca^{2+} sensitization to the increases in contractile state observed with these mixed myofilament Ca^{2+} sensitizer/phosphodiesterase III inhibitors remains somewhat controversial in vivo. Nevertheless, it appears likely that both mechanisms play a role in the positive inotropic effects of these drugs.

Clinical Pharmacology

Myofilament Ca^{2+} sensitizers have been shown to decrease LV filling pressure, mean arterial pressure, and pulmonary and systemic vascular resistances and to dramatically increase cardiac output in patients with end-stage heart failure[144,145] and coronary artery disease.[146] Modest reductions in arterial pressure observed with these drugs are similar to those produced by pure phosphodiesterase III inhibitors and respond to increases in LV preload. Myofilament Ca^{2+} sensitizers also improve LV-arterial coupling and mechanical efficiency,[101] while causing only minimal increases in heart rate and myocardial oxygen consumption.[147,148]

Pimobendan

Pimobendan is a benzimidazole pyridazine derivative myofilament Ca^{2+} sensitizer[149] that is currently used for treatment of heart failure in Japan. Pimobendan produces positive inotropic effects by increasing Ca^{2+} binding to troponin C[150] and inhibiting cardiac phosphodiesterase III.[151] Similar to pure phosphodiesterase III inhibitors, pimobendan enhances myocardial contractility without increasing myocardial oxygen consumption, because the vasodilating properties of the drug simultaneously improve LV loading conditions in the failing heart.[152] Pimobendan also increases myocardial blood flow[151] and may exert antiplatelet effects that potentially improve dysfunctional microcirculation.[153] Initial clinical trials of oral pimobendan indicated that this myofilament Ca^{2+} sensitizer increases exercise tolerance and improves quality of life in patients with heart failure.[154,155] However, further development of pimobendan as a chronic treatment for heart failure was halted in the United States because results of another multicenter clinical trial suggested that the drug was associated with an increase in mortality rates.[156]

Levosimendan

Levosimendan is a myofilament Ca^{2+} sensitizer that increases myocardial contractility by binding to troponin C and stabilizing the Ca^{2+}-bound conformational state of this protein without directly affecting actin/myosin interaction or altering the intracellular actions of the cAMP.[157-160] Unlike other drugs in this class of positive inotropic agents, enhanced Ca^{2+} binding to troponin C produced by levosimendan is dependent on the intracellular Ca^{2+} concentration. Myofilament Ca^{2+} sensitivity is augmented in the presence of greater systolic Ca^{2+} concentrations but is unaffected by the lower Ca^{2+} concentrations present during diastole.[143,161] This unique selectivity enhances contractility while simultaneously preserving relaxation.[159] Levosimendan augments myocardial contractility, improves indices of diastolic function, and reduces LV preload and afterload in the healthy,[162-164] cardiomyopathic,[148,165] and postischemic, reperfused heart.[142] Unlike other myofilament Ca^{2+} sensitizers, levosimendan also activates ATP-sensitive potassium (K_{ATP}) channels in arterial vascular smooth muscle[166] and ventricular myocardium.[167] Levosimendan-induced K_{ATP} channel activation may contribute to a reduction of myocardial ischemic injury[168] by stimulation of this endogenous cardioprotective mechanism.[169] Levosimendan has been shown to enhance cardiac performance in patients after cardiopulmonary bypass[170] and in those with congestive heart failure.[145,171,172] Further clinical trials are currently being conducted with levosimendan.

Thyroid Hormone

Abnormalities in thyroid hormone metabolism may occur in patients with congestive heart failure. Reversal of decreases in free triiodothyronine (T_3) concentration by administration of exogenous T_3 may enhance LV function and improve the short-term prognosis of patients with heart failure.[173] T_3 causes acute increases in myocardial contractility in papillary muscles[174] and in isolated[175] and intact hearts.[176] The positive inotropic effects of T_3 have been attributed to increases in sarcolemmal Ca^{2+} influx through the voltage-dependent Ca^{2+} channel[177,178] combined with enhanced activity of Ca^{2+}-ATPases in the sarcolemma and sarcoplasmic reticulum[179] independent of β adrenoceptor–mediated signal transduction.[180] However, T_3 may enhance β receptor density[181] and sensitivity[182] in hypothyroid states including those associated with heart failure. T_3 produces immediate and sustained improvements of LV systolic and diastolic function independent of alterations in the determinants of myocardial oxygen consumption in cardiomyopathic dogs.[176] The prolonged actions of T_3 correlate with the time-course of nuclear thyroid hormone receptor up-regulation[183] and the subsequent transcription and translation of sarcoplasmic reticular Ca^{2+}-ATPase.[184]

T_3 improves the functional recovery of stunned myocardium[185,186] and enhances contractility in experimental models of myocardial infarction and ventricular remodeling.[187,188] T_3 also produces beneficial hemodynamic effects in patients with acute myocardial infarction[189] and after sudden cardiac death,[190] and it may improve functional capacity in patients with idiopathic dilated cardiomyopathy.[191] T_3 concentrations have been shown to be reduced after cardiopulmonary bypass independent of hemodilution and systemic heparinization.[192] A decrease in T_3 levels was also observed in the setting of heart transplantation.[193] These observations encouraged exploration of the use of T_3 to improve contractile function during and after cardiac surgery. Current clinical evidence suggests that T_3 supplementation may acutely enhance cardiac performance, hasten the recovery of normal hemodynamics, and reduce the need for other inotropic support in patients with LV dysfunction after cardiopulmonary bypass,[194-196] but other studies have not supported these conclusions.[197-199] Thus the use of T_3 for inotropic support after cardiopulmonary bypass remains controversial and cannot be recommended for routine clinical practice.

Practical Aspects of Drug Administration

The combination of inotropic drugs is often used in an attempt to optimize the beneficial actions and minimize the adverse effects of each drug alone. Such a combination of drugs may produce an additive, synergistic, or antagonistic effect. Although dobutamine and epinephrine are each potent activators of the β_1 adrenoceptor, their combination has been shown not to enhance cardiac output beyond that observed with either drug alone.[200] These results were attributed to differences in β_1 adrenoceptor affinity between epinephrine and dobutamine. Calcium has also been shown to attenuate the effects of epinephrine in patients emerging from cardiopulmonary bypass after CABG.[42] These actions are probably mediated by direct inhibition of adenylyl cyclase by calcium.[201,202] In contrast, the combination of a β_1 adrenoceptor agonist and a phosphodiesterase III inhibitor enhances LV performance in an additive fashion.[203] This beneficial combination results from increases in intracellular cAMP concentration achieved through β_1 adrenoceptor–mediated activation of adenylyl cyclase and simultaneous reductions in the degradation of the second messenger by phosphodiesterase III inhibition. Combination therapy also facilitates a reduction in dose of the β_1 adrenoceptor agonist and may attenuate the down-regulation of the β_1 adrenoceptor observed during the administration of high doses of catecholamines. This combination of a β_1 adrenoceptor agonist and a phosphodiesterase III inhibitor is frequently used to improve contractile function after cardiopulmonary bypass in patients undergoing cardiac surgery.[203,204] Drugs that enhance myofilament Ca^{2+} sensitivity may also potentiate the positive inotropic effects of other agents that increase intracellular cAMP concentration.[164]

these drugs increase mortality rates.[205] New positive inotropic drugs that act directly on the contractile apparatus and that may increase myocardial contractility without causing adverse arrhythmogenesis are currently under clinical investigation. However, catecholamines and phosphodiesterase III inhibitors remain the most common drugs used to improve contractility in patients with acute LV dysfunction. A reduction in LV afterload using an arterial vasodilator should be initially considered to increase cardiac output before an inotropic drug is selected.[206] Use of a specific positive inotropic drug is highly dependent on the hemodynamic status of each patient, and a thorough knowledge of the cardiovascular pharmacology of these drugs is required to make the most rational choice.

Dosage and Administration

Digitalis Glycosides

Digoxin (Lanoxin; GlaxoSmithKline, Philadelphia, Pa): administered by mouth or intravenously. It is available as 0.125-, 0.25- or 0.5-mg tablets, as 0.05-, 0.1-, or 0.2-mg capsules, and as a 0.05-mg/mL elixir. The recommended dosage is 0.125 to 0.5 mg/day.

Digitoxin (Crystodigin; Merck, Whitehouse Station, Nj): administered by mouth. It is available as 0.05- or 0.1-mg tablets. The recommended dosage is 0.05 to 0.3 mg/day.

Phosphodiesterase Inhibitors

Milrinone (Primacor; Dow Chemical, Tarrytown, Ny): administered intravenously. It is available as 1-mg/mL solution for intravenous injection and as a 20-μg/mL solution for intravenous infusion. The loading dose is 50 μg/kg over 10 minutes, and the recommended infusion rate is 0.375 to 0.75 μg/kg per minute.

Inamrinone (Inocor): administered intravenously. It is available as a 5-mg/mL solution for intravenous injection. The loading dose is 0.75 mg/kg intravenously over 2 to 3 minutes, and the recommended infusion rate is 5 to 10 μg/kg per minute.

Catecholamines: see Chapter 34 for a detailed discussion.

Summary

The development of new drugs that enhance contractile performance in patients with acute and chronic heart failure remains an important pharmacologic objective. With the exception of the digitalis glycosides, all currently available catecholamines and phosphodiesterase III inhibitors cannot be used for the chronic treatment of heart failure because

References

1. Dougherty AH, Naccarelli GV, Gray EL, et al: Congestive heart failure with normal systolic function. Am J Cardiol 54:778–782, 1984.
2. Soufer R, Wohlgelernter D, Vita NA, et al: Intact systolic left ventricular function in clinical congestive heart failure. Am J Cardiol 55:1032–1036, 1985.
3. Pagel PS, Grossman W, Haering JM, Warltier DC: Left ventricular diastolic function in the normal and diseased heart: Perspectives for the anesthesiologist. (Second of two parts). Anesthesiology 79:1104–1120, 1993.
4. Pagel PS, Grossman W, Haering JM, Warltier DC: Left ventricular diastolic function in the normal and diseased heart: Perspectives for the anesthesiologist. (First of two parts). Anesthesiology 79:836–854, 1993.
5. Packer M: The neurohormonal hypothesis: A theory to explain the mechanism of disease progression in heart failure. J Am Coll Cardiol 20:248–254, 1992.
6. Komamura K, Shannon RP, Ihara T, et al: Exhaustion of Frank-Starling mechanism in conscious dogs with heart failure. Am J Physiol 265:H1119–H1131, 1993.
7. Armstrong PW, Moe GW: Medical advances in the treatment of congestive heart failure. Circulation 88:2941–2952, 1993.
8. van Zwieten PA: Current and newer approaches in the drug treatment of congestive heart failure. Cardiovasc Drugs Ther 10:693–702, 1996.
9. Eichhorn EJ, Bristow MR: Practical guidelines for initiation of beta-adrenergic blockade in patients with chronic heart failure. Am J Cardiol 79:794–798, 1997.
10. Pagel PS, Warltier DC: Mechanical function of the left ventricle. In Yaksh TL, Lynch III C, Zapol WM, et al (eds): Anesthesia: Biologic Foundations. Philadelphia, Lippincott-Raven, 1998, pp 1081–1133.
11. Feldman AM: Classification of positive inotropic agents. J Am Coll Cardiol 22:1223–1227, 1993.
12. Pagel PS, Haikala H, Pentikainen PJ, et al: Pharmacology of levosimendan: A new myofilament calcium sensitizer. Cardiovasc Drug Rev 14:286–316, 1996.
13. Johnston WE, Robertie PG, Butterworth IV JF, et al: Is calcium or ephedrine superior to placebo for emergence from cardiopulmonary bypass? J Cardiothorac Vasc Anesth 6:528–534, 1992.
14. Royster RL, Butterworth IV JF, Prielipp RC, et al: A randomized, placebo-controlled evaluation of calcium chloride and epinephrine for inotropic support after emergence from cardiopulmonary bypass. Anesth Analg 74:3–13, 1992.
15. Sanders MR, Kostis JB, Frishman WH: The use of inotropic agents in acute and chronic congestive heart failure. Med Clin N Am 73:283–314, 1989.
16. Applefeld MM, Roffman DS: Digitalis and other positive catecholamine-like inotropic agents in the management of congestive heart failure. Am J Med 80:40–45, 1986.
17. Hauptman PJ, Kelly RA: Digitalis. Circulation 99:1265–1270, 1999.

18. Blaustein MP: Physiological effects of endogenous ouabain: Control of intracellular Ca^{2+} stores and cell responsiveness. Am J Physiol 264:C1367–C1387, 1993.

19. Harrison SM, McCall E, Boyett MR: The relationship between contraction and intracellular sodium in rat and guinea-pig ventricular myocytes. J Physiol 449:517–550, 1992.

20. Schmidt TA, Allen PD, Colucci WS, et al: No adaptation to digitalization as evaluated by digitalis receptor (Na,K-ATPase) quantification in explanted hearts from donors without heart disease and from digitalized recipients with end-stage heart failure. Am J Cardiol 71:110–114, 1993.

21. Kulick DL, Rahimtoola SH: Current role of digitalis therapy in patients with congestive heart failure. JAMA 265:2995–2997, 1991.

22. Ferguson DW, Berg WJ, Sanders JS, et al: Sympathoinhibitory responses to digitalis glycosides in heart failure patients. Direct evidence from sympathetic neural recordings. Circulation 80:65–77, 1989.

23. Gheorghiade M: Digoxin therapy in chronic heart failure. Cardiovasc Drug Ther 11:279–283, 1997.

24. Newton GE, Tong JH, Schofield AM, et al: Digoxin reduces cardiac sympathetic activity in severe congestive heart failure. J Am Coll Cardiol 28:155–161, 1996.

25. Wang W, Chen JS, Zucker IH: Carotid sinus baroreceptor sensitivity in experimental heart failure. Circulation 81:1959–1966, 1990.

26. Uretsky BF, Young JB, Shahidi FE, et al: Randomized study assessing the effect of digoxin withdrawal in patients with mild to moderate chronic congestive heart failure: Results of the PROVED trial. PROVED Investigative Group. J Am Coll Cardiol 22:955–962, 1993.

27. Packer M, Gheorghiade M, Young JB, et al: Withdrawal of digoxin from patients with chronic heart failure treated with angiotensin-converting enzyme inhibitors. RADIANCE study. N Engl J Med 329:1–7, 1993.

28. Anonymous: The effect of digoxin on mortality and morbidity in patients with heart failure. The Digitalis Investigation Group. N Engl J Med 336:525–533, 1997.

29. Motulsky HJ, Insel PA: Adrenergic receptors in man: Direct identification, physiologic regulation, and clinical alterations. N Engl J Med 307:18–29, 1982.

30. Hoffman BB, Lefkowitz RJ: Catecholamines, sympathomimetic drugs, and adrenergic receptor antagonists. In Hardman JG, Limbird LE, Molinoff PB, et al (eds): Goodman and Gilman's The Pharmacological Basis of Therapeutics, 9th ed. New York, McGraw-Hill, 1996, pp 199–248.

31. Katz AM: Cyclic adenosine monophosphate effects on the myocardium: A man who blows hot and cold with one breath. J Am Coll Cardiol 2:143–149, 1983.

32. Bristow MR, Hershberger RE, Port JD, et al: Beta-adrenergic pathways in nonfailing and failing human ventricular myocardium. Circulation 82:I12-I25, 1990.

33. Post SR, Hammond HK, Insel PA: Beta-adrenergic receptors and receptor signaling in heart failure. Annu Rev Pharmacol Toxicol 39:343–360, 1999.

34. Booth JV, Landolfo KP, Chesnut LC, et al: Acute depression of myocardial beta-adrenergic receptor signaling during cardiopulmonary bypass: Impairment of the adenylyl cyclase moiety. Duke Heart Center Perioperative Desensitization Group. Anesthesiology 89:602–611, 1998.

35. Marty J, Nimier M, Rocchiccioli C, et al: Beta-adrenergic receptor function is acutely altered in surgical patients. Anesth Analg 71:1–8, 1990.

36. Cork RC, Azari DM, McQueen KA, et al: Effect of esmolol given during cardiopulmonary bypass on fractional area of contraction from transesophageal echocardiography. Anesth Analg 81:219–224, 1995.

37. Maze M, Buttermann A: G protein-coupled receptors. In Yaksh TL, Lynch III C, Zapol WM, et al (eds): Anesthesia: Biologic Foundations. Philadelphia, Lippincott-Raven, 1998, pp 55–64.

38. Warltier DC, Pagel PS, Kersten JR: Approaches to the prevention of perioperative myocardial ischemia. Anesthesiology 92:253–259, 2000.

39. DiSesa VJ: Pharmacologic support for postoperative low cardiac output. Semin Thorac Cardiovasc Surg 3:13–23, 1991.

40. Leenen FH, Chan YK, Smith DL, Reeves RA: Epinephrine and left ventricular function in humans: Effects of beta-1 vs nonselective beta blockade. Clin Pharmacol Ther 43:519–528, 1988.

41. Butterworth IV JF, Prielipp RC, Royster RL, et al: Dobutamine increases heart rate more than epinephrine in patients recovering from aortocoronary bypass surgery. J Cardiothorac Vasc Anesth 6:535–541, 1992.

42. Zaloga GP, Strickland RA, Butterworth IV JF, et al: Calcium attenuates epinephrine's β-adrenergic effects in postoperative heart surgery patients. Circulation 81:196–200, 1990.

43. Tinker J: Pro: strong inotropes (i.e., epinephrine) should be drugs of first choice during emergence from cardiopulmonary bypass. J Cardiothorac Anesth 1:256–258, 1987.

44. Bollaert PE, Bauer P, Audibert G, et al: Effects of epinephrine on hemodynamics and oxygen metabolism in dopamine-resistant septic shock. Chest 98:949–953, 1990.

45. Sung BH, Robinston C, Thadani U, et al: Effects of l-epinephrine on hemodynamics and cardiac function in coronary disease: Dose-response studies. Clin Pharmacol Ther 43:308–316, 1988.

46. Feigl EO: Coronary physiology. Physiol Rev 63:1–205, 1983.

47. Feigl EO: Adrenergic control of transmural coronary blood flow. Basic Res Cardiol 85:167–176, 1990.

48. Meadows D, Edwards JD, Wilkins RG, Nightingale P: Reversal of intractable septic shock with norepinephrine therapy. Crit Care Med 16:663–666, 1988.

49. Kristof AS, Magder S: Low systemic vascular resistance state in patients undergoing cardiopulmonary bypass. Crit Care Med 27:1121–1127, 1999.

50. Fullerton DA, Jones SD, Jaggers J, et al: Effective control of pulmonary vascular resistance with inhaled nitric oxide after cardiac operation. J Thorac Cardiovasc Surg 111:753–762, 1996.

51. Rich GF, Murphy Jr GD, Roos CM, Johns RA: Inhaled nitric oxide. Selective pulmonary vasodilation in cardiac surgical patients. Anesthesiology 78:1028–1035, 1993.

52. Ghignone M, Girling L, Prewitt R: Volume expansion versus norepinephrine in treatment of a low cardiac output complicating an acute increase in right ventricular afterload in dogs. Anesthesiology 60:132–135, 1984.

53. Richer M, Robert S, Lebel M: Renal hemodynamics during norepinephrine and low-dose dopamine infusions in man. Crit Care Med 24:1150–1156, 1996.

54. Post 4th JB, Frishman WH: Fenoldopam: A new dopamine agonist for the treatment of hypertensive urgencies and emergencies. J Clin Pharmacol 38:2–13, 1998.

55. Garwood S, Hines R: Perioperative renal preservation: Dopexamine and fenoldopam-new agents to augment renal performance. Semin Anesth Perioper Med Pain 17:308–318, 1998.

56. Desjars P, Pinaud M, Potel G, et al: A reappraisal of norepinephrine therapy in human septic shock. Crit Care Med 15:134–137, 1997.

57. Goldberg LI, Rajfer SI: Dopamine receptors: Applications in clinical cardiology. Circulation 72:245–248, 1985.

58. Bailey JM: Dopamine. One size does not fit all. Anesthesiology 92:303–305, 2000.

59. MacGregor DA, Smith TE, Prielipp RC, et al: Pharmacokinetics of dopamine in healthy male subjects. Anesthesiology 92:338–346, 2000.

60. Griffin MJ, Hines RL: Management of perioperative ventricular dysfunction. J Cardiothorac Vasc Anesth 15:90–106, 2001.

61. Davis RF, Lappas DG, Kirklin JK, et al: Acute oliguria after cardiopulmonary bypass: Renal functional improvement with low-dose dopamine infusion. Crit Care Med 10:852–856, 1982.

62. Notterman DA: Inotropic agents. Catecholamines, digoxin, amrinone. Crit Care Clin 7:583–613, 1991.

63. Frishman WH, Hotchkiss H: Selective and nonselective dopamine receptor agonists: An innovative approach to cardiovascular disease treatment. Am Heart J 132:861–870, 1996.

64. DiSesa VJ: The rational selection of inotropic drugs in cardiac surgery. J Card Surg 2:385–406, 1987.

65. DiSesa VJ, Gold JP, Shemin RJ, et al: Comparison of dopamine and dobutamine in patients requiring postoperative circulatory support. Clin Cardiol 9:253–256, 1986.

66. Steen PA, Tinker JH, Pluth JR, et al: Efficacy of dopamine, dobutamine, and epinephrine during emergence from cardiopulmonary bypass in man. Circulation 57:378–384, 1978.

67. Sterling RP, Taegtmeyer H, Turner SA, et al: Comparison of dopamine and dobutamine therapy during intraaortic balloon pumping for treatment of postcardiotomy low-output syndrome. Ann Thorac Surg 38:37–41, 1984.

68. Kabas JS, Spratt JA, Davis JW, et al: The effects of dopamine on

myocardial functional recovery after reversible ischemic injury. J Thorac Cardiovasc Surg 100:715–723, 1990.

69. Lekven J, Semb G: Effect of dopamine and calcium on lipolysis and myocardial ischemic injury following acute coronary artery occlusion in the dog. Circ Res 34:349–359, 1974.

70. Brown RA, Dixon J, Farmer JB, et al: Dopexamine: A novel agonist at peripheral dopamine receptors and beta2-adrenoceptors. Br J Pharmacol 85:599–608, 1985.

71. Tan LB, Littler WA, Murray RG: Comparison of the haemodynamic effects of dopexamine and dobutamine in patients with severe congestive heart failure. Int J Cardiol 30:203–208, 1991.

72. Fitton A, Benfield P: Dopexamine hydrochloride. A review of its pharmacodynamic and pharmacokinetic properties and therapeutic potential in acute cardiac insufficiency. Drugs 39:308–330, 1990.

73. Mousdale S, Clyburn PA, Mackie AM, et al: Comparison of the effects of dopamine, dobutamine, and dopexamine upon renal blood flow: A study in normal healthy volunteers. Br J Clin Pharmacol 85:555–560, 1988.

74. Hunter DN, Gray H, Mudaliar Y, et al: The effects of dopexamine hydrochloride on cardiopulmonary haemodynamics following cardiopulmonary bypass surgery. Int J Cardiol 23:365–371, 1989.

75. Santman FW: Prolonged infusion of varied doses of dopexamine hydrochloride for low cardiac output after cardiac surgery. J Cardiothorac Vasc Anesth 6:568–572, 1992.

76. MacGregor DA, Butterworth IV JF, Zaloga GP, et al: Hemodynamic and renal effects of dopamine and dobutamine in patients with reduced cardiac output following coronary artery bypass grafting. Chest 106:835–841, 1994.

77. Berendes E, Mollhoff T, Van Aken H, et al: Effects of dopexamine on creatinine clearance, systemic inflammation, and splanchnic oxygenation in patients undergoing coronary artery bypass grafting. Anesth Analg 84:950–957, 1997.

78. Cain SM, Curtis S: Systemic and regional oxygen uptake and delivery and lactate flux in endotoxic dogs infused with dopexamine. Crit Care Med 19:1552–1560, 1991.

79. Colardyn FC, Vandenbogaerde JF, Vogelaers DP, Verbeke JH: Use of dopexamine hydrochloride in patients with septic shock. Crit Care Med 17:999–1003, 1989.

80. Homoud MK, Chuttani K, Konstam MA: Positive inotropic agents in congestive heart failure. Coron Artery Dis 4:44–52, 1993.

81. Binkley PF, Van Fossen DB, Nunziata E, et al: Influence of positive inotropic therapy on pulsatile hydraulic load and ventricular-vascular coupling in congestive heart failure. J Am Coll Cardiol 15:1127–1135, 1990.

82. Keren G, Laniado S, Sonnenblick EH, LeJemtel TH: Dynamics of functional mitral regurgitation during dobutamine therapy in patients with severe congestive heart failure: A Doppler echocardiographic study. Am Heart J 118:748–754, 1989.

83. Ruffolo RR Jr: The pharmacology of dobutamine. Am J Med Sci 294:244–248, 1987.

84. Aronson S, Dupont F, Savage R, et al: Changes in regional myocardial function after coronary artery bypass are predicted by intraoperative low-dose dobutamine echocardiography. Anesthesiology 93:685–692, 2000.

85. Shoemaker WC, Appel PL, Kram HB, et al: Comparison of hemodynamic and oxygen transport effects of dopamine and dobutamine in critically ill surgical patients. Chest 96:120–126, 1989.

86. Amin DK, Shah PK, Shellock FG, et al: Comparative hemodynamic effects of intravenous dobutamine and MDL-17,043, a new cardioactive drug, in severe congestive heart failure. Am Heart J 109:91–98, 1985.

87. Kikura M, Levy JH: New cardiac drugs. Int Anesthesiol Clin 33:21–37, 1995.

88. Leier CV, Heban PT, Huss P, et al: Comparative systemic and regional hemodynamic effects of dopamine and dobutamine in patients with cardiomyopathic heart failure. Circulation 58:466–475, 1978.

89. Tinker JH, Tarhan S, White RD, et al: Dobutamine for inotropic support during emergence from cardiopulmonary bypass. Anesthesiology 44:281–286, 1976.

90. Cannom DS, Rider AK, Stinson EB, Harrison DC: Electrophysiologic studies in denervated transplanted human heart. II. Response to norepinephrine, isoproterenol and propranolol. Am J Cardiol 36:859–866, 1975.

91. Daoud FS, Reeves JT, Kelly DB: Isoproterenol as a potential pulmonary vasodilator in primary pulmonary hypertension. Am J Cardiol 42:817–822, 1978.

92. O'Connor SE, Langer SZ: Sympathomimetic amines and dopamine receptor agonists. In Singh BN, Dzau VJ, Vanhoutte PM, Woosley RL (eds): Cardiovascular Pharmacology and Therapeutics. New York, Churchill Livingstone, 1994, pp 63–83.

93. Movsesian MA, Smith CJ, Krall J, et al: Sarcoplasmic reticulum-associated cyclic adenosine 5'-monophosphate phosphodiesterase activity in normal and failing human hearts. J Clin Invest 88:15–19, 1991.

94. Kajimoto K, Hagiwara N, Kasanuki H, Hosoda S: Contribution of phosphodiesterase isozymes to the regulation of L-type calcium current in human cardiac myocytes. Br J Pharmacol 121:1549–1556, 1997.

95. Koss KL, Kranias EG: Phospholamban: A prominent regulator of myocardial contractility. Circ Res 79:1059–1063, 1996.

96. Luo W, Grupp IL, Harrer J, et al: Targeted ablation of the phospholamban gene is associated with markedly enhanced myocardial contractility and loss of β-agonist stimulation. Circ Res 75:401–409, 1994.

97. Auffermann W, Stefenelli T, Wu ST, et al: Influence of positive inotropic agents on intracellular calcium transients. Part I. Normal rat heart. Am Heart J 118:1219–1227, 1989.

98. Monrad ES, McKay RG, Baim DS, et al: Improvement in indexes of diastolic performance in patients with congestive heart failure treated with milrinone. Circulation 70:1030–1037, 1984.

99. Jiang H, Colbran JL, Francis SH, Corbin JD: Direct evidence for cross-activation of cGMP-dependent protein kinase by cAMP in pig coronary arteries. J Biol Chem 267:1015–1019, 1992.

100. Firth BG, Ratner AV, Grassman ED, et al: Assessment of the inotropic and vasodilator effects of amrinone versus isoproterenol. Am J Cardiol 54:1331–1336, 1984.

101. Pagel PS, Hettrick DA, Warltier DC: Comparison of the effects of levosimendan, pimobendan, and milrinone in canine left ventricular-arterial coupling and mechanical efficiency. Basic Res Cardiol 91:296–307, 1996.

102. Packer M: The development of positive inotropic agents for chronic heart failure: How have we gone astray? J Am Coll Cardiol 22(4 suppl A):119A–126A, 1993.

103. Konstam MA, Cohen SR, Salem DN, et al: Effects of amrinone on right ventricular function: Predominance of afterload reduction. Circulation 74:359–366, 1986.

104. Feneck RO: Intravenous milrinone following cardiac surgery: II. Influence of baseline hemodynamics and patient factors on therapeutic response. The European Milrinone Multicentre Trial Group. J Cardiothorac Vasc Anesth 6:563–567, 1992.

105. Doolan LA, Jones EF, Kalman J, et al: A placebo-controlled trial verifying the efficacy of milrinone in weaning high-risk patients from cardiopulmonary bypass. J Cardiothorac Vasc Anesth 11:37–41, 1997.

106. Chen EP, Bittner HB, Davis RD, Van Trigt P: Hemodynamic and inotropic effects of milrinone after heart transplantation in the setting of recipient pulmonary hypertension. J Heart Lung Transplant 17:669–678, 1998.

107. Prielipp RC, Butterworth IV JF, Zaloga GP, et al: Effects of amrinone on cardiac index, venous oxygen saturation and venous admixture in patients recovering from cardiac surgery. Chest 99:820–825, 1991.

108. Konstam MA, Cody RJ: Short-term use of intravenous milrinone for heart failure. Am J Cardiol 75:822–826, 1995.

109. Wilmshurst PT, Thompson DS, Jenkins BS, et al: Haemodynamic effects of intravenous amrinone in patients with impaired left ventricular function. Br Heart J 49:77–82, 1983.

110. Tisdale JE, Patel R, Webb CR, et al: Electrophysiologic and proarrhythmic effects of intravenous inotropic agents. Prog Cardiovasc Dis 38:167–180, 1995.

111. Lubbe WF, Podzuweit T, Opie LH: Potential arrhythmogenic role of cyclic adenosine monophosphate (AMP) and cytosolic calcium overload: Implications for prophylactic effects of beta-blockers in myocardial infarction and proarrhythmic effects of phosphodiesterase inhibitors. J Am Coll Cardiol 19:1622–1633, 1992.

112. Alhashemi JA, Hooper J: Treatment of milrinone-associated tachycardia with beta-blockers. Can J Anaesth 45:67–70, 1998.

113. Barradas MA, Jagroop A, O'Donoghue S, et al: Effect of milrinone in human platelet shape change, aggregation and thromboxane A$_2$ synthesis: An in vitro study. Thromb Res 71:227–236, 1993.

114. Kondo K, Umemura K, Miyaji M, Nakashima M: Milrinone, a phosphodiesterase inhibitor, suppresses intimal thickening after photochemically induced endothelial injury in the mouse femoral artery. Atherosclerosis 142:133–138, 1999.

115. Hayashida N, Tomoeda H, Oda T, et al: Inhibitory effect of milrinone on cytokine production after cardiopulmonary bypass. Ann Thorac Surg 68:1661–1667, 1999.

116. Salmenpera M, Levy JH: The in vivo effect of phosphodiesterase inhibitors on the human internal mammary artery. Anesth Analg 82:954–957, 1996.

117. Cracowski JL, Stanke-Labesque F, Chavanon O, et al: Vasorelaxant actions of enoximone, dobutamine, and the combination on human arterial coronary bypass grafts. J Cardiovasc Pharmacol 34:741–748, 1999.

118. Dubrey SW, Gnanasakthy A, Stein WK, et al: Enoximone in chronic stable angina: A double-blind, placebo-controlled cross-over trial. J Cardiovasc Pharmacol 23:532–538, 1994.

119. Feldman MD, Copelas L, Gwathmey JK, et al: Deficient production of cyclic AMP: Pharmacologic evidence of an important cause of contractile dysfunction in patients with end-stage heart failure. Circulation 75:331–339, 1987.

120. Gilbert EM, Hershberger RE, Wiechmann RJ, et al: Pharmacologic and hemodynamic effects of combined β-agonist stimulation and phosphodiesterase inhibition in the failing human heart. Chest 108:1524–1532, 1995.

121. Feldman AM, Cates AE, Veazey WB, et al: Increase of the 40,000-mol wt pertussis toxin substrate (G protein) in the failing human heart. J Clin Invest 82:189–197, 1988.

122. Packer M, Carver JR, Rodeheffer RJ, et al: Effect of oral milrinone on mortality in severe chronic heart failure. The PROMISE Study Research Group. N Engl J Med 325:1468–1475, 1991.

123. Uretsky BF, Jessup M, Konstam MA, et al: Multicenter trial of oral enoximone in patients with moderate to moderately severe congestive heart failure. Lack of benefit compared with placebo. Enoximone Multicenter Trial Group. Circulation 82:774–780, 1990.

124. Cohn JN, Goldstein SO, Greenberg BH, et al: A dose-dependent increase in mortality with vesnarinone among patients with severe heart failure. N Engl J Med 339:1810–1816, 1998.

125. Lowes BD, Higginbotham M, Petrovich L, et al: Low dose enoximone improves exercise capacity in chronic heart failure. Enoximone Study Group. J Am Coll Cardiol 36:501–508, 2000.

126. Shakar SF, Abraham WT, Gilbert EM, et al: Combined oral positive inotropic and beta-blocker therapy for the treatment of refractory Class IV heart failure. J Am Coll Cardiol 31:1336–1340, 1998.

127. Feneck RO: Effects of variable dose milrinone in patients with low cardiac output after cardiac surgery. Am Heart J 121:1995–1999, 1991.

128. Kikura M, Lee MK, Safon RA, et al: The effects of milrinone on platelets in patients undergoing cardiac surgery. Anesth Analg 81:44–48, 1995.

129. Feneck RO: Intravenous milrinone following cardiac surgery: I. Effects of bolus infusion followed by variable dose maintenance infusion. The European Milrinone Multicentre Trial Group. J Cardiothorac Vasc Anesth 6:554–562, 1992.

130. Rathmell JP, Prielipp RC, Butterworth IV JF, et al: A multicenter, randomized, blind comparison of amrinone and milrinone after elective cardiac surgery. Anesth Analg 86:683–690, 1998.

131. Butterworth IV JF, Hines RL, Royster RL, James RL: A pharmacokinetic and pharmacodynamic evaluation of milrinone in adults undergoing cardiac surgery. Anesth Analg 81:783–792, 1995.

132. Bailey JM, Levy JH, Kikura M, et al: Pharmacokinetics of intravenous milrinone in patients undergoing cardiac surgery. Anesthesiology 81:616–622, 1994.

133. Lobato EB, Florete Jr O, Bingham HL: A single dose of milrinone facilitates separation from cardiopulmonary bypass in patients with pre-existing left ventricular dysfunction. Br J Anaesth 81:782–784, 1998.

134. Prielipp RC, MacGregor DA, Butterworth IV JF, et al: Pharmacodynamics and pharmacokinetics of milrinone administration to increase oxygen delivery in critically ill patients. Chest 109:1291–1301, 1996.

135. LeJemtel TH, Keung E, Sonnenblick EH, et al: Amrinone: A new nonglycosidic, nonadrenergic cardiotonic agent effective in the treatment of intractable myocardial failure in man. Circulation 59:1098–1104, 1979.

136. Dupuis J-Y, Bondy R, Cattran C, et al: Amrinone and dobutamine as primary treatment of low cardiac output syndrome following coronary artery surgery: A comparison of their effects on hemodynamics and outcome. J Cardiothorac Vasc Anesth 6:542–553, 1992.

137. Butterworth IV JF, Royster RL, Prielipp RC, et al: Amrinone in

138. Kinney EL, Ballard JO, Carlin B, Zelis R: Amrinone-mediated thrombocytopenia. Scand J Haematol 31:376–380, 1983.

139. Gibelin P, Dadoun-Dybal M, Candito M, et al: Hemodynamic effects of prolonged enoximone infusion (7 days) in patients with severe chronic heart failure. Cardiovasc Drugs Ther 7:333–336, 1993.

140. Hajjar RJ, Gwathmey JK: Calcium-sensitizing inotropic agents in the treatment of heart failure: A critical view. Cardiovasc Drugs Ther 5:961–965, 1991.

141. Soei LK, Sassen LMA, Fan DS, et al: Myofibrillar Ca^{2+} sensitization predominantly enhances function and mechanical efficiency of stunned myocardium. Circulation 90:959–969, 1994.

142. Jamali IN, Kersten JR, Pagel PS, et al: Intracoronary levosimendan enhances contractile function of stunned myocardium. Anesth Analg 85:23–29, 1997.

143. Haikala H, Linden I-B: Mechanisms of action of calcium-sensitizing drugs. J Cardiovasc Pharmacol 26(suppl 1):S10–19, 1995.

144. Remme WJ, Wiesfeld ACP, Look MP, Kruyssen HACM: Hemodynamic effects of intravenous pimobendan in patients with left ventricular dysfunction. J Cardiovasc Pharmacol 14(suppl 2):S41–S44, 1989.

145. Lilleberg J, Sundberg S, Nieminen MS: Dose-range study of a new calcium sensitizer, levosimendan, in patients with left ventricular dysfunction. J Cardiovasc Pharmacol 26(suppl 1):S63–S69, 1995.

146. Thormann J, Kramer W, Schlepper M: Hemodynamic and myocardial energetic changes induced by the new cardiotonic agent, AR-L 115, in patients with coronary artery disease. Am Heart J 104:1294–1302, 1982.

147. Just H, Drexler H, Hasenfuss G: Pathophysiology and treatment of congestive heart failure. Cardiology 84(suppl 2):99–107, 1994.

148. Todaka K, Wang J, Yi G-H, et al: Effects of levosimendan on myocardial contractility and oxygen consumption. J Pharmacol Exp Ther 279:120–127, 1996.

149. Fujino K, Sperelakis N, Solaro RJ: Sensitization of dog and guinea pig heart myofilaments to Ca^{2+} activation and the inotropic effect of pimobendan: Comparison with milrinone. Circ Res 63:911–922, 1988.

150. Solaro RJ, Fujino K, Sperelakis N: The positive inotropic effect of pimobendan involves stereospecific increases in the calcium sensitivity of cardiac myofilaments. J Cardiovasc Pharmacol 14(suppl 2):S7–S12, 1989.

151. Verdouw PD, Hartog JM, Duncker DJ, et al: Cardiovascular profile of pimobendan, a benzimidazole-pyridazinone derivative with vasodilating and inotropic properties. Eur J Pharmacol 126:21–30, 1986.

152. Hasenfuss G, Holubarsch C, Heiss HW, Just H: Influence of UDCG-115 on hemodynamics and myocardial energetics in patients with idiopathic dilated cardiomyopathy. Am Heart J 118:512–519, 1989.

153. Sasayama S: Inotropic agents in the treatment of heart failure: Despair or hope? Cardiovasc Drugs Ther 10:703–709, 1996.

154. Kubo SH, Gollub S, Bourge R, et al: Beneficial effects of pimobendan on exercise tolerance and quality of life in patients with heart failure. Results of a multicenter trial. The Pimobendan Multicenter Research Group. Circulation 85:942–949, 1992.

155. Sasayama S, Asanoi H, Kihara Y, et al: Clinical effects of long-term administration of pimobendan in patients with moderate congestive heart failure. Heart Vessels 9:113–120, 1994.

156. Lubsen J, Just H, Hjalmarsson AC, et al: Effect of pimobendan on exercise capacity in patients with heart failure: Main results from the Pimobendan in Congestive Heart Failure (PICO) trial. Heart 76:223–231, 1996.

157. Pollesello P, Ovaska M, Kaivola J, et al: Binding of a new Ca^{2+} sensitizer, levosimendan, to recombinant human cardiac troponin C. A molecular modelling, fluorescence probe, and proton nuclear magnetic resonance study. J Biol Chem 269:28584–28590, 1994.

158. Edes I, Kiss E, Kitada Y, et al: Effects of levosimendan, a cardiotonic agent targeted to troponin C, on cardiac function and on phosphorylation and Ca^{2+} sensitivity of cardiac myofibrils and sarcoplasmic reticulum in guinea pig heart. Circ Res 77:107–113, 1995.

159. Haikala H, Nissinen E, Etemadzadeh E, et al: Troponin C-mediated calcium sensitization induced by levosimendan does not impair relaxation. J Cardiovasc Pharmacol 25:794–801, 1995.

160. Haikala H, Kaheinen P, Levijoki J, Linden I-B: The role of cAMP-

and cGMP-dependent protein kinases in the cardiac actions of the new calcium sensitizer, levosimendan. Cardiovasc Res 34:536–546, 1997.

161. Haikala H, Kaivola J, Nissinen E, et al: Cardiac troponin C as a target for a novel calcium sensitizing drug, levosimendan. J Mol Cell Cardiol 27:1859–1866, 1995.

162. Harkin CP, Pagel PS, Tessmer JP, Warltier DC: Systemic and coronary hemodynamic actions and left ventricular functional effects of levosimendan in conscious dogs. J Cardiovasc Pharmacol 26: 179–188, 1995.

163. Pagel PS, Harkin CP, Hettrick DA, Warltier DC: Zatebradine, a specific bradycardic agent, alters the hemodynamic and left ventricular mechanical actions of levosimendan, a new myofilament calcium sensitizer, in conscious dogs. J Pharmacol Exp Ther 275:127–135, 1995.

164. McGough MF, Pagel PS, Lowe D, et al: Levosimendan potentiates the inotropic actions of dopamine in conscious dogs. J Cardiovasc Pharmacol 28:36–47, 1996.

165. Pagel PS, McGough MF, Hettrick DA, et al: Levosimendan enhances left ventricular systolic and diastolic function in conscious dogs with pacing-induced cardiomyopathy. J Cardiovasc Pharmacol 29: 563–573, 1997.

166. Yokoshiki H, Katsube Y, Sunagawa M, Sperelakis N: Levosimendan, a novel Ca^{2+} sensitizer, activates the glibenclamide-sensitive K^+ channel in rat arterial myocytes. Eur J Pharmacol 333:249–259, 1997.

167. Yokoshiki H, Katsube Y, Sunagawa M, Sperelakis N: The novel calcium sensitizer levosimendan activates the ATP-sensitive K^+ channel in rat ventricular cells. J Pharmacol Exp Ther 283:375–383, 1997.

168. Kersten JR, Montgomery MW, Pagel PS, Warltier DC: Levosimendan, a positive inotropic agent, decreases myocardial infarct size *via* activation of K_{ATP} channels. Anesth Analg 90:5–11, 2000.

169. Kersten JR, Gross GJ, Pagel PS, Warltier DC: Activation of adenosine triphosphate-regulated potassium channels: Mediation of cellular and organ protection. Anesthesiology 88:495–513, 1998.

170. Nijhawan N, Nicolosi AC, Montgomery MW, et al: Levosimendan enhances cardiac performance after cardiopulmonary bypass in humans: A prospective, randomized double-blind trial. J Cardiovasc Pharmacol 34:219–228, 1999.

171. Lehtonen L, Mills-Owens P, Akkila J: Safety of levosimendan and other calcium sensitizers. J Cardiovasc Pharmacol 26(suppl 1):S70–S76, 1995.

172. Antila S, Eha J, Heinpalu M, et al: Haemodynamic interactions of a new calcium sensitizing drug levosimendan and captopril. Eur J Clin Pharmacol 49:451–458, 1996.

173. Hamilton MA: Prevalence and clinical implications of abnormal thyroid hormone metabolism in advanced heart failure. Ann Thorac Surg 56(suppl 1):S48–S52, 1993.

174. Murayama M, Goodkind MJ: Effect of thyroid hormone on the frequency-force relationship of atrial myocardium from the guinea pig. Circ Res 23:743–751, 1968.

175. Buccino RA, Spann Jr JF, Pool PE, et al: Influence of the thyroid state on the intrinsic contractile properties and energy stores of the myocardium. J Clin Invest 46:1669–1682, 1967.

176. Jamali IN, Pagel PS, Hettrick DA, et al: Positive inotropic and lusitropic effects of triiodothyronine in conscious dogs with pacing-induced cardiomyopathy. Anesthesiology 87:102–109, 1997.

177. Kim D, Smith TW, Marsh JD: Effect of thyroid hormone on slow calcium channel function in cultured chick ventricular cells. J Clin Invest 80:88–94, 1987.

178. Han J, Leem C, So I, et al: Effects of thyroid hormone on the calcium current and isoprenaline-induced background current in rabbit ventricular myocytes. J Mol Cell Cardiol 26:925–935, 1994.

179. Davis PJ, Davis FB: Acute cellular actions of thyroid hormone and myocardial function. Ann Thorac Surg 56(suppl 1):S16–S23, 1993.

180. Ririe DG, Butterworth 4th JF, Royster RL, et al: Triiodothyronine increases contractility independent of beta-adrenergic receptors or stimulation of cyclic-3′,5′-adenosine monophosphate. Anesthesiology 82:1004–1012, 1995.

181. Insel PA: Adrenergic receptors: Evolving concepts on structure and function. Am J Hypertens 2:112S–118S, 1989.

182. Polikar R, Kennedy B, Maisel A, et al: Decreased adrenergic sensitivity in patients with hypothyroidism. J Am Coll Cardiol 15:94–98, 1990.

183. Shanker R, Neeley WE, Dillmann WH: Time course of response of

individual messenger RNAs in the rat heart to T_3. J Mol Cell Cardiol 19:595–601, 1987.

184. Rohrer D, Dillmann WH: Thyroid hormone markedly increases the mRNA coding for sarcoplasmic reticulum Ca^{2+}-ATPase in the rat heart. J Biol Chem 263:6941–6944, 1988.

185. Novitzky D, Matthews N, Shawley D, et al: Triiodothyronine in the recovery of stunned myocardium in dogs. Ann Thorac Surg 51:10–16, 1991.

186. Kadletz M, Mullen PG, Ding M, et al: Effect of triiodothyronine on postishemic myocardial function in the isolated heart. Ann Thorac Surg 57:657–662, 1994.

187. Morkin E, Pennock GD, Raya TE, et al: Studies on the use of thyroid hormone and a thyroid hormone analogue in the treatment of congestive heart failure. Ann Thorac Surg 56(suppl 1):S54–S60, 1993.

188. Mahaffey KW, Raya TE, Pennock GD, et al: Left ventricular performance and remodeling in rabbits after myocardial infarction. Effects of a thyroid hormone analogue. Circulation 91:794–801, 1995.

189. Pedersen F, Perrild H, Rasmussen SL, Skovsted L: "Low T_3-syndrome" in acute myocardial infarction. Relationship to beta-adrenergic blockade and clinical course. Eur J Clin Pharmacol 26:669–673, 1984.

190. Wortsman J, Premachandra BN, Chopra IJ, Murphy JE: Hypothyroxinemia in cardiac arrest. Arch Intern Med 147:245–248, 1987.

191. Moruzzi P, Doria E, Agostoni PG, et al: Usefulness of L-thyroxine to improve cardiac and exercise performance in idiopathic dilated cardiomyopathy. Am J Cardiol 73:374–381, 1994.

192. Chu SH, Huang TS, Hsu RB, et al: Thyroid hormone changes after cardiovascular surgery and clinical implications. Ann Thorac Surg 52:791–796, 1991.

193. Novitzky D, Cooper DK, Human PA, et al: Triiodothyronine therapy for heart donor and recipient. J Heart Transplant 7:370–376, 1988.

194. Holland II FW, Brown Jr PS, Weintraub BD, Clark RE: Cardiopulmonary bypass and thyroid function: A "euthyroid sick syndrome." Ann Thorac Surg 52:46–50, 1991.

195. Novitzky D, Cooper DK, Barton CI, et al: Triiodothyronine as an inotropic agent after open heart surgery. J Thorac Cardiovasc Surg 98:972–977, 1989.

196. Dyke CM, Ding M, Abd-Elfattah AS, et al: Effects of triiodothyronine supplementation after myocardial ischemia. Ann Thorac Surg 56:215–222, 1993.

197. Bennett-Guerrero E, Jimenez JL, White WD, et al: Cardiovascular effects of intravenous triiodothyronine in patients undergoing coronary artery bypass graft surgery: A randomized, double-blind, placebo-controlled trial. Duke T_3 study group. JAMA 275:687–692, 1996.

198. Klemperer JD, Klein I, Gomez M, et al: Thyroid hormone treatment after coronary-artery bypass surgery. N Engl J Med 333:1522–1527, 1995.

199. Goarin J-P, Cohen S, Riou B, et al: The effects of triiodothyronine on hemodynamic status and cardiac function in potential heart donors. Anesth Analg 83:41–47, 1996.

200. Prielipp RC, MacGregor DA, Royster RL, et al: Dobutamine antagonizes epinephrine's biochemical and cardiotonic effects: Results of an in vitro model using human lymphocytes and a clinical study in patients recovering from cardiac surgery. Anesthesiology 89:49–57, 1998.

201. Prielipp RC, Hill T, Washburn D, Zaloga GP: Circulating calcium modulates adrenaline induced cyclic adenosine monophosphate production. Cardiovasc Res 23:838–841, 1989.

202. Abernethy WB, Butterworth IV JF, Prielipp RC, et al: Calcium entry attenuates adenylyl cyclase activity: A possible mechanism for calcium-induced catecholamine resistance. Chest 107:1420–1425, 1995.

203. Royster RL, Butterworth IV JF, Prielipp RC, et al: Combined inotropic effects of amrinone and epinephrine after cardiopulmonary bypass in humans. Anesth Analg 77:662–672, 1993.

204. Kikura M, Levy JH, Bailey JM, et al: A bolus dose of 1.5 mg/kg amrinone effectively improves low cardiac output state following separation from cardiopulmonary bypass in cardiac surgical patients. Acta Anaesthesiol Scand 42:825–833, 1998.

205. Teo KK, Ignaszewski AP, Gutierrez R, et al: Contemporary medical management of left ventricular dysfunction and congestive heart failure. Can J Cardiol 8:611–619, 1992.

206. Butterworth J: Selecting an inotrope for the cardiac surgery patient. J Cardiothorac Vasc Anesth 7(4 suppl 2):26–32, 1993.

38

Myocardial Protection

Charl de Wet, MB, ChB • Eric Jacobsohn, MB, ChB

Strategies to Improve Oxygen Supply/Demand
Balance
  β Adrenergic Receptor Antagonists
  α_2 Adrenoreceptor Agonists
  Thoracic Sympathectomy
  Adenosine and Nitric Oxide
  Endothelin
  Manipulation of the Hematocrit, Rheology of
    Hemoglobin, and Antiplatelet Drugs
Strategies Aimed at Preventing or Decreasing
Ischemia/Reperfusion Injury
  Cardioprotection before the Onset of Ischemia:
    Ischemic Preconditioning
  Drugs Acting Through the K^+_{ATP} Channel
  Potassium Channel Openers

Calcium Sensitizer: Levosimendan
Opioid Agonists
Volatile Anesthetics
Adenosine and Acadesine
Propofol: Cardioprotection during Reperfusion
Cardioprotection after Reperfusion: Inhibitors of
  Na^+/H^+ Exchanger
Oxidant Stress and Free Radicals
Anti-Inflammatory Strategies
  Corticosteroids
  Protease Inhibitors
Cardioplegia
  Inducing Cardiac Arrest
  Experimental Strategies with Cardioplegia

Inadequate myocardial protection rather than inadequate anatomic repair is recognized as the most common cause of low cardiac output after cardiac surgery.[1] Initially, hypothermia was the primary form of myocardial protection. During the last half century cardioplegia has been refined and has contributed immensely to the improved outcomes in modern-day cardiac surgery.[2–5] Although beating heart surgery has seen a return with the introduction of modern-day off pump beating heart coronary artery revascularization, there remains an ongoing search for better perioperative myocardial protection. Strategies for myocardial protection have been classified based on physiologic principles.[6] These strategies include: (1) interventions aimed at improving or optimizing the oxygen supply/demand ratio of the myocardium; (2) interventions aimed at preventing the additional injury and cell death that occurs in ischemic myocardium when blood flow is restored, referred to as *ischemia/reperfusion injury*[7,8]; and (3) interventions aimed at preventing the additional injury and cell death that occurs in an ischemic myocardium and peri-infarction zones caused by inflammation. This chapter is organized to sequentially address each of these strategies followed by a discussion of cardioplegia. Many of the novel pharmacologic approaches to alleviate myocardial injury and improve/restore endothelial myocyte function are still being developed or are

in clinical trials. For this reason, this chapter emphasizes drugs in the development stage, as well as existing pharmaceutical agents.

Strategies to Improve Oxygen Supply/Demand Balance

Myocardial oxygen delivery depends on blood flow (cardiac output and coronary artery perfusion pressure), oxygen saturation, and hemoglobin concentration. Myocardial blood flow in turn is controlled centrally and locally. The central vasomotor center responds to input from the baroreceptors and chemical receptors in the aortic arch and carotid sinus bifurcation, and through the cardiac sympathetic nervous outflow (low cervical and cardioaccelerator nerves, T1-4), causes the postsynaptic release of norepinephrine that reacts with α and β receptors. Local vasomotor control (i.e., coronary blood flow) is mediated through adenosine, nitric oxide (NO), and endothelin. Myocardial oxygen demand is also influenced by some of the same factors that affect oxygen delivery, and it is therefore imperative to understand this interaction to achieve an optimal supply demand ratio.[9–14]

β Adrenergic Receptor Antagonists

Mechanisms of Drug Action

(The molecular and cellular mechanisms of adrenergic agonists and antagonists are discussed in detail in Chapter 34.) β Adrenergic receptor blockers form the cornerstone of current perioperative myocardial protection and protection after myocardial infarction. Antagonists of β adrenergic receptors have also been shown to improve outcome among patients with acute myocardial infarction, silent ischemia, and heart failure. The anti-ischemic mechanism of β adrenergic blockers is related to reductions in heart rate and myocardial contractility. Beta-blockade may reduce myocardial oxygen consumption by suppressing lipolysis and thus causing the myocardium to metabolize more glucose in relation to free fatty acids. The decrease in heart rate increases the duration of diastole, enhances coronary perfusion time, increases subendocardial blood flow, and reduces myocardial oxygen consumption. β Adrenergic receptor blockers also reverse coronary steal by increasing coronary vascular tone in healthy regions by reducing oxygen demand. These drugs attenuate the adverse effects of sympathetic nervous system activation, including increases in heart rate and myocardial contractility, decreases in coronary blood flow secondary to constriction of large epicardial coronary vessels, coronary cyclical flow phenomena at the stenosis site generated by platelet aggregation and dispersion, and overall plaque instability. In addition, beta-blockers have important antiarrhythmic properties.

Preclinical and Clinical Pharmacology

Many β adrenergic antagonists (e.g., propranolol, metoprolol) are weak bases with large volumes of distribution and therefore may accumulate in organs such as the heart, liver, lungs, and brain depending on their water versus fat solubility. Water-soluble agents such as atenolol and sotalol are renally excreted without undergoing significant biotransformation and therefore have long plasma half-lives. Esmolol is an ultra-short–acting, cardioselective, water-soluble agent. It is rapidly hydrolyzed to inactive metabolites by red cell esterases. Water solubility also limits crossing of the blood–brain barrier, and therefore central nervous system side effects such as nightmares are infrequently seen with the water-soluble agents. Atenolol is both water-soluble and cardioselective. Bisoprolol is the most cardioselective agent available with a ratio of beta 1/beta 2 affinity of 147 (102-292).[15] Acebutolol, atenolol, and metoprolol have ratios of 1, 1-3, and 2.[16]

Beta-blockers have been found to reduce mortality and morbidity rates in patients with myocardial infarction and congestive heart failure. The beta-blockers with a proven effect on prognosis include two selective β_1 receptor block-ers—metoprolol and bisoprolol—and three nonselective beta-blockers—timolol, propranolol, and carvedilol. All beta-blockers with proven effect on mortality and on sudden death have one property in common: some degree of lipophilicity.[16] Like atenolol, sotalol is hydrophilic. Sotalol, a nonselective beta-blocker, which also has a pronounced class III antiarrhythmic effect, does not appear to have a significant effect on postinfarction mortality. Interestingly, sotalol reduced the incidence of reinfarction, but it had no influence on the incidence of sudden cardiac death. Beta-blockers such as metoprolol, bisoprolol, timolol, propranolol, and carvedilol reduce the incidence of both reinfarction and sudden cardiac death. Animal data suggest that beta-blockers with some lipophilicity penetrate the brain and have an indirect effect on vagal activity, which is of importance for prevention of ventricular fibrillation and sudden cardiac death.[16]

Some beta-blockers, including propranolol, metoprolol, carvedilol, labetalol, and the new generation beta-blocker celiprolol, have varying degrees of antioxidant activity that may play a role in preventing endothelial injury.[17] Atenolol and bisoprolol, do not to have any significant antioxidant properties,[18] whereas carvedilol appears to have the most antioxidant properties.[19] In a study of isolated rabbit hearts using an ischemia/reperfusion model, carvedilol counteracted the ischemia and reperfusion-induced oxidative stress and improved myocardial viability independent of its beta-blocking effect.[20]

Beta-blockers, when used as preoperative prophylaxis in patients with coronary artery disease, reduce both morbidity and mortality rates.[21,22] The ultra-short–acting beta-blocker, esmolol, significantly reduces postoperative myocardial ischemia.[23] In the initial study by Mangano and colleagues,[21] improvements in mortality rates occurred well beyond the perioperative period, suggesting that heart rate control alone was insufficient to explain the beneficial effects of beta-blockade. However, the Mangano study had some methodologic problems that make the interpretation of the results difficult. Subsequently, a well-controlled, clinical study by Poldermans and colleagues[24] studied the cardioprotective role of a selective β_1 receptor antagonist, bisoprolol, in high-risk patients undergoing major vascular surgery. The combined incidence rate of adverse cardiac events was 34% in the standard care group, compared with 3.4% in the bisoprolol group. On the basis of this study, surgical patients at high risk should receive beta-blockers perioperatively, beginning 1 to 2 weeks before surgery. The goal should be to reduce the heart rate to less than 70 beats per minute before surgery and to less than 80 beats per minute in the immediate postoperative period. In their long-term follow-up of these study patients, Poldermans and colleagues[25] examined the effect of prolonged bisoprolol therapy in the patients that survived the major vascular surgery. In this study, they showed that when followed for a mean of 22 months, the composite endpoint of cardiac events in the bisoprolol group was 12% versus 32% in the standard therapy group ($P = 0.025$). This is the first randomized study that shows that prolonged beta-blocker therapy reduces the incidence of late cardiac events in survivors of major vascular surgery who had received intraoperative and postoperative beta-blocker therapy.

α₂ Adrenoreceptor Agonists

Mechanisms of Drug Action

(The molecular and cellular mechanisms of α_2 adrenergic agonists are discussed in Chapters 28 and 34.) α_2 Adrenoreceptor agonists mimic baroreceptor stimulation and therefore decrease centrally mediated sympathetic norepinephrine release. This results in prevention of tachycardia and hypertension. Norepinephrine release is self-regulated through α_2 receptor–mediated norepinephrine release.

Preclinical and Clinical Pharmacology

Drugs such as clonidine, and more recently the more selective dexmedetomidine, have been used to treat hypertension and sympathetic symptoms that may occur with drug withdrawal. The selective α_2 adrenergic agonist dexmedetomidine decreases not only heart rate, myocardial contractility, and oxygen demand, but also cardiac output. In certain clinical situations, such as hypovolemia and sepsis, the reduction in cardiac output may be significant and may compromise perfusion of vital organs.[26] Also of concern is that dexmedetomidine[27] causes vasoconstriction by binding with peripheral α_2 receptors on coronary and cerebral vascular smooth muscle. This direct vasoconstrictor effect of α_2 adrenergic agonists may be opposed by release of endothelium-derived relaxing factor believed to be NO (nitric oxide).[28] The calcium channel blocker isradipine has also been shown to alleviate the peripherally-induced vasoconstriction without having any effect on the central actions of dexmedetomidine.[27] With dexmedetomidine, however, systemic and coronary vasoconstriction are short-lived, endocardial perfusion is maintained, myocardial energy requirements are decreased, and the balance between myocardial oxygen supply and demand is maintained.[29] Dexmedetomidine has been shown to have some antidysrhythmic effects, and these effects have been shown to be centrally mediated through nonadrenergic imidazoline receptors[30] and not through the α_2 receptor as was originally thought.

Mivazerol hydrochloride is a new α_2 adrenoreceptor agonist. In vitro and animal studies have demonstrated both sympatholytic and anti-ischemic properties.[31] Mivazerol has also been shown to produce a significant increase in exercise duration and time to the onset of angina when given before exercise tolerance testing to patients with stable angina[32] and reduces cardiac-related overall mortality rates in patients with coronary disease undergoing vascular surgery.[31,33–35]

Thoracic Sympathectomy

Thoracic epidural anesthesia (TEA) has clearly been shown to relieve refractory unstable angina[36] and may even be superior to medical therapy as measured by such indices as frequency of anginal episodes, duration of these episodes, and severity of ST-depression.[37] During ischemic chest pain, pulmonary artery and pulmonary capillary wedge pressures usually increase. With TEA, chest pain is relieved, and despite significant decreases in systolic arterial blood pressure, heart rate, and pulmonary artery and pulmonary capillary wedge pressures, TEA does not significantly change coronary perfusion pressure, cardiac output, stroke volume, or systemic or pulmonary vascular resistances. With exercise, TEA has been found to significantly decrease systolic arterial pressure, diastolic arterial pressure, and rate pressure product, but not heart rate. However, global and anterolateral ejection fractions were significantly greater and regional wall motion scores were significantly lower during TEA exercise than during control exercise. Despite decreases in blood pressure, ST-segment depression was significantly lower during TEA exercise.[38] During ischemic chest pain, TEA has beneficial effects on the major determinants of myocardial oxygen consumption, without jeopardizing coronary perfusion pressure.[39] TEA may therefore favorably alter the oxygen supply/demand ratio within ischemic myocardial areas. Beattie and colleagues[40] performed a meta-analysis to determine whether postoperative epidural analgesia for greater than 24 hours reduced perioperative myocardial infarction or death. Of 17 published studies, 11 were randomized controlled trials with a total of 1173 patients. The rate of perioperative myocardial infarction was 6.3%, with lower rates in the epidural group (rate difference, −3.8%; 95% confidence interval [CI], −7.4%, −0.2%; P = 0.049). The frequency of in-hospital death was 3.3%, with no significant difference between epidural and nonepidural groups (rate difference, −1.3%; 95% CI, −3.8%, 1.2%, P = 0.091). Subgroup analysis of postoperative thoracic epidural analgesia showed a significant reduction in myocardial infarction in the epidural group (rate difference, −5.3%; 95% CI, −9.9%, −0.7%; P = 0.04). However, in randomized trials by Rigg,[41] Park,[42] and Peyton,[43] epidural anesthesia was not superior to general anesthesia/parenteral analgesia in reducing the incidence of cardiac complications. However, as de Leon-Casasola[44] points out, there may be several methodologic concerns with these studies.

Whether TEA can be cardioprotective in the setting of patients undergoing cardiopulmonary bypass (CPB) for aortocoronary bypass grafting remains to be seen. Liem and colleagues[45] studied the hemodynamic results, postoperative outcome, and adrenergic responses to thoracic epidurals in patients undergoing CPB. Patients with TEA had more stable hemodynamics both before and after CPB. TEA continued into the postoperative period also resulted in earlier extubation and a lower incidence of myocardial ischemia.[46] Intraoperative adrenergic responses were suppressed with the use of TEA.[47] A recent study showed earlier extubation times in patients with TEA undergoing CPB. After surgery, there was no difference in the incidence of Q waves on electrocardiogram between the two groups. Although it did not reach statistical significance because of the small size of the study population, the investigators did note a trend toward a shorter ischemic time on Holter monitoring.[48] Scott and colleagues[49] performed an open, prospective, randomized, controlled study of the incidence of complications in 420 patients undergoing coronary artery bypass graft surgery with or without thoracic epidural anesthesia and analgesia. They found that new supraventricular arrhythmias occurred in 21 of 206 patients (10.2%) in the epidural group, compared with 45 of 202 patients (22.3%) in the group without an epidural ($P = 0.0012$).[49] More recently, Lee and colleagues[50] have shown that the administration of high-spinal spinal anesthesia with 37.5 mg spinal bupivacaine, combined with general anesthesia, results in less pre-CPB ischemia as measured by intraoperative transesophageal echocardiography (Fig. 38–1), less beta-receptor desensitization and down-regulation, and improves post-CPB hemodynamics.[50]

Adenosine and Nitric Oxide

Adenosine and NO are potent endogenous vasodilators; both traditionally thought to play a role in normal regulation of coronary blood flow. However, Tune and colleagues[51] have shown that whereas NO acts as a modest coronary vasodilator at rest, inhibition of NO synthesis does not significantly change coronary blood flow. This was hypothesized to be caused by cardiac adenosine concentration increases to compensate for the loss of NO vasodilation. Tune and colleagues[52] therefore investigated the role of adenosine in regulating coronary blood flow during exercise. Coronary blood flow, myocardial oxygen consumption, heart rate, and aortic pressure were measured in dogs at rest and during graded treadmill. Exercise increased myocardial oxygen consumption, coronary blood flow, and heart rate, whereas mean aortic pressure was unchanged. However, coronary venous plasma adenosine concentration was little changed with exercise, and the estimated interstitial adenosine concentration remained well below the threshold for coronary vasodilation. This suggested that adenosine played no role in the regulation of coronary blood flow during exercise. This was confirmed when adenosine receptor blockade did not significantly alter myocardial oxygen consumption or coronary blood flow at rest or during exercise. Furthermore, coronary venous and estimated interstitial adenosine concentration did not increase to overcome the receptor blockade, as would be predicted if adenosine were part of a high-gain, negative-feedback, local metabolic control mechanism. These results demonstrate that adenosine is not responsible for local metabolic control of coronary blood flow in dogs during exercise.

Although neither adenosine nor NO appear to be important in normal regulation of coronary blood flow, they may play a role in the response to myocardial ischemia. For example, NO does regulate coronary collateral growth, and ischemia-induced coronary collateral growth is dependent on NO and vascular endothelial growth factor.[53] NO also plays an important regulatory role in endothelial P-selectin expression that modulates early leukocyte/endothelial cell interactions.[54,55] P-selectin translocation to the surface of endothelial cells is increased after exposure to the NO synthase inhibitor, NG-nitro-L-arginine methyl ester, resulting in increased endothelial adhesiveness.[56] Endothelial dysfunction after reperfusion injury is heralded by an impairment of the synthesis or release of NO.[57] However, NO appears to be protective in reducing only postischemic polymorphonuclear leukocyte–mediated myocardial contractile dysfunction.[58] The formation and release of adenosine by cardiac muscle during periods of hypoxia or regional ischemia in the heart are well known to produce regional vasodilation and salvage of at-risk myocardium; however, this release is abluminal (endothelium independent), and intraluminal release is less well understood.[59] Overall, manipulation of NO or adenosine pathways is unlikely to be a viable strategy for preventing ischemia through improvement of oxygen supply/demand balance.

Endothelin

The endothelium is an important regulator of coronary vascular tone due to its ability to release potent vasoactive substances. These include vasodilators such as NO, endothelium-derived hyperpolarizing factor, prostacyclin, and the potent vasoconstrictor, endothelin. Endogenous endothelin-1 (ET-1) plays a role in the maintenance of basal vasomotor tone in patients with normal coronary arteries. During ischemia, the local release of ET-1 may also contribute to the impairment of the capacity of the coronary circulation to dilate and to a reduction in basal blood flow. This suggests a possible role for an ET-1 antagonist in improving oxygen supply/demand balance and treating myocardial ischemia. However, animal studies have shown that a specific endothelin receptor subtype A antagonist does not reduce ischemic injury when administered intravenously after experimental coronary artery occlusion.[60] This may be because the drug was unable to reach its target site.[60] Although ET-1 antagonists have not been shown to reduce ischemic injury, ET-1 treatment *before* ischemia has been

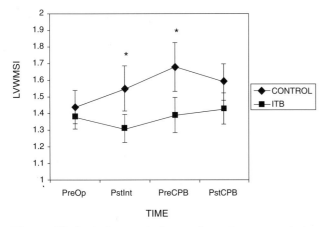

Figure 38–1. Left ventricular wall motion score index (LVWMSI) values. LVWMSI values were significantly lower in group ITB after intubation and preCPB, suggesting improved LVWM in the intrathecal bupivacaine group. 1, normal; 2, hypokinetic; 3, akinetic; 4, dyskinetic. PreOp, preoperative transesophageal echocardiography (TEE); PstInt, postintubation TEE; PreCPB, precardiopulmonary bypass (pre-CPB) TEE; PstCPB, post-CPB TEE. Results are expressed as mean ± SEM (*$P < 0.05$). (From Lee TW, Grocott HP, Schwinn D, et al: High spinal anesthesia for cardiac surgery: Effects on beta-adrenergic receptor function, stress response, and hemodynamics. Anesthesiology 98:499, 2003.)

shown to reduce infarct size. This effect occurs through a pathway involving protein kinase C (PKC) and K^+_{ATP} channels.[61] ET-1 also acts as a growth-promoting peptide and a potent survival factor against myocardial cell apoptosis.[62] Thus ET-1 is a complex mediator that may adversely affect coronary perfusion during an ischemic event, but may also have beneficial effects in providing protection against ischemic damage. Currently, neither ET-1 itself nor endothelin receptor antagonists are used in the treatment or prevention of myocardial injury.

Manipulation of the Hematocrit, Rheology of Hemoglobin, and Antiplatelet Drugs

Optimal oxygen delivery depends on cardiac output and arterial oxygen content (hemoglobin concentration and arterial oxygen saturation). It is known that blood viscosity is a determinant of resistance to blood flow at the arteriolar level and at areas of stenosis. Accordingly, a reduction in blood viscosity could exert a favorable influence on maximal myocardial oxygen delivery in the setting of stenosis, provided that the oxygen-carrying capacity of the blood is not excessively compromised. A reduction in blood viscosity by means of isovolumetric hemodilution will permit an increase in maximal oxygen delivery to myocardium distal to a moderate coronary arterial stenosis. This phenomenon has been described in dogs in which myocardial blood flow distal to an area of experimental stenosis increased in response to adenosine and after hemodilution.[63]

It may seem logical that optimization of hemoglobin concentration would improve myocardial oxygen delivery, and therefore decrease myocardial ischemia. However, one has to balance this with the known increase in viscosity accompanied by an increase in hematocrit. A greater hematocrit may not necessarily be better and may in fact worsen patient outcome as measured by left ventricular dysfunction and Q-wave infarction.[64] The "optimal" hematocrit remains unknown, and factors such as an increase in viscosity may play a role in negating the beneficial effect of improving the arterial oxygen content. In a landmark clinical trail, Hebert and the Canadian Critical Care Trials Group compared a liberal (hemoglobin maintained at 10–12 g/dL) versus restrictive (hemoglobin maintained 7.0–9.0 g/dL) transfusion strategy in critically ill patients.[65] They concluded that a restrictive transfusion strategy appears to be as effective or even superior to a liberal transfusion strategy in critically ill patients, with the possible exception of those with acute myocardial infarction or unstable angina. In another important recent study, Wu and colleagues studied transfusion in elderly patients after myocardial infarction and found that there may be a benefit in providing transfusions to elderly patients with myocardial infarction to hematocrit levels up to 33.0%.[66] In addition, they found that transfusion had a neutral effect on 30-day mortality rates among patients with hematocrit levels of 33.1% to 36.0%. Transfusion was associated with an increased risk for death within 30 days only among patients with hematocrit levels that exceeded 36.0%.

Inhibition of platelet function prevents clot formation, thereby protecting the myocardium by preserving myocardial blood flow. Aspirin has formed the mainstay of antiplatelet therapy. Currently, much interest is centered on newer drugs such as clopidogrel (a thienopyridine that inhibits adenosine diphosphate–mediated platelet aggregation) and the newer glycoprotein IIb/IIIa receptor inhibitors (tirofiban, and so on) with respect to their roles during the acute management of and prevention of myocardial ischemia. Drugs aimed at altering platelet function are discussed in detail in Chapter 53.

Strategies Aimed at Preventing or Decreasing Ischemia/Reperfusion Injury

Postischemic reperfusion may profoundly alter cardiac function. Principal mediators of this phenomenon are oxygen radicals and neutrophils. On reflow, oxygen radicals are generated in large amounts, overwhelming cellular defenses and inducing oxidative tissue damage. When neutrophils are reintroduced into postischemic tissues, they become activated and release lytic enzymes. These in turn induce tissue damage and proinflammatory mediators that amplify the local inflammatory reaction. Furthermore, neutrophils obstruct capillaries, further adding to ischemic injury. There are four basic forms of reperfusion injury.[67] Lethal reperfusion injury is described as necrosis of myocytes caused by reperfusion itself rather than to any existing preceding ischemia. Second, vascular reperfusion injury refers to progressive damage to the vasculature, which may include an expanding zone of no reflow and a deterioration of coronary flow reserve. Third, stunned myocardium refers to postischemic ventricular dysfunction of viable myocytes and probably represents a form of "functional reperfusion injury." Finally, reperfusion arrhythmias such as ventricular tachycardia and fibrillation can occur. They usually occur within seconds to minutes of restoration of coronary flow.[68] Cardioprotective strategies aimed at alleviating or preventing the ischemia/reperfusion injury may be targeted during three time intervals: before the onset of ischemia, after the onset of ischemic injury but prior to reperfusion, and after reperfusion.

Cardioprotection before the Onset of Ischemia: Ischemic Preconditioning

Murry and colleagues[69] were the first to describe ischemic preconditioning (IPC), which is an adaptive, cardioprotective response that follows a brief period of ischemia. Brief episodes of myocardial ischemia, followed by reperfusion of the ischemic tissue, paradoxically increase the resistance to further ischemic damage,[69] may slow ischemic injury, and may limit infarct size.[70] Two phases of IPC are recognized: an early phase and a delayed phase that may give protection for up to 3 days.[71] Yellon and colleagues[72] were the first to show that it may be possible to precondition and protect the *human* myocardium with short controlled periods of intermittent ischemia and reperfusion. They found two cycles of 3 minutes of ischemia, with 2 minutes of reperfusion, to be effective in protecting the myocardium during coronary artery bypass surgery. The exact duration of this immediate component of IPC in humans is unknown. This immediate protection can last up to 2 hours in dogs, but only 30 minutes in rabbits. Early preconditioning is mediated through the release of endogenous substances such as adenosine, bradykinin, and opioid peptides, which opens the mitochondrial K^+_{ATP} channel through a complex kinase-signaling cascade.[70]

Although a delayed component of IPC has been demonstrated in animal models,[73] it has not been clearly shown if the delayed IPC effect occurs in the human heart. Recently, however, the concept of the classic and delayed IPC effects was prospectively investigated in humans with acute myocardial infarction.[74] The beneficial effect of preinfarction angina on left ventricular wall motion, independent of collateral flow, seems to indicate the existence of the IPC effect in humans. In this study, the greater protective effect afforded by a longer time interval between angina pectoris and acute myocardial infarction suggests that this protection may be caused by a delayed IPC effect.

Drugs Acting Through the K^+_{ATP} Channel

Mechanisms of Drug Action

Ischemia results in the loss of adenosine triphosphate (ATP), which causes the ATP-regulated K^+ channels to open with subsequent hyperpolarization of the cell membrane. This results in shortening of the action potential, and therefore a decrease in inotropy. The shortened action potential also decreases effective time for Ca^{2+} entry into the cell. The cardioprotective effects of IPC are mediated by mitochondrial K^+_{ATP} channels.[75] These channels mediate the protective effects of IPC both during the onset of acute ischemia and during the reperfusion period.[76,77] In addition to being opened by ATP-depletion (ischemia), the K^+_{ATP} channel can be opened directly by drugs known as potassium channel openers or indirectly through the G protein–coupled adenosine receptor,[78] or by δ_1 opioid receptor agonists (e.g., morphine) acting through a PKC mechanism. Activation of PKC-linked receptors and subsequent opening of the mitochondrial ATP-sensitive K^+ channel leads to increased generation of NO and subsequent attenuation of the burst of reactive oxygen species seen within the first few minutes of reperfusion.[79] (Figure 38–2 also shows the differential effects of commonly used anesthetic agents on the mitochondrial K^+_{ATP} channel.[80])

NO seems to play an integral part in IPC. It limits the extension of a subsequent infarct and protects against ischemia/reperfusion–induced endothelial dysfunction, arrhythmias, and myocardial stunning. The protective activity occurs in both the first and the second window of protection. The antiarrhythmic effect is attributed to microvessel dilation and to the production of cyclic guanosine monophosphate in the myocardium. The endothelial protection involves an NO-mediated reduction in neutrophil adherence to the coronary endothelium and platelet aggregation and is accompanied by an enhanced response to vasodilator stimuli. During preconditioning ischemia, NO is released from the coronary endothelium as a result of bradykinin-induced activation of kinin B2 endothelial receptors. In addition to the early protection, endothelium-derived NO is also responsible for a signaling cascade, which leads to the activation of myocardial inducible NO synthase. Recently, however, it has been shown that the delayed phase of preconditioning induced by adenosine A1 receptor activation is independent of early generation of NO or late induction of inducible NO synthase.[73] The signaling cascade includes the activation of PKC-ε, tyrosine kinase, and mitogen-activated protein kinases.[81] Pharmacologic inhibition of the K^+_{ATP} channel with sulfonylureas[82,83] or the adenosine receptor with methylxanthines such as aminophylline,[84] has been shown to attenuate IPC.[85] Hyperglycemia, which also blocks the K^+_{ATP} channel, has been found to correlate linearly with infarct size regardless of whether the heart has been preconditioned.[86]

Potassium Channel Openers

Preclinical and Clinical Pharmacology

The ATP-sensitive mitochondrial K^+ channel openers include pinacidil[87] and nicorandil.[88] Nicorandil, an antianginal agent, is currently being evaluated in the Impact Of Nicorandil in Angina (IONA) study—a randomized, double-blind, placebo-controlled trial testing the hypothesis that nicorandil will reduce the incidence of cardiovascular events in patients with effort angina and additional risk factors.[89] Nicorandil is an antianginal agent that has been used in the United Kingdom for several years. It induces coronary and peripheral vasodilatation through a dual mode of action, mediated by the opening of K^+_{ATP} channels and by stimulation of adenyl cyclase, with a subsequent increase in cyclic guanosine monophosphate levels. Comparison to nitrates and other antianginal agents have shown it to be of equal efficacy in relieving ischemic symptoms. Recent evidence suggests a role for nicorandil as a myocardial-preconditioning agent, but this may be limited by systemic vasodilatation.[90]

Calcium Sensitizer: Levosimendan

Levosimendan (Simdax; Abbott Laboratories, Abbott Park, Ill.) is a new, experimental positive inotropic drug, which decreases myocardial infarct size through activation of K^+_{ATP} channels.[91] It is a novel calcium sensitizer developed for the treatment of decompensated or acute heart failure and is also an inodilator that increases coronary flow. In the presence of glibenclamide, a K^+_{ATP} channel inhibitor, the positive inotropic and chronotropic effects of levosimendan are unaltered. Coronary vasodilatation, however, is mediated through the opening of K^+_{ATP} channels, and diastolic coronary flow seems to be dose related. Levosimendan and pinacidil probably have different binding sites on K^+_{ATP} channels.[92] Because the inotropic action of levosimendan does not require an increase in cytosolic free calcium, it is less arrhythmogenic than the conventional parenteral

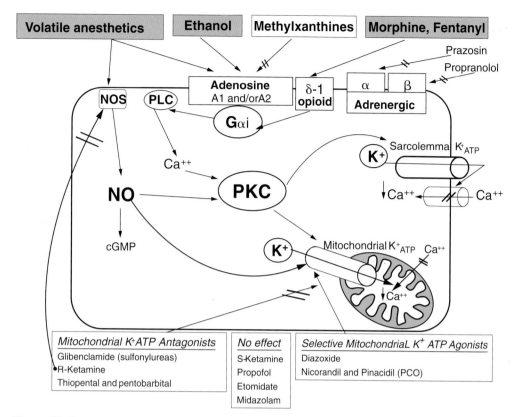

Figure 38–2. Cardioprotective role of the sarcoplasmic and mitochondrial K^+_{ATP} channel. Myocardial protection results from protein kinase C (PKC)-mediated opening or stimulation of the mitochondrial and sarcolemmal K^+_{ATP} channels. Nitric oxide (NO) can stimulate the mitochondrial K^+_{ATP} pump either directly or through PKC. The adrenergic system does not influence PKC-mediated cardioprotection. Graph shows several commonly used agents in current anesthetic practice and how they may ultimately influence PKC-mediated cardioprotection.[80] ATP, adenosine triphosphate; cGMP, cyclic guanosine monophosphate; $G\alpha_1$, G protein subunit; NOS, nitric oxide synthase; PLC, protein lipase C. (Modified from Zaugg M, Lucchinetti E, Spahn DR, et al: Volatile anesthetics mimic cardiac preconditioning by priming the activation of mitochondrial K(ATP) channels via multiple signaling pathways. Anesthesiology 97:4, 2002.)

β-agonist inotropes or phosphodiesterase III inhibiting drugs. Because of calcium-dependent binding of the drug to troponin C, levosimendan, unlike some other calcium-sensitizing drugs, does not prolong diastolic relaxation of the myocytes but acts in synergy with the intramyocellular calcium levels. Furthermore, because of its anti-ischemic effect, levosimendan could be used as an inotropic agent during myocardial ischemia. In clinical trials, levosimendan has dose-dependently increased cardiac output and decreased pulmonary capillary wedge pressure in patients with heart failure. Conversely, it also increases heart rate and decreases blood pressure. In major clinical trials, in which patients with decompensated heart failure have been treated with levosimendan, a reduction of overall mortality rates in comparison to placebo or dobutamine has been observed. The safety of levosimendan during myocardial ischemia will make this drug valuable in the short-term treatment of decompensated heart failure.[93]

The L-type Ca^{2+} channel also plays a role in IPC. Atrial muscle from patients taking L-type Ca^{2+} channel blockers cannot be preconditioned by transient ischemia, and the increased cardiovascular mortality rate historically associated with the use of calcium channel blockers in patients with coronary artery disease may be, in part, caused by the pharmacologic inhibition of IPC.[94]

Opioid Agonists

In human atrium, δ and μ have been shown to be the predominant opioid subtypes as compared with rat heart, which expresses κ and δ but not μ receptors. It has recently been shown that $δ_1$ opioid receptor stimulation is cardioprotective against myocardial ischemia and sublethal arrhythmias, and that its effect is mediated by PKC activation of the mitochondrial K^+_{ATP} channel.[95–97] In a swine model, stimulation of the δ opioid cardiac receptor leads to a reduction ion infarct size, which is abolished by a selective antagonist of the δ opioid receptor.[98]

There is evidence that κ opioid receptors mediate the cardioprotection in rat models of IPC, which may involve PKC.[99] Wang and colleagues showed in a rat model that κ opioid stimulation mediates the effects of IPC on both infarct size and arrhythmia, whereas δ opioid receptor stimulation only reduced infarct size.[100] In contrast, using a *swine* model, κ receptor activation during pharmacologic pre-conditioning was proarrhythmic.[101] This illustrates the differences in opioid subtype population and probable dose-related effect differences between different species. In an isolated human atrial muscle model, stimulation of the δ opioid receptor is cardioprotective, and antagonism of this receptor blocks the cardioprotective effect.[102]

Even though morphine and fentanyl are preferential μ receptor agonists, they are capable of binding to δ receptors and therefore mediate cardioprotection. The role of the μ receptor is unknown. The beneficial effects of opioids can be blocked by a G_i protein inhibitor, a PKC inhibitor, and a selective mitochondrial K^+_{ATP} channel blocker.[103]

Volatile Anesthetics

Volatile anesthetics such as isoflurane,[90,104,105] halothane,[78] desflurane,[106] and sevoflurane[107] mediate their cardioprotective effects through two pathways: adenosine receptor stimulation and through NO formation, converging on PKC, which then impacts on the primed mitochondrial K^+_{ATP} channel.

Volatile anesthetics mimic the effects of IPC, providing protection for the ischemic myocardium both experimentally and more recently in a placebo-controlled clinical study.[108] On initiation of CPB, patients were exposed to isoflurane at a minimum alveolar concentration of 2.5 for 5 minutes, followed by a washout of 10 minutes before cardioplegia and aortic cross-clamping. The activity of ecto-5′-nucleotidase, which contributes to adenosine production and is considered to be a marker of PKC activation, was assessed in right atrial biopsy samples taken before bypass and at the end of the preconditioning protocol. Patients who had their hearts preconditioned with isoflurane had statistically greater levels compared with the control group and also had lower levels of troponin I release. The likely site of action for volatile anesthetics is the K^+_{ATP} channel because the ability of volatile anesthetics to alter channel activity has been demonstrated in experiments on isolated myocytes. The effects of isoflurane on the K^+_{ATP} channel appear to be mediated through A1 receptors and the K^+_{ATP} channel, as isoflurane's effects are prevented by the A1 antagonist DPCPX and the K^+_{ATP} channel antagonist glibenclamide, respectively. Glibenclamide, a nonspecific inhibitor of the K^+_{ATP} channel, inhibits cardioprotection by isoflurane in a canine model of ischemia. The protection afforded by isoflurane is also inhibited by antagonists of adenosine receptors, suggesting that adenosine receptor activation may also be involved in the pathway linking isoflurane to cardioprotection.[109]

It is now evident that the IPC effect of the halogenated agents is mediated through the mitochondrial K^+_{ATP} channel and not through the sarcolemmal K^+_{ATP} channel.[106] Volatile anesthetics mimic cardiac preconditioning by priming the activation of mitochondrial K^+_{ATP} channels through multiple signaling pathways. Volatile anesthetics alone do not alter mitochondrial K^+_{ATP} channel activity, implying a *priming* effect of volatile anesthetics on mitochondrial K^+_{ATP} channels.[110] Even though protection of halogenated agents is not accompanied by augmented release of adenosine, cardio-

protection is dependent on the adenosine receptor, because blockade of this receptor abolishes halogenated-mediated cardioprotection.[111] It is therefore hypothesized that these agents stimulate adenosine receptors through a nonadenosine mechanism, or up-regulate the adenosine receptor/G protein complex to promote the signal transduction downstream.[103] Mechanisms other than preconditioning might be responsible for the cardioprotection of halogenated agents because they protect not only before ischemia, but they may also protect during ischemia or reperfusion.[112] They have also been shown to reduce myocardial stunning independent of the adenosine A1 receptor.[113] The volatile anesthetic agents appear to have different effects on reperfusion after regional myocardial ischemia. In an in vivo rabbit model of regional ischemia with reperfusion, desflurane, and sevoflurane markedly reduced infarct size. Enflurane had only a marginal effect and isoflurane offered no protection against reperfusion injury in vivo. These different effects suggest different protective mechanisms at the cellular level.[112]

The halogenated agents also have other beneficial effects during reperfusion—they decrease neutrophil adhesion to endothelium,[114] preserve the response to vasodilators through a *vasculature* IPC effect,[115] and selectively increase collateral flow with chronic left anterior descending coronary stenosis, independent of K^+_{ATP} channels.[116]

Adenosine and Acadesine

Adenosine is released locally during ischemia, and its cardioprotective properties are also mediated through the K^+_{ATP} channel.[117] This process is dependent on PKC.[118,119] Chronic ethanol consumption also activates adenosine receptors and PKC, which ultimately confers myocardial protection through opening of the K^+_{ATP} channel.[120] Acadesine (AICA-riboside), an adenosine-regulating agent, is a purine nucleoside analog with anti-ischemic properties that has been studied for the prevention of adverse cardiovascular outcomes in patients undergoing coronary artery bypass graft surgery.[121] It may confer cardioprotection before or during ischemia, or after the onset of reperfusion. In animal models, it has been found to improve the ability of the heart to recover from ischemia and reperfusion when administered before ischemia or when added to cardioplegia.[122,123] In addition, it also decreases the threshold for IPC.[124] This observation was thought to support the theory that endogenous adenosine that accumulates during IPC mediates these protective effects, and that this response could be augmented by acadesine.[124] However, the results from human trials have been mixed. Leung et al.[125] evaluated acadesine as a myocardial protectant when used intraoperatively or after surgery and also administered with cardioplegia. They showed no difference in ischemia detected by either continuous Holter electrocardiography or transesophageal echocardiography after CPB.[125] The same group subsequently reported that acadesine may reduce the incidence of large Q-wave infarctions after coronary artery bypass surgery.[126] Recently, Lasley and colleagues[127] have also showed that acadesine did not enhance myocardial adenosine levels, attenuate myocardial stunning, or potentiate the cardioprotective effects of adenosine in the pig. Smits and colleagues[128] showed that the novel adenosine A1/A2 receptor agonist (AMP579) produced marked cardioprotection whether administered before myocardial ischemia or with reperfusion. Cardioprotection was not dependent on changes in afterload or myocardial oxygen demand and was found to be a consequence of adenosine A2 receptor stimulation. Both acadesine, as an adenosine regulating agent, and selective A1 receptor agonist failed to reduce infarct size.[128] Endogenous adenosine is also an antiarrhythmic mediator that accumulates in acute ischemic myocardium. The decreased occurrence of ventricular fibrillation is mediated through A2 adenosine receptor activation.[129]

Other Agents That Modulate Ischemic Preconditioning

Postinfarct ventricular remodeling makes the myocardium refractory to IPC. Valsartan, an angiotensin II type 1 receptor blocker, is beneficial not only for suppression of ventricular remodeling but also for preservation of the IPC mechanism.[130] Chronic inhibition of the angiotensin-converting enzyme in a rabbit model has been shown to be beneficial in potentiating the anti-infarct effect of subthreshold IPC.[131] The angiotensin receptor and bradykinin B2 receptor also play a role in ischemia/reperfusion injury.[132] Bradykinin, released intracellularly during myocardial ischemia/reperfusion injury, mediates myocardial preservation by reducing angiotensin II formation. As with valsartan, the angiotensin II type 1 receptor blocker, losartan, has been shown in rat heart models to reduce myocardial ischemia/reperfusion injury and provide cardioprotection through both bradykinin-dependent and bradykinin-independent mechanisms.[133]

Propofol: Cardioprotection during Reperfusion

Propofol has a chemical structure similar to that of phenol-based free radical scavengers such as vitamin E. It reduces free radicals,[134] attenuates the concentration of intracellular calcium,[135] and suppresses the activity of neutrophils.[136] It therefore has beneficial effects during reperfusion, but does not confer preconditioning effects. Currently, there are no studies suggesting that it may have cardioprotection at doses currently used in clinical practice.

Cardioprotection after Reperfusion: Inhibitors of Na$^+$/H$^+$ Exchanger

Mechanisms of Action

The sarcolemmal Na$^+$/H$^+$ exchanger (NHE) or antiport membrane transport system is a major regulator of intracellular pH and is one of the major mechanisms for restoring intracellular pH after ischemia-induced intracellular acidosis (Fig. 38–3). It is quiescent during normal physiologic conditions but is activated when intracellular pH decreases to less than 6.19. Emerging evidence implicates the NHE-1 transport system in various cardiac disease states, and the

exchanger may be particularly critical to postinfarction remodeling responses resulting in development of hypertrophy and heart failure.[137] At the onset of ischemia, glucose metabolism is shifted to the anaerobic pathway. This reduces intracellular pH, which in turn activates the NHE. This 110-kDa glycoprotein extrudes protons concomitantly with Na$^+$ influx in a 1:1 stoichiometric relationship rendering the process electroneutral.[137] The ensuing high intracellular sodium concentration results in two major intracellular events. It leads to activation of the Na$^+$/K$^+$ ATPase, which leads to an increase in ATP consumption, depletion of cellular energy stores, and potentially to cell death. Because the Na$^+$/K$^+$ channel requires ATP to function, this membrane channel is unable to normalize intracellular sodium concentration, and therefore the excess sodium is exchanged for calcium through the Na$^+$/Ca^{2+} exchanger. This results in an increase of intracellular calcium concentrations, which may cause arrhythmias, myocardial necrosis, and contracture. The intracellular movement of sodium is also passively accompanied by water, which causes further cellular swelling and dysfunction. In addition to intracellular acidosis, other factors such as ET-1, angiotensin II, α_1 adrenergic agonists, and toxic agents, such as hydrogen peroxide and lysophosphatidylcholine, can also stimulate or modulate the Na$^+$/H$^+$ exchanger.[138,139]

Although at least six NHE isoforms have thus far been identified, it appears that NHE-1 is the predominant isoform in the mammalian myocardium. Effective pharmacologic inhibitors of NHE, including those that are NHE-1–specific, have been extensively demonstrated to protect the ischemic and reperfused myocardium in terms of improved systolic and diastolic function, preservation of cellular ultrastructure, attenuation of the incidence of arrhythmias, and reduction of apoptosis. The ability of these agents to reduce myocardial infarct size and stunning has been demonstrated using a variety of experimental models. This suggests that the role of NHE in mediating injury is not species-specific. These agents have a low potential for toxicity, which makes NHE inhibition an effective therapeutic strategy in ischemia and reperfusion.[139] Inhibition of proton-driven sarcolemmal sodium influx not only ameliorates ischemic injury in the quiescent myocardium, but also seems to protect the heart during ventricular fibrillation.[140] NHE inhibition leads to a decreased susceptibility to severe ventricular arrhythmias, attenuates contractile dysfunction, and decreases infarct size during myocardial ischemia and reperfusion. Such protection is likely to arise, at least in part, from attenuation of Ca^{2+} overload, which has been linked causally with all of these pathologic phenomena. The consistent and marked cardioprotective benefit that has been observed with cariporide, zoniporide, and related compounds in preclinical studies suggests that NHE inhibition may represent a novel and effective approach to the treatment of acute myocardial ischemia in humans.[138]

Preclinical and Clinical Pharmacology

Several NHE inhibitors have been developed. Most of them are amiloride derivatives including cariporide, eniporide, and zoniporide. A new benzodihydrofuranyl analogue 1 (BMS-284640) has recently been synthesized and shows

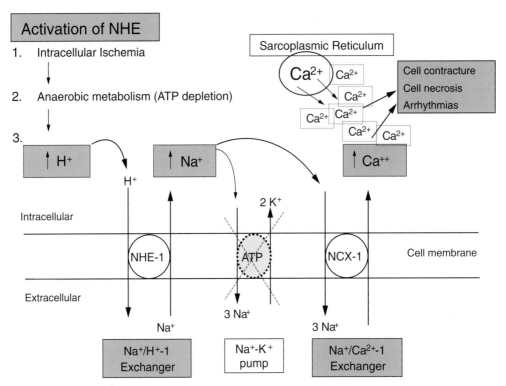

Figure 38–3. Na$^+$/H$^+$ Exchanger (NHE) function in ischemia/reperfusion injury. NHE-1 is activated during ischemia when anaerobic metabolism leads to a decrease in intracellular pH because of accumulation of hydrogen ions. *1,* Activation of NHE-1, attempts to decrease the intracellular hydrogen/ion concentration, but causes the accumulation of sodium in the intracellular space. *2,* With ongoing ischemia adenosine triphosphate (ATP) is depleted and the sodium potassium pump fails. *3,* The sodium/calcium exchanger (NCX-1) now exchanges sodium for calcium, which leads to accumulation of intracellular calcium. Calcium is also released from the sarcoplasmic reticulum. An increase in intracellular calcium is ultimately responsible for the deleterious side effects of ischemia. (Courtesy of R. Tracey, Pfizer, Inc)

greater than 380-fold increased NHE-1 inhibitory activity and improved selectivity for NHE-1 over NHE-2 compared with cariporide.[141] Cariporide is, however, the first of these agents to have been developed and subjected to clinical trial. Preclinical studies with cariporide revealed excellent protection against necrosis, apoptosis, arrhythmias, and mechanical dysfunction in hearts subjected to ischemia and reperfusion. Cariporide has recently been evaluated in a large dose-finding phase II/phase III clinical trial (GUARDIAN) to assess its efficacy in patients with acute coronary syndromes. Overall results failed to demonstrate protection, but subgroup analysis revealed significant risk reductions with the greatest cariporide dose (120 mg twice daily) especially in high-risk patients undergoing coronary artery bypass surgery. This suggests that insufficient dosage may have accounted, at least in part, for the less than optimum results. Another NHE-1 inhibitor, eniporide, is currently in phase II clinical trial (ESCAMI) in patients with acute myocardial infarction who require angioplasty or thrombolysis. Both drugs were well tolerated, produced no excess side effects compared with placebo, and there was a trend suggesting therapeutic benefit. TY-12533 is another compound currently being investigated. Its effect on arrhythmias and myocardial infarction has been compared with cariporide in a rat model of ischemia/reperfusion.

Inhibitory effects of TY-12533, TY-50893 (its metabolite), and cariporide on NHE-mediated platelet swelling in vitro were almost equal at pH 6.2 and decreased at pH 6.7; but TY-12533 was four times more potent than its metabolite and cariporide at pH 6.7. When administered before ischemia, all three drugs suppressed the ischemia/reperfusion–induced arrhythmias to the same extent in vivo, but TY-12533 was more effective than cariporide and TY-50893 when they were administered *during* ischemia. Similar results were obtained for the inhibitory effects of these drugs administered before ischemia and during ischemia on ischemia/reperfusion–induced myocardial infarction.[142]

The cardioprotective efficacy of zoniporide (CP-597,396), a novel, potent, and selective inhibitor of the NHE-1, has been evaluated both in vitro and in vivo using rabbit models of myocardial ischemia/reperfusion injury. Zoniporide elicited a concentration-dependent reduction in infarct size in the isolated heart preparation and produced a maximal reduction in infarct size of 83%. This compound is 2.5- to 20-fold more potent than either eniporide or cariporide, and reduced infarct size to a greater extent than eniporide (58% reduction in infarct size). In open-chest, anesthetized rabbits, zoniporide also elicited a dose-dependent reduction in infarct size and inhibited NHE-1–mediated platelet swelling. Furthermore, zoniporide did not cause any in vivo hemodynamic changes in parameters such as mean arterial pressure, heart rate, or rate pressure product.[143] It is currently undergoing clinical evaluation in patients undergoing vascular surgery and in patients undergoing cardiac bypass surgery.

Pharmacologic inhibition of the K^+_{ATP} channel with sulfonylureas, or the adenosine receptor with methylxanthines, has been shown to attenuate IPC. Both classes of compounds are widely used clinically, and several reports have demonstrated adverse outcomes in patients taking sulfonylureas. Recently, inhibition of NHE-1 has been shown to be equal to IPC at providing myocardial protection in dogs, and may be an alternative to IPC in patients taking sulfonylureas or methylxanthines.[144] In a rat heart model simulating cardiac allografts, cardioprotection conferred by the NHE inhibitor cariporide given during initial storage and perfusion was found to be additive to that of IPC and might effectively contribute to the improvement of donor heart preservation during cardiac transplantation.[145] It is also clear that the mitochondrial K^+_{ATP} channel plays a role in the cardioprotective effect of Na^+/H^+ exchange. In a recent study, it was shown that the cardioprotective effect of cariporide was abolished by glibenclamide, a nonselective K^+_{ATP} channel blocker. In vitro, the infarct-limiting effect of cariporide was blocked by 5-hydroxydecanoate (5-HD), a mitochondrial/K^+_{ATP} channel blocker, but not by HMR1098, a sarcolemmal/K^+_{ATP} channel blocker. Cariporide attenuated regional contractile dysfunction by stunning, and this protection was abolished by glibenclamide and 5-HD. Opening of the mitochondrial/K^+_{ATP} channel therefore contributes to cardioprotection by NHE inhibition, although the interaction between NHE and this K^+_{ATP} channel remains unclear.[146] IPC and NHE-1 inhibition provide comparable protection against 60 minutes of myocardial ischemia, but NHE-1 inhibition is more effective than IPC at protecting against a 90-minute ischemic insult. The combination of NHE-1 inhibition and IPC produces a greater than additive reduction in infarct size and area at risk, suggesting either that NHE activity limits the efficacy of IPC or that different mechanisms are involved in the cardioprotective effect of IPC and NHE-1 inhibition.[147]

Oxidant Stress and Free Radicals

Free radicals are highly reactive molecules formed during normal physiologic processes. Their formation is also seen with reperfusion of ischemic tissue, as may occur after myocardial infarction in patients undergoing thrombolysis and angioplasty, or after cardiac surgery. Free radicals are needed in normal homeostatic processes such as in the electron chain to form high-energy phosphates, or for the bactericidal function of macrophages and neutrophils. However, when excessive production of these oxygen-derived free radicals overwhelms the body's natural free radical scavenging mechanisms, cytotoxic damage may occur. Oxidants can also modulate various other pathophysiologic events such as NO formation, platelet-activating factor metabolism, tissue factor synthesis, and exposure of adhesion molecules.[7]

NO produced during ischemia/reperfusion produces local arterial vasodilatation and may increase the production of peroxynitrite, a physiologically active toxic metabolite of NO leading to vascular and myocardial dysfunction.[148,149] Recent evidence, however, has suggested that peroxynitrite may actually have antineutrophil and cardioprotective properties during in vivo biologic conditions when thiol-containing agents such as glutathione (GSH), albumin, or cysteine are available to convert the peroxynitrite anion to nitrosothiols and related products.[150] FK 409, the first spontaneous NO donor, increases the levels of cyclic guanosine monophosphate, and has been shown in orthotopic canine heart transplants to ameliorate ischemia/reperfusion injury and preserve cardiac function.[151]

Anti-Inflammatory Strategies

Corticosteroids

The inflammatory response to CPB, also known as the postperfusion syndrome, can be attenuated by the use of corticosteroids, aprotinin, anticytokine monoclonal antibodies, and by various modifications of the bypass circuit.[152] Corticosteroids may have beneficial effects on myocardial performance by reducing complement activation, reducing cytokine production, and reducing up-regulation in neutrophil adhesion molecules.[153] Recently, it has been demonstrated that pretreatment with methylprednisolone, through the induction of the cardioprotective heat shock protein 72, improved left ventricular function and coronary flow during reperfusion after 30 minutes of global ischemia and reduced infarct size in rat hearts.[154]

Protease Inhibitors

Aprotinin is a serine protease inhibitor that decreases the activation of plasminogen and the activity of plasmin. It has been shown to have anti-inflammatory properties, such as a reduction in interleukins and NO production, and is associated with a reduction in membrane injury associated with oxidant stress.[155] Its potential for myocardial protection may occur at different levels. It has the potential to decrease organ dysfunction by limiting or reducing the administration of blood products and platelets. It also preserves myocardial biochemical function during cold storage, as measured by preservation of ATP and protein synthesis, by inhibiting the release, uptake, and activity of tumor necrosis factor (TNF).[156] It has been postulated that microvascular blood flow might be improved by aprotinin, however, studies have yielded disparate results. A recent study in a rat model showed no difference in coronary blood flow or myocardial oxygen consumption with its use.[157] However, in a study of normothermic pentobarbital-anesthetized dogs, administration of clinically relevant doses of aprotinin before the onset of acute regional myocardial ischemia preserved regional systolic function and contractility at baseline values after re-establishment of myocardial perfusion.[158]

The CPB-related inflammatory response involves leukocyte activation and increased leukocyte/endothelial cell interaction. L-selectin, an adhesion molecule expressed on the surface of leukocytes, participates in the initial rolling step of the leukocyte/endothelial cell adhesion cascade. Leukocyte activation is heralded when L-selectin is cleaved off the surface of the leukocyte. Aprotinin inhibits shedding of L-selectin in a dose-dependent fashion and therefore contributes to the anti-inflammatory response.[159] During CPB, there is also a systemic increase in inflammatory cytokine levels, and there is sequestration of leukocytes within organs. Aprotinin exerts its anti-inflammatory effect in part by preventing transmigration of leukocytes through vascular endothelium. Aprotinin inhibits intercellular adhesion molecule-1 and vascular cell adhesion molecule-1 (but not E-selectin) expression on TNF-α–activated endothelial cells. Transendothelial migration by neutrophils is also specifically suppressed by aprotinin.[159] Intraoperative and postoperative infusion of aprotinin has resulted in more successful weaning from intra-aortic balloon counterpulsation[160] and has been shown to reduce troponin T release.[161] Because of the concern of graft patency with aprotinin, a large international multicenter study was undertaken, which did not show an association of aprotinin use with increased incidence of graft occlusion, myocardial infarction, or mortality.[162]

Cardioplegia

In cardiac surgery, a nonbeating, nonperfused flaccid heart provides optimal operating conditions. Arresting the heart for surgery is therefore the ultimate clinical application of the principles of cardiac protection. This section reviews the principles of cardiac protection as they relate to the clinical application of cardioplegia.

After the description of CPB in humans in 1953, methods evolved that would lead to protection of the arrested heart from ischemia. In 1955, Melrose and associates[163] first described chemical arrest of the heart using potassium citrate. Lam[164] subsequently coined the term *cardioplegia* after describing the arrest of the human heart using acetylcholine. However, because of early reports that chemical cardioplegia could damage the heart, cardioplegia solutions fell out of favor in the United States. Topical cooling of the heart, first described in 1959, became the standard method of protecting the heart during surgery.[165,166] However, it was subsequently established that hypothermia provided inadequate cardiac protection and that subendocardial necrosis occurred after topical cooling alone.[167,168] As a result, interest in chemically induced cardiac arrest resurfaced. It was shown that the earlier solutions used were inappropriately formulated, but that the concept of chemical arrest was sound. Subsequently, multiple solutions for arresting the heart safely have been introduced.[3,169] After crystalloid cardioplegia became established as a safe therapy, alternate chemical compositions and delivery methods were developed to improve cardiac protection. In 1978, the concept of cold, hyperkalemic blood cardioplegia was described.[4] The addition of blood to cardioplegic solutions improved oxygen-carrying capacity and buffering capacity.

The basic concepts of cardioplegia are: (1) to rapidly arrest the heart to create a still operative field and conserve cellular ATP stores; (2) to induce hypothermia to further reduce myocardial energy consumption; and (3) to provide other agents that further protect the heart from ischemia, edema formation, and reperfusion injury.

Inducing Cardiac Arrest

Cardiac arrest can be induced through one of two physiological mechanisms: depolarized cardiac arrest or hyperpolarized cardiac arrest.[170] Traditionally, myocardial protection during cardiac surgery has relied on hyperkalemic-depolarized arrest. However, hyperkalemia itself can lead to several problems related to the depolarization that causes ionic imbalances, continued metabolic activity, and the potential for reperfusion injury. This lead to the development of polarized or hyperpolarized arrest where the membrane potential (E_m) is kept close to, or more negative than the resting membrane potential. Maintaining the resting membrane potential close to normal levels should result in less ionic movement, maintenance of intracellular energy stores, and limited reperfusion injury.

Depolarizing Cardiac Arrest

Potassium is the agent most commonly used to induce cardiac arrest. Increasing the potassium concentration in the cardiac extracellular fluid decreases the resting membrane potential (i.e., brings it closer to 0 mV); at this potential, the myocytes become inexcitable and the heart becomes arrested in diastole. The concentration of potassium that is required to arrest the heart will depend on several factors, including the myocardial temperature, myocardial contractility, and use of ancillary agents that assist in the arrest. Typical commercial cardioplegia preparations, such as the modified St. Thomas Preparations (Plegisol; Abbott Laboratories), deliver between 15 and 20 mEq/L potassium to the coronary arteries to induce cardiac arrest. During the administration of potassium, the classical electrocardiogram changes of hyperkalemia occur. The administration of this concentration of potassium results in the depolarization of the E_m from a resting −80 to −50 mV. At this depolarized E_m, voltage-dependent Na^+ channels are inactivated and the heart becomes arrested in diastole. The main advantages of hyperkalemic arrest are rapidity of arrest and reversibility.

The reversal potential of the Na/Ca exchanger also occurs at −50 mV, therefore no net movement of Na^+ or Ca^{2+} should be occurring through the exchanger. There will, however, be an active Na^+ window current leading to an increase in the intracellular sodium concentration. This, in turn, leads to an increase in intracellular Ca^{2+} through the calcium window current and causes contracture of the muscle, even in the arrested state. Greater concentrations of potassium further depolarize the membrane (to about −40 mV), which will activate slow Ca^{2+} channels (which have a threshold of about −40 mV). This causes an influx of Ca^{2+} into the myocyte. At this Em, the Na^+/Ca^{2+} exchanger may be reversed resulting in net influx of Ca^{2+}, particularly if the intracellular Na^+ concentration is high as a result of sodium pump inhibition, hypothermia, or ischemia. This will lead to contracture, calcium overload, and subsequent myocardial injury, especially during reperfusion. These complex interactions between Na^+ and Ca^{2+} ion shifts, occurring as a result of hyperkalemic arrest, lead to a panoply of pathophysiologic processes, including Ca^{2+}-activated dysrhythmogenic currents, abnormal regulation of intracellular second messengers, activation of cytosolic and membrane-bound enzyme systems, impaired myocardial contraction, and the potential for Ca^{2+}-induced reperfusion injury. In addition, the use of potassium concentrations greater than 40 to 50 mEq/L are not advisable because there is a potential for direct tissue and vascular endothelial damage.[171] The main disadvantages of hyperkalemic arrest are therefore injury related to Ca^{2+} overload, the potential for endothelial damage at high potassium concentrations, temperature sensitivity requiring greater concentrations for normothermic arrest, the potential for systemic hyperkalemia, and sustained metabolic activity.

An alternative to hyperkalemic-induced depolarizing arrest is a hypocalcemic-induced depolarizing arrest.[172] In this technique, the arrest is induced with a solution containing zero calcium, combined with low sodium and procaine, which acts as a membrane stabilizer. However, a solution containing no calcium can induce a calcium paradox, although this is diminished by the solution containing a low sodium concentration and being hypothermic.[173] However, zero calcium and low sodium solutions appear to affect the cell membrane, leading to loosening of gap junctions and the intercalated disc, which can have adverse effects during the reperfusion phase.[173] As a result, this technique of cardioplegia is now rarely used.

Polarized or Hyperpolarized Cardiac Arrest

Because of the problems inherent in depolarized arrest, alternative techniques have evolved to induce electromechanical arrest of the heart. It has been shown experimentally that many of the problems inherent in the depolarized arrest can be avoided with hyperpolarizing agents.[170] The K^+_{ATP} channels were first described by Noma in 1983.[174] They are found in a variety of tissues, including cardiac myocytes, vascular smooth muscle, pancreatic beta cells, and neurons. Opening these channels induces myocardial relaxation by allowing K^+ efflux from the cell, which causes membrane hyperpolarization and decreases the probability that voltage-gated calcium channels will remain open. It has been shown that K^+_{ATP} channels mediate several important physiologic responses, including the cardiac and vascular response to hypoxemia,[175] basal coronary artery tone,[176] reactive hyperemia after brief coronary occlusion,[177,178] and coronary autoregulation.[178,179] In addition, it has been shown that K^+_{ATP} channels are critical in the cardiac protection mediated by IPC[180-182] and by adenosine.[180,183,184] In polarized or hyperpolarized arrest, the Em is kept at or close to the resting Em. This more physiologic state has several theoretic advantages. The transmembrane ion gradients remain balanced at or close to Em, which prevents the

ionic imbalance seen during hyperkalemic arrest. Few pumps or channels are activated, metabolic demand remains low, and myocyte energy stores are maintained. Importantly, the Na^+/Ca^{2+} channels are closed at these membrane potentials and hence the potential for Ca^{2+} and Na^+ overload are prevented. There are multiple potassium channel openers that have been studied in various models, including adenosine, diazoxide, nicorandil, minoxidil, pinacidil, cromakalim, lemakalim, and aprikalim.

K^+_{ATP} Channel Openers

Several studies have examined the efficacy of K^+ channel openers as agents for inducing cardiac arrest. Animal studies have shown that hearts arrested with aprikalim had better recovery than hearts arrested with potassium.[185,186] Despite the improved cardioprotection, hearts arrested with aprikalim had an increased incidence of postarrest arrhythmias. Further studies with pinacidil[187] and nicorandil[188] have shown that they are more protective in normothermic arrest than a depolarized potassium arrest. In rabbit[185] and canine[189] models, the protection afforded by K^+_{ATP} channel openers was equivalent to that of the commonly used St. Thomas Hospital cardioplegic solution. One of the main theoretic advantages of a hyperpolarized arrest is that ionic balances would be better maintained than a depolarized arrest. It has been shown that intercellular calcium rapidly increases when using a depolarizing potassium arrest, but that the increase can be avoided when the depolarizing solution is supplemented with a K^+_{ATP} channel opener.[190,191]

Sodium Channel Blockers

Sodium channel blockers (e.g., procaine or tetrodotoxin) produce a polarized arrest—that is, an arrest at the normal resting membrane potential. Chambers and colleagues have shown that hearts stored in a physiologic solution containing tetrodotoxin recovered better than hearts stored in a hyperkalemic solution.[192] They also showed that throughout the arrest the hyperkalemic-arrested hearts had an Em of about −50 mV (depolarized), and the hearts arrested with tetrodotoxin had a Em of −70 mV.

Adenosine

The intracoronary administration of adenosine was first shown to reduce reperfusion injury in 1987.[193] Adenosine produces its effects by interacting with a series of purigenic receptors, of which at least four are known: A1, A2a, A2b, and A3. A1 receptors are located on myocytes and neutrophils. The effector linked to the A1 receptors is the K^+_{ATP} channel. Stimulation of the A1 receptors leads to stimulation of the K^+_{ATP} channel, hyperpolarization of the cell, negative chronotropy, and negative dromotropy. Stimulation of A2 receptors, located on mainly on neutrophils, platelets, endothelium and vascular smooth muscle, leads to vasodilatation and decreased neutrophil free radical formation.[194,195] A3 receptors are also found on myocytes and also lead to stimulation of the K^+_{ATP} channel. In a recent study further examining the cardioprotective effect of adenosine in a rat cardioplegia model, adenosine supplementation improved myocardial functional recovery by preventing the depression in myofibrillar cooperative action that is known to occur after cardioplegic arrest and reperfusion.[196] In addition, there was an adenosine receptor–mediated increase in anaerobic glycolysis during cardioplegic arrest. It is well known that glycolysis is vital to protecting cardiac function during warm ischemia,[197] in conditions of reduced oxygen supply in relation to demand,[197] and during cardioplegic arrest. These protective effects were ablated with a nonspecific adenosine receptor blocker.

As discussed earlier, stimulation of each of the adenosine receptor subtypes may produce cardioprotection by distinct mechanisms.[195,198–201] Because the mechanisms involved in protection may be so different, stimulation of the various adenosine receptors may have the ability to confer protection at different stages of cardioplegia—i.e., before the arrest, during the cardioplegia, and after reperfusion. Adenosine has been shown to induce a hyperpolarized arrest in a rabbit heart,[202] adenosine cardioplegia more rapidly arrested rat hearts than did potassium cardioplegia.[203] In addition, recovery of the adenosine-arrested hearts was better than that of the potassium-arrested hearts. De Jong and colleagues[204] studied the electrophysiology of adenosine-supplemented cardiac arrest. They showed that the combination of adenosine and potassium induced an initial hyperpolarization, which led to arrest of the sinoatrial node, followed by depolarization arrest of the myocyte caused by the potassium. In a guinea pig model, adenosine-supplemented potassium cardioplegia was shown to reduce the rate of depolarization but not the overall level of depolarization achieved. However, adenosine attenuated the increased cytosolic Ca^{2+} levels induced by hyperkalemia. In a baboon model of CPB, adenosine was compared with hyperkalemic arrest with St. Thomas Hospital solution.[205] Adenosine caused a more rapid arrest, but the degree of cardiac protection conferred was equal. Several other models have examined the effect of adenosine on cardiac protection[206–208] and have shown that adenosine supplementation of blood cardioplegia improves postischemic cardiac function, reduces infarct size and myocyte edema, and reduces neutrophil myeloperoxidase activity. In a human phase I study, administering adenosine during cardioplegia was shown to be safe.[209] In a subsequent phase II study, adenosine appeared to confer no benefit versus routine antegrade warm cardioplegia.[210] However, in other studies with cold cardioplegia and much greater adenosine doses, adenosine supplementation reduced the need for post-CPB inotropic support[211] and reduced transfusion requirements.[212]

Experimental Strategies with Cardioplegia

Anticomplement Therapy

Complement activation, polymorphonuclear leukocytes, and increased circulating levels of various cytokines are three major causes of tissue damage and endothelial dysfunction after ischemia/reperfusion and CPB. Complement activation as a consequence of exposure of blood components to the CPB circuit occurs through both the classical and alternative pathways.[213] Many different strategies have been used to decrease complement activation including coating extracorporeal circuits with heparin to prevent activation and using leukocyte filters to reduce the number of neutrophils from the circulation. Another therapeutic modality has been monoclonal antibodies directed against the complement system itself.

Several complement inhibitors are being studied for potential applications during CPB. They include a recombinant soluble complement receptor-1 (sCR1),[214] a humanized single-chain anti-C5 antibody (h5G1.1-scFv),[215] a recombinant fusion hybrid (CAB-2) of human membrane cofactor protein and human decay accelerating factor,[216] and a 13-residue C3-binding cyclic peptide (Compstatin).[217] sCR1 and CAB-2 inhibit the classical and alternative complement pathways at the steps of C3 and C5 activation. Compstatin inhibits both complement pathways at the step of C3 activation, whereas h5G1.1-scFv does so only at the step of C5 activation. Factor D, one of the complement enzymes, is thought to be the rate-limiting enzyme for the activation and amplification of the alternative complement pathway.[218] Anti-factor D MAb is effective in inhibiting the activation of C3 and C5 and the other inflammatory responses in extracorporeal circulation. In a recent study using an anti-factor D Mab in a porcine model of CPB, a variety of cellular and humoral inflammatory responses to CPB were reduced.[219] However, the pattern of post-CPB inflammation is heterogeneous, and the results of animal work thus far have shown an inconsistent postcardioplegia contractile benefit. Human studies with anticomplement therapy are ongoing.

Nitric Oxide Therapy

During basal conditions, the intact vascular endothelium actively participates in protection of the vasculature by releasing NO synthesized through the L-arginine-NO synthase pathway, thereby functioning in a homeostatic capacity to prevent thrombus formation and neutrophil adherence. However, myocardial ischemia and reperfusion impair NO production,[220] thereby compromising this inherent protection. Several studies have shown that endothelial injury associated with prolonged ischemia or blood reperfusion is reduced by a NO donor (SPM-5185)[221] or L-arginine.[222] In another study by Sato and colleagues,[223] inhibition of endogenous NO synthase activity by L nitro-arginine in blood cardioplegic solution and during reperfusion, or during reperfusion only, was associated with a significant increase in infarct size and diastolic dysfunction. Also, L nitro-arginine treatment was associated with an increase in neutrophil accumulation within the area at risk. Inhibition of NO synthase–mediated protection may also damage both the coronary vascular endothelium and to a lesser extent the vascular smooth muscle. These data are consistent with the hypothesis that endogenous NO participates in the inherent protection of ischemic-reperfused and normal myocardium during cardiac operations.

There have been some conflicting data suggesting that NO-enhancing therapy in cardioplegia may be harmful. NO undergoes a rapid biradical reaction with superoxide anions to produce peroxynitrite. Peroxynitrite (ONOO-) in crystalloid cardioplegia induces injury to coronary endothelium and impairs systolic function after cardioplegia and reperfusion.[224] However, ONOO- may be degraded to less lethal or cardioprotective intermediates with GSH in reactions separate from its well-known antioxidant effects.[225] Endogenous thiol-containing substances such as GSH, albumin, and cysteine may convert ONOO- to less harmful or even cardioprotective byproducts. In addition to its potent antioxidant effects through the conversion of hydrogen peroxide to molecular oxygen and water through GSH peroxidase, GSH converts ONOO- into potential NO donors such as S-nitrosoglutathione and S-nitroglutathione, which exhibit physiologic and cardioprotective effects similar to those of NO. In a study examining GSH-enhanced cardioplegia.[226] Nakamura and colleagues[226] showed that GSH in crystalloid cardioplegia detoxifies ONOO- and forms cardioprotective nitrosoglutathione, resulting in attenuated neutrophil adherence and selective endothelial protection through the inhibition of neutrophil-mediated damage.

Insulin-Enhanced Cardioplegia

Glucose-insulin-potassium solutions have been commonly used to treat ischemic myocardium in a variety of medical and surgical settings. The results of earlier investigations were often conflicting, and interest in metabolic stimulation of the heart waned. One potential confounding factor in the early studies of glucose-insulin-potassium solutions was the routine use of moderate hypothermia during CPB. In retrospect, metabolic stimulation of the heart may not have been effective at temperatures that inhibit normal enzyme function. The advent of normothermic heart surgery prompted renewed interest in myocardial protection. In a rodent study, Kobayashi and Neely[227] demonstrated that the activity of a key mitochondrial enzyme, pyruvate dehydrogenase, was inhibited during early reperfusion. The recovery of postischemic myocardial function has also been shown to be dependent on the recovery of pyruvate dehydrogenase activity.[228] Rao and colleagues[229] reported that insulin was capable of stimulating mitochondrial pyruvate dehydrogenase activity in isolated human ventricular cardiomyocytes, which led to improved protection against ischemia and reperfusion. In a recent prospective study, patients undergoing elective coronary bypass surgery were given cardioplegia containing either 42 or 84 mmol/L glucose with or without 10 IU/L insulin.[230] Perioperative assessments of myocardial metabolism and left ventricular function were performed. In the insulin-enhanced groups, there were beneficial effects on both myocardial metabolic and functional recovery after cardioplegic arrest. The effect of insulin was independent of the glucose concentration. In another study by the same group, the incidence of atrial fibrillation was examined.[231] In this double-blinded, randomized, controlled clinical trial, 501 patients undergoing urgent coronary artery bypass graft received either insulin-enhanced or standard blood cardioplegia during CPB. Insulin-enhanced cardioplegia did not result in a significant reduction in postoperative atrial fibrillation and did not reduce the incidence of conduction defects, ventricular tachycardia, or pacemaker requirements among the groups.

Anti–Tumor Necrosis Factor α in Cardioplegia

TNF-α has been implicated in the pathogenesis of ischemia/reperfusion injury and heart failure.[232,233] Effects of TNF-α are initiated by membrane receptors coupled to sphingomyelinase signaling and include altered metabolism and calcium cycling, contractile dysfunction, and cell death. Stamm and colleagues[234] have shown that TNF-α is expressed in hearts with pressure-induced hypertrophy and contributes to reduced myocardial function after ischemia/reperfusion.[234] Neutralization of TNF-α, either by neutralizing antibody or inhibition of postreceptor signaling, led to improved contractile function in hearts with LV hypertrophy. Beneficial effects of TNF-α inhibition in hypertrophied hearts were associated with improved recovery of high-energy phosphates, pH, and intracellular calcium handling.

Practical Aspects of Drug Administration

Although there is an emerging pharmacologic armamentarium of cardioprotective drugs, few of these drugs are currently approved for routine use in the United States. A few drugs (e.g., nicorandil) are available and are in use in the United Kingdom. Nonetheless, the understanding of the mechanisms of cardioprotection is already beginning to have an impact on practice. There has been renewed interest in the cardiac protection afforded by total neuraxial blockade and its beneficial effects on ischemia and the prevention of β receptor desensitization and down-regulation. Preoperative beta-blockade has already become a standard of care for high-risk patients presenting for major surgery. Similarly, volatile anesthetics are now commonly used for cardioprotection during cardiac surgery, whereas once they were eschewed; this is in part because of the appreciation of the pre-IPC effects of these agents, which is seen at clinically relevant concentrations. Morphine in clinically relevant doses may be a good adjunct in this preischemic setting. (Neither morphine nor the halogenated agents though have been shown to be beneficial after the onset of ischemia.) Other opioids and propofol also have beneficial properties but may not be applicable because dosages studied thus far are not clinically relevant. As the new K^+_{ATP} openers and NHE inhibitors become available they are likely to have a major impact on preoperative and intraoperative management of patients undergoing cardiac surgery and patients with ischemic heart disease undergoing other major surgeries.

References

1. Shiroishi MS: Myocardial protection: The rebirth of potassium-based cardioplegia. Tex Heart Inst J 26:71, 1999.
2. Hearse DJ, Stewart DA, Braimbridge MV: Cellular protection during myocardial ischemia: The development and characterization of a procedure for the induction of reversible ischemic arrest. Circulation 54:193, 1976.

3. Gay WA Jr, Ebert PA: Functional, metabolic, and morphologic effects of potassium-induced cardioplegia. Surgery 74:284, 1973.

4. Follette DM, Mulder DG, Maloney JV, Buckberg GD: Advantages of blood cardioplegia over continuous coronary perfusion or intermittent ischemia. Experimental and clinical study. J Thorac Cardiovasc Surg 76:604, 1978.

5. Cordell AR: Milestones in the development of cardioplegia. Ann Thorac Surg 60:793, 1995.

6. Warltier DC, Pagel PS, Kersten JR: Approaches to the prevention of perioperative myocardial ischemia. Anesthesiology 92:253, 2000.

7. Ambrosio G, Tritto I: Reperfusion injury: Experimental evidence and clinical implications. Am Heart J 138:S69, 1999.

8. Collard CD, Gelman S: Pathophysiology, clinical manifestations, and prevention of ischemia-reperfusion injury. Anesthesiology 94:1133, 2001.

9. Sethna DH, Moffitt EA: An appreciation of the coronary circulation. Anesth Analg 65:294, 1986.

10. Schremmer B, Dhainaut JF: Regulation of myocardial oxygen delivery. Intensive Care Med 16:S157, 1990.

11. Muller JM, Davis MJ, Chilian WM: Integrated regulation of pressure and flow in the coronary microcirculation. Cardiovasc Res 32:668, 1996.

12. Krajcar M, Heusch G: Local and neurohumoral control of coronary blood flow. Basic Res Cardiol 88:25, 1993.

13. Heusch G: Control of coronary vasomotor tone in ischaemic myocardium by local metabolism and neurohumoral mechanisms. Eur Heart J 12:99, 1991.

14. Feigl EO: Coronary physiology. Physiol Rev 63:1, 1983.

15. Schliep HJ, Harting J: Beta 1-selectivity of bisoprolol, a new beta-adrenoceptor antagonist, in anesthetized dogs and guinea pigs. J Cardiovasc Pharmacol 6:1156, 1984.

16. Hjalmarson A: Cardioprotection with beta-adrenoceptor blockers. Does lipophilicity matter? Basic Res Cardiol 95:I41, 2000.

17. Lopez BL, Christopher TA, Yue TL, et al: Carvedilol, a new beta-adrenoreceptor blocker antihypertensive drug, protects against free-radical-induced endothelial dysfunction. Pharmacology 51:165, 1995.

18. Gao F, Chen J, Lopez BL, et al: Comparison of bisoprolol and carvedilol cardioprotection in a rabbit ischemia and reperfusion model. Eur J Pharmacol 406:109, 2000.

19. Feuerstein GZ, Yue TL, Cheng HY, Ruffolo RR Jr: Myocardial protection by the novel vasodilating beta-blocker, carvedilol: Potential relevance of anti-oxidant activity. J Hypertens Suppl 11:S41, 1993.

20. Cargnoni A, Ceconi C, Bernocchi P, et al: Reduction of oxidative stress by carvedilol: Role in maintenance of ischaemic myocardium viability. Cardiovasc Res 47:556, 2000.

21. Mangano DT, Layug EL, Wallace A, Tateo I: Effect of atenolol on mortality and cardiovascular morbidity after noncardiac surgery. Multicenter Study of Perioperative Ischemia Research Group. N Engl J Med 335:1713, 1996.

22. Wallace A, Layug B, Tateo I, et al: Prophylactic atenolol reduces postoperative myocardial ischemia. McSPI Research Group. Anesthesiology 88:7, 1998.

23. Raby KE, Brull SJ, Timimi F, et al: The effect of heart rate control on myocardial ischemia among high-risk patients after vascular surgery. Anesth Analg 88:477, 1999.

24. Poldermans D, Boersma E, Bax JJ, et al: The effect of bisoprolol on perioperative mortality and myocardial infarction in high-risk patients undergoing vascular surgery. Dutch Echocardiographic Cardiac Risk Evaluation Applying Stress Echocardiography Study Group. N Engl J Med 341:1789, 1999.

25. Poldermans D, Boersma E, Bax JJ, et al: Bisoprolol reduces cardiac death and myocardial infarction in high-risk patients as long as 2 years after successful major vascular surgery. Eur Heart J 22:1353, 2001.

26. Lawrence CJ, Prinzen FW, de Lange S: The effect of dexmedetomidine on nutrient organ blood flow. Anesth Analg 83:1160, 1996.

27. Roekaerts PM, Lawrence CJ, Prinzen FW, de Lange S: Alleviation of the peripheral hemodynamic effects of dexmedetomidine by the calcium channel blocker isradipine. Acta Anaesthesiol Scand 41:364, 1997.

28. Coughlan MG, Lee JG, Bosnjak ZJ, et al: Direct coronary and cerebral vascular responses to dexmedetomidine. Significance of endogenous nitric oxide synthesis. Anesthesiology 77:998, 1992.

29. Lawrence CJ, Prinzen FW, de Lange S: The effect of dexmedetomidine on the balance of myocardial energy requirement and oxygen supply and demand. Anesth Analg 82:544, 1996.

30. Khan ZP, Ferguson CN, Jones RM: Alpha-2 and imidazoline receptor agonists. Their pharmacology and therapeutic role. Anaesthesia 54:146, 1999.

31. Perioperative sympatholysis. Beneficial effects of the alpha 2-adrenoceptor agonist mivazerol on hemodynamic stability and myocardial ischemia. McSPI—Europe Research Group. Anesthesiology 86:346, 1997.

32. Fox K, Dargie HJ, de Bono DP, et al: Effect of an alpha(2) agonist (mivazerol) on limiting myocardial ischaemia in stable angina. Heart 82:383, 1999.

33. Wright RA, Decroly P, Kharkevitch T, Oliver MF: Exercise tolerance in angina is improved by mivazerol—an alpha 2-adrenoceptor agonist. Cardiovasc Drugs Ther 7:929, 1993.

34. Oliver MF, Goldman L, Julian DG, Holme I: Effect of mivazerol on perioperative cardiac complications during non-cardiac surgery in patients with coronary heart disease: The European Mivazerol Trial (EMIT). Anesthesiology 91:951, 1999.

35. Cohen AT: Prevention of perioperative myocardial ischaemia and its complications. Lancet 351:385, 1998.

36. Blomberg S, Curelaru I, Emanuelsson H, et al: Thoracic epidural anaesthesia in patients with unstable angina pectoris. Eur Heart J 10:437, 1989.

37. Olausson K, Magnusdottir H, Lurje L, et al: Anti-ischemic and anti-anginal effects of thoracic epidural anesthesia versus those of conventional medical therapy in the treatment of severe refractory unstable angina pectoris. Circulation 96:2178, 1997.

38. Kock M, Blomberg S, Emanuelsson H, et al: Thoracic epidural anesthesia improves global and regional left ventricular function during stress-induced myocardial ischemia in patients with coronary artery disease. Anesth Analg 71:625, 1990.

39. Blomberg S, Emanuelsson H, Ricksten SE: Thoracic epidural anesthesia and central hemodynamics in patients with unstable angina pectoris. Anesth Analg 69:558, 1989.

40. Beattie WS, Badner NH, Choi P: Epidural analgesia reduces postoperative myocardial infarction: A meta-analysis. Anesth Analg 93:853, 2001.

41. Rigg JR, Jamrozik K, Myles PS, et al: Epidural anaesthesia and analgesia and outcome of major surgery: A randomized trial. Lancet 359:1276, 2002.

42. Park WY, Thompson JS, Lee KK: Effect of epidural anesthesia and analgesia on perioperative outcome: A randomized, controlled Veterans Affairs cooperative study. Ann Surg 234:560, 2001.

43. Peyton PJ, Myles PS, Silbert BS, et al: Perioperative epidural analgesia and outcome after major abdominal surgery in high-risk patients. Anesth Analg 96:548, 2003.

44. de Leon-Casasola OA: When it comes to outcome, we need to define what a perioperative epidural technique is. Anesth Analg 96:315, 2003.

45. Liem TH, Booij LH, Hasenbos MA, Gielen MJ: Coronary artery bypass grafting using two different anesthetic techniques: Part I: Hemodynamic results. J Cardiothorac Vasc Anesth 6:148, 1992.

46. Liem TH, Hasenbos MA, Booij LH, Gielen MJ: Coronary artery bypass grafting using two different anesthetic techniques: Part 2: Postoperative outcome. J Cardiothorac Vasc Anesth 6:156, 1992.

47. Liem TH, Booij LH, Gielen MJ, et al: Coronary artery bypass grafting using two different anesthetic techniques: Part 3: Adrenergic responses. J Cardiothorac Vasc Anesth 6:162, 1992.

48. Priestley MC, Cope L, Halliwell R, et al: Thoracic epidural anesthesia for cardiac surgery: The effects on tracheal intubation time and length of hospital stay. Anesth Analg 94:275, 2002.

49. Scott NB, Turfrey DJ, Ray DA, et al: A prospective randomized study of the potential benefits of thoracic epidural anesthesia and analgesia in patients undergoing coronary artery bypass grafting. Anesth Analg 93:528, 2001.

50. Lee TW, Grocott HP, Schwinn D, Jacobsohn E: High spinal anesthesia for cardiac surgery: Effects on beta-adrenergic receptor function, stress response, and hemodynamics. Anesthesiology 98:499, 2003.

51. Tune JD, Richmond KN, Gorman MW, Feigl EO: Role of nitric oxide and adenosine in control of coronary blood flow in exercising dogs. Circulation 101:2942, 2000.

52. Tune JD, Richmond KN, Gorman MW, et al: Adenosine is not responsible for local metabolic control of coronary blood flow in dogs during exercise. Am J Physiol Heart Circ Physiol 278:H74, 2000.

53. Matsunaga T, Warltier DC, Weihrauch DW, et al: Ischemia-induced

coronary collateral growth is dependent on vascular endothelial growth factor and nitric oxide. Circulation 102:3098, 2000.

54. Lefer AM, Lefer DJ: The role of nitric oxide and cell adhesion molecules on the microcirculation in ischaemia-reperfusion. Cardiovasc Res 32:743, 1996.

55. Lefer AM: Nitric oxide: Nature's naturally occurring leukocyte inhibitor. Circulation 95:553, 1997.

56. Armstead VE, Minchenko AG, Schuhl RA, et al: Regulation of P-selectin expression in human endothelial cells by nitric oxide. Am J Physiol 273:H740, 1997.

57. Jones SP, Girod WG, Palazzo AJ, et al: Myocardial ischemia-reperfusion injury is exacerbated in absence of endothelial cell nitric oxide synthase. Am J Physiol 276:H1567, 1999.

58. Pabla R, Buda AJ, Flynn DM, et al: Nitric oxide attenuates neutrophil-mediated myocardial contractile dysfunction after ischemia and reperfusion. Circ Res 78:65, 1996.

59. Oxhorn BC, Cheek DJ, Buxton IL: Role of nucleotides and nucleosides in the regulation of cardiac blood flow. AACN Clin Issues 11:241, 2000.

60. Krause SM, Lynch JJ Jr, Stabilito II, Woltmann RF: Intravenous administration of the endothelin-1 antagonist BQ-123 does not ameliorate myocardial ischaemic injury following acute coronary artery occlusion in the dog. Cardiovasc Res 28:1672, 1994.

61. Bugge E, Ytrehus K: Endothelin-1 can reduce infarct size through protein kinase C and KATP channels in the isolated rat heart. Cardiovasc Res 32:920, 1996.

62. Kakita T, Hasegawa K, Iwai-Kanai E, et al: Calcineurin pathway is required for endothelin-1-mediated protection against oxidant stress-induced apoptosis in cardiac myocytes. Circ Res 88:1239, 2001.

63. Most AS, Ruocco NA Jr, Gewirtz H: Effect of a reduction in blood viscosity on maximal myocardial oxygen delivery distal to a moderate coronary stenosis. Circulation 74:1085, 1986.

64. Spiess BD, Ley C, Body SC, et al: Hematocrit value on intensive care unit entry influences the frequency of Q-wave myocardial infarction after coronary artery bypass grafting. The Institutions of the Multicenter Study of Perioperative Ischemia (McSPI) Research Group. J Thorac Cardiovasc Surg 116:460, 1998.

65. Hebert PC, Wells G, Blajchman MA, et al: A multicenter, randomized, controlled clinical trial of transfusion requirements in critical care. Transfusion Requirements in Critical Care Investigators, Canadian Critical Care Trials Group. N Engl J Med 340:409, 1999.

66. Wu WC, Rathore SS, Wang Y, et al: Blood transfusion in elderly patients with acute myocardial infarction. N Engl J Med 345:1230, 2001.

67. Mehta JL, Jayaram K: Reperfusion injury in humans: Existence, clinical relevance, mechanistic insights, and potential therapy. J Thromb Thrombolysis 4:75, 1997.

68. Kloner RA: Does reperfusion injury exist in humans? J Am Coll Cardiol 21:537, 1993.

69. Murry CE, Jennings RB, Reimer KA: Preconditioning with ischemia: A delay of lethal cell injury in ischemic myocardium. Circulation 74:1124, 1986.

70. Yellon DM, Baxter GF: Protecting the ischaemic and reperfused myocardium in acute myocardial infarction: Distant dream or near reality? Heart 83:381, 2000.

71. Dana A, Baxter GF, Walker JM, Yellon DM: Prolonging the delayed phase of myocardial protection: Repetitive adenosine A1 receptor activation maintains rabbit myocardium in a preconditioned state. J Am Coll Cardiol 31:1142, 1998.

72. Yellon DM, Alkhulaifi AM, Pugsley WB: Preconditioning the human myocardium. Lancet 342:276, 1993.

73. Dana A, Baxter GF, Yellon DM: Delayed or second window preconditioning induced by adenosine A1 receptor activation is independent of early generation of nitric oxide or late induction of inducible nitric oxide synthase. J Cardiovasc Pharmacol 38:278, 2001.

74. Noda T, Minatoguchi S, Fujii K, et al: Evidence for the delayed effect in human ischemic preconditioning: Prospective multicenter study for preconditioning in acute myocardial infarction. J Am Coll Cardiol 34:1966, 1999.

75. Gross GJ, Fryer RM: Sarcolemmal versus mitochondrial ATP-sensitive K+ channels and myocardial preconditioning. Circ Res 84:973, 1999.

76. Fryer RM, Hsu AK, Gross GJ: Mitochondrial K(ATP) channel opening is important during index ischemia and following myocar-

dial reperfusion in ischemic preconditioned rat hearts. J Mol Cell Cardiol 33:831, 2001.

77. Gross GJ: The role of mitochondrial KATP channels in cardioprotection. Basic Res Cardiol 95:280, 2000.

78. Cason BA, Gordon HJ, Avery EGt, Hickey RF: The role of ATP sensitive potassium channels in myocardial protection. J Card Surg 10:441, 1995.

79. Hoek TL, Becker LB, Shao Z, et al: Preconditioning antioxidant protection by katp channel opening requires nitric oxide synthase. Acad Emerg Med 8:548, 2001.

80. Zaugg M, Lucchinetti E, Spahn DR, et al: Differential effects of anesthetics on mitochondrial K(ATP) channel activity and cardiomyocyte protection. Anesthesiology 97:15, 2002.

81. Fryer RM, Schultz JE, Hsu AK, Gross GJ: Importance of PKC and tyrosine kinase in single or multiple cycles of preconditioning in rat hearts. Am J Physiol 276:H1229, 1999.

82. Cleveland JC Jr, Meldrum DR, Cain BS, et al: Oral sulfonylurea hypoglycemic agents prevent ischemic preconditioning in human myocardium. Two paradoxes revisited. Circulation 96:29, 1997.

83. Kersten JR, Lowe D, Hettrick DA, et al: Glyburide, a KATP channel antagonist, attenuates the cardioprotective effects of isoflurane in stunned myocardium. Anesth Analg 83:27, 1996.

84. Schaefer S, Correa SD, Valente RJ, Laslett LJ: Blockade of adenosine receptors with aminophylline limits ischemic preconditioning in human beings. Am Heart J 142:E4, 2001.

85. Liang BT: Direct preconditioning of cardiac ventricular myocytes via adenosine A1 receptor and KATP channel. Am J Physiol 271:H1769, 1996.

86. Kersten JR, Toller WG, Gross ER, et al: Diabetes abolishes ischemic preconditioning: Role of glucose, insulin, and osmolality. Am J Physiol Heart Circ Physiol 278:H1218, 2000.

87. Saltman AE, Krukenkamp IB, Gaudette GR, et al: Pharmacological preconditioning with the adenosine triphosphate-sensitive potassium channel opener pinacidil. Ann Thorac Surg 70:595, 2000.

88. Mizumura T, Saito S, Ozawa Y, et al: An ATP-sensitive potassium (KATP) channel opener, nicorandil, lowers the threshold for ischemic preconditioning in barbital-anesthetized dogs. Heart Vessels (suppl 12):175, 1997.

89. Trial to show the impact of nicorandil in angina (IONA): Design, methodology, and management. Heart 85:E9, 2001.

90. Kersten JR, Schmeling TJ, Pagel PS, et al: Isoflurane mimics ischemic preconditioning via activation of K(ATP) channels: Reduction of myocardial infarct size with an acute memory phase. Anesthesiology 87:361, 1997.

91. Kersten JR, Montgomery MW, Pagel PS, Warltier DC: Levosimendan, a new positive inotropic drug, decreases myocardial infarct size via activation of K(ATP) channels. Anesth Analg 90:5, 2000.

92. Kaheinen P, Pollesello P, Levijoki J, Haikala H: Levosimendan increases diastolic coronary flow in isolated guinea-pig heart by opening ATP-sensitive potassium channels. J Cardiovasc Pharmacol 37:367, 2001.

93. Lehtonen LA: Levosimendan: A parenteral calcium-sensitizing drug with additional vasodilatory properties. Expert Opin Invest Drugs 10:955, 2001.

94. Cain BS, Meldrum DR, Cleveland JC Jr, et al: Clinical L-type Ca(2+) channel blockade prevents ischemic preconditioning of human myocardium. J Mol Cell Cardiol 31:2191, 1999.

95. Huh J, Gross GJ, Nagase H, Liang BT: Protection of cardiac myocytes via delta(1)-opioid receptors, protein kinase C, and mitochondrial K(ATP) channels. Am J Physiol Heart Circ Physiol 280:H377, 2001.

96. Fryer RM, Hsu AK, Nagase H, Gross GJ: Opioid-induced cardioprotection against myocardial infarction and arrhythmias: Mitochondrial versus sarcolemmal ATP-sensitive potassium channels. J Pharmacol Exp Ther 294:451, 2000.

97. Liang BT, Gross GJ: Direct preconditioning of cardiac myocytes via opioid receptors and KATP channels. Circ Res 84:1396, 1999.

98. Sigg DC, Coles JA Jr, Oeltgen PR, Iaizzo PA: Role of delta-opioid receptor agonists on infarct size reduction in swine. Am J Physiol Heart Circ Physiol 282:H1953, 2002.

99. Wu S, Li HY, Wong TM: Cardioprotection of preconditioning by metabolic inhibition in the rat ventricular myocyte. Involvement of kappa-opioid receptor. Circ Res 84:1388, 1999.

100. Wang GY, Wu S, Pei JM, et al: Kappa- but not delta-opioid receptors mediate effects of ischemic preconditioning on both infarct and arrhythmia in rats. Am J Physiol Heart Circ Physiol 280:H384, 2001.

101. Coles JA Jr, Sigg DC, Iaizzo PA: The role of kappa-opioid receptor activation in pharmacological preconditioning of swine. Am J Physiol Heart Circ Physiol (in press).

102. Bell SP, Sack MN, Patel A, et al: Delta opioid receptor stimulation mimics ischemic preconditioning in human heart muscle. J Am Coll Cardiol 36:2296, 2000.

103. Kato R, Foex P: Myocardial protection by anesthetic agents against ischemia-reperfusion injury: An update for anesthesiologists. Can J Anaesth 49:777, 2002.

104. Roscoe AK, Christensen JD, Lynch C 3rd: Isoflurane, but not halothane, induces protection of human myocardium via adenosine A1 receptors and adenosine triphosphate-sensitive potassium channels. Anesthesiology 92:1692, 2000.

105. Toller WG, Kersten JR, Gross ER, et al: Isoflurane preconditions myocardium against infarction via activation of inhibitory guanine nucleotide binding proteins. Anesthesiology 92:1400, 2000.

106. Toller WG, Gross ER, Kersten JR, et al: Sarcolemmal and mitochondrial adenosine triphosphate-dependent potassium channels: Mechanism of desflurane-induced cardioprotection. Anesthesiology 92:1731, 2000.

107. Crystal GJ, Zhou X, Gurevicius J, et al: Direct coronary vasomotor effects of sevoflurane and desflurane in in situ canine hearts. Anesthesiology 92:1103, 2000.

108. Belhomme D, Peynet J, Louzy M, et al: Evidence for preconditioning by isoflurane in coronary artery bypass graft surgery. Circulation 100:II340, 1999.

109. Kersten JR, Orth KG, Pagel PS, et al: Role of adenosine in isoflurane-induced cardioprotection. Anesthesiology 86:1128, 1997.

110. Zaugg M, Lucchinetti E, Spahn DR, et al: Volatile anesthetics mimic cardiac preconditioning by priming the activation of mitochondrial K(ATP) channels via multiple signaling pathways. Anesthesiology 97:4, 2002.

111. Cope DK, Impastato WK, Cohen MV, Downey JM: Volatile anesthetics protect the ischemic rabbit myocardium from infarction. Anesthesiology 86:699, 1997.

112. Preckel B, Schlack W, Comfere T, et al: Effects of enflurane, isoflurane, sevoflurane and desflurane on reperfusion injury after regional myocardial ischaemia in the rabbit heart in vivo. Br J Anaesth 81:905, 1998.

113. Yao L, Kato R, Foex P: Isoflurane-induced protection against myocardial stunning is independent of adenosine 1 (A(1) receptor in isolated rat heart. Br J Anaesth 87:258, 2001.

114. Kowalski C, Zahler S, Becker BF, et al: Halothane, isoflurane, and sevoflurane reduce postischemic adhesion of neutrophils in the coronary system. Anesthesiology 86:188, 1997.

115. Rubino A, Yellon DM: Ischaemic preconditioning of the vasculature: An overlooked phenomenon for protecting the heart? Trends Pharmacol Sci 21:225, 2000.

116. Kersten JR, Schmeling T, Tessmer J, et al: Sevoflurane selectively increases coronary collateral blood flow independent of KATP channels in vivo. Anesthesiology 90:246, 1999.

117. Yao Z, Gross GJ: A comparison of adenosine-induced cardioprotection and ischemic preconditioning in dogs. Efficacy, time course, and role of KATP channels. Circulation 89:1229, 1994.

118. Cleveland JC Jr, Meldrum DR, Rowland RT, et al: The obligate role of protein kinase C in mediating clinically accessible cardiac preconditioning. Surgery 120:345, 1996.

119. Cleveland JC Jr, Meldrum DR, Rowland RT, et al: Adenosine preconditioning of human myocardium is dependent upon the ATP-sensitive K+ channel. J Mol Cell Cardiol 29:175, 1997.

120. Pagel PS, Toller WG, Gross ER, et al: K(ATP) channels mediate the beneficial effects of chronic ethanol ingestion. Am J Physiol Heart Circ Physiol 279:H2574, 2000.

121. Dixon R, Fujitaki J, Sandoval T, Kisicki J: Acadesine (AICA-riboside): Disposition and metabolism of an adenosine-regulating agent. J Clin Pharmacol 33:955, 1993.

122. Galinanes M, Mullane KM, Bullough D, Hearse DJ: Acadesine and myocardial protection. Studies of time of administration and dose-response relations in the rat. Circulation 86:598, 1992.

123. Vinten-Johansen J, Nakanishi K, Zhao ZQ, et al: Acadesine improves surgical myocardial protection with blood cardioplegia in ischemically injured canine hearts. Circulation 88:II350, 1993.

124. Tsuchida A, Liu GS, Mullane K, Downey JM: Acadesine lowers temporal threshold for the myocardial infarct size limiting effect of preconditioning. Cardiovasc Res 27:116, 1993.

125. Leung JM, Stanley T 3rd, Mathew J, et al: An initial multicenter, randomized controlled trial on the safety and efficacy of acadesine in patients undergoing coronary artery bypass graft surgery. SPI Research Group. Anesth Analg 78:420, 1994.

126. Effects of acadesine on the incidence of myocardial infarction and adverse cardiac outcomes after coronary artery bypass graft surgery. Multicenter Study of Perioperative Ischemia (McSPI) Research Group. Anesthesiology 83:658, 1995.

127. Lasley RD, Randhawa MP Jr, Hegge JO, Mentzer RM: Effects of adenosine and acadesine on interstitial nucleosides and myocardial stunning in the pig. Can J Physiol Pharmacol 77:259, 1999.

128. Smits GJ, McVey M, Cox BF, et al: Cardioprotective effects of the novel adenosine A1/A2 receptor agonist AMP 579 in a porcine model of myocardial infarction. J Pharmacol Exp Ther 286:611, 1998.

129. Schreieck J, Richardt G: Endogenous adenosine reduces the occurrence of ischemia-induced ventricular fibrillation in rat heart. J Mol Cell Cardiol 31:123, 1999.

130. Miki T, Miura T, Tsuchida A, et al: Cardioprotective mechanism of ischemic preconditioning is impaired by postinfarct ventricular remodeling through angiotensin II type 1 receptor activation. Circulation 102:458, 2000.

131. Nozawa Y, Miura T, Tsuchida A, et al: Chronic treatment with an ACE inhibitor, temocapril, lowers the threshold for the infarct size-limiting effect of ischemic preconditioning. Cardiovasc Drugs Ther 13:151, 1999.

132. Schoemaker RG, van Heijningen CL: Bradykinin mediates cardiac preconditioning at a distance. Am J Physiol Heart Circ Physiol 278:H1571, 2000.

133. Sato M, Engelman RM, Otani H, et al: Myocardial protection by preconditioning of heart with losartan, an angiotensin II type 1-receptor blocker: Implication of bradykinin-dependent and bradykinin-independent mechanisms. Circulation 102:III346, 2000.

134. Kahraman S, Demiryurek AT: Propofol is a peroxynitrite scavenger. Anesth Analg 84:1127, 1997.

135. Nakae Y, Fujita S, Namiki A: Propofol inhibits Ca(2+) transients but not contraction in intact beating guinea pig hearts. Anesth Analg 90:1286, 2000.

136. Skoutelis A, Lianou P, Papageorgiou E, et al: Effects of propofol and thiopentone on polymorphonuclear leukocyte functions in vitro. Acta Anaesthesiol Scand 38:858, 1994.

137. Karmazyn M, Gan XT, Humphreys RA, et al: The myocardial Na(+)-H(+) exchange: Structure, regulation, and its role in heart disease. Circ Res 85:777, 1999.

138. Avkiran M: Rational basis for use of sodium-hydrogen exchange inhibitors in myocardial ischemia. Am J Cardiol 83:10G, 1999.

139. Karmazyn M: Mechanisms of protection of the ischemic and reperfused myocardium by sodium-hydrogen exchange inhibition. J Thromb Thrombolysis 8:33, 1999.

140. Gazmuri RJ, Hoffner E, Kalcheim J, et al: Myocardial protection during ventricular fibrillation by reduction of proton-driven sarcolemmal sodium influx. J Lab Clin Med 137:43, 2001.

141. Ahmad S, Doweyko LM, Dugar S, et al: Arylcyclopropanecarboxyl guanidines as novel, potent, and selective inhibitors of the sodium hydrogen exchanger isoform-1. J Med Chem 44:3302, 2001.

142. Aihara K, Hisa H, Sato T, et al: Cardioprotective effect of TY-12533, a novel Na(+)/H(+) exchange inhibitor, on ischemia/reperfusion injury. Eur J Pharmacol 404:221, 2000.

143. Knight DR, Smith AH, Flynn DM, et al: A novel sodium-hydrogen exchanger isoform-1 inhibitor, zoniporide, reduces ischemic myocardial injury in vitro and in vivo. J Pharmacol Exp Ther 297:254, 2001.

144. Gumina RJ, Beier N, Schelling P, Gross GJ: Inhibitors of ischemic preconditioning do not attenuate Na+/H+ exchange inhibitor mediated cardioprotection. J Cardiovasc Pharmacol 35:949, 2000.

145. Kevelaitis E, Oubenaissa A, Mouas C, et al: Ischemic preconditioning with opening of mitochondrial adenosine triphosphate-sensitive potassium channels or Na/H exchange inhibition: Which is the best protective strategy for heart transplants? J Thorac Cardiovasc Surg 121:155, 2001.

146. Miura T, Liu Y, Goto M, et al: Mitochondrial ATP-sensitive K+ channels play a role in cardioprotection by Na+-H+ exchange inhibition against ischemia/reperfusion injury. J Am Coll Cardiol 37:957, 2001.

147. Gumina RJ, Buerger E, Eickmeier C, et al: Inhibition of the Na(+)/H(+) exchanger confers greater cardioprotection against 90 minutes of myocardial ischemia than ischemic preconditioning in dogs. Circulation 100:2519, 1999.

148. Ferdinandy P, Danial H, Ambrus I, et al: Peroxynitrite is a major contributor to cytokine-induced myocardial contractile failure. Circ Res 87:241, 2000.

149. Ferdinandy P, Schulz R: Peroxynitrite: Toxic or protective in the heart? Circ Res 88:E12, 2001.

150. Ronson RS, Nakamura M, Vinten-Johansen J: The cardiovascular effects and implications of peroxynitrite. Cardiovasc Res 44:47, 1999.

151. Mohara J, Oshima K, Tsutsumi H, et al: FK409 ameliorates ischemia-reperfusion injury in heart transplantation following 12-hour cold preservation. J Heart Lung Transplant 19:694, 2000.

152. Miller BE, Levy JH: The inflammatory response to cardiopulmonary bypass. J Cardiothorac Vasc Anesth 11:355, 1997.

153. Gal J, Smith A, Riedel B, Royston D: Preservation and protection of myocardial function. J Cardiothorac Vasc Anesth 14:22, 2000.

154. Valen G, Kawakami T, Tahepold P, et al: Glucocorticoid pretreatment protects cardiac function and induces cardiac heat shock protein 72. Am J Physiol Heart Circ Physiol 279:H836, 2000.

155. Tassani P, Augustin N, Barankay A, et al: High-dose aprotinin modulates the balance between proinflammatory and anti-inflammatory responses during coronary artery bypass graft surgery. J Cardiothorac Vasc Anesth 14:682, 2000.

156. Bull DA, Connors RC, Albanil A, et al: Aprotinin preserves myocardial biochemical function during cold storage through suppression of tumor necrosis factor. J Thorac Cardiovasc Surg 119:242, 2000.

157. Hoffmeister HM, Fischer M, Kazmaier S, et al: Action of aprotinin in myocardial ischemia—an investigation using a plasma-free model. Thorac Cardiovasc Surg 47:88, 1999.

158. McCarthy RJ, Tuman KJ, O'Connor C, Ivankovich AD: Aprotinin pretreatment diminishes postischemic myocardial contractile dysfunction in dogs. Anesth Analg 89:1096, 1999.

159. Asimakopoulos G, Lidington EA, Mason J, et al: Effect of aprotinin on endothelial cell activation. J Thorac Cardiovasc Surg 122:123, 2001.

160. Sunamori M, Suzuki A: Improved efficacy of intra-aortic balloon pumping by pharmacological myocardial protection for postoperative pump failure after coronary revascularization. Jpn J Surg 18:61, 1988.

161. Wendel HP, Heller W, Michel J, et al: Lower cardiac troponin T levels in patients undergoing cardiopulmonary bypass and receiving high-dose aprotinin therapy indicate reduction of perioperative myocardial damage. J Thorac Cardiovasc Surg 109:1164, 1995.

162. Alderman EL, Levy JH, Rich JB, et al: Analyses of coronary graft patency after aprotinin use: Results from the International Multicenter Aprotinin Graft Patency Experience (IMAGE) trial. J Thorac Cardiovasc Surg 116:716, 1998.

163. Melrose DG, Dreyer B, Bentall HH: Elective cardiac arrest. Lancet 2:21, 1955.

164. Lam CR, Gahagan T, Sergeant C, et al: Acetylcholine-induced asystole. In JG Allen (ed): Extracorporeal Circulation. Springfield, Ill, Charles C Thomas, 1958, p 451.

165. Shumway NE, Lower RR: Topical cardiac hypothermia for extended periods of anoxic arrest. Surg Forum 10:563, 1959.

166. Drew CE, Anderson IM: Profound hypothermia in cardiac surgery: Report of 3 cases. Lancet 1:748, 1959.

167. Buckberg GD: Left ventricular subendocardial necrosis. Ann Thorac Surg 24:379, 1977.

168. Taber RE, Morales AR, Fine G: Myocardial necrosis and the postoperative low-cardiac-output syndrome. Ann Thorac Surg 4:12, 1967.

169. Tyers GF, Manley NJ, Williams EH, et al: Preliminary clinical experience with isotonic hypothermic potassium-induced arrest. J Thorac Cardiovasc Surg 74:674, 1977.

170. Chambers DJ, Hearse DJ: Developments in cardioprotection: "Polarized" arrest as an alternative to "depolarized" arrest. Ann Thorac Surg 68:1960, 1999.

171. He GW, Yang CQ, Rebeyka IM, Wilson GJ: Effects of hyperkalemia on neonatal endothelium and smooth muscle. J Heart Lung Transplant 14:92, 1995.

172. Bretschneider HJ, Hubner G, Knoll D, et al: Myocardial resistance and tolerance to ischemia: Physiological and biochemical basis. J Cardiovasc Surg (Torino) 16:241, 1975.

173. Chapman RA, Tunstall J: The calcium paradox of the heart. Prog Biophys Mol Biol 50:67, 1987.

174. Noma A: ATP-regulated K+ channels in cardiac muscle. Nature 305:147, 1983.

175. Daut J, Maier-Rudolph W, von Beckerath N, et al: Hypoxic dilation of coronary arteries is mediated by ATP-sensitive potassium channels. Science 247:1341, 1990.

176. Samaha FF, Heineman FW, Ince C, et al: ATP-sensitive potassium channel is essential to maintain basal coronary vascular tone in vivo. Am J Physiol 262:C1220, 1992.

177. Aversano T, Ouyang P, Silverman H: Blockade of the ATP-sensitive potassium channel modulates reactive hyperemia in the canine coronary circulation. Circ Res 69:618, 1991.

178. Kanatsuka H, Sekiguchi N, Sato K, et al: Microvascular sites and mechanisms responsible for reactive hyperemia in the coronary circulation of the beating canine heart. Circ Res 71:912, 1992.

179. Komaru T, Lamping KG, Eastham CL, Dellsperger KC: Role of ATP-sensitive potassium channels in coronary microvascular autoregulatory responses. Circ Res 69:1146, 1991.

180. Hawaleshka A, Jacobsohn E: Ischaemic preconditioning: Mechanisms and potential clinical applications. Can J Anaesth 45:670, 1998.

181. Grover GJ, Sleph PG, Dzwonczyk S: Role of myocardial ATP-sensitive potassium channels in mediating preconditioning in the dog heart and their possible interaction with adenosine A1-receptors. Circulation 86:1310, 1992.

182. Gross GJ, Auchampach JA: Blockade of ATP-sensitive potassium channels prevents myocardial preconditioning in dogs. Circ Res 70:223, 1992.

183. Auchampach JA, Gross GJ: Adenosine A1 receptors, KATP channels, and ischemic preconditioning in dogs. Am J Physiol 264:H1327, 1993.

184. Toombs CF, McGee DS, Johnston WE, Vinten-Johansen J: Protection from ischaemic-reperfusion injury with adenosine pretreatment is reversed by inhibition of ATP sensitive potassium channels. Cardiovasc Res 27:623, 1993.

185. Cohen NM, Wise RM, Wechsler AS, Damiano RJ Jr: Elective cardiac arrest with a hyperpolarizing adenosine triphosphate-sensitive potassium channel opener. A novel form of myocardial protection? J Thorac Cardiovasc Surg 106:317, 1993.

186. Maskal SL, Cohen NM, Hsia PW, et al: Hyperpolarized cardiac arrest with a potassium-channel opener, aprikalim. J Thorac Cardiovasc Surg 110:1083, 1995.

187. Hosoda H, Sunamori M, Suzuki A: Effect of pinacidil on rat hearts undergoing hypothermic cardioplegia. Ann Thorac Surg 58:1631, 1994.

188. Qiu Y, Galinanes M, Hearse DJ: Protective effect of nicorandil as an additive to the solution for continuous warm cardioplegia. J Thorac Cardiovasc Surg 110:1063, 1995.

189. Chi L, Uprichard AC, Lucchesi BR: Profibrillatory actions of pinacidil in a conscious canine model of sudden coronary death. J Cardiovasc Pharmacol 15:452, 1990.

190. Lopez JR, Ghanbari RA, Terzic A: A KATP channel opener protects cardiomyocytes from Ca2+ waves: A laser confocal microscopy study. Am J Physiol 270:H1384, 1996.

191. Lopez JR, Jahangir R, Jahangir A, et al: Potassium channel openers prevent potassium-induced calcium loading of cardiac cells: Possible implications in cardioplegia. J Thorac Cardiovasc Surg 112:820, 1996.

192. Snabaitis AK, Shattock MJ, Chambers DJ: Comparison of polarized and depolarized arrest in the isolated rat heart for long-term preservation. Circulation 96:3148, 1997.

193. Olafsson B, Forman MB, Puett DW, et al: Reduction of reperfusion injury in the canine preparation by intracoronary adenosine: Importance of the endothelium and the no-reflow phenomenon. Circulation 76:1135, 1987.

194. Zhao ZQ, Sato H, Williams MW, et al: Adenosine A2-receptor activation inhibits neutrophil-mediated injury to coronary endothelium. Am J Physiol 271:H1456, 1996.

195. Cronstein BN, Levin RI, Belanoff J, et al: Adenosine: An endogenous inhibitor of neutrophil-mediated injury to endothelial cells. J Clin Invest 78:760, 1986.

196. Fogelson BG, Nawas SI, Law WR: Mechanisms of myocardial protection by adenosine-supplemented cardioplegic solution: Myofilament and metabolic responses. J Thorac Cardiovasc Surg 119:601, 2000.

197. Lasley RD, Mentzer RM Jr: Adenosine increases lactate release and delays onset of contracture during global low flow ischaemia. Cardiovasc Res 27:96, 1993.

198. Cronstein BN: Adenosine, an endogenous anti-inflammatory agent. J Appl Physiol 76:5, 1994.

199. Lasley RD, Mentzer RM Jr: Protective effects of adenosine in the reversibly injured heart. Ann Thorac Surg 60:843, 1995.

200. Thourani VH, Nakamura M, Ronson RS, et al: Adenosine A(3)-receptor stimulation attenuates postischemic dysfunction through K(ATP) channels. Am J Physiol 277:H228, 1999.

201. Thourani VH, Ronson RS, Jordan JE, et al: Adenosine A3 pretreatment before cardioplegic arrest attenuates postischemic cardiac dysfunction. Ann Thorac Surg 67:1732, 1999.

202. Belardinelli L, Giles WR, West A: Ionic mechanisms of adenosine actions in pacemaker cells from rabbit heart. J Physiol 405:615, 1988.

203. Schubert T, Vetter H, Owen P, et al: Adenosine cardioplegia. Adenosine versus potassium cardioplegia: Effects on cardiac arrest and postischemic recovery in the isolated rat heart. J Thorac Cardiovasc Surg 98:1057, 1989.

204. de Jong JW, van der Meer P, van Loon H, et al: Adenosine as adjunct to potassium cardioplegia: Effect on function, energy metabolism, and electrophysiology. J Thorac Cardiovasc Surg 100:445, 1990.

205. Boehm DH, Human PA, von Oppell U, et al: Adenosine cardioplegia: Reducing reperfusion injury of the ischaemic myocardium? Eur J Cardiothorac Surg 5:542, 1991.

206. Ledingham S, Katayama O, Lachno D, et al: Beneficial effect of adenosine during reperfusion following prolonged cardioplegic arrest. Cardiovasc Res 24:247, 1990.

207. Thelin S, Hultman J, Ronquist G: Effects of adenosine infusion on the pig heart during normothermic ischemia and reperfusion. Scand J Thorac Cardiovasc Surg 25:207, 1991.

208. Thourani VH, Ronson RS, Van Wylen DG, et al: Adenosine-supplemented blood cardioplegia attenuates postischemic dysfunction after severe regional ischemia. Circulation 100:II376, 1999.

209. Fremes SE, Levy SL, Christakis GT, et al: Phase 1 human trial of adenosine-potassium cardioplegia. Circulation 94:II370, 1996.

210. Cohen G, Feder-Elituv R, Iazetta J, et al: Phase 2 studies of adenosine cardioplegia. Circulation 98:II225, 1998.

211. Mentzer RM Jr, Rahko PS, Molina-Viamonte V, et al: Safety, tolerance, and efficacy of adenosine as an additive to blood cardioplegia in humans during coronary artery bypass surgery. Am J Cardiol 79:38, 1997.

212. Mentzer RM Jr, Rahko PS, Canver CC, et al: Adenosine reduces postbypass transfusion requirements in humans after heart surgery. Ann Surg 224:523, 1996.

213. Steinberg JB, Kapelanski DP, Olson JD, Weiler JM: Cytokine and complement levels in patients undergoing cardiopulmonary bypass. J Thorac Cardiovasc Surg 106:1008, 1993.

214. Chai PJ, Nassar R, Oakeley AE, et al: Soluble complement receptor-1 protects heart, lung, and cardiac myofilament function from cardiopulmonary bypass damage. Circulation 101:541, 2000.

215. Fitch JC, Rollins S, Matis L, et al: Pharmacology and biological efficacy of a recombinant, humanized, single-chain antibody C5 complement inhibitor in patients undergoing coronary artery bypass graft surgery with cardiopulmonary bypass. Circulation 100:2499, 1999.

216. Rinder CS, Rinder HM, Johnson K, et al: Role of C3 cleavage in monocyte activation during extracorporeal circulation. Circulation 100:553, 1999.

217. Nilsson B, Larsson R, Hong J, et al: Compstatin inhibits complement and cellular activation in whole blood in two models of extracorporeal circulation. Blood 92:1661, 1998.

218. Volanakis JE, Narayana SV: Complement factor D, a novel serine protease. Protein Sci 5:553, 1996.

219. Fung M, Loubser PG, Undar A, et al: Inhibition of complement, neutrophil, and platelet activation by an anti-factor D monoclonal antibody in simulated cardiopulmonary bypass circuits. J Thorac Cardiovasc Surg 122:113, 2001.

220. Ma XL, Weyrich AS, Lefer DJ, Lefer AM: Diminished basal nitric oxide release after myocardial ischemia and reperfusion promotes neutrophil adherence to coronary endothelium. Circ Res 72:403, 1993.

221. Nakanishi K, Zhao ZQ, Vinten-Johansen J, et al: Blood cardioplegia enhanced with nitric oxide donor SPM-5185 counteracts postischemic endothelial and ventricular dysfunction. J Thorac Cardiovasc Surg 109:1146, 1995.

222. Sato H, Zhao ZQ, McGee DS, et al: Supplemental L-arginine during cardioplegic arrest and reperfusion avoids regional postischemic injury. J Thorac Cardiovasc Surg 110:302, 1995.

223. Sato H, Zhao ZQ, Jordan JE, et al: Basal nitric oxide expresses endogenous cardioprotection during reperfusion by inhibition of neutrophil-mediated damage after surgical revascularization. J Thorac Cardiovasc Surg 113:399, 1997.

224. Lopez BL, Liu GL, Christopher TA, Ma XL: Peroxynitrite, the product of nitric oxide and superoxide, causes myocardial injury in the isolated perfused rat heart. Coron Artery Dis 8:149, 1997.

225. Ronson RS, Thourani VH, Ma XL, et al: Peroxynitrite, the breakdown product of nitric oxide, is beneficial in blood cardioplegia but injurious in crystalloid cardioplegia. Circulation 100:II384, 1999.

226. Nakamura M, Thourani VH, Ronson RS, et al: Glutathione reverses endothelial damage from peroxynitrite, the byproduct of nitric oxide degradation, in crystalloid cardioplegia. Circulation 102:III332, 2000.

227. Kobayashi K, Neely JR: Effects of ischemia and reperfusion on pyruvate dehydrogenase activity in isolated rat hearts. J Mol Cell Cardiol 15:359, 1983.

228. Lewandowski ED, White LT: Pyruvate dehydrogenase influences postischemic heart function. Circulation 91:2071, 1995.

229. Rao V, Merante F, Weisel RD, et al: Insulin stimulates pyruvate dehydrogenase and protects human ventricular cardiomyocytes from simulated ischemia. J Thorac Cardiovasc Surg 116:485, 1998.

230. Rao V, Borger MA, Weisel RD, et al: Insulin cardioplegia for elective coronary bypass surgery. J Thorac Cardiovasc Surg 119:1176, 2000.

231. Hynninen M, Borger MA, Rao V, et al: The effect of insulin cardioplegia on atrial fibrillation after high-risk coronary bypass surgery: A double-blinded, randomized, controlled trial. Anesth Analg 92:810, 2001.

232. Stamm C, Cowan DB, Friehs I, et al: Rapid endotoxin-induced alterations in myocardial calcium handling: Obligatory role of cardiac TNF-alpha. Anesthesiology 95:1396, 2001.

233. Irwin MW, Mak S, Mann DL, et al: Tissue expression and immunolocalization of tumor necrosis factor-alpha in postinfarction dysfunctional myocardium. Circulation 99:1492, 1999.

234. Stamm C, Friehs I, Cowan DB, et al: Inhibition of tumor necrosis factor-alpha improves postischemic recovery of hypertrophied hearts. Circulation 104:I350, 2001.

39

Vasodilators

Paul Zanaboni, MD, PhD • Laureen Hill, MD

The primary purpose of the circulatory system is to provide adequate blood flow to meet the metabolic demands of the tissues. The physical laws governing fluid dynamics are analogous to Ohm's law for electrical circuits and can be applied to the circulatory system as follows:

$$Q = (P_1 - P_2)/R$$

where Q is blood flow (mL/min), $P_1 - P_2$ is the pressure difference across a vascular bed (dyne/cm^2), and R is resistance to flow through the bed (dyne sec/cm^5). Application of Poiseuille's law further relates vascular resistance to blood flow directly to the blood viscosity and vessel length, and inversely to the vessel radius raised to the fourth power.[1] Changes in vascular smooth muscle tone have important implications for control of blood flow across a given vascular bed. Regulation of vascular smooth muscle is achieved through a complex interaction of humoral neural, and intrinsic vascular factors. Alterations in regulatory function may lead to pathologic conditions encountered in clinical medicine. Hypertension is one such cardiovascular disturbance with significant potential sequelae. Acutely, hypertensive crisis may lead to cerebral hemorrhage, cerebral edema, myocardial ischemia, and cardiogenic shock. Chronic hypertension increases the risk for atherosclerosis, stroke, heart failure, and renal insufficiency. Understanding the mechanisms of vasomotor control, and the pharmacologic

tools available to manipulate vascular smooth muscle tone is essential to the prevention and treatment of certain cardiovascular derangements and related complications. In this chapter, we will review the physiology of smooth muscle contraction, describe the neural and humoral factors involved in regulating vasomotor tone, define the mechanism of action for the different classes of vasodilators, and discuss the administration of vasodilating agents in clinical medicine.

Regulation of Vascular Tone

Neural regulation of vascular smooth muscle tone occurs predominately through sympathetic and parasympathetic postganglionic nerve fibers (see Chapter 19 for a more detailed discussion). Basal sympathetic nervous system activity keeps blood vessels partially constricted and is responsible for normal vascular tone.[2] Unlike skeletal muscle, which has neuromuscular junctions, smooth muscle is innervated by nerve fibers that branch diffusely in the perivascular space where they release neurotransmitters in response to nerve cell depolarization. The primary neurotransmitters involved in regulating vascular smooth muscle tone are norepinephrine and acetylcholine, but current evidence suggests individual neurons may release more than one transmitter substance including nonadrenergic, noncholinergic peptides and amines.[3-5] The net effect of neural input on vasomotor tone depends on the amount and type(s) of neurotransmitter(s) released after depolarization of the nerve ending and the response generated after stimulation of specific receptors in target vascular tissues. For example, sympathetic nervous system activation results in release of norepinephrine, which can produce vasoconstriction through α adrenergic receptors or vasodilation through β adrenergic receptors. Neurotransmitters can also act as neuromodulators by influencing the activity or subsequent release of other neurotransmitters.[6]

In addition to neural input, vascular smooth muscle responds to both circulating and local humoral factors, acting through specific membrane receptors to produce vasoconstriction or vasodilation. Vasoactive endocrine substances are produced in organs distant from the vascular tissues under regulatory control. Two classic examples include: epinephrine, produced and secreted by the adrenal medulla, and arginine vasopressin, produced in the hypothalamus and released into the circulation from the posterior pituitary gland. Other vasoactive agents may be produced and released within a given vascular bed to exert effects locally, including arachidonic acid metabolites, serotonin, adenosine, and histamine, among many others. Endothelial cells also play an important role in the regulation of vascular smooth muscle tone by producing and releasing vasoactive substances such as nitric oxide (NO) and endothelin in response to mechanical and chemical stimuli.[7] Similar to neural input, humral factors regulate vasomotor tone based on the degree and net effect of specific receptor binding. As discussed later in this chapter, receptors are coupled to second messenger systems, or specific ion channels, or both to ultimately affect intracellular calcium concentrations ($[Ca^{2+}]i$) and vascular smooth muscle tone.

Physiology of Muscle Contraction

The contractile machinery of vascular smooth muscle is composed of three elements: myosin (thick filaments), actin (thin filaments), and the regulatory proteins. Myosin is a hexamer composed of two heavy chains and two pairs of light chains (20 and 17 kDa). Actin that is involved in the contractile process is known as α–actin. The myosin and actin filaments are arranged in a diagonal pattern along the long axis of the cell; the α–actin is connected to the cytoskeleton at the dense bodies and to the cell membrane at dense plaques.[8] During contraction, the actin filaments slide along the myosin, resulting in cell shortening. This is an active process that translates chemical energy stored in the form of adenosine triphosphate (ATP) to mechanical force. The pivotal event in smooth muscle contraction is the increase in $[Ca^{2+}]i$. The two major sources of Ca^{2+} are from the extracellular space and the sarcoplasmic reticulum (SR). Extracellular Ca^{2+} enters the cell through voltage-dependent Ca^{2+} channels (VDCC).[9] These channels are activated by depolarization of the membrane and inactivated by repolarization and hyperpolarization. Two types of VDCC have been isolated in smooth muscle: L type and T type. The

T-type channel has not been well described, but it is transient in nature and may be related to phasically contracting smooth muscle.[9] The L type (found in vascular smooth muscle) has been extensively characterized. Its activity is enhanced by phosphorylation and is inhibited by $[Ca^{2+}]i$.[9]

Ca^{2+} is sequestered intracellularly in the SR. It serves as the major source of Ca^{2+} that participates in muscle contraction. Ca^{2+} is released from the SR by two mechanisms. Vasoconstrictor agonists combine with receptors in the cell membrane and activate phospholipase C (PLC) through a G protein. PLC, in turn, hydrolyzes phosphatidyl inositol-4,5-diphosphate to inositol 1,4,5-triphosphate (IP_3) and diacylglycerol (DAG). The increased IP_3 concentration results in the activation of IP_3-mediated channels in the SR, which allow for the release of the sequestered Ca^{2+}. Ca^{2+} is also released from the SR in response to the increase in $[Ca^{2+}]i$ through Ca^{2+}-dependent channels known as ryanodine receptors.[10]

Because Ca^{2+} acts as a second messenger in many cellular functions including muscle contraction, it is obvious that the $[Ca^{2+}]i$ is closely regulated. This is accomplished in two manners: the extrusion of Ca^{2+} from the cytoplasm to the extracellular space and the sequestration of Ca^{2+} in the SR. The extrusion of Ca^{2+} is accomplished in two manners: the sodium (Na)/Ca^{2+} exchanger and the Ca^{2+}/ATPase pump in the cell membrane.[9] Ca^{2+} is eliminated from the cytoplasm in exchange for Na and hydrogen ions, respectively. Ca^{2+}/ATPase (located in the SR membrane) activity sequesters Ca^{2+} in the SR. A protein, phospholamban, is a likely regulatory protein in this process. In its unphosphorylated state, phospholamban diminishes the Ca^{2+}/ATPase activity by decreasing its affinity for Ca^{2+}. However, phosphorylated phospholamban dissociates from the enzyme, and the activity of the pump increases such that Ca^{2+} reuptake into the SR is enhanced. Phosphorylation of phospholamban is mediated by the activity of cyclic guanosine monophosphate (cGMP)-dependent protein kinases. Vasodilator substances that increase cGMP may cause vasodilation by promoting the increased uptake of Ca^{2+} in the SR through phosphorylation of phospholamban.[11]

Smooth muscle is not associated with troponin as it is in striated muscle; rather, four Ca^{2+} ions bind to the regulatory protein, calmodulin. The Ca^{2+}/calmodulin complex then binds to myosin light chain kinase (MLCK). MLCK is a specific protein kinase that consists of a catalytic domain, a calmodulin-binding site, a putative autoinhibitory site, an actin-binding site, substrate (myosin and ATP) binding site, and sites for phosphorylation by other protein kinases.[12] The phosphorylation sites on MLCK provide for regulation of its activity; for example, the affinity of the Ca^{2+}/calmodulin complex for MLCK is decreased by phosphorylation of its binding site. This is a mechanism by which some vasodilatory drugs cause muscle relaxation (see later). Activated MLCK phosphorylates the regulatory myosin light chain at serine$_{19}$. This phosphorylation promotes the polymerization of myosin into filaments; it is this polymerized myosin that spontaneously binds to actin by the formation of crossbridges. The phosphorylation of the regulatory light chains also increases the ATPase activity of the myosin heads by 100-fold.[13] ATP is cleaved, resulting in the energy necessary for the lever action causing actin to slide across the myosin. This results in contraction of the smooth muscle cell. The mechanism of the increased ATPase activity induced by phosphorylation of the serine$_{19}$ residue of the myosin light chain is not clear; however, it is known that two myosin heads are necessary. In in vitro experiments, the phosphorylation of a single-headed myosin molecule is not associated with an increase in ATPase activity.[14]

Phosphorylation of the regulatory light chain is a major regulatory point in vascular smooth muscle contraction. Although the major pathway for this phosphorylation depends on free Ca^{2+} through MLCK, there are also calcium-independent pathways. Guanosine triphosphate (GTP) binding proteins can activate Rho-associated kinase (ROK)[15] and p21-activated kinase.[16] Both of these kinases are capable of phosphorylation of the serine$_{19}$ in the regulatory light chain, although the significance of these pathways is not clear. ROK inhibitors have been shown to decrease blood pressure.[17]

Vascular smooth muscle can sustain contraction for long periods. This is independent of the initial stimulus, increase in $[Ca^{2+}]i$, or phosphorylation of the myosin light chains, which return toward their baseline levels.[18] One possible explanation has been termed the *latch hypothesis*. In this scenario, the regulatory light chains are phosphorylated by MLCK in response to increased $[Ca^{2+}]i$. After the formation of the crossbridges and lever action, the myosin is associated with adenosine diphosphate (ADP) and inorganic phosphorus (Pi) (MYO-ADP-Pi). Dephosphorylation of the crossbridge results in MYO-ADP; this moiety has a high affinity for actin, thus forming a "latch." Thus there is a low cycling rate of the crossbridges, resulting in a prolonged contractile state.[19]

Control of the Contractile State

The force generated by the smooth muscle is not directly related to the $[Ca^{2+}]i$.[10] Several factors influence the force of contraction in response to an increase in $[Ca^{2+}]i$. The common pathway is the activation of myosin light chain phosphatase (MLCP). This enzyme dephosphorylates the regulatory light chains, thus decreasing the ATPase activity and lever action of the myosin heads and ultimately, contraction. The end result is the regulation of the contractile mechanism. Several intermediaries regulate MLCP. Of particular interest is the activation of MLCP by a cGMP-dependent kinase. This enzyme promotes dephosphorylation of the regulatory light chains and decreases the contractile state.[20] MLCP is also inhibited by other kinases that promote vasoconstriction; among these are ROK and members of the protein kinase C family.[9] Inhibition of MLCP by these enzymes may be part of the cascade that maintains the prolonged contractile state that is observed.

Another mechanism by which smooth muscle contraction is controlled is through the activity of other regulatory proteins. One such protein is caldesmon, which is associated with the thin filaments. It has binding sites for actin, tropomyosin (a component of the thin filament), myosin, and the calcium/calmodulin complex. In the presence of tropomyosin, caldesmon regulates the myosin/actin interaction by inhibiting the ATPase activity of the myosin head, resulting in decreased contraction.[9] This activity is promoted by the presence of tropomyosin and is inhibited in the presence of calcium/calmodulin.

MECHANISMS OF DRUG ACTION

All vasodilators ultimately work by decreasing $[Ca^{2+}]i$ or directly interfering with the phosphorylation of myosin necessary for contraction to occur.[21,22] Figure 39–1 demonstrates the variety of mechanisms by which this occurs and the sites at which various classes of vasodilators have their unique effects.

Calcium Channel Blockers

Calcium channel blockers inhibit the entry of calcium (Ca^{2+}) into the cell through the L-type VDCC on the cell membrane. The normal increase in $[Ca^{2+}]i$ in response to cell membrane depolarization and the secondary $[Ca^{2+}]$-dependent release of Ca^{2+} from intracellular stores are blunted. At low cytoplasmic concentrations of Ca^{2+}, contraction cannot occur. Three clinically useful classes of Ca^{2+} blockers are used as vasodilators. The first class is the dihydropyridine group, which includes nifedipine and nicardipine. These drugs bind to the external surface of the L-type VDCC and inhibit the influx of Ca^{2+}.[23] The second class is

the phenylalkylamines; the prototype is verapamil. The inhibition of the VDCC by verapamil is frequency-dependent. It appears as though this class of drugs must enter the cell and bind internally to have its effect.[24] The third class is the benzothiazepines, including the prototype, diltiazem. Its binding site is located on the extracellular side of the L-type channel.[25]

Membrane Hyperpolarization

Potassium channel openers target ATP-sensitive potassium channels (K_{ATP}) to permit potassium efflux from the smooth muscle cell to produce hyperpolarization and interfere with depolarization of the cell membrane necessary for Ca^{2+} influx and smooth muscle contraction.[26] Endogenous substances such as endothelium-derived relaxing factor, adenosine, and other factors including intracellular pH have been shown to influence smooth muscle tone through the K_{ATP} channel.[27–31]

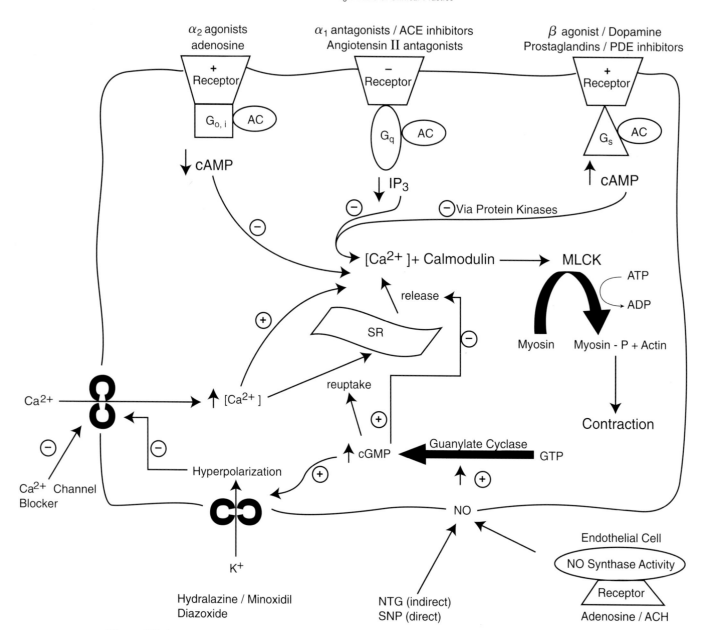

Figure 39–1. Mechanisms of vasodilator action. Figure illustrates drug targets for the various classes of vasodilators in a vascular smooth muscle cell and the signaling pathways they use to inhibit actin/myosin interaction and smooth muscle contraction. The targets include G protein—coupled receptors (α_2 and β adrenergic, prostaglandin, angiotensin II, adenosine), ion channels (Ca^{2+} channels, IK_{ATP}), and enzymes (guanylate cyclase, phosphodiesterase).

Angiotensin II Inhibition

Angiotensin-converting enzyme (ACE) inhibitors prevent the conversion of angiotensin I to angiotensin II, a potent vasoconstrictor responsible for arterial smooth muscle contraction, increased aldosterone secretion, and sympathetic nervous system stimulation. Angiotensin II binds to a specific cell membrane receptor, AT_1, which is coupled through the G_q protein to PLC, yielding increased levels of DAG and IP_3 and increased release of Ca^{2+} from the SR to produce vasoconstriction.[10] Decreased generation of angiotensin II leads to loss of this vasoconstrictive effect. Plasma aldosterone levels are reduced, decreasing sodium and water retention. ACE inhibitors also block the degradation of

bradykinin, an endogenous vasodilator substance, contributing to their antihypertensive effects. Bradykinin may produce unwanted side effects including dry cough and allergic reaction. An alternative approach to therapy is the use of angiotensin II receptor (AT_1) receptor inhibitors, which block the vasoconstrictive actions of angiotensin II without affecting ACE activity.[23]

Catecholamine Receptors

Catecholamines can increase or decrease smooth muscle tone depending on the type and density of adrenergic receptors involved. Adrenergic receptors are among the many G protein—coupled receptors. The numerous subtypes of G proteins and their second messenger systems are responsible for the diverse responses seen with receptor binding. Adding to the complexity is the presence of second messenger isoforms with differing tissue distributions and regulatory controls.[32,33]

α_1 Adrenergic receptors on vascular smooth muscle cells are linked to PLC through a G protein, G_q, resulting in the production of IP_3 and DAG with subsequent release of Ca^{2+} from the SR and smooth muscle contraction.[34] α Adrenergic receptor antagonists competitively bind to the α_1 adrenergic receptor and interfere with the ability of catecholamines to produce vasoconstriction through this mechanism. α_2 Adrenergic receptors are coupled to the G_i protein complex, which is involved in inhibition of adenylate cyclase, Ca^{2+}, and potassium channels. The net result of agonist binding to the α_2 adrenergic receptor is decreased cyclic adenosine monophosphate (cAMP), hyperpolarization, and decreased $[Ca^{2+}]i$. Presynaptic α_2 receptor stimulation results in decreased sympathetic output from the central nervous system, whereas agonist activity at the postsynaptic α_2 receptors in the central nervous system may be responsible for the sedative and analgesic properties of these drugs.[35]

Activated β adrenergic receptors in vascular smooth muscle stimulate adenylate cyclase to produce cAMP, which in turn activates several protein kinases that interfere with vasoconstriction. One of these kinases phosphorylates the Ca^{2+} channel, inhibiting the entry of Ca^{2+} into the cell. The phosphorylation of phospholamban by another protein kinase increases the reuptake of Ca^{2+} from the cytoplasm into the SR.[36] Cyclic AMP—dependent kinases also activate MLCP.[10] This enzyme dephosphorylates the regulatory myosin light chain to promote dissociation of myosin and actin, leading to smooth muscle relaxation.

Dopamine-1 receptors (D1) are postsynaptic receptors that mediate vasodilation through G protein/adenylate cyclase coupling to produce increased cAMP and $[Ca^{2+}]i$. Dopamine-2 receptors (D2) are presynaptic and are coupled to the inhibitory G protein complex that decreases cAMP levels and produces cell membrane hyperpolarization, reducing norepinephrine release. Dopamine produces its effects in a dose-dependent manner, with predominately D1 receptor stimulation at lower levels, β_1 receptor stimulation at moderate doses, and α_1 receptor activity at greater con-

centrations. A selective D1 receptor agonist is available for clinical use to mediate splanchnic vasodilation.[37]

Nitric Oxide

NO produces smooth muscle relaxation through the stimulation of guanylate cyclase to produce cGMP. cGMP activates protein kinases that phosphorylate various peptides leading to decreased $[Ca^{2+}]i$, similar to the effects of cAMP-dependent kinases.[10] NO is produced in endothelial cells from where it diffuses into vascular smooth muscle cells to modulate intrinsic vascular tone.[38] A number of compounds produce vasodilation through this route including organic nitrate compounds that "donate" or release NO. The nitrate group of nitroglycerin is biotransformed to NO through a glutathione-dependent pathway involving both glutathione and glutathione-S-transferase.[39] Sodium nitroprusside undergoes reduction to produce NO and cyanide. Adenosine stimulates purine receptors on endothelial cells to produce NO. Adenosine may also have direct effects on smooth muscle cells through a G protein pathway.[31,40]

Phosphodiesterase Inhibitors

Specific phosphodiesterase enzymes hydrolyze cAMP to 5′AMP, whereas other isozymes are responsible for the inactivation of cGMP. Selective phosphodiesterase inhibitors block the hydrolysis of either of these compounds, prolonging their vasodilatory effects in vascular smooth muscle.[38,41]

Eicosanoids

The eicosanoids (prostaglandins E_1, E_2, and prostacyclin) exert their vasodilating effects through receptor-mediated increases in cAMP, similar to the β adrenergic agonists. They are naturally occurring compounds derived from arachidonic acid metabolism and have a wide variety of physiologic effects including vasodilation, increased vascular permeability, and inhibition of platelet aggregation.

CLINICAL PHARMACOLOGY AND PRACTICAL ASPECTS OF DRUG ADMINISTRATION

The choice of drug and route of administration depend on a number of factors. Prompt control of blood pressure necessitates use of a rapid-acting intravenous agent, whereas management of chronic hypertension is likely to include use of long-acting oral preparations. Patient comorbidities and potential drug interactions or side effects will also influence

decisions regarding appropriate vasodilator therapy. The pharmacokinetics, actions, adverse effects, and interactions with other drugs and disease states will be discussed for the most frequently encountered agents within each drug category.

Nitrates

The metabolism of nitroglycerin yields NO, stimulating production of cGMP to cause vasorelaxation. The predominant effects are on the venous circulation, but it will produce dose-dependent arterial dilation. Nitroglycerin is an important coronary artery vasodilator and is used to promote coronary flow during myocardial ischemia. Increased venous capacitance leads to decreased preload, decreased left ventricular wall tension, and decreased myocardial oxygen consumption. Continuous intravenous infusion is recommended because of its immediate onset and short duration of action. Sublingual, oral, and topical preparations are available for outpatient treatment of angina, or myocardial ischemia, or both. Nitroglycerin should be avoided or used with extreme caution in patients with hypovolemia or hypotension. Use may cause flushing and headaches. Prolonged use or excessive dosing may cause methemoglobinemia. Tolerance develops rapidly to continuous exposure. Hypotensive effects may be potentiated by other vasodilatory agents or by sildenafil, a phosphodiesterase inhibitor that inhibits the metabolism of cGMP.

Sodium nitroprusside is a direct donor of NO that has potent effects on both arterial and venous smooth muscle tone. Like nitroglycerin, it has rapid onset and offset and is most effectively used as a continuous infusion. Its hypotensive effects may be potentiated by other vasodilators or sildenafil. Sodium nitroprusside rapidly interacts with red blood cell hemoglobin to produce cyanomethemoglobin and cyanide ions that combine with thiosulfate (produced in the liver) to generate thiocyanate, which is eliminated by the kidneys. The risk for thiocyanate or cyanide toxicity increases with prolonged or excessive use and in the setting of renal failure. Thiocyanate and cyanide levels can be monitored. Thiocyanate is potentially lethal in concentrations of 200 mg/L and can be cleared by dialysis. Cyanide toxicity can be manifest by venous hyperoxemia or metabolic acidosis. It should be promptly treated by discontinuing nitroprusside and administering sodium nitrite (5 mg/kg) to produce methemoglobinemia for combination with cyanide ions, followed by infusion of thiosulfate (200 mg/kg) to generate thiocyanate.

β Adrenergic Agonist

Isoproterenol is a synthetic catecholamine that binds to β_2 adrenergic receptors in vascular smooth muscle to produce vasodilation through G_s protein complexes that increase cAMP production, activate cAMP-dependent protein kinases, and thereby inhibit the cellular contractile machinery. It also possesses positive inotropic and chronotropic properties through β_1 adrenergic receptor binding in the heart and may be arrhythmogenic. Isoproterenol is the most potent of all agonists at the β_1 and β_2 receptors and has no activity at α adrenergic receptors. It is used clinically to improve myocardial contractility, decrease pulmonary vascular resistance, and increase heart rate in the setting of symptomatic bradycardia or heart block. It is rapidly metabolized in the liver to inactive metabolites and must be administered by continuous infusion. Sodium bicarbonate and other alkalinizing agents decrease efficacy.

Dopamine-1 Agonist

Fenoldopam selectively binds to D1 receptors, acting through G_s protein complexes to increase cAMP production, activate cAMP-dependent protein kinases, and thereby inhibit the cellular contractile machinery. The drug acutely decreases blood pressure and is administered through continuous infusion for the treatment of severe hypertension. It does not have D2 receptor or β adrenergic receptor activity, but does produce reflex-mediated increases in heart rate and cardiac index.[42] Therapeutic dosages of fenoldopam increase renal blood flow, creatinine clearance, urinary flow, and excretion of sodium.[43] It is extensively metabolized in the liver, but in patients with liver disease, plasma levels tend to be lower and clearance rates greater than in healthy volunteers, likely because of increased intrahepatic shunting and a greater volume of distribution. Although fenoldopam is given by continuous infusion, it has a relatively long duration of action (30–60 minutes); its actions can thus persist after discontinuation. Fenoldopam increases intraocular pressure and should be used with caution in patients with glaucoma or globe injury.

Angiotensin-Converting Enzyme Inhibitors

This class of drugs inhibits the activity of ACE, resulting in decreased levels of angiotensin II and aldosterone. They are most effective in treating hypertension secondary to high renin production, which may help explain some of the racial differences seen in clinical trials.[44] In addition to their antihypertensive effects, they have been shown to improve long-term outcomes in heart failure trials[45-47] and to slow renal dysfunction in diabetic nephropathy.[48] A decrease in glomerular filtration rate is seen in patients treated with ACE inhibitors, and caution must be used in patients with renal impairment. ACE inhibitors should be avoided in patients with renal artery stenosis. Hyperkalemia is possible because of reduced production of aldosterone, therefore potassium levels should be monitored. ACE inhibition inhibits bradykinin degradation, leading to increased bradykinin levels that may produce cough and limit patient tolerance. Fortunately, more serious side effects such as bronchospasm and angioedema are rare. Except for enalaprilat, all of the ACE inhibitors are administered orally. Many of the ACE inhibitors are designed as prodrugs to enhance their oral bioavailability, and they must undergo hepatic metabolism to the active form of the drug. Enalapril is the prodrug of the active ACE inhibitor, enalaprilat, and conversion may be affected in patients with hepatic dysfunction. Captopril and lisinopril are not prodrugs. Accumulation of these three drugs occurs in renal impairment, and dose adjustment is necessary. ACE inhibitors should not be used during pregnancy. Published experience in the pediatric population is limited, although captopril and enalapril have been used with no significant adverse effects reported.[49,50]

Angiotensin II Receptor Inhibitors

Losartan binds to the AT_1 receptor to inhibit vasoconstriction and secretion of aldosterone. It undergoes substantial first-pass metabolism through cytochrome P450 to an active metabolite. The parent drug exhibits reversible, competitive kinetics at the AT_1 receptor, whereas the active metabolite demonstrates reversible, noncompetitive kinetics. Patients with chronic heart failure have shown improved hemodynamics during treatment with this agent,[51] but the long-term benefits related to myocardial remodeling seen with ACE inhibitors have not yet been demonstrated with this class of agents. The undesirable cough related to bradykinin accumulation with ACE inhibition is significantly less problematic with losartan therapy.[52] Hyperkalemia is a potential side effect, especially with concomitant use of potassium-sparing diuretics. Both the parent compound and active metabolite undergo biliary excretion. Dosing requirements are lower in patients with hepatic dysfunction, but dosing adjustment is not necessary with renal impairment. Losartan should not be used during pregnancy or in children. As with ACE inhibitors, losartan is contraindicated in patients with renal artery stenosis. Fluconazole decreases cytochrome P450 activity and reduces active metabolite concentrations. Lithium reabsorption is increased, raising the possibility of lithium toxicity.

Eicosanoids

Prostaglandin E_1 (PGE_1) and prostacyclin (PGI_2) bind to specific prostanoid receptors coupled to G_s protein complexes that increase cAMP production, activate cAMP-dependent protein kinases, and inhibit the cellular contractile machinery to produce vasodilation. Although they produce reductions in systemic vascular tone, their most common clinical uses are related to their effects on the pulmonary vasculature. PGE_1 is used in neonates with congenital heart disease to maintain ductus arteriosus patency, and PGI_2 is used predominately for the treatment of primary pulmonary hypertension. Other important biologic effects include restoration of endothelial cell integrity, improved rheologic properties of red blood cells, decreased smooth muscle cell proliferation, and dose-dependent inhibition of platelet aggregation, making them useful in the treatment of occlusive peripheral arterial disease. They are rapidly metabolized in the lung and require administration by continuous infusion. Desensitization occurs with prolonged exposure to PGI_2 in the treatment of primary pulmonary hypertension, necessitating increasing doses to achieve the desired effect. These drugs may produce uterine smooth muscle contraction and should be avoided in pregnancy. Apnea occurs in ~10% of neonates receiving PGE_1, necessitating continuous respiratory monitoring. The potent antiplatelet effects may increase bleeding risk in surgical patients or those receiving anticoagulant/antithrombotic therapy.

Purinergic Agonists

Adenosine binds to specific purinergic receptors on vascular smooth muscle to open K_{ATP} channels, leading to membrane hyperpolarization and vasodilation. Adenosine also stimulates endothelial cells to produce NO and subsequent smooth muscle relaxation. It has an immediate onset and is rapidly metabolized to adenosine monophosphate, necessitating continuous intravenous infusion. Adenosine slows conduction through the atrioventricular node and may lead to heart block. Chest tightness and dyspnea have been reported, especially in patients with reactive airway disease. Dipyridamole potentiates the effects of adenosine, whereas theophylline and other methylxanthines antagonize its effects.

Calcium Channel Blockers

Verapamil is a phenylalkylamine that inhibits the influx of Ca^{2+} ions in cardiac muscle, cardiac conductive tissue, and vascular smooth muscle, producing decreases in cardiac contractility, heart rate, and both coronary and peripheral vascular tone. It is used clinically in the treatment of angina, tachydysrhythmia, and hypertension. Verapamil has a rapid onset when administered intravenously, with a duration of 20 to 30 minutes. Oral preparations vary in their duration of action depending on their formulation (i.e., sustained versus nonsustained). Verapamil is metabolized in the liver to norverapamil, an active metabolite with about 20% of the activity of the parent compound, which is renally excreted. Dosing adjustments are necessary in patients with renal or hepatic impairment. Caution must be used in patients with severe left ventricular dysfunction, second- or third-degree heart block, or in patients receiving other antiarrhythmic drugs, because of its negative inotropic and chronotropic effects. Verapamil may precipitate ventricular dysrhythmias in the setting of Wolff-Parkinson-White syndrome. Calcium channel blockers interfere with hepatic metabolism of a number of drugs, increasing the risk for important drug interactions. Neuromuscular blockade may be prolonged and the doses of sedative and analgesic drugs must be reduced with concomitant administration.

Nicardipine, nimodipine, and nifedipine are examples of dihydropyridine calcium channel blockers that inhibit the influx of Ca^{2+} ions in vascular smooth muscle with minimal effects on cardiac contractility or conduction. Cardiac output may increase because of reflex tachycardia and decreased afterload. Nifedipine is used to prevent vasospasm of arterial conduits in coronary artery bypass surgery, whereas nimodipine is used to treat or prevent cerebral arterial vasospasm in patients with subarachnoid hemorrhage. Nicardipine is available in intravenous and oral preparations, whereas the others are only available in oral form. Parenteral nicardipine is usually administered through continuous infusion because of its short biologic half-life. Nicardipine does undergo relatively slow terminal elimination and its effects can persist for several hours after discontinuation of a prolonged (e.g., >1 day) infusion. Again, the duration of oral agents varies depending on the type of preparation. Dose adjustments are necessary in patients with hepatic disease. Important drug interactions are possible secondary to interference with hepatic metabolism.

Diltiazem is a benzothiazepine that blocks Ca^{2+} influx in the myocardial conduction system and vascular smooth muscle. It causes mild to moderate decreases in myocardial contraction and decreases heart rate by decreasing both the automaticity of the sinoatrial node and rate of conduction in the atrioventricular node. It is indicated for treatment of tachydysrhythmia, angina, Raynaud syndrome, and hypertension. Diltiazem has a rapid onset when administered parenterally, and may be given by intermittent bolus or continuous infusion depending on the clinical circumstances. Diltiazem is also available in oral form with both sustained and nonsustained preparations. It is metabolized in the liver to an active metabolite. As with other calcium channel blockers, dose reductions are necessary in patients with hepatic dysfunction, and important drug interactions may occur.

Phosphodiesterase Inhibitors

Amrinone (inamrinone) and milrinone are bipyridine compounds that competitively inhibit phosphodiesterase III, increasing cAMP levels in myocardial and smooth muscle. In addition to their positive inotropic effects, amrinone and milrinone produce arterial and venous vasodilatation. Cardiac output is increased by improved contractility and decreased afterload, making these agents useful in the treatment of heart failure. They are administered by continuous intravenous infusion and have an elimination half-life of approximately 4 to 6 hours. Amrinone and milrinone undergo both hepatic and renal metabolism, and dosing must be adjusted for patients with significant renal or hepatic dysfunction. Both agents are associated with dose-dependent thrombocytopenia, however, the incidence is significantly less for milrinone. Platelet counts should be monitored during the treatment period. Amrinone and milrinone use is contraindicated during pregnancy. Furosemide and sodium bicarbonate should not be administered through the same infusion line because of precipitation risk.

Papaverine is a benzylisoquinoline alkaloid derivative of opium. It relaxes vascular smooth muscle by inhibiting phosphodiesterase. Cyclic AMP levels increase, protein kinases are activated, and Ca^{2+} entry into the cell is decreased. Because of poor gastrointestinal absorption, papaverine is rarely used in the chronic treatment of hypertension. Its major use is treatment of vasospasm in arterial or venous conduits used in coronary artery bypass surgery. It may also be used to treat cerebral vasospasm by selectively injecting papaverine into the affected vessel. Papaverine undergoes primarily hepatic metabolism.

Potassium Channel Openers

Hydralazine is included in this class of drugs that promote the influx of potassium into vascular smooth muscle cells, with resultant hyperpolarization and smooth muscle relaxation. It can be administered intravenously, intramuscularly, or orally and is useful in the treatment of severe hypertension, pre-eclampsia, and chronic heart failure. Onset of action may be as long as 20 minutes, even with intravenous administration, and caution must be used before re-dosing. It has a duration of action that varies from 3 to 8 hours. Metabolism is primarily hepatic by acetylation. The rate of acetylation varies among patients with about 30% of individuals undergoing rapid acetylation and 50% slow acetylation. This affects the bioavailability of the drug when orally administered. Rapid acetylators have lower bioavailability compared with slow acetylators. The acetylation rate does not appear to affect the drug concentration when administered intravenously. Reflex tachycardia may occur, thus special care must be taken if used in patients with coronary artery disease. Aplastic anemia and a lupus-like syndrome are associated with hydralazine use. Nonsteroidal anti-inflammatory drugs decrease the vasodilatory effect of hydralazine.

Like hydralazine, minoxidil increases the influx of potassium into vascular smooth muscle, resulting in hyperpolarization and vasodilation. It is administered orally and has a 30-minute onset, with a duration of about 24 hours. It is metabolized in the liver to minoxidil glucuronide with an elimination half-life of about 4 hours. Reflex tachycardia is common secondary to a baroreflex response and increased sympathetic activity. Likewise, renin levels are increased, leading to sodium and water retention. Minoxidil should be used in conjunction with a β adrenergic blocker and a diuretic. Minoxidil has been associated with the development of both pulmonary edema and pericardial effusion. It also causes electrocardiographic abnormalities, particularly T-wave flattening or inversion and increased QRS amplitude. Thrombocytopenia or leukopenia may occur, and Steven-Johnson syndrome has been associated with minoxidil use. Hypertrichosis is a common side effect.

α_2 Adrenergic Agonists

Clonidine is an α_2 adrenergic receptor agonist. It binds to the α_{2A} receptor in the locus ceruleus in the brain, which in turn inhibits the influx of Ca^{2+} into the cell and decreases neural activity. This results in decreased sympathetic tone, resulting in peripheral vasodilatation. When administered orally, peak concentrations are reached by about 90 minutes, and duration of activity is about 6 to 10 hours. It takes about 2 to 3 days for therapeutic levels to be reached after topical application, and levels are maintained for about 8 hours. Metabolism is approximately 50% hepatic and 50% renal. The half-life is prolonged in patients with renal insufficiency. Bradycardia and orthostatic hypotension are common secondary to the decreased sympathetic tone. Rebound hypertension may occur and may be severe. Clonidine may decrease minimum alveolar concentration by up to 50%, thus reducing anesthetic requirements. Sedation is a common side effect (see Chapter 28 for a more detailed discussion).

Dexmedetomidine is a highly selective α_2 adrenergic receptor agonist ($\alpha_2:\alpha_1$ selectivity ratio of 1600:1), which is seven times more selective than clonidine. Like clonidine,

TABLE 39–1.

Commonly Used Vasodilators: Doses and Routes of Administration

Drug	Dose
Nitrates	
Nitroglycerin	IV: 0.2–1 μg/kg/min; SL: 0.3–0.6 mg; TOP: 1–2 every 6–8 hr
Sodium Nitroprusside	IV: 0.2–1.0 μg/kg/min; maximum dose 2.0 μg/kg/min
β Agonists	
Dobutamine	IV: 1–20 μg/kg/min
Isoproterenol	IV: 0.02–0.5 μg/kg/min
Dopamine-1 Agonists	
Fenoldopam	IV: 0.1–0.5 μg/kg/min
ACE Inhibitors	
Captopril	PO: 6.25–12.5 mg twice daily initial dosage; maximum dose 150 mg/day
Enalapril	PO: 2.5 mg twice daily; maximum dose 40 mg/day;
	IV (as enalaprilat): 1.25 mg every 6 hr; maximum dose 20 mg/day
Angiotensin II Receptor Antagonists	
Losartan	PO: 25–50 mg daily; maximum dose 100 mg/day
Eicosanoids	
Prostaglandin E_1	IV: 0.05–0.1 μg/kg/min
Prostacyclin	IV: 2–3 ng/kg/min
Purinergic Agonists	
Adenosine	IV: 50 μg/kg/min
Calcium Channel Antagonists	
Verapamil	IV: 5–10 mg; may repeat 10 mg 30 min after initial dose
	PO: 180 to 360 mg/day for hypertension
Diltiazem	IV: 0.25 mg/kg then 5–15 mg/hr; may repeat a second bolus of 0.35 mg/kg 15 minutes after initial treatment;
	PO: 180 to 360 mg/day
Nicardipine	IV: Initial dose 5 μg/kg/min; decrease to 1–3 μg/kg/min;
	PO: 60–120 mg/day
Phosphodiesterase Inhibitors	
Amrinone	IV: 0.5–1.5 mg/kg bolus, then 2–10 μg/kg/min
Milrinone	IV: 50 μg/kg bolus; 0.5–1.0 μg/kg/min
Papaverine	Direct injection into the affected vessels
Potassium Channel Activators	
Hydralazine	IV: 2.5–10 mg every 20–30 min; max 30–40 mg
	IM: 10–20 mg every 4–6 hr;
	PO: 40–300 mg per day
Minoxidil	PO: 10–40 mg per day in two divided doses; max 100 mg/day
α_2 Adrenergic Agonists	
Clonidine	PO: 0.2–2.4 mg/day in two divided doses;
	TOP: 0.1–0.3 mg/hr every 7 days
Dexmedetomidine	IV: 1 μg/kg loading dose over 10 min, 0.2–0.7 μg/kg/hr
α_1 Adrenergic Antagonists	
Phentolamine	IV: 30–70 μg/kg bolus
Prazosin	PO: 3–20 mg per day in three divided doses

dexmedetomidine decreases sympathetic tone by inhibition of Ca^{2+} influx in the locus ceruleus. This results in decreased heart rate and vasodilation. Dexmedetomidine also possesses hypnotic, sedative, and analgesic properties while minimally affecting respiratory drive. It is administered intravenously with an onset of action of 2 to 5 minutes. Elimination half-life is about 2 hours. It is primarily metabolized in the liver by direct glucuronidation and the p450 enzyme system. The dose should be reduced in patients with hepatic failure. Bradycardia and hypotension are common secondary to decreased sympathetic tone; however, if infused too rapidly during the loading dose, hypertension may result secondary to direct activation of vascular α_2 adrenergic receptors. Caution must be used in hypovolemic patients. Rebound hypertension may occur after discontinuation. As with clonidine, dexmedetomidine may decrease minimum alveolar concentration by up to 50%, thus reducing anesthetic requirements. Sedative/hypnotic and opiate requirements are reduced with concomitant administration.

α_1 Adrenergic Antagonists

Phentolamine is a nonselective α adrenergic receptor antagonist. Its activity at the α_1 adrenergic receptor results in decreased $[Ca^{2+}]_i$ and vasorelaxation. It also blocks presynaptic α_2 receptors, where it interferes with the normal feedback inhibition of norepinephrine release. Plasma norepinephrine levels are increased in patients treated with phentolamine. It is used in the management of pheochromocytoma and as treatment for vasoconstriction secondary to drug extravasation (i.e., norepinephrine). It has an immediate onset with a duration of action of about 10 to 15 minutes, making it suitable for continuous infusion. Phentolamine undergoes primarily hepatic metabolism. Only 10% of the drug is excreted unchanged in the urine. Reflex tachycardia is common secondary to the baroreceptor reflex. Norepinephrine release is also enhanced from nerve terminals, which contributes to increased cardiac output. Caution must be used in patients with coronary artery disease.

Prazosin is a selective α_1 adrenergic antagonist that produces arterial and venous vasodilation. Because it does not inhibit the α_2 receptors, the feedback control of norepinephrine release is intact. Reflex tachycardia is relatively uncommon in patients treated with prazosin, and the cardiac output is increased to a lesser extent compared with phentolamine. It is administered orally and has an onset of action of about 30 minutes. Its half-life is about 3 hours, and the duration of activity is about 4 to 6 hours. Prazosin undergoes primarily hepatic metabolism. Caution must be used in hypovolemic patients because of increased venous capacitance and decreased preload. Patients treated with prazosin are prone to developing orthostatic hypotension.

Dosage and Administration

Table 39–1 lists the doses and administration of commonly used vasodilators.

References

1. Milnor W: Hemodynamics. Baltimore, Williams & Wilkins, 1989.
2. Burnstock G: Innervation of vascular smooth muscle: Histochemistry and electron microscopy [review]. Clin Exp Pharmacol Physiol (suppl 2):7–20, 1975.
3. Burnstock G: Do some nerve cells release more than one transmitter [review]? Neuroscience 1(4):239–248, 1976.
4. Burnstock G: Integration of factors controlling vascular tone. Overview [review]. Anesthesiology 79(6):1368–1380, 1993.
5. Rand MJ: Nitrergic transmission: Nitric oxide as a mediator of non-adrenergic, non-cholinergic neuro-effector transmission [review]. Clin Exp Pharmacol Physiol 19(3):147–169, 1992.
6. Stjarne L: Basic mechanisms and local modulation of nerve impulse-induced secretion of neurotransmitters from individual sympathetic nerve varicosities [review]. Rev Physiol Biochem Pharmacol 112:1–137, 1989.
7. Furchgott RF, Vanhoutte PM: Endothelium-derived relaxing and contracting factors [review]. FASEB J 3(9):2007–2018, 1989.
8. Murphy R: Smooth muscle. In Berne R, Levy M (eds): Physiology. St. Louis, Mosby Yearbook: St. Louis. 1993, pp 309–324.
9. Horowitz A, et al: Mechanisms of smooth muscle contraction [review]. Physiol Rev 76(4):967–1003, 1996.
10. Carpenter CL: Actin cytoskeleton and cell signaling [review]. Crit Care Med 28(4 suppl):N94–99, 2000.
11. Tada M: Molecular structure and function of phospholamban in regulating the calcium pump from sarcoplasmic reticulum. Ann NY Acad Sci 671:92–102; discussion, 102–103, 1992.
12. Walsh MP: Calmodulin and the regulation of smooth muscle contraction. Mol Cell Biochem 135(1):21–41, 1994.
13. Trybus KM: Regulation of expressed truncated smooth muscle myosins. Role of the essential light chain and tail length. J Biol Chem 269(33):20819–20822, 1994.
14. Cremo CR, Sellers JR, Facemyer KC: Two heads are required for phosphorylation-dependent regulation of smooth muscle myosin. J Biol Chem 270(5):2171–2175, 1995.
15. Van Eyk JE, et al: Different molecular mechanisms for Rho family GTPase-dependent, Ca2+-independent contraction of smooth muscle. J Biol Chem 273(36):23433–23439, 1998.
16. Chew TL, et al: Phosphorylation of non-muscle myosin II regulatory light chain by p21-activated kinase (gamma-PAK). J Muscle Res Cell Motil 19(8):839–854, 1998.
17. Uehata M, et al: Calcium sensitization of smooth muscle mediated by a Rho-associated protein kinase in hypertension [see comments]. Nature 389(6654):990–994, 1997.
18. Brophy CM: The dynamic regulation of blood vessel caliber [review]. J Vasc Surg 31(2):391–395, 2000.
19. Murphy RA: What is special about smooth muscle? The significance of covalent crossbridge regulation [review]. FASEB J 8(3):311–318, 1994.
20. Surks HK, et al: Regulation of myosin phosphatase by a specific interaction with cGMP-dependent protein kinase I alpha. Science 286(5444):1583–1587, 1999.
21. Rembold CM: Regulation of contraction and relaxation in arterial smooth muscle [review]. Hypertension 20(2):129–137, 1992.
22. Ruth P, et al: Transfected cGMP-dependent protein kinase suppresses calcium transients by inhibition of inositol 1,4,5-trisphosphate production. Proc Natl Acad Sci USA 90(7):2623–2627, 1993.
23. Kirsten R, et al: Clinical pharmacokinetics of vasodilators. Part I [review]. Clin Pharmacokinet 34(6):457–482, 1998.
24. Klockner U, Isenberg G: Myocytes isolated from porcine coronary arteries: Reduction of currents through L-type Ca-channels by verapamil-type Ca-antagonists. J Physiol Pharmacol 42(2):163–179, 1991.
25. Kurokawa J, Adachi-Akahane S, Nagao T: 1,5-benzothiazepine binding domain is located on the extracellular side of the cardiac L-type Ca2+ channel. Mol Pharmacol 51(2):262–268, 1997.
26. Leblanc N, et al: Electrophysiological mechanisms of minoxidil sulfate-induced vasodilation of rabbit portal vein. Circ Res 65(4):1102–1011, 1989.
27. Koyano T, et al: ATP-regulated K+ channels are modulated by intracellular H+ in guinea-pig ventricular cells. J Physiol 463:747–766, 1993.

28. Merkel LA, et al: Demonstration of vasorelaxant activity with an A1-selective adenosine agonist in porcine coronary artery: Involvement of potassium channels. J Pharmacol Exp Ther 260(2):437–443, 1992.

29. Miyoshi H, Nakaya Y, Moritoki H: Nonendothelial-derived nitric oxide activates the ATP-sensitive K+ channel of vascular smooth muscle cells. FEBS Lett 345(1):47–49, 1994.

30. Palmer RM, Ferrige AG, Moncada S: Nitric oxide release accounts for the biological activity of endothelium-derived relaxing factor. Nature 327(6122):524–526, 1987.

31. Hein TW, Kuo L: cAMP-independent dilation of coronary arterioles to adenosine: Role of nitric oxide, G proteins, and K(ATP) channels. Circ Res 85(7):634–642, 1999.

32. Krupinski J, et al: Molecular diversity in the adenylylcyclase family. Evidence for eight forms of the enzyme and cloning of type VI. J Biol Chem 267(34):24858–24862, 1992.

33. Tang WJ, Gilman AG: Adenylyl cyclases [review]. Cell 70(6):869–872, 1992.

34. Smiley RM, Kwatra MM, Schwinn DA: New developments in cardiovascular adrenergic receptor pharmacology: Molecular mechanisms and clinical relevance. J Cardiothorac Vasc Anesth 12(1):80–95, 1998.

35. Maze M, Tranquilli W: Alpha-2 adrenoceptor agonists: Defining the role in clinical anesthesia [review]. Anesthesiology 74(3):581–605, 1991.

36. Beall AC, et al: Cyclic nucleotide-dependent vasorelaxation is associated with the phosphorylation of a small heat shock-related protein. J Biol Chem 272(17):11283–11287, 1997.

37. Post JBT, Frishman WH: Fenoldopam: A new dopamine agonist for the treatment of hypertensive urgencies and emergencies. J Clin Pharmacol 38(1):2–13, 1998.

38. Kirsten R, et al: Clinical pharmacokinetics of vasodilators. Part II [review]. Clin Pharmacokinet 35(1):9–36, 1998.

39. Yamamoto T, Bing RJ: Nitric oxide donors. Proc Soc Exp Biol Med 225(3):200–206, 2000.

40. Sabouni MH, et al: G proteins subserve relaxations mediated by adenosine receptors in human coronary artery. J Cardiovasc Pharmacol 18(5):696–702, 1991.

41. Corbin JD, Francis SH: Cyclic GMP phosphodiesterase-5: Target of sildenafil. J Biol Chem 274(20):13729–13732, 1999.

42. Gombotz H, et al: DA1-receptor stimulation by fenoldopam in the treatment of postcardiac surgical hypertension. Acta Anaesthesiol Scand 42(7):834–840, 1998.

43. Brogden RN, Markham A: Fenoldopam: A review of its pharmacodynamic and pharmacokinetic properties and intravenous clinical potential in the management of hypertensive urgencies and emergencies [review]. Drugs 54(4):634–650, 1997.

44. Carson P, et al: Racial differences in response to therapy for heart failure: Analysis of the vasodilator-heart failure trials. Vasodilator-Heart Failure Trial Study Group. J Card Fail 5(3):178–187, 1999.

45. Pfeffer MA, et al: Effect of captopril on mortality and morbidity in patients with left ventricular dysfunction after myocardial infarction. Results of the survival and ventricular enlargement trial. The SAVE Investigators [see comments]. N Engl J Med 327(10):669–677, 1992.

46. Ray S, Dargie H: Infarct-related heart failure: The choice of ACE inhibitor does not matter [review]. Cardiovasc Drugs Ther 8(3):433–436, 1994.

47. Ball SG, Hall AS, Murray GD: ACE inhibition, atherosclerosis and myocardial infarction—the AIRE Study in practice. Acute Infarction Ramipril Efficacy Study. Eur Heart J 15(suppl B):20–25; discussion, 26–30, 1994.

48. Lewis EJ, et al: The effect of angiotensin-converting-enzyme inhibition on diabetic nephropathy. The Collaborative Study Group [see comments]. [erratum appears in N Engl J Med 1993 Jan 13;330(2):152]. N Engl J Med 329(20):1456–1462, 1993.

49. Miller K, et al: Enalapril: A well-tolerated and efficacious agent for the pediatric hypertensive patient. J Cardiovasc Pharmacol 10(suppl 7):S154–156, 1987.

50. Pereira CM, Tam YK, Collins-Nakai RL: The pharmacokinetics of captopril in infants with congestive heart failure. Ther Drug Monit 13(3):209–214, 1991.

51. Crozier I, et al: Losartan in heart failure. Hemodynamic effects and tolerability. Losartan Hemodynamic Study Group. Circulation 91(3):691–697, 1995.

52. Lacourciere Y, Lefebvre J: Modulation of the renin-angiotensin-aldosterone system and cough. Can J Cardiol 11(suppl F):33F–39F, 1995.

40

Bronchodilators, Corticosteroids, and Anti-inflammatory Agents

Charles Emala, MD

Bronchodilators
    β Adrenoceptor Agonists
    Methylxanthines
    Anticholinergics
    Volatile Anesthetics as Bronchodilators

Corticosteroids
Anti-Inflammatory Agents
    Nedocromil Sodium and Sodium Cromoglycate
    Leukotriene Antagonists and 5-Lipoxygenase
     Inhibitors

Bronchodilators

β Adrenoceptor Agonists

History and Background

β Adrenoceptor agonists, delivered through inhalation, are a mainstay in the treatment of asthma. Epinephrine was initially used systemically to achieve bronchodilation, but with the recognition of adrenoceptor classes (α and β),[1] the β-selective agonist isoproterenol evolved as the drug of choice.[2] However, its catecholamine structure rendered it unstable and it was replaced by the more chemically stable compound metaproterenol.[3] The discovery of subtypes of β adrenoceptors[4,5] led to the development of selective β₂ agonists devoid of the side effects of tachycardia that accompanied the nonselective β agonists. Metaproterenol was the first β₂-selective agonist introduced for asthma therapy followed by albuterol with increased β₂-selectivity, and despite the introduction of many other β₂-selective agonists (e.g., terbutaline, fenoterol, procaterol), albuterol has remained the most widely used β₂-selective agonist in the treatment of asthma. Attempts to further enhance the selectivity of β₂ agonists (and presumably decrease side effects such as vasodilation and skeletal muscle tremor) led to the recent introduction of levalbuterol, a pure R-isomer of the standard 50:50 racemic R- and S-mixture of albuterol. Despite their high efficacy in achieving bronchodilation, albuterol and terbutaline have a relatively short duration of action (up to 4–6 hours), which makes their clinical use in asthma maintenance therapy limited. Therefore, long duration β₂-selective agonists were introduced (salmeterol[6] and

formoterol[7]) in an attempt to maintain β agonist–mediated bronchodilation for up to 12 hours. Formoterol was developed because of its increased affinity for the β₂ adrenoceptor, whereas salmeterol contains a large lipophilic modification to facilitate binding to hydrophobic regions of the cell membrane. Although these long-acting formulations do provide extended relief, particularly useful in nocturnal asthma, they are not intended for acute rescue therapy during acute exacerbations of symptoms because of their slower onset of action in comparison with albuterol or terbutaline.

Mechanisms of Drug Action

β₂ Adrenoceptors belong to a large family of proteins structurally characterized by seven transmembrane-spanning regions with a carboxy-terminal intracellular tail. This family of proteins includes members that transduce such diverse cellular signals as odorant detection, light perception, and hormonal action. The β₂ adrenoceptor has served as the prototypical G protein–coupled receptor (GPCR) in the understanding of the mechanisms involved in receptor/G protein interaction for more than 100 different GPCRs. β₂ Adrenoceptors were classically described as coupling exclusively to the heterotrimeric stimulatory G protein, G_s, originally named for its stimulatory effect on adenylyl cyclase activity. Heterotrimeric G proteins are composed of three subunits denoted α, β, and γ. In the inactivated state, the three subunits form a heterotrimeric complex with guanosine diphosphate (GDP) bound to the α-subunit and the γ-subunit anchoring the complex to the cell membrane. After the binding of agonist to the β₂ adrenoceptor, interaction with an activated G_s protein (with guanosine triphosphate [GTP] displacing GDP) is favored, resulting in

703

disassociation of the α-subunit of G_s from the βγ dimer. The activated G_sα-subunit activates adenylyl cyclase resulting in the conversion of adenosine triphosphate (ATP) to cyclic adenosine monophosphate (cAMP), which in turn activates protein kinase A (PKA). PKA phosphorylates regulatory proteins (e.g., RhoA) involved in the control of smooth muscle tone (Fig. 40–1). In addition, cAMP inhibits calcium release from intracellular stores, reduces transmembrane calcium entry, and enhances intracellular calcium sequestration.[8] The hydrolysis of GTP to GDP results in the return of the α-subunit to an inactivated state and reassociation with the βγ dimer to reform the heterotrimer. In addition, $β_2$ adrenoceptors are also known to couple through G_s to cAMP-independent pathways, notably to direct G_s coupling to ion channels.[9–11]

Agonist binding to the $β_2$ adrenoceptor also initiates its own inactivation by phosphorylation. Receptor occupancy and the release of βγ-subunits from G_s recruits β adrenoceptor kinase (βARK) to the cellular membrane, which phosphorylates the $β_2$ adrenoceptor and allows the binding of β-arrestin, a protein that facilitates receptor desensitization and sequestration. Variation in the process of desensitization in various tissues has been attributed to variable amounts of βARK. The amount of mRNA encoding βARK in airway smooth muscle is only 11% of the amount expressed in mast cells.[12] This is consistent with isoproterenol-induced cAMP levels reaching maximum levels at 90 seconds in mast cells, whereas cAMP levels do not plateau in airway smooth muscle cells.[12] $β_2$ Adrenoceptor function is also attenuated by phosphorylation by PKA. It is now appreciated that the PKA-phosphorylated receptor selectively couples to the G_i protein to release βγ subunits, which couple through ras to activate mitogen-activated protein kinases.[13] Single nucleotide polymorphisms (SNPs) have been identified in both the promoter region and protein coding region of the human $β_2$ adrenoceptor gene. Nine different SNPs have been described[14] within the protein coding region with four of these SNPs resulting in changes in encoded amino acids, and three of these four resulting in changes in receptor protein function. The most frequent (30–45%) of these polymorphisms is the substitution of a glycine residue for an arginine residue at amino acid position 16 in the receptor protein resulting in an enhanced rate of receptor desensitization.[14,15] A second SNP results in the substitution of a glutamine residue for a glutamic acid residue at amino acid position 27, resulting in a decreased rate of receptor desensitization.[14,15] A less frequently occurring SNP (2–5%) results in the substitution of an isoleucine for a threonine residue at amino acid position 164 resulting in a receptor with reduced agonist binding affinity and reduced activation of its effector enzyme, adenylyl cyclase.[14,16]

An additional polymorphism has been described in the 5′ leader cistron region of the $β_2$ adrenoceptor gene within an open reading frame that encodes a 19-amino acid peptide that regulates $β_2$ mRNA translation. An Arg-Cys substitution resulting from this nucleotide polymorphism results in increased levels of $β_2$ adrenoceptor protein in both transfected COS-7 cells[17] and cultured human airway smooth muscle cells.[18]

Polymorphisms of the $β_2$ adrenoceptor gene encoding amino acid substitutions 16 and 27 have received the most

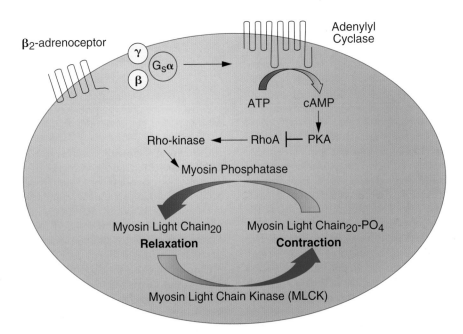

Airway Smooth Muscle Cell

Figure 40–1. β Adrenoceptor–mediated airway smooth muscle relaxation. Rho-kinase normally phosphorylates and thus inhibits myosin phosphatase favoring contraction. In the presence of β adrenoceptor agonists, increased cyclic adenosine monophosphate (cAMP) and protein kinase A (PKA) inhibit RhoA, which inhibits Rho-kinase increasing the activity of myosin phosphatase. The net result is dephosphorylation of myosin light chain$_{20}$ and relaxation. → Indicates activation; ⊥ indicates inhibition.

attention because of their high prevalence (30–45%) and have been evaluated as modifiers of several pathologic states including asthma, allergy, hypertension, and heart failure. The most comprehensive evaluation to date has been with asthma in which the incidence, severity, and response to therapy have been compared among patients with and without the Gly 16 and Glu 27 polymorphisms. Multiple studies have shown that the presence of polymorphisms at these sites can not alone account for the presence of asthma,[19–24] but that these polymorphisms are associated with the severity of airway hyper-responsiveness[20,25,26] and predict airway responses to histamine constriction[27] and β agonist–mediated airway relaxation.[28–30] Furthermore, the presence of the Arg 16 polymorphism appears to result in reduced airway relaxation during chronic use of β agonists[31,32] and to alter functional desensitization of β adrenoceptor function during chronic β agonist use.[33] The effects of these polymorphisms on β_2 adrenoceptor down-regulation were initially characterized in transfected cells,[15] but subsequently were shown to occur in human airway smooth muscle cells expressing native receptors.[34]

The general consensus that polymorphisms of the β_2 adrenoceptor gene are not linked directly to the cause of asthma but may modify the severity of the phenotype also holds true for allergy. Although the presence of these polymorphisms alone does not account for the presence of allergy,[35–37] the glu/gln 27 polymorphism was a modifier of total IgE levels.[35,36] Moreover, both the arg/gly 16 and glu/gly 27 polymorphisms affected the amount of desensitization induced by isoprenaline in human lung mast cells.[38]

A less frequently occurring SNP (2–5%) encodes the substitution of an isoleucine for a threonine residue at amino acid position 164 resulting in a receptor with reduced agonist binding affinity and reduced activation of its effector enzyme, adenylyl cyclase.[16] This Ile164 polymorphism is an attractive candidate to link to the causation of disease because it is the only known polymorphism that results in a direct effect on the β_2 adrenoceptor's ability to stimulate its target protein $G_s\alpha$ and subsequently adenylyl cyclase. However, the low frequency of even the heterozygous genotype (Thr/Ile164) in populations currently studied (2–5%) make the direct link of this polymorphism to a major proportion of pathologic states unlikely. Nonetheless, this polymorphism has been linked to decreased exercise performance,[39] an increased risk for death, and need for cardiac transplantation in congestive heart failure,[40] and has been listed as a criterion for indication for cardiac transplantation.[41]

Preclinical Pharmacology

Classical radioligand binding studies of β_2 adrenoreceptors have used ^{125}I-iodopindolol or ^{125}I-cyanopindolol, which bind to cell surface and internalized β_2 adrenoceptors. The availability of hydrophobic radioligands has allowed the study of internalization rates of β_2 adrenoceptors because the radioligand binds only to cell surface receptors. β_2 Adrenoceptors, like all GPCRs, display two affinity states for agonists in radioligand binding experiments. The low affinity state represents receptors not associated with G pro-

teins, whereas high affinity receptors are G protein–associated. Competitive binding of the radioligand by agonist results in a displacement curve with a biphasic shape reflecting these two affinity states. In the presence of saturating concentrations of GTP, favoring the activated state of the G protein, all β_2 adrenoceptors are disassociated from G_s proteins, resulting in a conversion of the displacement curve to a monophasic shape reflecting the low affinity state of the receptor.

β_2 Adrenoceptors are widely expressed in many cell types, and activation universally results in increases in cellular levels of cAMP. However, the downstream signaling events that result from increased cellular levels of cAMP are cell-type specific. For example, smooth muscle cells of the airway and uterus relax in response to cAMP,[42–45] whereas cardiac myocytes exhibit increased contractility.[46] Despite these cell-specific limitations, the β_2 adrenoceptor of the peripheral white blood cell has been used as a model of pulmonary β_2 adrenoceptors in many studies of human asthma because of the easy accessibility of the white blood cells.

Clinical Pharmacology

The dose of a β agonist aerosol deposited at the active site in the lungs (i.e., smooth muscle of large- and intermediate-sized airways) is a fraction of the inhaled dose, which in turn is a fraction of the dose delivered with each actuation. The determinants of the amount of drug that reaches target tissues include the particle size of the aerosol, the velocity at which it is released from the delivery device, the patient's inhalation technique, and the degree of airway narrowing. In some cases, the addition of a device-specific spacer increases the amount of aerosol reaching its airway target by keeping more of the drug aerosolized within the spacer, thus not allowing the drug to deposit in the oral cavity and oropharynx. The largest single factor that determines the amount and reproducibility of drug deposition at the smooth muscle target is the patient's technique of inhaler use. Approximately 90 μg albuterol is delivered per actuation of a metered dose inhaler, and it is estimated that with proper technique, approximately 18 μg is deposited in the lung. After its slow adsorption from the lung, aerosolized albuterol achieves peak serum concentrations in 2 to 4 hours. Urinary excretion studies reveal a half-life of 3.8 hours. Within 24 hours of an inhaled dose, 72% is excreted in the urine—28% as unchanged drug and 44% as metabolite. The time to onset of improved respiratory function after aerosolized albuterol is 15 minutes, as determined by improvements in both forced expiratory volume (FEV_1) and maximal mid-expiratory flow rate. Maximal improvement occurs within 60 to 90 minutes with duration of effect of 3 to 6 hours.

The primary action of β agonists is to stimulate adenylyl cyclase, the enzyme that synthesizes cAMP from ATP. Increased levels of cAMP mediate smooth muscle relaxation and inhibit the release of inflammatory mediators from cells, especially mast cells. Adverse effects of β agonists are attributable to increase of cAMP levels in nontarget tissues and are typical of effects of sympathomimetic agents. Although tremor and nervousness are the most frequently reported adverse effects, tachycardia, hypertension, palpitations, nausea, and vomiting have also been reported.

Until recently, all marketed β agonists were racemic preparations even though they were historically designed to mimic the bronchodilatory effect of endogenous epinephrine, which is an isomerically pure R-isomer (R-epinephrine). Indeed, the bronchodilatory effects of albuterol are mediated by the R-isomer, whereas the S-isomer has no therapeutic benefit. In fact, the S-isomer of albuterol has been shown to have effects on airway smooth muscle that would be expected to be detrimental to airway relaxation. The S-isomer of albuterol has been shown to increase intracellular calcium concentrations accompanied by increased cell shortening.[47,48] Eosinophils exposed to S-albuterol exhibited enhanced superoxide production, a potential proinflammatory effect[49]; this finding may partially account for the discrepancy between the anti-inflammatory action of β agonists in vitro and their lack of clinical anti-inflammatory effects.[50] The enhanced bronchodilatory effect of the R-isomer of albuterol on human airway smooth muscle[51-53] has led to the clinical introduction of levalbuterol. (R,R)-formoterol, the pure active enantiomer of formoterol, has been shown in phase II clinical trials to produce an increase in FEV$_1$ of 24 hours in duration.[54]

Practical Aspects of Drug Administration

β Agonists are indicated for the chronic maintenance, as well as the acute exacerbations, of asthmatic symptoms. Acute exacerbations are treated with rapidly acting agents (i.e., albuterol; onset 5–7 minutes); however, their duration is limited (4–6 hours). In contrast, improved duration can be achieved with salmeterol (>12 hours), but because of its slow onset (35 minutes), it is not useful during acute exacerbations. Formoterol, approved in 2001 by the Food and Drug Administration for use in the United States, combines rapid onset (5.3 minutes) with prolonged duration (10–12 hours), and the R,R-isomer of formoterol is currently being evaluated for U.S. release.

β Agonists are available as oral, intravenous, subcutaneous, and inhalational formulations. Inhalational administration is generally preferred because of the delivery of larger doses directly to the airways, minimizing the systemic toxicity, particularly on the cardiovascular system. Despite the relative β$_2$-selectivity of these agents, greater systemic doses can stimulate both β$_1$ and β$_2$ cardiac adrenoceptors. Inhalation of albuterol (Proventil or Ventolin) by metered dose inhaler results in the delivery of 90 to 108 μg albuterol per actuation. The speed of onset ranges from 6 to 15 minutes, with a duration of effect of 3 to 6 hours. Prophylactic administration of β agonists before exercise is beneficial in exercise-induced asthma. Prophylactic administration of β agonists or anticholinergic agents 1 hour before induction of general anesthesia results in reduced airway resistance after endotracheal intubation.[55]

Inhalational administration of β agonists can be achieved using a pressurized metered dose inhaler with or without a spacing device, a nebulizer, or a dry powder inhaler. Albuterol, metaproterenol, pirbuterol, and salmeterol are available in metered dose inhalers, whereas albuterol, pirbuterol, salmeterol, and formoterol are available in dry

powder inhalers. Albuterol, metaproterenol, and levalbuterol are available for nebulization. Metered dose inhalers have traditionally been powered by chlorofluorcarbons, but international agreements targeted at eliminating chlorofluorcarbons because of their detrimental effects on the earth's ozone layer have resulted in reformulations of several β agonists in metered dose inhalers powered by hydrofluoroalkane propellants. In addition, dry powder inhalers, actuated by the patient's inspiratory flow rate, are increasing in popularity for β agonist and inhaled steroid delivery because they do not require a propellant and they do not require close patient coordination between drug dispensing and the initiation of inspiration.

β Agonists are available for oral administration in both tablet and syrup formulations. Albuterol (4–8 mg), metaproterenol (10 mg), and terbutaline (5 mg) are available in standard and delayed-release tablet form, and albuterol and metaproterenol are also available in syrup formulation. β Agonists are rapidly and well absorbed after oral administration, but the time of onset for bronchodilating properties is 30 minutes (compared with 6–15 minutes through the aerosol route). Peak plasma levels after 2 and 4 mg albuterol doses are 6.7 and 14.8 ng/mL, respectively. Maximal serum levels occur 2 to 3 hours after dosing with an elimination half-life of 5 to 6 hours. Albuterol has been formulated to provide a duration of action of up to 12 hours (Proventil Repetabs).

Terbutaline is the only selective β$_2$ adrenoceptor agonist available for parenteral (subcutaneous) use. It may be advantageous in acute exacerbations of asthma in which inhaled β agonists have not adequately reversed bronchospasm and oral therapy is not appropriate (e.g., anesthetized patients). Subcutaneous terbutaline is most widely used as a tocolytic agent because of the relaxing effects of β agonists on the smooth muscle of the uterus. The usual initial dose is 0.25 mg subcutaneously, which can be repeated in 15 to 30 minutes if no clinical improvement is seen. The total dose within 4 hours should not exceed 0.5 mg subcutaneously.

Methylxanthines

Theophylline is a methylxanthine derivative that inhibits adenosine receptors facilitating release of catecholamines[56-58] and at very high concentrations inhibits phosphodiesterases, enzymes responsible for degradation of cAMP. Aminophylline is a water-soluble salt of theophylline that can be administered orally or intravenously. Theophylline remains the most widely prescribed medication for asthma in the world because it is inexpensive. However, in industrialized countries, theophylline is typically a third-line therapy for bronchodilation because of systemic toxicity and is reserved for patients with severe asthma not controlled with β agonists and steroids. Although theophylline is not typically the first choice for bronchodilating effects, the emerging understanding of theophylline's anti-inflammatory effects is contributing to a re-evaluation of the role of theophylline in chronic asthma management.

Acute asthmatic exacerbations in anesthetized patients are typically treated with β agonists and increased concentrations of volatile anesthetics. However, during emergence in patients that are not candidates for deep extubation, the addition of theophylline may be of theoretical benefit during awakening with an endotracheal tube in place. However, the combination of theophylline and halothane can be quite proarrhythmogenic because of halothane's ability to sensitize the myocardium to the catecholamines released by theophylline.[59,60] The use of theophylline during the maintenance phase of inhalational anesthesia appears to have no added bronchodilator affect over that of the volatile agents.[61]

Preclinical Pharmacology

Theophylline is a nonselective inhibitor of phosphodiesterases leading to increased cellular concentrations of cAMP and cyclic guanosine monophosphate. Despite more than 60 years of clinical use, the precise mechanism by which theophylline potentiates bronchodilation remains in debate. Theophylline is known to increase the secretion of adrenaline from the adrenal medulla, inhibit phosphodiesterase at high concentrations, inhibit adenosine receptors, and decrease airway inflammation. At therapeutic levels of theophylline, the predominant mechanism responsible for bronchodilation is uncertain. The release of epinephrine from the adrenal medulla results in an increase in plasma concentrations of epinephrine that may be too small to account for any bronchodilator effect. Theophylline, at therapeutic concentrations, inhibits only 5% to 10% of total phosphodiesterase activity in human lung extracts.[62] However, in vitro, the concentration of theophylline that inhibits phosphodiesterases is similar to the concentration that relaxes airway smooth muscle.[63] A theophylline derivative, 8-phenyltheophylline, inhibits adenosine receptors but does not inhibit phosphodiesterases and does not cause airway smooth muscle relaxation, suggesting that adenosine receptor antagonism is not a mechanism by which xanthines promote bronchodilation.[63] Thus it may be a combination of effects of theophylline including catecholamine release, phosphodiesterase inhibition, and inflammatory inhibition that contribute to smooth muscle relaxation and bronchodilation.

Clinical Pharmacology

Theophylline is rapidly and completely absorbed after oral administration, whether in solution or tablet form. The drug distributes freely into fat-free tissues and is extensively metabolized in the liver. Its pharmacokinetics vary widely among similar patients and cannot be predicted based on sex, age, body weight, or other demographic characteristics. Moreover, its metabolism and clearance is greatly affected by concurrent disease states and altered physiology including liver disease, cystic fibrosis, pulmonary edema, chronic obstructive pulmonary disease, thyroid disease, pregnancy, and sepsis with multiorgan failure. Multiple concurrent medications are known to enhance (carbamazepine, rifampin) or inhibit (cimetidine, erythromycin, tacrine) the liver metabolism of theophylline. Specific drug interactions with numerous anesthetic-related medications have been

described. There is an increased risk for ventricular arrhythmias when theophylline is used in the presence of halothane because of the sensitizing effects of halothane on the myocardium to increased catecholamines released by theophylline. Larger doses of benzodiazepines may be needed to achieve the desired effect in the presence of theophylline as benzodiazepines increase the central nervous system (CNS) concentrations of adenosine, a potent CNS depressant, whereas theophylline blocks adenosine receptors.[64] Ketamine may decrease the theophylline seizure threshold,[65] and theophylline can antagonize the effect of nonpolarizing muscle relaxants possibly because of phosphodiesterase inhibition.[66]

A single oral dose of 5 mg/kg will achieve a mean peak serum concentration of 10 μg/mL in adults 1 to 2 hours after dosing. Approximately 40% is bound to serum proteins, primarily albumin, whereas unbound drug distributes throughout body water and poorly in fat yielding an apparent volume of distribution of 0.45 L/kg. The apparent volume of distribution is increased in patients with hepatic cirrhosis, uncorrected acidemia, the elderly, premature neonates, and in women during the third trimester of pregnancy. In such cases, the patient may show signs of theophylline toxicity even though total serum concentrations are in the therapeutic range (10–20 μg/mL) because of increased levels of unbound drug.

Theophylline has effects on many physiologic processes including CNS stimulation, tachycardia, decreased peripheral vascular resistance, increased cerebral vascular resistance, smooth muscle relaxation, diuresis, and increased secretion by endocrine and exocrine tissues (e.g., gastrin, parathyroid hormone). Theophylline serum concentrations only slightly greater than recommended therapeutic ranges (10–20 μg/mL) can produce nervousness, restlessness, insomnia, tremors, and hyperesthesia. At greater serum concentrations, focal and generalized seizure activity can occur and have been reported at serum concentrations only 50% greater than the upper limit of the accepted therapeutic range. Methylxanthines stimulate the medullary respiratory centers by increasing the sensitivity of these centers to CO_2. Theophylline-induced emesis is common when serum concentrations exceed 15 μg/mL and this effect is likely centrally mediated. At therapeutic concentrations, theophylline produces a modest increase in heart rate.[67,68] At greater concentrations, tachycardia is experienced and some individuals may experience arrhythmias such as premature ventricular contractions. Therapeutic levels of theophylline reduce the left ventricular time index and isovolumetric contraction time, indicative of increased contractility and decreased preload.[67] Although some of these cardiac effects are likely caused by direct effects on the heart, they are likely augmented by theophylline-induced release of catecholamines from the adrenal glands.[68] Methylxanthines decrease peripheral vascular resistance[67,69] but increase cerebrovascular resistance with accompanying decreases in cerebral blood flow and brain oxygen tension.[70–73] This vasoconstriction is thought to account for the relief of hypertensive headaches by methylxanthines and the relief of postdural puncture headaches caused by intracranial arterial and venous dilatation.[74] In addition to the therapeutically exploited benefits of theophylline as a smooth muscle relaxant in the airways, it also relaxes smooth muscle of the ureter, bladder,[75] and at greater concentrations the rat uterus and guinea pig taenia coli.[76] Theophylline increases the production of urine by inhibiting solute reabsorption without changing total renal blood flow or glomerular filtration rate.[77]

Practical Aspects of Drug Administration

Theophylline preparations are indicated for the treatment of bronchospasm, but in developed countries, its use has been largely supplanted by inhaled β agonists and inhaled steroids. Its newly recognized effect as an anti-inflammatory agent have led some to suggest that it may reappear in the management of asthma. However, its narrow therapeutic index and serious systemic side effects may limit a renewed interest in this medication. Moreover, newer anti-inflammatory agents directed against selective components of inflammation may dampen the enthusiasm for reintroducing theophylline as an anti-inflammatory agent. Methylxanthines have also been used in various respiratory failure syndromes because of their effect on the medullary respiratory centers of the CNS, their improvement in respiratory muscle mechanics, and their improvement in blood flow to muscles of respiration.[78–81]

Anticholinergics

Introduction and Mechanism of Drug Action

Anticholinergic agents promote airway relaxation by inhibiting M2 and M3 muscarinic receptors on airway smooth muscle.[82,83] Normally, the release of acetylcholine from parasympathetic nerves activates muscle M3 muscarinic receptors, which couple through the G_q protein to activate phospholipase C, which in turn liberates inositol triphosphates increasing intracellular calcium and initiating muscle contraction. Acetylcholine also activates muscle M2 muscarinic receptors, which act through G_i proteins to inhibit G_s-mediated relaxation and also activate the small G protein RhoA that ultimately inactivates a myosin phosphatase, and maintains smooth muscle contraction. Interestingly, M2 muscarinic receptors also exist on the postganglionic prejunctional parasympathetic nerve itself where they function as an auto-feedback receptor inhibiting further acetylcholine release. The release of acetylcholine from parasympathetic nerves increases during exacerbations of asthma[84] and during the introduction of foreign substances into the well-innervated upper trachea (e.g., during endotracheal intubation).[85] The systemic administration of anticholinergics is limited by systemic side effects, and therefore ipratropium bromide and oxitropium bromide are commonly administered through inhalation using a metered dose inhaler.

Preclinical Pharmacology

At least one animal study has shown that lower doses of ipratropium may actually promote bronchoconstriction (presumably because of blockade of prejunctional M2 muscarinic autoreceptors on the parasympathetic nerve that normally function in an auto-feedback fashion to inhibit further acetylcholine release), whereas greater doses of ipratropium promote bronchodilation (presumably because of blockade of M3 muscarinic receptors on airway smooth muscle).[86]

Clinical Pharmacology

Most studies have suggested that inhaled anticholinergic agents supplement rather than replace other bronchodilators (such as β agonists). During acute exacerbations of asthma, the combination of nebulized ipratropium with β agonists has been shown in some studies to more quickly and completely relieve bronchoconstriction[87–98] than either agent alone, whereas other studies have failed to show a benefit.[99–104] A meta-analysis of 10 studies showed a small benefit of ipratropium when added to β agonists, but severe asthmatics benefited the most and the rate of hospital admissions from the emergency department was decreased.[105] Inhaled anticholinergics have a slower onset and slower time-to-peak effect than inhaled β agonists and are therefore not usually used alone to treat acute asthmatic exacerbations. It is not known if bronchoconstriction primarily induced by tracheal irritation and parasympathetic nerve acetylcholine release (as occurs with intubation) can be more effectively treated with anticholinergics than β agonists.

Practical Aspects of Drug Administration

Oral anticholinergics have only marginal antiasthma activity and intolerable side effects such as urinary retention and visual accommodation impairments. Therefore, only the inhaled formulations of anticholinergics (ipratropium and oxitropium) are practical antiasthma therapy. Inhaled anticholinergics have a slower time of onset and a slower time-to-peak effect than β agonists, such that β agonists are considered to be superior choices for acute rescue therapy. Anticholinergics may be used as rescue therapy in patients that experience side effects from traditional β agonist therapies or in patients who completely do not respond to β agonists. It might be expected that bronchospasm induced by the introduction of an endotracheal tube into the trachea, inducing an irritant reflex arc, may be more responsive to anticholinergic therapy, because this reflex is thought to be mediated by acetylcholine from parasympathetic nerves acting on muscarinic receptors of airway smooth muscle. Indeed, nine patients with asthma who developed bronchospasm after intubation improved with endotracheal ipratropium therapy[106] and prophylactic ipratropium before intubation was shown to reduce lung resistance following intubation in smokers.[107] However, in a separate study, patients with asthma treated after intubation with β agonists had more improvement in lung resistance than patients with asthma treated with ipratropium.[108] Viral infections have been shown to cause dysfunction of the M2 muscarinic autoreceptor of parasympathetic nerves resulting in increased release of acetylcholine.[109,110] Thus patients with recent upper respiratory tract infections may have a greater benefit from anticholinergics than β agonist therapy.

Volatile Anesthetics as Bronchodilators

Volatile anesthetics are such potent bronchodilators that they have been used when traditional therapies have failed to relieve status asthmaticus.[111,112] Animal studies have shown dose-dependent decreases in airway resistance with halothane and isoflurane.[113–115] The bronchodilatory effect of halothane has been shown to be additive to that of β agonists.[116] High resolution computer tomography of small canine airways (<3 mm) during inhalational anesthesia revealed halothane dilated histamine-constricted airways to a greater extent at 0.6 and 1.1 minimum alveolar concentrations (MACs) than isoflurane. At 1.7 MAC, the two agents dilated histamine-constricted airways to a similar extent.[113] One MAC of sevoflurane was shown to be as effective as 1 MAC of isoflurane in attenuating bronchoconstriction caused by induced anaphylaxis in dogs.[117] In individuals without asthma, 1.1 MACs of halothane, isoflurane, and sevoflurane decreased respiratory system resistance after tracheal intubation, with sevoflurane exhibiting the greatest effect.[118] In another study of individuals without asthma, 1 MAC of sevoflurane but not desflurane was shown to decrease respiratory system resistance after intubation. In contrast, in a subset of patients who smoked, respiratory system resistance actually *increased* in the presence of desflurane.[119]

The mechanism by which volatile anesthetics facilitate bronchodilation is incompletely understood. Relaxation is facilitated by both neural and direct muscle effects. Sevoflurane, desflurane, and halothane have been shown to attenuate guinea pig tracheal contractions in response to both electrical field stimulation and direct addition of acetylcholine in organ bath experiments, suggesting an effect on neural release of acetylcholine from parasympathetic nerves and a direct effect on muscarinic receptor modulation of contraction in the airway smooth muscle itself.[120] Halothane decreases calcium sensitivity of the contractile apparatus in airway smooth muscle,[121–125] at least in part, by increasing smooth muscle protein phosphatase activity and thus decreasing regulatory myosin light chain phosphorylation.[126] Halothane appears to have a greater effect on calcium sensitivity than either sevoflurane or isoflurane.[127] An additional mechanism by which volatile anesthetics directly facilitate airway smooth muscle relaxation is by impeding the entry of extracellular calcium through voltage-dependent calcium channels. Halothane, isoflurane, and sevoflurane dose-dependently inhibit the entry of extracellular calcium in airway smooth muscle through voltage-dependent calcium channels.[128] T-type, voltage-dependent calcium channels in bronchi have been shown to be more sensitive to isoflurane and sevoflurane than L-type channels in trachea.[129]

Corticosteroids

Inhaled corticosteroids are widely recommended as first-line therapy for persistent asthma. The benefits of steroids in asthma have been recognized for more than 40 years. It is widely accepted that asthma is an inflammatory disease of the lung, and it is now apparent that the inclusion of inhaled steroids in an asthma management regimen reduces both hospitalization rates and mortality rates from asthma.[130–132] The realization of the combined benefit of inhaled corticosteroids and inhaled β agonists has led to the development of inhalers that deliver both drugs simultaneously (e.g., budesonide/formoterol,[133] fluticasone/salmeterol).[134]

Mechanisms of Drug Action

Glucocorticoid molecules are thought to enter the cell by passive diffusion,[135,136] although some evidence suggests that an active membrane transport step may be involved.[137] Binding of intracellular glucocorticoid molecules to their target receptor first requires phosphorylation of the soluble receptor.[138–141] After phosphorylation the receptor binds to two heat shock protein-90 (HSP-90) molecules followed by the binding of one HSP56 molecule. This complex is then capable of binding to the glucocorticoid molecule with high affinity[142] (Fig. 40–2). A second form of the receptor, termed *glucocorticoid receptor β*, does not appear to bind hormone and may represent a mechanism of hormone resistance.[143] Before transport to the nucleus of the cell, the hormone/receptor complex must undergo a transformation that is thought to be a conformational change resulting from a change in the charge of the receptor. The precise mechanism of this transformation is incompletely understood but may involve dephosphorylation after which the hormone/receptor complex disassociates from its "chaperone" HSPs.[144] The transformed hormone/receptor complex is then translocated to the nucleus where the hormone/receptor complex binds to glucocorticoid response elements (GREs)—specific DNA consensus sequences located within the promoter regions of target genes[145] (see Fig. 40–2). GREs exist within a myriad of genes and binding of the hormone/receptor can result in expression or repression of transcription of a specific gene.[146] The transcription of mRNA encoding multiple cytokines known to be important in inflammation are inhibited by the interaction of hormone/receptor with GREs. These include interleukin-1 (IL-1), tumor necrosis factor-α, granulocyte-macrophage colony stimulating factor (GM-CSF), IL-3, IL-4, IL-5, IL-6, and IL-8.[147–149] Glucocorticoids can also inhibit several signaling pathways important in the activation of a diverse group of inflammatory mediators including leukotrienes, prostaglandins, platelet activating factor, inducible nitric oxide, and adhesion molecules.[149–153] Glucocorticoids can also interact directly with transcription factors such as activating protein 1, thereby inhibiting the expression of genes that rely on this transcription factor.[148,154] Nuclear factor kappa B is another transcription factor whose activity may be inhibited by its direct interaction with glucocorticoids.[155,156]

The availability of inhaled steroids was considered a major advance in the pharmacologic management of asthma because chronic use of systemic steroids contributes to a myriad of systemic complications. These complications are not toxicity but exaggerations of their hormonal actions and may lead to the clinical appearance of iatrogenic Cushing syndrome. Systemic corticosteroids used for short periods (less than a week), even at high doses, are unlikely to cause

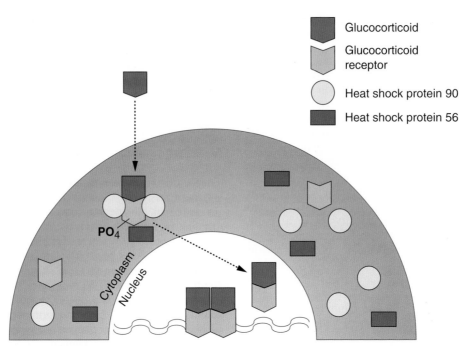

Figure 40–2. Mechanism of glucocorticoid action. After entry of the glucocorticoid molecule into the cell, its receptor must be phosphorylated and bind two large[90] and one small[56] molecules of heat shock proteins (HSP). This complex binds the corticosteroid molecule with high affinity and functions as a cytoplasmic chaperone. Disassembly of this glucocorticoid/receptor/HSP complex is required before nuclear entry where the glucocorticoid/receptor complex binds to specific DNA sequences to act as activators or repressors of transcription of specific genes.

serious side effects. When systemic steroids are chronically administered for periods of months to years, patients should receive supplemental therapy at times of severe stress such as surgery. Metabolic effects from chronic systemic steroid therapy include redistribution of fat from extremities to face and trunk, increased fine hair growth, acne, insomnia, increased appetite, protein breakdown, and increased gluconeogenesis leading to diabetes and osteoporosis. Other complications include peptic ulcers, infections, psychosis, cataracts, glaucoma, growth retardation in children with doses of 45 mg/m^2 per day or more, and hypokalemic/hypochloremic alkalosis.

Preclinical Pharmacology

Lymphocytes, eosinophils, neutrophils, macrophages, monocytes, mast cells, and basophils all have potential roles in the inflammatory response in the lung in asthma, and the contributions to inflammation of all of these cells are effected by steroids. Much attention has been focused on the role of cytokines liberated from specific subsets of T helper lymphocytes. Initially, studies in mice[157,158] and subsequently in humans revealed that at least a component of airway inflammation in asthma is orchestrated by CD$^+$ Th2 cells that secrete the cytokines IL-4, IL-5, and IL-13, whereas interferon γ secreted by Th1 cells suppresses the development and effector functions of Th2 cells. An attractive approach to modulating airway inflammation has been to selectively modulate the activity of Th1/Th2 lymphocytes.[159] The amount of eosinophils in peripheral blood and in bronchoalveolar lavage specimens has been correlated with the severity of asthma,[160–162] and corticosteroids reduce their numbers.[163] Glucocorticoids also inhibit IL-4- and IL-5-mediated survival[164] and enhance eosinophil apoptosis.[165] The role of neutrophils in asthma is less clear but infiltration of skin, airways, and mucosa has been demonstrated after antigen challenge. Oral corticosteroids inhibit the influx of cutaneous neutrophils during late-phase responses,[166] and neutrophil influx after nasal challenge was inhibited by topical corticosteroids.[167] Macrophages are found in increased numbers and altered phenotypes in bronchoalveolar specimens from patients with asthma[168] and glucocorticoids decrease the numbers of macrophages in skin and inhibit their release of numerous cytokines.[169] Mast cells are known to be increased in number[170] and to show enhanced release of inflammatory mediators in asthmatic airways.[171] Asthmatic airways are also more sensitive to the bronchospastic mediators released by mast cells.[172] Although a significant reduction was seen in mast cells in the epithelium and mucosa of patients with asthma after inhaled glucocorticoids, no effect of glucocorticoids was seen on mast cell release of inflammatory mediators. Mast cell apoptosis was increased after the withdrawal of IL-3 mediated by glucocorticoids.[173]

Numerous in vivo animal studies have evaluated the benefit of corticosteroids on airway responses. Chronic systemic steroids (4–7 weeks) have been shown to decrease methacholine-induced bronchoconstriction and to decrease propranolol-induced airway hyperresponsiveness in the Basenji-greyhound dog model of airway hyperresponsiveness.[174,175] These dogs also showed increased sensitivity to β adrenoceptor bronchodilation after 48 hours of systemic corticosteroid therapy.[176,177] At least part of this in vivo benefit of steroids on methacholine-induced bronchoconstriction may be accounted for by a reduced number of M2 and M3 muscarinic receptors in airway smooth muscle following 3 days of systemic corticosteroid but not mineralocorticoid therapy.[178] An additional mechanism that may contribute to improved β adrenoceptor responses after glucocorticoid therapy is an increased expression of β adrenoceptors[179–183] and coupling of these receptors to G$_s$ protein.[184] The inhaled corticosteroid budesonide was shown to reduce both ozone-[185] and allergen-induced[186] increases in airway hyper-responsiveness in dogs. In a model of antigen-challenged guinea pigs, whose airway dysfunction is mediated by eosinophil recruitment and neural M2 muscarinic receptor dysfunction, systemic dexamethasone reduced eosinophil recruitment and eliminated the neural M2 muscarinic receptor dysfunction.[187] Inhaled fluticasone decreased airway remodeling induced by ovalalbumin sensitization in rats.[188]

Clinical Pharmacology

Oral glucocorticoids are rapidly absorbed and approximately 90% bound to plasma proteins. In general, absorption is not affected by age, disease, or smoking but the concurrent use of oral antacids may reduce the bioavailability of prednisolone to as little as 57% to 74% of the level available in the absence of antacids.[189] Metabolism is principally in the liver where compounds are reduced and conjugated to form water-soluble compounds that are excreted in the urine. Prednisone is unique among the synthetic glucocorticoids in that it is a prodrug that must undergo an interconversion reaction to convert it to its active form prednisolone. A wide variety of synthetic steroids have been synthesized that vary in their relative glucocorticoid versus mineralocorticoid properties (Table 40–1). Serum half-lives of commonly used synthetic corticosteroids range from 90 to 240 minutes.[190] The rate of elimination is not affected by asthma but can be affected by liver disease. Concurrent medications that rely on liver metabolism can also alter the clearance of glucocorticoids. Phenytoin, phenobarbital, carbamazepine,[191,192] and rifampin can increase the elimination rate for dexamethasone, prednisolone, and methylprednisolone. Ketoconazole,[193,194] erythromycin, troleandomycin,[195] and oral contraceptives[196] can reduce clearance of glucocorticoids resulting in increased serum concentrations.

Numerous studies have evaluated the effectiveness of inhaled steroids and the reduced risk for systemic complications with inhaled versus systemic steroid administration. Efficacy of inhaled corticosteroids has been shown in many studies[197–200] and is usually comparable to benefits demonstrated with systemic steroids but with fewer long-term side effects. Studies have shown patients discharged from the

TABLE 40–1.

Relative Anti-inflammatory and Salt-Retaining Properties of Corticosteroids

Drug	Anti-Inflammatory	Salt-Retaining	Equivalent Oral Dose (mg)	Forms Available
Short-acting glucocorticoids				
Hydrocortisone	1	1	20	O, I, T
Cortisone	0.8	0.8	25	O, I, T
Prednisone	4	0.8	5	O
Prednisolone	4	0.8	5	O, I, T
Methylprednisolone	5	0.5	4	O, T
Intermediate-acting glucocorticoids				
Triamcinolone	5	0	4	O, I, T
Paramethasone	10	0	2	O
Long-acting glucocorticoids				
Betamethasone	25	0	0.75	O, I, T
Dexamethasone	25	0	0.75	O, I, T
Mineralocorticoids				
Fludrocortisone	10	250	2	O, I, T
Desoxycorticosterone	0	100	0	O, I
Aldosterone	?	3000		

I, injectable; O, oral; T, topical.

emergency room prescribed either 40 mg oral prednisone once a day or 600 µg budesonide through inhalation four times a day had similar relapse rates of asthma, similar improvements in FEV_1, asthma symptoms, and peak expiratory flow.[197] Inhaled steroids have also been shown to reduce or eliminate the need for systemic steroids in patients with severe asthma.[201]

It is generally accepted that inhaled corticosteroids use has reduced the systemic complications of chronic systemic steroids making routine steroids commonplace in the management of many adults with asthma. However, it should not be assumed that inhaled steroids are without possible detrimental systemic effects when chronically used. Although some studies report no or minimal effects on the hypothalamic-pituitary-adrenal axis, bone density, cataracts, or glaucoma,[202,203] other studies including a meta-analysis conclude that dose-related adrenal suppression, reduction in bone density, and posterior subcapsular cataracts occur with chronic use of all inhaled steroids.[204] The chronic effects of inhaled steroids in children with asthma is of particular concern because of possible effects on skeletal development. Children treated for 20 months with beclomethasone but not fluticasone showed reduced skeletal growth rates during the final months of the study.[205] Serum cortisol significantly decreased with beclomethasone but not with fluticasone.[206] A comparison of fluticasone and budesonide in adults with asthma in whom doses effective for improvement of asthma symptoms were accounted for along with changes in serum cortisol and calcitonin concluded that fluticasone had a more favorable therapeutic ratio.[190]

Practical Aspects of Drug Administration

Fluticasone and budesonide are more potent than beclomethasone, triamcinolone, and flunisolide. All five of these corticosteroids are available for inhalation. Drug delivery systems include both metered dose inhalers and dry powder inhalers. Inhaled glucocorticoids are typically used between 2 and 4 times per day, and like systemic steroids, the total dose of inhaled glucocorticoids that should be used is the minimum dose that maintains adequate control of asthmatic symptoms. Improvement in asthma symptoms can occur as quickly as 1 day after initiation of inhaled steroids, but maximum benefit may not be realized for 1 to 3 weeks. Inhaled steroids may be the sole drug therapy in asthma maintenance or more commonly they are combined with inhaled β agonists; several formulations are available that combine glucocorticoids and β agonist in the same inhalation delivery device.

Oral glucocorticoids are used to treat a wide variety of nonendocrine diseases that require anti-inflammatory and anti-immunologic therapy. In patients with asthma, the chronic use of systemic glucocorticoids is reserved for those patients who do not respond to combined therapy with inhaled steroids, inhaled β agonists, perhaps inhaled anticholinergics, oral methylxanthines and oral leukotriene antagonists, or 5-lipoxygenase inhibitors. Systemic steroids are a drug of last resort because of their devastating systemic effects with long-term use. Nonetheless, short courses (1–2 weeks) of oral steroids are extremely effective in treating acute asthma exacerbations.

The need for preoperative systemic corticosteroids in all patients with asthma before surgery is an important and unresolved clinical issue, especially for patients who are likely to have their airway instrumented with an endotracheal tube. Several studies have stressed the lack of serious side effects associated with prophylaxing all patients with asthma with systemic steroids before surgery. In one study of 68 patients with asthma, 100 mg hydrocortisone was administered intravenously beginning the night before surgery, and rates of wound infection and delayed wound healing were not different compared with historical control patient populations.[207] This study did not attempt to evaluate the rate of respiratory complications (i.e., bronchospasm) between patients with asthma receiving or not receiving steroid prophylaxis.[207] A second study evaluated the incidence of bronchospasm, infection, and adrenocortical insufficiency in patients with asthma treated before surgery with steroids and found no difference in infection rates between patients prophylactically treated with steroids and control patients not treated with steroids.[208] Again, this study did not compare patients with asthma with and without preoperative steroids to determine if steroids affected respiratory complications in the perioperative period. It is also unknown if patients already on inhaled steroids would benefit from systemic steroids in the perioperative period. Despite the absence of a randomized clinical trial to prove their effectiveness, these studies recommended that mild and moderate asthmatics receive 1 mg/kg prednisone orally (up to 60 mg) for 3 to 7 days before surgery and that patients with severe asthma (defined as those needing systemic steroids for asthma control) receive increased doses of systemic steroids.[207,208] The International Consensus Report on Diagnosis and Treatment of Asthma generated by the National Heart, Lung, and Blood Institute of the National Institutes of Health published guidelines in both U.S. and European literature. These guidelines are somewhat vague and reflect that no clinical trials have proven the benefit of preoperative steroids on respiratory complications. The guidelines recommend that: (1) all patients with asthma be seen before the day of surgery and that a measure of pulmonary function be performed; (2) if possible attempts should be made to improve lung function to their predicted values or their personal best level, a short course of systemic steroids may be necessary to optimize function; and (c) patients who have received systemic steroids within the past 6 months should receive 100 mg hydrocortisone intravenously every 8 hours during the surgical periods with a rapidly reduced dose within 24 hours of surgery.[209,210]

Anti-Inflammatory Agents

Nedocromil Sodium and Sodium Cromoglycate

One of the earliest clinical trials evaluating the effectiveness of sodium cromoglycate was carried out in ten severe, steroid-dependent asthmatics.[211] A larger study in 100 patients with a wider range of asthma severity and chronicity showed that cromolyn was of no benefit in patients without allergy, but that 89% of patients with allergic asthma had clinical improvement. In this study, younger patients tended to benefit more and 88% of all patients taking steroids improved with cromoglycate administration; approximately one third of these patients were able to reduce their average steroid dose by 40%.[212] In the more than 30 years since these original trials, the clinical profile and use of cromolyn has changed very little; cromolyn is most useful in younger patients who have an allergic basis for their asthma.

Sodium cromoglycate was synthesized in 1965 in an attempt to improve on the bronchodilating properties of khellin, a naturally occurring chromone derived from the plant *Ammi visnaga*, which has been known for centuries to function as a spasmolytic agent. Efforts to improve the therapeutic profile of sodium cromoglycate resulted in the synthesis of nedocromil sodium, which was released in the United States in 1992.[213]

Mechanism of Drug Action

Electrophysiologic studies have shown that antigen activation of mast cells results in intracellular influx of chloride through chloride channels, which in turn maintains activation of calcium channels, allowing intracellular entry of calcium leading to degranulation.[214] Sodium cromolyn[215,216] and nedocromil[214] have been shown to inhibit chloride channel activity in cultured mucosal-like mast cells and mouse 3T3 fibroblasts. It is unlikely that this fully explains the mechanism of action of these drugs because both can inhibit mediator release in the absence of extracellular calcium. Another signaling pathway that may be important in controlling mediator release involves a 78-kDa protein (resembling moesin), which is phosphorylated by protein kinase C (PKC) in rat peritoneal mast cells after nedocromil or sodium cromoglycate exposure. It is proposed that this phosphorylated protein, which contains actin binding domains,[217] attaches to the cytoskeleton preventing degranulation.[218] In addition to mast cells, sodium cromoglycate and nedocromil are known to inhibit mediator release from airway epithelial cells[219,220] and basophils and to inhibit eosinophil chemotaxis and adherence to endothelial cells.[221]

Preclinical Pharmacology

Mast cells are located in the respiratory epithelium of the nasal and airway mucosa. Increased mast cells are present in the nasal mucosa of patients with seasonal and perennial rhinitis.[222] Sodium cromoglycate and nedocromil inhibit histamine release from human bronchoalveolar mast cells.

Clinical Pharmacology

Both sodium cromoglycate and nedocromil sodium are administered by inhalation. Cromolyn inhibits both the immediate and late phase bronchoconstrictive response to inhaled antigen. It attenuates bronchospasm induced by exercise, aspirin, cold air, toluene diisocyanate, sulfur dioxide, and environmental pollutants. Approximately 8% of inhaled cromolyn is absorbed and is rapidly excreted unchanged in both urine and bile. The remainder is exhaled or deposited in the oropharynx, swallowed, and excreted in the alimentary tract. Systemic bioavailability of nedocromil sodium is low. Peak mean serum concentrations of 1.6 ng/mL occur 28 minutes after a 3.5-mg inhaled dose and have a half-life of 3.3 hours. Nedocromil is 89% protein bound and is not metabolized.

Adverse events with sodium cromoglycate or nedocromil sodium are uncommon and are usually mild. Nausea, vomiting, dyspepsia, and unpleasant taste occur more commonly with nedocromil than with placebo. Throat irritation or dryness, bad taste, cough, wheezing, and nausea are more common with sodium cromoglycate than placebo. Uncommonly and paradoxically severe asthma has been reported with sodium cromoglycate (presumably an airway irritant effect). Rarely laryngeal edema, nasal congestion, or pharyngeal irritation has been reported as an adverse effect of sodium cromoglycate.

Practical Aspects of Drug Administration

Cromolyn and nedocromil have found their greatest clinical use in the management of childhood asthma and exercise-induced asthma. Studies have shown an improvement in asthma symptom score and decreased use of albuterol in patients older than 12 years using cromolyn.[223] In children, cromolyn has been proposed as a first-line therapy to be used even before inhaled steroids[224,225] (because of concerns regarding effects of chronic inhaled steroids on skeletal development). Cromolyn is also known to reduce symptoms of exercise-induced bronchoconstriction in both children[226] and adults.[227] Despite these beneficial findings, the efficacy of cromolyn in childhood asthma has been questioned by some investigators.[228]

Sodium cromoglycate and nedocromil are indicated in the prophylactic management of asthma, and sodium cromoglycate nasal spray is indicated in the treatment of allergic rhinitis. Both medications are administered four times a day at regular intervals through inhalation, whereas sodium cromoglycate nasal spray is used once per day. Three clinical studies have compared sodium cromoglycate with nedocromil sodium in the management of asthma. One hundred thirty-two adults with moderately severe asthma had their inhaled glucocorticoid dose reduced by half and were then treated with either 16 mg/day nedocromil sodium, 8 mg/day sodium cromoglycate, or placebo. Both drugs were superior to placebo and nedocromil produced greater improvements than cromoglycate in asthma symptoms.[222] A comparison of 16 mg/day nedocromil sodium and 40 mg/day sodium cromoglycate in 77 patients already taking steroids and bronchodilators showed no difference between the two treatments.[229] Nedocromil sodium (16 mg/day), cromolyn sodium (8 mg/day), or placebo were compared in 306 patients during an 8-week period. Patients were selected who had a deterioration in their asthma symptoms after being switched from slow release theophylline to short-acting bronchodilators. Both drugs were better than placebo and cromolyn was more efficacious in night-time symptom control and in improving FEV_1 and forced expiratory flow rate between 25% and 75% of forced vital capacity (FVC) than nedocromil.[230]

Leukotriene Antagonists and 5-Lipoxygenase Inhibitors

The newest class of agents in the asthma armamentarium is inhibitors of the leukotriene pathway. Leukotrienes belong to a family of compounds known as eicosanoids, a large group of products synthesized from arachidonic acid (Fig. 40–3). Other family members include prostaglandins, thromboxanes, lipoxins, and isoprostanes. Leukotrienes are synthesized from arachidonic acid, which is released from membrane phospholipids by phospholipase A_2[231] when inflammatory cells are activated. The first leukotriene identified was leukotriene B_4 (LTB_4)[232] followed by the discovery that the LTC_4 was the slow reacting substance of anaphylaxis (SRS-A),[233] long presumed to be a mediator of asthma and inflammation. It was subsequently determined that SRS-A was also composed of LTD_4 and LTE_4, products of LTC_4.[234–236]

Mechanism of Drug Action

Two classes of leukotriene pathway inhibitors have been introduced for the clinical management of asthma. A 5-lipoxygenase inhibitor (zileuton) inhibits the conversion of arachidonic acid to leukotriene A_4, thus inhibiting the generation of LTB_4, LTC_4, LTD_4, and LTE_4. The second class of drugs is cysteinyl-leukotriene 1 ($CysLT_1$) antagonists, which competitively block the ability of LTD_4 to bind to the $CysLT_1$ receptor. Bronchospasm, plasma exudation, vasoconstriction, and eosinophil recruitment are at least in part mediated by LTD_4 binding to the $CysLT_1$ receptor, thus either blockade of the synthesis of LTD_4 (zileuton) or blockade of the $CysLT_1$ target receptor (zafirlukast, montelukast, pranlukast) are therapeutic targets.

The CysLT1 receptor is a glycosylated GPCR that initially had been identified as an orphan GPCR that could be activated by LTC_4 and LTD_4.[237] Molecular cloning and characterization of this receptor identified it as a 337-amino acid protein of approximately 38.5 kDa with seven putative transmembrane-spanning domains, potential N-glycosylation sites, and potential phosphorylation sites by PKA and PKC. When this receptor was expressed in oocytes, it exhibited dose-dependent increases in calcium-activated chloride conductance in response to LTD_4.[238] More recently, this receptor has been shown to respond to the pyrimidinergic agonist uridine diphosphate in addition to its classical activation by LTD_4.[239] Activation of $CysLT_1$ receptors by pyrimidines is consistent with its protein homology to the purinergic family of receptors.[239]

Preclinical Pharmacology

Research interests in leukotrienes and asthma extends from the original observations that slow reacting substance of anaphylaxis (now known to be a mixture of LTC_4, LTD_4, and LTE_4) is a potent bronchoconstrictor.[240–242] Subsequently, it was confirmed that the cysteinyl leukotrienes were potent constrictors of guinea pig airways in vivo and in vitro[243,244] and that they constricted human bronchi in vitro.[245,246] Leukotrienes (LTC_4 and LTD_4) were shown to increase plasma exudation in skin[243] and in the hamster cheek pouch.[247] LTC_4, LTD_4, and LTE_4 were each shown to increase extravasation of Evans blue dye in guinea pig airways, again supporting a role for leukotriene-mediated increases in vascular permeability.[248] In humans, inhalation of LTE_4 increased the infiltration of eosinophils into the airway mucosa,[249] whereas inhalation of LTD_4 increased eosinophil content of induced sputum from patients with asthma.[250] Leukotrienes may also be involved in airway smooth muscle hypertrophy and remodeling, hallmarks of chronic asthma.[251] Direct provocation of bronchoconstriction by leukotrienes in subjects with asthma has been confirmed in many clinical studies.[252–254]

Clinical Pharmacology

Montelukast and zafirlukast are the $CysLT_1$ receptor antagonists currently available in the United States. Montelukast and zafirlukast are rapidly absorbed after oral administration with mean peak plasma concentrations achieved in 3 to 4 hours. Montelukast is 99% bound to plasma proteins with a volume of distribution of 9 to 11 L. Montelukast and zafirlukast are extensively metabolized, and in vitro studies with human liver microsomal membranes indicate that cytochromes P450 3A4 and 2C9 are primarily responsible for liver metabolism.[255] Metabolites of both drugs are excreted almost entirely in bile. Mean plasma half-life is 2.7

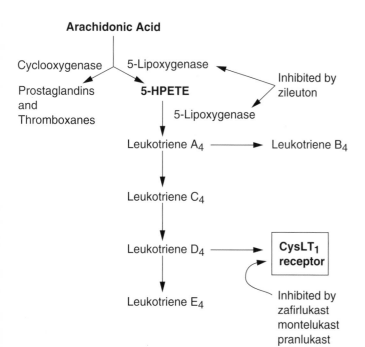

Figure 40–3. Biosynthetic pathway of leukotriene synthesis. Site of action of 5-lipoxygenase inhibitor (zileuton) and antagonists (zafirlukast, montelukast, pranlukast) of the cysteinyl/leukotriene 1 ($CysLT_1$) receptor are shown.

to 5.5 hours and pharmacokinetics remain linear for doses up to 50 mg/day. Although sex and age have not been shown to affect the pharmacokinetics of montelukast, clearance of zafirlukast decreases with age and hepatic insufficiency decreases the metabolism of both montelukast and zafirlukast; however, despite this no dosage adjustment is recommended in patients with mild-to-moderate hepatic insufficiency. Because montelukast, zafirlukast, and their metabolites are not excreted in urine, no changes in dosing are necessary in patients with renal failure.

Montelukast given at recommended amounts (10 mg/day) does not influence the metabolism of a single intravenous dose of theophylline, or a single oral dose (30 mg) of warfarin, digoxin, or terfenadine despite that all of these drugs depend on cytochrome P450 metabolism and warfarin and terfenadine are metabolized by the specific subclasses of cytochrome P450 implicated in the metabolism of montelukast (2C9 and 3A4, respectively). In contrast, the coadministration of zafirlukast and warfarin decrease the clearance of warfarin and increase prothrombin time.

Adverse effects of montelukast and zafirlukast are uncommon and typically are not severe, although severe liver injury has been reported with zafirlukast.[256] Most common side effects with montelukast in more than 2600 adults included headache (18.4% vs. 18.1% with placebo), cough/influenza symptoms (4.2% vs. 3.9% with placebo), abdominal pain/dyspepsia (2.9% vs. 2.5% with placebo), and elevation of alanine aminotransferase (2.1% vs. 2.0% with placebo). Adverse effects of zafirlukast were of similar quality and frequency.

Zileuton is the only currently available inhibitor of 5-lipoxygenase, an enzyme responsible for the conversion of arachidonic acid to 5-hydroperoxyeicosatetraenoic and subsequently to leukotriene A_4, a precursor to LTD_4. Zileuton is rapidly absorbed after oral administration with a peak serum concentration occurring at 1.7 hours. It is 93% bound to serum proteins and has a serum half-life of 2.5 hours. Zileuton is metabolized by cytochrome P450 isoenzymes 1A2, 2C9, and 3A4, and metabolites are found in both urine and bile. Sex, age, and renal failure do not require changes in dosing, but zileuton is contraindicated in patients with hepatic insufficiency. The most common adverse effect of zileuton is dyspepsia, but arthralgias, chest pain, conjunctivitis, constipation, dizziness, fever, hypertonia, insomnia, lymphadenopathy, malaise, neck rigidity, nervousness, pruritus, somnolence, urinary tract infections, vaginitis, and vomiting have all been reported at an incidence of greater than 1% and at a greater frequency than placebo.

Practical Aspects of Drug Administration

Corticosteroids do not suppress all inflammatory mediators involved in the asthmatic response. Patients with asthma demonstrate increased production of cysteinyl leukotrienes that enhance airway recruitment of eosinophils, produce bronchospasm, enhance airway hyper-responsiveness to other agents, and increase mucosal edema, mucus production, and airway smooth muscle cell proliferation.[257,258] The ability of steroids to modify the synthesis and release of leukotrienes is variable depending on the cell type studied.[258–261] Clinical studies have shown some benefit of

the 5-lipoxygenase inhibitors and leukotriene receptor antagonists in the management of asthma, and patients with exercise-induced asthma[262] and aspirin-sensitive asthma may benefit the most.[258]

Pranlukast plus bronchodilators reduced eosinophils in induced sputum and increased peak expiratory flow rates in patients with mild asthma compared with patients treated with either bronchodilators alone or bronchodilators plus inhaled steroids.[263] In a second clinical study, pranlukast improved asthma symptoms, increased peak expiratory flow rates, and reduced β agonist use but did not significantly change FEV_1 or FVC.[264] Montelukast was compared with inhaled fluticasone for asthma management in patients already taking β agonists. Patients receiving the inhaled steroid had greater improvements in FEV_1, FVC, and forced mid-expiratory flow.[265] In contrast, a second study comparing montelukast to inhaled beclomethasone showed similar improvements with either medication in several parameters of asthma control.[266] At least three studies have evaluated the addition of a leukotriene antagonist to a regimen that included high-dose inhaled steroids to question whether further improvement in asthma control could be achieved. Zafirlukast significantly improved peak expiratory flow rate, FEV_1, and β agonist use in two studies.[267,268] In contrast, montelukast did not improve peak expiratory flow or β agonist use in 100 patients with asthma over 14 days when added to various chronic medication regimens including β agonists and steroids.[269] The available data suggest that only subsets of individuals with asthma are likely to benefit from the leukotriene receptor antagonists, most notably those with aspirin-sensitive asthma and exercise-induced asthma.

Zileuton, a 5-lipoxygenase inhibitor, provided prophylaxis against exercise-induced asthma for 4 hours after administration, whereas the leukotriene receptor antagonists montelukast and zafirlukast provided protection for 12 hours.[262] The benefit of zileuton in aspirin-sensitive asthma has been evaluated in several studies. Whereas a small study of six patients taking zileuton for 1 week did not show protection from bronchospasm and naso-ocular reaction after oral aspirin ingestion,[270] a larger study of 40 patients over 6 weeks of zileuton use showed an improvement in FEV_1, peak expiratory flows, and reduced bronchodilator use.[271] A single dose of zileuton has been shown to attenuate bronchoconstrictive responses to acute challenges with histamine[272] and platelet-activating-factor.[273] Another study suggests that only subsets of patients known to have increased leukotrienes in bronchoalveolar lavage fluid after segmental ragweed challenge benefit from zileuton therapy as reflected in reduced eosinophils in bronchoalveolar lavage fluid.[274]

References

1. Ahlquist RP: A study of the adrenotropic receptors. Am J Physiol 153:586–600, 1948.
2. Gay LN, Long JW: Clinical evaluation of isopropylepinephrine in management of bronchial asthma. JAMA 139:452–457, 1949.
3. Engelhardt A, Hoefke W, Wick H: Zur pharmakologie des sympathomimeticums 1-(3,5-dihydroxylphenyl)-1-hydroxy-2-isopropyl aminoathan. Arzneimittel-Forschung 11:521–525, 1961.

4. Lands AM, Arnold A, McAuliff JP, et al: Differentiation of receptor systems activated by sympathomimetic amines. Nature 214:597–598, 1967.

5. Lands AM, Luduena FP, Buzzo HJ: Differentiation of receptors responsive to isoproterenol. Life Sci 6:2241–2249, 1967.

6. Ullman A, Svedmyr N: Salmeterol, a new long acting inhaled beta 2 adrenoceptor agonist: Comparison with salbutamol in adult asthmatic patients. Thorax 43:674–678, 1988.

7. Hekking PR, Maesen F, Greefhorst A, et al: Long-term efficacy of formoterol compared to salbutamol. Lung 168(suppl):76–82, 1990.

8. Johnson M, Coleman RA: Mechanisms of action of β_2-adrenoceptor agonists. In Busse WW, Holgate ST (eds): Asthma and Rhinitis. Malden, Mass, Blackwell Scientific Publications, pp 1278–1295, 1995.

9. Kume H, Hall IP, Washabau RJ, et al: Beta-adrenergic agonists regulate K_{Ca} channels in airway smooth muscle by cAMP-dependent and -independent mechanisms. J Clin Invest 93:371–379, 1994.

10. Kume H, Graziano MP, Kotlikoff MI: Stimulatory and inhibitory regulation of calcium-activated potassium channels by guanine nucleotide-binding proteins. Proc Natl Acad Sci USA 89:11051–11055, 1992.

11. Kim SJ, Yatani A, Vatner DE, et al: Differential regulation of inotropy and lusitropy in overexpressed Gsalpha myocytes through cAMP and Ca2+ channel pathways. J Clin Invest 103:1089–1097, 1999.

12. McGraw DW, Liggett SB: Heterogeneity in beta-adrenergic receptor kinase expression in the lung accounts for cell-specific desensitization of the beta2-adrenergic receptor. J Biol Chem 272:7338–7344, 1997.

13. Daaka Y, Luttrell LM, Lefkowitz RJ: Switching of the coupling of the beta2-adrenergic receptor to different G proteins by protein kinase A. Nature 390:88–91, 1997.

14. Reishaus E, Innis M, MacIntyre N, Liggett SB: Mutations in the gene encoding for the β_2-adrenergic receptor in normal and asthmatic subjects. Am J Respir Cell Biol 8:334–339, 1993.

15. Green SA, Turki J, Innis M, Liggett SB: Amino-terminal polymorphisms of the human β_2-adrenergic receptor impart distinct agonist-promoted regulatory properties. Biochemistry 33:9414–9419, 1994.

16. Green SA, Cole G, Jacinto M, et al: A polymorphism of the human β_2-adrenergic receptor within the fourth transmembrane domain alters ligand binding and functional properties of the receptor. J Biol Chem 268:23116–23121, 1993.

17. McGraw DW, Forbes SL, Kramer LA, Liggett SB: Polymorphisms of the 5′ leader cistron of the human beta2-adrenergic receptor regulate receptor expression. J Clin Invest 102:1927–1932, 1998.

18. McGraw DW, Liggett SB: Coding block and 5 leader cistron polymorphisms of the beta2-adrenergic receptor. Clin Exp Allergy 29(suppl 4):43–45, 1999.

19. Emala CW, McQuitty CK, Elleff SM, et al: Asthma, allergy and airway hyperresponsiveness are not linked to the β_2-adrenoceptor gene. Chest 121:722–731, 2002.

20. Weir TD, Mallek N, Sandiford AJ, et al: β_2-Adrenergic receptor haplotypes in mild, moderate and fatal/near fatal asthma. Am J Respir Crit Care Med 158:787–791, 1998.

21. Summerhill E, Leavitt SA, Gidley H, et al: β_2-Adrenergic receptor Arg 16/Arg 16 genotypes is associated with reduced lung function, but not with asthma in the Hutterites. Am J Respir Crit Care Med 162:599–602, 2000.

22. Ulbrecht M, Hergeth MT, Wjst M, et al: Association of beta(2)adrenoreceptor variants with bronchial hyperresponsiveness. Am J Respir Crit Care Med 161:469–474, 2000.

23. Dewar JC, Wheatley AP, Venn A, et al: Beta2-adrenoceptor polymorphisms are in linkage disequilibrium, but are not associated with asthma in an adult population. Clin Exp Allergy 28:442–448, 1998.

24. Turki J, Pak J, Green SA, et al: Genetic polymorphisms of the beta 2-adrenergic receptor in nocturnal and non-nocturnal asthma. Evidence that Gly16 correlates with the nocturnal phenotype. J Invest 95:1635–1641, 1995.

25. Holloway JW, Dunbar PR, Riley GA, et al: Association of beta2-adrenergic receptor polymorphisms with severe asthma. Clin Exp Allergy 30:1097–1103, 2000.

26. Hopes E, McDougall C, Christie G, et al: Association of glutamine 27 polymorphism of beta 2 adrenoceptor with reported childhood asthma: Population based study. BMJ 316:664, 1998.

27. Ramsay CE, Hayden CM, Tiller KJ, et al: Polymorphisms in the beta2-adrenoreceptor gene are associated with decreased airway responsiveness [see comments]. Clin Exp Allergy 29:1195–1203, 1999.

28. Martinez FD, Graves PE, Baldini M, et al: Association between genetic polymorphisms of the β_2-adrenoceptor and response to albuterol in children with and without a history of wheezing. J Clin Invest 100:3184–3188, 1997.

29. Kotani Y, Nishimura Y, Maeda H, Yokoyama M: Beta2-adrenergic receptor polymorphisms affect airway responsiveness to salbutamol in asthmatics. J Asthma 36:583–590, 1999.

30. Moore PE, Laporte JD, Abraham JH, et al: Polymorphism of the beta(2)-adrenergic receptor gene and desensitization in human airway smooth muscle. Am J Respir Crit Care Med 162:2117–2124, 2000.

31. Taylor DR, Drazen JM, Herbison GP, et al: Asthma exacerbations during long term beta agonist use: Influence of beta(2) adrenoceptor polymorphism. Thorax 55:762–767, 2000.

32. Israel E, Drazen JM, Liggett SB, et al: The effect of polymorphisms of the beta(2)adrenergic receptor on the response to regular use of albuterol in asthma. Am J Respir Crit Care Med 162:75–80, 2000.

33. Tan S, Hall IP, Dewar J, et al: Association between β_2-adrenoceptor polymorphism and susceptibility to bronchodilator desensitization in moderately severe stable asthmatics. Lancet 350:995–999, 1997.

34. Green SA, Turki J, Bejarano P, et al: Influence of beta 2-adrenergic receptor genotypes on signal transduction in human airway smooth muscle cells. Am J Respir Cell Mol Biol 13:25–33, 1995.

35. Dewar JC, Wilkinson J, Wheatley A, et al: The glutamine 27 β_2-adrenoceptor polymorphism is associated with elevated IgE levels in asthmatic families. J Allergy Clin Immunol 100:261–265, 1997.

36. Dewar J, Wheatley A, Wilkinson J, et al: Association of the Gln 27 beta 2-adrenoceptor polymorphism and IgE variability in asthmatic families. Chest 111:78S–79S, 1997.

37. Potter PC, Van Wyk L, Martin M, et al: Genetic polymorphism of the β-2 adrenergic receptor in atopic and non-atopic subjects. Clin Exp Allergy 23:874–877, 1992.

38. Chong LK, Chowdry J, Ghahramani P, Peachell PT: Influence of genetic polymorphisms in the beta2-adrenoceptor on desensitization in human lung mast cells. Pharmacogenetics 10:153–162, 2000.

39. Wagoner LE, Craft LL, Singh B, et al: Polymorphisms of the beta(2)adrenergic receptor determine exercise capacity in patients with heart failure. Circ Res 86:834–840, 2000.

40. Liggett SB, Wagoner LE, Craft LL, et al: The Ile164 beta2-adrenergic receptor polymorphism adversely affects the outcome of congestive heart failure. J Clin Invest 102:1534–1539, 1998.

41. Miller LW: Listing criteria for cardiac transplantation: Results of an American Society of Transplant Physicians-National Institutes of Health conference. Transplantation 66:947–951, 1998.

42. Emala CW, Black C, Curry C, et al: Impaired β-adrenergic receptor activation of adenylyl cyclase in airway smooth muscle in the basenji-greyhound dog model of airway hyperresponsiveness. Am J Respir Cell Mol Biol 8:668–675, 1993.

43. Bai TR: Abnormalities in airway smooth muscle in fatal asthma. Am Rev Respir Dis 141:552–557, 1990.

44. Bai TR, Mak JCW, Barnes PJ: A comparison of β-adrenergic receptors and in vitro relaxant responses to isoproterenol in asthmatic airway smooth muscle. Am J Respir Cell Mol Biol 6:647–651, 1992.

45. Goldie RG, Spina D, Henry PJ, et al: In vitro responsiveness of human asthmatic bronchus to carbachol, histamine, β-adrenoceptor agonists and theophylline. Br J Clin Pharmacol 22:669–676, 1986.

46. Dorn GW, Tepe NM, Lorenz JN, et al: Low- and high-level transgenic expression of beta2-adrenergic receptors differentially affect cardiac hypertrophy and function in Gαq-overexpressing mice. Proc Natl Acad Sci USA 96:6400–6405, 1999.

47. Mitra S, Ugur M, Ugur O, et al: (S)-Albuterol increases intracellular free calcium by muscarinic receptor activation and a phospholipase C-dependent mechanism in airway smooth muscle. Mol Pharmacol 53:347–354, 1998.

48. Yamaguchi H, McCullough JR: S-albuterol exacerbates calcium responses to carbachol in airway smooth muscle cells. Clin Rev Allergy Immunol 14:47–55, 1996.

49. Volcheck GW, Gleich GJ, Mita H: Pro- and anti-inflammatory effects of beta adrenergic agonists on eosinophil response to IL-5 [abstract]. J Allergy Clin Immunol 101:S35, 1998.

50. Handley DA, Anderson AJ, Koester J, Snider ME: New millennium bronchodilators for asthma: Single-isomer beta agonists. Curr Opin Pulm Med 6:43–49, 2000.

51. Templeton AG, Chapman ID, Chilvers ER, et al: Effects of S-

salbutamol on human isolated bronchus. Pulm Pharmacol Ther 11:1–6, 1998.

52. Cockcroft DW, Swystun VA: Effect of single doses of S-salbutamol, R-salbutamol, racemic salbutamol, and placebo on the airway response to methacholine. Thorax 52:845–848, 1997.

53. Handley DA, Tinkelman D, Noonan M, et al: Dose-response evaluation of levalbuterol versus racemic albuterol in patients with asthma. J Asthma 37:319–327, 2000.

54. Henriksen JM, Agertoft L, Pedersen S: Protective effect and duration of action of inhaled formoterol and salbutamol on exercise-induced asthma in children. J Allergy Clin Immunol 89:1176–1182, 1992.

55. Kil HK, Rooke GA, Ryan-Dykes MA, Bishop MJ: Effect of prophylactic bronchodilator treatment on lung resistance after tracheal intubation. Anesthesiology 81:43–48, 1994.

56. Higbee MD, Kumar M, Galant SP: Stimulation of endogenous catecholamine release by theophylline: A proposed additional mechanism of action for theophylline effects. J Allergy Clin Immunol 70:377–382, 1982.

57. Ishizaki T, Minegishi A, Morishita M, et al: Plasma catecholamine concentrations during a 72-hour aminophylline infusion in children with acute asthma. J Allergy Clin Immunol 82:146–154, 1988.

58. Fredholm BB, Hedqvist P: Modulation of neurotransmission by purine nucleotides and nucleosides. Biochem Pharmacol 29:1635–1643, 1980.

59. Zimmerman BL: Arrhythmogenicity of theophylline and halothane used in combination. Anesth Analg 58:259–260, 1979.

60. Stirt JA, Berger JM, Roe SD, et al: Halothane-induced cardiac arrhythmias following administration of aminophylline in experimental animals. Anesth Analg 60:517–520, 1981.

61. Tobias JD, Kubos KL, Hirshman CA: Aminophylline does not attenuate histamine-induced airway constriction during halothane anesthesia. Anesthesiology 71:723–729, 1989.

62. Polson JB, Krzanowski JJ, Goldman AL, Szentivanyi A: Inhibition of human pulmonary phosphodiesterase activity by therapeutic levels of theophylline. Clin Exp Pharmacol Physiol 5:535–539, 1978.

63. Rabe KF, Magnussen H, Dent G: Theophylline and selective PDE inhibitors as bronchodilators and smooth muscle relaxants. Eur Respir J 8:637–642, 1995.

64. Sierralta F, Miranda HF: Adenosine modulates the anti-nociceptive action of benzodiazepines. Gen Pharmacol 24:891–894, 1993.

65. Hirshman CA, Krieger W, Littlejohn G, et al: Ketamine-aminophylline-induced decrease in seizure threshold. Anesthesiology 56:464–467, 1982.

66. Daller JA, Erstad B, Rosado L, et al: Aminophylline antagonizes the neuromuscular blockade of pancuronium but not vecuronium. Crit Care Med 19:983–985, 1991.

67. Ogilvie RI, Fernandez PG, Winsberg F: Cardiovascular response to increasing theophylline concentrations. Eur J Clin Pharmacol 12:409–414, 1977.

68. Vestal RE, Eriksson Jr CE, Musser B, et al: Effect of intravenous aminophylline on plasma levels of catecholamines and related cardiovascular and metabolic responses in man. Circulation 67:162–171, 1983.

69. Starr I, Gamble CF, Margolies A, et al: A clinical study of the action of 10 commonly used drugs on cardiac output, work and size, on respiration, on metabolic rate and on the electrocardiogram. J Clin Invest 16:799–823, 1937.

70. Wechsler RL, Kleiss LM, Kety SS: The effects of intravenously administered aminophylline on cerebral circulation and metabolism in man. J Clin Invest 29:28–30, 1950.

71. Moyer JH, Tashnek AB, Miller SI, et al: The effect of theophylline with ethylenediamine (aminophylline) and caffeine on cerebral hemodynamics and cerebrospinal fluid pressure in patients with hypertension headaches. Am J Med Sci 224:377–385, 1952.

72. Robel-Tillig E, Vogtmann C: Aminophylline influences cerebral hyperperfusion after severe birth hypoxia. Acta Paediatr 89:971–974, 2000.

73. Motew SJ, Sam AD, Mourelatos MG, et al: Adenosine receptor antagonism affects regional resting vascular resistance during rat peritoneal sepsis. J Surg Res 80:326–332, 1998.

74. Fernandez E: Headaches associated with low spinal fluid pressure. Headache 30:122–128, 1990.

75. Zhou TJ, White PF, Chiu JW, et al: Onset/offset characteristics and intubating conditions of rapacuronium: A comparison with rocuronium. Br J Anaesth 85:246–250, 2000.

76. Zhou TJ, Coloma M, White PF, et al: Spontaneous recovery profile of rapacuronium during desflurane, sevoflurane, or propofol anesthesia for outpatient laparoscopy. Anesth Analg 91:596–600, 2000.

77. Brater DC, Kaojarern S, Chennavasin P: Pharmacodynamics of the diuretic effects of aminophylline and acetazolamide alone and combined with furosemide in normal subjects. J Pharmacol Exp Ther 227:92–97, 1983.

78. Heyman E, Ohlsson A, Heyman Z, Fong K: The effect of aminophylline on the excursions of the diaphragm in pre-term neonates. A randomized double-blind controlled study. Acta Paediatr Scand 80:308–315, 1991.

79. Sibert KS, Sladen RN: Impaired ventilatory capacity after recovery from Guillain-Barre syndrome. J Clin Anesth 6:133–138, 1994.

80. Derom E, Janssens S, Vanhaecke J, et al: Theophylline alters distribution of blood flow to respiratory muscles. Am J Respir Crit Care Med 150:941–946, 1994.

81. Rochester DF, Arora NS: Respiratory muscle failure. Med Clin North Am 67:573–597, 1983.

82. Jacoby DB, Fryer AD: Anticholinergic therapy for airway diseases. Life Sci 68:2565–2572, 2001.

83. Watson N, Eglen RM: Muscarinic receptor antagonists. Pulm Pharmacol Ther 12:115–118, 1999.

84. Costello RW, Jacoby DB, Fryer AD: Pulmonary neuronal M2 muscarinic receptor function in asthma and animal models of hyperreactivity. Thorax 53:613–616, 1998.

85. Dohi S, Gold MI: Pulmonary mechanics during general anaesthesia. The influence of mechanical irritation on the airway. Br J Anaesth 51:205–214, 1979.

86. Groeben H, Brown RH: Ipratropium decreases airway size in dogs by preferential M2 muscarinic receptor blockade in vivo. Anesthesiology 85:867–873, 1996.

87. Karpel JP, Schacter EN, Fanta C, et al: A comparison of ipratropium and albuterol vs. albuterol alone for the treatment of acute asthma. Chest 110:611–616, 1996.

88. Garrett JE, Town GI, Rodwell P, Kelly AM: Nebulized salbutamol with and without ipratropium bromide in the treatment of acute asthma. J Allergy Clin Immunol 100:165–170, 1997.

89. Lin RY, Pesola GR, Bakalchuk L, et al: Superiority of ipratropium plus albuterol over albuterol alone in the emergency department management of adult asthma: A randomized clinical trial. Ann Emerg Med 31:208–213, 1998.

90. Stoodley RG, Aaron SD, Dales RE: The role of ipratropium bromide in the emergency management of acute asthma exacerbation: A meta-analysis of randomized clinical trials. Ann Emerg Med 34:8–18, 1999.

91. Lanes SF, Garrett JE, Wentworth III CE, et al: The effect of adding ipratropium bromide to salbutamol in the treatment of acute asthma: A pooled analysis of three trials. Chest 114:365–372, 1998.

92. Nakano Y, Enomoto N, Kawamoto A, et al: Efficacy of adding multiple doses of oxitropium bromide to salbutamol delivered by means of a metered-dose inhaler with a spacer device in adults with acute severe asthma. J Allergy Clin Immunol 106:472–478, 2000.

93. Bryant DH: Nebulized ipratropium bromide in the treatment of acute asthma. Chest 88:24–29, 1985.

94. Rebuck AS, Chapman KR, Abboud R, et al: Nebulized anticholinergic and sympathomimetic treatment of asthma and chronic obstructive airways disease in the emergency room. Am J Med 82:59–64, 1987.

95. Leahy BC, Gomm SA, Allen SC: Comparison of nebulized salbutamol with nebulized ipratropium bromide in acute asthma. Br J Dis Chest 77:159–163, 1983.

96. O'Driscoll BR, Taylor RJ, Horsley MG, et al: Nebulized salbutamol with and without ipratropium bromide in acute airflow obstruction. Lancet 1:1418–1420, 1989.

97. Louw SJ, Goldin JG, Isaacs S: Relative efficacy of nebulized ipratropium bromide and fenoterol in acute severe asthma. S Afr Med J 77:24–26, 1990.

98. Teale C, Morrison JF, Muers MF, Pearson SB: Response to nebulized ipratropium bromide and terbutaline in acute severe asthma. Respir Med 86:215–218, 1992.

99. Craven D, Kercsmar CM, Myers TR, et al: Ipratropium bromide plus nebulized albuterol for the treatment of hospitalized children with acute asthma. J Pediatr 138:51–58, 2001.

100. Higgins RM, Stradling JR, Lane DJ: Should ipratropium bromide be

added to beta-agonists in treatment of acute severe asthma? Chest 94:718–722, 1988.

101. Summers QA, Tarala RA: Nebulized ipratropium in the treatment of acute asthma. Chest 97:425–429, 1990.

102. Fitzgerald JM, Grunfeld A, Pare PD, et al: The clinical efficacy of combination nebulized anticholinergic and adrenergic bronchodilators vs. nebulized adrenergic bronchodilator alone in acute asthma. Canadian Combivent Study Group. Chest 111:311–315, 1997.

103. McFadden ER Jr, el Sanadi N, Strauss L, et al: The influence of parasympatholytics on the resolution of acute attacks of asthma. Am J Med 102:7–13, 1997.

104. Weber EJ, Levitt MA, Covington JK, Gambrioli E: Effect of continuously nebulized ipratropium bromide plus albuterol on emergency department length of stay and hospital admission rates in patients with acute bronchospasm. A randomized, controlled trial. Chest 115:937–944, 1999.

105. Rodrigo G, Rodrigo C, Burschtin O: A meta-analysis of the effects of ipratropium bromide in adults with acute asthma. Am J Med 107:363–370, 1999.

106. Ho WM, Wong KC: Ipratropium bromide and intraoperative bronchospasm. Chung Hua I Hsueh Tsa Chih (Taipei) 55:319–324, 1995.

107. Kil HK, Rooke GA, Ryan-Dykes MA, Bishop MJ: Effect of prophylactic bronchodilator treatment on lung resistance after tracheal intubation. Anesthesiology 81:43–48, 1994.

108. Wu RS, Wu KC, Wong TK, et al: Effects of fenoterol and ipratropium on respiratory resistance of asthmatics after tracheal intubation. Br J Anaesth 84:358–362, 2000.

109. Fryer AD, Jacoby DB: Parainfluenza virus infection damages inhibitory M_2 muscarinic receptors on pulmonary parasympathetic nerves in the guinea pig. Br J Pharmacol 102:267–271, 1991.

110. Fryer AD, Adamko DJ, Yost BL, Jacoby DB: Effects of inflammatory cells on neuronal M2 muscarinic receptor function in the lung. Life Sci 64:449–455, 1999.

111. Parnass SM, Feld JM, Chamberlin WH, Segil LJ: Status asthmaticus treated with isoflurane and enflurane. Anesth Analg 66:193–195, 1987.

112. Johnston RG, Noseworthy TW, Friesen EG, et al: Isoflurane therapy for status asthmaticus in children and adults. Chest 97:698–701, 1990.

113. Brown RH, Zerhouni EA, Hirshman CA: Comparison of low concentrations of halothane and isoflurane as bronchodilators. Anesthesiology 78:1097–1101, 1993.

114. Brown RH, Mitzner W, Zerhouni E, Hirshman CA: Direct in vivo visualization of bronchodilation induced by inhalational anesthesia using high-resolution computed tomography. Anesthesiology 78:295–300, 1993.

115. Hermens JM, Edelstein G, Hanifin JM, et al: Inhalational anesthesia and histamine release during bronchospasm. Anesthesiology 61:69–72, 1984.

116. Tobias JD, Hirshman CA: Attenuation of histamine-induced airway constriction by albuterol during halothane anesthesia. Anesthesiology 72:105–110, 1990.

117. Mitsuhata H, Saitoh J, Shimizu R, et al: Sevoflurane and isoflurane protect against bronchospasm in dogs. Anesthesiology 81:1230–1234, 1994.

118. Rooke GA, Choi JH, Bishop MJ: The effect of isoflurane, halothane, sevoflurane, and thiopental/nitrous oxide on respiratory system resistance after tracheal intubation. Anesthesiology 86:1294–1299, 1997.

119. Goff MJ, Arain SR, Ficke DJ, et al: Absence of bronchodilation during desflurane anesthesia: A comparison to sevoflurane and thiopental. Anesthesiology 93:404–408, 2000.

120. Wiklund CU, Lim S, Lindsten U, Lindahl SG: Relaxation by sevoflurane, desflurane and halothane in the isolated guinea-pig trachea via inhibition of cholinergic neurotransmission. Br J Anaesth 83:422–429, 1999.

121. Kai T, Jones KA, Warner DO: Halothane attenuates calcium sensitization in airway smooth muscle by inhibiting G-proteins. Anesthesiology 89:1543–1552, 1998.

122. Bremerich DH, Hirasaki A, Jones KA, Warner DO: Halothane attenuation of calcium sensitivity in airway smooth muscle. Mechanisms of action during muscarinic receptor stimulation. Anesthesiology 87:94–101, 1997.

123. Kai T, Takahashi S, Kanaide H: Halothane counteracts acetylcholine-induced increase in Ca2+ sensitivity of the contractile apparatus in airway smooth muscle. Eur J Pharmacol 315:313–318, 1996.

124. Jones KA, Wong GY, Lorenz RR, et al: Effects of halothane on the relationship between cytosolic calcium and force in airway smooth muscle. Am J Physiol 266:L199–L204, 1994.

125. Yamakage M: Direct inhibitory mechanisms of halothane on canine tracheal smooth muscle contraction. Anesthesiology 77:546–553, 1992.

126. Hanazaki M, Jones KA, Perkins WJ, Warner DO: Halothane increases smooth muscle protein phosphatase in airway smooth muscle. Anesthesiology 94:129–136, 2001.

127. Kai T, Bremerich DH, Jones KA, Warner DO: Drug-specific effects of volatile anesthetics on Ca2+ sensitization in airway smooth muscle. Anesth Analg 87:425–429, 1998.

128. Yamakage M, Hirshman CA, Croxton TL: Volatile anesthetics inhibit voltage-dependent Ca2+ channels in porcine tracheal smooth muscle cells. Am J Physiol 268:L187–L191, 1995.

129. Yamakage M, Chen X, Tsujiguchi N, et al: Different inhibitory effects of volatile anesthetics on T- and L-type voltage-dependent Ca^{2++} channels in porcine tracheal and bronchial smooth muscles. Anesthesiology 94:683–693, 2001.

130. Suissa S, Ernst P: Inhaled corticosteroids: Impact on asthma morbidity and mortality. J Allergy Clin Immunol 107:937–944, 2001.

131. Laurie S, Khan D: Inhaled corticosteroids as first-line therapy for asthma. Why they work—and what the guidelines and evidence suggest. Postgrad Med 109:44–52, 55, 2001.

132. Littenberg B, Gluck EH: A controlled trial of methylprednisolone in the emergency treatment of acute asthma. N Engl J Med 314:150–152, 1986.

133. McGavin JK, Goa KL, Jarvis B: Inhaled budesonide/formoterol combination. Drugs 61:71–78, 2001.

134. Markham A, Adkins JC: Inhaled salmeterol/fluticasone propionate combination. A pharmacoeconomic review of its use in the management of asthma. Pharmacoeconomics 18:591–608, 2000.

135. Furu K, Kilvik K, Gautvik KM, Haug E: The mechanism of [3H]dexamethasone uptake into prolactin producing rat pituitary cells (GH3 cells) in culture. J Steroid Biochem 28:587–591, 1987.

136. Mendel DB, Orti E: Isoform composition and stoichiometry of the approximately 90-kDa heat shock protein associated with glucocorticoid receptors. J Biol Chem 263:6695–6702, 1988.

137. Johnson DM, Newby RF, Bourgeois S: Membrane permeability as a determinant of dexamethasone resistance in murine thymoma cells. Cancer Res 44:2435–2440, 1984.

138. Haske T, Nakao M, Moudgil VK: Phosphorylation of immunopurified rat liver glucocorticoid receptor by the catalytic subunit of cAMP-dependent protein kinase. Mol Cell Biochem 132:163–171, 1994.

139. Nielsen CJ, Sando JJ, Pratt WB: Evidence that dephosphorylation inactivates glucocorticoid receptors. Proc Natl Acad Sci USA 74:1398–1402, 1977.

140. Sando JJ, Hammond ND, Stratford CA, Pratt WB: Activation of thymocyte glucocorticoid receptors to the steroid binding form. The roles of reduction agents, ATP, and heat-stable factors. J Biol Chem 254:4779–4789, 1979.

141. Sando JJ, La Forest AC, Pratt WB: ATP-dependent activation of L cell glucocorticoid receptors to the steroid binding form. J Biol Chem 254:4772–4778, 1979.

142. Nemoto T, Ohara-Nemoto Y, Denis M, Gustafsson JA: The transformed glucocorticoid receptor has a lower steroid-binding affinity than the non-transformed receptor. Biochemistry 29:1880–1886, 1990.

143. Bamberger CM, Bamberger AM, de Castro M, Chrousos GP: Glucocorticoid receptor beta, a potential endogenous inhibitor of glucocorticoid action in humans. J Clin Invest 95:2435–2441, 1995.

144. Muller M, Renkawitz R: The glucocorticoid receptor. Biochim Biophys Acta 1088:171–182, 1991.

145. Bloom JW, Meisfeld RD: Molecular mechanisms of glucocorticoid action. In Szefler SJ, Leung DY (eds): Severe Asthma Pathogenesis and Clinical Management. New York, Marcel Dekker, pp 255–284, 1996.

146. Yamamoto KR: Steroid receptor regulated transcription of specific genes and gene networks. Annu Rev Genet 19:209–252, 1985.

147. Mozo L, Gayo A, Suarez A, Rivas D, et al: Glucocorticoids inhibit IL-4 and mitogen-induced IL-4R alpha chain expression by different posttranscriptional mechanisms. J Allergy Clin Immunol 102:968–976, 1998.

148. Guyre PM, Girard MT, Morganelli PM, Manganiello PD: Glucocor-

ticoid effects on the production and actions of immune cytokines. J Steroid Biochem 30:89–93, 1988.

149. Barnes PJ: Molecular mechanisms of steroid action in asthma. J Allergy Clin Immunol 97:159–168, 1996.

150. Radomski MW, Palmer RM, Moncada S: Glucocorticoids inhibit the expression of an inducible, but not the constitutive, nitric oxide synthase in vascular endothelial cells. Proc Natl Acad Sci USA 87:10043–10047, 1990.

151. Liu S, Adcock IM, Old RW, et al: Lipopolysaccharide treatment in vivo induces widespread tissue expression of inducible nitric oxide synthase mRNA. Biochem Biophys Res Commun 196:1208–1213, 1993.

152. Belvisi MG, Saunders MA, Haddad E, et al: Induction of cyclo-oxygenase-2 by cytokines in human cultured airway smooth muscle cells: Novel inflammatory role of this cell type. Br J Pharmacol 120:910–916, 1997.

153. Cronstein BN, Kimmel SC, Levin RI, et al: A mechanism for the anti-inflammatory effects of corticosteroids: The glucocorticoid receptor regulates leukocyte adhesion to endothelial cells and expression of endothelial-leukocyte adhesion molecule 1 and intercellular adhesion molecule 1. Proc Natl Acad Sci USA 89:9991–9995, 1992.

154. Adcock IM: Glucocorticoid-regulated transcription factors. Pulm Pharmacol Ther 14:211–219, 2001.

155. Scheinman RI, Gualberto A, Jewell CM, et al: Characterization of mechanisms involved in transrepression of NF-kappa B by activated glucocorticoid receptors. Mol Cell Biol 15:943–953, 1995.

156. Zhang HH, Kumar S, Barnett AH, Eggo MC: Dexamethasone inhibits tumor necrosis factor-alpha-induced apoptosis and interleukin-1 beta release in human subcutaneous adipocytes and preadipocytes. J Clin Endocrinol Metab 86:2817–2825, 2001.

157. Wills-Karp M, Ewart SL: The genetics of allergen-induced airway hyperresponsiveness in mice. Am J Respir Crit Care Med 156:S89–S96, 1997.

158. Wills-Karp M, Luyimbazi J, Xu X, et al: Interleukin-13: Central mediator of allergic asthma. Science 282:2258–2261, 1998.

159. Ray A, Cohn L: Altering the Th1/Th2 balance as a therapeutic strategy in asthmatic diseases. Curr Opin Invest Drugs 1:442–448, 2000.

160. Durham SR, Kay AB: Eosinophils, bronchial hyper-reactivity and late-phase asthmatic reactions. Clin Allergy 15:411–418, 1985.

161. Taylor KJ, Luksza AR: Peripheral blood eosinophil counts and bronchial responsiveness. Thorax 42:452–456, 1987.

162. Gibson PG, Saltos N, Borgas T: Airway mast cells and eosinophils correlate with clinical severity and airway hyperresponsiveness in corticosteroid-treated asthma. J Allergy Clin Immunol 105:752–759, 2000.

163. Robinson DS, Assoufi B, Durham SR, Kay AB: Eosinophil cationic protein (ECP) and eosinophil protein X (EPX) concentrations in serum and bronchial lavage fluid in asthma. Effect of prednisolone treatment. Clin Exp Allergy 25:1118–1127, 1995.

164. Wallen N, Kita H, Weiler D, Gleich GJ: Glucocorticoids inhibit cytokine-mediated eosinophil survival. J Immunol 147:3490–3495, 1991.

165. Zhang X, Moilanen E, Kankaanranta H: Enhancement of human eosinophil apoptosis by fluticasone propionate, budesonide, and beclomethasone. Eur J Pharmacol 406:325–332, 2000.

166. Oertel H, Kaliner M: The biologic activity of mast cell granules in rat skin: Effects of adrenocorticosteroids on late-phase inflammatory responses induced by mast cell granules. J Allergy Clin Immunol 68:238–245, 1981.

167. Bascom R, Pipkorn U, Lichtenstein LM, Naclerio RM: The influx of inflammatory cells into nasal washings during the late response to antigen challenge. Effect of systemic steroid pretreatment. Am Rev Respir Dis 138:406–412, 1988.

168. Lensmar C, Prieto J, Dahlen B, et al: Airway inflammation and altered alveolar macrophage phenotype pattern after repeated low-dose allergen exposure of atopic asthmatic subjects. Clin Exp Allergy 29:1632–1640, 1999.

169. Guyre PM, Munck A: Glucocorticoid actions on monocytes and macrophages. In Schleimer RP, Claman HN, Oronsky AR (eds): Anti-inflammatory Steroid Action: Basic and Clinical Aspects. New York, Academic Press, pp 199–225, 1991.

170. Kirby JG, Hargreave FE, Gleich GJ, O'Byrne PM: Bronchoalveolar cell profiles of asthmatic and non-asthmatic subjects. Am Rev Respir Dis 136:379–383, 1987.

171. Wardlaw AJ, Dunnette S, Gleich GJ, et al: Eosinophils and mast cells in bronchoalveolar lavage in subjects with mild asthma. Relationship to bronchial hyper-reactivity. Am Rev Respir Dis 137:62–69, 1988.

172. Boushey HA, Holtzman MJ: Experimental airway inflammation and hyper-reactivity. Searching for cells and mediators. Am Rev Respir Dis 131:312–313, 1985.

173. Yoshikawa H, Tasaka K: Suppression of mast cell activation by glucocorticoid. Arch Immunol Ther Exp (Warsz) 48:487–495, 2000.

174. Tobias JD, Sauder RA, Hirshman CA: Methylprednisolone prevents propranolol-induced airway hyper-reactivity in the Basenji-greyhound dog. Anesthesiology 74:1115–1120, 1991.

175. Darowski MJ, Hannon VM, Hirshman CA: Corticosteroids decrease airway hyperresponsiveness in the Basenji-Greyhound dog model of asthma. J Appl Physiol 66:1120–1126, 1989.

176. Sauder RA, Lenox WC, Tobias JD, Hirshman CA: Methylprednisolone increases sensitivity to beta-adrenergic agonists within 48 hours in Basenji greyhounds. Anesthesiology 79:1278–1283, 1993.

177. Sauder RA, Tobias JD, Hirshman CA: Methylprednisolone restores sensitivity to beta-adrenergic agonists in Basenji-Greyhound dogs. J Appl Physiol 72:694–698, 1992.

178. Emala CW, Clancy J, Hirshman CA: Glucocorticoid treatment decreases muscarinic receptor expression in canine airway smooth muscle. Am J Physiol 272:L745–L751, 1997.

179. Hadcock JR, Wang HY, Malbon CC: Agonist-induced destabilization of beta-adrenergic receptor mRNA. Attenuation of glucocorticoid-induced up-regulation of beta-adrenergic receptors. J Biol Chem 264:19928–19933, 1989.

180. Hadcock JR, Malbon CC: Regulation of beta-adrenergic receptors by "permissive" hormones: Glucocorticoids increase steady-state levels of receptor mRNA. Proc Natl Acad Sci USA 85:8415–8419, 1988.

181. Mak JC, Nishikawa M, Barnes PJ: Glucocorticosteroids increase beta 2-adrenergic receptor transcription in human lung. Am J Physiol 268:L41–L46, 1995.

182. Dangel V, Giray J, Ratge D, Wisser H: Regulation of beta-adrenoceptor density and mRNA levels in the rat heart cell-line H9c2. Biochem J 317(Pt 3):925–931, 1996.

183. Cao W, McGraw DW, Lee TT, et al: Expression of functional beta 2-adrenergic receptors in a rat airway epithelial cell line (SPOC1) and cell density-dependent induction by glucocorticoids. Exp Lung Res 26:421–435, 2000.

184. Jiang P, Arinze IJ: Developmental and glucocorticoid modulation of the expression of mRNAs for Gs alpha and G beta subunits in neonatal liver. Mol Cell Endocrinol 99:95–102, 1994.

185. Stevens WH, Adelroth E, Wattie J, et al: Effect of inhaled budesonide on ozone-induced airway hyperresponsiveness and bronchoalveolar lavage cells in dogs. J Appl Physiol 77:2578–2583, 1994.

186. Woolley MJ, Denburg JA, Ellis R, et al: Allergen-induced changes in bone marrow progenitors and airway responsiveness in dogs and the effect of inhaled budesonide on these parameters. Am J Respir Cell Mol Biol 11:600–606, 1994.

187. Evans CM, Jacoby DB, Fryer AD: Effects of dexamethasone on antigen-induced airway eosinophilia and M(2) receptor dysfunction. Am J Respir Crit Care Med 163:1484–1492, 2001.

188. Vanacker NJ, Palmans E, Kips JC, Pauwels RA: Fluticasone inhibits but does not reverse allergen-induced structural airway changes. Am J Respir Crit Care Med 163:674–679, 2001.

189. Uribe M, Casian C, Rojas S, et al: Decreased bioavailability of prednisone due to antacids in patients with chronic active liver disease and in healthy volunteers. Gastroenterology 80:661–665, 1981.

190. Ellul-Micallef R: Pharmacokinetics and pharmacodynamics of glucocorticoids. In Jenne JW, Murphy S (eds): Drug Therapy for Asthma: Research and Clinical Practice. New York, Marcel Dekker, pp 463–516, 1987.

191. Brooks SM, Werk EE, Ackerman SJ, et al: Adverse effects of phenobarbital on corticosteroid metabolism in patients with bronchial asthma. N Engl J Med 286:1125–1128, 1972.

192. Bartoszek M, Brenner AM, Szefler SJ: Prednisolone and methylprednisolone kinetics in children receiving anticonvulsant therapy. Clin Pharmacol Ther 42:424–432, 1987.

193. Glynn AM, Slaughter RL, Brass C, et al: Effects of ketoconazole on methylprednisolone pharmacokinetics and cortisol secretion. Clin Pharmacol Ther 39:654–659, 1986.

194. Zurcher RM, Frey BM, Frey FJ: Impact of ketoconazole on the metabolism of prednisolone. Clin Pharmacol Ther 45:366–372, 1989.

195. Szefler SJ, Ellis EF, Brenner M, et al: Steroid-specific and anticon-

vulsant interaction aspects of troleandomycin-steroid therapy. J Allergy Clin Immunol 69:455–460, 1982.

196. Boekenoogen SJ, Szefler SJ, Jusko WJ: Prednisolone disposition and protein binding in oral contraceptive users. J Clin Endocrinol Metab 56:702–709, 1983.

197. Fitzgerald JM, Shragge D, Haddon J, et al: A randomized, controlled trial of high dose, inhaled budesonide versus oral prednisone in patients discharged from the emergency department following an acute asthma exacerbation. Can Respir J 7:61–67, 2000.

198. Lawrence M, Wolfe J, Webb DR, et al: Efficacy of inhaled fluticasone propionate in asthma results from topical and not from systemic activity. Am J Respir Crit Care Med 156:744–751, 1997.

199. Pearlman DS, Noonan MJ, Tashkin DP, et al: Comparative efficacy and safety of twice daily fluticasone propionate powder versus placebo in the treatment of moderate asthma. Ann Allergy Asthma Immunol 78:356–362, 1997.

200. Chervinsky P, van As A, Bronsky EA, et al: Fluticasone propionate aerosol for the treatment of adults with mild to moderate asthma. The Fluticasone Propionate Asthma Study Group. J Allergy Clin Immunol 94:676–683, 1994.

201. Fish JE, Karpel JP, Craig TJ, et al: Inhaled mometasone furoate reduces oral prednisone requirements while improving respiratory function and health-related quality of life in patients with severe persistent asthma. J Allergy Clin Immunol 106:852–860, 2000.

202. Wong CA, Walsh LJ, Smith CJ, et al: Inhaled corticosteroid use and bone-mineral density in patients with asthma. Lancet 355:1399–1403, 2000.

203. Li JT, Ford LB, Chervinsky P, et al: Fluticasone propionate powder and lack of clinically significant effects on hypothalamic-pituitary-adrenal axis and bone mineral density over 2 years in adults with mild asthma. J Allergy Clin Immunol 103:1062–1068, 1999.

204. Lipworth BJ: Systemic adverse effects of inhaled corticosteroid therapy: A systematic review and meta-analysis. Arch Intern Med 159:941–955, 1999.

205. Rao R, Gregson RK, Jones AC, et al: Systemic effects of inhaled corticosteroids on growth and bone turnover in childhood asthma: A comparison of fluticasone with beclomethasone. Eur Respir J 13:87–94, 1999.

206. Nielsen LP, Dahl R: Therapeutic ratio of inhaled corticosteroids in adult asthma. A dose-range comparison between fluticasone propionate and budesonide, measuring their effect on bronchial hyperresponsiveness and adrenal cortex function. Am J Respir Crit Care Med 162:2053–2057, 2000.

207. Pien LC, Grammer LC, Patterson R: Minimal complications in a surgical population with severe asthma receiving prophylactic corticosteroids. J Allergy Clin Immunol 82:696–700, 1988.

208. Kabalin CS, Yarnold PR, Grammer LC: Low complication rate of corticosteroid-treated asthmatics undergoing surgical procedures. Arch Intern Med 155:1379–1384, 1995.

209. International Consensus Report on Diagnosis and Treatment of Asthma. Clin Exp Allergy 22(suppl 1):1–72, 1992.

210. International consensus report on diagnosis and treatment of asthma. National Heart, Lung, and Blood Institute, National Institutes of Health. Bethesda, Maryland 20892. Publication no. 92-3091, March 1992. Eur Respir J 5:601–641, 1992.

211. Howell JB, Altounyan RE: A double-blind trial of disodium cromoglycate in the treatment of allergic bronchial asthma. Lancet 2:539–542, 1967.

212. Altounyan RE, Howell JB: Treatment of asthma with disodium cromoglycate (FPL 670, 'Intal'). Respiration 26(suppl):40, 1969.

213. Eady RP: The pharmacology of nedocromil sodium. Eur J Respir Dis Suppl 147:112–119, 1986.

214. Paulmichl M, Norris AA, Rainey DK: Role of chloride channel modulation in the mechanism of action of nedocromil sodium. Int Arch Allergy Immunol 107:416, 1995.

215. Romanin C, Reinsprecht M, Pecht I, Schindler H: Immunologically activated chloride channels involved in degranulation of rat mucosal mast cells. EMBO J 10:3603–3608, 1991.

216. Reinsprecht M, Pecht I, Schindler H, Romanin C: Potent block of Cl—channels by anti-allergic drugs. Biochem Biophys Res Commun 188:957–963, 1992.

217. Wang L, Cornea L, Pang X, et al: Rat meosin: Cloning, phosphorylation and localization in mast cells [abstract]. FASEB J 9:A503, 1995.

218. Pestonjamasp K, Amieva MR, Strassel CP, et al: Moesin, ezrin, and

p205 are actin-binding proteins associated with neutrophil plasma membranes. Mol Biol Cell 6:247–259, 1995.

219. Correia I, Wang L, Pang X, Theoharides TC: Characterization of the 78 kDa mast cell protein phosphorylated by the anti-allergic drug cromolyn and homology to moesin. Biochem Pharmacol 52:413–424, 1996.

220. Marini M, Soloperto M, Zheng Y, et al: Protective effect of nedocromil sodium on the IL1-induced release of GM- CSF from cultured human bronchial epithelial cells. Pulm Pharmacol 5:61–65, 1992.

221. Vittori E, Sciacca F, Colotta F, et al: Protective effect of nedocromil sodium on the interleukin-1-induced production of interleukin-8 in human bronchial epithelial cells. J Allergy Clin Immunol 90:76–84, 1992.

222. Abdelaziz MM, Devalia JL, Khair OA, et al: The effect of nedocromil sodium on human airway epithelial cell-induced eosinophil chemotaxis and adherence to human endothelial cell in vitro. Eur Respir J 10:851–857, 1997.

223. Furukawa C, Atkinson D, Forster TJ, et al: Controlled trial of two formulations of cromolyn sodium in the treatment of asthmatic patients > or = 12 years of age. Intal Study Group. Chest 116:65–72, 1999.

224. Korhonen K, Korppi M, Remes ST, et al: Lung function in school-aged asthmatic children with inhaled cromoglycate, nedocromil and corticosteroid therapy. Eur Respir J 13:82–86, 1999.

225. Nathan RA, Minkwitz MC, Bonuccelli CM: Two first-line therapies in the treatment of mild asthma: Use of peak flow variability as a predictor of effectiveness. Ann Allergy Asthma Immunol 82:497–503, 1999.

226. Storm van's GK, Mattes J, Grossklauss E, et al: Preventive effect of 2 and 10 mg of sodium cromoglycate on exercise-induced bronchoconstriction. Eur J Pediatr 159:759–763, 2000.

227. Kelly KD, Spooner CH, Rowe BH: Nedocromil sodium versus sodium cromoglycate in treatment of exercise-induced bronchoconstriction: A systematic review. Eur Respir J 17:39–45, 2001.

228. Tasche MJ, Uijen JH, Bernsen RM, et al: Inhaled disodium cromoglycate (DSCG) as maintenance therapy in children with asthma: A systematic review. Thorax 55:913–920, 2000.

229. Bentley AM, Jacobson MR, Cumberworth V, et al: Immunohistology of the nasal mucosa in seasonal allergic rhinitis: Increases in activated eosinophils and epithelial mast cells. J Allergy Clin Immunol 89:877–883, 1992.

230. Lal S, Dorow PD, Venho KK, Chatterjee SS: Nedocromil sodium is more effective than cromolyn sodium for the treatment of chronic reversible obstructive airway disease. Chest 104:438–447, 1993.

231. Dennis EA: The growing phospholipase A2 superfamily of signal transduction enzymes. Trends Biochem Sci 22:1–2, 1997.

232. Borgeat P, Samuelsson B: Transformation of arachidonic acid by rabbit polymorphonuclear leukocytes. Formation of a novel dihydroxyeicosatetraenoic acid. J Biol Chem 254:2643–2646, 1979.

233. Murphy RC, Hammarstrom S, Samuelsson B: Leukotriene C: A slow-reacting substance from murine mastocytoma cells. Proc Natl Acad Sci USA 76:4275–4279, 1979.

234. Bach MK, Brashler JR, Brooks CD, Neerken AJ: Slow reacting substances: Comparison of some properties of human lung SRS-A and two distinct fractions from ionophore-induced rat mononuclear cell SRS. J Immunol 122:160–165, 1979.

235. Lewis RA, Austen KF, Drazen JM, et al: Slow reacting substances of anaphylaxis: Identification of leukotrienes C-1 and D from human and rat sources. Proc Natl Acad Sci USA 77:3710–3714, 1980.

236. Morris HR, Taylor GW, Jones CM, et al: Slow reacting substances (leukotrienes): Enzymes involved in their biosynthesis. Proc Natl Acad Sci USA 79:4838–4842, 1982.

237. Ellis C: EP874047A2: cDNA clone HMTMF81 that encodes a novel human 7-transmembrane receptor. Eur Patent ApplicEp0874047A2, 1998.

238. Heise CE, O'Dowd BF, Figueroa DJ, et al: Characterization of the human cysteinyl leukotriene 2 receptor. J Biol Chem 275: 30531–30536, 2000.

239. Mellor EA, Maekawa A, Austen KF, Boyce JA: Cysteinyl leukotriene receptor 1 is also a pyrimidinergic receptor and is expressed by human mast cells. Proc Natl Acad Sci USA 98:7964–7969, 2001.

240. Forsberg K, Sorenby L: The influence of a new corticosteroid, budesonide, on anaphylactic bronchoconstriction and SRS-A release in the guinea pig. Agents Actions 11:391–395, 1981.

241. Dahlen SE, Hedqvist P, Hammarstrom S, Samuelsson B: Leukotrienes are potent constrictors of human bronchi. Nature 288:484–486, 1980.

242. Burka JF, Eyre P: Effects of bovine SRS-A (SRS-Abov) on bovine respiratory tract and lung vasculature in vitro. Eur J Pharmacol 44:169–177, 1977.

243. Drazen JM, Austen KF, Lewis RA, et al: Comparative airway and vascular activities of leukotrienes C-1 and D in vivo and in vitro. Proc Natl Acad Sci USA 77:4354–4358, 1980.

244. Hedqvist P, Dahlen SE, Gustafsson L, et al: Biological profile of leukotrienes C4 and D4. Acta Physiol Scand 110:331–333, 1980.

245. Dahlen SE, Hedqvist P, Hammarstrom S, Samuelsson B: Leukotrienes are potent constrictors of human bronchi. Nature 288:484–486, 1980.

246. Hanna CJ, Bach MK, Pare PD, Schellenberg RR: Slow-reacting substances (leukotrienes) contract human airway and pulmonary vascular smooth muscle in vitro. Nature 290:343–344, 1981.

247. Dahlen SE, Bjork J, Hedqvist P, et al: Leukotrienes promote plasma leakage and leukocyte adhesion in postcapillary venules: In vivo effects with relevance to the acute inflammatory response. Proc Natl Acad Sci USA 78:3887–3891, 1981.

248. Jones TR, Davis C, Daniel EE: Pharmacological study of the contractile activity of leukotriene C4 and D4 on isolated human airway smooth muscle. Can J Physiol Pharmacol 60:638–643, 1982.

249. Laitinen LA, Laitinen A, Haahtela T, et al: Leukotriene E4 and granulocytic infiltration into asthmatic airways. Lancet 341:989–990, 1993.

250. Diamant Z, Hiltermann JT, van Rensen EL, et al: The effect of inhaled leukotriene D4 and methacholine on sputum cell differentials in asthma. Am J Respir Crit Care Med 155:1247–1253, 1997.

251. Wang CG, Du T, Xu, Martin JG: Role of leukotriene D4 in allergen-induced increases in airway smooth muscle in the rat. Am Rev Respir Dis 148:413–417, 1993.

252. Holroyde MC, Altounyan RE, Cole M, et al: Bronchoconstriction produced in man by leukotrienes C and D. Lancet 2:17–18, 1981.

253. Weiss JW, Drazen JM, Coles N, et al: Bronchoconstrictor effects of leukotriene C in humans. Science 216:196–198, 1982.

254. Barnes NC, Piper PJ, Costello JF: Comparative effects of inhaled leukotriene C4, leukotriene D4, and histamine in normal human subjects. Thorax 39:500–504, 1984.

255. Shader RI, Granda BW, von Moltke LL, et al: Inhibition of human cytochrome P450 isoforms in vitro by zafirlukast. Biopharm Drug Dispos 20:385–388, 1999.

256. Reinus JF, Persky S, Burkiewicz JS, et al: Severe liver injury after treatment with the leukotriene receptor antagonist zafirlukast. Ann Intern Med 133:964–968, 2000.

257. Bisgaard H: Pathophysiology of the cysteinyl leukotrienes and effects of leukotriene receptor antagonists in asthma. Allergy 56:7–11, 2001.

258. Salvi SS, Krishna MT, Sampson AP, Holgate ST: The anti-inflammatory effects of leukotriene-modifying drugs and their use in asthma. Chest 119:1533–1546, 2001.

259. Hood PP, Cotter TP, Costello JF, Sampson AP: Effect of intravenous corticosteroid on ex vivo leukotriene generation by blood leucocytes of normal and asthmatic patients. Thorax 54:1075–1082, 1999.

260. Sebaldt RJ, Sheller JR, Oates JA, et al: Inhibition of eicosanoid biosynthesis by glucocorticoids in humans. Proc Natl Acad Sci USA 87:6974–6978, 1990.

261. Powell WS, Xu LJ, Martin JG: Effects of dexamethasone on leukotriene synthesis and airway responses to antigen and leukotriene D4 in rats. Am J Respir Crit Care Med 151:1143–1150, 1995.

262. Coreno A, Skowronski M, Kotaru C, McFadden Jr ER: Comparative effects of long-acting beta2-agonists, leukotriene receptor antagonists, and a 5-lipoxygenase inhibitor on exercise-induced asthma. J Allergy Clin Immunol 106:500–506, 2000.

263. Yamauchi K, Tanifuji Y, Pan LH, et al: Effects of pranlukast, a leukotriene receptor antagonist, on airway inflammation in mild asthmatics. J Asthma 38:51–57, 2001.

264. Yoo SH, Park SH, Song JS, et al: Clinical effects of pranlukast, an oral leukotriene receptor antagonist, in mild-to-moderate asthma: A 4 week randomized multicentre controlled trial. Respirology 6:15–21, 2001.

265. Busse W, Raphael GD, Galant S, et al: Low-dose fluticasone propionate compared with montelukast for first-line treatment of persistent asthma: A randomized clinical trial. J Allergy Clin Immunol 107:461–468, 2001.

266. Williams B, Noonan G, Reiss TF, et al: Long-term asthma control with oral montelukast and inhaled beclomethasone for adults and children 6 years and older. Clin Exp Allergy 31:845–854, 2001.

267. Christian VJ, Prasse A, Naya I, et al: Zafirlukast improves asthma control in patients receiving high-dose inhaled corticosteroids. Am J Respir Crit Care Med 162:578–585, 2000.

268. Centanni S, Santus P, Casanova F, et al: Evaluation of the effects of zafirlukast 40 mg b.i.d. in addition to preexisting therapy of high-dose inhaled steroids on symptomatic patients with reversible respiratory obstruction: Preliminary data. Drugs Exp Clin Res 26:133–138, 2000.

269. Robinson DS, Campbell D, Barnes PJ: Addition of leukotriene antagonists to therapy in chronic persistent asthma: A randomized double-blind placebo-controlled trial. Lancet 357:2007–2011, 2001.

270. Pauls JD, Simon RA, Daffern PJ, Stevenson DD: Lack of effect of the 5-lipoxygenase inhibitor zileuton in blocking oral aspirin challenges in aspirin-sensitive asthmatics. Ann Allergy Asthma Immunol 85:40–45, 2000.

271. Dahlen B, Nizankowska E, Szczeklik A, et al: Benefits from adding the 5-lipoxygenase inhibitor zileuton to conventional therapy in aspirin-intolerant asthmatics. Am J Respir Crit Care Med 157:1187–1194, 1998.

272. Dekhuijzen PN, Bootsma GP, Wielders PL, et al: Effects of single-dose zileuton on bronchial hyperresponsiveness in asthmatic patients treated with inhaled corticosteroids. Eur Respir J 10:2749–2753, 1997.

273. Gomez FP, Iglesia R, Roca J, et al: The effects of 5-lipoxygenase inhibition by zileuton on platelet-activating-factor-induced pulmonary abnormalities in mild asthma. Am J Respir Crit Care Med 157:1559–1564, 1998.

274. Hasday JD, Meltzer SS, Moore WC, et al: Anti-inflammatory effects of zileuton in a subpopulation of allergic asthmatics. Am J Respir Crit Care Med 161:1229–1236, 2000.

41

Pulmonary Vasodilators

Sunita Sastry, MD • Ronald G. Pearl, MD, PhD

The pulmonary circulation is normally a low pressure, low resistance circulation. Pulmonary hypertension is frequently defined as a pulmonary artery systolic pressure greater than 30 mm Hg or a mean pressure greater than 20 mm Hg. In patients with pulmonary hypertension, altered vascular endothelial and smooth muscle function lead to a combination of vasoconstriction, localized thrombosis, and vascular growth and remodeling.[1] These processes increase pulmonary vascular resistance (PVR), resulting in right ventricular (RV) failure, inadequate oxygenation, and ultimately death.[2] Pulmonary vasodilator therapy is based on an understanding of the mechanisms of pulmonary hypertension.[1-5]

Etiologic Factors of Pulmonary Hypertension

The etiologic factors of pulmonary hypertension can be considered from the equation for PVR:

$$PVR = (PAP - LAP) \times 80/CO$$

where PVR represents pulmonary vascular resistance (in dynes $\cdot$ sec $\cdot$ cm^{-5}), PAP represents mean pulmonary artery pressure (in mm Hg), LAP represents left atrial pressure (in mm Hg), and CO represents cardiac output (in L $\cdot$ min^{-1}).
Rearranging this equation for PAP demonstrates that:

$$PAP = LAP + (CO \times PVR)/80.$$

Thus the three factors that cause pulmonary hypertension are increased LAP, increased CO, and increased PVR. For patients with chronic pulmonary hypertension, the common diagnoses can be considered in these three categories.

Increased LAP includes left ventricular (LV) failure and valvular heart disease (particularly mitral stenosis, or regurgitation, or both). Increased CO primarily refers to patients with congenital heart disease with cardiac shunts producing increased pulmonary blood flow such as ventricular septal defects. The major categories of chronically increased PVR are pulmonary disease (parenchymal or airway), hypoxia without pulmonary disease (hypoventilation syndromes, high altitude), pulmonary arterial obstruction (thromboembolism, schistosomiasis), and primary pulmonary hypertension (PPH). The 1998 World Symposium on PPH sponsored by the World Health Organization divided pulmonary hypertension into five diagnostic categories: pulmonary arterial hypertension (primary or related to collagen vascular disease, congenital systemic to pulmonary shunts, portal hypertension, human immunodeficiency virus infection, drugs/toxins, or persistent pulmonary hypertension of the newborn), pulmonary venous hypertension (left-sided heart disease, extrinsic compression of central pulmonary veins, pulmonary veno-occlusive disease), pulmonary hypertension associated with disorders of the respiratory system or hypoxemia, chronic thrombotic or embolic disease, and pulmonary hypertension caused by disorders directly affecting the pulmonary vasculature (schistosomiasis, sarcoidosis, pulmonary capillary hemangiomatosis).[6]

In addition to the etiologic factors of chronic pulmonary hypertension, acute increases in PVR may result from hypoxia, hypercarbia, acidosis, increased sympathetic tone, and endogenous or exogenous pulmonary vasoconstrictors (catecholamines, serotonin, thromboxane). Most patients with severe acute pulmonary hypertension will have a combination of chronic pulmonary hypertension with an acute increase in PVR; in general, therapy will be directed at reversing this acute increase in PVR.[7]

The pulmonary vascular endothelium is involved in the synthesis and removal of vasoactive substances that affect

723

pulmonary vascular tone. A variety of abnormalities in endothelial cell function have been demonstrated in vessels from patients with pulmonary hypertension, including decreased production of vasodilator and antiproliferative substances such as prostacyclin and nitric oxide (NO) and increased production of vasoconstrictors such as thromboxane A_2, endothelin, serotonin, and norepinephrine.[2,8–17] Changes in the synthesis and release of these substances may alter pulmonary vascular tone. The lung is responsible for synthesizing and inactivating eicosanoids, including prostaglandins (PGs), thromboxanes, and leukotrienes. Metabolism of the eicosanoids through the cyclo-oxygenase pathway produces $PGF_{2\alpha}$, PGE_2, and thromboxane A_2, which are pulmonary vasoconstrictors; other prostaglandins such as PGE_1 and prostacyclin (PGI_2) are vasodilators. Leukotrienes are products of the lipoxygenase pathway and produce pulmonary vasoconstriction. Thus a balance between the lipoxygenase and cyclo-oxygenase pathways may be an important determinant of the normally low resistance of the pulmonary circulation. Bradykinin is inactivated in the lungs by angiotensin-converting enzyme; bradykinin can produce direct pulmonary vasoconstriction through BK_2 receptors or indirect pulmonary vasodilation through endothelial NO production.[18] Histamine is produced by mast cells near the pulmonary arteries. Histamine is a strong pulmonary vasoconstrictor and systemic vasodilator. Histamine results in preferential pulmonary venoconstriction, thereby increasing capillary hydrostatic pressure and producing pulmonary edema.[19] Pulmonary vessels receive both sympathetic and parasympathetic innervation. α Adrenergic agonists such as norepinephrine produce pulmonary vasoconstriction, whereas β adrenergic agonists such as isoproterenol produce vasodilation.[17,20] Stimulation of the vagus nerve produces pulmonary vasodilation. Sympathetic nervous system stimulation from stress and pain may exacerbate pulmonary hypertension.[21]

Hypoxic Pulmonary Vasoconstriction

Acute hypoxia produces acute pulmonary hypertension caused by hypoxic pulmonary vasoconstriction (HPV). Chronic hypoxia produces chronic pulmonary hypertension caused by the combination of HPV, pulmonary vascular remodeling from release of hypoxia inducible factor-1,[22] and altered pulmonary vasoreactivity.[23] HPV was initially described by von Euler and Liljestrand in 1947[24] who demonstrated an increase in Ppa during hypoxic ventilation of the cat. HPV was demonstrated in humans the next year. Studies since then have attempted to define the sensor, transducer, and effector mechanisms of HPV.[25–31] Although HPV was initially described in vivo, subsequent studies demonstrated that vasoconstriction in response to hypoxia occurs in isolated perfused lungs, in pulmonary artery strips, and in cultured pulmonary artery smooth muscle cells (PASMCs). The small pulmonary arteries and arterioles (60–500 μm in diameter) have the strongest vasoconstrictor response and are primarily responsible for the increase in PVR. Large pulmonary arteries may not sense alveolar hypoxia in vivo because they receive perfusion with systemic blood through

the vasa vasorum. Studies that divide PVR into arteriolar, capillary, and venous components have demonstrated that resistance increases in all segments in response to hypoxia, but the arteriolar segment constitutes the majority of the total increase.[19] As a result, pulmonary capillary pressure remains relatively constant during HPV.[32]

The site of oxygen sensing for HPV is the small pulmonary arteries.[25,27,30] These are surrounded by alveolar gas and are perfused with mixed venous blood. Both the alveolar oxygen tension (PAO_2) and the mixed venous oxygen tension (PvO_2) contribute to the stimulus for vasoconstriction. The PAO_2 has a greater impact than the PvO_2 so that the integrated response occurs to a sensed oxygen tension (PsO_2) $= PAO_2^{0.6} + PvO_2^{0.4}$.[33] The arterial oxygen tension (PaO_2) has no effect on HPV. Vasoconstriction in response to the PsO_2 has a sigmoidal relationship similar to the oxyhemoglobin dissociation curve so that there is little effect until PsO_2 decreases to less than 70 mm Hg, a half-maximal effect at a PsO_2 of 30 mm Hg, and essentially complete effect at a PsO_2 of 10 mm Hg.[33]

Studies examining the mechanisms of HPV have often produced conflicting results.[25–27] There appear to be multiple redundant mechanisms and modulators of HPV so that results may depend on the species, the experimental preparation (intact subject, perfused lung, pulmonary vessel, cultured PASMC), the vessel size (proximal pulmonary artery, distal pulmonary artery), and the specific experimental conditions (duration of hypoxia, precontraction stimulus, presence or inhibition of modulators). In many studies, HPV has a triphasic response (early transient contraction, relaxation, late sustained contraction), and the mechanisms responsible for each phase may differ. The hypoxic relaxation is primarily endothelium-independent and the late hypoxic contraction is primarily endothelium-dependent with a major component from endothelin-1 and a requirement for superoxide anion. In preparations with intact endothelium, hypoxia decreases NO release from endothelium because of the role of oxygen as a substrate in NO synthesis from L-citrulline.

PASMCs rapidly contract in response to hypoxia, a phenomenon that does not occur in smooth muscle cells from systemic arteries. The standard view of the events responsible for HPV is that hypoxia inhibits voltage-gated potassium (K_v) channels, thereby producing membrane depolarization that activates voltage-dependent L-type calcium channels, resulting in increased calcium influx from the extracellular space. The increase in intracellular calcium results in calmodulin-mediated activation of myosin light chain kinase and contraction. Contraction is caused by increased intracellular calcium concentration with no significant change in sensitivity. Some studies suggest that calcium release may occur from ryanodine-sensitive stores in the sarcoplasmic reticulum. The mechanisms by which hypoxia inhibits K_v remains controversial.[26,28–30] The K_v channels in PASMCs are oxygen-sensitive, but whether the response is caused by decreased oxygen tension, by altered redox status, or by altered cellular energetic state is unresolved. K_v activity can be altered by oxidation of a cysteine residue in the N-terminal region. Hypoxia can alter the production of reactive oxygen species such as superoxide anion and hydrogen peroxide as a result of nicotinamide adenine dinucleotide or nicotinamide adenine dinucleotide phosphate oxidase activity. Studies suggest that the bioenergetic state of the cell is not a primary regulatory mechanism for HPV because the contraction significantly precedes any decline in adenosine triphosphate.

Hypoxia causing pulmonary hypertension is most commonly seen in patients with chronic lung disease.[34] Continuous prolonged administration of oxygen decreases or prevents the progression of pulmonary hypertension.[34,35] Treatment of patients in whom pulmonary hypertension either develops acutely or becomes intensified as a result of bronchitis or pneumonia is aimed at maintaining arterial oxygenation. Such patients may not need and indeed may not respond to pulmonary vasodilator therapy unless oxygen is appropriately administered and the underlying infection is adequately treated. In general, maintenance of PaO_2 at values greater than 50 to 60 mm Hg minimizes hypoxic pulmonary vasoconstriction. In patients with chronic lung disease, these levels can generally be achieved by administering oxygen at low flow rates through nasal cannula. Hypercarbia may develop with excessive oxygen administration in patients with chronic obstructive lung disease. This adverse effect is not primarily a result of decreased hypoxic respiratory drive, but instead results from worsened ventilation/perfusion mismatching during oxygen therapy.[36]

Evaluation of Pulmonary Hypertension

Evaluation of the patient with pulmonary hypertension should determine the underlying diagnosis and the severity of the disease.[6] History and examination should focus on issues such as underlying lung disease, congenital heart disease, myocardial or valvular heart disease, thromboembolic disease, connective tissue disease, liver disease, human immunodeficiency virus infection, prior intravenous drug use, prior use of appetite-suppressant drugs, and family history of pulmonary hypertension. Ventilation/perfusion lung scan, or spiral computed tomography of the lung, or both, can be used to demonstrate chronic thromboembolic pulmonary hypertension; patients with this disorder should be considered for surgical thromboendarterectomy.[37] Echocardiography with Doppler measurements can determine RV function and RV systolic pressure. Pulmonary artery catheterization will demonstrate pulmonary hemodynamics and whether the pulmonary circulation is reactive to vasodilators. Measurement of PAP, cardiac index, and right atrial pressure can be used to predict survival.[38] For evaluation of functional impairment and prognosis and in the evaluation of long-term treatment the 6-minute walk test is currently used.[39]

Therapy of Pulmonary Hypertension

In the face of increased impedance to RV ejection, compensatory reserves of RV are limited. Reduction in RV stroke volume and CO and ventricular interdependence with decreased LV filling and output occur.[40] RV dysfunction seen

after cardiopulmonary bypass (CPB) either from preexisting disease or inadequate myocardial RV protection can be exacerbated by an increase in PVR caused by pulmonary vasoconstrictors or by decreased endogenous NO production from pulmonary endothelial injury during CPB.[41] Traditional management of perioperative pulmonary hypertension involves optimization of acid-base status, oxygenation, ventilation, temperature, level of anesthesia, and use of systemic vasodilators. Treatment of secondary pulmonary hypertension involves treatment of the underlying etiologic factors. In patients with PPH, chronic anticoagulation therapy with a goal to achieve an international normalized ratio of 2 to 2.5 may improve survival.[42,43]

Pulmonary Vasodilator Therapy

Because pulmonary vasoconstriction is a major factor in the development of pulmonary hypertension, the traditional approach to the treatment of pulmonary hypertension has involved vasodilators to reverse any vasoconstriction. As a general rule, all systemic vasodilator agents are pulmonary vasodilators. Pulmonary vasodilators include: direct-acting nitrovasodilators such as hydralazine, nitroglycerin, and nitroprusside; α adrenergic blockers such as tolazoline and phentolamine; β adrenergic agents such as isoproterenol; calcium blockers such as nifedipine and diltiazem; prostaglandins such as PGE_1 and prostacyclin; adenosine; endothelin receptor antagonists; and indirect-acting vasodilators such as acetylcholine, which cause release of NO.[21-24]

Pulmonary vasodilator therapy frequently results in major adverse effects. These adverse effects can be considered in four categories.

1. Systemic hypotension: In pulmonary hypertension, CO varies with right heart function. Both the pulmonary and systemic vasodilator effects of drugs are dose-dependent. For the majority of drugs, systemic vasodilator effects occur at doses that do not produce pulmonary vasodilation. Thus with a decrease in systemic vascular resistance (SVR) and no change in PVR, CO cannot increase and systemic blood pressure must decrease ($BP = CO \times SVR$).
2. Pulmonary hypertension: A drug-induced decrease in systemic blood pressure may increase PAP by increasing CO and sympathetic tone.
3. Decreased contractility: This may occur either from reduced RV coronary perfusion as a result of drug-induced hypotension or from direct negative inotropic effects as seen with verapamil.
4. Hypoxemia: Pulmonary vasodilators may inhibit hypoxic pulmonary vasoconstriction and thereby adversely alter ventilation/perfusion matching. The degree of hypoxemia will depend on the degree of underlying ventilation/perfusion abnormalities.

All available intravenous vasodilators have one or more of these limitations. In general, the major limitation is the failure to produce selective pulmonary vasodilation.

Approaches to develop selective pulmonary vasodilators have attempted to exploit either pharmacokinetic or pharmacodynamic aspects. Adenosine has extensive red blood cell and pulmonary endothelial metabolism so that pulmonary blood levels may exceed systemic blood levels and thereby produce selective pulmonary vasodilation.[44,45] Acetylcholine (because of pseudocholinesterase) and PGE₁ (because of pulmonary metabolism) may have selective effects.[46–48] However, this selectivity is frequently lost at doses that are required to produce adequate pulmonary vasodilation. Nitroglycerin and prostacyclin appear to have the best ratio of pulmonary to systemic vasodilator effects and are frequently used in patients with perioperative pulmonary hypertension.[24,49–52]

Based on the adverse effects of vasodilators and the limited vasodilator capacity of many patients with chronic pulmonary hypertension, measurement of vasodilator responsiveness should be performed before initiating chronic vasodilator therapy. Although differences among acute vasodilator responses have been seen in some studies, most of the data suggest that assessment of vasodilator responsiveness can be performed equally well with any of several different agents. Measurement of vasodilator responsiveness should initially be performed with a short-acting vasodilator such as inhaled NO (INO), intravenous prostacyclin, acetylcholine, or intravenous adenosine.[1,2,6,23,45,46,52–56] The purpose of vasodilator testing is primarily to determine whether the patient will be responsive to calcium channel blockers. The majority of data suggest that all three of these vasodilators adequately predict response to calcium channel blockers. Vasodilator testing is currently performed during pulmonary artery catheterization, allowing measurement of PAP, pulmonary artery wedge pressure, CO, and PVR. Advances in echocardiography and noninvasive CO measurement may decrease the need for invasive hemodynamic monitoring in the future.

Calcium Channel Blockers

The calcium channel blockers, including nifedipine, diltiazem, and verapamil, have both systemic and pulmonary vasodilating effects.[57] Reports of the acute and chronic use of calcium channel blockers in pulmonary hypertension began in the early 1980s.[58] Subsequent studies demonstrated that high doses were required to produce acute pulmonary vasodilation during studies of pulmonary vascular responsiveness.[43,54,59,60] In patients with PPH who respond to acute therapy with calcium channel blockers, chronic therapy may result in sustained reduction of PAPs, regression of RV hypertrophy, and increased survival rates.[43,61] Most clinicians assume that patients who do not respond to acute calcium channel blocker therapy also will not respond to chronic therapy. Although initial reports indicated that approximately one third of patients were responsive to acute therapy with calcium channel blockers,[59] subsequent studies suggest that the actual number is approximately one fifth of patients.[6] Therefore an acute trial of a pulmonary vasodilator with invasive hemodynamic monitoring is generally used before chronic therapy. Nifedipine has been used empirically in the treatment of chronic pulmonary hypertension when invasive hemodynamic testing is not possible. Beneficial effects of calcium channel blockade occur in secondary, as well as primary, pulmonary hypertension.[62–64]

Although nifedipine is the most commonly used calcium channel blocker for pulmonary hypertension,[43,54,58–62] beneficial effects have been reported with diltiazem,[59,65,66] verapamil,[63,67] and amlodipine.[68] Adverse effects of calcium channel blockers include excessive systemic vasodilation, tachycardia, bradycardia, and negative inotropic effects.[64,69–71] These adverse effects, as well as the ratio of systemic to pulmonary vasodilation, may vary with the specific calcium channel blocker used.[59,64,69,71] Calcium channel blockers may also worsen ventilation/perfusion matching in patients with underlying lung disease.[66,67,72]

Nitrovasodilators

The nitrovasodilators include nitroprusside, nitroglycerin, and hydralazine. Nitrovasodilators produce both systemic and pulmonary vasodilatation through activation of guanylyl cyclase resulting in increased intracellular cyclic guanosine monophosphate (cGMP). The combination of pulmonary and systemic vasodilation unloads both the right and the left ventricle and is particularly useful for patients with pulmonary hypertension caused by cardiac failure. Combined vasodilators have been extensively studied in patients being considered for heart transplantation who have increased PVR because of remodeling. Nitroprusside is frequently used to determine pulmonary vasodilator responsiveness in this population.[73] Nitroprusside has a rapid onset of action and a short duration of effect because of the rapid breakdown of the unstable nitroprusside radical to produce cyanide.[74] Free cyanide ions are usually converted to thiocyanate in the liver and kidney. Free cyanide not converted to thiocyanate can inhibit cytochrome oxidase and prevent cellular aerobic respiration. Prolonged administration of nitroprusside at moderate doses may result in cyanide and thiocyanate toxicity. Nitroprusside is therefore not a suitable agent for long-term infusion in patients with chronic pulmonary hypertension. In patients with acute or chronic lung disease, nitroprusside may produce hypoxemia by inhibiting hypoxic pulmonary vasoconstriction.[75] The major limitation of the use of nitroprusside in patients with pulmonary hypertension is the potent systemic vasodilation that results in systemic hypotension and decreased RV coronary artery perfusion.[70,76]

Nitroglycerin is a nitrovasodilator with preferential effects on the venous capacitance vessels and the large coronary arteries. Nitroglycerin can produce pulmonary vasodilation equivalent to the degree of systemic arterial dilation.[49] Nitroglycerin may therefore be preferable to nitroprusside in patients with pulmonary hypertension.[49,77] The reduction in PVR that occurs with nitroglycerin is proportional to the baseline PVR. By decreasing PVR, RV output increases, allowing maintenance of blood pressure despite systemic vasodilation. However, if PVR is only slightly increased at baseline, the venodilating effect of nitroglycerin predominates, reducing left ventricle preload and CO. Nitroglycerin is effective in patients with pulmonary hypertension secondary to chronic left heart failure.[50] The major limitation in the use of nitroglycerin and the related nitrates for therapy of chronic pulmonary hypertension is the rapid development of tolerance.[78] Similar to other vasodilators, nitroglycerin will inhibit hypoxic pulmonary vasoconstriction and worsen gas exchange in patients with acute respiratory distress syndrome.[79] The excess systemic vasodilation and the adverse effects on ventilation/perfusion matching do not occur when nitroglycerin or related nitrates are administered by inhalation.[80-82] The degree of systemic and pulmonary vasodilation that occur in response to nitroglycerin and the related nitrovasodilators are dependent on endogenous NO production; therefore, inhibition (endogenous or exogenous) of NO synthase potentiates the effects of the nitrovasodilators.[83]

Hydralazine is a direct systemic arterial vasodilator that works primarily by activating guanylyl cyclase. The arterial vasodilation may produce reflex sympathetic activation with positive inotropic and chronotropic effects. The increased CO may increase PAP if pulmonary vasodilation does not occur. Hydralazine was one of the first vasodilators to be used in pulmonary hypertension.[84-86] However, hydralazine produces potent systemic vasodilation, which may result in severe hypotension and tachycardia.[76,87] As a result, hydralazine has not proven to be useful in patients with pulmonary hypertension.

Inhaled Nitric Oxide

NO is an endogenous vasodilator and inhibitor of platelet aggregation. NO is produced by the vascular endothelium, primarily in response to increased shear stress.[10] NO diffuses into the adjacent vascular smooth muscle cells, activating guanylyl cyclase, resulting in increased cGMP. NO also causes inhibition of phosphoinositide 3-kinase and cyclooxygenase and impairs calcium flux across cell membranes. Intravenous nitrovasodilators such as nitroprusside produce pulmonary and systemic vasodilation caused by release of NO in both the pulmonary and systemic circulations. In contrast, INO produces selective pulmonary vasodilation.[9,10,88,89] INO is lipid-soluble and diffuses across cell membranes from the alveoli into pulmonary vascular smooth muscle. INO diffuses from the alveoli to the adjacent pulmonary vascular smooth where it activates guanylyl cyclase, thereby increasing intracellular cGMP and producing pulmonary vasodilation. INO does not produce systemic vasodilation because any NO that is absorbed into the pulmonary circulation is inactivated by binding to hemoglobin. Patients with pulmonary hypertension have decreased endogenous NO production.[90-92] In addition to its beneficial effects on pulmonary hypertension, INO may improve ventilation/perfusion matching in patients with lung disease.[9,93-95] Unlike intravenous vasodilators that tend to increase blood flow to poorly ventilated alveoli, inhaled vasodilators are preferentially distributed to ventilated alveoli. By increasing blood flow to ventilated alveoli, there will be an improvement in ventilation/perfusion matching and a resulting improvement in gas exchange.[93] Although INO improves

oxygenation and decreases pulmonary hypertension in the acute respiratory distress syndrome, randomized studies have not demonstrated sustained improvement or improved outcome.[93,94,96-98]

In general, the INO dose-response curve in patients with pulmonary hypertension demonstrates maximal responses at doses of 10 ppm or less and clinically significant responses at doses of 10 to 100 ppb.[10,95] These doses of NO are physiologic because similar concentrations normally occur in the trachea as a result of production of NO by bacteria in the nasal mucosa and sinuses. In clinical practice, tracheal intubation bypasses the nasopharynx and sinuses and thereby prevents its inhalation.

INO is approved for therapy of pulmonary hypertension and hypoxemic respiratory failure in persistent pulmonary hypertension of the newborn (PPHN; persistent fetal circulation). In PPHN, pulmonary vasoconstriction and abnormal muscularization of peripheral pulmonary vessels lead to decreased pulmonary blood flow and increased anatomic shunting of desaturated venous blood across the ductus arteriosus or foramen ovale. The efficacy of INO in avoiding extracorporeal membrane oxygenation or death has been proven in multicenter, randomized, controlled trials.[88,99,100] NO doses used varied from 5 to 20 ppm to as high as 80 ppm. A response rate in these trials was usually more than 50%. In the Neonatal Inhaled Nitric Oxide Study trial, the effects of 20 ppm INO were investigated in more than 200 full-term and nearly full-term neonates with hypoxic respiratory failure; significant improvement in oxygenation and reduced need for extracorporeal membrane oxygenation (39% NO group vs. 54% control) were demonstrated.[101] There was no apparent effect on mortality rates.

INO effectively decreases perioperative pulmonary hypertension in multiple settings, particularly after CPB when PVR may be increased because of pulmonary endothelial dysfunction.[47,51,102] Selective pulmonary vasodilatation with maintenance of systemic blood pressure and therefore coronary perfusion pressure make INO an ideal agent in the setting of RV failure with increased PVR. INO may be useful in patients with allograft dysfunction after lung transplantation because NO may decrease pulmonary hypertension, improve ventilation/perfusion mismatch, and decrease ischemia/reperfusion lung injury. In pediatric cardiac surgery, INO has been used for preoperative assessment of PVR reactivity, diagnosis of anatomic obstructions leading to pulmonary hypertension, treatment of pulmonary hypertension when weaning from CPB, and after surgery.[103]

INO is an ideal agent for screening for pulmonary vascular reactivity in patients with pulmonary hypertension, because it may produce rapid, maximal pulmonary vasodilation without systemic vasodilation.[55,56,89] In patients with pulmonary hypertension, acute administration of INO can improve exercise tolerance.[104] Chronic INO has been used in selected patient populations for chronic pulmonary hypertension. Potential beneficial effects of INO include selective pulmonary vasodilatation, inhibition of platelet aggregation, and inhibition of cell proliferation. Pulsed delivery of INO through nasal prongs has been used for chronic outpatient use.[14,17]

Approximately one third of patients with perioperative pulmonary hypertension or acute respiratory failure have little or no response to INO. Possible explanations include an unreactive pulmonary circulation, rapid inactivation of NO, abnormalities in the guanylyl cyclase system, or rapid metabolism of cGMP. Inhibition of cGMP phosphodiesterase with zaprinast or dipyridamole can increase the frequency, the magnitude, and the duration of response to INO. Combination of INO with an intravenous vasodilator that is not dependent on cGMP may produce additive pulmonary vasodilator effects.[106,107] Because of the fixed pulmonary hypertension, INO produces acute pulmonary vasodilation in only a small minority of patients with PPH. However, chronic INO may produce pulmonary vascular remodeling in some of these patients.[14,105]

Adverse effects of INO include platelet inhibition and rebound hypoxemia and pulmonary hypertension. In patients with chronic obstructive pulmonary disease, INO can produce a paradoxical worsening of oxygenation by reversal of hypoxic pulmonary vasoconstriction in lung areas with low V/Q ratios. In patients with LV dysfunction, INO has been associated with episodes of LV failure and pulmonary edema. This occurs because the decrease of RV afterload augments pulmonary venous return to the left heart, thereby increasing LV filling pressures and precipitating LV failure. Multiple authors have reported severe rebound hypoxemia and pulmonary hypertension on INO withdrawal. The reasons for this phenomenon are not clear but may be related to suppression of endogenous NO synthase activity or down-regulation of guanylyl cyclase and subsequent mechanisms. Several methods are described to avoid clinical deterioration from this rebound effect. The easiest method is to withdraw INO after the patient has significantly improved and to increase the fraction of inspired oxygen (FIO_2) before discontinuation of INO. Dipyridamole, which inhibits phosphodiesterase, can attenuate rebound in patients with pulmonary hypertension. INO can produce toxicity caused by methemoglobin formation from NO, NO_2 production, peroxynitrite ($ONOO^-$)-related lung injury, and surfactant damage. Safe delivery of INO relies on monitoring of NO and NO_2 concentrations, analysis of methemoglobin levels, use of certified NO sources, and minimizing the delivered NO concentration.

Prostacyclin

Prostacyclin (epoprostenol, PGI_2, Flolan [GlaxoSmithKline, Philadelphia, Pa.) is a short-acting (half-life of 2–3 minutes) vasodilator produced by the vascular endothelium in response to increased shear stress. Prostacyclin infusion decreases PAP and PVR in patients with pulmonary hypertension.[46,53,85,108,109] Circulating concentrations of endogenous prostacyclin and prostacyclin synthase lung expression are decreased in patients with PPH.[11] Based on evidence that acute administration of intravenous prostacyclin produces pulmonary vasodilation, in 1984, Higenbottam and colleagues[110] demonstrated that continuous intravenous prostacyclin produced sustained beneficial effects in one patient with pulmonary hypertension. Current studies have demonstrated that continuous intravenous prostacyclin improves exercise tolerance, pulmonary hemodynamics, RV function, neurohumoral status, and survival in both primary and secondary pulmonary hypertension.[110–120] In the first of these reports, Rubin and colleagues[112] report that improvement in pulmonary resistance and CO persisted up to 18 months in patients treated with continuous infusion of prostacyclin, although dose requirements did increase in most cases. Although initial studies focused on chronic therapy in patients with an acute response to prostacyclin, subsequent studies have demonstrated that patients who do not acutely respond to intravenous prostacyclin have improvement after several weeks of chronic prostacyclin therapy. The beneficial chronic effects of prostacyclin may be related to pulmonary vascular remodeling, suggesting that prostacyclin may exert a remodeling effect on the pulmonary vasculature. Prostacyclin is also a potent inhibitor of platelet aggregation, which may explain the therapeutic benefit in patients with pulmonary hypertension secondary to thromboembolic diseases. Continuous intravenous prostacyclin has become standard therapy in patients with both primary and secondary pulmonary hypertension, particularly in patients who do not have an acute vasodilator response and are therefore not candidates for chronic oral calcium channel blocker therapy. Prostacyclin has been used as a long-term therapy in patients with pulmonary hypertension or as a bridge to transplantation.[121] Continuous intravenous infusion of prostacyclin is indicated in patients with pulmonary hypertension with New York Heart Association class III and IV severity. Failure to respond to prostacyclin is currently considered an indication for lung transplantation.[122]

Adverse effects of chronic prostacyclin therapy include systemic hypotension, flushing, jaw pain, gastrointestinal distress, diarrhea, rash, arthralgias, ascites, and life-threatening catheter infections; in addition, pump malfunction may result in ultra-rapid hemodynamic deterioration. Prostacyclin may cause pulmonary edema in patients with veno-occlusive disease because an increased pulmonary blood flow will increase pulmonary capillary pressures when there is venous obstruction. Prostacyclin therapy is not suitable for patients with pulmonary hypertension resulting from pulmonary parenchymal disease because it may increase intrapulmonary shunting from increased blood flow to poorly ventilated areas.[1]

Because of the difficulties in delivering intravenous prostacyclin, there has been considerable interest in alternative forms of this agent. Mikhail and colleagues[123] demonstrated that inhaled prostacyclin did not decrease systemic arterial pressure and did produce a greater reduction in PVR than either intravenous prostacyclin or INO. Other studies have demonstrated beneficial effects of inhaled prostacyclin.[124,125] Iloprost is a longer acting analog of prostacyclin and is effective in improving pulmonary hemodynamics and symptoms in patients with pulmonary hypertension.[126,127] Hoeper and colleagues used inhaled aerosolized iloprost to treat 24 patients with PPH and demonstrated significant improvements in pulmonary hemodynamics and exercise tolerance.[128] Benefits of inhaled iloprost in primary and secondary pulmonary hypertension have been confirmed in multiple studies.[89,129–131] Inhaled iloprost may have additive effects to intravenous prostacyclin[132] but may not necessarily be as effective during chronic administration.[133] Administration of iloprost requires a special inhalation device to produce particles of appropriate diameter and to prevent waste of the drug. Inhaled iloprost has a short duration of effect and necessitates up to 12 inhalations per day to achieve adequate and consistent effect in some patients.[128,129] Currently, more studies are underway to evaluate iloprost in a randomized, double-blind, placebo-controlled fashion.[134]

McLaughlin and colleagues[135] recently completed a study examining the subcutaneous analogue of prostacyclin, Uniprost (UT-15; Remodulin; United Therapeutics, Silver Spring, Md.), and reported improved exercise capacity and pulmonary hemodynamics compared with placebo. Uniprost is infused subcutaneously by portable pumps, similar to those used for administering insulin. The pump must be refilled every 3 days but requires no other management.[122] The most frequent side effect was pain and redness at the infusion site, which limited the dosage used in some patients and precluded the use of Uniprost in 8% of patients studied. Beraprost, an orally active and chemically stable analog of prostacyclin, was shown in an nonblinded, noncontrolled dosing study to improve pulmonary hemodynamics and New York Heart Association functional status in a group of 34 patients.[136] Beraprost may also improve survival rates for patients with PPH.[137]

Endothelin Antagonists

Endothelin-1 is a powerful vasoconstrictor and proliferative agent.[134] Patients with pulmonary hypertension may have enhanced pulmonary production and increased circulating concentrations of endothelin-1.[12,14,90] Intravenous infusion of bosentan, an endothelin receptor antagonist, produces pulmonary vasodilation in patients with pulmonary hypertension. In one study, oral bosentan improved pulmonary hemodynamics and increased exercise tolerance in patients with pulmonary arterial hypertension.[138] In the larger BREATHE-1 trial, which included 213 patients, bosentan at a dose of either 125 or 250 mg orally twice daily increased 6-minute walk times and delayed the time to clinical worsening. Because the greater dose resulted in more significant liver function test abnormalities, the study recommended 125 mg twice daily as the optimal dose. Bosentan was approved by the Food and Drug Administration in November 2001.

Phosphodiesterase Inhibitors

Nitrovasodilators produce pulmonary vasodilation by activating guanylyl cyclase and thereby increasing cGMP; prostacyclin, adenosine, and isoproterenol produce vasodilation by activating adenylyl cyclase and increasing cyclic adenosine monophosphate. Phosphodiesterases are enzymes that degrade cyclic nucleotides. The type V phosphodiesterase enzyme is selective for cGMP and is found in high concentrations in the lung. PDE V inhibitors therefore have the potential to produce pulmonary vasodilation when used as a single agent and to potentiate the magnitude and prolong the effect of pulmonary nitrovasodilators. The effects of phosphodiesterase (PDE) inhibitors have been demonstrated as selective pulmonary vasodilators in experimental pulmonary hypertension.[139–142] Sildenafil is a PDE V inhibitor

that is approved for the treatment of male erectile dysfunction. Sildenafil can improve symptoms and hemodynamics in PPH,[143] has additive effects with inhaled iloprost,[144] increases the response to INO,[145] and facilitates weaning of INO.[146]

Future Therapies

Future therapy of the patient with pulmonary hypertension may involve novel pulmonary vasodilators such as potassium channel openers, antiproliferative agents such as triptolide, rapamycin, and the statins,[147,148] and gene therapy to increase the production of pulmonary vasodilator substances (NO synthase or prostacyclin synthase gene therapy)[149,150] or to alter vascular proliferation.

References

1. Gaine S: Pulmonary hypertension. JAMA 284:3160, 2000.
2. Rubin LJ: Therapy of pulmonary hypertension: Targeting pathogenic mechanisms with selective treatment delivery. Crit Care Med 29:1086, 2001.
3. Gaine SP, Rubin LJ: Primary pulmonary hypertension. Lancet 29:719, 1998.
4. Klings ES, Farber HW: Current management of primary pulmonary hypertension. Drugs 61:1945, 2001.
5. Weinberger B, Weiss K, Heck DE, et al: Pharmacologic therapy of persistent pulmonary hypertension of the newborn. Pharmacol Ther 89:67, 2001.
6. Rich S (ed): Executive summary from the World Symposium on Primary Pulmonary. Available at: www.who.int/ncd/cvd/pph.html/, 1998.
7. Rodriguez RM, Pearl RG: Pulmonary hypertension and major surgery. Anesth Analg 87:812, 1998.
8. Chen YF, Oparil S: Endothelial dysfunction in the pulmonary vascular bed. Am J Med Sci 320:223, 2000.
9. Steudel W, Hurford WE, Zapol WM: Inhaled nitric oxide: Basic biology and clinical applications. Anesthesiology 91:1090, 1999.
10. Arnal JF, Dinh-Xuan AT, Pueyo M, et al: Endothelium-derived nitric oxide and vascular physiology and pathology. Cell Mol Life Sci 55:1078, 1999.
11. Christman BW, McPherson CD, Newman JH, et al: An imbalance between the excretion of thromboxane and prostacyclin metabolites in pulmonary hypertension. N Engl J Med 327:70, 1992.
12. Stewart DJ, Levy RD, Cernacek P: Increased plasma endothelin-1 in pulmonary hypertension: Marker or mediator of disease? Ann Intern Med 114:464, 1991.
13. Haynes WG, Webb DJ: Endothelin as a regulator of cardiovascular function in health and disease. J Hypertens 16:1081, 1998.
14. Giaid A, Yanagisawa M, Langleben D et al: Expression of endothelin-1 in the lungs of patients with pulmonary hypertension. N Engl J Med 328:1732, 1993.
15. MacLean MR, Herve P, Eddahibi S, et al: 5-hydroxytryptamine and the pulmonary circulation: Receptors, transporters and relevance to pulmonary arterial hypertension. Br J Pharmacol 131:161, 2000.
16. Egermayer P, Town GI, Peacock AJ: Role of serotonin in the pathogenesis of acute and chronic pulmonary hypertension. Thorax 54:161, 1999.
17. Salvi SS: Alpha1-adrenergic hypothesis for pulmonary hypertension. Chest 115:1708, 1999.
18. Fischer LG, Hollmann MW, Horstman DJ, et al: Cyclooxygenase inhibitors attenuate bradykinin-induced vasoconstriction in septic isolated rat lungs. Anesth Analg 90:625, 2000.

19. Dawson CA, Linehan JH, Rickaby DA, et al: Effect of vasoconstriction on longitudinal distribution of pulmonary vascular pressure and volume. J Appl Physiol 70:1607, 1991.

20. Ducas J, Duval D, Dasilva H, et al: Treatment of canine pulmonary hypertension: Effects of norepinephrine and isoproterenol on pulmonary vascular pressure-flow characteristics. Circulation 75:235, 1987.

21. Mathew R, Altura BM, et al: Physiology and pathophysiology of pulmonary circulation. Microcirc Endothelium Lymphatics 6:211, 1990.

22. Semenza GL: Hypoxia-inducible factor 1: Oxygen homeostasis and disease pathophysiology. Trends Mol Med 7:345, 2001.

23. Shimoda LA, Sham JS, Sylvester JT: Altered pulmonary vasoreactivity in the chronically hypoxic lung. Physiol Res 49:549, 2000.

24. von Euler US, Liljestrand G: Observations on the pulmonary arterial blood pressure in the cat. Acta Physiol Scand 12:301, 1946.

25. Weissmann N, Grimminger F, Olschewski A, et al: Hypoxic pulmonary vasoconstriction: A multifactorial response? Am J Physiol Lung Cell Mol Physiol 281:L314, 2001.

26. Ward JP, Aaronson PI: Mechanisms of hypoxic pulmonary vasoconstriction: Can anyone be right? Respir Physiol 115:261, 1999.

27. Dumas JP, Bardou M, Goirand F, et al: Hypoxic pulmonary vasoconstriction. Gen Pharmacol 33:289, 1999.

28. Coppock EA, Martens JR, Tamkun MM, et al: Molecular basis of hypoxia-induced pulmonary vasoconstriction: Role of voltage-gated K+ channels. Am J Physiol Lung Cell Mol Physiol 281:L1, 2001.

29. Archer SL, Weir EK, Reeve HL, et al: Molecular identification of O2 sensors and O2-sensitive potassium channels in the pulmonary circulation. Adv Exp Med Biol 475:219, 2000.

30. McCulloch KM, Osipenko ON, Gurney AM, et al: Oxygen-sensing potassium currents in pulmonary artery. Gen Pharmacol 32:403, 1999.

31. Madden JA, Vadula MS, Kurup VP: Effects of hypoxia and other vasoactive agents on pulmonary and cerebral artery smooth muscle cells. Am J Physiol 263:L384, 1992.

32. Siegel LC, Pearl RG: Measurement of the longitudinal distribution of pulmonary vascular resistance from pulmonary artery occlusion pressure profiles. Anesthesiology 68:305, 1988.

33. Marshall BE, Clarke WR, Costarino AT, et al: The dose-response relationship for hypoxic pulmonary vasoconstriction. Respir Physiol 96:231, 1994.

34. Pierson DJ: Pathophysiology and clinical effects of chronic hypoxia. Respir Care 45:39, 2000.

35. Tarpy SP, Celli BR: Long-term oxygen therapy. N Engl J Med 14:710, 1995.

36. Hanson CW 3rd, Marshall BE, Frasch HF, et al: Causes of hypercarbia with oxygen therapy in patients with chronic obstructive pulmonary disease. Crit Care Med 24:23, 1996.

37. Fedullo PF, Auger WR, Kerr KM, et al: Chronic thromboembolic pulmonary hypertension. N Engl J Med 345:1465, 2001.

38. D'Alonzo GE, Barst RJ, Ayres SM, et al: Survival in patients with primary pulmonary hypertension. Results from a national prospective registry. Ann Intern Med 115:343, 1991.

39. Miyamoto S, Nagaya N, Satoh T, et al: Clinical correlates and prognostic significance of six-minute walk test in patients with primary pulmonary hypertension. Comparison with cardiopulmonary exercise testing. Am J Respir Crit Care Med 161:487, 2000.

40. Belenkie I, Smith ER, Tyberg JV, et al: Ventricular interaction: From bench to bedside. Ann Med 33:236, 2001.

41. Riedel B: The pathophysiology and management of perioperative pulmonary hypertension with specific emphasis on the period following cardiac surgery. Int Anesthesiol Clin 37:55, 1999.

42. Fuster V, Steele PM, Edwards WD, Gersh BJ, et al: Primary pulmonary hypertension: Natural history and the importance of thrombosis. Circulation 70:580, 1984.

43. Rich S, Kaufmann E, Levy PS: The effect of high doses of calcium-channel blockers on survival in primary pulmonary hypertension. N Engl J Med 327:76, 1992.

44. Pearl RG: Adenosine produces pulmonary vasodilation in the perfused rabbit lung via an adenosine A2 receptor. Anesth Analg 79:46, 1994.

45. Nootens M, Schrader B, Kaufmann E, et al: Comparative acute effects of adenosine and prostacyclin in primary pulmonary hypertension. Chest 107:54, 1995.

46. Palevsky HI, Long W, Crow J, et al: Prostacyclin and acetylcholine as screening agents for acute pulmonary vasodilator responsiveness in primary pulmonary hypertension. Circulation 82:2018, 1990.

47. Schmid ER, Burki C, Engel MH, et al: Inhaled nitric oxide versus intravenous vasodilators in severe pulmonary hypertension after cardiac surgery. Anesth Analg 89:1108, 1999.

48. Tritapepe L, Voci P, Cogliati AA, et al: Successful weaning from cardiopulmonary bypass with central venous prostaglandin E1 and left atrial norepinephrine infusion in patients with acute pulmonary hypertension. Crit Care Med 27:2180, 1999.

49. Pearl RG, Rosenthal MH, Schroeder JS, et al: Acute hemodynamic effects of nitroglycerin in pulmonary hypertension. Ann Intern Med 99:9, 1983.

50. Bundgaard H, Boesgaard S, Mortensen SA, et al: Effect of nitroglycerin in patients with increased pulmonary vascular resistance undergoing cardiac transplantation. Scand Cardiovasc J 31:339, 1997.

51. Kieler-Jensen N, Lundin S, Ricksten SE: Vasodilator therapy after heart transplantation: Effects of inhaled nitric oxide and intravenous prostacyclin, prostaglandin E1, and sodium nitroprusside. J Heart Lung Transplant 14:436, 1995.

52. Murali S, Uretsky BF, Reddy PS, et al: Reversibility of pulmonary hypertension in congestive heart failure patients evaluated for cardiac transplantation: Comparative effects of various pharmacologic agents. Am Heart J 122:1375, 1991.

53. Raffy O, Azarian R, Brenot F, et al: Clinical significance of the pulmonary vasodilator response during short-term infusion of prostacyclin in primary pulmonary hypertension. Circulation 93:484, 1996.

54. Schrader BJ, Inbar S, Kaufmann L, et al: Comparison of the effects of adenosine and nifedipine in pulmonary hypertension. J Am Coll Cardiol 19:1060, 1992.

55. Sitbon O, Brenot F, Denjean A, et al: Inhaled nitric oxide as a screening vasodilator agent in primary pulmonary hypertension. A dose-response study and comparison with prostacyclin. Am J Respir Crit Care Med 151:384, 1995.

56. Ricciardi MJ, Knight BP, Martinez FJ, et al: Inhaled nitric oxide in primary pulmonary hypertension: A safe and effective agent for predicting response to nifedipine. J Am Coll Cardiol 32:1068, 1998.

57. Clusin WT, Anderson ME: Calcium channel blockers: Current controversies and basic mechanisms of action. Adv Pharmacol 46:253, 1999.

58. Rich S, Ganz R, Levy PS: Comparative actions of hydralazine, nifedipine and amrinone in primary pulmonary hypertension. Am J Cardiol 52:1104, 1983.

59. Rich S, Kaufmann E: High dose titration of calcium channel blocking agents for primary pulmonary hypertension: Guidelines for short-term drug testing. J Am Coll Cardiol 18:1323, 1991.

60. Rich S, Brundage BH: High-dose calcium channel-blocking therapy for primary pulmonary hypertension: Evidence for long-term reduction in pulmonary arterial pressure and regression of right ventricular hypertrophy. Circulation 76:135, 1987.

61. Malik AS, Warshafsky S, Lehrman S, et al: Meta-analysis of the long-term effect of nifedipine for pulmonary hypertension. Arch Intern Med 157:621, 1997.

62. Alpert MA, Pressly TA, Mukerji V, et al: Acute and long-term effects of nifedipine on pulmonary and systemic hemodynamics in patients with pulmonary hypertension associated with diffuse systemic sclerosis, the CREST syndrome and mixed connective tissue disease. Am J Cardiol 68:1687, 1991.

63. O'Brien JT, Hill JA, Pepine CJ: Sustained benefit of verapamil in pulmonary hypertension with progressive systemic sclerosis. Am Heart J 109:380, 1985.

64. Gassner A, Sommer G, Fridrich L: Differential therapy with calcium antagonists in pulmonary hypertension secondary to COPD. Chest 98:829, 1990.

65. Clozel JP, Delorme N, Battistella P: Hemodynamic effects of intravenous diltiazem in hypoxic pulmonary vasoconstriction. Chest 91:171, 1987.

66. Crevey BJ, Dantzker DR, Bower JS, et al: Hemodynamic and gas exchange effects of intravenous diltiazem in patients with pulmonary hypertension. Am J Cardiol 49:578, 1982.

67. Brzostek T, Dubiel JP, Zmudka K: Influence of verapamil and oxygen on pulmonary hypertension and right ventricular function. Cor Vasa 30:115, 1988.

68. Woodmansey PA, O'Toole L, Channer KS, et al: Acute pulmonary vasodilatory properties of amlodipine in humans with pulmonary hypertension. Heart 75:171, 1996.

69. Packer M, Medina N, Yushak M: Adverse hemodynamic and clinical effects of calcium channel blockade in pulmonary hypertension sec-

ondary to obliterative pulmonary vascular disease. J Am Coll Cardiol 4:890, 1984.

70. Cockrill BA, Kacmarek RM, Fifer MA, et al: Comparison of the effects of nitric oxide, nitroprusside, and nifedipine on hemodynamics and right ventricular contractility in patients with chronic pulmonary hypertension. Chest 119:128, 2001.

71. Packer M, Medina N, Yushak M, et al: Detrimental effects of verapamil in patients with primary pulmonary hypertension. Br Heart J 52:106, 1984.

72. Kennedy TP, Michael JR, Huang CK, et al: Nifedipine inhibits hypoxic pulmonary vasoconstriction during rest and exercise in patients with chronic obstructive pulmonary disease. A controlled double-blind study. Am Rev Respir Dis 129:544, 1984.

73. Costard-Jackle A, Fowler MB: Influence of preoperative pulmonary artery pressure on mortality after heart transplantation: Testing of potential reversibility of pulmonary hypertension with nitroprusside is useful in defining a high risk group. J Am Coll Cardiol 19:48, 1992.

74. Friederich JA, Butterworth JF 4th: Sodium nitroprusside: Twenty years and counting. Anesth Analg 81:152, 1995.

75. Adnot S, Radermacher P, Andrivet P, et al: Effects of sodium-nitroprusside and urapidil on gas exchange and ventilation-perfusion relationships in patients with congestive heart failure. Eur Respir J 4:69, 1991.

76. McLean RF, Prielipp RC, Rosenthal MH, et al: Vasodilator therapy in microembolic porcine pulmonary hypertension. Anesth Analg 71:35, 1990.

77. Packer M, Halperin JL, Brooks KM, et al: Nitroglycerin therapy in the management of pulmonary hypertensive disorders. Am J Med 76:67, 1984.

78. Parker JD, Parker JO: Nitrate therapy for stable angina pectoris. N Engl J Med 338:520, 1998.

79. Radermacher P, Santak B, Becker H, et al: Prostaglandin E1 and nitroglycerin reduce pulmonary capillary pressure but worsen ventilation-perfusion distributions in patients with adult respiratory distress syndrome. Anesthesiology 70:601, 1989.

80. Gong F, Shiraishi H, Kikuchi Y, et al: Inhalation of nebulized nitroglycerin in dogs with experimental pulmonary hypertension induced by U46619. Pediatr Int 42:255, 2000.

81. Adrie C, Ichinose F, Holzmann A, et al: Pulmonary vasodilation by nitric oxide gas and prodrug aerosols in acute pulmonary hypertension. J Appl Physiol 84:435, 1998.

82. Schutte H, Grimminger F, Otterbein J, et al: Efficiency of aerosolized nitric oxide donor drugs to achieve sustained pulmonary vasodilation. J Pharmacol Exp Ther 282:985, 1997.

83. Kavanagh BP, Thompson JS, Pearl RG: Inhibition of endogenous nitric oxide synthase potentiates nitrovasodilators in experimental pulmonary hypertension. Anesthesiology 85:860, 1996.

84. Rubin LJ, Peter RH: Oral hydralazine therapy for primary pulmonary hypertension. N Engl J Med 302:69, 1980.

85. Groves BM, Rubin LJ, Frosolono MF, et al: A comparison of the acute hemodynamic effects of prostacyclin and hydralazine in primary pulmonary hypertension. Am Heart J 110:1200, 1985.

86. Brent BN, Berger HJ, Matthay RA, et al: Contrasting acute effects of vasodilators (nitroglycerin, nitroprusside, and hydralazine) on right ventricular performance in patients with chronic obstructive pulmonary disease and pulmonary hypertension: A combined radionuclide-hemodynamic study. Am J Cardiol 51:1682, 1983.

87. Packer M, Greenberg B, Massie B, et al: Deleterious effects of hydralazine in patients with pulmonary hypertension. N Engl J Med 306:1326, 1982.

88. Kinsella JP, Abman SH: Clinical approach to inhaled nitric oxide therapy in the newborn with hypoxemia. J Pediatr 136:717, 2000.

89. Hoeper MM, Olschewski H, Ghofrani HA, et al: A comparison of the acute hemodynamic effects of inhaled nitric oxide and aerosolized iloprost in primary pulmonary hypertension. German PPH study group. J Am Coll Cardiol 35:176, 2000.

90. Endo A, Ayusawa M, Minato M, et al: Endogenous nitric oxide and endothelin-1 in persistent pulmonary hypertension of the newborn. Eur J Pediatr 160:217, 2001.

91. Cella G, Bellotto F, Tona F, et al: Plasma markers of endothelial dysfunction in pulmonary hypertension. Chest 120:1226, 2001.

92. Giaid A, Saleh D: Reduced expression of endothelial nitric oxide synthase in the lungs of patients with pulmonary hypertension. N Engl J Med 333:214, 1995.

93. Rossaint R, Falke KJ, Lopez F, et al: Inhaled nitric oxide for the adult respiratory distress syndrome. N Engl J Med 328:399, 1993.

94. Payen DM: Inhaled nitric oxide and acute lung injury. Clin Chest Med 21:519, 2000.

95. Iotti GA, Olivei MC, Palo A, et al: Acute effects of inhaled nitric oxide in adult respiratory distress syndrome. Eur Respir J 12:1164, 1998.

96. Lundin S, Mang H, Smithies M, et al: Inhalation of nitric oxide in acute lung injury: Results of a European multicentre study. The European Study Group of Inhaled Nitric Oxide. Intensive Care Med 25:911, 1999.

97. Sokol J, Jacobs SE, Bohn D: Inhaled nitric oxide for acute hypoxemic respiratory failure in children and adults. Cochrane Database Syst Rev (4):CD002787, 2000.

98. Dellinger PR, Zimmerman JL, Taylor R, et al: Effects of inhaled nitric oxide in patients with acute respiratory distress syndrome: Results of a randomized phase II trial. Crit Care Med 26:23, 1998.

99. Finer NN, Barrington KJ: Nitric oxide for respiratory failure in infants born at or near term (Cochrane Review). Cochrane Database Syst Rev (2):CD000399, 2001.

100. Clark RH, Kueser TJ, Walker MW, et al: Low-dose nitric oxide therapy for persistent pulmonary hypertension of the newborn. Clinical Inhaled Nitric Oxide Research Group. N Engl J Med 342:469, 2000.

101. Inhaled nitric oxide in full-term and nearly full-term infants with hypoxic respiratory failure. The Neonatal Inhaled Nitric Oxide Study Group. N Engl J Med 336:597, 1997.

102. Beck JR, Mongero LB, Kroslowitz, et al: Inhaled nitric oxide improves hemodynamics in patients with acute pulmonary hypertension after high-risk cardiac surgery. Perfusion 14:37, 1999.

103. Russell IA, Zwass MS, Fineman JR, et al: The effects of inhaled nitric oxide on postoperative pulmonary hypertension in infants and children undergoing surgical repair of congenital heart disease. Anesth Analg 87:46, 1998.

104. Hasuda T, Satoh T, Shimouchi A, et al: Improvement in exercise capacity with nitric oxide inhalation in patients with precapillary pulmonary hypertension. Circulation 101:2066, 2000.

105. Perez-Penate G, Julia-Serda G, Pulido-Duque J-M, et al: One year continuous inhaled nitric oxide for primary pulmonary hypertension. Chest 119:970, 2001.

106. Aranda M, Bradford KK, Pearl RG: Continuous therapy with inhaled nitric oxide and intravenous vasodilators during experimental pulmonary hypertension. Anesth Analg 89:152, 1999.

107. Kuhlen R, Walbert E, Frankel P, et al: Combination of inhaled nitric oxide and intravenous prostacyclin for successful treatment of severe pulmonary hypertension in a patient with acute respiratory distress syndrome. Intens Care Med 25:752, 1999.

108. Rubin LJ, Groves BM, Reeves JT, et al: Prostacyclin-induced acute pulmonary vasodilation in primary pulmonary hypertension. Circulation 66:334, 1982.

109. Montalescot G, Drobinski G, Meurin P, et al: Effects of prostacyclin on the pulmonary vascular tone and cardiac contractility of patients with pulmonary hypertension secondary to end-stage heart failure. Am J Cardiol 82:749, 1998.

110. Higenbottam TW, Wheeldon D, Wells FC, et al: Treatment of primary pulmonary hypertension with continuous intravenous epoprostenol (prostacyclin). Lancet I:1046, 1984.

111. Barst RJ, Rubin LJ, Long WA, et al: A comparison of continuous intravenous epoprostenol (prostacyclin) with conventional therapy for primary pulmonary hypertension: The primary pulmonary hypertension study group. N Engl J Med 334:296, 1996.

112. Rubin LJ, Mendoza J, Hood M: Treatment of primary pulmonary hypertension with continuous intravenous prostacyclin (epoprostenol). Ann Intern Med 112:485, 1990.

113. Badesch DB, Tapson VF, McGoon MD, et al: Effects of long-term infusion of prostacyclin on exercise performance in patients with primary pulmonary hypertension. Chest 116:914, 1999.

114. Hinderliter AL, Willis PW 4th, Barst RJ, et al: Effects of long-term infusion of prostacyclin (epoprostenol) on echocardiographic measures of right ventricular structure and function in primary pulmonary hypertension. Primary Pulmonary Hypertension Study Group. Circulation 95:1479, 1997.

115. Rich S, McLaughlin VV: The effects of chronic prostacyclin therapy on cardiac output and symptoms in primary pulmonary hypertension. J Am Coll Cardiol 34:1184, 1999.

116. Barst RJ, Rubin LJ, McGoon MD, et al: Survival in primary pulmonary hypertension with long-term continuous intravenous prostacyclin. Ann Intern Med 121:409, 1994.

117. McLaughlin VV, Genthner DE, Panella MM, et al: Compassionate use of continuous prostacyclin in the management of secondary pulmonary hypertension: A case series. Ann Intern Med 130:740, 1999.

118. Aguilar RV, Farber HW: Epoprostenol (prostacyclin) therapy in HIV-associated pulmonary hypertension. Am J Respir Crit Care Med 162:1846, 2000.

119. Robbins IM, Gaine SP, Schilz R, et al: Epoprostenol for treatment of pulmonary hypertension in patients with systemic lupus erythematosus. Chest 117:14, 2000.

120. Langleben D, Barst RJ, Badesch D, et al: Continuous infusion of epoprostenol improves the net balance between pulmonary endothelin-1 clearance and release in primary pulmonary hypertension. Circulation 99:3266, 1999.

121. Conte JV, Gaine SP, Orens JB, et al: The influence of continuous intravenous prostacyclin therapy for primary pulmonary hypertension on the timing and outcome of transplantation. J Heart Lung Transplant 17:679, 1998.

122. Galie N, Torbicki A: Pulmonary arterial hypertension: New ideas and perspectives. Heart 85:475, 2001.

123. Mikhail G, Gibbs J, Richardson M, et al: An evaluation of nebulized prostacyclin in patients with primary and secondary pulmonary hypertension. Eur Heart J 18:1499, 1997.

124. Haraldsson A, Kieler-Jensen N, Nathorst-Westfelt U, et al: Comparison of inhaled nitric oxide and inhaled aerosolized prostacyclin in the evaluation of heart transplant candidates with elevated pulmonary vascular resistance. Chest 114:780, 1998.

125. Della Rocca G, Coccia C, Costa MG, et al: Inhaled areosolized prostacyclin and pulmonary hypertension during anesthesia for lung transplantation. Transplant Proc 33:1634, 2001.

126. Higenbottam TW, Butt AY, McMahon A, et al: Long term intravenous prostaglandin (epoprostenol or iloprost) for treatment of severe pulmonary hypertension. Heart 80:151, 1998.

127. Higenbottam TW, Butt AY, Dinh-Xaun AT, et al: Treatment of pulmonary hypertension with the continuous infusion of a prostacyclin analogue, iloprost. Heart 79:175, 1998.

128. Hoeper MM, Schwarze M, Ehlerding S, et al: Long-term treatment of primary pulmonary hypertension with aerosolized iloprost, a prostacyclin analogue. N Engl J Med 342:1866, 2000.

129. Olschewski H, Ghofrani HA, Schmehl T, et al: Inhaled iloprost to treat severe pulmonary hypertension: An uncontrolled trial. German PPH Study Group. Ann Intern Med 132:435, 2000.

130. Olschewski H, Ghofrani HA, Walmrath D, et al: Inhaled prostacyclin and iloprost in severe pulmonary hypertension secondary to lung fibrosis. Am J Respir Crit Care Med 160:600, 1999.

131. Machherndl S, Kneussl M, Baumgartner H, et al: Long-term treatment of pulmonary hypertension with aerosolized iloprost. Eur Respir J 17:8, 2001.

132. Petkov V, Ziesche R, Mosgoeller W, et al: Aerosolized iloprost improves pulmonary haemodynamics in patients with primary pulmonary hypertension receiving continuous epoprostenol treatment. Thorax 56:734, 2001.

133. Schenk P, Petkov V, Madl C, et al: Aerosolized iloprost therapy could not replace long-term IV epoprostenol (prostacyclin) administration in severe pulmonary hypertension. Chest 119:296, 2001.

134. Bailey CL, Channick RN, Rubin LJ: A new era in the treatment of primary pulmonary hypertension. Heart 85:251, 2001.

135. McLaughlin VV, Hess DM, Sigman J, et al: Long term effects of UT-15 on hemodynamics and exercise tolerance in primary pulmonary hypertension. Eur Respir J 16:394S, 2000.

136. Vizza CD, Sciomer S, Morelli S, et al: Long term treatment of pulmonary arterial hypertension with beraprost, an oral prostacyclin analogue. Heart 86:661, 2001.

137. Nagaya N, Uematsu M, Okano Y, et al: Effect of orally active prostacyclin analogue on survival of outpatients with primary pulmonary hypertension. J Am Coll Cardiol 342:1188, 1999.

138. Channick RN, Simonneau G, Robbins IM: Effects of the dual endothelin receptor antagonist bosentan in patients with pulmonary hypertension: A placebo-controlled study. Circulation 98:1400, 1998.

139. Nagamine J, Hill LL, Pearl RG: Combined therapy with zaprinast and inhaled nitric oxide abolishes hypoxic pulmonary hypertension. Crit Care Med 28:2420, 2000.

140. Weimann J, Ullrich R, Hromi J, et al: Sildenafil is a pulmonary vasodilator in awake lambs with acute pulmonary hypertension. Anesthesiology 92:1702, 2000.

141. Schermuly RT, Ghofrani HA, Enke B, et al: Low-dose systemic phosphodiesterase inhibitors amplify the pulmonary vasodilatory response to inhaled prostacyclin in experimental pulmonary hypertension. Am J Respir Crit Care Med 160:1500, 1999.

142. Zhao L, Mason NA, Morrell NW, et al: Sildenafil inhibits hypoxia-induced pulmonary hypertension. Circulation 104:424, 2001.

143. Abrams D, Schulze-Neick I, Magee AG: Sildenafil as a selective pulmonary vasodilator in childhood primary pulmonary hypertension. Heart 84:E4, 2000.

144. Wilkens H, Guth A, Konig J, et al: Effect of inhaled iloprost plus oral sildenafil in patients with primary pulmonary hypertension. Circulation 104:1218, 2001.

145. Bigatello LM, Hess D, Dennehy KC, et al: Sildenafil can increase the response to inhaled nitric oxide. Anesthesiology 92:1827, 2000.

146. Mychaskiw G, Sachdev V, Heath BJ: Sildenafil (viagra) facilitates weaning of inhaled nitric oxide following placement of a biventricular-assist device. J Clin Anesth 13:218, 2001.

147. Nishimura T, Faul JL, Berry GJ: 40-O-(2-hydroxyethyl)-rapamycin attenuates pulmonary arterial hypertension and neointimal formation in rats. Am J Respir Crit Care Med 163:498, 2001.

148. Faul JL, Nishimura T, Berry GJ, et al: Triptolide attenuates pulmonary arterial hypertension and neointimal formation in rats. Am J Respir Crit Care Med 162:2252, 2000.

149. Champion HC, Bivalacqua TJ, D'Souza FM, et al: Gene transfer of endothelial nitric oxide synthase to the lung of the mouse in vivo. Effect on agonist-induced and flow-mediated vascular responses. Circ Res 84:1422, 1999.

150. Nagaya N, Yokoyama C, Kyotani S, et al: Gene transfer of human prostacyclin synthase ameliorates monocrotaline-induced pulmonary hypertension in rats. Circulation 102:2005, 2000.

42

Diuretics

Susan Garwood, MBChB, BSc, FRCA • Terri G. Monk, MD

Diuretics are used to increase the rate of urine formation and to adjust the composition of body fluids through the excretion of excess salts and ions by selective filtration in the kidney.[1,2] The earliest diuretics were natural substances such as caffeine, urea, sarsaparilla, theophylline, and theobromine.[3] It is believed that during the Paleolithic age humans discovered that caffeine-containing drinks could be prepared from the seeds and bark of various plants.[4] Ancient Egyptian medical papyri document that juniper berries were used for their mild diuretic action.[5] However, these natural diuretic agents were generally weakly effective and possessed unwanted side effects.[3]

The discovery of mercurial diuretics in 1919 introduced the era of modern diuretic therapy.[6] A young medical student in Vienna, A. Vogl, administered novasurol, a mercury derivative, to a young female patient with congenital syphilis and he observed that it increased urine output.[7] This was the beginning of mercurial drug use for the treatment of edema. During the next 30 years, hundreds of potent and effective diuretics were synthesized and physicians would never again be satisfied with the weak diuretics provided by nature.[3] The second half of the 20th century saw further advances in diuretic therapy including the development of carbonic anhydrase inhibitors, potassium-retaining diuretics, and nondiuretic ion transport modulators.[4,8,9]

Mechanisims of Action

Most diuretics act at specific segments of the nephron, the segment being determined by the mechanism of action and the distribution of the target sites along the nephron. This conveniently divides diuretics into a small number of classes of drugs, depending on their site of action. In this chapter,

the mechanisms of drug action, pharmacology, and practical aspects of drug administration are described for each class of diuretic. (For a discussion of renal physiology see Chapter 21.)

Osmotic Diuretics

Preclinical Pharmacology

Osmotic diuretics tend to be nonelectrolytes that are freely filtered by the glomerulus and are minimally reabsorbed. Mannitol stands as the archetypical osmotic diuretic, but others are clinically used and include urea, glycerin, and isosorbide. However, any nonabsorbed or poorly absorbed solute that exceeds its transport maximum can also act as an osmotic diuretic. Thus in hyperglycemia, once the transport maximum for glucose has been surpassed, an osmotic diuresis will ensue, demarking one of the hallmark symptoms of diabetes mellitus.

The primary sites for the action of osmotic diuretics are located in the segments of the nephron that are highly permeable to water: the proximal tubule and the thin descending part of the loop of Henle.[1,10] Water and solute reabsorption are coupled in these segments so that isotonicity is maintained, with the tubular fluid having the same tonicity as the interstitial fluid. In the presence of a nonreabsorbable osmotic diuretic, which increases the tonicity of the tubular fluid, an iso-osmotic fluid is achieved by retention of water and reabsorption of sodium from the tubular lumen. Therefore the clinical effect of administering mannitol is to increase urinary flow rate along with only a modest increase in natriuresis. Mannitol effectively causes an expansion of extracellular volume[11] with consequent increases in the renal tubular flow.[12] It has been shown to vasodilate afferent arterioles[13] and to increase renal blood flow (RBF),[14] intratubular pressure,[15] and glomerular filtration rate (GFR).[14] There is a preferential shift of RBF toward the medulla,[15] with medullary washout and the production of dilute urine. Other mechanisms of action attributed to mannitol include increased GFR, increased RBF, reduced cellular injury (swelling) during ischemia, prevention of tubular obstruction from cellular debris, and a degree of cellular protection.

The effects of mannitol are complex and related to actions not specific to the kidney. Because of its hypertonicity, mannitol extracts water from the intracellular space, leading to an increase in plasma volume and a reduction in hematocrit.[11] Infusion of mannitol is therefore accompanied by a decrease in arteriolar plasma oncotic pressure. Considering the determinants of glomerular filtration pressure (Fig. 42–1), this leads to an increase in GFR. Administration of mannitol to the hypoperfused rat kidney results in a vasodilatory response[13] that is inhibited by the prior administration of cyclo-oxygenase inhibitors, suggesting the response is mediated by prostaglandins. In fact, mannitol increases the excretion of prostaglandin E_2 in animal preparations.[16] The increased RBF secondary to the vasodilatory response and the increased plasma volume also enhances GFR (see Fig. 42–1). The effect of mannitol on RBF has also been attributed to release of atrial natriuretic peptide (ANP)[17] and to a decrease in renin production.[18]

The reduction in tubular obstruction that occurs after the administration of mannitol may be secondary to increased flow in the distal tubules and flushing out of cellular debris, but may also be a consequence of direct cellular protection. Schrier and colleagues investigated the effects of mannitol at the subcellular level in a dog model of renal ischemia.[19] In control dogs, renal ischemia produced cellular swelling associated with reduced mitochondrial adenosine triphosphate (ATP) and excessive accumulation of intramitochondrial calcium. In contrast, in dogs pretreated with mannitol, cellular respiration was preserved, with near normal levels of ATP, no mitochondrial sequestration of calcium, and normal cellular size and structure. Mannitol is also a scavenger of oxygen free radicals,[19] which have been implicated in the mechanism of renal ischemic injury; this may prevent cellular swelling and thus reduce tubular obstruction.[20] Further cellular protection may be afforded because mannitol reduces reabsorption of solute and water in the proximal tubule, sodium chloride in the thick ascending limb of the loop of Henle, and water in the collecting duct, all of which are energy demanding; mannitol may therefore preserve cellular integrity by maintaining a better oxygen balance by decreasing demand in times of ischemic stress.

Mannitol has been investigated in animal studies since the 1960s and has been successful as a renal protectant during a number of experimental conditions mimicking renal ischemia, namely renal artery occlusion or the infusion of high doses of vasoconstrictors.[21,22] It has proven to be protective particularly when given before the onset of ischemia.[22] There is also evidence that mannitol protects the kidneys when given after the insult, with the degree of protection waning with the increase in time between ischemia and administration.[22]

Clinical Pharmacology

Because mannitol is an old drug that has been in clinical use for decades, it suffers from an unfortunate lack of rigorous scientific investigation and much of its use relies on dogma. Mannitol is widely used in renal protection protocols in vascular and cardiac surgery, in transplantation surgery, and in nephrotoxic situations. The successes of the preclinical studies have not been duplicated convincingly in human trials, with mixed results depending on the particular situation.

The early reports of the use of mannitol in aortic surgery suggested a beneficial effect, but the evidence for this was based on uncontrolled data. Urine output was improved and hemodynamics appeared to be more stable.[23] Although a brisk diuresis is generally thought to be a sign of renal preservation, it has been demonstrated that intraoperative urine output per se is not an accurate predictor of renal function in the postoperative period.[24] Nevertheless, maintenance of urine output does allow for easier patient management, in terms of fluid balance and blood product administration. More recent studies conducted in a controlled and randomized manner demonstrate that neither serum creatinine nor creatinine clearance is improved after mannitol administration in aortic surgery.[25,26]

Mannitol is frequently used in cardiac surgery, either administered to the patient as an infusion or bolus or as part of the cardiopulmonary bypass prime. Fisher and colleagues[27] conducted a prospective randomized placebo-controlled trial of 10, 20, and 30 g mannitol in the cardiopulmonary bypass prime. Patients given the greater dose had significantly greater diuresis that was maintained longer into the postbypass period, even after the mannitol had been cleared from the circulation.[27] There is no question that mannitol behaves as an excellent diuretic in cardiac surgery, but the evidence for a renal protective effect is lacking. Ip-Yam and colleagues randomized patients to receive either placebo or 0.5 g/kg mannitol in the prime. Although diuresis was improved, other measures of renal glomerular or tubular function were unaffected.[28]

One area in which mannitol has had more success both as a diuretic and a renal protective agent is in renal transplant surgery. The incidence of acute renal failure is less in patients given mannitol before the revascularization of the graft.[29]

Glomerular filtration rate (GFR)

$$GFR = kS[(P_{GC} - P_T) - (p_{GC} - p_T)]$$

where   k   = capillary permeability
      S   = size of the capillary bed
      P_{GC} = mean hydrostatic pressure in glomerular capillaries
      P_T = mean hydrostatic pressure in tubule
      p_{GC} = osmotic pressure of plasma in glomerular capillaries
      p_T = osmotic pressure of filtrate in tubule

Figure 42–1. Determinants of glomerular filtration rate (GFR).

Until recently, mannitol was used routinely in the angiography suite for patients with or at risk for renal dysfunction. However, Solomon and colleagues noted in a prospective, randomized, placebo-controlled trial that mannitol is actually less effective than saline in preventing radiocontrast-induced decrements in renal function.[30]

Practical Aspects of Drug Administration

Mannitol administration often results in a brisk and prolonged diuresis, to such an extent that volume replacement is necessary. It may also be accompanied by hypokalemia. Patients who are given more than 1g/kg mannitol in the cardiopulmonary bypass prime are invariably volume and potassium depleted in the postoperative period.

Because mannitol is rapidly redistributed, it may paradoxically cause pulmonary or cerebral edema by translocation of fluid into the intracellular space. It should therefore be administered with extreme caution in patients with poor left ventricular function or prior history of congestive heart failure, head injury, or intracranial mass.

Loop Diuretics

Preclinical Pharmacology

As the name suggests, the main site of action for this class of diuretics is the loop of Henle, in particular the medullary thick ascending limb (mTAL; Fig. 42-2). The thick ascending limb reabsorbs 10% to 15% of the total filtered load of sodium chloride. Reabsorption of sodium across the luminal membrane is achieved by the electroneutral $Na^+/K^+/2Cl^-$ cotransport system. The continued entry of these ions across the membrane is dependent on the maintenance of (1) a low intracellular sodium concentration, which is achieved by the energy-dependent $Na^+/K^+/ATPase$ pump on the basolateral

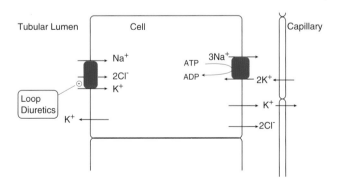

Figure 42-2. Cell from the medullary thick ascending loop of Henle. Loop diuretics are secreted into the tubular lumen where they inhibit the $Na^+/K^+/2Cl^-$ cotransport system; ADP, adenosine diphosphate; ATP, adenosine triphosphate; Cl^-, chloride; K^+, potassium; Na^+, sodium. (From Clarke P, Simpson KH: Diuretics and renal tubular function. Br J Anaesth—CEPD Reviews 1:100–102, 2001. © The Board of Management and Trustees of the British Journal of Anaesthesia. Reproduced by permission of Oxford University Press/British Journal of Anaesthesia.)

membrane, and (2) the recycling of potassium back to into the lumen through potassium channels. This recycling of potassium also generates an electrical current that results in a lumen-positive transepithelial voltage. This voltage drives the transport mechanism of paracellular pathways that carry sodium and other cations (potassium, calcium, magnesium, and ammonia) to the interstitial space. In principle, therefore, a loop diuretic could act at one or more of the sites that are involved (directly or indirectly) in the transport of sodium along the ascending limb:

1. The $Na^+/K^+/2Cl^-$ cotransport mechanism
2. The $Na^+/K^+/ATPase$ sodium pump
3. The potassium channels

In clinical practice the loop diuretics that are used are furosemide (Lasix), bumetanide (Bumex), ethacrynic acid, piretanide, and torsemide.

Early studies demonstrated that a loop diuretic was only effective when applied to the tubular lumen and not the basolateral aspect of tubular cells.[31] The primary action of loop diuretics appears to be the inhibition of the $Na^+/K^+/2Cl^-$ cotransport mechanism. Inhibition of solute reabsorption in the water-impermeable mTAL dilutes the concentration gradient of the countercurrent mechanism, thus reducing the concentrating capacity and the amount of water that can be absorbed in the collecting duct. Loop diuretics also have a site of action in the proximal tubule where they are thought to partially inhibit carbonic anhydrase. However, this may not account for all of the activity in the proximal tubule. Furosemide can reduce proximal reabsorption in tubules perfused with a bicarbonate-free solution,[32] and bumetanide, a very weak inhibitor of carbonic anhydrase, can still significantly reduce proximal reabsorption.[33] Further activity has been demonstrated in the distal tubule where furosemide has been shown to weakly inhibit the thiazide-sensitive Na^+/Cl^- cotransport system.[34] Activity of loop diuretics in the mTAL inhibits the reabsorption of approximately 30% of the filtered sodium load. The additive actions in the distal tubule blunt the expected increase in sodium reabsorption at that site, caused by the increased load. A reduction of the intracellular concentration of sodium by loop diuretics has two consequences. First, it reduces the requirement for activity of the $Na^+/K^+/ATPase$ in the basolateral membrane, thus reducing oxygen consumption in the mTAL, which is the most sensitive to hypoxic injury. Second, it produces the lumen-positive transepithelial potential that drives the paracellular reabsorption of calcium and magnesium.

Furosemide also increases renal elaboration of prostaglandins, producing renal vasodilatation (increased RBF), and inhibiting tubuloglomerular feedback.[35-37] These renovascular actions of furosemide produce redistribution of RBF from the inner to the outer cortex[38] and contribute to the diuretic actions of the drug. Furosemide-induced increases in RBF are prevented by nonsteroidal anti-inflammatory drugs leading to an attenuated diuretic effect.

Clinical Pharmacology

Furosemide is well absorbed from the stomach with an oral bioavailability of approximately 50%. About half of an oral dose is excreted by the kidneys (unchanged) and a lesser amount by the gut and liver. Metabolism takes place in the proximal tubule, where conjugation to an inactive glucuronide occurs. Furosemide is highly bound to albumin, which increases secretion into the proximal tubule by the probenecid-sensitive mechanism, thereby increasing the proportion of the drug that is metabolized. However, because the active site of furosemide is in the luminal membrane, secretion is required for activity. The excretion of water and electrolytes after a dose of furosemide is therefore related to the urinary concentration of furosemide rather than the serum concentration.

Loop diuretics are commonly used in the treatment of congestive heart failure, cirrhosis, and in patients with a low creatinine clearance. Loop diuretics are also used in the treatment of hypercalcemia, because they inhibit the paracellular uptake of calcium. In acute left ventricular failure, furosemide improves pulmonary edema before a noticeable diuretic effect by acute venodilation and a reduction in preload.

Although furosemide reduces the oxygen requirement in the mTAL, as described earlier, this does not appear to translate into pre-emptive protection against renal ischemia in clinical practice. In a study of cardiac surgery, 126 patients were randomized to receive furosemide (0.5 mg/kg for up to 48 hours after induction of anesthesia), dopamine, or placebo. In the postoperative period, the patients receiving furosemide had a greater serum creatinine, a greater increase from baseline to highest postoperative serum creatinine, and a greater reduction in creatinine clearance than either the dopamine or the placebo group.[39]

Practical Aspects of Drug Administration

Many patients follow a chronic oral furosemide dosing regimen, and it is prudent in these patients to check preoperative creatinine, urea, and electrolytes. Prolonged or excessive administration of furosemide may result in a hyponatremic, hypokalemic, and hypomagnesemic metabolic alkalosis.

Marked diuresis, especially after an intravenous dose of furosemide, can produce dehydration and hypotension, which if prolonged can result in prerenal failure. Although diuresis is observed in most patients after an intravenous dose, the duration or volume of diuresis is not predictable. A modest dose of furosemide during cardiopulmonary bypass to bring down a high serum potassium is frequently followed by a need for potassium supplementation within 1 or 2 hours, in addition to aggressive fluid replacement. Increased serum urate levels can be seen in chronic use. High doses, particularly if given rapidly or to patients with renal insufficiency, can produce ototoxicity. Rarely, loop diuretics can cause interstitial nephritis.

Tolerance to loop diuretics can occur with chronic use and is ascribed to compensatory hypertrophy of the distal tubule and collecting duct.[39] Patients with tolerance require greater doses of loop diuretics or the addition of a thiazide. Bumetanide is more extensively metabolized than furosemide and may be a better choice in patients with pre-existing renal insufficiency, especially if prolonged use is foreseen.

Thiazide Diuretics

Preclinical Pharmacology

The site of action of thiazides is the early distal convoluted tubule (Fig. 42–3). Thiazides block up to 40% of a filtered sodium load by inhibiting the coupled reabsorption of Na^+ and Cl^-.[34] An increase in the urine sodium concentration delivered to the collecting tubule enhances Na^+/K^+ exchange, inducing a kaliuresis. Like loop diuretics, thiazides also have a weak effect inhibitory effect on carbonic anhydrase.[41] Thiazides can also inhibit salt and water reabsorption in the medullary collecting ducts. Because the mTAL is unaffected by thiazides, maximal concentration may still take place.

The blockade of NaCl reabsorption in the distal tubule reduces the intracellular Na^+ to such an extent that basolateral Na^+/Ca^{2+} exchange is increased with a resulting modest increase in serum calcium, which is then regulated by parathyroid hormone. There is also some evidence that thiazides directly increase membrane permeability for Ca^{2+}. Thiazides have been demonstrated to have a direct vasodilatory effect by activating calcium-activated K^+ channels.

Clinical Pharmacology

The thiazides used in clinical practice are chlorothiazide, bendroflumethiazide, and metolazone. Oral availability is high, these drugs being readily absorbed from the gastrointestinal tract. They are highly protein bound and excreted mainly through the kidney. Thiazides are mainly used for maintenance treatment of hypertension, in which the dual actions of diuresis/natriuresis and vasodilation are synergistic. Other uses include hypercalciuria and nephrolithiasis.

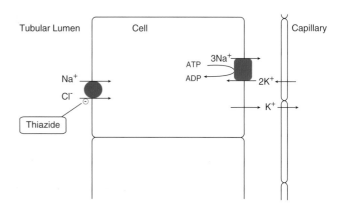

Figure 42–3. Thiazides are active at the luminal membrane of the distal convoluted tubule where they inhibit the Na^+/K^+ cotransport system. ADP, adenosine diphosphate; ATP, adenosine triphosphate; Cl^-, chloride; K^+, potassium; Na^+, sodium. (From Clarke P, Simpson KH: Diuretics and renal tubular function. Br J Anaes CEPD Reviews 1:100–102, 2001. © The Board of Management and Trustees of the British Journal of Anaesthesia. Reproduced by permission of Oxford University Press/British Journal of Anaesthesia.)

Practical Aspects of Drug Administration

Thiazides are not frequently used acutely in the perioperative period. However, this class of drug is commonly used in hypertension (often as a first-line treatment in the elderly or those with "borderline" hypertension). Patients taking these drugs should have appropriate blood work before surgery. In keeping with all diuretics, thiazides may cause azotemia if used excessively. Normally they are well tolerated, and GFR and RBF are maintained. Hypokalemia is a serious common side effect of thiazides, which are therefore usually prescribed along with potassium supplements. Chronic use interferes with lipid and carbohydrate metabolism and therefore their use requires careful monitoring in patients with diabetes or hyperlipidemia.

Dopamine

Preclinical Pharmacology

Dopamine was discovered in 1910[42] and was determined to be the precursor for noradrenaline. Dopamine has a unique effect on the kidney, which is separate from its inotropic effect.[43,44] The initial work on dopamine concentrated on the hydraulic effects of dopamine; animal studies demonstrated an increased peritubular hydrostatic pressure, changes in filtration fraction, and resultant decreases in efferent arteriolar oncotic pressure.[45] A direct renal vasodilatory effect was demonstrated in dogs.[46] By eliminating the direct and indirect sympathomimetic actions of dopamine with the use of specific α and β antagonists, it was demonstrated that increased RBF and excretion of sodium occurred in the absence of release of any known secondary renal vasodilator.[46,47] Thus the concept of a direct tubular effect through specific dopamine receptor activity was established.[48,49] Although a growing family of dopamine receptors has been demonstrated throughout the body, those specifically involved in renal function are the DA1 and DA2 receptors.

The receptor-signaling pathway has been established for dopamine and involves activity at both the basolateral and luminal membranes. Segments of rat tubule exhibit dose-dependent, reversible inhibition of $Na^+/K^+/ATPase$ when incubated with dopamine.[50,51] Stimulation of the DA1 receptor with dopamine activates membrane-associated phospholipase C,[52] resulting in a dose-dependent increase in the activity of protein kinase C,[53] and subsequent phosphorylation of the catalytic subunit of the $Na^+/K^+/ATPase$[54] (Fig. 42–4). On the luminal membrane, DA1 receptor activation stimulates the production of cyclic adenosine monophosphate,[55] activating protein kinase A, which in turn inhibits the Na^+/H^+ exchanger.[56] At this membrane, DA1 and DA2 activity are antagonistic, so that DA1 increases cyclic adenosine monophosphate production whereas pure DA2 activity reduces it.[57]

Clinical Pharmacology

In early studies in humans, using renal angiography and xenon washout techniques, Hollenberg showed that dopamine caused renal vasodilatation and increased RBF without concomitant cardiac changes at doses between 1 and 3 μg/kg per minute.[58] Further studies demonstrated a clear dose-dependent increase in GFR, RBF, urinary flow, natriuresis, and kaliuresis in healthy volunteers and in patients with normal renal function.[58,59] Dopamine also activates α and β adrenergic receptors in a dose-related manner.[60]

The enhanced GFR response to dopamine appears to be blunted in patients with poor renal reserve,[61] the reason for which is currently not established; possibly because of the pre-existing poor functional reserve or an already adaptive state consistent with high basal levels of catecholamines, including endogenous dopamine. Dopamine exhibits tachyphylaxis and is associated with a number of untoward side effects, most of which are associated with dose-dependent sympathomimetic activity (tachycardia and arrhythmia, a concomitant increased myocardial oxygen demand, increased vascular tone, reduced peripheral perfusion, depressed respiratory drive, and interference with the prolactin axis).[62,63]

Probably because it has been around for a long time, dopamine has come into clinical use on the basis of anecdotal reports and uncontrolled studies rather than through good scientific research. There is minimal evidence to support the use of dopamine in the perioperative period as a renal protective agent or even as a diuretic, with much of the current opinion against its routine use.[64–66]

A large number of studies have examined the actions of dopamine in patients undergoing cardiac surgery. In one well-designed study, Myles and colleagues[67] calculated that it would take a study of almost 1,000 patients to demonstrate even a diuretic effect for dopamine. These results were confirmed by Costa and coworkers.[68] Several studies have compared the renal effects of dopamine and dobutamine (no DA1 or DA2 action). In pediatric cardiac surgery patients, Wenstone and coworkers[69] showed no difference between dopamine and dobutamine in urine output, serum creatinine, fractional sodium excretion, and diuretic requirements. Hilberman and colleagues,[70] working in an adult cardiac surgery population, found that dopamine produced more diuresis, natriuresis, and kaliuresis than dobutamine, but had equivalent effects on GFR and effective renal plasma flow. Neither study investigated the effect of dopamine on long-term patient or renal outcome.

Dopamine is frequently used alone or in combination with other diuretics in aortic surgery, in an attempt to improve urine output during the ischemic period of cross clamping. The studies of dopamine in vascular surgery patients have revealed inconsistent results. Girbes and colleagues[71] demonstrated increased GFR and RBF in patients given dopamine before infrarenal clamping and a marked increase in cardiac output that more than accounted for the increase in RBF. Whereas Baldwin and coworkers[72] could not demonstrate a diuretic effect of dopamine in postoperative vascular patients, Schwartz and colleagues[73] did show a marked diuresis in his postoperative vascular patients, which bore no correlation to changes in GRF or RBF. Again, renal outcome and overall outcome were not part of the protocol in either study.

In a prospective, double-blinded, placebo-controlled study of dopamine in patients who received a liver

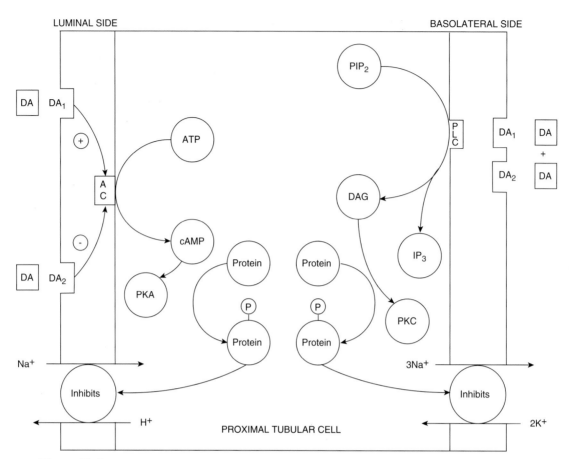

Figure 42–4. Intracellular signaling pathways for dopamine. AC, adenylate cyclase; ATP, adenosine triphosphate; cAMP, cyclic adenosine monophosphate; DA, dopamine; DAG, diacylglycerol; H^+, hydrogen; IP_3, inositol triphosphate; K^+, potassium; Na^+, sodium; P, phosphorylated; PIP_2, phophadtidyl-inositol-diphosphate; PKC, protein kinase C; PKA, protein kinase A; PLC, phospholipase C. (From Garwood S: The pathophysiology and pharmacology of renal protection. In Anaesthetic Pharmacology and Physiology Review. Kent, UK, Castle House Publications, p 49.)

transplant, there was no difference in the diuresis achieved during the neohepatic phase or in GFR at 1 month.[74]

Practical Aspects of Drug Administration

On the basis of the previous discussion, it is difficult to recommend the use of dopamine for any specific indication. Dopamine continues to be used routinely because of established protocols, but its use is questionable in many situations. Undoubtedly dopamine will induce a brisk diuresis in some patients, but potential side effects must first be assessed in critically ill patients. It has a tendency to be unpredictable in terms of its effects at any given dose, both in therapeutic activity and unwanted side effects. In a study of healthy male volunteers, a 75-fold intersubject variability of plasma dopamine concentrations occurred when subjects were infused with the same dose of dopamine, suggesting that there is great intraindividual and interindividual variability in dopamine distribution, metabolism, or both.[75] Although it may be reasonable to select dopamine as a diuretic when its other actions are also desired (e.g., inotrope, vasoconstrictor, chronotrope), there is some evidence from animal and patient studies that dopamine may be deleterious during circumstances of renal ischemia.[76–78]

In measuring retinal binding protein as a marker for renal tubular injury after cardiac surgery, Tang and colleagues[76] determined that dopamine not only did not offer renal protection, but it also increased the excretion of retinal binding protein, suggesting an exacerbation of tubular injury. Patients with preexisting renal dysfunction undergoing angiography actually had increased serum creatinine levels when given dopamine in comparison with saline.[77]

One can speculate why dopamine may enhance renal injury. Some authors have suggested that increased diuresis promotes hypovolemia with prerenal failure. Pure DA2 antagonism has been shown to elicit renal vasoconstriction and stimulation of the Na^+/H^+ exchanger.[59] Perhaps in some patients there is an unbalancing of the DA1 and DA2 effects so that the overall effect is of renal vasoconstriction. Gaudio and colleagues[78] demonstrated in the rat that unless renal ATP can be restored during or after ischemia, the increased RBF associated with dopamine is actually accompanied by loss of tubular integrity. This is speculated to be secondary to the increased Na^+ load presented to the mTal, which in the absence of regeneration of cellular ATP creates an oxygen imbalance, generating oxygen free radicals and causing the disruption of cellular integrity.

Dopamine is undoubtedly a useful drug in the treatment of cardiogenic shock and congestive heart failure and is often used as the inotrope of choice for separation from bypass. It is probably the preferred drug in most centers for cardiogenic shock where dopamine will induce a clinically significant diuresis on its own or in combination with furosemide. However, the medical community is divided as to whether dopamine is useful in the perioperative period. There is little support in the literature for its use as a renal protective agent, although it is often used routinely in patients at risk for renal injury. No large multicenter trial has addressed this question and it is unlikely that such a trial will be undertaken.

Other Dopaminergic Agents

A number of dopamine analogues have been produced and evaluated for their renal effects. Most of these agents were originally made for the treatment of congestive heart failure. Subsequently, two of these have been introduced into clinical practice: dopexamine and fenoldopam. Their relative potencies (as compared with dopamine) and receptor profiles are listed in Tables 42–1 and 42–2.

Dopexamine

Preclinical Pharmacology

The most interesting preclinical study suggesting that dopexamine has significant renal effects was a very elegant study of ischemia/reperfusion injury in rats.[79] To test whether dopexamine had any effect in this model, rats were pretreated with a series of agents including a DA1 agonist and antagonist, a β_2 agonist and antagonist, an oxygen free radical scavenger and dopexamine. Dopexamine and the β_2 agonist were both as effective as the free radical scavenger in promoting survival, an effect that was abolished by the addition of a β_2 antagonist. Simultaneous treatment with a DA1 antagonist and β_1 antagonist did not change the effect of dopexamine, leading the authors to conclude that the salutary effects of dopexamine were caused by β_2 activity. The same group also tested dopexamine in a dog model of hemorrhage and volume resuscitation. The placebo group demonstrated recovery of their circulatory profile but suffered renal shutdown, whereas the dopexamine group demonstrated return of renal circulation and function to baseline.

Clinical Pharmacology

In studies with healthy volunteers, infusions of dopexamine exhibit monoexponential elimination, with a half-life of 7 minutes. Plasma clearance is delayed in patients with low cardiac output, with an elimination half-life of 11 minutes. The rapid clearance is caused by extensive redistribution and extraneuronal catecholamine uptake. Metabolism is by O-methylation and O-sulphonation into inactive products. Drug and metabolites are excreted in urine and in stool.[80] Dopexamine does not cross the blood–brain barrier.

From Table 42–1 it can be inferred that the clinical effects of dopexamine are significant peripheral vasodilation, increased cardiac output and renal vasodilation. In healthy volunteers, dopexamine reduces renal vascular resistance in a dose-related manner over the dose range of 1 to $4\,\mu g/kg$ per minute.[81] Olsen and colleagues administered

TABLE 42–1.

Comparison of the Receptor Profiles of Dopamine, Fenoldopam, and Dopexamine

Receptor	Dopamine	Fenoldopam	Dopexamine
α_1	1	0	0
α_2	1	Minimal	0
β_1	1	0	0
β_2	1	0	60
DA1	1	10	1/3
DA2	1	0	Minimal
Other		Stimulates other neurohormonal parameters (see text)	Inhibits reuptake of norepinephrine

Source: From Garwood S, Hines R: Perioperative renal preservation: Dopexamine and fenoldopam—new agents to augment renal performance. Semin Anesth Periop Med Pain 17:311, 1998.

TABLE 42–2.

Comparison of the Renal Effects of Dopamine, Dopexamine, and Dobutamine

	Dopamine	Dopexamine	Dobutamine
Dose (µg/kg/min)	2.90 ± 0.19	1.00 ± 0.02	4.92 ± 0.40
ERFP	23% increase	10% increase	No change
Glomerular filtration rate	No change	7% increase	No change
C_{Li}	35% increase	30% increase	No change
APR	13% decrease	No change	No change
C_{Na}	103% increase	No change	No change
FDR	Reduced	No change	Increased
RVR	Reduced	No change	Increased
Renal fraction	No change	No change	Decreased

APR, absolute proximal reabsorption; C_{Na}, sodium clearance; C_{Li}, lithium clearance; ERFP, effective renal plasma flow; FDR, fractional distal reabsorption; RVR, renal vascular resistance.
Source: From Garwood S, Hines R: Perioperative renal preservation: Dopexamine and fenoldopam—new agents to augment renal performance. Semin Anesth Periop Med Pain 17:314, 1998.

dopexamine, dopamine, or dobutamine to volunteers in doses that were adjusted to achieve the same increase of 30% to 35% in cardiac output.[82] As can be seen from Table 42–2, the increase in effective renal plasma flow is only 10% compared with an increase in cardiac output of 30% for dopexamine. These results, along with similar data in other studies, have brought into question whether dopexamine has renal effects over and above the increase in cardiac output.[83-87] Several studies have, in fact, failed to demonstrate any direct renal effect. In adults undergoing cardiac surgery, dopexamine increased RBF to a significantly lesser extent than cardiac output, whereas renal vascular resistance decreased in parallel to systemic vascular resistance; this led to the conclusion that the vascular changes were caused by β_2 rather than DA1 stimulation.[86] In a postoperative study of children undergoing cardiac surgery, dopexamine produced an increased diuresis, GFR, and fractional excretion of sodium, but the fraction of the increased cardiac output delivered to the kidneys remained the same. Again the authors concluded that the effects of dopexamine on renal function were secondary to increased cardiac output.[88] Nevertheless, some evidence does exist for a specific dose-related renal effect of dopexamine. In a study of patients undergoing renal vein catheterization, Magrini and colleagues[89] reported an increase in RBF that was greater than could be accounted for by the increase in cardiac output.

Practical Aspects of Drug Administration

Dopexamine is currently only available commercially in Europe and Australia. It appears to be clinically useful in low output states as a positive inotrope and vasodilator ("inodilator"). There is also some interest in the free radical scavenger activity of dopexamine, which may be useful in preventing renal injury secondary to the release of these toxic metabolites.

Fenoldopam

Preclinical Pharmacology

Fenoldopam has a receptor profile that is consistent with both peripheral and renal vasodilation, with direct DA1 receptor activity at the proximal tubule. It has been used in animal preparations and in in vitro studies to examine the pure effects of DA1 stimulation as opposed to the mixed DA1 and DA2 effects seen with dopamine. Fenoldopam maintains or even augments RBF while reducing systemic blood pressure, unlike sodium nitroprusside, which redistributes blood flow away from the kidneys during blood pressure reduction.[90,91] To address the question of whether fenoldopam improves renal hemodynamics directly or secondarily to reduced systemic vascular resistance and enhanced forward flow, Kien and colleagues[92] induced hypotension in dogs with either fenoldopam or sodium nitroprusside and examined regional organ blood flow. While heart rate, systemic vascular resistance, cardiac output, and other measures of left ventricular systolic function did not differ between the two groups of animals, only those given fenoldopam exhibited an increase in RBF; sodium nitroprusside actually induced a reduction of RBF. Regional blood flow in other organs did not differ between the groups.

Clinical Pharmacology

Fenoldopam was first investigated as an oral dopamine analogue, for the treatment of congestive heart failure. However, a poor and unreliable bioavailablity limited the usefulness of the drug in this manner. It subsequently became approved as an intravenous antihypertensive agent for use in hypertensive urgencies and crises. Most of the early studies in humans reflect this indication.

Fenoldopam exhibits linear pharmacokinetics that are best described by a one-compartment model. The plasma half-life, which is not dose-dependent, is approximately 4 minutes. During continuous infusion, a steady state is achieved within 20 minutes and the plasma levels are proportional to the dose once steady state has been achieved.[93] Metabolism is hepatic and inactive metabolites are produced, with no cytochrome P450 involvement. In fact, fenoldopam clearance is not affected in patients with end-stage liver disease.[94] Only 4% of the drug is excreted unchanged. Onset and offset of the drug's actions are rapid after initiation and discontinuation of a continuous infusion.[93]

The pharmacologic effect of fenoldopam is dose-related. There are dose-related increases in RBF, diuresis, fractional excretion of sodium, and filtration fraction, and an associated decrease in renal vascular resistance[95]; GFR remains unchanged. At lower doses (0.001 to 0.05 µg/kg per minute) fenoldopam causes vasodilation of the renal vasculature without any peripheral effects.[95–97] Renal vasodilation is maximal at 0.5 µg/kg per minute, and at greater doses there is a generalized peripheral vasodilation.[98–103] There is, therefore, a dose-related reduction in total vascular resistance and systemic blood pressure that is associated with an increase in RBF. The reduction in systemic blood pressure is associated with increases in cardiac output and stroke volume in patients with hypertension or congestive heart failure,[92,101,102,104] which may account for some of the effects on renal hemodynamics.

Several authors have questioned whether fenoldopam increases RBF and other renal parameters directly or secondarily to improved hemodynamics. Most of these studies involve a head to head comparison between fenoldopam and sodium nitroprusside, in which the blood pressure is lowered to the same extent by both drugs. Fenoldopam has been repeatedly shown to improve renal performance (RBF, diuresis, natriuresis, kaliuresis) when used as an antihypertensive. These renal effects are greater than those seen with the same degree of hypotension and improved systemic hemodynamics during sodium nitroprusside administration.[98,101,105,106]

Both the hypotensive effects and the renal effects of fenoldopam appear to be more marked in patients with hypertension than in patients with normal blood pressure.[106] In a dose ranging study, patients with hypertension demonstrated a greater hypotensive effect than the control patients at peak doses (0.2 µg/kg per minute). Both groups of patients exhibited an increase in total and fractional excretion of sodium. Distal sodium delivery also increased only in the control patients, whereas distal fractional reabsorption of sodium and potassium decreased to a greater extent in the hypertensive group, suggesting that patients with hypertension have a blunted proximal tubular response to fenoldopam but an enhanced, compensatory distal tubular response.

Fenoldopam increases creatinine clearance, diuresis, and natriuresis in patients with impaired renal function[105] and restores RBF and urine output in patients receiving positive pressure ventilation.[107]

Practical Aspects of Drug Administration

Fenoldopam is currently marketed as an intravenous antihypertensive. Several abstracts have been presented at meetings that suggest fenoldopam may have renal salutary effects in the perioperative period. Most of these studies present preliminary data in high-risk populations such as patients undergoing aortic reconstruction surgery and cardiac surgery. However, the studies are mainly observational or at best compared with historic control subjects.

Anecdotally, fenoldopam acts as a reliable diuretic, often successful in patients that are resistant to high-dose furosemide infusions, dopamine, or both. Whether fenoldopam actually prevents renal injury or merely temporizes the situation until the kidneys are able to recover is currently unknown.

From experience in cardiac surgery, fenoldopam at doses of 0.01 to 0.03 µg/kg per minute induces a diuresis without affecting systemic blood pressure in most patients. However, there does appear to be patient variation in which even these lower doses will cause a significant decrease in systemic vascular resistance. Whether this is true patient variation or an interaction with other baseline cardiac drugs such as angiotensin-converting enzyme inhibitors or beta-blockers is also unknown. Fenoldopam has been recently shown to reduce cerebral blood perfusion in healthy volunteers.[108]

Atrial Natriuretic Peptides

Preclinical Pharmacology

ANP is recognized as an endogenous circulating hormone with powerful cardiovascular and renal regulating properties. Various molecules with ANP structure/activity relationships are produced in the cardiac atria and ventricles, the brain, and the kidneys. The pro-ANP molecule with 126 amino acids is cleaved at different positions at the carboxyl terminal to produce these various peptides. The circulating form of ANP produced in the atria is known as alpha-human ANP.[109] Although termed *brain natriuretic peptide*, BNP is also of myocardial cell origin and is produced primarily in the ventricle. C-type natriuretic peptide is of endothelial origin.[109,110] The peptide produced in the kidney is known as urodilatin.[111]

Two forms of ANP receptors exist; a high-affinity clearance receptor that is responsible for the short half-life (30 seconds to 3 minutes)[112] and the biologic receptor found on the glomerulus, inner medullary collecting ducts, and mesangial cells.[113,114]

The coupling of ANP with its receptor catalyzes the formation of intracellular cyclic guanosine monophosphate (cGMP).[115] Intracellular cGMP has a number of relevant actions (Fig. 42–5): namely it closes a calcium-dependent sodium channel in the medullary collecting tubules,[114] thereby decreasing sodium reabsorption; a cGMP-dependent protein kinase activates calcium-dependent ATPase,[116] blocking calcium entry into vascular smooth muscle and mesangial cells thereby inducing relaxation[116,117]; cGMP also directly blocks the contractile response by preventing phosphorylation of the myosin light chain.[118] cGMP-linked ANP activity also inhibits release of renin from the juxtaglomerular cells[119] and aldosterone from the adrenal cortex.[120]

The activation of ANP receptors along the nephron (glomerulus and inner medullary collecting ducts) causes a significant increase in GFR and decreased sodium resorption in single nephron preparations,[113] isolated perfused kidneys,[121] animal models,[113] and in humans.[122] ANP causes a simultaneous vasodilation of the afferent arteriole and a vasoconstriction of the efferent arteriole of the glomerulus,[113] thus increasing hydraulic pressure within the

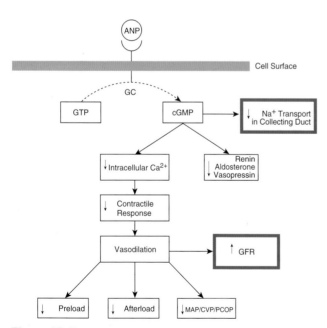

Figure 42–5. Signaling pathway and action of atrial natriuretic peptide (ANP). Ca²⁺, calcium; cGMP, cyclic guanosine monophosphate; CVP, central venous pressure; GC, guanylyl cyclase; GFR, glomerular filtration rate; GTP, guanosine triphosphate; MAP, mean arterial pressure; Na⁺, sodium; PCOP, pulmonary capillary occlusion pressure. (From Garwood S: The pathophysiology and pharmacology of renal protection. In Anaesthetic Pharmacology and Physiology Review. Kent, UK, Castle House Publications, p 51.)

glomerulus. Total vascular resistance,[123] overall RBF, and renal plasma flow therefore remain constant,[113] whereas filtration fraction increases.[113] A minor role is contributed by the increased coefficient of filtration, secondary to the relaxation of the mesangial cells.[124]

In experimental acute renal failure, ANP produced demonstrated renal protection with significantly increased renal plasma flow, GFR, diuresis, and sodium excretion, with lower serum creatinine levels in chronic preparations.[125,126] However, Nakamoto and colleagues[125] noted that the renal benefits were at the cost of a reduced systemic blood pressure and questioned whether this drug may, therefore, be limited in its clinical application. In a rat model of nephrotoxicity (cyclosporin), ANP restored GFR back to baseline and significantly increased urine flow and sodium excretion.[127]

Clinical Pharmacology

The physiologic role of ANP has been determined to be minor and secondary to the renin-aldosterone-angiotensin axis.[128] When exogenous ANP is infused in physiologic doses to healthy volunteers, there is little cardiovascular or renal response.[128] However, in pathophysiologic conditions, such as congestive heart failure, circulating levels of ANP are high and patients exhibit an exaggerated natriuretic response to infused ANP.[128]

Initial clinical trials with ANP were disappointing. Sands and colleagues[129] entered 20 renal transplant recipients (10 pairs of cadaveric kidneys) to receive either ANP or placebo in a paired fashion. ANP/placebo was given as a bolus on revascularization followed by a 4-hour infusion. Daily serum creatinine and weekly GFR did not differ between the two groups. Similarly ANP did not prove helpful in patients with cirrhosis.[130] All that could be demonstrated was a renal vasodilatory response but only if the baseline renal vascular resistance was high. The protocol was complicated by significant hypotension.

In a single center, open-label trial of 53 patients with acute renal failure,[131] ANP improved creatinine clearance and reduced the requirements for dialysis (23% for ANP-treated patients and 52% for control patients). The study was repeated as a multicenter trial,[132] with the study design as prospective, randomized, double blinded, and placebo controlled. More than 500 patients were enrolled. ANP did not change the overall dialysis-free survival. Patients with nonoliguric renal failure had a 59% dialysis-free survival when treated with ANP compared with 48% in control patients, but patients with oliguric renal failure appeared to do worse when treated with ANP (8% dialysis-free survival compared with 23% for control subjects). Subsequent analysis of the data concluded that those patients who converted from oliguric to nonoliguric renal failure in the ANP group had a better dialysis-free survival. This did not happen in the control group.

Urodilatin had a somewhat better initial clinical success, probably because it is resistant to degradation by endoproteases,[133] does not exhibit tachyphylaxis,[134] and has less of a hypotensive effect when compared with ANP.[135] Urodilatin is also a more potent diuretic and natriuretic agent than ANP.[135–137]

The first clinical trials of urodilatin were open trials with historical control patients. Cardiac transplant patients had lower peak creatinine levels, greater diuresis, and a lower incidence of dialysis than the control patients.[138,139] Cecedi and colleagues[140] infused urodilatin for 4 days in heart or liver transplant patients who had otherwise met the criteria for dialysis. All patients responded with a brisk diuresis; seven had significantly lower serum creatinine levels and only one patient required dialysis during the treatment period. The same group reported on eight liver transplant patients who were treated for 7 days with urodilatin after acute renal failure developed. Again patients had a prompt diuresis and six out of the eight patients avoided dialysis with maintenance of good renal function up to 3 months later.[141]

A series of small, prospective, randomized, double-blinded, placebo-controlled trials were conducted in similar patient populations, with mixed results. The Forssman group again studied cardiac transplant patients who were refractory to conventional diuretic therapy, randomizing them to 7 days of urodilatin versus placebo.[142] The patients receiving urodilatin diuresed well and none required dialysis, whereas the control group remained oliguric and six of the seven patients in the group required dialysis. At 3 months follow-up examination, all of the patients who received urodilatin were alive; four of the seven patients in the control group died while still receiving dialysis. Herbert and colleagues[143] used urodilatin in postoperative patients who fulfilled the requirements for dialysis, comparing them to placebo plus standard therapy of dopamine plus furosemide for 4 days. Five out of the six patients who received urodilatin maintained a good diuresis, compared with four out of the six control patients who became anuric. Overall serum creatinine levels were lower (but not statistically significant) in the urodilatin group, but total number of dialysis treatments did not differ between the two groups. In a group of liver transplant patients, patients who received urodilatin had lower serum creatinine levels and required lower total doses of furosemide to maintain the same urine output as placebo control patients.[144] The incidence of dialysis and number of dialysis treatments did not differ between the two groups.

Currently, interest has turned toward BNP and dendroais natriuretic peptide (DNP), another recently discovered peptide with natriuretic properties, as a treatment of congestive heart failure.[145] Both peptides exhibit increased GFR in association with natriuresis and diuresis. It is not yet clear whether BNP or DNP will prove to be more successful natriuretic peptides in the clinical arena than ANP and urodilatin.

Clinical Pharmacology and Practical Aspects of Drug Administration

Clinical use of ANP and to a lesser extent urodilatin is complicated by the accompanying hypotension secondary to peripheral vasodilation. This effect has limited the use of these peptides to such an extent that clinical and research protocols are difficult to carry out. It remains to be seen whether BNP and DNP will exhibit the same profile in clinical use.

Carbonic Anhydrase Inhibitors

Preclinical Pharmacology

Although not often used therapeutically in the perioperative period, carbonic anhydrase inhibitors will be briefly included because patients who routinely take these drugs (usually for glaucoma) will frequently present for surgery.

The enzyme carbonic anhydrase is present on the luminal membranes of the convoluted cells of the proximal tubule and in the cytoplasm of tubular cells. It catalyzes the reversible production of water and carbon dioxide from hydrogen ions and bicarbonate through the intermediate step of carbonic acid (Fig. 42–6). The luminal enzyme prevents acidification of tubular fluid by buffering secreted hydrogen ions with bicarbonate, whereas the cytoplasmic enzyme regenerates hydrogen ions for exchange with sodium; overall there is a net absorption of sodium bicarbonate. This also allows for a sparing of chloride, so that the concentration of sodium chloride increases along the proximal tubule, thereby enhancing passive absorption of sodium chloride at more distal sites.

When carbonic anhydrase is inhibited, carbonic acid accumulates in the tubular lumen. There are therefore less cytosolic-free hydrogen ions produced that can participate in Na^+/H^+ exchange. The result is an increased concentration of sodium bicarbonate in the tubular lumen. The chloride gradient is no longer allowed to build up, attenuating passive absorption of sodium chloride further along the nephron. Carbonic anhydrase inhibition results in a modest diuresis with an obligatory loss of sodium bicarbonate. The total sodium excretion overall is less than 5% of the filtered load, because of compensatory reabsorption in more distal parts of the nephron.

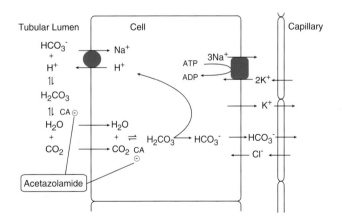

Figure 42–6. Actions of the carbonic anhydrase inhibitor (acetazolamide) in the proximal tubule. ADP, adenosine diphosphate; ATP, adenosine triphosphate; CA, carbonic anhydrase; Cl^-, chloride; CO_2, carbon dioxide; H^+, hydrogen; HCO_3^-, bicarbonate; H_2CO_3, carbonic acid; K^+, potassium; Na^+, sodium. (From Clarke P, Simpson KH: Diuretics and renal tubular function. Br J Anaesth—CEPD Reviews 1:100–102, 2001. © The Board of Management and Trustees of the British Journal of Anaesthesia. Reproduced by permission of Oxford University Press/British Journal of Anaesthesia.)

Clinical Pharmacology and Practical Aspects of Drug Administration

Carbonic anhydrase inhibitors are not frequently used for their diuretic activity. Their primary uses are in the treatment of glaucoma and altitude sickness. They may be encountered in critical care as a treatment for metabolic alkalosis or for alkalinization of the urine (e.g., in pigmenturias and forced excretion in drug overdose). Patients using carbonic anhydrase inhibitors chronically are liable to a hypokalemic metabolic acidosis.

Patients on carbonic anhydrase inhibitors, particularly if given intravenously in the perioperative period should have their acid-base status monitored.

Potassium-Sparing Diuretics

Potassium-sparing diuretics are active in the distal tubule and collecting ducts and fall into two classes: those that inhibit aldosterone (spironolactone) and those active at the amiloride-sensitive Na^+ channel (amiloride, triamterene). These drugs are not available as intravenous formulations and are therefore not frequently used in the perioperative period or in critically ill patients.

Preclinical Pharmacology

Potassium-sparing diuretics are weak diuretics because less than 5% of the filtered load of sodium is presented at their sites of action.

Aldosterone Inhibitors

The action of aldosterone involves intracellular receptor coupling in the cells of the distal tubule. The aldosterone/receptor complex then enters the nucleus-inducing mRNA and the synthesis of Na^+ and K^+ channels and the Na^+/H^+ cotransporter in the luminal membranes. Aldosterone also stimulates the turnover of ATP and thus increases the activity of Na^+/K^+/ATPase. Spironolactone inhibits all of the activities of aldosterone; the resulting effect is a weak diuresis, Na^+ excretion, and $K^+/Cl^-/H^+$ retention (Fig. 42–7).

Amiloride, Triamterene

In contrast to spironolactone, amiloride inhibits the sodium channel in the luminal membrane of the distal tubule by a nonaldosterone-dependent mechanism[146] (see Fig. 42–7). The decrease in intracellular Na^+ diminishes the activity of the basolateral Na^+/K^+/ATPase with a subsequent reduction in the electrochemical gradient for K^+ and H^+ secretion.[146] Amiloride can only act as a weak diuretic because the site of action is only associated with excretion of less than 5% of the filtered sodium load.

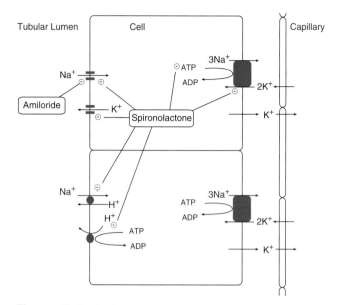

Figure 42–7. Actions of the potassium-sparing diuretics spironolactone and amiloride in the distal tuble and collecting ducts. ADP, adenosine diphosphate; ATP, adenosine triphosphate; H^+, hydrogen; K^+, potassium; Na^+, sodium. (From Clarke P, Simpson KH: Diuretics and renal tubular function. Br J Anaesth—CEPD Reviews 1:100–102, 2001. © The Board of Management and Trustees of the British Journal of Anaesthesia. Reproduced by permission of Oxford University Press/British Journal of Anaesthesia.)

Clinical Pharmacology and Practical Aspects of Drug Administration

Spironolactone is used in primary and secondary hyperaldosteronism (Conn's syndrome, chronic liver failure, and other refractory edematous states). Because spironolactone acts by inhibiting gene expression, the onset of action is measured in days. The metabolism of the drug itself is rapid, but its effects can last for 2 to 3 days after discontinuation, secondary to mRNA induction. Patients following a spironolactone dosing regimen are therefore prone to hyperkalemic, hyperchloremic acidosis. This is particularly the case in patients with renal insufficiency. The addition of thiazide may ameliorate these adverse effects.

Triamterene is readily absorbed from the gut, whereas amiloride is only incompletely absorbed. Both drugs are secreted into the tubular fluid. Triamterene is metabolized by the liver into active metabolites,[147] which are also secreted into the tubular lumen. The half-life for triamterene is 3 to 5 hours and 18 hours for amiloride.[148] Both drugs accumulate in renal failure and in the elderly. Triamterene will also accumulate in liver disease because of a reduction in hepatic metabolism, that is, hydroxylation and biliary secretion.[149]

Patients taking either triamterene or amiloride are also susceptible to hyperkalemia. Patients at greatest risk for this potentially lethal adverse effect are those with renal failure or those concurrently taking other drugs that are associated with an increase in serum K^+ (nonsteroidal anti-inflammatory drugs, angiotensin-converting enzyme inhibitors, beta-blockers). Acidotic states also worsen hyperkalemia.

TABLE 42–3.

Adult Dosing Guidelines for Commonly Administered Diuretics

Diuretic	Class	Indication	Dosage	Remarks
Mannitol	Osmotic	To promote diuresis in the prevention or treatment of the oliguric phase of acute renal failure	Test dose: 0.2 mg/kg IV over 3–5 min; May repeat one time Treatment of oliguria: 50–100 g of a 15–25% solution IV slowly	Include a filter when infusing concentrated mannitol
Furosemide	Loop	Treatment of edema associated with CHF, hepatic cirrhosis, or renal disease Treatment of hypertension	20–80 mg IM or IV slowly Dose may be increased by 20 mg and repeated in 2 hr; May dose 1–2 times daily 40 mg PO BID	Give intravenous injections slowly over 2 minutes For intravenous injections, do not exceed 1 g/day
Bumetanide	Loop	Same as furosemide	0.5–2 mg PO; may be repeated at 5-hr intervals up to a maximum dose of 10 mg/day; 0.5 to 1 mg IV or IM May be repeated at 3-hr intervals up to a maximum dose of 10 mg/day	Reserve intravenous or intramuscular use for patients with impaired GI absorption Can be used in patients allergic to furosemide at 1:40 ratio of bumetanide to furosemide
Ethacrynic acid	Loop	Same as furosemide	50–200 mg/day PO 50 mg IV or 0.5–1 mg/kg (usually only one intravenous dose necessary)	Do not give IM because of local pain and irritation. If second intravenous dose is necessary, use a new injection site to avoid thrombophlebitis
Chlorothiazide	Thiazide	Hypertension and edema associated with CHF, hepatic cirrhosis, or renal disease	0.5–1.0 g once or twice a day either PO or IV	Do not give IM IV; is reserved for patients unable to take oral medications of emergency situations
Hydrochlorothiazide	Thiazide	Hypertension Edema associated with CHF, hepatic cirrhosis, or renal disease	12.5–50 mg/day PO 25–100 mg/day PO until dry weight is obtained	
Acetazolamide	Carbonic anhydrase inhibitor	Glaucoma Diuresis in CHF	250–1 g/day PO or IV 5 mg/kg PO or IV	Intramuscular administration is painful
Spironolactone	Potassium-sparing	Treatment of edema associated with CHF, hepatic cirrhosis, or renal disease	25–200 mg/day PO	If diuretic response has not occurred after 5 days, add a second diuretic that acts more proximally in the renal tubule

TABLE 42–3.

Adult Dosing Guidelines for Commonly Administered Diuretics—cont'd

Diuretic	Class	Indication	Dosage	Remarks
Amiloride	Potassium-sparing	Adjunctive therapy with thiazide or loop diuretics in CHF or hypertension	5–10 mg/day	Useful for restoring normal serum potassium in patients with hypokalemia while taking diuretics
Triamterene	Potassium-sparing	Treatment of edema associated with CHF, hepatic cirrhosis, or renal disease	100–300 mg/day	May be used alone or with other diuretics for additive diuretic effect or antikaliuretic (potassium-sparing) effect

CHF, congestive heart failure; GI, gastrointestinal; IM, intramuscularly; IV, intravenously; PO, per os (by mouth).

General Comments on the Practical Aspects of Diuretic Use

Patients taking diuretics often exhibit an apparent tolerance or resistance, sometimes called the *braking phenomenon.* This can be seen after acute administration or chronic use. Acute tolerance is thought to be secondary to an acute reduction in extracellular volume (hypovolemia), which induces compensatory sodium retention through activation of the renal sympathetics and the rennin-angiotensin system. With chronic use, there is evidence of a compensatory hypertrophy of the sodium-retaining parts of the nephron at more distal sites. This has been demonstrated for furosemide, where hypertrophy of the distal convoluted tubule occurs and can be counteracted by the addition of a thiazide diuretic.

A further reason for resistance in chronic use is related to the disease state and is particularly seen in renal insufficiency and hepatic failure. In renal failure, the accumulation of organic acids compete for secretion in the proximal tubule with diuretics such as furosemide, so that less diuretic reaches the active site in the luminal membrane of the mTAL. In hepatic failure, the chronically contracted intravascular volume activates renal sympathetics and the Sp renin-angiotensin system, increasing proximal sodium resorption.

Understanding the possible reasons for diuretic resistance allows for a rational approach to the problem. Increasing sodium delivery to the tubule with judicious improvement in cardiovascular status may restore a reduced natriuresis secondary to hypotension or hypovolemia. Greater doses or continuous infusions of furosemide allow the drug to compete effectively for secretion in the proximal tubule. Continuous infusions also avoid the adverse effects of peak doses. Synergistic combinations of diuretics can restore a natriuretic and diuretic response in resistant states. This is effective if the individual drugs have different active sites. As noted earlier, addition of a thiazide to furosemide negates the compensatory reabsorption of sodium in the distal tubule. Smaller doses of the two drugs used in combination therapy also avoid the potential adverse side effects of a high dose of an individual drug.

Dosage and Administration

Diuretics can be administered orally (PO), intramuscularly (IM), or intravenously (IV). Adult dosing guidelines for the commonly administered diuretics are listed in Table 42–3.

Osmotic Diuretics: Mannitol is used to promote diuresis and to reduce intracranial and intraocular pressure. Urea is primarily used to reduce intracranial and intraocular pressure.

Mannitol—administered by IV infusion only and is available as 5% in 1000 mL, 10% in 500 and 1000 mL, 15% in 500 mL, 20% in 250 and 500 mL, or 25% in 50 mL.

Urea—40 g per 150 mL for IV infusion only.

Loop Diuretics:

Furosemide—administered PO, IM, or IV. It is available as 20-, 40-, and 80-mg tablets for oral use or oral solutions of 10 mg/mL or 40 mg/5 mL in 60 and 120 ml volumes. Injections are available as 10-mg/mL solutions in 2-, 4-, and 10-mL single-dose vials.

Bumetanide—administered PO, IM, or IV and available as 0.5-, 1-, and 2-mg tablets and as a 0.25-mg/mL solution in 2-mL ampules and 2-, 4-, 10-mL vials for injection.

Ethacrynic acid—administered PO or IV and available as 25- or 50-mg tablets and a 50-mg powder that is reconstituted in 50 mL of 5% dextrose or sodium chloride solution for injection.

Torsemide—administered PO or IV and available as 5-, 10-, 20-, and 100-mg tablets and a solution of 10 mg/mL in either 2- or 5-mL ampules for injection.

Thiazide Diuretics:

Chlorothiazide—administered PO or IV. It is available as 250- or 500-mg tablets, an oral suspension of 250 mg per 5 mL, and a lyophilized powder, 500 mg, which can reconstituted with 18 mL sterile water.

Hydrochlorothiazide—administered PO. It is available as 25-, 50-, and 100-mg tablets; 12.5-mg capsules; and a solution of 50 mg per 5 mL.

Bendroflumethiazide—available as 5- and 10-mg tablets for oral use.

Metolazone—available as 2.5-, 5-, and 10-mg tablets for oral use.

Carbonic Anhydrase Inhibitors:

Acetazolamide—administered PO or IV. It is available as 125- or 250-mg tablets, a 500-mg capsule, and a lyophilized powder, 500 mg, which can be reconstituted with 5 mL sterile water.

Potassium-Sparing Diuretics:

Spironolactone—available in 25-, 50-, and 100-mg tablets for oral administration.

Amiloride—available in 5-mg tablets for oral administration.

Triamterene—available in 50- and 100-mg capsules for oral administration.

References

1. Jackson EK: Diuretics. In Hardman JG, Limbird LE (eds): Goodman & Gilman's The Pharmacological Basis of Therapeutics, 10th ed. New York, McGraw-Hill, 2001.
2. Burger A: Drugs and People. Medications, Their History and Origins, and the Way They Act. Charlottesville, Va, University Press of Virginia, 1986.
3. Cragoe EJ: Diuretics—Chemistry, Pharmacology, and Medicine. New York, John Wiley & Sons, 1983.
4. Lang HJ, Hropot M: Discovery and development of diuretic agents. In Greger RF, Knauf H, Mutschler E (eds): Diuretics. Berlin, Springer-Verlag, 1995.
5. Leake CD: An Historical Account of Pharmacology. Springfield, Ill, Charles C Thomas, 1975.
6. Vogl A: On clinical medicine with notes from the diary of a part-time researcher. Bull NY Acad Med 46:39, 1970.
7. Vogl A: The discovery of organic mercurial diuretics. Am Heart J 39:881, 1950.
8. Hropot M, Muschaweck R: Chemistry and chemical classification of diuretics. In Reyes AJ (ed): Progress in Pharmacology and Clinical Pharmacology, Vol 9. Stuttgart, Fischer, 1992.
9. Kau ST: Basic pharmacology and pharmacological classification of diuretics. In Reyes AJ (ed): Progress in Pharmacology and Clinical Pharmacology, Vol 8. Stuttgart, Fisher, 1992.
10. Riley MR, Kastrup EK: Drug Facts and Comparisons. St. Louis, Wolters Kluwer Company, 2000.
11. Buerkert J, Martin D, Prasad J, Trigg D: Role of deep nephrons and the terminal collecting duct in a mannitol induced diuresis. Am J Physiol 240:F411–F422, 1981.
12. Behnia R, Koushanpoor E, Brunner EA: Effects of hyperosmotic mannitol infusion on hemodynamics of dog kidney. Anesth Analg 82:902–908, 1996.

13. Johnson PA, Barnard DB, Perrin NS, Levinsky NG: Prostaglandins mediate the vasodilatory effect of mannitol in the hypoperfused rat kidney. J Clin Invest 68:127–133, 1981.
14. Blantz CA: Effect of mannitol on glomerular ultrafiltration in the hydropenic rat. J Clin Invest 54:1135–1143, 1974.
15. Lang F: Osmotic diuresis. Renal Physiol 10:160–173, 1987.
16. Kirshenbaum MA, Serros ER: Effects of alterations in urine flow rate a on prostaglandin E in conscious dogs. Am J Physiol 238:F107–F111, 1980.
17. Kurnik BRC, Weisberg LS, Cuttler IM, Kurnik PB: Effects of atrial natriuretic peptide versus mannitol on renal blood flow during radio-contrast infusion in chronic renal failure. J Lab Clin Med 116:27–35, 1990.
18. Martinez-Maldonado M, Benabe JE, Garcia JC: Diuretics and renin release. In Puschett JB, Greenberg A (eds): Diuretics II. Chemistry, Pharmacology and Clinical Applications. New York, Elsevier, pp 497–502, 1987.
19. Schrier RW, Arnold PE, Gordon JA, Burke TJ: Protection of mitochondrial function by mannitol in ischemic acute renal failure. Am J Physiol 247:F365–F369, 1984.
20. Flores J, DiBona DR, Beck CH, Leaf A: The role of cell swelling in ischemic renal damage and the protective effect of hypertonic solute. J Clin Invest 51:118–126, 1972.
21. Hanley MJ, Davidson K: Prior mannitol and furosemide infusion in a model of ischemic acute renal failure. Am J Physiol 241:F556–F564, 1981.
22. Teschan PE, Lawson NL: Studies in acute renal failure. Prevention by osmotic diuresis and observations on the effect of plasma and extracellular volume expansion. Nephron 3:1–16, 1966.
23. Barry KG, Cohen A, Knochel JP, et al: Mannitol infusion. II. The prevention of acute functional renal failure during resection of an aneurysm of the abdominal aorta. N Engl J Med 264:967–971, 1961.
24. Alpert RA, Roizen MF, Hamilton WK, et al: Intraoperative urinary output does not predict postoperative renal function in patients undergoing abdominal aortic revascularization. Surgery 95:707–711, 1984.
25. Nicholson ML, Baker DM, Hopkinson BR, Wenham PW: Randomized controlled trial of the effect of mannitol on renal reperfusion injury during aortic surgery. Br J Surg 83:1230–1233, 1996.
26. Paul MD, Mazer D, Byrick RJ, et al: Influence of mannitol and dopamine on renal function during elective infrarenal aortic clamping in man. Am J Nephrol 6:427–434, 1986.
27. Fisher AR, Jones P, Barlow P, et al: The influence of mannitol on renal function during and after open-heart surgery. Perfusion 13:181–186, 1998.
28. Ip-Yam PC, Murphy S, Baines M, et al: Renal function and protein-uria after cardiopulmonary bypass. Anesth Analg 78:842–847, 1994.
29. Van Valenberg PLJ, Hoitsma AJ, Tiggeler RGWL, et al: Mannitol as an indispensable constituent of an intraoperative hydration protocol for the prevention of acute renal failure after renal cadaveric transplantation. Transplantation 44:784–788, 1987.
30. Solomon R, Werner C, Mann D, et al: Effects of saline, mannitol and furosemide to prevent acute decreases in renal function induced by radiocontrast agents. N Eng J Med 331:1416–1420, 1994.
31. Burg M, Stoner L: Renal tubular chloride transport and the mode of action of some diuretics. Annu Rev Physiol 38:37–45, 1976.
32. Radtke HW, Rumrich G, Kinne-Saffran E, et al: Dual action of acetazolamide and furosemide on proximal volume absorption in the rat kidney. Kidney Int 1:100–105, 1972.
33. Puschett JB, Sylk D, Teredesai PR: Uncoupling of proximal sodium bicarbonate from sodium phosphate transport by bemetanide. Am J Physiol 235:F403–F448, 1978.
34. Velazquez H, Wright FS: Effects of diuretic drugs on Na, Cl and K transport by rat renal distal tubule. Am J Physiol 250:F1013–F1023, 1986.
35. Gerber JG: Role of prostaglandins in the hemodynamic and tubular effects of furosemide. Fed Proc 42:1707–1710, 1983.
36. Gerber JG, Nies AS: Furosemide-induced vasodilation: Importance of the state of hydration and filtration. Kidney Int 18:454–459, 1980.
37. Wright FS, Schnermann J: Interference with feedback control of glomerular filtration by furosemide, triflucin and cyanide. J Clin Invest 53:1695–1708, 1974.
38. Epstein M, Hollenberg NK, Guttmann RD, et al: Effect of ethacrynic acid and chlorothiazide on intrarenal hemodynamics in normal man. Am J Physiol 220:482–487, 1971.

39. Kaissling B, Stanton BA: Adaptation of distal tubule and collecting duct to increased sodium delivery. I. Ultrastructure. Am J Physiol 248:F374–F381, 1985.

40. Lassnigg A, Donner E, Grubhofer G, et al: Lack of renoprotective effects of dopamine and furosemide during cardiac surgery. J Am Soc Nephrol 11:97–104, 2000.

41. Maren TH: The general physiology of reactions catalyzed by carbonic anhydrase and their inhibition by sulfonamides. Ann NY Acad Sci 429:568–579, 1984.

42. Mannich C, Jacobson W: Uber oxyphenylalkylamine und diophenyl-lalkylamine. Berichte Dtsch Chem Ges 43:189–197, 1910.

43. McNay JL, McDonald RH, Goldberg LI: Direct renal vasodilation produced by dopamine in the dog. Circ Res 16:510–517, 1965.

44. Goldberg LI: Cardiovascular and renal actions of dopamine: Potential clinical application. Pharmacol Rev 24:1–20, 1972.

45. Knox FG, Mertz JI, Burnett J Jr, Haramati A: Role of hydrostatic and osmotic pressure in renal sodium reabsorption. Circ Res 52:491–500, 1983.

46. Frederickson Ed, Bradley T, Goldberg LI: Blockade of renal effects of dopamine in the dog by the DA1 antagonist SCH 23390. Am J Physiol 249:F236–F240, 1985.

47. Jose PA, Eisner GM, Robillard JE: Renal hemodynamics and natriuresis induced by the dopamine agonist SKF 82526. Am J Med Sci 2944:181–186, 1987.

48. Goldberg LI, Yeh BK: Attenuation of dopamine induced renal vasodilation in the dog by phenothiazines. Eur J Pharmacol 15:36–40, 1971.

49. Yeh BK. McNay JL, Goldber LI: Attenuation of dopamine renal and mesenteric vasodilation by haloperidol: Evidence for a specific dopamine receptor. J Pharmacol Exp Ther 168:303–309, 1969.

50. Aperia A, Bertorello A, Seri I: Dopamine causes inhibition of Na$^+$K$^+$ ATPase activity in rat proximal convoluted tubule segments. Am J Physiol 252:F39–F45, 1987.

51. Bertorello A, Aperia A: Both DA$_1$ and DA$_2$ receptor antagonists are necessary to inhibit Na$^+$K$^+$ ATPase activity in proximal tubules from rat kidney. Acta Physiol Scand 132:441–443, 1988.

52. Felder CC, Blecher M, Jose PA: Dopamine-1 mediated stimulation of phospholipase C activity in rat renal cortical membranes. J Biol Chem 264:8739–8745, 1989.

53. Kansra V, Chen C, Lokhandwala MF: Dopamine causes stimulation of protein kinase C in rat renal proximal tubules by activating dopamine1 receptors. Eur J Pharmacol 289:391–394, 1995

54. Bertorello A, Aperia A, Walass SI, et al: Phosphorylation of the catalytic subunit of Na$^+$K$^+$ ATPase inhibits the activity of the enzyme. Proc Natl Acad Sci USA 88:1359–1362, 1991.

55. Baldi E, Pupilli C, Amenta F, Mannelli M: Presence of dopamine dependent adenylate cyclase activity in human renal cortex. Eur J Pharmacol 149:351–356, 1988.

56. Felder CC, Campbell T, Albrecht F, Jose PA: Dopamine receptors inhibit Na$^+$H$^+$ exchanger activity in renal BBMV by stimulation of adenylate cyclase. Am J Physiol 259:F297–F303, 1990.

57. Ricci A, Collier WL, Rossodivita I, Amenta F: Dopamine receptors mediating inhibition of the cyclic adenosine monophosphate generating system in the rat renal cortex. J Auton Pharmacol 11:121–127, 1991.

58. Hollenberg NK, Adams DF, Mendell P, et al: Renal vascular responses to dopamine: Haemodynamic and angiographic observations in man. Clin Sci Mol Med 45:733–742, 1973.

59. Carey RM, Siragy HM, Ragsdale NV, et al: Dopamine-1 and dopamine-2 mechanisms in the control of renal function. Am J Hypertens 3:59S–63S, 1990.

60. Goldberg LI, Rajafer SI: Dopamine receptors: Applications in clinical cardiology. Circulation 72:245–248, 1985.

61. Goldberg LI, McDonald RH Jr, Zimmerman AM: Sodium diuresis produced by dopamine in patients with congestive heart failure. N Eng J Med 269:1060–1064, 1963.

62. Bailey AR, Burchett KR: Effect of low-dose dopamine on serum concentrations of prolactin in critically ill patients. Br J Anaesth 78:97–99, 1997.

63. van den Berghe G, de Zegher F: Anterior pituitary function during critical illness and dopamine treatment. Crit Care Med 25:1580–1590, 1996.

64. Denton MD, Chertow GM, Brady HR: "Renal-dose" dopamine for the treatment of acute renal failure: Scientific rationale, experimental studies and clinical trials. Kidney Int 49:4–14, 1996.

65. Galley HF: Renal-dose dopamine: Will the message now get through? Lancet 256:2112–2113, 2000.

66. Perdue PW, Balser JR, Lipsett PA, Breslow MJ: "Renal dose" dopamine in surgical patients: Dogma or science? Ann Surg 227:470, 1998.

67. Myles PS, Buckland MR, Schnek NJ, et al: Effect of "renal-dose" dopamine on renal function following cardiac surgery. Anaesth Intens Care 21:56–61, 1993.

68. Costa P, Ottino GM, Matani A, et al: Low-dose dopamine during cardiopulmonary bypass in patients with renal dysfunction. J Cardiothoracic Anesth 4:469–473, 1990.

69. Wenstone R, Campbell JM, Booker PD, McKay R: Renal function after cardiopulmonary bypass in children: Comparison of dopamine with dobutamine. Br J Anaesth 67:591–594, 1984.

70. Hilberman M, Maseda J, Stinson EB, et al: The diuretic properties of dopamine in patients after open-heart operation. Anesthesiology 61:489–494, 1984.

71. Girbes ARJ, Lievers AG, Smit AJ, et al: Lack of specific renal haemodynamic effects of different doses of dopamine after infrarenal aortic surgery. Br J Anaesth 77:753–757, 1996.

72. Baldwin L, Henderson A, Hickman P: Effect of postoperative low-dose dopamine on renal function after elective major vascular surgery. Ann Intern Med 120:744–747, 1994.

73. Schwartz LB, Bissell MG, Murphy M, Gewertz BL: Renal effects of dopamine in vascular surgical patients. J Vasc Surg 8:367–374, 1988.

74. Swygert TH, Roberts LC, Valek TR, et al: Effects of intraoperative low-dose dopamine on renal function in liver transplant recipients. Anesthesia 75:571–576, 1991.

75. MacGregor DA, Smith TE, Prielipp RC, et al: Pharmacokinetics of dopamine in healthy male subjects. Anesthesiology 92:303–305, 2000.

76. Tang ATM, El-Gamel A, Keevil B, et al: The effect of 'renal-dose' dopamine on renal tubular function following cardiac surgery: Assessed by measuring retinol binding protein (RBP). Eur J Cardiothorac Surg 15:717–722, 1999.

77. Gare M, Haviv YS, Ben-yehuda A, et al: The renal effect of low-dose dopamine in high-risk patients undergoing coronary angiography. J Am Coll Cardiol 34:1682–1688, 1999.

78. Gaudio Km, Stromski M, Thulin G, et al: Postischemic hemodynamics and recovery of renal adenosine triphosphate. Am J Physiol 251:F603–F609, 1986.

79. Jacinto SM, Chintala MS, Lokhandwala MF, Jandhyala BS: Efficacy and mechanisms of dopexamine in the prevention of ischemia-reperfusion induced organ damage: Role of oxygen free radicals. Clin Exp Hypertens 19:181–190, 1997.

80. Fitton A, Benfield P: Dopexamine hydrochloride. A review of pharmacodynamic and pharmacokinetic properties and therapeutic potential in acute cardiac insufficiency. Drugs 39:308–330, 1990.

81. Foulds RA: Clinical development of dopexamine hydrochloride (dopacard) and an overview of its hemodynamic effects. Am J Cardiol 62:41C–45C, 1998.

82. Olsen NV, Lund J, Jensen PF, et al: Dopamine, dobutamine, and dopexamine: A comparison of renal effects in unanesthetized human volunteers. Anesthesiology 79:685–694, 1993.

83. Baumann G, Felix SB, Filcek SA: Usefulness of dopexamine hydrochloride versus dobutamine in chronic congestive heart failure and effects on hemodynamics and urine output. Am J Cardiol 65:748–754, 1990.

84. Atallah MM, Saied MM, El-Diasty TA, et al: Renal effect of dopexamine hydrochloride in patients with chronic renal dysfunction. Urol Res 20:419–424, 1992.

85. MacGregor DA, Butterworth JF, Zaloga GP, et al: Hemodynamic and renal effects of dopexamine and dobutamine in patients with reduced cardiac output following coronary artery bypass grafting. Chest 106:835–841, 1994.

86. Stephan H, Sonntag H, Henning H, Yoshimine K: Cardiovascular and renal haemodynamic effects of dopexamine: Comparison with dopamine. Br J Anaesth 65:380–387, 1990.

87. Sherry E, Tooley MA, Bolsin SN, et al: Effect of dopexamine hydrochloride on renal vascular resistance index and haemodynamic responses following coronary artery bypass graft surgery. Eur J Anesth 14:184–189, 1997.

88. Habre W, Beghetti M, Roduit C, et al: Haemodynamic and renal effects of dopexamine after cardiac surgery in children. Anaesth Intens Care 24:435–439, 1996.

89. Magrini F, Foulds R, Roberts N, et al: Human renovascular effects of dopexamine hydrochloride: A novel agonist of peripheral dopamine and beta$_2$-adreno-receptors. Eur J Clin Pharmacol 32:1–4, 1987.

90. Aronson S, Goldberg LI, Glock D, et al: Effects of fenoldopam on renal blood flow and systemic hemodynamics during isoflurane anesthesia. J Cardiothorac Vasc Anesth 5:29–32, 1991.

91. Aronson S, Goldberg LI, Roth S, et al: Preservation of renal blood flow during hypotension induced with fenoldopam in dogs. Can J Anaesth 37:380–384, 1990.

92. Kien ND, Moore PG, Jaffe RS: Cardiovascular function during induced hypotension by fenoldopam or sodium nitroprusside in anesthetized dog. Anesth Analg 74:72–78, 1992.

93. Weber RR, McCoy CE, Ziemniak JA, et al: Pharmacokinetic and pharmacodynamic properties of intravenous fenoldopam, a dopamine₁-receptor agonist, in hypertensive patients. Br J Clin Pharmacol 25:17–21, 1988.

94. Vlavianos P, Polson RJ, Settin A, et al: Haemodynamic and pharmacokinetic study of intravenous fenoldopam in patients with hepatic cirrhosis. Br J Clin Pharmacol 29:19–25, 1990.

95. Allison NL, Dubb JW, Ziemniak JA, et al: The effect of fenoldopam, a dopaminergic agonist, on renal hemodynamics. Pharmacol Ther 41:282–288, 1987.

96. Mathur VS, Carey RM, O'Connell DP: Renal and systemic hemodynamic effects of very-low dose fenoldopam in normotensive subjects. Anesth Analg 88:SCA85, 1999.

97. Mathur VS, Swan SS Lambrecht LJ, et al: The effects of fenoldopam, a selective dopamine receptor agonist, on systemic and renal hemodynamics in normotensive subjects. Crit Care Med 27:1832–1837, 1999.

98. Elliott WJ, Weber RR, Nelson KS, et al: Renal and hemodynamic effects of intravenous fenoldopam versus nitroprusside in severe hypertension. Circulation 81:970–977, 1990.

99. Munger MA, Benotti JR, Green JA, et al: Assessment of hemodynamic tolerance from a 24-hour intravenous infusion of fenoldopam mesylate in congestive heart failure. Am J Cardiol 65:206–210, 1990.

100. Murphy MB, McCoy CE, Weber RR, et al: Augmentation of renal blood flow and sodium excretion in hypertensive patients during blood pressure reduction by intravenous administration of the dopamine₁ agonist fenoldopam. Circulation 76:1312–1318, 1987.

101. White WB, Radford MJ, Gonzalez FM, et al: Selective dopamine-1 agonist therapy in severe hypertension: Effects of intravenous fenoldopam. J Am Coll Cardiol 11:1118–1123, 1988.

102. Young JB, Leon CA, Pratt CM, et al: Intravenous fenoldopam in heart failure: Comparing the hemodynamic effects of dopamine₁ receptor agonism with nitroprusside. Am Heart J 115:378–384, 1988.

103. Girbes ARJ, Smit AJ, Meijer S, Reitsma WD: Renal and endocrine effects of fenoldopam, and metodopramide in normal man. Nephrol 56:179–185, 1990.

104. Hackman BB, Griffin B, Mills M, Ramanathan KB: Comparative effects of fenoldopam mesylate and nitroprusside on left ventricular performance in severe systemic hypertension. Am J Cardiol 69:918–922, 1992.

105. Shusterman NH, Elliott WJ: Fenoldopam, but not nitroprusside, improves renal function in severely hypertensive patients with impaired renal function. Am J Med 95:161–168, 1993.

106. O'Connell D, Ragsdale V, Boyd D, et al: Differential human renal tubular responses to dopamine type 1 receptor stimulation are determined by blood pressure status. Hypertension 29:115–122, 1997.

107. Poinsot O, Romand J-A, Favre H, Suter PM: Fenoldopam improves renal hemodynamics impaired by positive end-expiratory pressure. Anesthesiology 79:680–685, 1993.

108. Prielipp RC, Wall MH, Groban L, et al: Reduced regional and global cerebral blood flow during fenoldopam-induced hypotension in volunteers. Anesth Analg 93:45–52, 2001.

109. Tanaka I, Misono KS, Inagami T: Atrial natriuretic factor in rat hypothalamus, atria and plasma: Determination by specific radioimmunoassay. Biochem Biophys Res Commun 124:663–668, 1984.

110. Sudoh T, Minamino N, Kangawa K, Matsuo H: C-type natriuretic peptide (CNP): A new member of the natriuretic family identified in porcine brain. Biochem Biophys Res Commun 168:863–870, 1990.

111. Schulz-Knappe P, Forssmann K, Herbst F, et al: Isolation and structural analysis of "Urodilatin," a new peptide of the cardiodilatin (ANP) family, extracted from human urine. Klin Wochenschr 66:752–759, 1988.

112. Maack T, Suzuki M, Almeda FA, et al: Physiological role of silent receptors of atrial natriuretic factors. Science 238:675–678, 1987.

113. Dunn BR, Ichikawa I, Pfeffer JM, et al: Renal and systemic effects of synthetic atrial natriuretic peptide in the anesthetized rat. Circ Res 59:237–246, 1986.

114. Light DB, Schweibert EM, Karlson KH, Stanton BA: Atrial natriuretic peptide inhibits a cation channel in renal inner medullary collecting duct cells. Science 242:383–385, 1989.

115. Schulze S, Chinkers M, Garbers DL: The guanylate cyclase receptor family of proteins. FASEB J 3:2026–2035, 1989.

116. Rashatwar S, Cornwell TL, Lincoln TM: Effects of 8 bromo cGMP on Ca²⁺ levels in vascular smooth muscle cells: possible regulation of Ca²⁺ ATPase by cGMP dependent protein kinase. Proc Natl Acad Sci USA 84:568–569, 1987.

117. Murad F: Cyclic guanosine monophosphate as a mediator of vasodilation. J Clin Invest 78:1–5, 1986.

118. Paglin S, Takuwa Y, Kainin KE, et al: Atrial natriuretic peptide inhibits the agonist induced increase in extent of myosin light chain phosphorylation in aortic smooth muscle. J Biol Chem 263:1317–1320, 1988.

119. Henrich WL, McAllister EA, Smith PB, Campbell WB: Guanosine 3′5′–cyclic monophosphate as a mediator of inhibition of rennin release. Am J Physiol 255:F474–F478, 1988.

120. Atarshi K, Mulrow PJ, Franco-Saenez R: Inhibition of aldosterone production by an atrial extract. Science 224:992–994, 1984.

121. Camargo MJF, Kleinert HD, Atlas SA, et al: Ca²⁺-dependent hemodynamic and natriuretic effects of atrial natriuretic extract in the isolated rat kidney. Am J Physiol 246:F447–F456, 1984.

122. Cody RJ, Atlas SA, Laragh JH, et al: Atrial natriuretic factor in normal subjects and heart failure patients. J Clin Invest 78:1362–1374, 1986.

123. Maack T, Marion DN, Camargo MJ, et al: Effects of auriculin (atrial natriuretic factor) on blood pressure, renal function and the rennin aldosterone system in dogs. Am J Med 77:1069–1075, 1984.

124. Freid TA, McCoy RN, Osgood RW, Stein JH: Effect of atriopeptin II on determinants of glomerular filtration rate in the in vitro perfused dog glomerulus. Am J Physiol 250:F1190–F1122, 1986.

125. Nakamoto M, Shapiro JI, Shanley PF, et al: In vitro and in vivo protective effect of atriopeptin III on ischemic acute renal failure. J Clin Invest 80:698–705, 1987.

126. Schafferhaus K, Heidbreder E, Grunin D, Heidland A: Norepinephrine induced acute renal failure: Beneficial effects of atrial natriuretic factor. Nephron 44:240–244, 1986.

127. Capasso G, Rosati C, Cianii F, et al: The beneficial effects of atrial natiuretic peptide on cyclosporin nephrotoxicity. Am. J Hypertens 3:204–210, 1990.

128. Cogan MG: Atrial natriuretic peptide. Kidney Int 37:1148–1160, 1990.

129. Sands Jm, Neylan JF, Olsen RA, et al: Atrial natriuretic factor does not improve the outcome of cadaveric renal transplantation. J Am Soc Nephrol 1:1081–1086, 1991.

130. Brenard R, Morean R, Pussard E, et al: Hemodynamic and sympathetic responses to human atrial natriuretic peptide infusion in patients with cirrhosis. J Hepatol 14:347–356, 1992.

131. Rahman SN, Conger JD: Glomerular and tubular factors in urine flow rates of acute renal failure patients. Am J Kidney Dis 23:788–793, 1994.

132. Allgren RL, Marbury TC, Rahman RS, et al: Anaritide in acute tubular necrosis. N Eng J Med 336:828–834, 1997.

133. Gagelmann M, Hock D, Forssmann W-G: Urodilatin (CDD/ANP-95-126) is not biologically inactivated by a peptidase from dog kidney cortex membrane in contrast to atrial natiuretic peptide/cardiodilatin (α-hANP/CDD-99-126). FEBS Lett 233:249–254, 1988.

134. Munzell T, Drexel H, Holtz J, et al: Mechanisms involved in the response to prolonged infusion of atrial natiuretic factor in patients with chronic heart failure. Circulation 83:191–201, 1991.

135. Saxenhoffer H, Rasellli A, Weidmann P, et al: Urodilatin, a new peptide from the kidneys can modify renal and cardiovascular function in men. Am J Physiol 259:F832–F838, 1990.

136. Hildebrandt DA, Mizelle HL, Brands MW, Hall JE: Comparison of actions of urodilatin and atrial natriuretic peptide. Am J Physiol 262:R395–399, 1992.

137. Elsner D, Muders F, Muntze A, et al: Efficacy of prolonged infusion of urodilatin (ANP-95-126) in patients with congestive heart failure. Am Heart J 129:766–773, 1995.

138. Hummel M, Kuhn M, Bub A, et al: Urodilatin: A new peptide with beneficial effects in the postoperative therapy of cardiac transplant recipients. Clin Invest 70:674–682, 1992.

139. Hummell M, Kuhn M, Bub A, et al: Urodilatin a new therapy to prevent kidney failure after heart transplantation. J Heart Lung Transplant 12:209–217, 1993.

140. Cecedi C, Kuse E-R, Meyer M, et al: Treatment of acute postoperative renal failure after liver and heart transplantation by urodilatin. Clin Invest 71:435–436, 1993.

141. Cecedi C, Meyer M, Kuse E-R, et al: Urodilatin: A new approach for the treatment of therapy resistant acute renal failure after liver transplantation. Eur J Clin Invest 24:632–639, 1994.

142. Wiebe K, Meyer M, Wahlers T, et al: Acute renal failure following cardiac surgery is reverted by administration of urodilatin. Eur J Med Res 1:259–265, 1996.

143. Herbert MK, Ginzel S, Muhlschlegel S, Weis KH: Concomitant treatment with urodilatin (ularitide) does not improve renal function in patients with acute renal failure after major abdominal surgery—a randomized controlled trial. Wiener Klin Wochenschrift 111:141–147, 1999.

144. Langrehr JM, Kahl A, Meyer M, et al: Prophylactic use of low-dose urodilatin for prevention of renal impairment following liver transplantation: A randomized placebo-controlled study. Clin Transplant 11:593–598, 1997.

145. Lisy O, Lainchbury JG, Leskinen H, Burnett JC Jr: Therapeutic actions of a new synthetic vasoactive and natriuretic peptide, dendroaspis natriuretic peptide, in experimental severe congestive heart failure. Hypertension 37:1089–1094, 2001.

146. Chambrey R, Achard J-M, St John PL, et al: Evidence for an amiloride-insensitive Na/H exchanger in rat renal cortical tubules. Am J Physiol 273:C1064–C1074, 1997.

147. Mutschler E, Gilfrich HJ, Knauf H, et al: Pharmacokinetics of triamterene. Clin Exp Hypertens 5:249–269, 1983.

148. Smith AJ, Smith RN: Kinetics and bioavailablity of two formulations of amiloride in man. Br J Pharmacol 48:646–649, 1973.

149. Villeneuve JP, Rocheleau F, Raymond G: Triamterene kinetics and dynamics in cirrhosis. Clin Pharmacol Ther 35:831–837, 1984.

43

Electrolytes Solutions and Colloids

Neil Soni, MB, ChB

History of Fluids

It would be hard to imagine daily medical practice without intravenous fluids, yet as a safe and dependable form of treatment it is a relatively new phenomenon. The need for fluid administration has always been a fundamental part of medical practice but caregivers before modern times had no recourse to intravenous administration. It is, however, clear that for some medical and nonmedical reasons blood and blood transfusion has intrigued the medical field for centuries. The first documented use of blood transfusion was in dogs in 1666 by Richard Lower, and this led to use in humans in 1667 by Jean Baptiste Denis, who was the physician to Louis XIV. In his first attempts, Denis used lambs' blood. This appeared to "work" in the first patient but then the next two patients died. It has been suggested that the cause of the deaths and in particular the issue of incompatibility might have been discussed in 1668 but the method fell into disrepute. There is little or no mention of blood transfusion until almost 150 years later when J. Blundell reported in 1818 on the first successful transfusion of human blood; the transfusion was performed at St. Thomas Hospital for a parturient. Vein to vein transfusion was described by James Hobson Aveling in 1819 and autotransfusion, introduced in 1874, was in common use at the end of the 19th century. At the time of World War I anesthesiologists such as G.W. Crile began involving themselves in maintaining the hemodynamic status of patients.

Growing interest in the use of fluids other than blood existed; subsequently, saline was first used in 1891 for the treatment of shock. A few years later "Hartmans" solution (a more "physiologic" approach) was hailed as a great advance. Technical advances in fluid administration spawned devices such as the drip chamber, which appeared in about 1909.

The first plasma substitutes were made from gum acacia in 1919, and polyvinyl pyrrolidone was developed in the 1940s by Helmut Wesse. The advent of plastics facilitated intravenous access and fluid administration and led to the development of a range of new colloids including the gelatins, dextrans, and starches. With these advances came the debate addressing the benefits of crystalloid versus colloid solutions, a debate that shows no signs of abating some 40 years later! More recent advances include hypertonic solutions and colloids formulated in a physiologic medium.

Physiology

The average adult ingests 2.5 L of fluids per day as both food and drink; water is also produced internally as a product of metabolism. Fluid is lost in the urine, feces, respiration, and through the skin. A range of pathologic conditions may increase losses from any of these sites. Mammals are extremely well adapted to manage their fluid homeostasis during normal conditions but the physiologic systems are compromised in pathologic circumstances.

The fundamental principle in fluid management is to maintain normovolemia (a state in which the patient **751** demonstrates hemodynamic stability) by delivering the physiologic requirements and replacing losses. The enormity of the physiologic mechanisms involved in maintaining normovolemia can be imagined where one considers that a 70-kg man flushes 200 L of fluid through the glomeruli containing 30,000 mmol sodium; a further 10 L of fluid and 1500 mmol of sodium are secreted into the gut each day. Almost all of these fluids are reabsorbed, but minor disruptions of these processes may rapidly create fluid and electrolyte imbalance.

In subacute loss, the clinical signs of dehydration are apparent when 6% total body fluid loss has occurred; severe dehydration is apparent with greater than 10% loss. In acute situations in which the patient is losing fluid rapidly, the physiologic mechanisms can usually compensate for a 15% to 25% loss of intravascular volume; beyond this hemodynamic decompensation occurs.

Electrolyte Balance

Sodium

The total body sodium is about 100 g with a normal daily replenishment requirement in an adult of about 2 g/day. Sodium achieves high concentrations (140 mmol/L) in the plasma compartment and in the interstitial space and lower concentrations intracellularly (4–15 mmol/L depending on the cell types).[1] As the intravascular and interstitial compartments are in equilibrium and constitute the main location of sodium, plasma sodium is a reasonable indicator of total body sodium.

Control of sodium (as well as fluid) balance is mediated through sensitive volume receptors and by osmoreceptors. A reduction in perceived blood volume or a decrease in osmotic pressure will result in sodium retention, which in turn will cause water to be retained.

Potassium

Total body potassium is approximately 3200 mmol with a daily turnover of 40 to 120 mmol. The serum value is between 3.5 and 5 mmol/L; however, only 2% of all potassium is in the intravascular compartment because potassium is predominantly intracellular when the concentration ranges from 135 to 150 mmol/L. Therefore, unlike sodium, the serum potassium value does not accurately reflect the total body potassium and thus reliance must be made on surrogate effects of deficiency rather than on serum potassium measurement. Potassium is lost from various sites, principally the gastrointestinal tract and the urine.

Intracellular versus extracellular levels of sodium and potassium are maintained by active transport mechanisms across the plasma membrane by energy-dependent pumps or exchangers. Potassium is interchangeable with both sodium and hydrogen; therefore, if potassium becomes depleted, hydrogen ions are secreted preferentially. To conserve potassium, a metabolic alkalosis will occur from hydrogen loss; thus alkalosis may be the earliest biochemical finding suggesting potassium deficiency (Table 43–1).

TABLE 43–1.

Electrolytes in Body Fluids

	Na	K	Cl
Stomach	60	9	84
Small intestine	111	4	104
Bile	148	5	100
Pancreatic juice	140	5	76
Ileostomy "new"	130	11	116
Ileostomy "old"	46	3	21
Cecostomy	52	8	42

Effects of "Injury"

Any major stress or injury threatens fluid homeostasis resulting in compensatory mechanisms to preserve the internal milieu through the secretion of adrenocortical hormones and of antidiuretic hormone. These humoral mechanisms impair sodium and water excretion at the expense of potassium and may continue for days after the initiating event.

Distribution of Fluids

Water, which constitutes 60% to 70% of total body volume, is distributed in a three-compartment model consisting of an intracellular space and two extracellular spaces composed of intravascular and interstitial spaces (Fig. 43–1).

The barriers between these spaces differentially impede water, electrolyte, and protein movement. There is an endothelial barrier between the intravascular and extravascular compartments and a cell wall barrier between the interstitial and the intracellular spaces. The physical barrier of the cell wall and the endothelium and the various, often energy-dependent processes that allow transfer across these are well reviewed in standard texts and therefore are not discussed in detail in this chapter.[1]

Movement between the intravascular and extravascular compartments is governed by the hydrostatic pressure gradient, the osmolar and oncotic gradients, and the integrity of the membrane as described by Starling (Fig. 43–2).

The osmotic pressure is determined by the molar concentrations of the ions across the membrane. If the membrane is semipermeable, the osmotic pressure across the membrane is determined by the difference in the total number of molecules on each side of the membrane. The oncotic pressure is determined by molecules (especially

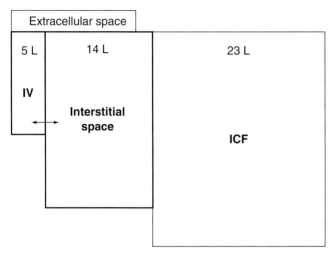

Figure 43–1. Idealized three-compartment model of fluid distribution. ICF, intracellular fluid; IV, intravascular space.

plasma proteins) that cannot traverse the membrane. Other factors affecting movement include molecular shape, molecular charge, and active transport mechanisms. Fluid transfer is governed by the pressure gradients rather than actual pressures. Within the capillaries a pressure-dependent process pushes fluid from intravascular to interstitial spaces. The electrolytes provide the effective oncotic gradient within the capillary to retain fluid; net movement of fluid is outward from the capillary. Within the interstitium lymphatic drainage clears excess fluid that becomes vulnerable in disease states. The oncotic gradient eloquently described in Starlings equation is dependent on the integrity of the endothelial barrier (Fig. 43–3).

If the capillary endothelium becomes defective, colloid moves freely across such that plasma albumin will decrease as the interstitial albumin increases. The increase in albumin in the interstitium causes the fluid to shift into this compartment by oncotic pressure, thereby increasing the volume of the interstitial space; the consequent dilution of albumin within the interstitial space reduces oncotic pressure, thereby establishing a new gradient.

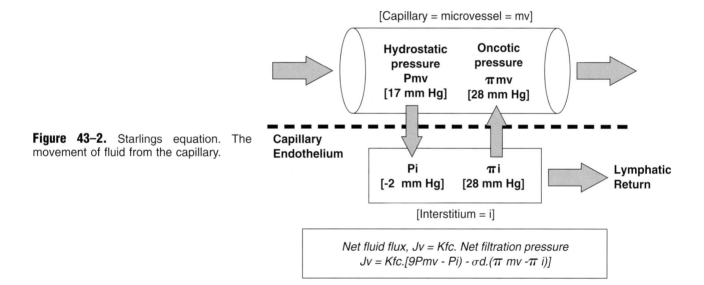

Figure 43–2. Starlings equation. The movement of fluid from the capillary.

Net fluid flux, Jv = Kfc. Net filtration pressure
$Jv = Kfc.[9Pmv - Pi) - \sigma d.(\pi\, mv - \pi\, i)]$

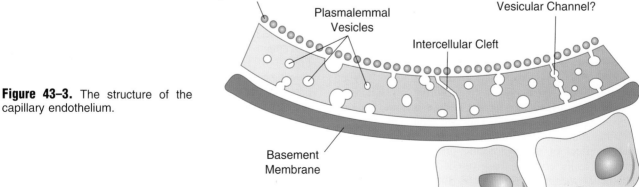

Figure 43–3. The structure of the capillary endothelium.

**Factors Controlling Albumin Distribution
in Plasma and Interstitium**

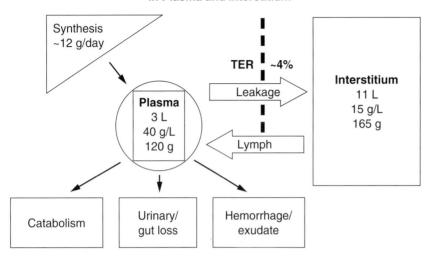

Figure 43–4. Movement of albumin from the intravascular to interstitial space. TER, transcapillary exchange rate.

Active Transport of Fluid Across Membranes

The role of active transport provided by the Na^+/K^+ pumps in the endothelium may play a bigger role than was previously appreciated and may be particularly important in disease states that predispose to pulmonary edema. Active fluid clearance from the alveoli across the alveolar membrane has been demonstrated both in animals and in humans.[2–6] When this mechanism fails, the balance of Starlings forces is disrupted.

Distribution of Crystalloids

Crystalloids consist of water and electrolytes or small molecules such as dextrose and freely distribute throughout the two extracellular spaces apart from the relative barrier presented by the endothelial barrier. Thus within 20 minutes an isotonic salt solution will have distributed to a degree that only about 20% of its volume will remain intravascularly!

When the administered crystalloid, such as a dextrose solution, is devoid of electrolytes it behaves similar to water because dextrose is taken up by cells and metabolized. Water is free to move across both the endothelial and cellular barriers and hence will distribute throughout the entire body. Even less of a dextrose solution will remain intravascularly at 20 minutes.[7]

The lungs are a model system in which to consider the factors influencing crystalloid fluid distribution. When crystalloids are given rapidly (e.g., during resuscitation), there will be a tendency for the colloid oncotic pressure to decrease through dilution. This will reduce the pressure returning fluid into the intravascular space, and hence the relative effect of the hydrostatic pressure will increase. However, as the crystalloid is given, it distributes across the endothelial membrane and dilutes the interstitial colloid oncotic pressure, and presumably increases the hydrostatic pressure in the interstitium. In this way the gradients will

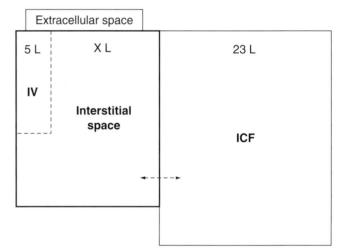

Figure 43–5. The two-compartment model of fluid compartments when the endothelium is incompetent. ICF, intracellular fluid; IV, intravascular space.

tend to equilibrate. Protection from excessive fluid accumulation in the interstitium is mediated by lymphatic flow, which can increase 10-fold.

Even though albumin is relatively large, it moves relatively freely between the intravascular and interstitial spaces by a mechanism that is poorly understood. This rate of movement, known as the transcapillary exchange rate (TER; Fig. 43–4), is slower than for crystalloids during normal circumstances possibly because of the molecular size. In a patient with sepsis, TER of albumin is enhanced through increased permeability. In effect the three-compartment model is reduced to two compartments as fluids given into the intravascular space partition out (Fig. 43–5). Although this has only been clearly demonstrated for albumin, it is likely that it happens with other colloid solutions too. Possibly there is an association between plasma half-life and molecular size, but this is not entirely linear and dynamically alters as the disease progresses or resolves.

Factors increasing endothelial permeability in the patient with sepsis are not well understood but probably involve activation and sequestration of passing neutrophils and activation of a complex cytokine-mediated cascade. The net result is that TER of larger molecules across the "endothelial barrier" is no longer retarded by the size of the molecules.[8]

Fluid Administration

Fluids are primarily administered to maintain homeostasis and standard electrolyte solutions are required to replenish daily requirements of water and electrolytes. Adequacy can be assessed by monitoring clinical symptoms and signs such as thirst, hemodynamic parameters, and urine output. Additional measurements of plasma electrolytes (especially sodium) and acid-base (indirectly reflecting the potassium status) are often necessary.

Volume replacement is required in pathologic states in which a loss of circulating volume impairs the delivery of substrates in particular oxygen. In these settings, the sympathetic nervous system compensates for fluid loss by reducing the effective intravascular space by differentially constricting capacitance vessels, thereby delivering the available intravascular volume to critical organs; also, increasing the cardiac output will deliver the available fluid more effectively.

In the setting of fluid loss, sufficient fluids are needed to fill and maintain the intravascular volume. Major red blood cell loss requires replacement with products to increase the oxygen-carrying capacity (see Chapter 52). During an emergency, any type of available fluid will initially suffice to accomplish the objectives of increasing circulating volume, increasing cardiac output, and ensuring adequate substrate delivery. Efficacy of resuscitation is determined by the time that the fluid remains in the relevant compartment.

Crystalloid solutions can only partially achieve these goals. For example, dextrose-containing solutions will fill the intravascular space but distribute rapidly and widely resulting in a transient intravascular effect. These solutions also provide a glucose load and excessive volumes of free water (the water content of a solution that is not matched by equivalent ions to make it isotonic with plasma) and are better suited to maintenance fluid roles. Ringers lactate will also achieve intravascular expansion, only transiently so that large volumes of fluid are required.

Hypertonic crystalloids "extract" fluid from the intracellular space. Although these do not provide free water, they do constitute a large osmotic load in the form of sodium. Its initial efficacy is useful for short-term resuscitation but at the risk for subsequent hypernatremia.

Colloid solutions contain larger molecules whose passage through the endothelium is retarded causing more fluid to remain intravascularly, and for longer in most nonpathologic situations. However, when the inflammatory process exceeds that seen after either minor or intermediate surgery, there may be increased permeability and hence more rapid distribution of the colloid out of the circulation.

Available Fluids

Crystalloids

Crystalloid solutions are free to move between compartments and will tend to distribute along a concentration gradient according to its composition. A sodium chloride solution will tend to disperse across the whole extracellular compartment almost intact while following a 5% dextrose solution water to distribute across all compartments equally; the dextrose component is distributed only into the intracellular compartment (Table 43–2).

Dextrose Solutions: High concentrations of dextrose can be used to administer glucose to patients in specific need because of hypoglycemia and is considered elsewhere (see Chapter 46). More commonly a 5% dextrose solution (5 g per 100 mL dextrose in water) is used; however, as the dextrose is removed, free water remains. The body has a daily requirement for free water and this is a useful source for replacing water across all compartments. If only water is given, and in larger than necessary volumes, this may result in hyponatremia, a far more common event than hyponatremia from inappropriate secretion of antidiuretic hormone (see Chapter 21). Another popular dextrose-containing solution is "dextrose-saline," a 4% dextrose in a dilute saline solution, containing approximately 30 mmol NaCl per liter. This solution can be considered to be composed of 200 mL normal saline with 800 mL "free water."

Normal saline contains equivalent molar concentrations (154 mM) of each of sodium and chloride and is isotonic. It is an unbuffered acidic solution able to cause a hyperchloremic acidosis,[9,10] but the clinical consequences are not profound.

Hartmans solution or Ringers lactate solution contains sodium lactate, a buffered physiologic solution. Lactate provides the buffering capacity by being metabolized in the liver to bicarbonate.[11] Lactate accumulation may occur if the lactate cannot be metabolized; however, much more commonly, lactate accumulates because of overproduction. Therefore, in situations in which production is ongoing, lactate-containing solutions should probably be avoided. This may be of greater relevance when lactate buffers are used in dialysis in which the potential for accumulation

TABLE 43–2.

	Na, mmol/L	K, mmol/L	Cl, mmol/L	Lactate, mmol/L
Hartmans	130	4	110	28
Normal saline	153	0	153	0
Extracellular fluid	140	5	103	<1

is greater and other buffers such as bicarbonate may be advantageous.[12,13] Concerning the distribution of lactate-containing solutions, after 30 minutes only 25% of the fluid will remain in the intravascular space.[14,15]

Efficacy of Crystalloids

In hypovolemia, the intravascular retention time of crystalloid may be longer, although the ability of crystalloid to fully restore perfusion in the microcirculation remains doubtful.[16-19] Furthermore, extravascular lung water may be greater even though oxygen delivery is maintained.[20]

Hypertonic Solutions

Hypertonic solutions have been used for a rapid effect on the intravascular volume during resuscitation. These include not only solutions with a range of saline concentrations from 1.85% to 7.2% but also the inclusion within these solutions of colloids such as starch. The high osmotic pressure generated by hypertonic solutions of the fluids encourages mobilization of fluid from the intracellular to extracellular spaces; hence smaller volumes are required to reduce the likelihood of edema.[21-25] The volume expansion may be as much as three to four times the infused volume of fluid and occurs almost immediately.[26] Beyond the volume itself, the hemodynamic improvement may also be attributed to the hypertonicity of the solutions increasing myocardial contractility and vasodilating the splanchnic and renal circulations.[27-29] Among possible deleterious effects of hypertonic solutions are increased risk for myocardial ischemia,[30] increased permeability,[31] and coagulopathies.[32]

Hypertonic solutions may have an effect on immune function as they appear to enhance T cell and monocyte function and to modify expression of adhesion molecules (L-selectin, CD11b, β_2-integrin).[33] Although there might be amelioration of the response to injury it might equally suggest that augmentation of both superoxide production and elastase release might occur and be deleterious.[33,34]

Hypertonic solutions have been used successfully in the setting of hemorrhagic and endotoxic shock.[35-39] The use of hypertonic solutions in the setting of burn injuries appears to be short-lived if administered as a large bolus, but clear benefit is obvious when given as two bolus doses (4 mL/kg) separated by an interval.[40] A further benefit seen with hypertonic solutions is a reduction in increased intracranial pressure changes where it compares favorably with mannitol.[37]

Generally speaking, the use of hypertonic solutions should be viewed as a short-term solution because hypertonicity and hypernatremia will ensue over time.[36] Hypotensive episodes, sudden increases in pulmonary capillary wedge pressure, and ventricular arrhythmias, cardiac failure, bleeding diathesis, and phlebitis, and a potential for rebound intracranial hypertension have all been reported.

With the exception of albumin no colloid solution occurs in physiologic systems. A major concern with the use of colloid solutions is its ability to affect coagulation; this occurs when the ratio of blood volume to colloid solution volume is less than 10:4[41] (Table 43–3).

Dextrans

Dextran is a single-chain polysaccharide derived from the bacterium, Leuconostoc mesenteroides. The dextrans are designated "70," "60," and "40" as their average molecular weight in daltons, 70,000, 60,000, and 40,000, respectively. Dextran 70 has a colloid osmotic pressure of 350 mOsm/L, whereas dextran 40 has a greater oncotic pressure and will help "extract" more fluid from the intracellular space. Dextrans are eliminated largely through the kidney, although small amounts are metabolized and even smaller amounts are eliminated in the gut.

Dextran 40 has been used extensively to reduce blood viscosity and also increase the time to red cell aggregation through an effect on rouleaux formation and has been used for prophylaxis against the development of thrombosis. There is a recent suggestion that dextrans may also influence leukocyte adherence and thereby may be of interest in ischemia/reperfusion injury.[42-44]

At dextran doses greater than 1.5 mL/kg, coagulation is impaired because of a reduction in factor VIII and an effect on the polymerization of fibrin. The effects are similar to von Willebrand disease and may be reversed in part with desmopressin.[45] The dextrans have been in clinical use for a considerable period in Europe and have a good safety record.

TABLE 43–3.

Principles for an Ideal Colloid

- Stable on the shelf

- Sterile, toxin free, antigen free, and devoid of active ingredients

- An adequate colloid oncotic pressure

- Long half-life in the circulation

- Easily cleared form the interstitium, e.g., lymph drainage

- Easily metabolized with no toxic metabolites

- No effect on the immune system

- No effects on coagulation

Gelatin

The average molecular weight of the gelatins is about 35,000 daltons, but there is a wide distribution in molecular size; thus the smaller molecules are easily removed from the intravascular compartment and can be detected in the urine. Even in healthy volunteers, gelatin solutions have a relatively short intravascular half-life albeit considerably longer than that seen with crystalloid solutions. This benefit may not be evident in the critically ill patient in whom endothelial permeability is increased.

There are at least two gelatin solutions in common use both of which are approximately isotonic. Hemaccel is a solution containing 3.5% gelatin derived by hydrolysis of animal collagen and is a di-isocyanate urea and contains high concentrations of calcium (6.25 mmol/L) and potassium (5.1 mmol/L). Gelofusin is a plasmion-succinylated gelatin and contains no calcium as it is in a 0.9% saline solution. Metabolism takes place in the liver and the gelatin is completely eliminated.

There are few documented problems with coagulation and those that occur are probably on the basis of "dilutional coagulopathy" (see Chapter 53). There is a small risk for true anaphylaxis; histamine release has been reported with polygelin and this may result in hypotension, bronchospasm, and skin rash; recent improvement in formulation have reduced the incidence of reactions to less than 1%.[46]

The clinical use of gelatins is widespread. It is relatively cheap and is easily metabolized and excreted producing an oncotic diuresis, although this is not evident in normovolemic patients. Being relatively small it will "leak" whenever the endothelial barrier is compromised.[47]

Hydroxy Ethyl Starch

Starch solutions were initially prepared by hydrolysis from corn. To prevent its further hydrolysis by alpha-amylase it is stabilized by hydroxylation or esterification. The hydroxy ethylation is usually at C2 but can be at C3 or C6. The resultant molecules are intrinsically hydrophilic and bind water with a capacity of 20 to 30 mL/kg. This combined with their oncotic pressure provides good volume expansion properties. The starches are now available in an ever-increasing array of configurations.

These are now conventionally described by the average molecular weight and then by the degree of molecular substitution. Hence hydroxy ethyl starch (HES) 6% 450/0.7 describes a starch with a molecular weight of 450,000 daltons and molecular substitution of 70%. The molecular weight is invariably less because of breakdown determined by the ratio of substitutions of anhydroglucose by hydroxyethyl groups at C2 and C6 (described as C2/C6) (Table 43–4).

Some of the starch will be sequestered in the reticuloendothelial system[48]; with repeated doses, accumulation and hence coagulopathies can occur, which is determined to a large extent by the degree of substitution and the ratio C2/C6. All of the starches discussed earlier are effective as plasma expanders and have reasonably long half-lives in the

TABLE 43–4.

Some of the Commercially Available Starches with Their Configurations

Hydroxy Ethyl Starch	
6%	450/0.7
3%	200/0.5
6%	200/0.62 (Elohes)
10%	200/0.45
6%	130/0.4 (Voluven)
Pentastarch	
	264/0.45

plasma in patients with "normal" endothelial permeability. The middle range starches such as HES 200/0.62 are effective in the maintenance of plasma volume expansion over 24 hours in routine surgical patients.[48] The low molecular weight-HES solution has been used effectively and safely for volume replacement in the prebypass period in small children undergoing cardiac surgery. The potential problems with the larger starches include coagulopathy, which has restricted their use. A 3% hetastarch has even been used in plasma exchange with no obvious deleterious effects.[49,50] The recommended limitations in dosing for 10% HES 200/0.5 is 20 mL/kg, whereas for the 6% HES 200/0.5 it is 33 mL/kg. The dose limitations were introduced to obviate the occurrence of coagulopathies. Lower molecular weight and lower substitution, such as HES 70/0.5, reduce this risk considerably.

Newer starches are being produced to overcome some of the perceived difficulties. A new product with a molecular weight of 130 kD ($\pm$20 kD) and with a narrow distribution of molecular size, a low degree of substitution, 0.4, and a C2/C6 ratio greater than 8 allows rapid elimination with minimal accumulation on multiple dosing.

Side effects are determined largely by the molecular weight of the starch, whereas pharmacokinetics is determined by the position of the hydroxy ethylation. Some studies have suggested that starches may have beneficial effects in patients undergoing major surgery. Gosling reported that Elohes 6% 200/0.62 appeared to have an anti-inflammatory action in patients undergoing aortic repair resulting in improved renal function. Another study using Hespan in trauma patients also showed less urinary albumin excretion, which again was taken as a surrogate for an improvement in capillary permeability.[51] There is also a report of a canine model of myocardial ischemia that suggests that the use of HES may reduce infarct size.[52] Hetastarch has also been shown to reduce the xanthine oxidase activity and hence exert an anti-inflammatory effect.[53,54]

Adverse side effects include pruritus in up to 22% of patients receiving Elohes.[55] The mechanism may relate to the storage of starches in various cells including macrophages, endothelial cells, and epithelial cells, and may be caused by direct stimulation of cutaneous nerves by HES deposits.[56,57]

The small starch molecules are eliminated through the kidneys and histology has revealed reversible swelling of tubular cells after starch administration. The mechanism is thought to be caused by reabsorption of macromolecules. Patients administered high molecular weight starches, 450 kD/0.7, show increased creatinine levels.[58] In some patients who received a transplant who were given high molecular weight starch, lesions were seen but these had no obvious effect on renal function.[59] It has also been suggested that lower molecular weight starches in high concentration might affect renal function. In a study of renal donors, the incidence of renal impairment was greater in the starch group (200/0.62) than the gelatin group, albeit in small numbers.[60] In contrast, in a study of renal allografts, starches had no obvious effect on renal function.[61] Similarly, there was no obvious renal problem in a group of critically ill patients.[62]

Immune Function: An adverse influence of starches on immune function has been reported including reduced leucocyte adherence in trauma patients.[63,64] There was no obvious effect of cell-mediated immunity in shocked mice.[65]

In many clinical situations for which patients are infused large volumes of colloid, there may already be underlying problems with hemostasis. Differentiating dilutional coagulopathy from effects of the colloid may prove difficult. Most of the initial coagulopathies were seen with the high molecular weight starches (such as 450 kD/0.7),[66,67] and considerably fewer coagulopathies are seen in patients treated with the newer starches.[62,68]

HES increases blood viscosity, decreases erythrocyte deformability, and increases erythrocyte aggregation when compared with saline.[69]

Higher molecular weight starches can cause a shortened thrombin time with decreased fibrinogen caused by increased polymerization of fibrinogen. Activated partial thromboplastin time is also prolonged because of a reduction in von Willebrand factor and also factor VIII,[70] possibly because these factors are complexed to the starch. The ratio of C2/C6 influences the breakdown of the starches and hence the tendency to accumulate. It is the accumulation of the larger molecules that leads to the impaired coagulation.[71-73]

Although the incidence of coagulopathies decreases with the reduction in molecular weight, these are still evident even when starches less than 70 kD are used.[74-76] Although effects may not be evident after a single dose, these may occur when the starch accumulates with repeated dosing.[77,78]

Colloids have now been formulated in a more physiologic medium. Hextend is 6% hetastarch in a balanced solution with a lactate buffer and physiologic levels of glucose. It is as effective as 6% hetastarch in saline for the treatment of hypovolemia but has a more favorable side effects profile in volumes of up to 5 L compared with 6% hetastarch in saline. Using TEG, there were less problems with clot formation than were seen with HES.[79]

Acetyl starch has been used and has the advantage of rapid and nearly complete enzymatic degradation.[80]

Albumin

Albumin is a naturally occurring protein with important biologic functions including binding because of its strong net negative charge. It is in effect a circulating depot and transport molecule for a large number of metabolites, including fatty acids, ions (especially Ca^{2+} and Cu^{2+}), thyroxine, bilirubin, and amino acids. It also binds covalently and irreversibly with Ag^{2+}, Hg^{2+}, D-glucose, and D-galactose. There are four discrete binding sites on the albumin molecule, with varying specificity for different substances. Ligands can compete at a single site or may compete by altering the affinity of remote sites through conformational changes to the tertiary structure of the molecule. Therefore, drugs that bind at the same site will compete for occupancy and are likely to displace one another (e.g., warfarin and Phenytoin); other drugs known to be highly albumin-bound in plasma may interact at separate sites and therefore will not displace one another (e.g., warfarin and diazepam). Pharmaceutical ligands (especially warfarin, phenytoin, nonsteroidal anti-inflammatory agents, and digoxin) binding to albumin are of particular clinical significance, because of their highly protein-bound state and low margin of safety. In the anesthetic and intensive care unit setting, midazolam, sodium pentothal, and several antibiotics can be considered in the same light.

Albumin comprises 50% of the normal intravascular protein mass; because of its relatively small size ($\pm67,000$ dalton) compared with other plasma protein, it represents some 75% of the total number of protein molecules and is responsible for 75% to 80% of the plasma colloid osmotic pressure. In fact, the rate of albumin synthesis is dependent on colloid osmotic pressure.

Albumin is a potential free radical scavenging agent and is the major intravascular source of reduced sulfhydryl groups because of the single exposed cysteine residue at position 31. These sulfhydryl groups are avid scavengers of reactive oxygen and nitrogen species, especially the superoxide, hydroxyl, and peroxynitrite radicals.[81] Albumin can also limit the production of these reactive species by binding free copper, an ion known to be particularly important in accelerating the production of free radicals.[82] It has been postulated that albumin has anticoagulant and antithrombotic function[83] mediated in part by its ability to bind nitric oxide radicals as S-nitrosothiols, thereby inhibiting their rapid inactivation and allowing a more prolonged antiaggregatory platelet effect.[84]

Albumin is used to prime the cardiopulmonary bypass circuits to reduce platelet deposition[85] especially in small volume circuits for children;[86,87] however, the functional advantage has yet to be clearly demonstrated.

Commercially produced albumin is available in several forms including 5% and 20% solutions; the latter is salt free but hypertonic. Albumin is prepared from pooled plasma, fractionated in ethanol, purified then heat treated for 10 hours at 60°C (to render it sterile and thereby obviating the risk for contamination by hepatitis or human immunodeficiency virus). It is already more expensive than the other available colloids and the yet more expensive recombinant albumin is priced too high for routine clinical use.

There are potential differences between the commercially available albumin and the natural substance. The preparative processes may affect charge, and a number of commercial albumins have been shown to contain significant quantities of residual ions from the separation and concentration processes, especially aluminium[70] and vanadium.[88] Potentially toxic levels of aluminium have been reported in patients after massive albumin infusion.[89]

Ever since the work by Demling established that reduced serum albumin is associated with increased capillary leakage that can be corrected by albumin administration,[90,91] albumin has been touted as having a more beneficial effect on membrane permeability than other colloid solutions.[92] Using radiolabeled albumin in patients with sepsis, no alteration in TER was observed after an albumin bolus.[93]

Albumin is an effective intravascular volume expanding agent; although the potential attributes listed earlier have been demonstrated in preclinical settings, it has not been shown to be superior to that seen with other colloid solutions when used for volume expansion.[94–96] In a poorly controlled study, marked benefit was seen in patients with liver failure and bacterial peritonitis who were treated with albumin; no volume expander was used in the control group![97] Hypertonic albumin has been advocated as a means of differentially affecting the intravascular and interstitial space; however, in the critically ill patient, the intravascular and interstitial compartments are not discrete and hence a beneficial effect seems unlikely.

Clinical Issues

In deciding the appropriate class of solution (crystalloid vs. colloid) to use a risk/benefit analysis one must consider whether the benefits of its long-lived efficacy as a plasma substitute is counteracted by the risks for edema, anaphylaxis, and coagulopathy. A further consideration is the cost/benefit analysis.

The low cost and incidence of anaphylactic reactions favor crystalloid solutions. If one considers short-term efficacy, then colloid solutions can be used in smaller volumes to achieve the same effect.[98] The most contentious issue is whether excessive fluid administration is more or less likely to result in the development of edema. Which of these two classes of solutions achieves this should be considered within the context of the goal of fluid resuscitation, i.e., the return of the circulating blood volume to normal as rapidly as possible. Achievement of this goal is signaled by restoration of normal hemodynamic parameters with warm and well-perfused peripheral tissues and maintenance of normal organ function (lucid mental state, satisfactory urine output with biochemical markers indicative of aerobic metabolism). These signs indicate that an effective cardiac output has been achieved and that the patient is perfusing and oxygenating his or her tissues well and providing a functional response to organ support and treatment. Use of surrogate hemodynamic end points such central venous pressure, pulmonary artery occlusion pressure, and cardiac output can be misleading and the clinical signs should not be disregarded as valid measures of physiologic well being simply because these are at variance with other parameters.

Studies addressing the influence of edema on oxygen delivery have provided equivocal data[99,100]; the confounding variable appears to be the precise constituents of the edema fluid and particularly the presence of albumin.[12]

A systematic review indicated a greater mortality rate with colloids than with crystalloids and a further review suggested that albumin caused harm.[101,102] However, the heterogeneity of the populations, the study designs, and the long-term consequence (beyond the impact on hemodynamic parameters), and the lack of "power" (less than 2,000 patients) make these analyses questionable. An effectively powered randomized control trial would need more than 5,000 patients to show a difference if one existed.[103,104] A more recent Cochrane review was considered in its conclusion and found no evidence of benefit of one class of solution over another.[105]

From a clinical viewpoint, resuscitation with crystalloid solutions require greater volumes to be administered, thereby increasing the risk for edema. However, colloid solutions do have occasional problems with anaphylaxis and are more expensive even though the cost of the fluids in the context of treating a severely ill patient is negligible.

Conclusion

Maintenance fluids should be appropriate to replenish the patient's daily losses. During resuscitation, clinical signs are the pre-eminent indicators supported if necessary by hemodynamic parameters and biochemical measurement. There is no clear advantage of any particular fluid. Hypertonic solutions are apparently useful in the short term but carry a potential price in terms of hypernatremia and of hyperosmolarity. Colloids are also effective but may have potential for anaphylaxis and have a cost implication. Both types of fluid are likely to reduce rather than to prevent edema. Crystalloids are inexpensive and effective but may require large volumes. Of all the fluids with which we replete the intravascular space, only albumin is supposed to have some of the intrinsic properties and qualities of plasma. The benign substitutes that are infused are not copies of plasma.

References

1. Ganong WF: The general and cellular basis of medical physiology. In Ganong WF (ed): Review of Medical Physiology, 17th ed. University of California: Prentice-Hall, pp 5–12, 1995.
2. Basset G, Crone C, Saumon G: Fluid absorption by rat lung in situ: Pathways for sodium entry in the luminal membrane of alveolar epithelium. J Physiol 384:325–345, 1987.
3. Verghese GM, Ware LB, Matthay BA, et al: Alveolar epithelial fluid transport and the resolution of clinically severe hydrostatic pulmonary edema. J Appl Physiol 87(4):1301–1312, 1999.
4. Suzuki S, Noda M, Sugita M, et al: Impairment of transalveolar fluid transport and lung Na(+)-K(+)-ATPase function by hypoxia in rats. J Appl Physiol 87(3):962–968, 1999.

5. Matthay MA, Wiener-Kronish JP: Intact epithelial barrier function is critical for the resolution of alveolar edema in humans. Am Rev Respir Dis 142(6 pt 1):1250–1257, 1990.

6. Pittet JF, Wiener-Kronish JP, McElroy MC, et al: Stimulation of lung epithelial liquid clearance by endogenous release of catecholamines in septic shock in anesthetized rats. J Clin Invest 94(2):663–671, 1994.

7. Twigley AJ, Hillman KM: The end of the crystalloid era? A new approach to peri-operative fluid administration. Anaesthesia 40(9):860–871, 1985.

8. Bone RC, Balk RA, Cerra FB, et al: Definitions for sepsis and organ failure and guidelines for the use of innovative therapies in sepsis. The ACCP/SCCM Consensus Conference Committee. American College of Chest Physicians/Society of Critical Care Medicine. Chest 101(6):1644–1655, 1992.

9. Alfaro VP, Palacios J: Acid-base disturbance during hemorrhage in rats: Significant role of strong inorganic ions. J Appl Physiol 86(5):1617–1625, 1999.

10. Waters JH, Bernstein CA: Dilutional acidosis following hetastarch or albumin in healthy volunteers. Anesthesiology 93(5):1184–1187, 2000.

11. Canizaro PC, Prager MD, Shires GT: The infusion of Ringer's lactate solution during shock. Changes in lactate, excess lactate, and pH. Am J Surg 122(4):494–501, 1971.

12. Kierdorf HP, Leue C, Arns S: Lactate- or bicarbonate-buffered solutions in continuous extracorporeal renal replacement therapies. Kidney Int 56(suppl 72):S32–S36, 1999.

13. Thongboonkerd V, Lumlertgul D, Supajatura V: Better correction of metabolic acidosis, blood pressure control, and phagocytosis with bicarbonate compared to lactate solution in acute peritoneal dialysis. Artif Organs 25(2):99–108, 2001.

14. Hauser CJ, Shoemaker WC, Turpin I, et al: Oxygen transport responses to colloids and crystalloids in critically ill surgical patients. Surg Gynecol Obstet 150(6):811–816, 1980.

15. Lamke LO, Liljedahl SO: Plasma volume changes after infusion of various plasma expanders. Resuscitation 5(2):93–102, 1976.

16. Cervera AL, Moss G: Crystalloid distribution following hemorrhage and hemodilution: Mathematical model and prediction of optimum volumes for equilibration at normovolemia. J Trauma 14(6):506–520, 1974.

17. Funk W, Baldinger V: Microcirculatory perfusion during volume therapy. A comparative study using crystalloid or colloid in awake animals. Anesthesiology 82(4):975–982, 1995.

18. Wang P, Hauptman JG, Chaudry IH: Hemorrhage produces depression in microvascular blood flow which persists despite fluid resuscitation. Circ Shock 32(4):307–318, 1990.

19. Svensen C, Sjostrand F, Hahn RG: Volume kinetics of intravenous fluid therapy in the prehospital setting. Prehospital Disaster Med 16(1):9–13, 2001.

20. Baum TD, Wang H, Rothschild HR, et al: Mesenteric oxygen metabolism, ileal mucosal hydrogen ion concentration, and tissue edema after crystalloid or colloid resuscitation in porcine endotoxic shock: Comparison of Ringer's lactate and 6% hetastarch. Circ Shock 30(4):385–397, 1990.

21. Rabinovici R, Gross D, Krausz MM: Infusion of small volume of 7.5 per cent sodium chloride in 6.0 per cent dextran 70 for the treatment of uncontrolled hemorrhagic shock. Surg Gynecol Obstet 169(2):137–142, 1989.

22. Croft D, Dion YM, Dumont M, et al: Cardiac compliance and effects of hypertonic saline. Can J Surg 35(2):139–144, 1992.

23. Diebel LN, Tyburski JG, Dulchavsky SA: Effect of hypertonic saline solution and dextran on ventricular blood flow and heart-lung interaction after hemorrhagic shock. Surgery 124(4):642–649, 1998.

24. Doucet JJ, Hall RI: Limited resuscitation with hypertonic saline, hypertonic sodium acetate, and lactated Ringer's solutions in a model of uncontrolled hemorrhage from a vascular injury. J Trauma 47(5):956–963, 1999.

25. Oi Y, Aneman A, Svensson M, et al: Hypertonic saline-dextran improves intestinal perfusion and survival in porcine endotoxin shock. Crit Care Med 28(8):2843–2850, 2000.

26. Dubick MA, Davis JM, Myers T, et al: Dose response effects of hypertonic saline and dextran on cardiovascular responses and plasma volume expansion in sheep. Shock 3(2):137–144, 1995.

27. Mouren S, Delayance S, Mion G, et al: Mechanisms of increased myocardial contractility with hypertonic saline solutions in isolated blood-perfused rabbit hearts. Anesth Analg 81(4):777–782, 1995.

28. Kien ND, Reitan JA, White DA, et al: Cardiac contractility and blood flow distribution following resuscitation with 7.5% hypertonic saline in anesthetized dogs. Circ Shock 35(2):109–116, 1991.

29. Kien ND, Antognini JF, Reilly DA, et al: Small-volume resuscitation using hypertonic saline improves organ perfusion in burned rats. Anesth Analg 83(4):782–788, 1996.

30. Kien ND, Moore PG, Pascual JM, et al: Effects of hypertonic saline on regional function and blood flow in canine hearts during acute coronary occlusion. Shock 7(4):274–281, 1997.

31. Zallen G, Moore EE, Tamura DY, et al: Hypertonic saline resuscitation abrogates neutrophil priming by mesenteric lymph. J Trauma 48(1):45–48, 2000.

32. Zoran DL, Jergens AE, Riedesel DH, et al: Evaluation of hemostatic analytes after use of hypertonic saline solution combined with colloids for resuscitation of dogs with hypovolemia. Am J Vet Res 53(10):1791–1796, 1992.

33. Patrick DA, Moore EE, Offner PJ, et al: Hypertonic saline activates lipid-primed human neutrophils for enhanced elastase release. J Trauma 44(4):592–597, 1998.

34. Ciesla DJ, Moore EE, Zallen G, et al: Hypertonic saline attenuation of polymorphonuclear neutrophil cytotoxicity: Timing is everything. J Trauma 48(3):388–395, 2000.

35. Shackford SR, Bourguignon PR, Wald SL, et al: Hypertonic saline resuscitation of patients with head injury: A prospective, randomized clinical trial. J Trauma 44(1):50–58, 1998.

36. Sirieix D, Hongnat JM, Delayance S, et al: Comparison of the acute hemodynamic effects of hypertonic or colloid infusions immediately after mitral valve repair. Crit Care Med 27(10):2159–2165, 1999.

37. Qureshi AI, Suarez JI: Use of hypertonic saline solutions in treatment of cerebral edema and intracranial hypertension. Crit Care Med 28(9):3301–3313, 2000.

38. Tollofsrud S, Noddeland H: Hypertonic saline and dextran after coronary artery surgery mobilizes fluid excess and improves cardiorespiratory functions. Acta Anaesthesiol Scand 42(2):154–161, 1998.

39. Simma B, Burger R, Falk M, et al: A prospective, randomized, and controlled study of fluid management in children with severe head injury: Lactated Ringer's solution versus hypertonic saline. Crit Care Med 26(7):1265–1270, 1998.

40. Elgjo GI, Traber DL, Hawkins HK, et al: Burn resuscitation with two doses of 4 mL/kg hypertonic saline dextran provides sustained fluid sparing: A 48-hour prospective study in conscious sheep. J Trauma 49(2):251–263, 2000.

41. Petroianu GA, Liu J, Maleck WH, et al: The effect of in vitro hemodilution with gelatin, dextran, hydroxyethyl starch, or Ringer's solution on Thrombelastograph. Anesth Analg 90(4):795–800, 2000.

42. Dewachter P, Laxenaire MC, Donner M, et al: In vivo rheologic studies of plasma substitutes. Ann Fr Anesth Reanim 11(5):516–525, 1992.

43. Steinbauer M, Harris AG, Leiderer R, et al: Impact of dextran on microvascular disturbances and tissue injury following ischemia/reperfusion in striated muscle. Shock 9(5):345–351, 1998.

44. Harris AG, Steinbauer M, Leiderer R, et al: Role of leukocyte plugging and edema in skeletal muscle ischemia-reperfusion injury. Am J Physiol 273(2 Pt 2):H989–H996, 1997.

45. Aberg M, Hedner U, Bergentz SE: Effect of dextran 70 on factor VIII and platelet function in von Willebrand's disease. Thromb Res 12(4):629–634, 1978.

46. Davies MJ: Polygeline. Dev Biol Stand 67:129–131, 1987.

47. Webb AR, Barclay SA, Bennett ED: In vitro colloid osmotic pressure of commonly used plasma expanders and substitutes: A study of the diffusibility of colloid molecules. Intensive Care Med 15(2):116–120, 1989.

48. Degremont AC, Ismail M, Arthaud M, et al: Mechanisms of postoperative prolonged plasma volume expansion with low molecular weight hydroxethyl starch (HES 200/0.62, 6%). Intensive Care Med 21(7):577–583, 1995.

49. Owen HG, Brecher ME: Partial colloid starch replacement for therapeutic plasma exchange. J Clin Apheresis 12(2):87–92, 1997.

50. Eastlund DT, Douglas MS, Choper JZ: Monocyte chemotaxis and chemotactic cytokine release after exposure to hydroxyethyl starch. Transfusion 32(9):855–860, 1992.

51. Allison KP, Gosling P, Jones S, et al: Randomized trial of hydroxyethyl starch versus gelatine for trauma resuscitation. J Trauma 47(6):1114–1121, 1999.

52. Zikria BA, Subbarao C, Oz MC, et al: Hydroxyethyl starch macro-

molecules reduce myocardial reperfusion injury. Arch Surg 125(7):930–934, 1990.

53. Nielsen VG, Tan S, Brix AE, et al: Hextend (hetastarch solution) decreases multiple organ injury and xanthine oxidase release after hepatoenteric ischemia-reperfusion in rabbits. Crit Care Med 25(9):1565–1574, 1997.

54. Nielsen VG, Baird MS, Brix AE, Matalon S: Extreme, progressive isovolemic hemodilution with 5% human albumin, PentaLyte, or Hextend does not cause hepatic ischemia or histologic injury in rabbits. Anesthesiology 90(5):1428–1435, 1999.

55. Morgan PW, Berridge JC: Giving long persistent starch as volume replacement can cause pruritus after cardiac surgery. Br J Anaesth 85(5):696–699, 2000.

56. Jurecka W, Szepfalusi Z, Parth E, et al: Hydroxyethylstarch deposits in human skin—a model for pruritus? Arch Dermatol Res 285(1-2):13–19, 1993.

57. Gall H, Schultz KD, Boehncke WH, et al: Clinical and pathophysiological aspects of hydroxyethyl starch-induced pruritus: Evaluation of 96 cases. Dermatology 192(3):222–226, 1996.

58. Haskell LP, Tannenberg AM: Elevated urinary specific gravity in acute oliguric renal failure due to hetastarch administration. NY State J Med 88(7):387–388, 1988.

59. Legendre C, Thervet E, Page B, et al: Hydroxyethyl staroh and osmotic-nephrosis like lesions in kidney transplantation. Lancet 342:248–249, 1993.

60. Cittanova ML, Leblanc I, Legendre C, et al: Effect of hydroxyethyl-starch in brain-dead kidney donors on renal function in kidney-transplant recipients. Lancet 348(9042):1620–1622, 1996.

61. Deman A, Peeters P, Sennesael J: Hydroxyethyl starch does not impair immediate renal function in kidney transplant recipients: A retrospective, multicentre analysis. Nephrol Dial Transplant 14(6):1517–1520, 1999.

62. Boldt J, Muller M, Mentges D, et al: Volume therapy in the critically ill: Is there a difference? Intensive Care Med 24(1):28–36, 1998.

63. Boldt J, Heesen M, Padberg W, et al: The influence of volume therapy and pentoxifylline infusion on circulating adhesion molecules in trauma patients. Anaesthesia 51(6):529–535, 1996.

64. Collis RE, Collins PW, Gutteridge CN, et al: The effect of hydroxyethyl starch and other plasma volume substitutes on endothelial cell activation an in vitro study. Intensive Care Med 20(1):37–41, 1994.

65. Schmand JF, Ayala A, Morrison MH, Chaudry IH: Effects of hydroxyethyl starch after trauma-hemorrhagic shock: Restoration of macrophage integrity and prevention of increased circulating inter-leukin-6 levels. Crit Care Med 23(5):806–814, 1995.

66. Warren BB, Durieux ME: Hydroxyethyl starch: Safe or not? Anesth Analg 84(1):206–212, 1997.

67. Cope JT, Banks D, Mauney MC, et al: Intraoperative hetastarch infusion impairs hemostasis after cardiac operations. Ann Thorac Surg 63(1):78–82, 1997.

68. Treib J, Haass A, Pindur G, et al: All medium starches are not the same: Influence of the degree of hydroxyethyl substitution of hydroxyethyl starch on plasma volume, hemorrheologic conditions, and coagulation. Transfusion 36(5):450–455, 1996.

69. Castro VJ, Astiz ME, Rackow EC: Effect of crystalloid and colloid solutions on blood rheology in sepsis. Shock 8(2):104–107, 1997.

70. Sanfelippo MJ, Suberviola PD, Geimer NF: Development of a von Willebrand-like syndrome after prolonged use of hydroxyethyl starch. Am J Clin Pathol 88(5):653–655, 1987.

71. Treib J, Baron JF, Grauer MT, Strauss RG: An international view of hydroxyethyl starches. Intensive Care Med 25(3):258–268, 1999.

72. Treib J, Baron JF: Hydroxyethyl starch: Effects on hemostasis. Ann Fr Anesth Reanim 17(1):72–81, 1998.

73. Treib J, Haass A, Pindur G, et al: HES 200/0.5 is not HES 200/0.5. Influence of the C2/C6 hydroxyethylation ratio of hydroxyethyl starch (HES) on hemorheology, coagulation and elimination kinetics. Thromb Haemost 74(6):1452–1456, 1995.

74. Stoll M, Treib J, Schenk JF, et al: No coagulation disorders under high-dose volume therapy with low-molecular-weight hydroxyethyl starch. Haemostasis 27(5):251–258, 1997.

75. Entholzner EK, Mielke LL, Calatzis AN, et al: Coagulation effects of a recently developed hydroxyethyl starch (HES 130/0.4) compared to hydroxyethyl starches with higher molecular weight. Acta Anaesthesiol Scand 44(9):1116–1121, 2000.

76. Jamnicki M, Bombeli T, Seifert B, et al: Low and medium molecular weight hydroxyethyl starches comparison of their effect on blood coagulation. Anesthesiology 95(5):1231–1237, 2000.

77. Medel J, Baron JF: A new hydroxyethyl starch for volume replacement: Elohes 6%. Rev Esp Anestesiol Reanim 45(9):389–396, 1998.

78. Baron JF: Pharmacology of low molecular weight hydroxyethyl starch. Ann Fr Anesth Reanim 11(5):509–515, 1992.

79. Gan TJ, Bennett Guerrero E, Phillips-Bute B, et al: Hextend, a physiologically balanced plasma expander for large volume use in major surgery: A randomized phase III clinical trial. Hextend Study Group. Anesth Analg 88(5):992–998, 1999.

80. Behne M, Thomas H, Bremerich DH, et al: The pharmacokinetics of acetyl starch as a plasma volume expander in patients undergoing elective surgery. Anesth Analg 86(4):856–860, 1998.

81. Halliwell B: Albumin—an important extracellular antioxidant? Biochem Pharmacol 37(4):569–571, 1988.

82. Strubelt O, Younes M, Li Y: Protection by albumin against ischaemia- and hypoxia-induced hepatic injury. Pharmacol Toxicol 75(5):280–284, 1994.

83. Dietrich G, Haupt W, Kretschmer V: Disorders of primary hemostasis caused by albumin infusion in hemodilution. Beitr Infusionsther 28:331–334, 1991.

84. Simon DI, Stamler JS, Jaraki O, et al: Antiplatelet properties of protein S-nitrosothiols derived from nitric oxide and endothelium-derived relaxing factor. Arterioscler Thromb 13(6):791–799, 1993.

85. Mulvihill JN, Faradji A, Oberling F, et al: Surface passivation by human albumin of plasmapheresis circuits reduces platelet accumulation and thrombus formation. Experimental and clinical studies. J Biomed Mater Res 24(2):155–163, 1990.

86. Marelli D, Paul A, Samson R, et al: Does the addition of albumin to the prime solution in cardiopulmonary bypass affect clinical outcome? A prospective randomized study. J Thorac Cardiovasc Surg 98(5 pt 1):751–756, 1989.

87. Tollofsrud S, Svennevig JL, Breivik H, et al: Fluid balance and pulmonary functions during and after coronary artery bypass surgery: Ringer's acetate compared with dextran, polygeline, or albumin. Acta Anaesthesiol Scand 39(5):671–677, 1995.

88. Quinlan GJ, Coudray C, Hubbard A, et al: Vanadium and copper in clinical solutions of albumin and their potential to damage protein structure. J Pharm Sci 81(7):611–614, 1992.

89. Koppel C, Baudisch H, Ibe K: Inadvertent metal loading of critically ill patients with acute renal failure by human albumin solution infusion therapy. J Toxicol Clin Toxicol 26(5-6):337–356, 1988.

90. Demling RH, Harms B, Kramer G, et al: Acute versus sustained hypoproteinemia and posttraumatic pulmonary edema. Surgery 92(1):79–86, 1982.

91. Harms BA, Kramer GC, Bodai BI, et al: Effect of hypoproteinemia on pulmonary and soft tissue edema formation. Crit Care Med 9(7):503–508, 1981.

92. Holbeck S, Grande PO: Effects on capillary fluid permeability and fluid exchange of albumin, dextran, gelatin, and hydroxyethyl starch in cat skeletal muscle. Crit Care Med 28(4):1089–1095, 2000.

93. Margarson MP: The Albumin Distribution Index [MD]. London: University of London, 2000.

94. Stockwell M, Soni N, Riley B: Colloid solutions in the critically ill. A randomized comparison of albumin and polygeline. 1. Outcome and duration of stay in the intensive care unit. Anaesthesia 47:3–6, 1992.

95. Stockwell M, Scott A, Riley B, et al: Colloid solutions in the critically ill. A randomized comparison of albumin and polygeline. 2. Serum albumin concentration and incidences of pulmonary edema and acute renal failure. Anaesthesia 47:7–9, 1992.

96. Golub R, Sorrento J, Cantu R, et al: Efficacy of albumin supplementation in the surgical intensive care unit: A prospective randomized study. Crit Care Med 22(4):613–619, 1994.

97. Sort P, Navasa M, Arroyo V, et al: Effect of intravenous albumin on renal impairment and mortality in patients with cirrhosis and spontaneous bacterial peritonitis. N Engl J Med 341(6):403–409, 1999.

98. Karanko MS, Klossner JA, et al: Restoration of volume by crystalloid versus colloid after coronary artery bypass: Hemodynamics, lung water, oxygenation, and outcome. Crit Care Med 15(6):559–566, 1987.

99. Ostgaard G, Reed RK: Interstitial fluid accumulation does not influence oxygen uptake in the rabbit small intestine. Acta Anaesthesiol Scand 39(2):167–173, 1995.

100. Rackow EC, Astiz ME, Schumer W, et al: Lung and muscle water after crystalloid and colloid infusion in septic rats: Effect on oxygen delivery and metabolism. J Lab Clin Med 113(2):184–189, 1989.

101. Schierhout G, Roberts I: Fluid resuscitation with colloid or crystalloid solutions in critically ill patients: A systematic review of randomized trials. BMJ 316:961–964, 1998.

102. Roberts I: Human albumin administration in critically ill patients: Systematic review of randomized controlled trials. BMJ 317:235–240, 1998.

103. Choi P, Yip G, Quinonez L, Cook D: Crystalloids vs colloids in fluid resuscitation: A systematic review. Crit Care Med 27:200–210, 1999.

104. Velanovich V: Crystalloid versus colloid resuscitation: A meta analysis of mortality. Surgery 105:65–71, 1989.

105. Bunn F, Alderson P, Hawkins V: Colloid solutions for fluid resuscitation. Cochrane Database Syst Rev (2):Cd001319, 2000.

44

Antimotility and Antisecretory Agents

Robert P. Walt, MD, FRCP • Eugene B. Campbell, MB, ChB

For decades the main therapies available to alter gut motility and secretion were opiates and antimuscarinic agents. In the 1970s, histamine-2 (H_2) receptor antagonists provided effective suppression of gastric acid secretion for the first time. A decade later, proton pump inhibitors (PPIs) went a step further in efficacy. With further recognition of the transmitters and receptors involved in secretion and motility, the promise of further advances seems likely.

Physiologic Targets for Drug Action

Motility

Transit of luminal contents depends on a series of contractions and relaxations of the smooth muscles. These are integrated to mix the bowel contents and propel them through the gut. This propulsion is under both central control through the vagus nerve and locally by the enteric nervous system. The enteric nervous system contains about 10^8 neurons, approximately the same number as in the spinal cord. These form neural circuits that control motor functions, blood flow, secretions, absorption, and interact with

TABLE 44–1.

Daily Fluid Turnover in the Gut (L)

Ingested	2
Endogenous secretions	
Saliva	1.5
Stomach	2.5
Bile	0.5
Pancreas	1.5
Intestine	1
Total input	9
Absorbed	
Jejunum	5.5
Ileum	2
Colon	1.3
Balance in stool	0.2

other organs such as the pancreas and gallbladder. There are many transmitters and receptors identified in the gut wall but their physiologic roles are not all understood.[1]

Secretions and Fluid Turnover

The normal small intestine is presented with about 9 L of fluid a day, 2 L from the diet and the rest are secretions. Net absorption is such that only 1.5 L reaches the colon (Table 44–1). The colon has a large capacity to absorb fluids—up to 6 L per 24 hours provided it is presented evenly and not in large fluxes.[2]

Gastric Acid Secretion

The human stomach contains 1 billion parietal cells, each capable of secreting 3.3 billion hydrogen ions per second. Hydrochloric acid is produced at a pH of 0.8 or 150 mmol/L. Gastric acid serves several purposes, including aiding digestion and preventing bacterial colonization of the small bowel.

Acid secretion is controlled by three pathways: neurocrine, paracrine, and endocrine. The major neurocrine transmitter is acetylcholine secreted from postganglionic vagal neurons. This acts through muscarinic receptors on the gastric parietal cell to stimulate hydrogen ion secretion. Histamine is the primary paracrine transmitter and binds to histamine receptors causing cyclic adenosine monophosphate levels within the cell to increase and acid secretion to begin. Endocrine control is mediated through gastrin secreted from the gastric antral cells. Gastrin causes acid secretion by stimulating histamine secretion from enterochromaffin-like cells and by binding to gastrin receptors on parietal cells.

The final step in acid production is the enzyme that secretes hydrogen ions. This is located on the tubulovesicular and canalicular structures and requires adenosine triphosphate (ATP) and K^+. This H^+K^+/adenosine triphosphatase (ATPase) is the proton pump. When acid secretion is stimulated, the H^+K^+/ATPase undergoes at least two conformational changes. First, the cytosolic side binds H^+ and transfers it to the luminal side. The H^+ is released and K^+ is grasped. A further conformational change translocates the K^+ intracellularly where it is released. Concurrently, Cl^- and K^+ channels are activated leading to efflux of these ions.[3]

Histamine Receptor Antagonists

Histamine was known to play a role in acid secretion but it was not until 1966 that H_1 and H_2 receptors were described.[4] Cimetidine, ranitidine, famotidine, and nizatidine are all competitive H_2 receptor antagonists.

Cimetidine

Early attempts at producing H_2 receptor antagonists used histamine analogues that contained a bulky side chain in place of the ethylamine moiety. The first H_2 antagonist burimamide was not suitable for oral use.[5] The next candidate, metiamide, was promising but caused neutropenia. Finally, cimetidine was produced and became the first commercially successful H_2 receptor antagonist.[6] Others followed but we describe cimetidine in more detail as the prototype drug.

Mechanism of Action

Cimetidine retains the imidazole ring of histamine but has a bulky side chain on the imidazole ring. It is a competitive antagonist for histamine at the H_2 receptor.

Clinical Pharmacology

After oral absorption, bioavailability is 60%, time to peak serum concentration is 1 to 2 hours, volume of distribution is 0.8 to 2.1 L/kg, serum half-life is 1.5 to 2.5 hours.

Elimination occurs by a combination of hepatic metabolism (60%) and renal clearance (40%) after oral doses. For intravenous doses, the percentages are 25% to 40% and 50% to 80%, respectively. No dose adjustment is normally needed in hepatic dysfunction.

In renal impairment, the dose should be halved if creatinine clearance is less than 15 mL/min.[7] Cimetidine crosses the placenta, the blood–brain barrier, and is excreted into breast milk.

Adverse Effects

CNS: Cimetidine interacts with cerebral H_2 receptors. Consequently, headaches, somnolence, confusion, and delirium may occur.[8] The distribution of cimetidine in cerebrospinal fluid is increased in severe hepatic dysfunction and dose reduction may be needed if confusion occurs.[9]

Cardiovascular: Bradycardia and hypotension may occur because of interactions with cardiac H_2 receptors. These events have generally been associated with rapid intravenous infusion and when used intravenously cimetidine should be given by slow infusion over 15 to 30 minutes.[10]

Endocrine: Cimetidine may cause impotence, loss of libido, gynecomastia, and a decrease in sperm counts in male patients. Hyperprolactinemia may occur in all patients. These effects may be caused by decreased testosterone synthesis, inhibition of oestradiol metabolism, or other mechanisms.[11]

Other reported effects include acute pancreatitis, reversible increases in transaminases, leucopenia, thrombocytopenia, pancytopenia and agranulocytosis, diarrhea, rash, dizziness, alopecia, and interstitial nephritis. Alcohol dehydrogenase may be inhibited by cimetidine and theoretically leads to greater plasma levels at lower doses of alcohol.[12]

Interactions

Cimetidine is metabolized in the liver where it binds to the heme group of cytochrome P450 and interferes with the metabolism of at least 41 drugs.[7] Only a few interactions are clinically relevant: the metabolism of warfarin, theophylline, phenytoin, carbamazepine, lidocaine, quinidine, tricyclic-antidepressants, and propanolol are reduced. Consequently, serum levels may increase and adverse effects may occur.

Concurrent sucralfate or antacid use decreases absorption of cimetidine by 10% to 30%. Because many people take H_2-blockers at night together with antacids effectiveness may be reduced.[13]

Practical Aspects

Cimetidine is indicated for benign gastric and duodenal ulceration, reflux esophagitis, and Zollinger-Ellison syndrome.

The longest period of basal acid secretion is at night. Nocturnal doses of H_2 antagonists suppress nocturnal acid secretion leaving daytime secretion virtually unchanged, yet ulcer healing is faster. Bedtime is the optimal time for giving H_2-blockers.[14]

Dosage and Administration

Benign gastroduodenal ulceration requires dosages of 400 mg twice daily or 800 mg at night for 4 to 8 weeks.

Reflux disease requires 400 mg four times daily for 4 to 8 weeks. An intravenous formulation is available in 200-mg ampoules. This is infused over 60 minutes in 100 mL sodium chloride 0.9%. Maximum daily dose by either route is 2.4 g.

Ranitidine

Mechanism of Action

The imidazole ring of histamine is replaced by a furan ring to produce ranitidine. It has a similar mechanism of action to cimetidine but is 5 to 10 times more potent.

Clinical Pharmacology

After oral administration, bioavailability is 50%, time to peak serum concentration is 1 to 3 hours, volume of distribution is 1.0 to 1.9 L/kg, and serum half-life is 1.6 to 3.1 hours.

Elimination occurs by a combination of hepatic metabolism (73%) and renal clearance (23%) after oral doses. For intravenous doses, the percentages are 30% and 50%, respectively. No dose adjustment is needed in hepatic dysfunction.

In renal impairment, the dose should be halved if creatinine clearance is less than 30 mL/min.[7]

Adverse Effects

Effects are similar to those for cimetidine. Ranitidine binds 5- to 10-fold less to cytochrome P450 than cimetidine and has no clinically significant interactions.

Practical Aspects

Practical aspects are similar to those for cimetidine.

Dosage and Administration

Benign gastric and duodenal ulceration require 150 mg twice daily or 300 mg at night for 4 to 8 weeks.

Reflux esophagitis requires 150 mg twice daily or 300 mg at night for up to 8 weeks. The dose can be doubled and course extended to 12 weeks in severe disease. For maintenance of reflux disease administer 150 mg twice daily.

Zollinger-Ellison syndrome requires 150 mg three times daily, but doses up to 6 g daily have been used.

An intravenous formulation is available in 50-mg ampoules. This should be diluted in 20 mL normal saline 0.9% or glucose 5% and given over 2 minutes by slow injection.

Nizatidine

Mechanism of Action

The imidazole ring of histamine is replaced by a thiazole ring to produce nizatidine, which is 5 to 10 times more potent than cimetidine.

Clinical Pharmacology

After oral administration, bioavailability is 95%. The greater bioavailability compared with the other H2-blockers is caused by lesser first-pass hepatic metabolism. Time to peak serum concentration is 1 to 3 hours. Volume of distribution is 1.2 to 1.6 L/kg. Serum half-life is 1.1 to 2 hours.

Elimination occurs by a combination of hepatic metabolism (22%) and renal clearance (65%) after oral doses. The percentages are similar after intravenous use. No dose reduction is needed for hepatic dysfunction.

In renal impairment, the oral dose should be halved if the creatinine clearance is less than 50 mL/min.[7]

Adverse Effects

Adverse effects are similar to those for cimetidine. There is no interference with cytochrome P450.

Practical Aspects

Practical aspects are similar to those for cimetidine.

Dosage and Administration

Nizatidine is supplied as 150- and 300-mg capsules.

Benign gastric and duodenal ulceration require 300 mg at night or 150 mg twice daily for 4 to 8 weeks.

Gastroesophageal reflux disease requires 150 to 300 mg twice daily for up to 12 weeks.

Famotidine

Mechanism of Action

The imidazole ring of histamine is replaced by a thiazole ring to produce famotidine, which is about 30 times more potent than cimetidine.

Clinical Pharmacology

After oral administration, bioavailability is 45%, time to peak serum concentration is 1 to 3.5 hours, volume of distribution is 1.1 to 1.3 L/kg, serum half-life is 2.5 to 4 hours.

Elimination occurs by a combination of hepatic metabolism (75%) and renal clearance (25%) after oral doses. After intravenous doses the percentages are 30% and 70%, respectively. No dose reduction is needed for hepatic dysfunction.

In renal impairment, the oral dose should be halved if the creatinine clearance is less than 50 mL/min.[7]

Adverse Effects

Adverse effects are similar to those for cimetidine. There is no interference with cytochrome P450.

Practical Aspects

The indications are similar to those for cimetidine.

Dosage and Administration

Benign gastric and duodenal ulceration requires 40 mg at night for 6 to 8 weeks.

Reflux esophagitis requires 20 to 40 mg twice daily for 6 to 8 weeks.

Zollinger-Ellison syndrome requires 20 mg every 6 hours.

Proton Pump Inhibitors

The final step in acid secretion is the $H^+K^+/ATPase$, the proton pump. PPIs bind irreversibly to the pump and inhibit acid secretion until new pumps become available. Omeprazole is the prototype PPI and will be described in more detail later.

Omeprazole (and Esomeprazole)

Omeprazole is a pyridyl methylsulphinyl benzimidazole. It is a lipophilic weak base, pKa 4, which is membrane permeable in the nonprotonated form but impermeable when protonated. Omeprazole preparations are produced with an enteric coat that releases the drug when the pH is above 6 in the small intestine. Otherwise, the acid environment of the stomach converts it to the nonabsorbable protonated form. Thus there is greater bioavailability after the first few doses than for the first dose. Esomeprazole is the S-isomer of omeprazole, which is a mixture of the S- and R-isomers. The S- and R-isomers are metabolized differently by the liver, resulting in greater plasma levels of the S- than of the R-isomer.[15]

Mechanism of Action

Omeprazole is absorbed in the small bowel and reaches the parietal cell from the circulation. It diffuses into the parietal cell and accumulates in the secretory canaliculus, where in the acid environment it is converted to a sulphenamide, the active component. This active molecule binds covalently to exposed cysteine residues on the luminal alpha domain of the $H^+K^+/ATPase$ and stops the pump functioning.[16] Three cysteine residues are accessible but cys 813 is critical to all PPIs. It is unclear whether binding to other cysteine residues is pharmacologically or clinically relevant.[17]

Preclinical Pharmacology

Animal studies demonstrated that omeprazole was a potent inhibitor of gastric acid secretion. Furthermore, in spite of a short half-life ($t_{1/2}$ = 60 minutes in dogs), omeprazole has a long duration of action and the acid-inhibitory effects increases with repeated dosing.[18]

Clinical Pharmacology

After oral administration, bioavailability is 60%. Time to peak serum concentration is 2 to 4 hours. More than 90% is bound to plasma proteins. Serum half-life is 0.5 to 1.0 hours.

Omeprazole is eliminated by cytochrome P450 in the liver. Metabolites are excreted in urine, feces, and breast milk. No dose reduction is needed in renal failure and omeprazole is not detected in dialysis fluid. Although hepatic dysfunction can prolong the elimination half-life slightly, no dose reduction is necessary.[19]

Contraindications

Contraindications include hypersensitivity to omeprazole. Caution should be used when prescribing omeprazole for pregnant women or women who are lactating.

Adverse Effects

CNS: Omeprazole crosses the blood–brain barrier and headache, dizziness, agitation, and confusion may occur.

Gastrointestinal tract (GIT): Three percent of patients taking omeprazole may experience GIT effects: nausea, vomiting, diarrhea, constipation, flatulence, or abdominal pain. Small bowel bacterial overgrowth may occur secondary to acid suppression.

Endocrine: An increase in serum gastrin is a consequence of acid suppression with omeprazole because the inhibitory effect of gastric acid is lost. Rat studies with high-dose omeprazole produced hyperplasia of enterochromaffin-like cells and carcinoid tumors. However, humans have lower gastrin secretion in response to acid inhibition compared with rats,[20] and despite omeprazole-doubling gastrin levels, no clinically significant enterochromaffin-like cell changes have been seen after long-term use and gastrin levels are usually maintained within the normal range.[21]

Interactions

Omeprazole is metabolized by cytochrome P450 in the liver. Despite a theoretic risk for drug interactions, in clinical practice these are rare. Metabolism of the R-isomer of warfarin may be inhibited but clinical studies suggest the effect is not great.[22] Similarly, omeprazole may reduce the metabolism of phenytoin and diazepam but in vivo studies show this to be minor.[23,24] Profound acid suppression may interfere with the absorption of certain drugs for which a low gastric pH is needed, for example, ketoconazole, itraconazole, ampicillin esters, and iron.

Practical Aspects

Omeprazole is indicated to heal benign gastroduodenal ulceration and maintenance to prevent recurrence, in combination with antibiotics in Helicobacter pylori eradication regimens, gastroesophageal reflux disease, Zollinger-Ellison syndrome, and prophylaxis for nonsteroidal antiinflammatory drug (NSAID)-induced ulceration.

The potency of omeprazole is theoretically reduced in patients who are fasting or concomitantly taking H_2-blockers because the initial dose of omeprazole will not inhibit all proton pumps, only those present and working on the luminal surface.[25] As pumps are generated and inserted into the membrane, further doses are required to inhibit these new pumps. Omeprazole thus takes several days to exert its maximal inhibitory effect on gastric acid secretion.[26] Once daily dosing gives 66% inhibition after 5 days. Likewise, once omeprazole has been stopped, acid secretion will not return to normal for several days until new pumps are generated.[27]

Dosage and Administration

Omeprazole is supplied as capsules containing 20 or 10 mg.

Benign gastroduodenal ulceration and NSAID-induced erosions and ulcers require 20 mg daily for 4 to 8 weeks; in severe cases, up to 40 mg daily may be required.

Zollinger-Ellison syndrome requires initially 60 mg daily, but up to 120 mg (in 2 divided doses) can be administered if needed.

Gastroesophageal reflux requires 20 mg daily for 4 weeks, but up to 40 mg in resistant cases; 10 mg daily can be prescribed for long-term maintenance.

Capsules can be opened and the granules passed down a nasogastric tube with a neutral liquid like water if capsules can not be swallowed.

An intravenous formulation is available in 40-mg vials. This requires reconstitution in normal saline 0.9% or glucose 5% solution and infused in 100 mL over 30 minutes.

Esomeprazole

Clinical Pharmacology

The clinical pharmacology of esomeprazole is similar to that of omeprazole, but the maximum daily dose is 20 mg for patients with severe hepatic insufficiency (Child Pugh Class C). A dose of 20 mg esomeprazole can be expected to produce greater inhibition of acidity than 20 mg omeprazole.

Contraindications

Contraindications are similar to those for omeprazole.

Adverse Effects

Adverse effects are similar to those for omeprazole.

Interactions

Interactions are similar to those for omeprazole.

Dosage and Administration

Gastroesophageal reflux disease requires 20 to 40 mg daily for 4 to 8 weeks.

Helicobacter eradication regimens recommend 40 mg twice daily.

Lansoprazole

Mechanism of Action

Lansoprazole is a substituted benzimidazole that inhibits the H$^+$K$^+$-ATPase. It is a weak base with a pKa ~4.0.

Clinical Pharmacology

After oral administration, bioavailability is 85%, time to peak serum concentration is 1.5 to 3 hours, 97% bound to plasma protein, serum half-life is 1.5 hours.

It is eliminated by cytochrome P450 in the liver. Lansoprazole induces some forms of P450 but rarely causes significant interactions. About 14% to 25% is excreted in urine as metabolites. Some is eliminated in bile, feces, and breast milk. No dose reduction is needed in patients with renal failure and hepatic dysfunction.[28]

Contraindications

Contraindications include hypersensitivity to lansoprazole. Caution should be used when prescribing lansoprazole for pregnant women or women who are lactating.

Adverse Effects

Adverse effects are similar to those for omeprazole.

Interactions

Lansoprazole may decrease theophylline levels and interfere with absorption of ketoconazole, digoxin, and ampicillin. Food reduces peak lansoprazole level by 50%. Sucralfate decreases bioavailability. No significant cytochrome P450 interactions occur.

Practical Aspects

It is indicated for treatment of benign gastroduodenal ulceration, Helicobacter eradication regimens, NSAID-induced ulcer healing, Zollinger-Ellison syndrome, and gastroesophageal reflux disease.

Dosage and Administration

Lansoprazole is supplied as capsules containing 30 or 15 mg.

Benign gastroduodenal ulceration requires 30 mg daily for 4 to 8 weeks.

Reflux disease requires 30 mg daily for 4 to 8 weeks; 15 mg daily may be prescribed for long-term maintenance.

Helicobacter eradication regimens recommend 30 mg twice daily.

Pantoprazole

Mechanism of Action

Pantoprazole is a substituted benzimidazole that inhibits the H$^+$K$^+$/ATPase. It is a weak base with a pKa ~4.0.

Clinical Pharmacology

After oral administration, bioavailability is 77%, time to peak serum concentration is 2.5 hours, 98% protein bound, serum half-life is 1.9 hours.

Pantoprazole is eliminated by cytochrome P450 in the liver. No clinically significant interactions have been reported. Metabolites are excreted in urine, feces, and breast milk. No dose reduction is needed for patients with renal failure or hepatic dysfunction.[28]

Contraindications

Contraindications include hypersensitivity to pantoprazole. Caution should be used when prescribing pantoprazole for pregnant women or women who are lactating.

Adverse Effects

Adverse effects are similar to those for omeprazole.

Interactions

Interactions are similar to those for omeprazole. No significant cytochrome P450 interactions occur.

Practical Aspects

Pantoprazole is indicated for benign gastroduodenal ulcer healing, Helicobacter eradication regimens, and gastroesophageal reflux disease.

Dosage and Administration

Pantoprazole is supplied as tablets containing 40 or 20 mg. An intravenous formulation is available in 40-mg vials. This requires reconstitution in normal saline 0.9% or glucose 5% and is infused in 100 mL over 2 to 15 minutes.

Benign gastroduodenal ulceration requires 40 mg daily for 4 to 6 weeks.

Reflux disease requires 40 mg daily for 4 to 8 weeks; 20 mg daily may be prescribed for long-term maintenance.

Helicobacter eradication regimens recommend 40 mg twice daily.

Rabeprazole

Mechanism of Action

Rabeprazole is a substituted benzimidazole that inhibits the $H^+K^+/ATPase$. It is a weak base with a pKa ~5.0.

Clinical Pharmacology

After oral administration, bioavailability is 85%, time to peak serum concentration is 2.9 to 3.8 hours, 96% bound to plasma protein, serum half-life is 1 hour.

Rabeprazole is eliminated by cytochrome P450 in the liver. No clinically significant interactions have been reported. Some is eliminated in bile, feces, and breast milk. No dose reduction is needed in patients with renal failure or hepatic dysfunction.[28]

Contraindications

Contraindications include hypersensitivity to rabeprazole. Caution should be used when prescribing rabeprazole for pregnant women or women who are lactating.

Adverse Effects

Adverse effects are similar to those for omeprazole.

Interactions

Rabeprazole may interfere with absorption of ketoconazole and digoxin.

Practical Aspects

Rabeprazole is indicated for benign gastroduodenal ulcer healing, Helicobacter eradication regimens, and gastroesophageal reflux disease.

Dosage and Administration

Rabeprazole is supplied as 20- or 10-mg tablets.

Benign gastroduodenal ulceration requires 20 mg daily for 4 to 6 weeks.

Reflux disease requires 20 mg daily for 4 to 8 weeks.

Helicobacter eradication regimens recommend 20 mg daily.

Comparing Histamine-2 Antagonist Versus Proton Pump Inhibitors for Clinical Applications

Gastroesophageal Reflux Disease

Gastroesophageal reflux disease covers a spectrum from symptoms and no endoscopic inflammation to complications such as ulcers, bleeding, and strictures. H_2 antagonists do alleviate symptoms and heal esophagitis but require greater doses than for peptic ulcer disease.[29] Moreover, tolerance develops and esophageal damage may occur despite absence of symptoms.[30] PPIs are more effective at healing esophagitis and preventing relapse compared with H_2 antagonists.[31-34] There are no significant differences among PPIs.[35-37] For patients with infrequent symptoms and no esophageal damage, an H_2 antagonist is probably the most cost-effective treatment. Otherwise, for patients with erosive esophagitis or frequent symptoms, PPIs are the treatment of choice.[38]

Gastroduodenal Ulcers

Duodenal ulcer healing is accelerated by H_2 receptor antagonists with no clinically significant differences among the H_2 receptor antagonists.[39-42] Healing rates for gastric ulcers are slower than for duodenal ulceration but again there are no major differences in healing rates among the four H_2 receptor antagonists when given over 8 weeks.[43,44]

PPIs are more effective at healing gastroduodenal ulcers compared with H_2 antagonists.[45-48] No one PPI is better than another.

The use of H_2 antagonists and PPIs for maintenance therapy has become obsolete since the role of H. pylori in gastroduodenal ulceration was discovered.[49] Eradication of H. pylori results in significantly fewer relapses and is more cost-effective than maintenance treatment.[50]

Helicobacter Eradication Regimens

Regimens include 7 days of treatment with:

- Amoxicillin 1 g twice daily (or metronidazole 400 mg twice daily if penicillin allergic) *plus*
- Clarithromycin 500 mg twice daily *plus*
- Omeprazole 20 mg twice daily or Lansoprazole 30 mg twice daily or Pantoprazole 40 mg twice daily or Rabeprazole 20 mg twice daily.
- Ranitidine 150 mg twice daily has also been shown to help in the eradication of H. Pylori in place of a PPI suggesting that such potent acid inhibition as provided by the

PPIs is not necessary and thus lower doses of PPIs would also be expected to work.

Zollinger-Ellison Syndrome

High doses of H[2] antagonists were used with some benefit but PPIs are the treatment of choice in Zollinger-Ellison syndrome because of their potent acid suppression.[51]

Acute Upper Gastrointestinal Hemorrhage

Studies have not conclusively demonstrated an important benefit from H[2] antagonists in upper gastrointestinal (GI) bleeding. A meta-analysis of 27 trials has been performed, with disappointing results and their routine use cannot be recommended.[52]

There are theoretical reasons why stronger acid suppression could be beneficial. Platelet aggregation is optimal at pH 7.4, whilst below pH 5.9 clot lysis occurs.[53] Dose-finding studies indicated that a bolus of 80 mg omeprazole, followed by continuous infusion of omeprazole 8 mg/h provided the required pH profile.[54,55] One trial suggests this regime for 72 hours offers benefits if used in conjunction with endoscopic heater probe and injection therapy in ulcers with visible vessels or active bleeding.[56] Currently, endoscopic therapy is the gold-standard and the evidence does not support the routine use of intravenous PPIs in acute upper GI hemorrhage.

NSAID-Associated Ulceration

NSAIDs may cause 30% of gastroduodenal ulcers. Risk factors are previous ulcer disease, age, particular "high risk" NSAIDs such as azapropazone and piroxicam, and concurrent use of warfarin or corticosteroids. Omeprazole can heal both gastric and duodenal ulcers despite continued NSAID use and it is superior to ranitidine. Omeprazole is also significantly better at preventing ulcer recurrence.[57,58] However, the optimal strategy to prevent NSAID-related ulceration is to avoid NSAIDs if possible.

Stress Ulcers

Stress ulcers are superficial erosions precipitated by reduced mucosal blood flow in critically ill patients. Those at greatest risk have a coagulopathy and require mechanical ventilation.[59] Several studies have examined H[2] antagonist use and have reported observing a benefit. A meta-analysis has suggested that they do reduce the incidence of bleeding but at increased risk for pneumonia.[60] Their use does not reduce mortality rates.

Although omeprazole reduced stress ulceration in animal experiments,[61] PPIs cannot currently be recommended for this role because there is a lack of evidence of benefit.[62]

Short Bowel Syndrome

H[2] antagonists may reduce enterostomy output by reducing the volume and osmolality of fluid entering the upper GIT. These effects may be enough to reduce jejunostomy output by up to 300 mL/day. High dose H[2] antagonists are normally required.[63] PPIs are more effective and are recommended over H[2]-blockers.

Aspiration Pneumonitis

Volume of aspirated contents and acidity of contents influences the severity of aspiration pneumonitis.[64] Cimetidine can reduce the volume and acidity of gastric contents when given electively and other H[2]-blockers have shown similar efficacy.[65,66]

There are theoretic reasons why omeprazole may not be effective, namely it takes up to 5 days to achieve full acid suppression. However, omeprazole can reduce acidity and volume if given at a high dose, 40 mg on the preceding evening and 40 mg 2 to 6 hours before surgery.[67] However, in emergency use, neither H[2] antagonists nor PPIs alter what is already present in the stomach and this still presents a risk for aspiration.

Somatostatin and Analogues

Somatostatin is a naturally occurring tetradecapeptide with many effects on the bowel. It stimulates water and salt absorption and inhibits small bowel motility and secretion of several gut hormones.[68-70] The short half-life of 2 to 3 minutes makes somatostatin unsuitable for many applications because it requires continuous intravenous infusion. Consequently, longer acting analogues were developed.

Octreotide

Studies of somatostatin analogues established that a four amino acid sequence was essential for biologic activity. This sequence, Phe-Trp-Lys-Thr, formed the basis for synthetic analogues. Furthermore, substituting the native L-amino acids for D-amino acids makes peptides more resistant to peptidases while retaining biologic activity. Substitution by D-Thr-ol at the carboxy terminal leads to an extra increase in in vitro and in vivo activity. This is the basis for octreotide acetate.[71]

Mechanism of Action

Octreotide activates the inhibitory G protein, G[i], thereby inhibiting adenylate cyclase.[72] Somatostatin and octreotide have slightly different affinities for somatostatin receptors that may account for differences in effects. There are five different receptors for somatostatin (sstr 1 to sstr 5). Octreotide is selective for sstr 2, less potent on sstr 3, and inactive on sstr 1 and 4.[73]

Clinical Pharmacology

Octreotide exerts a long-lasting inhibitory action on gastric acid secretion. It inhibits biliary secretion and gallbladder contraction. It inhibits the release of neuropeptides and hormones such as insulin, glucagon, pancreatic polypeptide, gastrin, and gastric inhibitory polypeptide. Octreotide reduces splanchnic blood flow and inhibits pancreatic exocrine function, diminishing secretions of amylase, trypsin, and lipase. It can prolong transit time and decrease fluid secretion in the jejunum and ileum, thus increasing the absorption of water and electrolytes.[74,75]

Pharmacokinetics

After subcutaneous injection, peak plasma concentrations are seen within 30 minutes with a half-life of about 100 minutes. After intravenous bolus injection, the elimination is biphasic, with half-lives of 10 and 80 minutes, respectively. About 65% octreotide is plasma protein bound. The volume of distribution is 0.27 L/kg. No dose adjustment is needed in patients with renal failure or hepatic dysfunction.[76]

Contraindications

Caution should be used when prescribing octreotide for pregnant women or women who are lactating.

Adverse Effects

When given subcutaneously, up to a third of patients experience side effects. Nausea, vomiting, pain, tingling at injection site, diarrhea, and abdominal discomfort occur in 10% of patients. Headaches, hyperglycemia, hypoglycemia, hair loss, increased transaminases, hyperbilirubinemia, steatorrhea, and increased risk for gallstone formation have been described. Side effects tend to improve with time or dose reduction.

Interactions

Octreotide may reduce intestinal absorption of cyclosporin.

Practical Aspects

Octreotide is indicated for relief of symptoms associated with gastroenteropancreatic endocrine tumors, including vipomas, glucagonomas, and carcinoid tumors with features of carcinoid syndrome.

Octreotide has been used in treatment of short bowel syndrome.[77,78] It successfully reduces enterostomy output but at the risk of retarding the physiologic process of adaptation.[79,80] Even so, it may still offer patients benefit in reducing stomal efflux and improving quality of life.

Dosage and Administration

Octreotide is supplied in vials with the following strengths: 0.05 mg/mL, 0.1 mg/mL, 0.2 mg/mL, and 0.5 mg/mL.

Initially, 50 μg once or twice daily by subcutaneous injection. Dosage increased gradually up to 200 μg three times daily, depending on response. Allowing the solution to reach room temperature before injection reduces local discomfort. For intravenous use, octreotide should be diluted with normal saline solution. Glucose solution is not recommended.

Antimuscarinic Agents

Antimuscarinic agents, also called anticholinergics, block the effects of acetylcholine and reduce secretory and motility responses. Their use is limited by side effects and there are doubts about their efficacy. Even so, they may prove beneficial in some patients.[81]

Dicyclomine Hydrochloride

Mechanism of Action

Dicyclomine is a synthetic tertiary amine. It is an antimuscarinic agent with an additional antispasmodic effect on smooth muscle.[82]

Pharmacology

Dicyclomine is absorbed in the gut. Time to peak serum concentration is 1.5 hours. Volume of distribution is 3.65 L/kg. Serum half-life is 4 to 6 hours.

The metabolism is uncertain but 80% of a dose appears in urine and 10% in feces. No dose adjustment is needed for renal and hepatic dysfunction. It has not been studied in pregnancy and lactation, therefore caution is advised before prescribing it for pregnant women or women who are lactating.

Contraindications

Contraindications include glaucoma, prostatism, and paralytic ileus. As mentioned earlier, caution is advised if prescribing for pregnant women or women who are lactating.

Adverse Effects

Adverse effects include dry mouth, pupillary dilatation, urinary urgency, and retention.

Practical Aspects

Dicyclomine hydrochloride may be a useful adjunct to treating irritable bowel syndrome (IBS).

Dosage and Administration

Dicyclomine hydrochloride is supplied as 10- and 20-mg tablets.

In adults, 10 to 20 mg three times daily can be administered.

Hyoscine Butylbromide

Mechanism of Action

Hyoscine butylbromide is a quaternary ammonium compound. It is an antimuscarinic agent. It does not cross the blood–brain barrier (unlike hyoscine hydrobromide).

Pharmacology

After oral administration, less than 10% is absorbed, 90% is lost in feces, and 2% in urine. After intravenous bolus, 42% is recovered in urine and 37% in feces. The serum half-life is 8 hours. There is no relation between plasma concentration and clinical activity. Liver metabolism produces unknown inactive compounds. No dose reduction is needed in renal and hepatic dysfunction.

Contraindications

Contraindications are similar to those for dicyclomine.

Adverse Effects

Adverse effects are similar to those for dicyclomine.

Practical Aspects

Hyoscine butylbromide may be used as an adjunct in IBS and as an aid to GI endoscopy. It may help cannulation of the ampulla during ERCP by producing a hypotonic duodenum.[83]

Dosage and Administration

Hyoscine butylbromide is supplied as 10-mg tablets and vial containing 20 mg for intravenous use.

In IBS, 20 mg up to four times daily is required.

In endoscopy, 20 mg by intravenous injection is required; dosage may be repeated as necessary.

Propantheline Bromide

Propantheline bromide is a synthetic quaternary ammonium compound. It is an antimuscarinic agent.

Pharmacology

Propantheline bromide is incompletely absorbed from the GIT. Time to peak serum concentration 2 hours and serum half-life is 1.6 hours.

The distribution and metabolism are not fully determined; 50% is metabolized in the GIT and is excreted primarily in urine. No dose adjustment is needed in patients with hepatic failure or renal dysfunction.

Contraindications

Contraindications are similar to those for dicyclomine.

Adverse Effects

Adverse effects are similar to those for dicyclomine.

Practical Aspects

Propantheline bromide may be useful in treatment of IBS.

Dosage and Administration

Propantheline bromide is supplied as 15-mg tablets.

It may be administered up to 15 mg three times daily and 30 mg nocte, taken an hour before meals; maximum dosage is 120 mg daily.

Serotonin Type 3 Receptor Antagonists

Serotonin type 3 receptors (5-HT$_3$) are nonselective cation channels that are extensively distributed on enteric neurones within the GIT and within the brain. The 5-HT$_3$ receptor antagonists have shown great efficacy in the treatment of chemotherapy-induced emesis and have been found to have effects on GI motility and visceral sensation (See also Chapter 45).

Alosetron

5-HT$_3$ antagonists cause constipation and increase thresholds for sensation and discomfort of the rectum.[84,85] These findings promoted the trial of 5-HT$_3$ receptor antagonists for IBS, particularly in diarrhea-predominant IBS. Alosetron was the first 5-HT$_3$ receptor antagonist licensed for use in IBS.

Preclinical Pharmacology

Alosetron has effects on visceral nociception in rats and dogs, attenuating the effects of rectal distension. These effects also occur in humans, in whom alosetron increases rectal compliance, delays colonic transit, and reduces visceral sensitivity to rectal distension.[86-88] Clinical trials have shown that alosetron is well tolerated and effective in alleviating pain and reducing bowel frequency in IBS, particularly in diarrhea-predominant IBS. These effects are mainly seen in women. It is not known if men derive equal benefit.[89,90]

Clinical Pharmacology

Alosetron has good oral bioavailability, approximately 50% to 60%. Peak plasma levels are reached within 1 hour and steady-state plasma levels are achieved within 1 day.

The elimination half-life is 93 hours. Alosetron is eliminated largely by the kidneys (73%) and the remainder is lost through fecal excretion. The long half-life allows for twice daily dosing. No dose adjustment is needed for elderly patients or for renal and hepatic impairment.

Animal studies show that alosetron is present in breast milk. No human studies have been done in women who are pregnant or lactating.

Contraindications

Alosetron is contraindicated with a history of intestinal obstruction, stricture, toxic megacolon, GI perforation, GI adhesions, ischemic colitis, active diverticulitis, and inflammatory bowel disease. Contraindications regarding women who are pregnant or lactating are mentioned earlier.

Interactions

No clinically important interactions have been reported for alosetron.

Adverse Reactions

Adverse reactions include headache, anorexia, nausea, dizziness, loose stools, abdominal cramping, and flatulence. Severe constipation, fecal impaction, and ischemic colitis have been reported and consequently alosetron should not be commenced when patients are constipated.

Practical Aspects

Alosetron is indicated for use in diarrhea-predominant IBS, where its effects on slowing bowel transit and reducing visceral pain sensation are helpful. Because of reports of ischemic colitis, alosetron has been voluntarily withdrawn by Glaxo Wellcome. It has been included here as an indication of future drug avenues.[91]

Dosage and Administration

Dosage and administration information is not available.

Opiates

Morphine and opiates produce constipation in all mammalian species, although there are variations in its actions between species. However, concern over addictive potential means synthetic alternatives have been sought.

Loperamide

Loperamide hydrochloride is a synthetic piperidine opioid used primarily for treatment of acute or chronic diarrhea.

Mechanism of Action

Animal experiments have shown opiates decrease luminal fluid content by actions on mucosal ion transport processes.[92] Loperamide may also have some nonopioid antidiarrheal effects: inhibiting calmodulin and preventing activation of Ca^{2+}/calmodulin–dependent protein kinases.[93]

Preclinical Pharmacology

Loperamide mediates most of its action through binding to the μ opioid receptor in the GIT, but also interacts with δ receptors.[94] Loperamide affects mucosal transport of water and solutes by slowing transit time, allowing lumen contents more time to be absorbed, and stimulates μ and δ receptors, resulting in decreased secretion of Na^+, K^+, and Cl^-, but not HCO_3^-.[95] This effect is maximal in the jejunum and colon. Loperamide also affects the rectum, increasing anal tone and decreasing urgency in patients with urge incontinence.[96]

Clinical Pharmacology

Loperamide is absorbed in the gut and is extensively metabolized by the liver. Because of its first-pass effects, peak plasma levels are low corresponding to less than 0.5% of the administered dose. Consequently, CNS side effects are rare.

The half-life of loperamide in humans is 10.8 hours with a range of 9 to 14 hours. Loperamide is metabolized in the liver where it is conjugated and excreted through bile. Loperamide is secreted in small amounts in breast milk.

Contraindications

Loperamide is contraindicated in children younger than 4 years. Caution is advised if prescribing for pregnant women or women who are lactating.

Adverse Effects

Abdominal cramps, nausea, vomiting, fatigue, drowsiness, dizziness, dry mouth, and skin reactions including urticaria have been reported. Paralytic ileus and bloating may occur.

Overdosage produces somnolence, myosis, and bradypnea, which responds to naloxone. The duration of loperamide is longer than naloxone, hence repeated doses or naloxone infusion may be required. In hepatic insufficiency, overdosage may occur because of decreased metabolism.

Reports of opiate toxicity symptoms means loperamide should not be prescribed to children younger than 4 years.[97]

Interactions

No interactions have been reported for loperamide.

Practical Aspects

Loperamide can be used for acute and chronic diarrhea. If used for diarrhea it is important to search for the underlying cause rather than just treat blindly. It can help in diarrhea-predominant IBS and short bowel syndrome. For short bowel syndrome, greater doses of loperamide have been used in some centers, up to 64 mg daily in combination with codeine phosphate to reduce stomal output and fluid losses.[98] Loperamide is not routinely advised in inflammatory bowel disease because it may precipitate toxic megacolon.[99]

Diphenoxylate is described in detail later, but briefly, two trials comparing loperamide and diphenoxylate have shown loperamide to be more effective at reducing diarrhea and better tolerated by patients with fewer side effects.[100,101]

Dosage and Administration

Loperamide is supplied as 2-mg tablets.

It is not recommended for children younger than 4 years. For children 4 to 8 years old, 1 mg three to four times daily for up to 3 days only is recommended. For 9- to 12-year-old children, 2 mg four times daily for up to 5 days is suggested. In adults with acute diarrhea, 4 mg initially followed by 2 mg after each loose stool is recommended. The usual dosage 6 to 8 mg daily, with a maximum of 16 mg daily. In adults with chronic diarrhea, up to 16 mg daily in divided doses is recommended. Adjust according to response. Loperamide is available as capsules and syrup, which can be given through nasogastric or PEG feeding tubes.

Diphenoxylate Hydrochloride and Atropine Sulphate

Diphenoxylate hydrochloride is a synthetic piperidine opioid used to treat diarrhea. The anticholinergic effects of atropine may help reduce GI motility and secretions, but the main reason for its addition is to discourage opiate abuse by causing unpleasant side effects such as dry mouth and blurred vision.

Mechanism of Action

The mechanism of action is similar to loperamide by binding to opiate receptors in the bowel.

Pharmacology

Peak plasma concentrations occur within 2 hours and plasma half-life is 2 hours. Diphenoxylate is metabolized to an active metabolite, diphenoxylic acid, which has a half-life of 3 to 14 hours. The clinical onset of action occurs within 45 minutes to 1 hour and duration of action is approximately 3 to 4 hours.

Diphenoxylate metabolites and their conjugates are excreted in bile. Smaller amounts appear in urine. Diphenoxylate is also excreted in breast milk and consequently infants may be affected.

No studies have looked at safety in pregnancy and the manufacturers advise caution. Both diphenoxylate and atropine are excreted in breast milk and infants may exhibit effects of the drugs.

Adverse Effects

Both diphenoxylate and atropine produce effects in overdoses. Diphenoxylate causes ileus and narcosis and will respond to naloxone. Onset may be delayed 12 to 30 hours after ingestion. Duration of action of naloxone is shorter than duration of diphenoxylate, and repeated doses or naloxone infusion may be necessary.

Atropine side effects include flushing, dry skin and mucous membranes, tachycardia, urinary retention, and hyperthermia; hyperthermia occurs especially in children.

Interactions

Because the chemical structure is similar to meperidine, concurrent use with monoamine oxidase inhibitors could precipitate a hypertensive crisis. Diphenoxylate may potentiate the action of CNS depressants such as barbiturates and alcohol.

Practical Aspects

Practical aspects include treatment of acute or chronic diarrhea.

Dosage and Administration

Diphenoxylate is supplied as tablets containing 2.5 mg diphenoxylate hydrochloride and 25 μg atropine sulphate. Administration in children younger than 4 years is not recommended. For children 4 to 8 years old, 1 tablet three times daily is recommended; for children 9 to 12 years old, 1 tablet four times daily is recommended; and for children 13 to 16 years old, 2 tablets three times daily is suggested. Initially,

4 tablets, followed by 2 tablets every 6 hours until diarrhea is controlled is recommended for adults.

References

1. Tack J: Receptors of the enteric nervous system: Potential targets for drug therapy. Gut 47(suppl IV):iv20–22, 2000.
2. Debongie JC, Phillips SF: Capacity of the human colon to absorb fluid. Gastroenterology 74:698–703, 1978.
3. Wallmark B, Lorentzon P, Sachs G: The gastric H$^+$,K$^+$-ATPase. J Intern Med 228(suppl 1):3–8, 1990.
4. Ash A, Schild H: Receptors mediating some of the actions of histamine. Br J Pharmacol 27:427–439, 1966.
5. Black JW, Duncan WAM, Durrant CJ, et al: Definition and antagonism of histamine H$_2$ receptor. Nature 263:385–390, 1972.
6. Molinder HK: The development of cimetidine: 1964–1976. A human story. J Clin Gastroenterol 19(3):248–254, 1994.
7. Feldman M, Burton ME: Histamine$_2$-receptor antagonists. Standard therapy for acid-peptic diseases. N Engl J Med 323(24):1672–1680, 1990.
8. Cantu TG, Korek JS: Central nervous system reactions to histamine-2 receptor blockers. Ann Intern Med 114:1027–1034, 1991.
9. Somogyi A, Gugler R: Clinical pharmacokinetics of cimetidine. Clin Pharmacokinet 8:463–495, 1983.
10. Hughes DG, Dowling EA, DeMeersman RE, et al: Cardiovascular effects of H$_2$-receptor antagonists. J Clin Pharmacol 29:472–477, 1989.
11. McGuigan JE: A consideration of the adverse effects of cimetidine. Gastroenterology 80:181–192, 1981.
12. Hernandez-Monoz R, Cabacleria J, Baraona E, et al: Human gastric alcohol dehydrogenase: Its inhibition by H$_2$-receptor antagonists, and its effect on the bioavailability of ethanol. Alcoholism 14:946–950, 1990.
13. Steinberg WM, Lewis JH, Katz DM: Antacids inhibit absorption of cimetidine. N Engl J Med 307:400–404, 1982.
14. Damman HG, Muller P, Simon B: 24 hour intragastric acidity and single night-time dose of three H$_2$ blockers. Lancet 2:1078, 1983.
15. Spencer CM, Foulds D: Esomeprazole (Review). Drugs 60(2):321–329, 2000.
16. Lorentzon P, Jackson R, Wallmark B, et al: Inhibition of H K-ATPase by omeprazole in isolated gastric vesicles requires proton transport. Biochem Biophys Acta 897:41–51, 1987.
17. Besancon M, Simon A, Sachs G, et al: Sites of reaction of the gastric H K-ATPase with extracytoplasmic thiol reagents. J Biol Chem 272:2438–2446, 1997.
18. Larsson H, Carlsson E, Junggren U, et al: Animal studies with omeprazole, a potent inhibitor of gastric acid secretion. Scand J Gastro 17(suppl 78), 1982.
19. Howden CW: Clinical pharmacology of omeprazole. Clin Pharmacokinet 20:38–49, 1991.
20. Carlsson E, Larsson H, Mattsson H, et al: Pharmocology and toxicology of omeprazole-with special reference to the effects on the gastric mucosa. Scand J Gastroenterol 118(suppl):31–38, 1986.
21. McCloy RF, Arnold KD, Bardhan KD, et al: Pathophysiological effects of long term acid suppression in man. Dig Dis Sci 42(suppl):96S–120S, 1995.
22. Unge P, Svedgerq LE, Nordgren A, et al: A study of the interaction of omeprazole and warfarin in anticoagulated patients. Br J Clin Pharmacol 34:509–512, 1992.
23. Pritchard PJ, Walt RP, Kitchingman DK, et al: Oral phenytoin pharmacokinetics during omeprazole therapy. Br J Clin Pharmacol 24:543–545, 1987.
24. Anderson T, Andren K, Cederberg C, et al: Effect of omeprazole and cimetidine on plasma diazepam levels. Eur J Clin Pharmacol 39:51–54, 1990.
25. Lindberg P, Brandstrom A, Wallmark B, et al: Omeprazole: The first proton pump inhibitor. Med Res Rev 10:1–54, 1990.
26. Howden CW, Forrest JAH, Reid JL: Effects of single and repeated doses of omeprazole on gastric and pepsin secretion in man. Gut 25:707–710, 1984.
27. Sachs G: Proton pump inhibitors and acid related diseases. Pharmacotherapy 17:22–37, 1997.
28. Richardson P, Hawkey CJ, Stack WA: Proton pump inhibitors. Pharmacology and rationale for use in gastrointestinal disorders. Drugs 56(3):307–335, 1998.
29. Feldman M, Burton ME: Histamine$_2$-receptor antagonists. Standard therapy for acid-peptic diseases. N Engl J Med 323(25):1749–1755, 1990.
30. Wilhelmsen I, Hatlebakk JG, Olaffson S: On demand therapy of reflux oesophagitis: A study of symptoms, patient satisfaction, and quality of life. Gastroenterology 114(4):A331, 1998.
31. Klinkenberg-Knol EC, Feston HPM, Jansen JM, et al: Double-blind multicenter comparison of omeprazole and ranitidine in the treatment of reflux esophagitis. Lancet 1:349–351, 1987.
32. Bardhan KD, Hawkey CJ, Long RG, et al: Lansoprazole versus ranitidine for the treatment of reflux oesophagitis. Aliment Pharm Ther 9:145–151, 1995.
33. Koop H, Schepp W, Dammann HG, et al: Comparative trial of pantoprazole and ranitidine in the treatment of reflux esophagitis: Results of a German multicenter study. J Clin Gastroenterol 20:192–195, 1995.
34. Humphries TJ, Spera A, Breiter J, et al: Rabeprazole sodium (E3810) once daily is superior to ranitidine 150 mg QID in the healing of erosive or ulcerative gastroesophageal reflux disease [abstract]. Gastroenterology 110(suppl):A139, 1996.
35. Petite JP, Salducci J, Grimaud JC, et al: Lansoprazole versus omeprazole in the treatment of reflux oesophagitis. Med Chir Dig 24:291–294, 1995.
36. Corinaldesi R, Valentini M, Belaiche J, et al: Pantoprazole and omeprazole in the treatment of reflux oesophagitis: A European multicenter study. Aliment Pharmacol Ther 9:667–671, 1995.
37. Thjodleifsson B, Beker JA, Dekkers C, et al: Rabeprazole versus omeprazole in preventing relapse of erosive or ulcerative gastroesophageal reflux disease. Dig Dis Sci 45:845–853, 2000.
38. Harris RA, Kuppermann M, Richter JE: Proton pump inhibitors or histamine-2 antagonists for the prevention of recurrence of erosive reflux oesophagitis: A cost-effectiveness analysis. Am J Gastroenterol 92:2179–2189, 1997.
39. Freston JW: Overview of medical therapy of peptic ulcer disease. Gastroenterol Clin North Am 19:121–140, 1990.
40. Walt RP, Trotman TF, Frost R, et al: Comparison of twice daily ranitidine with standard cimetidine treatment of duodenal ulcer. Gut 22:319–322, 1981.
41. Rohner HG, Gugler R: Treatment of active duodenal ulcers with famotidine: A double-blind comparison with ranitidine. Am J Med 81(suppl 4B):13–16, 1986.
42. Simon B, Cremer M, Damman HG, et al: 300 mg nizatidine at night versus 300 mg ranitidine at night in patients with duodenal ulcer. Scand J Gastro Suppl 136:61–70, 1987.
43. Dammann HG, Walter TA: Efficacy of continuous therapy for peptic ulcer in controlled clinical trials. Aliment Pharmacol Ther 7(suppl 2):17–25, 1993.
44. Howden CW, Jones DB, Peace KE, et al: The treatment of gastric ulcer with antisectory drugs. Relationship of pharmacological effect to healing rates. Dig Dis Sci 33:619–624, 1988.
45. Walan A, Bader JP, Classen M, et al: Effect of omeprazole and ranitidine on ulcer healing and relapse rates in patients with benign gastric ulcer. N Eng J Med 320:69–75, 1989.
46. Michel P, Lemaire M, Colin R, et al: Short report: Treatment of gastric ulcer with lansoprazole or ranitidine: A multicenter clinical trial. Aliment Pharmacol Ther 8:119–122, 1994.
47. Hotz J, Plein K, Schonekas H, et al: Pantoprazole is superior to ranitidine in the treatment of acute gastric ulcer. Scand J Gastroenterol 30:111–115, 1995.
48. Nakazawa S, Namiki M, Matsou Y, et al: Clinical utility of E3810 for the treatment of gastric ulcer: Comparison with famotidine by multicenter double-blind study. Rinsho Hyoka 21:337–359, 1993.
49. Marshall BJ, Warren JR: Unidentified curved bacilli in the stomach of patients with gastritis and peptic ulceration. Lancet Jun 16;1:1311–1315, 1984.
50. Sonnenberg A, Townsend WF: Costs of duodenal ulcer therapy with antibiotics. Ann Intern Med 155:922–928, 1995.
51. Hirschowitz BI, Maton PN, Freston J, et al: Zollinger-Ellison syndrome: Pathogenesis, diagnosis and management. Am J Gastroenterol 92(4 suppl):44S–50S, 1997.

52. Collins R, Langman M: Treatment with histamine H₂ antagonists in acute upper gastrointestinal hemorrhage: Implications of randomized trials. N Eng J Med 313:660–666, 1985.

53. Green FJ, Kaplan MM, Curtis LE, Levine PH: Effect of acid and pepsin on blood coagulation and platelet aggregation. A possible contributor to prolonged gastroduodenal hemorrhage. Gastroenterology 74:38–43, 1978.

54. Cederberg C, Thompson ABR, Kirkeikis P, Kristerson C: Effect of continuous intravenous infusion of omeprazole on 24-hour intragastric pH in fasting DU-patients: Comparison to repeated bolus doses of omeprazole or ranitidine. Gastroenterology 4:102, 1992.

55. Brunner G, Thiesemann C: The potential clinical role of intravenous omeprazole. Digestion 51(suppl 1):17–20, 1992.

56. Lau JYW, Sung JJY, Lee KKC, et al: Effect of intravenous omeprazole on recurrent bleeding after endoscopic treatment of bleeding peptic ulcers. N Engl J Med 343:310–316, 2000.

57. Hawkey CJ, Karrasch JA, Szczepanski L, et al: Omeprazole compared to misoprostol for ulcers associated with nonsteroidal antiinflammatory drugs. N Engl J Med 338:727–734, 1998.

58. Yeomans ND, Tulassay Z, Juhasz L, et al: A comparison of omeprazole with ranitidine for ulcers associated with nonsteroidal antiinflammatory drugs. N Engl J Med 338:719–726, 1998.

59. Cook DJ, Fuller HD, Guyatt GH, et al: Risk factors for gastrointestinal bleeding in critically ill patients. N Engl J Med 330:377–381, 1994.

60. Cook DJ, Reeve BK, Guyatt GH, et al: Stress ulcer prophylaxis in critically ill patients. Resolving discordant meta-analysis. JAMA 275:308–314, 1996.

61. Inaloz SS, Gloral V, Sari I, et al: Omeprazole, nitrendipine, famotidine and stress-induced ulcers. Acta Gastroenterol Belg 60:192–196, 1997.

62. Tryba M, Cook D: Current guidelines on stress ulcer prophylaxis. Drugs 54:581–596, 1997.

63. Cortot J, Fleming CR, Malagelada JR: Improved nutrient absorption after cimetidine in short-bowel syndrome with gastric hypersecretion. N Engl J Med 300:79–81, 1979.

64. Roberts RB, Shirley MA: Reducing the risk of acid aspiration during cesarian section. Anesth Analg 53:859–868, 1974.

65. Coomb DW, Hooper D, Colton T: Pre-anesthetic cimetidine alteration of gastric fluid volume and pH. Anesth Analg 58:183–188, 1979.

66. Toung T, Cameron JL: Cimetidine as a pre-operative medication to reduce the complications of aspiration of gastric contents. Surgery 87:205–208, 1980.

67. Ewart MC, Yau G, Gin T, et al: A comparison of the effects of omeprazole and ranitidine on gastric secretion in women undergoing elective caesarian section. Anesthesiology 45:527–530, 1990.

68. Ruskone A, Rene E, Chayvialle JA, et al: Effect of somatostatin on diarrhea and on small intestinal water and electrolyte transport in a patient with pancreatic cholera. Dig Dis Sci 27:459–466, 1982.

69. Efendic S, Mattson O: Effect of somatostatin on intestinal motility. Acta Radiol Diag 19:348–352, 1978.

70. Bloom SR: Somatostatin and the gut. Gastroenterology 75:145–147, 1978.

71. Pless J, Bauer W, Briner U, et al: Chemistry and pharmacology of SMS 201-995, a long-acting octapeptide analogue of somatostatin. Scand J Gastroenterol 119(suppl):54–64, 1986.

72. Yamada T: Local regulatory actions of gastrointestinal peptides. In Johnson LR (ed): Physiology of the Gastrointestinal Tract, 2nd ed. New York, Raven Press, p 131, 1987.

73. Viollet C, Prevost G, Maubert E, et al: Molecular pharmacology of somatostatin receptors. Fundam Clin Pharmacol 92(2):107–113, 1995.

74. Gyr KE, Meier R: Pharmacodynamic effects of Sandostatin in the gastrointetinal tract. Digestion 54(suppl 1):14–19, 1993.

75. Harris AG: Somatostatin and somatostatin analogues: Pharmacokinetics and pharmacodynamic effects. Gut 35(suppl 3):S1–S4, 1994.

76. Kutz K, Nuesch E, Rosenthaler J: Pharmacokinetics of SMS 201-995 in healthy subjects. Scand J Gastroenterol 119(suppl):65–72, 1986.

77. Cooper JC, Williams NS, King RF, Barker MCJ: Effects of a long-acting somatostatin analogue in patients with severe ileostomy diarrhoea. Br J Surg 73:128–131, 1986.

78. O'Keefe SJD, Peterson ME, Fleming CR: Octreotide as an adjunct to home parenteral nutrition in the management of permanent endjejunostomy syndrome. JPEN J Parenter Enteral Nutr 18:26–34, 1994.

79. Seydel AS, Miller JH, Sarac TP, et al: Octreotide diminishes luminal nutrient transport activity, which is reversed by epidermal growth factor. Am J Surg 172(3):267–271, 1996.

80. O'Keefe SJD, Haymond MW, Bennet WM, et al: Long-acting somatostatin analogue therapy and protein metabolism in patients with jejunostomies. Gastroenterology 107:379–388, 1994.

81. Klein KB: Controlled treatment trials in the irritable bowel syndrome: A critique. Gastroenterology 95:232–241, 1988.

82. McGrath WR, Lewis RE, Kuhn WL: The dual mode of the antispasmodic effect of dicyclomine hydrochloride. J Pharmacol Exp Ther 146:354–358, 1964.

83. Cotton PB: Progress report. ERCP. Gut 18:316–341, 1977.

84. Prior A, Read NW: Reduction of rectal sensitivity and post-prandial motility by granisetron, a 5-HT3 receptor antagonist, in patients with irritable bowel syndrome. Aliment Pharmacol Ther 7:175–180, 1993.

85. Goldberg PA, Kamm MA, Setti-Carraro P, et al: Modification of visceral sensitivity and pain and irritable bowel syndrome by 5-HT3 antagonism (ondansetron). Digestion 57:478–483, 1996.

86. Kozlowski CM, Green A, Grundy D, et al: The 5-HT₃ receptor antagonist alosetron inhibits the colorectal induced depressor response and spinal c-fos expression in the anaesthetized rat. Gut 46(4):474–480, 2000.

87. Balfour JA, Goa KL, Perry CM: Alosetron [review]. Drugs 59(3):511–518, 2000.

88. Miura M, Lawson DC, Clary DM, et al: Central modulation of rectal distension-induced blood pressure changes by alosetron, a 5HT₃ receptor antagonist. Dig Dis Sci 44:20–24, 1999.

89. Camilleri M, Mayer E, Drossman D, et al: Improvement in pain with alosetron, a 5-HT₃-receptor antagonist. Aliment Pharmacol Ther 14:1149–1151, 1999.

90. Camilleri M, Northcutt AR, Kong GE, et al: Efficacy and safety of alosetron in women with irritable bowel syndrome: A randomized, placebo-controlled trial. Lancet 355:1035–1040, 2000.

91. Friedel D, Thomas R, Fisher RS: Ischaemic colitis during treatment with Alosetron. Gastroenterology 120:557–560, 2001.

92. Coupar IM: Opioid action on the intestine: The importance of the intestinal mucosa. Life Sci 41:917–925, 1987.

93. Jaffe JH, Martin WR: Opioid analgesics and antagonists. In Gilman AG, Goodman, Rall TW, Murad F (eds): The Pharmacological Basis of Therapeutics, 7th ed. New York, Macmillan, pp 491–531, 1985.

94. Awouters F, Megens A, Verlinden M, et al: Loperamide: Surveys of studies on mechanism of its antidiarrheal activity. Dig Dis Sci 38:977–995, 1991.

95. Burleigh DE: Loperamide but not morphine has anti-secretory effects in human colon in vitro. Eur J Pharmacol 202:277–280, 1991.

96. Read M, Read NW, Barber DC, Duthie HL: Effects of loperamide on anal sphincter function in patients complaining of chronic diarrhea with faecal incontinence and urgency. Dig Dis Sci 27:807–814, 1982.

97. Minton NA, Smith PGD: Loperamide toxicity in a child after a single dose. BMJ 294:1383, 1987.

98. Forbes A: Clinicians Guide to Inflammatory Bowel Disease. Chapman & Hall Medical, 1997.

99. Brown JW: Toxic megacolon associated with loperamide therapy. JAMA 241:501–502, 1979.

100. Palmer KR, Corbett CL, Holdsworth CD: Double-blind crossover study comparing loperamide, codeine and diphenoxylate in the treatment of chronic diarrhea. Gastroenterology 79:1272–1275, 1980.

101. Pelemans W, Vantrappen G: A double blind crossover comparison of loperamide with diphehoxylate in the symptomatic treatment of chronic diarrhea. Gastroenterology 70:1030–1034, 1976.

45

Antiemetics

Jens Scholz, MD, PhD • Markus Steinfath, MD, PhD • Peter H. Tonner, MD, PhD

The decrease in the incidence of life-threatening anesthetic-related complications has led anesthesiologists to focus on the more common distressing symptoms including pain and nausea and vomiting after surgery. With respect to postoperative pain management, several convincing concepts have already been introduced into clinical practice, and postoperative pain should no longer be the most common sequel following surgery.[1] This chapter deals with antiemetics in the prevention and therapy of postoperative nausea and vomiting (PONV).

Nausea and vomiting have long been associated with anesthesia and surgery, as have attempts to alleviate them. In 1848, Snow recognized severe nausea and vomiting after ether inhalation and proposed wine and other pharmacologic solutions for postoperative treatment.[2] In 1991, PONV was described as the big "little problem"[3]—a comment on the dichotomy between the patients' and the physicians' perspectives. Surgical patients with previous experience of PONV invariably rate nausea and vomiting as the most unpleasant consequence of their surgery. This complication is not only unpleasant and aesthetically displeasing to patients and their caregivers, but can also be associated with stress on suture lines, wound dehiscence, bleeding,

electrolyte disturbances, dehydration, and pulmonary aspiration of gastric contents.[4] Frequently, PONV delays discharge from the ambulatory surgery center and results in an increased use of resources of both supplies and personnel, each of which have financial implications. Furthermore, after ambulatory surgery, PONV may occur at home resulting in an unplanned hospital admission.[4–6] Consequently, prevention and appropriate management of PONV are highly relevant.

Definitions

The terms *nausea, vomiting,* and *retching* are not synonymous. Nausea is a subjectively unpleasant sensation in the epigastrium and throat associated with the urge to vomit, whereas vomiting or emesis is the forceful expulsion of upper gastrointestinal contents through the mouth, caused by the powerful sustained contraction of the abdominal muscles. Retching refers to the labored rhythmic activity of the respiratory muscles, including the diaphragm and abdominal muscles, without expulsion of gastric contents. This sensation usually precedes vomiting.[6]

Incidence

During the early days of anesthesia with ether, the incidence rate of PONV is estimated at 75% to 80%.[6] Despite major advances in surgical techniques and the introduction of new anesthetic agents with reduced emetogenicity, the global incidence rates of PONV in an adult surgical population receiving general anesthesia has been estimated at 20% to 30%, differing considerably among institutions and even among anesthesiologists within the same hospital.[4-6] If less precise definitions are used, the incidence rates of PONV vary from 14% to 82%[5,7,8]; this wide range may also be because of the variety of anesthetic agents and different types of surgery or populations undergoing surgical procedures. In women undergoing laparoscopic procedures, the incidence rate of postoperative vomiting was found to be up to 54%.[5,9] Conversely, in patients undergoing short surgical procedures, including dental extraction, dilation and curettage of the uterus, or knee arthroscopy, PONV was observed in only 12% to 22%.[5,10]

Physiology

Vomiting is a complex process coordinated by the vomiting center in the lateral reticular formation of the medulla (Figs. 45–1 and 45–2).[4,10-12] Evidence for such a center is based on electrical stimulation and on brain stem lesion studies.[12] This center receives input from the chemoreceptor trigger zone in the area postrema in the floor of the fourth ventricle, from the vestibular apparatus through the nucleus vestibularis and cerebellum, from higher brain stem and cortical structures, and from visceral afferents that originate in peripheral structures including the gastrointestinal tract (see Figs. 45–1 and 45-2). The area postrema is highly vascular and the vessels terminate in fenestrated capillaries surrounded by large perivascular spaces. The blood–brain barrier is poorly developed in the area postrema; therefore, the chemoreceptor trigger zone is readily accessible to emetic substances in the circulation or cerebrospinal fluid. Some peripheral signals bypass the trigger zone, reaching the vomiting center through the nucleus tractus solitarius from the pharynx, stomach, and small intestine.

Knowledge of the neuropharmacology of pathways leading to and from the vomiting center is incomplete, but a picture is emerging that provides a rational basis for current antiemetic therapy. Serotonin (5-hydroxytryptamine [5-HT]), acting at serotonin subtype 3 (5-HT$_3$) receptors, is an important emetic signal and transmitter in the afferent pathways from the gastrointestinal tract terminating in the chemoreceptor trigger zone and in the nucleus tractus solitarius (see Fig. 45–2). Dopamine (acting at D$_2$ receptors), acetylcholine (acting through muscarinic [M] receptors), and histamine (acting at H$_1$ receptors) are also implicated in emetic signalling through the chemoreceptor trigger zone and in the nucleus tractus solitarius (see Fig. 45–2).[4,13-17] Antagonism of transmission through these pathways contributes to the antiemetic effects of especially 5-HT$_3$ and D$_2$ receptor antagonists. Cholinergic and histaminergic synapses seem to be involved in transmission from the vestibular apparatus to the vomiting center, suggesting a basis for the particular use of H$_1$ receptor–directed antihistaminic and muscarinic anticholinergic agents in motion sickness. Other useful antiemetic agents including corticosteroids do not fit into the scheme shown in Figure 45–2, but it is likely that such agents derive their antiemetic efficacy

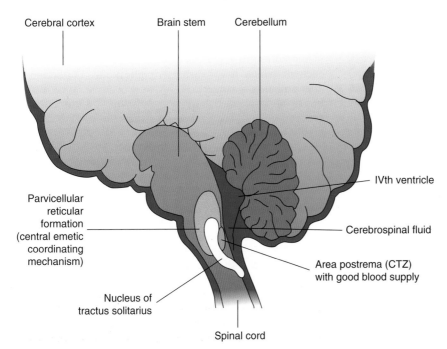

Figure 45–1. The structures within the brain involved in the control of emesis. (From Simpson KL, Lynch L: Physiology and pharmacology of nausea and comiting. In Hemmings H Jr, Hopkins P (eds): Foundations of Anesthesia: Basic and Clinical Sciences. London: Mosby, 2000, p 625.)

Cerebral cortex
Brain stem
Cerebellum
IVth ventricle
Parvicellular reticular formation (central emetic coordinating mechanism)
Cerebrospinal fluid
Nucleus of tractus solitarius
Area postrema (CTZ) with good blood supply
Spinal cord

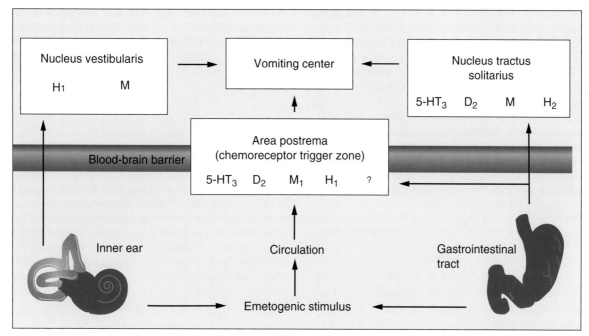

Figure 45–2. Schematic representation of the complex pathophysiology of postoperative nausea and vomiting. 5-HT$_3$, serotonin subtype 3 receptor; D$_2$, dopamine subtype 2 receptor; H$_1$, histamine subtype 1 receptor; M, muscarinic cholinergic receptor. (From Scholz J, Steinfath M, Tonner PH: Postoperative nausea and comiting. Curr Opin Anesthesiol 12:658, 1999.)

from other sites and mechanisms of action that have yet to be elucidated. Moreover, the role of specific opioid receptor subtypes within various brain stem structures in the genesis of the emetic response is not yet resolved.

After stimulation of the vomiting center either directly or indirectly through neural pathways, vomiting is mediated by various efferent pathways, including the vagus, the phrenic nerves, and innervation to the abdominal musculature. The initial manifestation often involves nausea, in which gastric tone is reduced, gastric peristalsis is reduced or absent, and the tone of the duodenum and upper jejunum is increased, so that, finally, gastric reflux occurs. Ultimately, the upper portion of the stomach relaxes whereas the pylorus constricts, and the coordinated contraction of the diaphragm and abdominal muscles leads to expulsion of gastric contents. Several risk factors for PONV have already been discovered in a large series of investigations.[4–6,10,18,19]

Patient- and Surgery-Related Risk Factors

Significant factors affecting PONV include patient characteristics, the nature of the underlying disease for which the surgical or diagnostic procedure is being performed, and the type and duration of surgery.

Age

A greater risk for PONV has been reported in pediatric patients than in adults.[10] Within the pediatric population,

postoperative emesis increases with age to reach a peak incidence in the preadolescent age group.[20] The incidence rates have been estimated at 5% in infants younger than 12 months old, 20% in children 1 to 5 years old, 34% in children 6 to 10 years old, and 32% in children older than 11 years.[21] Some investigators have suggested that increasing age during adulthood is associated with a decreased incidence of emesis.

Sex

PONV is approximately two to three times more prevalent in adult women than in men, and the severity of vomiting is greater.[10] There is no significant sex difference in children, but the incidence of PONV increases in girls as menarche approaches. Because PONV varies according to the phase of the menstrual cycle, with a fourfold increased incidence during menses,[22] it has been suggested that the increasing levels of estrogen, combined with decreasing levels of follicle-stimulating hormone, may sensitize chemoreceptors, or the vomiting center, or both.

Body Weight

Obesity, defined by a mass index greater than 30 kg/m^2 (weight divided by height squared), has been assumed to be associated with increased PONV in previous reports.[6,10,23,24] This correlation is explained by the fact that adipose tissue acts as a reservoir for anesthetic agents, from which they continue to enter the circulation even after their administration has been discontinued. Other explanations for an increased incidence of PONV in obese patients include a larger residual gastric volume, and increased incidence of esophageal reflux, gallbladder, and other gastrointestinal diseases. In addition, compared with nonobese subjects, these patients have a greater incidence of airway difficulties and more gastric insufflation occurs during attempts to maintain an adequate airway using a facemask.

Despite this a large retrospective analysis of clinical data, a systematic review failed to demonstrate a significant influence of body weight on frequency of PONV. Furthermore, several recent evaluations also failed to demonstrate obesity as a predictor for PONV.[25–27]

Smoking Status

Recent investigations have shown that PONV is more frequently observed in patients who do not smoke. Apfel and coworkers found a greater incidence for PONV in patients without history of smoking at two different centers that were evaluated independently.[28] In addition, Hennes and colleagues calculated similar odds ratios for the nonsmoking status and patient sex with respect to the occurrence of PONV.[29] The reason why nonsmoking status is a risk factor for PONV currently is not understood.

History of Motion Sickness or Previous Postoperative Nausea and Vomiting Sensations

Patients with a history suggesting that they have a low threshold for vomiting are at increased risk for development of emetic symptoms. These include patients with a prior history of PONV after surgical procedures or patients who experience motion sickness.[6,10]

Anxiety

Patients with undue anxiety about the forthcoming surgical procedure are at greater risk for emesis.[30] It has been suggested that PONV in anxious patients may be related to an increase in gastric fluid volume caused by increased circulating stress hormones[31]; also, anxiety may provoke air swallowing resulting in gut distension and activation of mechanoreceptors.[30] Others have not been able to correlate gastric volume with preoperative anxiety.[32] Decreased PONV was noted when hypnosis or relaxation techniques were used to reduce perioperative anxiety during plastic surgery operations performed under monitored anesthesia care.[33]

Presence and Absence of Food

Patients who have had recent food or fluid intake, e.g., emergency surgery patients, are often found to be at risk for PONV.[3] Apart from the high risk for aspiration into the bronchial tree, this is another reason to advocate fasting before elective surgery. However, prolonged fasting also tends to increase the incidence of nausea, particularly in women.[8] This may be related to hypoglycemia or ketonemia.

Gastroparesis

Patients with delayed gastric emptying secondary to an underlying disease (e.g., ileus) may be at increased risk for PONV after surgery.[5,10] These disease processes include gastrointestinal obstruction, chronic cholecystitis, neuromuscular disorder, and intrinsic neuropathies. Gastric hypomotility can complicate conditions such as scleroderma, myotonic dystrophy, and progressive muscular dystrophies, amyloidosis, and familial visceral myopathies. Gastroparesis also can be associated with pylorospasm and also isolated antral hypomotility in patients with diabetes mellitus.[10]

Type and Duration of Surgery

PONV is more often observed in patients undergoing abdominal versus nonabdominal surgery with a markedly increased incidence in women undergoing laparoscopic procedures.[8,34] Pediatric patients undergoing strabismus repair, adenotonsillectomy, orchiopexy, middle ear surgery, and laparotomy are also at increased risk.[10,35] The duration of surgery also has an effect on the incidence of PONV, with more frequent emesis being reported after longer operations because patients may receive a larger number and volume of potentially emetic anesthetic agents.[10,36,37]

Anesthesia-Related Risk Factors

Nitrous Oxide and Potent Inhalational Anesthetic Agents

The results of studies investigating the influence of nitrous oxide on PONV are inconsistent. Several fairly outdated studies suggest an independent contribution of nitrous oxide for PONV.[38] For example, the high incidence of PONV during laparoscopic procedures was thought to be further exacerbated by the introduction of nitrous oxide in this particular high-risk population.[39] Furthermore, after daycase gynecologic surgery, nitrous oxide in oxygen was associated with significantly more PONV than oxygen alone (29% vs. 9%, respectively[40]).

However, other investigators failed to demonstrate a significant increase in PONV after addition of nitrous oxide to other anesthetic agents.[5] For example, Kortilla and coworkers could not observe a significant increase in PONV in patients undergoing abdominal hysteroscopy receiving a balanced anesthesia with fentanyl and isoflurane and nitrous oxide in oxygen compared with oxygen in air.[41] In addition, in recent investigations dealing with the detection of relevant risk factors for PONV using multiple logistic regression analysis, nitrous oxide was not identified as a significant risk factor in this regard.[28]

Meta-analyses of existing studies support the view that addition of nitrous oxide will lead to increased nausea and vomiting.[42–44] Thus nitrous oxide has to be considered as a weak risk factor for PONV, and omitting nitrous oxide may decrease the incidence of PONV. Omitting nitrous oxide was also shown to be more effective in protecting against vomiting rather than from nausea; its prophylactic effect was most effective in patients at high risk for PONV.

Nitrous oxide may cause PONV through both central and peripheral mechanisms. This may involve stimulation of the sympathetic nervous system with catecholamine release, changes in middle ear pressure with stimulation of the vestibular system, and increased distension of the gastrointestinal tract.[5]

Only a few studies exist comparing volatile anesthetics with respect to their incidence of PONV, but the lack of consistent results suggests that there is probably little difference in associated PONV overall.[6] Retrospective analysis of data from a large multicenter trial involving more than 17,000 patients revealed no difference in the incidence of emesis among patients receiving halothane, enflurane, or isoflurane,[45] but there are some suggestions that sevoflurane is associated with a decreased PONV incidence.[46,47] Recently, it was reported that the early PONV rate in the postanesthetic care unit was significantly lower for isoflurane than for desflurane and sevoflurane in patients undergoing breast cancer surgery. Furthermore, desflurane had a markedly greater 24-hour PONV rate than isoflurane (67% vs. 22%).[48]

Opioid Analgesics

Opioids are well documented as powerful emetogenic agents.[5,6,18,49] Alfentanil infusions have been used instead of halothane for short surgical procedures in children and were associated with a greater incidence rate of PONV (45% vs. 15%). Forrest and coworkers found that fentanyl was associated with an incidence rate of approximately 25% and 18% of nausea and vomiting, respectively, compared with 18% and 12% with volatile anesthetics.[45] The more lipid-soluble agents, alfentanil and sufentanil, have also been associated with similar incidences of PONV.[51,52] Thus it seems insignificant which opioid is used because they are all associated with a similar incidence rates of PONV.[53]

Other Anesthetic Agents

Administration of traditional intravenous anesthetic agents, including barbiturates and etomidate, can also be associated with PONV.[5,6,10] Conversely, propofol has been shown to exhibit *antemetic* properties.[54] Watcha and White[10] mention a high incidence of PONV after ketamine administration;

however, Rabey and Smith[55] argue that there are no controlled data to support this contention.

Pharmacology of Antiemetics and Therapeutic Approach

Several strategies in PONV prophylaxis and therapy have been adopted from prevention to treatment of chemotherapy-induced emesis. A panel of clinical, health economic, and basic scientists with expertise in various oncology disciplines reviewed published literature to develop evidence-based consensus guidelines for the prevention and treatment of chemotherapy-induced emesis.[56] Currently, 5-HT receptor antagonists and corticosteroids are the two categories of antiemetics that are most effective; they have the fewest side effects and are the most convenient to use. Similar evidence-based consensus guidelines for the prevention and treatment of PONV are not yet available.

Currently, three major groups of agents—including benzamides, neuroleptics, and 5-HT$_3$ receptor antagonists—are most frequently used in the management of PONV in daily clinical practice. Other agents with antiemetic properties such as corticosteroids are also used but predominantly in combination. As mentioned earlier, muscarinic receptor antagonists and antihistaminics are effective in the prevention of motion sickness and treatment of postoperative vomiting related to vestibular stimulation, because the vestibular apparatus and the nucleus of the tractus solitarius are rich in muscarinic and histaminic receptors. The various antiemetic drugs are summarized in Table 45–1 in relation to their interaction with different specific receptor sites.

Benzamides

The substituted benzamides, particularly metoclopramide (Fig. 45–3), are widely used in chemotherapy-induced emesis and in some countries for the prevention and therapy of PONV. Although structurally related to procainamide, metoclopramide lacks significant local anesthetic or antiarrhythmic actions. Metoclopramide is rapidly and completely absorbed after oral administration, but hepatic first-pass metabolism reduces its bioavailability to about 75%. Metoclopramide is rapidly distributed into most tissues and readily crosses the blood–brain barrier and the placenta; the concentration of the drug in breast milk may exceed that in plasma. Up to 30% of metoclopramide is excreted unchanged in the urine, and the remainder is eliminated in

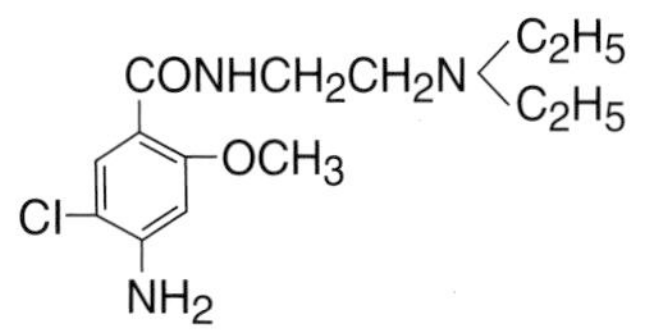

Figure 45–3. Chemical structure of metoclopramide.

TABLE 45–1.

Various Antiemetics and Their Interaction with Different Specific Receptor Sites

	Receptor Site of Action			
	H$_1$	M	D$_2$	5-HT$_3$
Antihistamines				
Promethazine	++++	++	++	−
Dimenhydrinate	++++	++	+	−
Anticholinergics				
Scopolamine	+	++++	+	−
Benzamides				
Metoclopramide	+	−	+++	++
Neuroleptics				
Droperidol	+	−	++++	+
Triflupromazine	+	−	++++	−
5-HT$_3$ Antagonists				
Ondansetron	−	−	−	++++
Tropisetron	−	−	−	++++
Granisetron	−	−	−	++++
Dolasetron	−	−	−	++++
Glucocorticoids				
Dexamethasone	−	−	−	−

(+), positive interaction; (−), no interaction; 5-HT$_3$, serotonin subtype 3 receptor; D$_2$, dopamine subtype 2 receptor; H$_1$, histamine subtype 1 receptor; M, muscarinic cholinergic receptor.

the urine and the bile after conjugation with sulfate or glucuronic acid. The half-life of the drug in the circulation is about 4 to 6 hours, but it may be as much as 24 hours in patients with impaired renal function.[18]

The efficacy of metoclopramide in preventing PONV is equivocal.[57] Nevertheless, some investigators found metoclopramide at doses of 0.25 mg/kg or 10 mg intravenously to be more effective in preventing PONV than 0.1 mg/kg tropisetron or 8 mg ondansetron, which are potent 5-HT$_3$ receptor antagonists. Other studies demonstrated metoclopramide to be of no or limited value when compared with other antiemetics including 5-HT$_3$ receptor antagonists and droperidol.[5,6] At high concentrations, metoclopramide has been shown to have a weak 5-HT$_3$ receptor antagonistic effect, which may account for some of its antiemetic properties,[38] when used at high doses in chemotherapy-induced emesis. However, the doses administered for PONV and the antiemetic effects of metoclopramide are likely to reside in its ability to antagonize the action of dopamine. In a systematic review of randomized, placebo-controlled studies,

metoclopramide was shown to have no clinically relevant antiemetic effect.[58]

Side effects typical of the dopamine antagonists, such as extrapyramidal reactions and sedation, may also occur in patients receiving metoclopramide.[18,59] Intravenous application may be associated with significant cardiovascular side effects, which include hypotension and bradycardia or tachycardia. Metoclopramide should not be used after gastrointestinal surgery, such as pyloroplasty or intestinal anastomosis, because it stimulates gastric motility and may delay healing.[18]

Other benzamide derivates have been synthesized (e.g., trimethobenzamide and cisapride) with the twin aims of increasing the antiemetic efficacy and reducing side effects; however, these hopes have not been realized.

Neuroleptics

The butyrophenones are potent neuroleptics that also have antiemetic properties mediated by their powerful D$_2$ receptor antagonism.[18] They were developed primarily for use in patients with schizophrenia and other psychoses, but droperidol (Fig. 45–4) has also been used extensively as an antiemetic in anesthesia.[57,60]

Other neuroleptic agents exhibiting antiemetic properties are the phenothiazines, triflupromazine, chlorpromazine, perphenazine, and levomepromazine.[18] Their antiemetic effects are primarily caused by an interaction with central dopaminergic receptors of the central nervous system (CNS). They seem to be most effective in preventing opioid-related nausea and vomiting. Although their antiemetic effects are achieved at low doses, all phenothiazines are capable of producing significant adverse effects, including extrapyramidal effects and sedation. Thus the phenothiazines may complicate postoperative care and result in prolonged hospitalization.[6] Conversely, in an investigation comparing the antiemetic efficacy of preoperative perphenazine (5 mg intravenously) with placebo, ondansetron (4 mg), droperidol (1.25 mg), and metoclopramide (10 mg) in 360 women undergoing transabdominal hysterectomy, perphenazine was the only agent free of side effects.[61]

Most studies involving dopamine antagonists have used droperidol. The total body clearance of droperidol is similar to hepatic blood flow, emphasizing the importance of hepatic metabolism in elimination of this drug (perfusion rather than capacity dependent); thus accumulation of droperidol is more likely to occur when the hepatic blood flow is decreased rather than with an alteration in hepatic enzyme activity. The elimination half-life of droperidol is about 100 minutes, the clearance is 14 mL/kg per minute, and the

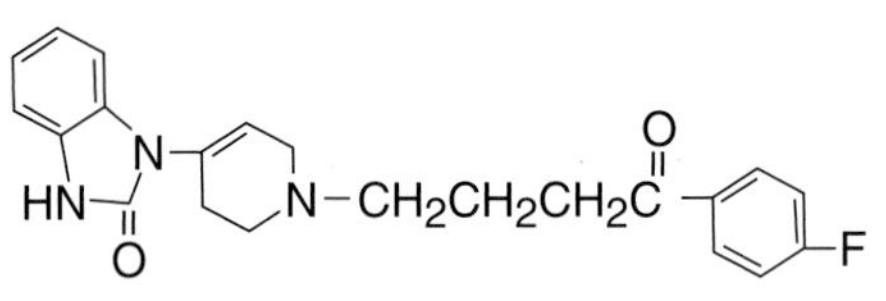

Droperidol

Figure 45–4. Chemical structure of droperidol.

volume of distribution 2 L/kg. The short elimination half-time is not consistent with the prolonged CNS effects of droperidol, which may reflect slow dissociation of the drug from receptors or retention of droperidol in the brain.[18]

Droperidol administered at a dose range between 1.25 to 2.5 mg intravenously before the conclusion of elective cesarean section surgery decreased the incidence of PONV; 0.02 mg/kg 2 minutes before the induction of anesthesia in female outpatients undergoing laparoscopy also reduces PONV. In unpremedicated children undergoing elective strabismus surgery, 0.075 mg/kg droperidol intravenously at the induction of anesthesia, greatly decreased the incidence of PONV and did not delay awaking from anesthesia.[62] In comparative studies, intravenous droperidol has been demonstrated to have greater prophylactic efficacy than metoclopramide.[63–66] In this regard, low doses of droperidol (0.01–0.02 mg/kg) have been used successfully in procedures associated with moderate emesis but have limited efficacy in more emetogenic procedures.[10] In outpatient gynecologic surgery, 0.625 mg droperidol intravenously provided antiemetic prophylaxis comparable to that of 4 mg ondansetron without increasing side effects or delaying discharge, and it was more cost-effective.[67] Grond and coworkers[68] found that 2.5 mg droperidol intravenously is more effective than 8 mg ondansetron for prevention of PONV after minor gynecologic surgery, but at the risk for delaying recovery from the effects of anesthesia.

Conversely, other studies failed to demonstrate an efficacy of droperidol administration in preventing PONV (see Scholz and Steinfath[5] and Rose and Watcha[6]). However, in these studies, droperidol was given during induction of anesthesia, and it was suggested that the efficacy might be improved if droperidol was to be administered toward the end of prolonged surgical intervention. Nevertheless, overall, most single studies found a beneficial effect of droperidol when compared with placebo in the prevention of PONV, and efficacy also has been demonstrated when droperidol was administered before and at the end of surgery. In a recent systematic review, Henzi and

coworkers[60] concluded that droperidol is antiemetic in the surgical setting, and the effect on nausea is short-lived but more pronounced than the effect on vomiting. Labyrinthine-induced vomiting (motion sickness) is not influenced by droperidol.

Neuroleptics can induce extrapyramidal side effects that are extremely unpleasant.[18,60] In addition, high doses of droperidol can cause hypotension (as a result of peripheral α adrenergic blockade), prolonged tiredness, or dysphoria. Anxiety and restlessness, developing after discharge, have also been reported, suggesting that droperidol may not be an appropriate prophylactic antiemetic for day-case and routine outpatient surgery.[18]

Although droperidol is a potent antiemetic drug, the use of this agent is likely to become more limited because oral administration of droperidol in a particular patient population was associated with QT interval prolongation in the electrocardiogram.

Serotonin Type 3 Receptor Antagonists

The role of 5-HT and 5-HT receptors in drug-induced emesis has received increased attention. As 5-HT is rapidly removed from plasma by platelets, endothelium, and the liver, peripheral 5-HT release is reflected by analyzing its major metabolite 5-hydroxyindole acetic acid (5-HIAA). In this regard it has been demonstrated that 5-HIAA levels showed a tendency to increase from 3 to at least 5 hours after cis-platinum administration (Fig. 45–5).[69] Furthermore, 5-HIAA levels are also significantly increased in patients with PONV sensations compared with patients without PONV.[70]

There are 14 5-HT receptor subtypes, among which the 5-HT$_3$ receptor occupies a special place (Fig. 45–6).[71] The 5-HT$_3$ receptor is phylogenetically much older than the other 5-HT receptors, all of which have developed from a single primordial 5-HT receptor and belong to the G

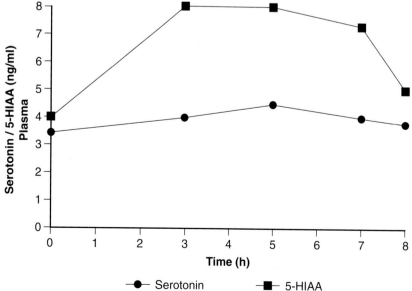

Figure 45–5. Serotonin and 5-hydroxyindole acetic acid (5-HIAA) plasma levels after cis-platinum administration.

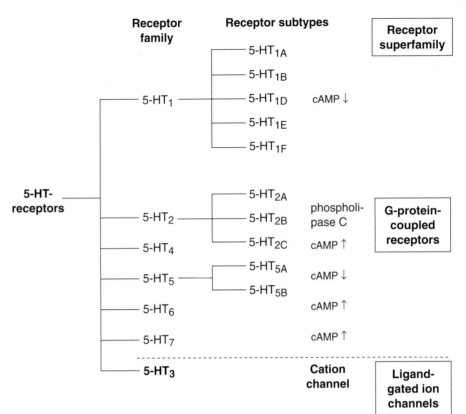

Figure 45–6. Serotonin (5-HT) receptor subtypes. (From Wolf H: Preclinical and clinical pharmacology of the 5-HT₃ receptor antagonists. Scand J Rheumatol 29(suppl 113):39, 2000.)

protein–coupled receptors. The 5-HT₃ receptor is a ligand-gated cation channel belonging to the nicotine/γ-aminobutyric acid (GABA) receptor superfamily (Fig. 45–7).[71] It is a pentamer consisting of five, possibly identical, monomers forming a central pore that can be readily penetrated by small cations. The 5-HT₃ receptors are present exclusively on neurons, both peripherally and centrally. In the periphery, these receptors have been detected on preganglionic and postganglionic autonomic neurons and on neurons of the sensory and enteric nervous system (myenteric and submucosal plexus). High densities of 5-HT₃ receptors have been identified at different CNS locations including the area postrema, nucleus tractus solitarii, and nucleus dorsalis nervi vagi.[71]

Agents such as ondansetron, tropisetron, granisetron, and dolasetron (Fig. 45–8),[5,6,10,18,71] which competitively antagonize the effect of 5-HT at 5-HT₃ receptor sites, have been shown to be extremely useful antiemetics in the prevention of chemotherapy-induced nausea and vomiting. 5-HT₃ receptor antagonists are very specific agents with almost no significant interaction with other 5-HT receptor subtypes or other specific receptor binding sites (Fig. 45–9).[71,72] The 5-HT₃ receptor antagonists represent a major advance in the management of emesis because they are highly effective and possess a low side effect profile, especially when compared with benzamides and neuroleptics.

Although the pharmacokinetic properties of the available 5-HT₃ receptor antagonists are similar, clinically relevant differences exist between their half-lives. Dolasetron also has a particular characteristic insofar as it is a prodrug that has to be reduced to its active metabolite hydrodolasetron

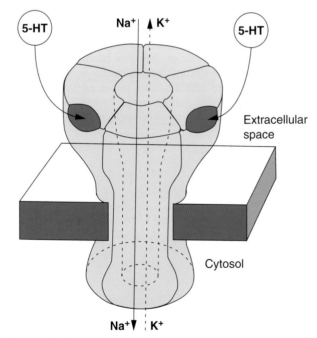

Figure 45–7. Schematic representation of the serotonin (5-HT) subtype 3 receptor. (From Wolf H: Preclinical and clinical pharmacology of the 5-HT₃ receptor antagonists. Scand J Rheumatol 29(suppl 113):38, 2000.)

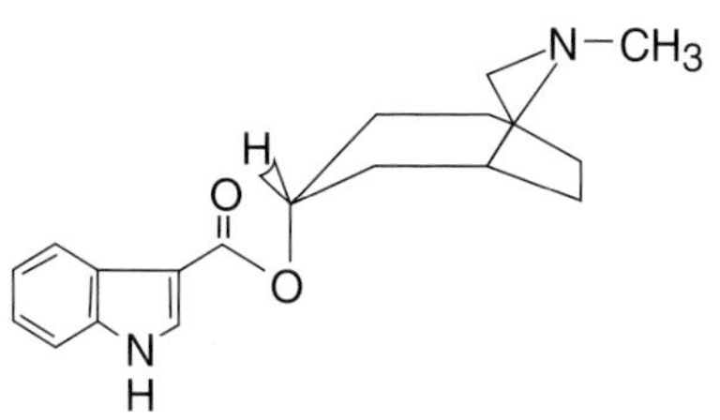

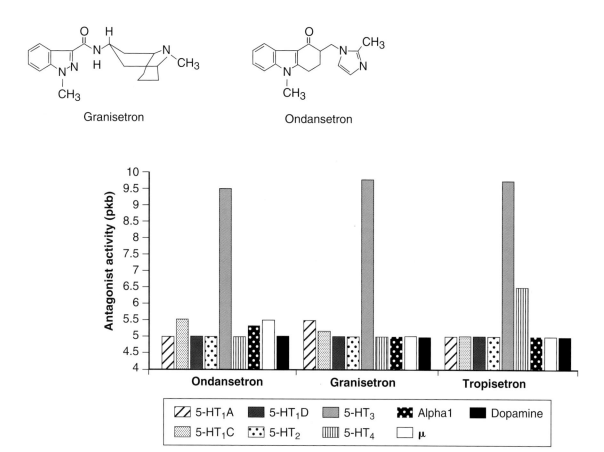

Figure 45–8. Chemical structures of serotonin subtype 3 (5-HT$_3$) receptor antagonists.

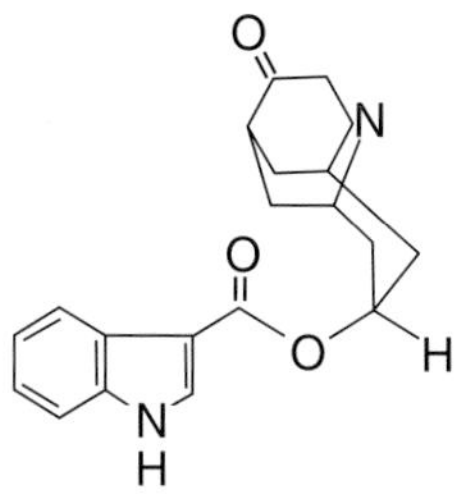

Figure 45–9. Interaction of ondansetron, granisetron, and tropisetron with various receptor sites. (Data from Scholz J, Steinfath M: Prophylaxis and therapy of postoperative nausea and vomiting. In Herbert MK, Holzer P, Roewer N (eds): Problems of the Gastrointestinal Tract in Anesthesia, the Perioperative Period, and Intensive Care. Heidelberg, Springer, 1999; Naylor RJ, Inall FC: The physiology and pharmacology of postoperative nausea and vomiting. Anesthesia 49:2–5, 1994.)

before exerting its effect. The 5-HT$_3$ receptor antagonists are readily absorbed after oral administration. The blood–brain barrier is easily crossed, and the maximum CNS concentration is reached within few minutes after intravenous injection. The compounds exhibit moderately strong protein binding of about 60% to 75%. The agents are metabolized by different subtypes of the cytochrome P450 enzyme system, and the biodegradation products are predominantly eliminated by the renal route.[71]

Ondansetron was the first drug of this class, and its efficacy has been established in large studies of various populations,[4–6,10,71] not only in chemotherapy-induced emesis but also in the prevention and therapy of PONV. Ondansetron is a carbazalone derivative that is structurally related to 5-HT and possesses specific 5-HT$_3$ subtype receptor antagonist properties, without affecting dopamine, histamine, adrenergic, or cholinergic receptor activity (see Table 45–1). It can be administered orally or intravenously and has an oral bioavailability of about 60%, with effective blood levels appearing 30 to 60 minutes after administration. This agent is metabolized extensively by the liver, with a plasma half-life of 3 to 4 hours.

Superior effects in the prevention of PONV have been observed after administration of ondansetron in comparison with droperidol and metoclopramide.[73–75] In a "dose-finding study" examining both antiemetic efficacy and side effects, it has been shown that ondansetron at a dose of 4 mg is associated with lowest emesis rate along with comparable side effect profiles at various doses ranging from 1 to 8 mg.[76] Four to 8 mg ondansetron intravenously administered over 2 to 5 minutes immediately before the induction of anesthesia is highly effective in decreasing the incidence of PONV in patients undergoing ambulatory gynecologic surgery or middle ear surgery. Oral (0.15 mg/kg) or intravenous (0.05–0.15 mg/kg) administration of ondansetron is effective in decreasing the incidence of PONV in preadolescent children undergoing ambulatory surgery including tonsillectomy and strabismus surgery. In addition to prophylaxis, 1 to 8 mg ondansetron is highly effective in the treatment of PONV. In a systematic review it has been demonstrated that ondansetron could prevent further PONV in one of four patients who would otherwise continue to have these symptoms. Whereas Tramer and colleagues[77] claim that ondansetron did not differ from metoclopramide or droperidol in controlling further emetic symptoms when administered to patients with established PONV, other studies[75] have shown ondansetron to provide better and longer-lasting control of PONV than metoclopramide. Although the antiemetic effects of ondansetron appear to be superior to those of other prophylactic antiemetics in many studies, more recent data suggest that small doses of droperidol (0.625 to 1.25 mg) may be equally effective. Other studies have also demonstrated that droperidol seems to be as effective as ondansetron in preventing PONV and that significant cost savings can be realized if droperidol is used rather than ondansetron.[67,78,79] Conversely, in pediatric surgical patients, prophylactic ondansetron (0.1 mg/kg intravenously) significantly decreased PONV compared with placebo and droperidol (0.75 mg/kg) and reduced hospital length of stay compared with droperidol (a drug whose distribution will in any event be limited in the future).

Ondansetron is generally well tolerated, causing only transient, mild adverse effects, including headache, constipation, and dizziness. Because this drug is not an antagonist of dopamine receptors, it does not cause the extrapyramidal side effects associated with metoclopramide or droperidol. In other words, the most significant feature of ondansetron prophylaxis and treatment is the relative freedom from side effects compared with other classes of antiemetic agents. Nevertheless, the cost of ondansetron is greater than that of other antiemetics such as metoclopramide or droperidol. Liver enzyme increases have been reported only in patients receiving antineoplastic drugs at the same time, and it is unclear whether this effect is a result of the chemotherapy or ondansetron. Ondansetron and other 5-HT$_3$ receptor antagonists such as tropisetron and granisetron can cause slight QT prolongation and reduced heart rate. In some cases, conduction disorders (atrioventricular block) and arrhythmias have been documented during treatment with 5-HT$_3$ receptor antagonists.[71]

Tropisetron is another highly potent and selective 5-HT$_3$ receptor antagonist developed by systematic methyl substitution of the 5-HT molecule (see Fig. 45–8).[71,80] In other words, it is an indoleacetic acid ester of tropine. Tropisetron is characterized by a longer half-life (7.3 hours for extensive metabolizers and 30.3 hours for poor metabolizers) when compared with ondansetron (3.5 and 5 hours, respectively).

The beneficial effect of tropisetron in chemotherapy-induced nausea and vomiting[81,82] and after gynecologic procedures[83] has also been reported. Additional investigations on patients undergoing gynecologic procedures, including laparoscopy, have suggested the administration of 2 mg tropisetron for the prevention of PONV.[84] In a recent multicenter trial it has been demonstrated that tropisetron has similar beneficial effects and side effect profiles when compared with ondansetron.[34] Both agents significantly reduced the rates of emetic episodes and nausea in the patient population undergoing abdominal surgery and were associated with low rates of minor side effects. Significant beneficial effects in patients undergoing nonabdominal surgical procedures were not observed for either ondansetron or tropisetron. Nevertheless, it has already been mentioned that patients undergoing abdominal surgery, especially laparoscopic procedures, are at much greater risk for PONV than patients undergoing nonabdominal surgery. In addition, in a recent article, Boogaerts and coworkers conclude that prophylactic tropisetron can reduce the incidence of PONV in selected high-risk inpatients undergoing various types of surgical procedures.[85] Furthermore, it has been shown that rescue treatment using a single dose of tropisetron is effective in reducing further nausea and vomiting, indicating its efficacy in the management of acute nausea and vomiting during the postoperative period.[86]

Granisetron is a 5-HT$_3$ receptor antagonist available for oral or intravenous administration to minimize chemotherapy-induced emesis and PONV.[5,71] This agent is more selective than ondansetron and is metabolized in the liver by N-demethylation, aromatic ring oxidation, and subsequent conjugation. Approximately 11% to 12% of the administered dose is eliminated unchanged in the urine; the rest is eliminated as metabolites in the urine (48%) and the feces (34%). The elimination half-time of granisetron is about 9 hours and 2.5 times longer than that of ondansetron and thus may require less frequent dosing.

In a dose-ranging study, a single doses of 0.04 mg/kg granisetron was as effective as 0.06 mg/kg, and both doses were better than placebo or 0.02 mg/kg granisetron.[87] Other investigators stated that 0.02 mg/kg granisetron provided adequate protection against PONV.[88] Concomitant administration of dexamethasone significantly improved the acute antiemetic efficacy of granisetron.[89] The mild adverse effects of this agent include headache, somnolence, and diarrhea or, conversely, in some patients, constipation.

Dolasetron is the most recent member in the class of 5-HT$_3$ receptor antagonist and has been demonstrated to reveal beneficial effects in the management of PONV.[71] After its administration, dolasetron is rapidly metabolized to hydrodolasetron, which is responsible for the antiemetic effect. The metabolite hydrodolasetron is approximately 100 times more potent as a 5-HT$_3$ receptor antagonist than the parent compound. Its elimination half-time is approximately 8 hours.

In a multicenter trial it has been shown that single oral doses of dolasetron, administered 1 to 2 hours before induction of anesthesia, are safe and effective for preventing PONV in patients undergoing gynecologic surgery.[90] A maximal antiemetic response was observed with the 50-mg oral dolasetron dose. Conversely, it has been demonstrated that doses of 25, 50, and 100 of dolasetron were equally effective in reducing PONV.[91] Moreover, it has also been observed that established PONV was effectively blunted by 12.5 mg intravenous dolasetron. However, usually half of the dose used for chemotherapy-induced nausea and vomiting is administered for PONV prophylaxis and therapy (e.g., 8 vs. 4 mg ondansetron and 4 vs. 2 mg tropisetron). Therefore, 50 mg dolasetron might be the adequate dose that should be administered for the prevention and therapy of PONV. Dolasetron is well tolerated in large doses, but dizziness, headache, light-headedness, and increased appetite occurred more often in dolasetron-treated patients than in the placebo group. After administration of dolasetron, an increase in heart rate is observed rather than a reduction. However, other investigators report that adverse events occurred in 3% of patients, regardless of whether they received dolasetron or placebo.[71]

Corticosteroids

Dexamethasone and other glucocorticoids (5–20 mg dexamethasone, 125–375 mg methylprednisolone) have significant antiemetic effects both when administered before chemotherapy and in the postoperative period.[6] Unlike other pharmacologic agents, efficacy in preventing PONV is still present for up to 24 hours.[92] In patients undergoing thyroidectomy, the minimum effective dose in preventing PONV was found to be 5 mg dexamethasone.[93] Although they are effective alone, corticosteroids are more commonly used in combination with other antiemetics.[6]

The administration of other antiemetic therapies enhances the overall antiemetic effect achieved and can reduce the severity and incidence of some adverse effects that are induced by other antiemetic drugs. It has been shown in chemotherapy-induced emesis that the combination of tropisetron plus dexamethasone is superior to tropisetron alone or tropisetron plus metoclopramide (Fig. 45–10).[94] Marked differences between tropisetron alone and tropisetron plus metoclopramide have not been observed (see Fig. 45–10). In pediatric patients undergoing tonsillectomy under general anesthesia, tropisetron (0.1 mg/kg up to 2 mg) plus dexamethasone (0.5 mg/kg up to 8 mg) was more effective than tropisetron alone in reducing the incidence of PONV.[95] The mechanisms by which corticosteroids exert their antiemetic effects currently are not completely understood. Nevertheless, dexamethasone is known to have multiple CNS effects, including effects on mood and sense of well-being.[6] However, with respect to side effects, it is still a matter of debate whether corticosteroids should be administered routinely in all patients at greater risk for PONV.

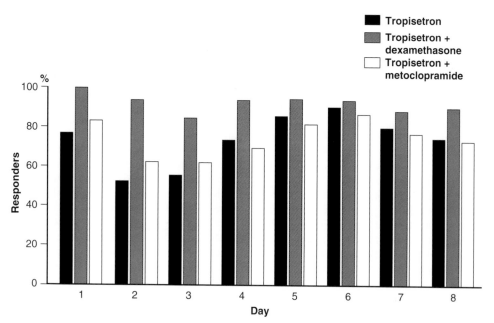

Figure 45–10. Antiemetic efficacy of tropisetron and its combinations with dexamethasone and metoclopramide during highly emetogenic chemotherapy. (Data from Wolf H: Preclinical and clinical pharmacology of the 5-HT₃ receptor antagonists. Scand J Rheumatol 29(Suppl 113):37–45, 2000; Drechsler S, Bruntsch U, Eggert J, et al: Comparison of three tropisetron-containing antiemetic regimens in the prophylaxis of acute and delayed chemotherapy-induced emesis and nausea. Support Care Cancer 5:387–395, 1997.)

Anesthetic and Pharmacologic Strategies in Postoperative Nausea and Vomiting Management

We have drawn attention to that PONV has a high incidence because of a variety of factors and that effective antiemetics are available for its prevention and therapy of PONV. Pharmacologic strategies in PONV management should be considered before submitting the patients to the recovery room or surgical ward.

Premedication

Anesthesiologists usually order a premedication for the patients that should be given before induction of anesthesia. Before the advent of benzodiazepines, it was traditional to use opioids for preanesthetic sedation, but this practice is associated with increased PONV. The benzodiazepines have become popular because they reduce anxiety, produce amnesia, and are associated with decreased PONV sensations,[96-98] possibly because of reduced anxiety. Similarly, the preoperative use of the α_2 receptor agonist clonidine for sedation seems to be associated with decreased PONV, perhaps as the need for anesthetic agents is reduced.[99]

Anesthesia

Regional anesthesia is usually associated with a lower incidence of PONV than general anesthesia.[10,100] A variety of techniques including inhaled anesthesia (potent-inhaled agent with or without nitrous oxide), balanced anesthesia (a combination of inhaled agents and opioid analgesics), and total intravenous anesthesia (TIVA) produce general anesthesia. If general anesthesia is essential, the anesthesiologist should use techniques known to reduce the risk for PONV. When antiemetic drugs have not been administered prophylactically, the incidence of PONV has been reported as greatest with balanced anesthesia, intermediate with inhaled anesthesia, and least with propofol-based TIVA (see article by Rose and Watcha[6]). This observation is supported by several additional investigations.

For example, Hennes and coworkers[29] found that TIVA with propofol is superior to balanced anesthesia with respect to PONV prevention in a variety of surgical patients. Watcha and colleagues[101] demonstrated that there was a lower incidence of PONV in children undergoing day-case strabismus surgery if propofol was used for both induction and maintenance of anesthesia than when administered for induction alone followed by maintenance with inhalational agents. In a study comparing TIVA with propofol and isoflurane anesthesia for major abdominal surgery, nausea during the first 2 hours after surgery was significantly decreased in the TIVA group. In a recent systematic review of randomized controlled trials of propofol, the authors conclude that propofol has a clinically relevant effect on PONV, but only in the short term, when given as a continuous infusion, and

only in settings where the rate for emesis was greater than 20%. Propofol may have a greater effect on the control of nausea than of emesis in low-risk patients. Conversely, it has been shown that the use of propofol for induction and maintenance of anesthesia may be as effective as ondansetron in preventing PONV (see article by Rose and Watcha[6]). Moreover, even subhypnotic doses of propofol administered after surgery have been shown to result in an antiemetic effect. No doubt, there is much evidence that propofol-based TIVA should be the principal anesthetic technique for general anesthesia in patients at high risk for PONV. However, it is still a matter of debate whether propofol has direct antiemetic properties.

There is some evidence that propofol has an antiemetic effect that may be mediated by GABA influences on the 5-HT system.[102] Propofol binds to a specific site on the $GABA_A$ receptor to potentiate GABA-activated chloride flux. In addition, 5-HT release is reduced by GABA-mediated inhibition. Cechetto and coworkers[102] postulate in a recent article that propofol inhibits the release of 5-HT from the dorsal raphe nucleus through an enhancement of the $GABA_A$ synaptic activity. This results in a reduction in the 5-HT released into the cerebrospinal fluid from the serotonergic supraependymal fibers that, in turn, causes a reduction in the 5-HT sequestered by the area postrema. In addition, the results with ondansetron, which would have antagonized the action of $5-HT_3$ receptors in the area postrema, indicates the possibility of a direct $GABA_A$-mediated action of propofol on $5-HT_3$ receptors in the area postrema.

Scoring Systems for Holistic Approach

Routine antiemetic prophylaxis is not warranted for all surgical patients because the global incidence of PONV is less than one third of the overall population scheduled for surgical and diagnostic procedures in anesthesia. However, it is still a matter of discussion which patients should receive an antiemetic prophylaxis, which antiemetic agents are most suitable, and when the drug should be administered.[6,103,104] Therefore, it might be helpful to have a scoring system that points out the probability of PONV and that leads the anesthesiologist to administer an adequate antiemetic prophylaxis. Some authors have quantified the risks for PONV for a given patient using statistical analyses that take into account the various risk factors and provide a risk score.

Koivuranta and coworkers published a simplified score based on the five strongest predictors of PONV, each having the same weight.[105] These factors were female sex, previous PONV, duration of operation over 60 minutes, history of motion sickness, and nonsmoking status. The presence of one of these factors increased the risk for nausea from 17% (no factor present) to 18%, 42%, 54%, 74%, and finally to 87%, when all five risk factors are present. Correspondingly, the risk for vomiting was 7%, 7%, 17%, 25%, 38%, and 61% for none up to five risk factors. The risk scores were based on surgical patients undergoing general anesthesia using an inhalational technique. This included a benzodiazepine for premedication, induction with 3 to 5 mg/kg thiopental and either up to 2 μg/kg fentanyl or up to 20 μg/kg alfentanil, and the use of a volatile anesthetic (isoflurane, enflurane, or sevoflurane). No prophylactic antiemetics were given. Post-operative pain was treated with nonsteroidal analgesic drugs or opioid analgesics if needed. The risk score evaluation published by Koivuranta and coworkers has been mentioned to be attractive for clinical practice.[105]

In a recent investigation, two centers have independently developed a risk score for predicting PONV.[28] The final score consisted of four predictors: female sex, history of motion sickness or PONV, nonsmoking status, and the use of postoperative opioids. If none, one, two, three, or four of these risk factors was present, the incidence rate of PONV was 10%, 21%, 39%, 61%, and 79%, respectively. Anesthesia was comparable to the strategy mentioned earlier. Finally, it could be demonstrated that risk scores derived from one center were able to predict PONV from the other center.

The odds ratios calculated from the equation given by Palazzo and Evans[107] are difficult to interpret, because they used the interaction of two factors as an additional factor in their model. Furthermore, the authors did not assess the smoking habits of their patients; consequently, this scoring system is unsuitable for clinical practice.

In a prospective evaluation including 17,638 consecutive outpatients undergoing surgical procedures, Sinclair and coworkers[108] found that a 10-year increase in age decreased the likelihood of PONV by 13%. A 30-minute increase in the duration of balanced general anesthesia increased the likelihood of PONV by 59%. Balanced general anesthesia increased the probability of PONV 11 times compared with other types of anesthesia.

Taken together, scoring systems, in fact, can give some information on the probability of PONV and clearly point out patients at high risk. But all score evaluations were based on general anesthesia using inhalational techniques. Therefore, additional evaluations are needed to reveal the risk for PONV in patients with multiple risk factors undergoing propofol-based TIVA.

Generally, routine antiemetic prophylaxis of all patients at high risk using either single or combined drug therapy administered at the optimal time using the smallest effective dose has been recommended. For patients at low risk (<10% risk for PONV), routine prophylaxis is difficult to justify. For adult patients with a 10% to 30% risk, prophylaxis with 5-HT$_3$ receptor antagonists has been recommended. However, others found that a PONV prophylaxis in these patients is not necessary when propofol-based anesthesia is being performed. For pediatric patients, 5-HT$_3$ receptor antagonists (e.g., 50–100 µg/kg ondansetron intravenously) have been shown to be useful. For patients at greater risk, a combined drug therapy using a 5-HT$_3$ receptor antagonist and a steroid (e.g., dexamethasone) has been recommended, whereas for patients at greatest risk, a two- or even three-drug regimen (e.g., 5-HT$_3$ receptor antagonist, dexamethasone, neuroleptic drug) might be justified. Combinations of different pharmacologic classes acting through different mechanisms produce a synergistic effect (see References 6, 28, 105, 106, and 109).

The timing of prophylactic antiemetic therapy is still a matter of debate. Some authors prefer the oral administration of 5-HT$_3$ receptor antagonists together with the premedication before induction of anesthesia, whereas others recommend intravenous administration of these agents near the end of surgery. Moreover, some authors administer neuroleptics as antiemetic agents during induction of anesthesia, whereas others give neuroleptics before cessation of the surgical procedure. Currently, a definitive recommendation when prophylactic antiemetic drugs should be administered is not warranted by scientific studies. Nevertheless, if patients experience breakthrough PONV despite prophylaxis, they should be treated with a drug from a group other than the one used for prophylaxis (see Rose and Watcha[6]).

Conclusion

Several antiemetics of different pharmacologic classes are available for the prophylactic use and therapy of nausea and vomiting. The 5-HT$_3$ receptor antagonists seem to be most attractive for the prevention and treatment of PONV, because they are usually superior to all other agents administered, especially when combined with corticosteroids (e.g., dexamethasone). Prophylactic approaches using 5-HT$_3$ receptor antagonists are quite expensive and not always wise, but it is justified in patients at high risk for PONV and in combination with other antiemetic drugs in patients at greatest risk for PONV. Unexpected hospital admission usually is more expensive than prophylactic therapy of PONV using antiemetics including 5-HT$_3$ receptor antagonists.

References

1. Rosen M, Camu F: Postoperative nausea and vomiting. Anesthesia 49:1–11, 1994.
2. Andrews PLR: Postoperative nausea and vomiting. In Herbert MK, Holzer P, Roewer N (eds): Problems of the gastrointestinal tract in anesthesia, the perioperative period, and intensive care. Berlin, Springer, pp 267–288, 1999.
3. Kapur PA: The big "little problem." Anesth Analg 73:243–245, 1991.
4. Scholz J, Steinfath M, Tonner PH: Postoperative nausea and vomiting. Curr Opin Anesthesiol 12:657–661, 1999.
5. Scholz J, Steinfath M: Prophylaxis and therapy of postoperative nausea and vomiting. In Herbert MK, Holzer P, Roewer N (eds): Problems of the gastrointestinal tract in anesthesia, the perioperative period, and intensive care. Berlin, Springer, pp 313–326, 1999.
6. Rose JB, Watcha MF: Postoperative nausea and vomiting. In Benumof JL, Saidman LJ (eds): Anesthesia and Perioperative Complications, 2nd ed. Mosby, St. Louis, pp 425–440, 1999.
7. Aitkenhead AR, Smith G: Textbook of Anesthesia. Edinburgh, Churchill Livingston, 1990.
8. Palazzo MAG, Strunin L: Anesthesia and emesis. I. Etiology. Can Anaesth Soc J 31:178–187, 1984.
9. Patasky AO, Kitz DS, Andrews RW, et al: Nausea and vomiting following ambulatory surgery: Are all procedures created equal? Anesth Analg 67:S163, 1988.
10. Watcha MF, White PF: Postoperative nausea and vomiting. Anesthesiology 77:162–184, 1992.
11. Andrews PLR, Davis CJ, Binham S, et al: The abdominal visceral innervation and the emetic reflex: Pathways, pharmacology and plasticity. Can J Physiol Pharmacol 68:325–345, 1990.
12. Borison HL: Area postrema: Chemoreceptor circumventricular organ of the medulla oblongata. Prog Neurobiol 32:351–390, 1989.
13. Stefanini E, Clement-Cormier Y: Detection of receptors in the area postrema. Eur J Pharmacol 74:257–260, 1981.

14. Atweh SF, Kuhar MJ: Autoradiographic localization of opiate receptors in the rat brain. II. The brain stem. Brain Res 129:1–12, 1977.

15. Waeber C, Dixon K, Hoyer D, et al: Localization by autoradiography of neuronal 5-HT$_3$ receptors in the mouse. Eur J Pharmacol 151:351–352, 1988.

16. Palacios JM, Wamsley JK, Kuhar MJ: The distribution of histamine H1-receptors in the rat brain: An autoradiographic study. Neuroscience 6:15–17, 1981.

17. Wamsley JK, Lewis MS, Young WS III, et al: Autoradiographic localization of muscarinic cholinergic receptors in rat brain stem. J Neurosci 1:176–191, 1981.

18. Hardman JG, Limbird LE: Goodman & Gilman´s The Pharmacological Basis of Therapeutics, 9th ed. New York, McGraw-Hill International Edition, 1996.

19. Simpson KH, Lynch L: Physiology and pharmacology of nausea and vomiting. In Hemmings H Jr, Hopkins P (eds): Foundations of Anesthesia–Basic and Clinical Sciences. St. Louis, Mosby, pp 623–630, 2000.

20. Rowley MP, Brown TCK: Postoperative vomiting in children. Anaesth Intensive Care 10:309–313, 1982.

21. Cohen M, Cameron CB, Duncan PG: Pediatric anesthesia morbidity and mortality in the perioperative period. Anesth Analg 70:160–168, 1990.

22. Beattie WS, Lindblad T, Buckley DN, et al: The incidence of postoperative nausea and vomiting in women undergoing laparoscopy is influenced by the day of the menstrual cycle. Can J Anaesth 38:298–302, 1991.

23. Bellville JW, Bross IDJ, Howland S: Postoperative nausea and vomiting IV: Factors related to postoperative nausea and vomiting. Anesthesiology 21:186–193, 1960.

24. Shankman Z, Shin Y, Brodsky JB: Perioperative management of the obese patient. Br J Anaesth 70:349–354, 1993.

25. Palazzo M, Evans R: Logistic regression analysis of fixed patient factors for postoperative sickness: A model for risk assessment. Br J Anaesth 75:301–304, 1995.

26. Haigh CG, Kaplan LA, Durham JM, et al: Nausea and vomiting after gynaecological surgery: A meta-analysis of factors affecting their incidence. Br J Anaesth 71:517–522, 1993.

27. Kranke P, Apfel CC, Papenfuss T, et al: An increased body mass index is no risk factor for postoperative nausea and vomiting. Acta Anesthesiol Scand 45:160–166, 2001.

28. Apfel CC, Läärä E, Koivuranta M, et al: A simplified risk score for predicting postoperative nausea and vomiting. Anesthesiology 91:693–700, 1999.

29. Hennes HJ, Scholz J, Kassabian T, et al: Incidence of nausea and vomiting after general anesthesia—a prospective study in 6705 patients. Anesthesiology 91:A394, 1999.

30. Andrews PLR: Physiology of nausea and vomiting. Br J Anaesth 69:2S–19S, 1992.

31. Ong BY, Palahniuk RJ, Cumming M: Gastric volume and pH in outpatients. Can Anaesth Soc J 25:36–39, 1978.

32. Haavik PE, Soreide E, Hofstad B, et al: Does preoperative anxiety influence gastric fluid volume and acidity? Anesth Analg 75:91–94, 1992.

33. Faymonville ME, Fissette J, Mambourg PH, et al: Hypnosis as an adjunct in conscious sedation for plastic surgery. Reg Anesth 20:145–148, 1995.

34. Scholz J, Hennes HJ, Steinfath M, et al: Tropisetron or ondansetron compared with placebo for prevention of postoperative nausea and vomiting. Eur J Anesthesiol 15:676–685, 1998.

35. Patel RI, Hannallah RS: Anesthetic complications following pediatric ambulatory surgery. Aesthesiology 69:1009–1012, 1988.

36. Cohen MM, Duncan PG, Tweed WA: The postoperative interview: Assessing risk factors for nausea and vomiting. Anesth Analg 78:7–12, 1994.

37. Larsson S, Lundberg D: A prospective survey of postoperative nausea and vomiting with special regard to incidence and relations to patient characteristics, anesthetic routines and surgical procedures. Acta Anesthesiol Scand 39:539–562, 1995.

38. Kenny GNC: Risk factors for postoperative nausea and vomiting. Anesthesia 49:6–10, 1994.

39. Lonie DS, Harper NJ: Nitrous oxide anesthesia and vomiting. The effect of nitrous oxide anesthesia on the incidence of vomiting following gynaecological laparoscopy. Anesthesia 41:703–707, 1986.

40. Felts J, Poler SM, Spitznagel EL: Nitrous oxide, nausea and vomiting after outpatient gynecologic surgery. J Clin Anesth 2:168–171, 1990.

41. Kortilla K, Hovorka J, Erkola O: Nitrous oxide does not increase the incidence of nausea and vomiting after isoflurane anesthesia. Anesth Analg 66:761–765, 1987.

42. Tramer M, Moore A, McQuay H: Meta-analytic comparison of prophylactic anti-emetic efficacy for postoperative nausea and vomiting: Propofol anesthesia vs omitting nitrous oxide vs total I.V. anesthesia with propofol. Br J Anaesth 78:256–259, 1997.

43. Divatia JV, Vaidya JS, Badwe RA, et al: Omission of nitrous oxide during anesthesia reduces the incidence of postoperative nausea and vomiting. Anesthesiology 85:1055–1062, 1996.

44. Hartung J: Twenty-four of twenty-seven studies show a greater incidence of emesis associated with nitrous oxide than with alternative anesthetics. Anesth Analg 83:114–116, 1996.

45. Forrest JB, Cahalan MK, Rehder K, et al: Multicenter study of general anesthesia. II. Results. Anesthesiology 72:262–268, 1990.

46. Johannesson GP, Floren M, Lindahl SG: Sevoflurane for ENT-surgery in children. Acta Anesthesiol Scand 39:546–549, 1995.

47. Hobbhahn J, Funk W: Sevoflurane in pediatric anesthesia. Anesthesia 45:22–25, 1998.

48. Lie Karlsen K, Persson E, Wennberg E, et al: Anesthesia, recovery and postoperative nausea and vomiting after breast surgery. A comparison between desflurane, sevoflurane and isoflurane anesthesia. Acta Anesthesiol Scand 44:489–493, 2000.

49. Clarke RSJ: Post-operative gastrointestinal complications. Curr Anaesth Crit Care 2:20–24, 1991.

50. Davis PJ, Chopyk JB, Nazif M, et al: Continuous alfentanil infusion in paediatric patients undergoing general anesthesia for complete oral restoration. J Clin Anesth 3:125–130, 1991.

51. White PF, Coe V, Shafer A, et al: Comparison of alfentanil with fentanyl for outpatient anesthesia. Anesthesiology 64:99–106, 1986.

52. White PF, Sung ML, Doze VA: Use of sufentanil in outpatient anesthesia: Determining an optimal preinduction dose. Anesthesiology 63:A202, 1995.

53. Unkel W, Peters J: Postoperative nausea and emesis: Mechanisms and treatment [review]. Anasthesiol Intensivmed Notfallmed Schmerzther 33:533–541, 1998.

54. Gan TJ, Ginsberg B, Grant AP, et al: Double-blind, randomized comparison of ondansetron and intraoperative propofol to prevent postoperative nausea and vomiting. Anesthesiology 85:1036–1042, 1996.

55. Rabey PG, Smith G: Anesthetic factors contributing to postoperative nausea and vomiting. Br J Anaesth 69:40S–45S, 1992.

56. Fauser AA, Fellhauer M, Hoffmann M, et al: Guidelines for anti-emetic therapy: Acute emesis. Eur J Cancer 35:361–370, 1999.

57. Rowbothan DJ: Current management of postoperative nausea and vomiting. Br J Anaesth 69:46S–59S, 1992.

58. Henzi I, Walder B, Tramer MR: Metoclopramide in the prevention of postoperative nausea and vomitng: A quantitative systematic review of randomized, placebo-controlled studies. Br J Anaesth 83:761–771, 1999.

59. Allen RW: Metoclopramide: A safe anti-emetic? S Afr Med J 77:219, 1990.

60. Henzi I, Sonderegger J, Tramer MR: Systematic review. Efficacy, dose-response, and adverse effects of droperidol for prevention of postoperative nausea and vomiting. Can J Anesth 47:537–551, 2000.

61. Desilva PH, Darvish AH, McDonald S, et al: The efficacy of prophylactic ondansetron, droperidol, perphenazine, and metoclopramide in the prevention of nausea and vomiting after major gynecologic surgery. Anesth Analg 81:139–144, 1995.

62. Tramer MR, Moore A, McQuay H: Prevention of vomiting after paediatric strabismus repair: A systematic review using the numbers-needed-to-treat methode. Br J Anaesth 75:556–562, 1995.

63. Kortilla K, Kauste A, Auvinen J: Comparison of domperidone, droperidol, and metoclopramide in the prevention and treatment of nausea and vomiting after balanced general anesthesia. Anesth Analg 66:761–765, 1979.

64. Cohen SE, Woods WA, Wyner J: Anti-emetic efficacy of droperidol and metoclopramide. Anesthesiology 60:67–69, 1984.

65. Kauste A, Tuominen M, Heikkinen H, et al: Droperidol, alizapride and metoclopramide in the prevention and treatment of postoperative emetic sequelae. Eur J Anaesth 3:1–9, 1986.

66. Pandit SJ, Kothary SP, Pandit UA, et al: Dose-response study of droperidol and metoclopramide as anti-emetics for outpatient anesthesia. Anesth Analg 68:798–802, 1989.

67. Tang J, Watcha MF, White PF: A comparison of costs and efficacy of ondansetron and droperidol as prophylactic anti-emetic therapy for elective outpatient gynecologic procedures. Anesth Analg 83:304–313, 1996.

68. Grond S, Lynch J, Diefenbach C, et al: Comparison of ondansetron and droperidol in the prevention of nausea and vomiting after inpatient minor gynecologic surgery. Anesth Analg 81:601–604, 1995.

69. Bruntsch U, Drechsler S, Eggert J, et al: Prevention of chemotherapy-induced nausea and vomiting by tropisetron (Navoban) alone or in combination with other anti-emetic agents. Semin Oncol 21:7–11, 1994.

70. Läer S, Scholz J, Ritterbach C, et al: Association between increased 5-HIAA plasma concentrations and postoperative nausea and vomiting in patients undergoing general anesthesia for surgery. Eur J Anesthesiol 18:833–835, 2001.

71. Wolf H: Preclinical and clinical pharmacology of the 5-HT3 receptor antagonists. Scand J Rheumatol 29(suppl 113):37–45, 2000.

72. Naylor RJ, Inall FC: The physiology and pharmacology of postoperative nausea and vomiting. Anesthesia 49:2–5, 1994.

73. Alon E, Himmelseher S: Ondansetron in the treatment of postoperative vomiting: A randomized, double-blind comparison with droperidol and metoclopramid. Anesth Analg 75:561–565, 1992.

74. Diemunsch P, Conseiller C, Clyti N, et al: Ondansetron compared with metoclopramide in the treatment of established postoperative nausea and vomiting. Br J Anaesth 79:322–326, 1997.

75. Polati E, Verlato G, Finco G, et al: Ondansetron versus metoclopramide in the treatment of postoperative nausea and vomiting. Anesth Analg 85:395–399, 1997.

76. Pearman MH: Single dose intravenous ondansetron in the prevention of postoperative nausea and vomiting. Anesthesia 49:11–15, 1994.

77. Tramer MR, Moore RA, Reynolds DJ, et al: A quantitative systematic review of ondansetron in treatment of established postoperative nausea and vomiting. BMJ 314:1088–1096, 1997.

78. Tang J, Watcha MF, White PF, et al: The effect of timing of ondansetron administration on its efficacy, cost-effectiveness, and cost-benefit as a prophylatic anti-emetic in the ambulatory setting. Anesth Analg 86:274–282, 1998.

79. Sniadach MS, Alberts MS: A comparison of the prophylactic anti-emetic effect of ondansetron and droperidol on patients undergoing gynecologic laparoscopy. Anesth Analg 85:797–783, 1997.

80. Richardson BP, Engel G, Donatsch P, et al: Identification of serotonin M-receptor subtypes and their specific blockade by a new class of drugs. Nature 316:126, 1985.

81. Sorbe BG, Högberg T, Glimelius B, et al: A randomized, multicenter study comparing the efficacy and tolerability of tropisetron, a new 5-HT$_3$ receptor antagonist, with a metoclopramide-containing anti-emetic cocktail in the prevention of cisplatin-induced emesis. Cancer 73:445–454, 1994.

82. Sorbe B, Högberg T, Himmelseher A, et al: Efficacy and tolerability of tropisetron in comparison with a combination of tropisetron and dexamethasone in the control of nausea and vomiting induced by cisplatin-containing chemotherapy. Eur J Cancer 30:629–634, 1994.

83. Zomers PJW, Langenberg CJM, DeBruijn KM: Tropisetron for postoperative nausea and vomiting in patients after gynecological surgery. Br J Anaesth 71:677–680, 1993.

84. Capouet V, Depauw C, Vernet B, et al: Single dose I.V. tropisetron in the prevention of postoperative nausea and vomiting after gynaecological surgery. Br J Anaesth 76:54–60, 1996.

85. Boogaerts JG, Bardiau FM, Seidel L, et al: Tropisetron in the prevention of postoperative nausea and vomiting. J Clin Anesth 12:402–408, 2000.

86. Alon E, Buchser E, Herrera E, et al: Tropisetron for treating established postoperative nausea and vomiting: A randomized, double-blind, placebo-controlled study. Anesth Analg 86:617–623, 1998.

87. Fuiji Y, Tanaka H, Toyooka H: Optimal anti-emetic dose of granisetron for prevention of postoperative nausea and vomiting. Can J Anaesth 41:794–797, 1994.

88. Mikawa K, Takao Y, Nishina K, et al: The anti-emetic efficacy of prophylactic granisetron in gynecologic surgery. Anesth Analg 80:970–974, 1995.

89. Fujii Y, Saitoh Y, Tanaka H, et al: Granisetron/dexamethasone combination for the prevention of postoperative nausea and vomiting after laparoscopic cholecystectomy. Eur J Anesthesiol 17:64–68, 2000.

90. Diemunsch P, Kortilla K, Leeser J, et al: Oral dolasetron mesylate for prevention of postoperative nausea and vomiting: A multicenter, double-blind, placebo-controlled study. J Clin Anesth 10:145–152, 1998.

91. Balfour JA, Goa KL: Dolasetron: A review of it's pharmacology and therapeutic potential in the management of nausea and vomiting induced by chemotherapy, radiotherapy or surgery. Drugs 273–282, 1997.

92. Henzi I, Walder B, Tramer MR: Dexamethasone for the prevention of postoperative nausea and vomiting: A quantitative systematic review. Anesth Analg 90:186–194, 2000.

93. Wang JJ, Ho ST, Lee SC, et al: The use of dexamethasone for preventing postoperative nausea and vomiting in females undergoing thyroidectomy: A dose-ranging study. Anesth Analg 91:1404–1407, 2000.

94. Drechsler S, Bruntsch U, Eggert J, et al: Comparison of three tropisetron-containing anti-emetic regimens in the prophylaxis of acute and delayed chemotherapy-induced emesis and nausea. Support Care Cancer 5:387–395, 1997.

95. Holt R, Rask P, Coulthard KP, et al: Tropisetron plus dexamethasone is more effective than tropisetron alone for the prevention of postoperative nausea and vomiting in children undergoing tonsillectomy. Paediatr Anaesth 10:181–188, 2000.

96. Khalil SN, Berry JM, Howard G, et al: The anti-emetic effect of lorazepam after outpatient strabismus surgery in children. Anesthesiology 77:915–918, 1992.

97. Splinter WM, MacNeill HB, Menard EA, et al: Midazolam reduces vomiting after tonsillectomy in children. Can J Anaesth 42:201–204, 1995.

98. Avramov MN, Smith I, White PF: Interaction between midazolam and remifentanil during monitored anesthesia care. Anesthesiology 85:1283–1286, 1996.

99. Mikawa K, Nishina K, Maekawa N, et al: Oral clonidine reduces vomiting after strabismus surgery. Can J Anaesth 42:977–979, 1995.

100. Mulroy MF: Regional anesthesia techniques. Int Anesthesiol Clin 32:81–84, 1994.

101. Watcha MF, Simeon RF, White PF, et al: Effect of propofol on the incidence of postoperative vomiting after strabismus surgery in paediatric outpatients. Anesthesiology 75:204–209, 1991.

102. Cechetto DF, Diab T, Gibson CJ, et al: The effects of propofol in the area postrema of rats. Anesth Analg 92:934–942, 2001.

103. Tramer MR: A rational approach to the control of postoperative nausea and vomiting: Evidence from systematic reviews. Part I. Efficacy and harm of anti-emetic interventions, and methodological issues. Acta Anesthesiol Scand 45:4–13, 2001.

104. Tramer MR: A rational approach to the control of postoperative nausea and vomiting: Evidence from systematic reviews. Part II. Recommendations for prevention and treatment, and research agenda. Acta Anesthesiol Scand 45:14–19, 2001.

105. Koivuranta M, Läärä E, Snare L, et al: A survey of postoperative nausea and vomiting. Anesthesia 52:443–449, 1997.

106. Eberhart LHJ, Högel J, Seeling W, et al: Evaluation of three risk scores to predict postoperative nausea and vomiting. Acta Anesthesiol Scand 44:480–488, 2000.

107. Palazzo M, Evans R: Logistic regression analysis of fixed patient factors for postoperative sickness: A model for risk assessment. Br J Anaesth 70:135–140, 1993.

108. Sinclair DR, Chung F, Mezei G: Can postoperative nausea and vomiting be predicted? Anesthesiology 91:109–118, 1999.

109. Watcha MF, White PF: Postoperative nausea and vomiting: Prophylaxis versus treatment. Anesth Analg 89:1337–1339, 1999.

Nutritional Supplements

Charles Weissman, MD

Eating and breathing are the essence of life. Eating an adequate and nutritious diet provides the body with substrates to generate energy and maintain structural and functional integrity. Breathing provides oxygen for oxidizing substrates and producing energy for aerobic metabolism. Breathing also eliminates carbon dioxide—a byproduct of metabolism. Yet illness often reduces food intake by inducing anorexia, malabsorption, maldigestion, nausea, vomiting, or simply not permitting the organism to forage for food. In addition, serious illness alters the underlying metabolic milieu changing substrate use and presenting a major obstacle to effective nutritional support. This spawned research aimed at elucidating the nature of these metabolic changes so that strategies could be developed to overcome these obstacles to effective nutrient intake and use.

Research after World War II detailed the obligate loss of muscle and fat during the initial convalescent period after major fractures, surgery, burns, and trauma (the catabolic [protein losing] phase[1]). Also described was the subsequent period where loss of muscle and fat abates and then reverses as patients began to eat and gain weight (the anabolic [protein synthesizing] phase). The challenge was developing nutrient strategies and delivery methods to attenuate the loss of muscle and fat during the catabolic phase. Initial methods used nasogastric and nasoduodenal tubes and food containing dried milk, nonfat milk solids, casein hydrolysates, and dextro-maltose. These attempts successfully fed patients with such diverse diseases as anorexia nervosa, cerebrovascular accidents, tuberculosis, and cancer. However, not all the patients who could not or would not eat could be nourished enterally. Therefore, parenteral feeding solutions were developed for patients with grossly dysfunctional gastrointestinal tracts (GITs), i.e., high-output

enteric-cutaneous fistulae and short bowel syndrome. Total parenteral nutritional (TPN) was a major advance in caring for patients unable to sustain adequate enteral intake.

Since the development of enteral and parenteral nutrition, nutrient formulas and delivery techniques have been refined. Simultaneously, there has been better understanding of the metabolic milieu during disease and how this milieu affects nutrient use.

Mechanisms of Drug Action

Nutrients, like drugs, act at various sites within the body and their actions often differ depending on the organ system or cell type. This section reviews normal nutrient metabolism and subsequent sections examine metabolism during various diseases.

Carbohydrate Metabolism

Glucose, the human body's main energy source, originates from food or endogenous sources, such as gluconeogenesis or glycogen breakdown (glycogenolysis). Glucose metabolic pathways are shown in Figure 46–1A. Control of glucose metabolism is partially dependent on blood glucose concentrations. Insulin, secreted by pancreatic β cells, is the major regulator of blood glucose concentrations. Epinephrine and norepinephrine block insulin secretion and together with glucagon and cortisol constitute the counter-regulatory

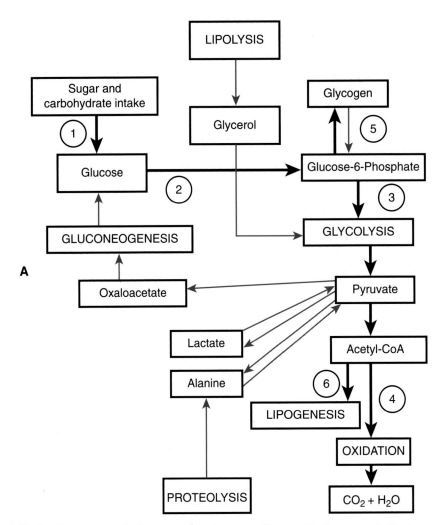

Figure 46–1. Glucose metabolism under various conditions. Black arrows indicate increased and blue arrows indicate decreased flux through a pathway. *A,* Glucose metabolism after a carbohydrate meal in a healthy individual. The carbohydrate intake (*1*) is converted to glucose, which is converted to glucose-6-phosphate (*2*). Most of the glucose undergoes glycolysis (*3*) to pyruvate, producing adenosine triphosphate (ATP). Pyruvate then enters the citric acid cycle (*4*) where more ATP is produced. Excess glucose is stored in the liver and muscles as glycogen (glycogenesis [*5*]) or is converted to fat (lipogenesis [*6*]).

(to insulin) hormones. These hormones act synergistically to counteract the hypoglycemic effects of insulin by stimulating glycogenolysis and gluconeogenesis.

Gluconeogenesis converts noncarbohydrates to glucose and supplies glucose when dietary carbohydrate intake is insufficient. At low and normal blood glucose concentrations, the liver is a net producer of glucose through gluconeogenesis, whereas at increased glucose concentrations, gluconeogenesis decreases. Gluconeogenesis clears metabolic products such as lactate from red blood cells and exercising muscles, glycerol from triglyceride breakdown, and amino acids from protein breakdown. Gluconeogenesis occurs mainly in the liver but up to 25% may occur in the kidneys.[2]

Lipid Metabolism

Triglycerols (glycerol + three fatty acids), the most common lipid in the body, may be of dietary origin or may be synthesized de novo from glycerol and fatty acids (esterification) derived from other lipids or carbohydrates (lipogenesis). Fatty acids may be long–chain fatty acids ($C_{16} – C_{24}$), which are the most common animal and plant fatty acids, or medium-chain fatty acids ($C_8 – C_{14}$), which are found in some plants.

Ingested long-chain triglycerides (LCTs) enter the lacteals and become components of chyle. Medium-chain triglycerides (MCTs) and free glycerol are absorbed directly into the portal system and are transported to the liver. Triglycerides transported in chyle and blood as chylomicrons and very low-density lipoproteins are hydrolyzed to free fatty acids and glycerol by endothelial-derived lipoprotein lipase. The free fatty acids are then either re-esterified to triglycerides in adipocytes where they are stored or are β-oxidized to acetyl-CoA, which then enters the citric acid cycle to yield energy (Fig. 46–2). Fatty acid-derived acetyl-CoA is the precursor of cholesterol, steroids, and ketone bodies.

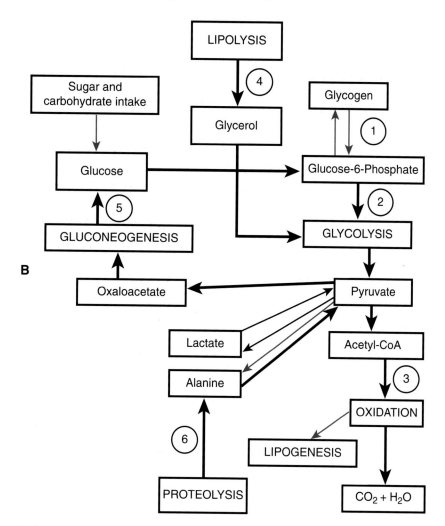

Figure 46–1. *B,* Initial response to starvation. Hepatic glycogen is converted to glucose-6-phosphate (glycogenolysis [*1*]), undergoes glycolysis (*2*) and enters the citric acid cycle (*3*). Fat stores are broken down into fatty acids (see Fig. 46–2) and glycerol (lipolysis [*4*]). Glycerol and alanine (from skeletal muscle proteolysis) enter the glycolytic pathway, are converted to pyruvate, and become glucose (gluconeogenesis [*5*]).

Protein Metabolism

Dietary protein provides the body with amino acids. Enough dietary protein/amino acids must be ingested to balance losses in the urine, feces, saliva, desquamated skin, hair, and nails. In healthy humans, 12% of the energy intake should be protein with the remainder being carbohydrate and fat. Inadequate nonprotein calories (fat and carbohydrates) may require exogenous or endogenous proteins/amino acids to be used as energy sources.

Dietary amino acids are the building blocks of proteins and are also precursors of special molecules. L-arginine is converted to nitric oxide, a neurotransmitter and smooth muscle vasodilator. Tryptophan, the precursor of serotonin, is another neurotransmitter. Tyrosine is metabolized by neural and adrenal tissues to form norepinephrine and epinephrine.

Energy Expenditure (Table 46–1)

Metabolism consumes fuel (nutrients). The amount of fuel burned is reflected directly by heat loss (direct calorime-

try) and indirectly by the amount of O_2 consumed, CO_2 produced, and urine urea nitrogen produced (indirect calorimetry).

Electrolytes (Macrominerals)

Maintaining electrolyte balance is a key homeostatic function. Therefore, adequate and correct electrolyte intake must be provided to replace urinary, fecal, and cutaneous losses. During illness, electrolytes may also be lost through vomiting, diarrhea, hemorrhage, nasogastric suction, drainage of surgical sites, and enterocutaneous fistulae. Sodium and potassium are the principal extracellular and intracellular cations and are balanced by the anions chloride and bicarbonate. Calcium regulates nerve and muscle function, whereas phosphorous is a component of adenosine triphosphate (ATP), nucleic acids, and enzymes. Magnesium is a kinase cofactor, whereas sulfur (as sulfate) is a component of glycoproteins and coenzymes.

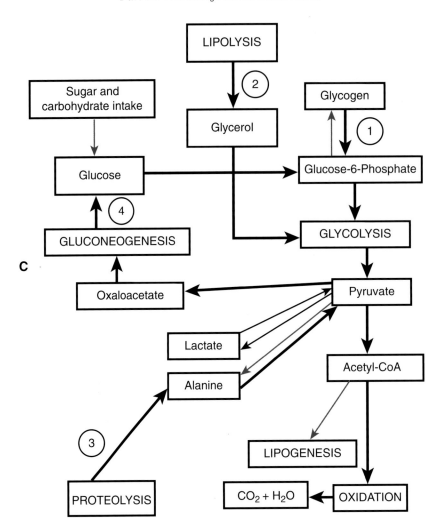

Figure 46–1. *C,* After the initial response to starvation, an adaptive process occurs. Glycogen stores are depleted within the first 24 to 36 hours of starvation (*1*). The rate of proteolysis decreases (protein-sparing effect) although it is still elevated, and lipolysis becomes the major energy-providing pathway (*2*). Fatty acids are converted to ketone bodies (see Fig. 46–2) and glycerol (*2*), and along with alanine from proteolysis (*3*), undergoes gluconeogenesis to glucose (*4*), which is used by tissues unable to use ketones.

Trace Elements (Microminerals)

See Table 46–2 for trace elements when designing nutritional support regimens.

Vitamins

See Table 46–2 for listing of vitamins when designing nutritional support regimens.

Water

Water is the solvent of the body and has been termed the "ideal biological solvent."[3] It constitutes 55% to 65% of the body weight of males and slightly less in females. Thirst controls the amount of water intake. The approximate daily fluid requirement of an adult patient = 1500 mL + 20 mL/kg for each kilogram more than 20 kg.

Clinical Pharmacology

In contrast to the efficient and orderly adaptive metabolic response to starvation (see Figs. 46–1*B* and *C*) that conserves body mass, the metabolic response to severe illness (stress) is quite the opposite. It involves the massive outpouring of the counter-regulatory (to insulin) hormones: glucagon, cortisol, and catecholamines that act synergistically to cause catabolism, hypermetabolism, glucose intolerance ("diabetes of injury"), accelerated gluconeogenesis, and increased lipolysis. These effects, augmented by the actions of cytokines, such as interleukin-1 (IL-1), tumor

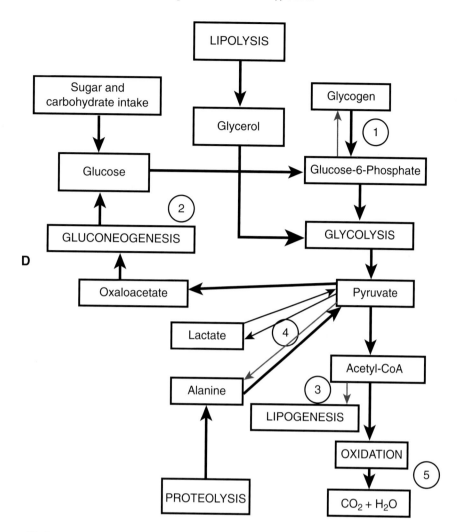

Figure 46–1. *D,* The stressed state: Hyperglycemia is seen because glucose clearance decreases because of insulin intolerance caused by a postreceptor defect and reduced glycogen synthesis (*1*). There is increased hepatic glucose production (gluconeogenesis [*2*]) using glycerol, alanine, and lactate as substrates. Lipogenesis (*3*) is reduced and, in sepsis, increased aerobic glycolysis increases lactate production (*4*). Because of reduced lipogenesis and glycogen synthesis, but intact glucose oxidation, the amount of CO_2 produced from a large glucose load may be increased to greater than normal production levels (*5*).

necrosis factor (TNF), and interleukin-6 (IL-6), activate proinflammatory responses causing fever, inflammation, catabolism, leukocytosis, and hepatic acute-phase protein production. The consequence of this metabolic disarray is loss of fat and lean (muscle) body mass coupled with inefficient substrate use, a problematic situation dubbed "autocannibalism."[4] It is thus not surprising that this abnormal metabolic milieu causes disordered use of exogenously administered nutrients. In general, the magnitude of the stress response is proportional to the intensity of the stress,[5] whereas the duration of the response is related to the magnitude and dura-tion of the initial stimulus. Therefore, the disruption of homeostatic mechanisms is greater after extensive burns than after minor extremity surgery. Traumatic injury causes a large, short-term response followed by a period of convalescence, whereas continuous sepsis causes more prolonged responses.

Conventional nutritional strategies, such as providing the equivalent of a usual human diet, frequently do not prevent or attenuate the loss of muscle and fat tissue during the period of stress. Therefore, the challenge is to develop nutritional strategies that overcome or circumvent the impediments to maintaining and restoring body mass induced by the disordered metabolic state.

Carbohydrates

Pathophysiology and Metabolism

Carbohydrate metabolism is significantly altered during stress by the increased secretion of cortisol, catecholamines, and glucagon.[6] These hormones increase endogenous glucose production (hepatic gluconeogenesis) in proportion to the degree of stress (see Fig. 46–1*D*). Insulin concentrations are normal or mildly increased but not sufficiently elevated to prevent hyperglycemia. Hyperglycemia is thought

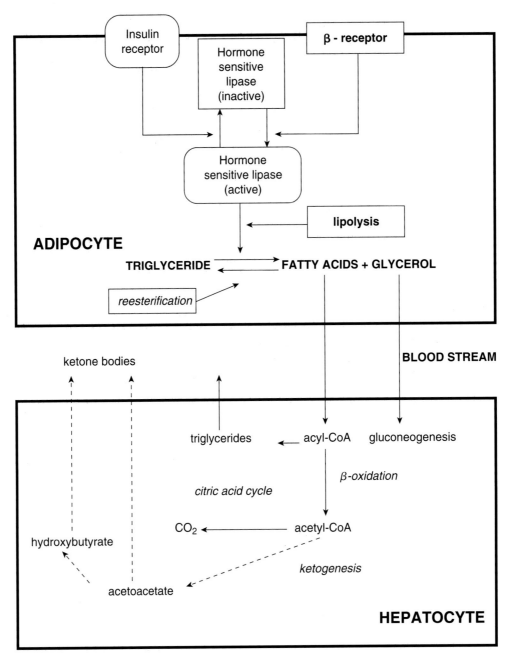

Figure 46–2. Lipid metabolism: Increased cathecholamines during stress stimulate β adrenergic receptors on adipocytes increasing lipolysis (breakdown of stored triglycerides into fatty acids and glycerol). Simultaneously, there is increased re-esterification of fatty acids and glycerol to triglycerides. Lipolysis is more rapid than re-esterification leading to net lipolysis. This accelerated lipolysis/re-esterification is a "futile cycle" and is a cause of hypermetabolism in stressed patients. Glycerol released by lipolysis is transformed in the liver to glucose (gluconeogenesis). Fatty acids transported to the liver are β-oxidized and enter the citric acid cycle to produce adenosine triphosphate. This is the major energy-producing pathway during stress. During starvation, lipolysis is the dominant energy pathway. Reduced insulin concentrations and mild cathecholamine stimulation increase hormone-sensitive lipase activity accelerating lipolysis. As in the stressed state, glycerol undergoes hepatic gluconeogenesis, whereas the fatty acids are used for energy. However, unlike stress in which insulin levels are normal or increased, the insulinopenic state found during starvation permits hepatic conversion of fatty acids to ketones. These enter the bloodstream and are used as an energy substrate by the tissues. Refeeding starved patients increases insulin concentrations, whereas slackening of the stress response reduces catecholamine concentrations leading to return of hormone-sensitive lipase to the inactive form, thus reducing the rate of lipolysis.

TABLE 46–1.

Energy Expenditure and Caloric Intake
CALORIC REQUIREMENTS

Estimating Resting Energy Expenditure (Harris-Benedict Equation)

Males: EBEE (kcal/day) = $66 + (13.7 \times W) + (5 \times H) - (6.8 \times A)$
Females: EBEE (kcal/day) = $655 + (9.6 \times W) + (1.7 \times H) - (4.7 \times A)$

Estimated Resting Energy Expenditure (EREE) = EBEE × stress factor
Estimated Total Energy Expenditure (ETEE) = EREE × activity factor

A, age (yr); EBEE, estimated basal energy expenditure; H, height (cm); W, weight (kg).

STRESS FACTORS		ACTIVITY FACTORS
Spontaneously breathing, nonsedated patients		
Major surgery: 15–25%	Burns: up to 120% depending on extent	Sedated mechanically ventilated patients: 0–5%
Infection: 20%	Sepsis: 30–55%	Bed-ridden, spontaneously breathing nonsedated patients: 10–15%
Long bone fracture: 20–35%	Major trauma: 20–35%	Sitting in chair: 15–20%
Malnutrition: subtract 10–15%	COPD: 10–15%	Ambulating patients: 20–25%

Note: Sedated mechanically ventilated patients: subtract 10–15%.

Measuring Energy Expenditure

Indirect calorimetry involves measuring oxygen consumption (VO_2) and carbon dioxide production (VCO_2).

Weir Equation: EE (kcal/day) = $1.44 (3.9 \times VO_2) + (1.1 \times VCO_2)$

Measurements made at rest provide the REE. To determine the Total Energy Expenditure: REE × Activity Factor

Continuous measurement made over 24 hours provides the Total Energy Expenditure

Measuring Nitrogen Balance

N balance = [N intake] − [N output]
Where: [N intake] = all protein/amino acid intake over 24 hours whether enteral or parenteral
[N output] = [UUN + 4 + EL]

UUN = Urine Urea Nitrogen over 24 hours; 4 g average fecal and cutaneous losses
EL = excessive losses, such as protein rich drainages (e.g., pus).

6.25 g protein/amino acids = 1 g nitrogen

TABLE 46–1.

Energy Expenditure and Caloric Intake
CALORIC REQUIREMENTS—cont'd

Daily Caloric Requirements

Sedated mechanically ventilated patients:	$1.0 - 1.2 \times$ REE
Nonsedated mechanically ventilated patients:	$1.2 \times$ REE
Spontaneously breathing critically ill patients:	$1.2 - 1.3 \times$ REE
Spontaneously breathing ward patients (maintenance):	$1.3 \times$ REE
Spontaneously breathing ward patients (repletion):	$1.5 - 1.7 \times$ REE

To gain 1 pound of body weight would need a cumulative excess greater than TEE of approximately 3500 kcal.

CALORIC PROPERTIES OF FOOD

	Energy (Kcal/g)
Carbohydrate	4.0
Dextrose (glucose monohydrate)	3.4
Fat	9.0
Protein	4.0
Alcohol	7.0

to ensure a ready supply of glucose to predominantly glucose-consuming cells, such as the wound, inflammatory cells, and immune cells.[7]

In addition to glucose intolerance, stressed patients have a reduced ability to achieve net lipogenesis, i.e., the ability to convert glucose to fat, which occurs in both liver[8] and adipose tissue.[9] When carbohydrate intake exceeds total energy expenditure, lipogenesis becomes significant and respiratory quotients may exceed 1.0, indicating net lipogenesis.[10] This is seen among patients with nutritional depletion receiving glucose infusions greater than 4 mg/kg per minute.[11] Critically ill patients administered intravenous glucose at a rate of 4 mg/kg minute as part of glucose-based TPN exhibited some increased hepatic lipogenesis but were unable to achieve net lipogenesis (respiratory quotient only 0.90[12,13]).

Glucose and Carbohydrate Nutrition

Administering exogenous glucose and carbohydrates to injured or septic patients minimally diminishes the rates of gluconeogenesis and lipolysis.[14] This contrasts with starvation during which carbohydrate administration reduces gluconeogenesis and lipolysis. Despite reduced glucose utilization, it is still important to administer carbohydrates because some body tissues are unable to readily use other substrates. Furthermore, glucose and carbohydrate intake stimulate the secretion of insulin, an anabolic hormone, that promotes protein synthesis[15] and has antilipolytic effects.[16,17] Yet hyperglycemia often limits the amount of glucose and carbohydrate that can be administered. The degree of TPN-induced hyperglycemia is directly proportional to the rate of glucose infusion and the degree of injury.[18] The elderly are more predisposed to the development of hyperglycemia.[19]

It is important to realize that critically ill patients often receive carbohydrates from sources other than the glucose in TPN or carbohydrates in enteral nutrition. Five percent dextrose infusions contain 170 kcal/L and lipid emulsions used in TPN contain 22 g/L glycerol. Overfeeding glucose (>4 mg/kg/min) to acutely stressed patients, receiving a total caloric intake greater than resting energy expenditure, results in further increase of blood glucose concentrations

TABLE 46–2.

Considerations When Designing Nutritional Support Regimens

Considerations	Issues	
1. Route of administration	Enteral vs. parenteral vs. both	
2. Caloric requirements	Measure energy expenditure using indirect calorimetry or estimate energy expenditure using established equations (see Table 46–1).	
3. Protein/amino acids	Evaluate degree of stress, measure nitrogen balance Parenteral nutrition: amino acid solutions Enteral nutrition: standard vs. high protein formulas; amino acids (elemental diet) peptides vs protein hydrolysates. If protein losses are excessive then need increased protein.	Unstressed patients: 0.8–1.2 g/kg/day protein Stressed patients: 1.0–1.5 g/kg/day protein
4. Calorie/Protein ratio	Expressed as calorie/nitrogen ratio: Standard enteral formulas 150:1 Enteral stress formulas 125–100:1	
5. Carbohydrates	Parenteral nutrition: glucose is only available nutrient Enteral nutrition: oligosaccharides and starches	Glucose intake not to exceed 4 mg/kg/min during stress
6. Lipid	Parenteral nutrition: LCT emulsions Enteral formulas: contain LCT or LCT/MCT; some enriched with ω–3 fatty acids	
7. Lipid/Carbohydrate ratio	Parenteral nutrition: lipid/CHO ratio 30:70 to 60:40 Enteral nutrition: depends on formula. Calorie-dense formulas have higher fat ratios	
8. Electrolytes	Parenteral nutrition: sodium (NaCl, Na acetate), potassium (KCL, K acetate), PO_4 (NaPO$_4$ KPO$_4$), MgSO$_4$, calcium (Ca-gluconate) Enteral nutrition: as per formulation. May add electrolytes, if needed.	K: 1–1.2 mEq/kg Mg: 8–20 mEq Ca: 10–15 mEq PO$_4$: 20–30 mmol/day
9. Trace elements	Trace elements are minerals with requirements <100 mg/d Parenteral nutrition: additives contain: Cu, Se, Zn, Mn, Cr. Co is given as vitamin B_{12}. Enteral nutrition: also contain Fe, Mo, I	
10. Vitamins	Parenteral nutrition: commercial preparations usually contain all vitamins (except vitamin K). Monitor PT weekly and give vitamin K, if indicated. Enteral nutrition: contain all vitamins including vitamin K; the volume of formula that provides the recommended daily requirements depends on the formula (see Table 46–4). Vitamin C: needs are increased during wound repair. Vitamin B (esp. Thiamine): important in alcoholics.	

TABLE 46–2.

Considerations When Designing Nutritional Support Regimens—cont'd

Considerations	Issues	
11. Water	Parenteral nutrition: dilute vs. concentrated formulas. Dilute for peripheral vein administration. Concentrated for fluid restriction and high caloric intakes. Standard enteral nutrition: (1.06 kcal/mL) vs. calorie dense (2.0 kcal/mL).	
12. Disease-specific considerations	Renal failure	See "Special Considerations"
	Hepatic failure	See "Special Considerations"
	Respiratory failure	May need to reduce absolute carbohydrate intake and substitute lipid for carbohydrates
	Burns	See "Special Considerations"
	Diabetes	Control blood glucose and monitor serum triglycerides.

and production of additional CO_2.[20] This CO_2 must be excreted through the lungs and, if inadequately excreted, can lead to increased $PaCO_2$. Such overfeeding is not uncommon. A survey of U.S. teaching hospitals demonstrated that many patients are fed with more than 4.5 mg/kg per minute glucose.[21]

Lipids

Pathophysiology and Metabolism

Lipid metabolism is substantially affected during stress,[22] most prominently by accelerated lipolysis because of increased β_2 adrenergic stimulation (see Fig. 46–2).[23] Glucagon, cortisol, TNF-α, IL-1, and interferon-γ may also stimulate lipolysis.[24–26]

During stress, the relative caloric contribution of fat oxidation to resting energy expenditure is increased while the contribution of glucose oxidation decreases.[27] Fatty acids released by lipolysis undergo β-oxidation, which in the stressed patient is the predominant ATP-producing pathway (see Fig. 46–2). This situation is seen after esophagectomy in which there is a gradual decrease in the contribution of fat oxidation and increase in glucose oxidation during convalescence.[28] Unlike starvation, ketone body formation is suppressed because of normal or increased insulin concentrations.

Lipid Nutrition

Intravenous lipid is most frequently administered as an emulsion of LCTs. These emulsions, available in 10%, 20%, and 30% solutions, contain soybean oil and an emulsifier (egg phospholipid). They are calorie dense (e.g., 10% and 20% solutions contain 1.0 and 2.0 kcal/mL, respectively). The lipid emulsion is converted in the blood to triglyceride-rich particles, the size of which approximates those of chylomicrons. These particles are hydrolyzed by lipoprotein lipase to fatty acids and glycerol. Lipid emulsions are also the vehicle for lipid-soluble drugs, such as propofol, amphotericin B, and etomidate.[29] In patients receiving infusions of propofol for sedation, the amount of lipid calories may be significant and should be included when calculating caloric intake.[30]

Exogenous lipid is needed to prevent essential free fatty acid deficiency, therefore patients receiving TPN should receive lipid emulsion infusions (500 mL of a 10% LCT emulsion) a minimum of 2 to 3 times a week. Lipid emulsion is also an energy substrate given that lipid oxidation is the predominant energy-producing pathway during stress. There has been debate whether exogenous lipids (LCT) are useful energy substrates occasioned by observations that, unlike in healthy subjects, exogenous LCT failed to suppress glucose oxidation in the critically ill so that 45% of the administered fat was stored.[31–34] Others observed that fat emulsions were well oxidized when administered to septic and trauma patients even when glucose was administered.[35,36] Current practice is to consider lipid emulsions as energy substrates and to administer them as 30% to 40% of total TPN calories.

Concern has been expressed over the possible immunosuppressive effects of lipid emulsions. Ex vivo studies demonstrated decreased neutrophil bacterial killing, depressed monokine expression, and other immunodepressant effects.[37] A study of trauma patients attributed increased infections to lipid emulsions.[38] This has led to recommendations to limit fat calories to 30% of total TPN calories.[39]

Because of the reported limitations of intravenous LCT emulsions, there has been interest in substituting MCT for some of the LCT. MCT do not require carnitine to enter the mitochondria and may be advantageous in situations where carnitine is reduced, such as some cases of sepsis. MCT are essentially an energy substrate[40]; it is unclear whether they can be stored. They may also cause less immunosuppression than LCT.[41-43] A small randomized trial failed to find any advantages of intravenous MCT/LCT over LCT.[44] Many enteral formulae contain both MCT and LCT, supposedly because MCT is better absorbed (Table 46–3). Intravenous MCT/LCT is not available in the U.S. It remains to be determined whether MCT or structured triglycerides (LCTs and MCTs bonded to a glycerol backbone[45]) actually confer advantages over LCT.

The soybean-derived fat emulsions traditionally used for parenteral nutrition contain high proportions of ω-6 polyunsaturated fatty acids, specifically linoleic acids (53%). Linoleic acid is the precursor of thromboxane A_2 and prostaglandin E_1, which cause platelet aggregation and inflammation. Alternately, fish oils containing ω-3 fatty acids (e.g., eicosapentaenoic and linolenic acids) are precursors of another class of prostaglandins, including thromboxane A_3, which have less platelet aggregating and inflammatory activity. Oral eicosapentaenoic acid intake improved lymphocyte proliferation and natural killer cell activity after surgery.[46-48] There has been interest in using ω-3 fatty acids in acute respiratory distress syndrome to reduce pulmonary microvascular permeability and alveolar macrophage prostaglandin and leukotriene synthesis.[49,50] Some enteral formulas are ω-3 fatty acid enriched (see Table 46–3).

Protein and Amino Acids

Metabolism and Pathophysiology

One of the hallmarks of the response to injury is catabolism caused by accelerated proteolysis of skeletal muscle thought to be modulated by cortisol and cytokines (TNF-α, IL-1, IL-6, and interferon-γ[51]). It is the balance between these catabolic substances and anabolic hormones, such as insulin and insulin growth factor-1 (IGF-1), that determine the degree of catabolism. The degree of nitrogen loss is proportional to the degree of stress and abates as patients convalesce.[52]

Protein and Amino Acid Nutrition

Amino acids and protein are basic ingredients of nutritional support regimens. TPN contains amino acid mixtures, whereas enteral formulas contain free amino acids, peptides, or whole proteins (see Table 46–3). The aim of administering protein or amino acids to stressed patients is to attenuate the breakdown of endogenous proteins by providing an alternate source of amino acids for gluconeogenesis and protein synthesis. Unfortunately, in the stressed state, exogenous amino acids and protein are not used well because proteolysis is relatively unresponsive to the usual negative feedback mechanisms, i.e., administration of exogenous

glucose or protein. Catabolism remains negative well into the convalescent period and may persist for as long as 9 months after severe (>40%) burns in children.[53] In the catabolic state, intake of 1.2 to 1.5 g/kg per day protein/amino acid is recommended. Greater amounts do not promote further nitrogen retention and are metabolized to urea, therefore the blood urea nitrogen may increase. Large external losses of protein, such as extensive burns and draining abscesses, make it necessary to increase protein/amino acid intake. Enough nonprotein calories, i.e., glucose and fat, must be concomitantly administered to prevent the use of protein/amino acids as energy sources.

The inability of the protein/amino acid intake to significantly attenuate nitrogen losses has led investigators to examine ways of either decreasing proteolysis or increasing protein synthesis. An initial attempt was to provide branched-chain-enriched amino acid solutions as a component of TPN. This resulted in some improvement in nitrogen balance but not in outcome. Some enteral formulations for very stressed patients are so enriched (see Table 46–3). More recent attempts focused on administering anabolic substances (e.g., insulin) to reduce protein oxidation and improve protein synthesis. At lower doses, insulin decreases protein breakdown, whereas at higher doses, it also stimulates protein synthesis.[54] Administering small doses of insulin to patients with burns increased skeletal muscle protein synthesis[55] and improved wound matrix formation.[56] Hypocaloric parenteral nutrition plus high-dose insulin improved nitrogen balance after surgery in patients with cancer.[57] However, the anabolic effects of insulin were not evident in enterally fed trauma patients. Therefore, the route of nutrient intake may play a role in the anabolic effects of insulin.[58]

Anabolic steroids have been tried as adjuncts to nutritional support but do not have beneficial effects.[59] The anabolic substances, growth hormone (GH) and IGF-1, have also been investigated. During catabolism, GH concentrations are reduced and there is resistance to its actions.[60] The aim of its administration is to increase nitrogen retention and promote wound healing. Small studies of GH administration to critically ill patients receiving nutritional support showed reduced nitrogen losses. However, a large randomized study showed that in critically ill patients, GH was associated with increased mortality because of infection and multiple organ failure attributed to its diabetogenic and lipolytic properties.[61] There remains interest in using GH during the anabolic phase. There is interest in giving IGF-1 to catabolic patients because of its insulin-like effects. IGF-1 stimulates protein synthesis at lower doses and at greater doses also reduces proteolysis.[62] When IGF-1 was administered for 3 days to burn patients, protein oxidation decreased, and when IGF-1 was administered with its binding protein, IGFBP-3, catabolism was attenuated.[63,64]

To help maintain gut integrity it has been recommended that glutamine be added to both enteral and parenteral nutrition regimens. Glutamine, the most abundant free amino acid in the blood and skeletal muscle, is a primary fuel for rapidly dividing cells such as enterocytes and immunocytes and is a precursor of purines, pyrimidines, and nucleotides.[65] Plasma glutamine concentration decreases during severe stress, likely because of decreased glutamine synthesis.[66,67] Animal studies indicate that glutamine may be an essential amino acid during catabolic illness when de novo synthesis

TABLE 46–3.

Enteral Nutrition Formulations

Classification	Calories (Kcal/ml) RDI (ml)	Protein (g/1000 mL)	Proportion PRO/CHO/FAT (% of calories)	Osmolality (mOsm/kg) NPcal:N	Indications	Comments
Isotonic e.g., Osmolite, Isocal	1.06 / 1890	34	13/50/37	270 / 168:1	General purpose isotonic tube feeding	Fat: 20% MCT + 80% LCT, Low residue
High nitrogen isotonic e.g., Isocal HN, Osmolite HN	1.06 / 1180	44	17/46/37	270 / 125:1	For mild-moderately stressed patients	Moderate high protein, isotonic
Isotonic w/fiber e.g., Jevity, Ultracal	1.06 / 1120	45	17/50/33	360 / 124:1	When fiber desired	Moderate high protein. Fat: 30% MCT
Supplement e.g., Ensure	1.06	35	14/64/22	590–640 / 150:1	Oral supplements for patients unable to eat sufficiently	Flavored
Calorie dense e.g., TwoCal HN, Nutren 2.0	2.0 / 750	84	17/43/40 16/39/45	730–745 / 125:1	Fluid restriction, e.g., CHF; high caloric needs, e.g., burns	High osmolality
Diabetic e.g., Glucotrol, Glucerna, Resource Diabetic	1.0 / 1400	45	17/34/49 18/40/42	320–355 / 79–125:1	Low CHO, high fat; fiber; follows ADA. Diabetic recommended	Fat: MCT, MUFA, PUFA. CHO: some fructose
Renal/Dialysis e.g., Nepro, Nutrirenal, Novasource Renal	2.0 / 750	70	14/40/46	665–700 / 140–154:1	*For dialysis patients:* moderate protein, high fat. Reduced electrolytes	Less vitamin A and D. Added vitamin B_6, folate. High osmolality

Type & Products	kcal/mL	mL to meet RDI	Protein (g)	%PRO/CHO/Fat	Osmolality	NPcal:N	Indications	Comments
Renal/no dialysis Suplena, RenalCal	2.0	1000	30–34	7/58/35 6/51/43	600	390:1	*For renal failure without dialysis:* Very low protein Reduced K, Mg, and PO_4 High osmolality	Some formulas enriched with essential amino acids
Elemental e.g., Vivonex TEN, *f-a-a*	1.0	1000	38	15/82/3 20/70/10	630–700	149:1	For malabsorption Free amino acids	Minimal fat High osmolality
Hepatic e.g., NutriHep	1.5	1000	40	11/77/12	790		For hepatic encephalopathy	Protein content: 50% branched-chain amino acids High osmolality
Stress e.g., TraumaCal, Perative	1.3–1.5	2000	67–82	21/55/25 22/44/38	385–560	91–97:1	For hypermetabolic stressed patients; High protein, BCAA enriched	May contain: Increased Arginine, vitamin B, C, E, Cu, Zn
Pulmonary e.g., Pulmocare, Respalor	1.5	1000	75	20/40/40 17/28/55	450–650	102–125:1	For pulmonary failure	High fat:CHO ratio to reduce CO_2 production
Peptide-based e.g., Sandosource Peptide, Vital HN	1.0	1750	42–50	20/65/15 17/74/9	490–500	125:1	For malabsorption	Low fat, high CHO
Immuno-nutrition Impact	1.0	1500	56	22/53/25	375	71:1		12.5% Arginine Purines, ω-3 fatty acids
"ARDS" diet e.g., Oxepa	1.5	1420	62.5	17/28/55	493	125:1	Mechanically ventilated patients with ARDS "anti-inflammatory"	High ω-3 fatty acid content

ADA, American Dietetic Association; CHO, carbohydrate; HN, high-nitrogen; LCT, long-chain triglycerides; MCT, medium-chain triglycerides; MUFA, monounsaturated fatty acids; N, nitrogen; NPcal, nonprotein calories; PRO, protein; PUFA, polyunsaturated fatty acids; RDI, recommended daily intake.
Adapted from references 182–184.

is insufficient. These studies also show that parenteral and enteral glutamine-supplemented nutrition may prevent gut bacterial translocation. The data in humans are less compelling.[68,69]

Glutamine is rather insoluble and is thus difficult to administer. Some success has been achieved infusing it as the L-amino acid, glutamine-dipeptides, alpha-ketoglutarate, or alanyl-glutamate.[70–72] TPN solutions enriched with glutamate, arginine, and aspartate increased glutamine concentrations.[73] Initial reports indicate that in some catabolic patients glutamine-containing nutrition may improve gut structure and function, exert an anabolic effect, and reduce morbidity rates, hospital costs, infection rates, and length of hospital stay.[74–77] Larger, multi-institutional studies are needed to ascertain whether glutamine administration improves outcome.[78]

Energy Expenditure

The response to stress is characterized by hypermetabolism.[79] After elective surgery, REE increases 10% to 20% above preoperative values. Septic patients have increases of 20% to 40%, whereas patients with burns have increases up to 120%, with the increase proportional to the extent of the burns.[80] Peak REE occurs about the third postoperative day and hypermetabolism may last up to 21 days in critically ill trauma[81] and burn[82] patients. Head injury and other neurologic problems increase REE secondary to marked outpouring of catecholamines. For at least 5 days after subarachnoid hemorrhage REE was 18% greater than predicted values.[83] Mechanically ventilated patients have lower increases in REE than spontaneously breathing patients because they are sedated and have no or minimal work of breathing.[84]

Practical Aspects of Drug Administration

Indications

The primary indication for initiating nutritional support is to avert or treat malnutrition among patients unable or unwilling to sustain sufficient oral intake. Furthermore, at least 20% to 35% of hospitalized patients experience malnutrition. A major consideration is whether the nutritional support will improve prognosis, or the quality of life, or both, because nutritional wasting is the inevitable consequence of many terminal diseases.

Preoperative malnutrition is associated with poor surgical outcome. Yet it has been difficult to demonstrate any benefit of preoperative parenteral nutrition in malnourished patients, except in those severely malnourished who had fewer noninfectious complications after 7 to 10 days of nutritional repletion. It is also beneficial to continue TPN during and after surgery in these patients.[85] Postoperative nutritional support is not indicated unless it is anticipated that patients will be unable to resume adequate oral feeding within 7 to 10 days of surgery. However, it is routine to administer at least 2 L/day of 5% dextrose solution, which has some protein sparing-effects. Patients not expected to resume adequate oral feedings within 7 to 10 days of surgery should begin nutritional support soon (2-4 days) after surgery. Evidence includes a study in which enteral nutrition started within 3 to 4 days of surgery reduced infectious complications after hepatectomy.[86] Sufficient early nutritional support of surgical patients not expected to eat soon after surgery reduced hospital length of stay and decreased costs.[87] Malnutrition was found in 38% to 100% of mechanically ventilated patients in the intensive care unit.[88] Therefore it is prudent to begin nutrition within 1 to 3 days of ICU admission to try to prevent further loss of lean body mass.

Route of Administration

A major decision in the nutritional support of seriously ill patients is the route of administration. If patients are eating on their own, it is necessary to monitor their actual intake to assess its adequacy. Many of these patients have little appetite and thus may need nutritional supplementation between meals (snacking) to increase their caloric intake. There are commercially available nutritional supplements that provide a balanced intake (see Table 46–3). Patients may be unable to feed themselves because of confusion or weakness and may need to be fed. The intake of patients with severe chronic obstructive pulmonary disease may be limited by desaturations during eating that cause fatigue. They may need supplemental oxygen through nasal cannula while eating. Patients who do not sustain adequate caloric intake by eating may require either supplemental enteral or parenteral nutrition.

The Enteral Route

The enteral route is preferred over the parenteral one because it is the natural portal for exogenous nutrients. The enteral route obviates the need for intravascular access and its attendant propensity for infections. Also, the variety of nutrients that can be administered through the (GIT) is greater than those available for parenteral use, allowing for better tailoring of nutrient intake. Other touted advantages of the enteral route include lower cost,[89] ease of administration, and maintenance of gut function. Regarding the latter, there has been much recent promotion of the enteral route occasioned by the desire to maintain gut integrity (the gut gets up to 70% of its nutrients from lumenal food) and therefore lessen the translocation of bacteria from the gut.[90] Animal experiments showed that translocation of bacteria from intestines with reduced integrity and increased permeability leads to local activation of the gut's immune inflammatory system (Peyer's patches and hepatic Kupffer cells[91]). The released cytokines then exacerbate the already existing systemic inflammatory response leading to multiple organ failure.[92] However, there is no overwhelming evidence of translocation in humans.[93] Lack of enteral intake, such as occurs among postoperative and critically ill patients receiving no nutrition or only TPN, is associated with small intestinal villus atrophy, decreased villous cell count, and reduced mucosal thickness.[94] Intestinal permeability, measured using the urinary lactulose/mannitol ratio, is increased.[94] These changes reversed with enteral feeding.[94,95] Interestingly, there was no evidence of mucosal atrophy among patients who had received 10 days of preoperative parenteral nutrition.[96] It is thought that atrophy itself does not lead to bacterial translocation, but that a further insult is needed such as ischemia/reperfusion injury to the small intestines after resuscitation from shock.[97] Moreover, during stress there is the possibility that constantly proliferating gut tissues (epithelial and lymphoid cells) may have an inadequate supply of nutrients, further compromising gut integrity.[98] This fear of reduced gut integrity[99] has been among the impeti for recommending that enteral nutrition should begin as soon as possible even if it is possible to administer only very small amounts. In the latter case, concomitant parenteral nutrition is indicated to provide adequate caloric intake.

A major consideration when using enteral nutrition is the delivery method. Most patients are fed through nasoenteric tubes. Some patients are fed initially through a conventional large-bore nasogastric tube. The advantages include the ability to quantify residual feedings and quickly reinitiate nasogastric suction. The disadvantages are the potential for pulmonary aspiration occasioned by gastroparesis and incompetence of the gastroesophageal junction because of the diameter of the tube. In addition, long-term use of large-bore tubes can lead to sinusitis and otitis media. Therefore, the type of feeding tube and the location of its distal end are major issues. For medium- and long-term feeding, it is best to use a small-bore (8-12 Fr), soft (e.g., silastic), long (to reach the jejunum) feeding tube with a weighted distal end. Such tubes reduce nasal and pharyngeal trauma, minimize incompetence of the gastroesophageal junction, and can reach the jejunum. Many critically ill patients have gastroparesis[100] so that placement of the tube distal to the ligament of Treitz (small intestinal function generally remains intact) prevents pooling of feeds in the stomach with its attendant risk for pulmonary aspiration. Yet there is controversy regarding whether jejunal feeding actually reduces the risk for aspiration.[101–103] Compared with gastric feedings, jejunal feedings facilitate greater caloric intakes.[104] Passing the tube through the pylorus is often problematic because of gastroparesis and a supine and immobile state. Therefore in patients undergoing abdominal surgery, the tube should be passed through the pylorus at the time of surgery. In nonsurgical situations, an attempt may be made to pass a weighted tube through the pylorus by placing the tube in the stomach, turning the patient on the right side, and administering a prokinetic drug such a metoclopramide. If that fails, the tube should be placed endoscopicaly[105] or fluoroscopically.[106] To reduce the possibility of aspiration, patients should be semirecumbent and not supine. Also, there are double-lumen tubes that allow the stomach to be suctioned while feeding into the jejunum. Such tubes may be especially useful in pancreatitis, duodenal fistulae, and gastric dilation.

Among the other enteral nutrition delivery methods is the placement of a jejunostomy during surgery in patients not expected to eat soon after surgery; such situations include patients with severe trauma, severe head injury, and

esophageal surgery. Patients being fed with a nasoenteric tube who will require prolonged enteral feeding (>4 weeks) should have either gastrostomies or jejunostomies placed surgically or percutaneously with endoscopic assistance.[107] Percutaneous endoscopic gastrostomies (PEG) are commonly performed and a modification of this procedure is to place a jejunal tube through the PEG.

Enteral nutrition is usually administered through continuous infusion. This tends to be better tolerated than bolus feeding, and reducing gastric volume may reduce aspiration.

The Parenteral Route

Parenteral nutrition is indicated when the enteral route cannot provide or sustain sufficient caloric intake. Although the current approach is to attempt to use the gut, there are situations in which parenteral nutrition is the mainstay of nutritional support. Patients with short bowel syndrome require parenteral nutrition after surgery and may require it for life if their remaining bowel does not undergo sufficient adaptation to sustain adequate oral intake. Other absolute indications for parenteral nutrition are small bowel obstruction, active gastrointestinal (GI) bleeding, pseudo-obstruction with complete intolerance to food, and high-output enterocutaneous fistulae (unless a feeding tube can be passed distal to the fistula). In partial large bowel obstruction it may or may not be possible to feed with a low residue diet. Relative indications for parenteral nutrition include nonhealing, moderate output, enterocutaneous fistulae; the need for bowel "rest" during inflammatory bowel flair-ups and acute radiation enteritis; marked abdominal distension and ileus caused by intra-abdominal sepsis; continued distention after relief of intestinal obstruction; and chylothorax unresponsive to MCT diet. Parenteral nutrition is also indicated when adequate nutrition cannot be sustained through the enteral route. In patients in the ICU this is often the case because of diarrhea, vomiting, poor stomach emptying, feeding tube dislodgement, and discontinuation of oral feeding for diagnostic tests, procedures, and operations.

Parenteral nutrition is administered through either central or peripheral venous catheters. Peripheral veins are unable to tolerate an osmolarity of more than 750 mOsm/L (the equivalent of 12.5% dextrose), consequently the fluid volume that can be tolerated limits the calories that can be administered. Therefore, this route is used mainly for supplementation or short-term feeding. Central venous catheters are the main route of TPN administration. The preferred entry is the subclavian vein, which provides a stable site, good patient acceptability, and lower infection rates than either the internal jugular or femoral routes. To minimize insertion and infectious complications, a skilled individual should insert subclavian catheters during sterile conditions. The catheter should be a single lumen catheter used only for TPN and should have antibacterial coatings (silver or antibiotics) to lessen the risk for infection. Multi-lumen catheters and multipurpose single-lumen catheters have high infection rates. For long-term use, silastic Hickman or Broviac catheters should be inserted using a subcutaneous tunnel. These catheters have a Dacron cuff at the proximal end of the tunnel to reduce infections.

Designing Nutrient Formulations

Nutritional regimens require many ingredients (see Table 46–2). The key decision is the route of administration because the composition of the feeding is wholly dependent on the route. With the parenteral route, protein intake is limited to commercial mixtures of amino acids, carbohydrate to glucose, and lipids to LCT emulsions (or LCT/MCT mixtures where available). There are many more options with enteral nutrition for which a variety of commercially available formulas exist (see Table 46–3). It is possible to supplement enteral formulas with modular protein, lipid, and carbohydrate products. Caloric intake may be determined by either measuring resting energy expenditure using indirect calorimetry or estimating requirements (see Table 46–1).

Nutrition support should be initiated slowly and increased only when the patient tolerates the regimen. Electrolytes and blood glucose must be closely monitored during this time and, if necessary, adjustments made to the formula. Insulin may be needed to control hyperglycemia. It is preferable to administer insulin than to reduce the glucose intake unless there is excessive hyperglycemia (>250 mg/dL).

Monitoring

In the acutely ill patient, the effects of enteral and parenteral nutrition must be monitored. The most basic monitoring is quantifying the actual caloric intake. This is especially important during enteral nutrition because it is difficult to achieve and maintain adequate intake using only the enteral route.[108] Monitoring also involves ensuring that access systems are functioning normally, are located in the correct anatomic locations, and are not infected. Electrolyte concentrations must be monitored, especially as the nutritional intake is being increased to reach the target caloric intake and whenever the clinical condition deteriorates. If there is a decrease in serum bicarbonate concentration, the cause of the acidosis must be ascertained and, with TPN, sodium or potassium acetate (which is metabolized to bicarbonate) substituted for some of the sodium or potassium chloride, respectively. Among patients receiving diuretics, nasogastric suction or steroids, metabolic alkalosis may occur and may need to be treated with increased KCl or acetazolamide. Calcium, phosphate, and magnesium should be monitored at least 2 to 3 times per week. With large losses of enteric content, serum zinc and selenium levels should be measured after a few weeks of nutritional support.

During the initial phase of parenteral support, plasma triglyceride should be monitored weekly in patients with potential fat clearance problems, such as those with hyperlipidemia, diabetes, sepsis, and impaired renal or hepatic function.[109] PT and PTT should also be monitored weekly, especially in patients with TPN, to ascertain whether additional vitamin K is needed. Liver function tests should be monitored weekly during the initial month of nutritional support. Increases of aminotransferases and alkaline phosphatase may occur secondary to hepatic steatosis, especially if large glucose loads are administered. Liver function tests should continue to be monitored monthly in patients with long-term TPN because intrahepatic cholestasis may develop.

It is imperative to monitor fluid balance among all patients receiving nutritional support. Critically ill patients have dynamic fluid shifts because of frequently changing extracellular ("third space") and intravascular volumes; reduced urinary output secondary to increased ADH, and reduced atrial natruetic factor; and nasogastric suction, diarrhea, and other fluid losses. Therefore accurate and frequent measurements of fluid intake and output, coupled with measurements of blood urea nitrogen, serum creatinine, and sodium are imperative. Patients unable to tolerate high fluid volumes may need diuretics and concentrated intakes (enteral: calorically dense formulas [see Table 46–3]; parenteral: 20% and 30% lipid emulsions plus solutions made with 70% dextrose and 15% amino acids). Alternately, patients may need added free water (as evidenced by hypernatremia and caused by osmotic diuresis secondary to glycosuria), which can be added by using dilute formulas and solutions. Among patients with frequent changes in fluid status, it is prudent to use concentrated formulas and add free water through other means, i.e., peripheral venous infusions, so that the caloric intake need not be changed.

Assessing the direct effects of nutritional support during the short-term (days to weeks) is difficult. In severely ill catabolic patients, the aim of feeding is not to restore lost body mass, but to attenuate further losses. Therefore, evidence of lean body mass restoration should not be expected. In one study, it took 2 weeks to show even a slight improvement in nutritional status.[110] Short-term changes in body weight in acutely ill patients reflect mainly fluid balance and anthropometric measurements (e.g., triceps skin thickness) often reflect the degree of edema. Measurements of nitrogen balance assess catabolic/anabolic state and guide adjustments in protein/amino acid intake. Serum albumin (normal $T^{1/2}$, 21 days) concentrations are decreased in acute illness because of decreased synthetic rate, shortened half-life, and redistribution into the extracellular fluid. The latter is caused by transcapillary escape facilitated by increased capillary permeability and extracellular expansion after fluid resuscitation. Therefore, acute changes in plasma albumin concentrations after surgery or trauma are caused by the redistribution of albumin into the expanded extracellular fluid. Proteins with short half-lives, e.g., prealbumin ($T^{1/2}$, 2–3 days) and transferrin ($T^{1/2}$, 8 days), are better indicators of protein synthesis.

As patients convalesce the type, amount, and composition of the nutritional support may need to be changed. TPN can be switched to enteral nutrition once the GIT begins to tolerate increased intake. The proportion of carbohydrate calories might be increased as glucose intolerance abates. Also, caloric intake should be adjusted as hypermetabolism lessens and anabolism appears. Overfeeding must be avoided (Table 46–4).

Complications

Complications of nutritional support can be caused by problems with the delivery system or the nutrition itself. A large

TABLE 46–4.

The Consequences of Overfeeding Parenteral and Enteral Nutrition

Caloric intake, >1.5–1.7 REE in stressed patients	Substrate in excess of energy needs and synthetic function. Increased fat storage, CO_2 production, urea production, and thermogenic effects
Carbohydrates	*Lungs:* Increased CO_2 production leads to: (1) increased VE that may lead to breathlessness: >4.5 mg/kg/min; (2) if insufficient increase in VE then increased $PaCO_2$. *Liver:* Fatty liver—increased AST, ALT, and Alk Phos, Hepatomegaly Hyperglycemia—may lead to osmotic diuresis and prerenal azotemia Increased intracellular K—decreased serum K Increased intracellular PO_4—decreased serum PO_4 Increased REE due to increase thermogenesis caused by increased catecholamine secretions
Lipids, >2 g/kg/day	*Liver:* (1) cholestasis, fatty liver; (2) increased congestion of RES with fat; (3) increased serum triglycerides
Protein, >2 g/kg/day	*Kidneys:* Increased ureagenesis (1) with decreased renal function BUN increases; (2) with normal renal function—diuresis may occur because of increased BUN secretion. This may lead to prerenal azotemia.
Fluid intake	If excessive may lead to fluid overload; is especially problematic with reduced cardiac or renal function.

BUN, blood urea nitrogen; REE, resting energy expenditure; RES, reticuloendothelial system; VE, minute ventilation.

study found more delivery system and feeding-related morbidity with enteral, than parenteral, nutrition.[111] However, infectious complications are greater with parenteral nutrition.

Delivery System: Parenteral Nutrition

Complications associated with parenteral nutrition delivery systems include those of central venous catheterization. These include pneumothorax secondary to subclavian or internal jugular vein catheterization. The pneumothorax rate for subclavian catheterization is approximately 1% to 5% and is lower if done by an experienced operator. Other complications include hemorrhage causing hemothorax, brachial plexus injury, and malposition (e.g., azygous vein, right ventricle or retrograde into the jugular vein). Peripherally inserted (through an arm vein) central venous catheters have the advantage of obviating the possibility of pneumothorax but are more difficult to place, have a greater incidence of malposition, and a tendency for skin site irritation.[112] The location of all catheter tips should be confirmed by chest radiograph before starting nutrition. Peripheral venous access, whether through a short peripheral venous catheter or a peripherally inserted central venous catheter line, is fraught with the possibility of thrombophlebitis.[113] In the former, the osmolarity of the solution must be limited to less than 750 mOsm to prevent phlebitis. Heparin and hydrocortisone may be added to the solution and a nitroglycerine patch placed over the catheter site.[114] It is imperative that all peripheral parenteral nutrition catheter sites be inspected

regularly and that catheters be changed when evidence of phlebitis develops.

Catheter-related infections are the major venous access complication encountered with TPN. Microbial colonization and bacteremias are caused by the interaction of four factors: the hydrophobicity and exopolysaccharide production of the microbe, the amount of fibrin and fibronectin attached to the catheter surface, the catheter material (hydrophobicity, thrombogenicity), and iatrogenic factors such as sterile technique and immunocompetence.[115] Infections are uncommon in the first 72 hours but then increase in incidence. The incidence of central venous catheter-related bloodstream infections ranges from 2 to 30 per 1000 catheter-days and is most often due to *Staphylococcus epidermidis* or *aureus* or *candida spp.* Mortality rates attributed to catheter-related infections are reported to be as high as 25%. The major thrust of TPN care is to reduce infection: solutions are prepared under laminar flow hoods, once prepared nothing is to be added to the solution, solutions must be refrigerated until use, any manipulation of the catheter or line must be done using sterile procedure, manipulation of the line should be kept to a minimum, and the site must be examined regularly for signs of erythema and infection.

Delivery System: Enteral Nutrition

Complications specific to enteral nutrition delivery systems include those of inserting nasoenteral tubes. It is important to confirm the location of feeding tubes by chest or abdominal radiographs, or both, before commencing feeding. This is because nasoenteric tubes can enter the pulmonary airways, coil and knot in the stomach, and be malpositioned in the esophagus. With nasoenteral tubes, pullback into the stomach (with jejunal feeding) or esophagus occurs increasing the risk for aspiration. This occurs because of pulling by the patient and during suctioning of the mouth. The tube thus should be securely fastened to the nose and if dislodgment is suspected a radiograph is obtained. However, the major problem with enteral nutrition is frequent decreases or discontinuations of the intake, which prevent administering of all the daily caloric requirements. These decreases and discontinuations have been ascribed to high gastric residuals, mechanical problems with the feeding tubes (e.g., dislodgment and obstruction), medical or surgical procedures, sepsis, and vomiting.[116,117] Up to a third of patients receiving enteral nutrition are unable to achieve a target intake of 25 kcal/kg per day.[110] Therefore, it is important to closely monitor the actual enteral nutrition intake so that measures can be taken to assure adequate caloric intake. These include establishing more secure access to obviate or prevent tube dislodgment (e.g., placing a PEG) and placing the tube tip distal to the ligament of Treitz to avoid gastric residuals. In cases in which the enteral intake remains inadequate, supplementation with parenteral nutrients should be considered.

PEGs are fraught with potential complications, yet the overall rate of complications is less than 2%. Complications include perforation of other visci, occlusions that may require tube replacement, cutaneous or intra-abdominal infections, balloon migration leading to pyloric obstruction, and peristomal leak.[118]

In general, surgically placed needle jejunotomies provide safe and effective access for postoperative enteral feeding.[119] Minor complications include tube dislodgment, local cellulitis, and blockage. The latter can be avoided by frequent flushing and limiting the viscosity of the feeds.[120] Major complications were seen in 4% of 220 trauma patients who had jejunostomies placed at the time of laparotomy. Major complications include small bowel perforations, small bowel volvulae with infarction, intraperitoneal leaks, and small bowel necrosis.[121] These occurred more often with larger diameter tubes than with needle jejunostomies.[121] Others reported intrabdominal and subcutaneous abscesses, small bowel obstruction, breaking of catheters (especially at the hub) and jejeuno-cutaneous fistulae on removal.[107,122]

Enteral and Parenteral Nutrition: Metabolic Complications

Metabolic complications of nutritional support occur with some frequency. Thus in acutely ill patients, it is important to monitor electrolytes and glucose daily especially when initiating the support. Hyperglycemia is a frequent problem especially with severe stress, steroid use, and diabetes mellitus. These patients often require insulin treatment. The initiation of insulin treatment can reduce serum K^+ and PO_4 concentrations, which require repletion. Importantly, as the stress response abates, the degree of glucose intolerance lessens and insulin requirements decrease. Therefore, it is imperative to monitor blood glucose closely to reduce insulin treatment and prevent hypoglycemia.

Hypoglycemia may occur on the abrupt discontinuation of continuous feedings containing significant amounts of carbohydrate. Continuous feedings result in high blood insulin concentrations so that hypoglycemia intervenes when the carbohydrate intake stops. Therefore, when stopping continuous parenteral and enteral nutrition, any concomitant insulin infusion should be stopped, intravenous glucose should be infused, and blood glucose monitored frequently. The practice of using TPN solutions containing lower glucose:lipid ratios (70:30 to 50:50) has reduced the incidence of hypoglycemia after abrupt discontinuation.[123–125] TPN should be continued during surgery, whereas enteral nutrition should be discontinued 8 hours before surgery and a glucose infusion should be started to prevent hypoglycemia.

Parenteral Nutrition: Gastrointestinal System Complications

Parenteral nutrition is associated with hepatobiliary complications whose causes may be multifactorial. The most important factors in the development of hepatobilliary dysfunction are the underlying disease and its severity, intercurrent sepsis, and drugs.[126] The role of TPN may be additive, if not primary. Large glucose loads (>4 mg/kg/min) can result in hepatic steatosis and steatohepatitis. The latter is accompanied by increases in ALT, AST, and alkaline phosphatase.[127] Intrahepatic cholestasis with increased alkaline phosphatase and bilirubin may occur 3 to 6 weeks after TPN is started. Large lipid loads (>2 g/day) administered for prolonged periods can also cause cholestasis.

Enteral Nutrition: Gastrointestinal System Complications

GIT complications of enteral nutrition occur frequently. Among patients fed intragastrically, gastric residuals, vomiting, and regurgitation occur more frequently than among those being fed into the small intestines. In a multicenter prospective study of 400 patients in the ICU fed mainly through nasogastric tubes, GI complications occurred in 63% and included diarrhea (15%), constipation (16%), high gastric residuals (39%), abdominal distention (13%), vomiting (12%), and regurgitation (6%). Enteral nutrition was withdrawn in 15% of patients because of GI complications.[128] With gastroparesis and large volume (150–220 mL) residuals, prokinetic agents (e.g., metoclopramide) should be considered. During enteral nutrition it is also important to be cognizant of the many drug/nutrient interactions that can occur.[129]

A frequent and particularly unpleasant (for patient and staff) complication of enteral nutrition is diarrhea. Its reported incidence rates, depending on the definition of diarrhea,[130] range from 2% to as high as 53% and 38% of feeding days.[131,132] The definition of diarrhea is important because many enteral products are "low-residual," i.e., they do not contain fiber and may not cause formed stools. Diarrhea is caused both by the feeds and by other factors.[133] Formula-related causes include hyperosmolar feeds and contamination of feedings with enterotoxigenic or pathogenic organisms. To prevent the latter, feeds should be sterile and not allowed to hang more than 8 hours. Nonformula-

811

Chapter 46 Nutritional Supplements

related causes include concomitant administration of drugs constituted in sorbitol elixirs, mannitol, or polyethylene glycol[131,134,135]; Clostridium difficile enterocolitis[136]; intra-abdominal infection[137]; broad spectrum antibiotics; and hypoalbuminemia. Diarrhea caused by hypoalbuminemia has been attributed to small bowel wall edema leading to malabsorption. Diarrhea-free feeding has been achieved in hypoalbuminemia by using elemental and peptide diets.[138] Fiber-containing formulations have been reported to reduce diarrhea in some studies.[139,140] Most enteral formulas are lactose free, which eliminates lactose intolerance as a problem. In patients without infectious diarrhea, pectin and antimotility drugs may reduce the diarrhea. Such patients must be monitored for the development of constipation. Repopulating the gut with *Saccharomyces boulardii*, a non-pathogenic yeast, was reported in a multicenter, randomized, double-blind placebo study to reduce the incidence of enteral nutrition associated diarrhea.[137] The incidence of hepatobilliary complications with enteral nutrition is rare (<5%[141,142]).

Enteral Nutrition, Stress Ulceration, and Pneumonia

Enteral nutrition affects the gastric environment. In some,[143] but not all,[144] investigations, enteral nutrition increased stomach pH by neutralizing gastric acidity. This may provide some protection against stress ulceration,[145] but may also increase colonization with gram-negative organisms.[144] Some authors surmise that these organisms are aspirated and cause nosocomial pneumonia. However, a critical review of randomized trials provided insufficient evidence concerning the association between enteral nutrition and nosocomial pneumonia.[146] To reduce gastric gram-negative bacterial colonization some authors have advocated acidifying enteral feeds.[147]

Refeeding

Refeeding nutritionally depleted patients must be done carefully to avoid overloading a metabolic system that has adapted to minimal or no food intake (see Table 46–4). Feeding must begin with a balanced diet of carbohydrates, fats, and proteins at intakes below resting energy expenditure and should be increased, stepwise, over 7 to 10 days.[148] Patients must be monitored for fluid overload, pulmonary edema, and electrolyte disturbances. Hypophosphatemia may occur if inadequate phosphate intake is provided as tissues begin to rebuild. It can lead to major (including respiratory) muscle weakness because phosphate is a vital component of tissue membranes, enzymes, and ATP. Concurrent hypomagnesemia, hypocalcemia, and hypokalemia may exacerbate the muscle weakness. Of 62 patients who received no nutrition for at least 48 hours after ICU admission, 34% developed hypophosphatemia on refeeding.[149]

Nitrogen balance may take time to turn positive because protein intake must be increased gradually and gluconeogenesis continues for some time after the beginning of refeeding. Generally, nutritionally depleted individuals efficiently replete their fat and glycogen stores and rebuild muscle tissue. Rebuilding muscles requires exercise, therefore it is virtually impossible to rebuild the muscles of bedridden or immobile patients.

Special Considerations

Burns

Patients with burns present special problems because of very high energy expenditures, large fluid requirements, and transcutaneous loss of protein. There is conflicting evidence whether enteral nutrition started within a few hours of admission reduces the magnitude of the stress response in these patients.[150] However, it is common practice with burns greater than 20% to begin nutrition within less than 16 hours of admission. If patients are unable to eat, enteral nutrition is preferred. To ensure success with the administration of many calories of a high-protein diet, the nasoenteric feeding tube should be placed into the jejunum. Caloric intake must be closely monitored. If inadequate calories are being ingested or administered, then supplementation is needed. In patients who are eating, this may be in the form of nutritional supplements ingested between meals. In enterally fed patients, supplementation can be provided with parenteral solutions.

Hepatic Dysfunction

Hepatic dysfunction, specifically cirrhosis, and intercurrent acute illness presents a complex scenario. Patients with cirrhosis are frequently nutritionally depleted secondary to anorexia,[151] lose large quantities of protein into ascites, and are hypermetabolic.[152] They also have hyperinsulinemia but with insulin resistance, accelerated gluconeogenesis and increased lipid oxidation; and, possibly, reduced glycogenesis[153–155] and essential fatty acid, zinc, and selenium deficiencies.[156] Interestingly, after liver transplantation, glucose clearance improves because of correction of the hyperinsulinemia and insulin resistance.[157–159] However, patients receiving corticosteroids as part of their immunosuppression continue to have abnormal glucose metabolism.[160]

Because of their depleted states, patients with cirrhosis would appear to be candidates for nutritional repletion. Yet because of the poor prognosis of cirrhosis, especially when complicated by serious illness, enteral nutritional support of seriously ill hospitalized patients with cirrhosis is associated with decreased survival.[161] However, the success of liver transplantation has renewed interest in nutritionally supporting candidates for transplantation.[162] These patients require fluid and sodium restriction and diuretics to control fluid overload. They need increased protein/amino acid intakes (1.0 to 1.5 g/kg/day) to replace the losses caused by ascites formation and high caloric intake to account for hypermetabolism (25–40 kcal/day[163]). Some patients with cirrhosis are susceptible to hepatic encephalopathy, limiting the amount of protein that can be ingested. When patients develop encephalopathy while receiving a standard protein intake of 0.8 g/day coupled with lactulose treatment, branched-chain amino acids-enriched nutrition should be used.

Renal Dysfunction

Preexisting chronic renal disease and newly developed acute renal failure present special nutritional challenges. Acute renal failure is especially problematic in the surgical arena because of its association with shock and sepsis. These patients are already catabolic and hypermetabolic and uremia adds another dimension because it exacerbates catabolism because of further insulin resistance, metabolic acidosis, and circulating proteases.[164] The kidney interconverts various amino acids and degrades specific peptides leading to major abnormalities in protein/amino acid handling.[164] Cytokine liberation during hemodialysis may further aggravate catabolism. Patients with renal failure do not tolerate large fluid loads, especially when oliguric; are unable to self-regulate electrolyte concentrations; and cannot tolerate large protein/amino acid loads because of an inability to excrete urea. Because these patients require about 30 kcal/kg per day and 1.0 to 1.5 g/kg per day of protein, frequent dialysis is needed to remove wastes and excess fluid.[165,166] The protein/amino acid intake may need to be increased (>1.5 g/kg) because of dialysis-related loss of amino acids.[164] Previously, essential amino acid–enriched solutions were used to reduce urea production. However, current recommendations are for a combination of essential and nonessential amino acids based on the theory that normally nonessential amino acids may become essential during disease.

Dialectic therapies include hemodialysis, veno-veno hemodiafiltration (CVVHD), and peritoneal dialysis. Dialysis facilitates enteral and parenteral nutrition by removing excess fluid and urea and balancing electrolyte concentrations, permitting patients to receive a full complement of calories and amino acids/protein. However, these therapies result in amino acid losses (10–15 g/d) unrelated to amino acid intake but related to plasma amino acid concentration, volume of dialysate effluent, and filter efficiency.[167] Therefore the amino acid/protein content of the nutritional support should be increased. With aggressive CVVHD, patients required as much as 2.5 g/kg per day of protein to achieve positive nitrogen balance.[168] Dialectic therapy also results in the loss of peptides, proteins (with peritoneal dialysis), and water-soluble vitamins that need to be replaced.[169] Therefore, some enteral nutrition formulations for these patients contain added B vitamins.

Solutions used for peritoneal dialysis and CVVHD usually contain 1.5% glucose and concentrations as high as 4.25% are used. Up to 35% to 45% of this glucose can be absorbed and it is a source of carbohydrate calories.[170] With peritoneal dialysis, as much as 500 g/day of dextrose may be absorbed.[171] Similarly, glucose-containing solutions used as replacement solutions during hemofiltration can be a source of glucose calories; one study reports these solutions providing 300 g/day of glucose.[172] This glucose load must be considered when designing nutritional regimens and glucose/carbohydrate contents must be reduced accordingly.

Generally, nutritional regimens for renal failure should not contain phosphate, potassium, or magnesium. Calcium intake may need to be increased, whereas sodium content should be nearly isotonic because of an inability to regulate serum sodium concentrations. During dialectic therapy, the serum electrolytes must be monitored and deficiencies corrected. In addition, glucose concentrations need to be monitored both because of the profound stress state (insulin resistance and increased gluconeogenesis) and dialysis-associated glucose absorption. Insulin therapy may be needed to reduce hyperglycemia, but such patients may be especially sensitive to insulin.

Pharmacologic Use of Nutritional Intake

Immunomodulation

Cellular immunity decreases during acute stress. This has led to interest in nutrient-induced immuno-enhancement using enteral diets containing added omega-3 fatty acids, arginine (enhances lymphocyte cytotoxicity), and purine nucleotides (precursors of RNA, DNA, and ATP to maintain competent immunity and cellular integrity in rapidly dividing cells[173]). A meta-analysis of 11 randomized trials of both critically ill and postoperative patients with GI cancer showed significant reductions in the risk for developing infectious complications and shorter hospital stays with immunonutrition compared with conventional nutrition.[174] However, no affect on mortality was observed. Further analysis of these and other studies hint that during severe sepsis, shock, or organ failure, immunonutrition may be detrimental by enhancing the inflammatory response, whereas less severely stressed postoperative patients and those convalescing from critical illness may benefit from immunonutrition.[173,175-178] Thus there has been a call for further study to delineate the specific patient populations most likely to benefit from these nutrients.[179]

The Bottom Line

The ultimate question is whether nutritional support improves patient outcome, i.e., whether it decreases morbidity and mortality rates. Unfortunately, no definitive large multicenter studies have examined this issue but a few meta-analyses have examined selected aspects of nutritional support. A meta-analysis using 26 studies performed in surgical and critically ill patients[180] found that TPN had no effect on mortality rates and only decreased complication rates in malnourished patients. Complication rates, but not mortality rates, were lower among those who did not receive lipids. This difference was confirmed by a meta-analysis of 27 trials in surgical patients.[180] It also showed no TPN affect on mortality, a possible reduction in complications with TPN, and no detrimental effects of lipids.[181] The five-center prospective SUPPORT study (6298 patients with serious illness) showed that nutritional support is not associated with improved survival rates in any group (chronic obstructive pulmonary disease, acute respiratory failure, multiple system organ failure, cirrhosis) except those in coma.[161]

There is a need for more study of the cost benefits and cost effectiveness of nutritional support in the critically ill. Until they are performed, nutritional support should continue to be viewed as an important adjunctive therapy and should be used in a manner that maximizes its positive effects and minimizes its detrimental effects.

Conclusion

Nutritional support is a supplemental therapy that attempts to provide seriously ill patients with metabolic disarray sufficient nutrients to forestall further loss of body tissue. However, its success in preventing such losses is dependent on successfully treating the underlying disease and reducing the ravages of the stress response. Only once the stress response has abated can repletion of depleted stores and tissues begin. Therefore, nutritional support must be considered in the context of the underlying metabolic milieu and only by better understanding the vast and complex metabolic changes that occur during stress can nutritional support regimens be improved so that they are more effective in stemming the losses of body tissues.

References

1. Moore FD: Metabolic Care of the Surgical Patient. Philadelphia, Saunders, 1959.
2. Stumvoll M, Meyer C, Mitrakou A, et al: Renal glucose production and utilization: New aspects in humans. Diabetologia 40:749–757, 1997.
3. Rodwell VW: Water and pH. In Murray RK, Graner DK, Mayes PA, Rodwell VW (eds): Harper's Biochemistry, 25th ed. Stamford, Conn, Appleton & Lange, p 16, 2000.
4. Cerra FB, Siegel JH, Coleman B, et al: Septic autocannibalism: Failure of exogenous nutritional support. Ann Surg 192:570–580, 1980.
5. Rolih CA, Ober KP: The endocrine response to critical illness. Med Clin N Am 79:211–224, 1995.
6. Wolfe RR: Herman Award Lecture 1996: Relation of metabolic studies to clinical nutrition—the example of burn injury. Am J Clin Nutr 64:800–808, 1996.
7. Chiolero R, Revelly JP, Tappy L: Energy metabolism in sepsis and injury. Nutrition 13(9 suppl):45S–51S, 1997.
8. Aarsland A, Chinkes D, Wolfe RR: Hepatic and whole body fat synthesis in humans during carbohydrate overfeeding. Am J Clin Nutr 65:1774–1782, 1997.
9. Wolfe RR: Substrate utilization/insulin resistance in sepsis/trauma. Ballieres Clin Endocrinol Metab 11:645–657, 1997.
10. Hellerstein MK: De novo lipogenesis in humans: Metabolic and regulatory aspects. Eur J Clin Nutr 53(suppl):S52–S65, 1999.
11. Guenst JM, Nelson LD: Predictors of total parenteral nutrition-induced lipogenesis. Chest 105:553–559, 1994.
12. Tappy L, Schwarz JM, Schneiter P, et al: Effects of isoenergetic glucose-based or lipid-based parenteral nutrition on glucose metabolism, de novo lipogenesis, and respiratory gas exchanges in critically ill patients. Crit Care Med 26:860–867, 1998.
13. Schwarz JM, Chiolero R, Revelly JP, et al: Effects of enteral carbohydrates on de novo lipogenesis in critically ill patients. Am J Clin Nutr 72:940–945, 2000.
14. Schricker T, Carli F, Lattermann R, et al: Glucose infusion does not suppress increased lipolysis after abdominal surgery. Nutrition 17:85–90, 2001.
15. Wolfe RR: Substrate utilization/insulin resistance in sepsis/trauma. Ballieres Clin Endocrinol Metab 11:645–657, 1997.
16. Fellander G, Nordenstrom J, Ungerstedt U, et al: Influence of operation on glucose metabolism and lipolysis in human adipose tissue: A microdialysis study. Eur J Surg 160:87–95, 1994.
17. Jeevanandam M, Shamos RF, Petersen SR: Substrate efficacy in early nutrition support of the critically ill multiple trauma victims. JPEN J Parenter Enteral Nutr 16:511–520, 1992.
18. Bjerke HS, Shabot MM: Glucose intolerance in critically ill surgical patients: Relationship to total parenteral nutrition and severity of illness. Am Surg 58:728–731, 1992.
19. Watters JM, Kirkpatrick SM, Hopbach D, et al: Aging exaggerates the blood glucose response to total parenteral nutrition. Can J Surg 39:481–485, 1996.
20. Rosemarin DK, Wardlaw GM, Mirtallo J: Hyperglycemia associated with high, continuous infusion rates of total parenteral nutrition dextrose. Nutr Clin Pract 11:151–156, 1996.
21. Schloerb PR, Henning JF: Patterns and problems of adult total parenteral nutrition use in US academic medical centers. Arch Surg 133:7–12, 1998.
22. Singer P, Bursztein S, Kirvela O, et al: Hypercaloric glycerol in injured patients. Surgery 112:509–514, 1992.
23. Carey GB: Mechanisms regulating adipocyte lipolysis. Adv Exp Med Biol 441:157–170, 1998.
24. Perea A, Clemente F, Martinell J, et al: Physiological effect of glucagon in human isolated adipocytes. Horm Metab Res 27:372–375, 1995.
25. Miles JM: Lipid fuel metabolism in health and disease. Curr Opin Gen Surg 78–84, 1993.
26. Doerrler W, Feingold KR, Grunfeld C: Cytokines induce catabolic effects in cultured adipocytes by multiple mechanisms. Cytokine 6:478–484, 1994.
27. Goldstein SA, Elwyn DH: The effects of injury and sepsis on fuel utilization. Ann Rev Nutr 9:445–473, 1989.
28. Sato N, Oyamatsu M, Tsukada K, et al: Serial changes in contribution of substrates to energy expenditure after thoracic esophagectomy for cancer. Nutrition 13:100–103, 1997.
29. Wood GC, Brown RO, Dickerson RN: Considerations in the use of lipid-based drug products. J Intraven Nurs 21:45–49, 1998.
30. Lowrey TS, Dunlap AW, Brown RO, et al: Pharmacologic influence on nutrition support therapy: Use of propofol in a patient receiving combined enteral and parenteral nutrition support. Nutr Clin Pract 11:147–149, 1996.
31. Stouthard JM, Endert E, Romiju Jam Sauerwein HP: Infusion of long-chain or medium-chain triglycerides inhibits peripheral glucose metabolism in men. JPEN J Parenter Enteral Nutr 18:436–441, 1994.
32. Haesler E, Schneiter P, Temler E, et al: Effects of infused amino acids on glucose metabolism in healthy lean humans. Int J Obes Relat Metab Disord 18:307–312, 1994.
33. Tissot S, Normand S, Khalfallah Y, et al: Effects of a continuous lipid infusion on glucose metabolism in critically ill. Am J Physiol 269:E753–E758, 1995.
34. Wolfe BM, Klein S, Peters EJ, et al: Effects of elevated free fatty acids on glucose oxidation in normal humans. Metabolism 37:323–329, 1988.
35. Nordenstrom J, Carpentier YA, Askanazi J, et al: Metabolic utilization of intravenous fat emulsion during total parenteral nutrition. Ann Surg 196:221–231, 1982.
36. Druml W, Fischer M, Ratheiser K: Use of intravenous lipids in critically ill patients with sepsis without and with hepatic failure. JPEN J Parenter Enteral Nutr 22:217–223, 1998.
37. Waitzberg DL, Bellinati-Pres R, Salgado MM, et al: Effect of total parenteral nutrition with different lipid emulsions on human monocyte and neutrophil functions. Nutrition 13:128–132, 1997.
38. Battistella FD, Widergren JT, Anderson JT, et al: A prospective, randomized trial of intravenous fat emulsion administration in trauma victims requiring total parenteral nutrition. J Trauma 43:52–60, 1997.
39. Chan S, McCowen KC, Blackburn GL: Nutritional management in the ICU. Chest 115:145S–148S, 1999.
40. Lai H, Chen W: Effects of medium-chain and long-chain triacylglyceroles in pediatric surgical patients. Nutrition 16:401–406, 2000.
41. Wanten GJ, Naber AH, Kruimel JW, et al: Influence of structurally different lipid emulsions on human neutrophil oxygen radical production. Eur J Clin Invest 29:357–363, 1999.
42. Heine J, Scheinichen D, Jaeger K, et al: In vitro influence of parenteral lipid emulsions on the respiratory burst of neutrophils. Nutrition 15:540–545, 1999.
43. Kruimel JW, Naber AH, Curfs JH, et al: With medium-chain triglycerides, higher and faster oxygen radical production by stimulated

polymorphonuclear leukocytes occurs. JPEN J Parenter Enteral Nutr 24:107–112, 2000.

44. Lindgren BF, Ruokonen E, Magnusson-Borg, et al: Nitrogen sparing effect of structured triglycerides containing both medium- and long-chain fatty acids in critically ill patients: A double blind randomized controlled trial. Clin Nutr 20:43–48, 2001.

45. Rubin M, Moser A, Vaserberg N, et al: Structured triacylglycerol emulsion, containing both medium- and long-chain fatty acids, in long-term home parenteral nutrition: A double-blind randomized cross-over study. Nutrition 16:95–100, 2000.

46. Roulet M, Frascarolo P, Pilet M, et al: Effects of intravenously infused fish oil on platelet fatty acid phospholipid composition and on platelet function in postoperative trauma. JPEN J Parenter Enteral Nutr 21:296–301, 1997.

47. Calder PC: n-3 polunsaturated fatty acids and cytokine production in health and disease. Ann Nutr Metab 41:203–234, 1997.

48. Furukawa K, Tashiro T, Yamamori H, et al: Effects of soybean oil emulsion and eicosapentanoic acid on stress response and immune function after a severely stressful operation. Ann Surg 229:255–261, 1999.

49. Mancuso P, Whelan J, DeMichele SJ, et al: Effects of eicosapentaenoic and gamma-linolenic acid on lung permeability and alveolar macrophage eicosanoid synthesis in endotoxic rats. Crit Care Med 25:523–532, 1997.

50. Planas M, Masclans JR, Iglesia R, et al: Eicosanoids and fat emulsions in acute respiratory distress syndrome patients. Nutrition 13:202–205, 1997.

51. Tashiro T, Yamamori H, Takagi K, et al: Effect of severity of stress on whole-body protein kinetics in surgical patients receiving parenteral nutrition. Nutrition 12:763–765, 1996.

52. Brown JA, Gore DC, Jahoor F: Catabolic hormones alone fail to reproduce the stress-induced efflux of amino acids. Arch Surg 129:819–824, 1994.

53. Hart DW, Wolf SE, Mlcak R, et al: Persistence of muscle catabolism after severe burn. Surgery 128:312–319, 2000.

54. Grizard J, Dardevet D, Balage M, et al: Insulin action on skeletal muscle protein metabolism during catabolic states. Reprod Nutr Dev 39:61–74, 1999.

55. Ferrando AA, Chinkes DL, Wolfe SE, et al: A submaximal dose of insulin promotes net skeletal muscle protein synthesis in patients with severe burns. Ann Surg 229:11–18, 1999.

56. Pierre EJ, Barrow RE, Hawkins HK, et al: Effects of insulin on wound healing. J Trauma 44:342–345, 1998.

57. Pearlstone DB, Wolf RF, Berman RS, et al: Effect of systemic insulin on protein kinetics in postoperative cancer patients. Ann Surg Oncol 1:321–332, 1994.

58. Clements RH, Hayes CA, Gibbs ER, et al: Insulin's anabolic effect is influenced by route of administration of nutrients. Arch Surg 134:274–277, 1999.

59. Gervasio JN, Dickerson RN, Swearingen J, et al: Oxandrolone in trauma patients. Pharmacotherapy 20:1328–1334, 2000.

60. Jenkins RC, Ross RJ: Acquired growth hormone resistance in catabolic states. Ballieres Clin Endocrinol Metab 10:411–419, 1996.

61. Takala J, Ruokonene E, Webster NR, et al: Increased mortality associated with growth hormone treatment in critically ill adults. N Engl J Med 341:785–792, 1999.

62. Miers WR, Barrett EJ: The role of insulin and other hormones in the regulation of amino acid and protein metabolism in humans. J Basic Clin Physiol Pharmacol 9:235–253, 1998.

63. Herndon DN, Ramzy PI, DebRoy MA, et al: Muscle protein catabolism after severe burn: Effects of IGF-1/IGFBP-3 treatment. Ann Surg 229:713–722, 1999.

64. Cioffi WG, Gore DC, Rue LW 3rd, et al: Insulin-like growth factor-1 lowers protein oxidation in patients with thermal injury. Ann Surg 220:310–319, 1994.

65. Hall JC, Heel K, McCauley R: Glutamine. Br J Surg 83:305–312, 1996.

66. Biolo G, Fleming RY, Maggi SP, et al: Inhibition of muscle glutamine formation in hypercatabolic patients. Clin Sci (Colch) 99:189–194, 2000.

67. Mittendorfer B, Gore DC, Herndon DN, et al: Accelerated glutamine synthesis in critically ill patients cannot maintain normal intramuscular free glutamine concentration. JPEN J Parenter Enteral Nutr 23:243–252, 1999.

68. Buchman AL: Glutamine: Is it a conditionally required nutrient for the human gastrointestinal system? J Am Coll Nutr 15:199–205, 1996.

69. Powell-Tuck J, Jaimeson CP, Bettany GE, et al: A double blind, randomized, controlled trial of glutamine supplementation in parenteral nutrition. Gut 45:82–88, 1999.

70. Cynober LA: The use of alpha-ketoglutarate salts in clinical nutrition and metabolic care. Curr Opin Clin Nutr Metab Care 2:33–37, 1999.

71. Jian ZM, Cao JD, Zhu XG, et al: The impact of alanyl-glutamine on clinical safety, nitrogen balance, intestinal permeability, and clinical outcome in postoperative patients: a randomized, double-blind, controlled study of 120 patients. JPEN J Parenter Enteral Nutr 23(5 suppl):S62–S66, 1999.

72. Morlion BJ, Stehle P, Wachtler P, et al: Total parenteral nutrition with glutamine dipeptide after major abdominal surgery: A randomized, double-blind, controlled study. Ann Surg 227:302–308, 1998.

73. Berard MP, Zazzo JF, Condat P, et al: Total parenteral nutrition enriched with arginine and glutamate generates glutamine and limits protein catabolism in surgical patients hospitalized in intensive care units. Crit Care Med 28:3637–3644, 2000.

74. Houdijk AP, Rijnsburger ER, Jansen J, et al: Randomized trial of glutamine-enriched enteral nutrition on infectious morbidity in patients with multiple trauma. Lancet 352:772–776, 1998.

75. Ziegler TR, Szeszycki EE, Estivariz CF, et al: Glutamine: From basic science to clinical applications. Nutrition 12(suppl):S68–S70, 1996.

76. Jones C, Palmer TE, Griffiths RD: Randomized clinical outcome study of critically ill patients given glutamine-supplemented enteral nutrition. Nutrition 15:108–115, 1999.

77. Mertes N, Schulzki C, Goeters C, et al: Cost containment through L-alanyl-L-glutamine supplemented total parenteral nutrition after major abdominal surgery: A protective randomized double-blind controlled study. Clin Nutr 19:395–401, 2000.

78. Sacks GS: Glutamine supplementation in catabolic patients. Ann Pharmacother 33:348–354, 1999.

79. Gil KM, Forse RA, Askanazi J, et al: Energy metabolism in stress. In Garrow JS, Halliday D (eds): Substrate and Energy Metabolism. London: John Libbey, pp 203–212, 1985.

80. Turner WW, Ireton CS, Hunt JL, et al: Predicting energy expenditures in burn patients. J Trauma 25:11–16, 1985.

81. Monk DN, Plank LD, Franch-Arcas G, et al: Sequential changes in the metabolic response in critically injury patients during the 25 days after blunt trauma. Ann Surg 223:395–405, 1996.

82. Khorram-Sefat R, Behrendt W, Heiden A, et al: Long-term measurements of energy expenditure in severe burn injury. World J Surg 23:115–122, 1999.

83. Hersio K, Takala J, Kari A, et al: Patterns of energy expenditure in intensive-care patients. Nutrition 9:127–132, 1993.

84. Brandi LS, Santini L, Bertolini R, et al: Energy expenditure and severity of injury and illness indices in multiple trauma patients. Crit Care Med 27:2684–2689, 1999.

85. Bozzetti F, Gavazzi C, Miceli R, et al: Perioperative total parenteral nutrition in malnourished, gastrointestinal cancer patients: A randomized, clinical trial. JPEN J Parenter Enteral Nutr 24:7–14, 2000.

86. Mochizuki H, Togo S, Tanaka K, et al: Early enteral nutrition after hepatectomy to prevent postoperative infection. Hepatogastroenterology 47:1407–1410, 2000.

87. Neumayer LA, Smout RJ, Jorn HG, et al: Early and sufficient feeding reduces length of stay and changes in surgical patients. J Surg Res 95:73–77, 2001.

88. Huang YC: Malnutrition in the critically ill. Nutrition 17:263–264, 2001.

89. Braga M, Gianotti L, Gentilini O, et al: Early postoperative enteral nutrition improves gut oxygenation and reduces costs compared with total parenteral nutrition. Crit Care Med 29:242–248, 2001.

90. Archer SB: Current uses and abuses of total parenteral nutrition. Adv Surg 26:165–189, 1996.

91. Hartung T, Sauer A, Hermann C, et al: Overactivation of the immune system by translocated bacteria and bacterial products. Scand J Gastroenterol Suppl 222:98–99, 1997.

92. Swank GM, Deitch EA: Role of the gut in multiple organ failure: Bacterial translocation and permeability changes. World J Surg 20:411–417, 1996.

93. Lipman TO: Bacterial translocation and enteral nutrition in humans: An outsider looks in. JPEN 19:156–165, 1995.

94. Buchman AL, Moukarzel AA, Bhuta S, et al: Parenteral nutrition is associated with intestinal morphologic and functional changes in humans. JPEN J Parenter Enteral Nutr 19:453–460, 1995.

95. Hadfield RJ, Sinclair DG, Houldsworth PE, et al: Effects of enteral and parenteral nutrition on gut mucosal permeability in the critically ill. Am J Respir Crit Care Med 152:1545–1548, 1995.

96. Groos S, Hunefeld G, Luciano L: Parenteral versus enteral nutrition: Morphological changes in human adult intestinal mucosa. J Submicrosc Cytol Pathol 26:61–74, 1996.

97. Kong SE, Blennerhassett LR, Heel KA, et al: Ischaemia-reperfusion injury in the intestine. Aust NZ J Surg 68:554–561, 1998.

98. McBurney MI: The gut: Central organ in nutrient requirements and metabolism. Can J Physiol Pharmacol 72:260–265, 1994.

99. Suchner U, Senftleben U, Eckart T, et al: Enteral versus parenteral nutrition: Effects on gastrointestinal function and metabolism. Nutrition 12:13–22, 1996.

100. Ritz MA, Fraser R, Tam W, Dent J: Impacts and patterns of disturbed gastrointestinal function in critically ill patients. Am J Gastroenterol 95:3044–3052, 2000.

101. Montecalvo MA, Steger KA, Farber HW, et al: Nutritional outcome and pneumonia in critical care patients randomized to gastric versus jejunal tube feedings. The Critical Care Research Team. Crit Care Med 20:1377–1387, 1992.

102. Fox KA, Mularski RA, Sarfati MR, et al: Aspiration pneumonia following surgically placed feeding tubes. Am J Surg 170:564–567, 1995.

103. Esparza J, Boivin MA, Hartshorne MF, et al: Equal aspiration rates in gastrically and transpylorically fed critically ill patients. Intensive Care Med 27:660–664, 2001.

104. Montecalvo MA, Steger KA, Farber HW, et al: Nutritional outcome and pneumonia in critical care patients randomized to gastric versus jejunal tube feedings. The Critical Care Research Team. Crit Care Med 20:1377–1387, 1992.

105. Napolitano LM, Wagle M, Heard SO: Endoscopic placement of nasoenteric feeding tubes in critically ill patients: Reliable alternative. J Laparoendosc Adv Surg Tech A 8:395–400, 1998.

106. Huerta G, Puri VK: Nasoenteric feeding tubes in critically ill patients (fluoroscopy versus blind). Nutrition 16:264–267, 2000.

107. Rumalla A, Baron TH: Results of direct percutaneous endoscopic jejunostomy, an alternative method for providing jejunal feeding. Mayo Clin Proc 75:807–810, 2000.

108. De Jonghe B, Appere-De-Vechi C, Fournier M, et al: A prospective survey of nutritional support practices in intensive care unit patients: What is prescribed? What is delivered? Crit Care Med 29:8–12, 2001.

109. Crook MA: Lipid clearance and total parenteral nutrition: The importance of monitoring plasma lipids. Nutrition 16:774–775, 2000.

110. Griffith RD: Nutrition in intensive care: Give enough but choose the route wisely? Nutrition 17:53–55, 2001.

111. Woodcock NP, Zeigler D, Palmer MD, et al: Enteral versus parenteral nutrition: A pragmatic study. Nutrition 17:1–12, 2001.

112. Cowl CT, Weinstock JV, Al-Jurf A, et al: Complications and cost associated with parenteral nutrition delivered to hospitalized patients through either subclavian or peripherally-inserted central catheters. Clin Nutr 19:237–243, 2000.

113. Cowl CT, Weinstock JV, Al-Jurf A, et al: Complications and cost associated with parenteral nutrition delivered to hospitalized patients through either subclavian or peripherally-inserted central catheters. Clin Nutr 19:237–243, 2000.

114. Tighe MJ, Wong C, Martin IG, et al: Do heparin, hydrocortisone, and glyceryl trinitrate influence thrombophlebitis during full intravenous nutrition via a peripheral vein? JPEN J Parenter Enteral Nutr 19:507–509, 1995.

115. Chatzinikolaou I, Raad II: Intravascular catheter-related infections: A preventable challenge in the critically ill. Semin Respir Infect 15:264–271, 2000.

116. Heyland D, Cook DJ, Winder B, et al: Enteral nutrition in the critically ill patient: A prospective survey. Crit Care Med 23:1055–1060, 1995.

117. Wolf SE, Jeschke MG, Rose JK, et al: Enteral feeding intolerance: An indicator of sepsis-associated mortality in burned children. Arch Surg 132:1310–1314, 1997.

118. Simon T, Fink AS: Recent experience with percutaneous endoscopic gastrotomy/jejunostomy (PEG/J) for enteral nutrition. Surg Endosc 14:436–438, 2000.

119. De Gottardi A, Krahenbuhl L, Farhadi J, et al: Clinical experience of feeding through a needle catheter jejunostomy after major abdominal operations. Eur J Surg 165:1055–1060, 1999.

120. Biffi R, Lotti M, Cenciarelli S, et al: Complications and long-term outcome of 80 oncology patients undergoing needle catheter jejunostomy placement for early postoperative enteral feeding. Clin Nutr 19:277–279, 2000.

121. Holmes JH IV, Brundage SI, Yuen P, et al: Complications of surgical feeding jejonostomy in trauma patients. J Trauma 47:1009–1012, 1999.

122. Eddy VA, Snell JE, Morris JA Jr: Analysis of complications and long-term outcome of trauma patients with needle catheter jejunostomy. Am Surg 62:40–44, 1996.

123. Krzywda EA, Andris DA, Whipple JK, et al: Glucose response to abrupt initiation and discontinuation of toal parenteral nutrition. JPEN J Parenter Enteral Nutr 17:64–67, 1993.

124. Eisenberg PG, Gianino S, Clutter WE, et al: Abrupt discontinuation of cycled parental nutrition is safe. Dis Colon Rectum 38:933–939, 1995.

125. Nirula R, Yamada K, Waxman K: The effect of abrupt cessation of total parenteral nutrition on serum glucose: A randomized trial. Am Surg 66:866–869, 2000.

126. Payne-James JJ, Silk DB: Hepatobiliary dysfunction associated with total parenteral nutrition. Dig Dis 9:106–124, 1991.

127. Martinez Tutor MJ, Alfaro Olea A, Brea Corral JM, et al: Liver dysfunction associated with total parenteral nutrition. Nutr Hosp 8:22–29, 1993.

128. Montejo JC: Enteral nutrition-related gastrointestinal complications in critically ill patients: A multicenter study. The Nutritional and Metabolic Working Group of the Spanish Society of Intensive Care Medicine and Coronary Units. Crit Care Med 27:1447–1453, 1999.

129. Lourenco R: Enteral feeding: Drug/nutrient interaction. Clin Nutr 20:187–193, 2001.

130. Bliss DZ, Guenter PA, Settle RG: Defining and reporting diarrhea in tube-fed patients—what a mess! Am J Clin Nutr 55:753–759, 1992.

131. Edes TE, Walk BE, Austin JL: Diarrhea in tube-fed patients: Feeding formula not necessarily the cause. Am J Med 88:91–93, 1990.

132. Medley F, Stechmiller J, Field A: Complications of enteral nutrition in hospitalized patients with artifical airways. Clin Nurs Res 2:21312–21323, 1993.

133. Heimburger DC, Sockwell DG, Geels WJ: Diarrhea with enteral feeding: Prospective reappraisal of putative causes. Nutrition 10:392–396, 1994.

134. Hill DB, Henderson LM, McClain CJ: Osmotic diarrhea induced by sugar-free theophylline solution in critically ill patients. JPEN J Parenter Enteral Nutr 15:332–336, 1991.

135. Shepherd MF, Felt-Gunderson PA: Diarrhea associated with lorazepam solution in a tube-fed patient. Nutr Clin Pract 11:117–120, 1996.

136. Bliss DZ, Johnson S, Savik K, et al: Acquisition of Clostridium difficile-associated diarrhea in hospitalized patients receiving tube feeding. Ann Intern Med 129:1012–1019, 1998.

137. Bleichner G, Blehaut H, Mentec H, et al: Saccharomyces boulardii prevents diarrhea in critically ill tube-fed patients. A multicenter, randomized, double blind placebo-controlled trial. Intensive Care Med 23:517–523, 1997.

138. Borlase BC, Bell SJ, Lewis EJ, et al: Tolerance to enteral tube feeding diets in hypoalbuminemic critically ill, geriatric patients. Surg Gynecol Obstet 174:181–188, 1992.

139. Reese JL, Means ME, Hanrahan K, et al: Diarrhea associated with nasogastric feedings. Oncol Nurs Forum 23:59–66, 1995.

140. Homann HH, Kemen M, Fuessenich C, et al: Reduction in diarrhea incidence by soluble fiber in patients receiving total or supplemental enteral nutrition. JPEN J Parenter Enteral Nutr 18:486–490, 1994.

141. Godeberge P: Hepato-biliary complications in enteral nutrition. Ann Gastroenterol Hepatol (Paris) 24:301–303, 1988.

142. Schwesinger WH, Page CP, Strodel WE, et al: Biliary sludge formation during enteral nutrition: Prevalence and nature history. Surgery 124:768–772, 1998.

143. Hsu TC, Leu SC, Su CF, et al: Assessment of intragastric pH value changes after early nasogastric feeding. Nutrition 16:751–754, 2000.

144. Bonten MJ, Gaillard CA, vand er Geest S, et al: The role of intragastric acidity and stress ulcus prophylaxis on colonization and infection in mechanically ventilated ICU patients. A stratified, randomized, double-blind study of sucralfate versus antacids. Am J Respir Crit Care Med 152:1825–1834, 1995.

145. Cook D, Jonghe BD, Heyland D: The relation between nutrition and nosocomial pneumonia: randomized trials in critically ill patients. Crit Care (Lond) 1:3–9, 1997.

146. Napolitano LM, Wagle M, Heard SO: Endoscopic placement of

nasoenteric feeding tubes in critically ill patients: Reliable alternative. J Laparoendosc Adv Surg Tech A 8:395–400, 1998.

147. Torres A, El-Ebiary M, Soler N, et al: Stomach as a source of colonization of the respiratory tract during mechanical ventilation: Association with ventilator-associated pneumonia. Eur Respir J 9:1729–1735, 1996.

148. Faintuch J, Garcia Soriano F, Ladeira JP, et al: Refeeding procedures after 43 days of total fasting. Nutrition 17:100–104, 2001.

149. Marik PE, Bedigian MK: Refeeding hypophosphatemia in critically ill patients in an intensive care unit. A prospective study. Arch Surg 131:1043–1047, 1996.

150. Noordenbos J, Hansbrough JF, Gutmacher H, et al: Enteral nutritional support and wound excision and closure do not prevent postburn hypermetabolism as measured by continuous metabolic monitoring. J Trauma 49:667–672, 2000.

151. Richardson RA, Davidson HI, Hinds A, et al: Influence of the metabolic sequelae of liver cirrhosis on nutritional intake. Am J Clin Nutr 69:331–337, 1999.

152. Muller MJ, Bottcher J, Selberg O, et al: Hypermetabolism in clinically stable patients with liver cirrhosis. Am J Clin Nutr 69:1194–1201, 1999.

153. Bugianesi E, Kalhan S, Burkett E, et al: Quantification of gluconogenesis in cirrhosis: Response to glucagon. Gastroenterology 115:1530–1540, 1998.

154. Petersen KF, Krssak M, Navarro V, et al: Contributions of net hepatic glycogenolysis and gluconeogenesis to glucose production in cirrhosis. Am J Physiol 276:E529–E535, 1999.

155. Schneider P, Gillet M, Jequier E, et al: Hepatic non-oxidative disposal of an oral glucose meal in patients with liver cirrhosis. Metabolism 48:1260–1266, 1999.

156. Clemmesen JO, Hoy CE, Jeppesen PB, et al: Plasma phospholipid fatty acid pattern in severe liver disease. J Hepatol 32:481–487, 1999.

157. Merli M, Leonetti F, Riggio O, et al: Glucose intolerance and insulin resistance in cirrhosis are normalized after liver transplantation. Hepatology 30:649–654, 1999.

158. Perseghin G, Mazzaferro V, Sereni LP, et al: Contribution of reduced insulin sensitivity and secretion to the pathogenesis of hepatogenous diabetes: Effect of liver transplantation. Hepatology 3:694–703, 2000.

159. Shetty A, Wilson S, Kuo P, Laurin JL, et al: Liver transplantation improves cirrhosis-associated impaired oral glucose tolerance. Transplantation 69:2451–2454, 2000.

160. Konrad T, Steinmuller T, Vicini P, et al: Evidence for impaired glucose effectiveness in cirrhotic patients after lifer transplantation. Metabolism 49:367–372, 2000.

161. Borum ML, Lynn J, Zhong Z, et al: The effect of nutritional supplementation on survival in seriously ill hospitalized adults: An evaluation of the SUPPORT data. Study to Understand Prognoses and Preferences for Outcomes and Risks of Treatments. J Am Geriatr Soc 48:S33–S38, 2000.

162. Manji S, Shikora S, McMahon M, et al: Peritoneal dialysis for acute renal failure: Overfeeding resulting from dextrose absorbed during dialysis. Crit Care Med 18:29–31, 1990.

163. Lochs H, Plauth M: Liver cirrhosis: Rationale and modalities for nutritional support—the European Society of Parenteral and Enteral Nutrition consensus and beyond. Curr Opin Clin Nutr Metab Care 2:345–349, 1999.

164. Druml W: Protein metabolism in acute renal failure. Miner Electrolyte Metab 24:47–54, 1998.

165. Alverstrand A: Nutritional aspects in patients with acute renal failure/multiorgan failure. Blood Purif 14:109–114, 1996.

166. Macias WL, Alaka KJ, Murphy MH, et al: Impact of the nutritional regimen on protein catabolism and nitrogen balance in patients with acute renal failure. JPEN J Parenter Enteral Nutr 20:56–62, 1996.

167. Frankenfield DC, Reynolds HN: Nutritional effect of continuous hemofiltration. Nutrition 11:388–393, 1995.

168. Druml W: Amino acid losses during intradialytic parenteral nutrition. Am J Clin Nutr 72:1237–1239, 2000.

169. Fortin MC, Amyot SL, Geadah D, et al: Serum concentrations and clearances of folic acid and pyridoxal-5-phosphate during venovenous continuous renal replacement therapy. Intensive Care Med 25:594–598, 1999.

170. Serna-Thome MG, Padilllla-Rosciano AE, Suchil-Bernal L: Practical aspects of intradialytic nutritional support. Curr Opin Clin Nutr Metab Care 5:293–296, 2002.

171. Manji S, Shikora S, McMahon M, et al: Peritoneal dialysis for acute renal failure: Overfeeding resulting from dextrose absorbed during dialysis. Crit Care Med 18:29–31, 1990.

172. Monaghan R, Watters JM, Clancey SM, et al: Uptake of glucose during continuous arteriovenous hemofiltration. Crit Care Med 21:1159–1163, 1993.

173. Rudolph FB, Van Buren T: The metabolic effects of enterally administered ribonucleic acids. Curr Opin Clin Nutr Metab Care 1:527–530, 1998.

174. Heys SD, Walker LG, Smith I, et al: Enteral nutritional supplementation with key nutrients in patients with critical illness and cancer: A meta-analysis of randomized controlled clinical trials. Ann Surg 229:467–477, 1999.

175. Jolliet P, Pichard C: Immunonutrition in the critically ill. Intens Care Med 25:631–633, 1999.

176. Galban C, Montejo JC, Mesejo A, et al: An immune-enhancing enteral diet reduces mortality rate and episodes of bacteremia in septic intensive care unit patients. Crit Care Med 28:643–648, 2000.

177. Beale RJ, Bryg DJ, Bihari DJ: Immunonutrition in the critically ill: A systemic review of clinical outcome. Crit Care Med 27:2799–2805, 1999.

178. Riso S, Aluffi P, Brugnani M, et al: Postoperative enteral immunonutrition in head and neck cancer patients. Clin Nutr 19:407–412, 2000.

179. Nutrition intervention in ICU improves outcomes. Health Benchmarks 5:175–176, 1998.

180. Heyland DK, MacDonald S, Keele L, et al: Total parenteral nutrition in the critically ill patient. JAMA 280:2013–2019, 1998.

181. Heyland DK, Montalvo M, MacDonald S, et al: Total parenteral nutrition in the surgical patient: A meta-analysis. Can J Surg 44:102–111, 2001.

47

Hypothalamic-Pituitary-Adrenal Axis

Christopher D. John, BSc, PhD • Elizabeth Theogaraj, BSc • Michael Schachter, BSc, MB • Julia C. Buckingham, BSc, PhD

Mechanisms of Action of Glucocorticoids
    Synthesis, Secretion, and Metabolism
    Molecular Basis of Glucocorticoid Action
    Systemic Effects of Glucocorticoids
Clinical Pharmacology of the Glucocorticoids
    Clinical Uses
    Selectivity and Unwanted Effects
    Pharmacokinetics of Glucocorticoids
    Anti-inflammatory and Immunosuppressive
        Actions
Mechanisms of Secretion of Glucocorticoids
    Role of the Hypothalamic-Pituitary Complex
    Stress-Induced Activation of the Hypothalamus
    Feedback Control of the Hypothalamic-Pituitary-
        Adrenal Axis
    Adaptive Responses to Repeated or Sustained
        Stress
Age- and Sex-Related Changes in Hypothalamic-
Pituitary-Adrenal Function
    Developmental Changes

Glucocorticoids and Perinatal Programming
Sex-Related Factors
Pregnancy-Related Factors
Age-Related Factors
Effect of Surgery on Hypothalamic-Pituitary-
Adrenal Function
    Serum Cortisol Levels During and After
        Surgery
    Adaptation of the Stress Response to
        Surgery
    Effect of Anesthesia on the HPA Axis
Practical Aspects of Drug Administration
    Hydrocortisone
    Prednisolone
    Betamethasone
    Dexamethasone
    Methylprednisolone
    Triamcinolone

The hypothalamic-pituitary-adrenal (HPA) axis is a hormonal circuit consisting of the hypothalamus in the brain, the pituitary gland, and the adrenal glands. This circuit is responsible for the production of glucocorticoids (principally cortisol in humans and corticosterone in rodents), and steroid hormones that exert widespread effects critical to the maintenance of homeostasis during physical and emotional stress. Cortisol (hydrocortisone), the principal glucocorticoid in man, and its synthetic analogs are widely used in clinical medicine mainly to suppress inflammation and immune function, and in replacement therapy for adrenocortical insufficiency. This chapter briefly reviews the physiologic and pharmacologic characteristics of glucocorticoids, in addition to the neuroendocrine mechanisms that control their secretion, with particular reference to the impact of surgery.

Mechanisms of Action of Glucocorticoids

Synthesis, Secretion, and Metabolism

Glucocorticoids are produced in the zona fasciculata of the cortex of the adrenal gland under the direction of adrenocorticotropic hormone (ACTH). This pituitary hormone facilitates the rate-limiting step in the biosynthetic pathway that governs conversion of cholesterol to pregnenolone, an intermediate compound in the synthesis of steroid hormones.[1,2] The newly synthesized steroid is not stored in the adrenal gland to any great degree but diffuses rapidly into the bloodstream where it is transported, bound largely to corticosteroid-binding globulin (CBG) (95%) and albumin. Cortisol (Fig. 47–1) is inactivated in the liver. The principal step is reduction of the A ring and, after other modifications, conjugation. The resulting tetrahydro-metabolites are excreted in the urine and through the bile. Although the serum half-life of cortisol is approximately 90 minutes, its biologic actions persist for several hours.[1,2]

Molecular Basis of Glucocorticoid Action

The actions of glucocorticoids are exerted largely through cytoplasmic receptors that belong to the superfamily of "nuclear receptors." When stimulated by ligand, these receptors initiate specific changes in the transcription of deoxyribonucleic acid (DNA) and, hence, the synthesis of proteins. In many instances, the activated steroid-receptor complex induces or represses transcription directly by binding to specific response elements on the promoter region of target genes.[3] In other instances, however, the activated receptor may interfere with the activity of other transcription factors,[3] for example, activator protein 1 or nuclear transcription factor κB. In addition, the activated receptor may regulate post-transcriptional events, including stability of the transcription of messenger ribonucleic acid (RNA), translation of RNA, and post-translational processing of the protein. In light of all these mechanisms, most of the biologic responses to glucocorticoids are slow to emerge. Some, however, are apparent almost immediately after steroid administration and may involve largely unexplored actions of the drugs on cell membranes.[1] For example, cortisol induces hyperpolarization of hippocampal neurons within 1 to 2 minutes of contact.

Two distinct subclasses of intracellular corticosteroid receptors have been identified: the mineralocorticoid receptor (MR) and the glucocorticoid receptor (GR). MRs have a discrete pattern of distribution (e.g., in the distal renal tubule and hippocampus) and a high and approximately equal affinity for cortisol and the mineralocorticoid aldosterone (dissociation constant [Kd] ≈1–2 nM). In contrast, GRs are widely expressed throughout the body, have only a low affinity for cortisol (Kd ≈10–20 nM), and do not bind aldosterone; the GR is, therefore, glucocorticoid selective.[4] A truncated form of this receptor, called GR-β, which binds DNA but not ligand, has also been identified.[3]

Because glucocorticoids in the systemic circulation are largely bound to proteins, in principle only free steroid has ready access to receptors in target cells. However, local mechanisms that "release" the steroid from its carrier protein(s) and thereby facilitate entry of the steroid into cells appear to exist in at least some target tissues, most notably areas of inflammation. Access of the steroids to their receptors is further regulated within the target cells by 11β-hydroxysteroid dehydrogenase (11β-HSD), an enzyme that controls the interconversion of cortisol (active) and cortisone (inert).[5] 11β-HSD exists in at least two isoforms, 11β-HSD-1 and 11β-HSD-2, both of which are expressed in a tissue-specific manner. 11β-HSD-2 acts primarily as a dehydrogenase and promptly inactivates cortisol when it enters target cells. It thus protects the high-affinity MRs in tissues such as the distal renal tubule, thereby permitting selective access of aldosterone to these receptors.[5] MRs not protected in this way (e.g., those in the hippocampus) are almost fully occupied by cortisol, even at the nadir of the circadian rhythm. They thus play an important role in mediating the actions of low levels of cortisol. In contrast, GRs, which have relatively low affinity, are normally only occupied when levels of glucocorticoids increase systemically (e.g., after stress or administration of glucocorticoids) or locally (i.e., in hepatocytes) through 11β-HSD-1–dependent conversion of cortisone to cortisol. A further important deter-

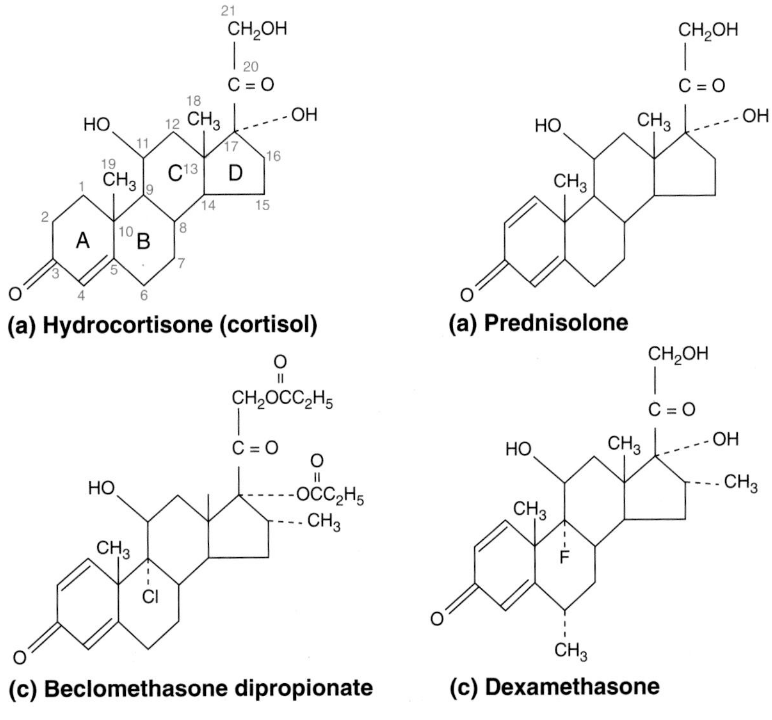

(a) Hydrocortisone (cortisol)

(a) Prednisolone

(c) Beclomethasone dipropionate

(c) Dexamethasone

Figure 47–1. Structures of selected glucocorticoids.

minant of the responsiveness of GRs is the concentration of receptors, which is known to fluctuate during development and the cell cycle and after disturbances in endocrine status.[3]

Systemic Effects of Glucocorticoids

The glucocorticoids produce diverse effects that influence a great variety of physiologic functions (Table 47–1).[1,3] These steroids are powerful catabolic agents that promote the breakdown of carbohydrates, proteins, and fats, and thus partially antagonize the physiologic effects of insulin. The glucocorticoids are also important regulators of the immune and inflammatory processes that are necessary for host defense. In addition, the glucocorticoids have complex effects on bone, they exert both positive and negative effects on cell growth, and they modulate blood pressure. Within the central nervous system, glucocorticoids target both neuronal and glial cells. During prenatal and postnatal development, they produce important organizational effects on the brain, and, in adulthood, they contribute to neuronal plasticity and the processes of neural degeneration. Other central effects include complex changes in mood and behavior, antipyresis, and modulation of neuroendocrine function.

In the last decade two types of activities have been ascribed to glucocorticoids with regard to their crucial role in maintenance of homeostasis during severe stress.[1,4,6,7] These are termed *permissive or proactive* and *suppressive or protective*. The permissive actions occur at low physiologic levels of the steroid and serve to prepare the body for responding to, and coping with, stress. Importantly, they

TABLE 47–1.

Responses to Acute and Long-Term Increases in Glucocorticoid Secretion/Activity

System	Acute	Long Term
a. Host defense	Protection from potentially harmful inflammatory mediators	Immunosuppression and vulnerability to infection Poor tissue repair/wound healing
b. Metabolism	Mobilization of energy stores ($\uparrow$ glycogen stores, $\uparrow$ gluconeogenes, $\uparrow$ blood glucose, $\uparrow$ lipolysis, $\uparrow$ protein catabolism, $\downarrow$ peripheral glucose uptake/utilization)	Insulin-resistant "steroid" diabetes mellitus Centripetal obesity, moonface Protein depletion in muscle, connective, and other tissues
c. Musculoskeletal	Protein catabolism Altered Ca^{2+} homeostatis	Increased serum lipids and cholesterol (see b.) Impaired growth Muscle wasting Loss of connective tissue (see a.) Osteoporosis and disturbed Ca^{2+} homeostasis
d. Central nervous system	Improved cognitive function	Mood changes (depression and psychotic episodes) Neurodegeneration
e. Cardiovascular	Salt and water retention Inhibition of the production of vasoactive inflammatory mediators (see a.)	Hypertension and other cardiovascular disease
f. Reproductive	Inhibition of hypothalamo-pituitary-gonadal function	Menstrual irregularities Infertility (male and female)
g. Gastrointestinal tract	Reduced bicarbonate and mucus production	Increased susceptibility to ulcers

maintain the basal activity of the HPA axis by providing negative feedback and by setting the threshold for a response to stress, thereby ensuring an appropriate cortisol response. Permissive actions also prime the human body's defense mechanisms. For example, permissive actions facilitate the effects of catecholamines on lipid and carbohydrate metabolism; up-regulate the expression of receptors for inflammatory mediators; and act centrally to aid the processes underlying selection attention, integration of sensory information, and response selection.

The "protective" mode is initiated when glucocorticoid levels become elevated. Key to this mode are the powerful anti-inflammatory and immunosuppressive actions of the steroids that prevent the host-defense mechanisms activated in stress from overshooting and damaging the organism.[6,7] Other important protective actions include the ability of the steroids to redirect metabolism to meet energy demands during stress, to exert important effects within the brain on memory processes, and to impair nonessential activities such as growth and reproduction.

The permissive and protective actions of the glucocorticoids are complementary and enable the organism to mount an appropriate stress response and to maintain homeostasis. Dysregulation of these actions by genetic, environmental, or other factors is potentially harmful and may predispose the individual to a variety of diseases. Long-term increases in serum glucocorticoids, which may result from chronic stress, Cushing syndrome, depression, drug therapy, and other events, are particularly hazardous and may have severe, deleterious effects on the body (see Table 47–1). Equally important is adrenal insufficiency—caused perhaps by Addison disease or congenital adrenal hyperplasia—which can lead to an increased white blood cell count, lymphoid tissue hypertrophy, hypotension, depression, weakness, lethargy, hypoglycemia, and other pathologic conditions. Patients with adrenal insufficiency are highly vulnerable to stress and, unless protected by administration of exogenous glucocorticoids, may experience a potentially fatal "adrenal crisis" characterized by a sudden decrease in blood pressure.

Clinical Pharmacology of the Glucocorticoids

Clinical Uses

Glucocorticoids are given principally for replacement therapy in adrenal insufficiency and for control of autoimmune and inflammatory disease. They also have an important place in the treatment of cerebral edema, anaphylactic shock, angioedema, and certain leukemias, and in the control of tissue rejection in patients who received a transplant. In addition, glucocorticoids are given acutely in surgery to protect patients at risk for adrenocortical insufficiency, and in high doses to mothers at risk for premature labor, to mature the fetal lung in preparation for extrauterine life. Table 47–2 provides details of steroid preparations commonly used in clinical medicine.

Selectivity and Unwanted Effects

Glucocorticoids produce few unwanted effects when given acutely or in appropriate doses for long-term replacement therapy. However, when given systemically in the relatively high doses required to quell inflammation or produce immunosuppression, these steroids cause a broad spectrum of detrimental effects (Table 47–3). In essence, they induce a dose-dependent "iatrogenic Cushing syndrome" and other effects that are not related to dose, for example, increased risk for peptic ulcers. Hydrocortisone (cortisol) is particularly problematic, because it has significant mineralocorticoid activity and therefore causes sodium and water retention and hypokalemia.

Studies on the relation between structure and activity (see Fig. 47–1) have shown that introduction of a double bond between C-1 and C-2 (prednisolone) and a methyl group at C-6α (methylprednisolone), C-16α (dexamethasone), or C-16β (betamethasone) reduces mineralocorticoid activity.[8] Further substitution of the fluoride (dexamethasone, betamethasone, or chloride beclomethasone) group at C-9α increases glucocorticoid activity. Dexamethasone, betamethasone, and beclomethasone are thus potent anti-inflammatory and immunosuppressive drugs that have negligible mineralocorticoid activity.[8]

Pharmacokinetics of Glucocorticoids

At low to moderate doses, hydrocortisone and prednisolone bind mainly to CBG and weakly to albumin; at greater doses, however, CBG becomes saturated, and the concentration of free steroid increases in the blood.[8] Conversely, methylprednisolone, dexamethasone, betamethasone, and beclomethasone do not bind to CBG, although they do bind weakly to albumin.[8] The presence of the double bond between C-1 and C-2 (prednisolone and methylprednisolone) provides resistance to degradation and thus extends the half-life of the molecule. Resistance to degradation is increased further by the introduction of a halogen group (fluoride or chloride) at C-9α (dexamethasone, betamethasone, and beclomethasone[8]).

Anti-inflammatory and Immunosuppressive Actions

Glucocorticoids attenuate both the early and the late stages of inflammation, i.e., they suppress not only initial vasodilation, infiltration of leukocytes, and pain but also the proliferative events associated with wound healing and tissue repair. These steroids also oppose the changes in vascular permeability that occur in inflammation and thus reduce edema formation. In addition, glucocorticoids are potent inhibitors of immune responses mediated by T cells and may also modulate humoral responses mediated by B cells.[9] These actions reflect the powerful influence of the steroids on the growth, differentiation, distribution, and function of monocytes, macrophages, polymorphonuclear leukocytes, and lymphocytes. At the cellular level, glucocorticoids

TABLE 47–2.

Steroid Preparations Commonly Used in Clinical Medicine

Drug	Dose	Duration	Administration	Indication	Side Effects
Dexamethasone sodium phosphate (4 mg/mL)	4 mg	4 times a day over 2–3 days	IV bolus or infusion IM (if vein cannot be found)	Symptoms of chemotherapy, e.g., nausea and vomiting	Prolonged use in intra-articular injections can lead to joint destruction and other systemic effects such as adrenal suppression.
	10 mg intravenously, then 4 mg intramuscularly every 6 hours	4 times a day between 2 and 10 days	IV bolus or infusion IM (if vein cannot be found)	Head injury with cerebral edema, also acute edema caused by tumors	Cardiovascular effects may include sodium and water retention and hypertension
	0.5–20 mg	4 times in 24 hours	IM, IV, or infusion	Suppression of inflammatory and allergic disorders; primary or secondary adrenocortical insufficiency; intra-articular disorders such as rheumatoid arthritis, skin disorders, infection, e.g., endotoxic shock. Neurologic disorders such as increased intracranial pressure secondary cerebral to cerebral tumors	Gastrointestinal effects include dyspepsia, peptic ulceration, esophageal ulceration Musculoskeletal effects include proximal myopathy, osteoporosis, and long bone fractures. Neuropsychiatric effects include depression, insomnia, psychosis, and aggravation of schizophrenia and epilepsy.
	200 µg/kg/day 100 µg/kg/day 50 µg/kg/day	*5-day course:* 3 days 1 day 1 day	IV IV IV	Wean babies off a ventilator	Endocrine effects include adrenal suppression, hirsutism, hypokalemia, diabetes, menstrual irregularities; increased susceptibility to and severity of infection. Ophthalmic effects include corneal and scleral thinning and glaucoma.

TABLE 47–2.

Steroid Preparations Commonly Used in Clinical Medicine—cont'd

Drug	Dose	Duration	Administration	Indication	Side Effects
Betamethasone sodium phosphate (4 mg/mL) Soluble in 1 in 2 of water, 1 in 470 of alcohol; insoluble in acetone or chloroform	12 mg	Twice a day to the mother	IM	Threatened premature delivery	General side effects include suppression of the mother's HPA axis.
	Betamethasone sodium phosphate (0.1%)	2–3 drops every 2–3 hours; frequency reduced when relief is seen	In the ear, eyes, and nose	Eczematous inflammation in otitis externa and other allergic or inflammatory conditions of the eyes and nose	
		0.5–5 mg daily	Mouth	Suppression of inflammatory and allergic disorders	
		4–20 mg repeated up to 4 times a day in 24 hours	IV, IM, or infusion		
		4–8 mg repeated 3 or 4 times in 24 hours depending on severity of condition	Local injection into soft tissues	Relieve the pain and stiffness of rheumatoid arthritis and other forms of joint inflammation	
Betamethasone benzoate dipropionate and valerate esters	Topical application 0.025% of betamethasone benzoate; 0.05% of dipropionate; and 0.025% or 0.1% valerate	As indicated by the physician	Cream or gel	Skin complaints as eczema and psoriasis	Other side effects include skin atrophy, acne, impaired healing.

	Dose	Route	Use	Comments
Beclomethasone Dipropionate	Starting dose is dependent on severity of their disease; usual starting dose for adults is 200 µg; in a severe case, dose can be increased to 600–800 µg	Oral inhalation (aerosol)	Preventative treatment for asthma, anti-inflammatory	Bronchospasm can occur with an immediate increase in wheezing after dosing. In some patients, candidiasis of the mouth and throat can occur. In overdose, temporary adrenal suppression may occur.
	400 µg	2 sprays into each nostril twice	Intranasal route (Aqueous nasal spray)	Prophylaxis and treatment of perennial and seasonal allergic rhinitis including hayfever, and vasomotor rhinitis	As with other nasal sprays, there can be dryness and irritation of the nose and throat. Overdose can rarely result in the suppression of the HPA axis.
Hydrocortisone Cream		A thin layer of cream applied to the affected area 2-3 times a day; treatment should be limited to 10–14 days and up to 7 days if applied to the face	Skin	Eczema and dermatitis of all types including atopic eczema, photodermatitis, primary irritant and allergic dermatitis, prurigo, and insect bite reactions.	Burning sensation and itching can occur at the site of application. Long-term use can lead to permanent thinning of the skin and rarely to adrenal suppression.
Hydrocortisone 10-mg tablets	20–30 mg	Daily	Mouth	Adrenal replacement therapy in deficiency states	Same as for Dexamethasone
Hydrocortisone sodium phosphate (100 mg/mL)	100–500 mg	3–4 times a day in 24 hr	IM, IV, or infusion	Injections may also be given to relieve severe attacks of asthma.	Same as for Dexamethasone

TABLE 47–2.

Steroid Preparations Commonly Used in Clinical Medicine—cont'd

Drug	Dose	Duration	Administration	Indication	Side Effects
Hydrocortisone acetate	adults 5–50 mg children 5–30 mg	daily	Intra-articular or periarticular injection	Arthritic conditions such as rheumatoid arthritis and osteoarthritis and also used for inflamed tendon sheaths	
Hydrocortisone succinate	100 mg	6–8 hours	IV	Acute adrenal insufficiency	
Prednisolone sodium phosphate	0.5% sodium phosphate w/v. Neomycin Sulphate EP 0.5% w/v	1 or 2 drops for the eye 6 times a day and 2 or 3 drops instilled into each ear 3 or 4 times daily	Drops applied to the eye and ear	Short-term treatment of steroid responsive conditions of the eye when prophylactic antibiotic treatment is also required, after excluding the presence of fungal and viral disease; also used to treat otitis externa	Same as for Dexamethasone
	20 mg	1 enema used nightly for 2–4 weeks	Rectal	Rectal and rectosigmoidal disease in ulcerative colitis and Chron disease	
	30–60 mg	Daily for a few days once the attack has been controlled	Oral taken in the morning after breakfast	Acute attacks of asthma	Same as for Dexamethasone
Prednisolone acetate	25–100 mg	Once or twice weekly	IM, injection into joints	Acute lymphoblastic leukemia; rheumatoid arthritis and other forms of arthritis	

It is very important that all patients carry "steroid treatment cards" that give clear guidance on the precautions to be taken to minimize risk and that provide details of prescriber, drug, dosage, and the duration of treatment. (ABPI Merck Sharp & Dohme).

HPA, hypothalamic-pituitary-adrenal; IM, intramuscular; IV, intravenous.

TABLE 47–3.

Unwanted Effects of Prolonged Systemic Treatment with Supraphysiologic Doses of Glucocorticoids

Dose-dependent effects
- Na^+ and H_2O retention, K^+ loss (mineralocorticoid action)
- Hyperglycemia, glucose intolerance, "steroid diabetes"
- Redistribution of fat, moon face, buffalo hump, centripetal obesity
- Muscle wasting, particularly in limbs
- Suppression of the HPA axis
- Collagen loss → thin skin, easy bruising
- Impaired wound healing
- Immunosuppression and increased susceptibility to infection
- Osteoporosis
- Menstrual irregularities
- Growth retardation

Dose-independent effects
- Mood swings, psychoses
- Increased risk for peptic ulcers
- Increased risk for cataracts and glaucoma
- Benign intracranial hypertension
- Hypertension
- Acute pancreatitis

Steroid withdrawal
- Withdrawal "syndrome" characterized by rheumatoid symptoms
- Sustained HPA suppression*

*The hypothalamic-pituitary-adrenal (HPA) axis may take weeks or even months to recover from long-term steroid treatment. During this phase, patients are unable to respond appropriately to stress and should if necessary be given exogenous steroids for "protection," for example, in surgery. If possible, steroid should be withdrawn slowly by reducing the dose over a period of months.

reduce the number of circulating lymphocytes, monocytes, and eosinophils by causing the cells to "marginate" to the lymphoid tissues, particularly the bone marrow. In contrast, the concentration of neutrophils in the blood increases as the steroids inhibit migration of the cells into inflamed tissues, apparently by reducing the expression of adhesion factors on the cell surface and thereby impairing the processes of adhesion and attachment. The profile of circulating white blood cells is also influenced by the fact that glucocorticoids induce apoptosis of thymocytes, mature T cells, and eosinophils, but not neutrophils.[2,9]

Glucocorticoids suppress cell-mediated immunity in three ways: (1) They direct the development of undifferentiated T helper (Th0) cells away from the Th1 phenotype, an action that is critical to cell-mediated responses, and toward the Th2 phenotype, an action that facilitates B

lymphocyte–dependent responses. (2) They inhibit the synthesis of interleukin (IL)-1 and IL-2 by antigen presentation and T cells, respectively; this impairs antigen presentation and T cell proliferation. (3) They induce T cell apoptosis.[9,10] The resulting inhibition of alloreactive and cytotoxic T cell proliferation provides the basis for treatment of allograft rejection, autoimmune disorders, and human leukemias with glucocorticoids. High doses of glucocorticoids may also depress the synthesis of cytokines required for synthesis of immunoglobulins and, with time, may decrease serum immunoglobulins. Lower doses of glucocorticoids may have a positive effect on production of antibodies, probably because of the positive effect of such doses on Th2 cells.

Other immune cell functions influenced by glucocorticoids include phagocytosis and processing of antigens. Glucocorticoids decrease expression of Fc receptors on macrophages and thus prevent the recognition of particulate antigens that are bound to antibodies or opsonized for subsequent clearance. Glucocorticoids also affect mast cell and basophil function by inhibiting IgE-dependent degranulation, and hence the release of histamine and leukotriene C4. In addition, the steroids impair fibroblast function, thereby reducing the production of collagen, glycosaminoglycans, and other components of the extracellular matrix.[9,10]

At the biochemical level, the diverse effects of glucocorticoids on immune and inflammatory cell function result from not only their impact on synthesis of cytokines but also their striking ability to inhibit the synthesis, release, and activity of the army of other mediators produced by activated immune or inflammatory cells. Particular emphasis has been placed on two of their abilities. First, glucocorticoids inhibit the generation of eicosanoids (prostanoids, leukotrienes, and epoxides) and platelet-activating factor by inhibiting the enzyme phospholipase A2. Second, glucocorticoids further suppress production of prostanoids by repressing the expression of the inducible form of cyclooxygenase, which is normally expressed in abundance by activated macrophages, fibroblasts, and endothelial cells. The release of other inflammatory mediators is also suppressed by the powerful actions of the steroids on the enzymes responsible for synthesis or degradation of the mediators. For example, glucocorticoids inhibit the generation of nitric oxide by suppressing the expression of the inducible form of nitric oxide synthase but promote the degradation of nonlipid inflammatory mediators by up-regulating the enzymes responsible for the breakdown of such mediators.[2,11] Further important actions of the glucocorticoids include reductions in the following: serum complement components, acute phase proteins and heat shock proteins (notably HSP70), release of mediators such as serotonin, and production or activity of proteolytic enzymes (e.g., elastase and collagenase), which occur in the late stages of inflammation.[2,10,11]

Mechanisms of Secretion of Glucocorticoids

Cortisol is released from the adrenal gland in an episodic manner. Although the frequency of pulses is normally fairly constant over a 24-hour period, the pulses change in amplitude; as a result, serum levels of cortisol follow a circadian rhythm. Increases in the amplitude of the pulses also underpin the increases in serum cortisol elicited by stressful stimuli, although, in some instances, the frequency of the pulses may also change.[11] This circadian rhythm is linked to the sleep/wake cycle, with maximal levels (140–180 ng/mL) occurring just before waking and the lowest levels (20–40 ng/mL) occurring 8 to 10 hours later. Significant changes in this profile occur in subjects whose sleep patterns have been disrupted, for example, by shift work or travel through time zones. Stress-induced changes in serum levels of cortisol are superimposed on the circadian tone and vary in onset, magnitude, and duration depending on the nature, intensity, and duration of the stress.[11]

Role of the Hypothalamic-Pituitary Complex

Synthesis of cortisol is governed mainly by ACTH, a polypeptide hormone secreted by the anterior pituitary gland. ACTH is synthesized in specialized cells (corticotrophs) by post-translational cleavage of a precursor molecule, pro-opiomelanocortin (POMC). POMC also gives rise to a number of other peptides that are released along with ACTH. Notably, some of these peptides (e.g., γ-melanocyte–stimulating hormone) also exert regulatory effects on adrenal function that augment the production of steroids.[11]

The secretion of ACTH by corticotrophs in the anterior pituitary gland is governed largely by two hypothalamic neurohormones that act synergistically: corticotropin-releasing hormone (CRH)[12] and arginine vasopressin (AVP)[13] (Fig. 47–2). These peptides are synthesized in parvocellular neurons that project from the median PVN (PVN) to the external lamina of the median eminence. The peptides are then secreted into the hypothalamo-hypophyseal portal vessels for transport to the anterior pituitary gland. The concentration of CRH and AVP in hypophyseal portal blood is thus high (compared with that in peripheral blood) and alters in parallel with perturbations of pituitary-adrenal function (e.g., stress). CRH and AVP show some degree of colocalization in secretory granules and may therefore be cosecreted. However, AVP is not normally expressed by all CRH-positive neurons, and the ratio of AVP:CRH released may thus vary in a stimulus-specific manner.[2,11]

The actions of CRH and AVP on the corticotrophs are brought about by specific, G protein–coupled receptors, i.e., type 1 CRH receptors and V1b AVP receptors, which are

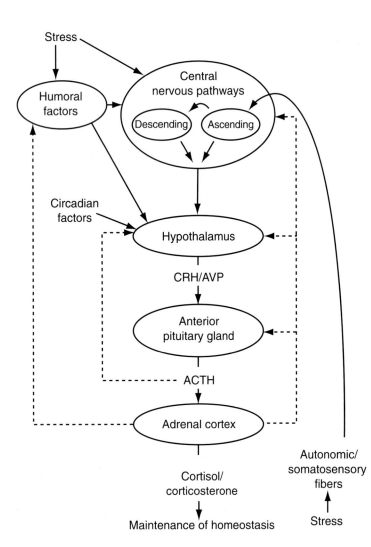

Figure 47–2. Schematic diagram illustrating the mechanisms controlling the activity of the hypothalamo-pituitary-adrenal (HPA) axis. CRH = corticotrophin releasing hormone; AVP = arginine vasopressin; ACTH = adrenocorticotrophic hormone; intact line = stimulatory pathway; dotted line = inhibitory pathway.

positively coupled to adenylyl cyclase and phospholipase C, respectively. Although release of ACTH is readily triggered by activation of either receptor, the response is modest compared with that from stimulation of both receptors. The biochemical basis of this synergism, which plays an important role in determining the level of ACTH release in vivo, is poorly defined. There is evidence, however, that activation of V1b AVP receptors potentiates CRH-induced cyclic adenosine monophosphate, possibly by a protein kinase C–dependent mechanism. Notably, the synergistic actions of CRH and AVP are directed only toward release of ACTH and the ability of CRH to augment POMC gene expression and, in the longer term, cause proliferation of corticotrophs is unaffected by AVP which, alone, does not affect these parameters.[2,11]

In addition to being expressed in the parvocellular neurons, which project from the PVN to the external lamina of the median eminence, CRH is expressed elsewhere in the central nervous system. Within the hypothalamus, it is found in magnocellular neurons that project from the posterior PVN and the supraoptic nucleus to the posterior pituitary gland and also at loci within the PVN that are concerned with the regulation of autonomic outflow. Other important sites of CRH production include the limbic system, particularly the amygdala, and the cortex. Functional studies have shown that, in addition to playing a key role in triggering ACTH release, CRH is critical to the manifestation of the behavioral and autonomic responses to stress and to the concomitant suppression of the growth hormone and pituitary gonadal axes. Indeed, CRH is sometimes termed the *executive organizer* of the stress response.

Stress-Induced Activation of the Hypothalamus

The parvocellular CRH and AVP neurons in the hypothalamus receive inputs from many ascending and descending nerve pathways. In addition, the neurons are sensitive to a variety of substances in the blood and cerebrospinal fluid (e.g., glucose and steroids) and to local factors released from glial cells or interneurons (e.g., eicosanoids and cytokines). Major roles in the stress-induced activation of the hypothalamus have been identified for the following: (1) pathways projecting to the PVN from the prefrontal cortex and the limbic system (hippocampus, amygdala, lateral septum, and the bed nucleus of the stria terminalis); and (2) inputs from the brain stem nuclei, in particular the nucleus tractus solitarius, which relay sensory information directly to the PVN (through the ventral noradrenergic bundle) and to other parts of the brain.[11,14] Other pathways—for example, those arising from the raphe nuclei—are also likely to contribute.[11]

The precise complement of neural pathways, humoral substances, and local mediators that orchestrates the release of CRH and AVP during stress almost certainly depends on the nature of the stimulus and the physical state of the individual at the time of stress. However, animal data now make it possible to classify the process according to the type of stress. For example, visceral "homeostatic" stressors that lack a cognitive component (e.g., acute hypotension) promote the release of ACTH by activating afferents fibers

that send signals to the PVN through the brain stem nuclei and ventral noradrenergic pathways. Stressors that have a significant cognitive component (e.g., foot shock, restraint, or cold) send additional signals to the PVN through the cortical-limbic system. The cortical-limbic system also plays a fundamental role in eliciting the HPA responses to emotional stressors. The role of the amygdala—a key area in coordinating the behavioral, autonomic, and neuroendocrine responses to fear or anxiety—is well documented in this regard, as is the importance of the hippocampus to cognitive function and particularly learning and memory. A further subgroup of homeostatic stressors also invoke humoral mechanisms; for example, the responses to hypertonicity and hypoglycemia involve intrahypothalamic osmotic- and glucose-sensitive neurons, respectively.

Challenges to the host defense system, such as those provoked by infection, injury, or inflammation, pose a major threat to homeostasis and thus constitute severe stresses. Not surprisingly, such challenges markedly increase activity of the HPA axis in both animals and humans. This response is triggered primarily by the army of products released from the activated immune or inflammatory cells (e.g., interleukins, eicosanoids, histamine, and phospholipase A_2). The mechanisms by which these products increase secretion of glucocorticoids are complex and varied. Some agents not only influence the HPA axis directly by acting mainly at the hypothalamic level to stimulate release of CRH and AVP, but also affect the anterior pituitary gland and adrenal cortex, to augment or sustain the adrenocortical response. Other agents may act at the site of the infection or inflammatory lesion or at the level of the blood–brain barrier to stimulate afferent fibers, possibly by local release of prostanoids, thereby activating the central pathways that precipitate release of CRH and AVP. In addition, many of the mediators provoke widespread pathologic effects in the body (e.g., hypotension, hypoglycemia) that themselves stimulate the HPA axis by the mechanisms described earlier. Recent review articles give a comprehensive description of this complex scenario[15,16] (see Fig. 47–2).

Feedback Control of the Hypothalamic-Pituitary-Adrenal Axis

The adrenocortical responses to incoming stimuli are tightly controlled by glucocorticoids and the other hormones of the HPA axis.[17,18] Thus the POMC-derived peptides ACTH and β-endorphin both inhibit secretion of CRH and AVP by the hypothalamus. In addition, CRH and AVP may modulate their own secretion. However, by far the most important feedback effects are those exerted by the glucocorticoids. Confirming this, increases in circulating glucocorticoids, possibly caused by adrenal tumors or administration of exogenous steroids, effectively suppress the circadian increase in pituitary-adrenocortical activity and the HPA responses to stress. Conversely, subjects with adrenocortical insufficiency (e.g., in Addison disease) show a sustained hypersecretion of ACTH and an exaggerated ACTH response to stress, both of which are readily corrected by glucocorticoid replacement therapy. The feedback actions of the steroids are extremely complex, because they affect multiple sites within the axis and involve multiple molecular mechanisms that operate over several time domains, termed (a) *rapid or fast,* (b) *early delayed,* and (c) *late delayed* feedback.

The hypothalamus and anterior pituitary gland are both important sites of glucocorticoid feedback. The steroids act directly on these tissues to suppress the genes encoding CRH/AVP and POMC and, thus with time reduce the store of peptides. The steroids also exert, on both tissues, more immediate effects that suppress the stimulus-evoked release of stored peptide. These actions depend in part on the translation of a protein, annexin 1 (also called lipocortin 1), that appears to interfere with the processes of exocytosis.[18] In addition, glucocorticoids produce further regulatory actions within the hippocampus and other parts of the central nervous system (e.g., amygdala, cerebral cortex, brain stem nuclei) that repress functional activity of the HPA axis. Finally, glucocorticoids may act within the periphery to quench the transmission of information to the brain by, for example, suppressing the generation of inflammatory mediators or limiting the passage of substances across the blood–brain barrier.[11] The suppression of HPA activity induced by increases in serum glucocorticoids resulting from stress or administration of exogenous steroids is mediated principally by GRs, which are expressed in abundance in the anterior pituitary gland, the hypothalamus, and elsewhere.[4] In contrast, feedback at the MRs, particularly at the level of the hippocampus, appears to be an important determinant of the basal output of the HPA axis.[4]

Adaptive Responses to Repeated or Sustained Stress

Most of the studies on stress and HPA function have focused on acute stresses, and relatively little is known about the characteristics of, or mechanisms controlling, the neuroendocrine responses to repeated or sustained stress.[11,19] Understanding such conditions and their influence on HPA function is highly desirable, not least because prolonged increases in circulating corticosteroids may initiate a wide range of disorders. However, for ethical and practical reasons, it is difficult to develop appropriate animal models. The limited data available suggest that some degree of adaptation may occur, but that this depends on the nature of the stress and the species concerned. Thus, in some instances, the HPA responses to repeated (successive or intermittent) or sustained (chronic) stressful stimuli are attenuated. For example, rodents develop a "tolerance" to stresses such as cold, handling, saline injection, and water deprivation. Some degree of "cross tolerance" may occur between stresses that invoke similar pathways or mechanisms to increase the release of CRH and AVP. For example, repeated handling of rats reduces their subsequent adrenocortical response to saline injection; however, rats tolerant to the C-fiber–dependent stress of exposure to cold respond to the novel stress of immobilization with a normal or even enhanced increase in serum corticosterone. In other situations, however, tolerance does not develop—for example, the HPA responses to the intermittent stresses of electric foot shock, insulin hypoglycemia, or administration of IL-1β and

to the chronic stress of septicemia were maintained or even enhanced.[20]

During acute stress, CRH appears to be the major hypothalamic factor governing release of ACTH, and AVP plays only a supporting role. In contrast, the sustained release of ACTH that occurs in certain repeated or chronic stress paradigms appears to be governed mainly by AVP.[20] Although it is not yet known how the "switch" to AVP takes place, that the expression of MRs in the hippocampus and GRs in the PVN decreases during chronic stress suggests disruption of the feedback action of the glucocorticoids.

AGE- and SEX-Related Changes in Hypothalamic-Pituitary-Adrenal Function

Developmental Changes

The glucocorticoids produce complex organizational effects both before and after birth, and thus play a key role in "developmental programming." Not surprisingly, the HPA axis is tightly regulated during fetal and perinatal life.[21] By mid-term the adrenal gland of the fetus is already producing appreciable amounts of cortisol and additional cortisol may enter the fetus from the maternal circulation. Much, however, is inactivated in the placenta and fetal tissues by 11β-HSD-2, the isozyme that converts cortisol to cortisone.

Serum cortisol levels increase progressively during the last trimester to reach a peak at term, and a concomitant decrease in 11β-HSD-2 increases the bioavailability of the steroid at the receptor. This increase in cortisol is critical because it permits the maturation of a number of systems that are essential for extrauterine survival.[22] These systems include the production of surfactant in the lung, the maturation of various enzymes in the liver, and the expression of phenylethanolamine *N*-methyltransferase, the enzyme that permits synthesis of epinephrine from norepinephrine in the adrenal medulla. Once the neonate separates from the placenta, the metabolic clearance of cortisol decreases dramatically. Thus despite an initial decrease in serum cortisol, basal-free cortisol levels remain fairly stable in the neonate, whereas total cortisol increases only as the liver begins to produce CBG.

The feedback control system matures progressively during the second half of pregnancy and early neonatal life. Stress-induced increases in ACTH and cortisol have been described in the neonate, although these are modest when compared with those of adults; the circadian rhythm does not emerge until about 6 months after birth.[23] The factors that determine the development of the axis are poorly understood, particularly in humans. In rodents, the activity of the axis regresses postnatally and a stress hyporesponsive period emerges at about Day 3 and persists for some 21 to 28 days. Moreover, although the hypothalamic suprachiasmatic nucleus that houses the circadian clock and receives important afferent projections from the retina and dorsal raphe nuclei (an area rich in GR) is evident at birth, oscillations in the activity of the AVP pathway that projects from the suprachiasmatic nucleus to the PVN do not emerge until about postnatal Day 10 to 12.

Glucocorticoids and Perinatal Programming

A growing body of evidence, drawn largely from animal studies, suggests that disturbances in the secretion or activity of glucocorticoids at critical stages of fetal or neonatal life may have a severe impact on developmental processes and may predispose the individual, in adulthood, to conditions as diverse as hypertension, insulin resistance, allergic or inflammatory disease, and cognitive and behavioral disorders.[24] These adverse effects of glucocorticoids appear to be caused in part by irreversible effects on the HPA axis that disrupt the negative feedback mechanisms and thereby alter the responsiveness of the HPA axis to stress throughout the lifetime of the individual. For example, rats exposed to exogenous glucocorticoids or stimuli that increase serum glucocorticoids (e.g., injection of lipopolysaccharide [endotoxin]) in neonatal life show reduced expression of GRs in the hippocampus and hypothalamus, reduced sensitivity of the HPA axis to negative feedback actions of the glucocorticoids, and exaggerated HPA responses to stress in adulthood.[25] Similar changes in HPA function emerge in adulthood in rats subjected to maternal separation in early life; these changes are associated with changes in T-cell antibody responses and in the incidence of age-related neuropathies.[26] Conversely, handling of the neonate, which increases expression of GRs in the hippocampus, reduces the magnitude and duration of the stress response in adulthood; maternal care may therefore help to program events that regulate responses to stress in the adult, and thus reduce vulnerability to disease.[26] Although the extent to which these data can be translated to humans remains to be determined, the data raise important questions about the long-term effects of glucocorticoids administered during perinatal life.

Sex-Related Factors

In adults, distinct sex-related patterns of glucocorticoid secretion emerge. The serum concentrations of glucocorticoids are consistently greater in female than male subjects, with additional increases occurring toward the middle of the menstrual or estrous cycle just before ovulation. These differences are attributable in part to the positive effects of estrogen on the expression of CBG.[27] In addition, estrogen exerts significant effects at the hypothalamic level, increasing the synthesis and the release of CRH. This phenomenon may account in part for the relatively high incidence in women of emotional disorders characterized by enhanced secretion of CRH (e.g., depression, anxiety).[28] Further modulation of the secretion of glucocorticoids may be brought about by progesterone because, when present in large amounts (e.g., in the premenstrual phase, in pregnancy, or in subjects taking oral contraceptives), progesterone binds readily to, but is only weakly active at, MRs in the hippocampus.[29]

Pregnancy-Related Factors

During pregnancy, serum cortisol levels increase markedly, particularly toward the end of gestation, the normal circadian rhythm becomes less pronounced, and the increased steroid levels are resistant to suppression with exogenous glucocorticoids, for example, dexamethasone.[30,31] These changes, which regress slowly postpartum, are not caused by increased secretion of cortisol but to a marked increase (governed by estrogen) in the synthesis of CBG and a resultant threefold to fourfold increase in serum CBG.[27,33] In addition, the hepatic metabolism of cortisol changes with a consequent reduction in glucuronidation and excretion of terahydro-metabolites and concomitant increase in the urinary excretion of unconjugated cortisol and cortisol sulphate.[30,32]

Even though most of the cortisol in the blood is bound, a small increase in the amount of unbound cortisol in the blood also occurs, so that maternal tissues are exposed to relatively high levels of cortisol.[32] Serum ACTH levels remain low throughout pregnancy,[30] and recent studies in rodents suggest that functional changes in the hypothalamus render the HPA axis refractory to stress.[34] Although the placenta produces substantial amounts of CRH (particularly during the last trimester), this has little effect on the pituitary gland, as such CRH is effectively sequestered by a specific binding protein.[35]

Age-Related Factors

For both sexes, serum levels of glucocorticoids tend to increase with age, particularly if disease states are present. In addition, the HPA response to stress may become slow in onset, exaggerated in magnitude, and prolonged in duration.[4] This "aging" process has been attributed in part to downregulation of the corticosteroid receptors (GRs and MRs) in the hippocampus and hypothalamus and the subsequent resistance of the HPA axis to negative feedback actions of the glucocorticoids.[4] The consequences are potentially significant, because abnormally high blood levels of glucocorticoids are important contributors to many age-related diseases, such as neurodegenerative conditions, cognitive dysfunction, osteoporosis, noninsulin-dependent diabetes mellitus, hypertension and other cardiovascular diseases, and the decline in immunocompetence.

Effect of Surgery on Hypothalamic-Pituitary-Adrenal Function

Major surgery represents a significant threat to homeostasis and triggers a substantial increase in HPA activity. The nature of the response is determined by the anesthetic regimen; the nature, duration, and severity of the operation; and the physical and mental health of the patient. Depending on those factors, cortisol secretion may increase before, during, and after an operative procedure. Indeed, recovery from surgery is an extensive endocrine adjustment that is analogous in scope, if not duration, to puberty, pregnancy, and other life events.

Serum Cortisol Levels During and After Surgery

Studies on the impact of surgery on the HPA axis began in the 1950s after reports that the metabolic changes observed during and after surgery were similar to those produced by administration of exogenous glucocorticoids.[36,37] A number of reports then described increases in plasma 17-hydroxy-corticosteroids after induction of anesthesia and during and after surgery, with the most marked effects occurring during and after reversal of anesthesia.[38] Also, the magnitude and duration of the glucocorticoid responses correlated roughly with the severity and duration of the operative procedure; minor operative procedures were essentially without effect.[39–42] Although there were contrary reports,[43] most of the data suggested that, as in other types of stress, the episodic profile of cortisol secretion was in effect both during and after surgery and the overall increase in serum cortisol levels reflected an increase in the amplitude but not the frequency of the cortisol pulses.[44]

Considerable interest has centered on the increase in serum cortisol that occurs with recovery from anesthesia and during the postoperative period. The increase appears to be caused in part by baroreceptor and spinal reflexes that "inform" the hypothalamus of the trauma associated with tissue injury and the current hemodynamic state[43,45] and by proinflammatory mediators released by the damaged tissue that, as discussed earlier, activate the HPA axis by other routes. In addition, postoperative pain is a highly significant factor.[46,47]

Although several studies have reported that serum cortisol levels return to normal within 24 hours of surgery,[47–51] others have reported increased steroid levels for up to 72 hours. These increases have varied in magnitude according to severity of the procedure, and this relation may also be associated with a significant shift in circadian rhythm.[52,53] Although the pattern of cortisol secretion is likely to reflect the metabolic needs of the patient in the postoperative phase,[44,54] the disturbance in circadian rhythm is less advantageous; it may lead to postoperative debility and fatigue[55] and, unless recognized, misinterpretation of the postsurgical activity of the HPA axis.

Restoration of normal cortisol levels after surgery does not follow a simple recovery course but has two phases. The first phase is characterized by high plasma levels of ACTH and cortisol and is thus consistent with sustained, stress-induced activation of the hypothalamus. In the second phase, however, plasma ACTH levels are low, and the increased cortisol levels must therefore be independent of activation of the hypothalamic-pituitary system. Reports that liver function decreases during and after surgery, and that the degree of impairment relates to the severity of the trauma, have suggested that clearance of cortisol is impaired. However, measures of cortisol clearance in the postsurgical phase,[56] and in subjects undergoing cholecystectomy or gastrectomy,[57] do not accord with this view. A more likely

explanation is that factors released from traumatized tissue, such as cytokines, may stimulate synthesis of adrenal glucocorticoids directly.[15,16,58] Alternatively, the earlier increase in ACTH may augment the expression of ACTH receptors in the adrenal gland, thereby enhancing the steroidogenic response.[59]

Adaptation of the Stress Response to Surgery

Taken together, these findings suggest that the stress response to major surgery adapts in such a way as to provide protection both during and after surgery. To test this concept, Udelsman and coworkers[60] examined hemodynamic responses during and after surgery in adrenalectomized primates treated with subphysiologic, physiologic, or supraphysiologic doses of cortisol. Animals given subphysiologic doses were unstable hemodynamically, both during and after surgery, and had a high mortality rate during the recovery phase. By contrast, those given physiologic or supraphysiologic doses of steroid coped well with surgery and were essentially indistinguishable from sham-operated control subjects. These findings and others[38] suggest that the basal (nonstress) level of cortisol production is both necessary and sufficient to produce tolerance to major surgery in primates, and that the "permissive" actions of the steroids may therefore be key in this regard.

The prospect of potentially life-threatening surgery is itself a major psychological stress that could be expected to activate the HPA axis before surgery. It is surprising, however, to find that serum cortisol levels remain within normal limits for most of the preoperative day and increase only when patients are being prepared for surgery (e.g., during washing and shaving of the body).[61] Moreover, it is not clear whether the trigger to the HPA response is nonspecific sensory (i.e., physiologic) stimulation or whether the preparative procedures themselves intensify anxiety about the forthcoming surgical procedure and therefore overcome the psychological defenses that keep adrenocortical secretion within normal range.

Effect of Anesthesia on the HPA Axis

The HPA response to surgery is influenced not only by the psychological and physical trauma associated with surgery but also by the choice of anesthetic regimen. Many drugs used as premedicants suppress HPA function (e.g., opioids, benzodiazepines, clonidine) and thus temper the cortisol response to surgery.[47,48] The impact on basal HPA activity of the various drug cocktails used for induction and maintenance of anesthesia and production of muscle relaxation is poorly researched. However, it is known that some inhalation anesthetics, such as ether and cyclopropane, themselves activate the HPA axis.[62–64] Others, such as the halogenated compounds halothane and enflurane, have an inhibitory influence,[65–67] as does the induction agent thiopental, which, like the benzodiazepines, increases transmission or secretion of γ-aminobutyric acid.[68] Nevertheless, regardless of the premedication or anesthetic agent used, transmission of information to the hypothalamus is impaired during general anesthesia. Thus increases in HPA activity during surgery are modest.[69]

Although general anesthesia permits a modest increase in plasma 17-hydroxycorticosteroid levels, spinal anesthesia and epidural block attenuate or prevent the cortisol response.[62,70] However, once the nerve block dissipates, the adrenocortical response ensues. Because high transection of the spinal cord prevents the normal adrenocortical response to abdominal surgery,[51] the cortisol responses appear to be mediated by neural mechanisms that link the operative site with the central nervous system. Such a mechanism is consistent with the view that cytokines and other proinflammatory mediators released from damaged neurons activate the HPA axis by stimulating local sensory neurons.[11] It also accords with the finding that in situations in which spinal anesthesia prevents an increase in plasma cortisol occurring during surgery HPA activity increases markedly during reversal of anesthesia and the immediate postoperative recovery period.

Practical Aspects of Drug Administration

Corticosteroids are administered by almost every possible route. Topical administration includes: drops for the eyes and ears; lozenges to dissolve in the mouth; skin creams, ointments and gels; aerosols for inhalation; and enemas and suppositories. This section focuses on the *systemic* administration of these drugs, by the oral and parenteral routes; doses are for adults.

The equivalent daily dosages of the different corticosteroid preparations for a generic "glucocorticoid and anti-inflammatory" effect:

hydrocortisone 120 mg = prednisolone 30 mg
= betamethasone 4 mg = dexamethasone 4 mg
= methylprednisolone 24 mg = triamcinolone 24 mg.

Healthy subjects secrete approximately 30 mg/day cortisol; these dosages are therefore approximately four times the amount produced endogenously each day. Thus corticosteroid side effects are more likely to occur when exceeding a threshold daily dosage of 7.5 mg prednisolone.

The following commentary relates to the specific preparations.

Hydrocortisone

The oral preparation is used for replacement therapy (10- and 20-mg tablets; 20 to 30 mg daily, usually in 2 doses).

The intravenous preparation is used in emergencies (100-mg/mL vials as sodium phosphate; 400–2000 mg daily, usually in 3–4 divided doses either by bolus or by continuous infusion). Although it is usual to give corticosteroids intravenously in emergencies, it is unlikely that the onset of action is significantly quicker than by oral administration. Administration by intramuscular injection is not recommended because absorption is unreliable.

Prednisolone

Prednisolone is the most widely used systemic corticosteroid for all indications other than replacement therapy. It is administered in 1-, 2.5-, and 5-mg tablets, with or without enteric coating. The prednisolone dosage may vary from 1 to 2 mg daily for conditions such as quiescent polymyalgia up to 100 mg daily in severe autoimmune disease. When dosages exceed 40 mg/day, it is recommended that prednisolone be administered in two doses, with the larger dose provided in the morning.

Betamethasone

Betamethasone is primarily used for suppression of inflammation and for cerebral edema and is also given parenterally in premature labour. It is dispensed in 0.5-mg tablets for oral use (daily dosage is usually 0.5–5 mg in 1 or 2 doses) or by injection in a vial containing 4-mg/mL injections (as sodium phosphate). The daily parenteral dosage is from 4 to 20 mg/day, in up to four divided doses.

Dexamethasone

Dexamethasone has similar indications to that for betamethasone; in addition, it has been used as adjuvant treatment of chemotherapy-induced nausea. It is dispensed orally as 0.5-mg tablets (dosage 0.5–10 mg daily in 1 or 2 doses); parenterally, it is dispensed as either 4-mg/mL injection or 24 mg/mL (as sodium phosphate) or 5 mg/mL (as phosphate). The daily dosage may be up to 0.5 to 24 mg. However, for septic shock, dosages as high as 6 mg/kg per day are prescribed. It is administered as bolus injections up to four times daily or by slow intravenous infusion.

Methylprednisolone

Methylprednisolone is used for each of the applications mentioned earlier and for acute graft rejection and acute relapses in multiple sclerosis. It is dispensed as 2-, 4-, 16-, and 100-mg tablets, and the daily dosage is between 2 and 40 mg. The parenteral preparation is dispensed as 40-, 125-, 500-mg, 1-, and 2-g vials of powder (as sodium succinate) for reconstitution with supplied solvent. The daily dosage is from 10 mg to 1 g either by intramuscular injection, intravenously by boluses (every 6 hours), or by continuous infusion. Methylprednisolone can also be dispensed as a 40-mg/ml aqueous suspension for intramuscular depot injection for which the daily dosage is between 40 and 120 mg.

Triamcinolone

Triamcinolone is not recommended for chronic dosage because of increased risk for myopathy compared with other corticosteroids. It is dispensed as 40- and 80-mg vials and prefilled syringes (as acetonide in aqueous suspension at 40 mg/mL). Typically, the aqueous suspension is administered by deep intramuscular injection to exploit the depot effect at dose of 40 to 100 mg in situations such as allergic rhinitis for which it is administered at the start of the hay fever season.

References

1. Buckingham JC: Glucocorticoids: Role in stress of. In Fink G (ed): The Encyclopaedia of Stress. New York, Academic Press, 1999.
2. Buckingham JC, Christian HC, Gillies GE, et al: The hypothalamo-pituitary-adrenocortical immune axis. In Marsh JA, Kendall MD (eds): The Physiology of Immunity. Boca Raton, Fla, CRC Press, 1996.
3. Oakley RH, Cidlowski A: The glucocorticoid receptor: Expression, function, and regulation of glucocorticoid responsiveness. In Goulding NJ, Flower RJ (eds): Glucocorticoids. Switzerland, Birkhauser Verlig, 2001.
4. de Kloet ER, Vreugdenhil E, Citzl MS, et al: Brain corticosteroid receptor balance in health and disease. Endocrine Rev 19:269, 1998.
5. Seckl JR: 11β-hydroxysteroid dehydrogenase in the brain: A novel regulator of glucocorticoid action? Front Neuroendocrinol 18:49, 1997.
6. Munck A, Guyre PM, Holbrook NJ: Physiological functions of glucocorticoids and their relation to pharmacological actions. Endocrine Rev 51:25, 1984.
7. Munck A, Naraj-Fejes-Toth A: The ups and downs of glucocorticoid physiology: Permissive and suppressive effects revisited. Mol Cell Endocrinol 90:25, 1992.
8. Parente L: The development of synthetic glucocorticoids. In Goulding NJ, Flower RJ (eds): Glucocorticoids. Switzerland, Birkhauser Verlig, 2001.
9. Rook GAW: Glucocorticoids and immune function. Balliere's Clin Endocrinol Met 13:567, 1999.
10. Paliogianni F, Boumpas DT: Molecular and cellular aspects of cytokine regulation by glucocorticoids. In Goulding NJ, Flower RJ (eds): Glucocorticoids. Switzerland, Birkhauser Verlig, 2001.
11. Buckingham JC: Glucocorticoids: Effects of stress on. In Fink G (ed): The Encyclopaedia of Stress. New York, Academic Press, 1999.
12. Vale W, Spiess J, Rivier L, et al: Characterization of a 41-residue ovine hypothalamic peptide that stimulates secretion of corticotropin and β-endorphin. Science 213:1394, 1981.
13. Gillies GE, Linton EA, Lowry PJ: Corticotropin releasing activity of the new CRH is potentiated several times by vasopressin. Nature 299:355, 1982.
14. Ericsson A, Arias C, Sawchenko PE: Evidence for an intramedullary prostaglandin-dependent mechanism in the activation of stress-related neuroendocrine circuitry by intravenous interleukin-1. J Neurosci 17:7177, 1997.
15. Turnbull A, Rivier C: Regulation of the hypothalamic-pituitary-adrenal axis by cytokines: Actions and mechanisms of action. Physiol Rev 79:1, 1999.
16. Mulla A, Buckingham JC: Regulation of the hypothalamo-pituitary-adrenal axis by cytokines. Balliere's Clin Endocrinol Met 13:503, 1999.
17. Keller-Wood ME, Dallman MF: Corticosteroid inhibition of ACTH secretion. Endocrine Rev 5:1, 1984.
18. Buckingham JC: Stress and the neuroendocrine immune axis: The pivotal role of glucocorticoids and lipocortin 1. Br J Pharmacol 118:1, 1996.
19. Aguilera G: Regulation of pituitary ACTH release during chronic stress. Front Neuroendocrinol 15:321, 1994.
20. Tilders FJ, Solimidt ED: Interleukin 1β-induced plasticity of hypothalamic CRH neurons and long-term hyperresponsivity. Ann NY Acad Sci 840:65, 1998.
21. Rosenfeld P, Suchecki AJ, Levine S: Multifactorial regulation of the hypothalamic-pituitary-adrenal axis during development. Neurosci Behav Rev 129:384, 1992.
22. Fisher D: Endocrinology of fetal development. In Wilson JD, Foster DW, Kronenberg HM, Larsen PR (eds): Williams Textbook of Endocrinology, 9th ed. Philadelphia, WB Saunders, 1998.
23. Liggins GC: The role of cortisol in preparing the fetus for birth. Reprod Fertil Devel 6:141, 1994.
24. Dodic M, Peers A, Coghlan, Wintour M: Can excess glucocorticoid *in utero* predispose to cardiovascular and metabolic disease in middle age? Trends Endocrinol Metab 10:86, 1999.
25. Shanks N, Larocque S, Meaney MJ: Neonatal endotoxin exposure alters the development of the hypothalamic-pituitary-adrenal axis: Early illness and later responsivity to stress. J Neurosci 15:376, 1995.
26. Liu D, Diorio J, Tannenbaum B, et al: Maternal care, hippocampal glucocorticoid receptors and hypothalamic-pituitary-adrenal responses to stress. Science 277:1659, 1997
27. Musa BU, Seal US, Doe RP: Elevation of certain plasma proteins in man following estrogen administration: a dose-response relationship. J Clin Endocrinol Metab 25:1163, 1965.
28. Vamvakopoulos NC, Chrousos GP: Hormonal regulation of human corticotropin releasing hormone gene expression: Implications for the sexual dimorphism of the stress response and immune inflammatory reaction. Endocrine Rev 15:409, 1994.
29. de Kloet ER, Rotd NY, van den Berg DTW, et al: Brain mineralocorticoid receptor function. Ann NY Acad Sci 746:8, 1994.
30. Mulay S, Solomon S: Adrenocortical function during pregnancy. In James VHT (ed): The Adrenal Cortex, 2nd ed. New York, Raven Press, 1992.
31. Nolten WE, Lindheimer MD, Rueckert PA, et al: Diurnal rhythm and regulations of cortisol secretion during pregnancy. J Clin Endocrinol Metab 51:466, 1980.
32. Bray HP, Hankin ME, Steinbeck AW: The urinary excretion of cortisol and cortisone sulphates in pregnancy. Med J Aust 2:259, 1977.
33. Robertson ME, Stiefel M, Laidlaw JC: The influence of oestrogen on the secretion, disposition and biological activity of cortisol. J Clin Endocrinol 19:1381, 1969.
34. Johnstone HA, Wigger A, Douglas AJ, et al: Attenuation of the hypothalamic-pituitary-adrenal axis stress response in late pregnancy: Changes in feed forward and feedback mechanisms. J Neuroendocrinol 12:811, 2000.
35. Linton EA, Perkins AV, Woods RJ, et al: Corticotropin-releasing-hormone-binding protein (CRHBP): Plasma levels decrease during the third trimester of normal human pregnancy. J Clin Endocrinol Metab 76:260, 1993.
36. Roche M, Thorn G, Hills AG: The levels of circulating eosinophils and their response to ACTH in surgery. N Engl J Med 242:307, 1950.
37. Moore FD, Ball MR: The metabolic response to surgery. Springfield, Ill, Charles C Thomas, 1952.
38. Udelsman R, Chrousos GP: Hormonal responses to stress. Adv Exp Med Biol 245:265, 1988.
39. Sandberg AV, Kristen E-N, Samuels LT: The effects of surgery on the blood levels and metabolism of 17-Hydroxycorticosteroids in man. J Clin Invest 33:1509, 1954.
40. Cooper CE, Nelson DH: ACTH levels in plasma in preoperative and surgically stressed patients. J Clin Invest 41:1599, 1962.
41. Thorn GW, Jenkins D, Laidlaw JC: The adrenal response to stress in man. In Pincus G (ed): Recent progress in hormone research. Proceedings of the Laurentian Hormone Conference. New York, Academic Press, 1953.
42. Uzunkey A, Coskun A, Akincl O, et al: Systemic stress responses after laproscopic or open hernia repair. Eur J Surg 116:467, 2000.
43. Udelsman R, Norton JA, Jelenich SE: Responses of the hypothalamic-pituitary-adrenal and rennin angiotensin exes and the sympathetic system during controlled surgical and anaesthesia stress. J Clin Endocrinol Metab 64:986, 1987.
44. Wise L, Margraf HW, Ballinger WF: A new concept on the pre- and postoperative regulation of cortisol secretion. Surgery 72:290, 1972.

45. Udelsman R, Holbrook NJ: Endocrine and molecular responses to surgical stress. Curr Prob Surg 31:653, 1994.

46. Yokoyama M, Itamo Y, Mizobuchi S, et al: The effects of epidural block on the distribution of lymphocyte subsets and natural killer cell activity in patients with and without pain. Anaesth Analg 92:463, 2001.

47. Solak M, Ulusey H, Sarihan H: Effects of caudal block on cortisol and prolactin responses to post-operative pain in children. Eur Pediatr Surg 10:219, 2000.

48. Franksson C, Gemzell CA: Blood levels of 17-hydroxycorticosteroids in surgery and allied conditions. Acta Chir Scand 106:24, 1954.

49. Elman R, Weichselbaum TE, Moncrief JC, et al: Adrenal cortical steroids following elective operations. Arch Surg 71:697, 1955.

50. Steenberg RW, Lennihan R, Moore FD: The free blood 17-hydroxycorticosteroids in surgical patients: Their relation to urine steroids, metabolism and convalescence. Ann Surg 2:180, 1956.

51. Hume DM, Bell CC, Bartter F: Direct measurement of adrenal secretion during operative trauma and convalescence. Surgery 52:174, 1962.

52. Cho Y, Lim SY, Cho BY, et al: Dissociation between plasma adrenocorticotrophin and serum cortisol levels during the early post-operative period after gastrectomy. Horm Res 55:246, 2000.

53. Mcintosh TK, Lothrop DA, Lee A, et al: Circadian rhythm of cortisol is altered in postsurgical patients. J Clin Endocrinol Metab 53:117, 1981.

54. Masden SN, Engquist A, Badani I, et al: Cyclic AMP, glucose and cortisol in plasma during surgery. Horm Metab Res 8:483, 1976.

55. Thomasson B: Studies on the content of 17-hydroxycorticosteroids and its diurnal rhythm in the plasma of surgical patients. Scand J Lab Invest 11(suppl 42):1, 1959.

56. Naito Y, Fukata J, Tamai S, et al: Biphasic changes in hypothalamo-pituitary-adrenal function during the early recovery period after abdominal surgery. J Clin Endocrinol Metab 73:11, 1991.

57. Kehlet H, Binder C: Alterations in distribution volume and biological half life of cortisol during major surgery. J Clin Endocrinol Metab 36:330, 1973.

58. Roh MS, Drazenovich KA, Barbose JJ, et al: Direct stimulation of the adrenal cortex by interleukin-1. Surgery 102:140, 1987.

59. Penhoat A, Jaillard C, Saez JM: Corticotrophin positively regulates its own receptors and cAMP response in cultured bovine adrenal cells. Proc Natl Acad Sci USA 86:4978, 1989.

60. Udelsman R, Goldstein DS, Loriaux DL, et al: Catecholamine-glucocorticoid interactions during surgical stress. J Surg Res 43:539, 1087.

61. Czeisler CA, Moore Ede MC, Regestein QR, et al: Epsiodic 24-hour cortisol secretory patterns in patients awaiting elective cardiac surgery. J Clin Endocrinol Metab 42:273, 1976.

62. Hammond WG, Aronow L, Moore FD: Studies in surgical endocrinology. III: Plasma concentrations of epinephrine and norepinephrine in anaesthesia, trauma and surgery, as measured by a modification of the method of Weilmalherbe and Bone. Ann Surg 144:715, 1956.

63. Oyama T, Shibata S, Matsumoto F, et al: Effects of halothane anaesthesia and surgery on adrenocortical function in man. Can Anaesth Soc J 15:258, 1968.

64. Oyama T, Takazawa T: Effect of cyclopropane anaesthesia and surgery on carbohydrate and fat metabolism in man. Anesth Analg Curr Res 48:1, 1972.

65. Werder KV, Stevens WC, Cromwell TH, et al: Adrenal function during long term anaesthesia in man. Exp Biol Med 135:854, 1970.

66. Oyama T, Matsuki A, Kudo T: Effect of enflurane anaesthesia and surgery on adrenocortical function. Can Anaesth Soc J 19:394, 1972.

67. Skovsted P, Sapthavichaikul S: The effects of isoflurane on arterial pressure, pulse rate, autonomic nervous activity and barostatic reflexes. Can Anaesth Soc 24:304, 1977.

68. Buckingham JC, Cowell AM, Gillies GE, et al: The neuroendocrine system: Anatomy, physiology and responses to stress. In Buckingham JC, Gillies GE, Cowell AM (eds): Stress, Stress Hormones and the Immune System. Chichester, UK, John Wiley and Sons, 1997.

69. Gordon NH, Scott DB, Percy Robb IW: Modification of plasma corticosteroid concentrations during and after surgery by epidural blockade. BMJ 1:581, 1973.

70. Oyama T, Matsuki A: Plasma levels of cortisol in man during spinal anaesthesia and surgery. Can Anaesth Soc J 17:234, 1970.

48

Insulin

Stephen Robinson, MD, FRCP • Martin Smith, BSc, MRCP

Diabetes was recognized in ancient times and is mentioned in ancient Egyptian texts. However, it was not until the 18th century that an association between diabetes mellitus and the pancreas was suggested when Thomas Cawley described pancreatic calcification in a patient with glycosuria. By the late 19th century, the link was demonstrated when Minkowski and Von Mering described diabetes having performed pancreatectomy in a dog. In 1864, Langerhans identified the aggregation of cells in the pancreas that are currently known as islets, but could not comment on their function. In 1909, Jean de Meyer suggested that these islets of Langerhans were responsible for the production of a substance that decreased blood glucose levels, naming it *insulin*, derived from the Latin for island.[1]

In 1921, Dr. Frederick Banting, working in Professor J. MacLeod's Toronto laboratory with Mr. Charles Best (a medical student), obtained an islet-rich pancreatic extract from dogs that 6 weeks earlier had their pancreatic duct ligated. This ligation caused degeneration of the exocrine pancreas, but with no deleterious effect on the islets. The resultant pancreatic extract was injected into a pancreatectomized dog and caused significant improvement of the animal's diabetes.[2] In January 1922, successful administration of the extract saved a child who was dying of diabetic ketosis. With the help of J.B. Collip, a biochemist, the extract was purified and mass production of insulin from the bovine pancreas for human administration was achieved by 1922–1923. Bovine insulin differs from human insulin by three amino acid substitutions and is still available outside of North America. The animal insulin currently preferred is porcine insulin, which differs from human insulin by one amino acid.

In 1954, Dr. Fred Sanger of Cambridge University identified the constituent amino acids of insulin. This intimate knowledge of the structure enabled industrial synthesis of insulin on a much larger scale than previously possible with early animal insulin extraction techniques. The first complete synthesis of insulin was achieved in 1963, and the first biosynthetic human insulin received U.S. Food and Drug Administration approval in 1982.

Human insulin is manufactured either by recombinant DNA technology using *Escherichia coli* or by enzymatic modification of porcine insulin. Currently, there are many available preparations of insulin, with the majority an exact biochemical match of endogenous human insulin. Further changes to the human insulin amino acid sequence have produced insulin analogues, which became available for prescription in 1996. These aim to mimic more accurately the postprandial profile of endogenous insulin and were designed to offer an advantage over conventional synthetic human insulin.[3]

Insulin is prescribed for the treatment of insulin deficiency and insulin resistance in diabetes mellitus. Type 1 and type 2 diabetes mellitus represent chronic disorders with symptoms associated with acute metabolic complications, chronic complications, and increased mortality rates. The chronic complications can be classified into microvascular (retinopathy, nephropathy, and neuropathy) and macrovascular (atherosclerosis causing coronary artery, cerebrovascular, and peripheral vascular disease). In addition, insulin is used in the treatment of acute hyperkalemia. The metabolic actions of insulin are summarized in Table 48–1.

Glucose Homeostasis

The endocrine pancreas is scattered throughout the substance of the gland as discrete islets of Langerhans representing 2% of pancreatic mass. Islets have three cell populations involved in the synthesis, storage, and secretion of hormones responsible for glucose homeostasis. The α cells synthesize glucagon, the β cells synthesize insulin, and the δ cells synthesize somatostatin. They possess a rich blood supply and are innervated by the parasympathetic and sympathetic nervous systems. During health, insulin and glucagon operate in a reciprocal manner to maintain blood glucose concentration within the physiologic range. They can directly modify the secretion of one another. Somatostatin inhibits the secretions of α and β cells from within the islet.

Intact homeostatic mechanisms maintain plasma glucose within the range of 4 to 8 mmol/L despite wide variation in dietary intake and metabolic expenditure[4] (Fig. 48–1). This is to ensure continuous delivery of glucose to the central nervous system because glucose is essential for brain function.[5] Glucose is taken up from the plasma in an insulin-independent manner by the Glucose 1 transporter (GLUT 1) within the blood–brain barrier. It enters the central nervous system along a concentration gradient. When plasma glucose decreases to less than 3.7 mmol/L, GLUT 1 activity becomes rate limiting for cerebral function.[6]

Postprandial State

The most potent stimulus for insulin secretion is an increase in plasma glucose. Insulin is the only hormone that will return this into the physiologic range. This is achieved through two mechanisms:

- Increased peripheral glucose uptake, predominately into muscle, mediated through the GLUT 4 transporter.
- Suppression of hepatic glucose output, because insulin inhibits gluconeogenesis and glycogenolysis.

The glucose taken up into muscle may be metabolized to generate adenosine triphosphate (ATP) or stored as glycogen. Insulin stimulates glucose uptake into adipose tissue where it may be metabolized to fatty acids. Lipogenesis is the combination of 2 or 3 fatty acids with glycerol to form diacylglycerol or triacylglycerol. This represents the most efficient and largest long-term energy source in humans.

Insulin is one of the principal anabolic hormones and is responsible for amino acid uptake into peripheral tissues and for the consequent increase in protein synthesis. Insulin suppresses proteolysis with a net effect of increasing amino acid incorporation into protein.

The insulin response to glucose is larger for an oral load than for an intravenous infusion—the "incretin" effect. This is because the oral load also causes the release of glucose-dependent insulinotropic polypeptide, which augments the β-cell response.

TABLE 48–1.

The Physiologic Effects of Insulin: Insulin Reduces Hepatic Glucose Output by the Inhibition of Gluconeogenesis and Glycogenolysis

Stimulation	Inhibition
1. Glucose uptake into skeletal muscle and adipose tissue (GLUT 4–mediated)	Gluconeogenesis
2. Amino acid uptake and protein synthesis in muscle	Proteolysis
3. Lipogenesis	Lipolysis and ketogenesis
4. Glycogen synthesis	Glycogenolysis
5. Activity of Na/K ATPase pump	Glucagon secretion
6. Nitric oxide synthesis	
7. Renal sodium reabsorption	

ATPase, adenosine triphophatase; GLUT, glucose transported.

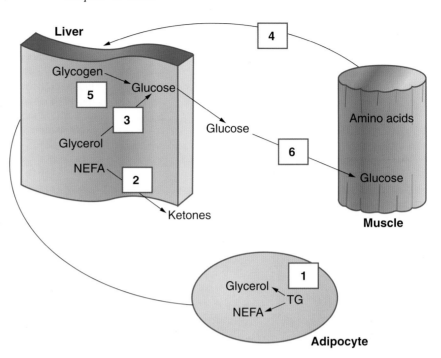

Figure 48–1. The regulation of glucose homeostasis: interrelation among carbohydrate, protein, and lipid metabolism. *1,* Lipolysis—triglyceride is broken down to glycerol and nonesterified fatty acids (NEFAs). *2,* Ketogenesis NEFAs are metabolized to ketoacids in the liver. *3,* Hepatic gluconeogenesis from glycerol. *4,* Hepatic gluconeogenesis from alanine derived from proteolysis of skeletal muscle. *5,* Glycogenolysis—hepatic glycogen is metabolized to glucose. *6,* Insulin-dependent uptake of glucose into skeletal muscle.

The Fasted State

During the fasted state, reduced insulin concentration and the counter-regulatory hormones to insulin are required for the maintenance of normoglycemia. Glucagon, epinephrine, growth hormone, and cortisol ensure plasma glucose remains at a concentration that will not compromise brain function. This is achieved through an increase in hepatic glucose production derived from an increase in glycogenolysis and an increase in gluconeogenesis from lactate, glycerol (from adipocytes), and alanine (and other gluconeogenic amino acids predominately from muscle). With prolonged fasting, or insulin deficiency, fat stores and muscle bulk are lost to maintain plasma glucose.

Glycogen provides the most immediately accessible source of nutrient storage that is consumed during fasting. A decrease in plasma glucose concentration inhibits insulin secretion and stimulates release of glucagon. This initial response to fasting increases hepatic glucose output by stimulation of hepatic glycogenolysis—glucagon acting through generation of cyclic adenosine monophosphate. Physical activity depletes muscle glycogen and increases the delivery of lactate to the liver where it is used as substrate for gluconeogenesis.

During a prolonged fast, hepatic glycogen stores become exhausted. The combination of increased concentrations of glucagon, epinephrine, growth hormone and cortisol, and a low concentration of insulin promotes lipolysis and proteolysis. Hormone-sensitive lipase is activated, which metabolizes triglyceride in adipose tissue to glycerol and free fatty acids. Glycerol is metabolized in the liver by gluconeogenic pathways, increasing hepatic glucose output. Free fatty acids are used as an alternative energy substrate to glucose by most tissues except the brain.

Ketoacids are produced from fatty acids, as a result of chronic lipolysis, when the capacity of Krebs' cycle to metabolize acetyl coenzyme A is reached.[7] During these circumstances, acetyl coenzyme A is metabolized to ketoacids—acetoacetate and 3-hydroxybutyrate; a small proportion of acetoacetate is spontaneously broken down to acetone, which is exhaled. Ketogenesis is important because during starvation the brain is *able* to use ketoacids as an *alternative* fuel source to glucose. This is a glucose-sparing and protein-conserving adaptation to starvation that compensates for the exhaustion of glycogen stores.

Proteolysis of skeletal muscle provides substrate for gluconeogenesis by increasing hepatic delivery of alanine. Significant gluconeogenesis occurs also in the kidney, but glutamine is the preferred substrate.

Therefore it should be appreciated that during fasting, counter-regulatory hormones to insulin operate to preserve glucose delivery to the brain specifically and to maintain the continuous production of ATP for cellular function in general. During a prolonged fast, exhaustion of glycogen is followed by the sacrifice of triglyceride and skeletal muscle protein.

Glucose Intolerance and Insulin Resistance

Glucose intolerance follows two process: insulin resistance and insulin deficiency. Insulin resistance is common in conditions such as hypertension and ischemic heart disease, or during such procedures as cardiac surgery. Type 2 diabetes may eventually develop in subjects who have impaired β-cell function.[8]

Insulin resistance (the inverse of insulin sensitivity) is when a cell, tissue, system, or whole body requires increased insulin concentration for a given effect. It is characterized by hepatic and peripheral insulin resistance and is associated with an increased cardiovascular risk[9] (Table 48–2). It

TABLE 48–2.

Clinical Features of the Insulin Resistance Syndrome

Glucose intolerance and hyperglycemia

Hypertension

Dyslipidemia
- Hypertriglyceridemia
- Low high-density lipoprotein cholesterol
- Small dense low-density lipoprotein particles

Postprandial lipemia

Visceral or generalized obesity

Diffuse atherosclerosis

Hyperuricemia

Increased plasminogen-activator inhibitor 1

Anovulatory polycystic ovary syndrome

Reduced postprandial thermogenesis

---

is associated also with polycystic ovary syndrome and reduced postprandial energy expenditure.[10,11] The main effect is an impaired intracellular insulin signal that leads to a decrease in the recruitment of glucose transport proteins to the plasma membrane and consequently reduced glucose uptake.[12,13] Therefore, compensatory hyperinsulinemia is required to overcome the peripheral resistance to insulin action and maintain normoglycemia.

Increased hepatic glucose production from glycogenolysis and gluconeogenesis leads to fasting hyperglycemia. This occurs because insulin resistance removes the feedback control of glucagon production. The increased glucagon concentration stimulates hepatic glycogenolysis and gluconeogenesis. In addition, insulin resistance leads to loss of insulin-induced suppression of hepatic glucose output.

Chronic hyperglycemia down-regulates the glucose transport system and exacerbates the tendency to hyperglycemia also.[14] This is glucose toxicity, which is alleviated by restoration to euglycemia.[15]

Metabolic Response to Surgery and Trauma

Trauma and surgery, changes in circulating volume with hemorrhage, and infection (local or systemic) all lead to a stress response. The increased concentrations of cate-

cholamines and glucocorticoids contribute to insulin resistance, whereas sympathetic activity (through stimulation of α_2 adrenoceptors) reduces insulin secretion. These lead to catabolism with lipolysis and ketogenesis, proteolysis, and a high hepatic glucose output from gluconeogenesis and glycogenolysis.[16] These changes are more pronounced in individuals with preexisting diabetes through the exacerbation of established insulin deficiency and insulin resistance.

Insulin Biosynthesis and Secretion

The mechanisms of insulin biosynthesis are outside the scope of this chapter. However, it is important in the investigation of hypoglycemia to recognize that insulin is cosecreted with C peptide. C peptide is secreted in equimolar concentrations with specific insulin after an appropriate stimulus. It is only specific insulin that has intrinsic biologic activity. Proinsulin, split fragments, and C peptide have no appreciable effect on glucose homeostasis.

Regulation of Insulin Action

Insulin Delivery to Target Tissues

Optimal delivery of insulin to target tissues is dependent on an adequate circulation to capillary beds, migration across the endothelium, and passage through interstitial fluid to the target insulin receptor. These are not thought to be significant determinants of insulin-stimulated glucose uptake. The major rate-limiting sites for insulin action are thought to be at the postreceptor level in the target cell.[17,18]

The Insulin Signal

Insulin's major actions on carbohydrate, lipid, and protein metabolism are initiated through binding to cell membrane insulin receptors in muscle, liver, and adipose tissue. This triggers a cascade of intracellular events, which, in insulin-stimulated glucose uptake, is dependent on the synthesis and transfer of the glucose transport protein, GLUT 4, to the plasma membrane.[19]

GLUT 4 is the insulin-responsive transporter, which is located in adipose tissue, skeletal, and cardiac muscle. The importance of GLUT 4 to glucose homeostasis was realized when 50% of GLUT 4 knockout mice developed diabetes and the other 50% became very insulin resistant.[20]

During fasting conditions, 90% of GLUT 4 resides in storage vesicles in the cytoplasm.[21] Insulin postreceptor signaling coordinates the mechanism for the transport of GLUT 4 from intracytoplasmic storage sites to the plasma membrane, where a hydrophilic pore increases glucose entry sevenfold.

Insulin Degradation

The plasma half-life of insulin, after endogenous β cell secretion, is estimated at 4 to 6 minutes with a plasma clearance of 8 to 18 mL/min per kilogram.[22] Metabolism of insulin by intracellular insulin degradation enzyme is the predominant method of elimination, because excretion of intact insulin by the kidney is minimal. Subsequent to the binding of insulin to its receptor, proteolysis occurs in liver (80%) and kidney (15%), with the liver removing 50% of the portal secreted load of insulin through a first-pass effect. The kidney, however, removes 50% of insulin that enters the systemic circulation, which is one reason why exogenous insulin requirements (administered into the systemic circulation) decrease in renal disease.[23] Skeletal muscle, adipose tissue, and skin also have minor contributions to insulin degradation.

Within the physiologic range, elimination of insulin is linear, but in the presence of persistently high concentrations of insulin (supraphysiologic or pharmacologic), the relation between clearance and concentration becomes nonlinear.[24] This is demonstrative of saturation kinetics and is indicative of a receptor-mediated process.

There is evidence that insulin resistance is associated with slower metabolic clearance of insulin, and this may contribute to the peripheral hyperinsulinemia seen in this context. This has been demonstrated in type 2 diabetes, obesity, and hypertension.[25-28] In obesity, reduction of body mass index is associated with reduced insulin concentration, predominantly through acceleration in metabolic clearance rather than significant reduction in insulin secretion.[29]

Insulin degradation plays a significant role in the termination of insulin action, because the major sites of insulin effect are responsible also for its degradation. The exact interrelation between the two has not been clarified.

Development and Administration of Insulin as a Drug

Insulin is manufactured in solution or suspension standardized to a concentration of 100 U/mL (U100), although more concentrated solutions (U500) are available for those whose insulin requirements are exceptionally high. Distribution is in vials or as "Pen" devices. Vials should be stored in a refrigerator. The biologic activities of the various manufactured types of insulin are not identical, and therefore the concentration of one insulin preparation in mass per unit volume is not predictive of its potency compared with other types of insulin. The "insulin unit" is an expression of bioequivalence among different insulin preparations, and one unit is defined as the amount of insulin necessary to reduce the fasting blood glucose of a rabbit to 2.5 mmol/L.

The manufacture of human insulin by recombinant DNA technology enables mass production of a variety of insulin on a scale not possible with the previous methods used in the extraction and purification of animal insulin. Human insulin causes less hypersensitivity reactions than animal insulin, and lipoatrophy of injection sites is not seen. The problem of lipoatrophy at injection sites is probably immunogenic in origin and was a recognized feature of animal insulin administration.

Routes of Administration

The major routes of administration of insulin are subcutaneous, intravenous, and intramuscular. Insulin is inactivated rapidly by proteases in the upper gastrointestinal tract and therefore cannot be given orally. The delivery of insulin into either the upper or lower respiratory tract can, at times, produce systemic insulin concentrations similar to subcutaneous administration, but currently there is marked variability of this effect.

Subcutaneous

This is the most widely used route of administration, and all insulin currently available can be given by subcutaneous bolus injection. Soluble insulin and the insulin analogues are licensed also for continuous subcutaneous infusion. Administration into the subcutaneous tissues differs from endogenous insulin secretion in two significant aspects: the kinetics does not mimic the normal rapid increase and decrease of native insulin secretion in response to ingestion of food, and the insulin diffuses into the systemic rather than the portal circulation. Therefore, the first-pass effects of insulin action on the liver during a meal do not occur.

The recommended sites for subcutaneous administration are the anterior abdominal wall, anterior or lateral aspect of the thigh, or the upper lateral aspect of the arm.[30] With repeated insulin administration into one site lipohypertrophy may develop in the patient; therefore, patients are recommended to rotate their injection sites on a daily basis. Significant lipohypertrophy may cause significant variability in insulin absorption. Mild lipohypertrophy is common in chronic subcutaneous insulin therapy. In the absence of hypertrophic injection sites, there remains mild variability in absorption between sites; insulin is absorbed quicker from the subcutaneous tissues of the anterior abdominal wall than from the thighs, with the slowest absorption seen from the upper arms. Exercise of a limb will also cause a mild increase in the absorption of subcutaneous insulin.

A subcutaneous bolus injection of insulin is administered using a conventional insulin syringe or Pen device with a needle. The syringe is graduated in insulin units so that the desired insulin dose can be drawn from a glass vial. There are many Pen devices, which are individual to the type of insulin contained, with both human and animal insulin Pens currently available. The desired dose of insulin is selected using a dial mechanism fitted in the body of the Pen. Pen devices are designed to be either disposable or fitted with replaceable 1.5- or 3-mL insulin cartridges. Most companies are moving exclusively to the manufacturing of 3-mL cartridges. Most patients prefer to use a Pen for insulin administration, because of the more acceptable appearance and the ease of use and storage. Pens do require a minimum standard of vision and manual dexterity, but have been adapted for visually or physically disabled patients.

Continuous subcutaneous insulin infusion (CSII) is achieved using a syringe pump, which delivers soluble regular insulin or an insulin analogue at a basal rate that attempts to mimic background endogenous insulin secretion.[31] This is typically within the range of 0.5 to 1.0 U/hr. In addition, the pump is able to administer intermittent bolus doses, which are given regularly before meal times or can be given to correct hyperglycemia at any time.[32] Both the basal infusion and bolus dose are programmable and readily adjustable by the patient in accordance with ambient glycemia. Because the insulin administered has a short duration of action and there is only a minimal amount of drug in the subcutaneous space at any one time, there is a faster onset of ketoacidosis should there be an unsuspected technical failure of insulin delivery.[33] Most pumps have alarms that warn the individual should this occur. No advantage of CSII over other insulin regimens has been demonstrated in a randomized trial.

Intravenous and Intramuscular

The intravenous route of administration is widely used in the management of diabetic hyperglycemic emergencies and the perioperative period, when the patient is unable, or not permitted, to take food by mouth. The continued administration of subcutaneous insulin when oral intake of food is insufficient increases the likelihood of hypoglycemia. Only soluble insulin is given intravenously, because the half-life of 4 to 6 minutes allows easy rapid adjustment of insulin requirements according to prevailing blood glucose concentration and the clinical condition. There is no advantage to giving insulin by intravenous bolus rather than continuous intravenous infusion.

The intramuscular route of administration of soluble insulin is considered for use in diabetic hyperglycemic emergency states, when there is unacceptable delay in the administration of intravenous insulin. The absorption of insulin from muscle can be compromised significantly in circulatory failure, therefore intravenous insulin should be preferred.

Pharmacokinetics of the Available Insulin

The kinetics of synthetic insulin can be altered either through changes to the insulin amino acid sequence or by the addition of a zinc salt or protamine to form an insulin suspension. Moreover, the degree of crystallization of a zinc insulin suspension is also important. These modifications have a major impact on the speed of onset, time-to-peak effect, and duration of action of subcutaneous insulin (Table 48–3).

Soluble Regular Insulin

Human, porcine, and bovine insulin are available as soluble insulin to be injected 30 minutes before meals. The time for

TABLE 48–3.

Pharmacokinetic Characteristics of the Commonly Used Insulins

	Onset (hr)	Peak (hr)	Duration (hr)
Soluble regular	0.5–1	2–3	4–6
Analogue	<0.25–0.5	0.5–1.5	2–3
Isophane	2–4	4–8	10–15
Insulin zinc suspension	2–4	7–15	15–24

dissociation of hexameric insulin aggregates into insulin monomers in the subcutaneous tissues, and their consequent absorption, is responsible for the delay in onset of action.[3]

Soluble regular insulin is used in subcutaneous multiple insulin injection regimens, when it is administered before meals and long-acting insulin is injected at night. In addition, soluble insulin can be drawn into a syringe containing isophane insulin for use in a twice daily insulin regimen. Soluble regular insulin is used also in continuous subcutaneous infusion pumps. Intravenous and intramuscular administration of soluble insulin is indicated in the management of hyperglycemic emergency states and to ensure adequate glycemic control during the perioperative period.

Insulin Analogues

Insulin analogues exist as monomeric insulin only; this ensures a faster onset of action and time-to-peak effect, with a shorter duration of action, than soluble regular insulin. Their kinetic profile is similar therefore to endogenous insulin. Insulin lispro and insulin aspart are the most widely prescribed analogues.

Analogues are used in multiple injection regimens, CSII, and twice-daily insulin regimens. They can be given intravenously, although this is not recommended because there is no advantage over regular soluble insulin when using this route. They are administered just before or up to 15 minutes after the start of a meal.

Isophane Protamine Insulin (NPH Insulin)

NPH (neutral protamine Hagedorn) insulin is a suspension of human, porcine, or bovine isophane insulin with protamine. The addition of protamine slows the speed of onset of action and lengthens the duration of effect of this insulin.

It may be given in isolation or mixed with soluble regular insulin drawn from a vial. However, human and porcine NPH are most commonly administered in a manufactured mixture with soluble regular insulin (biphasic isophane insulin) or human NPH can occur as a mixture with an analogue (biphasic isophane insulin analogue). When used in combination with an insulin analogue, there is a faster onset of action and time-to-peak effect, and administration should therefore occur within 15 minutes of starting a meal.

There is wide variety in the available ratios of isophane insulin to short duration insulin in these biphasic mixtures—from 90:10 to 50:50. There is no evidence of significant improvement in overall glycemic control with the use of different biphasic mixtures within the same subject or by switching from one mix to another. The 70:30 and 75:25 mixtures are the most commonly prescribed.

Insulin Zinc Suspension and Protamine Zinc Insulin Suspension

When human, porcine, or bovine insulin is mixed into a suspension with a zinc salt, this results in prolongation of insulin action to 24 to 30 hours. This insulin is used as a once daily subcutaneous injection in isolation or as part of a multiple injection regimen with soluble insulin. It must not be physically mixed with soluble insulin. There may be a greater risk for hypoglycemia when it is used in a multiple injection regimen, because of its longer duration of action and time-to-peak effect compared with isophane insulin.

Protamine zinc bovine insulin suspension has the longest duration of action of the available types of insulin and is therefore used once daily. It must not be physically mixed with soluble insulin, but can be used in a combination regimen. Currently, it is rarely prescribed.

Maintenance Treatment of Diabetes Mellitus

Type 1 Diabetes Mellitus

Type 1 diabetes mellitus is a state of absolute insulin deficiency caused by failure of the islet β cells, characterized by a predisposition to ketoacidosis. The incidence is currently less than 0.5% of the population, although the rate is increasing. All patients require life-long insulin therapy.

The destruction of the β-cell unit is a cell-mediated autoimmune response associated with circulating antibodies to its structural components and secretions. The precipitant of this autoimmune process is unknown, but there is a genetic susceptibility operating through the HLA-DR4 genotype.

The Diabetes Control and Complications Trial (DCCT) showed conclusively that intensive glycemic control with

either bolus subcutaneous insulin or CSII reduces the incidence rates of microvascular complications by 60% to 70%.[34]

There are four subcutaneous insulin regimens that attempt to achieve this goal:

Basal-bolus: Soluble insulin is given before meals and isophane protamine insulin at night.
Twice daily: Biphasic mixed insulin is given before breakfast and evening meal.
Three times daily: Soluble insulin is given before breakfast and lunch, and one dose of biphasic mixed insulin before the evening meal.
CSII: See earlier.

Patients are encouraged to perform home blood glucose monitoring with adjustment of insulin dosage to achieve fasting and preprandial glucose levels of less than 6 mmol/L. This is an ideal that can be difficult to achieve without hypoglycemia, and therefore some compromise of targets is inevitable within the lifestyle of each patient. Long-term metabolic control is best assessed with a measurement of glycosylated hemoglobin (HbA1c), which is DCCT aligned. This is representative of glycemia over the previous 8 weeks. A value less than 7.5% best reduces the risk for microvascular complications.[34]

The basal-bolus and CSII regimens are most likely to achieve the intensive glycemic control desired by DCCT to reduce microvascular complications. However, many patients have achieved the desired degree of control on alternative regimens.

Type 2 Diabetes Mellitus

Type 2 diabetes mellitus is a progressive metabolic disorder of peripheral insulin resistance, in association with hyperglycemia, which is accompanied commonly by progressive β-cell failure and relative insulin deficiency.[7,35] It is a genetic disorder with environmental factors also playing a significant role.[36,37] The mechanisms of the insulin resistance and later insulin deficiency are largely unknown. The prevalence varies with ethnic group from 2% in Europeans to 35% in Pima Indians.

Treatment consists initially of diet and weight reduction. If glycemic control is unsatisfactory, sulphonylureas or metformin are commonly prescribed as monotherapy. Some patients may come to combination therapy with these two agents. Acarbose is an α-glucosidase inhibitor that is helpful in some patients. Thiazolidinediones are insulin-sensitizing agents, which are agonists of peroxisome proliferator-activated receptors.[38] The therapeutic benefit of combination therapy with thiazolidinediones and other oral antidiabetic agents has been demonstrated.[39,40]

The United Kingdom Prospective Diabetes Study established that intensive glycemic control per se reduces the incidence of microvascular complications in type 2 diabetes, and intensive control achieved with metformin reduces macrovascular events.[41,42] In addition, intensive blood pressure treatment reduces the incidence of microvascular and macrovascular events.[43,44] The desired degree of metabolic control and blood pressure becomes increasingly difficult to achieve with time, despite stepped escalation in treatment.[45]

The principal indication for insulin therapy in type 2 diabetes is unsatisfactory glycemic control, despite attention to diet and compliance with maximal oral medication. Unexpected weight loss is a sign of insulin deficiency in type 2 diabetes.

Most patients with type 2 diabetes that require insulin therapy can be adequately managed with a twice daily insulin regimen of biphasic mixed insulin. However, insulin therapy is associated with weight gain, which is undesirable in the patient who is already overweight and insulin resistant. The introduction of insulin is not a guarantee of the achievement of satisfactory glycemic control. Insulin can be used in combination with metformin or a sulphonylurea, which may reduce insulin requirements.[46] Some countries have granted a license also for the combination of insulin and thiazolidinediones. In the patient who is overweight, the combination of metformin or an insulin sensitizer with one or two injections of insulin daily seems to be the best current treatment for patients requiring insulin.[47]

Perioperative Management of Diabetes Mellitus

In contrast to the patient with normal glucose tolerance, the patient with diabetes mellitus is at greater risk for an adverse event during the perioperative period. Some of this risk is predictable and is caused by preoperative factors that can be modified or assessed before surgery.

Preoperative Factors

Patients with diabetes carry a significant cardiovascular risk and are therefore more likely to suffer an acute coronary event, cardiac failure, or a stroke.[48] Attempts should be made to assess and minimize this risk before elective surgery with attention to blood pressure control, weight reduction, left ventricular function, coronary ischemia, renal function and proteinuria, and hyperlipidemia. Unless the medical and metabolic states are optimal, it is generally safer to delay surgery.

Obesity may lead to problems with intubation, ventilation, and postoperative atelectasis and pulmonary infection. There is the additional risk for thrombo-embolic disease and skin necrosis over pressure points, which should be anticipated with appropriate prophylaxis. The obese patient also will be slower to rehabilitate after major surgery.

Delayed wound healing and sepsis are more common in diabetes and relate in part to poor glycemic control and ischemia, but there is an increased susceptibility to wound complications per se from the diabetic state. Glycemic control should be optimized before surgery to minimize this risk, and optimal metabolic control should be the aim over the entire perioperative period.

Subjects with insulin-treated diabetes mellitus should be admitted 24 hours before elective major surgery. If metabolic control is poor, then admission may need to be earlier. Subjects taking long-acting sulphonylureas should be changed to short-duration agents to reduce the risk for fasting hypoglycemia in the preoperative period.

Perioperative and Postoperative Metabolic Control

The management of perioperative glycemic control is best considered according to the treatment used to manage diabetes before surgery, the nature of the surgical procedure, and its anticipated duration. The risk for hypoglycemia as a result of fasting on the day of surgery can be minimized. Not all patients require treatment with infusions of intravenous insulin and glucose. Some surgical procedures, particularly open-heart surgery, cause particular insulin resistance.[49] The glucose-rich solutions, inotropes, and metabolic consequences of hypothermia all contribute to this process.

If an intravenous insulin infusion is required (see later), two regimens are widely used. The most important aspect in the decision of which to select is local guidelines, knowledge, and expertise in the monitoring and adjustments required for each. Capillary glucose monitoring at least every 2 hours is essential with intravenous insulin infusions. Intravenous insulin should not be discontinued in insulin-treated patients; if hypoglycemia occurs despite low intravenous insulin infusion rates, the dextrose infusion should be changed from 5% to 10% solution.

- **Glucose-insulin-potassium infusion regimen** (Table 48–4): This is the simpler and easier to use of the intravenous regimens because the infusates are all contained within one infusion bag.[50] It is infused at a constant rate of 100 mL/hr without need for a pump. Because only one intravenous line is required, this eliminates the risk for an unidentified line or pump failure (increasing the risk for hypoglycemia or hyperglycemia) with the use of multiple

TABLE 48–4.

Glucose-Insulin-Potassium Regimen for the Perioperative Management of Diabetes. Further Adjustments Are Made in 5-U Increments

To a 500-mL bag of 10% dextrose, add 10 mmol KCl and 15 U soluble insulin.

Infuse at 100 mL/hr.

Check capillary glucose hourly.

Adjust infusion by making up a new mixture for infusion:
- If glucose > 12 mmol/L → 20 U soluble insulin
- If glucose < 5 mmol/L → 10 U soluble insulin

lines. If adjustments are required to achieve target glucose concentrations, a different glucose-insulin-potassium mixture is made up. It is the ideal regimen to choose for short surgical procedures that require fasting (e.g., endoscopy). Potassium is required to prevent insulin-induced hypokalemia.

■ **Intravenous insulin sliding scale** (Table 48–5): Intravenous soluble insulin (1 U/mL) is given as an infusion using a syringe-driver pump at a rate according to ambient capillary glucose measurements.[51] A total of 5% glucose solution at 100 mL/hr is infused either into a separate vein or into the same vein as the insulin infusion using a multiple connector to reduce the risk for hypoglycemia. This regimen provides more flexibility for insulin adjustment and is the ideal regimen if large fluctuations in blood glucose are anticipated (e.g., cardiopulmonary bypass surgery or parenteral nutrition therapy).[52]

Intravenous insulin requirements for sliding scales can be estimated in patients treated with insulin from the total daily maintenance subcutaneous dose. The intravenous insulin infusion rate per hour required for an ambient capillary glucose of 4 to 8 mmol/L approximates to the maintenance hourly subcutaneous insulin requirement. For example, a total daily dose of 24 U would approximate to an intravenous infusion rate of 1 U/hr for a capillary glucose of 4 to 8 mmol/L.

No Specific Medical Therapy (Diet Controlled)

If minor surgery is planned, and prior glycemic control is satisfactory, patients may require no specific intervention, other than capillary glucose monitoring, for a short procedure. With major surgery, blood glucose concentrations should be checked four times per hour; if persistent hyperglycemia develops (glucose >10 mmol/L), an intravenous insulin-glucose infusion should be commenced.

Oral Agents

Oral agents should be discontinued on the day of surgery. Long-duration oral agents should have been changed previously to short-duration agents.

If minor surgery is planned, and prior glycemic control is satisfactory, patients may require no specific intervention for a short procedure. Blood glucose concentrations should be checked four times per hour; if persistent hyperglycemia develops (glucose >10 mmol/L), an intravenous insulin-glucose infusion should be commenced. If major surgery is planned, an intravenous insulin-glucose infusion should be commenced at 8:00 AM or 2 hours before surgery. When the patient is eating and drinking normally after surgery, oral therapy can be restarted. Patients are more insulin resistant in the postoperative period and may require subcutaneous insulin for a short time if oral therapy does not ensure euglycemia.

Insulin Therapy

Ideally, patients treated with insulin should be first on a morning operating schedule. This reduces the inconvenience of an insulin-glucose infusion all morning and early afternoon in preparation for an afternoon surgery. In addition, the risk for overnight and early morning hypoglycemia should be reduced by a small meal at night if blood glucose levels are less than 8 mmol/L. If patients are scheduled for an afternoon surgery, an early light breakfast should be offered with administration of subcutaneous soluble insulin. An insulin-glucose infusion should be started from mid-morning.

The normal dose of subcutaneous insulin should be restarted when the patient is eating and drinking adequately. There should be an overlap of 30 minutes between the administration of subcutaneous insulin and the discontinuation of the intravenous infusion. Subcutaneous insulin requirements in the postoperative period can be estimated from the amount of intravenous insulin required during the previous 24 hours. A scale to plan subcutaneous insulin requirements can be used. The patient receives insulin twice daily or four time daily as prescribed, and in addition receives extra doses of soluble insulin before meals if the capillary glucose is greater than 12 mmol/L. Maintenance insulin can then be adjusted in accordance with the amount of additional soluble insulin required during the previous day.

TABLE 48–5.

Insulin Sliding Scale Regimen for the Perioperative Management of Diabetes

Capillary Glucose (mmol/L)	Infusion Rate for 1 U/mL Solution of Soluble Insulin
<4.0	0.5*
4.1–8.0	1.0
8.1–11.0	2.0
11.1–15.0	3.0
15.1–20.0	4.0
20.1–25.0	5.0
>25.1	6.0

The maximum insulin infusion rate can be increased (e.g., in extreme insulin resistance).

Infuse 5% dextrose solution at 100 mL/hr. Add 50 U soluble insulin to 50 mL of 0.9% saline. Infuse according to the variable rate above as dictated by capillary glucose.

*Ten percent dextrose should be substituted if capillary glucose measurements remain within this range. Insulin should **not** be discontinued.

Emergency Management of Diabetes Mellitus

The common metabolic emergencies of diabetes are:

- Diabetic ketoacidosis
- Hyperosmolar hyperglycemic state
- Hypoglycemia

Diabetic Ketoacidosis

Incidence and Prognosis

Diabetic ketoacidosis is a common medical emergency that still has a significant associated mortality. In North America, Europe, and Australia mortality rates have been quoted at 1% to 4% in unselected cases, but prognosis is significantly worse in advanced ketoacidosis with quoted mortality rates of 5% to 10% quoted.[53–56] Adverse outcomes are related to infection, multiple organ failure, adult respiratory distress syndrome, acute pancreatitis, cerebral edema, coronary heart and cerebrovascular disease, coma, or electrolyte disturbance.[57] In children, there is a greater frequency of cerebral edema as a cause of death.[58]

Seventeen percent of patients with diabetic ketoacidosis have new-onset type 1 diabetes.[59] The common causes of decompensation of known diabetes were cessation of insulin therapy, failure to increase insulin dosage in the presence of infection, and inadequate home blood glucose monitoring. These causes are more common in adolescents and young adults.[60] In middle age, acute coronary events and stroke also are significant causes. Patients using CSII are at risk for rapid-onset ketoacidosis in the event of pump or catheter failure.[33]

Ketogenesis to Ketoacidosis

With complete absence of insulin in type 1 diabetes, there is hyperglycemia and acceleration of lipolysis and proteoly-sis, which will lead to the clinical syndrome of ketoacidosis without urgent insulin replacement. Hyperglycemia may only be modest; it is the consequent metabolic acidosis and ketonemia that leads to the early presentation of decompensated type 1 diabetes compared with the relatively late presentation of the hyperosmolar hyperglycemic state of decompensated type 2 diabetes. Four clinical factors contribute to the development of ketoacidosis[61]:

1. Insulin deficiency occurs with β cell loss. Insulin deficiency causes hyperglycemia from increased hepatic glucose output (glycogenolysis and gluconeogenesis) and reduced peripheral glucose uptake.
2. Increased stress hormones (e.g., catecholamines, cortisol, glucagon, and growth hormone) may follow an infection or acute vascular event. Stress hormones exacerbate hepatic glucose output. The consequent hyperglycemia causes an osmotic diuresis with water and electrolyte loss.
3. The insulin deficiency and stress hormones accelerate lipolysis and ketogenesis, which in turn will be exacerbated by fasting.
4. The patient is able to buffer the acidic ketone bodies until dehydration leads to poor renal perfusion with failed distal convoluted tubule function. When ketosis and acidosis supervene, the patient cannot drink enough to maintain hydration. Vomiting exacerbates the deficit of water and electrolytes. Ketoacidosis causes vomiting both through a central effect and delayed gastric emptying.

With reference to Figure 48–1 the metabolic consequences of insulin deficiency can be understood, namely increased hepatic glucose output, lipolysis, and proteolysis. Figure 48–2 summarizes the clinical features of ketoacidosis. All four factors contribute to varying degrees.

Hyperkalemia results from the systemic acidosis and sodium-potassium/ATPase pump failure. There will be a total body deficit of potassium that must be addressed.

Ketoacidosis can occur also in type 2 diabetes and is therefore not entirely indicative of the true insulin dependency of type 1 diabetes.[54,62] In Afro-Caribbean and Chinese patients, ketoacidosis as the presentation of type 2 diabetes is being increasingly recognized.[63,64] This syndrome is more

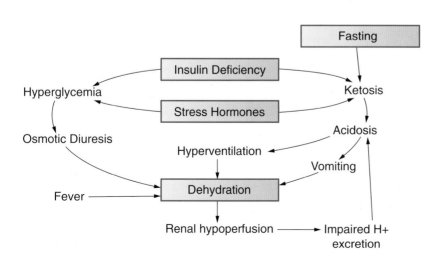

Figure 48–2. Principal factors involved in the development of diabetic ketoacidosis.

common in obese patients and in the presence of acanthosis nigricans. It is causally linked to preexisting severe insulin resistance that is heightened during an acute medical illness (e.g., sepsis). Hyperosmolality, hyperglycemia, and insulin counter-regulatory hormones increase insulin resistance further to a point where ketogenesis ceases to be inhibited. With medical intervention, these patients may eventually be treated with diet alone or oral hypoglycemic agents. In this instance, ketoacidosis does not predict true insulin dependency.

Clinical Management: General Aspects

The management of the patient with diabetic ketoacidosis involves general aspects in the resuscitation of the unwell or patients in coma, in addition to the specific management of hyperglycemia, electrolyte disturbances, and metabolic acidosis.

The assessment of airway protection, oxygenation, gas exchange, and adequacy of the circulation should proceed as for any acutely ill patient. History, clinical examination, initial laboratory investigations, and radiology should be directed toward the identification of a precipitant of the decompensation (e.g., infection, myocardial infarction, stroke, or pancreatitis) and complications of the adverse clinical state (e.g., arrhythmia, organ failure, aspiration, electrolyte disturbance, and metabolic acidosis) (Table 48–6). In 30% of admissions, the precipitant is unidentified. Sepsis is the most common precipitating factor that is identified.

Increased concentrations of amylase and lipase are seen in up to 30% of presentations with ketoacidosis; however, only one third of these patients have acute pancreatitis confirmed in one study on computed tomography.[65] Computed tomography confirmed acute pancreatitis does relate to an adverse outcome more than the absolute degree of hyper-amylasemia, hyperlipidemia, or Ranson's criteria prognostic score, which overestimates the severity of pancreatitis in diabetic ketoacidosis. Whether acute pancreatitis is a cause or effect of ketoacidosis is unclear. In some individuals, hypertriglyceridemia and alcohol are important precipitants.

1. Saline Replacement

The osmotic diuresis and vomiting of advanced diabetic ketoacidosis lead to profound deficiencies principally of sodium, potassium, and fluid, with significant losses of phosphate, calcium, and magnesium also. These total body deficits on average amount to 7 L water, 700 mEq sodium, 350 mEq potassium, 500 mEq phosphate, 100 mEq magnesium, and 100 mEq calcium in a 70-kg individual.[66] Most patients will have prerenal failure related to the degree of fluid loss, although the osmotic diuresis may protect against the development of intrinsic renal dysfunction.

An outline for the rate of rehydration with 0.9% saline is suggested (Table 48–7). In the past, faster rates have been

TABLE 48–6.

Initial Investigations in the Management of Diabetic Ketoacidosis

Full blood count and differential

Electrolytes and renal function

Plasma glucose

Arterial blood gases and bicarbonate

Blood cultures

Urine microscopy and culture

Electrocardiography

Chest radiograph

TABLE 48–7.

Electrolyte Replacement Rates in the Early Management of Diabetic Ketoacidosis

Intravenous Saline (0.9%) Replacement*

- 1 L over 15 minutes

- 1 L over 1 hour

- 1 L over 2 hours

- 1 L over 4 hours

- 1 L 6–8 hours, hourly thereafter

Intravenous Potassium Replacement†

Serum Potassium Concentration (mmol/L)	Concentration of KCl Infusion (mmol/L in Saline or Dextrose)
>5.5	Nil
4.0–5.4	20
<3.9	40

*This should be replaced with 5% or 10% dextrose when the blood glucose falls to less than 12 mmol/L.
†Intravenous potassium should be infused at no more than 10 mmol/hr.

suggested, but there have been concerns regarding the incidence of pulmonary edema and cerebral edema. Generally, 4 L saline should be given in the first 7 to 8 hours, and then a further 3 to 4 L per 24 hours with strict monitoring of fluid balance and urine output.[67] Central venous pressure measurements are justified in elderly patients or those in whom there is concern regarding cardiac, renal, or fluid status. The use of intravenous colloid in preference to crystalloid infusions in initial fluid resuscitation is not advocated.

2. Insulin Therapy

Diabetic ketoacidosis is treated optimally with a continuous intravenous infusion of soluble insulin through a delivery system that allows easy and frequent adjustments of the infusion rate. The most convenient method is the use of a syringe-driver pump administering a 1 U/mL solution of soluble insulin. Significant hypokalemia should be treated before any intravenous bolus of insulin is administered. Insulin will cause a rapid decrease in serum potassium concentration, which may precipitate cardiac arrhythmia if there is significant preexisting hypokalemia. The rate of infusion should be guided by hourly capillary glucose measurements, and a suggested variable insulin infusion rate appropriate to these glucose measurements is presented (Table 48–8). Insulin requirements can be large during the initial stage of treatment because of insulin resistance caused by metabolic acidosis, high concentrations of counter-regulatory hormones, infection, tissue hypoxia, and glucose toxicity.[68] If glucose concentrations do not decrease after the start of the infusion, the rate of infusion should be increased. Once blood glucose concentrations are persistently less than

TABLE 48–8.

Insulin Infusion Rate for Diabetic Ketoacidosis

Capillary Glucose (mmol/L)	Infusion Rate for 1 U/mL Solution of Soluble Insulin
<4.0	0.5
4.1–8.0	1.0
8.1–11.0	2.0
11.1–15.0	3.0
15.1–20.0	4.0
20.1–25.0	5.0
>25.1	6.0

Insulin should **not** be discontinued. Normoglycemia is maintained with a dextrose infusion when glucose is <12 mmol/L.

12 mmol/L, the intravenous crystalloid should be changed from 0.9% saline to 5% dextrose to maintain normoglycemia in the presence of continuous intravenous insulin. Some patients may require a greater concentration of intravenous dextrose.

If intravenous insulin therapy is difficult to achieve during the initial treatment phase, 10 U soluble insulin can be administered intramuscularly every 2 hours, with capillary glucose monitoring, until intravenous delivery is sustained.

The initiation of intravenous insulin therapy for diabetic ketoacidosis immediately terminates ketogenesis; however, ketones can persist in the urine for a further 72 hours before they are metabolized and excreted completely. Insulin will immediately inhibit glycogenolysis and gluconeogenesis and stimulate glucose uptake into muscle and adipose tissue, which will correct hyperglycemia. Correction of dehydration and restoration of renal perfusion pressure with fluid replacement will encourage excretion of ketones and hydrogen ions, the generation of bicarbonate and, therefore, restoration of normal blood and cellular pH.

When acidosis has been corrected and the patient is eating and drinking normally, subcutaneous insulin can be started.

3. Potassium Replacement

One of the principal causes of early morbidity and mortality in diabetic ketoacidosis is cardiac arrhythmias caused by hypokalemia. At presentation with ketoacidosis, all patients have a whole body deficit of potassium. Insulin deficiency and metabolic acidosis cause redistribution of potassium across plasma membranes, which may result in hyperkalemia. Consequent hesitation about replacing potassium in the initial stages of management can rapidly cause life-threatening hypokalemia. This is because insulin replacement drives potassium back into cells and causes an immediate rapid decrease in the serum potassium concentration. Intravenous potassium replacement is usually essential after the first 500 mL of 0.9% saline. Obviously, oliguria and hyperkalemia will dictate a different strategy.

Potassium requirements are considerable in the initial stages of management of ketoacidosis to restore and maintain normokalemia. To ensure adequate rates of replacement, serum electrolytes need to be checked frequently (2–4 hourly) in the first 24 to 48 hours and infusion rates adjusted accordingly.

An outline for intravenous potassium replacement is suggested (see Table 48–7).

4. Use of Sodium Bicarbonate

Adequate intravenous insulin therapy and fluid replacement will correct the metabolic acidosis of diabetic ketoacidosis. During the last 5 to 10 years, there has been less enthusiasm for the previous widespread administration of intravenous sodium bicarbonate to rapidly increase the arterial pH in cases of advanced ketoacidosis. The concerns regarding bicarbonate therapy were the exacerbation of hypokalemia and hyperosmolality, and an increase in intracellular acidosis (especially within the central nervous system) despite an increase in arterial pH—paradoxic cerebrospinal fluid acidosis (Table 48–9). The administration of bicarbonate may also delay recovery from ketosis by the stimulation of hepatic ketogenesis.[69]

Clinical studies, examining the administration of bicarbonate to patients with advanced diabetic ketoacidosis (pH 6.9–7.1), have shown neither an improvement in morbidity or mortality rates nor an increase in the frequency of adverse outcomes compared with those cases when bicarbonate was withheld.[70] Therefore, we would advocate its use only if the pH is less than 6.9 with no improvement in the metabolic parameters during the early stages of insulin and fluid therapy. Failure to improve acidosis despite an increase in the rates of replacement is usually related to an unidentified source of sepsis or tissue necrosis; management should be directed toward its identification (e.g., intra-abdominal abscess, foot sepsis, bowel infarction, pancreatitis, and others).

If bicarbonate is deemed necessary, 100 to 150 mmol sodium bicarbonate should be given as a solution in saline or water over 2 to 3 hours.

5. Other Measures

The identification of sepsis may be difficult during the initial clinical and biochemical assessment of patients with diabetic ketoacidosis. Ketoacidosis can cause pyrexia, increased C reactive protein, and leucocytosis, which may be difficult to differentiate from infection. It may be associated also with peripheral vasodilatation, which can cause hypothermia and can mask the presence of infection. Because sepsis is an important precipitant of increasing insulin requirements and consequent metabolic decompensation, most patients with ketoacidosis receive broad spectrum antibiotics while bacteriologic results are pending.

TABLE 48–9.

Issues with the Use of Bicarbonate in Management of Diabetic Ketoacidosis

Risk-Benefit Considerations in the Use of Bicarbonate

Dangers of Acidemia	Dangers of NaHCO₃
■ Negative inotropism	■ Hypokalemia
■ Peripheral vasodilatation	■ Hypernatremia
■ Cerebral depression	■ Cerebrospinal acidosis
	■ Impaired oxyHb dissociation

A nasogastric tube should be passed and aspirated in the patient in coma. Gastric stasis and reduced gastric emptying consequent to ketoacidosis make the risk for vomiting, with consequent inhalation, considerable in the absence of stomach aspiration.

Continuous bedside cardiac monitoring is advised during the initial treatment phase of electrolyte replacement because arrhythmias are most common at this time.

Phosphate deficiency is commonly seen at presentation with ketoacidosis, but there is no evidence that replacement improves outcome. Severe deficiency of phosphate per se is associated with respiratory and skeletal muscle weakness and reduced cardiac function.[71] Some authors advocate phosphate replacement in diabetic ketoacidosis if there was associated cardiorespiratory failure. It is administered as 20 to 30 mEq/L potassium phosphate added to solutions of crystalloid and infused over several hours. Hypocalcemia can occur during replacement.

Prevention and Counseling

An important aspect to be addressed with the patient before discharge from the hospital is the reason for the development of ketoacidosis and how it could be avoided in the future. This may involve improvements in the day-to-day management and monitoring of diabetes, the management of "sick days" and reiteration of the signs of imminent metabolic decompensation, and when to seek medical assistance.[72]

Hyperglycemic Hyperosmolar State

The hyperglycemic hyperosmolar state describes the metabolic decompensation of type 2 diabetes. It is characterized by severe hyperglycemia, hyperosmolality of the plasma (>330 mOsm/kg), and dehydration sufficient to cause renal failure. It is differentiated clinically from diabetic ketoacidosis by an arterial pH greater than 7.30 and the presence of no more than mild dipstick ketonuria. It is not exclusive to type 2 diabetes because some patients with type 1 diabetes can present with a similar syndrome.[54] This illustrates the concept that diabetic ketoacidosis and hyperglycemic hyperosmolar syndrome represent the spectrum of hyperglycemic crises in diabetes, and that there is potential for overlap between types 1 and 2 diabetes in their clinical and metabolic presentation.

Precipitants induce hyperglycemic crises by increasing insulin resistance. Common precipitants include sepsis, acute coronary syndromes, stroke, trauma, and alcohol abuse.[73]

Incidence and Prognosis

Hospital admissions because of hyperglycemic hyperosmolar state are less common than diabetic ketoacidosis. Among patients with diabetes, ketoacidosis accounts for 4% to 9% of admissions, whereas the hyperglycemic hyperosmolar state accounts for less than 1%.[59,66] The prognosis for hyperglycemic hyperosmolar state is worse than ketoacidosis because patients are typically older and more hyperglycemic, dehydrated, and hyperosmolar. They are likely to have significant coexisting disease that contributes to an adverse clinical course (e.g., diffuse atherosclerosis, coronary insufficiency, cerebrovascular disease, and pulmonary embolism).[74,75] Mortality rates have been quoted from 15% to 50% compared with the less than 5% mortality rate of ketoacidosis.[55,75]

Pathogenesis

The development of the hyperglycemic hyperosmolar state results from the combination of inadequate insulin action and increased concentrations of the counter-regulatory hormones, glucagon, epinephrine, cortisol, and growth hormone.[61] There may be also an additional defect of sodium reabsorption in the kidney. The ambient concentration of insulin is able to prevent the transition from ketogenesis to ketoacidosis. It is not clear whether there are differences in the concentrations of counter-regulatory hormones, which may also contribute to the differences in degree of ketogenesis between ketoacidosis and the hyperglycemic hyperosmolar state. There is some evidence that lower concentrations of cortisol, growth hormone, and glucagon are present in the latter.[76,77]

In the absence of ketoacidosis, patients present with the symptoms of hyperglycemia. The degree of hyperglycemia can be extreme, and the chronic osmotic diuresis leads to dehydration, significant loss of electrolytes, and renal failure. The combination of hyperglycemia, uremia, and hypernatremia (from water depletion) results in plasma hyperosmolality, and this is a major contributing factor toward the high mortality rate of this condition.[54] Severe hyperosmolality leads to altered consciousness and coma.[74] Elderly patients may have dehydration exacerbated by hypodipsia. Coexisting disease contributes to their adverse prognosis.

Clinical Management: General Aspects

The general aspects of management and supportive care are as for ketoacidosis. Precipitants for the decompensation should be identified and treated; pneumonia and urinary tract sepsis remain the most common. Abdominal pain is less common than in ketoacidosis and its presence is more indicative of underlying pathology. Drowsiness or coma occurs more frequently and focal neurologic signs may be apparent, although these can be transient (e.g., hemiparesis).

1. Electrolyte and Fluid Replacement

The dehydration and electrolyte losses of the hyperglycemic hyperosmolar state are greater than for diabetic ketoacidosis. This relates to the longer passage of time before disease presentation. Average fluid depletion is 9 L. Average electrolyte losses are: 5 to 13 mEq/kg sodium, 4 to 6 mEq/kg potassium, 3 to 7 mEq/kg phosphate, 1 to 2 mEq/kg magnesium, and 1 to 2 mEq/kg calcium.[66]

Fluid replacement should commence with isotonic 0.9% saline. The estimated fluid deficit and the consequent improvements in hemodynamic parameters and urine output should guide the rate of fluid replacement. Central venous pressure monitoring should be considered in all patients to ensure optimal rates of fluid replacement. After the first 1 to 2 L of 0.9% saline, differing opinions exist as to whether hypotonic 0.45% saline should be substituted.[73] There is agreement that isotonic saline restores circulating volume, which independently improves insulin sensitivity and reduces the concentration of the counter-regulatory hormones. Rapid correction of plasma hyperosmolality with hypotonic saline may cause a significant cerebrospinal fluid/plasma osmotic gradient that may precipitate cerebral o.

Hypotonic saline is thought to reduce the risk for hypernatremia. Hypernatremia could be viewed as a compensatory response to a rapid decrease in plasma glucose (caused by intravenous insulin), whose role is to prevent rapid correction of plasma hyperosmolality, which would increase the risk for cerebral edema. Hypernatremia would be better avoided by rehydration with isotonic saline and slow correction of hyperglycemia with low-dose intravenous insulin. Hypotonic saline can be used on an empirical basis only, if the plasma sodium increases to greater than 160 mmol/L during treatment and only after initial treatment with isotonic saline. The rates of electrolyte and fluid replacement are similar to those advised for ketoacidosis (see Table 48–7).

When plasma glucose concentration decreases to less than 12 mmol/L, 5% dextrose should be substituted for saline to reduce the risk for hypoglycemia and to enable the continuation of intravenous insulin.

2. Insulin Therapy

Fluid replacement and gradual correction of plasma hyperosmolality is of greater importance than rapid achievement of euglycemia. Fluid replacement and treatment of precipitants of the hyperglycemic state will cause improvement in insulin sensitivity.

An intravenous insulin infusion regimen is suggested that aims to achieve a reduction in plasma glucose to no more than 70 mg/mL per hour (Table 48–10).

When the patient can eat and drink, and the metabolic and hemodynamic parameters are clearly improving, intravenous fluids can be discontinued. Oral rehydration should continue. Patients are likely to require subcutaneous insulin during the acute illness because of significant insulin resistance. However, most can be managed with oral hypoglycemic agents or diet alone at the time of discharge from hospital.

3. Potassium Replacement

If serum potassium is less than 3.3 mmol/L at presentation, insulin should be withheld until this is corrected by intravenous replacement. The replacement regimen is similar to that advised for ketoacidosis (see Table 48–7).

TABLE 48–10.

Insulin Infusion Rate for the Hyperglycemic Hyperosmolar State

Capillary Glucose (mmol/L)	Infusion Rate for 1 U/mL Solution of Soluble Insulin
<4.9	0.5
5.0–9.9	1.0
10–19.9	2.0
>20	3.0

Normoglycemia is maintained with a dextrose infusion when glucose is <12 mmol/L.

4. Other Measures

The risk for venous or arterial thromboembolic events in the hyperglycemic hyperosmolar state is significant and is a cause of the heightened mortality of the condition.[61,73] Consequently, patients are at increased risk for myocardial infarction, cerebral thrombosis, pulmonary embolism, and systemic arterial thromboembolism. Most physicians would advocate systemic anticoagulation with low molecular weight or intravenous heparin in all patients with plasma osmolality greater than 330 mOsm/kg.[78] This advice also should apply to diabetic ketoacidosis. When plasma osmolality is restored to normal and the patient is mobile, this can be discontinued. If there is delay in the return to full mobility, anticoagulant therapy should continue at a dose sufficient for prophylaxis of thromboembolic events.

Sepsis is the most common precipitant of the hyperglycemic hyperosmolar state. Patients should receive antibiotics appropriate to the likely source.

Lactic Acidosis

Lactic acidosis is defined as metabolic acidosis with a blood lactate concentration greater than 5 mmol/L. Two types of lactic acidosis are recognized: type A and type B. Type A is more common and occurs with hypoxia and reduced oxidative phosphorylation. It is seen in shock, cardiac failure, and as a preterminal event. Type B lactic acidosis occurs with:

- Systemic disorders including diabetes (particularly ketoacidosis) and liver failure
- Drug toxicity including aspirin and the older biguanide, phenformin (it may rarely occur with metformin)
- Inborn errors of metabolism
- Malignancy

No specific therapy for lactic acidosis is indicated. Treatment is of the underlying cause, although drug toxicity may require systemic alkalinization with intravenous bicarbonate and hemodialysis to enhance drug elimination. The lactic acidosis accompanying some episodes of diabetic ketoacidosis responds to insulin, fluid, and electrolyte replacement.

Hypoglycemia

Hypoglycemia is the most common metabolic emergency in diabetes. Fear of hypoglycemia or recurrent, unpredictable hypoglycemia is one of the major limiting factors for the achievement of desirable glycemic control.[79]

For ease of description, hypoglycemia can be classified as:

- *Asymptomatic:* this requires the confirmation of a low plasma glucose in the absence of symptoms.
- *Mild to moderate:* recognition of symptoms of hypoglycemia that allows self-treatment.
- *Severe:* the help of another individual is required in the treatment of hypoglycemia.

There is not a clear relation between plasma glucose concentration and the clinical features in any individual.

The intensive treatment group in the DCCT trial had 62 episodes of severe hypoglycemia per 100 patient-years.[34] The conventional treatment group had 19 episodes. The true prevalence may be greater because those with recurrent episodes were excluded from the main study.[80]

The prevalence of hypoglycemia in type 2 diabetes is less than in type 1.[81] The rate of severe hypoglycemia with sulphonylurea treatment is approximately 2 episodes per 100 patient years.[82] With treatment comparable to the intensive treatment group of DCCT, rates of severe hypoglycemia increase, although they remain at least 20% less than the annual rates seen in type 1 diabetes.[83]

Causes of Hypoglycemia

Hypoglycemia relates to physicians' inability to administer insulin with normal feedback control. It is defined as a plasma glucose less than 2.5 mmol/L; symptoms relating to hypoglycemia may not be experienced. The common causes are[6]:

1. Food intake is insufficient or ill-timed for the amount of insulin administered.
2. Insulin dose is excessive or ill-timed for a given meal.
3. Glucose consumption is excessive for given doses of insulin (e.g., exercise).
4. Hepatic glucose production is reduced (e.g., alcohol).
5. Insulin resistance is reduced (e.g., weight loss, thiazolidinediones, hypopituitarism, hypoadrenalism).
6. Insulin elimination rate is reduced (e.g., chronic renal failure).

In type 1 diabetes, the best predictive factors for severe hypoglycemia were a previous episode (relative risk 2.2) and 9- to 12-year duration of diabetes.[84]

Mechanisms for recurrent severe hypoglycemia may involve dysfunctional counter-regulatory hormones. In type 1 diabetes, the glucagon and epinephrine response to acute hypoglycemia is defective after 5- to 10-year duration of disease.[85] This is a selective glucose-sensing defect because other stimuli remain able to provoke a normal physiologic response from the α cells and adrenal medulla.

Clinical Features

When plasma glucose concentration decreases to less than 4.6 mmol/L, the brain initiates counter-regulatory responses that aim to maintain normoglycemia and glucose delivery to the central nervous system. In individuals with diabetes these involve inhibition of insulin secretion initially. When plasma glucose decrease to less than 70 mg/mL, secretion of glucagon, epinephrine, growth hormone, and cortisol begins.[86] Recruitment of these hormones causes the neurogenic symptoms of hypoglycemia: anxiety, sweating, tremor, palpitations, pallor, pilo-erection, mydriasis, and hunger. When plasma glucose decrease to less than 50 mg/mL, cognition and the sensorium become impaired. These neuroglycopenic symptoms include confusion, disorientation, agitation, poor concentration, incoordination, speech disturbance, automatism, and personality and behavioral changes. Seizures may occur while irreversible severe hypoglycemia leads to coma and death.

Hypoglycemia unawareness in type 1 diabetes is common and may affect up to 25% of all patients at some stage during insulin therapy.[87] Patients do not experience the neurogenic symptoms, and hypoglycemia becomes apparent only with the appearance of neuroglycopenic symptoms. It seems related to metabolic factors and autonomic neuropathy.[83] There are no good data to suggest that it is related to insulin species.[88]

Treatment of Hypoglycemia

The treatment route of hypoglycemia is dependent on the patient's ability to protect his or her airway. In the alert, cooperative individual, hypoglycemia can be treated by the consumption of a rapid-acting source of glucose (e.g., sugary drink). This should be followed by a meal of complex carbohydrate to replete hepatic glycogen stores.

Third-party assistance will be required if neuroglycopenic symptoms render the patient unable to self-treat. With an uncooperative patient or if the airway is compromised, intravenous glucose should be given as a 10% to 20% solution. Extravasation of 50% glucose can cause loss of tissue or even a limb.

When it proves difficult or impossible to secure venous access, 1 mg glucagon can be given by intramuscular injection. This stimulates hepatic glucose production through glycogenolysis. Improvement in the clinical condition should occur within 5 to 10 minutes. If hepatic glycogen stores are depleted (e.g., catabolic state, prolonged fasting, alcohol excess, or eating disorders), glucagon will be ineffective. The most common adverse effect of glucagon is nausea and vomiting.

All patients should eat a substantive meal to prevent recurrence of hypoglycemia. The possible precipitants should be examined. Hospital admission should be arranged if the patient is taking sulphonylureas with a long duration of action, because there is significant risk for recurrence of hypoglycemia. Patients treated with insulin do not require admission unless there are confounding factors such as advanced age, complex psychosocial factors, or lack of supervision. With repeated hypoglycemic episodes, the diabetologist will review diet, lifestyle, and treatment.

Additional Indications for Insulin Therapy

Hyperkalemia

The sodium-potassium/ATPase cotransporter of plasma membranes is important in the maintenance of the transmembrane electrochemical gradient. Insulin stimulates activity of this pump in the liver and in muscle, which drives potassium into cells. This action is used in the treatment of acute hyperkalemia because intravenous insulin will cause a significant rapid decrease in serum potassium concentration. A total of 15 U of soluble insulin is added to 250 mL of 10% dextrose and infused over 30 minutes. This will reduce the serum potassium concentration by 1 to 1.5 mmol/L over 60 to 120 minutes, but the effect is temporary.

Acute Myocardial Infarction in Diabetes

It has been proposed that the prognosis of acute myocardial infarction in diabetes can be improved with insulin therapy initiated during the immediate postinfarction period. The use of a continuous intravenous insulin infusion during the acute treatment phase and treatment with subcutaneous insulin for a further 12 months caused a 30% reduction in mortality.[89] Benefit continued for up to 3 years.[90] This was attributed to a reduced incidence of cardiac failure after infarction. The mechanism proposed was that early insulin therapy reduced the extent of myocardial damage. Similar benefit was seen also in patients without diabetes with an admission blood glucose greater than 200 mg/mL. The findings of this study have not been universally practiced, but most physicians would agree that insulin therapy has important advantages over sulphonylureas and metformin during the acute stage of myocardial infarction.[91] There is no consensus regarding whether insulin should be continued after hospital discharge.

References

1. Schadewaldt H: The history of diabetes mellitus. In von Engelhardt D (ed): Diabetes, Its Medical and Cultural History. Berlin Heidelberg, Springer-Verlag, 1989.

2. Banting FG, Best CH: The internal secretion of the pancreas. J Lab Clin Med 7:256, 1922.

3. Brange J, Owens DR, Kang S, et al: Monomeric insulins and their experimental and clinical implications. Diabetes Care 13:923–954, 1990.

4. Robinson S, Johnston DG: Metabolic disorders: Diabetes. In Tomlinson S, Heagerty AM, Weetman AP (eds): Mechanisms of Disease: An Introduction to Clinical Science. Cambridge, Cambridge University Press, 1997.

5. McCall AL: Effects of glucose deprivation on glucose metabolism in the central nervous system. In Frier BM, Fisher BM (eds): Hypoglycemia and Diabetes. London, Edward Arnold, 1993.

6. Cryer PE, Fisher JN, Shamoon H: Hypoglycemia. Diabetes Care 17:734–755, 1994.

7. Laffel L: Ketone bodies: A review of physiology, pathophysiology and application of monitoring to diabetes. Diabetes Metab Res Rev 15:412–426, 1999.

8. Ward WK, Beard JC, Halter JB, et al: Pathophysiology of insulin secretion in non-insulin-dependent diabetes mellitus. Diabetes Care 7:491–502, 1984.

9. Reaven GM: Pathophysiology of insulin resistance in human disease. Physiol Rev 75: 473–486, 1995.

10. Franks S, Gilling-Smith C, Watson H, et al: Insulin action in the normal and polycystic ovary. Endocrinol Metab Clin North Am 28:361–378, 1999.

11. Robinson S, Niththyananthan R, Anyaoku V, et al: Reduced postprandial energy expenditure in women predisposed to type 2 diabetes. Diabet Med 11:545–550, 1994.

12. Hunter SJ, Garvey WT: Insulin action and insulin resistance: Diseases involving defects in insulin receptors, signal transduction and the glucose transport effector system. Am J Med 105:331–345, 1998.

13. Cheatham B, Kahn CR: Insulin action and the insulin signalling network. Endocrin Rev 16:117–142, 1995.

14. Yki-Jarvinen H: Acute and chronic effects of hyperglycemia on glucose metabolism. Diabetologia 33:579–585, 1990.

15. Yki-Jarvinen H: Glucose toxicity. Endocrin Rev 13:415–431, 1992.

16. Elliott MJ, Alberti KGMM: Carbohydrate metabolism—effects of pre-operative starvation and trauma. Clin Anaesthesiol 1:527–550, 1983.

17. Ziereth JR, He L, Guma A, et al: Insulin action on glucose transport and plasma membrane GLUT 4 content in skeletal muscle from patients with NIDDM. Diabetologia 39:1180–1189, 1996.

18. Cline GW, Petersen KF, Krssak M, et al: Impaired glucose transport as a cause of decreased insulin-stimulated muscle glycogen synthesis in type 2 diabetes. N Eng J Med 341:240–246, 1999.

19. Shepherd PR, Kahn BB: Glucose transporters and insulin action. Implications for insulin resistance and diabetes mellitus. N Eng J Med 341:248–257, 1999.

20. Stenbit AE, Tsao TS, Li J, et al: GLUT 4 heterozygous knockout mice develop muscle insulin resistance and diabetes. Nat Med 3:1096–1101, 1997.

21. Kandror KV, Pilch PF: Compartmentalization of protein traffic in insulin-sensitive cells. Am J Physiol 271:E1–E14, 1996.

22. Castillo MJ, Scheen AJ, Letiexhe MR, et al: How to measure insulin clearance. Diabetes Metab Rev 10:119–150, 1994.

23. Duckworth WC, Bennett RG, Hamel FG: Insulin degradation: Progress and potential. Endocrin Rev 19:608–624, 1998.

24. Ferrannini E, Cobelli C: The kinetics of insulin in Man. General aspects. Diab Metab Rev 3:335–363, 1987.

25. Bonora E, Zavaroni I, Coscelli C, et al: Decreased hepatic insulin extraction in subjects with mild glucose intolerance. Metabolism 32:438–436, 1983.

26. Giugliano D, Quatraro A, Minei A, et al: Hyperinsulinemia in hypertension: Increased secretion, reduced clearance or both? J Endocrinol Invest 16:315–321, 1993.

27. Lender D, Arauz-Pacheco C, Adams-Huet B, et al: Essential hypertension is associated with decreased insulin clearance and insulin resistance. Hypertension 29:111–114, 1997.

28. Jiang X, Srinivasan SR, Berenson GS: Relation of obesity to insulin secretion and clearance in adolescents: The Bogalusa Heart Study. Int J Obes Relat Metab Disord 20:951–956, 1996.

29. Letiexhe MR, Scheen AJ, Gerard PL, et al: Insulin secretion, clearance and action before and after gastroplasty in severely obese subjects. Int J Obes Relat Metab Disord 18:295–300, 1994.

30. American Diabetes Association: Insulin administration (Position Statement). Diabetes Care 24(suppl 1):S94–S98, 2001.

31. Pickup JC, Keen H, Parsons JA: Continuous subcutaneous insulin infusion: An approach to achieving normoglycemia. BMJ 1:204–207, 1978.

32. Boland EA, Grey M, Oesterle A, et al: Continuous subcutaneous insulin infusion. A new way to lower risk of severe hypoglycemia, improve metabolic control and enhance coping in adolescents with type 1 diabetes. Diabetes Care 22:1779–1784, 1999.

33. Mecklenburg RS, Benson EA, Benson JW, et al: Acute complications associated with insulin pump therapy. Report of experience with 161 patients. JAMA 252:3265–3269, 1984.

34. The Diabetes Control and Complications Trial Research Group: The effect of intensive treatment of diabetes on the development and progression of long-term complications in insulin-dependent diabetes mellitus. N Eng J Med 329:977–986, 1993.

35. Ferrannini E: Insulin resistance versus insulin deficiency in non-insulin dependent diabetes mellitus: Problems and prospects. Endocr Rev 19:477–490, 1998.

36. McCarthy MI, Froguel P, Hitman GA: The genetics of non-insulin-dependent diabetes mellitus: Tools and aims. Diabetologia 37:959–968, 1994.

37. Hattersley AT: Maturity-onset diabetes of the young: Clinical heterogeneity explained by genetic heterogeneity. Diabet Med 17:15–24, 1998.

38. Saltiel AR, Olefsky JM: Thiazolidinediones in the treatment of insulin resistance and type 2 diabetes. Diabetes 45:1661–1669, 1996.

39. Fonseca V, Rosenstock J, Patwardhan R, et al: Effect of metformin and rosiglitazone combination therapy in patients with type 2 diabetes mellitus: A randomized controlled trial. JAMA 283:1695–1702, 2000.

40. Wolffenbuttel BHR, Gomis R, Squatrito S, et al: Addition of low-dose rosiglitazone to sulphonylurea therapy improves glycaemic control in type 2 diabetic patients. Diabet Med 17:40–47, 2000.

41. UK Prospective Diabetes Study Group: Intensive blood glucose control with sulphonylureas or insulin compared with conventional treatment and risk of complications in patients with type 2 diabetes (UKPDS 33). Lancet 352:837–853, 1998.

42. UK Prospective Diabetes Study (UKPDS) Group: Effect of intensive blood glucose control with metformin on complications in overweight patients with type 2 diabetes (UKPDS 34). Lancet 352:854–865, 1998.

43. UK Prospective Diabetes Study Group: Efficacy of atenolol and captopril in reducing risk of macrovascular and microvascular complications in type 2 diabetes: UKPDS 39. BMJ 317:713–720, 1998.

44. UK Prospective Diabetes Study Group: Tight blood pressure control and risk of macrovascular and microvascular complications in type 2 diabetes: UKPDS 38. BMJ 317:703–713, 1998.

45. Turner RC: The UK Diabetes Prospective Study. A review. Diabetes Care 21(suppl 3): C35–C38, 1998.

46. Bell DSH: Prudent utilization of the presently available treatment modalities for type 2 diabetes. Endocrinologist 8:332–341, 1998.

47. Robinson A, Burke J, Robinson S, et al: The effects of metformin on glycaemic control and serum lipids in insulin treated NIDDM patients with suboptimal metabolic control. Diabetes Care 21:701–705, 1998.

48. Haffner SM, Lehto S, Ronnemaar T, et al: Mortality from coronary heart disease in subjects with type 2 diabetes and in nondiabetic subjects with or without prior myocardial infarction. N Engl J Med 339:229–234, 1998.

49. Crock PA, Ley CJ, Martin IK, et al: Hormonal and metabolic changes during hypothermic coronary artery bypass surgery in diabetic and non-diabetic subjects. Diabet Med 5:47–52, 1988.

50. Thompson J, Husband DJ, Thai AC, et al: Metabolic changes in the non-insulin dependent diabetic undergoing minor surgery: Effect of glucose-insulin-potassium infusion. Br J Surg 73:301–304, 1986.

51. Podolsky S: Management of diabetes in the surgical diabetic patient. Med Clin N Am 66:1361–1372, 1982.

52. Elliott MJ, Gill GV, Home PD, et al: A comparison of two regimes for the management of diabetes during open heart surgery. Anaesthesiology 60:364–368, 1984.

53. Bagg W, Sathu A, Streat S, et al: Diabetic ketoacidosis in adults at Auckland Hospital, 1988–1996. Aust N Z J Med 28: 604–608, 1998.

54. Wachtel TJ, Tetu-Mouradjian LM, Goldman DL et al: Hyperosmolarity and acidosis in diabetes mellitus: A three year experience in Rhode Island. J Gen Intern Med 6:495–502, 1991.

55. Levetan BN, Levitt NS, Bonnici F: Hyperglycaemic emergencies are a common problem. S Afr Med J 87 (3 suppl):368–370, 1997.

56. Wagner A, Risse A, Brill HL, et al: Therapy of severe diabetic ketoacidosis. Zero-mortality under very-low-dose insulin application. Diabetes Care 22:674–677, 1999.

57. Oschatz E, Mullner M, Herkner H, et al: Multiple organ failure and

prognosis in adult patients with diabetic ketoacidosis. Wien Klin Wochenschr 111:590–595, 1999.

58. Edge JA: Cerebral o during treatment of diabetic ketoacidosis: Are we any nearer finding a cause? Diabetes Metab Res Rev 16:316–324, 2000.

58. Umpierrez GE, Kelly JP, Navarette JE, et al: Hyperglycaemic crises in urban blacks. Arch Intern Med 157:669–675, 1997.

60. Gill GV, Lucas S, Kent LA: Prevalence and characteristics of brittle diabetes in Britain. QJM 89:839–843.

61. Delaney MF, Zisman A, Kettyle WM: Diabetic ketoacidosis and hyperglycaemic hyperosmolar nonketotic syndrome. Endocrinol Metab Clin North Am 29:683–705, 2000.

62. Gomez Diaz RA, Rivera Moscoso R, Ramos Rodriguez R, et al: Diabetic ketoacidosis in adults: Clinical and laboratory features. Arch Med Res 27:177–181, 1996.

63. Balasubramanyam A, Zern JW, Hyman DJ, et al: New profiles of diabetic ketoacidosis: Type 1 vs. type 2 diabetes and the effect of ethnicity. Arch Intern Med 159:2317–2322, 1999.

64. Yan SH, Sheu WH, Song YM, et al: The occurrence of diabetic ketoacidosis in adults. Intern Med 39:10–14, 2000.

65. Nair S, Yadav D, Pitchumoni CS, et al: Association of diabetic ketoacidosis and acute pancreatitis: Observation in 100 consecutive episodes of DKA. Am J Gastroenterol 95:2795–2800, 2000.

66. Kitabchi AE, Umpierrez GE, Murphy MB, et al: Management of hyperglycaemic crises in patients with diabetes. Diabetes Care 24:131–153, 2001.

67. Adrogue HJ, Barrero J, Eknoyan G: Salutary effects of modest fluid replacement in the treatment of adults with diabetic ketoacidosis. Use in patients without extreme volume deficit. JAMA 262:2108–2113, 1989.

68. Barrett EJ, DeFronzo RA, Bevilacqua S, et al: Insulin resistance in diabetic ketoacidosis. Diabetes 31:923–928, 1982.

69. Okuda Y, Adrogue HJ, Field JB, et al: Counterproductive effects of sodium bicarbonate in diabetic ketoacidosis. J Clin Endocrinol Metab 81:314–320, 1996.

70. Viallon A, Zeni F, Lafond P, et al: Does bicarbonate therapy improve the management of severe diabetic ketoacidosis? Crit Care Med 27:2690–2693, 1999.

71. Miller DW, Slovis CM: Hypophosphatemia in the emergency department therapeutics. Am J Emerg Med 18:457–461, 2000.

72. Laffel L: Sick-day management in type 1 diabetes. Endocrinol Metab Clin North Am 29:707–723, 2000.

73. Lorber D: Nonketotic hypertonicity in diabetes mellitus. Med Clin North Am 79:39–52, 1995.

74. Pinies JA, Cairo G, Gaztambide S, et al: Course and prognosis of 132 patients with diabetic nonketotic hyperosmolar state. Diabetes Metab 20:43–48, 1994.

75. Rimailho A, Riou B, Dadez E, et al: Prognostic factors in hyperglycaemic hyperosmolar nonketotic syndrome. Crit Care Med 14:552–554, 1986.

76. Gerich JE, Martin MM, Recant LL: Clinical and metabolic characteristics of hyperosmolar nonketotic coma. Diabetes 20:228–238, 1971.

77. Lindsey Ca, Faloona GR, Unger RH: Plasma glucagon in nonketotic hyperosmolar coma. JAMA 229:1771–1773, 1974.

78. Rolfe M, Ephraim GG, Lincoln DC, et al: Hyperosmolar non-ketotic coma as a cause of emergency hyperglycaemic admission to Baragwanath hospital. S Afr Med J 85:173–176, 1995.

79. Cox DJ, Gonder-Frederick L, Antoun B, et al: Psychobehavioral metabolic parameters of severe hypoglycaemic episodes. Diabetes Care 13:458–459, 1990.

80. The Diabetes Control and Complications Trial research Group: Diabetes Control and Complications Trial (DCCT): Results of feasibility study. Diabetes Care 10:1–19, 1987.

81. Bell DSH, Yumuk V: Frequency of severe hypoglycemia in patients with non-insulin dependent diabetes mellitus treated with sulphonylureas or insulin. Endocr Pract 3:281–283, 1997.

82. Berger W: Incidence of severe side effects during therapy with sulfonylureas and biguanides. Horm Metab Res Suppl 15:111–115, 1985.

83. Fox C, Cull CA, Holman RR: Three year response to randomly allocated therapy with diet, sulphonylurea or insulin in 1592 diabetic patients. Diabet Med 8(suppl 1):8A, 1991.

84. The Diabetes Control and Complications Trial research Group: Epidemiology of severe hypoglycemia in the Diabetes Control and Complications Trial. Am J Med 90:450–459, 1991.

85. Bolli G, DeFreo P, Compagnucci P, et al: Abnormal glucose counterregulation in insulin-dependent diabetes mellitus: Interaction of anti-insulin antibodies and impaired glucagon and epinephrine secretion. Diabetes 32:134–141, 1983.

86. Thompson CJ, Baylis PH: Endocrine changes during insulin-induced hypoglycemia. In Frier BM, Fisher BM (eds): Hypoglycemia and Diabetes. London, Edward Arnold, 1993.

87. Gerich JE, Mokan M, Veneman T, et al: Hypoglycemia unawareness. Endocrin Rev 12:356–371, 1991.

88. Colagiuri S, Miller JJ, Petocz P, et al: Double blind crossover comparison of human and porcine insulins in patients reporting hypoglycemia unawareness. Lancet 339:1432–1435, 1992.

89. Malmberg K, Ryden L, Efendic S, et al: Randomized trial of insulin-glucose infusion followed by subcutaneous insulin treatment in diabetic patients with acute myocardial infarction (DIGAMI study): Effects on mortality at 1 year. J Am Coll Cardiol 26:57–65, 1995.

90. Malmberg K, Norhammar A, Wedel H, et al: Glycometabolic state at admission: Important risk factor of mortality in conventionally treated patients with diabetes mellitus and acute myocardial infarction: Long term results from the Diabetes and Insulin-Glucose Infusion in Acute Myocardial Infarction (DIGAMI) study. Circulation 99:2626–2632, 1999.

91. Yudkin JS: Managing the diabetic patient with acute myocardial infarction. Diabet Med 15:276–281, 1998.

49

Drugs Affecting Lipid Metabolism

Anne Carol Goldberg, MD

The relation between the risk for atherosclerotic heart disease and serum lipoproteins is now well established.[1] Increased levels of total cholesterol[2] and low-density lipoprotein (LDL) cholesterol, and low levels of high-density lipoprotein (HDL) cholesterol,[3] are associated with increased risk. Decreasing total and LDL cholesterol levels has been shown to decrease the risk for coronary events and procedures in patients with and without coronary artery disease.[4-9]

HDL cholesterol level is inversely related to the risk for coronary artery disease.[3] Because most agents affecting HDL cholesterol also have effects on other lipoproteins, the issue of whether primarily increasing HDL cholesterol will decrease risk for coronary disease is less clear. At least one trial of increasing HDL cholesterol and decreasing triglycerides showed a decreased risk for atherosclerotic vascular events in men.[10]

The relation of triglyceride levels to coronary disease risk is not as strong as cholesterol. Some analyses of epidemiologic data have shown a lack of correlation between triglyceride levels and risk. Other analyses have shown that increasing triglyceride levels are correlated with risk.[11,12] Results of trials with triglyceride lowering drugs have been mixed, with some showing and others not showing decreased event rates.[10,13-15]

Understanding of the relation of cholesterol and lipids to atherosclerosis has evolved over the last century and especially during the last 50 years.[1] The "lipid hypothesis"—that decreasing cholesterol levels would decrease the risk for atherosclerotic vascular disease—was not accepted for many years.[1,16] Data from population studies, animal studies, cell culture experiments, and eventually clinical trials of lipid-lowering interventions have made the therapy of hyperlipidemia an accepted part of decreasing cardiovascular risk.[1,16]

The National Cholesterol Education Program of the National Heart, Lung, and Blood Institute (part of the National Institutes of Health of the United States) has published guidelines to help physicians detect, evaluate, and treat patients with dyslipidemia. The Adult Treatment Panel has published three sets of guidelines: the first in 1988,[17] the second in 1993,[18] and the third in 2001.[19,20] The guidelines have used the accumulating evidence from clinical trials and other studies to outline an approach to treatment for patients with increased cholesterol levels and other disorders of lipoprotein metabolism. The major focus is on decreasing LDL cholesterol because the data from clinical trials are strongest for a benefit of therapy, but the report also considers HDL cholesterol, triglycerides, and other clinical situations.[19,20]

Basics of Cholesterol and Triglyceride Metabolism

Cholesterol and triglycerides (Fig. 49-1) are fatty substances carried in the blood by complexes of free and **853**

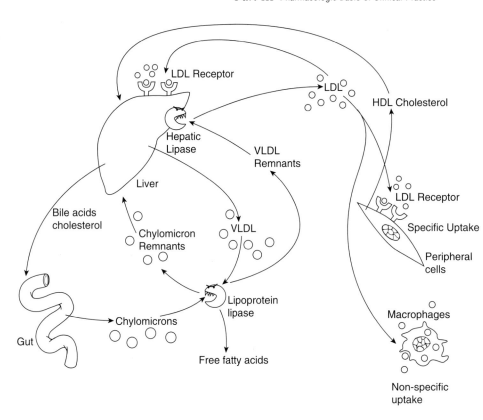

Figure 49–1. Cholesterol and triglyceride metabolism. HDL, high-density lipoprotein; LDL, low-density lipoprotein; VLDL, very low-density lipoprotein. (Adapted from a design by John Guyton, M.D., with permission.)

esterified cholesterol, triglycerides, phospholipids, and proteins called apolipoproteins. Chylomicrons carrying triglycerides and small amounts of cholesterol are produced in the intestine and enter the circulation where they interact with the endothelial-bound enzyme, lipoprotein lipase. Lipoprotein lipase hydrolyzes the triglycerides, delivering free fatty acids to cells. The depleted lipoproteins, called chylomicron remnants, interact with receptors on hepatic cells, delivering the remaining triglycerides and cholesterol. In the liver, free fatty acids are esterified and combined with cholesterol and apolipoproteins to form very low-density lipoprotein (VLDL) particles. These particles also interact with lipoprotein lipase, and some of the triglycerides and apolipoproteins are removed leaving a VLDL remnant particle. The remnants interact with another enzyme, hepatic lipase, with the resulting particle being LDL. LDL can be recognized by specific cell surface receptors known as the LDL receptor, which accounts for removal of most of the LDL from the circulation. LDL receptors also contribute to the clearance of some VLDL remnants. If LDL receptors are insufficient in number or activity, LDL accumulates in the blood where it can be modified by oxidation and taken up by scavenger receptors on macrophages, a process that contributes to the development of atherosclerotic plaques. Cholesterol is accepted from cells by HDL particles, which start as biconcave discs that change size and composition as they accept cholesterol. They participate in a process called reverse cholesterol transport by delivering cholesterol to the liver. Cholesterol can leave the liver in the bile as cholesterol or bile acids.[21-23]

Atherogenic lipoproteins include VLDL, VLDL remnants, chylomicron remnants, and LDL, particularly small, dense LDL particles.[22,23] The most convincing randomized, clinical trial data exist for LDL reduction, but there may be multiple mechanisms involved in the effect of any intervention. With the publication of five major randomized, placebo-controlled, 5-year event, statin trials—the Scandinavian Simvastatin Study,[5] the Cholesterol and Recurrent Events study,[7] the West of Scotland trial,[6] the Air Force/Texas Cholesterol Atherosclerosis Prevention Study,[8] and the Long-Term Intervention with Pravastatin in Ischemic Disease Study[9]—it became clear that use of statins can decrease the risk for death and major cardiovascular events. For the most part, the National Cholesterol Education Program Adult Treatment Panel III (NCEP ATP III) guidelines focus on LDL but also discuss the varying levels of evidence available for a variety of interventions including diet and drug therapy.[20]

Mechanisms of Drug Action

Statins

The statins work by inhibiting hydroxymethylglutaryl-coenzyme A (HMG-CoA) reductase. This enzyme catalyzes the conversion of the substrate, HMG-CoA, to mevalonate, which is an early and rate-limiting step in the biosynthesis of cholesterol.[24] The statins, which are also called HMG-CoA reductase inhibitors, are structurally similar to HMG-CoA and occupy a portion of the active binding site on the enzyme, blocking access of the substrate to the binding site.[25] This competitive inhibition leads to decreased production of cholesterol, and thus a decrease of intracellular cholesterol levels. This causes up-regulation of LDL receptors and a reduction in LDL cholesterol levels because of their increased clearance by LDL receptors.[26] Statins also reduce the release of lipoproteins from the liver into the circulation.[27,28] At high doses, the statins also decrease triglyceride levels because of clearance of VLDL and decreased production of lipoproteins.

Bile Acid Sequestrants

The bile acid sequestrants work by binding bile acids in the intestine. This interrupts the enterohepatic circulation of bile acids leading to increased conversion of cholesterol into bile within the liver.[29,30] The resulting decreased hepatocyte cholesterol content promotes an increase in LDL receptors and increased clearance of LDL from the circulation.[31] Hepatic synthesis of cholesterol increases as well, increasing the secretion of VLDL into the circulation and limiting the LDL-lowering effect of the resins, as well as raising serum triglyceride levels.[32]

Niacin

The mechanism of action of niacin, also known as nicotinic acid, is not completely understood. Nicotinic acid inhibits the mobilization of free fatty acids from peripheral tissues, which leads to a reduction of hepatic synthesis of triglycerides and decreased secretion of VLDL.[33] It may also decrease the conversion of VLDL to LDL.[34] Niacin increases HDL by unknown mechanisms.

Fibrates

Part of the mechanism of action of the fibrates, derivatives of fibric acid, may involve activation of specific transcription factors called peroxisome proliferator-activated receptors (PPARs). PPARs bind as heterodimers with another nuclear receptor, the retinoic receptor RXR, to specific response elements called peroxisome proliferator response elements and alter the transcription rate of target genes. The PPARα form of this receptor mediates the effect of fibrates on lipoprotein metabolism. Possible mechanisms include the up-regulation of genes for lipoprotein lipase, apolipoprotein A1, fatty acid transport protein, and fatty acid oxidation, and down-regulation of the apolipoprotein *CIII* gene.[35] Induction of lipoprotein lipase contributes to lipolysis of the triglyceride-rich lipoproteins, VLDL and chylomicrons. Apolipoprotein CIII is an inhibitor of lipoprotein lipase activity; a decreased amount of this protein leads to decreased inhibition of lipoprotein lipase activity and increased catabolism of VLDL. There is also increased hepatic fatty acid uptake and fatty acid oxidation, decreased synthesis of fatty acids and triglycerides, and decreased production of VLDL. Fibrates increase the production of apolipoproteins AI and AII in the liver, which may contribute to the increase in plasma HDL seen with fibrate therapy.[36]

Clinical Pharmacology

Statins

Randomized clinical trials using lovastatin, pravastatin, and simvastatin have demonstrated reductions of atherosclerotic event rates in patients with and without evidence of atherosclerosis, including total mortality, death from coronary heart disease, revascularization procedures, stroke, and peripheral vascular disease. Men and women, patients with diabetes or hypertension, and middle-aged or older patients have all experienced benefits in the trials.[5–9,37,38] In addition, angiographic studies have shown benefit on coronary stenosis in native vessels or grafts with the use of statins, and also have shown beneficial effects after acute coronary syndromes.[39,40]

Five statins are currently available (Fig. 49–2). Lovastatin is a naturally occurring cholesterol-lowering agent isolated from a strain of *Aspergillus terreus*. Simvastatin is derived synthetically from a fermentation product of the same fungus. Pravastatin is also derived from a fungal fermentation product. All three have structures similar to mevastatin, previously called compactin, which was derived from *Penicillium citrinum*.[24] Lovastatin, simvastatin, and pravastatin have structures similar to each other, but fluvastatin and atorvastatin are synthetic drugs with structures that are quite different from each other and from the other three statins. Lovastatin became available commercially in the

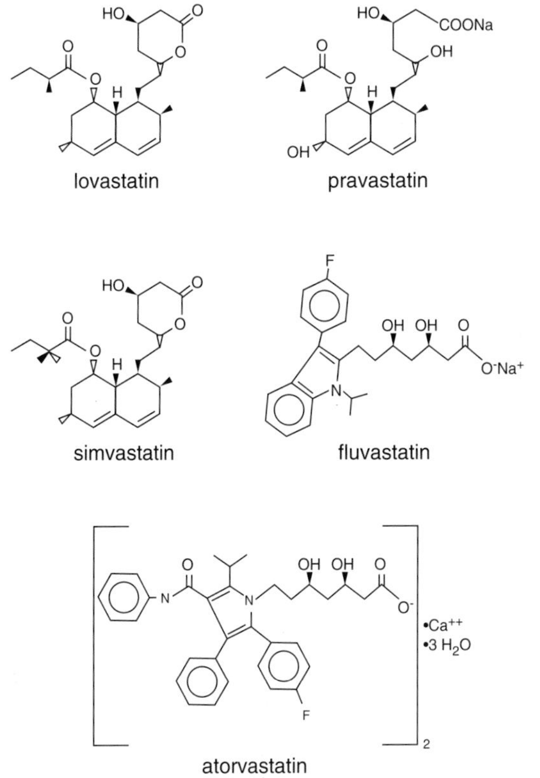

Figure 49–2. Chemical structures of statins.

United States in 1987. Cerivastatin, another synthetic statin, was removed from the market in the United States in August 2001.

Lovastatin and simvastatin are prodrugs with lactone rings that require metabolism to the open β-hydroxyacid form to be active. Pravastatin, atorvastatin, and fluvastatin are given as the active β-hydroxyacid form. Fluvastatin has two optical enantiomers, one of which is active while the other is inactive. All of the statins are absorbed rapidly after oral administration with variable extent of absorption. Food intake increases plasma levels of lovastatin, has no effect on simvastatin, has a slight effect on atorvastatin and fluvastatin, and decreases bioavailability of pravastatin.[41] All of the statins except for pravastatin are extensively protein bound. Pravastatin is approximately 50% protein bound.

Except for pravastatin, all of the statins are highly extracted by the liver. Pravastatin and fluvastatin are more hydrophilic, whereas atorvastatin, lovastatin, and simvastatin are lipophilic.[42,43] The clinical significance of this difference is unclear. Atorvastatin, lovastatin, and simvastatin undergo metabolism by cytochrome P450 3A4 enzymes. Fluvastatin is metabolized predominantly through cytochrome P450 2C9 activity, but pravastatin does not have significant cytochrome P450 metabolism. Lovastatin, pravastatin, simvastatin, and fluvastatin have half-lives of approximately 1 to 4 hours, whereas atorvastatin has a half-life of 14 hours.[43] Although all the statins except for atorvastatin have short half-lives and do not accumulate in plasma, the duration of their pharmacodynamic effect is approximately 24 hours. Atorvastatin can accumulate in the plasma.[44] The statins are excreted through urine and feces, but atorvastatin and fluvastatin have minimal renal excretion and generally do not need dose adjustment in patients with renal insufficiency. Dosages of pravastatin and to a lesser extent simvastatin and lovastatin may need to be adjusted in patients with significant renal insufficiency.[43] Because of their extensive first-pass clearance by the liver, all of the statins carry warnings about use in patients with active liver disease or heavy alcohol consumption.[45–49] The statins should not be used in pregnant women because they are teratogenic in high doses in animals.

The major effect of the statins is a reduction in serum levels of LDL cholesterol by 18% to 60% from baseline levels.[50–54] The percent changes in LDL cholesterol are mean reductions; individual patients may have greater or lesser decreases in LDL.[55] Typically every doubling of the dose of a statin gives a further 6% reduction of LDL cholesterol. The dose response curves for the statins are thus curvilinear.[22] The statins increase HDL modestly, typically by 5% to 15%, and decrease triglycerides by 7% to 30%. The reduction of triglycerides is primarily seen in patients with triglycerides greater than 250 mg/dL (2.82 mmol/L) and is dose dependent. The magnitude of triglyceride reduction is proportional to the percent reduction of LDL.[56]

Simvastatin and lovastatin appear more efficacious than fluvastatin at the higher end of their dose-response ranges. Atorvastatin at 10 mg daily produces a decrease in LDL cholesterol similar to that of simvastatin 20 mg/day,[57] and at 80 mg daily, atorvastatin may decrease LDL by as much as 60%.[54] The decrease in LDL cholesterol is seen within 1 to 2 weeks[50,54,58,59] with maximum effect and stability of LDL reduction at about 4 to 6 weeks. The reduction of LDL is

generally maintained while the patient continues taking the statin.[52,60,61]

The statins are usually well tolerated. The most common adverse effects are gastrointestinal upset including abdominal pain, bloating, diarrhea, and constipation, which are often transient, and muscle pain. Patients can have muscle pain or weakness with or without increases of serum creatine kinase (CK). Other complaints include fatigue, malaise, sleep disturbances, headache, loss of concentration, rash, and peripheral neuropathy.[22,62] A lupus-like syndrome has been reported with several of the drugs.[22,62] Potential side effects of statin therapy causing the most fear are liver enzyme increases and severe myopathy with the possibility of rhabdomyolysis, myoglobinuria, and acute renal failure. Increases in serum liver transaminases to 2 to 3 times the upper limit of normal occur in 0.5% to 2% of cases and are dose dependent.[63,64] The increases reverse with discontinuation of the drugs. They may occur transiently and resolve even if the patient continues taking the medication. Progression to liver failure is extremely rare.[20] Patients who have increases of transaminases with one drug may not have them with another drug in the same class.

Myopathy can have several manifestations. Mild to severe myalgias or weakness can occur without CK increases. The incidence of myositis, typically defined as muscle pain accompanied by greater than 10-fold increases in CK levels, is low. Cases of rhabdomyolysis have been reported with all the statins. An excess number of deaths from rhabdomyolysis and renal failure led to the withdrawal of cerivastatin from the market in the United States in August 2001. Myopathy is more likely to occur in patients with multiple medical problems and patients taking multiple drugs. Small-framed, older patients with impaired renal function may also be more susceptible.[65] The use of statins in combination with a number of other medications increases the risk for myopathy. Among these are fibric acid derivatives, niacin, and drugs metabolized by the cytochrome P450 enzyme system including itraconazole, ketoconazole, erythromycin, clarithromycin, nefazodone, cyclosporine, and several protease inhibitors, especially ritonavir.[62,65–68] Although agents used during anesthesia have not been shown to increase the incidence of statin-induced myopathy, it is recommended that statins be discontinued 48 hours before surgery. There is also a possible interaction of statins with large quantities of grapefruit juice, which inhibits intestinal cytochrome P450 3A4, but how much this contributes to the risk for myopathy is unclear.[69–71]

In addition to interactions mediated by cytochrome P450 enzymes, there may be an increase in the anticoagulant effect of warfarin in patients taking lovastatin, simvastatin, or fluvastatin. The bile acid binding resins, cholestyramine and colestipol, can decrease the absorption of the statins.[22]

Bile Acid Sequestrants

In the Lipid Research Clinics Coronary Primary Prevention Trial, therapy with cholestyramine reduced the risk for coronary heart disease.[4,72] In other trials, resins alone or in combination with other agents showed beneficial effects on coronary disease.[73,74]

The bile acid sequestrants, cholestyramine resin and colestipol hydrochloride, are large, nonabsorbed anion-exchange resins. Colesevelam hydrochloride is a nonabsorbed hydrophilic polymer. Cholestyramine and colestipol have been in use since the 1970s. Colesevelam is a more recent agent, which has greater bile acid binding efficacy than cholestyramine.[75,76] Used alone, bile acid sequestrants decrease LDL by 10% to 30% in a dose-dependent manner.[72,75–79] The effect is seen within 4 weeks of the start of therapy and generally remains stable over time.[76,80] The combination of sequestrant and statin can decrease LDL cholesterol levels by up to 60%.[59,81–83] HDL cholesterol may increase modestly, but triglycerides may increase[80] because of increased production of VLDL.[32] In patients with elevated triglycerides, the increase in serum triglyceride levels can be substantial.[84]

There is no systemic absorption of the bile acid sequestrants, but the tolerability of the two older drugs is often poor. They are bulky and can be inconvenient to take. Patients must either drink suspensions of powder or granules or take a large number of large pills. The usual side effects are gastrointestinal including constipation, abdominal pain, bloating, fullness, nausea, and flatulence.[4] Serum transaminases can increase slightly.[4] Gastrointestinal symptoms are dose dependent and seem to be less common with colesevelam.[85]

Cholestyramine and colestipol can have significant interactions with many other medications, including warfarin, thyroid hormone, thiazide diuretics, propranolol, statins, gemfibrozil, and antibiotics. Colesevelam did not show interactions in studies with quinidine, valproic acid, digoxin, warfarin, or metoprolol.[86] Cholestyramine can cause hyperchloremic acidosis in patients with renal failure.

Niacin

Niacin reduced the risk for recurrent myocardial infarction in the Coronary Drug Project[87] and decreased mortality in the 15-year follow-up of the study.[88] In angiographic trials, niacin combined with a resin or statin showed decreased progression of atherosclerosis.[73,89]

Niacin or nicotinic acid is a water-soluble, B-complex vitamin. Its cholesterol-lowering effect was first reported in 1955.[90] Its effects on lipid occur at doses many times the required vitamin dose. Nicotinamide (or niacinamide) has activity as a vitamin but no effect on lipids. The doses required to effect changes of lipid levels range from 1 to 8 g/day. Niacin is readily absorbed from the gastrointestinal tract after oral administration. It reaches a peak level in plasma between 30 and 60 minutes. Niacin undergoes extensive first-pass metabolism through various pathways. The primary route of metabolism is by methylation to *N*-methylnicotinamide, which is oxidized to *N*-methyl-2-pyridone and *N*-methyl-4-pyridone carboxamides. Nicotinic acid is conjugated with glycine to produce nicotinuric acid. The metabolites are excreted in the urine. Nicotinuric acid may be a detoxification product, and its production rate appears to be saturable. When the production rate of the various

pathways are saturated at high doses of niacin, niacin is excreted unchanged in the urine.[91,92]

Niacin has favorable effects on several lipoproteins. Niacin decreases serum total cholesterol and triglyceride levels, decreases LDL cholesterol, and increases HDL cholesterol. It also decreases remnant lipoproteins and lipoprotein (a), a lipoprotein that may be a contributor to increased risk for coronary disease. Doses of 1000 to 1500 mg/day decrease triglycerides and increase HDL, but most patients require 1500 to 2000 mg/day or more to reduce LDL-cholesterol levels by 15% or more. The effects are rapid and dose dependent. Niacin can increase HDL by up to 35% and decrease triglycerides by 20% to 50%.[33,91,93–95] The effect is maintained with continued use.[96]

Side effects and toxicity limit the use of niacin. The most common side effect is cutaneous flushing, which about 10% of patients find intolerable.[22] Other side effects include pruritus, heartburn, diarrhea, nausea, abdominal discomfort, hyperglycemia, increase of serum transaminases, and hyperuricemia (occasionally leading to acute gouty arthritis). Rare side effects include acanthosis nigricans, ichthyosis, conjunctivitis, and cystoid macular edema. Hepatotoxicity can be a significant problem. This is partly dose dependent but is more prevalent with some preparations of time-release niacin. There is often less flushing with time-release or sustained-release preparations compared with non–time-release or crystalline niacin,[33] but more hepatotoxicity occurs.[97–100] A case of fulminant hepatic failure with high-dose sustained-release niacin has been reported.[101] Some of the hepatotoxicity of niacin may be related to constant exposure of the liver to circulating niacin.[94] A prescribed extended-release niacin preparation appears to have similar efficacy to crystalline niacin and is not associated with increased hepatotoxicity at usually prescribed doses.[94–96] Niacin should not be used in patients with significant liver disease because of its potential for hepatotoxicity.

Hyperglycemia is common with up to 16% increases in mean plasma glucose concentration and glycosuria reported in some studies.[102] Niacin was considered to be contraindicated in patients with diabetes, but a recent study in well-controlled patients with type 2 diabetes suggests that some patients with diabetes may benefit from the lipid-modifying effects of niacin without major loss of glycemic control.[103]

Aspirin decreases the flushing seen with niacin if administered 30 minutes in advance. Administration of niacin with food can also decrease flushing. Alcohol potentiates the flushing effect. The combination of niacin and statins has been associated with an increased risk for myopathy, but to a lesser extent than that seen with statin/fibrate combinations.[22]

Fibrates

Clofibrate and gemfibrozil were used in two large clinical trials showing a decreased risk for fatal and nonfatal myocardial infarction.[13,14] In a secondary prevention trial, treatment with gemfibrozil reduced death from coronary heart disease (CHD), nonfatal myocardial infarction, and nonfatal stroke.[10] Decreased progression of atherosclerosis was seen in a trial with bezafibrate.[104] No decrease in risk was seen in the clofibrate arm of the Coronary Drug Project[87] or in the Bezafibrate Infarction Prevention Study.[15]

The fibrates are the most effective drugs for decreasing triglyceride levels. Clofibrate, gemfibrozil, and fenofibrate are available in the United States, and bezafibrate and ciprofibrate are available outside of the United States. Use of clofibrate has declined because of its lesser efficacy and the increased rate of noncardiovascular mortality seen in the World Health Organization study.[13,62] Gemfibrozil is well absorbed from the gastrointestinal treat if given before meals and has a half-life of 1.5 hours. Plasma levels do not accumulate across time with multiple doses. Gemfibrozil is metabolized by oxidation of a ring methyl group to form a hydroxymethyl and then a carboxyl metabolite. It is extensively protein bound. Excretion is primarily through the kidney with 70% of administered dose excreted in the urine, primarily as a glucuronide.[105] Absorption of fenofibrate is increased when administered with food. Protein binding is approximately 99%. Fenofibrate is a prodrug. It is hydrolyzed by esterases to the active metabolite, fenofibric acid. Fenofibric acid is metabolized by conjugation with glucuronic acid. Approximately 60% to 88% of administered drug is excreted in the urine. There is no cytochrome P450 metabolism. The half-life is 20 hours.[106]

The major action of the fibric acid derivatives is a reduction in triglyceride levels. HDL cholesterol is increased. LDL cholesterol may decrease by approximately 5% to 25% in patients who have increased LDL cholesterol and normal triglycerides, but usually increases in patients with elevated triglycerides.[107–109] Triglyceride levels may decrease by 20% to 50% and HDL cholesterol levels increase by 10% to 35%.[107–112] The decrease in LDL cholesterol levels in patients with hypercholesterolemia appears to be greater with fenofibrate, bezafibrate, and ciprofibrate than with gemfibrozil.[113–115] Changes in lipoprotein levels occur within 2 weeks.[108,114] There may be further change with continued therapy.[116]

The main side effects seen with the fibrates are gastrointestinal, including abdominal pain, dyspepsia, bloating, flatulence, nausea, vomiting, diarrhea, and constipation. Less frequent are muscle pain (particularly in patients with renal insufficiency), rash, headache, and impotence.[22,108,116,117] Serum transaminases may increase, and increases in creatinine have been seen with fenofibrate, without apparent change in renal function.[116] Because of their excretion by the kidney, the fibrates can accumulate in serum in patients with renal failure. Their significant protein binding causes displacement of warfarin from albumin-binding sites so that patients on fibrates may require 30% less warfarin.[22] Combinations of fibrates with statins have been associated with an increase of myalgias and myopathy including rhabdomyolysis.[22,62,65,67,68]

Fibric acid derivatives increase the cholesterol concentration of bile and decrease the bile acid concentration of bile leading to an increase in the cholesterol saturation level.[118] Increased prevalence of surgery for gallstones was seen in the World Health Organization Clofibrate Study with clofibrate and the Helsinki Heart Study with gemfibrozil.[13,14] Fibrates are contraindicated in severe hepatic or renal insufficiency.

Although lipid-lowering drugs should generally not be used in women who are pregnant, to prevent pancreatitis gemfibrozil can be used starting in the second trimester in women who have severely increased triglyceride levels, greater than 1000 mg/dL (11.28 mmol/L), and who do not respond to dietary measures.

Practical Aspects of Drug Administration

The National Cholesterol Education Program Adult Treatment Panel III guidelines provide an approach to detection, evaluation, and treatment of hyperlipidemia. The guidelines define thresholds and goals for treatment of increased levels of LDL cholesterol as the primary goal of therapy and treatment of hypertriglyceridemia and low HDL cholesterol levels. Decisions about intervention are based on the patient's risk status. Risk assessment is based on LDL levels, the presence or absence of atherosclerotic disease, risk factors, and assessment of 10-year risk based on Framingham formulas.[19,20]

A fasting lipid profile should be obtained in all adults aged 20 years and over every 5 years, and evaluation of risk factors should be performed. Patients who are admitted to the hospital with an acute coronary syndrome should have a lipid profile performed in the hospital. Fasting profiles done within 24 hours of an acute myocardial infarction will generally reflect the patient's usual profile. Severe illness including surgery, acute febrile illnesses, and poor intake of food may affect lipid levels. Acute febrile illnesses and acute inflammatory states may increase triglycerides and decrease cholesterol levels. Nevertheless, for patients with coronary disease, it is useful to obtain a lipid profile and start therapy during the hospitalization if the patient is not currently receiving therapy. An acute event or intervention such as angioplasty is a chance to make lifestyle changes such as diet improvements, smoking cessation, and exercise. Patients need to start lipid-lowering therapy while in the hospital to avoid gaps in therapy.

Patients are divided into three levels of risk: those with established CHD or risk for CHD equivalent to that of people with established disease, those with multiple (two or more) risk factors, and those with one or no risk factors (Table 49–1). For patients with two or more risk factors, a further calculation of risk score based on Framingham scoring is performed.[19] This gives an estimation of the patient's 10-year risk of a major coronary event. Clinical atherosclerotic disease includes clinical CHD and CHD risk equivalents: symptomatic carotid artery disease, peripheral arterial disease, and abdominal aortic aneurysm. Diabetes mellitus and a 10-year risk of greater than 20% are also considered CHD risk equivalents, requiring more aggressive treatment.

Patients with certain inherited dyslipidemias such as familial hypercholesterolemia and familial combined hyperlipidemia are at particularly increased risk and may require intensive therapy. Familial hypercholesterolemia is a disorder of LDL receptors in which patients with the heterozygous form (one abnormal allele of the LDL receptor gene) have cholesterol levels of 250 to 500 mg/dL (6.45 to

TABLE 49–1.

National Cholesterol Treatment Program Adult Treatment Panel III Guidelines: Major Risk Factors (Exclusive of LDL Cholesterol) That Modify LDL Goals

Cigarette smoking

Hypertension (blood pressure ≥ 140/90 mm Hg or on antihypertensive medication)

Family history of premature CHD (CHD in male first-degree relative < 55 years old; CHD in female first-degree relative < 65 years)

Low HDL cholesterol (<40 mg/dL [1.03 mmol/L])*

Age: men ≥ 45 years; women ≥55 years

*HDL cholesterol level ≥ 60 mg/dL (1.55 mmol/L) counts as a "negative" risk factor; its presence removes one risk factor from the total count.
CHD, coronary heart disease; HDL, high-density lipoprotein; LDL, low-density lipoprotein.
From reference 19.

12.91 mmol/L). The incidence is approximately 1 in 500, and the disorder is associated with increased risk for atherosclerotic vascular, even in the absence of other risk factors. Patients who have two abnormal alleles for the abnormal LDL receptor gene have cholesterol levels of 600 to 1000 mg/dL (15.5 to 25.8 mmol/L) and may develop symptomatic coronary artery disease in early childhood. Familial combined hyperlipidemia is a disorder of overproduction of VLDL, occurs in 1% to 2% of the population, and is associated with increased risk for atherosclerosis. Increases of VLDL, LDL, or both occur. HDL is often low.[22] Patients with severe hypertriglyceridemia are at risk for pancreatitis and require therapy. Patients with hypertriglyceridemia from underlying genetic abnormalities such as familial combined hyperlipidemia may develop the chylomicronemia syndrome, characterized by triglyceride levels greater than 1000 mg/dL (11.29 mmol/L), lipemic plasma, and a risk for pancreatitis. They may also have enlargement of the liver or spleen, eruptive xanthomas, lipemia retinalis, paresthesias, and abdominal pain.

Part of the initial evaluation of patients with hyperlipidemia should include evaluation for secondary dyslipidemias. Acquired dyslipidemia can be caused by diabetes mellitus, renal failure, systemic lupus erythematosus, nephrotic syndrome, alcohol intake, dysgammaglobulinemias, glucocorticoid excess, acromegaly, anorexia nervosa, acute intermittent porphyria, lipodystrophy (including human immunodeficiency virus) and medications. Medications that can increase triglycerides include retinoids, estrogen (taken orally), thiazide diuretics, and occasionally β-adrenergic-blocking agents.[21] Beta-blockers can decrease HDL cholesterol. Treatment of diabetes mellitus with good control of blood sugars is particularly important if reasonable control of hypertriglyceridemia is to be achieved.

Women with triglyceride levels greater than 300 mg/dL (3.39 mmol/L) may be at risk for development of severe hypertriglyceridemia and pancreatitis when taking oral estrogen preparations.

Thresholds for therapy and goals of therapy are shown in Table 49–2. Initial therapy is known as therapeutic lifestyle change and includes dietary intervention, moderate exercise, and weight loss. Lifestyle changes may be sufficient therapy for mild to moderate hypercholesterolemia and hypertriglyceridemia. All other treatment should build on therapeutic lifestyle changes. Many patients will have a 10% to 15% decrease in LDL levels with diet; this may be enough to reach goal levels in some patients and is important in patients in whom the ultimate LDL cholesterol reduction needs to be 30% to 60%. Hypertriglyceridemia often responds quite well to decreased dietary intake of fats, sugar, alcohol, and calories in overweight people. Response to lipid-lowering drugs may be disappointing in patients who continue to consume high fat diets. Patients who have LDL cholesterol levels greater than 190 mg/dL (4.9 mmol/L) or multiple risk factors should have only 6 to 12 weeks of intensive diet therapy before proceeding to drug therapy. Patients with CHD or CHD risk equivalents who have LDL cholesterol levels greater than 130 mg/dL (3.36 mmol/L) should start drug therapy at the same time as nonpharmacologic therapy. CHD patients with LDL levels greater than 100 mg/dL (2.58 mmol/L) also can be considered for immediate drug therapy.

LDL is the primary target of intervention, but triglycerides require treatment in some patients. NCEP definitions of triglyceride levels are shown in Table 49–3. Patients with triglycerides less than 200 mg/dL (2.26 mmol/L) may respond to lifestyle changes and use of a statin for treatment if LDL is not at goal. Patients with triglycerides remaining greater than 200 mg/dL (2.26 mmol/L) after LDL goal is reached may have a secondary goal of non-HDL cholesterol used in management. This number is the total cholesterol minus HDL and gives an approximation of LDL, VLDL, and remnant lipoproteins. Goals are 30 mg/dL (0.78 mmol/L) greater than LDL goals. Weight loss, use of greater doses of statins, or the addition of niacin or a fibrate may help achieve better results. Patients with very high triglycerides need intensive dietary therapy, weight loss, and exercise and may require treatment with a fibrate or niacin.

The best drugs for decreasing LDL cholesterol are the statins, the bile acid sequestrant resins, and niacin in high doses. Niacin and the fibrates are useful for hypertriglyceridemia. For increased LDL cholesterol combined with triglyceride levels less than 500 mg/dL (5.64 mmol/L), the statins, niacin, or a fibrate may provide acceptable results.

Statins

Statins are now the first choice for decreasing LDL cholesterol in most patients. They are particularly useful when a substantial reduction in LDL is required such as for patients with CHD and patients with moderately high LDL

TABLE 49–2.

National Cholesterol Education Program Adult Treatment Panel III Guidelines: Treatment Decisions Based on LDL Cholesterol

Risk Category	LDL Goal	LDL Level at Which to Initiate Therapeutic Lifestyle Changes	LDL Level at Which to Consider Drug Therapy
CHD or CHD risk equivalents (10-year risk > 20%)	<100 mg/dL (2.58 mmol/L)	≥100 mg/dL (2.58 mmol/L)	≥130 mg/dL [3.36 mmol/L] (100–129 mg/dL [2.58–3.33 mmol/L]: drug optional)
2+ Risk factors (10-year risk ≤ 20%)	<130 mg/dL (3.36 mmol/L)	≥130 mg/dL (3.36 mmol/L)	10-year risk 10–20%: ≥130 mg/dL (3.36 mmol/L) 10-year risk <10%: ≥160 mg/dL (4.13 mmol/L)
0–1 Risk Factor	<160 mg/dL (4.13 mmol/L)	≥160 mg/dL (4.13 mmol/L)	≥190 mg/dL [4.91 mmol/L] (160–189 mg/dL [4.13–4.88 mmol/L]: LDL-lowering drug optional)

CHD, coronary heart disease; LDL, low-density lipoprotein. Modified from reference 19.

TABLE 49–3.

National Cholesterol Education Program Adult Treatment Panel III Guidelines: Definition of Triglyceride Levels

Normal triglycerides	<150 mg/dL (1.69 mmol/L)
Borderline high triglycerides	150–199 mg/dL (1.69–2.25 mmol/L)
High triglycerides	200–499 mg/dL (2.26–5.63 mmol/L)
Very high triglycerides	≥500 mg/dL (5.64 mmol/L)

Modified from reference 19.

cholesterol levels. Patients with familial hypercholesterolemia benefit from high doses of statins as their first therapy, although more than one medication is usually necessary. The risk for significant liver toxicity is low with the statins, but measurements of hepatic transaminases should be obtained before starting therapy and generally at 6- to 12-week intervals after initiation of therapy and dose escalation. After a patient has been taking a statin at a stable dose for 6 months, monitoring can be done at 6-month intervals. If transaminases are increased to 2 to 3 times the upper limit of normal, they should be repeated. In many cases, the transaminases will decrease while the patient is receiving therapy. If the patient has malaise or nausea and increased transaminases, the statin should be discontinued. Most patients who have increased transaminases have no symptoms. If liver enzymes remain elevated greater than three times the upper limit of normal, the statin should be discontinued and the enzymes followed until they return to normal, usually in 4 to 8 weeks.

Complaints of muscle discomfort or weakness may be difficult to manage in patients on statins. It is useful to obtain baseline levels of CK, but routine monitoring of CK levels is not useful in most patients. In the Expanded Clinical Evaluation of Lovastatin study, a placebo-controlled lovastatin study, a high proportion of patients taking placebo had an increased CK level at some time during the study.[60] It is useful to check CK if patients are known to have high levels or if symptoms such as myalgias or muscle weakness occur. It is not necessary to discontinue the medication for a mildly abnormal CK level (twice the upper limit of normal) in the absence of any symptoms, especially if there is a clear reason for the increased CK such as a change in exercise regimen or minor injury. Most patients with muscle complaints do not have increased CK levels.

Importantly, serious myopathy can occur with statin therapy. Rhabdomyolysis can occur when statins are combined with fibrates or gemfibrozil or in the presence of other drugs that affect metabolism of statins. Serious illness, renal insufficiency, general debility, congestive heart failure, and the use of multiple medications can contribute to an increased risk for myopathy and rhabdomyolysis. Statins should be discontinued temporarily in patients who are seriously ill. Patients undergoing surgery with general anesthesia should hold the dose of statin for 1 or preferably 2 days before surgery. The statin can be resumed when the patient is eating.

Bile Acid Sequestrants

The bile acid sequestrants are used to treat patients with increased LDL cholesterol levels who do not have increased triglycerides. The most common side effects of the resins are bloating, hard stools, and constipation. Because of their effects on the gastrointestinal tract, the bile acid sequestrants should be discontinued several days before planned surgery. They should not be resumed until patients are eating normally and have resumed normal bowel function.

Niacin

At dosages of 1000 to 2000 mg/day, niacin decreases triglycerides and increases HDL cholesterol. These are secondary goals of therapy according to the NCEP guidelines. A total of 1500 to 2000 mg daily or more decreases LDL cholesterol levels. Since the statin drugs became available, dosages greater than 3000 mg/day are used infrequently. The effects of niacin on VLDL and remnant lipoproteins make it useful in many clinical situations. It is the most effective drug for increasing HDL.

The major side effect of niacin is flushing. Patients unaware of the typical flushing response will assume they are having an allergic reaction to the niacin or other serious illness. Other important side effects include hepatotoxicity, increased uric acid, and impaired glucose tolerance. Uric acid, blood glucose, and liver transaminases should be checked before the start of therapy and every 6 to 8 weeks while dosage is being adjusted. After patients are on a stable dose of niacin, they can be checked every 4 months. Patients who are taking niacin can have sudden problems with abnormal liver enzymes.

Niacin should not be given to acutely ill patients or to those who may be exposed to hepatotoxins. It is prudent to discontinue niacin the day before exposure to general anesthesia.

Fibrates

The fibrates are the most useful drugs for treatment of hypertriglyceridemia. They may also be useful in combined hyperlipidemia. Abnormalities of liver enzymes can be seen with all fibrates but are more common with fenofibrate. Baseline liver enzymes and creatinine should be obtained before starting therapy and repeated after about 6 to 8 weeks. Myalgias are infrequent on monotherapy with fibrates, but are more likely in patients with decreased renal function. The combination of fibrates with statin drugs increases the risk for myopathy and rhabdomyolysis. Patients who are taking warfarin will need to have more frequent monitoring of the blood clotting measurements when starting treatment with a fibrate, and the dose of warfarin may need to be

decreased. Fibrates should be used with caution in patients with renal insufficiency. It is possible to treat patients with renal failure with low doses of fibrates, but myalgias or rashes may be seen more frequently. Because of their possible gastrointestinal effects and renal clearance, fibrates should be held before surgery and not restarted after surgery until patients are well hydrated and eating normally.

Combination Therapy

The use of two or more lipid-lowering medications may be needed to obtain improved serum levels of LDL cholesterol, triglycerides, and HDL cholesterol. Various drug combinations are used including statin/resin combinations, statin/fibrate combinations, and statin/niacin combinations. The risk for myopathy and rhabdomyolysis is increased in patients receiving combination therapy, particularly with statin/fibrate combinations. Patients on this combination should be warned about the risks for myopathy and the signs of rhabdomyolysis and myoglobinuria.. Patients who have acute illnesses or who are receiving general anesthesia should have the medications discontinued temporarily.

Dosage and Administration

Availability applies to the United States only.

Statins

As of June 2002, there are five available statins. Lovastatin is available in 10-, 20-, and 40-mg tablets. The usual starting dose is 20 mg daily, given with the evening meal. The maximum dosage is 80 mg/day, usually given as 40 mg twice a day. Pravastatin is available in 10-, 20-, 40-, and 80-mg tablets. The usual starting dose is 20 mg/day, and the maximum dosage is 80 mg/day, usually given once a day in the evening. Simvastatin is available in 5-, 10-, 20-, 40-, and 80-mg tablets. The usual starting dosage is 20 mg/day, and the maximum dosage is 80 mg/day, usually given once a day in the evening. Fluvastatin is available in 20- and 40-mg capsules, and 80-mg XL tablets. The usual starting dosage is 20 mg/day, and the maximum dosage is 80 mg/day. Doses are usually given in the evening. Atorvastatin is available in 10-, 20-, 40-, and 80-mg doses. The usual starting dosage is 10 mg/day, although 20 mg can be started in patients requiring greater LDL lowering. The maximum dosage is 80 mg/day. Atorvastatin can be given at any time of the day.

Bile Acid Sequestrants

Cholestyramine is available as a regular and a "light" preparation. Regular cholestyramine is available in 9-g packets containing 4 g anhydrous cholestyramine with most of the rest of the material being sucrose. The light preparation also contains 4 g anhydrous cholestyramine with most of the sucrose removed and aspartame included. Both the regular and light forms are available in bulk form. A can of regular cholestyramine contains 378 g and a can of the light cholestyramine contains 210 g. The usual daily dose of cholestyramine is from 4 to 16 g (1–4 packets or scoops). The maximum dose is 24 g/day. Colestipol is available in 5-g packets, 500-g bottles, and 1-g tablets. The usual daily dosage is from 4 to 20 g/day in the form of tablets, packets, or scoops of granules. The maximum dosage is 30 g/day. Colesevelam is available in 625-mg tablets and the usual dosage is 2.6 to 3.3 g/day with the maximum dosage of 7 tablets (4.3 g) per day. The sequestrants are given close to meals once or twice a day depending on the total dose.

Niacin

There are many over-the-counter preparations of crystalline and time-release (or sustained-release) niacin. Typically, crystalline niacin is available in 100-, 250-, and 500-mg tablets, and sustained-release niacin in 250 and 500-mg capsules or tablets. Prescription extended-release niacin, Niaspan®, is available in 500-, 750-, and 1000-mg tablets. The usual dosage of plain niacin is 1000 to 2000 mg/day, up to a maximum of 4.5 g/day. The maximum amount of over-the-counter sustained-release niacin that should be used is 1500 to 2000 mg/day. The maximum dose of Niaspan is 2000 mg/day.

Fibrates

Clofibrate is available in 500-mg tablets. The usual dosage is 1000 mg twice a day. Gemfibrozil is available as 600-mg tablets, and the usual and maximum dosage is 600 mg twice a day. Fenofibrate is available as 54- and 160-mg tablets. The usual dosage is 160 mg/day, but 54 mg/day is available for patients who need a smaller dosage. The maximum dosage is 160 mg/day.

Fixed-Dose Combinations

A fixed-dose combination of lovastatin and extended-release niacin is available. Available strengths are tablets containing 500 mg niacin with 20 mg lovastatin, 750 mg niacin with 20 mg lovastatin, and 1000 mg niacin with 20 mg lovastatin. The starting dosage is 500/20, and the maximum dose is two 1000/20 tablets. The drug is given at bedtime.

References

1. Steinberg D, Gotto AM: Preventing coronary artery disease by lowering cholesterol levels. Fifty years from bench to bedside. JAMA 282:2043, 1999.
2. Stamler J, Wentworth D, Neaton JD: Is the relationship between serum cholesterol and risk of premature death from coronary hear disease continuous and graded? Findings in 356,222 primary screenees of the Multiple Risk Factor Intervention Trial (MRFIT). JAMA 256:2823, 1986.
3. Castelli WP, Garrison RJ, Wilson PW, et al: Incidence of coronary heart disease and lipoprotein cholesterol levels. The Framingham Study. JAMA 256:2835, 1986.
4. Lipid Research Clinics Program: The Lipid Research Clinics Coronary Primary Prevention Trial results, I: reduction in the incidence of coronary heart disease. JAMA 251:351, 1984.
5. Scandinavian Simvastatin Survival Study Group: Scandinavian Simvastatin Survival Study. Lancet 344:1383, 1994.
6. Shepherd J, Cobbe SM, Ford I, et al: Prevention of coronary heart disease with pravastatin in men with hypercholesterolemia. N Engl J Med 333:1301, 1995.
7. Sachs FM, Pfeffer MA, Moye LA, et al: The effect of pravastatin on coronary events after myocardial infarction in patients with average cholesterol levels. N Engl J Med 335:1001, 1996.
8. Downs JR, Clearfield M, Weis S, et al., for the AFCAPS/TexCAPS Research Group: Primary prevention of acute coronary events with lovastatin in men and women with average cholesterol levels. Results of AFCAPS/TexCAPS. JAMA 279:1615, 1998.
9. The Long-Term Intervention with Pravastatin in Ischemic Disease (LIPID) Study Group: Prevention of cardiovascular events and death with pravastatin in patients with coronary heart disease and a broad range of initial cholesterol levels. N Eng J Med 339:1349, 1998.
10. Rubins HB, Robins SJ, Collins D, et al: Gemfibrozil for the secondary prevention of coronary heart disease in men with low levels of high-density lipoprotein cholesterol. N Engl J Med 341:410, 1999.
11. Hokanson JE, Austin MA: Plasma triglyceride level is a risk factor for cardiovascular disease independent of high-density lipoprotein cholesterol level: A meta-analysis of population-based prospective studies. J Cardiovasc Res 3:213, 1996.
12. Sprecher DL: Triglycerides as a risk factor for coronary artery disease. Am J Cardiol 82:49U, 1998.
13. Committee of Principal Investigators: A co-operative trial in the primary prevention of ischaemic heart disease using clofibrate. Br Heart J 40:1069, 1978.
14. Frick M, Elo O, Haapa K, et al: Helsinki Heart Study: Primary-prevention trial with gemfibrozil in middle-aged men with dyslipidemia. N Engl J Med 317:1237, 1987.
15. The BIP Group: Secondary prevention by raising HDL cholesterol and reducing triglycerides in patients with coronary artery disease. Circulation 102:21, 2000.
16. Thompson GR: The proving of the lipid hypothesis. Curr Opin Lipidol 10:201, 1999.
17. The Expert Panel Report of the National Cholesterol Education Program Expert Panel on Detection, Evaluation, and Treatment of High Blood Cholesterol in Adults. Arch Intern Med 148:36, 1988.
18. Summary of the Second Report of the National Cholesterol Education Program (NCEP) Expert Panel on Detection, Evaluation, and Treatment of High Blood Cholesterol in Adults (Adult Treatment Panel II). JAMA 269:3015, 1993.
19. Executive Summary of the Third Report of the National Cholesterol Education Program (NCEP) Expert Panel on Detection, Evaluation, and Treatment of High Blood Cholesterol in Adults (Adult Treatment Panel III). JAMA 285:2486, 2001.
20. Third Report of the Expert Panel on Detection, Evaluation, and Treatment of High Blood Cholesterol in Adults (Adult Treatment Panel III) Full Report. Online at http://www.nhlbi.nih.gov. Accessed June 22, 2002.
21. Chait A, Brunzell JD: Acquired hyperlipidemia (secondary dyslipoproteinemias). Endocrinol Metab Clin North Am 19:259, 1990.
22. Knopp RH: Drug treatment of lipid disorders. N Engl J Med 341:498, 1999.
23. Kwiterovich PO: The metabolic pathways of high-density lipoprotein, low-density lipoprotein, and triglycerides: A current review. Am J Cardiol 86(suppl):5L, 2000.
24. Endo A: The discovery and development of HMG-CoA reductase inhibitors. J Lipid Res 33:1569, 1992.
25. Istvan ES, Deisenhofer J: Structural mechanism for statin inhibition of HMG-CoA reductase. Science 292:1160, 2001.
26. Bilheimer DW, Grundy SM, Brown MS, et al: Mevinolin and colestipol stimulate receptor-mediated clearance of low density

lipoprotein from plasma in familial hypercholesterolemia heterozygotes. Proc Natl Acad Sci USA 80:4124, 1983.

27. Arad Y, Ramakrishnan R, Ginsberg HN: Effects of lovastatin therapy on very-low density lipoprotein triglyceride metabolism in subjects with combined hyperlipidemia: Evidence for reduced assembly and secretion of triglyceride-rich lipoproteins. Metabolism 41:487, 1992.

28. Arad Y, Ramakrishnan R, Ginsberg HN: Lovastatin therapy reduces low density lipoprotein apoB levels in subjects with combined hyperlipidemia by reducing the production of apoB-containing lipoproteins: Implications for the pathophysiology of apoB production. J Lipid Res 31:567, 1990.

29. Grundy SM, Ahrens EH, Salen G: Interruption of the enterohepatic circulation of bile acids in man: Comparative effects of cholestyramine and ileal exclusion on cholesterol metabolism. J Lab Clin Med 78:94, 1971.

30. Shepherd J, Packard CJ, Bicker S, et al: Cholestyramine promotes receptor-mediated low-density-lipoprotein catabolism. N Engl J Med 302:1219, 1980.

31. Rudling MJ, Reihner E, Einarsson K, et al: Low density lipoprotein receptor-binding activity in human tissues: Quantitative importance of hepatic receptors and evidence for regulation of their expression *in vivo*. Proc Natl Acad Sci USA 87:3469, 1990.

32. Beil U, Crouse JR, Einarsson K, et al: Effects of interruption of the enterohepatic circulation of bile acids on the transport of very low density-lipoprotein triglycerides. Metabolism 31:438, 1982.

33. Knopp RH, Ginsberg J, Albers JJ, et al: Contrasting effects of unmodified and time-release forms of niacin on lipoproteins in hyperlipidemic subjects: Clues to mechanism of action of niacin. Metabolism 34:642, 1985.

34. Grundy SM, Mok HYI, Zech L, et al: Influence of nicotinic acid on metabolism of cholesterol and triglycerides in man. J Lipid Res 22:24, 1981.

35. Schoonjans K, Staels B, Auwerx J: Role of the peroxisome proliferator-activated receptor (PPAR) in mediating the effects of fibrates and fatty acids on gene expression. J Lipid Res 37:907, 1996.

36. Fruchart JC, Brewer HB, Leitersdorf E: Consensus for the use of fibrates in the treatment of dyslipoproteinemia and coronary heart disease. Am J Cardiol 81:912, 1998.

37. MRC/BHF Heart Protection Study Collaborative Group: MRC/BHF Heart Protection Study of cholesterol-lowering therapy and of antioxidant vitamin supplementation in a wide range of patients at increased risk of coronary heart disease death: Early safety and efficacy experience. Eur Heart J 20:725, 1999

38. MRC/BHF Heart Protection Study. Online at http://www.hpsinfo.org. Accessed June 9, 2002.

39. Jukema JW, Bruschke AVG, van Boven AJ, et al., on behalf of the REGRESS Study Group: Effects of lipid lowering by pravastatin on progression and regression of coronary artery disease in symptomatic men with normal to moderately elevated serum cholesterol levels. The Regression Growth Evaluation Statin Study (REGRESS). Circulation 91:2528, 1995.

40. Schwartz G, Olsson AG, Ezekowitz MD, et al: Effects of atorvastatin on early recurrent ischemic events in acute coronary syndromes: The MIRACL Study: A randomized controlled trial. JAMA 285:1711, 2001.

41. Corsini A, Bellosta S, Baetta R, et al: New insights into the pharmacodynamic and pharmacokinetic properties of statins. Pharmacol Ther 84:413, 1999.

42. Lennernäs H, Fager G: Pharmacodynamics and pharmacokinetics of the HMG-CoA reductase inhibitors. Similarities and differences. Clin Pharmacokinet 32:403, 1997.

43. Chong PH, Seeger JD, Franklin C: Clinically relevant differences between the statins: Implications for therapeutic selection. Am J Med 111:390, 2001.

44. Cilla DD, Whitfield LR, Gibson DM, et al: Multiple-dose pharmacokinetics, pharmacodynamics, and safety of atorvastatin, an inhibitor of HMG-CoA reductase, in healthy subjects. Clin Pharmacol Ther 60:687, 1996.

45. Mevacor [package insert]. West Point, PA: Merck & Co, Inc., 2001.

46. Pravachol [package insert]. Princeton, NJ: Bristol-Myers Squibb Company, 2000.

47. Zocor [package insert]. West Point, PA: Merck & Co, Inc., 2002.

48. Lescol [package insert]. East Hanover, NJ: Novartis Pharmaceuticals Corporation, 2001.

49. Lipitor [package insert] Morris Plains, NJ: Parke-Davis, 2000.

50. The Lovastatin Study Group II: Therapeutic response to lovastatin (mevinolin) in nonfamilial hypercholesterolemia. A multicenter study. JAMA 256:2829, 1986.

51. Hunninghake DB, Knopp RH, Schonfeld G, et al: Efficacy and safety of pravastatin in patients with primary hypercholesterolemia. I. A dose-response study. Atherosclerosis 85:81, 1990.

52. Mol MJTM, Erkelens DW, Gevers Leuven JA, et al: Simvastatin (MK-733): A potent cholesterol synthesis inhibitor in heterozygous familial hypercholesterolemia. Atherosclerosis 69:131, 1988.

53. Insull W, Black D, Dujovne C, et al: Efficacy and safety of once-daily vs twice-daily dosing with fluvastatin, a synthetic reductase inhibitor, in primary hypercholesterolemia. Arch Intern Med 154:2449, 1994.

54. Nawrocki JW, Weiss SR, Davidson MH, et al: Reduction of LDL cholesterol by 25% to 60% in patients with primary hypercholesterolemia by atorvastatin, a new HMG-CoA reductase inhibitor. Arterioscler Thromb Vasc Biol 15:678, 1995.

55. Davidson MH, Stein EA, Dujovne CA, et al: The efficacy and six-week tolerability of simvastatin 80 and 160 mg/day. Am J Cardiol 79:38, 1997.

56. Stein EA, Lane M, Laskarzewski P: Comparison of statin in hypertriglyceridemia. Am J Cardiol 81(4A):66B, 1998.

57. Jones P, Kafonek S, Laurora I, et al., for the CURVES Investigators: Comparative dose efficacy study of atorvastatin versus simvastatin, pravastatin, lovastatin, and fluvastatin in patients with hypercholesterolemia (the CURVES) study. Am J Cardiol 81:582, 1998.

58. Tobert JA, Bell GD, Birtwell J, et al: Cholesterol-lowering effect of mevinolin, an inhibitor of 3-hydroxy-3-methylglutaryl-coenzyme A reductase, in healthy volunteers. J Clin Invest 69:913, 1982.

59. Pan HY, DeVault AR, Swites BJ, et al: Pharmacokinetics and pharmacodynamics of pravastatin alone and with cholestyramine in hypercholesterolemia. Clin Pharmacol Ther 48:201, 1990.

60. Bradford RH, Shear CL, Chremos A, et al: Expanded clinical evaluation of lovastatin (EXCEL) study results. I. Efficacy in modifying plasma lipoproteins and adverse event profile in 8245 patients with moderate hypercholesterolemia. Arch Intern Med 151:43, 1991.

61. Heinonen TM, Stein E, Weiss SR, et al: The lipid-lowering effects of atorvastatin, a new HMG-CoA reductase inhibitor: Results of a randomized, double-masked study. Clin Ther 18:853, 1996.

62. Choice of lipid-regulating drugs. Med Lett 43:43, 2001.

63. Hsu I, Spinler SA, Johnson NE: Comparative evaluation of the safety and efficacy of HMG-CoA reductase inhibitor monotherapy in the treatment of primary hypercholesterolemia. Ann Pharmacother 29:743, 1995.

64. Bradford RH, Shear CL, Chremos AN, et al: Expanded Clinical Evaluation of Lovastatin (EXCEL) Study results: Two-year efficacy and safety follow-up. Am J Cardiol 74:667, 1994.

65. Pierce LF, Wysowski DK, Gross TP: Myopathy and rhabdomyolysis associated with lovastatin-gemfibrozil combination therapy. JAMA 262:71, 1990.

66. Goldman JA, Fishman AB, Lee JE, et al: The role of cholesterol-lowering agents in drug-induced rhabdomyolysis and polymyositis [letter]. Arthritis Rheum 32:358, 1989.

67. Duell PB, Connor WE, Illingworth DR: Rhabdomyolysis after taking atorvastatin with gemfibrozil. Am J Cardiol 81:368, 1998.

68. Omar MA, Wilson JP: FDA adverse event reports on statin-associated rhabdomyolysis. Ann Pharmacother 36:288, 2002.

69. Kantola T, Kivisto KT, Neuvonen PJ: Grapefruit juice greatly increases serum concentrations of lovastatin and lovastatin acid. Clin Pharmacol Ther 63:397, 1998.

70. Rogers JD, Zhao J, Liu L, et al: Grapefruit juice has minimal effects on plasma concentrations of lovastatin-derived 3-hydroxy-3-methylglutaryl coenzyme A reductase inhibitors. Clin Pharmacol Ther 66:358, 1999.

71. Bailey DG, Malcolm J, Arnold O, et al: Grapefruit juice-drug interactions. Br J Clin Pharmacol 52:216, 2001.

72. Lipid Research Clinics Program: The Lipid Research Clinics Coronary Primary Prevention Trial results, II: The relationship of reduction in incidence of coronary heart disease to cholesterol lowering. JAMA 251:365, 1984.

73. Blankenhorn DH, Nessim SA, Johnson RL, et al: Beneficial effects of combined colestipol-niacin therapy on coronary atherosclerosis and coronary venous bypass grafts. JAMA 257:3233, 1987.

74. Brown G, Albers JJ, Fisher LD, et al: Regression of coronary artery disease as a result of intensive lipid-lowering therapy in men with high levels of apolipoprotein B. N Engl J Med 323:1289, 1990.

75. Davidson MH, Dillon MA, Gordon B, et al: Colesevelam hydrochloride (Cholestagel). A new, potent bile acid sequestrant associated with

a low incidence of gastrointestinal side effects. Arch Intern Med 159:1893, 1999.

76. Insull W, Toth P, Mullican W, et al: Effectiveness of colesevelam hydrochloride in decreasing LDL cholesterol in patients with primary hypercholesterolemia: A 24-week randomized controlled trial. Mayo Clin Proc 76:971, 2001.

77. Lyons D, Webster J, Fowler G, et al: Colestipol at varying dosage intervals in the treatment of moderate hypercholesterolemia. Br J Clin Pharmacol 37:59, 1994.

78. Hunninghake DB, Probstfield Jl, Crow LO, et al: Effect of colestipol and clofibrate on plasma lipid and lipoproteins in type IIa hyperlipoproteinemia. Metabolism 30:605, 1981.

79. Hunninghake DB, Bell C, Olson L: Effect of colestipol and clofibrate, singly and in combination, on plasma lipid and lipoproteins in type IIb hyperlipoproteinemia. Metabolism 30:610, 1981.

80. Vecchio TJ, Linden CV, O'Connell JMJ, et al: Comparative efficacy of colestipol and clofibrate in type IIa hyperlipoproteinemia. Arch Intern Med 142:721, 1982.

81. Davidson MH, Toth P, Weiss S, et al: Low-dose combination therapy with colesevelam hydrochloride and lovastatin effectively decreases low-density lipoprotein cholesterol in patients with primary hypercholesterolemia. Clin Cardiol 24:467, 2001.

82. Hunninghake D, Insull W, Toth P, et al: Coadministration of colesevelam hydrochloride with atorvastatin lowers LDL cholesterol additively. Atherosclerosis 158:407, 2001.

83. Knapp HH, Schrott H, Ma P, et al: Efficacy and safety of combination simvastatin and colesevelam in patients with primary hypercholesterolemia. Am J Med 110:352, 2001.

84. Crouse JR: Hypertriglyceridemia: A contraindication to the use of bile acid binding resins. Am J Med 83:243, 1987.

85. Adridge MA, Ito MK: Colesevelam hydrochloride: A novel bile acid-binding resin. Ann Pharmacother 35:898, 2001.

86. Donovan JM, Stypinski D, Stiles MR, et al: Drug interactions with colesevelam hydrochloride, a novel, potent lipid-lowering agent. Cardiovasc Drugs Ther 14:681, 2000.

87. Coronary Drug Project Research Group: Clofibrate and niacin in coronary heart disease. JAMA 231:360, 1975.

88. Canner PL, Berge KG, Wenger NK, et al: Fifteen year mortality in Coronary Drug Project patients: Long-term benefit with niacin. J Am Coll Cardiol 8:1245, 1986.

89. Brown BG, Zhao X-Q, Chait A, et al: Simvastatin and niacin, antioxidant vitamins, or the combination for the prevention of coronary disease. N Engl J Med 345:1583, 2001.

90. Altshul R, Hoffer A, Stephen JD: Influence of nicotinic acid on serum cholesterol in man. Arch Biochem Biophys 54:558, 1955.

91. Drood JM, Zimetbaum PJ, Frishman WH: Nicotinic acid for the treatment of hyperlipoproteinemia. J Clin Pharmacol 31:641, 1991.

92. Morgan JM, Capuzzi DM, Guyton JR: A new extended-release niacin (Niaspan): Efficacy, tolerability, and safety in hypercholesterolemic patients. Am J Cardiol 82:29U, 1998.

93. Luria MH: Effect of low-dose niacin on high-density lipoprotein cholesterol and total cholesterol/high-density lipoprotein cholesterol ratio. Arch Intern Med 148:2493, 1988.

94. Morgan JM, Capuzzi DM, Guyton JR, et al: Treatment effect of Niaspan, a controlled-release niacin, in patients with hypercholesterolemia: a placebo-controlled trial. J Cardiovasc Pharmacol Therapeut 1:195, 1996.

95. Knopp RH, Alagona P, Davidson M, et al: Equivalent efficacy of a time-release form of niacin (Niaspan) given once-a-night versus plain niacin in the management of hyperlipidemia. Metabolism 47:1097, 1998.

96. Capuzzi DM, Guyton JR, Morgan JM, et al: Efficacy and safety of an extended-release niacin (Niaspan): A long-term study. Am J Cardiol 82:74U, 1998.

97. McKenney JM, Proctor JD, Harris S, et al: A comparison of the efficacy and toxic effects of sustained- vs immediate-release niacin in hypercholesterolemia patients. JAMA 271:672, 1994.

98. Etchason JA, Miller TD, Squires RW, et al: Niacin-induced hepatitis: A potential side effect with low-dose time-release niacin. Mayo Clin Proc 66:23, 1991.

99. Rader JI, Calvert RJ, Hathcock JN: Hepatic toxicity of unmodified and time-release preparations of niacin. Am J Med 92:77, 1992.

100. Gray DR, Morgan T, Chretien SD, et al: Efficacy and safety of controlled-release niacin in dyslipoproteinemic veterans. Ann Intern Med 121:252, 1994.

101. Mullin GE, Greenson JK, Mitchell MC: Fulminant hepatic failure after ingestion of sustained-release nicotinic acid. Ann Intern Med 111:253, 1989.

102. Garg A, Grundy SM: Nicotinic acid as therapy for dyslipidemia in non-insulin-dependent diabetes mellitus. JAMA 264:723, 1990.

103. Elam MB, Hunninghake DB, Davis KB, et al: Effect of niacin on lipid and lipoprotein levels and glycemic control in patients with diabetes and peripheral arterial disease. The ADMIT Study: A randomized trial. JAMA 284:1263, 2000.

104. Ericsson CG, Hamsten A, Nilsson J, et al: Angiographic assessment of effects of bezafibrate on progression of coronary artery disease in young male postinfarction patients. Lancet 347:849, 1996.

105. Lopid package insert. Physician's Desk Reference. 2002.

106. Chapman MJ: Pharmacology of fenofibrate. Am J Med 83(suppl 5B):21, 1987.

107. Leaf DA, Connor WE, Illingworth R, et al: The hypolipidemic effects of gemfibrozil in type V hyperlipidemia. JAMA 262:31564, 1989.

108. Goldberg AC, Feldman EB, Ginsberg HN, et al: Fenofibrate for the treatment of type IV and V hyperlipoproteinemias: A double-blind, placebo-controlled multicenter US study. Clin Ther 11:69, 1989.

109. Pauciullo P, Marotta G, Rubba P, et al: Serum lipoproteins, apolipoproteins and very low density lipoprotein subfractions during 6-month fibrate treatment in primary hypertriglyceridaemia. J Intern Med 228:425, 1990.

110. Steinmetz A, Schwartz T, Hehnke U, et al: Multicenter comparison of micronized fenofibrate and simvastatin in patients with primary type IIA or IIB hyperlipoproteinemia. J Cardiovasc Pharmacol 4:563, 1996.

111. Farnier M, Bonnefous F, Debbas N, et al: Comparative efficacy and safety of micronized fenofibrate and simvastatin in patients with primary type IIa or IIb hyperlipidemia. Arch Intern Med 154:441, 1994.

112. Miller M, Bachorik PS, McCrindle BW, et al: Effect of gemfibrozil in men with primary isolated low high-density lipoprotein cholesterol: A randomized, double-blind, placebo-controlled, crossover study. Am J Med 94:7, 1993.

113. Illingworth DR, Olsen GD, Cook SR, et al: Ciprofibrate in the therapy of type II hyperlipoproteinemia. A double-blind trial. Atherosclerosis 44:211, 1982.

114. Brown WV, Dujovne CA, Farquhar JW, et al: Effects of fenofibrate on plasma lipids. Double-blind multicenter study in patients with type IIA or IIB hyperlipoproteinemia. Arteriosclerosis 6:670, 1986.

115. Gavish D, Oschry Y, Fainaru M, et al: Change in very low-, low-, and high-density lipoproteins during lipid lowering (bezafibrate) therapy: Studies in type IIA and type IIb hyperlipoproteinemia. Eur J Clin Invest 16:61, 1986.

116. Adkins JC, Faulds D: Micronised fenofibrate. Drugs 54:615, 1997.

117. Blaine GF: Comparative toxicity and safety profile of fenofibrate and other fibric acid derivatives. Am J Med 83(suppl5B):26, 1987.

118. Palmer RH: Effects of fibric acid derivatives on biliary lipid composition. Am J Med 83(suppl 5B):37, 1987.

50

Antimicrobial Therapy

Richard Teplick, MD • Lindsey Baden, MD • Robert H. Rubin, MD

Antimicrobials are used in surgical patients either prophylactically, to prevent infection, or therapeutically, to treat ongoing infection. In the latter instance, initial therapy is often empirical, directed against the most likely organisms and their antimicrobial resistance patterns in a particular hospital or area within the hospital such as an intensive care unit (ICU). In prophylaxis, antimicrobial use is directed against the organisms most likely associated with a particular type of surgery. Other important considerations in selecting a prophylactic antimicrobial agent are its toxicity, its spectrum, its antimicrobial properties (e.g., bacteriostatic or bacteriocidal), postantibiotic effect (PAE), the presumed site of infection (e.g., abdomen, cerebrospinal fluid), and the agent's pharmacokinetics and pharmacodynamics.

It is of great concern that a significant proportion of antimicrobial use, particularly broad-spectrum agents, both in the inpatient and outpatient setting are often inappropriate.[1,2] Antibiotic use has been clearly associated with the emergence and dissemination of antibiotic-resistant organisms, with this occurring far more commonly in ICUs than in non-ICU inpatient wards, and more commonly on inpatient wards than in the outpatient setting.

In general, antimicrobials may be used in three different modes. In the therapeutic mode, they are prescribed to treat established clinical infection. The appropriate therapeutic use of antimicrobial drugs requires the prompt diagnosis of clinical infection and a clear understanding of the pharmacologic principles governing treatment of such infections. In the prophylactic mode, antimicrobials are prescribed to all members of a given population before an event to prevent the occurrence of clinical infection. Successful prophylactic programs require that the antimicrobial therapy be sufficiently nontoxic and inexpensive to justify the intervention. Finally, in the pre-emptive mode, antimicrobial therapy is administered to the subgroup of individuals based on either laboratory markers or clinical epidemiologic characteristics that place them at significant risk for a serious clinical infection. Effective pre-emptive therapy requires the careful delineation of the factors that justify antimicrobial intervention at a point when clinical disease is not yet manifest.[3,4] The purpose of this chapter is to present the pharmacologic and clinical principles that underlie all three forms of antimicrobial use, carefully distinguishing between that which is known and that which needs further study. Reviews of specific antibiotics can be found in a recent series published in the Mayo Clinics Proceedings.[5-14] However, there are important differences among different classes of antibiotics, which are discussed later. First, some antibiotics are bacteriostatic (e.g., tetracyclines), that is, they prevent bacteria from growing but generally do not kill them; this is accomplished by leukocytes. Another important distinction is their mechanism of action, especially the distinction between antimicrobials that affect cell wall synthesis and those that affect protein or nucleic acid synthesis. β-Lactams and vancomycin are examples of the former, whereas aminoglycosides and fluoroquinolones are examples of the latter. There are other important distinctions such as the rate of development of resistance, presence of PAE, and pharmacokinetics and pharmacodynamics.

General Principles

Minimum Inhibitory Concentration, Minimum Bacteriocidal Concentration

When exposed to antibiotics, bacteria may be killed or their growth may be inhibited without being killed. The minimum inhibitory concentration (MIC) of an antibiotic is the lowest concentration required to prevent growth, whereas the minimum bacteriocidal concentration is the concentration required to kill 99.9% of the inoculum used for the test. The minimum bacteriocidal concentration is technically much more difficult and time-consuming to determine than the MIC, is subject to multiple potential errors and is not needed for routine clinical care.[15]

Most clinical laboratories now use the disk diffusion technique to determine bacterial sensitivity to antibiotics. Multiple disks, each impregnated with a different antibiotic, are placed over a growth medium that is then covered with a fixed inoculum of the bacteria of interest. The antibiotics diffuse outward from the disks with concentrations that decrease with increasing radii from each disk. Susceptibility to an antibiotic is determined by the radius around each disk that inhibits bacterial growth. Based on the size of the zone that inhibits growth, the bacterium is considered susceptible, intermediately susceptible, or resistant to the antimicrobial. These zones are determined for each antibiotic disk and each bacterium.

A susceptible strain implies that an infection caused by that particular bacterium may "be appropriately treated with the dosage of antimicrobial agent recommended for that type of infection and infecting species." Intermediate sensitivity means that antimicrobial MICs "usually approach attainable blood and tissue levels and for which response rates may be lower than for susceptible isolates." Intermediate sensitivity implies that the antibiotic may be clinically useful in body sites where it is concentrated such as β-lactams in urine or when greater than usual doses of the antibiotic may be used. Resistant means that the bacterium is "not inhibited by usually achievable systemic concentrations of the agent with normal dose schedules and/or fall in the range where specific microbial resistance mechanisms are likely" and when "clinical efficacy has not been reliable in treatment studies."[16]

Time- Versus Dose-Dependent Killing

Some antibiotics, notably aminoglycosides and fluoroquinolones, increase the rate and extent of bacterial killing with increasing concentrations. This is known as concentration-dependent killing. The pharmacologic parameters that best relate to the clinical efficacy of this phenomenon are either the ratio of the maximum concentration to the MIC or the ratio of the area under the 24-hour concentration curve to the MIC. In contrast to concentration-dependent killing, many antibiotics, notably most β-lactams, monobactams such as aztreonam, and macrolides such as erythromycin and clindamycin, increase their rate of microbial killing with concentrations up to about four times the MIC. Greater concentrations do not kill bacteria faster or in greater numbers. The clinical efficacy of these antibiotics is related to the duration for which these levels are maintained; hence this is referred to as *time-dependent killing.*

Postantibiotic Effect

Some antibiotics continue to suppress the growth of certain bacteria after the antibiotic is no longer detectable in the media; a phenomenon termed the *postantibiotic effect.* For example, after a 2-hour exposure of susceptible staphylococcal cultures to penicillin, growth is still inhibited for 1.4 to 1.6 hours after multiple washings removed the penicillin.[17] Although PAE can be demonstrated for virtually all antimicrobials, the bacteria affected and the duration of the effect is highly variable.[15] β-Lactam antibiotics, with the exception of carbapenems such as imipenem, have significant PAEs only for some gram-positive bacteria. In contrast, most antimicrobials that inhibit protein or nucleic acid synthesis in gram-negative bacteria generally exhibit a PAE for these organisms. For example, for gram-negative bacteria, aminoglycosides and fluoroquinolones produce PAEs varying from approximately 1 to 4 hours, whereas β-lactams, with the exception of carbapenems such as imipenem or meropenem, have no PAEs. Importantly, the PAE duration tends to be reduced for aminoglycosides and fluoroquinolones in acidic media as might be encountered in necrotic tissue. A related but poorly understood phenomenon is that during the PAE phase, bacteria are more susceptible to killing by leukocytes, an effect termed *postantibiotic leukocyte enhancement.*[18] In addition, the PAE itself may be prolonged by leukocytes.

Pharmacokinetics and Pharmacodynamics

The distinction between time-dependent and concentration-dependent killing and the presence or absence of the PAE have important clinical ramifications.[19–21] The most clinically relevant aspects relate to dosing intervals of antibiotics. For antimicrobial/bacteria combinations that exhibit time-dependent killing, especially when there is no PAE, the duration that the antimicrobial level is greater than the lethal range theoretically should be important. There is general agreement that for β-lactams to be effective, their concentration must be well above the MIC for most of the dosing interval. This is especially true for gram-negative bacteria, which usually do not exhibit PAE for β-lactams. However, there are few human studies with continuous infusions, and it is puzzling that continuous infusions of β-lactams have not uniformly proven superior to more conventional dosing schedules in animal models of infection.[22]

In contrast, for antibiotic/bacteria combinations that do exhibit concentration-dependent killing and significant PAEs, it may be more important to achieve very high peak levels and allow the trough to decrease to less than the MIC because efficacy will still be maintained by the PAE. This is the theoretic basis for the success of once daily dosing of aminoglycosides. For combinations of antibiotics, the situation is more complicated. The PAEs for gram-positive bacteria were increased either additively or synergistically when aminoglycosides were added to cell wall active antibiotics.[23] In contrast, this did not occur with gram-negative bacteria except when imipenem was used with an aminoglycoside.[24]

These considerations led to the concept that administering aminoglycosides in large doses once daily would prove more beneficial and less toxic than the usual standard of three times daily.[25] In particular, because aminoglycosides exhibit concentration-dependent killing, concentrations that achieve 8 to 10 times the MIC will rapidly kill all susceptible bacteria and suppress the survival of higher MIC mutants. Because of the PAE, suppression can be sustained during the period that the concentration decreases to less than the MIC. The maintenance of drug-free intervals for a period before the next dose may also help prevent adaptive resistance, which is a decreased aminoglycoside uptake by bacteria exposed to smaller levels of the drug. Finally, because renal uptake is saturable, the high initial levels are not accompanied by proportionally increased renal uptake. Consequently, renal toxicity should not increase. Numerous studies show that in most patients and even in febrile neutropenic patients these tenets seem to hold: efficacy is at least equal to multiple daily dosing and renal toxicity is not increased.[26]

Three pharmacokinetic issues should be considered in the choice of antimicrobial therapy: the ability of the drug to penetrate to the site of presumed infection, the presence of local factors at the site of infection that might modify the efficacy of particular antimicrobial agents, and the route of delivery that should be used. Thus if infection of the central nervous system (CNS) is suspected, drugs that reach effective concentrations within the CNS should be used in doses adequate to achieve this objective (Table 50–1). However, there are exceptions. For example, meningitis from high-level, penicillin-resistant *Streptococcus pneumococcus* has been successfully treated with antibiotics that typically do not penetrate the CNS well. This may be a result of increased penetration resulting from inflammation. Local factors that modify the effectiveness of particular antimicrobial agents include the following: inadequately drained infections will limit the effectiveness of aminoglycoside therapy, even if the organisms present are sensitive in vitro, because these drugs are far less effective in the presence of pus (both aminoglycosides and vancomycin are bound by pus, limiting their antimicrobial activity) and in conditions of low pH and low oxygen tensions.[27] The requirement for oxygen-dependent transport for aminoglycosides to penetrate the outer membranes of susceptible bacteria explains the latter point and why they are generally ineffective against anaerobic bacteria.[8] In the presence of mixed infections, β-lactamase pro-

TABLE 50–1.

Penetration of the Cerebrospinal Fluid by Different Antimicrobial Agents

Penetration	Antimicrobial Agents
Penetrate noninflamed meninges	Chloramphenicol, trimethoprim-sulfamethoxazole, isoniazid, rifampin, pyrazinamide, flucytosine, fluconazole
Penetrate to therapeutic levels in the presence of inflammation	Penicillin, ampicillin, oxacillin, nafcillin, ticarcillin, azlocillin, mezlocillin, piperacillin, cefuroxime, cefotaxime, ceftriaxone, ceftizoxime, ceftazidime
Penetrate poorly or unreliably even in the presence of inflammation	Cephalothin, cefazolin, cephapirin, cefoxitin, cefotetan, all aminoglycosides, vancomycin, fluoroquinolones, ketoconazole, itraconazole, amphotericin B

duced by such organisms as *Bacteroides fragilis* can cause local inactivation of β-lactam antibiotics and failure to clear organisms from the site that are sensitive in vitro to the β-lactam drug.[28] Penicillins and tetracyclines bind to hemoglobin, thus rendering therapy with these drugs less effective when infection is complicating hematoma formation.[29] In most instances, the continuing presence of a foreign body at the site of infection will prevent the elimination of the microbial invaders even with the best antimicrobial regimen available.[30] Finally, antimicrobials such as trimethoprim-sulfamethoxazole, fluoroquinolones, and fluconazole can be administered orally and still achieve blood levels that are comparable to those obtained with parenteral therapy, provided gastrointestinal function is adequate and, at least in the case of levofloxacin, food or substances containing divalent metal ions are not given at the same time. In addition, even if therapy is initiated intravenously, completion of a course of treatment can be accomplished with a more cost-effective oral regimen when the patient stabilizes.

Resistance

General Concepts

Bacteria may be intrinsically resistant to antimicrobials or they may acquire resistance. Intrinsic resistance reflects a natural resistance to an antimicrobial. For example, vancomycin is ineffective against gram-negative bacteria because it cannot penetrate their outer membrane. Acquired resistance reflects a genetic alteration in the bacteria that renders a once effective antimicrobial ineffective. The general mechanisms for bacterial resistance to antimicrobials are: (1) decreased permeability to the antimicrobial preventing its entry; (2) increased efflux pumps that keep the antimicrobial concentrations in the space between the inner and outer membranes of gram-negative bacteria or the cytoplasmic spaces low; (3) antimicrobial inactivation; (4) modification of the antimicrobial target; and (5) development of pathways that bypass the target. The genes encoding these phenotypes may be chromosomal or plasmid in origin, inducible, or constitutive. With broad use of antibiotics, multiple resistant determinants have been selected. A detailed review of antimicrobial resistance mechanisms can be found elsewhere.[31–33] Methicillin resistance in *Staphylococcus*, vancomycin resistance in *Enterococcus*, and broad-spectrum β-lactam resistance in gram-negative organisms have important diagnostic and therapeutic implications in the hospital setting.[34–36]

In gram-negative bacteria, antimicrobials usually must penetrate the outer membrane through specialized channels termed *porins*. Alterations in the permeability of porins to antimicrobials can either prevent sufficient quantities from entering the bacteria or limit the rate of entry to the extent that even a relatively low inactivation rate is sufficient to render them ineffective. The former is a frequent cause of *Pseudomonas aeruginosa* resistance to aminoglycosides and imipenem and the latter allows many gram-negative bacteria to inactivate β-lactams through β-lactamases. Increased active efflux of antimicrobials is a less common mechanism of resistance but can be important for macrolides, fluoroquinolones, and some β-lactams. Inactivation is the predominant mechanism of resistance for several classes of antimicrobials. Aminoglycosides can be inactivated by both gram-positive and gram-negative bacteria, usually by plasmid-mediated enzymes. Perhaps the most comprehensively studied and categorized inactivating enzymes are the β-lactamases. There are an enormous number of these enzymes. They are often characterized by their genomic sequence and the β-lactams they can hydrolyze. Virtually every β-lactam, monobactam, or carbapenem can be inactivated by one or more of these enzymes. Target modifications in penicillin-binding proteins account for methicillin resistance in staphylococci and penicillin resistance in pneumococci and enterococci. Finally, bypass pathways account for vancomycin resistance in *Enterococcus faecium* and resistance of many bacteria to folate antagonists such as trimethoprim-sulfamethoxazole.

Specific Mechanisms

Perhaps the best-studied and most problematic mechanism of antimicrobial resistance is the β-lactamases. There are at least 340 different β-lactamases; one or more of which can inactivate virtually any β-lactam–based antimicrobial. The classification of β-lactamases is constantly evolving and is based both on phenotype and genotype.[37] Class C β-lactamases can inactivate virtually all classes of β-lactams except the carbapenems and are not inhibited by β-lactamase inhibitors. These enzymes are largely derived from the chromosomal *Escherichia coli ampC* gene but they may also be plasmid borne. They tend to be produced by *Enterobacter, Citrobacter, Serratia, Pseudomonas,* and some species of *Proteus.* Certain β-lactam antibiotics induce this enzyme. Chow and colleagues[38] demonstrated that clinical failure associated with the emergence of resistance often occurs when serious *Enterobacter* infections were treated with a cephalosporin despite initial cephalosporin susceptibility. Thus cephalosporins should be used carefully in the setting of infection with the gram-negative pathogens mentioned earlier.[34,38]

The class A β-lactamases comprise the largest group and include the extended spectrum β-lactamases, which can inactivate third-generation cephalosporins and aztreonam.[39] Fortunately, most of these enzymes can be inhibited by β-lactamase inhibitors that may be used in conjunction with the selected β-lactams.

Although β-lactamases are produced by some gram-positive bacteria, notably staphylococci (but not streptococci) and many anaerobes, the problem is a bit different. The efficacy of these β-lactamases is limited because they are diluted by the extracellular space as opposed to being confined in the periplasmic space in gram-negative bacteria.[40] Although plasmid-encoded β-lactamases cause staphylococcal resistance to many penicillins, resistance of some staphylococci and other gram-positive bacteria also occur by completely different mechanisms. For example, methicillin resistance in *Staphylococcus aureus* is caused by the chromosomal presence of the *mecA* gene, which decreases the binding affinity of methicillin to penicillin-binding proteins. Similarly, ampicillin-resistant *Enterococcus faecium* has an altered penicillin-binding protein that has a greatly reduced affinity for these antibiotics. In contrast, vancomycin resistance in enterococci is related, in the majority of cases, to a multigene plasmid, which is easily spread among enterococci. This plasmid alters a terminal amino acid group in one of the crosslinking amino acids that prevents vancomycin from binding to the growing cell membrane.[41,42] It is astonishing that the first time vancomycin-resistant enterococci (VRE) were observed was in 1986[43] and within 15 years it has come to represent 23.9% of U.S. ICU enterococcal isolates. Unfortunately, there are limited options for the treatment of severe infections related to VRE, which are typically also resistant to ampicillin and aminoglycosides. Several new agents have recently been FDA approved: quinupristin/dalfopristin, a streptogramin, and linezolid, an oxazolidinone, with promising clinical use against resistant gram-positive organisms.[44]

There is great concern that *S. aureus* will acquire the vancomycin resistance determinant from enterococci. Although this has been shown to be possible in the laboratory,[45] it has not yet happened clinically. However, prolonged use of vancomycin in patients with MRSA has led to the emergence of MRSA strains with decreased vancomycin susceptibility known as vancomycin-intermediate *S. aureus*. The mechanism for this diminished susceptibility appears to be caused by a thickening of the cell wall leading to decreased antibiotic penetration, rather than the transfer of vancomycin-resistant genes from enterococcus leading to an altered vancomycin binding target.[46–48]

Emerging Bacterial Resistance

During the last decade, there has been a dramatic increase in the development and dissemination of antibiotic-resistant organisms. In 1998, 23.9% of enterococci were found to be vancomycin resistant, 46.7% of *S. aureus* and 85.7% of *Staphylococcus epidermidis* were methicillin resistant, 10.7% of *K. pneumoniae* and 34% of *Enterobacter* were resistant to third-generation cephalosporins, 17.1% of *P. aeruginosa* were resistant to imipenem, and 23.3% of *P. aeruginosa* were found to be resistant to fluoroquinolones. Comparing the increase in resistance from 1993 to 1997 with 1998, there have been increases of 55% in VRE, 31% in MRSA, 32% in imipenem-resistant *P. aeruginosa*, and 89% in fluoroquinolone-resistant *P. aeruginosa*.[49] Many factors have contributed to the marked increase in resistance, however, indiscriminate broad-spectrum antibiotic use is an important factor.[50] Thus it is critically important to use antimicrobials judiciously because overuse will facilitate the propagation of pathogens that are difficult or impossible to treat.

Multidrug Therapy

There are several reasons for using more than one antimicrobial to treat infections including:

1. *Polymicrobial infections:* To cover all of the bacteria in polymicrobial infections, such as those related to abdominal contamination with colonic contents, more than one antimicrobial may be required. For example, three drugs may be required to cover gram-positive cocci, gram-negative bacilli, and anaerobic bacteria. However, as newer broad-spectrum agents, such as ampicillin-sulbactam, piperacillin-tazobactam, ticarcillin-clavulanate, imipenem, meropenem, and others, have become available for clinical use, the need for broad-spectrum coverage can now often be satisfied with a single agent. Technically, these drugs actually are combinations—ampicillin and piperacillin with β-lactamase inhibitors (other examples of this being amoxicillin and ticarcillin with clavulanate) to prevent destruction of the β-lactam that actually has the desired antibacterial activity, and imipenem with cilastin to inhibit the metabolism of the drug to nephrotoxic metabolites.

2. *Emergence of resistance:* It is logical that if two different antimicrobials with different mechanisms of action such as a β-lactam and an aminoglycoside are used to treat a given bacterium, emergence of resistant strains of that organism will be inhibited because strains that evolve resistance to one of the drugs will still be sensitive to the other. For example, it is true in the case of tuberculosis for which the prescription of multiple drugs to prevent the emergence of resistance by a single step mutation is well established both in the laboratory and clinically. Although it is logical, evidence is currently lacking to support "double coverage" to suppress the emergence of resistance for other forms of infection, for which mechanisms for developing resistance are far more complex.

3. *Synergy:* A third justification for prescribing antibiotic combinations is the possibility of synergy, the most important benefit stemming from this being enhanced killing of the invading organisms. However, the term synergy is often used without a clear understanding of its meaning. In general, a combination of drugs can produce a variety of responses ranging from antagonistic when the combination is less effective than either drug alone to indifferent when the response to the combination is no different from either drug alone to additive when the combined effect equals the sum of the effect of each drug alone. A combination may also produce an effect that is greater than either drug alone, but less than additive. Finally, a combination of drugs may be synergistic, producing an effect that is greater than the sum of the effects of each drug alone. Unfortunately, this terminology has been used in a confusing and sometimes arbitrary manner for antimicrobials, yet it has provided the rationale for some antimicrobial combinations.

The two techniques most commonly used to determine synergy are the checkerboard and time-kill methods. Unfortunately, synergy studies tend to yield different results depending on the method used to determine the effects of antimicrobial combinations.[51] Although there is little doubt that synergy exists for some combinations of antimicrobials against some strains of some bacteria, the concept seems often to be extrapolated to any combination of antimicrobials and any gram-negative bacteria, especially *Pseudomonas aeruginosa*.

The clearest example of the use of synergistic antimicrobial therapy is in the treatment of enterococcal endocarditis. Treatment with penicillin or ampicillin alone has a high rate of relapse, as predicted by in vitro tests that show only a bacteriostatic effect. In contrast, penicillin (or ampicillin or vancomycin) combined with streptomycin or gentamicin is bactericidal in action and has a bacteriologic cure rate of more than 90%.[52–54] Indeed, the appearance of enterococcal strains with high-level resistance to aminoglycosides (MIC > 2000 μg/mL) has incited great concern because it means loss of the ability to prescribe bactericidal therapy when such resistance is present.[55] Optimal therapy for such strains has yet to be determined, but it is clear that more aggressive surgery in combination with bacteriostatic treatment with high-dose ampicillin or vancomycin is now necessary.[56–59]

Checkerboard or time-kill methods have indicated that combinations of β-lactams with aminoglycosides seem to be synergistic in vitro against some species of a variety of organisms, especially nonenterococcal streptococcal species including *Streptococcus pneumoniae*, *S. aureus*, Enterobacteriaceae, and *Pseudomonas aeruginosa*. Direct translation of such in vitro results to clinical therapy, however, has not been very convincing. Unless relative penicillin resistance is present, the addition of an aminoglycoside to penicillin in the treatment of nonenterococcal streptococcal infection may allow a decrease in the duration of therapy but otherwise does not add significantly to the excellent results achieved with penicillin alone for the great majority of isolates.[60] Similarly, the addition of gentamicin to nafcillin therapy of *S. aureus* appears to clear the bacteremia faster but does not change the mortality rate in staphylococcal endocarditis.[61] The combination of an antipseudomonal β-lactam antibiotic with an aminoglycoside appears to be more effective than either drug by itself in the treatment of *Pseudomonas* infection in neutropenic patients and in serious *Pseudomonas* infections in normal hosts, although whether such therapy is more effective than single drug therapy with ceftazidime or imipenem in these patients is unclear. However, synergy has been demonstrated between β-lactams and aminoglycosides in certain circumstances,[62,63] and clinical experience suggests this to be the optimal combination for serious Pseudomonal infections, especially in neutropenic patients. Nonetheless, recent studies have questioned the necessity of this practice in most other patient populations. The major potential disadvantage to such combination therapy is that the nephrotoxicity of aminoglycosides is enhanced by hypotension and endotoxin; the conditions in which the temptation to use them is greatest.

It has become common practice at some centers to substitute a fluoroquinolone for the aminoglycoside; however, there is no compelling evidence that this combination is advantageous. Similarly, although some data are consistent with an added benefit from combination therapy for life-threatening *Klebsiella* infection, again this concept remains controversial.[64] Finally, the combination of amphotericin plus flucytosine can be shown to be synergistic in vitro and in vivo in the treatment of cryptococcal meningitis.[65] Other instances in which "test tube synergy" without defined clinical correlations has been reported include aztreonam with other β-lactams and fluoroquinolones with aminoglycosides.[66]

Thus the situations in which synergistic killing effects of combination therapy that have been demonstrated in vitro are of proven clinical benefit are quite limited. However, the clinical use and the in vitro measurement of synergy currently should be regarded as unsettled. Nonetheless, many skilled clinicians recommend the use of both a β-lactam and an aminoglycoside for gram-negative coverage in critically ill patients, especially for *P. Aeruginosa, Klebsiella,* and in the treatment of rapidly progressive staphylococcal infection. However, it is precisely these patients, especially those who are hypotensive or septic, who have the greatest risk for aminoglycoside-induced renal failure. The issue in these very ill patients is if the potential benefits of adding an aminoglycoside to a β-lactam with an adequate antimicrobial spectrum outweighs the risk for aminoglycoside nephrotoxicity. Data to answer this question are not available.

One potential disadvantage of whimsically combining antimicrobial drugs is the possibility of antagonism. This has been a major concern since the report in 1951 that penicillin alone was significantly better than penicillin plus chlortetracycline in the treatment of pneumococcal meningitis (mortality rate 21% vs. 79%).[67] The validity of this study was strengthened by the observation that children with bacterial meningitis treated with ampicillin alone fared better than those treated with ampicillin plus chloramphenicol and streptomycin.[68] Common to both of these studies was the combination of a bacteriostatic agent (chlortetracycline and chloramphenicol) with bacteriocidal β-lactams. Such antagonism is probably important in the treatment of meningitis and in the severely neutropenic patients[69] but is relatively unimportant in the management of most other infections. Thus combinations of bacteriostatic and bacteriocidal antimicrobials should be avoided in those circumstances. However, this is not an important issue in the treatment of such other infections as peritonitis, where such regimens as penicillin or ampicillin plus chloramphenicol have a long record of clinical success, although seldom used anymore.

Clinical Pharmacology: General Principles of Therapeutic Antimicrobial Use

Treatment of established infection with an effective therapeutic course of antimicrobial agents is based on the delivery of a concentration of drug to the site of infection that exceeds the concentration of drug necessary to kill (bacteriocidal therapy) or inhibit the growth (bacteriostatic therapy) of the infecting organism(s) for a sufficient period to eradicate the infection. Although it would seem reasonable to postulate that bacteriocidal therapy is inherently superior to bacteriostatic therapy, there are only five clinical situations in which bacteriocidal therapy has been shown to be essential for clinical cure: (1) cardiovascular infection, particularly endocarditis;[70] (2) meningitis and cerebral abscess;[71] (3) invasive bacterial infection in the severely neutropenic patient;[72] (4) staphylococcal (and presumably other forms of) osteomyelitis;[73] and (5) the attempted treatment of prosthesis- (or vascular access) related infections without removing the device.[74–77] If one of these forms of infection is present and the organism(s) identified preclude using bacteriocidal therapy, then ablative surgical therapy under coverage of bacteriostatic antibiotics is indicated.

Effective antimicrobial therapy requires the integration of a sizable body of information regarding the patient, the invading microbe(s), and the antimicrobial agents themselves into an effective antimicrobial prescription. The factors that must be considered are discussed in the following section.

The identity of the infecting organism(s) must be known, or at the very least, it must be possible to make a high probability assessment of the most likely culprit(s). That is, the initial choice of antimicrobial agents is usually based on probability assessments of the most likely pathogens causing a particular clinical syndrome, with subsequent adjustment of the regimen once specific microbiologic information becomes available. Important factors to be weighed in determining the likely infecting organism include the likely source, e.g., vascular access device, lung, or urinary tract, and whether the infection is likely to be community-acquired or nosocomial.

To assist in the initial choice of antimicrobial therapy, the following must be kept in mind. First, the patient must be kept stable until the etiologic factors and antimicrobial susceptibility of the invading pathogens are known. Therefore, a key question is whether one is dealing with a therapeutic emergency or a diagnostic dilemma. In the former case, the broadest possible regimen should be used initially with later modifications based on precise microbiologic information. This is often termed "front loading" of the antimicrobial regimen. In the latter case, narrower spectrum initial therapy is possible, with fine-tuning of the regimen when specific information is available.

Epidemiologic considerations must also be factored into antimicrobial decision-making. When dealing with primary illnesses acquired in the community, the nature and timing of possible exposures must be considered. Important exposures include the geographically restricted systemic mycoses (*Blastomyces dermatitidis*, *Coccidioides immitis*, and *Histoplasma capsulatum*), *Mycobacterium tuberculosis*, influenza, group A streptococci, legionella, and meningococcus. Even more important is the special epidemiology of the nosocomial environment, be it a nursing home, a hospital, or a specialized area of the hospital such as an ICU. Specifically, the microbiologic flora within a hospital or even a particular ICU within the hospital and their respective resistance patterns are essential information. The increasing incidence of infection with difficult to treat organisms such as methicillin-resistant *Staphylococcus aureus,* vancomycin-resistant Enterococci, and multiply resistant gram-negative bacilli is already having a profound influence on the initial choice of antibiotics. For example, vancomycin is usually preferred over nafcillin as initial therapy for suspected staphylococcal infection, and advanced-spectrum β-lactam agents such as imipenem rather than cefazolin or gentamicin for gram-negative infection that could be caused by highly resistant Klebsiella species.[64,78] It is likely that these problems with antibiotic resistance will increase, not just in terms of these organisms but also with increasing incidences of infections with penicillin-resistant pneumococci[79] and ampicillin, vancomycin, and gentamicin-resistant enterococcal.[56–59] These considerations highlight the importance of the reservoir of a given organism and the selective pressure that reservoir is experiencing, e.g., *Salmonella* and *Campylobacter* in domestic animals vs. *S. pneumoniae* in the community at large vs. resistant gram-negative rods in the nosocomial environment.[80,81] By understanding the reservoir, the prevalence of antimicrobial resistance in the reservoir, and the risk for exposure of a patient to a given organism, one can determine appropriate initial antimicrobial therapy. The implication of these principles is twofold. First, every hospital and patient area within the hospital must engage in ongoing surveillance of the most common organisms and antimicrobial susceptibility patterns causing nosocomial infection in their particular units. Second, decisions about antimicrobial use should take into consideration such information, particularly in patients who have been subjected to the selection pressures of previous courses of antibiotics that will have rendered them more vulnerable to colonization or invasion with resistant flora, or both.

Host Factors

A number of host factors must be considered in formulating an antimicrobial regimen. These can be divided into three groups: those that increase a patient's risk for a specific type of infection; those that increase a patient's risk for complications from an infection such as the presence of prostheses such as artificial joints, synthetic vascular grafts, or cardiac valves; and those that increase the risks of treating an infection with specific drugs.

In relation to the latter, perhaps the most important consideration is the history of previous adverse reactions to the drugs in question. Great precision is needed in defining the nature of the adverse reaction. For example, nausea, vomiting, and diarrhea, particularly after oral administration, do not preclude the use of an antimicrobial agent, especially intravenously. In contrast, a history of anaphylaxis, Stevens-Johnson syndrome, or allergic interstitial nephritis does preclude further use. Commonly, the exact nature of the allergy is unclear. In this circumstance, either the class of drug implicated should be avoided or skin testing with a subsequent desensitization regimen should be performed. The presence of renal dysfunction in the patient being treated can also have a profound effect on antimicrobial therapy (Table 50–2). Antimicrobials cleared by the kidney require an alteration in the dosage regimen with renal impairment. Unless such adjustments are made, toxic side effects may occur, such as injury to the eighth cranial nerve or renal injury with aminoglycosides,[82] seizures with penicillin and imipenem,[83,84] and bleeding caused by platelet dysfunction (added to that already caused by the uremic state) induced by ticarcillin, mezlocillin, and piperacillin.[85] Although many drugs are cleared or metabolized by the liver, hepatic dysfunction usually requires less adjustment of antimicrobial therapy than renal dysfunction. In general, little dosage adjustment is required until the bilirubin exceeds 5 mg/dL (see Table 50–2). With hepatic dysfunction, chloramphenicol, clindamycin, the tetracyclines, and the antituberculous drugs isoniazid and rifampin should be avoided, if possible (in the case of the antituberculous drugs, if they are required for emergency therapy, then special effort should be made to monitor blood levels in the face of serious hepatic dysfunction).[86] When both renal and hepatic dysfunction are present, then therapy with essentially all β-lactam antimicrobial agents should be carried out with great care.[87]

Special considerations need to be extended to those patients who have specific impairments in host defenses. Impairment may be anatomic such as cutaneous ulcerations or mucosal abnormalities or it may be secondary to functional host defense defects such as neutropenia, asplenia, malignancy, immunosuppressive therapy, and human immunodeficiency virus (HIV) infection. A detailed discussion of the infectious implications of the various alterations of host defenses is beyond the scope of this chapter; however, it is well reviewed elsewhere. Patients with prosthetic heart valves, prosthetic joints, vascular grafts, or other prosthesis can experience dire consequences from metastatic spread of infection if initial therapy is inadequate. Therefore, these patients should be considered for frontloading of the regimen, ideally with a bacteriocidal drug, even if their initial clinical state would not normally require it.

A critically ill patient who is pregnant, and for whom termination of the pregnancy is not an option, represents a particular challenge. First, the pharmacokinetics of many antibiotics are altered in pregnancy because of a larger volume of distribution and increased glomerular filtration rate. Second, the database on the safety of different antibiotics during pregnancy is woefully incomplete. However,

TABLE 50–2.

Use of Antimicrobial Agents in the Presence of Renal or Hepatic Dysfunction

Use	Antimicrobial Agents
Contraindicated in the presence of renal failure	Tetracyclines (except doxycycline), nitrofurantoin, cephaloridine, long-acting sulfonamides, methenamine, paraaminosalicylic acid
Require no dosage change in the presence of renal failure	Erythromycin, azithromycin, clarithromycin, clindamycin, chloramphenicol, doxycycline, cefoperazone, nafcillin, oxacillin, rifampin, amphotericin B, ceftriaxone, metronidazole, grepafloxacin, minocycline, linezolid, quinupristin/dalfopristin
Require dosage adjustment with moderate renal failure	Carbenicillin, ticarcillin, cefazolin, all aminoglycosides, vancomycin, imipenem, flucytosine, penicillin G, 5-fluorocytosine, fluconazole
Require dosage adjustment only with severe renal failure	Ampicillin, cefoxitin, cefotaxime, ceftizoxime, piperacillin, isoniazid, ethambutol, trimethoprim-sulfamethoxazole, cefotetan, ceftazidime, cefuroxime, mezlocillin, meropenem, nalidixic acid, ciprofloxacin, ofloxacin, levofloxacin, norfloxacin, itraconazole
Avoid or dose adjust in the setting of significant hepatic dysfunction (e.g., bilirubin > 5 mg/dL)	Quinupristin/dalfopristin, chloramphenicol, clindamycin, lincomycin, all the tetracyclines, cefoperazone, ceftriaxone, metronidazole, nafcillin, nitrofurantoin, fusidic acid, isoniazid, rifampin, rifabutin, pyrazinamide, rimantadine, ketoconazole, fluconazole, itraconazole

Data from Moellering RCJ: Principles of anti-infective therapy. In Mandell BJ, Dolin R (eds): Principles and Practice of Infectious Diseases. Philadelphia, Churchill Livingstone, 2000.

the following currently appear reasonable. Penicillins (except ticarcillin, which is teratogenic in rodents), cephalosporins, and erythromycin appear to be relatively safe. Aminoglycosides and isoniazid should only be prescribed if absolutely necessary because the former may be associated with eighth cranial nerve dysfunction in the infant and the latter with an increased incidence of psychomotor retardation, myoclonus, and seizures. Metronidazole, ticarcillin, rifampin, trimethoprim, the fluoroquinolones, and the tetracyclines should be avoided completely because of the potential for injuring the developing fetus. In addition, tetracycline use in the pregnant woman is associated with acute fatty necrosis of the liver, pancreatitis, and possibly renal injury.[88]

Practical Aspects of Drug Administration: Antimicrobial Therapy of Particular Clinical Situations

General

When choosing the appropriate antibiotic therapy it is critical to decide if the infectious process is nosocomially acquired or present at admission, i.e., community acquired. Of the nosocomially acquired infections, the National Nosocomial Infections Surveillance system has demonstrated that almost 80% occur in three sites: 24% in the respiratory system, 17% in the bloodstream, and 36% in the urinary track. The majority of the remaining 19% of nosocomial-acquired infections are associated with the gastrointestinal tract, cardiovascular system, skin and soft tissue, surgical site, or ear, eye, nose, and throat as shown in Figure 50–1. The primary pathogens associated with these various sites are outlined in Table 50–3. It is important to recognize that gram-positive pathogens, particularly *S. epidermidis, S. aureus,* and *Enterococcus* are the leading bloodstream pathogens, whereas *S. aureus* and gram-negatives, particularly *P. aeruginosa,* are the predominant pathogens associated with nosocomial pneumonia. In addition to *S. aureus* and *P. aeruginosa, E. coli* and *Candida albicans* are the primary pathogens found in urinary tract infections, with the great majority of these being associated with urinary tract instrumentation.[49,89–93] These data are consistent across continents.[94]

The incidence of nosocomial infections is highly associated with the use of devices such as ventilators, vascular access catheters, and urinary catheters. This is likely caused by the breakdown of normal host defenses and clearance mechanisms. In addition, the various devices may support various microorganisms differently. For example, the

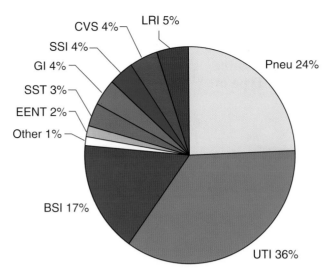

Figure 50–1. Site distribution of 2321 nosocomial infections in coronary care units, National Nosocomial Infections Surveillance System, 1992–1997. BSI, primary bloodstream infection; CVS, cardiovascular system infection; EENT, eye, ear, nose, throat infection; GI, gastrointestinal infection; LRI, lower respiratory tract infection other than pneumonia; PNEU, pneumonia; SSI, surgical site infection; SST, skin and soft tissue infection; UTI, urinary tract infection. (From National Center for Infectious Diseases, Centers for Disease Control and Prevention. National Nosocomial Infections Surveillance (NNIS) System Report, Data, Summary from October 1986-April 1998, Issued June 1998. 1998:1–25.)

development of biofilms on urinary and central venous catheters enhances the adherence of certain microorganisms such as *E. coli* and impairs the penetration of antimicrobials, whereas the condensation of water in ventilator circuits is a conducive environment for *Pseudomonas* and *Acinetobacter*.[92] The rate of device-related infections per 1000 device days also varies by type of ICU from 3.3 (cardiothoracic) to 10.0 (burn) for urinary catheter–associated urinary tract infections; from 2.8 (cardiothoracic) to 12.8 (burn) for central line–associated bloodstream infections; and from 8.5 (medical) to 21.1 (burn) for ventilator-associated pneumonia.[49]

Catheter-Related Infections

Intravascular access devices are common causes of bacteremia and fungemia. A catheter-related infection is defined as a bacteremia or fungemia in a patient with a central venous catheter who has at least one positive blood culture drawn from both the catheter and a peripheral site, clinical manifestations of an infection, and no apparent source for the infection.[95] The most widely used diagnostic technique to assay for catheter infection is a semiquantitative method, which involves rolling the catheter tip across an agar plate and then counting the number of colony-forming units after overnight incubation. More than 15 colony-forming units found using this technique suggests a catheter-related infection. A positive culture drawn through a catheter is relatively nonspecific, but a negative culture generally rules out a

catheter-related infection because of the low false-negative rate.[96] However, it is recommended that if catheter-related infection is suspected, at least one blood culture should be drawn percutaneously. Table 50–4 outlines the risks for septicemia associated with various vascular devices. To put this risk in perspective, it is worth noting that 50,000 to 100,00 patients in U.S. hospitals develop nosocomial bloodstream infections (BSI) each year, with 70% to 90% of these infections being related to central venous catheters of various types.[49,97] Such infections are associated with mortality rates of 25% to 35% and a twofold to threefold increase in attributable mortality. The Infectious Diseases Society of America has recently published guidelines for the management of intravascular catheter–related infections.[95] Although the guidelines state, "there is a notable absence of compelling clinical data to make firm recommendations for an individual patient," understanding the pathogenesis and virulence of the typical organisms involved still permits this problem to be approached rationally. For nontunneled central catheters, the organism usually comes from a colonized catheter, often the hub or lumen. These organisms usually reflect the flora of the skin. As shown in Table 50–3, *S. epidermidis, S. aureus, Enterococcus,* and *Candida* are the prime culprits, but gram-negative bacilli also cause infection. The latter is particularly true when there is gram-negative infection of the respiratory tract or of surgical wounds and drains as they increase incidence of gram-negative skin colonization, and hence the reservoir of organisms from which infection is derived. This pathogenic mechanism explains the increasing infection rate associated with central line position (femoral > internal jugular > subclavian). Presumably, internal jugular catheter infection is more likely than subclavian catheter infection because the former is more likely to be exposed to orotracheal secretions. One solution has been to use antibiotic-impregnated catheters, which have been shown to prevent microbial contamination of the catheter and subsequent bacteremia in some, but not all, studies. In one study, catheter associated bacteremia decreased from 3.4% to 0.3% with the use of a minocycline and rifampin impregnated catheter.[98] However, these results should be interpreted cautiously because these coatings may lead to false-negative culture results.

Initial therapy of suspected intravascular catheter infection usually includes vancomycin because of the high prevalence, in the nosocomial environment, of methicillin-resistant *S. aureus* and *epidermidis*. Additional coverage directed at gram-negative organisms should be considered if gram-negative infection is present at other bodily sites or if the patient manifests cardiovascular instability that is thought to be caused by infection. Empiric therapy directed at vancomycin-resistant enterococci is rarely indicated, because this organism is an unusual cause of acute hemodynamic instability. Antifungal therapy is also not initiated unless there is microbiologic evidence of fungal infection (see later). When the offending bloodstream pathogen is identified and its resistance profile known, focused antimicrobial therapy should be used. There are several important issues to consider in the treatment of the common BSI pathogens. *Staphylococcus epidermidis* is often a contaminant. However, when it does cause a BSI it typically behaves as a relatively avirulent pathogen. Consequently, it usually can be treated with removal of the catheter and a short

TABLE 50–3.

Data Derived from the NNIS Database Elucidating the Relative Frequency of Various Pathogens by Site of Infection by Type of ICU (MICU vs. CCU)

Pathogen	Bloodstream Infection		Pneumonia		Urinary Tract Infection	
	CCU n = 1159	MICU n = 2971	CCU n = 1635	MICU n = 4389	CCU n = 2321	MICU n = 4956
CNS	37	36	2	1	3	2
SA	24	13	21	20	3	2
Enterococcus	10	16	2	2	14	14
E. coli	3	3	4	4	28	14
Enterobacter	3	3	9	9	4	5
C. albicans	2	6	6	5	10	21
K. pneumoniae	2	4	8	8	6	6
S. marcescens	2	1	4	4	1	0.7
P. aeruginosa	2	3	14	21	7	10
Other Candida	2	3	0.2	1	4	5
C. glabrata	2	2	3	0.2	3	5
Acinetobacter	1	2	3	6	0.2	1
Other fungi	1	0.8	2	1	5	8
P. mirabilis	0.6	0.5	2	2	4	2
Citrobacter		0.5		2		1
S. pneumoniae	0.4		2		0	
H. influenzae	0.1		3		0	
Other	7	6	16	14	8	3

Data was obtained between 1992 and 1997.

CCU, coronary care unit; CNS, coagulase-negative Staphylococcus; ICU, intensive care unit; MICU, medical intensive care unit; NNIS, National Nosocomial Infections Surveillance; SA, *Staphylococcus aureus*.

Data from National Center for Infectious Diseases, Centers for Disease Control and Prevention. National Nosocomial Infections Surveillance (NNIS) System Report, Data, Summary from October 1986–April 1998, Issued June 1998. 1998:1–25; Richards MJ, Edwards JR, Culver DH, et al: Nosocomial infections in coronary care units in the United States. National Nosocomial Infections Surveillance System. Am J Cardiol 82:789–793, 1998; Richards MJ, Edwards JR, Culver DH, et al: Nosocomial infections in medical intensive care units in the United States. National Nosocomial Infections Surveillance System (see comments). Crit Care Med 27:887–892, 1999.

TABLE 50–4.

Approximate Risks for Septicemia Associated with Various Types of Intravascular Access Devices

Type of Device	Representative Rate
Short-term temporary access (no. septicemias per 100 device-days)	
Peripheral intravenous cannulas	
Winged steel needles	<0.2
Peripheral intravenous catheters	
Percutaneously inserted	0.2
Cut down	6
Arterial catheters	1
Central venous catheters	
All-purpose, multilumen	3
Swan-ganz	1
Hemodialysis	10
Long-term indefinite access (no. of septicemias per 100 device-days)	
Peripherally inserted central venous catheters	0.2
Cuffed central catheters (e.g., Hickman, Broviac)	0.2
Subcutaneous central venous ports (e.g., Infusaport, Port-a-cath)	0.04

Data from Pfaller MA, Jones RN, Messer SA, et al: National surveillance of nosocomial bloodstream infection due to *Candida albicans:* frequency of occurrence and antifungal susceptibility in the SCOPE Program. Diagn Microbiol Infect Dis 31:327–332, 1998.

course of antibiotics. Nonetheless, this organism has a propensity to adhere to prosthetic devices such as cardiac valves and artificial joints. Therefore, when *S. epidermidis* bacteremia occurs, one must carefully evaluate prosthetic devices for evidence of superinfection. In light of these considerations, patients with indwelling prostheses should be considered at greater risk for central catheter placement, and they should be discontinued at the earliest opportunity.

Conversely, *S. aureus* is an extremely virulent organism, which in the setting of bacteremia, often disseminates and causes osteomyelitis, endocarditis, and other severe, destructive infections. Thus when a bacteremia with this organism is confirmed, a careful evaluation for metastatic infection should occur and prolonged therapy (2 to 4 weeks) is indicated.[99] Enterococcal BSI behaves in a similar manner

as *S. epidermidis* and typically responds to removal of the catheter. However, endocarditis may occur, particularly in the setting of prolonged bacteremia. The optimal therapy for this organism is ampicillin plus an aminoglycoside. In the setting of multidrug-resistant VRE, the therapeutic options are quite limited (see later). When *C. albicans* is cultured from the blood, the patient should be evaluated for metastatic infectious foci (e.g., hepatic, ocular, and skin), and if none are found, the catheter should be removed followed by antifungal therapy typically with fluconazole.[100] If metastatic foci of candidal infection are found, then the optimal management of these complications will determine the duration of therapy.

Prophylaxis

Surgical

Need for Prophylaxis

The need for antibiotic prophylaxis for surgery depends on the risk for infection, which is related to the wound classification, patient-related factors such as immunocompetence, the bacterial milieu, and hospital infection rate for various procedures and factors relating to the wound itself. Wounds are usually classified as Clean (Class I), Clean-Contaminated (Class II), Contaminated (Class III), and Dirty-Infected (Class IV). A clean wound is atraumatic in which there has been no break in sterile technique and the respiratory, alimentary, or genitourinary tracks have not been entered. Clean-Contaminated wounds result from surgery in areas known to harbor bacteria such as the biliary, respiratory, alimentary, and genitourinary tracts, when there is no spillage of contents. Contaminated wounds occur with a major break in sterile technique, or with surgery on a traumatic wound, or gross gastrointestinal spillage, or entrance into an infected biliary or genitourinary tract. Dirty-Infected wounds are those for which infection existed before the surgery, e.g., old wounds with devitalized tissue or surgery for patients with perforated viscera. This classification scheme relates to the risk for postoperative infection and is thought to be related to the bacterial burden except for Dirty-Infected wounds, which are, by definition, already infected. However, careful microscopic examination shows that even clean wounds are contaminated with skin flora.[101] Apparently then, the distinction between the wound classifications are more related to the quantity of bacteria contaminating the wound than the presence or absence of bacteria.

Staphylococcal species are the most common wound pathogens for clean wounds. Prophylaxis is debatable for some clean procedures such as an inguinal hernia repair or mastectomy. However, for other clean procedures, especially for median sternotomies, gram-positive coverage with cefazolin is recommended. Prophylactic antibiotics should be administered for all clean contaminated and contaminated wounds, as well as for hysterectomies and most urologic procedures. Sterilization of the urinary tract is recommended before any urologic procedure if possible. Prophylaxis is advised for patients at high or moderate risk undergoing procedures involving infected tissues. Prophylaxis should include antistaphylococcal antibiotics for cellulitis and osteomyelitis. Similar coverage is advised for patients receiving prosthetic cardiac valves. Patients with urinary tract infections should receive antibiotics active against gram-negative bacilli such as fluoroquinolones, third-generation cephalosporins, or an aminoglycoside. Convincing evidence of prophylactic antimicrobial benefit is also found in association with procedures: the use of antibiotics (such as ampicillin-sulbactam and piperacillin-tazobactam) to prevent biliary sepsis in patients undergoing endoscopic manipulation of the biliary tree or urosepsis in patients undergoing manipulation of an infected urinary tract.

Comparable successes with prophylactic antimicrobial regimens in patients in the ICU have been more difficult to find. Thus attempts to prevent infection with selective gut decontamination regimens remain controversial. These involve using either nonabsorbable antimicrobial agents or fluoroquinolones and aiming to eliminate the aerobic gram-negative flora while leaving the anaerobic flora intact, which provides some protection against colonization with a variety of potential pathogens, so-called *colonization resistance*. Similarly, aerosolized antibiotics, particularly polymyxin or aminoglycosides, have not been shown to prevent pneumonia. Topical antibiotic ointments have not been shown to decrease the incidence of intravenous access-related bloodstream infection.

Recently, the concept of pre-emptive therapy has come to the forefront. Pre-emptive therapy was initially defined in patients who received transplants, where the initiation of ganciclovir therapy in patients with bone marrow transplant with evidence of cytomegalovirus (CMV) replication either in the blood or in the respiratory secretions, at a time when they were asymptomatic, prevented the development of otherwise life-threatening CMV pneumonia. In patients with organ transplant, the initiation of pre-emptive ganciclovir during intensive antirejection therapy markedly decreases the incidence of systemic CMV infection normally associated with such therapy.[3,4]

The efficacy of prophylaxis for fungal infection is difficult to prove. The diagnosis of invasive candidal infection is often difficult, even with modern blood culturing techniques, and the ability of the clinician to distinguish between Candidal colonization and invasion is not great. Several studies have shown that when a patient is colonized at three or more sites, there is a 30% to 60% incidence of invasive disease, with a high associated mortality rate. The question that should be answered is whether the institution of fluconazole pre-emptively will improve this situation, thus bypassing our currently inadequate diagnostic techniques.[102–104] An analogous situation is the patient who has surgery for a gastric or upper small bowel perforation, which are the anatomic sites where large numbers of *Candida* species are normally found. There is some agreement that pre-emptive therapy should be initiated only after recent abdominal surgery with recurrent gastrointestinal perforations or anastomotic leaks, and it is not necessary for the initial surgery even if there is soilage, so long as it has not been present for a relatively long period.[105] However, this issue is further complicated by the emergence of fluconazole-resistant *C. albicans* and the change in common

fungal species to more resistant yeast such as *C. krausei* and *C. glabrata*.

Timing of Prophylaxis.

It is generally believed that prophylactic antibiotics should be administered intravenously shortly before the time of incision—i.e., no more than 2 hours before incision with the infusion completed before the time of incision. The major impetus for this practice comes from a study that looked retrospectively at the timing of prophylactic antibiotic administration in patients with a reported wound infection.[106] The investigators found that patients who developed wound infections were more likely to have received prophylaxis between 24 and 2 hours before surgery or after surgery. Interestingly, the incidence was not increased for patients receiving prophylaxis intraoperatively. When the data were subjected to a multiple logistic regression, the only variables related to wound infection were underlying disease, nursing service, type of surgery, duration of surgery, and time after the start of surgery for the first dose of prophylactic antibiotics. Notably, of the 41 wound infections, 58% were resistant to the antimicrobial drug used. Thus although this study is widely quoted as showing that prophylaxis must be given within 2 hours of the incision, the data do not really support this conclusion. Moreover, a prospective study validating these retrospective findings has not been published. Finally, an animal study widely cited as documenting the need to have the antimicrobial given before the incision lacks statistical testing and uses high inocula and varying doses of antimicrobials.[107] Therefore, although it seems logical to have adequate tissue levels of prophylactic antimicrobials before skin incision, supporting data are only inferential and it is likely that the importance depends on the size of the inoculum.

Bacterial Endocarditis

Although there are generally agreed on guidelines for surgical prophylaxis for bacterial endocarditis, there are not any studies that definitively show that antibiotic prophylaxis prevents bacterial endocarditis during procedures that can produce a bacteremia. Nonetheless, given the consequences of endocarditis and the minimal risk associated with prophylaxis, the use of antibiotics to prevent cardiac infection is sensible in high-risk procedures. The following is a summary of the most recent recommendations by the American Heart Association.[108] These recommendations are based on the risk of a procedure producing a significant bacteremia with an organism likely to produce endocarditis and the risk for development of bacterial endocarditis with such a bacteremia. They are also predicated on cardiac conditions that are associated with an increased risk for endocarditis even without surgery. Patients considered to be at highest risk for endocarditis are those with prosthetic heart valves, a previous history of endocarditis, complex cyanotic heart disease, and those with surgical systemic-pulmonary shunts or conduits. Moderate risk patients include those with uncorrected ventricular septal defects, primum atrial septal defects, patient ductus arteriosus, aortic coarctation, bicuspid aortic valves, acquired valvular dysfunction, and hypertrophic cardiomyopathy. Prophylaxis for mitral valve prolapse is an enlightening controversy for several reasons. First, prolapse can occur in normal mitral valves during conditions that reduce the end-diastolic volume of the left ventricle such as hypovolemia or enhanced contractility, especially in young adults. Second, prolapse without regurgitation is not thought to increase the risk for bacterial endocarditis because the regurgitant jet seems to produce the valvular abnormalities that make bacteria more likely to adhere to the valve. Thus it is thought that only patients with mitral valve prolapse who also have mitral regurgitation should receive antibiotic prophylaxis. However, this is further complicated by the observation that regurgitation may occur only with exercise. Consequently, it might be missed on routine examination. In addition, men older than 45 years with mitral valve prolapse are at greater risk for bacterial endocarditis development.

Procedures such as central catheter placement through skin that is otherwise healthy and has been cleansed with povidone-iodine or chlorhexidine are not associated with significant bacteremias, and therefore do not warrant prophylaxis. In contrast, patients undergoing dental procedures associated with bleeding or patients with poor dental hygiene should receive prophylaxis. Streptococcus viridans (α-hemolytic streptococci) is the most common cause of endocarditis in dental or oral surgical procedures. A single oral dose of 2 g amoxicillin given 1 hour before the procedure is the recommended prophylaxis. If oral medications cannot be used, intravenous ampicillin or penicillin is recommended. Clindamycin or azithromycin are alternatives for patients allergic to penicillin. Other procedures for which similar prophylaxis is recommended include rigid (but not flexible) bronchoscopy, esophageal stricture dilatation, and sclerotherapy (but not banding). Surgery that involves the biliary tree or intestinal mucosa or endoscopic procedures of the pancreatic or biliary tree are also associated with bacteremia with organisms that cause endocarditis, especially enterococcus faecalis. The recommended prophylaxis for high-risk patients undergoing such procedures is ampicillin and gentamicin. Vancomycin may be substituted for ampicillin in patients allergic to penicillin. Gentamicin may be omitted in patients at medium risk.

Endocarditis prophylaxis is recommended for some clean procedures such as abdominal and lower extremity vascular procedures, craniotomies, orthopedic procedures with hardware insertion, and any procedure that includes implantation of permanent prosthetic material. In contrast, the need for prophylactic antibiotics for orthopedic procedures such as laminectomies and spinal fusions is controversial.

The rate of endocarditis-causing bacteremia with genitourinary tract surgery or instrumentation is high in patients with urinary tract infections, prostatitis, and with prostatic surgery. Enterococcus faecalis is the most common bacteria but Klebsiella is also common. Prophylaxis recommendations are the same as for intestinal or biliary tract surgery, but attempted sterilization of the urinary tract before any procedure is also thought to be beneficial. Prophylaxis is not recommended for uncomplicated vaginal delivery, cervical biopsy, or manipulation of an intrauterine device in the absence of infection. However, because bacteremia after removal of an intrauterine device is thought to be relatively common, prophylaxis similar to that used for other genitourinary procedures is recommended.

Pneumonia

Patients with pneumonia can be divided into two general categories: those with community-acquired pneumonia and those with nosocomial pneumonia (particularly acquired in the ICU).

It is useful to consider community-acquired pneumonias in three different categories. First are the typical pneumonias of conventional bacterial origin, which are characterized by the abrupt onset (over <24 hours) of fever, chills, systemic toxicity, cough, purulent sputum production, and dyspnea, often after a preceding viral illness. Second are the atypical pneumonias characterized by a subacute onset of fever, nonproductive cough and malaise, with a gradual progression over several days. The third category is legionnaires' disease, which combines features of both, has an abrupt onset of fever, rigors, nonproductive cough, systemic toxicity, and increasing dyspnea (often after a several day prodrome of gastrointestinal upset, headache, malaise, and encephalopathy). Although there is considerable overlap among these presentations, initial therapy can be guided by such categorization and by considering the different etiologic factors within each category (Table 50–5).

The choice of appropriate antimicrobial therapy is helped by Gram stain of sputum; urinary Legionella antigen assays, which detect more than 80% of cases of pneumonia caused by *Legionella pneumophila* type I but not other Legionella species or types; polymerase chain reaction test for Mycoplasma and Chlamydia; rapid viral antigen panel for respiratory viruses; and special studies for other pathogens. However, in 20% to 50% of cases, antimicrobial therapy needs to be initiated in the absence of clear-cut microbiologic information. Patients without a predisposing host defense defect or history of a gross aspiration episode, in whom a typical pneumonia is suspected as a cause of respiratory failure, should have initial therapy especially directed against *S. pneumoniae, Haemophilus influenzae, S. aureus*, and the Enterobacteriaceae. Thus such drugs as ampicillin-sulbactam, cefuroxime, and ceftriaxone are useful as initial therapy. If atypical pneumonia is suspected, then a fluoroquinolone (such as levofloxacin) or erythromycin (or one of the newer macrolides, azithromycin and clarithromycin, with or without trimethoprim-sulfamethoxazole), would constitute reasonable initial therapy. For patients with a Legionella-like presentation, high-dose erythromycin has been the traditional therapy of choice; however, azithromycin or levofloxacin may be preferable combined with of one of the regimens used for the treatment of typical bacterial pneumonia such as ampicillin-sulbactam or ceftriaxone if resistant pathogens are a concern. It is also important to consider viral pathogens because they are a common cause of community-acquired pneumonia; rapid diagnostic tests are available, and the possibility of antiviral therapy exists. Although the initiation of empiric therapy is often obligatory, invasive diagnostic techniques such as bronchoalveolar lavage or lung biopsy should be considered for any patient with respiratory failure in whom the etiologic

TABLE 50–5.

Etiology of Community Acquired Pneumonia

	Incidence (%)
Typical (acute onset or abrupt deterioration after viral prodrome, with productive cough, systemic toxicity, and a lobar infiltrate)	
Streptococcus pneumoniae	20–60
Haemophilus influenzae	5–20
Staphylococcus aureus	2–10
Enterobacteriaceae	4–8
Others (*B. catarrhalis*, anaerobes, *P. aeruginosa*)	5–10
Atypical (subacute onset, nonproductive cough, interstitial infiltrate)	
Viral (influenza, RSV, parainfluenza, adenovirus)	30–60
Mycoplasma pneumoniae	20–40
Chlamydia pneumoniae	4–15
Others (PCP, Q fever, psittacosis)	1–2
Legionella	1–15

The pathogens involved in community acquired pneumonia are very different from those involved in nosocomial pneumonia. Compare these data to the data in Table 50–3.
RSV, respiratory syncytial virus.

diagnosis is not quickly apparent or if the patient does not respond to therapy. This is especially important for individuals with underlying conditions that predispose them to a broader range of pathogens than those listed in Table 50–3.

The etiology of nosocomial pneumonia, especially that acquired within the ICU, is vastly different from the etiology of community-acquired infection. The pathogenesis is typically an extension of a tracheobronchitis into a bronchopneumonia. In the hospital setting, relatively antibiotic-resistant, aerobic, gram-negative bacilli are the most frequent invading pathogens. This is thought to be because of the increased rate of oropharyngeal and gastric colonization with these organisms, with such colonization serving as a reservoir for the introduction of this flora into the lower respiratory tract (usually caused by aspiration), and the impaired ability to clear these organisms. This is especially true among intubated patients, those with previous lung injury or significant atelectasis, and immunocompromised patients.

Although Table 50–3 lists the etiology of nosocomial pneumonias caused by different bacteria nationally, it should be emphasized that the etiologic factors of nosocomial pneumonia in each individual hospital may be very different from the national average. Although gram-negative bacillary pneumonia remains the major problem, the nature of the gram-negatives causing infection and their antibiotic sensitivity patterns will vary widely in different hospitals and even in different areas within a hospital. Thus precise antibiotic recommendations for initiating therapy must be based on ongoing surveillance of the resident bacterial flora in the particular hospital area. Surveillance is necessary to identify and appropriately treat infection caused by the evolving resident flora and to identify rapidly the introduction of possible epidemic strains, both to treat patients infected with these organisms and to prevent spread to other patients.

Initial therapy should reflect the ongoing surveillance information and should be modified on the basis of sputum examinations including Gram stains, which provide important information about the relative importance of a particular organism found on culture. Initial therapy is usually accomplished with a single advanced-spectrum anti–gram-negative drug such as ceftazidime, piperacillin-tazobactam, imipenem, ciprofloxacin, or levofloxacin for less severe disease, and perhaps one of these drugs with an aminoglycoside for patients with more severe illness.[109,110] As noted previously, clear-cut evidence in humans that two-drug, potentially synergistic therapy is more effective than a single drug is not available, but such therapy would be considered by many clinicians in the face of rapidly progressive *Pseudomonas* or *Klebsiella* infection.[111] In the case of *Klebsiella* infection, cefazolin can be substituted for the more expensive advanced-spectrum drugs previously listed if the organism is susceptible to cefazolin.

In immunocompromised patients, pulmonary infection is the most common form of life-threatening infection. Although a detailed discussion of the approach to pulmonary infection in these patients is beyond the scope of this chapter, certain principles are worth noting here in terms of antimicrobial strategies. As outlined in Table 50–6, particular host defense defects are associated with particular infections, and initial therapy should reflect these associations. Even more than other ICU patients, these immunocompromised individuals are especially susceptible to nosocomial infection, both with the resident gram-negative flora and with *Aspergillus* species. Because of the importance of such infections in these patients, precise diagnosis is essential, using invasive techniques if necessary.

Bacteremia

Bacteremia occurring in hospitalized patients can be considered as arising from two separate pathogenic routes. One is a consequence of definable tissue infection at an anatomic

TABLE 50–6.

Frequent Causes of Pneumonia in Patients with Various Defects in Host Defenses and Initial Antimicrobial Therapy

Host Defense Defect	Pulmonary Infection	Initial Therapy
Impaired antibody formation or splenectomized	Streptococcus pneumoniae, Haemophilus influenza type B	Levofloxacin, azithromycin or ampicillin + β-lactamase inhibitor
Depressed cell-mediated immunity	Pneumocystis carinii, Mycobacteria species, fungi, Nocardia, Legionella, herpes group viruses, Strongyloides stercoralis	Trimethoprim-sulfamethoxazole
Decrease in the number and/or function of granulocytes	Oral bacterial flora, Enterobacteriaceae, *Pseudomonas aeruginosa*, *Aspergillus*	Ceftazidime, imipenem, ± an aminoglycoside
Oral and tracheobronchial ulcerations	Oral bacterial flora, Enterobacteriaceae	Ceftazidime, imipenem

site. Common causes of bacteremia of this type are biliary and urinary tract sepsis (usually caused by gram negative bacilli, or enterococci, or both); peritonitis caused by a disruption of bowel integrity (mixed infection caused by such anaerobic organisms as *B. fragilis*, the Enterobacteriaceae, especially *E. coli*, and bowel streptococci, especially enterococci); and pneumonia. The incidence of bacteremia with pneumonia varies according to which organism is causing the infection. For example, 30% to 50% of patients with pneumococcal infection will have demonstrable bacteremia compared with less than 10% with gram-negative or aspiration pneumonia. In pneumococcal infection, the bacteremia is typically caused by hematogenous seeding from the pulmonary infection, whereas in gram-negative VAP, the bacteremia is likely related to heavy oropharyngeal colonization leading to skin contamination with consequent seeding of a central venous catheter. Thus in the setting of VAP, all vascular access devices should be carefully evaluated especially for duration of implantation, exit site erythema and drainage, and by blood cultures. The initial antimicrobial therapy of bacteremia secondary to invasive tissue infection is identical to that which would be prescribed in the absence of bacteremia.

Urinary Tract Infection

Urosepsis is relatively uncommon unless complicating factors such as obstruction to urine flow are present. In this circumstance, infection under high pressure can develop, producing high-level bacteremia and an increased risk for septic shock. Therapy with broad-spectrum antibiotics (usually with fluoroquinolones or advanced-spectrum β-lactam agents such as ceftazidime, ampicillin-sulbactam, ticarcillin-clavulanate, aztreonam, or imipenem), in conjunction with relief of the obstruction, is the initial treatment of choice. When the identity of the invading pathogen is known, modification of the antimicrobial regimen is then carried out. Although there is little indication that one or another drug is superior in terms of control of the initial symptom complex, there is an increasing body of evidence that fluoroquinolones and trimethoprim (or trimethoprim-sulfamethoxazole) are particularly effective in eradicating bacteria from kidney and prostatic tissue, presumably because of their ability to achieve high tissue and intracellular concentrations.[112]

A more common problem in hospitalized patients, especially those with urinary catheters, is nosocomial bacteriuria. The cause of such infections is far different from that observed in community-acquired infections. Whereas *E. coli* accounts for more than 85% of community-acquired urinary tract infections, it is responsible for only one third of nosocomial infections. Enterococci, *P. aeruginosa*, relatively antibiotic-resistant Enterobacteriaceae such as *Klebsiella, Proteus, Enterobacter,* and *Serratia* species, as well as *Candida* species, currently account for the majority of these infections.[113] Antibiotic therapy can delay the appearance of bacteriuria for a short time, but the price to be paid if catheterization is maintained is that when infection does occur it will be relatively resistant. Treatment of asymptomatic positive cultures when the catheter is still present is not indicated, because this represents colonization rather than invasive infection and long-term benefits of such therapy are unlikely. Treatment if symptoms develop or instrumentation of the urinary tract is to be carried out is indicated, with the choice of antibiotic dictated by the results of culture.

Other Syndromes

Clostridium Difficile

Clostridium difficile is the leading cause of gastrointestinal infection in the nosocomial environment. This pathogen is an important cause of fever and leukocytosis, which may precede the diarrheal phase. The pathogenesis of this disease is typically toxin-mediated (enterotoxin A or cytotoxin B), with bacteremia extremely rare. The diagnosis is confirmed with the detection of either of the aforementioned toxins. The spores from *C. difficile* are extremely hearty and impervious to antimicrobial therapy, which explains the 10% relapse rate in successfully treated patients. Metronidazole is the therapy of choice even in relapsing cases; however, in recalcitrant cases where there is no response to metronidazole therapy, oral vancomycin can be considered. In patients being treated for an ongoing pyogenic process, the treatment of *C. difficile* is particularly vexing. In this setting, where continued broad-spectrum antibiotic use is required, we recommend continuing the *C. difficile* therapy in parallel with the other antimicrobial agents and extend the course of therapy for *C. difficile* for several days after completion of the other antibiotics, typically 5 to 10 days. The extended *C. difficile* course of therapy is required because of the role of antibiotic therapy in provoking *C. difficile* disease by altering the normal bowel flora. Future antibiotic therapy needs to be considered with great care in a previously infected patient, because *C. difficile* can be provoked with subsequent antibiotic courses, in part because of the latent spores. In patients who are severely ill from *C. difficile,* several adjuvant approaches should be considered including minimization of other antimicrobial therapy, toxin-binding resins such as cholestyramine, fecal enemas, and, in severe cases, surgical resection of the colon (e.g., in the setting of toxic megacolon). In a patient who undergoes a colectomy for *C. difficile* toxic megacolon, the rectal stump, if one is left behind, may be a source of residual disease. Patients receiving immunosuppressive therapy appear to be at particularly high risk for severe *C. difficile* disease.

Acute Pancreatitis

Antibiotic management in acute pancreatitis is challenging because the severity of illness often indicates a therapeutic emergency; the traditional markers of infection are of no value and there are limited clinical data. Depending on the degree of pancreatic injury, these patients may have septic physiology, including hypotension, tachycardia, hypoxemia, tachypnea, metabolic acidosis, leukocytosis with a left shift, thrombocytopenia, and coagulopathy. These findings are all consistent with the pathogenesis of this disease in which an inciting event such as alcohol, gallstones, or trauma leads to pancreatic injury and inflammation, which in turn leads to autodigestion, liquefaction, and necrosis. This tissue necrosis results in a cytokine release syndrome, which can mimic all aspects of septic physiology. If the necrotic pancreatic tissue becomes infected, by biliary reflux (often polymicrobial), colonic bacterial translocation, or hematogenous seeding, there is an associated increased morbidity and mortality rate.[114] Notably, infection is rarely the inciting event but rather a consequence of pancreatitis and often occurs weeks into the hospital course. Abdominal imaging, with a contrast computed tomography scan, has enabled stratification of those patients at risk for superimposed infection with increasing degree of pancreatic necrosis. Infection of the pancreatic bed is extremely rare in the absence of necrosis.[114] Unfortunately, imaging, like the physical examination and laboratory evaluation, cannot reliably distinguish an infectious from sterile inflammation. The only reliable means of making this determination is through a Gram stain and culture of the peripancreatic fluid. Because an infected necrotic pancreas requires surgical debridement, in addition to antibiotic therapy and supportive care, a diagnostic procedure, such as an ultrasound-guided, fine-needle aspirate is extremely helpful before initiating antimicrobial therapy.[115] When cultures have been obtained, the microbiologic results should guide antibiotic therapy, given the high sensitivity of the Gram stain from the pancreatic aspirate (>90% in one study).[116]

In the critically ill patient in whom it is too risky to delay antimicrobial therapy, targeting the typical infecting organisms, which includes aerobic enteric gram-negative rods and gram-positive cocci, is appropriate. Two reasonable combinations are: ceftazidime, a fluoroquinolone or piperacillin plus metronidazole; or imipenem or meropenem.[117] If empiric antibiotics were initiated, the Gram stain is negative, and the microbiologic cultures are sterile, typically at 48 to 72 hours, then antimicrobial therapy should be discontinued. Otherwise therapy should be directed at the pathogens identified.[115] The role of empiric antibiotic therapy to either prevent infection or treat early infection is controversial, with no convincing evidence for a mortality benefit, less multiorgan failure, diminished operative intervention, or shortened duration of hospitalization; empiric antibiotics may promote colonization with resistant organisms that may subsequently seed the inflamed pancreatic bed.[118–123]

Fungal Infection

By far the most important fungal infections occurring in the hospital are those caused by yeast species, with *C. albicans*, *C. glabrata*, and *C. tropicalis* accounting for more than 75% of these infections. The isolation of *Candida* species from the sputum is a common event, although candidal pneumonia is quite rare, even in immunocompromised patients.[124–126] Thus antifungal therapy is not indicated for positive sputum cultures, even in patients with abnormal chest radiographs. Candiduria is also an extremely common event, typically representing colonization or contamination, and rarely representing disseminated disease or an established urinary tract infection. In addition, candiduria rarely poses a risk for systemic dissemination. A recent large multicenter study reports a 1.3% rate of candidemia associated with candiduria in high-risk patients.[127] Therapy for isolated candiduria should rarely be instituted. However, an important exception is the need to instrument a colonized urinary tract. If antifungals are used, fluconazole for 5 days or a single dose of 0.3 mg/kg amphotericin B[128] is preferable to intravesicular therapy with amphotericin B.[129,130] However, recrudescence typically occurs within a few days of cessation of therapy if the urinary catheter is not discontinued.[128,131,132]

In contrast, candidemia, often because of contaminated intravascular access devices, is an uncommon event. However, even a transient episode of candidemia in immunocompromised patients carries a significant risk for visceral seeding. For example, in patients who received an organ transplant or neutropenic patients undergoing cancer chemotherapy, there is a greater than 50% incidence of metastatic infection if a transient episode of candidemia remains untreated.[133,134] Therefore, all such episodes in immunocompromised patients warrant systemic antifungal therapy.[102]

Candidemia carries a significant morbidity and mortality in the non-neutropenic host.[135] The incidence of metastatic complications of transient candidemia in patients with intact host defenses is probably 5% to 10%, often presenting 1 to 6 months later as candidal endophthalmitis, hepatosplenic candidiasis, skeletal infection, and other forms of metastatic infection. Because of the these late consequences of candidemia, we strongly recommend systemic antifungal therapy in patients with candidemia even when only transient.[100,136] Fluconazole (400 mg/day) and amphotericin B (0.5–0.6 mg/kg/day have been shown to be equally effective therapy in this setting.[137–140] Amphotericin B is the preferred therapy in patients in whom candidemia develops in the setting of azole use or when an azole resistant species is identified. This highlights the importance of performing yeast speciation as 100% of *C. krausei* and 10% to 30% of *C. glabrata* are azole resistant. In uncomplicated cases of transient candidemia, the vascular access device should be removed[141] and 2 weeks of systemic therapy should be instituted from the date of the last positive blood culture.

Amphotericin B requires prolonged intravenous administration, and its use is associated with a high incidence of side effects: fever, chills, malaise, and possibly hypotension caused by cytokine release; and dose-related renal and bone marrow toxicity. By administering the drug over 4 to 6 hours, diluting it in 500 mL of 5% dextrose in water, and pretreating with acetaminophen, small doses of steroids, and other agents, the cytokine release syndrome can be overcome. The dose-related nephrotoxicity of amphotericin remains the major limitation to its use. Amphotericin, however, remains the one broadly active fungicidal drug and is the standard against which all new therapies should be measured. The infusion-related toxicity and the nephrotoxicity of amphotericin have been significantly reduced by the successful development of liposomally encapsulated forms.[142–145] The efficacy of these agents appears to be equal to that of conventional amphotericin.

A major advance in recent years with antifungal therapy has been the advent of the azole antifungal agents: ketoconazole, itraconazole, and fluconazole. Ketoconazole, which has significant hepatic toxicity and may interfere with mammalian steroid synthesis, is administered orally, is relatively inexpensive, and has been particularly useful in the treatment of mucocutaneous candidal infections. Its pharmacokinetic properties are less than ideal, requiring a low pH in the stomach for reliable absorption to occur and achieving relatively low levels in the urinary tract and CNS. Because of the unreliability of its absorption, it has little role

in the critically ill patient, many of whom are receiving therapies that increase the gastric pH to prevent gastrointestinal hemorrhage. Itraconazole is somewhat better in this regard, but again, penetration into the CNS and urinary tract is limited, making it a less attractive drug in the ICU. Oral absorption of this drug can also be unreliable; with the same gastric pH issues as ketoconazole. Its major use has been in immunocompromised patients with invasive aspergillosis, where itraconazole has found a niche as "consolidation therapy" after initial control with amphotericin.[146]

Fluconazole has a number of advantages over other azoles in the ICU setting. It can be administered orally or intravenously as a single dose once daily; its volume of distribution is such that therapeutic levels are achieved in essentially all tissues, including the urinary tract and CNS; its absorption is not significantly affected by gastric pH and it is far less toxic than any other antifungal drug. Both the incidence and type of toxicities are comparable to those observed with a β-lactam antibiotic. The limitations of fluconazole are that its effects are fungistatic rather than fungicidal, and its spectrum is limited practically to *C. albicans*, *C. tropicalis*, a variety of other candidal strains, and *Cryptococcus neoformans*.[147] Nearly all *Candida krusei* and 10% to 30% of *Candida glabrata* are resistant to fluconazole.[136]

A recent multicenter study of nonimmunocompromised patients with candidemia compared 14 days of 0.5 mg/kg amphotericin per day to 14 days of 400 mg/day fluconazole. These regimens were found to be of equal efficacy in terms of both mortality and incidence of metastatic infection, but there was a significantly greater incidence of toxicity in the amphotericin group. Such results make it easier to recommend systemic antifungal therapy for all individuals with documented fungemia. Our current approach is as follows: patients with candidemia who are toxic, hypotensive, and critically ill are treated initially with amphotericin and then switched to fluconazole when clinical control has been achieved. Subacutely ill patients are treated with fluconazole as primary therapy, with oral therapy being substituted for parenteral therapy once reliable gastrointestinal function is present. The optimal duration of therapy remains unclear for both drugs. Rather than recommend a fixed duration of therapy, our preference is to treat for 14 days beyond the point when clinical and microbiologic evidence is present.

New Diagnostics

One of the greatest frustrations when caring for a potentially septic patient is having to wait 1 to 2 days for culture results to find out if the patient is infected, and then to wait another day or two to discover the identity and later the susceptibility profile of the infecting organism. With the molecular biologic revolution, new tests have emerged, typically polymerase chain reaction–based technology, enabling the rapid identification of specific pathogens directly from the infected body site. Nonetheless, this technology is prone to many of the same interpretation challenges. For example, does a positive result represent colonization or disease? To help both diagnostically and prognostically, the development of new assays are focusing on the levels (or presence) of mediators in the inflammatory cascade or on circulating bacterial moieties, such as endotoxin or NFκB, to improve our ability to risk stratify patients or determine the infecting pathogen.[148–151]

A broad array of pathogens currently can be identified by molecular techniques, including viruses (HIV, CMV), fungi *(Candida, Aspergillus)*, and bacteria (VRE, *E. coli, M. tuberculosis, Bacteroides)*.[152–155] As learned for patients who are HIV positive, monitoring the HIV viral load has become an important parameter in gauging the success of therapy. The development of technology may allow us to provide pathogen-directed therapy earlier in a patient's illness, enabling more focused narrow-spectrum antimicrobial use. This would diminish the selective pressure, which leads to the emergence and dissemination of resistance and yielding novel markers to gauge the duration and intensity of therapy.

Conclusion

Antimicrobial therapy is complicated by the increasing incidence of antibiotic resistance. As a result, a broader range of antimicrobial agents has come into use, with the basic approach to antimicrobial therapy in these patients being front-loading, broad-spectrum antimicrobials. This therapy is then modified to relatively narrow-spectrum specific therapy. The regimens chosen and the doses prescribed are based on the principle that effective therapy is dependent on the delivery of a level of antimicrobial agent to the site of infection that significantly exceeds the MIC of the invading organism. Bacteriocidal therapy is essential when dealing with cardiovascular infection, CNS infection, prosthesis-associated infection, osteomyelitis, and infection in the neutropenic patient. Synergistic therapy may be important when dealing with life-threatening enterococcal, *P. aeruginosa*, and perhaps other gram-negative infections, but the definition of synergy varies and the clinical efficacy is not firmly established. Finally, it is hoped that a better definition of high-risk patients will permit the more effective use of pre-emptive antimicrobial regimens. It is clear that many questions remain unanswered and that many therapeutic decisions must be based on a thorough understanding of the properties of antimicrobials and the pathogenesis of infections rather than efficacy demonstrated in clinical studies.

References

1. Gonzales R, Steiner JF, Sande MA: Antibiotic prescribing for adults with colds, upper respiratory tract infections, and bronchitis by ambulatory care physicians [see comments]. JAMA 278:901–904, 1997.
2. McCaig LF, Hughes JM: Trends in antimicrobial drug prescribing among office-based physicians in the United States [see comments]. JAMA 273:214–219, 1995. [published erratum appears in JAMA Feb 11;279(6):434, 1998].
3. Rubin RH, Tolkoff-Rubin NE: Antimicrobial strategies in the care of organ transplant recipients. Antimicrob Agents Chemother 37:619–624, 1993.
4. Rubin RH: Preemptive therapy in immunocompromised hosts [editorial; comment]. N Engl J Med 324:1057–1059, 1991.
5. Estes L: Review of pharmacokinetics and pharmacodynamics of antimicrobial agents. Mayo Clin Proc 73:1114–1122, 1998.
6. Thompson RL, Wright AJ: General principles of antimicrobial therapy. Mayo Clin Proc 73:995–1006, 1998.
7. Alvarez-Elcoro S, Enzler MJ: The macrolides: Erythromycin, clarithromycin, and azithromycin. Mayo Clin Proc 74:613–634, 1999.
8. Edson RS, Terrell CL: The aminoglycosides. Mayo Clin Proc 74:519–528, 1999.
9. Kasten MJ: Clindamycin, metronidazole, and chloramphenicol. Mayo Clin Proc 74:825–833, 1999.
10. Marshall WF, Blair JE: The cephalosporins. Mayo Clin Proc 74:187–195, 1999.
11. Smilack JD: Trimethoprim-sulfamethoxazole. Mayo Clin Proc 74:730–734, 1999.
12. Smilack JD: The tetracyclines. Mayo Clin Proc 74:727–729, 1999.
13. Wilhelm MP, Estes L: Symposium on antimicrobial agents—Part XII. Vancomycin. Mayo Clin Proc 74:928–935, 1999.
14. Wright AJ: The penicillins. Mayo Clin Proc 74:290–307, 1999.
15. Lorian V: Antibiotics in Laboratory Medicine. Baltimore, Williams & Wilkins, 1996.
16. Standards NCfCL. Performance Standards for Antimicrobial Susceptibility Testing; Eleventh Informational Supplement. 21:27–30, 2001.
17. Wilson DA, Rolinson GA: The recovery period following exposure of bacteria to penicillins. Chemotherapy 25:14–22, 1979.
18. McDonald PJ, Pruul WB: Postantibiotic leukocyte enhancement: Increased susceptibility of bacteria pretreated with antibiotics to activity of leukocytes. Rev Infect Dis 3:38–44, 1981.
19. Craig WA: Pharmacokinetic/pharmacodynamic parameters: Rationale for antibacterial dosing of mice and men. Clin Infect Dis 26:1–12, 1998.
20. Turnidge JD: The pharmacodynamics of β-lactams. Clin Infect Dis 27:10–22, 1998.
21. DiPiro JT, Edmiston CE Jr, Bohnen JMA: Pharmacodynamics of antimicrobial therapy in surgery. Am J Surg 171:615–622, 1996.
22. MacGowan AP, Bowker KE: Continuous infusion of β-lactam antibiotics. Clin Pharmacokinet 35:391–402, 1998.
23. Fuursted K: Comparative killing activity and postantibiotic effect of streptomycin combined with ampicillin, ciprofloxacin, imipenem, piperacillin or vancomycin against strains of *Streptococcus faecalis* and *Streptococcus faecium*. Chemotherapy 24:229–234, 1988.
24. Gudmundsson A, Gottfredsson M, Gudmundsson S: The postantibiotic effect induced by antimicrobial combinations. Scand J Infect Dis Suppl 74:80–93, 1991.
25. Lacy MK, Nicolau DP, Nightingale CH, Quintiliani R: The pharmacodynamics of aminoglycosides. Clin Infect Dis 27:23–27, 1998.
26. Freeman CD, Nicolau DP, Belliveau PP, Nightingale CH: Once-daily dosing of aminoglycosides: Review and recommendations for clinical practice. J Antimicrob Chemother 39:677–686, 1997.
27. Verklin RM Jr, Mandell GL: Alteration of effectiveness of antibiotics by anaerobiosis. J Lab Clin Med 89:65–71, 1977.
28. O'Keefe JP, Tally FP, Barza M, Gorbach SL: Inactivation of penicillin G during experimental infection with Bacteroides fragilis. J Infect Dis 137:437–442, 1978.
29. Craig WA, Kunin CM: Significance of serum protein and tissue binding of antimicrobial agents. Annu Rev Med 27:287–300, 1976.
30. Dickinson GM, Bisno AL: Infections associated with indwelling devices: Concepts of pathogenesis; infections associated with intravascular devices [see comments]. Antimicrob Agents Chemother 33:597–601, 1989.
31. Jones RN, Pfaller MA, Marshall SA, et al: Antimicrobial activity of 12 broad-spectrum agents tested against 270 nosocomial bloodstream infection isolates caused by non-enteric gram-negative bacilli: Occurrence of resistance, molecular epidemiology, and screening for metallo-enzymes. Diagn Microbiol Infect Dis 29:187–192, 1997.
32. Virk A, Steckelberg JM: Clinical aspects of antimicrobial resistance. Mayo Clin Proc 75:200–214, 2000.
33. Medeiros AA: Evolution and dissemination of beta-lactamases accelerated by generations of beta-lactam antibiotics. Clin Infect Dis 24(suppl 1):S19–S45, 1997.
34. Pfaller MA, Jones RN, Marshall SA, et al: Inducible amp C beta-lactamase producing gram-negative bacilli from bloodstream infec-

tions: Frequency, antimicrobial susceptibility, and molecular epidemiology in a national surveillance program (SCOPE). Diagn Microbiol Infect Dis 28:211–219, 1997.

35. Pitout JD, Sanders CC, Sanders WE Jr: Antimicrobial resistance with focus on beta-lactam resistance in gram-negative bacilli. Am J Med 103:51–59, 1997.

36. Gold HS, Moellering RC Jr: Antimicrobial-drug resistance. N Engl J Med 335:1445–1453, 1996.

37. Bush K: New B-lactamases in gram-negative bacteria: Diversity and impact on the selection of antimicrobial therapy. Clin Infect Dis 32:1085–1089, 2001.

38. Chow JW, Fine MJ, Shlaes DM, et al: Enterobacter bacteremia: Clinical features and emergence of antibiotic resistance during therapy [see comments]. Ann Intern Med 115:585–590, 1991.

39. Pitout JD, Moland ES, Sanders CC, et al: Beta-lactamases and detection of beta-lactam resistance in Enterobacter spp. Antimicrob Agents Chemother 41:35–39, 1997.

40. Lee NL, Yuen KY, Kumana CR: Beta-lactam antibiotic and beta-lactamase inhibitor combinations. JAMA 285:386–388, 2001.

41. Kaye KS FH, Abrutyn E: Pathogens resistant to antimicrobial agents. Epidemology, molecular mechanisms and clinical management. Infect Dis Clin North Am 14:475–487, 2000.

42. Cunha BA: Antibiotic resistance. Med Clin North Am 84:1407–1429, 2000.

43. Leclercq R, Derlot E, Duval J, Courvalin P: Plasmid-mediated resistance to vancomycin and teicoplanin in Enterococcus faecium. N Engl J Med 319:157–161, 1988.

44. Murray BE: Vancomycin-resistant enterococcal infections. N Engl J Med 342:710–721, 2000.

45. Noble WC, Virani Z, Cree RG: Co-transfer of vancomycin and other resistance genes from Enterococcus faecalis NCTC 12201 to Staphylococcus aureus. FEMS Microbiol Lett 72:195–198, 1992.

46. Smith TL, Pearson ML, Wilcox KR, et al: Emergence of vancomycin resistance in Staphylococcus aureus. Glycopeptide-Intermediate Staphylococcus aureus Working Group [see comments]. N Engl J Med 340:493–501, 1999.

47. Wong SS, Ho PL, Woo PC, Yuen KY: Bacteremia caused by staphylococci with inducible vancomycin heteroresistance [see comments]. Clin Infect Dis 29:760–767, 1999.

48. Moellering RC Jr: Editorial response: Staphylococci vs. glycopeptides—how much are the battle lines changing? [editorial; comment]. Clin Infect Dis 29:768–770, 1999.

49. NNIS HIP, National Center for Infectious Diseases, Centers for Disease Control and Prevention: National Nosocomial Infections Surveillance (NNIS) System Report, Data, Summary from October 1986-April 1998, Issued June 1998. pp 1–25, 1998.

50. Fridkin SK, Steward CD, Edwards JR, et al: Surveillance of antimicrobial use and antimicrobial resistance in United States hospitals: Project ICARE phase 2. Project Intensive Care Antimicrobial Resistance Epidemiology (ICARE) hospitals. Clin Infect Dis 29:245–252, 1999.

51. White RL BD, Manduru M, Bosso JA: Comparison of three different in vitro methods of detecting synergy: Time-kill, checkerboard and E test. Antimicrob Agents Chemother 40:1914–1918, 1996.

52. Mandell GL, Kaye D, Levison ME, Hook EW: Enterococcal endocarditis. An analysis of 38 patients observed at the New York Hospital-Cornell Medical Center. Arch Intern Med 125:258–264, 1970.

53. Moellering RC Jr, Wennersten C, Weinberg AN: Studies on antibiotic synergism against enterococci. I. Bacteriologic studies. J Lab Clin Med 77:821–828, 1971.

54. Rahal JJ Jr: Antibiotic combinations: The clinical relevance of synergy and antagonism. Medicine (Baltimore) 57:179–195, 1978.

55. Krogstad DJ, Korfhagen TR, Moellering RC Jr, et al: Aminoglycoside-inactivating enzymes in clinical isolates of Streptococcus faecalis. An explanation for resistance to antibiotic synergism. J Clin Invest 62:480–486, 1978.

56. Jacoby GA, Archer GL: New mechanisms of bacterial resistance to antimicrobial agents. N Engl J Med 324:601–612, 1991.

57. Moellering RC Jr: The Garrod Lecture. The enterococcus: A classic example of the impact of antimicrobial resistance on therapeutic options. J Antimicrob Chemother 28:1–12, 1991.

58. Vemuri RK, Zervos MJ: Enterococcal infections. The increasing threat of nosocomial spread and drug resistance. Postgrad Med 93:121–124, 127–128, 1993.

59. Eliopoulos GM: Increasing problems in the therapy of enterococcal infections [editorial]. Eur J Clin Microbiol Infect Dis 12:409–412, 1993.

60. Wilson WR, Karchmer AW, Dajani AS, et al: Antibiotic treatment of adults with infective endocarditis due to streptococci, enterococci, staphylococci, and HACEK microorganisms. American Heart Association [see comments]. JAMA 274:1706–1713, 1995.

61. Ribera E, Gomez-Jimenez J, Cortes E, et al: Effectiveness of cloxacillin with and without gentamicin in short-term therapy for right-sided Staphylococcus aureus endocarditis. A randomized, controlled trial. Ann Intern Med 125:969–974, 1996.

62. Klastersky J, Hensgens C, Meunier-Carpentier F: Comparative effectiveness of combinations of amikacin with penicillin G and amikacin with carbenicillin in gram-negative septicemia: Double-blind clinical trial. J Infect Dis 134(suppl):S433–S440, 1976.

63. Lau WK, Young LS, Black RE, et al: Comparative efficacy and toxicity of amikacin/carbenicillin versus gentamicin/carbenicillin in leukopenic patients: A randomized prospective trail. Am J Med 62:959–966, 1977.

64. Meyer KS, Urban C, Eagan JA, et al: Nosocomial outbreak of Klebsiella infection resistant to late-generation cephalosporins [see comments]. Ann Intern Med 119:353–358, 1993.

65. Bennett JE, Dismukes WE, Duma RJ, et al: A comparison of amphotericin B alone and combined with flucytosine in the treatment of cryptoccal meningitis. N Engl J Med 301:126–131, 1979.

66. Neu HC: Synergy and antagonism of combinations with quinolones. Eur J Clin Microbiol Infect Dis 10:255–261, 1991.

67. Lepper MH: Treatment of pneumococcal meningitis with penicillin compared with penicillin plus aureomycin. Arch Intern Med 88:489, 1951.

68. Mathies AW Jr, Leedom JM, Ivler D, et al: Antibiotic antagonism in bacterial meningitis. Antimicrob Agents Chemother 7:218–224, 1967.

69. Sande MA, Overton JW: In vivo antagonism between gentamicin and chloramphenicol in neutropenic mice. J Infect Dis 128:247–250, 1973.

70. Coleman DL, Horwitz RI, Andriole VT: Association between serum inhibitory and bactericidal concentrations and therapeutic outcome in bacterial endocarditis. Am J Med 73:260–267, 1982.

71. Tauber MG, Sande MA: Principles in the treatment of bacterial meningitis. Am J Med 76:224–230, 1984.

72. Ceftazidime combined with a short or long course of amikacin for empirical therapy of gram-negative bacteremia in cancer patients with granulocytopenia. The EORTC International Antimicrobial Therapy Cooperative Group. N Engl J Med 317:1692–1698, 1987.

73. Weinstein MP, Stratton CW, Hawley HB, et al: Multicenter collaborative evaluation of a standardized serum bactericidal test as a predictor of therapeutic efficacy in acute and chronic osteomyelitis. Am J Med 83:218–222, 1987.

74. Lucet JC, Herrmann M, Rohner P, et al: Treatment of experimental foreign body infection caused by methicillin-resistant Staphylococcus aureus. Antimicrob Agents Chemother 34:2312–2317, 1990.

75. Chuard C, Herrmann M, Vaudaux P, et al: Successful therapy of experimental chronic foreign-body infection due to methicillin-resistant Staphylococcus aureus by antimicrobial combinations. Antimicrob Agents Chemother 35:2611–2616, 1991.

76. Mont MA, Waldman B, Banerjee C, et al: Multiple irrigation, debridement, and retention of components in infected total knee arthroplasty. J Arthroplasty 12:426–433, 1997.

77. Zimmerli W, Widmer AF, Blatter M, et al: Role of rifampin for treatment of orthopedic implant-related staphylococcal infections: A randomized controlled trial. Foreign-Body Infection (FBI) Study Group [see comments]. JAMA 279:1537–1541, 1998.

78. Brun-Buisson C, Legrand P, Philippon A, et al: Transferable enzymatic resistance to third-generation cephalosporins during nosocomial outbreak of multiresistant Klebsiella pneumoniae. Lancet 2:302–306, 1987.

79. Appelbaum PC: World-wide development of antibiotic resistance in pneumococci. Eur J Clin Microbiol 6:367–377, 1987.

80. Fey PD, Safranek TJ, Rupp ME, et al: Ceftriaxone-resistant Salmonella infection acquired by a child from cattle. N Engl J Med 342:1242–1249, 2000.

81. Molbak K, Baggesen DL, Aarestrup FM, et al: An outbreak of multidrug-resistant, quinolone-resistant Salmonella enterica serotype typhimurium DT104. N Engl J Med 341:1420–1425, 1999.

82. Appel GB, Neu HC: The nephrotoxicity of antimicrobial agents (first of three parts). N Engl J Med 296:663–670, 1977.

83. Fossieck B Jr, Parker RH: Neurotoxicity during intravenous infusion of penicillin. A review. J Clin Pharmacol 14:504–512, 1974.

84. Tse CS, Hernandez Vera F, Desai DV: Seizure-like activity associated with imipenem-cilastatin [letter]. Drug Intell Clin Pharm 21:659–660, 1987.

85. Burroughs SF, Johnson GJ: Beta-lactam antibiotic-induced platelet dysfunction: Evidence for irreversible inhibition of platelet activation in vitro and in vivo after prolonged exposure to penicillin. Blood 75:1473–1480, 1990.

86. Davey PG: Pharmacokinetics in liver disease. J Antimicrob Chemother 21:1–5, 1988.

87. Singh N, Yu VL, Mieles LA, Wagener MM: Beta-Lactam antibiotic-induced leukopenia in severe hepatic dysfunction: Risk factors and implications for dosing in patients with liver disease [see comments]. Am J Med 94:251–256, 1993.

88. Chow AW, Jewesson PJ: Pharmacokinetics and safety of antimicrobial agents during pregnancy. Rev Infect Dis 7:287–313, 1985.

89. Fridkin SK, Gaynes RP: Antimicrobial resistance in intensive care units. Clin Chest Med 20:303–316, viii, 1999.

90. Pittet D, Wenzel RP: Nosocomial bloodstream infections. Secular trends in rates, mortality, and contribution to total hospital deaths. Arch Intern Med 155:1177–1184, 1995.

91. Richards MJ, Edwards JR, Culver DH, Gaynes RP: Nosocomial infections in coronary care units in the United States. National Nosocomial Infections Surveillance System. Am J Cardiol 82:789–793, 1998.

92. Richards MJ, Edwards JR, Culver DH, Gaynes RP: Nosocomial infections in medical intensive care units in the United States. National Nosocomial Infections Surveillance System [see comments]. Crit Care Med 27:887–892, 1999.

93. Richards MJ, Edwards JR, Culver DH, Gaynes RP: Nosocomial infections in pediatric intensive care units in the United States. National Nosocomial Infections Surveillance System. Pediatrics 103:e39, 1999.

94. Spencer RC: Predominant pathogens found in the European Prevalence of Infection in Intensive Care Study. Eur J Clin Microbiol Infect Dis 15:281–285, 1996.

95. Mermel LA, Farr BM, Sheretz RJ, et al: Guidelines for the management of intravascular catheter-related infections. Clin Infect Dis 32:1249–1268, 2001.

96. DesJardin JA, Falagas JM, Ruthazer R, et al: Clinical utility of blood cultures drawn from indwelling central venous catheters in hospitalized patients with cancer. Ann Intern Med 131:641–647, 1999.

97. Wenzel RP, Edmond MB: The evolving technology of venous access [editorial; comment]. N Engl J Med 340:48–50, 1999.

98. Darouiche RO, Raad II, Heard SO, et al: A comparison of two antimicrobial-impregnated central venous catheters. Catheter Study Group [see comments]. N Engl J Med 340:1–8, 1999.

99. Jernigan JA, Farr BM: Short-course therapy of catheter-related Staphylococcus aureus bacteremia: A meta-analysis. Ann Intern Med 119:304–311, 1993.

100. Edwards JE Jr, Bodey GP, Bowden RA, et al: International Conference for the Development of a Consensus on the Management and Prevention of Severe Candidal Infections [see comments]. Clin Infect Dis 25:43–59, 1997.

101. Howe CW: Bacterial flora of clean wounds and its relation to subsequent sepsis. Am J Surg 107:696–700, 1964.

102. Edwards JE Jr, Lehrer RI, Stiehm ER, et al: Severe candidal infections: Clinical perspective, immune defense mechanisms, and current concepts of therapy. Ann Intern Med 89:91–106, 1978.

103. Solomkin JS, Flohr AB, Quie PG, Simmons RL: The role of Candida in intraperitoneal infections. Surgery 88:524–530, 1980.

104. Peoples JB: Candida and perforated peptic ulcers. Surgery 100:758–764, 1986. [published erratum appears in Surgery 1988 Feb;103(2):270.]

105. Eggimann P, Francioli P, Bille J, et al: Fluconazole prophylaxis prevents intra-abdominal candidiasis in high-risk surgical patients. Crit Care Med 27:1066–1072, 1999.

106. Classen DC, Evans RS, Pestotnik SL, et al: The timing of prophylactic administration of antibiotics and the risk of surgical-wound infection. N Engl J Med 326:281–286, 1992.

107. Burke JF: The effective period of preventive antibiotic action in experimental incisions and dermal lesions. Surgery 50:161–168, 1961.

108. Dajani AS, Taubert KA, Wilson W, et al: Prevention of bacterial endocarditis. Recommendations by the American Heart Association. JAMA 277:1794–1801, 1997.

109. Bartlett JG, Breiman RF, Mandell LA, File TM Jr: Community-acquired pneumonia in adults: Guidelines for management. The Infectious Diseases Society of America. Clin Infect Dis 26:811–838, 1998.

110. Hospital-acquired pneumonia in adults: Diagnosis, assessment of severity, initial antimicrobial therapy, and preventive strategies. A consensus statement, American Thoracic Society, November 1995. Am J Respir Crit Care Med 153:1711–1725, 1996.

111. Korvick JA, Bryan CS, Farber B, et al: Prospective observational study of Klebsiella bacteremia in 230 patients: Outcome for antibiotic combinations versus monotherapy. Antimicrob Agents Chemother 36:2639–2644, 1992.

112. Rubin RH, Shapiro ED, Andriole VT, et al: Evaluation of new anti-infective drugs for the treatment of urinary tract infection. Infectious Diseases Society of America and the Food and Drug Administration. Clin Infect Dis 15(suppl 1):S216–S227, 1992.

113. Haley RW, Culver DH, White JW, et al: The nationwide nosocomial infection rate. A new need for vital statistics. Am J Epidemiol 121:159–167, 1985.

114. Isenmann R, Rau B, Beger HG: Bacterial infection and extent of necrosis are determinants of organ failure in patients with acute necrotizing pancreatitis [see comments]. Br J Surg 86:1020–1024, 1999.

115. Rau B, Pralle U, Mayer JM, Beger HG: Role of ultrasonographically guided fine-needle aspiration cytology in the diagnosis of infected pancreatic necrosis. Br J Surg 85:179–184, 1998.

116. Banks PA, Gerzof SG, Langevin RE, et al: CT-guided aspiration of suspected pancreatic infection: Bacteriology and clinical outcome. Int J Pancreatol 18:265–270, 1995.

117. Kramer KM, Levy H: Prophylactic antibiotics for severe acute pancreatitis: The beginning of an era. Pharmacotherapy 19:592–602, 1999.

118. Finch WT, Sawyers JL, Schenker S: A prospective study to determine the efficacy of antibiotics in acute pancreatitis. Ann Surg 183:667–671, 1976.

119. Pederzoli P, Bassi C, Vesentini S, Campedelli A: A randomized multicenter clinical trial of antibiotic prophylaxis of septic complications in acute necrotizing pancreatitis with imipenem. Surg Gynecol Obstet 176:480–483, 1993.

120. Delcenserie R, Yzet T, Ducroix JP: Prophylactic antibiotics in treatment of severe acute alcoholic pancreatitis. Pancreas 13:198–201, 1996.

121. Schwarz M, Isenmann R, Meyer H, Beger HG: [Antibiotic use in necrotizing pancreatitis. Results of a controlled study]. Dtsch Med Wochenschr 122:356–361, 1997.

122. Sainio V, Kemppainen E, Puolakkainen P, et al: Early antibiotic treatment in acute necrotizing pancreatitis [see comments]. Lancet 346:663–667, 1995.

123. de Vera F, Martinez JF, Clara Verdu R, et al: [Pancreatic abscess caused by Candida following wide-spectrum antibiotic treatment]. Gastroenterol Hepatol 21:188–190, 1998.

124. Haron E, Vartivarian S, Anaissie E, et al: Primary Candida pneumonia. Experience at a large cancer center and review of the literature. Medicine (Baltimore) 72:137–142, 1993.

125. Masur H, Rosen PP, Armstrong D: Pulmonary disease caused by Candida species. Am J Med 63:914–925, 1977.

126. el-Ebiary M, Torres A, Fabregas N, et al: Significance of the isolation of Candida species from respiratory samples in critically ill, non-neutropenic patients. An immediate postmortem histologic study. Am J Respir Crit Care Med 156:583–590, 1997.

127. Kauffman CA, Vazquez JA, Sobel JD, et al: Prospective multicenter surveillance study of funguria in hospitalized patients. The National Institute for Allergy and Infectious Diseases (NIAID) Mycoses Study Group. Clin Infect Dis 30:14–18, 2000.

128. Leu HS, Huang CT: Clearance of funguria with short-course antifungal regimens: A prospective, randomized, controlled study. Clin Infect Dis 20:1152–1157, 1995.

129. Trinh T, Simonian J, Vigil S, et al: Continuous versus intermittent bladder irrigation of amphotericin B for the treatment of candiduria [see comments]. J Urol 154:2032–2034, 1995.

130. Sanford JP: The enigma of candiduria: Evolution of bladder irrigation with amphotericin B for management—from Anecdote to Dogma and a lesson from Machiavelli [see comments]. Clin Infect Dis 16:145–147, 1993.

131. Sobel JD, Kauffman CA, McKinsey D, et al: Candiduria: A randomized, double-blind study of treatment with fluconazole and placebo.

The National Institute of Allergy and Infectious Diseases (NIAID) Mycoses Study Group. Clin Infect Dis 30:19–24, 2000.

132. Jacobs LG, Skidmore EA, Freeman K, et al: Oral fluconazole compared with bladder irrigation with amphotericin B for treatment of fungal urinary tract infections in elderly patients [see comments]. Clin Infect Dis 22:30–35, 1996.

133. Fraser VJ, Jones M, Dunkel J, et al: Candidemia in a tertiary care hospital: Epidemiology, risk factors, and predictors of mortality [see comments]. Clin Infect Dis 15:414–421, 1992.

134. Leccines JA, Lee JW, Navarro EE, et al: Vascular catheter-associated fungemia in patients with cancer: Analysis of 155 episodes. Clin Infect Dis 14:875–883, 1992.

135. Wey SB, Mori M, Pfaller MA, et al: Hospital-acquired candidemia. The attributable mortality and excess length of stay. Arch Intern Med 148:2642–2645, 1988.

136. Rex JH, Walsh TJ, Sobel JD, et al: Practice guidelines for the treatment of candidiasis. Clin Infect Dis 30:662–678, 2000.

137. Rex JH, Bennett JE, Sugar AM, et al: A randomized trial comparing fluconazole with amphotericin B for the treatment of candidemia in patients without neutropenia. Candidemia Study Group and the National Institute [see comments]. N Engl J Med 331:1325–1330, 1994.

138. Phillips P, Shafran S, Garber G, et al: Multicenter randomized trial of fluconazole versus amphotericin B for treatment of candidemia in non-neutropenic patients. Canadian Candidemia Study Group. Eur J Clin Microbiol Infect Dis 16:337–345, 1997.

139. Anaissie EJ, Rex JH, Uzun O, Vartivarian S: Predictors of adverse outcome in cancer patients with candidemia. Am J Med 104:238–245, 1998.

140. Nguyen MH, Peacock JE Jr, Tanner DC, et al: Therapeutic approaches in patients with candidemia. Evaluation in a multicenter, prospective, observational study. Arch Intern Med 155:2429–2435, 1995.

141. Rex JH, Bennett JE, Sugar AM, et al: Intravascular catheter exchange and duration of candidemia. NIAID Mycoses Study Group and the Candidemia Study Group. Clin Infect Dis 21:994–996, 1995.

142. Gallis HA, Drew RH, Pickard WW: Amphotericin B: 30 years of clinical experience. Rev Infect Dis 12:308–329, 1990.

143. Walsh TJ, Hiemenz JW, Seibel NL, et al: Amphotericin B lipid complex for invasive fungal infections: Analysis of safety and efficacy in 556 cases. Clin Infect Dis 26:1383–1396, 1998.

144. Leenders AC, Daenen S, Jansen RL, et al: Liposomal amphotericin B compared with amphotericin B deoxycholate in the treatment of documented and suspected neutropenia-associated invasive fungal infections [see comments]. Br J Haematol 103:205–212, 1998.

145. Walsh TJ, Finberg RW, Arndt C, et al: Liposomal amphotericin B for empirical therapy in patients with persistent fever and neutropenia. National Institute of Allergy and Infectious Diseases Mycoses Study Group [see comments]. N Engl J Med 340:764–771, 1999.

146. Graybill JR: New antifungal agents. Eur J Clin Microbiol Infect Dis 8:402–412, 1989.

147. Galgiani JN: Fluconazole, a new antifungal agent. Ann Intern Med 113:177–179, 1990.

148. Romaschin AD, Harris DM, Ribeiro MB, et al: A rapid assay of endotoxin in whole blood using autologous neutrophil dependent chemiluminescence. J Immunol Methods 212:169–185, 1998.

149. Carlet J: Rapid diagnostic methods in the detection of sepsis. Infect Dis Clin North Am 13:483–494, xi, 1999.

150. Arnalich F, Garcia-Palomero E, Lopez J, et al: Predictive value of nuclear factor kappaB activity and plasma cytokine levels in patients with sepsis. Infect Immun 68:1942–1945, 2000.

151. Bohrer H, Qiu F, Zimmermann T, et al: Role of NFkappaB in the mortality of sepsis. J Clin Invest 100:972–985, 1997.

152. Dutka-Malen S, Evers S, Courvalin P: Detection of glycopeptide resistance genotypes and identification to the species level of clinically relevant enterococci by PCR. J Clin Microbiol 33:1434, 1995.

153. Einsele H, Hebart H, Roller G, et al: Detection and identification of fungal pathogens in blood by using molecular probes. J Clin Microbiol 35:1353–1360, 1997.

154. Flahaut M, Sanglard D, Monod M, et al: Rapid detection of Candida albicans in clinical samples by DNA amplification of common regions from C. albicans-secreted aspartic proteinase genes. J Clin Microbiol 36:395–401, 1998.

155. Kane TD, Alexander JW Johannigman JA: The detection of microbial DNA in the blood: A sensitive method for diagnosing bacteremia and/or bacterial translocation in surgical patients [see comments]. Ann Surg 227:1–9, 1998.

51

Chemotherapeutic Agents

Howard L. McLeod, PharmD • Chris Papageorgio, MD

Cancer is a major public health problem throughout the world. An estimated 1,268,000 new cases of cancer will be diagnosed in the United States in the year 2001, and an estimated 553,400 Americans will die of cancer during that year.[1] Cancer of the prostate, lung and bronchus, colon and rectum, bladder, and lymphatic system are the most common sites for men, whereas breast, lung and bronchus, colon and rectum, uterus, and lymphatic system are the most common sites in women.[1] Although there are many distinct molecular differences among cancers from various anatomic locations, there are some basic tenets of tumor biology that influence therapeutic strategies.[2-5] A tumor cell is more than just a normal cell with an abnormal ability to proliferate, with changes in genetic stability, angiogenesis, tissue invasion capacity, cell death, sensitivity to growth signals, and ability to sustain limitless replicative potential (Fig. 51–1). The same set of functional capabilities seems to be acquired during the development of a tumor cell, albeit through various mechanisms.[3] The observation of greater proliferation in tumor cells led to the development of the current armamentarium of DNA alkylators, mitotic inhibitors, and antimetabolites for the treatment of cancer. It is the clearer understanding of these various important biologic processes that will spawn the next generation of antitumor molecules.[6-11]

The majority of human cancers arise from solid organs, rather than lymphatics or bone marrow (BM), and surgery remains the only consistently curative approach. Chemotherapy and radiation therapy are useful in the adjuvant setting, where the goal is the eradication of residual microscopic disease, or in palliation, where the goal is focused on symptom control and increased quality and quantity of life.[12-15] The timing of chemotherapy is dependent on the clinical intent. Induction chemotherapy is used as initial therapy for leukemia to achieve significant cytoreduction (complete remission) of disease. This is then followed by consolidation/intensification chemotherapy, during which postremission treatment is given with the same drugs used in induction (consolidation) or drugs that are non–cross-resistant to the induction drugs (intensification). Postremission chemotherapy is necessary to prolong remission duration and overall survival in certain hematologic malignancies such as acute lymphoblastic leukemia (ALL) and acute myelogenous leukemia (AML). Adjuvant chemotherapy is given after eradication of disease with local treatment (surgical or radiation) to treat putative microscopic disease and prevent local or distant relapse. This differs from neoadjuvant chemotherapy, which is given before local therapy (primarily surgery) in hopes of reducing the extent of local treatment or increasing its effectiveness. For example, neoadjuvant combination chemotherapy and radiation therapy is given for T_3/T_4 rectal cancer to allow for a greater chance of definitive surgery and a lower incidence of local disease recurrence. Maintenance chemotherapy is the use of chronic, low-dose, outpatient chemotherapy intended to prolong the duration of remission and achieve cure in patients in remission. Salvage chemotherapy is used after the failure of other treatments (surgery, radiation, or prior chemotherapy) to control disease or provide palliation.

The clinical end points in evaluating response to chemotherapy differ based on the approach taken to treatment. For induction chemotherapy, a complete response is defined as disappearance of disease on imaging studies for at least 1 month. A partial response is decrease of 50% or more in the sum of the products of the biperpendicular diameters with no new sites of disease for at least 1 month. In hematologic malignancies (e.g., AML), a complete response is defined as less than 5% blasts in the BM, no circulating blasts in the peripheral blood, and no extramedullary disease by Day 14 after induction. A partial response in hematologic malignancies is defined as 5% to 20% blasts in the BM by Day 14 after induction or less than 4% blasts in the BM for

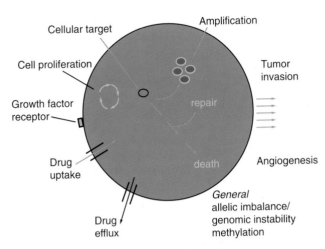

Figure 51–1. Cellular targets for chemotherapy.

- Only drugs known to be partially effective against the same tumor when used alone should be selected for use in combination.
- When several drugs of a class are available and are equally effective, a drug should be selected on the basis of toxicity that does not overlap with the toxicity of other drugs to be used in the combination.
- Drugs should be used in their optimal dose and schedule.
- Drug combinations should be given at consistent intervals. Because long intervals between cycles negatively affect dose intensity, the treatment-free interval between cycles should be the shortest possible time necessary for recovery of the most sensitive normal target tissue, which is usually the BM.

Response to Chemotherapy and the Biology of Human Tumor Growth

Skipper and colleagues[17] developed the L1210 rodent leukemia model, a rapidly growing tumor with nearly all cells actively synthesizing DNA as measured by the uptake of tritiated thymidine (the labeling index). The L1210 leukemia has a growth fraction of 100% (i.e., all of its cells are actively progressing through the cycle), and hence its life cycle is consistent and predictable, enabling Skipper and colleagues to show that this rodent leukemia could be cured by specifically designed doses and schedules tied to tumor volume and growth characteristics. Although the killing effects of cancer drugs in this model tumor followed log-kill kinetics (i.e., if a particular dose of an individual drug kills three logs of cells and reduces tumor burden from 10^{10} to 10^7 cells, then the same dose will reduce the tumor burden from 10^5 to 10^2 cells), human tumors appeared to follow a Gompertzian model of growth and regression. The critical distinction between Gompertzian and exponential growth is that in Gompertzian kinetics the growth fraction of the tumor is not constant, but decreases exponentially with time (exponential growth is matched by exponential retardation of growth). The growth fraction peaks when the tumor size is about 37% of its maximum size. In a Gompertzian model, when a patient with advanced cancer is treated the tumor mass is larger, its growth fraction is low and the fraction of cells killed therefore is small, because response to chemotherapy depends on whether the tumor is in its phase of exponential growth. This information has been useful in the design of adjuvant chemotherapy because it impacts on the patterns of regrowth of residual tumor cells.

less than 30 days. No response (stable disease) is declared when a patient has less than 50% response or actual progression of disease, and disease progression is when there is a greater than 25% increase in the sum of the products of the biperpendicular diameters of known lesions or any new sites of disease. For adjuvant chemotherapy, the primary end point is relapse-free survival, which is the time from start of therapy to regrowth of tumor to detectable levels. This end point is also used for primary (neoadjuvant) chemotherapy. However, the unique feature of primary chemotherapy is the ability to delineate partial responders with variable degrees of prognosis because removal of residual tumor mass and histologic examination of the tissue allow determination of the viability and character of the remaining tumor cells (pathologic response). With salvage chemotherapy, progression-free survival remains the major end point in patients with advanced disease and is the equivalent of relapse-free survival in the adjuvant setting.

Combination Chemotherapy

With rare exceptions (e.g., Burkitt lymphoma), single drugs in standard doses do not cure cancer. Combination chemotherapy accomplishes not only maximal cell kill within the range of toxicity tolerated by the host for each drug, but also it provides a broader range of coverage of resistant cell lines, thus preventing or slowing the development of new resistant cells. The development of resistance by cancer cells to anticancer drugs without prior exposure to these drugs has been predicted, by the Goldie and Coldman mathematical model, to occur at population sizes between 10^3 and 10^6 tumor cells, much less than the mass of cells considered to be clinically detectable (i.e., 10^9 cells or a 1-cm mass).[16] Hence, as per the "Goldie-Coldman hypothesis," resistance should be a problem even with small tumors, and the maximal chance for cure occurs when all effective drugs are given simultaneously. The following principles have been useful in the selection of drugs in the most effective drug combinations.

General Mechanism of Action

Cell Cycle and Therapeutic Targets

The eukaryotic cell cycle is divided into four stages: G_1, S, G_2, and M.[6] The mechanisms that allow normal renewing cell populations of the body, like hematopoietic and GI precursors, to monitor and repair damaged DNA or undergo cell cycle arrest/apoptosis are responsible for the phenomenon called *the therapeutic index*. The disruption of this cycle, which is a hallmark of cancer, presents numerous opportunities for targeting checkpoint controls to develop new therapeutic strategies for this disease. Such strategies include either induction of arrest at the G_1/S and/or G_2/M checkpoints (leading to cytostasis and ultimately apoptosis), or abrogation of arrest at the G_2/M checkpoint in p53-deficient cells (leading to progression of cells with damaged DNA through the cell cycle beyond the G_2/M checkpoint and ultimately apoptosis or sensitization to genotoxic stresses such as radiation). The G_1/S checkpoint can occur only by p53-dependent mechanisms, whereas the G_2/M checkpoint can occur by either p53-dependent or p53-independent mechanisms.[4-6] However, p53 can also activate an apoptotic response to DNA damage, especially in hematopoietic cells, which often overrides the checkpoint response. Hence in cell types programmed for apoptosis, loss of p53 function decreases sensitivity to a wide variety of DNA-damaging agents, whereas in cell types of some solid tumors not inherently programmed for apoptosis, a clear relation between *p53* gene status and radiosensitivity or chemosensitivity has been more difficult to establish.

Categories of Drugs by Their Activities Relative to the Cell Cycle

Cytotoxic agents can be roughly categorized by their activities relative to the cell generation cycle (Table 51–1).[18]

Phase-Specific Agents

Phase-specific agents are effective only if present in the cancer cell during a particular phase of the cell cycle (Fig. 51–2). Over a certain dosage level, further increases in drug dose will not result in more cell killing. If the drug concen-

TABLE 51–1.

Common Classes of Anticancer Therapy

Class	Target	Cell Cycle Specificity	Examples	Limiting Toxicities*
Alkylators	DNA	Nonspecific	Cyclophosphamide nitrogen mustard	Neutropenia, alopecia, mucositis
Antimetabolites	DNA synthesis	S phase	Methotrexate 5-Fluorouracil Mercaptopurine Gemcitabine	Mucositis, diarrhea
Vinca alkaloids	Tubulin	M phase	Vincristine Vinblastine	Neurotoxicity (vincristine) Neutropenia
Epipodophyllotoxins	Topoisomerase II	$S-G_2$	Etoposide	Neutropenia
Anthracycline	DNA	Nonspecific	Doxorubicin	Neutropenia Cardiomyopathy
Bleomycin	DNA	Nonspecific	Bleomycin	Pulmonary
Camptothecins	Topoisomerase I	S phase	Topotecan	Neutropenia Irinotecan-induced diarrhea
Taxanes	Tubulin	M phase	Paclitaxel Docetaxel	Neutropenia neurotoxicity
Platinum agents	DNA	Nonspecific	Cisplatin Carboplatin	Nephrotoxicity (cisplatin) Neutropenia Thrombocytopenia (carboplatin)

*Toxicities common to most or all members of the class.

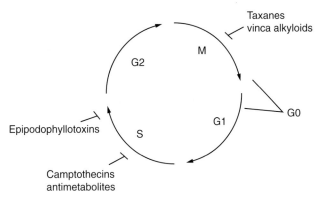

Figure 51–2. Cell cycle specificity of commonly used anticancer agents.

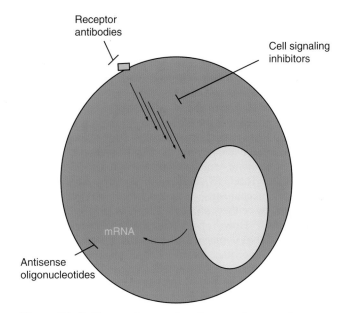

Figure 51–3. Targets for novel anticancer therapeutics.

tration is maintained over time, however, more cells will enter the specific lethal phase of the cell cycle and will die.

- In the G_0 phase (gap 0 or resting phase), cells are for the most part refractory to chemotherapy.
- In the G_1 phase (gap 1 or interphase), cells synthesize proteins and RNA for specialized cell functions. In late G_1, a burst of RNA synthesis occurs and many of the enzymes necessary for DNA synthesis are manufactured. G_1 phase–specific drugs: L-asparaginase, antisense therapies.
- In the S phase (DNA synthesis), the cellular content of DNA doubles. S phase–specific drugs: procarbazine, antimetabolites, hydroxyurea, camptothecins.
- In the G_2 phase (gap 2), DNA synthesis ceases, protein and RNA synthesis continues, and the microtubular precursors of the mitotic spindle are produced. G_2 phase–specific drugs: bleomycin, vinca alkaloids, taxanes.
- In the M phase (mitosis), the rates of protein and RNA synthesis diminish abruptly while the genetic material is segregated into daughter cells. After completion of mitosis, the new cells enter either the G_0 or G_1 phase. M phase–specific drugs: vinca alkaloids, taxanes.

Phase Nonspecific Agents

These agents can kill either dividing cells at any point in the cell cycle (e.g., alkylating agents, platinum compounds, cell signaling inhibitors) or nondividing cells ($\Rightarrow$cycle nonspecific; e.g., steroid hormones, antitumor antibiotics except bleomycin) (Fig. 51–3). All phase nonspecific drugs generally have a linear dose-response curve: the greater the amount of drug administered the greater the fraction of cells killed.[18]

Obstacles to Clinical Success

Multiple Drug Resistance

There are several ways in which tumor cells can express or acquire resistance to chemotherapeutic agents. These methods are described in the following sections.

Transporter-Mediated Resistance

Tumor cells selected for resistance to a particular drug in the class of "natural product" or their semisynthetic analogs (topoisomerase I inhibitors, vinca alkaloids, taxanes, anthracyclines) display cross-resistance to these and other agents that have in common the following features: they are in general lipophilic, they range in molecular weight from 300 to 900 daltons, and they appear to enter cells by passive diffusion.[19] The accumulation and retention of these drugs is less in the multidrug resistance (MDR) cells than in the drug-sensitive cells from which they were derived. This alteration in cellular activity is mediated by P-glycoprotein. It is hypothesized that the drug molecule binds to a specific site on P-glycoprotein within the lipid bilayer of the cell plasma membrane and by an adenosine triphosphate (ATP)-dependent process and is transported out of the cell. P-glycoprotein belongs to the superfamily of ATP-binding cassette transporters, which include MDR-associated protein, breast cancer resistance protein, and a host of other family members with a putative role in drug resistance.[20] In addition to membrane transporters, cytoplasmic vault proteins, such as lung resistance protein, may also contribute to resistance by diverting the chemotherapy from having its desired effect.

Intrinsic MDR

Untreated carcinomas of the colon, kidney, hepatomas, adrenal tumors, pheochromocytomas, and some other malignancies demonstrate high levels of *MDR1* gene expression. Some hematologic malignancies (acute myeloid leukemia, chronic lymphocytic leukemia, adult T-cell lymphomas) also express MDR based on the type of cells from which the malignancy arose.

MDR Mediated by Detoxification of the Drug in the Cell

Glutathione, a nonprotein thiol can interact with the reactive site of a drug resulting in conjugation of the drug with glutathione. The conjugate is less active and more water-soluble and it is excluded from the cell with the participation of transporter proteins named GS-X pumps (including MDR-associated protein). Increased levels of glutathione (GSH) were found in cell lines resistant to alkylating agents (e.g., nitrogen mustard, chlorambucil, melphalan, cyclophosphamide, carmustine [BCNU]). Alkylating agents share in common an electrophilic nature and ability to spontaneously interact with the thiol of reduced GSH. Glutathione-*S*-transferases (GST) catalyze the interactions between GSH and alkylating agents increasing the rate of a drug detoxification. Activation of these enzymes can therefore cause cellular drug resistance. Enzymes that catalyze GSH synthesis could also mediate drug resistance; however, their role in this phenomenon is not yet clear.

MDR Mediated by Enhanced DNA Repair

ALKYLATING AGENTS (NITROSOUREAS)

Resistance to the chloroethylating agents such as BCNU that exert cytotoxicity by the formation of intrastrand crosslinks is well understood. Bifunctional intrastrand crosslinks are gradually formed over time from the precursor monofunctional DNA adduct, O^6 chloroethylguanine.[21] Resistance to these agents occurs when there is repair of the O^6 chloroethylguanine lesion before the bifunctional alkylator DNA adduct forms. Hence BCNU resistance has been correlated with tumor expression of the DNA repair enzyme O^6-alkylguanine-DNA alkyltransferase (AT), also known as methylguanine methyltransferase, which removes alkyl adducts at the O^6 position of guanine before crosslink formation occurs and thereby prevents nitrosourea-induced cytotoxic DNA damage. The strong correlation between AT expression and BCNU resistance has led to the development of strategies to deplete AT to reverse nitrosourea resistance. Thus to circumvent this form of resistance, one approach has been to deplete AT through the use of a methylating agent, such as streptozotocin, to form O^6-methylguanine DNA adducts, which in turn are repaired by AT and deplete the enzyme. Streptozotocin administered before BCNU was shown to decrease AT activity in peripheral mononuclear cells and to decrease colon cancer metastasis. However, residual AT levels appear to be sufficient to maintain resistance to BCNU. Therefore, more potent modulators of AT in tumor cells are needed to reverse clinical resistance to BCNU.

PLATINATING AGENTS

Cisplatin and analogues cause interstrand cisplatin (CDDP)-DNA and intrastrand crosslinks.[22] Changes in the quantities of proteins recognizing and repairing DNA injury (ERCC1, ERCC2, and ERCC3/XPB) were found in cultured cells with altered sensitivity to platinum complexes. However, resistance to these agents has been shown to be multifactorial: altered expression of oncogenes; increased repair of intrastrand crosslinks; association of proteins (e.g., high-mobility group proteins HMG1 and HMG2) with CDDP-modified DNA: inactivation in the cytosol by either increased levels of metallothionein or increases in GSH, and decreased cellular accumulation of CDDP.

MDR Mediated by Alteration of Drug Targets

TOPOISOMERASES AND THEIR INHIBITORS

Two types of topoisomerases exist in mammalian cells. The type I enzymes (molecular weight about 100 kD) cut and pass single-stranded DNA, are thought to play a prominent role in transcription, and are specifically inhibited by camptothecin and derivatives currently in clinical use: topotecan and irinotecan (CPT-11). All of these agents inhibit topoisomerase I by blocking the relegation step. The type II enzymes exist as two forms, both the products of separate genes: α (molecular weight about 170 kD), located on chromosome 17; and β (molecular weight about 180 kD), located on chromosome 3. For the type II enzymes "classic" anthracyclines (e.g., doxorubicin and daunorubicin), the epipodophyllotoxins (etoposide and teniposide), and aminoacridines (e.g., amsacrine) all block strand relegation and stabilize DNA-protein complexes. In general, resistance to topoisomerase inhibitors manifests itself in two forms: decreased enzyme amount or mutation in specific domains, with the net result being a decrease in topoisomerase II activity.

ANTIMETABOLITES

Both the dihydrofolate reductase (DHFR) inhibitors and fluoropyrimidines target the thymidylate synthesis (TS) cycle and induce a "thymineless death" in cancer cells.

METHOTREXATE

Methotrexate is transported into cells by reduced folate carriers and consequently reduction in carrier-mediated transport is frequently seen as a basis of resistance to this drug in tumor cells.[23] Other mechanisms of resistance to methotrexate include impaired polyglutamination and increased levels of DHFR. Methotrexate is polyglutamylated in the cell by folyl polyglutamate synthetase allowing for its longer intracellular retention. Decreased levels of folyl polyglutamate synthetase can therefore lead to methotrexate resistance. Decreased polyglutamination of methotrexate has been observed in adult patients with B-cell acute lymphoblastic leukemia. Increased levels of the target enzyme DHFR often by gene amplification is a well documented basis of resistance to methotrexate. Also, mutations in the *DHFR* gene also have been observed to confer resistance to methotrexate by decreasing binding affinity of the drug to DHFR.

5-FLUOROURACIL

5-Fluorouracil (5-FU) has multiple mechanisms of action all of which require metabolism of 5-FU to active species. Uridine, the natural nucleoside, may compete for the same metabolizing enzymes that convert 5-FU into the active moiety responsible for binding TS. Decreasing levels of the competing natural uridine nucleotides by removing the feedback inhibition of de novo pyrimidine synthesis may result in enhanced 5-FU activity.

Classes of Chemotherapeutic Agents

There are more than 70 anticancer agents approved by the U.S. Food and Drug Administration, ranging from cytotoxic DNA alkylators to cytostatic antibodies. The following sections focus on the major classes of chemotherapeutic agents, omitting comment on antiendocrine agents and biologics such as interleukins and monoclonal antibodies.

Alkylating Agents

All these agents have in common the property of becoming strong electrophiles through the formation of carbonium ion intermediates. As a result, they form covalent linkages by alkylation of various nucleophilic moieties such as phosphate, amino, sulfhydryl, hydroxyl, carboxyl, and imidazole groups. The chemotherapeutic and cytotoxic effects, however, are directly related to the alkylation of the 7 nitrogen atom of guanine, which becomes a quaternary ammonium nitrogen, thus leading to either base pairing with thymine (substitution of AT for GC) or labilization and opening of the imidazole ring (depurination by excision of guanine residues). It appears that the selectivity of certain alkylating agents against specific malignancies may result from the capacity of normal tissues such as liver to protect themselves against cytotoxicity by further degrading the activated intermediates.

The pharmacokinetics of these drugs are characterized by linear dose-response curves; more cells are killed with increasing doses (these drugs are effective only if the cells proceed through the cell cycle, but they can inflict injury at any phase of the cycle).

Nitrogen Mustards

Mechlorethamine (HN2, Mustargen)

a. **Indications:** Lymphomas, malignant pleural, pericardial and peritoneal effusions
b. **Pharmacology**
   1. Mechanism: Alkylation of DNA. With intracavitary use, mechlorethamine causes sclerosis and inflamma-

tory reaction of serous membranes leading to adherence of serosal surfaces.
   2. Metabolism: The native drug is highly active and is rapidly deactivated within the blood by spontaneous hydrolysis; the elimination half-life is 15 minutes. Metabolites are mostly excreted in the urine.
c. **Toxicity**
   1. Dose-limiting: Myelosuppression
   2. Common: Severe nausea and vomiting beginning 1 hour after administration, skin necrosis if extravasated (sodium thiosulfate may be tried), metallic taste, and discoloration of the infused vein
   3. Occasional: Alopecia, sterility, diarrhea, and thrombophlebitis
   4. Rare: Neurotoxicity (including hearing loss), angioedema, and secondary neoplasms
d. **Administration:** Patients should always be premedicated with antiemetics. The drug should be administered through the tubing of a running intravenous line, using extravasation precautions. The drug is supplied as 10-mg vials. Dose modification needs to be made for hematologic toxicity, but is not required for hepatic or renal impairment (apparently <0.01% of the drug remains unchanged). A typical dose is 0.2 to 0.4 mg/kg (10 mg/m^2) as a single or divided dose monthly, or 6 mg/m^2 on Day 1 and 8 of the MOPP regimen.

Cyclophosphamide (Cytoxan)[24–26]

a. **Indications:** Used in a wide variety of conditions including ALL, AML, chronic myeloid leukemia (CML), chronic lymphocytic leukemia (CLL), ovarian and breast cancer.
b. **Pharmacology**
   1. Mechanism: Alkylation of DNA.
   2. Metabolism: The native drug is inactive and requires activation by the liver microsomal oxidase system to form an aldehyde that decomposes in plasma and peripheral tissues to yield acrolein and an alkylating metabolite, phosphoramide mustard. The liver also metabolizes metabolites to inactive compounds. Drugs that induce microsomal enzymes (e.g., barbiturates, anticonvulsants) may enhance toxicity, whereas liver disease may decrease toxicity. The native drug is not protein bound but active products are 50% protein bound. Active and inactive metabolites are excreted in urine.
c. **Toxicity**
   1. Dose limiting: Myelosuppression. Leukopenia develops 8 to 14 days after administration. Degradative products are responsible for hemorrhagic cystitis, which is prevented by maintaining a high urine output. Hemorrhagic cystitis is more common and can be severe when massive doses are used (e.g., for BM transplantation). Bladder fibrosis with telangiectasia of the mucosa can occur (usually after long-term oral therapy) without episodes of cystitis.
   2. Common: Alopecia, stomatitis, aspermia, amenorrhea, and headache (fast onset, short duration).

Nausea and vomiting are common after doses greater than or equal to 700 mg/m^2 beginning 6 to 10 hours after administration.

3. Occasional: Skin or fingernail hyperpigmentation, metallic taste during injection, sneezing or a cold sensation in the nose after injection, allergy, fever, dizziness, and abnormal liver function tests

4. Rare: Transient syndrome of inappropriate antidiuretic hormone secretion (SIADH), hypothyroidism, cataracts, jaundice, cardiac necrosis and acute myopericarditis, and secondary neoplasms (acute leukemia, bladder cancer)

d. Administration: The drug should be administered with a large volume of fluid to avoid cystitis. The drug is supplied as 25- or 50-mg tablets and vials contain 100 to 1000 mg. Dose modification needs to be made for hematologic toxicity and may be required for hepatic functional impairment. Cyclophosphamide is frequently used as part of combination chemotherapy regimens. Some common dosages are 0.5 to 1.5 g/m^2 intravenously (IV) every 3 weeks or 50 to 200 mg/m^2 orally for 14 days every 28 days. BMT regimens use up to 2 gm/m^2 IV daily for 3 days.

Ifosfamide (Isophosphamide, Ifex)[24]

a. Indications: A wide variety of neoplasms including lymphomas, sarcomas, head and neck carcinomas, breast carcinoma, and germ cell testicular tumors

b. Pharmacology

1. Mechanism: Metabolites are alkylating agents that are similar to cyclophosphamide but not cross-resistant

2. Metabolism: Like cyclophosphamide, the drug undergoes hepatic activation to an aldehyde form that decomposes in plasma and peripheral tissues to yield acrolein and its alkylating metabolite. Acrolein is highly toxic to urothelial mucosa. The chloroacetaldehyde metabolite may be responsible for the neurotoxic effects, particularly in patients with renal dysfunction. Metabolites and unaltered drug (15–55%) are excreted in the urine.

c. Toxicity

1. Dose-limiting: Myelosuppression and hemorrhagic cystitis

2. Common: Alopecia, nausea and vomiting, neurotoxicity, lethargy, dizziness, confusion, and ataxia

3. Occasional: Salivation, stomatitis, diarrhea, constipation, urticaria, hyperpigmentation, nail ridging, abnormal liver function tests, phlebitis, fever; hypotension, hypertension, hyponatremia, hypokalemia, and renal tubular acidosis

d. Administration: Aggressive concomitant hydration (2–4 L/day) and mesna are given to reduce the incidence of hemorrhagic cystitis. The drug is supplied as 1- and 3-g vials; mesna is available in 400-mg vials. Dose modification is required for hematologic and renal dysfunction. A typical dose is 1000 to 1200 mg/m^2 IV over 30 minutes for 5 days every 3 to 4 weeks. The total dosage of mesna is 60% of the isophosphamide dosage.

Melphalan (Alkeran, L-sarcolysin)

a. Indications: Multiple myeloma, ovarian cancer, breast cancer, melanoma (the parenteral form is used for limb perfusion for melanoma and in BM transplantation studies)

b. Pharmacology

1. Mechanism: Alkylation of DNA

2. Metabolism: Acts directly. Ninety percent of the drug is bound to plasma proteins and undergoes spontaneous hydrolysis in the bloodstream to inert products. Melphalan is excreted in the urine as unchanged drug and metabolites.

c. Toxicity

1. Dose-limiting: Myelosuppression, which may be cumulative and recovery may be prolonged

2. Occasional: Anorexia, nausea, vomiting, mucositis, and sterility

3. Rare: Alopecia, pruritus, rash, hypersensitivity, secondary malignancies (acute leukemia), pulmonary fibrosis, vasculitis, and cataracts

d. Administration: The drug is supplied as 2-mg tablets and 50-mg vials. Dose modification is required for hematologic toxicity. The drug should be administered cautiously in patients with azotemia. If no myelosuppression is observed after oral dosing, poor oral absorption should be suspected. Continuous therapy: 0.10 to 0.15 mg/kg orally daily for 2 to 3 weeks; no therapy for 2 to 4 weeks, then 2 to 4 mg orally daily; or pulse therapy: 0.25 mg/kg (10 mg/m^2) orally daily for 4 days every 4 to 6 weeks (with prednisone for myeloma).

Chlorambucil (Leukeran)

a. Indications: CLL, Waldenstrom macroglobulinemia, indolent lymphomas, Hodgkin lymphoma, ovarian carcinoma, hairy cell leukemia, and trophoblastic tumors

b. Pharmacology

1. Mechanism: Alkylation of DNA

2. Metabolism: Does not require metabolism for activity and is spontaneously hydrolyzed to inactive and active products; some is also metabolized in the liver. Native drug and metabolic products are excreted in urine.

c. Toxicity

1. Dose-limiting: Myelosuppression (usually moderate, gradual, and reversible)

2. Occasional: Gastrointestinal (GI) upset, mild liver function test abnormalities, and sterility

3. Rare: Rash, alopecia, fever, cachexia, pulmonary fibrosis, neurologic or ocular toxicity, cystitis, and acute leukemia

d. Administration: The drug is supplied as 2-mg tablets. Dose modification is required for hematologic toxicity. It is recommended that chlorambucil be withdrawn if signs of pulmonary toxicity or severe skin reaction occur.

Ethyleneimines

Thiotepa (Triethylenethiophosphoramide, Thio-TEPA)

a. **Indications:** Breast, ovarian and bladder cancers; Hodgkin lymphoma; pleural and pericardial effusions
b. **Pharmacology**
   1. Mechanism: Alkylation of DNA
   2. Metabolism: Rapidly decomposed in plasma and excreted largely as metabolites in the urine
c. **Toxicity**
   1. Dose-limiting: Myelosuppression
   2. Common: GI upset, abnormal liver function tests, rash and hives
   3. Rare: Alopecia, fever, and angioedema
d. **Administration:** Thiotepa may be administered IV, intramuscularly (IM), intracavitary, intrathecally, intra-arterially, intravesicularly and as an ophthalmic installation. Thiotepa is supplied as a 15-mg vial. Dose modification is required for hematologic toxicity. Typical doses are: IV: 12 to 16 mg/m^2 every 1 to 4 weeks; intravesicular: 15 to 60 mg every week for 4 weeks.

Alkyl Sulfonates

Busulfan (Myleran)

a. **Indications:** CML (not in the blastic crisis phase), myeloproliferative disorders, BM transplantation (high doses)
b. **Pharmacology**
   1. Mechanism: Alkylation of DNA
   2. Metabolism: Acts directly; catabolized in the liver to inactive products that are excreted in the urine
c. **Toxicity**
   1. Dose-limiting: Myelosuppression with slow recovery; blood counts decrease for about 2 weeks after discontinuation of drug
   2. Common: GI upset and sterility
   3. Occasional: Skin hyperpigmentation, alopecia, rash, gynecomastia, cataracts, liver function test abnormalities (sometimes fatal hepatovenoclusive disease)
   4. Rare: Pulmonary fibrosis ("busulfan lung"), retroperitoneal fibrosis, endocardial fibrosis, Addisonian-like asthenia (without biochemical evidence of adrenal insufficiency), impotence, hemorrhagic cystitis, and secondary neoplasms.
d. **Administration:** The drug is supplied as a 2-mg tablet. Dose modifications need to be made for hematologic toxicity. A typical dosage is 2 to 8 mg daily orally or 0.05 mg/kg per day.

Nitrosoureas

Carmustine (BCNU), Lomustine (CCNU)

a. **Indications:** Brain cancer, lymphomas, multiple myeloma (in combination with prednisone)
b. **Pharmacology**
   1. Mechanism: Alkylation of DNA
   2. Metabolism: BCNU and CCNU are highly lipid-soluble drugs that cross the blood–brain barrier. They are rapidly biotransformed in the liver into active and inactive products that are excreted in the urine (some products have an enterohepatic cycle).
c. **Toxicity**
   1. Dose-limiting: Myelosuppression is prolonged and cumulative
   2. Common: Nausea and vomiting
   3. Occasional: Stomatitis, esophagitis, diarrhea, liver function test abnormalities, alopecia, facial flushing, brown discoloration of skin, pulmonary fibrosis (with prolonged therapy and higher doses), dizziness, optic neuritis, ataxia, organic brain syndrome, and renal insufficiency
d. **Administration:** The drug is supplied as 100-mg vials of BCNU and 10-, 40-, and 100-mg capsules of CCNU. Dose modifications are required for hematologic or renal insufficiency. Typical doses are: (i) BCNU: 150 to 200 mg/m^2 IV every 6 to 8 weeks; (ii) CCNU: 100 to 130 mg/m^2 orally every 6 to 8 weeks.

Antimetabolites

General Mechanism of Action

Antimetabolites are generally either structural analogues of the purines and pyrimidines or inhibitors of their synthesis. They therefore inhibit DNA synthesis and their activity is greatest in the S phase of the cell cycle.

Folic Acid Analogs

Methotrexate (MTX, Amethopterin)[23]

a. **Indications**
   1. Carcinomas of head and neck, breast, and lung
   2. Leukemias: acute and meningeal
b. **Pharmacology**
   1. Mechanism: MTX, the 4-amino, 10-methyl analog of folic acid, is a tight-binding inhibitor of DHFR, a critical enzyme in maintaining the intracellular folate pool in its reduced form. Tetrahydrofolate serves as a 1-carbon carrier for the de novo synthesis of thymidine 5′-monophosphate (thymidylate, dTMP) and purine nucleotides, as well as for certain amino acids. TS catalyzes the formation of dTMP from 2′-deoxyuridine-5′-monophosphate (deoxyuridylate, dUMP). This reaction uses 5,10-methylenetetrahydrofolate as a methyl donor and results in the oxidation of the reduced folate to dihydrofolate. The activity of the TS reaction thus creates the requirement for DHFR to maintain the intracellular reduced folate pool. Inhibition of DHFR results in accumulation of oxidized folates at the expense of reduced folates because of the continued synthetic function of TS. Additional metabolic effects of MTX result from

its transformation to polyglutamate forms (80% of intracellular MTX), which are potent direct inhibitors of several folate-dependent enzymes including DHFR and TS. Polyglutamation occurs in tumor cells and to a lesser extent in healthy tissue. Hence metabolic inhibition caused by MTX depends not only on partial depletion of reduced folates, but also on direct inhibition of folate-dependent enzymes by the polyglutamates of both MTX and dihydrofolate that accumulate after inhibition of DHFR. The cytotoxic action of methotrexate has been referred to as "self-limiting," because MTX is also capable of inhibiting RNA and protein synthesis and thus slowing the entry of cells into S phase.

2. Metabolism: MTX is readily absorbed from the GI tract at doses less than 25 mg/m^2, but larger doses are absorbed incompletely and are routinely administered IV. It enters cells by the same active transport mechanisms used by physiologic folates. Approximately 35% of MTX is bound to plasma proteins and may be displaced from plasma albumin by a number of drugs, including sulfonamides, salicylates, tetracycline, chloramphenicol, and phenytoin. It is metabolized minimally and once absorbed, from 50% of a lower dose to 90% of a greater dose, is excreted unchanged in the urine within 48 hours. Administration of reduced folates, such as 5-formyltetrahydrofolate (Leucovorin; LV), after high-dose MTX therapy can prevent toxicity to the BM and GI epithelium. LV is converted intracellularly to reduced folates that compete with the polyglutamates of both MTX and dihydrofolate to overcome the inhibition of TS and de novo purine synthesis. In addition, MTX and reduced folates compete for transport into cells and for subsequent intracellular polyglutamation. The portion of each dose of methotrexate that normally is excreted rapidly gains access to the urine by a combination of glomerular filtration and active tubular secretion. Therefore, the concurrent use of drugs that reduce renal blood flow (e.g., nonsteroidal anti-inflammatory drugs), that are nephrotoxic (e.g., cisplatin), or that are weak organic acids (e.g., ASA or piperacillin) can delay drug excretion and lead to severe myelosuppression. MTX is entrapped in cells as polyglutamates for long periods, e.g., for weeks in the kidneys and for months in the liver. Third body spaces, such as pleural or peritoneal cavities, when expanded can act as a site of storage and release methotrexate with resultant prolonged elevation of plasma concentrations and more severe toxicity.

c. **Toxicity:** LV can reverse the immediate cytotoxic effects of MTX; generally, 1 mg LV is given for each 1 mg MTX.
1. Dose-limiting: Myelosuppression, stomatitis (may be preventable by sucking ice during the injection), and renal dysfunction (especially in patients with dehydration or pre-existing renal dysfunction)
2. High dose regimens: Nausea, vomiting, renal tubular necrosis, and cortical blindness. In previously irradiated areas, additional toxicities are encountered including skin erythema, pulmonary fibrosis, transverse myelitis, and cerebritis

3. Chronic therapy: Patients receiving chronic MTX therapy also can get hepatic cirrhosis (subclinical and reversible hepatic dysfunction occurs with short-term intermittent therapy) and osteoporosis (in children)

Pyrimidine Analogs

Fluorouracil (5-FU)[27]

a. **Indications:** Carcinomas of the breast, stomach, pancreas, colon, rectum
b. **Pharmacology**
1. Mechanism of action: 5-FU undergoes conversion to 5-fluorouridine-5′-monophosphate (5-F-UMP or 5-F-uridylate) by either reacting directly with 5′-phosphoribosyl-1-pyrophosphate (PRPP) in the salvage pathway for purines or first being converted to 5-fluorouridine and then monophosphorylated in the salvage pathway for pyrimidines (5-F-UMP may be phosphorylated to the nucleoside triphosphate 5-F-UTP and then incorporated into RNA where it may have an inhibitory effect). Subsequently, 5-F-UMP is phosphorylated to the nucleoside diphosphate 5-F-UDP, which is then reduced by NDP reductase to the deoxynucleoside diphosphate 5-F-dUMP, which is eventually dephosphorylated to the deoxynucleoside monophosphate 5-F-dUMP. 5-F-dUMP is the critical form of the drug that reacts with thymidylate synthase. The fluorine atom blocks the transfer of a methylene group to the pyrimidine ring from N^5,N^{10}-methylenetetrahydrofolate. LV enhances 5-FU cytotoxicity by stabilizing the covalent ternary complex of thymidylate synthase and 5-F-dUMP. The mechanism of "thymineless death" is purportedly secondary to dUMP accumulation and eventually formation of dUTP, which can be used by DNA polymerase with the same efficiency as for dTTP. Uracil in DNA is excised rapidly by uracil glycosylate leaving an apyrimidinic site. During repair of apyrimidinic sites, in the presence of unbalanced dUTP/dTTP ratios, uracil is likely to be reinserted causing a futile cycle of excision, repair, and reinsertion, leading to DNA strand breakage and ultimately cell death.
2. Metabolism: 5-FU is administered parenterally, because absorption after ingestion is unpredictable and incomplete. 5-FU is inactivated by reduction of the pyrimidine ring by dihydrouracil dehydrogenase, which is found in the liver, intestinal mucosa, and other tissues. The product of this reaction, 5-F-5,6-dihydrouracil, is ultimately degraded to α-F-β-alanine plus CO_2 in the pyrimidine degradation pathway. The primary route of elimination of this drug is therefore respiratory (as CO_2). Dosage does not have to be modified in patients with hepatic dysfunction, presumably because of degradation of the drug at extrahepatic sites. 5-FU rapidly enters all tissues, including spinal fluid and malignant effusions.

c. **Toxicity:** Toxicity is more common in patients with inherited deficiency of dihydrouracil dehydrogenase.

1. Dose-limiting: Myelosuppression (more common with rapid injection), mucositis, and diarrhea (more common with 5-day infusion; diarrhea may be cholera-like with high doses of LV).

Cytarabine (Ara-C)[28]

a. **Indications:** Leukemia: AML, ALL, CML (blast phase), meningeal (prevention and treatment; intrathecal administration). Lymphomas. Carcinomatous meningitis.
b. **Pharmacology**
   1. Mechanism of action: Cytarabine (1-β-D-arabinofuranosylcytosine) is an analog of 2′-deoxycytidine with the 2′-hydroxyl in position trans to the 3′-hydroxyl of the sugar. The 2′-hydroxyl causes steric hindrance to the rotation of the pyrimidine base around the nucleosidic bond, thus the bases of the polyarabinonucleotides cannot stack normally. As with most purine and pyrimidine antimetabolites, Ara-C must be "activated" to the 5′-monophosphate nucleotide (AraCMP), in this case catalyzed by deoxycytidine kinase. AraCMP can then react with appropriate nucleotide kinases to form the diphosphate and triphosphate nucleotides (AraCDP and AraCTP). Accumulation of AraCTP causes potent inhibition of DNA synthesis in many cells. The incorporation of about 5 molecules of AraC per 10^4 bases in DNA decreases cellular clonogenicity by about 50%. Thus inhibition of DNA synthesis by AraC without concomitant inhibition of protein and RNA syntheses can result in "unbalanced growth"—i.e., marked increases in cellular volume and in cellular death.
   2. Metabolism: AraC and AraCMP are converted to nontoxic metabolites AraU and Ara-UMP by deoxycytidine deaminase and deoxycytidylate deaminase, respectively, whereas other catabolic enzymes like 5′-nucleotidase affect Ara-C metabolite levels. When compared with other cell types, lymphocytes have high levels of deoxycytidine kinase, for which the purine deoxyribonucleosides are also substrates, and low levels of 5′-nucleotidase. The appreciation of these pathways has prompted the development of 3 antilymphocyte agents that are all purine analogs: 2′-chlorodeoxyadenosine (2CDA; Cladribine), 2′-fluoroadenine-arabinoside-5′-monophosphate (Fludarabine), and 2′-deoxycoformycin (Pentostatin).
c. **Toxicity**
   1. Dose-limiting: Myelosuppression (nadir is expected in 5–7 days and recovery in 2–3 weeks).

Gemcitabine (Gemzar)[29]

a. **Indications:** Pancreatic adenocarcinoma and non–small cell lung cancer. Also, carcinoma of the urinary bladder.
b. **Pharmacology**
   1. Mechanism: Gemcitabine (2′,2′-difluorodeoxycytidine; dFdC) is a 2′-deoxycytidine in which the deoxy-cytidine moiety contains 2 fluorine atoms at the 2′-position. It is metabolized by the same salvage enzyme pathways as AraC, i.e., it is phosphorylated by deoxycytidine kinase to dFdCMP and subsequently by monophosphate and diphosphate kinases to dFCDP and dFCTP, respectively. dFdCDP is an inhibitor of ribonucleotide reductase and thus decreases the pools of dATP, dCTP, dGTP, and dTTP. Depletion of dCTP as a consequence of ribonucleotide reductase inhibition leads to decreased feedback inhibition of deoxycytidine kinase and increased phosphorylation of dFdC. DFdCTP competes with dCTP for incorporation into DNA, by DNA polymerase, and depletion of dCTP favors incorporation dFdCTP. DNA polymerase ε is unable to remove the incorporated dFdCTP and repair the DNA strands. Thus inhibition of DNA synthesis may result from both perturbations of deoxyribonucleotide pools and inhibition of DNA synthesis.
   2. Metabolism: dFdC undergoes deamination to an inactive uracil metabolite that is excreted through the kidneys. As is true for many other antimetabolites, the volume of distribution of dFdC is significantly affected by the duration of its infusion.
c. **Toxicity**
   1. Dose-limiting: Myelosuppression
   2. Common: Edema/peripheral edema, fever, proteinuria, skin rash, increased liver function tests, nausea and vomiting.
   3. Occasional: Bronchospasm, cardiovascular effects, and cerebrovascular accident
   4. Rare: Alopecia, constipation or diarrhea, and stomatitis
d. **Administration:** Gemcitabine is supplied as 200-mg or 1-g single-dose vial, respectively. Dose modifications are required for myelosuppression. The usual dose in pancreatic cancer is 1000 mg/m^2 as an intravenous bolus weekly for up to 7 weeks, followed by a week of rest before another cycle is begun.

Purine Analogues

6-Thiopurines[30–32]

a. **Indications:** Acute leukemia.
b. **Pharmacology**
   1. Mechanism: 6-Mercaptopurine (6-MP) and 6-thioguanine (6-TG) are together called the 6-thiopurine analogues because they have a single substitution of a thiol group in place of the keto group on carbon 6 of the purine ring. 6-MP and 6-TG are structural analogues of hypoxanthine and guanine, respectively. Both of them are excellent substrates for hypoxanthine-guanine phosphoribosyltransferase (HGPRT; salvage pathway for purine nucleotides inosine monophosphate and guanosine monophosphate) and are converted to the ribonucleotides 6-thioguanosine-5′-monophosphate (6-thioGMP) and 6-thioinosine-5′-monophosphate (T-IMP). Because T-IMP is a poor substrate for guanyl kinase, the enzyme

that converts GMP to GDP, T-IMP accumulates intracellularly. The accumulation of T-IMP may inhibit several vital metabolic reactions in the de novo pathway of purine synthesis, e.g., the oxidation of inosinate (IMP) to xanthylate (XMP). Conversely, 6-thioGMP is slowly converted by guanyl kinase to 6-thioGDP and 6-thioGTP, which gets incorporated into DNA causing DNA synthesis inhibition. Both 6-thioGMP and I-IMP can cause "pseudofeedback inhibition" of the first committed step in the de novo purine biosynthesis pathway. Inhibitors of de novo purine biosynthesis, such as MTX, are synergistic with 6-thiopurines because the MTX-induced block expands the PPRP required for 6-thiopurine activation in the purine salvage pathway.

2. Metabolism: They are degraded largely by xanthine oxidase in the liver to 6-thiouric acid, an inactive metabolite. Allopurinol, a xanthine oxidase inhibitor, increases the toxicity without apparent improvement in the therapeutic index. The polymorphic enzyme thiopurine methyltransferase (TPMT) plays a major role in 6-MP inactivation.[30] Approximately 90% of patients have "high" TPMT activity, 10% are intermediate, and 1/300 are deficient (and at risk of severe toxicity with normal doses).

c. Toxicity
1. Dose-limiting: Myelosuppression and gastrointestinal toxicity
2. Common: Reversible cholestasis
3. Rare: Stomatitis, dermatitis, fever, hematuria, Budd-Chiari-like syndrome. and hepatic necrosis

d. Administration: Mercaptopurine is supplied as 50-mg tablets, whereas thioguanine is a 40-mg tablet. The dose of either drug must be reduced with impaired liver function and coadministration of allopurinol or hepatotoxic drugs. A typical dose is: (i) 6-MP: 70 to 100 mg/m^2 orally daily until patient responds or toxic effects are seen; then adjust for maintenance therapy; (ii) 6-TG: 100 mg/m^2 orally twice daily for 5 days or 2 to 3 mg/kg orally daily until toxic effects are seen.

Pentostatin (2-deoxycoformycin, dCF)[33]

a. Indications: Hairy cell leukemia; possibly cutaneous T-cell lymphoma.
b. Pharmacology
1. Mechanism: As a natural product derived from Streptomyces, Pentostatin structurally resembles the transition state of adenosine as it is hydrolyzed by adenosine deaminase (ADA) in the purine nucleotide degradation pathway. As a result, it is a potent inhibitor of ADA, the greatest activity of which is found in cells of the lymphoid system. T cells have greater ADA activity than B cells, and T-cell malignancies have greater activity than B-cell malignancies. The cytotoxicity that results from prevention of catabolism of adenosine or deoxyadenosine is thought to be caused by increased intracellular levels of dATP, which can block DNA synthesis through inhibition of ribonucleotide reductase.

2. Metabolism: The majority of dCF is excreted unchanged in the urine.
c. Toxicity
1. Dose-limiting: Myelosuppression.
2. Common: Immunosuppression, nausea and vomiting, diarrhea, altered taste, fatigue, and fever
3. Occasional: Chills, myalgias, arthralgias, abnormal liver function tests, keratoconjunctivitis, photophobia, and renal failure
4. Rare: Hepatitis, pulmonary infiltrates, and pulmonary insufficiency
d. Administration: The drug is supplied in 10-mg vials. A typical dose is 4 mg/m^2 IV infusion over 20 minutes with 1 or 2 L hydration every 2 weeks. Dosing is reduced for renal impairment.

Cladribine (2-chloro-2-deoxyadenosine; 2-CdA)[34]

a. Indications: Hairy cell leukemia, indolent lymphomas, chronic lymphocytic leukemia, mycosis fungoides
b. Pharmacology
1. Mechanism: Antimetabolite. It blocks adenosine deaminase and inhibits RNA synthesis.
2. Metabolism: Plasma half-life is 7 hours
c. Toxicity
1. Dose-limiting: Myelosuppression
2. Common: Nausea, skin reactions at injection site, fever, and chills
3. Occasional: Headache and fatigue
4. Rare: Neurotoxicity and pancreatitis
d. Administration: The drug is supplied in 20-mg vials. Doses need to be modified with hematologic toxicity. A typical dose is either 0.10 mg/kg per day IV for 7 days or 0.14 mg/kg per day IV over 2 hours for 5 days.

Fludarabine (2-fluoroadenine arabinoside; Fludara)[35]

a. Indications: Chronic lymphocytic leukemia and low-grade lymphoma
b. Pharmacology
1. Mechanism: Its active metabolite, 2-fluoro-ara-A appears to inhibit DNA primase, DNA polymerase alpha, and ribonucleotide reductase
2. Metabolism: The plasma half-life is 9 to 10 hours; metabolites are excreted primarily in the urine.
c. Toxicity
1. Dose-limiting: Myelosuppression
2. Common: Nausea and vomiting
3. Occasional: Alopecia and the tumor lysis syndrome
4. Rare: Stomatitis, diarrhea, dermatitis, neurotoxicity, and chest pain
d. Administration: Drug is supplied as a 50-mg vial. A typical dose is 25 mg/m^2 IV over 30 minutes daily for 5 consecutive days every 4 weeks. Doses need to be adjusted for patients with renal insufficiency.

Natural Products

Vinca Alkaloids[36–38]

GENERAL MECHANISM OF ACTION

Vinca alkaloids bind to tubulin and block its ability to polymerize into microtubules. Through disruption of the microtubules of the mitotic apparatus, cell division is arrested in metaphase. The inability to segregate chromosomes correctly during mitosis presumably leads to cell death. In addition to the formation of mitotic spindles, microtubules are involved in many other cellular functions, e.g., axonal transport of subcellular organelles, which explains some of the other effects of vinca alkaloids (colchicine, taxanes, and podophyllotoxin also bind to tubulin but apparently at a different site from that bound by the vinca alkaloids).

Vinblastine (VBL)

a. **Indications:** Lymphomas, testicular carcinomas, a variety of other tumors, histiocytosis
b. **Pharmacology**
   1. Mechanism: It arrests cells at the G_2-M interface of the cell cycle.
   2. Metabolism: Vinblastine is highly bound to plasma proteins and to formed blood elements, especially platelets. It is metabolized in the liver and excreted in bile.
c. **Toxicity**
   1. Dose-limiting: Neutropenia
   2. Common: Cramps or severe pain in jaw, pharynx, back or limbs after injection; local vesicant if extravasated
   3. Occasional: Thrombocytopenia, anemia.
   4. Rare: Nausea, vomiting, diarrhea, mucositis, abdominal cramps, acute interstitial pneumonitis, especially when administered with mitomycin C; ischemic cardiotoxicity
d. **Administration:** Drug is supplied in 10-mg vials. Dose needs to be modified in patients with liver dysfunction. A typical dose is 5 mg/m² IV every 1 or 2 weeks; greater doses at 3-week intervals are used for testicular carcinomas. As a continuous infusion, 1.7 to 2 mg/m² per day is given over a 96-hour period.

Vincristine (VCR)

a. **Indications:** A wide variety of malignancies
b. **Pharmacology:** Same as vinblastine
c. **Toxicity:** A dose-dependent peripheral neuropathy universally develops. It usually reverses within several months. Jaw, throat, or anterior thigh pain occurring within hours of injection disappears within days and usually does not recur.
   1. Dose-limiting: Severe paresthesias, ataxia, foot drop (slapping gait), muscle wasting, cranial nerve palsies, paralytic ileus, obstipation, abdominal pain, optic atrophy, cortical blindness, seizures

   2. Common: Tissue necrosis if extravasated, alopecia
   3. Occasional: Mild leukopenia, SIADH
   4. Rare: Nausea, vomiting, pancreatitis, fever
d. **Administration:** Patients receiving vincristine should be given bulk laxatives routinely. Drug is supplied in 1-, 2-, and 5-mg vials. Dose needs to be modified in patients with liver dysfunction. A typical dose is 1.0 to 1.4 mg/m² IV every 1 to 4 weeks; continuous infusion regimens involve 0.5 mg/m² per day for 4 days.

Vinorelbine (VRL; Navelbine)

a. **Indications:** Non–small cell lung cancer; metastatic breast cancer
b. **Pharmacology:** Same as vinblastine
c. **Toxicity**
   1. Dose-limiting: Myelosuppression
   2. Occasional: Chest pain, mild to moderate peripheral neuropathy, pulmonary reactions, stomatitis
   3. Rare: Hemorrhagic cystitis, skin rash, anorexia, constipation
d. **Administration:** Drug is supplied in 1- and 5-mL vials. Dose modification is required with hematologic toxicity or hepatic insufficiency. A typical dose is 30 mg/m² once a week as a single agent. The same dose is used in combination therapy with cisplatin.

Epipodophyllotoxins[39,40]

GENERAL MECHANISM OF ACTION

Unlike podophyllotoxin, these agents do not cause mitotic arrest by binding to microtubules. Rather, at low concentrations they block cells at the S-G_2 interface of the cell cycle and at greater concentrations they cause G_2 arrest. They interact with the topoisomerase II/DNA complex (topoisomerase II or topotecan II is a chromatin scaffold protein that during replication projects from the scaffold and causes DNA double-strand breaks moving the cleaved ends apart). This interaction prevents the resealing of the topotecan II–mediated DNA double-strand breaks. These breaks result in cell death only if DNA synthesis is ongoing.

Etoposide (VP-16)

a. **Indications:** Testicular carcinoma, lung cancer, lymphoma, and a variety of other malignancies
b. **Pharmacology**
   1. Mechanism: As described earlier
   2. Metabolism: VP-16 is highly bound (~95%) to plasma proteins and is metabolized in the liver by cytochrome P450 3A4.
c. **Toxicity**
   1. Dose-limiting: Neutropenia
   2. Common: Nausea and vomiting (with oral dosing, but uncommon with intravenous dosing), alopecia, hypotension if rapidly infused

3. Occasional: Anemia, thrombocytopenia, pain at injection site, phlebitis, abnormal liver function tests, peripheral neuropathy.
4. Rare: Stomatitis, dysphagia, diarrhea, constipation, parotiditis, rash, radiation recall reaction, hyperpigmentation, anaphylaxis, somnolence, vertigo, and transient cortical blindness
d. **Administration:** Drug is supplied as 50-mg capsules and 100-mg vials. Dose modification is required for renal insufficiency. Typical doses are: 50 mg/m^2 orally daily for 21 days or 50 to 120 mg/m^2 IV daily for 3 to 5 days.

Teniposide (VM-26)

a. **Indications:** Acute lymphoblastic leukemia
b. **Pharmacology**
1. Mechanism: As described earlier
2. Metabolism: Virtually all (>97%) of the drug is protein bound in plasma. Systemic metabolism is significant but metabolites have not been identified. Renal excretion is only a small fraction of its clearance (<10%).
c. **Toxicity**
1. Dose-limiting: Neutropenia
2. Common: Thrombocytopenia, hypotension with too rapid an infusion
3. Occasional: Nausea and vomiting, alopecia, abnormal liver function tests, phlebitis
4. Rare: Diarrhea, stomatitis, anaphylaxis, azotemia, fever, paresthesias, seizures
d. **Administration:** The drug is administered by slow intravenous infusion over at least 30 minutes. Drug is supplied as a 50-mg vial. A typical dose is 20 to 60 mg/m^2 per day for 5 days or 100 mg/m^2 once or twice weekly.

Enzymes

L-Asparaginase (Elspar; Kidrolase)[41]

a. **Indications:** Acute lymphocytic leukemia
b. **Pharmacology**
1. Mechanism: Most healthy tissues synthesize L-asparagine in amounts sufficient for protein synthesis. Certain neoplastic tissues, including acute lymphocytic leukemic cells, requires an exogenous source of this amino acid. L-Asparaginase deprives these cells of the asparagine available from extracellular fluid by catalyzing the hydrolysis of asparagine to aspartic acid and ammonia. There may be striking synergistic effects when L-asparaginase is used in combination with drugs such as methotrexate or cytarabine. The sequence of the administration is crucial, e.g., synergistic cytotoxicity is seen when methotrexate is administered before L-asparaginase. It appears to be cell cycle–specific for the G$_1$ phase of cell division.
2. Metabolism: Unknown; only trace amounts are recovered in the urine
c. **Toxicity**

1. Dose-limiting: Allergic reactions usually develop within 1 hour of dosing and are most likely to occur after several doses are given, particularly if the last dose was given more than 1 month previously and if the drug is administered IV rather than IM. Patients who respond to E. coli asparaginase but develop allergic reactions may be treated relatively safely with another source of the enzyme.
2. Common: Encephalopathy occurs in 25% to 50% of patients. Lethargy, somnolence, and confusion tend to occur within the first few days of therapy and reverse after completion of therapy; encephalopathy is rarely a cause for discontinuing treatment. Hemorrhagic and thrombotic CNS events occur later and are associated with the induced imbalances in the coagulation and fibrinolytic systems. Nausea, anorexia, and vomiting; hepatitis, pancreatitis, coagulation defects (associated with decreased synthesis of clotting factors, especially fibrinogen and antithrombin III), prerenal azotemia, hyperglycemia.
3. Rare: Myelosuppression, diarrhea, severe renal failure, hyperthermia
d. **Administration:** Administer a small (2-unit) intradermal test dose to check for hypersensitivity. Epinephrine (1 mg, 1:1000), hydrocortisone (100 mg), and diphenhydramine (50 mg) should be readily available to treat anaphylaxis each time the drug is given. Drug is supplied as 10,000-U vials. Dose modification is required for hepatic dysfunction or pancreatitis. Drug is usually administered in combination with vincristine and prednisone at a dose of 6000 U/m^2 IM three times weekly for nine doses.

Antibiotics

General Mechanism of Action

Antitumor antibiotics generally are drugs derived from micro-organisms. They usually are not cell cycle–specific agents, and they are especially useful in slow-growing tumors with low growth fractions.

Actinomycin D (Dactinomycin)

a. **Indications:** Ewing sarcoma, testicular carcinoma, Wilms' tumor, rhabdomyosarcoma, and trophoblastic tumors
b. **Pharmacology**
1. Mechanism: Actinomycin D intercalates between base pairs and inhibits DNA-dependent RNA synthesis.
2. Metabolism: It is extensively bound to tissues resulting in long (36 hours) half-life in plasma and tissue. The drug is excreted unchanged in bile and urine.
c. **Toxicity**
1. Dose-limiting: Myelosuppression
2. Common: Nausea and vomiting, alopecia, acne, erythema, desquamation, hyperpigmentation, radiation recall reaction (i.e., darkening of skin if patient has received previous radiation therapy). It is a vesicant that can cause necrosis if extravasated.

3. Occasional: Stomatitis, cheilitis, glossitis, proctitis, diarrhea, vitamin K antagonism
4. Rare: Hepatitis, anaphylaxis, hepatoxicity including ascites, hepatomegaly, hyperuricemia (joint pain; lower back or side pain), hypocalcemia, and lethargy

d. **Administration:** Premedication with antiemetics and extravasation precautions are of utmost importance. Drug is supplied as a 0.5-mg vial. Dose modification is required in the presence of renal or hepatic functional impairment. Typical doses are: (i) 0.25 to 0.60 mg/m^2 IV daily for 5 days every 3 to 4 weeks, or (ii) 1 to 2 mg/m^2 IV single dose every 3 to 4 weeks.

Daunorubicin[42]

a. **Indications:** ALL or AML
b. **Pharmacology**
   1. Mechanism: Daunorubicin is an anthracycline glycoside. It is most active in the S phase of cell division, but it is not cell cycle phase–specific. Its exact mechanism of antineoplastic action is unknown but may involve binding to DNA by intercalation between base pairs and inhibition of DNA and RNA synthesis by template disordering and steric obstruction.
   2. Metabolism: It is rapidly biotransformed in the liver to produce an active metabolite, daunorubicinol. Further metabolism is hepatic and an estimated 40% is eliminated by biliary excretion.
c. **Toxicity**
   1. Dose-limiting: Myelosuppression, esophagitis, or stomatitis. Cardiotoxicity in the form of congestive heart failure (irregular heart beat, shortness of breath, swelling of feet and lower legs) can also occur. The incidence of cardiotoxicity is more frequent in adults receiving a total cumulative dosage of more than 550 mg/m^2 of body surface (450 mg/m^2 in patients who have received previous chest irradiation), in the elderly, and in patients with a history of cardiac disease or mediastinal radiation. It usually appears within 1 to 6 months after initiation of therapy. It may develop suddenly and may not be detected by routine electrocardiogram (ECG). It may be irreversible and fatal but responds to treatment if detected early.
   2. Common: Hyperuricemia, uric acid nephropathy, nausea and vomiting, alopecia and reddish urine (reddish urine usually clears within 48 hours)
   3. Occasional: Allergic reactions and cardiotoxicity in the form of pericarditis-myocarditis
   4. Rare: Radiation recall reaction, diarrhea
d. **Administration:** It is recommended that patients be hospitalized during initial treatment. Care must be taken to avoid extravasation during intravenous administration. Drug is supplied as a 20-mg vial. The maximum recommended total lifetime dosage is 550 mg/m^2 of body surface or 450 mg/m^2 of body surface in patients who have received previous chest irradiation (to reduce risk for cardiotoxicity). Typical doses are: (i) ALL: 45 mg/m^2 of body surface on Days 1, 2, and 3 of a 32-day course in combination with vincristine, prednisone, and asparaginase. (ii) AML: 45 mg/m^2 of body surface on Days 1, 2,

and 3 of the first course and Days 1 and 2 of the second course in combination with cytarabine.

Doxorubicin (adriamycin)[42,43]

a. **Indications:** ALL, AML, breast cancer, gastric cancer, small cell lung cancer, epithelial ovarian cancer, thyroid cancer, neuroblastoma, Wilms' tumor, or bladder carcinoma
b. **Pharmacology**
   1. Mechanism: Doxorubicin is an anthracycline glycoside. It is cell cycle–specific for the S phase of cell division. Its mechanism of action may involve binding to DNA by intercalation between base pairs and inhibition of DNA and RNA synthesis by template disordering and steric obstruction. Other possible mechanisms of action may include binding to cell membrane lipids and interacting with topoisomerase II to form DNA-cleavable complexes.
   2. Metabolism: It is biotransformed rapidly in the liver to produce an active metabolite doxorubicinol. The enzymatic reduction of doxorubicin by oxidases, reductases, and dehydrogenases results in the production of free radicals, which may contribute to cardiotoxicity.
   3. Excretion: An estimated 40% of the drug is excreted unchanged in the bile over 5 days. An estimated 5% to 12% of doxorubicin and metabolites appear in urine over 5 days imparting a red tinge to the urine.
c. **Toxicity**
   1. Dose-limiting: Myelosuppression and cardiomyopathy are the two major toxicities of adriamycin. Cardiomyopathy with congestive heart failure is more frequent in patients receiving total dosages greater than 550 mg/m^2 of body surface area (400 mg/m^2 of body surface area in patients who have previously received chest irradiation or medication increasing cardiotoxicity, and in patients with a history of cardiac disease or mediastinal radiation). Cardiotoxicity usually appears within 1 to 6 months after initiation of therapy. Cardiomyopathy has been reported to be associated with persistent voltage reduction of the QRS complex, systolic interval prolongation, and reduction of ejection fraction. It may develop suddenly and may not be detected on routine ECG. It may be irreversible and fatal but responds to treatment if detected early. Monitoring the left ventricular ejection fraction with radionuclide techniques is mandatory particularly when the cumulative dose exceeds 300 mg/m^2. Current data suggest that when the maximum cumulative dose has been reached the drug can never be safely resumed. The drug should be discontinued if any of the following occurs: congestive heart failure, ECG changes, decreased left ventricular ejection fraction to less than 50% or at least by 10%.
   2. Common: Alopecia (in nearly 100% of patients when administered as a bolus every 3–4 weeks, but minimal when the dose is divided and given weekly), nausea and vomiting, stomatitis, and radiation recall reaction. Extravasation of the drug results in severe ulceration and necrosis

3. Occasional: Diarrhea, hyperpigmentation of nail beds and dermal creases, facial flushing, conjunctivitis, lacrimation, and red urine
4. Rare: Anaphylaxis, activation of fibrinolysis, fever, chills

d. **Administration:** The drug must be slowly pushed through a running intravenous line over 2 to 5 minutes or continuously infused through a central venous line. Rapid infusion may induce serious arrhythmias, flushing, or syncope.. The drug is supplied as 10-, 20-, 50-, 100-, and 150-mg vials. The risk for congestive heart failure is estimated to be 1% to 2% at a total cumulative dosage of 300 mg/m^2 of body surface area, 2% to 3% at a total cumulative dosage of 400 mg/m^2 of body surface area, 5% to 8% at a total cumulative dosage of 450 mg/m^2 and 6% to 20% at a total cumulative dosage of 500 mg/m^2. This toxicity may develop at lower cumulative dosages in patients who have previously received chest irradiation, patients who have received medications increasing cardiotoxicity, or patients with pre-existing heart disease. Doxorubicin should not be given to patients with congestive heart failure from any cause. Typical doses are: (i) 50 to 75 mg/m^2 intravenous bolus or continuous infusion over 2 to 4 days every 3 to 4 weeks; (ii) 30 mg/m^2 IV daily for 3 days every 3 to 4 weeks; (iii) 10 to 20 mg/m^2 IV weekly.

Idarubicin (Idamycin)/Epirubicin (Ellence)[44,45]

a. **Indications:** AML
b. **Pharmacology:** Idarubicin and epirubicin are anthracycline glycosides. They may intercalate between DNA strands, inhibit DNA synthesis, interact with RNA polymerases, and inhibit topoisomerase II. It is more lipophilic than other anthracycline antibiotics.
c. **Toxicity:** Similar to doxorubicin
d. **Administration:** Like doxorubicin, a slow intravenous injection over 5 minutes using extravasation precautions is required. Idarubicin is supplied as 5- and 10-mg vials and epirubicin as 50- and 200-mg vials. A typical dose of idarubicin is 12 mg/m^2 IV daily for 3 days and epirubicin 100 mg/m^2 every 21 days.

Bleomycin (Blenoxane)

a. **Indications:** Head and neck carcinoma, laryngeal carcinoma, vulvar carcinoma or testicular carcinoma, Hodgkin lymphoma, and non–Hodgkin lymphomas
b. **Pharmacology**
   1. Mechanism: Although bleomycin is effective against both cycling and noncycling cells, it seems to be most effective in the G$_2$ phase of cell division. It causes DNA strand cleavage by free radicals and inhibits DNA repair by marked inhibition of DNA ligase.
   2. Metabolism: Biotransformation is probably by enzymatic degradation in tissues. It is not known if any metabolites are active. Both free drug and metabolic products are excreted in the urine.

c. **Toxicity**
   1. Dose-limiting:
   i. Fever and chills occur in approximately 20% to 60% of patients, usually 3 to 6 hours after administration; they last 4 to 12 hours and become less frequent with continued use. An unusual idiosyncratic reaction (confusion, faintness, fever and chills, wheezing) occurs in approximately 1% of treated patients, but in approximately 1% to 6% of patients with lymphoma! If not promptly treated, it may progress to sweating, dehydration, hypotension, and renal failure or cardiorespiratory collapse. It usually occurs at doses of 25 U/m^2 or greater. This reaction may be immediate or delayed by several hours and occurs after the first or second dose.
   ii. Pulmonary toxicity occurs in 10% to 40% of treated patients, usually 4 to 10 weeks after initiation of treatment; approximately 1% of treated patients have died of pulmonary fibrosis. Pulmonary toxicity is age- and dose-related, occurring most frequently in patients older than 70 years or patients receiving a total dose of greater than 400 units (although it has been reported with doses as low as 20–60 units). It may be irreversible and fatal; however, there is some evidence that in patients who survive, symptoms and pulmonary function parameters return to normal in approximately 2 years. Pulmonary toxicity occurs at lower doses in patients who have received other antineoplastics or thoracic irradiation; mortality rates may be as high as 10% in patients who have received pulmonary irradiation. A low-dose allergic pneumonitis has also been reported. The earliest signs of pulmonary toxicity are a decrease in diffusion capacity and fine rales. On chest radiograph, pneumonitis is seen as nonspecific patchy opacities, usually in the lower lung fields. Pulmonary function tests show a decrease in total lung volume and a decrease in vital capacity.
   2. Common: Sensitizes tumor and healthy tissues to radiation. Dermatologic abnormalities occur frequently and include: hyperpigmentation of skin stretch areas (e.g., knuckles, elbows); hardening tenderness or loss of fingernails; hyperkeratosis of palms and fingers, scleroderma-like changes; skin tenderness, pruritus or urticaria, erythroderma, desquamation, and alopecia.
   3. Occasional: Nausea, vomiting, mild reversible myelosuppression, Raynaud's phenomenon, phlebitis, and pain at the injection site
d. **Administration:** A 2-unit test dose is given before the first treatment followed by a 1- to 2-hour observation period. Drug is supplied as a 15-unit vial. It is recommended that the dosage of bleomycin be reduced in patients with renal function impairment (creatinine clearance <25 to 35 mL/min). It is also recommended that equipment and medications (including epinephrine, oxygen, diphenhydramine, and intravenous corticosteroids) necessary for treatment of a possible anaphylactic reaction be readily available at each administration of bleomycin. The drug should not be given to patients with symptomatic chronic obstructive lung disease. It must be discontinued in patients who have erythroderma (contin-

ued treatment may lead to fatal exfoliative dermatitis). The drug must also be discontinued if there are symptoms or signs of interstitial lung disease. Routine pulmonary functions are generally not helpful; some authorities recommend monitoring carbon monoxide diffusing capacity. Avoid cumulative dosage of greater than 400 units; some physicians limit the total dosage to 300 units. Typical doses include: (i) 10 to 20 U/m^2 IM, IV, or subcutaneously once or twice weekly; (ii) 15 to 20 U/m^2 daily for 3 to 7 days by continuous infusion; or (iii) 60 U/m^2 dissolved in 100 mL normal saline for intracavitary therapy.

Camptothecin Analogues[46,47]

General Mechanism of Action

The two camptothecin analogues approved for clinical use are topotecan and irinotecan. They contain the camptothecin pentacyclic structure with a closed lactone ring moiety in the E ring, which is essential for cytotoxicity. They both interact with topoisomerase I and prevent the resealing of the topotecan I–mediated, DNA, single-strand breaks. These strand breaks result in cell death only if DNA synthesis is ongoing—a division between the advancing replication fork and the drug-stabilized, single-strand break in DNA result in replication fork breakage and double-strand breaks in the DNA. Treatment of mammalian cells with topoisomerase I inhibitors induces inhibition of DNA synthesis, cell cycle arrest in G_2, and cell death by apoptosis. Drug-induced G_2 arrest has been associated with a failure to activate cdc2 kinase. Because the cytotoxicity associated with topotecan I interactive agents is highly dependent on DNA synthesis; any deregulation of cyclins, cell cycle–regulated kinases, or phosphatases may influence the cytotoxicity of topotecan I interactive agents.

Topotecan (Hycamtin)

a. **Indications:** Ovarian carcinoma, small cell lung carcinoma
b. **Pharmacology**
  1. Mechanism: Topotecan I inhibitor as outlined earlier.
  2. Metabolism: Topotecan undergoes reversible, pH-dependent hydrolysis of the active lactone moiety forming an open ring hydroxy acid, which is inactive. Neither the lactone nor the hydroxy acid form of topotecan is metabolized to a significant extent. Approximately 30% of the dose is eliminated through the kidneys and a lower percentage of the dose through the biliary route.
c. **Toxicity**
  1. Dose-limiting: Myelosuppression
  2. Common: Nausea or vomiting, anorexia, constipation or diarrhea, neurologic effects including muscle weakness or paresthesia
  3. Rare: Allergic reactions including anaphylactoid reactions
d. **Administration:** Drug is supplied in 4-mg vials and should only be administered IV. Dose modification is

required for patients with renal insufficiency. Doses include (i) ovarian carcinoma: 1.5 mg/m^2 daily for 5 consecutive days repeated every 21 days; (b) small cell lung carcinoma: 1.25 to 2 mg/m^2 daily for 5 consecutive days repeated every 21 days.

Irinotecan (Camptosar or CPT-11)

a. **Indications:** Colorectal carcinoma (metastatic)
b. **Pharmacology**
  1. Mechanism: Irinotecan and its active metabolite, SN-38, inhibit the action of topotecan I. The precise contribution of the metabolite to the activity of irinotecan in humans is not known because its protein binding is significantly greater and its area under the plasma concentration-time curve is much lower than those of irinotecan (although SN-38 is approximately 2 to 2000 times more potent than the parent compound in various in vitro toward cytotoxicity assays).
  2. Metabolism: Primarily hepatic. Up to 11% to 20% of a dose is excreted through the kidneys as unchanged irinotecan, whereas less than 1% of a dose is excreted as SN-38. The effect of hepatic or renal function impairment on elimination of irinotecan and its metabolites has not been formally studied.
c. **Toxicity**
  1. Dose-limiting: Myelosuppression, diarrhea possibly proceeded by abdominal cramping, sweating, or both
  2. Common: Dyspnea, nausea and vomiting, weakness, constipation
  3. Occasional: Abdominal bloating, flatulence, headache, indigestion, rhinitis, skin rash, flushing
d. **Administration:** It is recommended that irinotecan be administered to patients only under the supervision of a physician experienced in cancer chemotherapy and only by intravenous infusion, taking extravasation precautions. Drug is supplied as 40 mg/2 mL and 100 mg/5 mL single use vials. A typical dose is 100 mg/m^2 IV once a week for 4 weeks followed by a rest period of 2 weeks.

Taxanes[48–52]

General Mechanism of Action

The taxanes bind to tubulin polymers (microtubules) at binding sites that are distinct from exchangeable GTP, colchicine, podophyllotoxin, and vincalkaloids. Paclitaxel binds preferentially to the N-terminal 31 amino acids of the β-tubulin subunit. Docetaxel, which most likely shares the same tubulin-binding site as paclitaxel, appears to have a 1.9-fold greater affinity for this site. However, this difference might not translate into greater therapeutic index for docetaxel in the clinic as greater potency may also portend more severe toxicity at identical drug concentrations in vivo. Nevertheless, the results of both preclinical and clinical studies suggest that the taxanes may not be completely cross-resistant. Although the precise mechanism by which microtubule disturbances lead to apoptosis has not been determined, the taxanes interact with numerous substances including regulatory molecules and oncogenes that bind to the mitotic apparatus.

Paclitaxel (Taxol)

a. **Indications:** Ovarian carcinoma, breast carcinoma, Kaposi's sarcoma, non–small cell lung carcinoma
b. **Pharmacology**
   1. Mechanisms: Antimicrotubule agent as outlined earlier
   2. Metabolism: Taxol is almost totally protein bound and distributed well to body fluids (including effusions) with a plasma half-life of about 5 hours. It has substantial hepatic metabolism, biliary excretion, and fecal elimination.
c. **Toxicity**
   1. Dose-limiting: Neutropenia, particularly in patients who were previously heavily treated or who received cisplatin just prior to Taxol. Hypersensitivity (3%) is manifested by cutaneous flushing, hypotension, bronchospasm, urticaria, diaphoresis, pain, or angioedema. Reactions usually develop within 20 minutes of starting the treatment; 90% of hypersensitivity reactions develop after the first or second dose. Peripheral neuropathy occurs particularly in the higher dosage ($>170\,mg/m^2$) schedules and in patients with concomitant etiologies for peripheral neuropathy. The distribution is usually "stocking-glove" and consists of dysesthesias, paresthesias, and loss of proprioception.
   2. Common: Alopecia, thrombocytopenia, transient arthralgias and myalgias, and transient bradycardia (usually asymptomatic)
   3. Occasional: Nausea and vomiting, taste changes, mucositis, diarrhea; atrioventricular conduction defects, ventricular tachycardia, cardiac angina; skin necrosis when extravasated
   4. Rare: Paralytic ileus, generalized weakness, seizures, myocardial infarction
d. **Administration:** Taxol should be given before cisplatin, in combination regimens where both are administered. Patients who were previously treated may require support with granulocyte-colony stimulating factor. Cardiac monitoring is recommended for patients taking cardiac medications or with a history of cardiac disease. The drug is supplied in 30-mg vials and dose modifications are required for hematologic toxicity. A typical dose is 135 to $175\,mg/m^2$ infused over 3 to 24 hours.

Docetaxel (Taxotere)

a. **Indications:** Breast carcinoma
b. **Pharmacology:** As outlined for Paclitaxel
c. **Toxicity**
   1. Dose-limiting: Anemia and neutropenia, hypersensitivity reactions, edema and peripheral neuropathy are the severe, dose-limiting toxicities of docetaxel.

Edema usually begins in the lower extremities but may become generalized and lead to pleural effusions, pericardial effusions, or ascites (prophylactic corticosteroid administration decreases incidence and severity of this complication and increases the median cumulative dose at which moderate or severe edema occurs). Edema is caused by increased capillary permeability rather than hypoalbuminemia or cardiac, hepatic, or renal damage. Fluid retention is usually reversible after treatment is discontinued. Peripheral neuropathy can result in decreased dexterity or disturbances in gait, usually after cumulative dosages of $600\,mg/m^2$.
   2. Common: Mild cutaneous reactions, diarrhea, stomatitis
   3. Occasional: Arthralgias or myalgias, headache, infusion site reactions, nail discoloration, and vomiting
   4. Rare: Cardiovascular effects, including angina, arrhythmia, heart failure, hypertension
d. **Administration:** Docetaxel should be administered only under the supervision of a physician experienced in cancer chemotherapy. Pretreatment administration of an oral corticosteroid is recommended to decrease the frequency and severity and delay the onset of docetaxel-induced fluid retention. Pretreatment administration of an oral corticosteroid with or without antihistamines also reduces the severity of docetaxel-induced hypersensitivity reactions and cutaneous toxicity. Drug is supplied as 20 mg/0.5 mL vial and 80 mg/2 mL vial. Dose modification is required for patients in whom severe neutropenia develops. Docetaxel is not recommended for patients with hepatic dysfunction, because of the considerably greater risk for severe toxicity. A typical dose is 60 to 100 mg/m^2 IV administered as a 1-hour infusion every 3 weeks.

Miscellaneous

Platinum Coordination Complexes[53]

CISPLATIN (PLATINOL; PLATINOL-AQ)

a. **Indications:** Bladder carcinoma, ovarian carcinoma, testicular carcinoma. Cisplatin is used for a wide variety of malignancies such as breast, gastric, lung; however, these indications are not included in the U.S. product labeling.
b. **Pharmacology**
   1. Mechanism of action: Cisplatin resembles an alkylating agent. Although the exact mechanism of action is unknown, action is thought to be similar to that of the bifunctional alkylating agents. It is cell cycle phase nonspecific. Stimulation of the host immune system is also possible.
   2. Metabolism: Cisplatin is metabolized by rapid nonenzymatic conversion to inactive metabolites. It is eliminated up to 27% to 43% through the kidneys. (Platinum may be detected in tissues for 4 months or more after administration).

c. **Toxicity**

1. Dose-limiting: Renal insufficiency occurs in about 5% of patients with adequate hydration measures and in 25% to 45% without hydration measures. Nephrotoxicity (and perhaps ototoxicity) is increased by concurrent administration of nephrotoxic drugs such as aminoglycoside antibiotics, methotrexate, or amphotericin B. Peripheral sensory neuropathy develops after administration of 200 mg/m^2 and can become dose-limiting when the cumulative cisplatin dose exceeds 400 mg/m^2. Symptoms may progress after treatment is discontinued and include loss of proprioception and vibratory senses. Symptoms may resolve slowly after many months but are aggravated by further dosing. Ototoxicity with tinnitus and high-frequency hearing loss occurs in 5% of patients. Ototoxicity occurs more commonly in patients receiving doses more than 100 mg/m^2 by rapid infusion or high cumulative doses.

2. Severe nausea and vomiting occur in all treated patients and last more than 24 hours without use of effective preventative antiemetic regimens. Hypokalemia, hypomagnesia, and mild myelosuppression also occur.

3. Occasional: Alopecia, loss of taste, vein irritation, abnormal liver function tests, SIADH, hypophosphatemia, myalgias, and fever

4. Rare: Altered color perception and reversible focal encephalophyma that often causes cortical blindness; Raynaud phenomenon, bradycardia, bundle-branch block, congestive heart failure; anaphylaxis, and tetany

d. **Administration:** The drug is supplied as 10- and 50-mg vials. Renal function must return to normal before cisplatin can be given. Many physicians avoid using cisplatin when the creatinine clearance is less than 40 mL/min. Cisplatin is relatively contraindicated in patients with documented hearing impairment. Doses include: (i) 40 to 120 mg/m^2 or more IV every 3 to 4 weeks or (ii) 20 to 40 mg/m^2 IV daily for 3 to 5 days every 3 to 4 weeks. The principles of cisplatin administration are:

(a) Monitoring—serum creatinine, electrolytes, and magnesium and calcium levels should be measured daily during therapy.

(b) Antiemetics—patients should be given antiemetics such as ondansetron and dexamethasone before, during, and after cisplatin infusion.

(c) Hydration and diuresis is required when 40 mg/m^2 or more of cisplatin is given as a short infusion to maintain a urine output of 100 to 150 mL/hr before administration of the drug.

CARBOPLATIN (PARAPLATIN; PARAPLATIN-AQ)

a. **Indications:** Ovarian carcinoma; other indications such as endometrial or lung carcinoma are not included in the U.S. product labeling. Carboplatin may be an alternative to cisplatin when renal or neural toxicity are dose-limiting considerations.

b. **Pharmacology**

1. Mechanism: Similar to cisplatin. Cisplatin and carboplatin exhibit substantial clinical cross-resistance.

2. Metabolism: The plasma half-life of carboplatin is only 2 to 3 hours. It is excreted in the urine as unchanged drug (60%) and metabolites.

c. **Toxicity**

1. Dose-limiting: Myelosuppression, especially thrombocytopenia with cumulative suppression of erythropoiesis

2. Common: Nausea and vomiting (less severe than with cisplatin), pain at injection site

3. Occasional: Abnormal liver function test and azotemia

4. Rare: Alopecia, rash, flulike syndrome, hematuria, hyperamylasemia; peripheral neuropathy (especially in patients older than 65 years), hearing loss, optic neuritis

d. **Administration:** Drug is supplied as 50-, 150-, 450-mg vials. Dose modification is required for patients with renal insufficiency. Typical dosages include 300 to 400 mg/m^2 IV over 15 to 60 minutes every 4 weeks.

Anthracenedione

MITOXANTRONE (NOVANTRONE)

a. **Indications:** Advanced hormone-refractory prostate cancer, AML

b. **Pharmacology**

1. Mechanism of action: Mitoxantrone appears to be most active in the late S phase of cell division, but is not cycle phase specific. Although the exact mechanism of action is unknown, evidence seems to indicate involvement of 2FX binding to DNA by intercalation between base pairs and a nonintercalative electrostatic interaction resulting in inhibition of DNA and RNA synthesis. Mitoxantrone is in the anthracenedione class of compounds, which are analogues to the anthracyclines.

2. Metabolism: Mitoxantrone is metabolized in the liver and is excreted into bile and urine as metabolites and unchanged drug.

c. **Toxicity:** Compared with the anthracyclines, mitoxantrone is associated with less cardiotoxicity and less nausea and vomiting.

1. Dose-limiting: BM suppression

2. Common: Mild nausea and vomiting, mucositis; alopecia (usually mild); blue discoloration of the urine, sclera, fingernails, and over venous site of injection that may last 48 hours

3. Occasional: Cardiomyopathy (most well defined for patients who have previously received doxorubicin; appears to be less cardiotoxic than doxorubicin), pruritus, abnormal liver function tests, and allergic reactions

4. Rare: Jaundice, seizures, pulmonary toxicity

d. **Administration:** Drug is supplied as 20-, 25-, and 30-mg vials. Typical dosage is 10 to 12 mg/m^2 IV given every 3 weeks for solid tumors or daily for 5 days in combination with cytarabine for acute leukemia.

Substituted Urea

HYDROXYUREA (HYDREA)

a. Indications: Epithelial ovarian carcinoma, CML

b. Pharmacology

1. Mechanism: Hydroxyurea can also be classified as an antimetabolite. It is thought to be cell cycle-specific for the S phase of cell division. The exact mechanism of antineoplastic activity is unknown but it is thought to involve interference with synthesis of DNA with no effect on the synthesis of RNA or protein.
2. Metabolism: Half of the drug is rapidly degraded into inactive compounds. Inactive products and unchanged drug (50%) are excreted in urine. Hydroxyurea readily crosses the blood–brain barrier.

c. Toxicity

1. Dose-limiting: Myelosuppression, which recovers rapidly when treatment is stopped (prominent megaloblastosis resembling pernicious anemia, probably caused by delaying of the rate of iron utilization by erythrocytes)
2. Occasional: Nausea and vomiting, skin rash, facial erythema, hyperpigmentation, azotemia or uric acid nephropathy transient liver function test abnormalities, and radiation recall reactions
3. Rare: Alopecia, mucositis, diarrhea, constipation; neurologic events; pulmonary edema; flulike syndrome

d. Administration: Drug is supplied as 500-mg capsules. The drug should be given cautiously in the presence of liver dysfunction or when combined with other antimetabolites. Dosages should be reduced in patients with renal insufficiency. Dosages include: (i) CML: 15 to 30 mg/kg orally every day; or (ii) solid tumors: 80 mg/kg orally every 3 days.

Methylhydrazine Derivative

PROCARBAZINE (MATULANE; NATULAN)

a. Indications: Hodgkin lymphoma

b. Pharmacology:

1. Mechanism: DNA alkylation and depolymerization. It is cell cycle specific for the S phase of cell division. Inhibits DNA, RNA and protein synthesis.
2. Metabolism: The drug is metabolized in liver into active compounds which are subsequently excreted in urine. The drug readily enters the CSF.

c. Toxicity

1. Dose-limiting. Myelosuppression, which may not begin until several weeks after starting treatment
2. Common: Nausea and vomiting, which decrease with continued use; myalgias, arthralgias; sensitizes tissue to radiation
3. Occasional: Dermatitis, hyperpigmentation, photosensitivity; stomatitis, dysphagia, diarrhea; hypotension, tachycardia; urinary frequency, hematuria, and gynecomastia
4. Neurologic: Procarbazine may result in disorders of consciousness or mild peripheral neuropathies in about 10% of cases. These abnormalities are reversible and rarely serious enough to alter drug dosage. Manifestations of toxicity include sedation, depression, agitation, psychosis, decreased deep-tendon reflexes paresthesias, myalgias, and ataxia.
5. Rare: Xerostomia, retinal hemorrhage, photophobia, papilledema; allergic pneumonitis, secondary malignancy

d. Administration: Drug is supplied as 50-mg capsules. Dose should be reduced in patients with hepatic, renal, or BM dysfunction. Dosages include 100 mg/m^2 orally daily for 14 days in combination regimens. Procarbazine is a monoamine oxidase inhibitor and interacts with a number of molecules, including:

(i) Alcohol causing disulfiram (Antabuse)-like reactions
(ii) CNS depressants synergistically (antihistamines, phenothiazines, barbiturates)
(iii) Tricyclic antidepressants and monoamine oxidase inhibitors causing hyperpyrexia or convulsions
(iv) Meperidine and other narcotics causing hypertension, hypotension, and coma
(v) Hypoglycemic agents increasing hypoglycemia
(vi) Levodopa causing hypertensive crisis (nullified by carbidopa)
(vii) Sympathomimetic amines and tyramine-containing foods causing hypertensive crisis (after dosage is stopped monoamine oxidase inhibitor effects of this medication may persist for up to 2 weeks.

Practical Aspects of Drug Administration

Practitioners of anesthesia rarely administer chemotherapeutic agents, but often must assess and respond to the short- and long-term toxicity of these agents (see Table 51–1). This is particularly important in patients presenting for surgery after neoadjuvant chemotherapy. Many of the chemotherapeutic agents produce BM depression, which can be manifest as anemia, neutropenia, or thrombocytopenia. This is an important consideration for planning blood component replacement therapy, particularly as patients recently treated with chemotherapy may have relatively normal blood counts, but a diminished ability to mount a BM response to blood loss or surgical stress. It is also important to assess patients before surgery for the unique toxic effects of several of the chemotherapeutics agents. Patients with a history of treated malignancy should be specifically questioned about what chemotherapeutic drugs they have received and assessed accordingly. Special attention should be given to the following:

1. Patients treated with vinca alkaloids (particularly vincristine) or platinum agents should be examined and questioned for evidence of peripheral neuropathy. Evidence of peripheral neuropathy should be fully documented and extraordinary attention should be given to patient positioning.

2. Patients treated with anthracyclines (particularly doxorubicin/adriamycin) should be examined, questioned, and assessed for evidence of cardiomyopathy. The cardiomyopathy is related to total cumulative dose and is generally not reversible. Therefore patients who have received a large dose of doxorubicin/adriamycin (>450 mg/m^2) should have an assessment of cardiac function before major surgery.

3. Patients exposed to bleomycin or busulfan should be questioned and examined for evidence of pulmonary dysfunction. Patients recently treated with bleomycin should not be exposed to high oxygen tensions (>30%) because there is some evidence that this can promote lung injury.

4. Patients treated with cisplatin should be assessed for evidence of renal insufficiency. Several other chemotherapeutic agents including the nitrosoureas, hydroxyurea and methotrexate, are also commonly nephrotoxic.

Conclusion

Chemotherapy has achieved an important place in the management of human cancer, with clear antitumor activity and benefit to many patients. However, the problem of tissue selectivity remains. New approaches that use antibodies against tumor antigens, antitumor vaccines, growth factor cell signaling inhibitors, antiangiogenesis agents, and other antitumor strategies are in clinical use or late clinical development. This makes anticancer therapy an exciting area of medicine for the near future.

References

1. Greenlee RT, Hill-Harmon MB, Murray T, Thon M: Cancer statistics, 2001. CA Cancer J Clin 51:15–36, 2001.
2. Weinberg RA: How cancer arises. Sci Am 275:62–70, 1996.
3. Hanahan D, Weinberg RA: The hallmarks of cancer. Cell 100:57–70, 2000.
4. Lundberg AS, Weinberg RA: Control of the cell cycle and apoptosis. Eur J Cancer 35:531–539, 1999.
5. Blagosklonny MV, Pardee AB: Exploiting cancer cell cycling for selective protection of normal cells. Cancer Res 61:4301–4305, 2001.
6 Shah MA, Schwartz GK: Cell cycle-mediated drug resistance: An emerging concept in cancer therapy. Clin Cancer Res 7:2168–2181, 2001.
7. Adjei AA: Blocking oncogenic Ras signaling for cancer therapy. J Natl Cancer Inst 93:1062–1074, 2001.
8. Pritchard SC, Nicolson MC, Lloret C, et al: Expression of matrix metalloproteinases 1, 2, 9 and their tissue inhibitors in stage II non-small cell lung cancer: Implications for MMP inhibition therapy. Oncol Rep 8:421–424, 2001.
9. McLeod HL, McKay JA, Collie-Duguid ES, Cassidy J: Therapeutic opportunities from tumour biology in metastatic colon cancer. Eur J Cancer 36:1706–1712, 2000.
10. McKay JA, Douglas JJ, Ross VG, et al: Expression of cell cycle control proteins in primary colorectal tumors does not always predict expression in lymph node metastases. Clin Cancer Res 6:1113–1118, 2000.
11. McLeod HL, Murray GI: Tumour markers of prognosis in colorectal cancer. Br J Cancer 79:191–203, 1999.
12. Nieto Y: Pharmacodynamics of high-dose chemotherapy. Curr Drug Metab 2:53–66, 2001.
13. Porrata LF, Adjei AA: The pharmacologic basis of high dose chemotherapy with haematopoietic stem cell support for solid tumours. Br J Cancer 85:484–489, 2001.
14. Hogberg T, Glimelius B, Nygren P: A systematic overview of chemotherapy effects in ovarian cancer. Acta Oncol 40:340–360, 2001.
15. Rodman JH, Relling MV, Stewart CF, et al: Clinical pharmacokinetics and pharmacodynamics of anticancer drugs in children. Semin Oncol 20:18–29, 1993.
16. Coldman AJ, Goldie JH: Impact of dose-intense chemotherapy on the development of permanent drug resistance. Semin Oncol 14:29–33, 1987.
17. Skipper HE, Schabel FM Jr, Lloyd HH: Experimental therapeutics and kinetics: Selection and overgrowth of specifically and permanently drug-resistant tumor cells. Semin Hematol 15:207–219, 1978.
18. Shah MA, Schwartz GK: The relevance of drug sequence in combination chemotherapy. Drug Resist Update 3:335–356, 2000.
19. McLeod HL: Clinical reversal of the multidrug resistance phenotype: True tumour modulation or pharmacokinetic interaction? Eur J Cancer 30A:2039–2041, 1994.
20. Borst P, Evers R, Kool M, Wijnholds J: A family of drug transporters: The multidrug resistance-associated proteins. J Natl Cancer Inst 92:1295–1302, 2000.
21. Dolan ME, Pegg AE: O6-benzylguanine and its role in chemotherapy. Clin Cancer Res 3:837–847, 1997.
22. Kelland LR: Preclinical perspectives on platinum resistance. Drugs 59(suppl 4):1–8, 2000.
23. Evans WE, Pui CH, Relling MV: Defining the optimal dosage of methotrexate for childhood acute lymphoblastic leukemia. New insights from the lab and clinic. Adv Exp Med Biol 457:537–541, 1999.
24. Huitema AD, Smits KD, Mathot RA, et al: The clinical pharmacology of alkylating agents in high-dose chemotherapy. Anticancer Drugs 11:515–533, 2000.
25. Colvin OM: An overview of cyclophosphamide development and clinical applications. Curr Pharm Des 5:555–560, 1999.
26. Petros WP, Colvin OM: Metabolic jeopardy with high-dose cyclophosphamide?—not so fast. Clin Cancer Res 5:723–724, 1999.
27. Wang W, Marsh S, Cassidy J, McLeod HL: Pharmacogenomic dissection of resistance to thymidylate synthase inhibitors. Cancer Res 61:5505–5510, 2001.
28. Plunkett W, Gandhi V: Pharmacology of purine nucleoside analogues. Hematol Cell Ther 38(suppl 2):S67–S74, 1996.
29. Heinemann V: Gemcitabine: Progress in the treatment of pancreatic cancer. Oncology 60:8–18, 2001.
30. McLeod HL, Krynetski EY, Relling MV, Evans WE: Genetic polymorphism of thiopurine methyltransferase and its clinical relevance for childhood acute lymphoblastic leukemia. Leukemia 14:567–572, 2000.
31. Relling MV, Hancock ML, Boyett JM, et al: Prognostic importance of 6-mercaptopurine dose intensity in acute lymphoblastic leukemia. Blood 93:2817–2823, 1999.
32. Relling MV, Hancock ML, Rivera GK, et al: Mercaptopurine therapy intolerance and heterozygosity at the thiopurine S-methyltransferase gene locus. J Natl Cancer Inst 91:2001–2008, 1999.
33. Johnson SA: Clinical pharmacokinetics of nucleoside analogues: Focus on haematological malignancies. Clin Pharmacokinet 39:5–26, 2000.
34. Liliemark J: The clinical pharmacokinetics of cladribine. Clin Pharmacokinet 32:120–131, 1997.
35. Galmarini CM, Mackey JR, Dumontet C: Nucleoside analogues: Mechanisms of drug resistance and reversal strategies. Leukemia 15:875–890, 2001.
36. Chan JD: Pharmacokinetic drug interactions of vinca alkaloids: Summary of case reports. Pharmacotherapy 18:1304–1307, 1998.
37. Dumontet C: Mechanisms of action and resistance to tubulin-binding agents. Exp Opin Investig Drugs 9:779–788, 2000.
38. Leveque D, Jehl F: Clinical pharmacokinetics of vinorelbine. Clin Pharmacokinet 31:184–197, 1996.
39. McLeod HL, Evans WE: Clinical pharmacokinetics and pharmacodynamics of epipodophyllotoxins. Cancer Surv 17:253–268, 1993.
40. Relling MV, Pui CH, Sandlund JT, et al: Adverse effect of anticonvulsants on efficacy of chemotherapy for acute lymphoblastic leukaemia. Lancet 356:285–290, 2000.
41. Woo MH, Hak LJ, Storm MC, et al: Hypersensitivity or development of antibodies to asparaginase does not impact treatment outcome of childhood acute lymphoblastic leukemia. J Clin Oncol 18:1525–1532, 2000.

42. Danesi R, Conte PF, Del Tacca M: Pharmacokinetic optimisation of treatment schedules for anthracyclines and paclitaxel in patients with cancer. Clin Pharmacokinet 37:195–211, 1999.

43. Perez EA: Doxorubicin and paclitaxel in the treatment of advanced breast cancer: Efficacy and cardiac considerations. Cancer Invest 19:155–164, 2001.

44. Coukell AJ, Faulds D: Epirubicin. An updated review of its pharmacodynamic and pharmacokinetic properties and therapeutic efficacy in the management of breast cancer. Drugs 53:453–482, 1997.

45. Ormrod D, Holm K, Goa K, Spencer C: Epirubicin- a review. Drugs Aging 15:389–416, 1999.

46. Ormrod D, Spencer CM: Topotecan: A review of its efficacy in small cell lung cancer. Drugs 58:533–551, 1999.

47. Mathijssen RH, van Alphen RJ, Verweij J, et al: Clinical pharmacokinetics and metabolism of irinotecan (cpt-11). Clin Cancer Res 7:2182–2194, 2001.

48. Earhart RH: Docetaxel (Taxotere): Preclinical and general clinical information. Semin Oncol 26(suppl 17):8–13, 1999.

49. Cabral F, Trimble E, Reed E, Sarosy G: Future directions with taxane therapy. Hematol Oncol Clin North Am 13:21–41, 1999.

50. Goldspiel BR: Clinical overview of the taxanes. Pharmacotherapy 17(5 pt):110S–125S, 1997.

51. McLeod HL, Kearns CM, Kuhn JG, Bruno R: Evaluation of the linearity of docetaxel pharmacokinetics. Cancer Chemother Pharmacol 42:155–159, 1998.

52. Vaishampayan U, Parchment RE, Jasti BR, Hussain M: Taxanes: An overview of the pharmacokinetics and pharmacodynamics. Urology 54(suppl):22–29, 1999.

53. O'Dwyer PJ, Stevenson JP, Johnson SW: Clinical pharmacokinetics and administration of established platinum drugs. Drugs 59(suppl 4):19–27, 2000.

52

Red Blood Cell Substitutes

Brian Woodcock, MB ChB, MRCP, FRCA • Kevin K. Tremper, PhD, MD

Although blood performs a variety of physiologic functions, the most basic of these is to provide a circulating volume to transport substrate and metabolites and to transport the most valuable of substrates: oxygen. Supplementing intravascular volume with crystalloid and colloid has been part of medical practice for nearly a century. For more than 50 years efforts have been directed toward developing a substitute for the red blood cell's function of transporting oxygen. The U.S. Army, before World War II, initiated early work on blood substitutes. It was known that approximately 30% of all battlefield deaths occurred because of the inability to effectively treat hemorrhage. During combat conditions, the logistics of collecting, storing, transporting and cross-matching blood were too difficult and many soldiers died of treatable injuries because of lack of an adequate resuscitation fluid.

Initially, the defense department sought a powdered form of hemoglobin solution that could be stored indefinitely at room temperature and subsequently dissolved in normal saline and transfused without a need for cross-matching. Currently, there are several hemoglobin-based products that are in various stages of clinical testing that are described in this chapter.

Another method of transporting oxygen has been through the use of emulsions of perfluorochemicals (PFCs). PFCs are inert liquids that have a solubility for oxygen and carbon dioxide 20 times that of water. These liquids are immiscible with water and therefore have been used in an emulsion form dispersed in normal saline. Both of these oxygen-carrying substrates, solutions of hemoglobin and emulsions of PFCs,

have completed animal testing and have been investigated in the clinical setting. Both of these types of red blood cell substitutes have limitations, and currently neither has been made available for routine use.

In the current civilian setting, the Red Cross, the American Blood Centers, and the blood banking system make typed and cross-matched blood and blood product readily available in most surgical settings. In a time when blood usage is increasing and blood donations are declining,[1] the possibility of blood shortages is also driving the search for alternatives. In the past two decades there has also been tremendous concern regarding the infectious risks for blood-borne pathogens.[2,3] Although the 1990s saw a dramatic improvement in blood safety to the point in which contracting human immunodeficiency virus (HIV) from a unit of blood is approaching 1 in 1,000,000, there are still substantial concerns regarding transmission of HIV, hepatitis viruses, and other as of yet undetectable diseases. Religious concerns lead some groups, e.g., Jehovah's Witnesses, to refuse all blood products. Two thirds of blood transfusions are given in the surgical setting and banked blood is often wasted while active bleeding continues. Blood substitutes could be used as a resuscitation bridge until bleeding is controlled.[4] These concerns have further stimulated efforts to develop red cell substitutes for use in the routine clinical setting. Advances have been made and multiple large-scale phase II and III clinical trials are proceeding.[5]

This chapter reviews the development, physiology, and pharmacology of both types of red blood cell substitutes. The chapter concludes with a discussion of the current clinical studies of each of these products. To provide a context for this discussion, the current risks for allogeneic blood transfusion and then oxygen transport physiology are reviewed first.

Current Risks of Banked Blood

Risks of Transfusion

Blood transfusion is safer today than it has ever been. This complex logistical and technical process is performed approximately 20 million times per year in the United States, with an impressive safety record.[6] The acute death rate associated with a blood transfusion is approximately 1 in 300,000.[7] Two thirds of these deaths are the result of clerical errors (i.e., the wrong blood given to the patient). Other risks associated with blood transfusion include infection and immune reactions.[8,9]

Infection

The risk for infection encompasses the risk for transmitting viral agents, other exotic infectious agents, and bacterial contamination of blood products (Table 52–1). Preventing infections is first accomplished by carefully noting the donor's history and excluding donors with risk factors.

Testing donated units and eliminating units that contain these infectious agents further reduces the risk. It is difficult to accurately assess the true risk of transmission because the risk is small and can be determined only after a significant delay. The public is most anxious regarding the potential transmission of HIV. In March 1996, HIV antigen p24

TABLE 52–1.

Infectious Agents Occurring in Blood Products

Viral Infections	Nonviral	Bacterial Contamination
Hepatitis A	Malaria	Enterobacter
Hepatitis B	Trypanosomiasis:	Pseudomonas
Hepatitis C	Chagas' disease	Yersinia E
Hepatitis G	Sleeping sickness	Spirochetes:
HTLV I	Leishmaniasis	Lyme disease
CMV	Toxoplasmosis	Syphilis
HIV	Babesiosis	Rickettsia
	Microfilariasis	

CMV, cytomegalovirus; HIV, human immunodeficiency virus; HTLV I, human T-cell lymphotrophic virus I.

testing was instituted in the United States. After 18 months, 18 million units of blood had been collected, and only 3 units were identified as antigen-positive and antibody-negative units.[10] Blood donations are now tested for HIV-1 and HIV-2.[11] The apparent risk for HIV transmission is currently about 1 in 1,000,000. Hepatitis is more prevalent, but less feared. With the advent of more sophisticated tests for antigens, the current aggregate risk for post-transfusion hepatitis (B or C) is estimated to be fewer than 1 in 34,000.[12] Hepatitis G has recently been recognized, and there is currently no screening test. It may be identified by the polymerase chain reaction test, but this has not been implemented as a routine screening test. Fortunately, the sequelae of infection appear to be minimal, although there is a weak link between hepatitis G and fulminant hepatitis in rare cases.[13]

Of recent interest is the potential transmission of Creutzfeldt-Jakob disease. Although more than 100 cases of transmissible Creutzfeldt-Jakob disease have been reported, all have involved central nervous system tissue (or extract) transfer. No case has been definitively linked to blood transfusion.[14]

In the United Kingdom, an outbreak of bovine spongiform encephalopathy (BSE) or "Mad Cow disease" has led to concern that a new variant Creutzfeldt-Jacob disease has been transferred to the human population through consumption of contaminated beef products. Transmission of BSE by blood transfusion has been demonstrated to occur in sheep.[15] In the United Kingdom, blood transfusions are leucodepleted, which is thought to reduce the risk for transmission of variant Creutzfeldt-Jacob disease by blood transfusion. The possibility that transmission may occur has led the U.S. Food and Drug Administration (FDA) to institute a policy "deferring" (i.e., declining) blood donations from anyone who has lived in the United Kingdom for a cumulative period of more than 6 months during the years 1980 to 1996.[16]

Bacterial contamination of stored blood is rare (1/500,000), but it is associated with a mortality rate of 25% to 80%. Because platelets are stored at room temperature, allowing rapid bacterial proliferation, the risk for bacterial infection is greatest with these units (1:3000–7000), and the bacteria are typically gram-positive staphylococci. The most common infectious contaminants in red cells are gram-negative psychrophilic species such as Pseudomonas or Yersinia.[17]

Immune Reactions

The risk for immune reactions is small but real. The majority of acute hemolytic reactions are caused by clerical errors because cross-matching should predict these events. However, immune reactions are the most common cause of fatality associated with transfusions, and the current risk exceeds that of HIV transmission. Minor reactions, such as common febrile reactions, are discomforting to the patient but are not associated with significant morbidity, although the transfusion may need to be stopped and the product discarded. Graft-versus-host disease may occur rarely after transfusion, most commonly after transfusion of nonirradi-

TABLE 52–2.

Infectious Risks

Viral Infections	Risk
HIV	1 : 1,000,000
Hepatitis B	1 : 60,000
Hepatitis C	1 : 103,000
Hepatitis G	?
Bacterial	1 : 500,000

HIV, human immunodeficiency virus.

ated blood components to patients with immunodeficiency. Transfusion-associated, graft-versus-host disease results in an overall mortality rate of 84% at a median of 21 days after transfusion. Patients with an immunodeficiency disorder should receive irradiated units. Immunocompetent individuals may develop graft-versus-host disease if the donor and recipient share histocompatibility leukocyte antigen haplotype. This situation can occur between first-degree family members; therefore, relative-to-patient directed donations may carry an increased risk for initiating transfusion-associated graft-versus-host disease.

Transfusion-related immunomodulation has been recognized since the mid-1970s but is not well quantified. Exposure to allogeneic blood can cause both allosensitization and immunosuppression. Clinical studies have demonstrated a beneficial effect of allogeneic blood transfusion on transplant organ survival, but an adverse effect on cancer recurrence and postoperative infection.[18,19] Leukocyte depletion through filtration may ameliorate these effects.

Allogeneic blood transfusion is currently safer than it has ever been (Table 52–2). However, these risks for infection and concerns regarding immune reactions and immunomodulation signify that the development of oxygen-carrying colloids remains an important objective.

Mechanisms of Action of Oxygen-Carrying Colloids

Oxygen Transport

Oxygenation is adequate when oxygen is being supplied to the tissues at a sufficient rate to maintain aerobic metabolism. The primary oxygen transport variable is the arterial oxygen content (CaO_2), which is defined as the volume of oxygen (mL) carried in 100 mL of blood (Vol%).

Hemoglobin carries most of the oxygen, with little dissolved in the plasma. When the hemoglobin is fully saturated at a PaO_2 level of approximately 90 mm Hg, no additional oxygen is added to the hemoglobin phase, whereas additional oxygen is dissolved in the plasma phase as oxygen tension increases.

Assuming a hemoglobin level of 15 mg/100 mL, the arterial oxygen content can be calculated as follows:

$$CaO_2 = (Hb \times 1.34 \times SaO_2) + (0.003 \times PaO_2)$$
$$\approx 20 \, mL/100 \, mL \qquad (1)$$

where Hb is hemoglobin; SaO_2 is arterial oxygen saturation; and PaO_2 is arterial oxygen tension.

With a normal 15 g hemoglobin and normal PaO_2 and SaO_2 values of 90 mm Hg and 97%, respectively, an arterial oxygen content of 20 mL/dL is obtained. This is similar to the oxygen content of room air at sea level. Therefore, the cardiovascular system produces the same oxygen content near each cell that would exist if the cells were surrounded by room air.

Oxygen delivery is the oxygen content multiplied by blood flow: because cardiac output is usually calculated as liters of blood per minute and CaO_2 in milliliters O_2/100 mL blood, the product is multiplied by 10 to allow the liter and deciliter to cancel out. Assuming a cardiac output of 5 L/min, the oxygen delivery can be calculated as follows:

$$Oxygen \, delivery = (CaO_2) \, (cardiac \, output) \times 10$$
$$\approx 20 \times 5 \times 10$$
$$\approx 1000 \, mL/min \qquad (2)$$

Therefore, the healthy 70-kg adult has an oxygen delivery of one liter per minute to the tissues.

Perfluorochemical Emulsions

In 1965, Clark and Gollan[20] performed an ingenious experiment that spawned the development of a new concept in oxygen transport. They were experimenting with a new series of compounds known as PFCs that have unique properties as chemically inert liquids with high solubilities for gases.

These PFCs consisted of 8 to 10 carbon structures that were completely fluorinated and, therefore, were chemically inert, clear, odorless liquids with a density of nearly twice that of water. Because the solubility of PFCs for oxygen was nearly 20 times that of water, Clark and Gollan questioned whether an animal could survive if it breathed this liquid equilibrated with one atmosphere of oxygen.

They submerged a rat beneath the liquid for 30 minutes (Fig. 52–1) and the rat was retrieved having experienced no apparent harm (Fig. 52–2). Because these liquids are completely immiscible with water, an intravenous injection is immediately lethal because the injection forms a liquid embolus. In 1968, Gehes and colleagues[21] produced a microemulsion (particle size: 0.1 micron) of a PFC in normal saline. They conducted a complete exchange

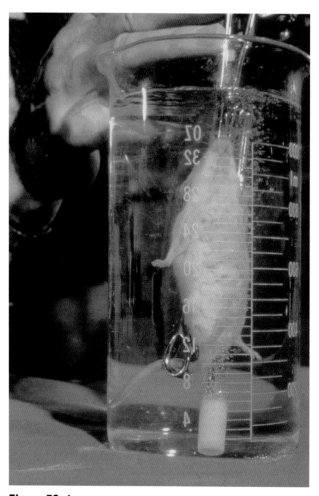

Figure 52–1. A rat immersed in, and breathing, oxygenated perfluorochemical.

transfusion with a rat, and it survived breathing 100% oxygen with a hematocrit of 0% (Fig. 52–3). Because of the inert nature of these compounds, they are not metabolized but are cleared from the vascular space by the reticuloendothelial system (RES) and ultimately collect in the liver

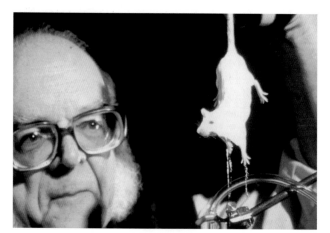

Figure 52–2. The rat after retrieval.

and spleen. Eventually, the PFC slowly leaves the body as vapor in the respiratory gas. Because PFCs transport oxygen by simple solubility, the amount of oxygen they carry is directly proportional to the percentage of PFC in the bloodstream and to the PaO_2.

Perfluorochemical Oxygen Content

Figure 52–4 shows that PFCs carry oxygen by direct solubility, as does plasma. The oxygen content equation requires a third term to represent the contribution from perfluorocarbon.

$$CaO_2 = (Hb \times 1.34 \times SaO_2) + (0.003 \times PaO_2) + (0.057 \times Fct/100 \times PaO_2) \quad (3)$$

where Fct is fluorocrit, which is the fraction of the blood volume that is PFC (analogous to hematocrit).

Note that the solubility factor in the third term (0.057) is nearly 20 times that of the solubility factor for oxygen in plasma (0.003). As with plasma, the greater the PaO_2, the

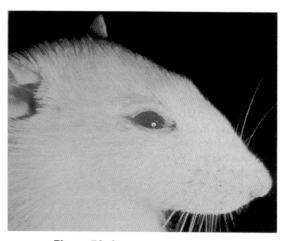

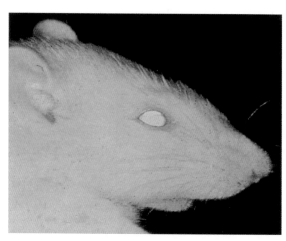

Figure 52–3. A rat before and after complete exchange transfusion. The red reflex of the retina is replaced by a white reflex when the hematocrit is zero.

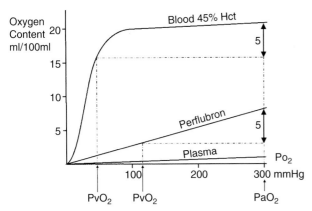

Figure 52–4. Oxygen content plotted against P_{O_2} for whole blood, plasma, and a perfluorochemical emulsion, with a 45% content of perfluorochemical (PFC; e.g., Perflubron). Hemoglobin saturates at a P_{O_2} of 100 mm Hg, but the curve continues to rise because of the dissolved oxygen in plasma, therefore the whole blood and plasma lines are parallel above a P_{O_2} of 100. The line for perflubron is similar to plasma but has a higher slope because of the greater affinity for oxygen. Content lines for hemoglobin are similar to whole blood, but slightly displaced to the right or left if the P_{50} is greater or lower than 27. At an arterial P_{O_2} (Pa_{O_2}) of 300 mm Hg, blood has an oxygen content of 21 mL/100 mL if 5 mL/100 mL are extracted the venous P_{O_2} (Pv_{O_2}) will be less than 50 mm Hg. Although perflubron has a lower content of 7.7 mL/100 mL at a Pa_{O_2} of 300 mm Hg, if 5 mL/100 mL is extracted, then the Pv_{O_2} will be greater than 100 mm Hg. This greater Pv_{O_2} will increase the oxygen pressure gradient into the tissues and cells.

larger the contribution of the PFC-delivered oxygen. The factor 0.057 is the solubility of O_2 in PFC minus the solubility of O_2 in plasma. The correction is required because as PFC is added to the plasma there is less plasma available to carry O_2.

The amount of oxygen carried by a PFC emulsion is substantially less than the amount carried by blood with a normal hematocrit. Because the PFC carries oxygen by direct solubility, it also releases it in direct proportion to the P_{O_2}, unlike the cooperative binding effect of hemoglobin. Thus PFCs have a linear oxygen dissociation curve unlike the sigmoid curve for hemoglobin. We may assess the potential contribution of PFCs to oxygen transport by looking at mixed venous values of P_{O_2} and the quantity of oxygen consumed by the tissue. The content of oxygen extracted from the arterial blood or arteriovenous difference in oxygen content (A–V_{DO_2}) can be calculated as follows:

$$A–V_{DO_2} = Ca_{O_2} – Cv_{O_2}$$
$$= 5 \, mL/dL \qquad (4)$$

where Cv_{O_2} is mixed venous oxygen content.

If we assume a mixed venous oxygen tension (Pv_{O_2}) level of 40 mm Hg and an oxygen extraction of 5 mL/dL, a bloodless animal could survive with fluorocrits of 10%, 20%, and 45% with Pa_{O_2} values of 920, 480, and 235 mm Hg, respectively. Any increase in Pa_{O_2} above these values would increase the Pv_{O_2} by the same amount (see Fig. 52–4). The increased Pv_{O_2} in these circumstances could increase the pressure gradient for oxygen diffusion from the vascular space into the tissues and cells, theoretically increasing tissue oxygenation. From these calculations, it would appear that a patient could survive with a PFC emulsion without red blood cells. In practice, this would be difficult. The emulsion is cleared from the vascular space within 24 hours, and because of the long tissue half-life of a PFC in the body (months to years depending on the PFC compound), it would not be feasible to continuously redose the patient.

The initial technical problem in producing a clinically usable product was the development of a stable emulsion that contained sufficient PFC. In the late 1970s, the Green Cross Corporation in Japan developed a product called Fluosol DA 20%, which was an emulsion composed of two PFCs: perfluorodecalin and perfluorotripropylamine[22] (Fig. 52–5). This combination of PFCs was used to take advantage of the emulsion stability of perfluorodecalin and the shorter tissue half-life of perfluorotripropylamine. Even with this mixture, the solution contained only 10% PFC (Fluosol DA 20% is 20% by weight, 10% by volume). The surfactant used to maintain this emulsion was Pluronic F68, an emulsifier used in other medical products. To maintain stability, the product needed to be frozen until use.

In spite of these limitations, the product was used in early clinical studies and will be described in the next section on clinical pharmacology. The general limitations of PFCs as red cell substitutes—i.e., short endovascular half-life of less than 24 hours and that they require high Pa_{O_2} values to carry significant oxygen—will likely never be circumvented. The principal limitation of Fluosol-DA 20% was the difficulty in producing a stable emulsion. Because of this difficulty, the product had little perfluorochemical in it (10% by volume) and required freezing for the emulsion to remain stable. Second-generation PFC emulsions have been under development over the past decade (Table 52–3). One of these uses the perfluorocarbon perflubron (perfluorooctyl bromide).[23] This PFC is unique because it has one bromine replacing a fluorine making it radiopaque (Fig. 52–6). This emulsion, perflubron (Oxygent; Alliance Pharmaceuticals, San Diego, Calif), contains 90% PFC by weight or 45% by volume and is emulsified with lecithin from egg yolk. Perflubron emul-

Figure 52–5. Structures of perfluorodecalin *(A)* and perfluorotripropylamine *(B)*, constituents of Fluosol DA.

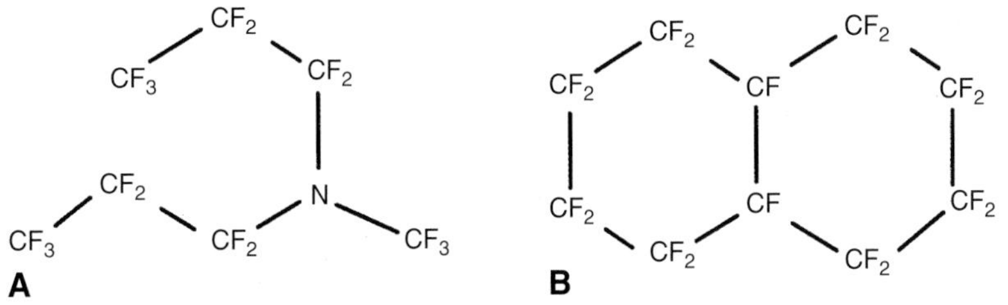

TABLE 52–3.

Perfluorochemical Emulsions

Product (Manufacturer)	Perfluorochemical	Concentration	Surfactant
Fluosol DA 20% (Green Cross Corp., Osaka, Japan)*	Perfluorodecaline and perfluorotripoplyamine	14 g/100 mL 6 g/100 mL	Pluronic F68
Oxygent (Alliance Pharmaceutical, San Diego, Calif)	Perfluorooctyl bromide (Perflubron)	90 g/100 mL	Lecithin
Oxyfluor (Hemagen, St. Louis, Mo)*	Perfluordichlorooctane (HM 351)	80 g/100 mL	Lecithin and safflower oil

*Product is discontinued.

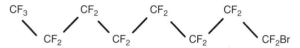

Figure 52–6. Structure of perfluorooctyl bromide (Perflubron, Oxygent).

sion has optimal properties pharmaceutically, it has as high an emulsion concentration as can be achieved, and it is stable at room temperature for more than 6 years. Nevertheless, the two inherent limitations of a short endovascular half-life and the requirement for high-inspired oxygen limit the use of these emulsions to acute settings in which supplemental oxygen is readily available.

The primary toxicity concern of these compounds is their effect on the RES as they are cleared. No long-term toxicity has been noted, but there is concern about RE cell "blockade" and effects on the liver because the capacity of the RES may be overwhelmed as a result of clearing the PFC from the vascular space. An influenza-like syndrome[24] and sequestration of circulating platelets are commonly seen with perfluorocarbons.[25–27]

Hemoglobin Solutions

Originally, hemoglobin solutions were made by obtaining outdated human blood, lysing the red cells, filtering the hemoglobin, and resuspending it in normal saline, thereby producing a free hemoglobin solution. There have been a series of difficulties in developing a nontoxic clinical product that is effective in transporting oxygen. The first problem encountered was acute renal failure, which was assumed to be caused by the free hemoglobin. As noted by Rabiner and Friedman[28] in the 1960s, this problem was actually caused by residual red blood cell membranes (stroma) and not the hemoglobin molecule itself. For the next few decades the primary goal was to produce a pure hemoglobin solution, thereby eliminating the toxicity associated with this residual red cell membrane (i.e., stroma-free hemoglobin).[29] When hemoglobin is lysed from the red cells, two other problems occur. First, the tetrameric structure of the hemoglobin molecule breaks down into dimers. Second, the 2,3-DPG is lost and the P_{50} of the hemoglobin decreases from the normal level of 26 mm Hg to the range of 12 to 14 mm Hg. The low P_{50} means that the hemoglobin dimers will pick up oxygen aggressively but not release it in the normal ranges of physiologic P_{O_2}. Therefore, the hemoglobin would pick up oxygen in the lungs, and then circulate through the arteries and capillary and back to the venous system without releasing it.

In addition, the dimer is approximately 32,000 daltons and is therefore small enough to cross the renal capillary basement membrane. Consequently, when the purified hemoglobin solution is infused intravascularly, it will pick up oxygen and then act as an osmotic diuretic, ultimately reducing the intravascular volume and causing the patient to lose not only hemoglobin, but also oxygen attached to it in the urine. This "red mannitol effect" of the early hemoglobin solutions could be resolved by increasing the molecular size.

The correction of the hemoglobin size problem has four possible methods of attack. First, the dimers could be crosslinked to produce a tetramer. Second, the dimers could be polymerized to form larger, roughly octameric molecules (Fig. 52–7). Polymerization of hemoglobin also has other beneficial effects: the P_{50} is increased to a greater level than free dimers of hemoglobin, there is an increase in plasma half-life, and a high concentration can be achieved without creating an excessively high colloid oncotic pressure.[30] Free hemoglobin molecules act as colloidal particles producing oncotic pressure. If hemoglobin solutions are produced as dimers and a solution contains 15 g total hemoglobin, the oncotic pressure is well above the normal value of 25 mm Hg. In fact, the technique of polymerization used by Gould and colleagues[31] and Sehgal and coworkers[32] continues the polymerization process until the oncotic pressure has decreased to about 25 mm Hg, thereby using the oncotic pressure as a parameter for titrating the polymerization process. Perfluorochemical emulsions achieve normal oncotic pressure by the addition of hydroxyethyl starch to the solution.

Figure 52–7. Hemoglobin dimer subunits *(A)* can be crosslinked to form tetramers *(B)*, the tetramers can be polymerized to form larger units *(C)*. The resulting solution has the same hemoglobin concentration but has a lower colloid oncotic pressure and will not cross the kidney basement membrane.

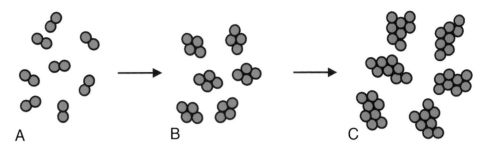

A third way to increase the size of the hemoglobin molecule is to attach the dimer to a large nonhemoglobin molecule, such as polyethylene glycol used in polyethylene glycol (PEG) hemoglobin. A final method is to encapsulate hemoglobin in phospholipid vesicles or liposomes.[33]

The first two methods have been used in commercial products. Crosslinking the molecule with pyridoxal-5-phosphate, which acts as an artificial 2,3-DPG, can increase the P_{50}. This technique is used in PolyHeme (Northfield Pharmaceutical, Chicago, Ill) polymerized hemoglobin solution[32] and pyridoxylated hemoglobin polyoxyethylene conjugate (or PHP hemoglobin).[34]

Other sources of hemoglobin can be used that do not have the problem of a low P_{50}. Hemoglobin can not only be obtained from outdated human blood, but also from bovine blood or by manufacture using recombinant techniques. The use of bovine hemoglobin has two advantages over outdated human blood as a source of hemoglobin. First, there is a

tremendous supply, because almost 1 million U/day are produced as a byproduct of meat production. Second, bovine hemoglobin does not contain 2,3-DPG, and therefore maintains a P_{50} in the range of 32 mm Hg even as a dimer.[35] Concern over the spread of BSE may impact the development of bovine products.[36] The FDA has restricted the import of bovine products from Europe because of the outbreak of Mad Cow disease there.[37] In April 2000, the Center for Biologics Evaluation and Research sent a letter to manufacturers requesting that ruminant-derived material from Europe not be used in the manufacture of FDA-regulated products for humans.

Recombinant hemoglobin can also be engineered to have a P_{50} in the normal range. However, manufacture of Optro (Somatogen), the sole recombinant hemoglobin, has been discontinued.[36]

There are a variety of hemoglobin solutions that have undergone clinical trial (Table 52–4). Because these prod-

TABLE 52–4.

Hemoglobin Solutions

Product (Manufacturer)	Hb Source	Configuration	Concentration	P_{50} (mm Hg)
HBOC201 Hemopure (Biopure, Cambridge, Mass)	Bovine	Polymerized with glutaraldehyde	13 g/dL	34
PolyHeme (Northfield Pharmaceutical, Chicago, Ill)	Human	Polymerized, tetramer-free	10 g/dL	30
Optro (Somatogen)*	Recombinant	Genetically fused	5 g/dL	17.2
Hemolink (Hemosol, Toronto, Ontario, Canada)	Human	Polymerized with o-raffinose	10 g/dL	32
PEG-hemoglobin (Enzon, Piscataway, NJ)	Bovine	PEG conjugated noncrosslinked	6 g/dL	20
DCLHb (Baxter Pharmaceutical, Chicago, Ill)*	Human	Crosslinked with diaspirin	10 g/dL	32
PHP (Apex Bioscience, Research Triangle Park)	Human	Pyridoxylated	8 g/dL	

*Product is discontinued.
Hb, hemoglobin; PEG, polyethylene glycol.

ucts are produced from different hemoglobin sources, have different sizes, and have different P_{50}, each needs to be evaluated as a separate drug with its own effectiveness and toxicity profile. In general, there are common problems to all hemoglobin solutions that must be considered. All of these products have a relatively short intravascular half-life and are cleared from the vascular space by the RES, as are the perfluorochemical emulsions, with a half-life of approximately 24 hours. Second, the shelf-life of hemoglobin solutions is limited by the rate of conversion of the hemoglobin to methemoglobin. Finally, a problem of pulmonary and systemic hypertension has been observed in animal[38-42] and clinical studies.[43-52] The cause of this was not clarified until the early 1990s. It was at this time that the role of nitric oxide in controlling vascular resistance was elucidated. Nitric oxide is produced in the endothelial cells of blood vessel walls, and produces smooth muscle relaxation, thereby causing vasodilatation. As blood flow increases, nitric oxide is carried away, reducing its concentration and causing vasoconstriction.[53] It was noted during early studies with hemoglobin solutions that an infusion was associated with an acute increase in blood pressure and pulmonary vascular resistance. It is now known that binding to hemoglobin plays an important role in the removal of nitric oxide and thereby the control of the pulmonary vasculature. It appears that nitric oxide binds more avidly to free hemoglobin in the plasma than to hemoglobin within the red cell, and nitric oxide clearance is increased.[54] It may also be true that as hemoglobin molecule size decreases nitric oxide clearance increases and pulmonary hypertension becomes more problematic. The severity of this side effect needs to be evaluated with each product. A summary of the hemodynamic effects of hemoglobin solutions is shown in Table 52-5.

Oxygen Content

When the free hemoglobin solution (FHb) has the same P_{50} as blood (27 mm Hg), there is no difference between the hemoglobin solution oxygen-content curve and the curve for normal whole blood.

$$CaO_2 = (FHb \times 1.34 \times FSaO_2) + (Hb \times 1.34 \times SaO_2) + (0.003 \times PaO_2) \quad (5)$$

FHb is the concentration of free hemoglobin solution in blood (g/dL), and $FSaO_2$ is the saturation of FHb.

Using a separate hemoglobin term and a separate saturation for the free hemoglobin is more of a theoretical concern than a practical one. For clinical purposes, when total hemoglobin is measured spectrophotometrically, the total hemoglobin present is measured, and the saturation is measured by an oximeter. The effective weighted mean saturation is then achieved, because the device measures the amount of oxyhemoglobin and divides it by total hemoglobin to achieve the calculated saturation. Therefore for practical uses the oxygen content equation in the presence of a hemoglobin solution is the same as that for normal blood. The important clinical point is that the oxygen-carrying capacity of blood cannot be determined by using a measurement of hematocrit, for it will not account for the free hemoglobin in the plasma.

Just as perfluorochemical solutions are recognized as abnormal by the body, the RES scavenges the particles of the hemoglobin solution from the bloodstream. The effective intravascular life of the hemoglobin solution is approximately 24 to 48 hours, depending on the dose.[35] Therefore, these solutions, like the PFCs, will find their greatest applicability in acute, limited, blood loss situations, perhaps associated with an autologous hemodilution scheme during surgery.[55,56] Because hemoglobin solutions deliver oxygen in a manner similar to that of hemoglobin in red blood cells, they offer no benefit at low temperatures (i.e., cardioplegia). However, unlike PFCs, hemoglobin solutions may have an added advantage to compensate for the problem of limited intravascular retention. Animals that are hemodiluted to low hematocrits and given transfusions of hemoglobin solutions dramatically exceed the reticulocytosis expected even with the administration of exogenous erythropoietin. Beagles that were bled to a hematocrit of 5% required only two doses of a hemoglobin solution during an 8-day period. By the eighth day, the average hematocrit had returned to 15% because of significant red blood cell production.[57] Lamy and colleagues used diaspirin crosslinked hemoglobin (DCLHb) to transfuse cardiac surgery patients in the postbypass period.[48] A total of 19% of patients given DCLHb were able to avoid packed red blood cell (PRBC) transfusion; despite the relatively short duration of DCLHb in the plasma, the free iron liberated when it is metabolized may stimulate erythropoiesis and reticulocytosis, reducing the requirement for subsequent red cell transfusion.[58] Although nearly one fifth of patients were able to avoid red cell transfusion, the total cumulative amounts of red cell product given to the DCLHb and red cell transfused groups were the same after 7 days.

Microcirculation and Oxygen-Carrying Colloids

Oxygen-carrying colloids differ from red cells in terms of size. Free hemoglobin molecules in solution range in size from 68,000 to 500,000 daltons, and the fluorochemical emulsion particles are approximately 0.2 microns. This size range is within the range of many of the plasma proteins. Therefore, these particles can be expected to participate in extravascular circulation, as do plasma proteins. Animal data indicate that these oxygen-carrying colloids leave the intravascular space and rejoin it through lymphatic circulation.[57] This raises noteworthy questions about the ability of these colloids to provide increased oxygen delivery to the extravascular space.[50,59] In addition, studies on microcirculation have shown that capillaries can open and close to red cell flow, but plasma flow continues even when red cells are not traversing the capillary. Again, because the oxygen-carrying colloids travel in the plasma space, they can provide oxygen delivery to tissues even though red cells are not present in the capillaries. It has been speculated that oxygen-carrying colloids will provide enhanced oxygen delivery to tissues, especially in tissues where red cell flow is limited.

TABLE 52–5.

Hemodynamic Effects of Hemoglobin Solutions

Author	Subjects	Solution	Hemodynamic Effects
Krieter et al. (40)	Dogs	Bovine HBOC	SVR increased 130% PVR increased 129% CO decreased 32%
Ulatowski et al. (42)	Cats	Bovine HBOC	BP increased 25%
Maxwell et al. (41)	Swine	Bovine polymerized	BP 20 mm Hg greater than control CO 40% less than control
DeAngeles et al. (38)	Sheep	DCLHb	BP 37 mm Hg greater than control
Ning et al. (39)	Rats	Hemolink	Increased BP Bradycardia
LaMuraglia et al. (46)	Human	HBOC-201	BP increased 15%
Standl et al. (47)	Human	HBOC-201	BP increased 18% CO decreased
Kasper et al. (43)	Human	HBOC-201	BP increased 59% SVR increased 121% PVR increased 170%
Wahr et al. (45)	Human	HBOC-201	BP unchanged
Lamy et al. (48)	Human	DCLHb	BP 10 mm Hg greater than control SVR 50% greater than control CO 20% less than control
Saxena et al. (44)	Human	DCLHb	BP 23% greater than control
Reah et al. (50)	Human	DCLHb	Reduced norepinephrine requirement in septic shock
Carmichael et al. (51)	Human	Hemolink	BP increased 14%
Cheng et al. (52)	Human	Hemolink	BP increased 7–10%
Johnson et al. (90)	Human	PolyHeme	BP, PAP, CO, SVR, PVR unchanged
Gould et al. (91)	Human	PolyHeme	BP unchanged

BP, systemic blood pressure; CO, cardiac output; DCLHb, diaspirin crosslinked hemoglobin; HBOC, hemoglobin-based oxygen carrier; PAP, pulmonary artery blood pressure; PVR, pulmonary vascular resistance; SVR, systemic vascular resistance.

This potential application of blood substitutes, as "therapeutic oxygenating agents" for ischemic tissue, has been investigated for myocardial ischemia[30,60,61] and for enhancing the effectiveness of radiation therapy and chemotherapy of ischemic tumors.[62,63] Clinical trials resulted in FDA approval for use of a perfluorochemical emulsion during coronary angioplasty,[64] which is discussed in the following section.

Clinical Pharmacology

Clinical Trials: Monitoring Adequacy of Oxygen Delivery

For a new drug to be approved for clinical use, it must prove itself to be more effective than the currently available products or of similar effectiveness with an improved side effect profile. For red blood cell substitutes, this is challenging for a variety of reasons. First, the only competitor is blood itself, which even with all its problems is considered to be a very effective treatment for acute severe anemia. Unfortunately, there is not a consensus on the specific indications for red blood cell transfusion, other than the physiologic signs of inadequate oxygen-carrying capacity.[65] It is difficult to select one variable to assure that the tissues are adequately oxygenated. Given that there is significant controversy and there is no definitive consensus regarding the indication for an individual transfusion, proving that a red cell substitute is equal to or superior to red blood cells is a daunting task.

During normal circumstances, only 25% of the oxygen delivered is actually consumed, and there can be adequate tissue oxygenation at lower than normal oxygen delivery rates. On average, tissues require approximately 30 to 40 mm Hg interstitial oxygen tension for adequate cellular oxygenation, whereas intracellular PO_2 only needs to be maintained in the single digit range to ensure aerobic metabolism. The clinically available physiologic variable that correlates most closely with tissue oxygenation is mixed venous PO_2. Because mixed venous PO_2 has been used as a sentinel variable to continuously monitor adequate oxygen transport, it has been used in many studies as an indicator of the effectiveness of red cell or red cell substitute transfusions.[66]

As shown in Figure 52–4, the hemoglobin in blood normally unloads 5 mL/dL oxygen as it passes through the tissue to support metabolic needs. Dissolved oxygen in the plasma contributes little during these circumstances, but if PO_2 was increased to 1500 mm Hg, a patient could theoretically survive on the oxygen dissolved in the plasma alone. In this situation, although the plasma carries only a little more than 5 mL/dL oxygen, but because it is released to the tissues in direct proportion to the oxygen tension, nearly all the oxygen is extracted. Understanding these two methods of oxygen transport (hemoglobin carriage vs. dissolved carriage) becomes important when the two types of blood substitutes are discussed and compared.

Clinical Trials: Perfluorochemicals Emulsions

Fluosol DA

Clinical studies were initiated in the late 1970s in patients who were actively bleeding, required surgery, and refused blood transfusion. In this unique patient population, 20 mL/kg body weight of Fluosol DA 20% PFC emulsion was transfused before surgery with a maximum of one additional dose after surgery.[22,67] The patients achieved a maximal fluorocrit of less than 3% with an intravascular half-life of approximately 19 hours. Subsequent studies confirmed the oxygen-carrying contribution of the PFC, but could not show a beneficial effect on patient outcome.[68] Another problem with Fluosol DA 20% was the appearance of an acute complement-mediated reaction caused by the surfactant, Pluronic F68, which necessitated pretreatment of all patients with corticosteroids.[25]

Despite these shortcomings, Fluosol DA 20% is the only oxygen-carrying colloid to gain FDA approval. However, approval was not for use as a red cell substitute but for intracoronary infusion in patients undergoing angioplasty. Fluosol DA 20% has been shown to improve myocardial recovery in an isolated neonatal pig heart model.[69] However, a trial of Fluosol as adjunct reperfusion therapy, aimed at preventing reperfusion injury for patients with acute myocardial infarction, failed to show any decrease in infarct size or improvement in myocardial function. The incidence of recurrent ischemia was decreased in patients who received Fluosol.[64] Fluosol is no longer being manufactured because of low demand.

Perflubron

Second-generation PFC emulsions have been developed (see Table 52–3). One of these, Oxygent, uses the perfluorocarbon, perfluoro-octylbromide, or perflubron[70] (see Fig. 52–6). This PFC is unique because it has one bromine replacing fluorine, making it radiopaque. This emulsion (Oxygent) contains 90% PFC by weight or 45% by volume. It is emulsified with lecithin (egg yolk phospholipids) and is stable at room temperature for more than 6 years. It is the only perfluorochemical currently being studied for use as a blood substitute.

Because of a short intravascular half-life and the need for a high FiO_2, it has been suggested that these PFC solutions should be used in conjunction with acute normovolemic hemodilution. In this setting, patients who are expected to have significant surgical blood loss have 2 to 4 units of blood removed before surgery. Initial volume expansion is with crystalloid or colloid. As surgical bleeding continues, the PFC is administered at the first transfusion trigger, allowing for adequate oxygen delivery at low hemoglobin levels. When surgical bleeding stops, the patient receives their autologous blood.

The ultimate use of PFC emulsions in the perioperative period is yet to be determined, although a study by Wahr and colleagues[71] in surgical patients showed enhanced mixed venous PO_2 in patients who received perflubron.

The European Perflubron Emulsion Study Group looked at perflubron administration in response to transfusion triggers after normovolemic hemodilution during orthopedic surgery. This study had two control and two treatment groups. The control groups were patients that received blood or colloid, whereas the two treatment groups were given two doses of perfluorochemical (0.9 and 1.8 g/kg). The triggers of tachycardia—hypotension, increased cardiac and decreased mixed venous PO_2—were at least as effectively reversed by perflubron with 100% oxygen ventilation as by autologous transfusion or colloid administration.[23] Patients who received perflubron had greater mixed venous PO_2 levels, which continued for longer than the other treatment groups. Allogeneic blood transfusion requirements were not reduced by perflubron administration. The same group has presented preliminary results in a group of 492 general surgery patients with a reduction in usage and an increase in avoidance of blood product administration.

A phase III cardiac surgery study of perflubron was voluntarily suspended in 2001 because of an increased incidence of stroke, but it has not been determined if this was caused by PFC administration (Alliance Pharmaceuticals press release, available online at: www.allp.com).

The increased oxygen delivery conferred by PFCs may be more effectively used in other settings. In particular, situations in which regional oxygen delivery is not sufficient may benefit from the enhanced tissue oxygenation that is possible with PFCs. During cardioplegia for cardiac surgery, for example, the myocardium is essentially ischemic. Although red cells may be present in the cardioplegia solution, the 9° C temperature results in a low P_{50} and little release of oxygen to the myocardium. Solubility of oxygen in PFCs and therefore oxygen delivery are affected by high but not low temperature. Multiple laboratory studies of transplantation have shown increased organ survival if the transplanted organ was preserved with a Wisconsin solution modified to include PFC.[72-74] Isolated Langendorff heart models have shown enhanced function of the heart after global ischemia if PFC was included in the cardioplegia solution.[69]

Animal models of regional myocardial or cerebral ischemia also exist. In many of these studies, administration of PFCs before ischemia or reperfusion with a PFC solution results in smaller infarct size and better functional recovery.[72,75,76] There are no clinical trials currently underway to evaluate the efficacy of PFCs in ameliorating global or regional ischemia.

PFCs have also been studied extensively for the treatment of tumors. Cancer patients are often anemic and their tumors are hypoxic. The level of cellular oxygenation is an important factor in the sensitivity of many tumors to radiation or chemotherapy. Although numerous trials have been undertaken to study the adjuvant benefit of PFCs with radiation or chemotherapy, FDA approval has not yet been given for this indication.[62,63]

Liquid Ventilation with Perfluorochemicals

In addition to their use as blood substitutes, PFCs have been used to treat acute respiratory distress syndrome when used in liquid ventilation. Clark's original experiment demonstrated that mammals could breath pure perfluorochemical when equilibrated at high PaO_2.[20]

Over the past 20 years there have been multiple studies evaluating the efficacy of liquid ventilation with perflubron (LiquiVent, Alliance Pharmaceuticals) at improving oxygenation while avoiding high peak airway pressures in patients with adult respiratory distress syndrome. This method (partial liquid ventilation) entails instillation of perflubron through the endotracheal tube followed by mechanical ventilation with an oxygen-rich gas mixture.[77] The PFC collects in the alveoli and stents them open, thereby improving their compliance,[78-80] while transporting oxygen and decreasing pulmonary shunt. This effect of recruiting collapsed alveoli and decreasing shunt has been called "liquid PEEP" or "PEEP in a bottle,"[81] for it has the effect of PEEP without requiring additional airway pressure, which may be damaging to the lung.

The perfluorocarbons have a low surface tension, which gives them excellent surfactant properties that may also be of benefit in the treatment of adult respiratory distress syndrome. The pulmonary lavage that occurs with liquid breathing may help to mobilize secretions into the central airways. It has also been suggested that perfluorocarbons may have direct anti-inflammatory effects.[82-84]

Partial liquid ventilation is an interesting application of these unique liquids, but until prospective, randomized, controlled studies compare outcomes with conventional gas ventilation its clinical use is unclear.[85]

Oxyfluor

Perfluorodichlorooctane (Oxyfluor; Hemagen, St. Louis, Mo) has been assessed as a cardiopulmonary bypass pump prime in animals,[86] and oxygen delivery was increased during bypass; however, increases in tissue and brain acidosis also occurred. Production of Oxyfluor has been discontinued.

Contrast Agents

PFCs have been used as echocardiographic contrast agents. Perflenapent (EchoGen; SONUS Pharmaceuticals, Bothell, Wash) is an emulsion of dodecafluoropentane that becomes a dispersion of microbubbles with hypobaric activation and is highly echogenic to ultrasound. It has been used to delineate the left ventricle in echocardiography.[87]

Perflubron has been studied as a contrast agent for computed tomography, ultrasound, and magnetic resonance imaging[88]; the vascular persistence of PFCs gives them ideal properties for imaging vessels and cardiac chambers.

Clinical Trials: Hemoglobin Solutions

Several types of hemoglobin solution have proceeded to clinical trial. One of the products is produced from modified polymerized bovine hemoglobin (Hemopure, HBOC-201;

Biopure, Cambridge, Mass).[43,89] Other products have been developed from outdated human blood: PolyHeme,[90,91] DCLHb (Baxter Healthcare, Chicago, Ill),[38,44] and Hemolink (Hemosol, Toronto, Ontario, Canada). All of these products have a P_{50} within the normal range and have an increased size because of crosslinking or polymerization. PolyHeme is also filtered to remove the smaller molecular weight tetrameric hemoglobin molecules.

HBOC-201 (Hemopure)

The bovine product HBOC-201 has been studied in patients undergoing abdominal aortic aneurysm surgery. Treatment with the hemoglobin solution produced an increase in pulmonary and systemic vascular resistance and an associated decrease in cardiac output.[43] In a similar study by LaMuraglia and colleagues,[46] HBOC-201 given in aortic surgery eliminated the need for blood transfusion in 27% of patients, but the median transfusion requirement was not decreased. Mean arterial blood pressure increased by 15% in this study. Another study by Standl and colleagues,[47] examining preoperative hemodilution with bovine HBOC-201 before liver resection, showed an increase in systemic vascular resistance and a decrease in cardiac output. More recently, a study by Wahr and colleagues[45] found this product to be useful in reducing the amount of allogeneic blood in surgical patients. This study did not note increases in pulmonary or systemic resistance, but a mild increase in blood pressure occurred.

A case report of reversal of myocardial ischemia with administration of HBOC-201 was attributed to the hemodynamic effects and improvement of oxygen delivery.[92]

HBOC-201 has been administered to patients with sickle cell anemia and may have a role in the treatment of vaso-occlusive or aplastic crises in this disease.[93,94] A case report also described life-saving administration of HBOC-201 to a young woman with severe autoimmune hemolytic anemia.[95] The hemoglobin solution reversed both lactic acidosis and myocardial ischemia in the presence of a hematocrit of 4.4%.

It has been suggested that degradation of hemoglobin solutions after administration may have hematopoietic effects.[96] A study by Hughes and colleagues[97] in healthy volunteers showed that after acute normovolemic hemodilution with HBOC-201 there were increases in serum iron, ferritin, and erythropoietin, which did not occur after acute normovolemic hemodilution with Ringer's lactate solution.

HBOC-201 has been licensed to treat anemia in surgical patients in South Africa, the first time a hemoglobin solution has reached the market for humans. It is also licensed, as Oxyglobin, for veterinary use in the United States and Europe.

Diaspirin Cross-Linked Hemoglobin

Current clinical studies have had varying results with DCLHb. It was investigated in a randomized study of patients with acute ischemic stroke.[44] Unfortunately, it was found that the patients receiving the hemoglobin solution had worse outcome scale scores, more serious adverse outcomes, and a higher mortality rate.

In animal studies, this product was also noted to increase pulmonary and systemic vascular resistance in the hemodilution model to the point of reducing cardiac index and oxygen delivery relative to a test band control.[38] In human studies of DCLHb given after cardiac surgery, pulmonary and systemic hypertension occurs with increases in SVR and PVR and decreased cardiac output compared with patients given red cell transfusion.[48] Another study by Shubert and colleagues[98] showed that DCLHb reduced the number of patients requiring PRBC transfusions after vascular, orthopedic, and abdominal surgery compared with patients randomized to PRBC transfusions during the perioperative period. Over 7 days the total PRBC and other blood product requirements of the two groups were similar. Side effects of hypertension, jaundice, and hemoglobinuria were noted. One death from respiratory distress syndrome was attributed to DCLHb, although this was not statistically significant, and the study was terminated early. Because of these results, Baxter Healthcare has discontinued further work with DCLHb. Baxter has acquired Somatogen, manufacturer of Optro, a first-generation recombinant hemoglobin, and has shifted its research-and-development efforts to a second-generation product based on recombinant technology.

Treatment of Septic Shock

The observed vasoconstriction with hemoglobin solutions has led to the evaluation of DCLHb solution as a vasopressor in critically ill patients with septic shock or systemic inflammatory response syndrome.[50] In septic shock, excessive synthesis of nitric oxide may occur and the scavenging effect of the hemoglobin solution may be beneficial in restoring vascular tone in this setting. The smaller size of the hemoglobin molecules compared with red blood cells may also improve oxygen delivery through the microcirculation, thereby improving tissue perfusion. The combination of these effects with the properties of oxygen carriage, improved distribution of blood flow, and high colloid osmotic pressure make hemoglobin solutions attractive as an "all-in-one" therapeutic strategy in vasodilated shock states.[59] However, in a study of a mouse model of gramnegative sepsis, hemoglobin solution increased lethality and was associated with increased circulating tumor necrosis factor.[99] Kupffer cells, which release tumor necrosis factor, may be sensitized by hemoglobin. Further work is required to determine the use of hemoglobin solutions in critical illness.[100]

PolyHeme

PolyHeme has been used in a trial treating acute trauma patients. Gould and colleagues[91] randomly assigned 44 trauma patients to either receive blood (23 patients) or up to 6 units of PolyHeme (21 patients). They found no adverse effects on pulmonary and systemic vascular resistance or cardiac output in the patients who received PolyHeme.

There were no differences in patient outcomes, although there was a reduced need for red blood cells in the Poly-Heme group at Day 1, which was no longer seen by Day 3. The authors of this study, and a preliminary study using the same protocol,[101] attribute lack of effect of PolyHeme on systemic and peripheral vascular resistance to its manufacturing process, which filters out the smaller tetrameric hemoglobin.[90,91] They speculate that the smaller size hemoglobin constituents defuse through the vessel wall, thereby increasing nitric oxide scavenging and producing vasoconstriction. The PolyHeme product is manufactured as a 10-gm/dL solution (i.e., 50 g in 500 mL), and therefore is equivalent to transfusing blood with a hematocrit of 30%. These studies found an intravascular half-life of 24 hours, which is longer than previous studies that found half-lives in a range of 9 to 12 hours. Many studies have found that the half-life of these products is dose dependent (i.e., a larger dose produces a longer half-life). Trauma patients who were given up to 20 U PolyHeme[102] showed less priming of polymorphonuclear neutrophil cells, which may reduce post-traumatic hyperinflammatory response and multiple organ failure. If these preliminary studies with Poly-Heme are confirmed with larger studies in the perioperative setting, then this product may have a role in future clinical practice.

Hemolink

Hemolink is an O-raffinose, crosslinked, human hemoglobin that has been shown to cause vasoconstriction in animals.[39] As with other crosslinked hemoglobin solutions, the hemodynamic effects are less pronounced than with unmodified hemoglobin solutions,[103] but exceeds that of polymerized hemoglobin solutions.

A phase I study in healthy volunteers showed the solution was well tolerated apart from some moderate to severe abdominal pain, which occurred in all subjects at greater doses. Blood pressure increased by 14% after administration and with greater doses this increase lasted 24 hours.[51] The initial findings of a phase III study in coronary artery bypass surgery[52] showed a 7% to 10% increase in blood pressure, which was not statistically significant, and a reduction in the number of patients requiring red cell transfusion from 57% to 10%.

Hemolink is being reviewed for approval by the drug agencies in the United States, Canada, and the United Kingdom.

Polyethylene Glycol Hemoglobin

PEG hemoglobin (Enzon, Piscataway, NJ) does not use crosslinking between molecules but is conjugated with polyethylene glycol to increase the molecular size of bovine hemoglobin. This increases retention in the circulation and reduces immune reaction to the molecule. In canine administration, there was no increase of blood pressure and it was well tolerated.[104]

PEG hemoglobin has been used to sensitize tumors to chemotherapy[105] and radiotherapy in rodents.[106] Hypoxic tumors are less responsive to chemotherapy and radiother-apy; using hemoglobin solutions with a small molecular size, compared with red cells, allows an improvement in microvascular oxygenation and increases the response to treatment.

PEG hemoglobin has also been studied as a constituent of cardioplegic preservative for transplanted hearts in rabbits with improvement in cardiac function after surgery.[107]

PHP

Pyridoxylated hemoglobin polyoxyethylene conjugate (PHP; Apex Bioscience, Research Triangle Park, NC) is a human hemoglobin solution, crosslinked by pyridoxal-5-phosphate, which is being developed as a nitric oxide scavenger for use in septic shock and systemic inflammatory response syndrome.[34] A phase II study has been completed and a phase III study is in progress investigating PHP for the treatment of nitric oxide–induced shock.

Encapsulated Hemoglobin

Encapsulated hemoglobin solutions, sometime referred to as *neo red cells,* mimic the natural presentation of hemoglobin in whole blood.[108] Recent work has used liposome-encapsulated hemoglobin, but phospholipid vesicles have also been used. There is significant accumulation of liposomes in the liver and spleen, when liposome-encapsulated hemoglobin is administered, causing vacuolization and an elevation in liver transaminases.[30] Circulation time of the hemoglobin is increased by encapsulation and can be increased further, from 18 hours to 65 hours, by PEG modification[109]; these long-lasting derivatives have been named "stealth" liposomes.

Effects on Clinical Laboratory Tests

Hemolysis causing hemoglobinemia[110] and lipemia[111] are recognized causes of interference in laboratory assays.

Lipemia causes light scattering, which can affect colorimetric and spectrophotometric laboratory tests. Plasma samples from patients receiving perfluorocarbons appear lipemic. All hemoglobin solutions interfere with spectrophotometric laboratory determinations of the concentrations of certain plasma constituents.[57] Because of optical absorbance between 400 and 600 nm, plasma hemoglobin, in concentrations of approximately 2 g/mL, interferes significantly with a wide variety of serum chemistry determinations. Most electrolyte assays are unaffected by hemoglobin or PFCs because ion-specific electrodes are used that are unaffected by light absorbance, colored substances, or light scatter from emulsion particles.

Table 52–6 shows the possible effects of hemoglobin solutions and perfluorocarbons on laboratory assays as demonstrated by several studies.[111–116] Different laboratory analyzers use varying techniques and reagents and this accounts for some of the variation in effects solutions can have on a particular assay. The concentration of hemoglobin solution present may also affect the degree of interference—

TABLE 52–6.

Effects of Hemoglobin Solutions and Perfluorocarbons on Laboratory Tests

Assay	Hemoglobin Solution	Perfluorocarbon
Sodium	None	None
Potassium	None	None
Chloride	None	None
Urea	None or ↑	None
Total carbon dioxide	None or ↑	None
Phosphate	None, ↑, ↓ or unreadable result	↑
Uric acid	None, ↑ or unreadable result	None
Magnesium	None, ↑ or unreadable result	None
Calcium	None or ↑	None
Creatinine	None, ↑, ↓ or unreadable result	None
Glucose	None or ↓	None
Ammonia		↑
Total protein	None	None
Albumin	↑ or ↓	None
Lactate dehydrogenase	↑, ↓ or unreadable result	None
Aspartate aminotransferase	None or ↑	None
Alanine aminotransferase	↑ or ↓	None
Gamma-glutamyltransferase	↑ or ↓ or unreadable result	None
Alkaline phosphatase	↓ or unreadable result	None
Amylase	↑ or unreadable result	↓
Lipase	None or ↓	None
Bilirubin	↑, ↓ or unreadable result	None
Iron	↑	↓
Cholesterol	None or ↑	None

TABLE 52–6.

Effects of Hemoglobin Solutions and Perfluorocarbons on Laboratory Tests—cont'd

Assay	Hemoglobin Solution	Perfluorocarbon
Creatine kinase-MB	None, ↓ or unreadable result	None
Coagulation tests	None or unreadable result	
Hemoglobin	None	
Coulter blood count variables	None	
Platelet count		↑
Reticulocyte count	None	
Gentamycin	↑	None
Vancomycin	↓	None
Phenytoin	None or ↓	

at lower levels there may be no effect on the assay level on an analyzer, which is influenced by greater concentrations.[116] Immunoassays unaffected by hemoglobin solutions include troponin I, troponin T, thyroid-stimulating hormone, digoxin, lidocaine, procainamide and *N*-acetyl-procainamide, quinidine, and theophylline. Notably, creatine kinase-MB is adversely affected on some analyzers but troponin T remains reliable and should be used when myocardial infarction is suspected in a patient receiving a hemoglobin solution. Coagulation tests are unaffected if electrical clot detection is used but analyzers that use optical detection of clot formation fail completely. All Coulter blood count variables were unaffected by the presence of free hemoglobin. Cross-matching is unaffected by hemoglobin solutions.

A study of eight co-oximeters with five hemoglobin solutions[117] showed that the total hemoglobin level was uninfluenced by the hemoglobin solutions, but fractional readings of oxyhemoglobin, deoxyhemoglobin, carboxyhemoglobin, and methemoglobin showed greater variability between oximeters; the results were less accurate but still clinically useful.

Pulse oximetry is not affected by administration of HBOC-201 (Hemopure) when compared with arterial blood gas analysis with co-oximetry.[118]

The emulsion particles in perfluorodichlorooctane (Oxyfluor) emulsion appear as platelets in automated cell counters and can cause a spurious increase in the platelet count.[119]

Although other means of determining these affected laboratory values may be available, spectrophotometric methods are so ubiquitous that the widespread use of hemoglobin solutions would require some adaptation. Laboratories will have to be aware of which analyzers and reagents are affected and use alternatives if available. Hemoglobind (LigoChem, Fairfield, NJ), an insoluble anionic polyelectrolyte that selectively binds and removes free hemoglobin, has been used to remove Hemolink hemoglobin solution from serum,[120] but it is unable to reduce the concentration sufficiently to allow accurate performance of affected laboratory tests. Filtration of sera-containing hemoglobin solution can eliminate interference with some creatinine assays.[116]

Conclusion

Any of these products may find a useful niche in clinical settings in which an oxygen-carrying drug may be beneficial for a specific organ or clinical situation. Hemoglobin solutions may be more useful as field resuscitation fluids before hospital admission or as hematopoietic drugs, whereas PFCs may be useful intraoperatively or for cardioplegia or organ preservation. Neither hemoglobin emulsions nor PFC solutions in current development will provide prolonged benefit after a single dose, and they may only be useful to reduce the amount of homologous blood required, not to replace it. Neither of these products will benefit or supplement the coagulation cascade, and they may have a detrimental effect, at least by dilution. Ultimately, a combination of homologous and autologous blood products, intraoperative and postoperative blood salvaging techniques, and these oxygen-carrying solutions may provide an overall system for reducing mortality, morbidity, and costs associated with blood transfusions.

References

1. Epstein JS: The US blood supply. Am Fam Physician 61(2): 549–550,2000.

2. American Society of Anesthesiologists Task Force on Blood Component Therapy: Practice Guidelines for blood component therapy. Anesthesiology 84(3):732–747, 1996.

3. Spahn DR, Cassutt M: Eliminating blood transfusions: New aspects and perspectives. Anesthesiology 93(1):242–255, 2000.

4. Cohn SM: Blood substitutes in surgery. Surgery 127:599–602, 2000.

5. Ketcham EM, Cairns CB: Hemoglobin-based oxygen carriers: Development and clinical potential. Ann Emerg Med 33(3):326–337, 1999.

6. Newman RJ, Podolsky D, Loeb P: Bad blood. US News World Rep 116:68–70, 72–78, 1994.

7. Myhre BA, Bove JR, Schmidt PJ: Wrong blood—a needless cause of surgical deaths. Anesth Analg 60:777–778, 1981.

8. Nichollis MD: Transfusions: Morbidity and mortality. Anaesth Intensive Care 21:15–19, 1993.

9. Sazama K: Reports of 355 transfusion-associated deaths: 1976 through 1985. Transfusion 30:583–590, 1990.

10. Lackritz EM: Prevention of HIV transmission by blood transfusion in the developing world: Achievements and continuing challenges. AIDS 12(suppl A):581–586, 1998.

11. Chamberland M, Khabbaz RF: Emerging issues in blood safety. Infect Dis Clin North Am 12(1):217–229, 1998.

12. Dodd RY: The risk of transfusion-transmitted infection. N Engl J Med 327:419–421, 1992.

13. Karayiannis P, Thomas HC: Current status of hepatitis G virus (GBV-C) in transfusion: Is it relevant? Vox Sang 7:3:155–163, 1997.

14. Ricketts MN, Cashman NR, Stratton EE, et al: Is Creutzfeldt-Jakob disease transmitted in blood? Emerg Infect Dis 3:155–163, 1997.

15. Houston F, Foster JD, Chong A, et al: Transmission of BSE by blood transfusion in sheep. Lancet 356(9234):999–1000, 2000.

16. Mitka M: Blood groups differ on donor deferral. JAMA 285(13):1694–1695, 2001.

17. Blumberg N: Allogeneic transfusion and infection: Economic and clinical implications. Semin Hematol 34:34–40, 1997.

18. Blumberg N, Triulzi DJ, Heal JM: Transfusion-induced immunomodulation and its clinical consequences. Transfus Med Rev 4:24–35, 1990.

19. Bordin JO, Blajchman MA: Immunosuppressive effects of allogeneic blood transfusions: Implications for the patient with a malignancy. Hematol Oncol Clin North Am 9:205–218, 1995.

20. Clark LC Jr, Gollan F: Survival of mammals breathing organic liquids equilibrated with oxygen at atmospheric pressure. Science 152: 1755–1756, 1966.

21. Gehes RP, Monroe RG, Taylor K: Survival of rats having red cells totally replaced with emulsified fluorocarbon. Fed Proc 27:384, 1968.

22. Tremper KK, Friedman AE, Levine EM, et al: The preoperative treatment of severely anemic patients with perfluorochemical oxygen-transport fluid, Fluosol-DA. N Engl J Med 307:277–283, 1982.

23. Spahn DR, van Brempt R, Theilmeier G, et al: Perflubron emulsion delays blood transfusions in orthopedic surgery. Anesthesiology 91(5):1195–1208, 1999.

24. Noveck RJ, Shannon EJ, Leese PT, et al: Randomized safety studies of intravenous perflubron emulsion II: Effects on immune function in healthy volunteers. Anesth Analg 91(4):812–822, 2000.

25. Tremper KK, Vercellotti GM, Hammerschmidt DE: Hemodynamic profile of adverse clinical reactions to Fluosol-DA 20%. Crit Care Med 12:428–431, 1984.

26. Klein HD: The prospects for red-cell substitutes. N Engl J Med 342(22):1666–1668, 2000.

27. Geyer RP: Perfluorochemicals as oxygen transport vehicles. Biomater Artif Cells Artif Organs 16(1–3):31–49, 1988.

28. Rabiner SF, Friedman L: The role of intravascular hemolysis and the reticuloendothelial system in production of the hypercoagulable state. Brit J Haematol 14:105, 1968.

29. Rabiner SF, Helbert JR, Lopas H, et al: Evaluation of a stroma-free hemoglobin solution for use as a plasma expander. J Exp Med 126:1127–1142, 1967.

30. Creteur J, Sibbald W, Vincent JL: Hemoglobin solutions—not just red blood cells substitutes. Crit Care Med 28(8):3025–3034, 2000.

31. Gould SA, Sehgal LR, Rosen AL, et al: The development of polymerized pyridoxylated hemoglobin solution as a red cell substitute. Ann Emerg Med 15(12):1416–1419, 1986.

32. Sehgal LR, Rosen AL, Gould SA, et al: Preparation and in vitro characteristics of polymerized pyridoxylated hemoglobin. Transfusion 23(2):158–162, 1983.

33. Rudolph AS: Encapsulated hemoglobin: Current issues and future goals. Artif Cells Blood Substit Immobil Biotechnol 22(2):347–360, 1994.

34. Privalle C, Talarico T, Keng T, et al: Pyridoxylated hemoglobin polyoxyethylene: A nitric oxide scavenger with antioxidant activity for the treatment of nitric oxide-induced shock. Free Radic Biol Med 28(10):1507–1517, 2000.

35. Hughes GS Jr, Antal EJ, Locker PK, et al: Physiology and pharmacokinetics of a novel hemoglobin-based oxygen carrier in humans. Crit Care Med 24:756–764, 1996.

36. Winslow RM: Blood substitutes. Adv Drug Deliv Rev 40:131–142, 2000.

37. USDA Interim Rule on Import Restrictions of Ruminant Material from Europe. Fed Reg 63(3):406–408, 1998.

38. DeAngeles DA, Scott AM, McGrath AM, et al: Resuscitation from hemorrhagic shock with diaspirin cross-linked hemoglobin, blood, or hetastarch. J Trauma 42(3):406–412, discussion 412–414, 1997.

39. Ning J, Wong LT, Christoff B, et al: Haemodynamic response following a 10% top load infusion of Hemolink™ in conscious, anaesthetized and treated spontaneously hypertensive rats. Transfus Med 10(1):13–22, 2000.

40. Krieter H, Hagan G, Waschke KF, et al: Isovolemic hemodilution with a bovine hemoglobin-based oxygen carrier: Effects on hemodynamics and oxygen transport in comparison with a nonoxygen-carrying volume substitute. J Cardiothorac Vasc Anesth 11:3–9, 1997.

41. Maxwell RA, Gibson JB, Fabian TC, et al: Resuscitation of severe chest trauma with four different hemoglobin-based oxygen carrying solutions. J Trauma 49:200–211, 2000.

42. Ulatowski JA, Nishikawa T, Matheson-Urbaitus B, et al: Regional blood flow alterations after bovine fumaryl beta beta-cross-linked hemoglobin transfusion and nitric oxide synthase inhibition. Crit Care Med 24(4):558–565, 1996.

43. Kasper SM, Grune F, Walter M, et al: The effects of increased doses of bovine hemoglobin on hemodynamics and oxygen transport in patients undergoing preoperative hemodilution for elective abdominal aortic surgery. Anesth Analg 87(2):284–291, 1998.

44. Saxena R, Wijnhoud Ad, Carton H, et al: Controlled safety study of a hemoglobin-based oxygen carrier, DCLHb, in acute ischemic stroke. Stroke 30(5):993–996, 1999.

45. Wahr JA, Levy JH, Kindscher, J, et al: Hemodynamic effects of a bovine based oxygen carrying solution in surgical patients. Anesthesiology 85(3A):A347, 1996.

46. LaMuraglia GM, O'Hara PJ, Baker WH: The reduction of the allogenic transfusion requirement in aortic surgery with a hemoglobin-based solution. J Vasc Surg 31(2):299–308, 2000.

47. Standl T, Wilhelm S, Horn EP, et al: Preoperative hemodilution with bovine hemoglobin. Acute hemodynamic effects in liver surgery patients. Anaesthetsist 46(9):763–770, 1997.

48. Lamy ML, Daily EK, Brichant JF, et al: Randomized trial of diaspirin cross-linked hemoglobin solution as an alternative to blood transfusion after cardiac surgery. Anesthesiology 92(3):646–656, 2000.

49. Schubert A, Mascha E, O'Hara JF, et al: Synthetic hemoglobin reduces perioperative blood transfusions in vascular, orthopedic and abdominal surgery. Anesthesiology 93(3A):A-180, 2000.

50. Reah G, Bodenham AR, Mallick A, et al: Initial evaluation of diaspirin cross-linked hemoglobin (DCLHb) as a vasopressor in critically ill patients. Crit Care Med 25(9):1480–1488, 1997.

51. Carmichael FJ, Ali AC, Campbell JA, et al: A phase I study of oxidized raffinose cross-linked human hemoglobin. Crit Care Med 28(7):2283–2292, 2000.

52. Cheng DC, Ralph-Edwards A, Mazer CD, et al: The hemodynamic effects of the red cell substitute Hemolink™ (o-rafinose cross-linked

human hemoglobin) on vital signs in patients undergoing CABG surgery. Anesthesiology 93(3A):A-180, 2000.

53. Patel RP: Biochemical aspects of the reaction of hemoglobin and NO: Implications for Hb-based substitutes. Free Radic Biol Med 28(10):1518–1525, 2000.

54. Kim HW, Greenberg AG: Ferrous sulphate scavenging of endothelium derived nitric oxide is a principal mechanism for hemoglobin mediated vasoactivities in isolated rat thoracic aorta. Artif Cells Blood Substit Immobil Biotechnol 25(1):121–133, 1997.

55. Lee R, Neya K, Svizzero TA, et al: Limitations of the efficacy of hemoglobin-based oxygen-carrying solutions. J Appl Physiol 79:236–242, 1995.

56. Slanetz PJ, Lee R, Page R, et al: Hemoglobin blood substitutes in extended preoperative autologous blood donation: An experimental study. Surgery 115:256–254, 1994.

57. Wahr JA, Levy JR, Kindscher J, et al: Hemodynamic effects of a bovine hemoglobin-based oxygen-carrying solution in surgical patients. Anesthesiology 85(3A):A347, 1996.

58. Levy JH: Hemoglobin-based oxygen-carrying solutions: Close but still so far. Anesthesiology 92(3):639–641, 2000.

59. Creteur J, Vincent JL: Hemoglobin solutions: An "all-in-one" therapeutic strategy in sepsis? Crit Care Med 28(3):894–896, 2000.

60. Kent KM, Cleman MW, Cowley MJ, et al: Reduction of myocardial ischemia during percutaneous transluminal coronary angioplasty with oxygenated Fluosol. Am J Cardiol 66(3):279–284, 1990.

61. Robalino BD, Marwick T, Lafont A, et al: Protection against ischemia during prolonged balloon inflation by distal coronary perfusion with use of an autoperfusion catheter or Fluosol. J Am Coll Cardiol 20(6):1378–1384, 1992.

62. Teicher BA, Schwartz GN, Dupuis NP, et al: Oxygenation of human tumor xenografts in nude mice by a perfluorochemical emulsion and carbogen breathing. Artif Cells Blood Substit Immobil Biotechnol 22:1369–1375, 1994.

63. Teicher BA: An overview on oxygen carriers in cancer therapy. Artif Cells Blood Substit Immobil Biotechnol 23:395–405, 1995.

64. Wall TC, Califf RM, Blankenship J, et al: Intravenous Fluosol in the treatment of acute myocardial infarction. Results of the thrombolysis and angioplasty in myocardial infarction 9 trial. TAMI 9 Research Group. Circulation 90:114–120, 1994.

65. Tremper KK: Perfluorochemical "blood substitutes." Anesthesiology 91(5):1185–1187, 1999.

66. McFarland JG: Perioperative blood transfusions: Indications and options. Chest 115(5 suppl):113S–121S, 1999.

67. Tremper KK, Levine EM, Waxman K: Clinical experience with Fluosol-DA (20%) in the United States. Int Anesthesiol Clin 23:185–197, 1985.

68. Gould SA, Rosen AL, Sehgal LR, et al: Fluosol-DA as a red-cell substitute in acute anemia. N Engl J Med 314:1653–1656, 1986.

69. Martin SM, Laks H, Drinkwater DC, et al: Perfluorochemical reperfusion yields improved myocardial recovery after global ischemia. Ann Thorac Surg 55:954–960, 1993.

70. Keipert PE, Faithfull NS, Bradley JD, et al: Oxygen delivery augmentation by low-dose perfluorochemical emulsion during profound normovolemic hemodilution. Adv Exp Med Biol 345:197–204, 1994.

71. Wahr JA, Trouwborst A, Spence RK, et al: A pilot study of the effects of a perflubron emulsion, AF 0104, on mixed venous oxygen tension in anesthetized surgical patients. Anesth Analg 82:103–107, 1996.

72. Kloner RA, Hale S: Cardiovascular applications of fluorocarbons in regional ischemia/reperfusion. Artif Cells Blood Substit Immobil Biotechnol 22:1069–1081, 1992.

73. Segel LD, Follette DM, Iguidbashian JB, et al: Post-transplantation function of hearts preserved with fluorochemical emulsion. J Heart Lung Transplant 13:669–680, 1994.

74. Grunert A, Qui H, Muller I, et al: A new extracorporeal perfusion system: prolongation of liver organ vitality beyond 24 hours. Ann NY Acad Sci 723:488–490, 1994.

75. Premaratne S, Harada RN, Chun P, et al: Effects of perfluorocarbon exchange transfusion on reducing myocardial infarct size in a primate model of ischemia-reperfusion injury: A prospective randomized study. Surgery 117:670–676, 1995.

76. Cole DJ, Schell RM, Drummond JC, et al: Focal cerebral ischemia in rats: Effect of hemodilution with alpha-alpha cross-linked hemoglobin on brain injury and edema. Can J Neurol Sci 20:30–36, 1993.

77. Wiedemann HP: Partial liquid ventilation for acute respiratory distress syndrome. Clin Chest Med 21(3):543–554, 2000.

78. Gauger PG, Overbeck MC, Chambers SD, et al: Partial liquid ventilation improves gas exchange and increases EELV in acute lung injury. J Appl Physiol 84:1566–1572, 1998.

79. Hirsch RB, Pranikoff T, Wise C, et al: Initial experience with partial liquid ventilation in adult patients with the acute respiratory distress syndrome. JAMA 275(5):383–389, 1996.

80. Gauger PG, Pranikoff T, Schreiner RJ, et al: Initial experience with partial liquid ventilation in pediatric patients with the acute respiratory distress syndrome. Crit Care Med 24(1):16–22, 1996.

81. Wong DH: Liquid ventilation: More than "PEEP in a bottle"? Crit Care Med 27(6):1052–1053, 1999.

82. Colton DM, Hirsch RB, Johnson KJ, et al: Neutrophil accumulation is reduced during partial liquid ventilation. Crit Care Med 26(10):1716–1724, 1998.

83. Smith TM, Steinhorn DM, Thusu K, et al: A liquid perfluorochemical decreases the in vitro production of reactive oxygen species by alveolar macrophages. Crit Care Med 23(9):1533–1539, 1995.

84. Mrozek JD, Smith KM, Bing DR, et al: Exogenous surfactant and partial liquid ventilation: Physiologic and pathologic effects. Am J Respir Crit Care Med 156:1058–1065, 1997.

85. Hirschl RB, Conrad S, Kaiser R, et al: Partial liquid ventilation in adult patients with ARDS: A multicenter phase I-II trial. Adult PLV study group. Ann Surg 228(5):692–700, 1998.

86. Briceno JC, Rincon IE, Velez JF, et al: Oxygen transport and consumption during experimental cardiopulmonary bypass using oxyfluor. ASAIO J 45(4):322–327, 1999.

87. Kitzman DW, Wesley DJ: Safety assessment of perflenapent emulsion for echocardiographic contrast enhancement in patients with congestive heart failure or chronic obstructive pulmonary disease. Am Heart J 139(6):1077–1080, 2000.

88. Mattrey RF: Perfluorooctylbromide: A new contrast agent for CT, sonography, and MR imaging. AJR Am J Roentgenol 152(2):247–252, 1989.

89. Standl T, Burmeister MA, Horn EP, et al: Bovine haemoglobin-based oxygen carrier for patients undergoing haemodilution before liver resection. Br J Anaesth 80(2):189–194, 1998.

90. Johnson JL, Moore EE, Offner PJ, et al: Resuscitation of the injured patient with polymerized stroma free hemoglobin dues not produce systemic or pulmonary hypertension. Am J Surg 176(6):612–617, 1998.

91. Gould SA, Moore EE, Hoyt DB, et al: The first randomized trial of human polymerized hemoglobin as a blood substitute in acute trauma and emergent surgery. J Am Coll Surg 187(2):113–120; discussion 120–122, 1998.

92. Niquille M, Touzet M, Leblanc I, et al: Reversal of intraoperative myocardial ischemia with a hemoglobin-based oxygen carrier. Anesthesiology 92(3):882–885, 2000.

93. Gonzalez P, Hackney AC, Jones S, et al: A phase I/II study of polymerized bovine hemoglobin in adult patients with sickle cell disease not in crisis at the time of study. Invest Med 45(5):258–264, 1997.

94. Feola M, Simoni J, Angelillo R, et al: Clinical trial of a hemoglobin based blood substitute in patients with sickle cell anemia. Surg Gynecol Obstet 174(5):379–386, 1992.

95. Mullon J, Giacoppe G, Clagett C, et al: Transfusions of polymerized bovine hemoglobin in a patient with a severe autoimmune hemolytic anemia. N Engl J Med 342(22):1638–1643, 2000.

96. Vlahakes GJ: Hemoglobin solutions come of age. Anesthesiology 92(3):637–638, 2000.

97. Hughes GS, Francome SF, Antal EJ, et al: Hematologic effects of a novel hemoglobin-based oxygen carrier in normal male and female subjects. J Lab Clin Med 126:444–451, 1995.

98. Shubert A, Maascha E, O'Hara JF, et al: Synthetic hemoglobin reduces perioperative blood transfusions in vascular, orthopedic and abdominal surgery. Anesthesiology 93(3A):A-180, 2000.

99. Su D, Roth RI, Levin J: Hemoglobin infusion augments the tumor necrosis factor response to bacterial endotoxin (lipopolysaccharide) in mice. Crit Care Med 27(4):771–778, 1999.

100. Zimmerman JJ: Deciphering the dark side of free hemoglobin in sepsis. Crit Care Med 27:685–686, 1999.

101. Gould SA, Moore EE, Moore FA, et al: Clinical utility of human polymerized hemoglobin as a blood substitute after acute trauma and urgent surgery. J Trauma 43:325–331, 1997.

102. Johnson J, Moore EE, Offner PJ, et al: Resuscitation with a blood substitute abrogates pathologic post injury neutrophil cytotoxic function. J Trauma 50(3):449–455, 2001.

103. Lieberthal W: O-raffinose cross-linking markedly reduces systemic

and renal vasoconstrictor effects of unmodified human hemoglobin. J Pharmacol Exp Ther 288(3):1278–1287, 1999.

104. Conover CD, Lejeune L, Shum K, et al: Physiological effect of polyethylene glycol conjugation on stroma-free bovine hemoglobin in the conscious dog after partial exchange transfusion. Artif Organs 21(5):369–378, 1997.

105. Teicher BA, Ara G, Herbst, R, et al: PEG-hemoglobin: Effects on tumor oxygenation and response to chemotherapy. In Vivo 11(4): 301–311.

106. Linberg R, Conover CD, Shum KL, et al: Increased tissue oxygenation and enhanced radiation sensitivity of solid tumors in rodents following polyethylene glycol conjugated bovine hemoglobin administration. In Vivo 12(2):167–173, 1998.

107. Serna DL, Powell LL, Kahwaji C, et al: Cardiac function after eight hour storage by using polyethylene glycol hemoglobin versus crystalloid perfusion. ASAIO J 45(5):547–552, 2000.

108. Rudolph AS: Encapsulated hemoglobin: Current issues and future goals. Artif Cells Blood Substit Immobil Biotechnol 22(2):347–360, 1994.

109. Phillips WT, Klipper RW, Awasthi VD, et al: Polyethylene glycol-modified liposome-encapsulated hemoglobin: A long circulating red cell substitute. J Pharmacol Exp Ther 288(2):665–670, 1999.

110. Sonntag O: Haemolysis as an interference factor in clinical chemistry. J Clin Chem Clin Biochem 24(2):127–139, 1986.

111. Ma Z, Monk TG, Goodnough LT, et al: Effect of hemoglobin and Perflubron-based oxygen carriers on common clinical laboratory tests. Clin Chem 43(9):1732–1737.

112. Ali AC, Campbell JA: Interference of o-raffinose cross-linked hemoglobin with routine Hitachi 717 assays. Clin Chem 43(9):1794–1796, 1997.

113. Wolthuis A, Peek D, Scholten R, et al: Effect of the hemoglobin-based oxygen carrier HBOC-201 on laboratory instrumentation: Cobas integra, Chiron blood gas analyzer 840, Sysmex SE-9000 and BCT. Clin Chem Lab Med 37(1):71–76, 1999.

114. Eldridge J, Russell R, Christenson R, et al: Liver function and morphology after resuscitation from severe hemorrhagic shock with hemoglobin solutions or autologous blood. Crit Care Med 24(4):663–671, 1996.

115. Ali AC, Mihas CC, Campabell JA: Interferences of o-raffinose cross-linked hemoglobin in three methods for serum creatinine. Clin Chem 43(9):1738–1743, 1997.

116. Callas DD, Clark TL, Moreira PL, et al: In vitro effects of a novel hemoglobin-based oxygen carrier on routine chemistry, therapeutic drug, coagulation, hematology, and blood bank assays. Clin Chem 43(9):1744–1748, 1997.

117. Ali AA, Ali GS, Steinke JM, et al: Co-oximetry interference by hemoglobin-based blood substitutes. Anesth Analg 92(4):863–869, 2001.

118. Hughes GS, Francom SF, Antal EJ, et al: Effects of a novel hemoglobin-based oxygen carrier on percent oxygen saturation as determined with arterial blood gas analysis and pulse oximetry. Ann Emerg Med 27(2):164–169, 1996.

119. Cuignet OY, Wood BL, Chandler WL, et al: A second-generation blood substitute (Perfluorodichlorooctane emulsion) generates spurious elevations in platelet counts from automated hematology analyzers. Anesh Analg 90(3):517–522.

120. Balion CM, Champagne PA, Ali AC, et al: Evaluation of Hemoglo-Bind for removal of o-raffinose cross-linked hemoglobin (Hemolink) from serum. Clin Chem 43(9):1796–1797, 1997.

Agents Affecting Coagulation and Platelet Function

Michael Avidan, MD • Susan McDonald, MD • George Despotis, MD

Antifibrinolytic Agents: Synthetic Lysine Analogs
Mechanisms of Action
Clinical Pharmacology
Practical Aspects of Drug Use
Dosage and Administration

Aprotinin
Mechanisms of Action
Clinical Pharmacology
Practical Aspects of Drug Use
Dosage and Administration

Physiology of the Hemostatic System

The hemostatic system limits hemorrhage when vascular integrity is compromised and includes several major components: platelets, von Willebrand factor (vWF), coagulation and fibrinolytic factors, and the blood vessel wall (Fig. 53–1). The endothelium normally serves as a protective layer and prevents hemostatic activation. When endothelium is denuded, activated platelets adhere to exposed subendothelium, a reaction largely mediated by vWF, and then

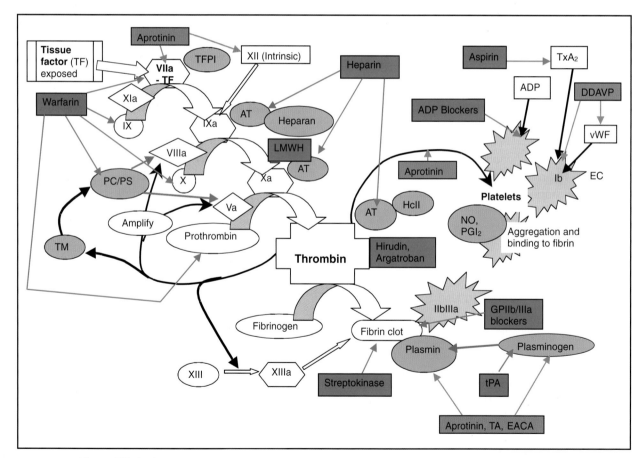

Figure 53–1. Sites of action of some key drugs that affect clotting, platelet function, and fibrinolysis. *Roman numerals* represent the factors in the coagulation cascade; *light green ovals* represent physiologic anticoagulants; *red rectangles* represent exogenous anticoagulants, platelet antagonists, and fibrinolytics; *purple rectangles* represent drugs that tend to promote hemostasis. a, activated; ADP, adenosine diphosphate; AT III, antithrombin III; EACA, epsilon amino caproic acid; DDAVP, desmopressin; EC, endothelial cells; HcII, heparin cofactor II; NO, nitric oxide; PC/PS, protein C/protein S; PGI_2, prostacyclin; TA, tranexamic acid; TFPI, tissue factor pathway inhibitor; TM, thrombomodulin; tPA, tissue plasminogen activator; TxA_2, thromboxane A_2; vWF, von Willebrand Factor. Ib and IIb/IIIa are platelet glycoprotein receptors.

aggregate to provide initial hemostasis (Figs. 53–1 and 53–2). Platelets also provide an active phospholipid surface for interaction with coagulation factors that are activated by tissue factor. The coagulation system consists of a number of clotting active zymogens and cofactors and is subdivided into the intrinsic, extrinsic, and common pathways that lead to formation of a fibrin clot (see Fig. 53–1). Tissue factor activates the extrinsic pathway to form fibrin, which stabilizes the hemostatic platelet plug. Prostacyclin (PGI$_2$) and nitric oxide (NO) inhibit platelets, whereas proteins C and S, antithrombin III, heparin-cofactor II, and tissue factor pathway inhibitor inhibit or degrade coagulation proteins. The fibrinolytic system consists of several plasmatic factors including tissue plasminogen activator (tPA) and plasminogen that interact to produce plasmin, which lyses clots and potentially prevents vaso-occlusion at the site of vessel injury. The fibrinolytic system is regulated by factors such as plasminogen activator inhibitor and α-1-antiplasmin that bind and inhibit tPA and plasmin, respectively.

There are many congenital and acquired causes of hemostatic abnormalities including deficiencies or abnormal function of platelets, vWF, coagulation proteins, anticoagulants, or fibrinolytic peptides. With disseminated intravascular coagulopathy (DIC), excessive bleeding occurs after consumption of clotting factors. Thrombotic complications can also result from DIC-related excessive activation of the hemostatic system. Congenital abnormalities of platelets or coagulation factors are rare with the most common involving defects in factor VIII (1 in 10,000 individuals) and vWF, which has been estimated to be present in as much as 1.5% of the general population. Acquired abnormalities of the hemostatic system occur with liver, renal, bone marrow or B-cell dysfunction, deficiencies of key nutrients such as proteins, folate, vitamin K, consumption of clotting factors or

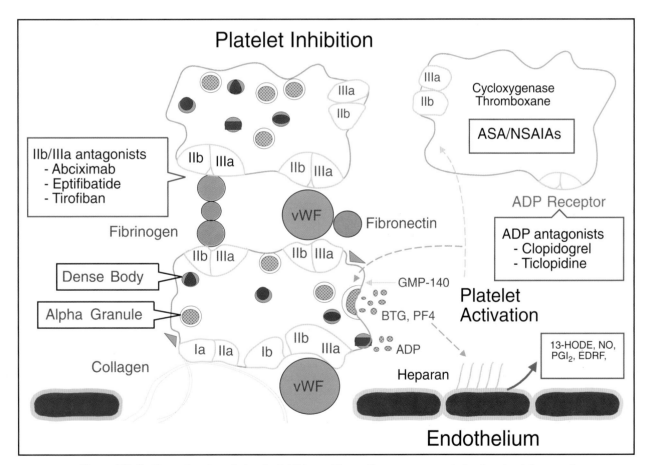

Figure 53–2. Sites of action of platelet inhibitors. Figure illustrates normal platelet physiology and the sites of action of four major categories of platelet inhibitors: endogenous inhibitors such as nitric oxide (NO), heparan, 13-HODE, prostacyclin (PGI$_2$), adenosine, and endothelial-derived relaxant factor (EDRF) versus cyclo-oxygenase inhibitors such as aspirin (ASA), nonsteroidal anti-inflammatory agents (NSAIAs) versus adenosine diphosphate (ADP)-receptor blockers such as ticlopidine and clopidogrel versus IIb/IIIa receptor antagonists such as abciximab, eptifibatide, or tirofiban. Also shown are the normal mechanisms of platelet adhesion mediated by the Ia receptor and collagen or the Ib receptor and high-molecular weight multimers of von Willebrand Factor (vWF) or platelet aggregation mediated by the IIb/IIIa receptor and either vWF or fibrinogen. Alpha and dense granules that promote secondary aggregation also are shown. (Modified from Fuster V, Badimon L, Cohen M, et al: Insights into the pathogenesis of acute ischemic syndromes. Circulation 77:1213–1220, 1988.)

platelets with DIC, and with therapeutic use of anticoagulant or antiplatelet agents. Significant hepatic dysfunction can result in reduced synthesis of all of the coagulation proteins with the exception of factor VIII, accelerated clearance of platelets (i.e., with hepatosplenomegaly), or abnormal platelet function related to reduced hepatic clearance of fibrinogen/fibrin split products. Uremia related to significant renal impairment can affect platelet function and interaction of platelets with vWF. Impairment of hepatic or renal function may affect the clearance of drugs that affect clotting and bleeding. Deficiency of a protein substrate or key cofactors (such as vitamin K) impairs coagulation factor synthesis, whereas vitamin B_{12} and folate are required for platelet production. In certain clinical situations, there is a loss of platelets and coagulation factors that are not related to DIC. Such circumstances include volume resuscitation for

bleeding and pre-eclampsia. Other clinical conditions such as abruptio placentae, hypoperfusion, organ ischemia, ABO-incompatible transfusion, trauma, and use of cardiopulmonary bypass (CPB) with cardiac surgery can result in development of a consumptive process (i.e., DIC) that ultimately depletes coagulation factors and platelets.

Numerous pharmacologic agents have been developed to modify the hemostatic system. Warfarin prevents coagulation factor synthesis; heparin and thrombin inhibitors oppose coagulation factor activity (Fig. 53–3); and aspirin, adenosine diphosphate (ADP) receptor blockers and glycoprotein IIb/IIIa (GPIIb/IIa) antagonists inhibit platelet function (see Fig. 53–2), whereas tPA and streptokinase (SK) accelerate clot lysis (see Fig. 53–1). Agents that inhibit coagulation factors or platelet function are administered to prevent thromboses or complications relating to existing

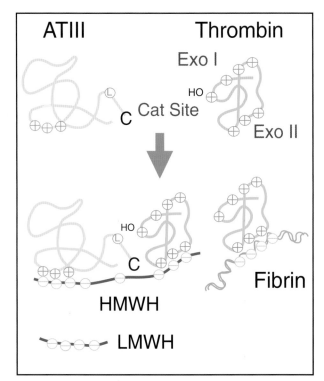

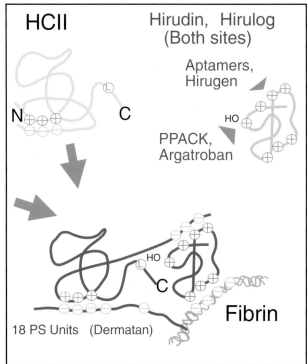

Figure 53–3. Inhibition of thrombin activity. *Left,* Normal physiologic inhibition of fluid phase thrombin by high molecular weight heparin (HMWH) molecules and the limitations of heparin in inhibiting clot-bound thrombin. The thrombin molecule has three major binding sites: the fibrinogen binding site (Exo I), the fibrinogen catalytic site (Cat Site), and the fibrin binding site (Exo II). After binding of heparin to the antithrombin (III) molecule through a critical pentasaccharide sequence, a conformational change in the C-terminal portion of the ATIII molecule is induced. Inhibition of the thrombin molecule requires heparin molecules with a critical oligosaccharide chain length of 18 units that serve as a template for the binding of ATIII with thrombin. However, thrombin inhibition through the ATIII-heparin mechanism is limited by availability of the Exo II site, which can also be occupied by fibrin. Although low molecular weight (LMW) fractions of heparin induce a conformational change in the C-terminal portion of the ATIII molecule, they cannot serve as a template for ATIII and thrombin because of their short chain length. *Right,* Figure depicts the normal inhibition of clot-bound thrombin by the heparin cofactor II (HCII)-heparin complex and the sites of action of various direct thrombin inhibitors. A minimum chain length of 6 units for the heparin oligosaccharide is required to activate HCII, however, 20- to 24-unit chain lengths result in a substantially greater thrombin inhibition through HCII. Direct thrombin inhibitors such as hirudin and Hirulog bind to both the Exo I and catalytic sites of the thrombin molecule. In contrast, polypeptide aptamers and hirugen bind to the Exo I site, whereas D-Phe-L-Pro-L-Arg-chloromethyl (PPACK) and argatroban bind to the fibrinogen catalytic site of thrombin. (Modified from Tollefson D, et al: Thromb Hemostas 96:120–129, 1995.)

clots. Patients with established thromboses in the deep veins, arteries, and the heart require anticoagulant medication. In addition, patients who are at high risk for thromboses require anticoagulation—for example, patients with a history of recurrent thromboses, those with known thrombophilia, patients undergoing orthopedic surgery or other operative procedures that involve an extended period of immobilization (i.e., 50% incidence of calf vein thrombosis and 1-5% incidence of fatal pulmonary embolus in patients undergoing total hip arthroplasty), patients with prosthetic cardiac valves or with abnormal cardiac function (e.g., dilated or dyskinetic cardiac chambers, arrhythmias), patients with acute ischemic stroke (i.e., deep venous thrombosis [DVT] occurs in 60–70% of patients with dense hemiplegia with 1–2% incidence of fatal pulmonary embolism), patients with arterial vaso-occlusive disease, patients with acute coronary syndromes, patients undergoing either percutaneous angioplasty or stenting procedures, and patients undergoing operative revascularization procedures (e.g., carotid endarterectomy, coronary revascularization) or other cardiac surgical procedures (e.g., valve repair/replacement, aortic reconstruction). The intensity of anticoagulation (e.g., heparin concentration: 0.5–5 U/mL; International Normalized Ratio [INR]: 2–4) required the specific use of either anticoagulant, antiplatelet, or fibrinolytic agent, and the route of drug administration (e.g., intravenous [IV], subcutaneous, oral) depends on the specific clinical indications. In the United States alone, there are 300,000 patient admissions for DVT and 500,000 cardiac surgical revascularization procedures performed annually.

There are also several medications that oppose the actions of anticoagulants or prevent excessive bleeding. Protamine reverses the anticoagulant properties of heparin, epsilon amino caproic acid or tranexamic acid (TA) inhibit physiologic or excessive fibrinolysis, and desmopressin (DDAVP) augments endothelial release of vWF, vWF/platelet interactions, or platelet function (enhanced platelet microtubule function, platelet expression of Ib receptors). Aprotinin is a broad-spectrum agent that affects hemostatic system function in multiple ways, including reduction of contact and tissue factor activation, inhibition of platelets, fibrinolysis, complement, and leukocyte function. Aprotinin is probably the most effective agent available to reduce perioperative bleeding, re-exploration, and transfusion.

Heparin and Related Compounds

Unfractionated heparin was first isolated by Howell in 1922. Standard unfractionated heparin is by far the most commonly used anticoagulant in the hospital-based setting.

Mechanisms of Action

Heparin, a glycosaminoglycan, is contained within mast cell secretory granules and requires a cofactor, antithrombin III (currently referred to as antithrombin or ATIII), to inhibit acti-

vated coagulation factors and result in anticoagulation (see Fig. 53–3).[1] Unfractionated heparin is a mixture of low and high molecular weight fractions that range from 3000 to 30,000 daltons, whereas low molecular weight heparin (LMWH) consists of molecular weight fractions ranging from 2,000 to 10,000 daltons. Greater molecular weight fractions (with minimum chain length of 18 oligosaccharide units) preferentially inhibit thrombin (factor IIa).[2] Oligosaccharide chain length (>18 saccharide units) is important because thrombin inhibition requires simultaneous binding of thrombin and ATIII by heparin, which acts as a template (see Fig. 53–3). Because inhibition of factor Xa does not require simultaneous binding of Xa and ATIII through a heparin template, lower molecular weight fractions of unfractionated heparin easily inhibit factor Xa (see Fig. 53–3).

The antithrombotic properties of heparin are predominantly mediated by the binding of a specific pentasaccharide sequence on heparin to ATIII; this complex then inhibits both factor Xa and thrombin.[3] Although the binding of heparin to ATIII most importantly inhibits thrombin and factor Xa,[4] this complex also inhibits several other sites in the intrinsic coagulation pathway including factors IXa, XIa, and XIIa. Heparin indirectly suppresses thrombin-induced activation of factors V and VIII by binding thrombin.

A minimum chain length of 6 oligosaccharide units is essential for heparin to catalyze the inhibition of thrombin by heparin cofactor II, another important in vivo inhibitor of the hemostatic system (see Fig. 53–3). Inhibition of thrombin through heparin cofactor II is optimal with a chain length of 20 to 24 oligosaccharide units.[5] The ability of heparin cofactor II to inhibit clot-bound thrombin (at greater heparin concentrations) may be important in some clinical settings (i.e., during extracorporeal circulation with cardiac surgery).[6] The extrinsic pathway can also be inhibited by heparin-mediated release of tissue factor pathway inhibitor.[7] Unfractionated heparin may also inhibit[8–10] or activate[8] platelets, affect endothelial function or vessel wall permeability, initiate fibrinolysis,[10] and may also augment inhibition of fibrinolysis by plasminogen activator inhibitor 1.

Preclinical Pharmacology

The dose of unfractionated heparin used to manage patients with venous thromboembolism or unstable angina is based on maintenance of activated partial thromboplastin time (aPTT) values in the range of 1.5 to 2.5 × control. This therapeutic range of heparin[11,12] for venous thromboembolism or unstable angina is based on early animal studies.[13] With respect to coronary interventions such as angioplasty or stenting procedures, activated coagulation time (ACT) values that approximate 350 seconds are considered to be therapeutic.[14] Anticoagulation is used during cardiac surgery to prevent overt thrombosis of the extracorporeal circuit and to minimize excessive CPB-related activation of the hemostatic system. In this setting, greater heparin concentrations (3–7 U/mL) are generally maintained to offset the extraordinary activation of the hemostatic system that occurs. Early studies in humans[15] demonstrated that fibrin formation during extracorporeal circulation could be avoided when

ACT values exceeded 280 to 300 seconds; in an attempt to provide a margin of safety, this led to the recommendation that ACT values exceed 480 seconds in this setting.[15,16] Subsequent studies have demonstrated that ACT values can be extremely misleading during CPB with respect to heparin-mediated anticoagulation based on the effects of hypothermia and hemodilution on this test system.[17]

Clinical Pharmacology

Unfractionated heparin is normally present within mast cells and is synthesized from UDP-sugar precursors as a polymer of alternating *N*-acetyl-D-glucosamine and D-glucuronic acid residues. The commercial heparin preparations are derived from either bovine lung or porcine intestinal mucosa and have biologic activities similar to those of endogenous heparin. Although unfractionated heparin is metabolized in the reticuloendothelial system and liver, at least 50% is eliminated unchanged through a slower first-order process through the kidneys. Generally, the plasma elimination half-life of unfractionated heparin is 1 to 2 hours; however, the half-life increases with significant hepatic or renal dysfunction or with heparin doses greater than 100 U/kg.[18] In contrast to unfractionated heparin, LMWH compounds such as enoxaparin or dalteparin, which are derived from unfractionated heparin, have a longer half-life (i.e., 4–5 hours). These agents also have a more consistent pharmacokinetic profile between patients because of the lower protein-binding affinity for platelets,[9] vWF[9] and endothelial cells, and clearance, which is primarily renal.[19] A new preparation that consists of very LMWH fragments (pentasaccharide sequence only) and has a much longer half-life (24 hours) is currently being investigated with respect to safety and efficacy.[20]

Practical Aspects of Drug Use

Heparin is generally administered either through deep subcutaneous injection or IV bolus or infusion because it is not absorbed through the gastrointestinal (GI) tract. The mode of administration and dose of heparin used depends on the clinical indication. When administered parenterally, heparin has an immediate onset of action, whereas subcutaneous administration results in variable bioavailability with a delay in the onset of action (1–2 hours). IV heparin is used when rapid or therapeutic anticoagulation is needed and during specific procedures. Deep venous thrombosis, pulmonary embolism, interventional cardiology, and cardiac or vascular surgery are typical examples. Heparin loading doses between 80 and 400 U/kg vary substantially depending on the clinical setting. Because of heparin's relatively short half-life and the importance of maintenance of anticoagulation, infusions are generally used to maintain steady-state levels when heparin is administered intravenously in the settings of DVT or acute coronary syndromes. Monitoring systems are generally not used for monitoring of subcutaneous administration of unfractionated heparin or LMWH compounds unless substantial renal dysfunction is present,

in which case chromogenic assays or protamine titration assays are used to measure or quantify heparin concentration. Several different tests are used to monitor the extent of anticoagulation or levels of unfractionated heparin such as aPTT, ACT, and automated protamine titration methods. Monitoring of unfractionated heparin is essential to confirm adequacy of anticoagulation, which can minimize recurrent venous thromboembolism,[11,12] left ventricular thrombosis,[15] recurrent angina in the setting of an acute myocardial infarction (AMI),[21] or thrombosis within extracorporeal circuits.[22]

The anticoagulant properties of unfractionated heparin are monitored with tests that assess the intrinsic coagulation pathway. The specific test used depends on the relative dose/concentration required for any particular clinical situation. The aPTT monitoring is generally maintained at 1.5 to 2.5 × control values, which is consistent with heparin levels of 0.3 to 0.7 U/mL (antifactor Xa) or 0.2 to 0.4 U/L (protamine titration) in patients receiving heparin for the management of DVT/pulmonary embolism, as well as with noninterventional acute coronary syndromes (e.g., unstable angina).[23] The ACT or heparin concentration methods (e.g., Hepcon automated protamine titration) are used when greater heparin concentrations are required for interventional cardiology procedures (ACT values of 200–400 seconds, heparin concentrations of 1–3 U/mL) or cardiac surgical procedures (ACT values >400–500 seconds, heparin concentrations of 2–8 U/mL).[24]

There is substantial variability of heparin anticoagulant responsiveness in patients receiving either low- or high-dose heparin therapy. Impaired heparin responsiveness (also termed *heparin resistance*) is often attributed to ATIII deficiency.[25] ATIII activity levels as low as 40% to 50% of normal, which are similar to those observed in patients with heterozygotic hereditary deficiency,[26] are commonly seen during cardiac surgery.[27–29] Acquired perioperative reductions in plasma ATIII concentrations have been related to preoperative heparin use, hemodilution, or consumption during extracorporeal circulation. The heparin tissue source (intestinal vs. lung, porcine vs. bovine), method of preparation, molecular weight distribution of heparin used,[31,32] and possibly the use of nitroglycerin infusions[33,54] (for which the mechanisms are unknown) may also contribute to impaired responsiveness. In addition to congenital deficiency, ATIII levels may be lower than normal in patients with nephrotic syndrome, hepatic cirrhosis, with prolonged infusion of heparin, or with DIC.

Adverse Effects

With respect to adverse effects, it is well-established that heparin or any related compound can result in bleeding complications. The risk for these complications increases with the intensity of anticoagulation required, the pre-existing state of the patient with respect to defects in the hemostatic system, concurrent use of other antithrombotic or antiplatelet agents, and instrumentation as related to biopsies, surgery, or neuroaxial anesthetic techniques. Distinct advantages of unfractionated heparin are that its anticoagulant properties can be easily assessed with routine tests (e.g., aPTT, thrombin time), its short half-life, and the availability of an immediate reversal agent (i.e., protamine). LMWH, the new pentasaccharide, and danaparoid do not have these advantages; this has proven to be important in patients receiving LMWH in whom there have been multiple reports of epidural/spinal hematomas leading to paraplegia, the setting of neuroaxial anesthetic blocks.[34]

Another serious complication of treatment with heparin is immune-mediated, heparin-induced thrombocytopenia (HIT). In approximately 5% to 10% of patients receiving unfractionated heparin, HIT develops within 3 to 15 days after first exposure or as early as 12 to 24 hours with repeated exposure.[35] In addition to thrombocytopenia, HIT can lead to thrombosis in 0.75% of patients.[36]

Dosage and Administration

Lower heparin doses (e.g., 5000 U every 12 hours) are administered subcutaneously to prevent DVT, whereas higher subcutaneous doses (e.g., 17,000 U every 12 hours) can be used for long-term anticoagulation when warfarin is contraindicated. Generally, monitoring is not used in these two scenarios.

An initial bolus dose (5000 U or 80 U/kg) followed by a continuous IV infusion (1200–1600 U/hour) is used when immediate anticoagulation is required. Greater initial IV doses are administered for interventional cardiology procedures (100–200 U/kg) and during cardiac surgery (300–400 U/kg); subsequent doses of 5,000 to 10,000 units are administered to maintain sufficient anticoagulation. This is usually guided by near patient anticoagulation assessment using monitoring systems such as ACT or heparin concentration through an automated protamine titration method.

Danaparoid

Because of the recognition of HIT, investigators and clinicians have pursued alternative anticoagulant agents. Danaparoid, derived from porcine intestinal mucosa, is a glycosaminoglycuronan that consists of a mixture of heparan sulfate (84%), dermatan sulfate (12%), and chondroitin sulfate (4%). This low molecular weight heparinoid compound has a molecular weight of approximately 5500 to 6000 daltons. Although 5% of the heparan molecules within danaparoid have a high affinity for ATIII, this compound does not contain any heparin or heparin fragments.

Mechanisms of Action

Similar to heparin, the antithrombotic properties of danaparoid relate to its ability to attenuate fibrin formation through inhibition of Xa and thrombin. The main anti-Xa activity of danaparoid is related to binding of ATIII by heparin, whereas its anti-IIa activity is related to dermatan sulfate, which binds to ATIII and heparin cofactor II.[37] Dana-

paroid has substantially greater inhibitory effects on Xa activity than either standard unfractionated heparin or LMWH.

Clinical Pharmacology

Subcutaneous administration of danaparoid is associated with 100% bioavailability. The volume of distribution is 9 L and peak plasma levels are achieved within 4 to 5 hours (maximum anti-Xa activity in 2–5 hours) with linear kinetics. Elimination of danaparoid is predominately through the kidneys and the terminal half-lives for anti-factor Xa and anti-IIa activity are 24 and 7 hours, respectively.[38]

Practical Aspects of Drug Use

Compared with placebo, danaparoid has been shown to reduce the incidence of DVT from 57% to 15% in the setting of total hip arthroplasty.[39] In a recent randomized trial, there was a 17% incidence of DVT with danaparoid compared with a 32% incidence with unfractionated heparin.[40] In the setting of hip fracture surgery, danaparoid was shown to reduce the incidence of DVT from 35% to 13% compared with dextran[41] and from 21% to 7% compared with warfarin[42] without an increase in bleeding complications. Less impressive reductions in the incidence of perioperative DVT were observed when danaparoid was compared with heparin in the setting of abdomino-thoracic surgery.[43] After ischemic stroke, danaparoid has been shown to reduce DVT occurrence from 28% to 4% compared with placebo[44] and from 31% to 9% compared with heparin.[37]

There is some experience with use of danaparoid on a "compassionate use" basis during cardiac surgery in patients with HIT despite early case reports of increased bleeding in this setting.[45,46] In a series of 47 patients who received danaparoid during cardiac surgery, either resistance, thrombotic, or bleeding complications developed in 20%.[47]

The antithrombotic effects of danaparoid should be monitored using an anti-factor Xa method because routine tests that assess ATIII activity such as aPTT and the thrombin time are minimally affected by danaparoid.

Dosage and Administration

The recommended dosage of danaparoid for prevention of DVT is 750 anti-Xa units by subcutaneous injection before surgery, 2 hours after surgery, and then daily for 7 to 14 days. Dosage should be adjusted for patients with significant renal insufficiency. As with LMWH, no agents are currently available to reverse danaparoid.

Protamine

Protamine sulfate is a low-molecular weight cationic protein that is derived from salmon sperm.

Mechanisms of Action

Protamine is the principal agent used to reverse unfractionated heparin and does so by ionically binding to acidic polyanionic heparin to form a stable salt without any anticoagulant activity. Protamine has two active binding sites. One binds to heparin and the other exerts a mild anticoagulant effect. Every milligram of protamine neutralizes approximately 80 to 100 USP units of unfractionated heparin. Of importance, protamine inadequately and inconsistently reverses the anticoagulant (anti-factor Xa) activity of LMWH. If protamine is administered alone or in excess to what is needed to reverse heparin, it has antiplatelet activity.[48] This is evident with circulating levels as low as 30 μg/mL, which can be attained with as little as 50 to 60 mg protamine. At doses in excess of 600 to 800 mg, protamine also displays anticoagulant activity.

Clinical Pharmacology

Protamine has a rapid onset of action with neutralization of heparin occurring within 5 minutes. The fate of the heparin/protamine complex has not been clearly elucidated. Protamine is cleared rapidly through the reticulo-endothelial system within 20 minutes,[49] which is more rapid than heparin clearance. This finding may in part explain the phenomenon of "heparin rebound." Heparin rebound has been described predominately after cardiac surgery and consists of heparin-related anticoagulation and bleeding that occurs 30 minutes to 9 hours after protamine administration. The etiology of heparin rebound is most likely related to release of heparin from intravascular or extravascular protein binding sites or from the heparin/protamine complex.

Practical Aspects of Drug Use

The full protamine dose should be administered slowly through an IV catheter over 20 to 30 minutes (about 5 mg/min) after confirming that there is no reaction when a small (10 mg) test dose is administered. The patient should be carefully observed for development of any hypersensitivity or nonimmunologic reactions. Several reports have summarized relatively uncommon (<1%) immunologic reactions involving classic anaphylaxis (mediated through antiprotamine IgE). Other reports have described catastrophic hemodynamic reactions (possibly mediated through antiprotamine IgG or complement activation) consisting of thromboxane-mediated development of noncardiogenic pulmonary edema, severe pulmonary vasoconstriction, right heart decompensation, hypotension, and on occasion cardiovascular collapse. This immunologic reaction may be more common in patients who have received insulin that contains protamine (NPH, isophane), those with a previous exposure to protamine, those with fish allergies, or in male vasectomized patients, of whom 22% to 33% have antiprotamine antibodies. Protamine has also been shown to result in activation of the complement cascade and can lead to development of noncardiogenic pulmonary edema. More commonly, protamine-induced hypotension and bronchospasm may be related to nonimmunologic (direct physiochemical displacement of histamine from mast cells) mechanisms that are generally related to total dose and rate of administration.

Dosage and Administration

When heparin has been administered by deep subcutaneous injection, 1 to 1.5 mg protamine should be administered for every 100 U heparin given over an extended period. When heparin has been given intravenously, 1 to 1.5 mg protamine should be administered for every 100 U heparin administered at the last dose, or 1 mg protamine for every 100 U heparin administered over the last 4 hours. If 30 to 60 minutes have elapsed since the last dose of IV heparin, then 0.5 to 0.75 mg protamine should be administered for every 100 U heparin, whereas 0.25 to 0.375 mg protamine should be administered if 2 hours have lapsed since the last IV injection of heparin. During cardiac surgery, several different approaches have been used. Empiric dosing schedules such as administration of 0.5 to 1.0 mg protamine for every 100 U heparin administered throughout the procedure or 1 mg protamine for every 100 U heparin administered initially before initiation of CPB have been described. Ideally, test systems, such as the Hepcon automated protamine titration method, that quantify the circulating concentration of heparin should be used to identify the accurate dose of protamine required to neutralize heparin. Although not consistently observed within the literature, optimizing protamine dose seems to be supported by several studies that have demonstrated either reduced bleeding or transfusion when lower doses of protamine are administered.[50,51] The decreases in perioperative blood loss associated with reduced doses of protamine may be related to less complement activation, protamine-induced platelet dysfunction, or inhibition of thrombin with high protamine levels.

Tests that are sensitive to low concentrations (0.1 U/mL) of heparin such as the aPTT, the thrombin time, the automated protamine titration, the heparinase ACT, and the heparin-neutralized thrombin time should be used to confirm adequacy of heparin reversal in the operating room or to assess heparin rebound in the postoperative setting. When patients (those receiving NPH insulin) are at increased risk for an adverse hemodynamic reaction to protamine, antihistamine blockers and steroids should be considered in addition to a protamine test dose.

Argatroban

Argatroban is an arginine derivative that is a highly specific thrombin inhibitor.[52] Argatroban's binding site on thrombin and pharmacologic characteristics are different from those of hirudin (see Fig. 53–3). Argatroban is undergoing evaluation in numerous clinical contexts. It is particularly promising for patients with HIT and for use with extracorporeal circuits. Direct thrombin inhibitors do not stimulate formation of the antibody that causes HIT.[53]

Mechanisms of Action

Argatroban is an arginine derivative, synthetic, small molecule that binds to the catalytic but not the exo 1 or exo 2 sites (see Fig. 53–3) of thrombin and inhibits its activity. In addition to its antithrombin activity, argatroban has also been shown to promote NO release, which may partially explain the improved perfusion seen when it is administered to patients with peripheral vascular disease.[54]

Preclinical Pharmacology

In rabbit models of arterial but not venous thrombosis, argatroban is a more potent antithrombotic agent than heparin, with antithrombotic effects at a much lower degree of systemic anticoagulation.[55] Argatroban was compared with heparin for anticoagulation in a dog model of CPB. There were no clots in the extracorporeal circuit. There was less activation of coagulation and fibrinolysis and better preservation of platelet number and function in the argatroban group.[56]

Clinical Pharmacology

The pharmacokinetics of argatroban is well described by a two-compartment model with first-order or concentration-dependent elimination.[57] Plasma drug concentrations increase linearly with dose, and weight-adjusted plasma clearance is dose-independent.[58] The elimination half-life is 40 to 50 minutes. Argatroban is distributed mainly in the extracellular space and is readily metabolized in the liver to an active M1-metabolite that has pharmacologically distinct characteristics.[59] In patients with liver dysfunction, the half-life is increased twofold to threefold and clearance is 25% that of healthy volunteers.[57] Renal function, age, and sex do not significantly affect the pharmacokinetics of argatroban.[57]

Practical Aspects of Drug Use

Argatroban anticoagulation, compared with historical control subjects, was found to improve clinical outcomes in patients diagnosed with HIT, without increasing bleeding risk.[60]

Argatroban has been proposed as an alternative to heparin for anticoagulation during CPB. One of the main disadvantages with argatroban, as with the other direct thrombin inhibitors, is that there is no available drug that rapidly reverses its anticoagulant action. Nonetheless, its reversible binding to thrombin, coupled with its rapid clearance from circulation, suggest that it may be a viable anticoagulant in this setting.[61] Experiments showing that argatroban preserves platelet function and fibrinogen concentrations when blood flows through extracorporeal circuits provide further impetus for evaluating its possible role.[61] Safety studies are required before routine use in this setting.

Monitoring

A bolus dose argatroban produces dose-related increases in ACT and aPTT within 10 minutes of administration.[58] After infusion, the effects of argatroban on the ACT and the aPTT are dose-related and are more consistent than those of heparin.[58]

Dosage and Administration

For thrombosis prophylaxis in patients with HIT, an initial infusion of 2 μg/kg per minute is recommended. This may be adjusted according to clinical effect (aPTT, ACT, or ecarin clotting time). For patients with hepatic dysfunction, the initial infusion rate should be decreased to 0.5 μg/kg per minute. The maximum advisable dose is 10 μg/kg/min.

Hirudin and Bivalirudin

Hirudin is a direct-acting thrombin inhibitor derived from the leech, *Hirudo medicinalis*. Using polymerase chain reaction technology, recombinant hirudin (desirudin, lepirudin) has been synthesized in yeast. Bivalirudin or Hirulog is a synthetic peptide based on hirudin.[62] Unlike unfractionated heparin, direct thrombin inhibitors such as hirudin and bivalirudin inhibit both clot-bound and free thrombin, are not neutralized by platelet products such as platelet factor 4, and are not associated with immune thrombocytopenia.[63] Hirudin is indicated for anticoagulation in patients with HIT, where in whom a rapid and sustained increase in platelet number has been demonstrated.[64] Bivalirudin in combination with aspirin has been approved for use in patients with unstable angina who are undergoing percutaneous transluminal coronary angioplasty.

Mechanisms of Action

Hirudin and bivalirudin are direct thrombin inhibitors that bind thrombin itself and do not depend on ATIII for their anticoagulant activity. Although hirudin and Hirulog both inhibit thrombin by attaching to the exo I (fibrinogen binding site) and catalytic sites (see Fig. 53–3), Hirulog has a shorter biologic half-life, which is in part related to disinhibition through the catalytic site secondary to enzymatic digestion by thrombin. One molecule of hirudin binds to one molecule of thrombin. Hirudin has also been found to stimulate PGI_2 production, which may contribute to its antithrombotic activity because PGI_2 promotes vasodilatation and prevents platelet aggregation.[65]

Clinical Pharmacology

Hirudin and bivalirudin are administered by IV infusion. Onset of action is rapid and the peak effect occurs after about 4 hours. Distribution is mainly to the extracellular fluid space. There is some metabolism by hydrolysis, but the drugs are mainly excreted unchanged in the urine. When renal function is normal, plasma clearance is rapid and both drugs obey a first-order or concentration-dependent pharmacokinetic model. The plasma half-lives of hirudin and bivalirudin are about 1.5 hours and 30 minutes, respectively. As with other small polypeptides, bivalirudin is filtered at the glomerulus, secreted in the proximal convoluted tubule, reabsorbed in the distal convoluted tubule, and degraded within intracellular lysosomes to constituent amino acids.[66] When there is severe renal impairment (creatinine clearance <15 mL/min), elimination half-life may be extended to days. These drugs can be cleared from plasma by hemodialysis.

Hirudin has been used successfully for the management of HIT in several cardiac surgical series without evidence of increased bleeding.[67–70] However, these agents should be used with caution in patients who are at increased risk for perioperative bleeding (e.g., repeat or combined procedures, procedures involving long CPB intervals) or in patients with renal insufficiency.

Practical Aspects of Drug Use

The clinical niche for hirudin has yet to be determined. Hirudin may be an alternative to heparin when there is heparin resistance or HIT.[71,72] There have been several reports of successful anticoagulation for CPB using hirudin for patients with HIT. The main disadvantage with hirudin in this setting is that there is no agent available currently to reverse the anticoagulation. For both hirudin and bivalirudin, there is a correlation between plasma concentrations and the aPTT and the ACT.[66]

The Thrombin Inhibition in Myocardial Ischemia (TIMI-7) trial demonstrated that bivalirudin was a valuable adjunct to aspirin in the treatment of unstable angina.[62] In the Global Use of Strategies to Open Occluded Coronary Arteries (GUSTO 2b) trial, patients treated with SK and adjunctive hirudin after myocardial infarction had a reduction in death or myocardial infarction of 40% at 30 days compared with adjunctive heparin.[73,74] The Hirulog/Early Reperfusion Occlusion (HERO-1) study similarly showed improved arterial patency and decreased bleeding when bivalirudin was used as opposed to heparin in combination with aspirin and SK for AMI.[75]

Adverse Effects

Use of these agents may increase the risk for bleeding. Liver dysfunction and skin rashes have been reported. Severe hypersensitivity reactions can also occur. Because they are excreted largely unchanged in urine, hirudin and bivalirudin are best avoided in the setting of renal failure. Bleeding is significantly increased when hirudin or bivalirudin are administered to patients with impaired renal function.[66] Antihirudin antibodies develop in 40% of patients, but this has not been associated with adverse events.

Monitoring

In the noncardiac surgical setting, prothrombin time (PT) values are maintained at 2 to 3 × control, and these values are generally associated with hirudin levels of approximately 1 to 1.5 µg/mL.[76] With cardiac surgery, maintenance of levels of 4 to 5 µg/mL has been suggested.[76] A plasma-modified ACT may be useful in monitoring hirudin anticoagulation during CPB.[77]

Dosage and Administration

In view of the extracellular distribution, dosage should be calculated according to lean body mass. The suggested hirudin dose for thrombosis prophylaxis is 400 µg/kg followed by an infusion at a rate of 150 µg/kg per hour. The dosage for anticoagulation for CPB is not well established. In one study with eight patients, an initial dose of 250 µg/kg was administered followed by 5-mg increments as needed.[64] Others have recommended an initial bolus of 0.25 mg/kg, 0.25 mg/kg in the CPB circuit, and an infusion of 0.5 mg/min.[76] With bivalirudin, an initial 1-mg/kg dose followed by 2.5 mg/kg per hour for 4 hours is advocated. The infusion may be continued at 200 µg/kg per hour for up to 20 hours. Dosages of both drugs should be decreased for patients with renal failure.

Warfarin and Related Compounds

Schofield first reported hemorrhage in cattle secondary to ingestion of spoiled sweet clover silage; Roderick traced the cause of bleeding to reduced levels of prothrombin; and Link determined that bishydroxycoumarin (dicoumarol) formed in the spoilage process of sweet clover, was responsible for development of hypoprothrombinemia, and that this effect could be reversed by vitamin K.[78] The coumarin agents were introduced into clinical practice in the early 1940s for the management of myocardial infarction and cerebral embolism, and a derivative of dicoumarol (i.e., warfarin) was introduced in 1948 as a rodenticide. Warfarin is the most commonly used oral anticoagulant in North America because of its predictable onset of action, superb bioavailability, and predictable duration of action.[79,80]

Mechanisms of Action

The 4-hydroxycoumarin compounds (warfarin, aceno-coumarol, ethyl biscoumacetate, and phenprocoumon), as well as dicumarol, inhibit the hepatic conversion of four vitamin K–dependent coagulation proteins (i.e., factors II, VII, IX, and X) and two anticoagulant proteins (i.e., protein C and S) to active forms. Specifically, these agents inhibit the cyclic interconversion of vitamin K and vitamin K epoxide. Vitamin K plays an essential role in the synthesis of the vitamin K–dependent coagulant proteins by acting as a cofactor for the post-translational carboxylation of glutamate residues to gamma-carboxyglutamate on the N-terminal regions of these proteins. Gamma-carboxylation is essential in that it enables these coagulation proteins to undergo a conformational change in the presence of calcium, which is critical for their biologic activity and binding of these proteins to their cofactors on phospholipid surfaces.[81,82]

The therapeutic anticoagulant effect of warfarin is achieved after several days when the vitamin K–dependent procoagulant proteins (factors II, VII, IX, and X) are reduced by 30% to 50% of normal, which is consistent with INR values in the range of 2 to 3. The antithrombotic effects of warfarin are predominately mediated by reduction in plasma concentrations of factor II and, to a lesser extent, factor X. Because warfarin and related compounds have no effect on carboxylated coagulation factors, the time required for each vitamin K–dependent protein to be substantially reduced and reach a steady state depends on the half-lives of the respective protein. The half-lives of the vitamin K–dependent procoagulant and anticoagulant proteins vary substantially as follows: factor VII: 6 hours; factor IX: 24 hours; factor X: 36 hours; factor II: 40 hours; protein C: 8 hours; protein S: 30 hours.

Clinical Pharmacology

Warfarin consists of a racemic mixture of similar amounts of two active optical isomers—designated R and S forms—which have different pharmacologic properties. These two forms are cleared by different pathways and *S*-warfarin is five times more potent with respect to vitamin K antagonism.[83] After rapid absorption in the GI tract, which may be slowed by food, blood concentrations usually peak 2 to 8 hours after ingestion[79,84] and the plasma half-life is approximately 40 hours.[83] Warfarin is an organic acid (pKa, 5.1), which accumulates rapidly in the liver, is highly protein bound (99%) to plasma albumin, and has a volume of distribution similar to albumin (12% to 13% of body weight or 0.14 L/kg). Plasma concentrations of warfarin within a fetus approximate maternal levels, whereas warfarin, unlike other coumarins, is not present in breast milk.

Warfarin is metabolized into byproducts that have little anticoagulant activity. The average rate of clearance from plasma is 0.045 mL/min per kilogram, the biologic half-life ranges from 25 to 60 hours (mean = 40 hours), and the duration of action is 2 to 5 days. The metabolic byproducts are excreted in the urine or stool after some degree of conjugation with glucuronic acid.

Highly variable between-subject and within-subject dose-response relations are frequently observed with warfarin, which necessitates ongoing monitoring of anticoagulant response. The intensity of anticoagulation induced by warfarin can be affected by several factors. These include differences in absorption or clearance, differences in warfarin protein binding, differences in the hemostatic response to a given concentration of warfarin, inaccuracies in laboratory testing, poor patient compliance, and poor communication between the patient and physician.

Practical Aspects of Drug Use

Although warfarin is almost always administered orally, an injectable preparation is available. Several factors affect the pharmacokinetic and pharmacodynamic profiles of warfarin including the metabolic clearance of warfarin, the pharmacologic profile of vitamin K (intake, absorption, concurrent use of antibiotics), factors that influence the vitamin K–dependent clotting factors (synthesis, clearance, liver disease) and numerous causes of hemostatic system malfunction (drugs, acquired and inherited disorders). The significance of these factors cannot be overemphasized based on the potential for both bleeding (supratherapeutic anticoagulation) and thrombotic (subtherapeutic anticoagulation) complications that can develop as a result. This emphasizes the importance of monitoring the anticoagulant properties of warfarin and related compounds, especially when the status of the patient changes.

The anticoagulant effects of warfarin are routinely assessed using the prothrombin time (PT). Prolongation of the PT depends on the stage of therapy (initiation vs. maintenance) based on the different half-lives of the respective vitamin K–dependent coagulation factors (factor VII: 6 hours; factor X: 36 hours; factor II: 40 hours). A major limitation of the PT relates to the variability in responsiveness to different thromboplastins or specific methods of clot detection to reduce levels of clotting factors.[85] To standardize the PT, the World Health Organization has used a reference preparation of thromboplastin to develop an INR, which can be reliably used to measure warfarin anticoagulation.[86] The optimal INR depends on the clinical indication for warfarin therapy and accordingly, guidelines by several organizations have been generated. The American College of Chest Physicians has suggested INR values ranging from 1.5 to 2.5 to as high as 3.0 to 4.5 based on the intensity of anticoagulation required for different clinical situations. For example, the target INR varies widely for treatment of venous thromboembolism, patients with mechanical heart valves, atrial fibrillation, and after AMI.[87] Several randomized trials have been pursued to establish the optimal intensity for warfarin-induced anticoagulation (i.e., therapeutic INR range) for venous thromboembolism.[88] Based on efficacy coupled with lower bleeding rates, an INR of 2.0 to 3.0 is currently recommended.[88] There is emerging evidence that even lower INR values may be effective for patients receiving primary prophylaxis.[89–91]

Although prolongation of the PT or INR is frequently observed within 1 to 2 days after initiation of therapy, reflecting the reduction in factor VII, it generally takes an additional 2 to 3 days to achieve therapeutic anticoagulation based on the slower reductions in factors X and II. Because protein C and S have shorter half-lives compared with factors X and II, initiation of warfarin therapy may result in a period of hypercoagulability in the first 24 to 48 hours. This has led to the recommendations that heparin therapy should be initiated before administration of warfarin or related compounds and then discontinued when the INR is in the therapeutic range.

Complications Related to Warfarin Use

Bleeding is the most common complication related to warfarin therapy. Several studies have demonstrated that greater intensity anticoagulation with warfarin may result in increases in bleeding rates when INR values range from 3 to 4.5.[92-94] Although periprocedure-related bleeding secondary to warfarin therapy can occur, empiric reversal of warfarin anticoagulation with plasma is not indicated based on several studies that have not demonstrated a relation between low coagulation factor levels and bleeding.[95-97] Reversal of warfarin-induced anticoagulation depends on the relative urgency, which is predominately driven by presence or absence of clinical bleeding or the requirement for a surgical procedure. In nonurgent situations, discontinuation of warfarin will result in normalization of the INR in 3 days unless the patient has substantial liver disease or vitamin K deficiency. When warfarin reversal is required more rapidly, administration of vitamin K (either orally or parenterally) can result in normalization of INR values within 12 to 24 hours. Low doses of vitamin K (0.5–1.0 mg) should be used if moderate decreasing of the INR is required or if warfarin therapy is to be reinitiated. Otherwise, 5 to 10 mg vitamin K can be administered. Urgent reversal of warfarin anticoagulation caused by warfarin overdosage, active or life-threatening bleeding, or high-risk surgical procedures such as craniotomy procedures can be achieved by administering 2 to 4 units of fresh frozen plasma, which should increase coagulation factor levels by 20% to 30% or 0.2 to 0.3 U/mL.

An uncommon, nonhemorrhagic side effect of warfarin, which may be more likely in patients with either protein C[98] or protein S deficiency,[99] involves skin necrosis caused by extensive thrombosis of the venules and capillaries within subcutaneous fat in the third to eighth day after initiating therapy. This complication can be managed with heparin or alternative therapy (direct thrombin inhibitors), whereas restoration of protein C or S levels can be achieved with fresh-frozen plasma.

Dosage and Administration

The initial dosage of warfarin is 5 to 10 mg/day for the first 2 to 4 days, followed by 2 to 10 mg/day as directed by prolongation of the INR. Although the average dose of warfarin required to maintain an INR of 2 to 3 is 4 to 5 mg/day, a small percentage of patients may require substantially less (1 to 3 mg/day) based on slower hepatic metabolism.

Agents Affecting Platelet Function

Platelet Physiology

Platelets are integrally involved in the initial response to vessel injury and play a pivotal role in hemostasis. Inactivated, they float inert as smooth discs in the blood. In response to numerous stimuli, they change shape, form pseudopods, extrude their granular contents, and bind avidly both to subendothelial surfaces and to one another (see Figs. 53–1 and 53–2). Platelet receptors are membrane GPs that bind to vWF (GPIb), collagen (GPIa), and fibrinogen (GPIIb/IIIa) (see Fig. 53–2).

The intact endothelium repels platelets and opposes their activation through the secretion of several mediators including NO and PGI_2. When the endothelium is breached, underlying collagen is exposed and both thromboxane A_2 (TxA_2) and vWF are released; all three are powerful promoters of platelet activation, adhesion, and aggregation. Endothelial cells also release PGI_2 and NO in response to shearing forces; these mediators are labile vasorelaxant and antiaggregatory substances.[100]

Activated platelets express adhesins and integrins, members of the superfamily of adhesion molecules (see Fig. 53–2). Collagen binds to the platelet GPIa receptor and vWF to the GPIb receptor, both located on the surface of the activated platelet. The platelet, once activated, initiates an amplification process of further platelet aggregation and binding. There is release of platelet agonists from dense storage granules in the platelet. These include ADP, serotonin, and TxA_2. Thrombin, a key regulator of the coagulation cascade, is one of the most powerful platelet activators. The platelet GPIIb/IIIa receptor acts as a binding site for fibrinogen and fibrin, which facilitate the linkage of platelets to one another and stabilizes the platelet plug.

As the physiology of platelets has been elucidated, targets for therapeutic intervention have been realized (see Fig. 53–2). There has been an explosion of agents that work in concert with aspirin to prevent or attenuate platelet activation by acting on different pathways. Examples include ticlopidine and clopidogrel, which block the platelet ADP receptor. The recently developed glypoprotein IIb/IIIa (GPIIb/IIIa) receptor blockers result in virtually complete inhibition of platelet to fibrinogen and platelet-to-platelet binding. This has been invaluable for interventional cardiology in which early restenosis was a common event after coronary angioplasty. With GPIIb/IIIa receptor blockers, coronary angioplasty and stenting has become as successful in treating coronary artery disease in many instances as bypass surgery at a fraction of the cost and with considerably less morbidity.[101-103]

Aspirin

Aspirin is the prototype nonsteroidal anti-inflammatory drug. There are also wide-ranging anticoagulant indications for aspirin therapy including AMI, unstable angina, prevention of both arterial and venous thromboses, interventional cardiology after cardiac surgery, transient ischemic attacks, atrial fibrillation, indwelling prostheses, and for platelet disorders such as essential thrombocytosis and idiopathic thrombotic thrombocytopenia. Aspirin is useful for the treatment of angina and generally for those at risk for vascular morbidity. (See Chapter 26 for additional information regarding the mechanism of action, analgesic and anti-inflammatory effects of aspirin, and the nonsteroidal anti-inflammatory agents.)

Mechanisms of Action

PGI_2 is the major eicosanoid synthesized by endothelial cells and TxA_2 is the chief eicosanoid produced by platelets. Endothelial production of PGI_2 and platelet TxA_2 synthesis are blocked by aspirin; but because of the rapid turnover of endothelial cells, PGI_2 production is quickly restored. TxA_2 synthesis is inhibited for the lifetime (about 10 days) of the platelet. The net result is that at low doses, aspirin inhibits TxA_2 production without affecting PGI_2.[104] Aspirin also inhibits the second phase of platelet aggregation by preventing release of ADP from platelets. The overall effect of aspirin is antithrombotic because of its inhibition of platelet function. (See Chapter 26 for a detailed discussion of the molecular aspects of aspirin's mechanism of action.)

Clinical Pharmacology

Aspirin is available in oral and rectal formulations. Ingested aspirin has a systemic bioavailability of 40% to 50%.[105] Aspirin undergoes extensive first-pass metabolism and is rapidly hydrolyzed to salicylic acid in the liver, plasma, and red blood cells. Salicylate has less pharmacologic activity than aspirin.[106] After oral aspirin administration, salicylate is detected in serum within 5 to 30 minutes, and peak serum salicylate concentrations occur within 0.25 to 2 hours. A high proportion of aspirin in the blood is bound to albumin.

Aspirin is rapidly and widely distributed, apparently into most body tissues and fluids. The volume of distribution of aspirin is approximately the same as that of salicylate (about 0.15–0.2 L/kg). Aspirin and its metabolites are excreted in the urine. Only about 1% of an oral dose of aspirin is excreted unchanged in urine. The remainder is excreted in urine as salicylate and its metabolites. The plasma half-life of aspirin is 15 minutes and that of salicylate is dose-dependent ranging between 2 and 12 hours. Thus aspirin has a brief pharmacokinetic half-life, but a long pharmacodynamic half-life, because the duration of platelet inhibition far outlasts the physical presence of the drug in the body.[107]

Practical Aspects of Drug Use

Aspirin is indicated for the prevention of myocardial infarction and strokes in patients with known vascular disease. The ISIS 2 study showed that aspirin improves short-term and long-term mortality rates when given to patients pre-

senting with AMI.[108] The combination of aspirin and SK improved morbidity significantly compared with either agent alone.

Aspirin is also useful in conjunction with other antiplatelet agents for coronary angioplasty. There is controversy surrounding the benefit of aspirin for patients with atrial fibrillation. No real benefit has been shown in this setting. Adding low-dose aspirin to warfarin decreases the risk for systemic embolism and death among patients with prosthetic heart valves.[109]

A large randomized prospective study recently suggested that aspirin decreases the incidence of venous thrombosis after major orthopedic surgery.[110] Aspirin reduces the risk for pulmonary embolus and DVT by at least one-third in different surgical and medical groups, largely irrespective of the use of any other antithrombotic agents. Hence, there is now good evidence for considering aspirin use routinely in a wide range of patients at high risk for venous thromboembolism, and for continuing it throughout the period of increased risk.[110]

Aspirin and Surgery

There are important debates surrounding the use of anticoagulants in the perioperative period. These include whether the agent should be stopped before surgery, when the agent should be started after surgery, and whether neuraxial anesthesia is safe for patients taking the drug. Aspirin protects against both arterial and venous thromboses. Given that postoperative thromboses may have devastating consequences, such as pulmonary emboli, myocardial infarction, and stroke, it is probably beneficial to continue aspirin therapy until the time of surgery and to restart it in the postoperative period.[110] Excessive bleeding is a theoretical concern with aspirin, but aspirin, unlike the GPIIb/IIIa receptor blockers, only blocks one pathway of platelet activation, namely TxA_2. When there is a significant tissue injury, such as occurs with surgery, there is major release of thrombin and ADP, which activate platelets allowing clotting to occur. For surgeries during which increased bleeding has devastating consequences, such as eye surgery and neurosurgery, aspirin may be stopped 5 to 7 days before surgery. A recent study suggests that despite individual variability, the defect in primary hemostasis after aspirin disappears 48 hours after the last dose.[111] Although a topic of considerable controversy, aspirin does not appear to be associated with increased bleeding after cardiac surgery. Aspirin has not been implicated in an increased incidence of epidural hematoma after neuraxial blockade, and most practitioners would not consider aspirin therapy alone to be a contraindication to spinal or epidural anesthesia.[112,113] However, there is a small subgroup of aspirin hyper-responders, who may be at increased risk for postoperative bleeding and spinal or epidural hematoma.[114] Caution should be exercised when patients receiving aspirin therapy provide a history of excessive bleeding.

Adverse Effects

Aspirin's adverse effects relate predominantly to its mechanisms of action. (These adverse effects including erosion of the GI mucosa, decreased renal blood flow leading to acute tubular necrosis, and bleeding are discussed in detail in Chapter 26.) The inhibition of cyclo-oxygenase may also increase the generation of lipoxygenase metabolites of arachidonic acid. Increased leukotriene synthesis through the lipoxygenase pathway can precipitate bronchospasm in patients with aspirin sensitivity or asthma.[115] Finally, aspirin is not licensed for use in children because it has been associated with Reye syndrome; life-threatening acute liver failure after the use of aspirin.[116]

Patients who have had an aspirin overdose may present with renal failure, complex acid-base abnormalities, dehydration, deranged blood glucose, seizures, or coma. Treatment should be in an intensive care unit and includes forced alkaline diuresis to promote salicylate excretion.[117] Emergency hemodialysis may be required.[117] Activated charcoal may prevent the systemic absorption of ingested aspirin.[118]

Monitoring

The effects of aspirin on platelet function are not detected by routine laboratory tests of coagulation. The template bleeding time has been advocated, but results have been inconsistent.[119,120] Platelet aggregometry induced by epinephrine and low concentrations of collagen, but not induced by thrombin or high concentrations of collagen, detect an aspirin effect.[121] The ACT and thromboelastography are unaffected by aspirin.[122] The PFA-100 platelet function analyzer detects the antiplatelet effect of aspirin.[123,124]

Dosage and Administration

For almost all of its indications, a daily dose of aspirin of 80 to 325 mg is recommended. The antithrombotic effect of aspirin does not appear to be dose-related over a wide range of daily doses, an observation consistent with saturability of platelet cyclo-oxygenase-1 inhibition by aspirin at very low doses. In contrast, GI toxicity of the drug does appear to be dose related. Across a broad range of aspirin doses, from 50 to 1500 mg/day, aspirin uniformly reduces the relative risk for stroke by approximately 15%. There is a subgroup of people who are aspirin resistant[240,244] and a subgroup who are ultrasensitive.[114] To decrease the incidence of GI effects, aspirin and other nonsteroidal anti-inflammatory drugs should be taken with meals. Enteric coating and limiting daily dosage are also effective strategies. Histamine 2 antagonists and proton pump inhibitors are helpful in decreasing GI tract mucosal damage and upper GI bleeding in the high-risk patient taking aspirin.[126]

Dipyridamole

Dipyridamole is both an antiplatelet agent and a vasodilator, which is usually combined with another antiplatelet or anti-coagulant agent for optimum therapeutic effect. It may be

most useful in preventing clotting associated with artificial surfaces, such as vascular grafts and prosthetic valves.[127] It has also been used in combination with aspirin to prevent clotting of saphenous vein cardiac bypass grafts.[127] Dipyridamole improves claudication symptoms when given together with aspirin to patients with peripheral vascular disease.[128]

Mechanisms of Action

Dipyridamole increases the concentrations of adenosine, possibly by decreasing its breakdown or its reuptake.[129] Adenosine stimulates adenylate cyclase activity, leading to increased cyclic adenosine monophosphate (cAMP) synthesis.[130] The increase in platelet cAMP inhibits calcium release and decreases secretion of serotonin and ADP. Dipyridamole has various actions, including vasodilatation, inhibition of platelet adhesion, PGI_2 potentiation, phosphodiesterase inhibition, and enhanced action of cAMP.[131] These actions result in a greater inhibition of platelet adhesion than aspirin, but much less effect on aggregation. Dipyridamole also enhances the effects of NO in opposing platelet aggregation and promoting vasorelaxation.[132]

Clinical Pharmacology

Oral absorption is slow and dipyridamole is extensively protein bound, mainly to α_1 acid GP.[131] Dipyridamole is metabolized in the liver through glucuronic acid conjugation and is excreted in bile.[131] There is minimal urinary excretion. The time to peak effect is rapid (<5 minutes) after IV administration and takes about 1.5 hours after ingestion. Elimination half-life is 10 hours.

Practical Aspects of Drug Use

The main indications for dipyridamole are for prevention of thrombosis in combination with warfarin for patients with prosthetic heart valves and for additive protection against ischemic neurologic events in combination with aspirin. When adenosine is administered to patients taking dipyridamole, it should be given in reduced doses because dipyridamole may lead to an accumulation of adenosine.

Adverse Effects

Adverse effects include hypotension, headache, bronchospasm, nausea, vomiting, and diarrhea. Cardiac ischemia, arrhythmias, and angina pectoris may be precipitated by dipyridamole, possibly as a result of coronary steal.[129]

Dosage and Administration

The adult dosage of dipyridamole in patients with prosthetic heart valves is 75 to 100 mg four times daily. When dipyridamole is used together with aspirin to prevent perioperative thrombosis (for cardiac or vascular surgery), the usual dose is 150 to 400 mg/day. The usual dose for stroke prophylaxis is 200 mg twice daily in combination with another antiplatelet agent.

Prostacyclin

PGI_2 is an important physiologic inhibitor of platelet activation and aggregation (see Fig. 53–2). The triad of PGI_2, NO, and tPA constitute key endothelial mediators that inhibit platelet activation and intravascular thrombosis.[133] The recent development of stable PGI_2 analogues has facilitated the exogenous administration of this crucial prostaglandin.

Mechanisms of Action

PGI_2 binds to receptors on platelets that activate adenylate cyclase and increase intracellular cAMP. This in turns leads to a decrease in intracellular free calcium and inhibition of platelet activity.

Practical Aspects of Drug Use

PGI_2 has a half-life of only 3 minutes in plasma and is thus given by continuous IV infusion. PGI_2 is a potent vasodilator and its side effects include flushing, headache, nausea, vomiting, and hypotension. Epoprostenol (PGI_2) can be given to inhibit platelet aggregation during renal dialysis either alone or with heparin. The use of exogenous PGI_2 as an antithrombotic agent is limited by its chemical instability and its vasodilatory actions.[134]

Dosage and Administration

PGI_2 may be initiated at a rate of 2 ng/kg per minute and increased in increments of 2 ng/kg per minute every 15 minutes. Infusion rate may be limited by hemodynamic instability or other side effects.

Nitric Oxide and Nitrates

In addition to its actions as a powerful vasorelaxant, NO also has potent antiplatelet action. Many drugs, such as the nitrates, either promote NO release or generate NO as their active metabolites. NO is released from platelets and from the endothelium.[135]

Mechanisms of Action

NO inhibits platelet activation, adhesion, and aggregation by activating guanylyl cyclase, inhibiting phosphoinositide 3-kinase, impairing calcium influx, and inhibiting cyclooxygenase-1. Endothelial cells and platelets are both important sources of NO. Platelet-derived NO limits recruitment of further platelets to the platelet-rich clots.[136] NO decreases platelet GPIIb/IIIa receptor activation in response to thrombin and ADP stimulation.[137] NO also increases platelet cAMP production, which acts synergistically with cyclic 3',5'-guanosine monophosphate in decreasing platelet responsiveness.[138]

Practical Aspects of Drug Use

Patients with symptomatic ischemic heart disease have decreased platelet responsiveness to NO donors (nitrates).[139] Treatment with hydroxymethylglutaryl-CoA reductase inhibitors, the so-called *statins,* may amplify NO-induced platelet inhibition.[139] Experimental work suggests that there is long-lasting inhibition of platelet responsiveness after sodium nitroprusside and continued infusion does not appear to lead to a desensitization of the platelet response.[138] *N*-acetyl-L-cysteine exerts antiaggregating effects through an increased bioavailability of platelet NO.[140] Losartan, the angiotensin II receptor blocker, reduces platelet adhesion to collagen in a dose-dependent manner. The observed action of losartan seems to be mediated mainly by endothelium- and platelet-derived NO.[141]

Ticlopidine and Clopidogrel

The thienopyridine ADP receptor blockers prevent a pathway of platelet activation parallel to the TxA_2 pathway. Drugs in this class include ticlopidine and clopidogrel. These can be used together with aspirin producing additive antiplatelet effects. Indications include prophylaxis for myocardial infarction, ischemic stroke, and progression of peripheral vascular disease.[142]

Mechanisms of Action

Ticlopidine and clopidogrel are prodrugs. Their active metabolites block ADP receptors expressed on the platelet surface membrane (see Fig. 53–2). As such, they block the actions of ADP on platelets, namely promotion of platelet activation, aggregation, and degranulation.[143–145] ADP-induced binding of fibrinogen to the platelet GPIIb/IIIa receptor is inhibited.[145] Clopidogrel irreversibly modifies the

ADP receptor resulting in lifelong platelet inhibition. Platelet aggregation induced by agonists other than ADP is also inhibited by blocking the amplification of platelet activation by released ADP. Ticlopidine may also block the binding of vWF to platelets and increases NO generation in recipients of a heart transplant.[146]

Clinical Pharmacology

Clopidogrel and ticlopidine are prodrugs that are metabolized in the liver to pharmacologically active compounds.[147] Clopidogrel has an onset about 2 hours after ingestion. Peak effect occurs 3 days after initiation of therapy, and the duration of action is about 5 days. The peak effect of ticlopidine after oral administration occurs several days after initiation, and its duration of action is 7 to 10 days, the lifespan of the platelet.[148] Both drugs are more than 98% protein bound and are metabolized in the liver followed by excretion in the urine and feces. Ticlopidine has an elimination half-life between 8 and 13 hours after a single dose and 4 to 5 days with repeated dosing.

Practical Aspects of Drug Use

The CAPRIE study demonstrated that clopidogrel is more efficacious than aspirin for patients with ischemic heart disease, cerebrovascular disease, and peripheral vascular disease. Treatment with clopidogrel results in a significant decrease in the need for rehospitalization for ischemic events or bleeding compared with aspirin.[149] Clopidogrel may be of particular benefit compared with aspirin after coronary artery surgery, where one study has shown a decreased risk for recurrent ischemia without an increase in bleeding.[149] The efficacy of aspirin and ticlopidine were compared in survivors of AMI treated with thrombolysis. No difference was found between the ticlopidine and aspirin groups in the rate of the primary combined end point of death, recurrent AMI, stroke, and angina.[150] Clopidogrel and ticlopidine act in concert with aspirin and therefore have been used with aspirin to prevent the clotting of coronary stents.[151]

Surgery and Anesthesia

The ADP receptor blockers should be stopped at least a week before elective major surgery until there are more data about their safety with respect to bleeding complications. Platelet transfusion may be effective in improving hemostasis. Regional anesthesia is best avoided until the effects of these agents have dissipated.

Adverse Effects

Both clopidogrel and ticlopidine may cause neutropenia or agranulocytosis. There have also been reports of fatal aplastic anemia thought to be attributable to clopidogrel.[152] Ticlopidine may cause hepatic impairment and life-threatening thrombotic thrombocytopenic purpura. These drugs should be avoided in patients with hepatic insufficiency. Intracranial and GI bleeding are also potential serious complications.

Dosage and Administration

Clopidogrel: 75 mg orally once a day. A larger initial (300 mg) dose has been administered to accelerate the onset of peak effect.
Ticlopidine: 250 mg orally twice daily with food.

Glycoprotein IIb/IIIa Receptor Blockers

The introduction of the GPIIb/IIIa receptor blockers has had a profound effect on clinical practice. These drugs are indicated for acute coronary syndromes, apart from myocardial infarction with ST-segment elevation. In a meta-analysis involving more than 32,000 patients, use of GPIIb/IIIa antagonists was associated with a 30% decrease in short-term mortality rates in the setting of acute coronary syndromes. The biggest impact has been for interventional cardiology. Abciximab (ReoPro) has consistently reduced the incidence of myocardial infarction after percutaneous coronary interventional procedures.[153,154] The presumed mechanism is prevention of platelet thrombus formation associated with vessel wall injury and downstream embolization into the microcirculation.[153] Early administration of abciximab to patients undergoing coronary stenting with AMI improves coronary patency before stenting, the success rate of the stenting procedure, the rate of coronary patency at 6 months, left ventricular function, and other clinical outcomes.[155] The use of GPIIb/IIIa blockers for angioplasty and for percutaneous coronary stent placement has resulted in decreased restenosis and long-term outcomes comparable with coronary artery bypass surgery.[101–103]

Mechanisms of Action

Abciximab is a chimeric human-murine monoclonal antibody that binds avidly to the platelet GPIIb/IIIa receptor (see Fig. 53–2). Eptifibatide (Integrilin) is a reversible peptide antagonist of the GPIIb/IIIa receptor. Tirofiban (Aggrastat) is a reversible nonpeptide antagonist of the GPIIb/IIIa receptor. The GPIIb/IIa receptor is the major surface receptor that is responsible for platelet aggregation.[156] All three agents prevent binding of fibrinogen, vWF, and other adhesive molecules to activated platelets. Pharmacologically, these agents do not all have equal efficacy, with abciximab displaying the greatest antiplatelet effect.[157]

Clinical Pharmacology

All three drugs are administered by IV infusion. Abciximab has the highest affinity for the IIb/IIIa receptor, whereas eptifibatide has the lowest affinity of the three agents. The onset of action of abciximab is almost immediate, and although its duration of action after cessation of the infusion is up to 48 hours, most of its platelet inhibition wears off after about 12 hours.[158] Abciximab is cleared by the kidneys. Whereas the onset of action of eptifibatide is within 15 minutes, the time to reach peak effect may be as long as 6 hours, and clinical effect continues for 4 to 6 hours after discontinuation. Up to 50% of the drug is excreted unchanged in the urine. Tirofiban achieves peak platelet inhibition within 0 minutes and lasts between 4 and 8 hours after discontinuation. The elimination half-life of tirofiban is 2 hours, and it is mainly excreted unchanged in urine and feces. Eptifibatide and tirofiban may be cleared from plasma by dialysis. Oral short-acting GPIIb/IIIa blockers have been developed. These include orbofiban, sibrafiban, and xemilofiban. Studies with these agents, such as the OPUS, SYMPHONY, and EXCITE trials, have been disappointing because these agents may be associated with an increased risk for thrombosis.[159–162]

Practical Aspects of Drug Use

Clinical benefits of the GPIIb/IIIa blockers have been demonstrated in several large clinical studies. The EPIC, EPILOG, CAPTURE, and EPISTENT studies provide support for abciximab.[156,163–167] IMPACT-II, PURSUIT and ESPRIT demonstrated the benefits of eptifibatide.[168–170] PRISM, PRISM-Plus, and RESTORE showed the efficacy of tirofiban.[171–173] Interestingly, recent comparisons among the various GPIIb/IIIa receptor blockers suggest that abciximab may be associated with the greatest clinical benefit, such as reduction in myocardial infarction.[154,174] This may relate to its greater potency or more sustained platelet inhibition.

The GPIIb/IIIa blockers do not prevent platelet adhesion or the secretion of platelet mediators. They only partially block the responsiveness of platelets to TxA_2 and arachidonic acid.[175] Current evidence supports the use of these drugs in combination with other agents, such as aspirin, ticlopidine, or clopidogrel.[175,176]

Adverse Effects

Bleeding represents the most likely complication encountered with any of the GPIIb/IIIa receptor blockers, but may occur most frequently with abciximab.[177] Acute severe thrombocytopenia is a class effect of these drugs and occurs in 0.5% of cases. This risk may be compounded when they are given together with other drugs that carry this risk, such as ticlopidine or clopidogrel.[178] Thrombocytopenia can reportedly be treated successfully with a combination of platelet and steroid therapy.[179]

Monitoring

The ACT has generally been recommended for near patient monitoring of GPIIb/IIIa receptor blockers. Target ACT values for percutaneous interventional procedures range between 200 and 400 seconds. Recently, the PFA-100 platelet function analyzer has been described in this setting and may be more specific as a monitor of platelet function.[180] Platelet counts should be checked regularly and therapy should be discontinued if thrombocytopenia (platelet count <100 000/mm^3) develops.

Surgery and Anesthesia

Increasing numbers of patients presenting for surgery will have received GPIIb/IIIa receptor blockers. Their effects may be reversed with platelet transfusions or potentially cryoprecipitate (tirofiban, eptifibatide) or may be allowed to dissipate. An early report indicated that the use of abciximab may increase perioperative bleeding especially if administered within 12 hours of surgery.[181] There are, however, other data suggesting that there is no increased bleeding during cardiac surgery after administration of GPIIb/IIIa receptor blockers.[182] Although abciximab may be associated with increased hemorrhage,[181] the GPIIb/IIIa receptor blockers may protect platelets, preventing sequestration during CPB.[182,183] There is a suggestion that heparin dosage for CPB should be reduced in patients who have received GPIIb/IIIa receptor blockers.[181] The combination of unfractionated heparin with GPIIb/IIIa receptor blockers during CPB may be an alternative to other anticoagulation strategies in patients with HIT.[184] Regional anesthesia is best avoided when patients have recently received GPIIb/IIIa antagonists.

Dosage and Administration

The GPIIb/IIIa antagonists are not intended as monotherapy and should be given in conjunction with other agents, such as aspirin and heparin. For thrombosis prophylaxis during percutaneous coronary intervention, the following guidelines may be applied:

Abciximab: Loading dose of 250 μg/kg administered 10 to 60 minutes before the start of the procedure followed by an infusion of 0.125 μg/kg per minute for 12 hours.

Eptifibatide: Loading dose of 180 μg/kg followed by an infusion of 2 μg/min for up to 72 hours. The dosage should be adjusted in renal failure.

Tirofiban: IV infusion of 0.4 μg/kg per minute for 30 minutes followed by 0.1 μg/kg per minute. Decrease the infusion rate by 50% in patients with creatinine clearance less than 30 mL/min.

Thrombolytic Agents

Fibrinolytic drugs such as SK, urokinase, anisoylated plasminogen activator complex (APSAC), and tPA are used for thrombolysis of arterial or venous clots in a variety of clinical settings. In the past decade, fibrinolytic agents have revolutionized the treatment of AMI as it has been decisively established that these drugs can significantly improve survival. Although also suggested as a therapy for acute ischemic stroke and pulmonary embolism, the efficacy and improvement of outcome has not been clearly established. Thrombolysis initiated by these drugs is not without risk for significant bleeding complications and allergic reactions.

Mechanisms of Action

Fibrinolysis occurs when circulating and fibrin-bound plasminogen activators enzymatically convert plasminogen into plasmin. Plasmin, a serine protease, hydrolyzes fibrin to dissolve clot. All fibrinolytic agents promote thrombolysis through this plasmin-mediated degradation of fibrinogen, circulating fibrin monomers/polymers, and clot-bound fibrin. Plasminogen activators act either directly (tPA) or indirectly (SK) and are much more capable of dissolving newly formed "white" clot—that is, platelet-rich (formed by weaker fibrinogen bonds)—than the older, more stable "red" clot that is tightly bound with fibrin.[185] Therefore, to be most effective, fibrinolytic agents must be given soon after thrombus formation.

SK is a protein that forms a complex with the proactivator plasminogen to catalyze uncomplexed plasminogen's conversion to plasmin. This indirect action makes SK much less fibrin-specific by combining with free as well as clot-bound plasminogen. In contrast, tPA and its genetically engineered cousins, are enzymes that cleave plasminogen into plasmin directly. Its activity is preferential to plasminogen already bound to fibrin, and thus makes tPA more clot-specific than SK. When interacting within a clot, their presence effectively shields plasmin from circulating plasmin inhibitors.[185]

Other related fibrinolytic agents are used in clinical practice. Urokinase is an enzyme derived from the human fetal renal cell lines. It is not antigenic like SK and has a direct action on fibrin/fibrinogen. Anisoylated plasminogen activator complex (or anistreplase) is the preformed complex that SK forms in vivo and has the same mechanism of action as SK.

Preclinical Pharmacology

Development of Genetically Engineered Mutants

In an effort to provide more rapid, more specific, and longer-acting thrombolytic agents, researchers have created a number of new plasminogen activators by genetically engineering human tPA with sequence deletions and substitutions. The first commercially available agent was reteplase (rPA), a deletion mutant, that has a longer half-life than human tPA.[186] Another genetic variation is tenecteplase (TNK-tPA), offering a 14-fold increase in fibrin specificity in vitro, which theoretically should reduce systemic plasminogen activation.[186] Both have equivalent infarct-artery patency rates and patient survival data as human tPA (alteplase), but have the advantage of administration as a bolus injection and thus may provide faster onset in clinical settings.

Laboratory Evaluation of Therapy

The fibrinolytic state created by these drugs affects the coagulation system and consequently its laboratory tests. This activity results in a depletion of plasma fibrinogen levels, factor V, and factor VIII. The low levels of fibrinogen (as low as 50 mg/dL or less) can persist for more than 24 hours. Laboratory evaluation has demonstrated increased levels of fibrinogen degradation products and prolonged thrombin time, PT, and aPTT. Such laboratory tests are nonspecific and generally are not useful in guiding therapy. It is recommended, however, that patients receiving SK have fibrinogen and aPTT levels drawn several hours after administration; if there is no significant change, then the patient is likely resistant to treatment secondary to preformed antistreptococcal antibodies, and another drug should be selected. This testing is unnecessary in the setting of AMI because the initial dose is large enough to overcome most resistance.

Clinical Pharmacology

Each agent has relative advantages and disadvantages based on its fibrin specificity, biologic half-life, cost, ease of administration, and risk for allergic and other adverse reactions. U.S. Food and Drug Administration–approved indications for usage include the treatment of AMI and acute pulmonary embolism. SK is also approved for the treatment of DVT and arterial thrombosis; tPA is the only approved drug for the treatment of acute ischemic stroke. The novel genetically engineered versions of tPA have only been studied in the setting of AMI.

Pharmacokinetics

For the treatment of AMI, fibrinolytic agents can be delivered through the coronary arteries or the venous system. Although intracoronary administration provides rapid, reliable thrombolysis and minimizes bleeding risks, the IV route is more suitable for rapid delivery within the first hours of symptoms and provides fibrinolytic therapy without the added procedural risks.

SK has a half-life of approximately 23 minutes, and its infusion may decrease vascular resistance and cause hypotension. SK is eliminated by the liver without detectable metabolites. Antistreptococcal antibodies contribute significantly to its inactivation. Alteplase (recombinant human tPA) is cleared from the plasma primarily by the liver, with a half-life of 5 minutes and a volume of distribution approximating plasma volume.

Adverse Effects

All fibrinolytic agents may cause major bleeding complications, including intracranial hemorrhage. Severe bleeding can be treated with transfusions of fresh-frozen plasma, cryoprecipitate, or platelets and agents that have antifibrinolytic properties (e.g., epsilon aminocaproic acid [EACA] or aprotinin).[187] Other adverse reactions include reperfusion arrhythmias, hypotension, cholesterol embolism, and allergic reaction. Allergic reactions are most commonly seen with SK (1–4% develop fever and shivering, whereas <0.5% develop true anaphylaxis), because many patients have varying levels of antistreptococcal antibodies from previous bacterial infections; repeat administration of SK carries greater risk for allergic reaction, including serum sickness and hypersensitivity vasculitis.[188] Risk for allergic reaction to tPA is less than 0.2%.

Practical Aspects of Drug Use

Acute Myocardial Infarction

Survival is the primary end point of all trials investigating fibrinolytic agents in AMI. Clinical trials have clearly established that any form of early reperfusion therapy (whether fibrinolytic drugs or percutaneous coronary interventions) improves patient survival. The key to improving survival is related to reducing infarct size by rapidly restoring arterial patency and normal antegrade flow.[189,190] Patients with the greatest mortality rate reduction are those who present within 6 hours and have electrocardiogram evidence of bundle branch block or ST-segment elevation and those with anterior infarct.[191,192] Thrombolysis provides no survival benefit to patients with persistent unstable angina or non–Q-wave myocardial infarction.[193,194]

The concept that thrombolytic therapy needs to be initiated early has also been clearly established. The GISSI-1 trial demonstrated that SK given within 1 hour of symptom onset reduced mortality rates by 47%, but that survival benefit decreased to 23% and 17% if therapy was initiated after 1 to 3 hours or 3 to 6 hours after onset of symptoms, respectively.[195] These findings were confirmed in the ISIS-2 trial.[188]

Clinical trials have been designed to determine which fibrinolytic regimen can provide the most rapid, most complete, and most sustained patency rates with the smallest risk. One of the most widely cited investigations is the GUSTO trial. Patients (n = 41,022) with ST-segment elevations within 6 hours of symptom onset were randomized into four groups: SK plus subcutaneous heparin, SK plus IV heparin, accelerated tPA plus IV heparin, or combined mid-dose accelerated tPA plus SK. Data revealed an immediate reduction in mortality rate of 19% in the tPA group versus either SK group; 30-day mortality rate was reduced by 14% in the tPA group and by 10% in the combined therapy group. These results translated into an absolute mortality rate reduction of 1% with tPA, equaling 10 lives saved per 1000 treated.[196] However, the rate of hemorrhagic stroke was significantly increased in the tPA group, with an excess of 2 per 1000 patients treated when compared

with SK and an excess of 4 per 1000 in patients treated with combined therapy. Nevertheless, when combining outcomes of death and disabling stroke, tPA still showed greater benefit than SK.[196]

The GUSTO trials findings are in contrast to two other multicentered, randomized, controlled studies: the GISSI-2[197] and the ISIS-3[198] trials. Both studies showed no difference in overall survival benefit between tPA and SK, despite evidence that the tPA group had lower reinfarction rates in ISIS-3. They also demonstrated an increased risk for stroke in patients receiving tPA (although the differentiation of hemorrhagic stroke was unclear).

Acute Pulmonary Embolism

Large randomized controlled studies regarding the treatment of acute pulmonary embolism with fibrinolytic drugs are lacking. Therefore, it has not been determined that thrombolytic treatment definitively reduces the mortality rates or the development of chronic pulmonary hypertension.

Acute Ischemic Stroke

Currently, only tPA (alteplase) is approved by the U.S. Food and Drug Administration for the treatment of acute ischemic stroke. The guidelines for treatment, however, are strict. The patient's symptoms must have a definitive onset of less than 3 hours. Other patient-related criteria include: a computed tomography scan without evidence of early infarct signs, noncomatose mental status, and the absence of rapidly improving symptoms. In addition, there are strict admission blood pressure, coagulation, and glucose parameters. These criteria are derived from the National Institute of Neurological Disorders and Stroke study, which demonstrated a trend toward overall improved outcome at 3 months with intravenous tPA versus placebo plus an approximately 30% greater chance of having no or minimal neurologic deficit with thrombolysis. Notably, the tPA group had a 6.4% rate of symptomatic intracranial hemorrhage when compared with a 0.6% incidence in control patients.[199] The risk/benefit ratio between severe bleeding and cerebral reperfusion appears to have a narrow margin. A European study using greater dose tPA and a 6-hour window showed symptomatic intracranial hemorrhage in 8.8% of the patients receiving tPA versus 3.4% in the placebo group, in the setting of no significant change in mortality rate or neurologic outcome.[200] More recent studies have failed to show that thrombolytic therapy offers significant improvement in outcome; however, these studies did not have similar study designs.[201]

Dosage and Administration

Streptokinase

In the setting of AMI, dosage for IV administration is 1,500,000 U over 60 minutes; intracoronary delivery is 20,000 U bolus followed by a 2,000 U/min infusion for

60 minutes. For pulmonary embolism, DVT, or arterial thrombosis, the loading dose is 250,000 U IV infusion over 30 minutes followed by a 100,000 U infusion for 24 to 72 hours. To treat occlusion of arteriovenous cannulae, 250,000 U in 2 mL of solution should be instilled and left in the clamped-off cannula for 2 hours. Then the contents of the cannula should be aspirated—not flushed—and then, if clear, flushed with saline and reconnected.

Alteplase

For the treatment of AMI, alteplase can be delivered intravenously using either the conventional 3-hour infusion or the accelerated infusion, which involves administration of two thirds of the dose over the first 30 minutes.[196] The recommended dose is based on patient weight and should not exceed 100 mg because of the increased risk for intracranial hemorrhage. For pulmonary embolism, infusion of 100 mg over 2 hours is recommended, followed by therapeutic heparinization. For the treatment of acute ischemic stroke, alteplase should be given in a total dose not to exceed 90 mg, with 10% of the dose given as an IV bolus followed by a 60-minute infusion of the remaining 90%.[201]

Desmopressin

DDAVP is a synthetic polypeptide structurally related to arginine vasopressin (antidiuretic hormone). As a hemostatic agent, it is indicated for the treatment of bleeding associated with mild hemophilia, von Willebrand disease, uremia, antiplatelet drugs, and platelet dysfunction after surgery.[202–204]

Mechanisms of Action

DDAVP causes a dose-dependent increase in clotting factor VIII, plasminogen activator, factor VIII-related antigen, and vWF activity. DDAVP increases plasma vWF concentrations through receptor-mediated release from endothelial cells.[205]

Although increases in vWF can improve platelet/subendothelium and platelet/platelet interactions,[206] other mechanisms may occur, such as DDAVP-mediated generation of platelet microparticles or enhanced procoagulant activity,[207] improvement of platelet retention,[208] increased release of vWF from platelets, and increased expression of GPIb receptors.[209]

Clinical Pharmacology

After intranasal administration of DDAVP, 10% to 20% is absorbed through the nasal mucosa. Bioavailability is 3.3% to 4.1% and peak plasma concentrations are attained after 40 to 45 minutes. After both intranasal and IV administration, increases in plasma concentrations of factor VIII and vWF are evident within 30 minutes and peak between 90 minutes and 3 hours. Plasma concentrations of DDAVP decline in a biphasic manner with a mean initial plasma half-life of 8 minutes and a mean plasma elimination half-life of 75 minutes. The metabolic fate of DDAVP is unknown. Large IV doses of DDAVP increase factor VIII activity in healthy individuals, in patients with mild hemophilia A and B, in patients with certain types of von Willebrand disease, and in patients with uremia. The effect of DDAVP effect on platelet function lasts for about 3 hours, but may be prolonged by a repeat dose.[210]

Practical Aspects of Drug Use

The increase in factor VIII activity is dose-dependent, with a 300% to 400% maximum increase occurring after IV administration of a 0.4-μg/kg dose. DDAVP is only beneficial for treatment of hemophilia A when baseline plasma factor VIII activity is greater than 5%. DDAVP should be used judiciously in patients with type 2B von Willebrand disease, because there may be an increased risk for thrombocytopenia or thrombosis. DDAVP is ineffective for type 3 von Willebrand disease. Tachyphylaxis occurs if the DDAVP is administered more than once within a 48-hour period.

Adverse Effects

In patients with type 2B and pseudo–von Willebrand disease, DDAVP may induce platelet aggregation and thrombocytopenia secondary to release of abnormal forms of high molecular weight multimers. With large doses administered rapidly, tachycardia, hypotension, facial flushing, headache, water retention, and hyponatremia have been reported.[211] Hypotension may be related to the rate of administration and release of vasodilating prostaglandins from endothelial cells.[212] The risk for water intoxication and hyponatremia increases with doses greater than 0.5 μg/kg. Hemodynamic side effects can be attenuated by slow IV drug administration.[203]

Dosage and Administration

The intranasal dosage of DDAVP for the management of hemophilia A or type 1 von Willebrand disease is 300 μg (0.1 mL or 1 spray from the spray pump into each nostril of a solution containing 1.5 mg/mL). A dosage of 150 μg may be sufficient in patients who weigh less than 50 kg. The usual parenteral dose for those older than 3 months with hemophilia A or type 1 von Willebrand disease is 0.3 to 0.4 μg/kg given by slow IV infusion over 30 minutes.[203]

Monitoring

In patients with hemophilia A, factor VIII and vWF activities, factor VIII antigen levels, and aPTT should be monitored during DDAVP therapy. In patients with von Willebrand disease, factor VIII and vWF antigen and activities should be monitored. Tests of platelet function such as the bleeding time, platelet aggregometry, the HemoSTA-TUS,[203] and the PFA-100 platelet function analyzer may be useful.

Surgery and Anesthesia

If DDAVP is used before surgery for bleeding prophylaxis, the nasal drug should be administered 2 hours before surgery and the IV infusion 30 minutes before surgery. DDAVP is well established in the prevention of bleeding for patients with inherited bleeding abnormalities, especially von Willebrand disease.[213] In the perioperative period, patients are particularly vulnerable to electrolyte and fluid imbalances. DDAVP increases these risks. Hyponatremia should be treated and diuretic therapy may prevent fluid overload.

There is much controversy surrounding the ability of DDAVP to decrease perioperative bleeding when patients are not known to have a specific bleeding diathesis. Most of the studies, including spinal, aortic, and liver surgery, have not shown a reduction in blood loss after routine DDAVP administration.[214–216] The composite evidence does not support the routine use of DDAVP, unless there is a specific indication such as von Willebrand disease, patients at high-risk for bleeding (e.g., uremia, long CPB intervals), or in vitro evidence of platelet dysfunction.[203,217,218]

Antifibrinolytic Agents: Synthetic Lysine Analogs

The fibrinolytic pathway is important in that it results in clot lysis, which potentially prevents vaso-occlusion at sites of vessel injury. However, excessive fibrinolysis can lead to a bleeding diathesis by depleting fibrinogen, factors V, and VIII, and by leading to increases in circulating fibrinogen/fibrin degradation products that can inhibit platelet function. Surgery, organic diseases, and drugs can initiate and promote fibrinolysis, with CPB representing the most extensively studied clinical situation. Antifibrinolytic agents can inhibit this activity and aid in reducing the associated bleeding. These agents include the synthetic lysine analogs—EACA and TA—and the nonspecific serine protease inhibitor—aprotinin. Although their mechanisms of action, efficacy, adverse effects, and cost have been extensively studied in the cardiac surgical setting, they have also been evaluated in various other clinical settings.

Mechanisms of Action

All antifibrinolytic agents competitively inhibit the degradation of fibrin and fibrinogen by plasmin. The method of inhibition differs between the lysine analogs and aprotinin, and their effects may be additive or even synergistic.

EACA is a synthetic chemical analog of the amino acid lysine. It acts by binding to the kringles, or lysine-binding sites, of plasminogen and plasmin. Once bound, EACA displaces plasminogen from fibrin, thus inhibiting its ability to split fibrinogen.[219] Another proposed mechanism of action involves the ability of EACA to bind to fibrin and protect it from plasmin degradation. The mechanism of action of TA is identical to EACA, but it is approximately 10 times more potent on a molar basis. Both TA and EACA preferentially inhibit the cleavage of plasminogen to plasmin by clot-bound tPA rather than circulating tPA; accordingly, they may not be as effective as aprotinin in inhibiting systemic fibrinolysis when high levels of tPA result in systemic plasmin generation and prolongation of bleeding times secondary to increased fibrinogen degradation products.[220]

Clinical Pharmacology

EACA is a water-soluble drug with a volume of distribution of approximately 30 L. It is primarily eliminated unchanged (65%) in urine and has a terminal half-life of approximately 2 hours.[221]

TA has a volume of distribution of about 9 to 12 L. Of the TA found circulating, about 3% is bound to plasminogen. It is almost entirely excreted unchanged through the kidney (90–95%), with little undergoing metabolism. Its terminal elimination half-life is also about 2 hours.[221,222] Given the high degree of renal excretion, the doses of both EACA and TA should be reduced in patients with renal insufficiency.

Adverse Effects

Although antifibrinolytic agents have been implicated with thrombotic complications, meta-analyses and randomized clinical trials have not revealed any increased incidence of thrombotic complications when routine dosing has been used.[219,221–224] However, in specific clinical situations such as ongoing DIC or concomitant treatment with coagulation factor concentrates, such as factor IX concentrate in patients with hemophilia, an increased incidence of thrombotic complications has been observed.

Other rare but serious adverse effects have been reported. Hyperkalemic arrest after CPB has been attributed to the structural similarity of EACA with the cationic amino acid lysine. Lysine has been shown in isolated rat muscle and intact animals to increase serum potassium by an electroneutral exchange of intracellular potassium for extracellular lysine. The resultant increase in potassium can be rapid and can be worse in patients with significant reduction in renal function.[225] Intravenous EACA has been linked with postoperative proteinuria and with skeletal muscle injury, ranging from myalgias to myonecrosis and rhabdomyolysis.[226,227]

Practical Aspects of Drug Use

EACA and TA have been used in treatment and prophylaxis of bleeding in numerous clinical situations. They have been helpful as adjunctive therapy in disease states such as hemophilia, von Willebrand disease, and uremia.[228] They have been administered to reduce risk for rebleeding in upper GI bleeding, severe epistaxis, menorrhagia, hemorrhagic laryngitis/tonsillitis, traumatic hyphema, and subarachnoid hemorrhage from cerebral aneurysm.[229] In the surgical setting, these drugs have been given to reduce perioperative bleeding in major orthopedic joint replacement, liver transplantation, and most extensively with cardiac surgery and use of ECMO.

In many of these situations, these agents have been used to inhibit primary fibrinolysis. Concerns have been raised regarding the use of these agents in settings involving secondary fibrinolysis such as DIC. The administration of antifibrinolytic drugs in this setting can potentially lead to be catastrophic thrombotic complications, especially if given without concomitant heparin. However, these agents have been extensively used in cardiac surgery (which routinely leads to secondary fibrinolysis) without an apparent increased risk for thrombotic complications. This may be because of the routine use of high-dose heparin for systemic anticoagulation and the hypocoagulable state associated with CPB. TA is approved by the U.S. Food and Drug Administration only for the prophylaxis of patients with hemophilia undergoing tooth extraction.[221] Outside the United States, TA has been used extensively in the perioperative setting for reduction of blood loss.

EACA and TA have little effect on the laboratory evaluation of coagulation. Tests of platelet function, including aggregation and thromboelastograph curves, are unchanged in vivo when standard dosing is used.[230,231] Intraoperative point-of-care testing with ACTs is also unaffected by EACA.[222,232] EACA activity can be demonstrated ex vivo by a decrease in circulating fibrin degradation products when compared with placebo.[222,230]

Cardiac Surgery

Numerous studies have been performed to evaluate the efficacy of EACA and TA in reducing blood loss during and after cardiac surgery. Meta-analyses of these studies conclude that both TA and EACA can reduce blood loss after cardiac surgery, but are inconclusive regarding reduction of transfusion rates. These studies and those comparing the two lysine analogs overall favor TA in its ability to decrease blood loss and transfusion rates.[217,219,233] This difference may be related to potency or equivalent dosing issues.

Orthopedic Surgery

There are conflicting reports regarding the benefit of antifibrinolytics in major joint replacement surgery. TA and EACA have been used in total knee and total hip arthroplasty procedures. Proponents theorize that use of tourniquet and traumatic exposure of marrow can promote fibrinolysis. The conclusions of these studies range from no difference in blood loss,[234] to reduction in blood loss but not transfusion rate,[235] to significant decreases in both postoperative blood loss and need for transfusion.[236,237] None of the studies, however, reports an increased incidence in thromboembolic events.

Other Clinical Uses

Antifibrinolytic agents have been administered to neurosurgical patients to decrease the risk for rebleeding from cerebral aneurysm while awaiting surgery. In patients with subarachnoid hemorrhage, antifibrinolytic therapy reduced the risk for rebleeding by 45% when compared with placebo. The beneficial effect on rebleeding is, however, offset by an increased risk for cerebral ischemia, and there is no overall improvement in mortality rate.[229] In addition, Kang and colleagues[238] demonstrated that an EACA-modified thromboelastograph can be used to identify patients with hyperfibrinolysis during the anhepatic stage of liver transplantation. These authors also demonstrated that use of this technique reduced bleeding when EACA was administered on the basis of thromboelastogram results.[239]

Dosage and Administration

EACA is available as a 250-mg/mL injectable solution, with benzyl alcohol as a preservative (thus not recommended for use in newborns). For oral administration, EACA is available as a 25% syrup and as 500-mg tablets. TA is available in injectable form, in a 100 mg/mL concentration, and in 50-mg tablets.

For the control of local fibrinolysis, the recommended dosing regimen for EACA is a 4- to 5-g loading dose infused intravenously over 1 hour followed by a 1-g/hr infusion for 8 hours or until the bleeding is controlled. TA dosing has been recommended as 0.5- to 1-g slow IV infusion twice daily or as 1 to 1.5 g orally twice daily or three times daily. TA, as indicated for tooth extraction prophylaxis, is a 10-mg/kg IV bolus given just before surgery, followed by 25 mg/kg orally or 10 mg/kg IV three or four times daily for 2 to 8 days.

For the inhibition of general fibrinolysis associated with CPB, EACA can be given as a 75- to 150-mg/kg IV loading dose over 15 to 30 minutes, followed by a 10 to 15 mg/kg per hour infusion.[221] More recent evidence indicates that to maintain a reasonable level of this agent, the bolus dose should be reduced to 50 mg/kg and the infusion rate should be increased to 25 mg/kg per hour.[240] The most common TA dosing for cardiac surgery is a 10- to 15-mg/kg IV loading dose with a 1-mg/kg per hour infusion.[219,221,222]

Aprotinin

Although aprotinin has antifibrinolytic properties, it is clearly a broad-spectrum agent on the basis of its anticoagulant and anti-inflammatory properties. Although widely used abroad for the prevention and treatment of bleeding associated with cardiac surgery, it was not until 1989 that it was approved for use in the United States.[242]

Mechanisms of Action

Aprotinin is a strongly basic polypeptide isolated from bovine lung that has a molecular weight of 6512 daltons and belongs to the Kuntz family of serine protease inhibitors.[241,242] In addition to its antifibrinolytic properties (plasmin inhibition), aprotinin also inhibits trypsin, chymotrypsin, thrombin, kallikrein, bradykinin, elastase, activated protein C, and urokinase.[221–243] Overall, aprotinin is categorized as an antifibrinolytic, anticoagulant, platelet-protective, and anti-inflammatory agent.

Aprotinin has its strongest affinity for plasmin, based on in its derived in vitro inhibition constant, making plasmin its strongest target and aprotinin's major site of action.[221,241,242] Aprotinin binds plasmin bound to fibrin and to cell receptors, where plasmin is usually protected from the body's naturally occurring inhibitors (such as α_2-antiplasmin and α_2-macroglobulin). Aprotinin can also prevent fibrinolysis by a nonplasmin pathway by inhibiting kallikrein (and therefore the contact activation coagulation system).[221,241,242]

Aprotinin may also reduce tissue factor–mediated activation of the hemostatic system by directly inhibiting the tissue factor—factor VIIa complex and factor VIII.[243,244] This action on the coagulation cascade is also intertwined with aprotinin's other mechanisms: decreasing thrombin-induced platelet activation and inhibiting kallikrein activation of fibrinolysis. By acting on plasmin, aprotinin can protect platelets because plasmin and thrombin can induce platelet activation, release, and aggregation. Potential explanations for the ability of aprotinin to preserve platelets include attenuation of TxA₂ release, inhibition of thrombin formation, preservation of GPIIb/IIIa receptors, and protection against heparin-induced platelet dysfunction.[241,242,245] In addition, aprotinin can inhibit thrombin-mediated platelet activation through a dose-dependent inhibition of the platelet PAR1 receptor.[246]

Clinical Pharmacology

After IV injection, aprotinin is rapidly distributed throughout the extracellular compartment. This distribution phase has a half-life of approximately 0.3 to 0.5 hour.[242] Aprotinin has a plasma half-life of approximately 150 minutes and a terminal elimination half-life of 7 to 10 hours. Aprotinin requires repeated boluses or maintenance infusion to maintain therapeutic plasma concentrations.

Aprotinin is reabsorbed by the renal proximal tubular system, with 80% to 90% stored in phagosomes found in the tubules' ciliated border cells. The remainder is excreted unchanged in the urine, with the excreted fraction increasing as the dose increases. These border cells accumulate aprotinin for the first 12 to 24 hours to be later metabolized and eliminated during the next 4 to 5 days.[242,247]

Potential Adverse Effects

Thrombotic Complications

Thrombosis is a serious concern when using any drugs that inhibit fibrinolysis. Unlike the lysine analogs, high concentrations of aprotinin can inhibit activated protein C, which is an important step in limiting thrombin formation by inactivating factors Va and VIIIa.[241,248] This theoretical link to thrombotic complications currently is unsubstantiated. Studies in cardiac surgical patients show no increased risk for graft thrombosis in the early postoperative period. However, most of the studies evaluating early graft patency have enrolled small numbers of patients, leading to possibly underpowered analyses.[249–251]

Despite the potential risk for thrombosis, the incidence of stroke appears to be reduced in patients treated with aprotinin.[252,253] This benefit has been confirmed in a extensive analysis of the U.S. aprotinin database by Smith.[253]

Renal Function

Aprotinin does accumulate in the proximal tubular cells and this can lead to a phenomenon known as *tubular overloading*, in which normally filtered proteins are spilled into the urine.[241,247] Aprotinin can cause mild increases in serum creatinine, which are usually well tolerated.[247,254]

Allergic Reactions

Because aprotinin is a foreign protein, allergic reactions are another concern. The overall risk for allergic reaction has been estimated to be about 2.8%.[256,257] There is strong evidence that re-exposure within 3 to 6 months carries the greatest risk for reaction: 4.5% to 6.5% within 6 months versus 0.9% to 1.8% for less than 6 months.[256] Pretesting for IgG and IgE leads to nonspecific results and is not recommended as a screening tool.[257] Administering a test dose of 10,000 kallikrein inhibiting units (KIU) before IV or CPB prime bolus is strongly recommended.

Practical Aspects of Drug Use

Therapeutic Range

Most studies have demonstrated that aprotinin can reduce both perioperative blood loss and transfusion requirements by 40% to 80% in cardiac surgical patients undergoing CPB. This reduction is most evident in the full-Hammersmith dosing regimen, but has also been widely shown in the half-Hammersmith dosage. Because its antifibrinolytic activity is responsible for part of this effect, ultralow doses (2×10^5 KIU IV load plus 2×10^5 KIU CPB prime plus 1×105 KIU/hr infusion) have also produced significant decreases in blood loss and donor exposure.[189]

Patients at high risk may benefit the most from aprotinin therapy. This category would include reoperations, complex cases or combined procedures, patients with bleeding disorders related to drug therapy (e.g., LMWH, IIb/IIIa inhibitors, ADP antagonists) or disease states (e.g., renal or hepatic insufficiency), and patients with congenital hemostatic system disorders (e.g., factor deficiencies, platelet of vWF defects).[258-260]

Use With Deep Hypothermic Circulatory Arrest

The use of aprotinin in deep hypothermic circulatory arrest remains one area of significant controversy. Theoretically, the combination of a stasis-induced hypercoagulable state and aprotinin could promote thrombosis. However, aprotinin may also have a positive effect in its attenuation of hypothermia-induced anticoagulation, fibrinolysis, and platelet deformation.[248] Conflicting evidence has been presented concerning increased risk for thrombotic complications and mortality in this subset of cardiac patients.

Pediatric Cardiac Surgery

The use of aprotinin has been studied in children. No adverse effects have been observed with aprotinin use in the setting of deep hypothermic circulatory arrest in more than 500 cases involving children.[248] For other types of cardiac surgery, aprotinin appears to be safe and to have some benefit in reducing blood loss and donor exposures,[261-263] although this has not been universally observed. In children, aprotinin is dosed by weight—a high-dose regimen would be $240 \, mg/m^2$ IV load and CPB prime with $56 \, mg/m^2$ per hour infusion intraoperatively.[262]

Other Surgical Procedures

Aprotinin has also been used to reduce postoperative bleeding and transfusion rates in total hip arthroplasty procedures.[264,265] The incidence of DVT tended to be lower in the aprotinin-treated patients, although the small enrollment limits conclusions to be drawn. Further studies are needed to determine whether aprotinin can reduce the risk for postoperative thrombotic complications.

Effect on Monitoring (ACT)

Aprotinin prolongs whole blood activated or non-ACTs in a dose-dependent manner.[266,267] When heparin dosing is guided by celite ACT protocols during aprotinin administration, patients receive smaller heparin doses and have lower blood heparin concentrations.[248,268] The concern, therefore, is maintaining adequate heparinization in this setting of increased ACT values and thus reducing the risk for thromboembolic complications.[248,267] Celite ACT is affected considerably more by aprotinin than kaolin ACT, but both result in values greater than with those achieved with heparin alone.[267] In patients receiving aprotinin and heparin anticoagulation for CPB, celite ACT values should exceed 750 seconds and kaolin ACT should be more than 450 seconds.[267]

Dosage and Administration

Aprotinin or Trasylol (Bayer Corporation, West Haven, Conn) is administered intravenously. It is available in a clear, isotonic, pH-adjusted, sterile solution with a concentration of 10,000 KIU/mL and is supplied in 100- and 200-mL vials. Aprotinin dosing is expressed in KIU with 1 mg aprotinin equal to 7143 KIU. For cardiac surgery with CPB, aprotinin is typically given as a Hammersmith dose: 2×10^6 KIU IV bolus administered at the beginning of surgery followed by 5×10^5 KIU/ hr infusion throughout surgery plus 2×10^6 KIU in the CPB prime.[269] Two lower dose schemes have been used in an effort to reduce cost and to adjust for weight and renal function. The half-Hammersmith dose is simply half of the full-Hammersmith dose: 1×10^6 KIU intravenous bolus administered at the beginning of surgery followed by 2.5×105 KIU/hr infusion throughout surgery plus 1×10^6 KIU in the CPB prime. The "pump-prime" dose calls for 2×10^6 KIU aprotinin to be placed in the CPB priming solution with no additional IV dosing.

References

1. Brinkhous KM, Smith HP, Warner ED: The inhibition of blood clotting: An unidentified substance which acts in conjunction with heparin to prevent the conversion of prothrombin into thrombin. Am J Physiol 125:683–687, 1939.
2. Bray B, Lane DA, Freyssinet JM, et al: Anti-thrombin activities of heparin. Effect of saccharide chain length on thrombin inhibition by heparin cofactor II and by antithrombin. Biochem J 262:225–232, 1989.
3. Choay J, Petitou M, Lormeau JC, et al: Structure-activity relationship in heparin: A synthetic pentasaccharide with high affinity for antithrombin III and eliciting high anti-factor Xa activity. Biochem Biophys Res Commun 116:492–499, 1983.
4. Hirsh J, Raschke R, Warkentin TE, et al: Heparin: Mechanism of action, pharmacokinetics, dosing considerations, monitoring, efficacy, and safety. Chest 108:258S–275S, 1995.
5. Tollefsen DM: Insight into the mechanism of action of heparin cofactor II. Thromb Haemost 74:1209–1214, 1995.
6. Tollefson FA, Fernandez F, Gauthier D, Buchanan MR: Heparin cofactor II and other endogenous factors in the mediation of the antithrombotic and anticoagulant effects of heparin and dermatan sulfate. Semin Thromb Hemost 86:385–391, 1985.
7. Abildgaard U: Heparin/low molecular weight heparin and tissue factor pathway inhibitor [review]. Haemostasis 23(suppl 1):103–106, 1993.
8. John LC, Rees GM, Kovacs IB: Inhibition of platelet function by heparin. An etiologic factor in post bypass hemorrhage. J Thorac Cardiovasc Surg 105(5):816–822, 1993.
9. Sobel M, McNeill PM, Carlson PL, et al: Heparin inhibition of von Willebrand factor-dependent platelet function in vitro and in vivo. J Clin Invest 87(5):1787–1793, 1991.
10. Khuri SF, Valeri CR, Loscalzo J, et al: Heparin causes platelet dysfunction and induces fibrinolysis before cardiopulmonary bypass. Ann Thorac Surg 60:1008–1014, 1995.
11. Hull RD, Raskob GE, Hirsh J, et al: Continuous intravenous heparin compared with intermittent subcutaneous heparin in the initial treatment of proximal-vein thrombosis. N Engl J Med 315(18):1109–1114, 1986.
12. Basu D, Gallus A, Hirsh J, Cade J: A prospective study of the value of monitoring heparin treatment with the activated partial thromboplastin time. N Engl J Med 287(7):324–327, 1972.
13. Chiu HM, Hirsh J, Yung WL, et al: Relationship between the anticoagulant and antithrombotic effects of heparin in experimental venous thrombosis. Blood 49(2):171–184, 1977.

14. Chew DP, Bhatt DL, Lincoff AM, et al: Defining the optimal activated clotting time during percutaneous coronary intervention: Aggregate results from 6 randomized, controlled trials. Circulation 103(7):961–966, 2001.

15. Bull BS, Korpman RA, Huse WM, Briggs BD: Heparin therapy during extracorporeal circulation. I. Problems inherent in existing heparin protocols. J Thorac Cardiovasc Surg 69(5):674–684, 1975.

16. Bull BS, Huse WM, Brauer FS, Korpman RA: Heparin therapy during extracorporeal circulation. II. The use of a dose-response curve to individualize heparin and protamine dosage. J Thorac Cardiovasc Surg 69(5):685–689, 1975.

17. Despotis GJ, Summerfield AL, Joist JH, et al: Comparison of activated coagulation time and whole blood heparin measurements with laboratory plasma anti-Xa heparin concentration in patients having cardiac operations. J Thorac Cardiovasc Surg 108(6):1076–1082, 1994.

18. de Swart MAC, Nijmeyer B, Roelofs JMM, Sixma JJ: Kinetics of intravenously administered heparin in normal humans. Blood 60: 1251–1258, 1982.

19. Boneu B, Caranobe C, Cadroy Y, et al: Pharmacokinetic studies of standard unfractionated heparin, and low molecular weight heparins in the rabbit. Semin Thromb Hemost 14:18–27, 1988.

20. Turpie AG, Gallus AS, Hoek JA: A synthetic pentasaccharide for the prevention of deep-vein thrombosis after total hip replacement. N Engl J Med 344(9):619–625, 2001.

21. Kaplan K, Davison R, Parker M, et al: Role of heparin after intravenous thrombolytic therapy for acute myocardial infarction. Am J Cardiol 59(4):241–244, 1987.

22. Cheung AT, Levin SK, Weiss SJ, et al: Intracardiac thrombus: A risk of incomplete anticoagulation for cardiac operations. Ann Thorac Surg 58:541–542, 1994.

23. Cruickshank MK, Levine MN, Hirsh J, et al: A standard heparin nomogram for the management of heparin therapy. Arch Intern Med 151(2):333–337, 1991.

24. Despotis GJ, Gravlee GP, Filos KS, Levy JH: Anticoagulation monitoring during cardiac surgery: A review of current and emerging techniques. Anesthesiology 91:1122–1151, 1999.

25. Despotis GJ, Levine V, Joist JH, et al: Antithrombin III during cardiac surgery: Effect on response of activated clotting time to heparin and relationship to markers of hemostatic activation. Anesth Analg 85: 498–506, 1997.

26. Schwartz RS, Bauer KA, Rosenberg RD, et al: Clinical experience with antithrombin III concentrate in treatment of congenital and acquired deficiency of antithrombin. The Antithrombin III Study Group. Am J Med 87:53S–60S, 1989.

27. Hashimoto K, Yamagishi M, Sasaki T, et al: Heparin and antithrombin III levels during cardiopulmonary bypass: Correlation with subclinical plasma coagulation. Ann Thorac Surg 58:799–805, 1995.

28. Zaidan JR, Johnson S, Brynes R, et al: Rate of protamine administration: Its effect on heparin reversal and antithrombin recovery after coronary artery surgery. Anesth Analg 65:377–380, 1986.

29. Dietrich W, Spannagl M, Schramm W, et al: The influence of preoperative anticoagulation on heparin response during cardiopulmonary bypass. J Thorac Cardiovasc Surg 102(4):505–514, 1991.

30. Lane DA, Pejler G, Flynn AM, et al: Neutralization of heparin-related saccharides by histidine-rich glycoprotein and platelet factor 4. J Biol Chem 261:3980–3986, 1986.

31. Hirsh J: Heparin [review]. N Engl J Med 324(22):1565–1574, 1991.

32. Thomas DP, Barrowcliffe TW, Johnson EA: The influence of tissue source, salt and molecular weight and heparin activity [review]. Scand J Haematol Suppl 36:40–49, 1980.

33. Anderson EF: Heparin resistance prior to cardiopulmonary bypass. Anesthesiology 64(4):504–507, 1986.

34. Wysowski DK, Talarico L, Bacsanyi J, Botstein P: Spinal and epidural hematoma and low-molecular-weight heparin. N Engl J Med 338(24): 1774–1775, 1998.

35. Shorten GD, Comunale ME: Heparin-induced thrombocytopenia. J Cardiothorac Vasc Anesth 10:521–530, 1997.

36. Singer RL, Mannion JD, Bauer TL, et al: Complications from heparin-induced thrombocytopenia in patients undergoing cardiopulmonary bypass. Chest 104(5):1436–1440, 1993.

37. Turpie AG, Gent M, Cote R, et al: A low-molecular-weight heparinoid compared with unfractionated heparin in the prevention of deep vein thrombosis in patients with acute ischemic stroke. A randomized, double-blind study. Ann Intern Med 117(5):353–357, 1992.

38. Bradbrook ID, Magnani HN, Moelker MC, et al: ORG 10172: A low

molecular weight heparinoid anticoagulant with a long half-life in man [abstract]. Br J Clin Pharmacol 23:667–668, 1987.

39. Hoek JA, Nurmohamed MT, Hamelynck KJ, et al: Prevention of deep vein thrombosis following total hip replacement by low molecular weight heparinoid. Thromb Haemost 67(1):28–32, 1992.

40. Leyvraz P, Bachmann F, Bohnet J, et al: Thromboembolic prophylaxis in total hip replacement: A comparison between the low molecular weight heparinoid Lomoparan and heparin-dihydroergotamine. Br J Surg 79(9):911–914, 1992.

41. Gerhart TN, Yett HS, Robertson LK, et al: Low-molecular-weight heparinoid compared with warfarin for prophylaxis of deep-vein thrombosis in patients who are operated on for fracture of the hip. A prospective, randomized trial. J Bone Joint Surg Am 73(4):494–502, 1991.

42. Bergqvist D, Kettunen K, Fredin H, et al: Thromboprophylaxis in patients with hip fractures: A prospective, randomized, comparative study between Org 10172 and dextran 70. Surgery 109(5):617–622, 1991.

43. Gallus A, Cade J, Ockelford P, et al: Orgaran (Org 10172) or heparin for preventing venous thrombosis after elective surgery for malignant disease? A double-blind, randomized, multicentre comparison. ANZ-Organon Investigators' Group. Thromb Haemost 70(4):562–567, 1993.

44. Turpie AG, Levine MN, Hirsh J, et al: Double-blind randomized trial of Org 10172 low-molecular-weight heparinoid in prevention of deep-vein thrombosis in thrombotic stroke. Lancet 1(8532):523–526, 1987.

45. Doherty DC, Ortel TL, de Bruijn N, et al: "Heparin-free" cardiopulmonary bypass: First reported use of heparinoid (Org 10172) to provide anticoagulation for cardiopulmonary bypass. Anesthesiology 73:562–565, 1990.

46. Magnani HN: Heparin-induced thrombocytopenia (HIT): An overview of 230 patients treated with orgaran (Org 10172). Thromb Haemost 70:554–561, 1993.

47. Magnani HN, Beijering RJR, Ten Cate JW, Chong BH: Orgaran anticoagulation for cardiopulmonary bypass in patients with heparin-induced thrombocytopenia. In Pifarre R (ed): New Anticoagulants for the Cardiovascular Patient. Philadelphia, Hanely & Belfus, pp 487–500, 1997.

48. Ammar T, Fisher CF: The effects of heparinase 1 and protamine on platelet reactivity. Anesthesiology 86:1382–1386, 1997.

49. DeLucia A III, Wakefield TW, Kadell AM, et al: Tissue distribution, circulating half-life, and excretion of intravenously administered protamine sulfate. ASAIO J 39(3):M715–M718, 1993.

50. Guffin AV, Dunbar RW, Kaplan JA, Bland JW Jr: Successful use of a reduced dose of protamine after cardiopulmonary bypass. Anesth Analg 55(1):110–113, 1976.

51. Jobes DR, Schaffer GW, Aitken GL: Increased accuracy and precision of heparin and protamine dosing reduces blood loss and transfusion in patients undergoing primary cardiac operations. J Thorac Cardiovasc Surg 110:36–45, 1995.

52. Fitzgerald D, Murphy N: Argatroban: A synthetic thrombin inhibitor of low relative molecular mass. Coron Artery Dis Jun;7(6):455–458, 1996.

53. Matthai WH: Use of argatroban during percutaneous coronary interventions in patients with heparin-induced thrombocytopenia. Semin Thromb Hemost 25(suppl 1):57–60, 1999.

54. Ueki Y, Matsumoto K, Kizaki Y, et al: Argatroban increases nitric oxide levels in patients with peripheral arterial obstructive disease: placebo-controlled study. J Thromb Thrombolysis Aug;8(2):131–137, 1999.

55. Berry CN, Girard D, Girardot C, et al: Antithrombotic activity of argatroban in experimental thrombosis in the rabbit. Semin Thromb Hemost 1996;22(3):233–241, 1996.

56. Sakai M, Ohteki H, Narita Y, et al: Argatroban as a potential anticoagulant in cardiopulmonary bypass-studies in a dog model. Cardiovasc Surg Mar;7(2):187–194, 1999.

57. Swan SK, Hursting MJ: The pharmacokinetics and pharmacodynamics of argatroban: Effects of age, gender, and hepatic or renal dysfunction. Pharmacotherapy Mar;20(3):318–329, 2000.

58. Swan SK, St Peter JV, Lambrecht LJ, Hursting MJ: Comparison of anticoagulant effects and safety of argatroban and heparin in healthy subjects. Pharmacotherapy Jul;20(7):756–770, 2000.

59. Ahmad S, Ahsan A, George M, et al: Simultaneous monitoring of argatroban and its major metabolite using an HPLC method: potential clinical applications. Clin Appl Thromb Hemost Oct;5(4):252–258, 1999.

60. Lewis BE, Wallis DE, Berkowitz SD, et al: Argatroban anticoagulant therapy in patients with heparin-induced thrombocytopenia. Circulation Apr 10;103(14):1838–1843, 2001.

61. Kawada T, Kitagawa H, Hoson M, et al: Clinical application of argatroban as an alternative anticoagulant for extracorporeal circulation. Hematol Oncol Clin North Am Apr;14(2):445–457, 2000.

62. Fuchs J, Cannon CP: Hirulog in the treatment of unstable angina. Results of the Thrombin Inhibition in Myocardial Ischemia (TIMI) 7 trial. Circulation Aug 15;92(4):727–733, 1995.

63. White HD, Ellis CJ, French JK, Aylward P: Hirudin (desirudin) and Hirulog (bivalirudin) in acute ischaemic syndromes and the rationale for the Hirulog/Early Reperfusion Occlusion (HERO-2) Study. Aust N Z J Med Aug;28(4):551–554, 1998.

64. Greinacher A, Völpel H, Janssens U, et al: Recombinant hirudin (lepirudin) provides safe and effective anticoagulation in patients with heparin-induced thrombocytopenia: A prospective study. Circulation 99(1):73–80, 1999.

65. Turunen P, Mikkola T, Ylikorkala O, Viinikka L: Hirudin stimulates prostacyclin but not endothelin-1 production in cultured human vascular endothelial cells. Thromb Res 81(6):635–640, 1996.

66. Robson R: The use of bivalirudin in patients with renal impairment. J Invasive Cardiol Dec;12(suppl F):33F–36F, 2000.

67. Riess FC, Kormann J, Poetzsch B: Recombinant hirudin as anticoagulant during cardiopulmonary bypass. Anesthesiology Dec;93(6):1551–1552, 2000.

68. Riess FC, Bleese N, Kormann J, et al: Recombinant hirudin is a heparin alternative in cardiac surgery. J Cardiothorac Vasc Anesth 11(4):538–539, 1997.

69. Koster A, Kuppe H, Crystal GJ, Mertzlufft F: Cardiovascular surgery without cardiopulmonary bypass in patients with heparin-induced thrombocytopenia type II using anticoagulation with recombinant hirudin. Anesth Analg 90(2):292–298, 2000.

70. Koster A, Pasic M, Hetzer R, et al: Hirudin as anticoagulant for cardiopulmonary bypass: Importance of preoperative renal function. Ann Thorac Surg 69(1):37–41, 2000.

71. Chamberlin JR, Lewis B, Leya F, et al: Successful treatment of heparin-associated thrombocytopenia and thrombosis using Hirulog. Can J Cardiol Jun;11(6):511–514, 1995.

72. Sun Y, Greilich PE, Wilson SI, et al: The use of lepirudin for anticoagulation in patients with heparin-induced thrombocytopenia during major vascular surgery. Anesth Analg Feb;92(2):344–346, 2001.

73. A comparison of recombinant hirudin with heparin for the treatment of acute coronary syndromes. The Global Use of Strategies to Open Occluded Coronary Arteries (GUSTO) IIb investigators. N Engl J Med 335(11):775–782, 1996.

74. Metz BK, White HD, Granger CB, et al: Randomized comparison of direct thrombin inhibition versus heparin in conjunction with fibrinolytic therapy for acute myocardial infarction: Results from the GUSTO-IIb Trial. Global Use of Strategies to Open Occluded Coronary Arteries in Acute Coronary Syndromes (GUSTO-IIb) Investigators. J Am Coll Cardiol 31(7):1493–1498, 1998.

75. White HD, Aylward PE, Frey MJ, et al: Randomized, double-blind comparison of hirulog versus heparin in patients receiving streptokinase and aspirin for acute myocardial infarction (HERO). Hirulog Early Reperfusion/Occlusion (HERO) Trial Investigators. Circulation Oct 7;96(7):2155–2161, 1997.

76. Greinacher A: Treatment of heparin-induced thrombocytopenia. Thromb Haemost 82(2):457–467, 1999.

77. Despotis GJ, Hogue CW, Saleem R, et al: The relationship between hirudin and activated clotting time: implications for patients with heparin-induced thrombocytopenia undergoing cardiac surgery. Anesth Analg 93(1):28–32, 2001.

78. Link KP: The discovery of dicoumarol and its sequels. Circulation 19:97–107, 1959.

79. Breckenridge A: Oral anticoagulant drugs: Pharmacokinetic aspects. Semin Hematol 15(1):19–26, 1978.

80. O'Reilly RA: Vitamin K and the oral anticoagulant drugs. Annu Rev Med 27:245–261, 1976.

81. Nelsestuen GL: Role of gamma-carboxyglutamic acid. An unusual protein transition required for the calcium-dependent binding of prothrombin to phospholipid. J Biol Chem 251(18):5648–5656, 1976.

82. Borowski M, Furie BC, Bauminger S, Furie B: Prothrombin requires two sequential metal-dependent conformational transitions to bind phospholipid. Conformation-specific antibodies directed against the phospholipid-binding site on prothrombin. J Biol Chem 261(32):14969–14975, 1986.

83. Breckenridge A, Orme M, Wesseling H, et al: Pharmacokinetics and pharmacodynamics of the enantiomers of warfarin in man. Clin Pharmacol Ther 15(4):424–430, 1974.

84. Kelly JG, O'Malley K: Clinical pharmacokinetics of oral anticoagulants. Clin Pharmacokinet 4(1):1–15, 1979.

85. Poller L, Taberner DA: Dosage and control of oral anticoagulants: An international collaborative survey. Br J Haematol 51(3):479–485, 1982.

86. Taberner DA, Poller L, Thomson JM, Darby KV: Effect of international sensitivity index (ISI) of thromboplastins on precision of international normalized ratios (INR). J Clin Pathol 42(1):92–96, 1989.

87. ACCP-NHLBI National Conference on Antithrombotic Therapy. American College of Chest Physicians and the National Heart, Lung and Blood Institute. Chest 89(2 suppl):1S–106S, 1986.

88. Hirsh J, Dalen JE, Deykin D, Poller L: Oral anticoagulants. Mechanism of action, clinical effectiveness, and optimal therapeutic range. Chest 102(4 suppl):312S–326S, 1992.

89. Poller L, McKernan A, Thomson JM, et al: Fixed minidose warfarin: A new approach to prophylaxis against venous thrombosis after major surgery. Br Med J (Clin Res Ed) 295(6609):1309–1312, 1987.

90. Bern MM, Lokich JJ, Wallach SR, et al: Very low doses of warfarin can prevent thrombosis in central venous catheters. A randomized prospective trial. Ann Intern Med 112(6):423–428, 1990.

91. Levine M, Hirsh J, Gent M, et al: Double-blind randomized trial of a very-low-dose warfarin for prevention of thromboembolism in stage IV breast cancer. Lancet 343(8902):886–889, 1994.

92. Altman R, Rouvier J, Gurfinkel E, et al: Comparison of two levels of anticoagulant therapy in patients with substitute heart valves. J Thorac Cardiovasc Surg 101(3):427–431, 1991.

93. Hull R, Hirsh J, Jay R, et al: Different intensities of oral anticoagulant therapy in the treatment of proximal-vein thrombosis. N Engl J Med 307(27):1676–1681, 1982.

94. Saour JN, Sieck JO, Mamo LA, Gallus AS: Trial of different intensities of anticoagulation in patients with prosthetic heart valves. N Engl J Med 322(7):428–432, 1990.

95. Ewe K: Bleeding after liver biopsy does not correlate with indices of peripheral coagulation. Dig Dis Sci 26(5):388–393, 1981.

96. Friedman EW, Sussman II: Safety of invasive procedures in patients with the coagulopathy of liver disease. Clin Lab Haematol 11(3):199–204, 1989.

97. Foster PF, Moore LR, Sankary HN, et al: Central venous catheterization in patients with coagulopathy. Arch Surg 127(3):273–275, 1992.

98. Broekmans AW, Bertina RM, Loeliger EA, et al: Protein C and the development of skin necrosis during anticoagulant therapy. Thromb Haemost 49(3):251, 1983.

99. Grimaudo V, Gueissaz F, Hauert J, et al: Necrosis of skin induced by coumarin in a patient deficient in protein S. BMJ 298(6668):233–234, 1989.

100. Vane JR, Botting RM: Formation by the endothelium of prostacyclin, nitric oxide and endothelin. J Lipid Mediat 6(1-3):395–404, 1993.

101. Dzavik V, Ghali WA, Norris C, et al: Long-term survival in 11,661 patients with multivessel coronary artery disease in the era of stenting: A report from the Alberta Provincial Project for Outcome Assessment in Coronary Heart Disease (APPROACH) Investigators. Am Heart J 142(1):119–126, 2001.

102. Pell JP, Walsh D, Norrie J, et al: Outcomes following coronary artery bypass grafting and percutaneous transluminal coronary angioplasty in the stent era: A prospective study of all 9890 consecutive patients operated on in Scotland over a two year period. Heart 85(6):662–666, 2001.

103. Rodriguez A, Bernardi V, Navia J, et al: Argentine Randomized Study: Coronary Angioplasty with Stenting versus Coronary Bypass Surgery in patients with Multiple-Vessel Disease (ERACI II): 30-day and one-year follow-up results. ERACI II Investigators. J Am Coll Cardiol 37(1):51–58, 2001.

104. Vane J: The evolution of non-steroidal anti-inflammatory drugs and their mechanisms of action. Drugs 33(suppl 1):18–27, 1987.

105. Pedersen AK, FitzGerald GA: Dose-related kinetics of aspirin. Presystemic acetylation of platelet cyclooxygenase. N Engl J Med 311(19):1206–1211, 1984.

106. Higgs GA, Salmon JA, Henderson B, Vane JR: Pharmacokinetics of aspirin and salicylate in relation to inhibition of arachidonate cyclooxygenase and antiinflammatory activity. Proc Natl Acad Sci USA 84(5):1417–1420, 1987.

107. Pedersen AK, FitzGerald GA: The human pharmacology of platelet

inhibition: Pharmacokinetics relevant to drug action. Circulation 72(6):1164–1176, 1985.

108. Randomized trial of intravenous streptokinase, oral aspirin, both, or neither among 17,187 cases of suspected acute myocardial infarction: ISIS-2. ISIS-2 (Second International Study of Infarct Survival) Collaborative Group. Lancet 2(8607):349–360, 1988.

109. Massel D, Little SH: Risks and benefits of adding anti-platelet therapy to warfarin among patients with prosthetic heart valves: A meta-analysis. J Am Coll Cardiol Feb;37(2):569–578, 2001.

110. Prevention of pulmonary embolism and deep vein thrombosis with low dose aspirin: Pulmonary Embolism Prevention (PEP) trial. Lancet 355(9212):1295–1302, 2000.

111. Sonksen JR, Kong KL, Holder R: Magnitude and time course of impaired primary haemostasis after stopping chronic low and medium dose aspirin in healthy volunteers. Br J Anaesth 82(3):360–365, 1999.

112. Wulf H: Epidural anaesthesia and spinal haematoma. Can J Anaesth 43(12):1260–1271, 1996.

113. Horlocker TT, Wedel DJ, Schroeder DR, et al: Preoperative antiplatelet therapy does not increase the risk of spinal hematoma associated with regional anesthesia. Anesth Analg 80(2):303–309, 1995.

114. Barbui T, Buelli M, Cortelazzo S, et al: Aspirin and risk of bleeding in patients with thrombocythemia. Am J Med 83(2):265–268, 1987.

115. Babu KS, Salvi SS: Aspirin and asthma. Chest 118(5):1470–1476, 2000.

116. Heubi JE, Partin JC, Partin JS, Schubert WK: Reye's syndrome: Current concepts. Hepatology 7(1):155–164, 1987.

117. Higgins RM, Connolly JO, Hendry BM: Alkalinization and hemodialysis in severe salicylate poisoning: comparison of elimination techniques in the same patient. Clin Nephrol 50(3):178–183, 1998.

118. Barone JA, Raia JJ, Huang YC: Evaluation of the effects of multiple-dose activated charcoal on the absorption of orally administered salicylate in a simulated toxic ingestion model. Ann Emerg Med 17(1): 34–37, 1988.

119. Michelson AD, Barnard MR, Khuri SF, et al: The effects of aspirin and hypothermia on platelet function in vivo. Br J Haematol 104(1): 64–68, 1999.

120. Pogliani EM, Fowst C, Bregani R, Corneo G: Bleeding time and antiplatelet agents in normal volunteers. Int J Clin Lab Res 22(1):58–61, 1992.

121. Sathiropas P, Marbet GA, Sahaphong S, Duckert F: Detection of small inhibitory effects of acetylsalicylic acid (ASA) by platelet impedance aggregometry in whole blood. Thromb Res 51(1):55–62, 1988.

122. Orlikowski CE, Payne AJ, Moodley J, Rocke DA: Thrombelastography after aspirin ingestion in pregnant and non-pregnant subjects. Br J Anaesth 69(2):159–161, 1992.

123. Gum PA, Kottke-Marchant K, Poggio ED, et al: Profile and prevalence of aspirin resistance in patients with cardiovascular disease. Am J Cardiol 88(3):230–235, 2001.

124. Homoncik M, Jilma B, Hergovich N, et al: Monitoring of aspirin (ASA) pharmacodynamics with the platelet function analyzer PFA-100. Thromb Haemost 83(2):316–321, 2000.

125. Szczeklik A, Undas A, Sanak M, et al: Relationship between bleeding time, aspirin and the PlA1/A2 polymorphism of platelet glycoprotein IIIa. Br J Haematol 110(4):965–967, 2000.

126. Lanas AI: Current approaches to reducing gastrointestinal toxicity of low-dose aspirin. Am J Med Jan 8;110(1A):70S–73S, 2001.

127. 2nd ACCP Conference on Antithrombotic Therapy. American College of Chest Physicians. June 21, 1988. Proceedings. Chest 95(2 suppl): 1S–169S, 1989.

128. Hess H, Mietaschk A, Deichsel G: Drug-induced inhibition of platelet function delays progression of peripheral occlusive arterial disease. A prospective double-blind arteriographically controlled trial. Lancet 1(8426):415–419, 1985.

129. Younis LT, Chaitman BR: Update on intravenous dipyridamole cardiac imaging in the assessment of ischemic heart disease. Clin Cardiol 13(1):3–10, 1990.

130. Harker LA, Fuster V: Pharmacology of platelet inhibitors. J Am Coll Cardiol 8(6 suppl B):21B–32B, 1986.

131. FitzGerald GA: Dipyridamole. N Engl J Med 316(20):1247–1257, 1987.

132. Bult H, Fret HR, Jordaens FH, Herman AG: Dipyridamole potentiates the anti-aggregating and vasodilator activity of nitric oxide. Eur J Pharmacol 199(1):1–8, 1991.

133. Gryglewski RJ: Interactions between endothelial secretogogues. Ann Med 27(3):421–427, 1995.

134. Saniabadi AR, Belch JJ, Lowe GD, et al: Comparison of inhibitory actions of prostacyclin and a new prostacyclin analogue on the aggregation of human platelet in whole blood. Haemostasis 17(3):147–153, 1987.

135. Freedman JE, Parker C III, Li L, et al: Select flavonoids and whole juice from purple grapes inhibit platelet function and enhance nitric oxide release. Circulation 103(23):2792–2798, 2001.

136. Loscalzo J: Nitric oxide insufficiency, platelet activation, and arterial thrombosis. Circ Res 88(8):756–762, 2001.

137. Keh D, Kurer I, Dudenhausen JW, et al: Response of neonatal platelets to nitric oxide in vitro. Intensive Care Med 27(1):283–286, 2001.

138. Anfossi G, Russo I, Massucco P, et al: Studies on inhibition of human platelet function by sodium nitroprusside. kinetic evaluation of the effect on aggregation and cyclic nucleotide content. Thromb Res 102(4):319–330, 2001.

139. Chirkov YY, Holmes AS, Willoughby SR, et al: Stable angina and acute coronary syndromes are associated with nitric oxide resistance in platelets. J Am Coll Cardiol 37(7):1851–1857, 2001.

140. Anfossi G, Russo I, Massucco P, et al: N-acetyl-L-cysteine exerts direct anti-aggregating effect on human platelets. Eur J Clin Invest 31(5):452–461, 2001.

141. Matys T, Chabielska E, Pawlak R, et al: Losartan inhibits the adhesion of rat platelets to fibrillar collagen—a potential role of nitric oxide and prostanoids. J Physiol Pharmacol 51(4 Pt 1):705–713, 2000.

142. Hass WK, Easton JD, Adams HP Jr, et al: A randomized trial comparing ticlopidine hydrochloride with aspirin for the prevention of stroke in high-risk patients. Ticlopidine Aspirin Stroke Study Group. N Engl J Med 321(8):501–507, 1989.

143. Gachet C, Cazenave JP, Ohlmann P, et al: The thienopyridine ticlopidine selectively prevents the inhibitory effects of ADP but not of adrenaline on cAMP levels raised by stimulation of the adenylate cyclase of human platelets by PGE1. Biochem Pharmacol 40(12): 2683–2687, 1990.

144. Defreyn G, Gachet C, Savi P, et al: Ticlopidine and clopidogrel (SR 25990C) selectively neutralize ADP inhibition of PGE1-activated platelet adenylate cyclase in rats and rabbits. Thromb Haemost 65(2):186–190, 1991.

145. Defreyn G, Bernat A, Delebassee D, Maffrand JP: Pharmacology of ticlopidine: A review. Semin Thromb Hemost 15(2):159–166, 1989.

146. de Lorgeril M, Bordet JC, Salen P, et al: Ticlopidine increases nitric oxide generation in heart-transplant recipients: A possible novel property of ticlopidine. J Cardiovasc Pharmacol 32(2):225–230, 1998.

147. Savi P, Herbert JM, Pflieger AM, et al: Importance of hepatic metabolism in the antiaggregating activity of the thienopyridine clopidogrel. Biochem Pharmacol 44(3):527–532, 1992.

148. McTavish D, Faulds D, Goa KL: Ticlopidine. An updated review of its pharmacology and therapeutic use in platelet-dependent disorders. Drugs 40(2):238–259, 1990.

149. Bhatt DL, Chew DP, Hirsch AT, et al: Superiority of clopidogrel versus aspirin in patients with prior cardiac surgery. Circulation Jan 23;103(3):363–368, 2001.

150. Scrutinio D, Cimminiello C, Marubini E, et al: Ticlopidine versus aspirin after myocardial infarction (STAMI) trial. J Am Coll Cardiol Apr;37(5):1259–1265, 2001.

151. Cadroy Y, Bossavy JP, Thalamas C, et al: Early potent antithrombotic effect with combined aspirin and a loading dose of clopidogrel on experimental arterial thrombogenesis in humans. Circulation Jun 20; 101(24):2823–2828, 2000.

152. Trivier JM, Caron J, Mahieu M, et al: Fatal aplastic anaemia associated with clopidogrel. Lancet Feb 10;357(9254):446, 2001.

153. Anderson KM, Califf RM, Stone GW, et al: Long-term mortality benefit with abciximab in patients undergoing percutaneous coronary intervention. J Am Coll Cardiol 37(8):2059–2065, 2001.

154. Brown DL, Fann CS, Chang CJ: Meta-analysis of effectiveness and safety of abciximab versus eptifibatide or tirofiban in percutaneous coronary intervention. Am J Cardiol Mar 1;87(5):537–541, 2001.

155. Montalescot G, Barragan P, Wittenberg O, et al: Platelet glycoprotein IIb/IIIa inhibition with coronary stenting for acute myocardial infarction. N Engl J Med 344(25):1895–1903, 2001.

156. Topol EJ, Califf RM, Weisman HF, et al: Randomized trial of coronary intervention with antibody against platelet IIb/IIIa integrin for reduction of clinical restenosis: results at six months. The EPIC Investigators. Lancet 343(8902):881–886, 1994.

157. Lages B, Weiss HJ: Greater inhibition of platelet procoagulant activity

by antibody-derived glycoprotein IIb-IIIa inhibitors than by peptide and peptidomimetic inhibitors. Br J Haematol 113(1):65–71, 2001.

158. Ellis SG, Bates ER, Schaible T, et al: Prospects for the use of antagonists to the platelet glycoprotein IIb/IIIa receptor to prevent postangioplasty restenosis and thrombosis. J Am Coll Cardiol 17(6 suppl B):89B–95B, 1991.

159. Cannon CP, McCabe CH, Wilcox RG, et al: Oral glycoprotein IIb/IIIa inhibition with orbofiban in patients with unstable coronary syndromes (OPUS-TIMI 16) trial. Circulation 102(2):149–156, 2000.

160. O'Neill WW, Serruys P, Knudtson M, et al: Long-term treatment with a platelet glycoprotein-receptor antagonist after percutaneous coronary revascularization. EXCITE Trial Investigators. Evaluation of Oral Xemilofiban in Controlling Thrombotic Events. N Engl J Med 342(18):1316–1324, 2000.

161. Randomized trial of aspirin, sibrafiban, or both for secondary prevention after acute coronary syndromes. Circulation 103(13):1727–1733, 2001.

162. Comparison of sibrafiban with aspirin for prevention of cardiovascular events after acute coronary syndromes: A randomized trial. The SYMPHONY Investigators. Sibrafiban versus Aspirin to Yield Maximum Protection from Ischemic Heart Events Post-acute Coronary Syndromes. Lancet 355(9201):337–345, 2000.

163. Cho L, Topol EJ, Balog C, et al: Clinical benefit of glycoprotein IIb/IIIa blockade with Abciximab is independent of gender: pooled analysis from EPIC, EPILOG and EPISTENT trials. Evaluation of 7E3 for the Prevention of Ischemic Complications. Evaluation in Percutaneous Transluminal Coronary Angioplasty to Improve Long-Term Outcome with Abciximab GP IIb/IIIa blockade. Evaluation of Platelet IIb/IIIa Inhibitor for Stent. J Am Coll Cardiol Aug;36(2):381–386, 2000.

164. Topol EJ, Mark DB, Lincoff AM, et al: Outcomes at 1 year and economic implications of platelet glycoprotein IIb/IIIa blockade in patients undergoing coronary stenting: Results from a multicentre randomized trial. EPISTENT Investigators. Evaluation of Platelet IIb/IIIa Inhibitor for Stenting. Lancet 354(9195):2019–2024, 1999.

165. Randomized placebo-controlled and balloon-angioplasty-controlled trial to assess safety of coronary stenting with use of platelet glycoprotein-IIb/IIIa blockade. The EPISTENT Investigators. Evaluation of Platelet IIb/IIIa Inhibitor for Stenting. Lancet 352(9122):87–92, 1998.

166. Kereiakes DJ, Lincoff AM, Miller DP, et al: Abciximab therapy and unplanned coronary stent deployment: Favorable effects on stent use, clinical outcomes, and bleeding complications. EPILOG Trial Investigators. Circulation 97(9):857–864, 1998.

167. Van de WF: More evidence for a beneficial effect of platelet glycoprotein IIb/IIIa-blockade during coronary interventions. Latest results from the EPILOG and CAPTURE trials. Eur Heart J 17(3):325–326, 1996.

168. Randomized placebo-controlled trial of effect of eptifibatide on complications of percutaneous coronary intervention: IMPACT-II. Integrilin to Minimise Platelet Aggregation and Coronary Thrombosis-II. Lancet 349(9063):1422–1428, 1997.

169. Inhibition of platelet glycoprotein IIb/IIIa with eptifibatide in patients with acute coronary syndromes. The PURSUIT Trial Investigators. Platelet Glycoprotein IIb/IIIa in Unstable Angina: Receptor Suppression Using Integrilin Therapy. N Engl J Med 339(7):436–443, 1998.

170. Novel dosing regimen of eptifibatide in planned coronary stent implantation (ESPRIT): A randomized, placebo-controlled trial. Lancet 356(9247):2037–2044, 2000.

171. A comparison of aspirin plus tirofiban with aspirin plus heparin for unstable angina. Platelet Receptor Inhibition in Ischemic Syndrome Management (PRISM) Study Investigators. N Engl J Med 338(21):1498–1505, 1998.

172. Effects of platelet glycoprotein IIb/IIIa blockade with tirofiban on adverse cardiac events in patients with unstable angina or acute myocardial infarction undergoing coronary angioplasty. The RESTORE Investigators. Randomized Efficacy Study of Tirofiban for Outcomes and REstenosis. Circulation 96(5):1445–1453, 1997.

173. Inhibition of the platelet glycoprotein IIb/IIIa receptor with tirofiban in unstable angina and non-Q-wave myocardial infarction. Platelet Receptor Inhibition in Ischemic Syndrome Management in Patients Limited by Unstable Signs and Symptoms (PRISM-PLUS) Study Investigators. N Engl J Med 338(21):1488–1497, 1998.

174. Topol EJ, Moliterno DJ, Herrmann HC, et al: Comparison of two platelet glycoprotein IIb/IIIa inhibitors, tirofiban and abciximab, for the prevention of ischemic events with percutaneous coronary revascularization. N Engl J Med 344(25):1888–1894, 2001.

175. Scazziota A, Altman R, Rouvier J, et al: Abciximab treatment in vitro after aspirin treatment in vivo has additive effects on platelet aggregation, ATP release, and P-selectin expression. Thromb Res Dec 15;100(6):479–488, 2000.

176. Kleiman NS, Grazeiadei N, Maresh K, et al: Abciximab, ticlopidine, and concomitant abciximab-ticlopidine therapy: Ex vivo platelet aggregation inhibition profiles in patients undergoing percutaneous coronary interventions. Am Heart J Sep;140(3):492–501, 2000.

177. Jong P, Cohen EA, Batchelor W, et al: Bleeding risks with abciximab after full-dose thrombolysis in rescue or urgent angioplasty for acute myocardial infarction. Am Heart J Feb;141(2):218–225, 2001.

178. Dillon WC, Eckert GJ, Dillon JC, Ritchie ME: Incidence of thrombocytopenia following coronary stent placement using abciximab plus clopidogrel or ticlopidine. Catheter Cardiovasc Interv Aug;50(4):426–430, 2000.

179. Nguyen N, Salib H, Mascarenhas DA: Acute profound thrombocytopenia without bleeding complications after re-administration of abciximab. J Invasive Cardiol Jan;13(1):56–58, 2001.

180. Madan M, Berkowitz SD, Christie DJ, et al: Rapid assessment of glycoprotein IIb/IIIa blockade with the platelet function analyzer (PFA-100) during percutaneous coronary intervention. Am Heart J 141(2):226–233, 2001.

181. Gammie JS, Zenati M, Kormos RL, et al: Abciximab and excessive bleeding in patients undergoing emergency cardiac operations. Ann Thorac Surg 65:465–469, 1998.

182. Lincoff AM, LeNarz LA, Despotis GJ, et al: Abciximab and bleeding during coronary surgery: Results from the EPILOG and EPISTENT trials. Improve Long-term Outcome with Abciximab GP IIb/IIIa blockade. Evaluation of Platelet IIb/IIIa Inhibition in STENTing. Ann Thorac Surg 70(2):516–526, 2000.

183. Silvestry SC, Smith PK: Current status of cardiac surgery in the abciximab-treated patient. Ann Thorac Surg Aug;70(2 suppl):S12–S19, 2000.

184. Koster A, Kukucka M, Bach F, et al: Anticoagulation during cardiopulmonary bypass in patients with heparin-induced thrombocytopenia type II and renal impairment using heparin and the platelet glycoprotein IIb-IIIa antagonist tirofiban. Anesthesiology 94(2):245–251, 2001.

185. Tsikouris JP, Tsikouris AP: A review of available fibrin-specific thrombolytic agents used in acute myocardial infarction. Pharmacotherapy 21(2):207–217, 2001.

186. Ross AM: New plasminogen activators: A clinical review. Clin Cardiol 22(3):165–171, 1999.

187. Iqbal O: New anticoagulants for adjunct use in angiography. In Pifarre R (ed): New anticoagulants for the cardiovascular patient. Philadelphia, Hanley & Belfus, pp 471–480, 1997.

188. International Study of Infarct Survival (ISIS-2) Investigators: Randomized trial of intravenous streptokinase, oral aspirin, both, or neither among 17,187 cases of suspected acute myocardial infarction: ISIS-2. ISIS-2 (Second International Study of Infarct Survival) Collaborative Group. Lancet 2(8607):349–360, 1988.

189. Holmes JH, Jones MF, Anderson RP, et al: The use of micro-dose aprotinin with continuous infusion in coronary artery bypass surgery. J Cardiovasc Surg (Torino) 40(5):621–626, 1999.

190. Simes RJ, Topol EJ, Holmes DR Jr, et al: Link between the angiographic substudy and mortality outcomes in a large randomized trial of myocardial reperfusion. Importance of early and complete infarct artery reperfusion. GUSTO-I Investigators. Circulation 91(7):1923–1928, 1995.

191. Califf RM, Woodlief LH, Harrell FE Jr, et al: Selection of thrombolytic therapy for individual patients: Development of a clinical model. GUSTO-I Investigators. Am Heart J 133(6):630–639, 1997.

192. Fibrinolytic Therapy Trialists' (FTT) Collaborative Group: Indications for fibrinolytic therapy in suspected acute myocardial infarction: Collaborative overview of early mortality and major morbidity results from all randomized trials of more than 1000 patients. Fibrinolytic Therapy Trialists' (FTT) Collaborative Group. Lancet 343(8893):311–322, 1994.

193. The Thrombolysis in Myocardial Ischemia (TIMI IIIA) Investigators: Early effects of tissue-type plasminogen activator added to conventional therapy on the culprit coronary lesion in patients presenting with ischemic cardiac pain at rest. Results of the Thrombolysis in Myocardial Ischemia (TIMI IIIA) Trial. Circulation 87(1):38–52, 1993.

194. The Thrombolysis in Myocardial Ischemia (TIMI IIIB) Investigators: Effects of tissue plasminogen activator and a comparison of early invasive and conservative strategies in unstable angina and non-Q-wave myocardial infarction. Results of the TIMI IIIB Trial. Thrombolysis in Myocardial Ischemia. Circulation 89(4):1545–1556, 1994.

195. Gruppo Italiano per lo Studio della Streptochinasi nell' Infarto Miocardico (GISSI) Investigators. Long-term effects of intravenous thrombolysis in acute myocardial infarction: Final report of the GISSI study. Gruppo Italiano per lo Studio della Streptochi-nasi nell'Infarto Miocardico (GISSI). Lancet 2(8564):871–874, 1987.

196. Global utilization of streptokinase and t-PA for occluded coronary arteries (GUSTO) investigators: An international randomized trial comparing four thrombolytic strategies for acute myocardial infarction. N Engl J Med 329(10):673–682, 1993.

197. Gruppo Italiano per lo Studio della Streptochinasi nell' Infarto Miocardico (GISSI-2) Investigators: GISSI-2: A factorial randomized trial of alteplase versus streptokinase and heparin versus no heparin among 12,490 patients with acute myocardial infarction. Gruppo Italiano per lo Studio della Sopravvivenza nell'Infarto Miocardico. Lancet 336(8707):65–71, 1990.

198. International Study of Infarct Survival (ISIS-3) Investigators: ISIS-3: A randomized comparison of streptokinase vs tissue plasminogen activator vs anistreplase and of aspirin plus heparin vs aspirin alone among 41,299 cases of suspected acute myocardial infarction. ISIS-3 (Third International Study of Infarct Survival) Collaborative Group. Lancet 339(8796):753–770, 1992.

199. The National Institute of Neurological Disorders and Stroke rt-PA Stroke Study. Tissue plasminogen activator for acute ischemic stroke group. N Engl J Med 333(24):1581–1587, 1995.

200. Hacke W, Kaste M, Fieschi C, et al: Randomized double-blind placebo-controlled trial of thrombolytic therapy with intravenous alteplase in acute ischaemic stroke (ECASS II). Second European-Australian Acute Stroke Study Investigators. Lancet 352(9136):1245–1251, 1998.

201. Alberts MJ: Diagnosis and treatment of ischemic stroke. Am J Med 106(2):211–221, 1999.

202. Mannuccio PM, Altieri D, Faioni E: Vasopressin analogues. Their role in disorders of hemostasis. Ann NY Acad Sci 509:71–81, 1987.

203. Despotis GJ, Levine V, Saleem R, et al: Use of point-of-care test in identification of patients who can benefit from desmopressin during cardiac surgery: A randomized controlled trial. Lancet 354(9173):106–110, 1999.

204. Lethagen S: Desmopressin—a haemostatic drug: State-of-the-art review. Eur J Anaesthesiol Suppl 14:1–9, 1997.

205. Czer LS, Bateman TM, Gray RJ, et al: Treatment of severe platelet dysfunction and hemorrhage after cardiopulmonary bypass: Reduction in blood product usage with desmopressin. J Am Coll Cardiol 9(5):1139–1147, 1987.

206. Cattaneo M, Mannucci PM: Desmopressin and blood loss after cardiac surgery. Lancet 342(8874):812, 1993.

207. Horstman LL, Valle-Riestra BJ, Jy W, et al: Desmopressin (DDAVP) acts on platelets to generate platelet microparticles and enhanced procoagulant activity. Thromb Res 79:163–174, 1995.

208. Lethagen S, Nilsson IM: DDAVP-induced enhancement of platelet retention: Its dependence on von Willebrand factor and the platelet receptor GP IIb/IIIa. Eur J Haematol 49:7–13, 1992.

209. Sloand EM, Alyono D, Klein HG, et al: 1-Deamino-8-D-arginine vasopressin (DDAVP) increases platelet membrane expression of glycoprotein Ib in patients with disorders of platelet function and after cardiopulmonary bypass. Am J Hematol 46(3):199–207, 1994.

210. Lethagen S, Olofsson L, Frick K, et al: Effect kinetics of desmopressin-induced platelet retention in healthy volunteers treated with aspirin or placebo. Haemophilia 6(1):15–20, 2000.

211. Humphries JE, Siragy H: Significant hyponatremia following DDAVP administration in a healthy adult. Am J Hematol 44:12–15, 1993.

212. Johns RA: Desmopressin is a potent vasorelaxant of aorta and pulmonary artery isolated from rabbit and rat. Anesthesiology 72:858–864, 1990.

213. Nitu-Whalley IC, Griffioen A, Harrington C, Lee CA: Retrospective review of the management of elective surgery with desmopressin and clotting factor concentrates in patients with von Willebrand disease. Am J Hematol 66(4):280–284, 2001.

214. Alanay A, Acaroglu E, Ozdemir O, et al: Effects of deamino-8-D-arginin vasopressin on blood loss and coagulation factors in scoliosis surgery. A double-blind randomized clinical trial. Spine 24(9):877–882, 1999.

215. Theroux MC, Corddry DH, Tietz AE, et al: A study of desmopressin and blood loss during spinal fusion for neuromuscular scoliosis: a randomized, controlled, double-blinded study. Anesthesiology 87(2):260–267, 1997.

216. Clagett GP, Valentine RJ, Myers SI, et al: Does desmopressin improve hemostasis and reduce blood loss from aortic surgery? A randomized, double-blind study. J Vasc Surg 22:223–229, 1995.

217. Laupacis A, Fergusson D: Drugs to minimize perioperative blood loss in cardiac surgery: meta-analyses using perioperative blood transfusion as the outcome. The International Study of Peri-operative Transfusion (ISPOT) Investigators. Anesth Analg 85:1258–1267, 1997.

218. Henry DA, Moxey AJ, Carless PA, et al: Desmopressin for minimizing perioperative allogeneic blood transfusion (Cochrane Review). Cochrane Database Syst Rev 2:CD001884, 2001.

219. Attar S, Hammon JW: Pharmacologic agents in perioperative bleeding. In: Attar S (ed): Hemostasis in Carrdiac Surgery. Armonk, NY, Futura Publishing Company, pp 203–214, 1999.

220. de Bono DP, Pringle S: Local inhibition of thrombosis using urokinase linked to a monoclonal antibody which recognizes damaged endothelium. Thromb Res 61(5–6):537–545, 1991.

221. Levy JH, Morales A, Lemmer JH: Pharmacologic approaches to prevent or decrease bleeding in surgical patients. In Speiss BD, Counts RB, Gould SA (eds): Perioperative Transfusion Medicine. Baltimore, Williams & Wilkins, pp 383–397, 1998.

222. Dunn CJ, Goa KL: Tranexamic acid: A review of its use in surgery and other indications. Drugs 57(6):1005–1032, 1999.

223. Munoz JJ, Birkmeyer NJ, Birkmeyer JD, et al: Is epsilon-aminocaproic acid as effective as aprotinin in reducing bleeding with cardiac surgery?: A meta-analysis. Circulation 99(1):81–89, 1999.

224. Bennett-Guerrero E, Spillane WF, White WD, et al: Epsilon-aminocaproic acid administration and stroke following coronary artery bypass graft surgery. Ann Thorac Surg 67(5):1283–1287, 1999.

225. Perazella MA, Biswas P: Acute hyperkalemia associated with intravenous epsilon-aminocaproic acid therapy. Am J Kidney Dis 33(4):782–785, 1999.

226. Stafford-Smith M, Phillips-Bute B, Reddan DN, et al: The association of epsilon-aminocaproic acid with postoperative decrease in creatinine clearance in 1502 coronary bypass patients. Anesth Analg 91(5):1085–1090, 2000.

227. Britt CW Jr, Light RR, Peters BH, Schochet SS Jr: Rhabdomyolysis during treatment with epsilon-aminocaproic acid. Arch Neurol 37(3):187–188, 1980.

228. Mezzano D, Panes O, Munoz B, et al: Tranexamic acid inhibits fibrinolysis, shortens the bleeding time and improves platelet function in patients with chronic renal failure. Thromb Haemost 82(4):1250–1254, 1999.

229. Roos Y: Antifibrinolytic treatment in subarachnoid hemorrhage: A randomized placebo-controlled trial. STAR Study Group. Neurology 54(1):77–82, 2000.

230. Vander Salm TJ, Kaur S, Lancey RA, et al: Reduction of bleeding after heart operations through the prophylactic use of epsilon-aminocaproic acid. J Thorac Cardiovasc Surg 112(4):1098–1107, 1996.

231. Troianos CA, Sypula RW, Lucas DM, et al: The effect of prophylactic epsilon-aminocaproic acid on bleeding, transfusions, platelet function, and fibrinolysis during coronary artery bypass grafting. Anesthesiology 91(2):430–435, 1999.

232. Saleem R, Bigham M, Spitznagel E, Despotis GJ: The effect of epsilon-aminocaproic acid on HemoSTATUS and kaolin-activated clotting time measurements. Anesth Analg 90(6):1281–1285, 2000.

233. Casati V, Guzzon D, Oppizzi M, et al: Hemostatic effects of aprotinin, tranexamic acid and epsilon-aminocaproic acid in primary cardiac surgery. Ann Thorac Surg 68(6):2252–2256, 1999.

234. Engel JM, Hohaus T, Ruwoldt R, et al: Regional hemostatic status and blood requirements after total knee arthroplasty with and without tranexamic acid or aprotinin. Anesth Analg 92(3):775–780, 2001.

235. Ido K, Neo M, Asada Y, et al: Reduction of blood loss using tranexamic acid in total knee and hip arthroplasties. Arch Orthop Trauma Surg 120(9):518–520, 2000.

236. Zohar E, Fredman B, Ellis M, et al: A comparative study of the postoperative allogeneic blood-sparing effect of tranexamic acid versus acute normovolemic hemodilution after total knee replacement. Anesth Analg 89(6):1382–1387, 1999.

237. Jansen AJ, Andreica S, Claeys M, et al: Use of tranexamic acid for an effective blood conservation strategy after total knee arthroplasty. Br J Anaesth 83(4):596–601, 1999.

238. Kang Y, Lewis JH, Navalgund A, et al: Epsilon-aminocaproic acid for treatment of fibrinolysis during liver transplantation. Anesthesiology 66(6):766–773, 1987.

239. Kang YG, Martin DJ, Marquez J, et al: Intraoperative changes in blood coagulation and thrombelastographic monitoring in liver transplantation. Anesth Analg 64:888–896, 1985.

240. Butterworth J, James RL, Lin Y, et al: Pharmacokinetics of epsilon-aminocaproic acid in patients undergoing aortocoronary bypass surgery. Anesthesiology 90:1624–1635, 1999.

241. Dobkowski WB, Murkin JM: A risk-benefit assessment of aprotinin in cardiac surgical procedures. Drug Saf 18(1):21–41, 1998.

242. Levy JH: Hemostatic agents and their safety. J Cardiothorac Vasc Anesth 13(4 suppl 1):6–11, 1999.

243. Fareed J, Koza M, Walenga JM, et al: Anti-inflammatory effects of serine protease inhibitors. In Wechsler AS (ed): Pharmacologic management of perioperative bleeding. Southhamptom, NY, CME Network, pp 150–161, 1996.

244. Menichetti A, Tritapepe L, Ruvolo G, et al: Changes in coagulation patterns, blood loss and blood use after cardiopulmonary bypass: aprotinin vs tranexamic acid vs epsilon aminocaproic acid. J Cardiovasc Surg 37:401–407, 1996.

245. Lavee J, Savion N, Smolinsky A, et al: Platelet protection by aprotinin in cardiopulmonary bypass: Electron microscopic study. Ann Thorac Surg 53(3):477–481, 1992.

246. Poullis M, Manning R, Laffan M, et al: The antithrombotic effect of aprotinin: actions mediated via the protease activated receptor 1. J Thorac Cardiovasc Surg 120(2):370–378, 2000.

247. Feindt PR, Walcher S, Volkmer I, et al: Effects of high-dose aprotinin on renal function in aortocoronary bypass grafting. Ann Thorac Surg 60(4):1076–1080, 1995.

248. Smith CR, Spanier TB: Aprotinin in deep hypothermic circulatory arrest. Ann Thorac Surg 68(1):278–286, 1999.

249. Lass M, Welz A, Kochs M, et al: Aprotinin in elective primary bypass surgery. Graft patency and clinical efficacy. Eur J Cardiothorac Surg 9(4):206–210, 1995.

250. Lemmer JH Jr, Stanford W, Bonney SL, et al: Aprotinin for coronary bypass operations: Efficacy, safety, and influence on early saphenous vein graft patency. A multicenter, randomized, double-blind, placebo-controlled study. J Thorac Cardiovasc Surg 107(2):543–553, 1994.

251. Bidstrup BP, Underwood SR, Sapsford RN, Streets EM: Effect of aprotinin (Trasylol) on aorta-coronary bypass graft patency. J Thorac Cardiovasc Surg 105:147–153, 1993.

252. Levy JH, Ramsay JG, Murkin JM: Aprotinin reduces the incidence of stroke following cardiac surgery [abstract]. Circulation 94:I-535, 1996.

253. Smith PK: Aprotinin: Safe and effective only with the full-dose regimen. Ann Thorac Surg 62:1575–1577, 1996.

254. Lemmer JH Jr, Stanford W, Bonney SL, et al: Aprotinin for coronary artery bypass grafting: Effect on postoperative renal function. Ann Thorac Surg 59(1):132–136, 1995.

255. D'Ambra MN, Akins CW, Blackstone EH, et al: Aprotinin in primary valve replacement and reconstruction: A multicenter, double-blind, placebo-controlled trial. J Thorac Cardiovasc Surg 112(4):1081–1089, 1996.

256. Dietrich W, Spath P, Ebell A, Richter JA: Prevalence of anaphylactic reactions to aprotinin: Analysis of two hundred forty-eight reexposures to aprotinin in heart operations. J Thorac Cardiovasc Surg 113(1):194–201, 1997.

257. Dietrich W, Spath P, Zuhlsdorf M, et al: Anaphylactic reactions to aprotinin reexposure in cardiac surgery: Relation to antiaprotinin immunoglobulin G and E antibodies. Anesthesiology 95(1):64–71, 2001.

258. Wong BI, McLean RF, Fremes SE, et al: Aprotinin and tranexamic acid for high transfusion risk cardiac surgery. Ann Thorac Surg 69(3):808–816, 2000.

259. Nuttall GA, Oliver WC, Ereth MH, et al: Comparison of blood-conservation strategies in cardiac surgery patients at high risk for bleeding. Anesthesiology 92(3):674–682, 2000.

260. Bennett-Guerrero E, Sorohan JG, Gurevich ML, et al: Cost-benefit and efficacy of aprotinin compared with epsilon-aminocaproic acid in patients having repeated cardiac operations: A randomized, blinded clinical trial. Anesthesiology 87:1373–1380, 1997.

261. Tweddell JS, Berger S, Frommelt PC, et al: Aprotinin improves outcome of single-ventricle palliation. Ann Thorac Surg 62(5):1329–1335, 1996.

262. D'Errico CC, Shayevitz JR, Martindale SJ, et al: The efficacy and cost of aprotinin in children undergoing reoperative open heart surgery. Anesth Analg 83(6):1193–1199, 1996.

263. Dietrich W, Mossinger H, Spannagl M, et al: Hemostatic activation during cardiopulmonary bypass with different aprotinin dosages in pediatric patients having cardiac operations. J Thorac Cardiovasc Surg 105(4):712–720, 1993.

264. Murkin JM, Shannon NA, Bourne RB, et al: Aprotinin decreases blood loss in patients undergoing revision or bilateral total hip arthroplasty. Anesth Analg 80:343–348, 1995.

265. Janssens M, Joris J, David JL, et al: High-dose aprotinin reduces blood loss in patients undergoing total hip replacement surgery. Anesthesiology 80:23–29, 1994.

266. Despotis GJ, Filos KS, Levine V, et al: Aprotinin prolongs activated and nonactivated whole blood clotting time and potentiates the effect of heparin in vitro. Anesth Analg 82:1126–1131, 1996.

267. Hunt BJ, Segal H, Yahoub M: Aprotinin and heparin monitoring during cardiopulmonary bypass. Circulation 86SII:410–412, 1992.

268. Feindt P, Volkmer I, Seyfert U, et al: Activated clotting time, anticoagulation, use of heparin, and thrombin activation during extracorporeal circulation: changes under aprotinin therapy. Thorac Cardiovasc Surg 41(1):9–15, 1993.

269. van Oeveren W, Jansen NJ, Bidstrup BP, et al: Effects of aprotinin on hemostatic mechanisms during cardiopulmonary bypass. Ann Thorac Surg 44(6):640–645, 1987.

Immunosuppressants

Nándor Marczin, MD, PhD

The immune system protects the internal milieu by developing a tolerance to the "inner self" while recognizing and effectively eliminating foreign tissue, which may threaten the homeostasis of the organism. The importance of this system in survival is highlighted by the fact that even primitive multicellular organisms have devised an intricate system of innate or natural immunity. Despite a genetically limited number of recognition molecules, these primitive organisms are capable of recognizing invading pathogens despite their variability, molecular heterogeneity, and mutagenic potential.[1] The innate immunity provides a rapid antimicrobial host defense, which is based on selective recognition of the non-self only through a few, relatively inflexible cell populations together with soluble components. Consequently, this system is incapable of initiating an immune response against itself.

In vertebrates, this primitive system is supplemented by the acquired immune system, which exhibits almost infinite capacity by rearranging genes that encode specific, clonally distributed receptors toward individual antigenic sites. Unfortunately, self-antigens can initiate this process and require additional mechanisms to put a break on self-destruction initiated by an immune response against self-antigens. Clonal elimination in the thymus and in the peripheral lymphatic organs represents an effective mechanism to induce self-tolerance in most but not all healthy individuals.[2] The presence of autoreactive T cells in healthy individuals highlights the imperfect nature of negative selection and also suggests that there are active peripheral mechanisms responsible to maintain tolerance to self. Not surprisingly, failure of any of these control mechanisms results in self-destruction leading to organ-selective or generalized autoimmune diseases such as multiple sclerosis, insulin-dependent diabetes mellitus, glomerulonephritis, and rheumatoid arthritis.[3]

Despite major advances in general and specialized medicine in the last century, there is no definite cure for most degenerative diseases. Many of the patients with these conditions present with end-stage organ failure, and for a significant number only organ transplantation provides hope for increased survival and temporary improvement in quality of life. The transplant of a tissue from one individual to another with a fully functional immune system, however, is followed almost invariably by rejection of the graft. This is because of the relentless aggression of immunocompetent cells against the foreign tissue, followed by a massive inflammatory reaction resulting in acute damage, loss of function, and death in most instances. For many years this response was attenuated by using general anti-inflammatory and antiproliferative agents. Serendipitously, certain xenobiotics inhibited different aspects of the immune response and are currently being evaluated as immunosuppressants in both transplantation and autoimmune disease. These discoveries have stimulated research into cellular signaling of immune cell activation and molecular targets of immunosuppressant substance action. The use of novel immunosuppressive agents has resulted in significant improvements of both graft and patient survival. Stimulated by the clinical demand and improvement in our knowledge of the molecular and cellular biology, the pharmaceutical industry continues to develop new and more specific molecules with immunosuppressant activity and to develop them into clinically useful drugs.

Mechanisms of Drug Action Based on Principal Events of T-Cell Activation

The pivotal event in the initiation of the complex immunologic process that ultimately leads to destruction of invading foreign pathogen or recognized self-antigen is antigen-induced activation, proliferation, and differentiation of T lymphocytes. The engagement between the antigen and T-cell receptor is followed by activation of the T cells, which involves intricate signal transduction mechanisms leading to up-regulation of T cell–derived cytokines, among them the potent T-cell growth factor interleukin-2 (IL-2).[4] These in turn initiate a series of events underlying proliferation and differentiation of T cells to helper and effector cells, which in concert with B-cell–mediated humoral response results in elimination of the initiating antigen.

During transplant rejection and autoimmunity, these cellular mechanisms are exaggerated either because of continuous presence of alloantigens in the transplanted organs or problems in the regulation of self-tolerance. Although there are several endogenous mechanisms to attenuate the ongoing immune response, drug-mediated immunosuppression is the reason for the current level of success observed with organ transplantation and also remains the mainstream therapy of autoimmune diseases.[5]

Antigen Presentation and Cell Surface Events in T Lymphocytes

The principal immune reaction after allograft engraftment is the recognition and response to donor antigens, which are part of the major histocompatibility complex (MHC). There appear to be two major mechanisms whereby recipient T cells interact with donor MHC peptide antigens and recent studies suggest that these distinct mechanisms might play a crucial and distinctive role in the initiation of the acute or chronic rejection process.[6] Generally, T cells recognize the donor MHC antigens through antigen-presenting cells (APCs). In the process of direct allorecognition, T cells recognize determinant peptides on the intact donor MHC molecules on the surface of the transplanted donor cells. There is, however, an alternative mechanism in which the *donor's* MHC molecules are processed and presented as peptides by the *recipient's* MHC molecules at the surface of the *host's* APCs, thereby eliciting a T-cell response that is restricted to the host rather than donor ("indirect pathway"). Increasing evidence suggest that although direct antigen recognition is responsible for the initial in vivo sensitization of recipient T cells to allograft MHC antigens on the surface of "professional" bone marrow–derived donor APCs, the indirect pathway might play a key role in the actual rejection process at the site of the graft, especially after the grafted tissues becomes devoid of donor APCs.[7]

During the recognition step, the MHC antigen becomes engaged with the T-cell antigen receptor complex (TCR). This is composed of a clonally variant, immunoglobulin-like, binding chain that recognizes the antigenic peptide in the context of MHC proteins, and a clonally invariant subunit that initiates intracellular signals originating from antigenic recognition.[4] Allorecognition stimulates a redistribution of cell-surface proteins and co-clustering of the TCR complex. This multimeric complex includes additional surface proteins and signaling molecules and functions as a unit in initiating T-cell activation.[8]

Engagement of the donor MHC antigenic peptides and the TCR, however, only results in weak stimulation of T-cell responses and anergy or paralysis in most instances.[9] Sufficient T-cell activation requires the presence of supplementary costimulatory signals in addition to the antigenic signals. This is usually brought about by cell-to-cell interactions among the antigen-specific T cells and APCs because of interactions of a number of cognate cell surface proteins on both.[10] In addition to direct cell/cell interactions, APC-derived soluble cytokines such as IL-1β and IL-6 provide costimulatory signals that result in T-cell activation in vitro, resulting in effective signal transduction in the T cells and up-regulation of pivotal T-cell activation genes such as *IL-2*.[11]

T-Cell Receptor Signaling

IL-2 gene expression is controlled in part by its 5′ flanking sequences, which contain critical regulatory regions corresponding to binding sites for various transcription factors. Mutation of these regulatory regions results in a variable degree of loss of induction of *IL-2* gene transcription confirming that functional binding of enhancer proteins is obligatory for gene transcription. Although transcription factor Oct-1 and factors interacting with the costimulatory CD28 response element (CD28RE) are involved in *IL-2* gene transcription, nuclear factor of activated T cells (NF-AT), nuclear factor kappa B (NF-κB), and activator protein 1 (AP-1) are of paramount importance.[12] A Ca-calmodulin and calcineurin pathway is the major determinant of NF-AT activation, whereas mitogen-activated protein kinase (MAPK) pathways have been implicated in AP1 and NF-κB-activation, nuclear translocation, and binding to a promoter element of the *IL-2* gene.[13]

One of the most interesting features of T-cell activation is that gene transcription is not merely the sum of multiple independent interactions of transcription factors with the basal transcription complex. Rather, transcription is driven by the formation of highly cooperative protein complexes containing a precise arrangement of many components, including the transcription factors, DNA-binding proteins that serve an architectural function, and linker proteins that provide a bridge between the inducible transcription factors and the basal transcription complex.[13,14] This is shown in in vivo footprinting experiments in which coordinate occupancy of all sites is observed as early as 1 hour after T-cell stimulation. The functional consequence of this is that interference with any one component may abolish formation of the entire enhancer complex with resultant attenuation of T-cell activation and immunosuppression.

Calcium/Calmodulin/Calcineurin–Induced Nuclear Factor of Activated T Cells

Within 1 to 100 seconds of T-cell receptor engagement, tyrosine kinases become activated leading to the generation of inositol 1,4,5-trisphosphate (IP_3) and subsequent intracellular release of Ca^{2+} and the increase in cytoplasmic Ca^{2+} concentration $[Ca^{2+}]i$.[15] The increase in intracellular calcium activates calmodulin, a Ca^{2+}-binding protein, which in turn interacts with calcineurin that belongs to a superfamily of protein serine/threonine phosphatases.[16,17] Calcineurin consists of two subunits, a catalytic subunit (calcineurin A [CnA]) and a regulatory subunit. Binding of activated calmodulin to CnA releases the autoinhibitory domain of CnA from its active site and brings about increase of its phosphatase activity. One of the substrate of calcineurins phosphatase activity is the NFAT family of transcription factors.[18] Dephosphorylation of NFAT allows translocation of NFAT into the nucleus with activation of gene expression through the cis-acting element called NF-AT (Fig. 54–1).

Role of Mitogen-Activated Protein Kinase

In addition to calcium signaling, a number of other events occur after allorecognition and engagement of TCR and costimulation receptors. Recent studies highlight the role of the MAPK and NF-κB activation pathways in cell activation, which might be crucial in activation of additional transcription factors capable to cooperatively regulate T-cell cytokine gene induction.

As detailed elsewhere in this book, the MAPK pathway is a conserved eukaryotic signaling cascade consisting of hierarchically organized kinases termed *MAPK, MAPK*

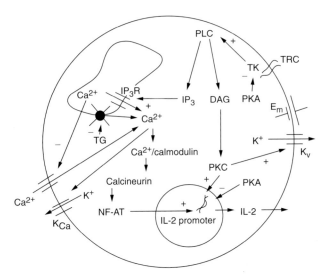

Figure 54–1. Signaling pathways in T cells. A signal transduction cascade leading from the T-cell receptor (TCR) to interleukin (IL)-2 secretion. (+), activation and minus signs indicate inhibition; DAG, diacylglycerol; E_m, plasma membrane potential; IP_3R, inositol 1,4,5-trisphosphate receptor; NF-AT, nuclear factor of activated T cells; PKA, protein kinase A; TG, thapsigargin; TK, tyrosine kinase. (From Cahalan MD, Chandy KG: Ion channels in the immune system as targets for immunosuppression. Curr Opin Biotechnol 8(6):749–756, 1997.)

kinase (MAPKK), and *MAPKK kinase* (MAPKKK).[19] All of the three major subgroups of the MAPK superfamily—extracellular signal-regulated kinases (ERK), c-jun N-terminal kinase (JNK), and p38—have been defined in T cells and have been shown to be activated by various stimuli relevant to T-cell activation. One of the most exciting aspects of these investigations is the relation among the combination of stimuli necessary to induce full T-cell activation, activation of MAPK subgroups, and efficient gene induction of IL-2.[20]

Several studies have demonstrated that activation of ERK pathway after TCR stimulation alone does not lead to *IL-2* gene transcription, suggesting that ERK activation is not sufficient to drive full T-cell activation. However, when the costimulus was provided, there was evidence of JNK activation associated with *IL-2* gene transcription. Similar findings were reported with the p38 pathway. Interestingly, pharmacologic inhibition of either JNK, p38, ERK, or molecular strategies to attenuate these pathways all result in inhibition of IL-2 transcription. Thus ERK activation cannot confer but is obligatory for full T-cell activation and integration of the signals at the level of p38 and JNK appears to be required to elicit gene transcription.[20] Cooperative activation of JNK and p38 in conjunction with ERK leads to activation of transcription factors including AP-1.[21] Because AP-1 binding is important in both NF-AT and IL-2 promoter function, proper activation of the MAPK after TCR engagement and costimulation might provide a critical second transcription factor to interact with the calcineurin-induced NF-AT proteins to build the necessary protein complex at the promoter region of IL-2.[22,23] Activation and nuclear translocation of NF-κB, another cytosolic protein involved in gene regulation, appears to be another component of this machinery.[13]

Role of Nuclear Factor kappa B

This transcription factor is held in the cytoplasm of unstimulated cells by association with an inhibitory I-κB protein. T-cell costimulation leads to the activation of NF-κB, which appears to play an important role in IL-2 transcription.[24,25] This appears to be mediated by two homologous kinases, which are contained in the I-κB kinase complex (IKC). These phosphorylate I-κB proteins and allow ubiquitinylation and degradation of I-κB, which results in the subsequent activation of NF-κB. Recent progress has uncovered additional proximal kinases in this system such as IKKs, which are in turn activated by IKK kinases (IKKKs).[26] This area is rapidly developing and is likely to answer many important aspects of signaling in T lymphocytes such as convergence of multiple signals, links between the MAPK and NF-κB pathways, and differential mechanisms of TCR-mediated and costimulus-mediated events.[27]

Interleukin-2 Receptor Signaling

Secreted IL-2 from activated T cells acts as a major growth factor producing mitogenesis and proliferation of T cells. This involves entry from a resting G_0 cell cycle phase into a cell cycle progression through G_1 phase and DNA synthesis followed by cell division.

Mechanism of this mitogenic effect of IL-2 involves activation of IL-2 receptor (IL-2R) and signaling events activating a distinct set of transcription factors leading to up-regulation of genes responsible for G_0/G_1 transition and progression through G_1 phase.[28] Three critical events have been identified in the generation of the IL-2R signal for cell cycle progression: heterodimerization of the cytoplasmic domains of the IL-2R beta and gamma(c) chains, activation of the tyrosine kinase Jak3, and phosphorylation of tyrosine residues on the IL-2R beta chain.[29] These proximal events lead to the creation of an activated receptor complex, to which various cytoplasmic signaling molecules are recruited and become substrates for regulatory enzymes (especially tyrosine kinases) that are associated with the receptor.[30] Among these, phosphorylation and nuclear translocation of STAT-3 and STAT-5—two members of the transcription factor family known as signal transducers and activators of transcription (STATs)—appear to be the most important.[31,32]

Cell Cycle Regulation in T Cells

The biologic consequence of the signaling discussed earlier is up-regulation of genes involved in cell cycle progression. Using candidate gene approaches, a number of such genes have been identified.[33] Recently, large-scale screening methods allow a more global understanding of gene expression modulation by *IL-2*. These studies indicate that *IL-2* modulates the expression of gene clusters that constitute a complex multifaceted program allowing dynamic regulation of both cellular proliferation and survival.[34] This includes both up-regulation of genes that promote cell cycle progression, control cell survival, and increase synthetic and metabolic processes during proliferation, as well as suppression of genes that block cell cycle progression and promote cell death.

Cellular proliferation not only depends on the appropriate genetic environment of the cells but also on increased metabolism including appropriate rate of synthesis of nucleic acid building blocks such as purine and pyrimidine nucleotides.[5] Particularly, dividing lymphocytes increase both their pyrimidine and purine pools dramatically after stimulation.[35] All cells in the body are able to synthesize nucleotides by two pathways: de novo synthesis and the salvage pathway.[4] There are indications that lymphocytes might become more dependent on the de novo purine and pyrimidine pathway during proliferation. This might offer important opportunities for immunosuppression based on inhibitors of crucial enzymes in the de novo nucleotide synthetic pathways such as inosine monophosphate dehydrogenase (IMPDH) and dihydroorotate dehydrogenase for purine and pyrimidine nucleotides, respectively.[5]

Preclinical Pharmacology

The past decade has seen important progress in the field of immunosuppressive drug development for transplantation. Two main classes of drugs have been the focus of this intense endeavor: biologics and xenobiotics. Biologics are naturally occurring mammalian proteins or peptides or modified forms of these, whereas xenobiotics are drugs produced from micro-organisms or chemically synthesized molecules that are structurally dissimilar from naturally occurring mammalian molecules. Although xenobiotics have proven to be the most efficacious in the clinical practice, biologics are now beginning to fulfill the promise afforded by careful molecular design and application of biotechnology on the basis of better understanding and targeting molecular events in lymphocyte activation.

There are two major strategies to control the accelerated immune response to transplantation donor antigens and recognized self-antigens. One strategy involves the establishment of tolerance toward the specific donor and self-antigens or control of the subsets of T cells specifically engaged in the specific immune response against these antigens. This approach would be extremely desirable because it would not compromise the function of the immune system guarding against infection and malignant cells in the body. The strategy that currently dominates clinical practice involves global suppression of immune system, which carries the considerable risk for increased infection and immunosuppression-related neoplasms. Table 54–1 summarizes potential events to interfere with untoward T-cell activation, drugs affecting these events that are already in clinical use, and molecules in development that target these steps.

TABLE 54–1.

Immunosuppressants and Their Molecular and Physiologic Targets

Targets	Immunosuppressants
Antigen presentation and allorecognition	MHC protein, peptides, anti–T-lymphocyte globulin, mAb OKT3, mAb CD4
Costimulation	Anti-CD 40, CTLA4-Ig, Anti-monokine Abs, glucocorticoids
TCR signaling	Cyclosporin, tacrolimus, MAPK inhibitors, NF-κB inhibitors
IL-2 binding	mAb-IL2R, Daclizumab
IL-2R signaling	Rapamycin, JAK 3 inhibitors
Clonal expansion	Azathioprine, mycophenolate mofetil, leflunomide

IL-2R, interleukin-2 receptor; mAb, monoclonal antibody; MAPK, mitogen-activated protein kinase; MHC, major histocompatibility complex; NF-κB, nuclear factor kappa B; TCR, T-cell receptor.

Drugs Affecting Antigen Presentation and Alloregulation

Recent insight into the underlying mechanisms of allorecognition may allow novel strategies to maneuver the alloresponse toward tolerance or ineffectiveness.[7] The direct alloresponse is characterized by the high frequency of polyclonal alloreactive T cells recognizing multiple antigen peptides and displaying a large variety of T-cell surface receptors. It is therefore likely that devising selective antigen- or TCR-based immunotherapy to block such a polyclonal T-cell response would be difficult. In contrast, T-cell response to donor MHC peptides involved in the indirect allorecognition pathway is mediated by a limited set of oligoclonal T cells responding to a single or a few dominant donor MHC determinants. This suggests that selective immune intervention could be designed to interfere with the indirect rejection process. A number of studies have demonstrated that immunologic tolerance to MHC-derived peptides can be achieved by selecting appropriate routes and forms of administration of these peptides in recipient rodents. Benichou and colleagues showed that intravenous administration of high doses of MHC class I and II peptides given in saline leads to complete and sustained state of in vivo T-cell unresponsiveness to these peptides in mice.[36,37] Important studies by Sayegh and colleagues have shown the successful induction of long-term, alloantigen-specific, graft survival by intrathymic injection and oral administration of rat recipients with a mixture of peptides corresponding to different polymorphic regions of donor MHC molecules.[38]

Aligned to these efforts is the infusion of donor bone marrow cells.[39,40] This represents the transplantation of the regulatory components of the donor immune system and professional donor APCs that may produce in the recipient a state of specific tolerance to any tissue transplanted from the bone marrow donor.[41] Initial experience in kidney transplantation suggests that although having no major influence on acute rejection episodes, biopsy-proven chronic rejection and loss of graft were greatly reduced in the bone marrow–infused group (2/63 vs. 41/219).[42] Although the mechanisms involved in MHC peptide or bone marrow–induced tolerance are not fully defined, these strategies represents a promising approach for ensuring long-lasting graft acceptance in the absence of widespread immunosuppression.[41]

Drugs Affecting the T-Cell Receptor Complex

The T-cell antigen receptor is a complex of two with variable regions for antigen binding and four conserved proteins, one of which is targeted by the monoclonal antibody (mAb) OKT3. When given in vivo, OKT3 causes profound immunosuppression by three basic mechanisms: reduction in T-cell numbers, modulation of the T-cell receptor (TCR), and blocking the T-cell response through transient activation followed by unresponsiveness or anergy.[43] Within 5 minutes of the first dose, the number of T cells decreases to nearly undetectable levels and remains low throughout a 2-week course of therapy. Furthermore, the remaining T cells have greatly reduced numbers of receptors per cell, sufficient to suppress their responsiveness.[44]

As discussed earlier, engagement of the TCR by antigen does not directly result in T-cell activation. Rather, it is the rearrangement of membrane proteins in the area of contact between the T cell and the APC and the formation of contact cap that is the critical event.[45] This specific rearrangement of the T-cell surface is critical for signaling because it recruits and induces the apposition of protein kinases with their substrates at the cell contact and excludes negative regulators such as tyrosine phosphatases from the contact.[46]

CD4 and CD8 proteins bind to the monomorphic component of human leukocyte antigen class II and class I molecules, respectively, and are important in stabilizing the TCR APC contact, the interaction between the TCR-MHC peptide complexes, and in the initiation of signal transduction after antigenic recognition. Prevention of CD4 and MHC class II interaction by mAbs have been shown to prolong graft survival and to cause tolerance induction in different animal models.[47] Clinical studies have borne out the prediction that these mAbs induce a long-lasting, nonspecific immunosuppression suggesting that it might be useful as an adjuvant therapy.[48]

Drugs Affecting Costimulation

Some of the costimulatory signals for T-cell activation are provided at least in part by the T cell–based CD28 molecule when bound to its counter receptors CD80 or CD86 on APCs.[49] The interaction of CD40 and its T cell–based ligand CD40L also plays an important role in T-cell activation at least in part by up-regulating CD80/86. In addition, CD40 and CD40L play a fundamental role in establishing T cell–dependent B-cell activity. Interestingly, endogenous inhibitor proteins also exist, and it has been shown that the T-cell molecule CTLA4 down-regulates costimulation and TCR-mediated activation.[50] These mechanisms have been exploited to devise strategies to down-regulate T-cell activation either by using blocking mAbs against CD40 or CD40L or by delivering a fusion protein CTLA4-Ig to augment the negative signal. Following promising results in rodent models, a combination therapy has provided impressive results in that it not only prevented but also reversed acute kidney allograft rejection in primates even in the absence of other forms of chronic immunosuppression.[51,52] Unfortunately, a recent clinical study had to be stopped because of an unexpected high incidence of thromboembolic events.[41]

Because APC-derived cytokines including IL-1β and IL-6 can also provide costimulatory signals that result in T-cell activation, monokine release and action represents an important target of immunosuppressive strategies using glucocorticoids (GCs).

It is widely accepted that the potent anti-inflammatory and immunomodulatory actions of GCs are caused by inhibition of the activity of transcription factors, such as NF-κB and AP-1. Because of their lipophilic nature, GCs freely enter the cells, where they exert their effects by binding to the glucocorticoid receptor (GR), a transcription factor. In the absence of GCs, this intracellular receptor protein is sequestered in the cytoplasm in a complex with two heat shock protein 90, one heat shock protein 70, and one p56 immunophilin molecule. Binding of GCs is thought to induce a conformational change in GR, which releases it from its chaperones, thereby allowing its translocation to the nucleus.[53] Genes positively regulated by GR are characterized by GR-responsive elements in the promoter. However, the anti-inflammatory potential of GR is thought to be mediated through negative modulation of transcription of the various proinflammatory cytokines through interference with NF-κB and AP-1 pathways.[54–56]

Although there are several hypotheses to explain the negative "cross-talk" between NF-κB and GR, the favored models suggests a negative physical interaction between GC-activated GR and NF-κB subunit in the nucleus through protein/protein interactions.[57] Supporting this idea, the p65 subunit of NF-κB and GR have been found to associate both in vitro and in vivo. The transcriptional inhibition by GR might be the result of masking the p65 transactivating domains, the induction of post-translational modifications, and conformational changes within the transcription initiation complex. The exact mechanisms remain highly controversial, and it is likely that more than one mechanism is responsible for the gene-repressive effect of GCs in different cell types and tissues.

Drugs Affecting Signaling Underlying Interleukin-2 Gene Transcription

Cyclosporine (cyclosporin A [CsA]), a neutral lipophilic cyclic undecapeptide isolated from the fungus *Tolypocladium inflatum,* has revolutionized treatment of allograft rejection since the late 1970s, when studies revealed that CsA inhibits T-cell activation by blocking the transcription of cytokine genes, including those of *IL-2* and *IL-4*.[58–61] On entering T cells, CsA binds with high affinity to cyclophilins, especially to the cytosolic 17-kD cyclophilin A, which is the most abundant cyclophilin in T cells.[62,63] These molecules are ubiquitous cytosolic proteins that possess peptidyl-proline-cis-trans isomerase (PPIase) activity, an enzymatic activity involved in protein folding.[64] CsA inhibits the PPIase activity of cyclophilins, however, inhibition of PPIase is not involved in the mechanism of immunosuppression because some of CsA analogues that fail to block T-cell activation are still able to inhibit the PPIase activity.[22,65]

The major mechanism of action of CsA has been uncovered by observations showing that the cyclophilin/CsA complex, but not cyclophilin alone, can associate with calcineurin and that this direct binding to calcineurin A (CnA) inhibits the phosphatase activity of calcineurin.[66,67] By preventing their calcineurin-mediated dephosphorylation of NFAT transcription factor, CsA inhibits the nuclear translocation of NFAT family members and subsequent gene expression in activated T cells. Undoubtedly, inhibition of the calcineurin/NFAT pathway is one of the mechanisms of CsA-mediated immunosuppression.

Complicating the issue is the finding that CsA affects the activities of AP-1 and NF-κB transcription factors, implying the presence of additional target(s) of CsA.[22] The results of recent studies raise the possibility that the immunosuppressive effect of CsA is attributed, at least in part, to the inhibition of JNK and p38 pathways.[20,23] Interestingly, this was restricted to JNK and p38 activation initiated by the T cell–specific signaling pathway triggered by the TCR and CD28 costimulatory molecules but not those activated by cellular stresses.[22] This implies that proximal signal transduction mechanisms specifically positioned in between the TCR and MAPK pathways are sensitive to CsA. Most recent studies propose that the Rho subfamily of small G proteins such as Rac1 and Vav1, a guanine nucleotide exchange factor for Rac1, would be the molecular target of CsA (Fig. 54–2).[68] Whether this is a direct action of CsA or represents "cross- talk" between the MAPK and calcineurin pathway remains to be established.

In addition to inhibition of T-cell mitogen expression, CsA might constrain cell growth by promoting the production of growth-inhibitory cytokines, such as transforming growth factor.[69,70] Indeed, TGF mRNA and secretion has been shown to be increased in stimulated T cells exposed to the immunosuppressant CsA. Because this is not restricted to T cells, such an action in other tissues might represent one of the principal mechanisms of CsA side effects and toxicity.[71] CsA-induced up-regulation of TGF might stimulate cells to increase their extracellular matrix composition and decrease the production of extracellular matrix–degrading proteases, thereby inducing a profibrogenic state. This is in keeping with that the CsA-induced nephrotoxicity has the characteristics of interstitial fibrosis. Alternatively, CsA nephrotoxicity has been related to endothelin release and the consequent vasoconstriction and vascular remodeling caused by smooth muscle cell proliferation.[72] Furthermore, it has also been reported that TGF produced by CsA administration directly promotes cancer progression.[73]

Although structurally different from CsA, tacrolimus (FK506) also binds to immunophilins, termed FK506 binding proteins, and shares with CsA the inhibition of calcineurin as a molecular mechanism underlying its immunosuppressant activity.[74–76] As a side effect it also induces endothelin release from mesangial cells potentially contributing to nephrotoxicity.[77] Contrary to CsA, however, tacrolimus has been shown to activate NF-κB resulting in *IL-6* gene induction and release in the kidneys.[78,79] This has

been implicated in mesangial cell inflammation and proliferation and is thought to be involved in tacrolimus-induced nephrotoxicity.

Drugs Affecting the Interleukin-2 Receptor Complex

IL-2 and IL-2R are not expressed by resting T cells, but are expressed by T cells activated by interaction with alloantigens.[80] Murine mAbs directed against this inducible IL-2R inhibit the proliferation of alloantigen-activated T cells and prevent generation of cytotoxic T cells in vitro and have been proven effective in animal models of transplantation. In the initial clinical trials of anti-IL-2R–directed therapy in the transplant setting, the murine antibody was well tolerated; it was effective and as part of a combined immunosuppression, the addition of murine anti-Tac significantly delayed the time until the first rejection episode.[81,82] Similar to other monoclonal or murine antibodies, this antibody induced a host immune response against the murine protein and exhibited a short half-life. To overcome this problem, molecularly engineered humanized antibodies were introduced with better pharmacokinetics and exhibiting little immunogenicity and a longer half-life.[83,84] Following encouraging results in preclinical models, Daclizumab was evaluated for its capacity to prevent allograft rejection. In placebo-controlled, randomized, phase III trials (when added to standard cyclosporin-based immunosuppression), Daclizumab significantly reduced the frequency of renal allograft rejection when compared with a placebo.[85] The incidence of adverse events related to treatment was not increased compared with placebo recipients. These data led to U.S. Food & Drug Administration approval for the use of Daclizumab in the prevention of acute kidney transplant rejection.

Daclizumab is now being evaluated as an agent to prevent acute rejection of other organ transplants such as heart and lung and in autoimmune disorders. Furthermore, a series of IL-2R–directed agents are being developed to increase therapeutic efficacy by "armed" anti–IL-2R molecules including a bispecific mAb (combining anti-CD3 and anti-IL-2R), antibodies armed with toxins such as ricin or Pseudomonas exotoxin, or antibodies armed with radioisotopes.[80]

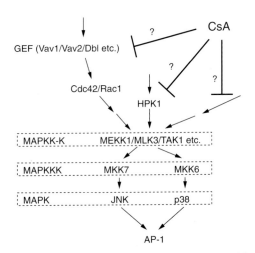

Figure 54–2. Potential target sites of cyclosporin A (CsA) for c-jun N-terminal kinase (JNK) and p38 activation pathways. Guanine nucleotide exchange factors (GEF) for Rac1 and/or Cdc42, such as Vav1, Vav2, and Dbl, are candidates for the target of CsA. Another candidate is an HPK1 (a hematopoietic protein kinase) pathway, which functions as an activator for mitogen-activated protein kinase kinase kinases (MAPKKKs) such as MLK3 and TAK1. It is also possible that the CsA-sensitive JNK and p38 activation in T cells is mediated by unidentified molecule(s). (From Matsuda S, Koyasu S: Mechanisms of action of cyclosporine. Immunopharmacology 47(2-3):119–125, 2000.)

Drugs Affecting T-Cell Clonal Proliferation

Rapamycin (Sirolimus) is a macrolide structurally related to tacrolimus. Like FK506, it binds to FKBP but it does not inhibit calcineurin and does not block cytokine release from activated T cells.[86–88] Rapamycin is able to block signal transduction mediated by IL-2 through the IL-2R complex. The cellular receptor(s) for the rapamycin/FKBP complex is beginning to be characterized. Two cellular proteins, 245 kD and 34 kD in size having sequence similarities to yeast TOR1 and TOR2 (which are homologous to the catalytic domain of p110 subunit of PI-3 kinase), have recently been identified as putative targets for the drug/immunophilin complex.[89] The antiproliferative activity of rapamycin appears to be a consequence of the rapamycin/FKBP complex blocking the activation of the 70-kD S6 protein kinases that are involved in cell proliferation.[90] Rapamycin selectively inactivates p70s6k activity, resulting in selective inhibition of the synthesis of several ribosomal proteins and the inhibition of the induction of mRNA for new ribosomal proteins. The effect of rapamycin on protein synthesis, rather than its direct effects on cell cycle proteins, is thought to be the primary cause of the prolongation of cell cycle progression in rapamycin-treated cells.

In addition to the influence of rapamycin on T-cell signaling, treatment of vascular smooth muscle cells resulted in reduced growth factor–stimulated proliferation in vitro.[91,92] This represents an additional therapeutic potential of rapamycin to control the intimal thickening of graft vascular disease and potentially prevent chronic rejection in other forms of organ transplantation.[5]

Another class of drugs, which interferes with proliferation of T cells, targets nucleotide metabolism necessary to provide building blocks for the DNA synthetic phase of cell cycle.

The antimetabolite azathioprine is a thioguanine derivative of 6-mercaptopurine. This purine analog acts as a purine antagonist and is the oldest but still effective antiproliferative agent.[4,93]

Mycophenolate mofetil (MMF) is rapidly converted after oral or intravenous administration to its active metabolite: mycophenolic acid (MPA). MPA inhibits IMPDH activity and thus disables the de novo pathway for purine biosynthesis.[5,94,95] In cultured cells, the addition of MPA leads to a decrease in intracellular guanosine triphosphate (GTP) and dGTP levels, particularly in activated lymphocytes, whereas ATP levels are not affected.[96,97] In addition, GTP levels in human polymorphonuclear cells are unaffected, which suggests some specificity to lymphocytes. The strongest evidence that a reduction in guanine nucleotide levels is responsible for the antiproliferative effect of MPA comes from the observation that antiproliferative activity of MPA is fully reversed by exogenous guanine, guanosine, or

deoxyguanosine, each of which allows purine nucleotides to be synthesized through the salvage pathway (Fig. 54–3).

After MMF was first shown to prolong organ allograft survival, additional studies in experimental animal models confirmed its therapeutic efficacy for suppression of allograft and xenograft rejection and control of autoimmune diseases.[98] Similarly to rapamycin, MMF appears to suppress arterial intimal thickening associated with chronic organ allograft rejection.[99] This might be caused by a combination of its antiproliferative effects on immune cells and its direct effects on smooth muscle cells. These have been seen in vitro and also in balloon catheter-induced arterial injury.

Leflunomide (LFM) is rapidly converted to A77 1726 in vivo, which is believed to be responsible for the drug's immunosuppressive effects.[5] A77 1726 reversibly inhibits proliferation of both T and B cells stimulated by a variety of mitogens and inhibits antibody production.[100] LFM appears to elicit this response by inhibiting dihydroorotate dehydrogenase, the rate-limiting step in de novo pyrimidine nucleotide synthesis.[101,102]

In addition to its effectiveness in several animal models of arthritis, autoimmune disease, and allograft and xenograft rejection, particularly those in which antibody plays a prominent role, LFM also inhibits chronic rejection manifested by vascular and airway narrowing.[101,103,104] This may be explained by directly inhibition of the proliferation of stimulated smooth muscle cells in vitro.[105]

Anesthetic Agents as Immunosuppressants

The evidence to support a clinically significant direct immunosuppressant effect of inhalation or intravenous anesthetics after surgery is inconclusive.[106–108] There is evidence that a variety of anesthetics produce a considerable suppression of both nonspecific and antigen-specific cellular

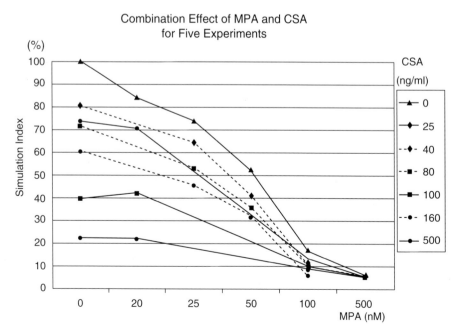

Figure 54–3. Cyclosporin A (CSA) and mycophenolic acid (MPA) inhibition of Staphylococcus enterotoxin B (SEB) stimulation of normal peripheral blood leukocytes (PBL) after 4 days of culture. SEB was chosen as a physiologic and polyclonal MHC-based superantigen stimulus. Note concentration-dependent inhibition of proliferation by CSA alone and potentiation of CSA effect by MPA. The stimulation is only suppressed below 20% with added MPA. (From Ogawa N, Nagashima N, Nakamura M, et al: Measurement of mycophenolate mofetil effect in transplant recipients. Transplantation 72(3):422–427, 2001.)

immune mechanisms in vitro. However, in clinically used concentrations, these negative effects are rapidly and completely reversible.[109] No clinically relevant adverse actions on the immune system have ever been conclusively identified that have been shown to be attributable to short-term anesthesia.[110] However, the situation might be different with high doses of anesthetic in long-term sedation, during which thiobarbiturates or diazepam can reach tissue concentrations sufficient to cause suppression of cellular immune mechanisms. This has been shown in patients with craniocerebral trauma who received high doses of thiopental associated with increased incidence of bacterial pneumonias.[111]

The relative contribution of anesthesia itself and the surgical trauma and stress in causing immunosuppression remains controversial. Many findings seem to point to an essential role played by surgical factors, as well as by the preoperative immune status of the patient, in the occurrence of subsequent infectious complications.[109,112]

Clinical Pharmacology

The following section reviews clinical pharmacology of the most important immunosuppressants approved by the U.S. Food and Drug Administration with special reference to how these compare with cyclosporine, the "gold standard." To avoid repetition, we refer to other chapters in this book regarding the clinical pharmacology of corticosteroids as anti-inflammatory agents.

Cyclosporine

Pharmacokinetics

Cyclosporine has a complex pharmacokinetic profile with poor absorption, formulation-dependent bioavailability, extensive metabolism to more than 30 metabolites, and considerable interpatient and intrapatient variability.[113,114] It has a narrow therapeutic range with adverse clinical consequences after either underdosing or overdosing.

Published studies suggest that a correlation exists between cyclosporine blood levels and acute rejection. Monitoring of cyclosporine levels is, therefore, essential to determine the optimum therapeutic dose in each patient.[115] Although it is generally accepted that drug exposure is best estimated by the full 12-hour area under the curve, this method is limited by the practical effort and cost implications.[116] Trough whole blood levels before administration of a new dose or blood levels 2 hours after administration are, therefore, used by most centers as a guide to dosing and are accepted as a useful and practical method of monitoring drug levels.[117]

Because of the limitations in the bioavailability and pharmacokinetics of cyclosporine that were associated with the original formulation, a microemulsion formulation was developed to improve bioavailability.[118] Neoral, the microemulsion formulation, exhibits significantly faster and more extensive absorption than the original oil-based formulation. Because of the more rapid and complete absorption of cyclosporine from Neoral, patients are exposed to greater peak blood concentrations and to greater areas under the curve of the drug. Several comparative trials have found that this increased exposure does not produce augmented nephrotoxicity and is not associated with an increased incidence of adverse side effects. The more efficient immunosuppression, however, resulted in lower incidence of acute rejection episodes in patients receiving Neoral compared with those on the older oral formulation of Sandimmune (solution or capsule).[119]

Cyclosporine is primarily eliminated through biotransformation by cytochrome P450 (CYP)3A in the gut wall and liver.[120] In addition, P glycoprotein (mdr-1) located in the gastrointestinal epithelium can affect blood concentrations of the drug after oral administration of cyclosporine, presumably by countertransporting the drug from the systemic circulation back into the gastrointestinal lumen. CYP3A4 oxidizes a broad spectrum of drugs by a number of metabolic processes. The location of CYP3A4 in the small bowel and liver permits both to exert an effect on orally administered drugs. Thus drugs inhibiting or inducing CYP activity are expected to interact and modulate CsA levels. The implications of these interactions are twofold: they might increase CsA levels to reach toxic concentrations, and they might be used to allow a reduction in the dosage of cyclosporine while maintaining therapeutic blood cyclosporine (cyclosporine-sparing agents).[121] Included in this list are the azole antifungal drugs: ketoconazole, fluconazole and itraconazole; the calcium channel blockers: diltiazem, verapamil, and nicardipine; and the macrolide antibacterials: erythromycin and related compounds.[122] Studies of various regimens involving the combined use of ketoconazole and cyclosporin have shown that cyclosporin dosages can be reduced by approximately 70% to 85% while maintaining therapeutic blood concentrations in patients who received kidney, heart, or liver transplant.[123] The calcium channel blocker, diltiazem, allows a decrease in cyclosporin dosage by approximately 30% to 50% in this same group of patients who received an organ transplant.

Contrastingly, CYP inhibitors, rifampicin, and the majority of anticonvulsants can decrease cyclosporine blood concentrations to undetectable levels.[124] Other drugs that have been reported to decrease cyclosporine concentration include sulfadimidine, trimethoprim, nafcillin, and octreotide. Because of the numerous interactions with cyclosporine, clinicians should monitor the concentration of this agent more frequently when another drug is added or discontinued and cyclosporine dosage should be adjusted when appropriate because sustained departure from optimal concentrations can result in either graft rejection or increased renal toxicity.

Pharmacodynamics

Pharmacodynamic assays of orally active immunosuppressants either measure the drug effect on a discrete molecule that is important for lymphocyte activation or measure more complex biologic events required for normal immune functions.[125] Assays that evaluate drug-mediated changes in the activity of a specific target molecule presume that the target for that drug is known and that it is essential for the drug's relevant pharmacologic effects. In the case of CsA and tacrolimus, these appear to be inhibition of calcineurin phosphatase activity.

A direct relation has been shown between cyclosporine blood concentrations and the extent of calcineurin inhibition.[126] Single- and multiple-dose studies show that the maximum cyclosporine concentrations occurred 1 to 2 hours after the cyclosporine dose and that they were paralleled by a maximum inhibition of calcineurin activity. As cyclosporine levels decreased there was a spontaneous recovery of calcineurin activity. Thus there is a close temporal relation between changes in cyclosporine whole blood concentrations and immunosuppressive efficacy as estimated from calcineurin activity. In a further study, cyclosporine inhibition of phytohemagglutinin-stimulated, IL-2 production was investigated by using an ex vivo whole blood assay.[127] Once again there was a close temporal relation between cyclosporine whole blood concentrations and the degree of inhibition of IL-2 production.

Adverse Effects

The arterial blood pressure increases soon after administration of immunosuppressive regimens containing cyclosporine. Characteristic vascular changes lead to systemic and renal vasoconstriction, associated with disturbed circadian regulation.[128] The mechanisms underlying this disorder are complex and include altered vascular endothelial function. Vasodilators such as prostacyclin and nitric oxide are suppressed, whereas vasoconstrictors, including endothelin, are increased.

Changes in the kidney include vasoconstriction, reduced glomerular filtration, and sodium retention.[129] Pathologic alterations show chronic progressive tubulointerstitial fibrosis and arteriopathy. Calcineurin inhibitor-induced acute renal failure may occur as early as a few weeks or months after initiation of cyclosporine therapy and has become the "Achilles heel" of this class of immunosuppressive agents.

Between 10% and 28% of patients who receive cyclosporine experience some form of neurotoxic adverse event.[130,131] Both sensory and motor functions may be adversely affected, and thus patients present with a wide range of neurologic and psychiatric disorders. Mild symptoms are common and include tremor, neuralgia, and peripheral neuropathy. Severe symptoms affect up to 5% of patients and include psychoses, hallucinations, blindness, seizures, cerebellar ataxia, motor weakness, or leukoencephalopathy. Occipital white matter appears to be uniquely susceptible to the neurotoxic effects of CsA; injury to both the major and minor vasculature may cause hypoperfusion or ischemia and local secondary toxicity in this area.

Although obesity, steroid use, and reduced renal function contributes to metabolic alterations in transplant recipients, cyclosporine appears to play an independent role in increasing cholesterol levels, which relates to the modulation of the low-density lipoprotein receptor.[132]

Pharmacologic management in general revolves around the HMG coenzyme A reductase drugs, which can be used safely if liver function tests and muscle enzymes are monitored. CsA can also worsen glucose tolerance to unmask a genetic predisposition to type II diabetes or even create glucose intolerance in otherwise healthy individuals. Management is based on dietary manipulations and the judicious use of oral hypoglycemic agents. Half of these recipients may ultimately need to be converted to receive insulin.

Gingival hyperplasia appears in 8% to 85% of patients treated with cyclosporine.[133,134] Most studies show an association between oral hygiene status and the prevalence and severity of this gingival overgrowth. Thus in addition to attention to CsA dosage and drug interactions, treatment usually involves maintenance of strict oral hygiene. Sometimes a second treatment phase involving periodontal surgery is necessary. In addition to cosmetic appearance, de novo malignancies have been reported arising in areas of gingival hyperplasia, in a group already at high risk for malignancy.

Tacrolimus

Tacrolimus is a very potent immunosuppressant, with a 10- to 100-fold greater in vitro immunosuppressive activity compared with cyclosporine.[114] Consistent with its greater potency, therapeutic whole blood trough concentrations for tacrolimus are ~20-fold less than the corresponding cyclosporine concentrations.[135]

In general, the clinical efficiency of tacrolimus is similar to cyclosporine. Both agents provide comparable 1-year graft and patient survival rate. However, in patients who received renal transplant tacrolimus is more powerful in preventing severe and refractory rejections, even when compared with the new cyclosporine microemulsion formulation. Both drugs are equally nephrotoxic, but tacrolimus induces less hypertension, less pronounced hyperlipidemia, gingival hyperplasia, and hirsutism.[129]

Initial pharmacokinetic studies failed to establish a relation between tacrolimus blood levels and rejection episodes. However, recent studies appear to advocate a correlation between low or increased tacrolimus whole blood trough concentrations and rejection or toxicity, respectively.[114] On the basis of international pharmacodynamic/pharmacokinetic efforts, optimal therapeutic ranges have now been proposed for whole blood tacrolimus concentrations in patients who received kidney, liver, or heart transplant.[136] In the initial post-transplant phase (<3 months), the recommended therapeutic ranges are 10 to 15 μg/L for recipients of kidney or liver transplant and 10 to 18 μg/L for recipients of heart transplant. The recommended ranges during maintenance therapy are 5 to 10 μg/L for liver and kidney and somewhat greater for the heart (8–15 μg/L).

Azathioprine

Azathioprine is a prodrug that is converted in vivo to 6-mercaptopurine, which is subsequently metabolized to the pharmacologically active 6-thioguanine nucleotides. The latter is also responsible for the cytotoxic side effects associated with this drug, which includes bone marrow depression.[137] Measuring blood counts has, therefore, been a part of routine monitoring during azathioprine therapy. However, blood counts do not provide information on immunosuppressive efficacy. More pertinent information can be obtained through pharmacodynamic measurements such as thiopurine S-methyltransferase activity and the quantification of intracellular 6-thioguanine nucleotide concentrations in red blood cells.

Azathioprine is largely inactivated by xanthine oxidase and the product, 6-thiouric acid, is excreted by the kidneys. Toxicity is increased by twofold in renal failure and fourfold by inhibiting xanthine oxidase. Thus one of the most important drug interaction of azathioprine with allopurinol in patients treated for hyperuricemia.[138]

Rapamycin

Similar to animal models (Fig. 54–4), rapamycin has been shown to produce a significant reduction in acute rejection (7% vs. 36%) in clinical trials, when used in combination with other immunosuppressants such as CsA and prednisone.[139] It also allowed early withdrawal of steroid therapy in a large number of patients (78%), demonstrating a great clinical impact.[140,141]

Pharmacokinetic studies in adult patients who received a kidney transplant have shown that rapamycin may be characterized as a drug with rapid gastrointestinal absorption reaching peak concentrations within 1 hour in 70% of patients. Its systemic availability is low (14%).[142] The majority of drug is sequestered in red blood cells causing plasma concentrations to be less than in the whole blood. It is primarily metabolized by the same CYP3A4 enzyme involved in the metabolism of calcineurin inhibitors, thus exhibiting large intersubject and intrasubject variability because of

genetic differences in the activity of this system. The drug has a relatively long half-life (62 hours). A whole-blood rapamycin therapeutic window of 5 to 15 ng/mL is recommended for patients at standard risk for rejection. The large intrapatient variability observed in trough rapamycin concentrations indicates that dose adjustments should be optimally based on more than a single trough sample. Because of the time required to reach steady state, Sirolimus dose adjustments would optimally be based on trough levels obtained less than 5 to 7 days after a dose change.

Available data regarding the side effect profile in stable patients who received kidney transplant suggest that rapamycin is a safe adjuvant immunosupressant.[143] Although hypertension, nephrotoxicity, and hepatotoxicity do not appear to occur, rapamycin causes leukopenia, thrombocytopenia, and a marked hyperlipidemia as side effects.[144] It interferes with lipid clearance by inhibiting lipoprotein lipase and blocking insulin growth factor–induced signaling underlying uptake of fatty acids.[41] In addition, platelet and white blood cell counts were significantly decreased with return to normal after discontinuation of rapamycin.

Mycophenolate Mofetil

Similar to preclinical studies, promising data were observed in initial multicenter clinical studies in renal transplantation showing a reduction of acute rejection episodes by 40% in patients treated with mycophenolate; histology showed less extensive disease.[145,146] Recent randomized clinical trials also have demonstrated that mycophenolate, when used with cyclosporine and steroids, reduces the frequency and severity of acute rejection episodes in kidney, heart, and lung transplants (Fig. 54–5)[147]; it also improved patient and graft survival rates in heart allograft recipients and increased renal allograft survival at 3 years.[148] In addition, mycophenolate

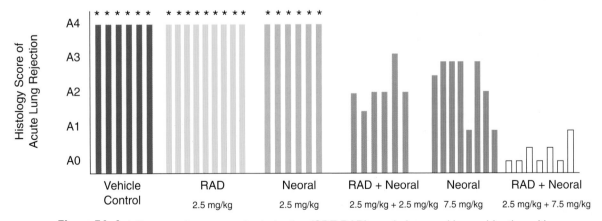

Figure 54–4. Influence of a rapamycin derivative (SDZ RAD) used alone and in combination with a microemulsion formulation of cyclosporine (Neoral) on histology scores of acute lung rejection in individual rats. *Hemorrhagic infarction. One-way analysis of variance on ranks: Control (Group I) vs. Neoral (7.5 mg/kg/day) + RAD (Group IV), $P < 0.02$; Neoral (7.5 mg/kg/day) + RAD (Group IV) vs. RAD (2.5 mg/kg/day; Group III), $P < 0.001$; Neoral (7.5 mg/kg/day) + RAD (Group IV) vs. Neoral (2.5 mg/kg/day; Group V), $P < 0.001$. (From Hausen B, Boeke K, Berry GJ, et al: Suppression of acute rejection in allogeneic rat lung transplantation: A study of the efficacy and pharmacokinetics of rapamycin derivative (SDZ RAD) used alone and in combination with a microemulsion formulation of cyclosporine. J Heart Lung Transplant 18(2):150–159, 1999.)

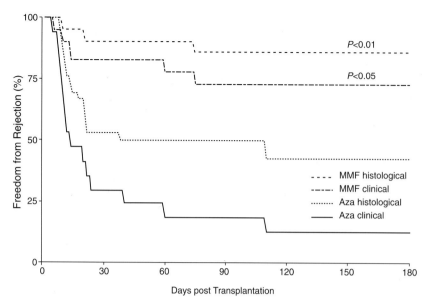

Figure 54–5. Actuarial freedom from acute rejection after lung transplantation. Over the first 6 months patients treated with mycophenolate mofetil (MMF) had significantly less clinical rejection episodes ($P <$ 0.05) and histologically verified rejection episodes ($P <$ 0.01) than azathioprine (Aza)-treated patients. (From Zuckermann A, Klepetko W, Birsan T, et al: Comparison between mycophenolate mofetil- and azathioprine-based immunosuppressions in clinical lung transplantation. J Heart Lung Transplant 18(5):432–440, 1999.)

has been effective in reversing acute and resistant rejection episodes in patients who received heart, kidney, or liver transplants. The ability of MMF to facilitate sparing of other immunosuppressive agents, particularly in CsA-related nephrotoxicity, is also promising. By permitting reduction in CsA doses, MMF may stabilize or improve renal graft function in patients with CsA-related nephrotoxicity or chronic allograft nephropathy. Regarding mycophenolate-induced toxicity, the main adverse effects included gastrointestinal and hematologic complications.

The conversion of MPA to the pharmacologically inactive phenolic acid glucuronide (MPAG) is catalyzed by uridine 5′-diphosphate-glucuronosyltransferase.[149,150] The most likely sites for this conversion are in the gastrointestinal tract, liver and possibly kidney. This metabolic step is generally regarded quantitatively as the most important and rate-limiting one. An important pathway linking the metabolism and the pharmacokinetic profile for MPA is enterohepatic circulation, whereby MPAG formed in the liver is excreted into bile and is converted back to MPA on delivery to the gastrointestinal tract. The latter conversion is thought to occur through the action of glucuronidase shed by gastrointestinal tract bacteria. Another important property of MPA is its tight and extensive binding to human serum albumin.[151] Inhibition of human IMPDH and suppression of proliferation in mitogen-stimulated lymphocytes in pharmacodynamic assays was dependent on free MPA concentration suggesting that this is the pharmacologically active fraction of the drug.[125]

Practical Issues

Immunosuppression Protocols

Current protocols rely on combinations of immunosuppressive agents to produce an additive or synergistic effect while minimizing toxicity. Agents with different mechanisms of action and preferentially nonoverlapping toxicity are

combined so that the doses of the individual drugs can be reduced to levels below toxicity. A strict initial immunosuppression is needed in the immediate and critical postoperative period followed by a more relaxed regimen, termed *maintenance immunosuppression.*

On arrival to the transplant ward, the patient usually receives the loading dose for immunosuppression and prophylactic treatment. In general, the induction immunosuppression involves larger doses of immunosuppressive drugs to minimize the initial immune response. Cyclosporin is the first line of immunosuppression regimens in most centers apart from surgery in which perioperative renal dysfunction is likely to occur, such as kidney and heart transplantation. This is followed by intravenous administration of a loading dose of methylprednisolone during the operation, usually before reperfusion of the implanted graft. The author, however, prefers administration of methylprednisolone to the donors before harvesting to minimize cytokine induction within the graft during ischemia and also before cardiopulmonary bypass in operations such as heart and lung transplantation to decrease systemic inflammatory response to bypass. In many situations, anti–T-cell agents including polyclonal anti–T-cell immunoglobulins or mAbs against T-cell receptor are important components of the induction immunosuppression.

Maintenance immunosuppression refers to lifelong prophylactic therapy against rejection. The most commonly used protocol is the three-drug combination of a calcineurin inhibitor such as cyclosporine, a nucleotide inhibitor such as azathioprine or mycophenolate, and corticosteroids. Breakthrough acute rejection is usually treated with high-dose steroids with or without supplemental anti–T-lymphocyte agents.

Anesthetic Implications of Immunosuppressive Agents

Anesthesia for patients with an organ transplant organ or with autoimmune disease is complicated first by physiologic changes caused by the transplantation or the nature of autoimmune disease onto which is superimposed the alterations caused by the immunosuppression therapy. Safe conduct of anesthesia thus requires understanding, thorough preoperative evaluation of the organ systems involved, interpretation of necessary laboratory tests, and appropriate modification of anesthetic administration, monitoring, and postoperative care.

Detailed and systematic analysis of individual organ dysfunction after transplantation is beyond the scope of this chapter, but there are excellent anesthetic reviews available on the topic.[152–154] Here we will emphasize the influence of immunosuppressants on different organ function and potential drug interactions, which might be important to the anesthesiologist.

Cyclosporine causes at least 20% decrease in renal function in almost all patients, an effect shared with tacrolimus. This is associated with slightly increased serum urea nitrogen, creatinine, and potassium. Hypertension might be caused by renal mechanisms but could be related to generalized vasoconstriction caused by interference with endogenous nitric oxide mechanisms or overproduction of vasoconstrictor endothelins or angiotensins. Immunosuppressant-induced liver disease can be a major problem in many patients who received transplant, and preoperative checks should include assessment of cellular integrity, synthetic, detoxification, and excretion capacity. This can be done by measuring aminotransferases, bilirubins, and clotting profile. This is especially important in anesthesia for surveillance or diagnostic biopsy procedures. As discussed earlier, several of the immunosuppressants influence bone marrow function and a full blood count is required to assess acceptable reserve. A leukocyte count of less than 2000/μL in patients receiving azathioprine is usually a contraindication to surgery, which should be postponed until recovery is achieved after dose adjustment. Special consideration should be given to metabolic changes caused by immunosuppressants such as increased glucose tolerance and hyperlipidemia.

It is advisable to maintain the patient's regular medications until surgery because sudden changes might greatly influence serum levels of immunosuppressants. Usual premedication is appropriate in most cases. Most intravenous anesthetic agents can be used and isoflurane is commonly and safely delivered as the primary inhalation agent. Repeated use of halothane is probably best avoided and there is theoretical reason to avoid enflurane and sevoflurane because of potential liberation of nephrotoxic inorganic fluoride.

Among muscle relaxants, succinylcholine is appropriate for short procedures if serum potassium levels are in the normal range, whereas atracurium is useful for longer procedures. Renal dysfunction and cyclosporine might increase the duration of pancuronium and vecuronium-induced neuromuscular blockade, and liver dysfunction should be taken into consideration in dosing vecuronium. Regarding postoperative pain control, nonsteroidal anti-inflammatory drugs should be totally avoided because together with cyclosporine they might precipitate renal failure. Perhaps the best solution is an opiate-based, patient-controlled anesthesia for intermediate and painful operations.

One of the most important aspects of the conductance of anesthetic is infection control and prophylaxis. Invasive

monitoring should be used judiciously when hemodynamic instability is anticipated but limited to a minimum. Most centers have relaxed extra measures for sterility but anesthetic personnel should adapt to strict asepsis. Masks and gloves should be worn all the time, all ports and syringes should be kept capped and sterile, and the use of bacterial filters is recommended. Most of these patients are already receiving antibacterial, viral, and fungal prophylaxis, but if bacteriemia is anticipated during the surgery, extra-antibiotic prophylaxis is recommended with the initial dose given before surgery and cover for the postoperative period. In this regard, potential drug interactions with cyclosporin should be taken into account.

Dosage and Administration

Cyclosporin

Cyclosporin is available for oral use in capsule and oral solution. In oral administration, total daily dose should be taken in two divided doses. Grapefruit juice should be avoided because it increases plasma concentrations. As a single immunosuppressant for adult transplantation, the usual preoperative cyclosporin dose is 10 to 15 mg/kg by mouth 4 to 12 hours before transplantation, followed by the same daily dosage for 1 to 2 weeks after surgery with reduction to 2 to 6 mg maintenance dosage thereafter. These dosages should be reduced in cases of combined therapy and should be adjusted according to stable preoperative creatinine levels. At our institution, the preoperative dose is omitted in recipients of heart transplant to minimize perioperative nephrotoxicity, and cyclosporin is started on the second day of uneventful heart transplantation. If needed, the oral solution can be administered through a nasogastric tube. Cyclosporin levels should be monitored throughout and if therapeutic levels are not achieved poor absorption should be considered and intravenous supplementation of the drug should be initiated. If the patient is fully converted from oral to parenteral administration, the approximate equivalent intravenous dose is one third of the total daily oral dose. When converting back to oral route, intravenous administration cannot be stopped suddenly but should be reduced gradually with increasing the oral dose until therapeutic levels are achieved.

The Sandimmune intravenous formulation contains polyethoxylated castor oil, which has been associated with anaphylaxis. Thus careful patient monitoring is required when initiating intravenous cyclosporin treatment.

Tacrolimus

Tacrolimus is used as primary immunosuppression in patients who received liver and kidney allograft and as a rescue therapy in resistant allograft rejection. Tacrolimus is usually started 6 hour after liver and 24 hours after renal transplantation. If oral preparation is used perioperatively, nasogastric feeding should be stopped because of potential interference with tacrolimus absorption. The oral dosage is usually 100 to 300 μg/kg daily in 2 divided doses. Because there is wide variability in perioperative tacrolimus absorption, intravenous administration is preferable usually at 10 to 100 μg/kg over 24 hours.

Azathioprine

Azathioprine is widely used as a first-line agent for transplant recipients and a number of autoimmune conditions. Treatment is usually provided in tablets (1–4 mg/kg daily). Intravenous injection at the same doses should only be used if oral route is not feasible because the preparation is very alkaline and very irritant.

Mycophenolate Mofetil (MMF)

MMF is used for prophylaxis of acute renal, cardiac, and hepatic transplant rejection, generally in combination with cyclosporin and corticosteroids under specialist supervision. It is available in tablets, capsules, and as an intravenous infusion. In liver and renal transplantation, the usual intravenous dose is 1 g twice daily starting 1 to 3 days after the operation up to a maximum 14 days followed by transfer to oral administration at the same dose. For cardiac transplantation, the recommended dose is slightly greater at 1.5 g starting within 5 days of transplantation.

Rabbit and Horse Antithymocyte Globulins

At some institutions (including Harefield Hospital), rabbit and horse antithymocyte globulins are routinely used as induction therapy in heart transplant recipients and during resistant rejection episodes at 100 and 400 mg daily doses, respectively, for 3 days. These doses should be diluted in 250 saline and given only after a test dose by the doctor and under constant medical supervision by slowly increasing infusion rate from 10 mL/hr to a maximum of 50 mL/hr. Hemodynamic instability should be anticipated, which could range from mild hypotension only requiring dose reduction to anaphylaxis, a true emergency. Although these reactions are much less frequent with mAb administration such as Muromonab, Basiliximab, and Daclizumab, care must be exercised even with these agents.

References

1. Medzhitov R, Janeway CA Jr: Innate immunity: Impact on the adaptive immune response. Curr Opin Immunol 9:4–9, 1997.
2. King C, Sarvetnick N: Organ-specific autoimmunity. Curr Opin Immunol 9:863–871, 1997.
3. Mason D: T-cell-mediated control of autoimmunity. Arthritis Res 3:133–135, 2001.
4. Sharma VK, Li B, Khanna A, et al: Which way for drug-mediated immunosuppression? Curr Opin Immunol 6:784–790, 1994.
5. Brazelton TR, Morris RE: Molecular mechanisms of action of new xenobiotic immunosuppressive drugs: Tacrolimus (FK506), sirolimus (rapamycin), mycophenolate mofetil and leflunomide. Curr Opin Immunol 8:710–720, 1996.
6. Benichou G, Malloy KM, Tam RC, et al: The presentation of self and allogeneic MHC peptides to T lymphocytes. Hum Immunol 59:540–548, 1998.
7. Benichou G: Direct and indirect antigen recognition: The pathways to allograft immune rejection. Front Biosci 4:D476–D480, 1999.
8. Weiss A, Littman DR: Signal transduction by lymphocyte antigen receptors. Cell 76:263–274, 1994.
9. Schwartz RH: T cell clonal anergy. Curr Opin Immunol 9:351–357, 1997.
10. Suthanthiran M: Signaling features of T cells: Implications for the regulation of the anti-allograft response. Kidney Int Suppl 43:S3–S11, 1993.
11. Williams JM, Deloria D, Hansen JA, et al: The events of primary T cell activation can be staged by use of Sepharose-bound anti-T3(64.1) monoclonal antibody and purified interleukin 1. J Immunol 135:2249–2255, 1985.
12. Lin X, Cunningham ET Jr, Mu Y, et al: The proto-oncogene Cot kinase participates in CD3/CD28 induction of NF-kappaB acting through the NF-kappaB-inducing kinase and IkappaB kinases. Immunity 10:271–280, 1999.
13. Jain J, Loh C, Rao A: Transcriptional regulation of the IL-2 gene. Curr Opin Immunol 7:333–342, 1995.
14. Chen D, Rothenberg EV: Interleukin 2 transcription factors as molecular targets of cAMP inhibition: Delayed inhibition kinetics and combinatorial transcription roles. J Exp Med 179:931–942, 1994.
15. Cahalan MD, Chandy KG: Ion channels in the immune system as targets for immunosuppression. Curr Opin Biotechnol 8:749–756, 1997.
16. Crabtree GR, Clipstone NA: Signal transmission between the plasma membrane and nucleus of T lymphocytes. Annu Rev Biochem 63:1045–1083, 1994.
17. Clipstone NA, Crabtree GR: Identification of calcineurin as a key signalling enzyme in T-lymphocyte activation. Nature 357:695–697, 1992.
18. Flanagan WM, Corthesy B, Bram RJ, Crabtree GR: Nuclear association of a T-cell transcription factor blocked by FK-506 and cyclosporin A. Nature 352:803–807, 1991.
19. Su B, Karin M: Mitogen-activated protein kinase cascades and regulation of gene expression. Curr Opin Immunol 8:402–411, 1996.
20. Su B, Jacinto E, Hibi M, et al: JNK is involved in signal integration during costimulation of T lymphocytes. Cell 77:727–736, 1994.
21. Karin M: The regulation of AP-1 activity by mitogen-activated protein kinases. J Biol Chem 270:16483–16486, 1995.
22. Matsuda S, Koyasu S: Mechanisms of action of cyclosporine. Immunopharmacology 47:119–125, 2000.
23. Matsuda S, Moriguchi T, Koyasu S, Nishida E: T lymphocyte activation signals for interleukin-2 production involve activation of MKK6-p38 and MKK7-SAPK/JNK signaling pathways sensitive to cyclosporin A. J Biol Chem 273:12378–12382, 1998.
24. Garrity PA, Chen D, Rothenberg EV, Wold BJ: Interleukin-2 transcription is regulated in vivo at the level of coordinated binding of both constitutive and regulated factors. Mol Cell Biol 14:2159–2169, 1994.
25. Kang SM, Tran AC, Grilli M, Lenardo MJ: NF-kappa B subunit regulation in nontransformed CD4+ T lymphocytes. Science 256:1452–1456, 1992.
26. Huxford T, Malek S, Ghosh G: Structure and mechanism in NF-kappa B/I kappa B signaling. Cold Spring Harb Symp Quant Biol 64:533–540, 1999.
27. Voll RE, Ghosh S: Role of NF-kappa B in T-lymphocyte development. Cold Spring Harb Symp Quant Biol 64:485–490, 1999.
28. Taniguchi T, Minami Y: The IL-2/IL-2 receptor system: A current overview. Cell 73:5–8, 1993.
29. Gaffen SL: Signaling domains of the interleukin 2 receptor. Cytokine 14:63–77, 2001.
30. Johnston JA, Kawamura M, Kirken RA, et al: Phosphorylation and activation of the Jak-3 Janus kinase in response to interleukin-2. Nature 370:151–153, 1994.
31. Johnston JA, Bacon CM, Finbloom DS, et al: Tyrosine phosphorylation and activation of STAT5, STAT3, and Janus kinases by interleukins 2 and 15. Proc Natl Acad Sci USA 92:8705–8709, 1995.
32. Welte T, Leitenberg D, Dittel BN, et al: STAT5 interaction with the

T cell receptor complex and stimulation of T cell proliferation. Science 283:222–225, 1999.

33. Martino A, Holmes JH, Lord JD, et al: Stat5 and Sp1 regulate transcription of the cyclin D2 gene in response to IL-2. J Immunol 166:1723–1729, 2001.

34. Nelson BH, Willerford DM: Biology of the interleukin-2 receptor. Adv Immunol 70:1–81, 1998.

35. Fairbanks LD, Bofill M, Ruckemann K, Simmonds HA: Importance of ribonucleotide availability to proliferating T-lymphocytes from healthy humans. Disproportionate expansion of pyrimidine pools and contrasting effects of de novo synthesis inhibitors. J Biol Chem 270:29682–29689, 1995.

36. Benichou G, Takizawa PA, Ho PT, et al: Immunogenicity and tolerogenicity of self-major histocompatibility complex peptides. J Exp Med 172:1341–1346, 1990.

37. Benichou G, Fedoseyeva E, Olson CA, et al: Disruption of the determinant hierarchy on a self-MHC peptide: Concomitant tolerance induction to the dominant determinant and priming to the cryptic self-determinant. Int Immunol 6:131–138, 1994.

38. Sayegh MH, Khoury SJ, Hancock WW, et al: Induction of immunity and oral tolerance with polymorphic class II major histocompatibility complex allopeptides in the rat. Proc Natl Acad Sci USA 89:7762–7766, 1992.

39. Ildstad ST, Sachs DH: Reconstitution with syngeneic plus allogeneic or xenogeneic bone marrow leads to specific acceptance of allografts or xenografts. Nature 307:168–170, 1984.

40. Fontes P, Rao AS, Demetris AJ, et al: Bone marrow augmentation of donor-cell chimerism in kidney, liver, heart, and pancreas islet transplantation. Lancet 344:151–155, 1994.

41. Ciancio G, Burke GW, Miller J: Current treatment practice in immunosuppression. Exp Opin Pharmacother 1:1307–1330, 2000.

42. Ciancio G, Miller J, Garcia-Morales RO, et al: Six-year clinical effect of donor bone marrow infusions in renal transplant patients. Transplantation 71:827–835, 2001.

43. Bonnefoy-Berard N, Revillard JP: Mechanisms of immunosuppression induced by antithymocyte globulins and OKT3. J Heart Lung Transplant 15:435–442, 1996.

44. Norman DJ: Mechanisms of action and overview of OKT3. Ther Drug Monit 17:615–620, 1995.

45. Grakoui A, Bromley SK, Sumen C, et al: The immunological synapse: A molecular machine controlling T cell activation. Science 285:221–227, 1999.

46. Shaw AS, Dustin ML: Making the T cell receptor go the distance: A topological view of T cell activation. Immunity 6:361–369, 1997.

47. Saitovitch D, Bushell A, Mabbs DW, et al: Kinetics of induction of transplantation tolerance with a nondepleting anti-Cd4 monoclonal antibody and donor-specific transfusion before transplantation. A critical period of time is required for development of immunological unresponsiveness. Transplantation 61:1642–1647, 1996.

48. Tak PP, van der Lubbe PA, Cauli A, et al: Reduction of synovial inflammation after anti-CD4 monoclonal antibody treatment in early rheumatoid arthritis. Arthritis Rheum 38:1457–1465, 1995.

49. Salomon B, Bluestone JA: Complexities of CD28/B7: CTLA-4 co-stimulatory pathways in autoimmunity and transplantation. Annu Rev Immunol 19:225–252, 2001.

50. Chambers CA, Kuhns MS, Egen JG, Allison JP: CTLA-4-mediated inhibition in regulation of T cell responses: Mechanisms and manipulation in tumor immunotherapy. Annu Rev Immunol 19:565–594, 2001.

51. Kirk AD, Harlan DM, Armstrong NN, et al: CTLA4-Ig and anti-CD40 ligand prevent renal allograft rejection in primates. Proc Natl Acad Sci USA 94:8789–8794, 1997.

52. Larsen CP, Elwood ET, Alexander DZ, et al: Long-term acceptance of skin and cardiac allografts after blocking CD40 and CD28 pathways. Nature 381:434–438, 1996.

53. Reichardt HM, Schutz G: Glucocorticoid signalling—multiple variations of a common theme. Mol Cell Endocrinol 146:1–6, 1998.

54. DiDonato JA, Saatcioglu F, Karin M: Molecular mechanisms of immunosuppression and anti-inflammatory activities by glucocorticoids. Am J Respir Crit Care Med 154:S11–S15, 1996.

55. Adcock IM, Ito K: Molecular mechanisms of corticosteroid actions. Monaldi Arch Chest Dis 55:256–266, 2000.

56. Karin M, Chang L: AP-1—glucocorticoid receptor crosstalk taken to a higher level. J Endocrinol 169:447–451, 2001.

57. De Bosscher K, Vanden Berghe W, Haegeman G: Mechanisms of anti-inflammatory action and of immunosuppression by glucocorticoids:

Negative interference of activated glucocorticoid receptor with transcription factors. J Neuroimmunol 109:16–22, 2000.

58. Borel JF, Feurer C, Gubler HU, Stahelin H: Biological effects of cyclosporin A: A new antilymphocytic agent. 1976. Agents Actions 43:179–186, 1994.

59. Kronke M, Leonard WJ, Depper JM, et al: Cyclosporin A inhibits T-cell growth factor gene expression at the level of mRNA transcription. Proc Natl Acad Sci USA 81:5214–5218, 1984.

60. Herold KC, Lancki DW, Moldwin RL, Fitch FW: Immunosuppressive effects of cyclosporin A on cloned T cells. J Immunol 136:1315–1321, 1986.

61. Granelli-Piperno A: In situ hybridization for interleukin 2 and interleukin 2 receptor mRNA in T cells activated in the presence or absence of cyclosporin A. J Exp Med 168:1649–1658, 1988.

62. Handschumacher RE, Harding MW, Rice J, et al: Cyclophilin: A specific cytosolic binding protein for cyclosporin A. Science 226:544–547, 1984.

63. Schreiber SL: Chemistry and biology of the immunophilins and their immunosuppressive ligands. Science 251:283–287, 1991.

64. Schmid FX: Protein folding. Prolyl isomerases join the fold. Curr Biol 5:993–994, 1995.

65. Sigal NH, Dumont F, Durette P, et al: Is cyclophilin involved in the immunosuppressive and nephrotoxic mechanism of action of cyclosporin A? J Exp Med 173:619–628, 1991.

66. Liu J, Albers MW, Wandless TJ, et al: Inhibition of T cell signaling by immunophilin-ligand complexes correlates with loss of calcineurin phosphatase activity. Biochemistry 31:3896–3901, 1992.

67. Liu J, Farmer JD Jr, Lane WS, et al: Calcineurin is a common target of cyclophilin-cyclosporin A and FKBP-FK506 complexes. Cell 66:807–815, 1991.

68. Wu J, Katzav S, Weiss A: A functional T-cell receptor signaling pathway is required for p95vav activity. Mol Cell Biol 15:4337–4346, 1995.

69. Roberts AB, Sporn MB: Physiological actions and clinical applications of transforming growth factor-beta (TGF-beta). Growth Factors 8:1–9, 1993.

70. Khanna A, Li B, Stenzel KH, Suthanthiran M: Regulation of new DNA synthesis in mammalian cells by cyclosporine. Demonstration of a transforming growth factor beta-dependent mechanism of inhibition of cell growth. Transplantation 57:577–582, 1994.

71. Islam M, Burke JF Jr, McGowan TA, et al: Effect of anti-transforming growth factor-beta antibodies in cyclosporine-induced renal dysfunction. Kidney Int 59:498–506, 2001.

72. Gonzalez-Santiago L, Lopez-Ongil S, Lamas S, et al: Imbalance in endothelial vasoactive factors as a possible cause of cyclosporin toxicity: A role for endothelin-converting enzyme. J Lab Clin Med 136:395–401, 2000.

73. Hojo M, Morimoto T, Maluccio M, et al: Cyclosporine induces cancer progression by a cell-autonomous mechanism. Nature 397:530–534, 1999.

74. Goto T, Kino T, Hatanaka H, et al: Discovery of FK-506, a novel immunosuppressant isolated from Streptomyces tsukubaensis. Transplant Proc 19:4–8, 1987.

75. Ochiai T, Nakajima K, Nagata M, et al: Effect of a new immunosuppressive agent, FK 506, on heterotopic cardiac allotransplantation in the rat. Transplant Proc 19:1284–1286, 1987.

76. Griffith JP, Kim JL, Kim EE, et al: X-ray structure of calcineurin inhibited by the immunophilin-immunosuppressant FKBP12-FK506 complex. Cell 82:507–522, 1995.

77. Goodall T, Kind CN, Hammond TG: FK506-induced endothelin release by cultured rat mesangial cells. J Cardiovasc Pharmacol 26(suppl 3):S482–S485, 1995.

78. Muraoka K, Fujimoto K, Sun X, et al: Immunosuppressant FK506 induces interleukin-6 production through the activation of transcription factor nuclear factor (NF)-kappa(B). Implications for FK506 nephropathy. J Clin Invest 97:2433–2439, 1996.

79. Zhang Y, Sun X, Muraoka K, et al: Immunosuppressant FK506 activates NF-kappaB through the proteasome-mediated degradation of IkappaBalpha. Requirement for IkappaBalpha n-terminal phosphorylation but not ubiquitination sites. J Biol Chem 274:34657–34662, 1999.

80. Waldmann TA, O'Shea J: The use of antibodies against the IL-2 receptor in transplantation. Curr Opin Immunol 10:507–512, 1998.

81. Soulillou JP, Cantarovich D, Le Mauff B, et al: Randomized controlled trial of a monoclonal antibody against the interleukin-2 receptor (33B3.1) as compared with rabbit antithymocyte globulin for

prophylaxis against rejection of renal allografts. N Engl J Med 322:1175–1182, 1990.

82. Kirkman RL, Shapiro ME, Carpenter CB, et al: A randomized prospective trial of anti-Tac monoclonal antibody in human renal transplantation. Transplant Proc 23:1066–1067, 1991.

83. Queen C, Schneider WP, Selick HE, et al: A humanized antibody that binds to the interleukin 2 receptor. Proc Natl Acad Sci USA 86:10029–10033, 1989.

84. Junghans RP, Waldmann TA, Landolfi NF, et al: A humanized antibody to the interleukin 2 receptor with new features for immunotherapy in malignant and immune disorders. Cancer Res 50:1495–1502, 1990.

85. Vincenti F, Kirkman R, Light S, et al: Interleukin-2-receptor blockade with daclizumab to prevent acute rejection in renal transplantation. Daclizumab Triple Therapy Study Group. N Engl J Med 338:161–165, 1998.

86. Calne RY, Collier DS, Lim S, et al: Rapamycin for immunosuppression in organ allografting. Lancet 2:227, 1989.

87. Morris RE, Meiser BM, Wu J, et al: Use of rapamycin for the suppression of alloimmune reactions in vivo: Schedule dependence, tolerance induction, synergy with cyclosporine and FK 506, and effect on host-versus-graft and graft-versus-host reactions. Transplant Proc 23:521–524, 1991.

88. Sehgal SN, Camardo JS, Scarola JA, Maida BT: Rapamycin (sirolimus, rapamune). Curr Opin Nephrol Hypertens 4:482–487, 1995.

89. Lorenz MC, Heitman J: TOR mutations confer rapamycin resistance by preventing interaction with FKBP12-rapamycin. J Biol Chem 270:27531–27537, 1995.

90. Terada N, Takase K, Papst P, et al: Rapamycin inhibits ribosomal protein synthesis and induces G1 prolongation in mitogen-activated T lymphocytes. J Immunol 155:3418–3426, 1995.

91. Morris RE, Cao W, Huang X, et al: Rapamycin (Sirolimus) inhibits vascular smooth muscle DNA synthesis in vitro and suppresses narrowing in arterial allografts and in balloon-injured carotid arteries: Evidence that rapamycin antagonizes growth factor action on immune and nonimmune cells. Transplant Proc 27:430–431, 1995.

92. Gregory CR, Huang X, Pratt RE, et al: Treatment with rapamycin and mycophenolic acid reduces arterial intimal thickening produced by mechanical injury and allows endothelial replacement. Transplantation 59:655–661, 1995.

93. Elion GB: Symposium on immunosuppressive drugs. Biochemistry and pharmacology of purine analogues. Fed Proc 26:898–904, 1967.

94. Ransom JT: Mechanism of action of mycophenolate mofetil. Ther Drug Monit 17:681–684, 1995.

95. Shaw LM, Sollinger HW, Halloran P, et al: Mycophenolate mofetil: A report of the consensus panel. Ther Drug Monit 17:690–699, 1995.

96. Allison AC, Eugui EM: Purine metabolism and immunosuppressive effects of mycophenolate mofetil (MMF). Clin Transplant 10:77–84, 1996.

97. Allison AC, Eugui EM: Mycophenolate mofetil and its mechanisms of action. Immunopharmacology 47:85–118, 2000.

98. Sollinger HW: From mice to man: The preclinical history of mycophenolate mofetil. Clin. Transplant 10:85–92, 1996.

99. Fraser-Smith EB, Rosete JD, Schatzman RC: Suppression by mycophenolate mofetil of the neointimal thickening caused by vascular injury in a rat arterial stenosis model. J Pharmacol Exp Ther 275:1204–1208, 1995.

100. Cherwinski HM, McCarley D, Schatzman R, et al: The immunosuppressant leflunomide inhibits lymphocyte progression through cell cycle by a novel mechanism. J Pharmacol Exp Ther 272:460–468, 1995.

101. Morris RE, Huang X, Cao W, et al: Leflunomide (HWA 486) and its analog suppre. Transplant Proc 27:445–447, 1995.

102. Silva HT Jr, Cao W, Shorthouse RA, et al: In vitro and in vivo effects of leflunomide, brequinar, and cyclosporine on pyrimidine biosynthesis. Transplant Proc 29:1292–1293, 1997.

103. Breedveld FC, Dayer JM, Leflunomide: Mode of action in the treatment of rheumatoid arthritis. Ann Rheum Dis 59:841–849, 2000.

104. Bartlett RR, Anagnostopulos H, Zielinski T, et al: Effects of leflunomide on immune responses and models of inflammation. Springer Semin Immunopathol 14:381–394, 1993.

105. Nair RV, Cao W, Morris RE: The antiproliferative effect of leflunomide on vascular smooth muscle cells in vitro is mediated by selective inhibition of pyrimidine biosynthesis. Transplant Proc 28:3081, 1996.

106. Thomson DA: Anesthesia and the immune system. J Burn Care Rehabil 8:483–487, 1987.

107. Hunter JD: Effects of anaesthesia on the human immune system. Hosp Med 60:658–663, 1999.

108. Galley HF, Webster NR: Effects of propofol and thiopentone on the immune response. Anaesthesia 52:921–923, 1997.

109. Procopio MA, Rassias AJ, DeLeo JA, et al: The in vivo effects of general and epidural anesthesia on human immune function. Anesth Analg 93:460–465, 2001.

110. Kress HG, Eberlein T: (Effect of anesthesia and operation on essential immune functions). Anasthesiol Intensivmed Notfallmed Schmerzther 27:393–402, 1992.

111. Nadal P, Nicolas JM, Font C, et al: Pneumonia in ventilated head trauma patients: The role of thiopental therapy. Eur J Emerg Med 2:14–16, 1995.

112. Brocker EB, Macher E: (The effect of anaesthesia and surgery on immune function. A review (author's transl)). Klin Wochenschr 59:1297–1301, 1981.

113. Tsunoda SM, Aweeka FT: The use of therapeutic drug monitoring to optimise immunosuppressive therapy. Clin Pharmacokinet 30:107–140, 1996.

114. Armstrong VW, Oellerich M: New developments in the immunosuppressive drug monitoring of cyclosporine, tacrolimus, and azathioprine. Clin Biochem 34:9–16, 2001.

115. Kahan BD, Welsh M, Schoenberg L, et al: Variable oral absorption of cyclosporine. A biopharmaceutical risk factor for chronic renal allograft rejection. Transplantation 62:599–606, 1996.

116. Kahan BD, Welsh M, Rutzky LP: Challenges in cyclosporine therapy: The role of therapeutic monitoring by area under the curve monitoring. Ther Drug Monit 17:621–624, 1995.

117. Oellerich M, Armstrong VW, Kahan B, et al: Lake Louise Consensus Conference on cyclosporin monitoring in organ transplantation: Report of the consensus panel. Ther Drug Monit 17:642–654, 1995.

118. Ritschel WA: Microemulsion technology in the reformulation of cyclosporine: The reason behind the pharmacokinetic properties of Neoral. Clin Transplant 10:364–373, 1996.

119. Keown P, Niese D: Cyclosporine microemulsion increases drug exposure and reduces acute rejection without incremental toxicity in de novo renal transplantation. International Sandimmun Neoral Study Group. Kidney Int 54:938–944, 1998.

120. Fahr A: Cyclosporin clinical pharmacokinetics. Clin Pharmacokinet 24:472–495, 1993.

121. Grinyo JM: Progress with cyclosporine-sparing regimens. Transplant Proc 31:11S–16S, 1999.

122. Trotter JF: Drugs that interact with immunosuppressive agents. Semin Gastrointest Dis 9:147–153, 1998.

123. Martin JE, Daoud AJ, Schroeder TJ, First MR: The clinical and economic potential of cyclosporin drug interactions. Pharmacoeconomics 15:317–337, 1999.

124. Campana C, Regazzi MB, Buggia I, Molinaro M: Clinically significant drug interactions with cyclosporin. An update. Clin Pharmacokinet 30:141–179, 1996.

125. Dambrin C, Klupp J, Morris RE: Pharmacodynamics of immunosuppressive drugs. Curr Opin Immunol 12:557–562, 2000.

126. Halloran PF, Helms LM, Kung L, Noujaim J: The temporal profile of calcineurin inhibition by cyclosporine in vivo. Transplantation 68:1356–1361, 1999.

127. van den Berg AP, Twilhaar WN, van Son WJ, et al: Quantification of immunosuppression by flow cytometric measurement of intracellular cytokine synthesis. Transpl Int 11(suppl 1):S318–S321, 1998.

128. MacDonald AS: Impact of immunosuppressive therapy on hypertension. Transplantation 70:SS70–SS76, 2000.

129. Olyaei AJ, de Mattos AM, Bennett WM: Immunosuppressant-induced nephropathy: Pathophysiology, incidence and management. Drug Saf 21:471–488, 1999.

130. Bechstein WO: Neurotoxicity of calcineurin inhibitors: Impact and clinical management. Transpl Int 13:313–326, 2000.

131. Gijtenbeek JM, van den Bent MJ, Vecht CJ: Cyclosporine neurotoxicity: A review. J Neurol 246:339–346, 1999.

132. Ballantyne CM, el Masri B, Morrisett JD, Torre-Amione G: Pathophysiology and treatment of lipid perturbation after cardiac transplantation. Curr Opin Cardiol 12:153–160, 1997.

133. Meraw SJ, Sheridan PJ: Medically induced gingival hyperplasia. Mayo Clin Proc 73:1196–1199, 1998.

134. Oettinger-Barak O, Machtei EE, Peled M, et al: Cyclosporine

A-induced gingival hyperplasia pemphigus vulgaris: Literature review and report of a case. J Periodontol 71:650–656, 2000.

135. Jusko WJ, Thomson AW, Fung J, et al: Consensus document: Therapeutic monitoring of tacrolimus (FK-506). Ther Drug Monit 17:606–614, 1995.

136. Oellerich M, Armstrong VW, Schutz E, Shaw LM: Therapeutic drug monitoring of cyclosporine and tacrolimus. Update on Lake Louise Consensus Conference on cyclosporin and tacrolimus. Clin Biochem 31:309–316, 1998.

137. Schutz E, Gummert J, Armstrong VW, et al: Azathioprine pharmacogenetics: The relationship between 6-thioguanine nucleotides and thiopurine methyltransferase in patients after heart and kidney transplantation. Eur J Clin Chem Clin Biochem 34:199–205, 1996.

138. el Gamel A, Evans C, Keevil B, et al: Effect of allopurinol on the metabolism of azathioprine in heart transplant patients. Transplant Proc 30:1127–1129, 1998.

139. Kahan BD, Podbielski J, Napoli KL, et al: Immunosuppressive effects and safety of a sirolimus/cyclosporine combination regimen for renal transplantation. Transplantation 66:1040–1046, 1998.

140. Mahalati K, Kahan BD: Sirolimus permits steroid withdrawal from a cyclosporine regimen. Transplant Proc 33:1270, 2001.

141. Podbielski J, Schoenberg L: Use of sirolimus in kidney transplantation. Prog Transplant 11:29–32, 2001.

142. MacDonald A, Scarola J, Burke JT, Zimmerman JJ: Clinical pharmacokinetics and therapeutic drug monitoring of sirolimus. Clin Ther 22(suppl B):B101–B121, 2000.

143. Meier-Kriesche HU, Kaplan B: Toxicity and efficacy of sirolimus: Relationship to whole-blood concentrations. Clin Ther 22(suppl B):B93–B100, 2000.

144. Hong JC, Kahan BD: Immunosuppressive agents in organ transplantation: Past, present, and future. Semin Nephrol 20:108–125, 2000.

145. Sollinger HW: Mycophenolate mofetil. Kidney Int Suppl 52:S14–S17, 1995.

146. Sollinger HW: Mycophenolate mofetil for the prevention of acute rejection in primary cadaveric renal allograft recipients. U.S. Renal Transplant Mycophenolate Mofetil Study Group. Transplantation 60:225–232, 1995.

147. Mele TS, Halloran PF: The use of mycophenolate mofetil in transplant recipients. Immunopharmacology 47:215–245, 2000.

148. Mycophenolate mofetil in renal transplantation: 3-Year results from the placebo-controlled trial. European Mycophenolate Mofetil Cooperative Study Group. Transplantation 68:391–396, 1999.

149. Bullingham RE, Nicholls A, Hale M: Pharmacokinetics of mycophenolate mofetil (RS61443): A short review. Transplant Proc 28:925–929, 1996.

150. Shaw LM, Korecka M, DeNofrio D, Brayman KL: Pharmacokinetic, pharmacodynamic, and outcome investigations as the basis for mycophenolic acid therapeutic drug monitoring in renal and heart transplant patients. Clin Biochem 34:17–22, 2001.

151. Bullingham RE, Nicholls AJ, Kamm BR: Clinical pharmacokinetics of mycophenolate mofetil. Clin Pharmacokinet 34:429–455, 1998.

152. Toivonen HJ: Anaesthesia for patients with a transplanted organ. Acta Anaesthesiol Scand 44:812–833, 2000.

153. Sharpe MD: Anaesthesia and the transplanted patient. Can J Anaesth 43:R89–R98, 1996.

154. Kostopanagiotou G, Smyrniotis V, Arkadopoulos N, et al: Anesthetic and perioperative management of adult transplant recipients in nontransplant surgery. Anesth Analg 89:613–622, 1999.

Index

Page numbers followed by "t" denote tables; those followed by "f" denote figures

Index